Second Edition

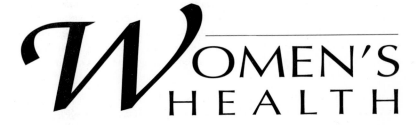

WOMEN'S HEALTH

A Primary Care Clinical Guide

Ellis Quinn Youngkin, PhD, RNC, ARNP
Professor and Graduate Program Coordinator
Women's Health Care Nurse Practitioner
College of Nursing
Florida Atlantic University
Boca Raton, Florida

Marcia Szmania Davis, MS, MS ED, RNC, WHCNP, ANP
Women's Health Care Nurse Practitioner
Virginia Women's Center
Adjunct Clinical Assistant Professor
School of Nursing
Virginia Commonwealth University
Medical College of Virginia
Richmond, Virginia

APPLETON & LANGE
Stamford, Connecticut

Cover art: Photomicrograph of an estrogen crystal. Copyright © Dennis Kunkel, PhD, University of Hawaii. This image of an estrogen (estradiol) crystal viewed under polarized light was part of a display of Dr. Kunkel's photomicrography published in the May 1993 issue of Smithsonian *magazine.*

Copyright © 1998 by Appleton & Lange
A Simon & Schuster Company
Copyright © 1994 by Appleton & Lange

98 99 00 01 02 / 10 9 8 7 6 5 4 3 2 1

Prentice-Hall International (UK) Limited, *London*
Prentice-Hall of Australia Pty. Limited, *Sydney*
Prentice Hall Canada, Inc., *Toronto*
Prentice Hall Hispanoamericana, S.A., *Mexico*
Prentice Hall of India Private Limited, *New Delhi*

Prentice Hall of Japan, Inc., *Tokyo*
Simon & Schuster Asia Pte. Ltd., *Singapore*
Editora Prentice Hall do Brasil Ltda., *Rio de Janeiro*
Prentice Hall, *Upper Saddle River, New Jersey*

Library of Congress Cataloging-in-Publication Data

Women's health : a primary care clinical guide / [edited by] Ellis
    Quinn Youngkin, Marcia Szmania Davis.—2nd ed.
        p.   cm.
    Includes bibliographical references and index.
    ISBN 0–8385–9640–1 (pbk. : alk. paper)
    1. Women—Health and hygiene—Sociological aspects.   2. Women—
Diseases.   3. Women's health services.   4. Gynecology.
5. Obstetrics.   I. Youngkin, Ellis Quinn.   II. Davis, Marcia
Szmania.
    [DNLM: 1. Women's Health.   2. Primary Health Care.   WA 309 W8712
1998]
    RA564.85.W6668   1998
    613´.04244—dc21
    DNLM/DLC
    for Library of Congress   97–42654

ISBN 0-8385-9640-1

90000
9 780838 596401

Editor-in-Chief: Sally J. Barhydt
Production Editor: Jeanmarie Roche
Production Service: Shepherd, Inc.

PRINTED IN THE UNITED STATES OF AMERICA

▪ ▪ ▪ ▪ ▪ CONTENTS

▪ ▪ ▪ ▪ ▪ CONTRIBUTORS

Kathleen M. Akridge, MS, RNC, WHCNP
Drs. Dineen and Wetchler
Newport News, Virginia
Adjunct Clinical Faculty
School of Nursing
Virginia Commonwealth University
Medical College of Virginia
Richmond, Virginia

Cynthia W. Bailey, MS, RNC, WHCNP
Drs. Fiedler and Smith
Richmond, Virginia

Sharon Baker, MN, RNC, WHCNP
President
The Women's Information Network, Inc.
Rome, Georgia

Lynette Galloway Branch, MS, RNC, FNP
Richard W. Dunn Family Practice
Petersburg, Virginia

Brenda T. Brickhouse, RNC, MS, WHCNP, CNM
Virginia Women's Center
Richmond, Virginia

Mary Beth Bryant McGurin, RNS, MS, WHCNP
Kaiser Permanente
Washington, D.C.

Kathryn A. Caufield, MS, RN, CFNP
Sentara Medical Group
Old Hampton Family Practice
Hampton, Virginia

Judith B. Collins, MS, RNC, WHCNP, FAAN
Director Women's Center
Virginia Commonwealth University
Medical College of Virginia
Richmond, Virginia

Joan Corder-Mabe, RNC, MS, WHCNP
Nurse Consultant
Virginia Department of Health
Richmond, Virginia

Valerie T. Cotter, MSN, RN, CS
Lecturer and Associate Director
Gerontological Nurse Practitioner Program
University of Pennsylvania
Philadelphia, Pennsylvania

Judy Parker-Falzoi, RNC/FNP, BS, BSN, MS
South Richmond Health Center
Adjunct Clinical Instructor
School of Nursing
Virginia Commonwealth University
Richmond, Virginia

Elaine Ferrary, MS, RN, CFNP
Primary Care
Adjunct Clinical Faculty
Virginia Commonwealth University
Richmond, Virginia

Catherine Ingram Fogel, PhD, RNC, FAAN, WHCNP
Professor, School of Nursing
University of North Carolina
Chapel Hill, North Carolina

Donna E. Forrest, RNC, MS, FNP, WHCNP
Women's Health Care
Riverside Physician Associates
Newport News, Virginia

Marion Herndon Fuqua, MS, RNC, WHCNP
Gynecology Associates
Paducah, Kentucky

Martha Edwards Hart, MS, RNC
Pediatric and Neonatal Nurse Practitioner
Clinical Faculty
School of Nursing
Virginia Commonwealth University
Richmond, Virginia

Cathy A. James, RNC, MS, WHCNP
Commonwealth Physicians for Women
Richmond, Virginia

Judith A. Lewis, PhD, RNC, FAAN
Associate Professor and Chair
Maternal Child Nursing Department
Virginia Commonwealth University
Richmond, Virginia

Angela Carter Martin, MS, RN, CFNP, CS
Old Dominion University
Lecturer and Director of the Distance Learning
Program/Family Nurse Practitioners
Norfolk, Virginia

Deborah A. Raines, PhD, RNC, CNS
Assistant Professor
School of Nursing
Virginia Commonwealth University
Richmond, Virginia

Maryellen C. Remich, RNC, MSN, WHCNP
The Group for Women
Norfolk, Virginia

Kathleen J. Sawin, DNS, RN, CS, FAAN
Pediatric and Family Nurse Practitioner
Associate Professor, School of Nursing
Virginia Commonwealth University
Richmond, Virginia

Susan D. Schaffer, PhD, RN, CFNP
Associate Professor
Old Dominion University
Norfolk, Virginia

Nancy J. Sharp, RN
President
Sharp & Associates
Bethesda, Maryland

CONTRIBUTORS TO FIRST EDITION

A special thank you and recognition go to those who contributed to the first edition of this book:

Emily Coogan Bennett
Vaginitis and Sexually Transmitted Diseases

Catherine H. Garner
The Climacteric, Menopause, and the Process
of Aging

Linda C. Hancock and Patricia M. Selig
Common Medical Problems in Primary Care

Nancy L. Harris and Belinda Seimer
Psychosocial Health Problems

Valerie Johnson South
Assessing Health During Pregnancy

Sue C. Wood
Infertility

■ ■ ■ ■ ■ REVIEWERS

Rebecca Donohue, PhD, RN, CS
Assistant Professor
Graduate Program in Primary Health Care
Nursing
Graduate School for Health Studies
Simmons College
Boston, Massachusetts

Susan C. Rawlins, MS, RNC
Director of Women's Health Care Nurse
Practitioner Program
University of Texas
Southwestern Medical Center at Dallas
Dallas, Texas

Marjorie J. Smith, PhD, RN, CNM
Professor and Director
Masters Program in Nursing
Winona State University
Winona, Minnesota

■ ■ ■ ■ ■ PREFACE

Many women, by choice or by necessity, will seek out the women's health care provider as their source of primary care. This second edition of *Women's Health: A Primary Care Clinical Guide* is designed to help meet the needs of these providers who offer women more than basic reproductive health care. It covers the traditional reproductive content as well as selected common medical, psychosocial, developmental, and political problems, issues, and needs. We have updated every chapter, and added new chapters in subject areas needing specific attention.

Part I, Women, Health, and the Health Care System, begins with a chapter on the major historical and contemporary changes in health care relating to women, focusing on the important societal, economic, and political factors that will affect health needs for the end of this century and into the next. Chapter 2, which is new to this edition, addresses legal issues in the primary care of women. Chapter 3 discusses women's health and development through the life cycle, followed by a new chapter specific to the adolescent woman. Chapter 5 deals with incidences of diseases, general guidelines for health care screening, and interventions. Chapter 6 covers sexuality facts and issues and is followed by another new chapter concerning the health needs of lesbians.

Part II, Promotion of Gynecologic Health Care, delves into the more traditional health problems and needs of women related to the reproductive systems. Chapters 8 through 15 cover menstrual concerns, fertility management, infertility, sexually transmitted diseases and vaginitis, pelvic and abdominal diseases, breast concerns, and the special needs of perimeno-pausal and older women. A new chapter addressing the special health needs of women with HIV has been added to this second edition. With the numbers of women with HIV anticipated to equal that of men by the year 2000, providers in every setting should be aware of the often complex treatment issues.

Part III, Promotion of Women's Health Care During Pregnancy, details uncomplicated and complicated pregnancy care, postpartum needs and problems, lactation issues, and fetal surveillance.

Primary Care Problems Affecting Women's Health, Part IV, has been significantly expanded to address even more of the medical problems frequently encountered in primary care of women such as headaches, anemia, hypertension, asthma, and dermatologic conditions. Chapters 21 and 22 are both dedicated to common medical problems, rather than only a single chapter as in the first edition. Selected psychosocial problems, such as violence, depression, and eating disorders and their impacts on women, with insights into related health care needs and therapies are discussed in Chapter 23. Chapter 24 reviews unique care concerns of women with disabilities and chronic illness. The appendices address emergency childbirth (Appendix A), assessment of the newborn (Appendix B), and selected laboratory values commonly referenced in women's health (Appendix C).

We particularly want this book to be a handbook, a resource that allows any primary health care provider to retrieve basic information easily. We see it as a reference with enough depth to be useful in a clinical setting, serving as a source of teaching advice for clients, including nursing diagnoses as well as differential medical diagnoses, screening and early intervention measures, and guidelines for referral. Some of the chapters fit more easily into an outline format for diseases or other conditions, whereas many chapters conform to a more traditional text format or a combination format for presentation of issues.

We wish to remind the reader that the scope of advanced practice nursing varies from state to state, and the individual practitioner is responsible for knowing his or her legal limits of practice. Also, recognizing the rapidity with which new knowledge becomes available and standards change, the practitioner must stay ever alert.

Women's health care providers are continuously challenged to expand their knowledge and ability to help women fulfill a wide spectrum of needs, both physical and psychosocial. Women's health is no longer limited to reproductive organs. The broadening scope of women's health care is a critically important issue in this period of rapidly changing health care systems. Resources are burgeoning, empowering women to become more informed consumers in the health care arena, yet attaining holistic care to meet basic needs remains a struggle for many. We, with the contributing authors, hope that you as primary care providers in a rapidly changing world of health care will find this book a useful and an effective resource in your endeavors to provide women with the health care they need and deserve.

Our sincere thanks go to our excellent contributing authors. Their outstanding expertise and effort have made this book the useful clinical reference we envisioned. We extend a special thank you to Mimi Coogan Bennett, MS, RNC, WHNP, a certified colposcopist, for her expert consultation on Pap smears and interpretation of reports. Ms. Bennett is a nurse practitioner at the Medical College of Virginia Women's Center, Virginia Commonwealth University, Richmond, Virginia. We also wish to thank the fine editors and staff at Appleton & Lange for their support and many hours of work on this project. Lastly, our deep appreciation goes out to our families who encouraged us during the months of preparation and work. A special note goes to our inspiring "little women," Alicia and Valarie, who will be the women of the twenty-first century needing the best health care of that new age.

Ellis Quinn Youngkin
Marcia Szmania Davis

▪ ▪ ▪ ▪ ▪ FOREWORD

For many years, women's health issues were not a priority in research and clinical practice. This lack of attention to women's health resulted in serious gaps in knowledge about the causes, treatment, and prevention of diseases in women. Currently, there is heightened awareness about women's health issues in the United States, and improving women's health is a top priority at the U.S. Department of Health and Human Services. Yet despite all these efforts to increase awareness and funding for women's health issues, women in this country continue to face serious threats to their mental and physical well being.

The "corporatization" of health delivery is proving to be a challenge for providing quality health care for women. Managed care organizations have defined a leaner standard of care by attempting to restrict the types and amounts of clinical services available to patients, many of whom are women. This was most evident in the political and legislative debate surrounding hospital length of stay for maternity services as well as the debate over when a woman should receive a mammogram. Although health care costs have dropped in recent years, nurses, physicians, and women worry that the quality of the care may be suffering due to these cost-saving efforts. The challenge for nurses and other health care providers caring for women is to continue to improve women's health in the midst of an evolving health care delivery system.

In addition to efforts at the Department of Health and Human Services (HHS), the National Institutes of Health (NIH) continues to support research on women's health through the Office of Research on Women's Health as well as the National Center for Health Statistics, Centers for Disease Control and Prevention, the Food and Drug Administration, and the Agency for Health Care Policy and Research. The U.S. Public Health Service's (PHS) Office of Women's Health, under the direction of Susan J. Blumenthal, MS, MPA, Deputy Assistant Secretary for Health, is charting an impressive, comprehensive agenda for women's health this year. Major initiatives include: 1) applying imaging technologies used for intelligence and defense purposes to improve the early detection of breast cancer; 2) establishing a National Women's Health Information Center; 3) developing and supporting six National Model Centers of Excellence in Women's Health; 4) implementing the National Action Plan on Breast Cancer; and 5) organizing several Healthy Women 2000 conferences, the first National Leadership Conference on Physical Activity and Women's Health, and a national minority women's health conference.

"From Missiles to Mammograms: New Frontiers in Breast Cancer Early Detection" is a unique partnership between the PHS Office of Women's Health, the Central Intelligence Agency, the Department of Defense (DOD), and the National Aeronautic and Space Administration. A contract of $1.98 million has been awarded to these sites to develop and to improve early detection of breast cancer by applying imaging technologies used for intelligence and defense purposes. The PHS Office of Women's

Health is also continuing to implement the National Action Plan on Breast Cancer (NAPBC). NAPBC is a public and private partnership that is increasing knowledge about the causes of breast cancer and using new information technologies, such as the Internet, to bring resources about breast cancer to women and their health care providers. NAPBC is also decreasing some of the barriers to women's participation in clinical trials and discussing the legal and ethical issues associated with the discovery of hereditary susceptibility genes.

In addition to improving breast cancer imaging technologies with DOD, the PHS Office of Women's Health is also collaborating with DOD to establish the National Women's Health Information Center (NWHIC). The Center will serve as a "women's health central" providing a user-friendly single point of entry to federal information and private-sector resources on women's health for consumers, clinicians, and researchers. The Center will be available by a toll-free telephone line and on the Internet. The projected launch date for the NWHIC is Winter 1997.

In the past year, six National Centers of Excellence in Women's Health have been developed and supported by the PHS Office of Women's Health. The Centers will serve as national models that can be evaluated and duplicated across the country. These Centers of Excellence will provide state-of-the-art comprehensive and integrated health care services, multidisciplinary research, and public and health care professional education targeted toward the unique needs of women.

The HHS is also taking action to improve the health of minority women. Minority women experience the same health problems as other women in our nation; however, their health outcomes are less favorable than those of Caucasian women. It is estimated that almost 35 million American women, which is 26 percent of the total female population, are members of culturally and ethni-

cally diverse groups. Of these, African Americans are the largest population in the United States followed by Hispanics, Asian/Pacific Islanders, and American Indians.

In an effort to bridge the gap and to enhance partnerships to improve minority women's health, the PHS Office of Women's Health sponsored a comprehensive conference in January 1997. The Minority Women's Health Conference focused on special health issues affecting women from culturally and ethnically diverse populations. The conference also developed partnerships throughout the nation with health care providers, educators, and researchers to improve the health of minority women.

Improving women's health in a comprehensive, science-based manner is critical in addressing the long-standing inequities in women's health. *Women's Health: A Primary Care Clinical Guide,* second edition, continues to provide an excellent vehicle for the transfer of such knowledge, not only for nurses but also for other health care providers caring for women. This book promotes comprehensive and culturally appropriate health promotion/disease prevention and diagnostic and treatment modalities for women across the life span. It also presents a wide spectrum of physical and psychosocial factors that can impact the health of women in a holistic, comprehensive, and practical manner. Once again, nurses have accepted the challenge to provide optimal health care for women in the nation's rapidly changing health care delivery system. The nurses who have written this book exemplify the type of knowledge, expertise, and commitment essential to improving the health of all women.

Stephanie L. Ferguson, PhD, RN
1996–1997 White House Fellow
Immediate Office of the Secretary
U.S. Department of Health
and Human Services

WOMEN, HEALTH, AND THE HEALTH CARE SYSTEM

I

WOMEN AND THE HEALTH CARE SYSTEM

Judith B. Collins • Nancy J. Sharp

*T*his spotlight of at-
tention on women's
health issues has ener-
gized women and or-
ganizations across the
United States and em-
powered them to speak
out with new force
about inequities.

Highlights

- Historical Perspective
- Societal Barriers to Quality Health Care
- Other Influences on Women's Health
- Political Action
- Health Care Policies
- Predictions for the Future

► INTRODUCTION

Many authors have noted that women enter the health care system by their reproductive organs. Often health care for women has focused on the reproductive system to the exclusion of other health needs, leading to the emergence of a narrow definition of women's health care centered on the breasts and the pelvis. A comprehensive approach to women's health care, on the other hand, addresses the physical, social, emotional and spiritual needs of women. This holistic approach is sensitive to women's *dis-ease,* not just their *diseases.* Some women may seek care only in a women's health care setting; therefore, health care providers in that setting must think beyond the breasts and the pelvis.

The U.S. Department of Health and Human Services (HHS), at the benchmark National Conference on Women's Health in 1986, defined a women's health issue as "any matter that affects the health of women exclusively, that impacts predominately on women's health (at any age), or that affects women's health differently from that of men."[1] This definition of women's health, it is pointed out, is based on a male norm. Thus, "by limiting women's health to consideration of ways that women are different from men, this definition not only defines women's health incompletely—to the detriment of women—but also ensures that no beneficial effects can accrue to men, because only women's differences from men are legitimate areas of concern."[2] Alternatively, a "woman centered" definition addressing all of women's needs would provide for broader societal changes to benefit everyone.[2]

A comprehensive view of women's health care moves beyond the biomedical approach to the concepts of totality, centrality, and diversity.[2] *Totality* includes women's many roles and contexts. The Rodriquez-Trias totality concept "defines the health problems of women as deeply implanted in the statuses that derive from their multiple social relations."[3] Totality calls for women to be viewed as inextricably connected with their families and communities, not separate from the multiple roles as mothers, sisters, wives, workers, and caretakers.[3]

Centrality denotes care that is woman centered. One view of centrality "defines health problems as women themselves experience those problems."[3] This view casts women as "active decision makers in their own lives" and thus rejects and reshapes "the all too common view of women as passive recipients of health care and public health action."[3]

Diversity entails meeting the needs of all women. It "requires recognizing not only women's different social roles but also their different races, economic conditions, sexual orientations, and cultures and how these relate to health."[2] Diversity is manifested in "varying rates of diseases among ethnic groups" as well as "in different understandings of what health is and what health needs are, and [these] are shaped by socioeconomic status and social roles."[3]

McBride also advocates a broader view of women's health by refocusing gynecology to "Gyn-ecology," to acknowledge the fit between a woman and her environment.[4]

Historical perspective

Throughout the ages, an evolution of the health care of women has occurred, often paralleling the changing roles of women in society. Women's consumer health activities began in the United States during the 1830s and 1840s. Suffrage during the mid-19th century was accomplished by the Popular Health Movement, which demanded a total redefinition of health itself and health care. Abrums'[5] historical perspective on women's health care discusses Naphey's 1870 work entitled *The Physical Life of Women: Advice to Maiden, Wife, and Mother.* Although the book was widely acclaimed as valuable scientific literature, it identified only three phases in a woman's life: maidenhood, matrimony, and maternity.[6]

About the turn of the 20th century, it was believed that the ovaries and uterus were the controlling organs and the center of all disease in a woman's body, thus the etiology of most female complaints, including headaches, indigestion, and sore throats.[7] Consequently, the stage was set for decades during which women's health care would be plagued with sexism and ageism. Women felt that they lacked control of their bodies, and many normal physiological processes were viewed by medicine and society as diseases. For example, menstruation was seen as a chronic problem, and pregnancy and menopause as disorders requiring intervention.[7] Sexism in the health care system provided the basis for "oppression of women derived from her 'womanness': her biologic differences and her ability to bear children."[8] These differences have been used to build social structures and a supportive ideology of female submissiveness and to "permit condescension toward women."[8] Further reinforcing this ideology, in 1905, the president of the Oregon State Medical Society stated, "Educated women could not bear children with ease because study arrested the development of the pelvis at the same time it increased the size of the child's brain, and therefore its head."[9]

This ideology was also extended to mature women. In the popular 1970 book *Everything You Always Wanted to Know about Sex,* Dr. David Reuben described the menopausal woman:

> As the estrogen is shut off, a woman comes as close as she can to being a man. Increased facial hair, deepened voice, obesity, and the decline of breasts and female genitalia all contribute to a masculine appearance. Coarsened features, enlargement of the clitoris, and gradual baldness complete the picture. Not really a man but no longer a functional woman, these individuals live in a world of intersex . . . sex no longer interests them. To many women the menopause marks the end of their useful life. They see it as the onset of old age, the beginning of the end. They may be right. Having outlived their

> ovaries, they may have outlived their usefulness as human beings. The remaining years may be just marking time until they follow their glands into oblivion.[10]

THE 1960s AND 1970s

Many social changes erupted in the 1960s fueled by societal unrest about the lack of equality for all citizens. Most notable and visible was the civil rights movement. Major changes for women also evolved, catalyzed in 1963 by Betty Friedan's historic book *The Feminine Mystique,* which told of women's disenchantments with their relationships, both personal and institutional.[11] This disenchantment developed into the women's liberation movement, which addressed the cause of equal rights for women. Health care system change was strategic to women's liberation, because the system is an agent of social control equally as restrictive as any political or economic system.[8]

The women's health movement grew from the women's liberation movement in the early 1970s as a grassroots organization with a common uniting goal: "a demand for improved health care for all women and an end to sexism in the health system."[8]

"Activities centered around abortion law reform provided the initial cohesion from which the women's health movement could emerge."[8] In January 1973, the landmark Supreme Court decision in *Roe v. Wade* provided a legal right to abortion.

The women's health movement focused on "changing consciousness, providing health related services, and struggling to change established health institutions."[8] The major thrust of concern was that women wanted to own and control their bodies, not just to be cured. In a landmark book published by the Boston Women's Health Collective, *Our Bodies, Ourselves,* women spoke out and asked for something different and better from health care providers.[12]

The women's health movement also raised issues of childbirth education, natural methods of childbirth, and birthing options, including father participation in labor and delivery and home births. Spurred by consumer education in books, magazines, and networking meetings, women's requests from the health care system then grew beyond childbearing issues. Hospitals, awakened to the fact that women were their major customers, began to market women's services by establishing women's health resource centers (either within the hospital or as a freestanding center) to provide specialized care and education in homelike surroundings.

THE 1980s AND 1990s

More recently, women have demanded participatory health care decision making, humanistic and holistic preventive care, and a wellness, rather than illness, orientation to care. In the sociopolitical arena women have been advocating for health services and policies that address reproductive freedom, contraceptive options, domestic violence, and research on women's special health problems (e.g., breast disease, menopause, osteoporosis, hormonal replacement therapy, premenstrual syndrome, heart disease, human immunodeficiency virus/acquired immunodeficiency syndrome, depression and stress related illnesses).

Abortion rights remain a major emotional and legal issue for the nation. Since the *Roe v. Wade* decision in 1973, abortion has been legal in all 50 states. Some states have implemented laws such as twenty-four hour waiting periods, parental notification, and other restrictions. The court system uses an undue burden measure to determine if such restrictions are legal. Access to abortion services is a critical issue. In many areas of the country, women have to travel hundreds of miles to find qualified abortion providers.

Betty Friedan, speaking out on the new feminine mystique,[13] asserted that the women's movement had been halted by the general reversal of social progress in the United States during the 1980s and 1990s. She felt that the rights women had won during the past 20 years were in "grave danger."[13]

Women are the preeminent consumers of health care in the United States, measured by standards such as doctors' visits, medication prescriptions, surgery, hospitalization, and nursing home care.[14] Women are also responsible for spending two of every three health care dollars.[15] Seventy to 90 percent of all health care decisions are made by women for themselves and their families, and 60 to 70 percent of all hospital beds are filled by women. The National Center for Health Statistics (NCHS) reports, as mentioned in McKinnon, that of the 20 most frequently performed surgeries, 11 are performed exclusively on women; none are performed exclusively on men.[16] Women account for 63 to 66 percent of all surgeries.[16] Women, therefore, should have the best health care that the U.S. system can offer.

SOCIETAL BARRIERS TO QUALITY HEALTH CARE

Not all American women are getting quality health care. Clancy and Massion view American women's health care as "a patchwork quilt with gaps."[17] For many women, access to care still has many barriers, including excessive costs; limited availability of providers and services; some insensitive attitudes and paternalism in the medical profession; lack of transportation; poorly coordinated and disorganized systems for referral; and problems with insurance and managed care.

DISCOUNTING OF WOMEN'S SYMPTOMS

Women's symptoms, rather than being taken seriously, often are ascribed to hormonal or psychiatric causes. This delays diagnosis and treatment and may have serious consequences. According to Paula Doress, co-author of *Ourselves, Growing Older,* as reported in Southwick's article, "If a man comes in with certain symptoms, it's diabetes or heart disease. For women, menopause is the wastebasket diagnosis for everything."[14] The combination of social inequities and a historically male-dominated medical profession has had a major effect on women's health referred to as "gender bias." Fortunately, this is changing as more women are entering medicine and there is increasing research on health issues and diseases in women.

OVERUSE OF SURGICAL PROCEDURES

The most common surgical procedures in the United States are cesarean birth and hysterectomy. The rate of cesarean births has increased steadily: from 5 percent in 1970 to 23.5 percent in

1991.[18] Thus, in the United States, almost one infant in four is delivered by cesarean.

RESTRICTED ACCESS TO PRENATAL CARE

Despite technological advances in perinatal health care, many women are still unable to access routine care. In 1993, 21 percent of women who had a live birth did not receive prenatal care in the first trimester,[19] and the United States ranked behind 21 other nations in infant mortality.[20]

In 1994, the overall U.S. infant mortality rate was 8.0 per 1000 live births. Among African American infants, the rate was 15.8 per 1000, 2.4 times that of white infants at 6.6.[21] Historically, the rate of infant mortality among African American infants has been more than double that of white infants.

Multiple social and health problems contribute to these tragic statistics, but to a great extent the dismal record can be attributed to severely inadequate access to prenatal care. The poor health status among rural mothers and infants is indicative of limited availability of obstetric providers and limited access to specialized care for complicated pregnancies and deliveries.[22] In the United States, a large number of counties have no private or clinic-based provider of prenatal care, which in some states has left a significant number of women with reduced access to care.[18] As a nation, we spent nearly one trillion dollars for health care in 1995,[23] yet we made no commitment to ensuring prenatal care for every pregnant woman in the United States. This is a significant political issue because women and children—who represent more than half of the population—are not our policymakers and often do not vote.

Politics also plays a role in other health issues for women, such as problems with health insurance coverage for infertility and bone marrow transplant for breast cancer and the ongoing challenge of abortion rights.

INADEQUATE INSURANCE

Approximately 40 million Americans were uninsured in 1995.[24] Between 1991 and 1993, 27 percent of the population was uninsured for at least one month.[25] The number of Americans without health insurance is growing as more employers shift workers to temporary or part-time positions and reduce insurance to existing employees. Families of workers most often will lose coverage when employers tighten health care benefits and increase the employee insurance contributions. It is estimated that the number of uninsured will increase to 45.6 million by the year 2000.[26] Despite recent increases in Medicaid benefits for women and children, 14 million women of childbearing age have no coverage, and 5 million have insurance that excludes coverage for prenatal care and delivery.[27] Most of the uninsured do not qualify for Medicaid either because they are not eligible to receive AFDC or state welfare, or because they do not meet other categorical or financial standards.[28] Sixty million Americans are underinsured or have inadequate coverage that is often comparable to no insurance.[29]

Being underinsured is especially difficult for women. It can include high cost sharing, lengthy waiting periods, restricted coverage for preexisting conditions, and limited services or exclusion from some services that are important to women (e.g., Papanicolaou smears, mammograms, bone densitometry, infertility services, and family planning services). In addition, lack of long-term care insurance is a special threat to older women, who "live longer than men and suffer more chronic disorders as they age."[30]

LACK OF RESEARCH

Though often viewed as a major disease in men, heart disease is the leading cause of death among all American women.[19] Each year cardiovascular disease claims the lives of nearly half a million U.S. women.[18] In the past, too little research has focused on women's unique response to disease and common health issues, especially studies of chronic diseases and their prevention in older women.

A study of women's health research revealed three points that were especially disturbing.

- Historically, women have been excluded from large clinical trials, such as the study of aspirin and heart disease. Even when women were included, study results were not routinely analyzed for general differences.

- No gynecologic unit existed within the entire structure of the National Institutes of Health (NIH) nor was there any central coordinating office for women's health matters.
- Few women have achieved the top echelons of medicine and scientific research.[31]

Thus, even though women make up 51 percent of the U.S. population, research on major diseases and the drugs to treat them has been done mostly on "mice and men." Researchers, until recently, had excluded women, arguing that pregnancy and women's fluctuating hormone levels could alter study results.[32]

In the 1990s, however, a time of major political activity and regulatory change, the national research agenda on women's health has been invigorated. A study indicates there is evidence that women are being included in studies; however, the "potential differences in response to treatment are not being addressed vigorously by researchers or research organizations. In addition, even in the small number of articles that provide evidence of some form of gender analysis, almost all treatment recommendations are gender neutral."[33]

OTHER INFLUENCES ON WOMEN'S HEALTH

POVERTY

Poverty and health are significantly interrelated. Low income women are in poorer health and have greater difficulty accessing health care services than do affluent women. Poor women face the inability to pay for care. Pregnant women eligible for Medicaid, however, may find improved access to care with the increase in reimbursement to providers. Child care, time off from work, and transportation are other issues they still face.[30]

Inequities in income between men and women persist. "Women are poorer than men regardless of age, race, ethnicity, education or employment status."[30] Even though women's salaries are starting to catch up and sometimes surpass men's pay, more typically women still earn 5 cents to 15 cents less on the dollar than do men working in similar jobs. The Bureau of Labor Statistics determined that women earn 74 cents to a man's dollar when all jobs are included as comparison of like jobs.[34] Furthermore, nearly three-fourths of elderly Americans living in poverty are women.[35]

In addition, after divorce or separation, the average family income of mothers with child custody drops by 23 percent. Families headed by a mother alone are six times as likely to be poor as those with two parents.[36] Women and children are the fastest growing segment of the homeless population.

MARITAL STATUS

Marital status, standard of living, and health status are also interrelated. Public policy is often developed on the outdated concept of the American family headed by a male wage earner with a spouse at home. Social Security, private pension, and health insurance plans are notable examples.[30] Only about one U.S. family in four, however, conforms to this model.[37]

LONGEVITY

Since the turn of the century, women's life expectancy has increased from 48.3 years to 78.8 years. While living longer, women are not necessarily living better. Women represent 51 percent of the total U.S. population, 60 percent over age 65 and more than 70 percent above age 85.[38] By living longer, women may have an increased incidence of chronic diseases that require long-term care. It is estimated that more than half of the women who have reached age 85 are living in nursing homes.[39]

CAREGIVING

Women, providing the majority of paid and unpaid family care, have become the safety net for our health care system. Women make up three-fourths of the unpaid caregivers of the elderly.[40] Without these family caregivers, many more elderly would be in health care institutions. "Almost two million women, the 'sandwich generation,' have both elder and child care responsibilities."[30] Women's health can be impacted by the stress of juggling employment, homemaking, and child and elder care. One caregiver in three is age

65 or over, and the impact on one's health may be severe.[41] Because women are nurturers and caregivers, their state of health can also affect their families and society.

POLITICAL ACTION

THE PAST IN REVIEW

In 1983, Dr. Edward N. Brandt, Jr., assistant secretary of health, commissioned a Public Health Services (PHS) task force to examine the status of women's health. This action acknowledged that cultural, economic, social, and environmental factors make it necessary to develop approaches and strategies to provide adequate health care services that meet woman's needs. In 1985, the task force findings were published in *Women's Health: Report of the Public Health Service Task Force on Women's Health Issues.*[42] Academics and government policymakers agreed, for the first time, that women were disadvantaged in terms of health care. The task force report made 15 recommendations that focused on six major areas:

- Promoting physical and social environments that are safe and healthful.
- Providing services to prevent and treat disease.
- Conducting research and evaluation.
- Recruiting and training women health care personnel.
- Education and informing the public and disseminating research information.
- Designing guidance for legislative and regulatory measures.

CONGRESSIONAL CAUCUS ON WOMEN'S ISSUES

Despite the startling conclusions of the PHS task force report, little action was taken, especially in eliminating the inequities in women's health research. In 1989, the Congressional Caucus on Women's Issues (CCWI), a bipartisan group of more than 125 members of Congress, was formed and officially requested an audit of the inclusion of women by the NIH in clinical trials (a policy adopted as a result of the PHS task force recommendations in 1985). The report, issued in June

1990, found that the NIH had failed in several serious ways: policy not well communicated or understood, study results not being analyzed by gender, and policy only applied to extramural, not intramural, research.

When the NIH, Congress, the media, and the public reacted to this report, changes began to occur. Multimedia coverage showed women's omission from research, and reports focused on women's diseases. Meanwhile, the CCWI developed a women's health legislative agenda for research, prevention, and services. It was introduced in Congress in The Women's Health Equity Act (WHEA) in 1990 and has continued to the present.

The WHEA is a package of individual bills introduced as omnibus legislation that presents a forward looking agenda for women's health. Title I addresses research on women's health, and Title II addresses the delivery of health services. More than a dozen WHEA provisions have been enacted since the bill was introduced in 1990, resulting in signficant progress toward redressing inequities in medical research and health care delivery, and helping improve the health of American women. The omnibus package also serves an important purpose in educational and health policy agenda setting. In addition, at the end of each congressional session, a review of the WHEA provides a means of measuring action on issues important to women.[43]

RECENT MILESTONES IN WOMEN'S HEALTH

Background/Historical Perspective

Recent milestones that have contributed to a focus on women's health during the 1990s include the following.

Office of Research on Women's Health (ORWH) at the National Institutes of Health (NIH) (1990)

Established in 1990 within the Office of the Director of NIH, ORWH serves as a focal point for women's health research at NIH in setting and monitoring policy, promoting, and enhancing scientific career development and ensuring that women's health research becomes an integral part of the scientific fabric at NIH and the scientific community. The ORWH has a threefold mandate:

1. To strengthen and enhance research related to diseases, disorders, and conditions that affect women and to ensure that research conducted and supported by NIH adequately addresses issues regarding women's health;
2. To ensure that women are appropriately represented in biomedical and behavioral research studies supported by NIH; and
3. To develop opportunities and support for recruitment, retention, re-entry, and advancement of women in biomedical careers.

The office continues to revise and update its agenda based on deliberations with the NIH, congressional directives and hearings, discussions with women's health experts and advocates, and scientific literature and advances.[44]

The ORWH plays a collaborative advisory role in the NIH's Women's Health Initiative (WHI), the largest disease-prevention study ever conducted in the United States.[45] The WHI has three major components:

1. A prospective surveillance study of over 100,000 women to examine specific risk factors and biomarkers for disease.
2. A randomized clinical trial in 40 centers across the United States with approximately 64,500 postmenopausal women to examine the effects of diet modifications, hormonal replacement therapy, and dietary supplementation with calcium and vitamin D on the prevention of cardiovascular disease, breast and colorectal concerns, and osteoporosis.
3. A multicommunity prevention study to examine risk factor modification among women.

The WHI will span approximately 15 years and cost more than $628 million.[46]

Office of Women's Health (OWH) of the U.S. Public Health Service (1991)

Established in 1991, the OWH is the champion and cornerstone for women's health activities within the Department of Health and Human Services (DHHS) by administering cross cutting initiatives across the agencies and offices of the Public Health Services including the following: NIH, Substance Abuse and Mental Health Services Administrations (SAMHSA) Office, CDC, FDA, Agency for Health Care Policy and Research, Health Resources and Services Administration, and the Indian Health Service.[47]

The OWH was instrumental in the development of the PHS Action Plan for Women's Health (1991), a key document outlining national strategies for women's health. The OWH serves to advise the Assistant Secretary for Health, the Secretary of HHS, the White House, and Members of Congress on scientific, medical, legal, ethical, and policy issues relating to the advancement of women's health. In addition, the Office has established widespread public/private partnerships to set women's health policy into action at all levels. Some areas of activity include the following: National Action Plan on Breast Cancer and Breast Cancer Imaging, regional women's health initiatives, Federal Interagency Coordinating Committee on Women's Health and the Environment, model women's health curricula, Healthy Women 2000 Initiative, and domestic violence.[47]

Food and Drug Administration (FDA) Office of Women's Health (1994)

During the past decade, there has been growing concern that the drug development process does not produce adequate information about the effects of drugs in women. The 1977 FDA Guidelines, which excluded women of childbearing potential from drug study participation, seen from the viewpoint of the 1990s appear "rigid and paternalistic, leaving virtually no room for the exercise of judgment by responsible female research subjects, physicians, investigators, and IRBs"[48] (institutional review boards). The new FDA guidelines (1993) provide for "inclusion of patients of both genders in drug development, analyses of clinical data by gender, assessment of potential pharmacokinetic differences between genders, and conduct of specific additional studies in women when indicated."[48]

Women's Policy, Inc. (1995)

In January, 1995, the House of Representatives abolished Legislative Service Organizations and Caucuses including the Caucus on Women's Issues (CCWI). The Women's Policy, Inc. formed with the mission of providing nonpartisan research and information on legislative actions affecting women and families. WPI was established by former staff of the CCWI, with support from its congressional members to carry on the informational services previously provided by the CCWI.[43]

This spotlight of attention on women's health issues has energized women and organizations across the United States and empowered them to speak out with new force. For example, the National Breast Cancer Coalition and advocacy groups across the nation have been a powerful force in increasing breast cancer awareness—the tragedy for women and families, the need for more research dollars and changes in health insurance coverage, the launching of a U.S. postage stamp for breast cancer awareness, and the risks and benefits of the identification of the breast cancer genes. Though the National Cancer Institute announced a decline in the breast cancer rate probably due to earlier detection and changes in breast cancer management, it was projected 44,300 women would die of breast cancer in 1996. Inequities are still noted, with the age adjusted mortality rates falling approximately 6 percent in white women but rising 1 percent in African American women, possibly related to lack of access to regular exams, mammograms, and state-of-the-art treatment.[49] Despite decades of research, breast cancer continues to present the scientist with a challenge to explain the steady increase in the disease over the past years. "The lifetime risk of developing breast cancer has increased from one in 20 two decades ago to one in eight today."[43] Truly the "public policy response to breast cancer in recent years has been more elaborate than to any other women's health issue,"[43] in major part due to women and coalitions becoming a grassroots political force.

The 1990s viewed as a decade of women's health is expected to continue into the next century with even greater momentum.

HEALTH CARE POLICIES

MANAGED CARE AND IMPLICATIONS FOR WOMEN'S HEALTH

Viewed as the "health care reformer," managed care is considered the most important factor in the health care marketplace for the future and has important implications for women's health. A dramatic growth in managed care entities has occurred with approximately 51 percent of all employees in employer-sponsored health insurance enrolled in manage care plans.[50] A paradigm shift has occurred in providing care with managed care from the traditional fee-for-service medical model that reimbursed for high-tech medical intervention to preventive services.[51] See definitions relevant to managed care (Table 1–1).

Managed care was designed initially as a system of organizing *care* and not a financing mechanism of managing *cost*.[51] The best managed care initiatives value a comprehensive approach to care with a focus on prevention, early intervention, and continuity of care.[51,52]

The worst managed care creates incentives to provide inadequate care, less time with patients to meet increasing productivity standards, frequent change of providers, too early discharge of hospital patients, and impingement of professional judgment with preauthorization/review of every clinical service.[52] All this leads to a lack of continuity of care, with care more fragmented and decreased opportunity for holistic care, and accessible care potentially compromised by financial incentives.

Health policy proposals being considered or adopted to adjust managed care impact are the following:

- Postpartum stay—must cover hospital stay for mother and newborn for at least 48 hours after normal delivery.
- Any willing provider—must accept providers with appropriate credentials who agree to abide by contract considerations/terms.
- Emergency care—must pay whenever a prudent lay person would consider a situation an emergency; care may not be delayed to get authorization.

TABLE 1–1. RELEVANT MANAGED CARE DEFINITIONS

HMO

A health care delivery system that gives enrollees health coverage for a prepaid, fixed fee. The HMO may directly employ physicians or contract with them and other providers such as hospitals and other health care professionals. Enrollees must select from these approved providers for all of their health care services. Five models of HMOs: staff, group, network, mixed, and independent (or individual practice/physician association) (IPA).

IPA

An association of physicians who may practice as part of a medical group or individually. Created with the purpose of contracting with HMOs and other managed care organizations.

PPO

A plan or a benefit arrangement where services are supplied to plan members at a discount by providers who contract with the PPO. A variety of incentives, such as lower co-payments and limits on out-of-pocket expenses, are used to encourage members to use the preferred providers. PPOs are not insurers and are not prepaid plans.

Providers

A provider is any individual that provides health care services to patients. Provider is most often used to denote the physician, but it also may refer to other individuals such as nurse practitioners, physical therapists, psychologists, etc. or to an institution such as a hospital or an organization such as a pharmacy.

Capitation

A form of payment where the physician agrees to a set fee per month (or quarter) for each subscriber assigned by the MCO. The fee is received whether or not the patient comes to the office. There is no additional income if the patient is seen on more than one occasion during the period.

The Ortho Institute of Physician Development. (1994.) "Glossary of Terms." Understanding Managed Care. Raritan, NJ: Ortho Pharmaceuticals Corporation.

- No gag rules—cannot restrict what information providers can give patients about care choices.
- Incentive disclosures—patients and state regulators must be informed of financial incentives networks to providers.[53]

The rapid growth and shift to managed health care has important implications for women's health including the following:

- Cost-cutting strategies that influence the visible and measured cost of managed care may be based on hidden costs to women, i.e., decreased length of hospital stay for children and the elderly are often met by increased at-home care given by women as caregivers.[54] In addition, with the gatekeeper referral system and the frequent need to go to multiple sites for diagnostic tests, an additional burden is placed on the patients and on women who are principally the care coordinators helping family members obtain health care.[54]
- Loss of continuity of care and an established trust relationship for a woman when her plan does not include her current provider.[54]
- Potential prohibition of Ob/Gyn physicians from making referrals for services, i.e., surgical consult after abnormal mammography.[54]
- Constraining clinical judgment that may affect individualization of care and increase patient morbidity, i.e., dictating length of stay for mothers and newborns who may require more observation and nursing care.[54]
- Attempts to cut costs by excluding the sickest or most troublesome populations from coverage, i.e., the uninsured with a high proportion of women and children.[54]

INFLUENCES ON HEALTH POLICY AND WOMEN'S HEALTH CARE

To understand health policy as it relates to women, the subject must be viewed in the context of all health policy, including the major influencing economic, social, and political forces.

Health Care Costs

- National health care expenditures in 1995 were $988.5 billion and 13.6 percent of the gross domestic product (GDP).[23]
- The growth rate for health spending was slightly higher than 5.1 percent increase in 1994 with an estimated average of $3621 per person.[23]

Corporate Influence on the Health Industry

- In today's market, a business approach is taken to health care delivery, with a focus on marketing services and the financial bottom line. Women's health care is viewed as a tremendous source of revenue for health care organizations. Exploitation of women's services as simply a hospital marketing strategy, without provision of quality services, must be guarded against.

- Economic good competes with social good; emphasis can be on paying for care or on providing care.

Competition

- Players in the health care marketplace—patients, providers, payers, purchasers, and policymakers—have competing objectives.
- Prices and costs of services should decrease with competition, but this principle is not reflected in the health care industry.

Care of the Poor

- The gap between the "haves" and the "have nots" in American society is increasing.
- Women are especially vulnerable to a market oriented system with health insurance linked to employment. Many women work in jobs without health benefits; others do not work outside the home while caring for children and aging relatives.
- Debate is increasing about health care as a right or a privilege for all, including the poor.

Reproductive Freedom

- A public spotlight is on this women's issue.
- *Roe v. Wade,* which was the basis of the 1973 Supreme Court decision on abortion, is constantly challenged in test cases that seek to limit or reverse it.
- Title X, the nation's family planning program, faces challenges every year. Although the program has never funded abortion services, amendments that would require parental notification for contraception, gags on counseling concerning reproductive choices, and others are brought up at each appropriation cycle.
- Parental notification and/or consent for abortion is a national issue.
- Funding for and availability of abortion services are major health policy issues.
- Limited contraceptive options for women remain an issue.
  - A National Academy of Science report stated that contraceptive research in the United States had come to a virtual halt and that the United States had fallen far behind other countries in developing new techniques.[55]

- Up to 15 years and $50 million are required for a new contraceptive to move from the laboratory through the U.S. Food and Drug Administration (FDA) approval process.[55]
- A study published in the *American Journal of Public Health* demonstrated that preventing unintended pregnancy saves a health care system at least three thousand dollars per woman per year.[56]
- Two recommendations by the FDA's Advisory Committee on Reproductive Health Drugs should increase reproductive health options for women. The first is a June, 1996 decision to recommend the oral contraceptives containing levonorgestrel are safe and effective as emergency contraception. The second is a July, 1996 decision to recommend mifepristone (RU 486) as a safe and effective drug for early medical abortion.

Technological Advances

Medical

- Advancing technology in areas such as bioengineering, transplantation, cloning, and use of fetal tissue raises issues of who shall live, who shall die, and who shall decide.
- With increasing technological ability to save and prolong life, discussions of health care rationing arise, requiring explicit policy decisions of who gets advanced technology care based on age, illness, and so on.

Information Systems and Telemedicine

- Push-button telephones, fax machines, computers and electronic mail are now the current standard for transmitting messages and information. Computers have now moved into our daily lives. Computing is not just about computers anymore. It is about living. In 1995, 35 percent of American families and 50 percent of American teenagers had a personal computer at home; 30 million people are estimated to be on the Internet; and 65 percent of new computers sold worldwide in 1994 were for the home.[57]
- Women and their families are now able to access, from their own home or work desktop computer, libraries (i.e., National Library of Medicine in Bethesda, MD), schools and

universities (i.e., University of Washington, Seattle, WA), corporate giants (i.e., ATT, NYLife Managed Care Co., Starbucks Coffee), professional and voluntary organizations (i.e., American Heart Association, American Cancer Society, and American Medical Association). Health information can be accessed either on a specific disease condition and/or health promotion activities such as exercise and antismoking programs.

- Primary care providers soon will all be connected to the Internet, where they also can access the World Wide Web to obtain health information to discuss with women and their families. Health care providers may also have access to high resolution x-ray transmission equipment that can send an x-ray image across town or across several states to consult with a clinical expert on a particular diagnosis. Pictures of skin conditions or an EKG strip can be sent via high speed telecommunications equipment to receive consultation from a clinical expert not available in the patient's hometown.

- Telemedicine is defined simply as removing distance and time barriers to the provision of health services or health information. To survive, telemedicine must become the "embedded technology" that supports more effective health care and health service delivery, not an end in itself.[58]

Aging/Migrant Populations

- The number of elderly and the number of migrants in the United States are growing. Each group has very different needs for health care services.

- The "intergenerational war," or competition for funding of programs and services for the elderly and children, is a major political issue.

Primary Care and Prevention

- The Institute of Medicine's Committee on the Future of Primary Care defines primary care as the provision of *integrated,* accessible health care services by *clinicians* who are *accountable* for addressing a large majority of personal health care needs, developing a *sustained part-*nership with patients, and practicing in the context of *family and community.* A key term in this definition is *integration,* which encompasses the provision of *comprehensive, coordinated,* and *continuous* services.[59]

- For women, having a primary care clinician means that they have a place to bring a wide range of health problems for appropriate attention—a place where they can expect, in most instances, that their problems will be resolved, or the primary care clinicians will guide women through the health system, referring them to specialists when appropriate. Primary care facilitates an ongoing relationship between women and their clinicians and fosters participation by women in decision making about their health care. Such continuing relationships provide opportunities for health promotion and disease prevention as well as for early detection of problems.[59]

- The IOM committee recognizes and supports interdisciplinary teams being used increasingly to deliver primary care. Such teams may include nurse practitioners, physicians, and physician assistants, as well as other health care professionals. The committee urges review of state restrictions on the scope of practice of these health care professionals and the elimination or modifications of those restructions that impede collaborative practice and reduce access to primary care. The state restrictions currently in place impede women from fully accessing all qualified primary care providers and services.[60]

Long-Term Care/Home Health Care

- Women provide the majority of paid and unpaid family care in the United States, including that for elders and children.[30]

- The rate of home health care utilization is 36 percent higher for women than for men age 65–74 and 65 percent higher among those age 85 and older.[19]

- 93 percent of the 1.5 million workers in long-term care facilities in the United States are women.[61]

- Women are the primary users of long-term services.[18]

- Approximately two-thirds of persons over age 65 who require nursing home care are women.[18]

HIV/AIDS

- HIV/AIDS is a major public health issue; and public policy and political forces are pushing for funding for research, prevention, education, and treatment.
- In the United States, nearly 90,000 women between ages 15 and 44 are infected; this is the fastest growing group with HIV/AIDS in the country.[43]
- HIV/AIDS is the third leading cause of death among women ages 25 to 44.[43]
- The rate of AIDS among minority women in the United States is high; one in five African American women between 25–44 years old is expected to die from AIDS, compared with one in 17 Caucasian women in the same age group.[43]
- The majority of AIDS cases in women occur as a result of heterosexual transmission or intravenous drug use.[43]
- Infected women die sooner than infected men. This may be related to delay in diagnosis, treatment later in the disease progression, HIV/AIDS affecting women in fundamentally different ways than men, or possibly lack of access to health care.[43]

Substance Abuse

- Substance abuse is a major public health and public safety issue.
- Alcohol use by women in the United States is prevalent, but less than in men. Of approximately 11 million heavy drinkers, 2 percent are women and 10 percent are men. Since women consuming alcohol has been stigmatized since ancient times, unwillingness to report makes it difficult to estimate the magnitude of the problem.[18]
- Illicit drug use in the United States is estimated at 11.7 million with women at 4.1 percent use versus men at 7.4 percent. In women age 35 and older, the rate is 1.4 percent whereas among young women age 12–17, the rate is 6 percent for both women and men.[18]
- Women are more likely than men to become addicted to prescription drugs and use them often with alcohol, for medication to cope with anxiety, depression, and painful reactions to life stress.[18]

- Approximately one in four women in the United States currently smokes. The rate of cigarette smoking for women and men is declining but is less dramatic for women. Tobacco use has been identified as the chief preventable cause of premature death and disease. More than 140,000 women's deaths in the United States in 1990 were attributed to smoking: 21 percent of coronary heart disease, 82 percent of chronic obstructive pulmonary disease, and 87 percent of lung cancer.[18]

Domestic Violence

- Domestic violence is now recognized as a major hazard to the health of women.[62]
- It is the single largest cause of injury to women in the United States—more common than automobile accidents, muggings, and rapes combined.[63]
- Four million women are abused each year,[62] and battered women account for 21 percent of the women who use emergency room services.[42]

Consumerism

- The American public has an increasing knowledge of health issues and is demanding quality health care services.
- Consumer advocates are lobbying at the local, state, and national levels for special interest needs, such as breast cancer, HIV/AIDS, domestic violence, infant mortality, and aging.
- Women are becoming more vocal and active, especially regarding reproductive rights and research on women's diseases.

Complementary and Alternative Medicine

- The Office of Alternative Medicine started in 1993 at the National Institutes of Health (NIH) to provide research funding to complementary and alternative health care providers to study the effectiveness of alternative treatment therapies, such as biofeedback, acupuncture, massage therapy, nutrition counseling, herbal/ vitamin therapies, chiropractic, and reflexology.
- Columbia University College of Physicians and Surgeons, New York, NY, received over $1 million dollars to study the effectiveness of

alternative therapies in conditions relative to women's health. This research study is co-funded by the Office of Research on Women's Health at NIH and will help promote scholarly research and education in this area.[64]

- Unconventional, alternative, or unorthodox therapies are used by one in three people. Among those who used unconventional therapy for serious medical conditions, the vast majority (83 percent) also sought treatment for the same condition from a medical doctor; however, 72 percent of the respondents to the survey who used unconventional therapy did not inform their medical doctor that they had done so, which may suggest a deficiency in current patient-doctor relations.[65]

- More women are asking for alternative natural therapies such as herbs and vitamins to address PMS and menopausal symptoms versus standard hormonal or medicinal approaches.

Liability Insurance

- Increased lawsuits have led to increased defensive medical practices by physicians to protect themselves. Hence a major increase in the cost of liability insurance to providers has occurred.

- High liability insurance premiums have caused some obstetricians to eliminate maternity care or reduce services for high risk women, leaving many women unserved.

- Contrary to public opinion, the American College of Obstetricians and Gynecologists reports that poor women do not sue more often than other patient groups.[66]

- Tort reform is being addressed throughout the nation, e.g., caps on malpractice awards.

PREDICTIONS FOR THE FUTURE

The United States has never enjoyed a comprehensive, internally consistent national health policy. Instead, the nation has been a "clumsy juggler" of diverse policies and objectives, trying to achieve equilibrium in access, quality, and cost-effectiveness.[67] A scenario for health policy in the year 2000 has been predicted.

- Cost effectiveness versus access or quality will remain the most urgent and dominant issue influencing health policy decisions. The aims of cost effectiveness include the provision of medically appropriate care in the least costly way.

- A mixture of regulatory and market-based approaches will be evident in emerging health policy. The regulatory approach encompasses governmental regulations, certificates of need, rate review/rate-setting programs, and peer review organizations. The market-based approach encourages competition, alternative delivery systems, and use of management programs.

- Incremental (minor) policy changes will be made rather than fundamental (major) policy changes in response to powerful advocate groups, such as hospitals, professional organizations, consumer organizations, and insurance companies.

- A continuing shift will occur, from treating health care as a social good to treating it as an economic good. Thus, policy emphasis will be on the purchasing and financing of health care versus the provision of accessible quality care to all individuals.[67]

Health care reforms are being proposed and occurring in incremental steps on both the national and state arenas. Portability of health insurance with geographic or job changes has been passed by Congress and signed by the President. Other major issues being addressed include no discrimination for pre-existing conditions of mental health services, focus on managed care for Medicaid and Medicare programs, and carve-outs for special vulnerable populations. In the health care reform proposals, benefits for pregnant women and children to age eighteen are protected. With a focus on quality and access to care and prevention, women's health care needs must be addressed.

CONCLUSION

Providers involved in women's health care have a professional responsibility to know the issues and be involved in the political process to exert positive influence over state and national health policy for women, infants, and their families.

The U.S. health care system is in transition and the nation is focused on evolving reform. Women's health care is spotlighted in Congress, the U.S. Public Health Service, the academic and research arena, the health care marketplace, and the media.

Providers of women's health care have an unprecedented opportunity to enter the public policy debate and advocate for quality and access to services, new care delivery approaches in a managed care world, and more research in women's health. Vigilance will be important to foster the momentum of real changes for women and their families. With attention on prevention and personal responsibility, health care providers can also help empower women to become partners in self-care and health care decision making.

REFERENCES

1. Young, F. E. (1987). Proceedings of the national conference on women's health. *Public Health Reports: Journal of the U.S. Public Health Service, 4*(Suppl. 1).

2. Dan, A. J., & Hemphill, S. T. (1992). Women's health. In *Medical and health annual*. Chicago: Encyclopedia Britannica.

3. Rodriquez-Trias, H. (1992). Women's health, women's lives, women's rights. *American Journal of Public Health, 82*(5).

4. McBride, A. (1993). From gynecology to gynecology: Developing a practice-research agenda for women's health. *Health Care of Women International, 14,* 315–325.

5. Abrums, M. (1986). Health care for women. *Journal of Obstetrics, Gynecologic and Neonatal Nursing, 3,* 250–255.

6. Naphey, G. (1870). *The physical life of women: Advice to maiden, wife, and mother* (4th ed.). Philadelphia: George Maclean.

7. Ehrenreich, B., & English, D. (1973). *Complaints and disorders: The sexual politics of sickness.* New York: Feminist Press.

8. Marieskind, H. (1975). The women's health movement. *International Journal of Health Services, 5*(2), 217–223.

9. Bullough, V., & Vought, M. (1973). Women, menstruation, and nineteenth century medicine. *Bulletin of Historical Medicine, 47*(1).

10. Reuben, D. (1970). *Everything you always wanted to know about sex.* New York: David McKay.

11. Friedan, B. J. (1963). *The feminine mystique.* New York: W. W. Norton.

12. Boston Women's Health Collective. (1971). *Our bodies, ourselves.* New York: Simon & Schuster.

13. Friedan, B. (1991, November). The dangers of the new feminine mystique. *McCall's,* 78–86.

14. Southwick, K. (1990, August). Women confront second-class care. *Healthweek,* 1, 40–42.

15. Day, K. (1997, June 26). A fever for women's health care. Washingtonpost.com.

16. McKinnon, S. (1990, June/July). Women's control of health care dollars. *Richmond Surroundings,* 34–73.

17. Clancy, C. M., & Massion, C. T. (1992). American women's health care: A patchwork quilt with gaps. *Journal of American Medical Association, 268*(14).

18. Horton, J. A. (ed.). (1995). *The women's health data book: A profile of women's health in the United States.* (2nd ed.). Washington, DC: Jacobs Institute of Women's Health.

19. National Center for Health Statistics. (1996). *Health, United States, 1995 chartbook.* Hyattsville, MD: Public Health Service.

20. Cunningham, F. G., MacDonald, P. C., Gant, N. F., Leveno, K. J., Gilstrap, L. C., III, Hankins, G. D. V., & Clark, S. L. (1997). *Williams obstetrics, 20th Edition.* Stamford, CT: Appleton and Lange.

21. National Center for Health Statistics. (1995). Monthly vital statistics report. *Births and Deaths: United States, 45,* 3–52.

22. Office of Technology Assessment. (1990, September). *Health care in rural America* (OTA Publication No. H435). Washington, DC: U.S. Government Printing Office.

23. Health Care Financing Press Office. (1997, January). *HHS News.* Press Release: World Wide Web.

24. Employee Benefits Research Institute. (1996). Notes: a monthly newsletter. Washington, DC. *EBRI Education and Research Fund, 17*(1), 1–7.

25. Department of Commerce. (1995). Insurance coverage—who had a lapse between 1991 and 1993? *Statistical Brief 95-21.* Washington, DC: Urban Institute.

26. Auerback, S. (1996, September). Number of uninsured growing. *The Washington Post,* p. F 1.

27. Lemcke, D. P. & Pattison, J. (Eds.). (1995). *Primary Care of Women.* Norwalk, CT: Appleton & Lange.

28. Schroeder, S. A. (1996). The medically uninsured—will they always be with us? *The New England Journal of Medicine, 334*(17), 1130–1133.

29. U.S. Senate Committee on Labor and Human Resources. (1990). *The health care crisis: A report to the American People* (p. 3). Washington, DC: U.S. Government Printing Office.

30. Campaign for Women's Health. (1991). *A challenge for the 1990's: Improving health care for American women.* Washington, DC: Older Women's League.

31. Bass, M., & Howes, J. (1992). Women's health: The making of a powerful new public issue. *Women's Health Issues, 2*(1), 3.

32. Bhargaua, S. W. (1992, July). Finally, a health interest in women. *Business Week,* 88–89.

33. Merkatz, R. (1996). Promoting gender analysis in peer-reviewed scientific journals: A call to publisher. *Journal of Women's Health, 5*(6), 525–527.

34. The Associated Press. (1996, January). Study finds women still earn less than men. *The Richmond Times Dispatch,* p. A1.

35. Older Women's League. (1990, May). *Heading for hardship: Retirement income for American women in the next century.* Washington, DC: Author.

36. Waldman, S. (1992, May). Deadbeat dads. *Newsweek,* 46–52.

37. Hartmann, H., & Spalter-Roth, R. (1990, November). *Working parents: Differences, similarities and the implications for a policy agenda.* Paper presented at a meeting on women, work, and the family: Advancing the Policy and Research Agenda, Institute for Research on Women and Center. Columbia University, New York.

38. Office on Women's Health. (1995). *Women's health issues fact sheet.* U.S. Public Health Service.

39. Agency for Health Care Policy and Research. (1990, October). *Research Activities,* 134.

40. Raymon, R., & Allshouse, K. (Undated). *Resiliency amidst inequity: Older women workers in an aging U.S.* (pp. 1–4). Southport, CT: Southport Institute for Policy Analysis, Project for Women and Population Aging.

41. Older Women's League. (1989, May). Failing America's caregivers: A status report on women who care. *Mother's Day Report,* 3.

42. U.S. Public Health Service. (1985). *Women's health: Report of the public health service task force on women's health issues: Vol II* (DHHS Publication No. PHS 85-50206). Washington, DC: U.S. Government Printing Office.

43. Women's Policy, Inc. (1996). *The Women's Health Equity Act of 1996, Legislative summary and overview.* Washington, DC: Women's Policy, Inc.

44. Office of Research on Women's Health. (1996, April). *Overview: Office of research on women's health.* National Institutes of Health, 1–4.

45. Pinn, V. (1994). The role of the NIH office of Research on Women's Health. *Academic Medicine, 69*(9), 698–702.

46. Office of Research on Women's Health. (1996, March). *Overview statement on the women's health initiative.* National Institutes of Health, 1–2.

47. Office of Women's Health. (1996). *Fact sheet: What is the office on women's health?* U.S. Public Health Service, 1–4.

48. U.S. Department of Health and Human Services. (1993, July). Food & Drug Administration. Guidelines for the study and evaluation of gender differences in the clinical evaluation of drugs: Part IV. *Federal Register, 58*(139), 39406–39407.

49. National Cancer Institute Cancer Information Service. (1996, May). Press Release.

50. Igelhart, J. (1994). Health policy reports physicians and the growth of managed care. *The New England Journal of Medicine, 331,* 1167–1171.

51. Himali, W. (1995, June). Managed care: Does the promise meet the potential? *The American Nurse,* 14, 16.

52. Hadley, E. H. (1996). Nursing in the political and economic marketplace: Challenges for the 21st century. *Nursing Outlook, 44*(1), 6–10.

53. Freudenheimc, M. (1996, May). HMOs cope with a backlash of cost cutting. *The New York Times.*

54. American College of Obstetricians and Gynecologists. (1996, April). *Committee opinion— Physician responsibility under managed care: Patient advocacy in a changing health environment.* Washington, DC: American College of Obstetricians and Gynecologists.

55. Elmer-DeWitt, P. (1990, February). A better pill to swallow. *Time,* 44.

56. Trussell, J., et al. (1995). The economic value of contraception: A comparison of 15 methods. *The American Journal of Public Health, 85*(4), 494–503.

57. Negroponte, N. (1995) *Being digital.* New York: Random House/Vintage Books.

58. Bashsuhr, R. & Puskin, D. (1995). General introduction: Consumers process and background of August conference. *Telemedicine Journal, 1*(4), 340.

59. Institute of Medicine. (1996). *Primary care: American's health in a new era.* Washington, DC: National Academy of Medicine.

60. Vanselow, N.A. (1996, March). Opening statement at press briefing on report, *Primary care: America's Health is in a new era.* Washington, DC.

61. Loeb, L. (1990). *Caring for caregivers: Addressing the employment needs of long term care workers.* Washington, DC: Older Women's League.

62. Crisso, J. A. & Ness, R. B. (1996). Update in women's health. *Annuals of Internal Medicine, 125*(3), 213–220.

63. Novello, A. C., & Soto-Torres, L. E. (1992). Women and hidden epidemics: HIV/AIDS and domestic violence. *Female Patient, 17,* 17–31.

64. National Institute of Health, Office of Alternative Medicine. (1995, December). *Complementary and Alternative Medicine at NIH Newsletter, 2*(5, 6), 8.

65. Eisenberg, D.M., et al. (1993). Unconventional medicine in the United States: Prevalence, costs, and patterns of use. *New England Journal of Medicine, 328*(1), 246–252.

66. Opinion Research Corporation. (1988, February). Hospital survey on obstetric claim frequency by patient category, prepared for the American College of Obstetricians and Gynecologists, Washington, DC.

67. Longest, B. B. (1988). American health policy in the year 2000. *Hospital and Health Services Administration, 33*(4), 419–434.

CHAPTER 2

LEGAL ISSUES IN THE PRIMARY CARE OF WOMEN

Judith A. Lewis

*T*he scope of professional practice, relationships with other providers, and environmental factors that affect our ability to provide care are variables subject to constant change. Practice settings, reimbursement arrangements, and regulatory authorities all have a major impact on the nurse-patient relationship. Individual nurses and organized nursing associations need to reflect upon these issues and develop strategies for professional practice that maximize nursing's ability to contribute to improved patient outcomes in an environment that challenges all of us on a daily basis.

Highlights

- Scope of Practice
- Licensure, Certification, and Credentialing
- Health Care Delivery Team: Relationships
- Reimbursement and Managed Care
- Prescriptive Privileges
- Professional Liability

► INTRODUCTION

The role of the advanced practice nurse as a member of the primary health care delivery team has been clearly established. The relationships among members of the various disciplines comprising the health care delivery team are less clearly defined. Pearson notes that the most serious challenges facing nurse practitioners are the limits being placed upon them by the restructuring of the private sector health care delivery system. Limits placed upon advanced practice nurses' ability to perform the role of the nurse practitioner and lack of universal access of patients to nurse practitioner services are results of this restructuring.[1]

Laws, rules, and regulations play increasingly important roles in our personal and professional lives. The purpose of this chapter is to discuss several important areas where laws and regulations affect the way we practice. These areas include defining the scope of practice; licensure, certification, and credentialing; relationships with other members of the health-care delivery team; third-party reimbursement for services; prescriptive privileges; and professional liability insurance. The further purpose of the chapter is to promote thoughtful reflection about these issues, discussion of possible solutions among nurse practitioners, and identification of actions that might be taken by organized nursing associations to bring about change. Questions and concerns about specific individual situations may require legal consultation, and no material presented in this chapter can substitute for such counsel.

Scope of practice

The practice of professional nursing and the expanded role of the advanced practice nurse have grown during the last quarter of the 20th century. In some states, this has happened by amending or altering state nurse practice acts. In other jurisdictions, state boards of nursing have expanded the scope of practice by promulgating additional rules and regulations. It is important for each advanced practice nurse to know which statutes apply in her or his own practice site. For the past nine years, *Nurse Practitioner,* in its January issue, has provided an annual update that displays a state-by-state analysis, including the legal authority for advanced practice nursing, information on reimbursement for services by advanced practice nurses, and a summary of regulations governing prescriptive authority.[1]

Although the scope of practice is defined by state laws and regulations, the standards of practice are defined by the profession, often through professional associations. The American Nurses Association (ANA) publishes a document defining the scope and standards of advanced nursing practice that are generic to advanced practice nurses in all clinical specialties.[2] The Association of Women's Health, Obstetric, and Neonatal Nurses (AWHONN) has promulgated generic standards for the nursing care of women and children[3] and has published guidelines for practice and education for women's health nurse practitioners in collaboration with the National Association of Nurse Practitioners in Reproductive Health (NANPRH).[4]

Documents such as those just cited provide valuable information regarding the scope of professional practice and are the gold standards by which individual clinicians' practice may be measured. They are invaluable resources when interdisciplinary health care teams are writing clinical protocols defining the scope and responsibilities of the various members of the practice team.

LICENSURE, CERTIFICATION, AND CREDENTIALING

Many different types of advanced practice nurses may participate in providing primary health care to women. Depending on their age, health status, health care plan, and personal preference, women may be cared for by pediatric, adult, family, women's health, perinatal or gerontologic nurse practitioners, certified nurse midwives, or clinical nurse specialists. The scope of practice of each group of providers is regulated on a state-by-state basis.

Licensure is granted by the individual state, province, or territory. Most states currently have three categories of nursing licensees: licensed practical nurses, registered nurses, and advanced practice registered nurses.[5] Each jurisdiction has unique requirements, although there are clear similarities. The purpose of mandatory licensure falls under the general area of consumer protection. The best source of information about licensure requirements is the State Board of Nursing.

Certification is a national process. The original intent of certification was that it be a voluntary process designed to differentiate and recognize those individuals who displayed excellence in clinical practice. As originally conceptualized, certification was never intended to be mandatory, nor was it ever intended that all nurses in any area would seek, or achieve, certification.

Many states have adopted certification as a mandatory prerequisite to licensure as an advanced practice nurse. State boards of nursing, in an attempt to define characteristics that would protect consumers without requiring yet another licensure examination, adopted regulations that, in essence, made the certification process mandatory, rather than voluntary.

Because the certification movement arose from professional nursing associations' efforts to provide recognition to outstanding practitioners, there are several certification agencies. Although each certification agency has autonomy, many have close relationships with the organizations from which they arose. Each certification agency sets its own eligibility requirements for initial certification as well as certification maintenance.

Some advanced practice nurses have more than one option for certification, whereas other specialties, such as women's health, have but a single agency from which to choose. Specific certification offered, eligibility requirements, and certification maintenance requirements change frequently. Requirements and regulations are published annually by certification agencies such as the American Nurses' Credentialing Center; the National Certification Corporation for the Obstetric, Gynecologic and Neonatal Nursing Specialties; the National Certification Board of Pediatric Nurse Practitioners and Nurses; the American Academy of Nurse Practitioners; and the American College of Nurse-Midwives.[6]

Many advanced practice nurses seek hospital privileges, including the right to admit patients to inpatient facilities, to serve as members of the attending staff, and to write progress notes or orders in the medical record. Because hospital privileges are the purview of the individual institution, no state or federal statutes pertain. When granted, the extent of these privileges may vary widely and may include some, but not all, of the items listed previously.[7]

The question of a second level of licensure for advanced practice nurses has been raised and has been hotly debated at the national level. The purpose of such a second licensure process would be to ensure that all nurse practitioners could demonstrate achievement of selected core competencies. Those agencies responsible for the certification process believe that the current certification process provides such safeguards and that such an advanced practice licensure examination is unnecessary. The issue continues to be debated at many levels and a definitive answer has yet to be negotiated.

RELATIONSHIPS WITH OTHER MEMBERS OF THE HEALTH CARE DELIVERY TEAM

Since only Alaska and New Mexico permit totally independent practice, essentially all nurse practitioners practice as a part of a team.[8] It is important to understand the parameters of legal relationships as defined by the laws governing the jurisdiction in which the practice occurs.

Most employer-employee relationships are defined by a written letter of agreement, or contract. Contracts are legally binding documents that outline the duties and responsibilities of all parties.[9] The process of negotiating a contract is as important as the contract itself, because this process often serves to stimulate discussion and clarify issues of concern to either or both parties. Placing the relationship on a business level is especially important. A clearly defined administrative structure with mutually agreed upon roles and responsibilities will go far in avoiding broken partnerships and animosity. Another important reason to have a clearly defined written agreement is to minimize the risk for unpleasant contact with the Internal Revenue Service, which has rules and regulations defining differences between employees and those who consider themselves independent contractors.[10]

Each agreement covers issues important to the parties involved. Topics that may be addressed by such a contract may include salary arrangements, fringe benefits such as sick leave, educational leave, continuing education reimbursement, dues for professional associations, vacation and holiday arrangements, as well as the roles and responsibilities of the employer and employee.[9] Table 2–1 presents information on non-salary benefits that may be considered when negotiating a contract.

When negotiating a contract for the first time, it is helpful to talk with other advanced practice nurses in the vicinity. Since salary is often determined by the local market, knowing the range of salary agreements in the local area is important. Local nurse practitioner organizations often have performed surveys of their members that provide valuable information about what typical regional employment agreements include and exclude.

It is important to remember that this is a negotiated agreement. Flexibility and compromise are important negotiation skills. Skilled negotiators compromise and concede in order to achieve gains in areas that are of strategic importance to them. Those individuals who end up with personally satisfying agreements look for are as where they can concede on minor issues, emphasize those points on which they have made con-

TABLE 2–1. NON-SALARY BENEFITS TO DISCUSS WHEN NEGOTIATING AN EMPLOYMENT CONTRACT

Vacation   Negotiate for an annual increase. For example, start with two weeks plus holidays; negotiate for additional days each year up to one month total.

Sick Leave   Eight hours per month is usual for full-time employees; may be prorated for part-time employment.

Continuing Professional Education   Negotiate for time and money to attend defined activities annually. If the employer wants you to learn a special skill or have some other development activity, then a general statement to the effect that the cost for this education should be borne by the employer should be in the contract. This section may be called professional development.

Leave of Absence   Negotiate for a clause granting leave of absence for family illnesses, deaths, or family crises without penalty to you when you return.

Personal Business Days   Negotiate for days to manage personal business that do not need to be counted against vacation days.

Retirement Plans   If inadequate, negotiate to pay into your own retirement plan.

Health Benefits   Negotiate for health, dental, vision, or disability plans. If the plans are inadequate, negotiate to pay for an alternate plan with pre-tax dollars.

Life Insurance   Some type of group term life insurance is common.

Malpractice Insurance   Rates vary by specialty.

Evaluation   Negotiate for established times for written evaluation of your work.

Grievance Procedure   Negotiate for a time frame and arbitration plan in case of dispute.

Resignation or Termination Notice Time   Negotiate time frame for both resignation and termination.

Severance Pay in the Event of Termination   Negotiate for some amount, such as six months of salary or one month of salary for every year of employment, whichever is greater.

Duration of Contract   One year is common; negotiate for time to renegotiate, renew, or terminate contract that provides for sufficient time for these negotiations, such as three months.

Jury Duty   Negotiate to receive the difference between jury pay and regular salary.

cessions, and look for areas that are suitable for compromise.[9] It may be helpful to have a contract reviewed by a legal or financial advisor before finalizing the terms and signing the document to ensure that no important issues have been overlooked.

Most nurse practitioners regularly seek consultation from, and refer patients to, other members of the health care team. When seeking consultation from another member of the health care delivery team, the original provider retains the ultimate responsibility for treatment decisions.[8] The consultant's role is that of an advisor. Although a clinician may seek consultation from any number of sources, the final decision for treatment rests with the original clinician.

When a patient referral is made, this responsibility is shifted from the original clinician to the clinician who has accepted the referral.[8] The original clinician's responsibility to the patient is to seek a competent source for the referral. It is important to document the recommendation for referral in the patient's record. Some clinicians prefer to provide the patient with a list of competent sources and leave the choice of the specific provider to the patient. Most referral centers provide reports to the referring clinicians informing them of patient progress, but until the patient's care is transferred back to the original clinician, the responsibility for treatment decisions remains with the provider who has accepted the referral. Guido notes that most malpractice actions brought against advanced practice nurses are because of alleged failure of the nurse to refer the patient to another provider.[7]

REIMBURSEMENT AND MANAGED CARE

Reimbursement for care is defined by the patient's health care insurance carrier. Regulations for Medicare reimbursement are determined federally; each state determines its own Medicaid policies; and, although private insurers often follow the federal lead, they are free to make whatever rules they wish, knowing that their ability to compete successfully for contracts will be enhanced or hindered by their reimbursement policies.

Nurses have been lobbying to have legislation passed that would mandate Medicare and Medicaid reimbursement to all advanced practice nurses; this has yet to become a reality. Although the cost effectiveness of this initiative has been clearly demonstrated, the loss of potential income to other providers has proved to provide sufficient pressure to block passage of legislation at the federal level. It seems likely that, in the current fiscal climate, the private sector may provide the impetus to reimburse non-physician providers at a lower rate, thus achieving cost savings for their health plans.

This may turn out to be a mixed blessing. Although it would be a major coup for nurses to receive direct reimbursement for services rendered, to be paid less than other providers for the same services reinforces the gender discrimination and comparable worth issues that have plagued women and women's work for centuries.

Managed care arrangements have, in many cases, shifted the locus of control for clinical decision making from the provider-patient relationship to the administrator of the health care insurance plan, whose responsibility is at the systems, rather than the individual, level.[11] Clinicians may be informed by third party payors that only certain options are covered by patients' insurance plans. Although insurance plans have always had limits on and exclusions to coverage, the pressure to control escalating health care costs has increased the level of involvement of non-medically trained personnel in clinical decision making at the individual level.

In the fee-for-service arrangement, individual clinicians made decisions about treatment, often realizing that some patients would be unable to pay; uncompensated care to some was factored into the fee schedule and, in some cases, contributed to the escalation of costs that the current health care delivery system is attempting to control. Unfortunately, some clinicians are experiencing subtle or not-so-subtle pressure to present only the most fiscally attractive options for treatment to their patients.

The American College of Obstetricians and Gynecologists (ACOG) is but one of many professional associations whose leaders have gone on record stating that part of the health care professional's responsibility is to advocate for patients by appealing such rulings to health care plan directors.[11] In addition, ACOG's Committee on Ethics has recommended that ACOG fellows become involved in policymaking. ACOG's Ethics Committee further suggests that patients be informed of all viable treatment options, regardless of whether they are covered by insurance; that third party payors be required to justify the rationale for denial of services; that providers not be penalized if they advocate for their patients; and that clinicians continue to contribute uncompensated care. Finally, ACOG recommends that its fellows refuse to participate in health care insurance plans that are unethical in their treatment of subscribers.[11]

PRESCRIPTIVE PRIVILEGES

Prescriptive privileges vary from state to state. Some states allow great flexibility to advanced practice nurses, other states require strict physician collaboration or supervision, while yet others have no statutory prescriptive authority.[1] Some states limit practice by limiting the categories of drugs that advance practice nurses are allowed to prescribe; others limit practice by requiring physician supervision or cosignature on prescriptions.[12] In states where nurses have been most successful in obtaining broad prescriptive authority, the sustained efforts of organized groups of advanced practice nurses, consumers, and other health care professionals were clearly evident. It is clear that the lack of full prescriptive privileges is one of the strongest barriers to independent practice.[12]

PROFESSIONAL LIABILITY

A comprehensive data base of malpractice claims yielding financial settlements and adverse actions since September, 1990 is maintained in the National Practitioner Data Bank (NPDB). Analysis of these data shows that successful claims against advanced practice nurses are rare in comparison with claims against physician providers. During the initial 33 months of operation of the NPDB, 2.5 percent of the claims paid were for nurses, while 97.5 percent of the payment reports named physician providers. Of the 999 claims paid for nurses, only 73 were for nurse practitioners or nurse midwives. While the data are old, underreporting has been documented, malpractice payment reports do not represent all malpractice settlements, and the increase in prescriptive roles may increase the exposure for malpractice, it is clear that advanced practice nurses are far less vulnerable to malpractice suits resulting in payment than are their physician counterparts.[13] There are, however, important issues related to malpractice and legal liability that require the attention of advanced practice nurses in primary care settings.

Employment contracts and collaboration agreements create legal relationships between the nurse practitioner and the other parties to these contracts or agreements. The type of liability created is dependent upon the type of agreement.[8]

When the contract establishes an employer-employee relationship, the employer is assumed to be liable for actions that the employee performs within the scope of the employment agreement. The employer does not assume liability for those actions that deviate from, or go beyond, those established protocols that guide the actions of the advanced practice nurse.[8] It is evident that both parties are best served by written employment agreements, job descriptions that delineate the scope of practice of the employee, and appropriate clinical protocols.

Each member of a joint, or collaborative, practice arrangement is liable for her or his own actions. In a formal partnership, each partner is liable for the actions of other partners.[8] In such arrangements, written agreements among partners should define the structure of the arrangement, the roles and responsibilities of all members of the practice, and the protocols guiding the practice of each partner.

Informed consent and informed refusal are issues often raised in malpractice cases. Consent must be gained before any treatment is delivered. Indeed, inferred fear of such may be construed as assault, and actual physical contact without such consent may be construed as battery. Those who have authority to give consent include competent adults, adults who have authority to consent for minor children, court appointed guardians for adults or children, and persons designated in health care proxies, living wills, or power of attorney agreements.[14]

Most states do not recognize spousal consent; thus, it is important that couples have mutually executed health care powers of attorney or health care proxies. Likewise, some states do not recognize the rights of emancipated minors to provide consent.[14] In many states, emergency treatment decisions are handled differently, but the definition of what constitutes a medical emergency may vary. It is important to know the statutes governing the jurisdiction in which the clinician is practicing.

The right to refuse treatment can be as problematic as the right to consent to care. ACOG's Committee on Professional Liability notes that, once informed of the risks and benefits of any procedure or treatment, the patient has the right to choose among a variety of acceptable options, as well as the right to forego any treatment at all. ACOG's committee opinion further notes that, if the refusal is based on lack of insurance coverage, the physician has the obligation to advocate for the patient with the third party payor.[15]

Yet another area of concern is that of giving free or social advice. When one ventures an opinion on a health care matter affecting a friend, colleague, or family member, the potential for exposure to a malpractice claim is there. Although it is easy to offer a suggestion, critique a plan of care, or proffer a professional opinion, these are potential pitfalls that should be avoided.[10]

The debate about whether to carry individual professional and personal liability insurance is a multifaceted argument, and there is no clear cut answer. Employers' contracts may provide adequate coverage of all employees in many situations; individual policies in those instances may be unnecessarily duplicative. It is also possible that duplicate coverage can lead to lack of clarity about which insurer should assume primary responsibility for coverage, tendency of plaintiffs' attorneys to seek deep pockets with the purpose of maximizing the likelihood of large awards, and a false sense of security on the part of the policyholder. Those in favor of individual policies voice concern that employers' contracts may not provide adequate coverage for nonemployment related professional liability. The individual nurse is well advised to consult a personal legal advisor if she or he wishes additional advice on this topic.

SUMMARY

Advanced practice nurses who provide primary care to women work in an environment that is changing rapidly. The scope of professional practice, relationships with other providers, and environmental factors that affect our ability to provide care are variables subject to constant change. Practice settings, reimbursement arrangements, and regulatory authorities all have a major impact on the nurse-patient relationship. Individual nurses and organized nursing associations need to reflect upon these issues and develop strategies for professional practice that maximize nursing's ability to contribute to improved patient outcomes in an environment that challenges all of us on a daily basis.

REFERENCES

1. Pearson, L. J. (1996). Annual update of how each state stands on legislative issues affecting advanced nursing practice. *Nurse Practitioner, 21*(1), 10, 12–14, 16, 21–22, 25–26, 28–30, 34, 36, 39–40, 43–45, 49–50, 52–54, 57–58, 60–62, 65–66, 68–70.
2. American Nurses Association. (1996). *Scope and standards of advanced practice registered nursing.* Washington, DC: Author.
3. Association of Women's Health, Obstetric and Neonatal Nurses. (1997, in press). *Standards for the nursing care of women and newborns* (5th ed). Washington, DC: Author.
4. Association of Women's Health, Obstetric and Neonatal Nurses, and National Association of Nurse Practitioners in Reproductive Health. (1996). *The women's health nurse practitioner: Guidelines for practice and education.* Washington, DC: Author.
5. Bullough, B. (1995). State nurse practice acts. In M. D. Mezey & D. O. McGivern (Eds.), *Nurses, nurse practitioners.* (pp. 267–280) New York: Springer.
6. Hahn, M. S. (1995, October). The ABCs of credentialing choices. *ADVANCE for Nurse Practitioners, 37–39.*
7. Guido, G. W. (1995). Advanced nursing practice: Legal concerns. *AACN Clinical Issues, 6*(1), 99–104.
8. Henry, P. F. (1996). Analysis of the nurse practitioner's legal relationships. *Nurse Practitioner Forum, 7*(1), 5–6.

9. Mackey, T. A. (1996). Compensation for nurse practitioners. *ADVANCE for Nurse Practitioners, 4*(6), 47–48.

10. Buppert, C. (1996). Nurse practitioner private practice: Three legal pitfalls to avoid. *Nurse Practitioner, 21*(4), 32, 34, 37.

11. American College of Obstetricians and Gynecologists Committee on Ethics. (1996). Physician responsibility under managed care: Patient advocacy in a changing health care environment. *Committee Opinion #170*. Washington, DC: Author.

12. Mirr, M. P. (1995). Legal issues: Licensure and certification, prescriptive privileges, and reimbursement. In M. Snyder & M. P. Mirr (Eds.), *Advanced practice nursing: A guide to professional development* (pp. 39–53). New York: Springer.

13. Birkholz, G. (1995). Malpractice data from the national practitioner data bank. *Nurse Practitioner, 20*(3), 32–35.

14. Cummings, C. (1996, May). More on informed consent doctrine. *ADVANCE for Nurse Practitioners,* 18.

15. American College of Obstetricians and Gynecologists Committee on Professional Liability. (1996). Informed refusal. *Committee Opinion #166*. Washington, DC: Author.

CHAPTER 3

HEALTH AND DEVELOPMENT THROUGH THE LIFE CYCLE

Marcia Szmania Davis • Ellis Quinn Youngkin

*P*erhaps as more emphasis is given to female perspectives, society can move toward more acceptance of power-with, rather than power-over, which would help facilitate a more peaceful environment on a larger scale.[22]

Highlights

- Stage Theories of Development
- Historical Psychoanalytic Influence
- Erikson's Stages
- Levinson's Model
- Life Cycle Concepts
- Current Views on Women's Development
- A New Psychology of Women
- Societal Issues
- Major Periods and Tasks: The Women's Perspective

▶ INTRODUCTION

In order to define and understand women's development, one must address the societal norms that prevail over time (see Chapter 1). One important change during the late 1960s and early 1970s was women's realization that many important individual concerns they had previously been hesitant to discuss were actually widespread and political in nature. "The personal is political" slogan reflected an energy borne out in consciousness-raising groups where women talked about their lived experiences, learning that their innermost feelings were shared by women in general. A period of self-discovery began as women began to break out of socially constrictive stereotypes.

Earlier, in the 1950s, remarkable changes in women's lives were associated with fewer births, extended longevity, greater acceptance of lifestyle options in marriage and family formation, and attachment to the labor force.[1] Affirmative action movements eventually developed into academic programs in women's studies beginning in the 1960s, often with reluctant acceptance by universities.[2] These courses reflected limitations set on women by patriarchal societies, and women contemplated the reasons. Recent history books celebrated women's influences that had largely been ignored or downplayed. In today's world, women, compared with their mothers, are better educated, spend more of their adult life living alone, and participate more consistently in the labor force.[3]

Is the contemporary view of society toward women indeed different, however, from the past? The answer must be an equivocal yes, in part because traditional sex role stereotypes continue to pervade the thinking of many men and women. Women who do not marry and reproduce may be viewed as having failed to develop their fullest potential. Moreover, femininity has long been, and to a great extent continues to be, equated with passivity, dependency, and pleasing men.[3]

GROWTH AND DEVELOPMENT

Growth and development are often viewed according to a person's stage in the life cycle. Whereas *growth* refers to quantitative physical and physiological changes, *development* encompasses more qualitative changes, including functional, psychosocial, and cognitive behaviors.[5] Both areas need to be assessed so that the health care provider can offer anticipatory guidance to women as they adapt to personal and environmental changes. Providers must also understand contemporary women's roles and expectations as well as their stressors within a social context in order to assist women that develop health promotion behaviors.[3] The developmental theories most closely linked to sequential ages and life stages have frequently been used for clinical evaluation.

Controversy exists, however, about the applicability of such theories to women, particularly because cultural biases may be a problem. For example, Erikson studied primarily white, middle-class males. Also, developmental norms may not apply to all cultural backgrounds; and stage theories may promote ageism if one does not fulfill expectations, such as marriage, by a given point in life.[5]

Today, women's lives are very complex. Numbers of different life cycles and lines of development exist, overlap, conflict, and perhaps enhance each other. Seiden whimsically refers to a "life pretzel" where the biologic-reproductive circle, the family-marital circle, and the educational-vocational circle are all bound together. A simple circle tied to a reproductive life cycle will simply no longer suffice (if it ever did).[6]

STAGE THEORIES OF DEVELOPMENT

Investigation of developmental change across the life span has gained prominence over the past 50 years, largely as a result of psychoanalytic influence. The resulting developmental theories emerged from the body of knowledge in child psychology. Although the life span developmental framework focused primarily on men, the resulting theories were generalized to apply to all adults. Women's development, which was seldom alluded to, was viewed narrowly and judged aberrant if gender development did not conform to the accepted male pattern.[7]

Characteristics commonly attributed to women, such as being less aggressive, more emotional, and less independent, were seen to be less healthy. Although the majority of psychoanalytic clients were women, little was known about their experiences as women. Virtually no attention was directed towards the effects of the societal environment on women. Feminists thus came to view traditional psychotherapy as an agent of social control, reinforcing the traditional sex roles and traditional values that led to a devaluation of women.

HISTORICAL PSYCHOANALYTIC INFLUENCE

Freudian psychosexual theory and practice—the largest influence on psychotherapeutic knowledge—gave therapists a largely antifeminine orientation.[8,9] Freud espoused that biological drives influence a person's psychological and personality development. In his view, superiority of men was largely derived from the possession of a penis. Penis envy purportedly led to feminine aggression. According to Freud, limitations of women inherent in their biology ("anatomy is destiny") included women's innate dependency, passivity, and masochism, which were required for their primary fulfilling role, successful motherhood. Compared with men, women were viewed as more narcissistic, more prone to jealousy, and having a weaker sense of justice.[10] Women were labeled "frigid" if they were incapable of mature (phallocentric) vaginal orgasm, versus clitoral orgasm. The studies of Masters and Johnson proved this concept incorrect.[7]

FEMINIST VIEWS ON PSYCHOANALYSIS

Critics condemned Freud for deriding women who displayed qualities that would be lauded in men, primarily boldness and independence.[2] Many women also voiced resentment toward the implied foreclosure on women's opportunities.

- Karen Horney (1920s and 1930s) proposed that if penis envy existed, it was because the penis symbolized the social and political power of men.[9]
- Simone de Beauvoir (*The Second Sex,* 1949) caused a great deal of controversy by challenging the ideation of biological and psychological determination of roles for women.
- Betty Friedan (*The Feminine Mystique,* 1963) attempted to broaden society's narrow role of women's place being in the home.
- Kate Millet (*Sexual Politics,* 1969) continued to scorn Freud for upholding the male body as the norm and questioned the validity of Freud's concept of female fear of castration while ignoring issues such as rape.

ADULT DEVELOPMENTAL THEORIES

Although developmental changes during childhood and adolescence have been studied, relatively little attention has been paid to the adult years,[11] and the study of women's development is still in its infancy and is controversial. The climate exists for an interdisciplinary approach to the study of human development, and social scientists have shown us that societal issues must be closely addressed.

ERIKSON'S STAGES OF PSYCHOSOCIAL DEVELOPMENT (1950s TO 1960s)

One of the earliest contributors to the study of adult development, Erikson suggested the normalcy and necessity of growth and change during adult years and not just in childhood.[12,13] His theories, grounded in conceptions of the life cycle and the life course, addressed stages in ego development. According to Erikson,

- Each stage is primary at a particular age level, or segment of the life cycle, from infancy to old age.
- If a task that is appropriate to a given phase of life is not resolved, then development in subsequent phases of life may be impaired.
- A patterned sequence of stages occurs, each with appropriate physical, emotional, and cognitive tasks.
- A person who successfully passes through each stage eventually attains ego integrity, which is associated with high self-esteem and a positive outlook on life.
- A major difference for a woman is that her identity is enmeshed in a married state, wherein the task of her mate is to provide her with an adult identity, a necessary step in her mature integration of personality (see Chapter 1, Other Influences on Women's Health, Marital Status).

Erikson's eight stages of development, composed of bipolar tasks at various stages of life, include *Trust versus Mistrust,* infancy; *Autonomy versus Shame and Doubt,* early childhood; *Initiative versus Guilt,* preschool age; *Industry versus Inferiority,* school age; *Identify versus Identity Diffusion,* adolescence; *Intimacy versus Isolation or Self-Absorption,* young adulthood; *Generativity versus Stagnation,* middle adulthood; and *Integrity versus Despair and Disdain,* late adulthood.

LEVINSON'S MODEL OF ADULT DEVELOPMENT (1970s TO PRESENT)

This well-known model of adult development, which is grounded in psychoanalytic theory, is applied in research and psychotherapy.[14] Levinson believes that there is a single human life cycle through which both men and women evolve (the life structure). Tremendous variation exists related to gender, class, race, culture, historical epoch, specific circumstances, and genetics.[15] Levinson expanded on Erikson's notion of development and characterized each segment of adulthood in terms of intrinsic tasks.[12,14,15] This theory proposes an underlying set of developmental periods and tasks along with transition crises that involve reassessment of one's life.

Adult development is an evolving process of mutual interaction between self and the world, of which family and work are central components. Career choice and work are paramount in terms of goals, social roles, ethical standards and values, and development of self-concept. The assumption is that we desire self-actualization, which requires psychological and realistic change in controllable measures. To this extent, men and women are similar.

Levinson uses a central concept of gender splitting, which views a sharp division between feminine and masculine permeating every aspect of human life from cultural to individual. He also describes the current existence in the early stages of a vast historical transition where traditional patterns are eroding but satisfactory new ones have not been discovered and legitimized.[15] (Women's adult development is addressed later in this chapter in Major Periods and Tasks: The Women's Perspective.)

Early Adult Transition (Ages 17 to 22). The shaky start toward maturity involves taking new steps in individuation. Choices are made concerning career, lifestyle, and modification of existing family and social relationships. This is the adult era of greatest energy and abundance—and of greatest contradiction and stress.

Entering the Adult World (Ages 22 to 28). Through the establishment of an independent living situation, exploration, and commitment to adult roles, the 20s reflect structure building.

Age 30 Transition (Ages 28 to 33). During the transition period, the sense of being young, especially in terms of options, is given up. Current lifestyles, values, family situations, and career choices are evaluated. Biologically, the 20s and 30s are the peak years of life.

Settling Down (Ages 33 to 40). Affirming personal integrity, realizing oneself as a full-fledged adult, and goal achievement are characteristic of this period.

Midlife Transition (Ages 40 to 45). Lifestyle is critically examined, and the need arises to recognize time limitations for goal achievement. Polarities, including young—old and destruction—creation, are integrated. Levinson believes that the character of living always changes appreciably between early and middle adulthood.

Entering Middle Adulthood (Ages 45 to 50). Undergoing restabilization after midlife transition, individuals in middle adulthood have biological capacities below earlier years but normally are still sufficiently fit for energetic, personally satisfying, and socially valuable lives.

Age 50 Transition (Ages 50 to 53). Once more, lifestyle and major goals are reevaluated.

Middle Adulthood Culmination (Ages 53 to 60). Work continues toward achieving life goals and contributing to society.

Late Adulthood (Ages 60 to 80) and the Late Adult Transition (60 to 65). Although the character of one's life is fundamentally altered as a result of biological, psychological, and social changes, the individual recognizes that this period can be distinctive and fulfilling.

Late, Late Adulthood (Age 80 and Older). At this time, the process of aging may be more obvious than the process of growth. The individual must make peace with dying; development occurs as one gives new meaning to life and death. These oldest adults may be an example for others by demonstrating wisdom and personal nobility.[15]

LIFE CYCLE CONCEPTS

Several intersecting normative life cycles exist for women. As women's lives and roles are changing, pulls from traditional definitions of role exist.[6]

BIOLOGIC-REPRODUCTIVE LIFE CYCLE

This cycle encompasses one's own birth, menarche, possible pregnancies and births, child rearing, and menopause during which rearing of children may still occur. Women have growing choices in reproduction, including newer options in contraception and, if necessary, abortion. Women are having babies well into their 40s. The sense of control based on these growing choices

may make infertility even more difficult for women to accept if it occurs. Women may blame themselves for delaying childbirth, for contracting a sexually transmitted disease, and so forth. Technology seems to promise perfect babies, making the potential unexpected reality more difficult to accept.

FAMILY-MARITAL LIFE CYCLE

This cycle is no longer assured to be linked to the reproductive life cycle. A woman's historical major interpersonal investment in family of origin and procreation may be redefined since marriage, divorce, single parenting, step parenting, and other choices exist.

The stigma of single parenting as well as remaining single or choosing to be a child-free couple has lessened. Many married women acknowledge that divorce or early widowhood may occur. Fewer women live within extended families as individual independence is more prized and more achievable.

Extended families may grow with former spouses, in-laws, grandparents, and half-siblings. Expanding circumstances such as artificial insemination and surrogate motherhood challenge traditional "family" definitions. Women who define themselves as lesbian may or may not have children and if they do, they may be single parents or in stable or unstable relationships.[6]

EDUCATIONAL-VOCATIONAL LIFE CYCLE

More and more, today's job market requires higher levels of education or specialized training. Gaps in education and work history may be looked upon suspiciously. It is not commonplace to experience midlife change of careers or reentry into education or the job market.

Women may still enter the job market without the education or vision equal to their talents due to deterrence by early marriage and/or responsibilities to child care or limited concepts of their opportunities. Women are becoming more effectively involved in mentoring and networking as part of their careers, versus putting time into more limited "jobs."[6]

CURRENT VIEWS ON WOMEN'S DEVELOPMENT

WOMEN'S CONTRIBUTIONS

Women's influence has been largely absent in many areas, including art, literature, social sciences, and psychological research.[8,16] Even though women have devoted their lives to supporting the lifelong development of others, their own development experiences are still essentially untold.[16] Women's life experiences and viewpoints may indeed be different from men's as a result of complex factors such as social status, power and reproductive biology.[8,17]

Gilligan's Theory of Moral Development

Gilligan, a clinical psychologist, traced women's voices as she studied the development of morality.[8] She found that existing psychological accounts failed to describe the progression of relationships toward a maturity of interdependence, or to trace the evolution of the capacity for responsible care. Gilligan challenged Freud, Piaget, and Kohlberg, who studied boys and men and then assumed that women's ability to make moral judgments was inferior.[18] Gilligan's work asserts that

- Women have learned, from their early socialization, to place priority on responsibility toward others in important relationships (the ethics of care) rather than on individual welfare and concerns. Identity and intimacy are not separate stages of development for women.
- When faced with a dilemma, women are interested in understanding individual circumstances and in obtaining the best possible solution for all concerned, rather than using more abstract universal justice principles employed by men.
- The standard of moral judgment that women use for self-assessment also has to do with relationships: the ability to nurture, to care for others, and to bear responsibility.
- Women's differing modes of moral reasoning lead to different forms of self-definition and different views of relationships.[8] Gilligan's work has been criticized as perpetuating gender stereotypes during the socially conservative 1980s.[19]

Bardwick's Model of Human Development

Bardwick's model addresses women's adult development while incorporating much of Levinson's model of adult maturation. Bardwick maintains that psychological growth and change are intertwined and never cease.[20] Moreover, the goals and values of one's life reflect changing societal and cultural values.[11] The transition from one developmental stage to the next includes a process of self-evaluation. For women, transitions to new values and lifestyles are likely to be more extreme and more emotionally volatile than in previous generations, as options provided to women become more numerous.[20]

Bardwick defines the self in terms of dependent, interdependent, and egocentric mental stances. A woman may maintain a *dependent* sense of self, which is basically relational, or move toward a more *interdependent* stance, in which a sense of self exists simultaneously with a keen awareness of being a contributing and receiving member of an affectional relationship. Bardwick, however, contends that for a woman to develop a permanent *egocentric* stance is rare, because socialization of women in our society and the definition of femininity tend much more toward an interdependent or dependent sense of self.

A NEW PSYCHOLOGY OF WOMEN

Equality

Caring for others is valued less in our society than are individuation and individual achievement; thus women's concern with relationships is often viewed as a weakness.[17] The need for social equality is reflected in problems that arise when affiliation and relationships are molded by domination and subordination.[17] A new language in psychology should describe the structuring of women's sense of self, that is, the need to make and then maintain relationships. Caring and connection must be separated from the resulting inequality and oppression. Women judge themselves in terms of their ability to care, so much so that professional and academic endeavors may be seen as jeopardizing their own sense of themselves.[8] Personal conflict may arise when women have to choose between achievement and caring, if being successful is at the expense of another's failure.

Valuing Self

The psychology of women is distinct in relationships of temporary and permanent inequality.[18] A woman may be temporarily dominant in relationships of nurturance, yet subservient in relationships of permanently unequal social status and power. Women are subordinate in social position to men, yet at the same time entwined with them in the intimate and intense relationships of adult sexuality and family life. Feminist therapy involves the individual's recognition of the restrictive social binds that influence many women, including an overdependence on men for self-esteem and financial, psychological, and social needs.[7] Women with less traditional sex role norms have reported better mental health and more health promoting lifestyles.[3] Women traditionally have taken care of men, but men have tended to assume or devalue that care.[8] Women need to learn to nurture and value themselves and other women, rather than nurturing only men and children. Women's psychology reflects both sides of relationships of interdependence.

Empowerment

Women need power to advance their own development and maintain an identity characterized by self-determination and a diminished need for continuous approval.[17] Too often women find their lives being dominated by prevalent societal values.[17] Often, women and men experience enormous differences in access to power and control of resources,[21] and for women, a stance of less power may result in an emphasis on relatedness to others and compassion.[19] Powerlessness, or learned helplessness, in femininity may be exhibited in relationships of battering and more subtly as depression.[7] Perhaps as more emphasis is given to female perspectives, society can move toward more acceptance of power-with rather than power-over, which would help facilitate a more peaceful environment on a larger scale.[22] Mutuality in relationships would help foster efforts toward elimination of many social maladies such as violence against women and discrimination based on ethnicity and

gender. Women could make significant steps toward healthier lives, as stressors compromising many intimate affiliations diminish.

Many women have learned to demystify aspects of their lives, finding strength in the shared experiences of other women. Their strength is reflected in greater self-sufficiency, assertiveness, and self-knowledge. Consider the example of violence against women. Issues such as rape, battering of women, child sexual abuse, and incest were largely ignored, or their existence disbelieved before the collected efforts of enraged women.[17] Women have effected changes in medical/gynecologic care and will no longer accept care that is limited to their reproductive organs to the exclusion of concerns such as cardiac disease or to the discounting of entities such as premenstrual syndrome (PMS).

A Different Starting Point in Defining Women's Development

Women essentially develop in a context of their attachment to others. The cornerstone of a new psychology of women is the appreciation of the power of relationship and connection in women's lives.[22] Women's sense of self, as well as their perceived strength, is based on the ability to form affiliations and relationships.[8,17] Although this experience of attachment to others provides women with more opportunities for interpersonal pleasure, there is the concurrent fear of separation.[22] Many women perceive the threat of a disrupted affiliation as a total loss of self. Perhaps there is a more ideal midpoint where affiliation is valued along with self-sufficiency. Possibilities exist for a more advanced approach to living and functioning in which affiliation is valued as highly, or more highly, than self-enhancement.[17]

Traditional developmental models define growth and psychological maturity in linear, incremental movement toward more independence and autonomy. In a relational model, a girl's developmental quest is more realistically portrayed as a spiraling process of self-definition within important relationships. Therapists now perceive as ego strengths the intellectual and emotional qualities necessary to engage in meaningful, personal, nurturing, reciprocal relationships.[23]

THE WAYS THAT WOMEN KNOW

The intellectual development of women has become another topic of study.[16,24] The inability for women to gain a voice reflects their image of being powerless, subjugated, and inadequate. Indeed, more women than men pose questions, listen to others, and refrain from speaking out, but women's pattern of discourse may be suitable for a maternal, caring, relationship-oriented role. For example, a mother may refrain from sharing ideas too quickly with her child in order to foster the child's own ability to form ideas. Thus, women may value drawing out the voices of others as a means of enhancing others' development. This mode of discourse, similar to Socratic thinking, could serve as a model for promoting human development.[23]

SOCIETAL ISSUES

Ambiguity in the language of adult development stems from the lack of a cultural definition of *adulthood* and how people's lives evolve within it.[11] Controversies in the study of adult development include whether the use of separate, gender-specific, and age-status criteria is still relevant.[25] In fact, age norms today are more fluid than in the past; for example, many people divorce, or never marry, and many adults choose to have no children or to have children later in life.

Furthermore, in our society women as well as men are economically productive and not isolated in the home. The 1980s witnessed a remarkable increase in the number of employed women, especially married working mothers. Both men and women may aspire for social power, social privileges, and dominant social status. Meanwhile, many of the baby boomer generation, born during the 1950s and 1960s, men and women alike, are taking another look at the importance of work and family life.[26] A substantial portion claim that family life will become more important to them, a trend sometimes referred to as "downshifting," including earlier retirement for both men and women and more leisure activities for greater family contact.

An alternative approach to the study of adult development is to focus on changing social contexts surrounding human development and the normative life crises marking individual and family lifestyle.[25] The individual's inner developmental changes and outer contextual life changes can be viewed as dynamically interdependent; consequently, age diminishes as the focus of our attention in a complex social structure.

WOMEN'S ISSUES AND CONFLICTING VALUES

Value Changes

The value changes that occurred most dramatically during the 1970s redefined and expanded choices for women in their roles related to work and family.[20] Many women must now address both modern and traditional patterns of lifestyle in their decision making. Facing conflicting life choices and societal norms, women grapple with cultural ambiguity and personal uncertainty. Traditional norms regarding femininity prevail, even for women in less traditional roles. For example, despite reduced gender separation of work and family roles in the 1990s, couples still tend to make decisions concerning geographical locations and timing of major family events according to the husband's career needs. On the other hand, women are choosing to have fewer children. This fact, combined with increasing longevity, means that a substantially shorter percentage of women's lives are spent childrearing.

Cultural Ambiguity and Personal Uncertainty

Although women's choices can create ambiguity and uncertainty, the freedom of choice is perhaps less frustrating then the restrictions of the recent past.[20] Often, however, change may be an illusion for women; the reality of the social foundation of power still leans strongly toward enhanced status for traditional feminine values.[19] Modern women also face significant challenges to have it all, as the social changes necessary to allow for ample choices have not been resolved. Barriers still exist to equitable pay, adequate child care, and breaking through old boy networks. Women may have adequate drive to achieve; however, they may feel limited to a level of achievement that society deems appropriate for their gender difference or, some would argue, their social status.[20] Conflict may arise between the need for affiliation or the desire for approval from other people, and the pursuit of achievement for its own sake. Competition may be viewed as contrary to the traditional feminine ideal and may lead to social rejection. Although women and men tend to be compared favorably in neutral situations, women tend to have less internal hope for success in more competitive situations. A particular dilemma for women has been to achieve success in a traditionally male occupation.

Gender Issues

Levinson believes that the timing of developmental periods and tasks are similar for women and men,[11,15] while giving weight to how men's and women's lives are affected by gender splitting issues, creating in human life a rigid division between male and female, masculine and feminine. To a much greater extent than we have previously been comfortable acknowledging, women and men have lived in different social worlds with very different social roles, identities, and psychological attributes.

Levinson identifies four basic forms of gender splitting: 1) the domestic sphere and the public sphere; 2) the traditional marriage enterprise (homemaker and provider); 3) "women's work" and "men's work"; and 4) the feminine and masculine psyches. As this century has seen an increasing number of single parent (mother) households, the traditional source of women's identity and meaningful family activity has been altered, bringing both satisfaction and dissatisfaction.

The historical process within postindustrial conditions has included a gender revolution. Many social changes have reduced women's involvement in the family and have increased involvement in outside work. Some of these changes include 1) the sharp rise of human longevity; 2) the decreasing demand for women's work in the family, concomitant with smaller family size (contraception options); and 3) the growing incidence of divorce. More than 50 percent of all American women are now in the labor force—part time or full time, paid or volunteer, continuously or sporadically.[15]

Other developmental themes hold that gender differences exist in movement through developmental periods.[8,9,20] Furthermore, women, more than men, tend to avoid evaluating their own lives. Perhaps this is because self-assessment may heighten women's awareness of their lack of self-determination and relative powerlessness, revealed in their tendency to respond to the directives and initiative of others.[20] Women's self-esteem and identity also depend more heavily on validation by others.

Life Events, Options, and Stress

Along with more options, women may also experience discontent, as it is less clear what is expected of them. Stressors occur in traditional homemaker choices, in career options, and in attempts to combine the two. In addition, women may experience developmental periods at later ages and in more irregular sequences, while focusing on different aspects of their life structure.[27] Moreover, developmental tasks may be dealt with very differently at different times, as women themselves may change psychologically over time.

MAJOR PERIODS AND TASKS: THE WOMEN'S PERSPECTIVE

A well-formed body of knowledge on women's development does not exist; however, issues in women's development are discussed here, using Levinson's framework, where feasible, and other authors' contributions, especially those of Bardwick.[20] The novice phase of early adulthood—individuals as apprentice adults, ages 17 to 33—encompasses several large tasks, including forming a dream, a mentor relationship, an occupation, and an enduring relationship. Women and men may have significant differences in accomplishing these tasks.[28] Timing of major life events is not as important as understanding the importance in forming the life structure. A discussion of key transition periods follows.

EARLY ADULT TRANSITION (AGES 17 TO 22)

Major tasks for women in this period include value assessment; goal setting for education and work; formation of important peer relationships that focus on sex, love, commitment; formation of relationships to occupation; and separation from parents. The task is not to end the relationship, but rather to reject certain aspects (e.g., submission, defiance), sustain more valued aspects, and build in new qualities such as mutual respect.[15] Individuation may be reflected in great differences in values between parents and young adults in areas such as politics and career choices. Values may more strongly reflect identification with peer groups, however, than true individuation or autonomy.

A major conflict exists between making commitments and avoiding them in order to keep options open.[13] Commitments are more easily made if one's peers are doing so. The early adult is often egocentric as she progresses through rapid emotional and physical changes. She may believe that she is invulnerable, unique, and immune, and hence be prone to misconceptions, for example, that sexual activity will not lead to pregnancy.[29]

Gender Identity

A crucial task is to internalize a sense of gender, which encompasses a sense of one's body in relation to sexuality. To traditional young women, this focus may mean marriage, the prime example of moving into an adult sexual role. Women are essentially dependent at this time, and occasionally interdependent, as the need to form relationships dominates. A great deal of psychological fluidity exists with some sense of egocentrism. Men at this time exhibit comparatively less fluidity and interpersonal dependence and more egocentricity.

Traditional sex role expectations are still prominent in adolescence and early adulthood.[23] For example, a woman may fear that her own ambitions will cost a relationship. A conflict exists between fulfillment of egocentric and interpersonal/dependent priorities as the early adult tries to define the sense of self.

Identity and Adult Commitments

Erikson describes the male adolescent as developing an autonomous, initiating, industrious self through the forging of an identity based on the ideal image—ability to support and justify adult commitments.[13] He describes the female adoles-

cent as holding her identity in abeyance while preparing to attract the man she will marry and by whose status she will be defined.[13] Such attitudes predominated well into the 1960s and, to a great degree, still exist. Many women, however, have begun to emerge as breadwinners in their own right, often choosing professions once thought of as strictly in the man's domain. These women may have more confusing choices as they struggle with career decisions that will affect their family's life.

Identity and Intimacy

For men, identity precedes intimacy and generativity in the traditional view of the optimum cycle of human separation and attachment. For women, these tasks are fused, developing together as the woman comes to know herself as she is known, primarily through her relationships with others.[8,30] Most men in their 20s are not ready to form loving, emotionally intimate relationships, or to make an enduring commitment to wives and families.[11] Whereas women resolve the intimacy issue by their 20s,[31] men are still engaged in this task well into their 30s. Traditionally, men view attachment as a developmental impediment. Hence, married women may be intimacy mentors to their husbands.

Factors Influencing Identity

Identity development in women is influenced by communion, connection, relation (to friends and all significant others) embeddedness, spirituality, and affiliation.[32] Men and women differ significantly in the separation—individuation process. Some women may never completely individuate from their mothers. Often they transfer their dependence onto a boyfriend, as their vision of themselves is relational. A process of anchoring in the family of origin, with a partner and children, in a career, or with friends is critical to women's identity formation and provides the anchor for growth, change, or new directions in life. For women, identity and intimacy are developed at the same time.[8]

Challenges to Women's Independent Goals

Women now in their 20s have grown up in a society different from that of their mothers.[20] A growing number of women today focus on their own careers, as independent goals are articulated more freely. During this period as a woman deals with the demands of egocentric children, it is possible to become engulfed and lose a sense of self, especially if her marital partner is also demanding. More than one-fifth of women are now the sole parent for their children. The typical homeless woman is a 27-year-old mother of two facing incredible challenges associated with acute and chronic medical problems, risk of violence and sexual abuse, depression, and substance abuse.[22] Although the majority of women who divorce in their 20s do remarry, they may become more egocentric, unwilling to give anyone else that much power over them again.

Identity and Parenthood

Women, especially working women or those with difficult infants, experience appreciably more change than do men in the transition to parenthood.[33] Women tend to feel responsible for their children's success and happiness. They also experience the contagion of stress as they internalize the distress experienced by those to whom they are closest, particularly family members. During this period, however, if work serves as a visible marker of achievement, it may lessen stress. Indeed, women with multiple roles may be the most well adjusted. The supportive family buffers a woman from endless demands of child care and other family responsibilities.

ENTRY LIFE STRUCTURE FOR EARLY ADULTHOOD (AGES 22 TO 28)

Life structures for women tend to be less stable than those for men, essentially because of more diverse concerns involving marriage, motherhood, and career.[28] The primary tasks of this period are to build and maintain a first adult life structure and to enrich one's life within that structure.[15]

AGE THIRTY TRANSITION AND THE SETTLING DOWN PERIOD OF EARLY ADULTHOOD (AGES 28 TO 39)

Both sexes in settling down must give up a youthful self-image and the idea that involvements are tentative and options still open. Priorities of the 20s may be reversed; choices and their consequences may be reassessed; and options regarding marriage and especially childbearing may not exist much longer.[11] A bewildering discovery occurring at about age 30 is that the life one has arduously constructed has major imperfections and that there is still some growing up to do.[15]

- *Men's Success.* Success in work is imperative to men's timetable. A shift in centrality by men—from work to family—may be a reaction to a combination of stress, age, or failure in work. Men sever ties with mentors in order to be seen as knowledgeable and successful in their own right of becoming one's own man.[11]
- *Women's Success.* In contrast, few women would define becoming one's own woman primarily through success in their work.[20] Those who are successful in their careers may still be anxious about their femininity unless they are also involved in significant relationships and have experienced motherhood. Women may sacrifice success in careers and attain lower financial status as they compromise to maintain relationships. Sadness and depression may develop as women suppress their authentic selves and make repeated compromises.[34] Factors leading to a sense of independence in men, such as career success, may instead highlight the dependent needs in women. Her success includes becoming more fully adult by dealing with the child in herself and with the cultural assumption that an adult female is still a girl.[15]
- *Prolonged Transition.* Women in their 30s are likely to experience a more prolonged and profound transition period than men are, perhaps most importantly linked to the age limits for childbearing (the biological clock). Current technology may permit women to become pregnant well beyond their earlier expectations, however. The age thirty transition can be a time of increased individuation that is self-generated rather than relational. During the period of evaluation and reappraisal (ages 28 to 33), married women may demand that husbands recognize and accommodate their aspirations and interests outside of the home.[28]
- *Career versus Family.* Women reappraise the relative importance of career and family, often

adding the missing component rather than reversing priorities (e.g., a mother may begin a career).[20] Women may attempt to lead a life in which they do it all. The mental health stressors of women's multiple roles may be influenced more by marital factors than by work factors. Work often buffers some marital stress, but parenthood exacerbates occupational stress, especially if responsibilities are not shared in the home.[33]

- *Multiple Roles.* Having multiple roles may counterbalance some negative effects of a particular role. Thus, the healthiest women may be those with multiple roles, including having a career, a husband, and often children.[33] "Having it all" may mean "doing it all," and women may experience strain in attempting to fulfill multiple role obligations. American society does not yet support working women with child care options or pay that is comparable to men's. Often they must choose between family and career. Women's ability to cope with the stresses has been associated with having a high income and job satisfaction, marrying later, and arranging time for family activities.[33]

- *American Values and Women's Sexuality.* The American culture values youth and beauty, and often by age 35, a woman is no longer considered young.[35] Women are labeled old 10 to 15 years earlier than men are, with resulting psychological, sexual, and economic disadvantages.[35]

- *Confusing Choices.* Women in their 30s are facing the growing influence of feminist thinking and more egalitarian life patterns. At the same time they are confronted by others who tell them that their behaviors should be more traditional. Women also struggle with their own psychological tendencies regarding more traditional values, which they internalized early in life.

- *Readjustment in the Thirties.* Demographically, most women now in their 30s are married with school-age children. Those who are employed are not necessarily on a career path. Others who are unemployed have been out of school for about 10 years.[20] As women reach ages 35 to 40, their husband's tremendous involvement in their own careers and children's decreasing dependence on them may provide the opportunity for personal change. Women may return to

work or school, or look for other relationships in the community. Family members may initially agree to change their lifestyles in order to accommodate the women's needs; however, when changes impact them directly, they may become resentful or confused.

- *Stress.* Stress is inherent in the reality or the illusion of choice. Some women may sacrifice personal relationships to achieve career success; others may be doing it all with very little support from their partners. Partners' expectations of each other in their relationship are not always clear. Many women who divorce in their 30s may become more confident and perhaps more angry. Anger may lead to egocentricism that enables women to formulate obtainable objectives. For married women, responsibilities outside the home—community and career involvement—may help them become less dependent economically, socially, and psychologically. Most women in this age group tend toward interdependence.

MIDLIFE TRANSITION AND MIDDLE ADULTHOOD (AGES 39 TO 60)

An appreciable change in the character of living occurs between early and middle adulthood. The main tasks of entering middle adulthood are making crucial choices, giving those choices meaning and commitment, and building a life structure around them.[11]

Midlife Transitions

- Assessment for both men and women may have a sense of urgency; they wish to accomplish their life goals as they confront mortality. Those who do not assess their lives at this point may feel frightened and unable to make changes in their lifestyles or careers. Men assess what they receive and what they give to work, family, friends, and community as they reach the symbolically powerful age of 40.[11,14] Their established autonomy now allows greater compassion, more reflection, less tyranny by inner conflicts and external demands, and more genuine love of self and others. Middle aged men may experience this as their fullest and most creative period.

By the end of middle adulthood, problems may include declining health, aging or death of parents, spousal death, and stagnation at work with no viable options. Although the relationship with one's spouse may only be comfortable, the option of ending it means losing crucial roots. Nonetheless, divorce has increased markedly for both men and women in their 40s. One may see a partner as a reason for discontent or as someone to blame for perceived losses. A new relationship may be viewed as a way to recoup the feelings and pleasure of youth.

- Growth can be seen in women who become more autonomous as they succeed in relationships; both sexes may become more interdependent.[20] Women may grow more comfortable as initiators and become gratified functioning as individuals. Most women now in their 40s grew up in traditional environments in which choices were limited. Consequently, few have been seriously involved in a career. Becoming involved in a career after 40 can be an opportunity for real beginnings, but it also can be frightening. This may be a time for women to generate new values internally, reflecting who they are rather than what they do.
- Losses or adjustments in relationships may cause depression in women beginning the midlife phase; they may experience loneliness as children leave home or they become widowed or divorced.[20] The empty nest concept is not totally supported by national data; a dependent woman who faces the loss of her children and her husband at this time may be more vulnerable. Women, but not men, tend to define their age status in terms of the timing of events within their family; even unmarried career women often discuss middle age in terms of the family they might have had. Women with more complex lives may experience sadness and joy in this time of readjustment as they face losses along with new beginnings. Many more men than women remarry at this age.

A majority of women have made a reality transition, as evidenced by a high employment rate.[20] The expansion of activities, maturing, and increased self-confidence lead many of these women to be more interdependent rather than dependent, as compared with women in

their 30s. This is perhaps the most complex of all developmental periods because women are given social permission to work at precisely the time their traditional responsibilities decline.

Middle Adulthood

Although Levinson's studies ended with men and women in their 40s, he believed that a major transition phase occurs from ages 50 to 55. A stable period follows from ages 55 to 60, during which rejuvenation in some can result in achieving significant fulfillment and enrichment.[11,14] For men especially whose connection with others depends largely on their jobs, retirement may be associated with a loss of prestige and decreased self-esteem. Women tend to face this loss much earlier if their primary role in life is that of mother, their secondary role that of homemaker, and their tertiary role that of sexual partner. As family becomes less central to women's lives, other sources of satisfaction can be significant. Often, the marital relationship has to be modified as women strive to create better lives for themselves. Career promotions are less common and may be disappointing compared with what was hoped for. Accomplishments in careers may not bring the same satisfaction or sense of accomplishment as in earlier years. The question "How successful am I in the eyes of the world?" may be less important than "What do I give and receive from my work? How satisfying is my relationship with work?"[15]

- The aging process traditionally has been symbolized as retirement for men and menopause for women, although the formerly predominant views regarding women and the menopause have been challenged.[31] Anticipating menopause is often more dreadful than the difficulty experienced with its actual occurrence. Women often feel relief with the loss of menses as well as the loss of tasks associated with rearing young children. The real difficulty may be adjusting to the aging process—a continuum that does not just begin after menses ends. Other changes associated with aging are socially more apparent, such as graying hair and wrinkles. Bifocal glasses and hearing aids may be a threat to self-esteem and a visible admission of aging, which may cause problems in intimate relationships.[31,36]

- "The sandwich generation" refers to the women who are caretakers for their children as well as for their aging parents.

  Aging is a gradual process, and changes of aging are adaptive across the life span. During middle age, women may to some extent lose their roles of mother and sex partner, especially through divorce or death. A partner's retirement may force another adaptation. Distancing from parents in the middle years is replaced by establishing a commitment for parents' care, which allows some women who see themselves primarily as homemakers to reestablish that lifestyle.

- Readjustment in the 50s may be necessary because today's women in that age group were in their 20s when new options for women gained momentum.[20] A few will feel the need to change or reassess values or direction at this stage in their lives; others will reject new values, believing themselves incapable of achieving different goals. Women most at risk for psychological dependence are traditional housewives who lack involvement or outside commitments. Interdependence is more likely to occur among older women who have found fulfillment in their traditional roles and who have assumed varied roles, whether or not through employment. A few older women are egocentric as a result of being widows, divorced, displaced homemakers, or having never married.

- Societal views of aging women include negative stereotypes such as being inactive, unhealthy, asexual, unattractive, and ineffective—despite the diversity of older women who lead interesting, productive lives.[21] Revising expectations about advancing age requires that society move beyond these stereotypes and overcome ageist and sexual biases.[29] Health care providers need to recognize the diversity among women as they age. Older women receive messages that growing older is a process to be prevented (with face lifts or antiaging facial creams) rather than to be enjoyed. Even professional women view aging as a serious impairment. Discrimination in employment is particularly harmful for women reentering the work force after their children leave home or when

the loss of a spouse decreases their income and security. Throughout adulthood, women are increasingly threatened by poverty as a result of greater numbers of female-headed households and the continuing disparity in salaries between men and women. Older women are particularly affected by inadequate spousal retirement plans, especially if they themselves have a history of unemployment. As women live longer, they have more opportunity to develop illness, another stress on their finances.

LATE ADULT TRANSITION

Ages 60 to 65 mark the end of middle life and entry into the late adult transition.[15] Overall, women feel good about themselves and what they are accomplishing as they use time freed by retirement or other life changes to pursue creative activities, community work, and self-development.[27] When women outlive their husbands, creativity may develop as a response to loss and loneliness, including social and emotional isolation. Women may also return to creative activities they enjoyed in earlier years. During their 60s women are most likely to experience transitions relating to their own illness and the illness and death of significant others.

Behavioral Shifts with Age

In the last decades, studies have addressed endocrine changes as they affect the physiological and psychological aspects of life, as well as the relationships between women and men, and women and women, and the changes that occur in those relationships over time. The studies are controversial.[31] Some authors propose that a shift to more assertive or controlling behavior among women beginning in midlife is the result of a change in the androgen-estrogen ratio toward more biologically active androgens of greater influence. The reverse pattern is observed in men, with estrogens affecting affiliative and nurturing aspects as androgens drop. Thus, while aging women may become more tolerant of their own aggressive and egocentric impulses, aging men may become more accepting of their nurturant and affiliative impulses.

LATE ADULTHOOD AND LATE, LATE ADULTHOOD

Women can expect to live well into their 70s and 80s. Ages 76 to 80 may represent a transition toward wisdom as women are challenged to adapt to a number of changes, including loss of health, friends, and family.[27] A surge of creativity may continue as women find pleasurable ways to enrich their lives. Relationships and affiliation with others remain important for women, and their creativity may take the form of altruistic responses to the needs of others. Successful or creative aging may be associated with maintaining meaningful activities, keeping close relationships with persons of all ages, and remaining flexible and adaptable. Nonconformists who are willing to take risks and who sustain a positive outlook on life perhaps experience the greatest success in aging. Psychological development never ends as long as the individual engages in reality; thus the potential for growth and change is always present.[20,27]

REFERENCES

1. O'Rand, A. M., & Henrette, J. C. (1982). Women at middle age: Development and transitions. *Annals of the American Academy of Political and Social Sciences.* Beverly Hills, CA: Sage.
2. Grosskurth, P. (1991). The new psychology of women. *New York Review of Books, 38*(17).
3. Woods, N. F., Lentz, M., & Mitchell, E. (1993). The new woman: Health promoting and health damaging behaviors. *Health Care for Women International, 14,* 389–405.
4. Barnard, J. (1982). Women's educational needs. In A. W. Chickering and Associates (Eds.), *The modern American college: Responding to the new realities of diverse students and a changing society.* San Francisco: Jossey-Bass.
5. Fuller, J., & Schaller-Ayers, J. (1990). *Health assessment: A nursing approach.* Philadelphia: Lippincott.
6. Seiden, A. M. (1989). Psychological issues affecting women throughout the life cycle. *Psychiatric Clinics of North America, 12*(1), 1–24.
7. Kaschak, E. (1981). Feminist psychotherapy: The first decade. In S. Cox (Ed.), *Female psychology* (pp. 387–401). New York: St. Martin's Press.
8. Gilligan, C. (1982). *In a different voice: Psychological theory and women's development.* Cambridge, MA: Harvard University Press.
9. Hyde, J. S. (1985). *Half the human experience: The psychology of women* (3rd ed.). Lexington, MA: D.C. Heath.
10. Strachey, J. (Ed. and Trans.). (1961). *The standard edition of the complete psychological works of Sigmund Freud.* London: Hogarth Press.
11. Levinson, D. J. (1986). A conception of adult development. *American Psychologist, 41*(1), 3–13.
12. Erikson, E. H. (1950). *Childhood and society.* New York: Norton.
13. Erikson, E. H. (1968). *Identity, youth and crises.* New York: Norton.
14. Levinson, D. J. (1978). *The seasons of a man's life.* New York: Alfred A. Knopf.
15. Levinson, D. J. (1996). *The seasons of a woman's life.* New York: Alfred A. Knopf.
16. Belenky, M. F., et al. (1985). Epistemological development and the politics of talk in family life. *Journal of Education, 167*(3).
17. Miller, J. B. (1986). *Toward a new psychology of women* (2nd ed.). Boston: Beacon Press.
18. Gilligan C. (1982). New maps of development: New visions of maturity. *American Journal of Orthopsychiatry, 52*(2), 199–212.
19. Mednick, M. T. (1989). On the politics of psychological constructs: Stop the bandwagon, I want to get off. *American Psychologist, 44*(8), 1118–1123.
20. Bardwick, J. M. (1980). The seasons of a woman's life. In D. G. McGuigan (Ed.), *Women's lives: New theory, research, and policy.* Ann Arbor: University of Michigan, Center for Continuing Education of Women.
21. Lott B. (1987). *Women's lives: Themes and variations in gender learning.* Pacific Grove, CA: Brooks/Cole.
22. Lewis, J. A. & Bernstein, J. (1996). *Women's health: A relational perspective across the life cycle.* Sudbury, MA: Jones and Bartlett.
23. Rosenblatt, E. A. (1995). Emerging concept of women's development. Implications for psychotherapy. *The Psychiatric Clinics of North America, 18*(1), 95–106.
24. Belenky, M. F., et al. (1986). *Women's ways of knowing. The development of self, voice, and mind.* New York: Basic Books.
25. Steitz, J. A. (1982). The female life course: Life situations and perception of control. *International Journal of Aging and Human Development, 14*(3).
26. Hueber, G. (1991, April 7). Baby boomers heading for earlier retirement. *Richmond Times-Dispatch,* p. H 8.

27. Mercer, R. T., Nichols, E. G., & Doyle, G. C. (1989). *Transitions in a woman's life: Major life events in developmental context.* New York: Springer.

28. Roberts, P., & Newton, P. M. (1987). Levinsonian studies of women's adult development. *Psychology & Aging, 2*(2), 154–163.

29. Lichtman, R., & Papera, S. (1990). *Gynecology: Well woman care.* Norwalk, CT: Appleton & Lange.

30. Evans, N. J. (1985, March). Women's development across the life span. In N. J. Evans (Ed.), *Facilitating the development of women: New directions for student services,* No. 29. San Francisco: Jossey-Bass.

31. Rossi, A. S. (1980). Life span theories and women's lives. *Signs: Journal of Women in Culture and Society, 6*(1).

32. Josselson, R. (1987). *Finding herself: Pathways to identity development in women.* San Francisco: Jossey-Bass.

33. McBride, A. B. (1990). Mental health effects of women's multiple roles. *American Psychologist, 45*(3), 381–384.

34. Jack, D. (1991). *Silencing the self: Women and depression.* Cambridge, MA: Harvard University Press.

35. Bell, I. P. (1979). The double standard: Age. In Freeman (Ed.), *Women: A feminist perspective* (pp. 145–155). Palo Alto, CA: Mayfield.

36. Eliopoulos, C. (1990). *Health assessment of the older adult* (2nd ed.). Redwood City, CA: Addison-Wesley.

SELECTED BIBLIOGRAPHY

Bem, S. L. (1993). *The lenses of gender: Transforming the debate on sexual inequality.* New Haven: Yale University Press.

Brown, L., & Gilligan, C. (1992). *Meeting at the crossroads: Women's psychology and girls' development.* Cambridge, MA: Harvard University Press.

Eisler, R. (1988). *The chalice and the blade.* San Francisco: Harper.

Friedan, B. (1993). *The fountain of age.* New York: Simon & Schuster.

Lott, B. (1981). *Becoming a woman: The socialization of gender.* Springfield, IL: Charles C. Thomas.

Matlin, M. W. (1987). *The psychology of women.* New York: CBS College Publishing.

McGuigan, D. G. (Ed.). (1980). *Women's lives: New theory, research and policy.* Ann Arbor: University of Michigan, Center for continuing Education of Women.

Pipher, M. (1994). Reviving Ophelia: Saving the selves of adolescent girls. New York: Ballantine Books.

Rossi, A. S. (1985). *Gender and the life course.* Hawthorne, NY: Aldine.

CHAPTER 4

ASSESSING ADOLESCENT WOMEN'S HEALTH

Deborah A. Raines

*A*dolescence offers unique opportunities for investment in the health and well-being of future generations.

Highlights

- Growth and Development of Puberty
- Developmental Tasks of Adolescence
- Health Issues and Risks
- Caring for Adolescents
- Sexual Behavior Decisions

▶   INTRODUCTION

Adolescence is considered a critical period in human development. The adolescent is an individual in transition between childhood and adulthood, and this transition is a complex process. Adolescent transitions include the completion of gender-specific physical growth and development resulting in reproductive maturity and the achievement of developmental tasks resulting in the establishment of a personal identity. Adolescence offers unique opportunities for investment in the health and well-being of future generations. Adolescence, however, is also a time of high risk behaviors and involvement in conduct often disturbing to society. According to Hechinger, the state of adolescent health in America has reached crisis proportions and adolescents' glaring need for health care is largely ignored.[1] The 1995 adolescent report card from the Carnegie Corporation revealed the following startling statistics:

- Every 22 seconds, an American teenager becomes pregnant
- Every 67 seconds, an American teenager has a baby
- Every day, six teenagers commit suicide
- Every day, 623 teenagers get a sexually transmitted disease.[2]

As these data indicate, the adolescent's behavior has long-term implications for individual and societal health and well-being. Consequently, understanding the unique physical and developmental needs of the adolescent is important.

ADOLESCENCE

In the past, puberty and adolescence were considered synonymous. They are separate entities, however, encompassing the biological and psychological responses to this critical transition. Puberty is focused on physical changes culminating in the functional ability to engage in sexual reproduction. For the female, puberty begins with a physical growth spurt and ends with the onset of menstruation signifying the achievement of biological maturity. Adolescence is a broader concept based on the individual's progressive psychological maturation and readiness to assume adult responsibilities. Although chronologic age plays a role in definitions of adolescence and the anticipation of the events of puberty, the process of physical and psychological development is highly individualized and variable. Adolescence is typically defined as the period of life beginning with puberty and extending for an average of eight to ten years.[3] Females experience the adolescent period an average of two years earlier than males, due in part to earlier onset of physical changes and development. The psychological responses of the adolescent are often delineated by chronologic age. Psychosocial development is frequently categorized as behaviors of early, middle or late adolescence. Similar to the biological growth variation during puberty, however, individual differences manifest themselves in the achievement of the developmental tasks of adolescence as well.

HYPOTHALAMIC-PITUITARY-GONADAL DEVELOPMENT

The growth and development changes evident in the adolescent are attributable to the Hypothalamic-Pituitary-Gonadal (HPG) axis and the presence of sex hormones. The HPG axis is a cyclic phenomenon: the activity of gonadotrophic releasing hormone, the pituitary secretion of gonadotropins, and the estradiol positive feedback triggering the preovulatory luteinizing hormone (LH) surge, follicular rupture, and corpus luteum formation.[4] The HPG axis is established during in utero development, becomes dormant or suspended during childhood, and is reactivated during the second decade of life by an as yet unidentified mechanism.[5]

Gonadotropin-releasing hormone (GnRH), LH, follicle stimulating hormone (FSH), and estrogen are detectable in the female fetus by 10 weeks' gestation. The episodic release of GnRH and gonadotropins (FSH and LH), with an intact negative feedback mechanism, demonstrates that the hypothalamic-pituitary-gonadal system is functional at a mature level prior to birth. The presence of the negative feedback response of the hypothalamus and pituitary in response to circulating estrogen prevents the development of mature, gender-specific sexual characteristics in the fetus.

During puberty, there is a resurgence of GnRH, LH and FSH, and sex steroid (estrogen) secretion. It has been suggested that the time frame of puberty is controlled by blood borne substances that convey metabolic information related to carbohydrate or protein utilization as an indicator about the growth and nutrition of the body and that these signals influence the hormonal biochemistry of the body, thereby directing the activity of the GnRH secretory system.[6] Although the exact mechanism of this reactivation of the HPG axis is not well explicated, sequential maturation of the central nervous system and decreased sensitivity of the hypothalamus and pituitary to circulating levels of estradiol are thought to play a significant role.[7] Consequently, puberty is a brain driven event controlled by maturation of the somatic component of the axis and not maturation of the gonad.

The increased secretion of hormones is initiated by release of GnRH in a pulsatile fashion coincident with sleep. Eventually, the pulsatile pattern increases in frequency and magnitude, extending beyond sleep time to encompass the entire 24-hour period.[6] Gonadotrophic secretion causes progressive changes in the morphology of the ovarian follicles and an increase in estrogen secretion. In the female, the development of a positive feedback system, in which critical levels of estrogen trigger a large release of GnRH, stimulating LH to initiate ovulation, is the final stage of axis development during the adolescent years.[5]

Reactivation of the HPG axis is responsible for the physical changes evident during puberty. After the completion of reproductive maturity, the HPG axis is replaced, however, as the mediator of hormone secretion. The mature ovary, with positive and negative feedback loops based on the secretion of estrogen and progesterone, takes over control of hormone levels. Thus, the gonadal component of the axis becomes the regulating force. The female gonad remains in control throughout the reproductive years.

GROWTH AND DEVELOPMENT OF PUBERTY

Physical changes during puberty are typified by growth spurts, development of secondary sexual characteristics, maturation of genital organs, and the onset of menstruation. These events occur in an orderly and sequential pattern. In the female, the onset of puberty is signaled by the initiation of rapid physical growth, and the end point of puberty is menarche. The mean age for the initiation of puberty is 11.2 years but can range from 9.0 to 13.4 years.[5] The duration of puberty for the female ranges from 18 months to 5 years.[7] The time of onset is not related to the duration of puberty.

Chronologic age and physical growth are closely linked with the concept of puberty. Age, height, and weight alone, however, are not the best indicators of physical maturity. To specifically classify the level of physical maturation and to determine normality of development, a sexual maturity rating (SMR) scale is essential. For females, sexual maturity rating scales are based on five stages of breast and genital hair development, correlating with prepubescent (stage I) through adult characteristics (stage V) (see Chapter 5).

GROWTH SPURT

After infancy, adolescence is the most rapid period of physical growth. In the female, onset of the growth spurt is between age 8 and 17 years. The mean age for peak height velocity growth is 12 years.[5] The average duration of this growth spurt is three years in females.[3] Females grow approximately 2 1/2 to 5 inches (6–12.5 cm) in height per year and gain 8–20 pounds (3.5–4.5 kg) per year.[3] Consequently, the pubertal growth spurt contributes a significant proportion of adult body size. Initially, the increase in height is due to lengthening of the long bones in the legs and arms, often resulting in poor posture and decreased co-ordination. Later, growth is in trunk length resulting in adult body proportions. Following menarche, growth rate slows, due to epiphyseal fusion secondary to elevated estrogen levels. Females also experience growth and reshaping of the pelvis during puberty. The bony pelvis grows into the gynecoid shape characteristic of the mature female. Accelerated growth involves an interaction between the endocrine and skeletal systems. Human growth hormone (hGH), thyroxine, insulin, and corticosteroid are growth promoting, while parathyroid hormone, 1,25-dihydroxy-vitamin D and, calciton affect skeletal mineralization.[5] HGH is the key hormone released by the pituitary gland and is the primary influence of adolescent growth. Activity of the pituitary gland is influenced by the multifocal effects of rising estrogen levels. The effect of hGH is modulated through somatomedins or a class of peptide hormones known as insulin-like growth factors (IGF I and IGF II).[8] IGFs, as their names imply, have a biological effect similar to insulin, leading to stimulation of lipid and carbohydrate (CHO) metabolism resulting in fat deposits and development of the female body form.

Weight gain is related to an increase in total body size but, more significantly, is attributable to an increase in the percent of body fat from 15.7 percent to 26.7 percent and a lower percentage of lean body mass.[5] In general, females add more adipose tissue as a result of estrogenic influence. Subcutaneous deposits of adipose tissue are evident in the female hips and breasts.

THELARCHE

Initiation of the female growth spurt precedes thelarche, or breast development, by approximately one year.[5,6] The stimulus for breast development is estrogen. Breast growth is due to extensive fat depositions as well as growth and branching of the ductal system and development of small solid cell masses (potential alveoli) at the duct endings. During puberty, breast size varies and asymmetry is common.

The prepubertal breast has no glandular tissue, and the areola conforms to the general chest line. As puberty progresses, a breast bud with a small amount of glandular tissue and widening of the areola develops. The breast tissue grows larger and the elevation from the chest wall is more pronounced. In sexual maturity rating IV, the areola forms a projecting mound, also known as a double hump, from the contour of the breast. The final or adult stage of breast development is characterized by protrusion of the nipple, but the areola becomes congruent with the remainder of the breast tissue (see Chapter 5).

ADRENARCHE

Concurrent with breast development is pubic hair growth or adrenarche. Prepubescent females have no hair growth in the pubic area. Initial hair growth is a small amount of slightly pigmented, straight, vellus hair on the labia majora. As maturity progresses, the quantity of hair growth increases and the distribution spreads from the labia to the mons veris. The texture also becomes coarser, curlier, and more darkly pigmented. The final stage of pubic hair development is established in about two years and is characterized by an abundant quantity of coarse, curly hair in the typical female triangular distribution with a horizontal upper border. Approximately 2 years after the first appearance of pubic hair, axillary hair growth begins.

EXTERNAL AND INTERNAL GENITALIA

While thelarche and adrenarche are the most obvious of the physical changes associated with puberty, a number of maturational changes are occurring in other structures as well. In addition to pubic hair growth, the vulva is changing in shape and enlarging. The labia majora develop as fat is deposited in the subcutaneous tissue beneath them. Subcutaneous fat deposits also develop over the mons veris and the pubic symphysis. As the labia majora increase in size, they fall inward and tend to obscure the labia minora, which become more vascular and well rounded. The clitoris becomes larger and more erectile and the entire introitus appears larger.

Before puberty, the vaginal epithelium is only a few cells thick, is incapable of glycogen production, has scant secretions, and has an alkaline pH. With the influence of increasing estrogen levels, the vaginal lining is transformed to a layer of thick, stratified squamous epithelial cells containing glycogen. The thickness of the vaginal lining varies with the cyclic circulating levels of female sex hormones. With decreased hormone stimulation, the vaginal epithelium exfoliates, resulting in increased vaginal secretions. During early adolescence, the presence of leukorrhea, or a white mucoid discharge, often precedes menarche by approximately one year.[9] Cellular exfoliation results in the conversion of the intracellular glycogen to lactic acid. Lactic acid formation results in the establishment of Doderlein's bacilli as a component of the normal vaginal flora making the environment more hostile to foreign bacteria and viruses.[9]

The uterus changes from the tubular formation of childhood to a hollow, muscular adult organ. The uterus prior to puberty is characterized by an elongated cervix with a small fundus. Under estrogenic stimulation, both the cervix and the fundus enlarge, but the major change is seen in the fundus. The size of the fundus increases in all dimensions, so that eventually the fundus accounts for three-fourths of the total uterine size.[4] Concurrent with uterine growth, the endometrial lining proliferates, under the influence of cyclic circulating hormone levels, in preparation for menarche.

The ovaries and fallopian tubes also grow, but their growth is slower. The ovaries increase in size and the tubes enlarge and lose some of their tortuousness. The final stage of ovarian development, however, is attained only after the ovary is capable of reacting to both FSH and LH. While uterine and ovarian development begin in parallel, the ovary must develop an adequate vascular system to transport the stimulus for FSH to the follicle cell. The development of a vascular system begins with the onset of puberty but proceeds at a slower rate than does uterine development. Consequently, with increased FSH secretion, estrogen is produced, which leads to gradual proliferation of vascular channels. With fully developed vascular channels, ovarian estrogen secretion is elevated to levels adequate to trigger the release of luteinizing hormone and to initiate ovulation.[4] The slower development of ovarian function, as compared with endometrial function, is the rationale for early menstrual cycles being anovulatory.

MENARCHE

Menarche is the final major landmark of puberty. Menarche occurs after a series of the physical changes of puberty have occurred. In general, menarche occurs approximately 1 to 3 years after initiation of thelarche and during sexual maturity rating 3 or 4. The initial menstrual cycles may be irregular not only in frequency but in duration and quantity. Early menstrual cycles are frequently anovulatory, secondary to the immaturity of ovarian function. Immature ovarian function results in lack of progesterone secretions. Therefore, the endometrial lining is in the proliferative phase. For the first year after menarche, the interval between periods varies widely. The variability decreases with time and establishment of pulsatile secretion of FSH and LH and mature ovarian response, including the secretion of estrogen and progesterone.[7] A woman's interval pattern is usually set about 3 or 4 years after menarche. Establishment of a rhythmic menstrual pattern is thought to be associated with the initiation of ovulation and ovarian control of hormone secretion.[6]

DEVELOPMENTAL TASKS OF ADOLESCENCE

Psychosocial development is a sequential process including the stages of early, middle, and late adolescence. Psychosocial developmental tasks are delineated by chronologic age, in part related to the influence of cultural and social norms that influence their resolution. The developmental tasks of adolescence include the following: accepting one's mature body and sexual identity, developing a personal value system, preparing for productive function, achieving independence from parents, and developing an adult identity. The achievement of psychological maturity is progressive as the individual attains greater physical, cognitive, and social skills. Erikson labeled adolescence the stage of identity versus role confusion, or a time when individuals face identity crisis from which they will emerge with either a clear sense of identity or a state of confusion about their future roles and purpose.[10]

EARLY ADOLESCENCE

Early adolescence is the period between ages 11 and 13 years. Interests focus on same gender peer group identification. Peer acceptance and conformity are important and are often the source of parental conflicts. At this stage, the adolescent wishes to be more grown-up and is concerned with developing into a physically mature adult and with being normal. The adolescent's definition of normal is in relation to the peer group. Therefore, individual variation in physical development can be a source of distress. Questions related to physical development are highly mechanistic in nature, focusing on concern and curiosity about their own and peers' bodies. During the early adolescent stage, the individual's thinking is concrete and lacks the ability for abstract thinking or introspection.[11] Because of the concrete thinking pattern and the limited reasoning capacities, the early adolescent is easily overwhelmed and overruled.

The early adolescent has an increased interest in sexual processes but has no direct sexual ambitions. She frequently finds sexual behaviors such as kissing or intercourse disgusting. Sexual fantasies are common, however, and may be a source of guilt. Desired sexual activities are of a nonphysical nature during this period. The early adolescent is most likely to express her sexual urges through dress, body language, and curiosity about sexual acts.[3,12]

MIDDLE ADOLESCENCE

The most turbulent stage is age 14 to 16 years or middle adolescence. During this period, the adolescent is becoming psychologically egocentric and is preoccupied with self.[10] Self-esteem is established through recognition of the peer group. Behavior is characterized by rebellion and profound mood swings as the adolescent struggles to establish independence. The middle adolescent begins to use abstract reasoning and introspection to develop a better understanding of herself and others. The middle adolescent often exhibits a feeling of immortality or indestructibility, however, as a result of increasing intellect, physical size, and peer identity. This false sense of security can contribute to impulsive and risk-taking behaviors, with no thought of the danger or the sequelae.[11,13]

By middle adolescence, physical maturation is well established and menarche has occurred in the majority of females. Sexual energy is high with an emphasis on physical contact.[3] Sexual behavior, however, is primarily explorative and exploitative in nature. Dating leads to casual relationships with both coital and noncoital contacts.[12] Sexual interests continue to grow and heterosexual relationships become important but are of short duration and erratic. Asynchrony between physical maturity and psychological immaturity in the middle adolescent leads to denial of the potential consequences of sexual behavior. Typically, she believes that the complications of sexual activity, such as sexually transmitted diseases (STDs) or pregnancy, cannot happen to her.[13]

Middle adolescence may also mark the adolescent's realization that she is attracted to members of her own gender.[13] The heterosexual orientation of societal expectations can result in confusion and anxiety for the lesbian adolescent (see Chapter 7). The process of establishing a healthy individual identity, or the fusion of emotions and sexuality into a meaningful whole, is an important developmental task.[14]

LATE ADOLESCENCE

Late adolescence or ages 17 to 21 coincides with full sexual maturity for most individuals. The individual has developed a sense of self and purpose to her life. Sexual behavior is more expressive and less exploitative.[3] Relationships that are monogamous and intimate are developed. Abstract reasoning skills are fully operational, and the individual is able to interact in the adult world and consider the long-term implications of her actions.[11] She also achieves sociolegal maturity during this stage.

Health issues and risks

A major focus of health care for the adolescent is on the physical changes resulting in reproductive maturity and on the psychosocial changes resulting in the establishment of independence. There are a number of other issues and risks that need to be considered in the care of the adolescent, however, to assure adaptive coping and positive growth.

NUTRITION AND EATING DISORDERS

The adolescent's nutritional needs are increased as a result of the increased metabolic processes associated with accelerated growth. The female adolescent between ages 11 and 14 years needs 2200 kcal/day while the 15–18-year-old needs 2400 kcal/day.[3] Nutrient intake should include good dietary sources of protein, calcium, and zinc to meet rapid growth and development demands. In addition, the female adolescent requires an adequate intake of iron. Dietary iron is necessary for the increasing blood volume that accompanies growth as well as to replace the iron lost during menstrual bleeding.

Eating disorders during adolescence include compulsive overeating, anorexia nervosa, and bulimia. Overeating resulting in obesity is the most common malnutrition problem among adolescents and is demonstrating a rising incidence. The prevalence of obesity and overweight in American teens ranges from 16–22 percent, varying by sex, race, family history, and physical activity.[15] Eating disorders can be associated with the individual's anxiety about weight, distortion of body image, and desire to exert control. Therefore, eating disorders are often symptoms of an underlying problem, rather than a primary disease entity. Food has come to be associated with more than a source of nutrition; it is a source of celebration, consolation, punishment, or reward.[3] Adolescent eating disorders frequently begin subsequent to an emotional trauma and are the manifestation of an overwhelming feeling of helplessness, dissatisfaction, or unattractiveness.[13] Feelings of low self-esteem and negative self-image may trigger eating disorders, but may also be exacerbated as the eating disorder progresses. Critical to the prevention and resolution of eating disorders is the promotion of self-esteem and a positive self-image. Consequently, the primary goal in managing the adolescent's nutritional well-being is based on understanding the adolescent's perception and the underlying pressures that influence the meaning of food to the adolescent. Establishing a healthy lifestyle including healthy eating habits and exercise during the adolescent period can influence the individual's nutritional habits throughout her lifetime (see Chapter 23 for further discussion of eating disorders).

MENSTRUAL DISORDERS

Menstrual complaints of the adolescent are primarily related to abnormal bleeding or painful bleeding. Prior to maturation of the HPG axis, disorders manifested as abnormal menstrual bleeding are usually related to the anovulatory nature of the menstrual cycle in the adolescent.[16] Menstrual irregularities in adolescents can also be related to stress, weight changes, change in level of physical activity, pregnancy, and trauma.[17]

Acute adolescent menorrhagia can present as a minor deviation in the amount of blood loss to life threatening hemorrhage.[18] Due to lack of cognitive maturity manifested as embarrassment or fear of being different, the adolescent may attempt to ignore or hide an episode of excessive blood loss. Consequently, menorrhagia can lead to excessive blood loss and a clinical presentation of a pale, anxious girl presenting with heavy bleeding of several days or weeks duration. The primary etiology of acute adolescent menorrhagia is an anovulatory menstrual cycle. Pregnancy related complications also should be explored and ruled out, however. After anovulatory uterine bleeding, pregnancy related states, such as spontaneous abortion, complications of an elective termination, and ectopic pregnancy are the leading etiologies.[18]

Therapy for acute adolescent menorrhagia is focused on controlling bleeding, restoring circulating volume, and preventing recurrence. In anovulatory cycles, the main cause of bleeding is extreme endometrial proliferation secondary to fluctuating estrogen levels and the lack of progesterone secretion. Consequently, a primary component of treatment is exogenous hormones to stabilize circulating levels of estrogen and to stabilize the endometrium with progestogen.[18] Long-term follow-up includes surveillance for the spontaneous onset of ovulatory cycles, through measurement of basal body temperature, a difficult monitoring parameter to implement with the adolescent population. Individuals with acute adolescent menorrhagia are at greater risk for chronic anovulation disorders (see Chapter 8).

Dysmenorrhea is one of the most common complaints of adolescent women and accounts for a large number of days lost from work or school. The typical presentation is an adolescent 1 to 3 years following menarche, complaining of cramps and lower abdominal pain coinciding with the first day of the menses. Dysmenorrhea may be experienced as an isolated symptom or as a component of premenstrual syndrome (PMS). The onset of pain occurs within 1–4 hours of the beginning of the menses and lasts for 24–48 hours and can be mild to severe in intensity.[18] The adolescent usually presents with primary or functional dysmenorrhea, that is, painful menstruation with a nonpathological etiology. In the adolescent, dysmenorrhea is usually associated with the onset of ovulatory menses. Ovarian maturation and cyclic progestogen secretions are associated with the myometrial spasms characteristic of dysmenorrhea. The adolescent with severe dysmenorrhea should be thoroughly evaluated, however, to rule out a pathological etiology such as endometriosis. In sexually active adolescents, dysmenorrhea may be symptomatic of pelvic inflammatory disease. Treatment of primary dysmenorrhea is usually symptomatic (see Chapter 8).

SEXUALLY TRANSMITTED DISEASES

Sexually transmitted diseases (STDs) are a significant source of potentially reversible morbidity in the adolescent population. Individuals under age 25 account for two-thirds of all STDs.[19] Prevalence rates for most STDs peak during the adolescent and young adult years.[20] Data may underestimate the actual prevalence rate in adolescents, however, since the most frequently occurring sexually transmitted infections in this population, chlamydia and HPV infections, are not routinely reportable.[21] The presence of STDs accelerates the risk for HIV infection, and the incidence of HIV is increasing most rapidly among young women age 13 to 24 years.[17]

The reasons adolescents engage in sexual activity are varied. The individual's ability to physically engage in sexual activity does not correspond with cognitive or social maturity. This disparity between physiologic ability and cognitive understanding is often a contributing factor in unprotected sexual practices. A study examining safer sexual practices among adolescents found there to be a low rate of barrier contraceptive use and poor knowledge about the acquisition and prevention of sexually transmitted diseases.[21] Another study reported that approximately 50 percent of sexually active teens engage in risk behaviors that leave them susceptible to STD.[22]

The clinical presentation of STDs in the adolescent is essentially the same as in the adult: abnormal vaginal discharge, vulvar irritation, perianal sores, ulceration, dysuria or lower abdominal pain. There are some special considerations in the etiology and the implications of STDs in the adolescent population, however.

Physiologically, two factors, transitional vaginal epithelium and the lack of cervical mucous production, make the adolescent more susceptible to sexually transmitted bacterial and viral organisms. During puberty, the vaginal epithelium is in continual transition. The everted columnar cells on the portico of the cervix are preferentially attached to by organisms such as gonorrhea neisseria, chlamydia, and trachomatis.[17] The metamorphosis of the vaginal mucosa and the establishment of an acidic environment serve as protective mechanisms in the mature female. The second factor is the lack of cervical mucosa production. Cervical mucosa is the result of cyclic progesterone production from the mature ovary. Cervical mucosa forms a protective barrier to exclude pathogens from the internal reproductive structures and has specific protective properties including phagocytic cell production. These protective mechanisms are not functional, however, until after ovarian maturation, establishment of ovulation, and ovarian progesterone secretion. As previously discussed, ovarian maturation usually does not occur until 1–2 years after menarche.

For many sexually transmitted infections, the time from infection to diagnosis and treatment is influential of the prognosis. The lack of adequate or prompt treatment can result in the development of long-term sequelae. Women are at particular risk for complications from untreated or inadequately treated STDs. The long-term complications include sterility, ectopic pregnancy, fetal or infant death, and chronic pelvic inflammation.[17]

The progressively earlier age of first sexual intercourse is associated with an increased number of life time sexual partners and an increased risk of exposure to STDs. In addition, many adolescents become sexually active prior to seeking professional guidance related to safe sexual behaviors. Recognizing the significance of the problem and the future implications, guidelines for Adolescent Preventive Services (GAPS) recommend that health care providers screen all adolescents for risk specific behaviors, educate patients about transmission, and counsel adolescents about reducing their risk for contracting a sexually transmitted disease.[23]

ADOLESCENT PREGNANCY

Adolescent pregnancy has become a major concern for all sectors of society. Adolescents who become parents tend to have less formal education, lower paying jobs, and higher rates of unemployment, as compared with their childless peers.[24] Among adolescents ages 15–19 years in the United States, 12 percent become pregnant each year and 21 percent of all sexually active teens become pregnant annually.[24] A majority of teen pregnancies are unintentional.[25] An unintended pregnancy can be a crisis for the adolescent and her family. A minority of adolescent pregnancies are intended. The adolescent's desire to conceive usually emerges from the desire to please her partner or to solidify a relationship, to have someone to love and to take care of, to change her status in the family or to assert her independence, and to establish her fertility. Whether a pregnancy is accidental or intended, the normal process of adolescent maturation is interrupted. In addition, a pregnancy can exacerbate an adolescent's feeling of loss of control.

Presenting symptoms of an adolescent pregnancy—secondary amenorrhea, breast ten-derness, morning nausea and weight gain—are typical of any pregnancy. Many adolescents may deny their concern about an unplanned pregnancy, however, by presenting with alternative complaints such as fatigue, weight changes, abdominal pain or a request for contraception. Consequently, careful history and physical examination by the provider are essential to an accurate diagnosis. As a result of denial, fear, or lack of recognition of existing signs and symptoms, adolescents often present for diagnosis of the pregnancy and initiation of prenatal care after the completion of the first trimester. Late prenatal care limits both the quality and quantity of prenatal care services and may also limit the woman's options related to the disposition of her pregnancy.

Following the confirmation of a pregnancy, the adolescent must make a decision about the disposition of the pregnancy. It is important that the decision is made by the adolescent; the role of the health care provider is to offer supportive counseling and information about all options and resources. Of 1,040,000 adolescent pregnancies in 1990, 51 percent delivered, 35 percent aborted and 14 percent miscarried.[24] If abortion is the option of choice, the adolescent not only needs information about the procedure but needs appropriate follow-up care for both physical and emotional adaptation. Another option is adoption. Prior to 1970, the majority of unmarried, white adolescents chose adoption, but by 1990, less than 5 percent of teens selected adoption.[26] Adoption has never been a highly chosen option by African American teens. The third option is parenthood. When parenthood is chosen, the adolescent needs high quality prenatal care as well as preparation for the emotional, financial, and physical demands of parenting. Adolescents attempting to establish their own independence and to formulate their personal identity have difficulty balancing their own psychological responses with the demands of an infant.

If the adolescent chooses to continue the pregnancy, she is at greater risk for perinatal complications than the pregnant nonadolescent. Females under age 17 years have a high incidence of pregnancy related iron deficiency anemia, pregnancy induced hypertension, operative births, preterm delivery, and low birth weight infants.[26]

In part, the increase in perinatal complications is related to competition between the adolescent's growth needs and the fetal demands on the maternal system for metabolic support. From a dietary perspective, additional amounts of protein, iron, and calcium are necessary for individual growth and fetal development. The role of folate in prevention of neural tube defects and promotion of DNA synthesis is becoming widely publicized. Current recommendation is for folic acid supplementation of 800–1000 micrograms daily.[27]

Adolescents who conceive within 2 years of menarche are at particular risk. Pregnant adolescents of young gynecologic age have not completed their physical growth. Consequently, fetal distress and cephalopelvic disproportion during labor account for an increased risk for cesarean births among young adolescents. In addition, there is an increased incidence of low birth weight among infants born to adolescent mothers, related to competition between mother and fetus for nutritional resources.[28] Recent reports indicate that the increased morbidity seen in adolescent pregnancy is related more to socioeconomic factors than the chronologic age at conception, particularly, the lack of early and adequate prenatal care.[29] Many adolescents receive late or inadequate care either because the pregnancy was denied or the resources were lacking to access prenatal care. The adolescent's access to prenatal care is further complicated by factors including lack of money, transportation, knowledge, and not valuing prenatal care as contributing to a healthy pregnancy outcome. Adolescents who lack early and adequate obstetrical care have a higher incidence of spontaneous abortions, placental disorders, low birth weight, PIH, and prolonged labors.[28]

Although there are physical risks associated with an adolescent pregnancy, most pregnant adolescents do well physically. The biggest risk to both the adolescent and the infant, however, is the lack of parenting skills. Inadequate parenting skills predispose the adolescent to an increased risk of frustration, feeling of failure and social isolation, and negative self-image. Furthermore, these inadequate skills place the infant at great risk for physical and emotional developmental delay and, in extreme situations, an increased risk of injury or abuse.[26]

SMOKING

Smoking has been listed as the most important source of preventable morbidity and premature death in every report of the surgeon general since 1964.[30] Despite these warnings, data indicate that initiation of tobacco use rapidly increases after age 11 years and peaks between age 17 to 19 years.[31] In fact, most adults who smoke regularly started during adolescence.[32] Reasons adolescents begin to smoke include peers and parents or siblings who smoke. Adolescents with high exposure to cigarette advertising and role models are significantly more likely to be smokers than those with low exposure.[33] One study of smoking behaviors suggested that self-esteem may be a factor in the smoking behavior of female adolescents, but not for males. Therefore, female adolescents may have unique motivations to initiate tobacco use, making them more susceptible to advertising and media portrayals. Adolescents frequently do not enjoy smoking but report doing it to "fit in."[3] A study of 155 adolescent smokers found that 95 percent knew the health risks and hazards associated with smoking, but those risks were of little concern to 70 percent of participants.[32] Adolescent smoking has a negative correlation with academic performance and a positive correlation with use of alcohol and illicit drugs.[32]

It is estimated that 5.5 minutes of life is lost for each cigarette smoked.[30] Adolescents also need to be aware of the addictive effects of nicotine, the effects on the cardiovascular and respiratory systems, the alterations of blood coagulation and the use of oral contraceptives, an increased incidence of cervical cancer, as well as the effect of passive smoke on pregnancies, infants, and children. Interventions focused on preventing initiation of smoking or cessation of smoking need to include more than giving the facts. The provider must explore the individual's idea of health and the social dynamics of smoking. Smoking cessation is a loss. The provider needs to aid the individual to recognize what is gained by not maintaining a smoking habit.

SUICIDE

Suicide is the second leading cause of death, after accidents, in 13–24-year-olds.[34] While male suicides are more successful, females attempt suicide four times more frequently than males.[35] Adolescent suicide is often associated with impulsivity and anger.[3] Suicide attempts in adolescents correlate with depression including lack of parental support, lack of attachment to a peer group, and low self-esteem. Neinstein, Julian, and Shapario have identified a four-step progressive behavioral pattern, evident in suicidal adolescents:

- Long-Standing problem: lack of social connections or problems that create vulnerabilities,
- Escalation: childhood problems exacerbate during adolescent development,
- Progressive social isolation: failure of available adaptive techniques leading to social isolation and depression,
- Final state: the attempt preceded by increased despair.[36]

Asking adolescents about suicide doesn't give them the idea. Asking key questions as part of health care visits can identify the adolescent in trouble and open the opportunity to secure help and counseling.

CARDIOVASCULAR DISEASE RISK

The pathogenesis of atherosclerosis begins in childhood and results from the interaction of genetic and environmental factors.[37] Although genetics cannot be altered, environmental factors such as dietary intake of saturated fats and cholesterol, exercise patterns, and smoking patterns, can be modified during the adolescent years.

The adolescent's blood pressure should be evaluated annually. Ninety-one percent of hypertension in adolescents is of a primary etiology, and more than half of hypertensive adolescents are obese.[37] Usual interventions include low-salt diet, weight reduction, exercise, and relaxation as the foundation of a healthy lifestyle.

SEXUAL ASSAULT

Female adolescents are the most likely victims of sexual assault. Fifty percent of rape victims are between 10 and 19 years.[38] The perpetrator is an acquaintance in 78 percent of cases.[39] Sexual assault or rape with a known perpetrator can lead to self-blame and guilt.

The adolescent who is assaulted or raped is the object of hostile, dehumanizing attacks that may have long standing effects on the victim's self-worth and identity. These effects are particularly difficult for the adolescent still dealing with issues of separation, independence, and development of sexual identity.[40] Helton found that asking two questions about the possibility of abuse increased the opportunity for positive responses and communicated that the provider was concerned and committed.[41] Once abuse is identified, the adolescent needs to hear that she is not alone, it is not her fault, she needs to talk about it, and she needs help and support.

CARING FOR ADOLESCENTS

Providing health care for the adolescent can present complex and difficult situations. Strategies for promoting adolescent health care need to emphasize helping the individual to adapt to the physical and psychological changes, to become aware of the risk and negative consequences of behaviors, and to help her to engage in responsible decision making processes. Although many of the physical problems experienced by the adolescent are similar to problems seen in the adult population, the adolescent presents with emotional characteristics that require special attention. The adolescent is often confused and ambivalent about her feelings and may be unable or unwilling to share her concerns, needs, or questions. Therefore, providers need to allot adequate time and use language appropriate to the adolescent's developmental and cultural background.

During adolescence, the individual makes the transition from patterns of child health care to adult health management and care systems. During childhood, health care providers primarily work with parents to make decisions related to health care as well as to educate and counsel parents about the intervention implemented for their child. The child is primarily a passive recipient of health evaluation and management. During adolescence, the emerging woman needs to become an active participant in her health care. The adolescent's activities have consequences that may impact current and future health care status. Thus, she not only becomes an active participant in health care choices but also learns to accept responsibility for the consequences of a choice. The adolescent should perceive that she is in partnership with the health care provider. Empowering the adolescent in the delivery of health care enhances compliance and further open, honest communication between the client and the provider.[42]

Adolescents have reported that they would find it helpful to talk with a health care provider about health related topics.[43] Adolescents also report, however, that one of the barriers to communication is failure of the provider to raise a subject or the provider's lack of response when the adolescent asks about a subject.[43] Consequently, the adolescent needs to be seen by a provider who will obtain a thorough assessment of sexual knowledge and behaviors, and who has the time to listen and respond to the adolescent's needs with satisfactory explanations and to answer questions in a manner appropriate to her level of development and comprehension. The interaction between the adolescent and the health care provider provides an opportunity for the adolescent to establish an important relationship outside the family and peer group structure.

SEXUAL BEHAVIOR DECISIONS

Adolescents need to discuss issues of sexuality and their decisions related to sexual activity. The United States Preventive Health Care Services Task Force recommends that a sexual history be taken and risk prevention discussed with all adolescents.[44] The sexual history should use language understandable to the adolescent and should progress from least to most intimate areas to establish a sense of respect and trust between the provider and the adolescent. A well conducted sexual history allows the provider to gather data and to facilitate expression by the adolescent in a direct but nonconfrontational manner. Based on the information obtained in the sexual history, the provider is able to identify areas of counseling, education, prevention, and referral. It is important to acknowledge the adolescent's desire for autonomy and to encourage and support the adolescent's values and choices throughout this process.

Educational and counseling strategies need to focus on safer sexual practices and contraception to prevent sexually acquired diseases and pregnancy. In addition, female adolescents need information focused on decisions regarding becoming sexually active, empowering women to say no, and helping women in abusive or coercive relationships. Strategies and awareness of situational factors leading to sexual violence may foster preparedness in this at-risk population. Two point three percent of girls between ages 12 and 15 years and 4.8 percent of women between 16 and 19 years of age have been victims of sexual assault, making the female adolescent the most likely victim of sexual violence.[17]

Promotion of school based clinics, distribution of condoms, and family life programs are efforts to provide education and resources for health enhancing and risk avoiding behaviors. All adolescents have a right to and a need for information about healthy and responsible sexual behavior. Without factual information, the young woman is denied her right to protect herself and to make decisions within the framework of her emerging personal identity. Information and resources should be accessible and provided in an accepting, supportive, and nonjudgmental environment. Providing supportive and honest information and feedback to the adolescent will enhance her development of self-esteem, acceptance of responsibility for her actions, and the establishment of a values system.[42] Support must also exist for the adolescent who chooses virginity or not to become sexually active. The adolescent needs to be reassured about the acceptability of abstinence. Support includes discussion of how to effectively say no and how to interact with pressure from peers or acquaintances who may not understand or want to accept her decision. Respecting and supporting the choice of the adolescent and promoting a healthy adolescence are the interventions that promote the emergence of a healthy adult.[42]

PELVIC EXAMINATION

The first pelvic examination should be approached with care and gentleness. The provider should be aware of the adolescent's developmental level since the internal examination is a source of anxiety for many adolescents. Common concerns include the fear of pain, embarrassment, or discovery of an anomaly as well as inadequate knowledge of the vaginal anatomy and physiology. The impact of the first examination can leave long-term positive or negative effects that can impact the individual's future health care practices. Basically, the indications for a pelvic examination include symptoms specific to the female reproductive system, initiation of sexual activity, or age 18 years at which time annual examination should commence[45] (see Chapter 5). Virginal females find the gynecologic examination particularly distressing. In nonsexually active, younger adolescents, a recto-vaginal examination is an alternative that may provide information about the status of the external genitalia and may assist in identifying possible abnormalities of the vaginal, uterine, and adnexal structures.[45] When an internal examination is necessary, younger adolescents and virginal girls prefer a female family member to be present during the examination, whereas older or sexually active adolescents prefer a female chaperone to be present.[46] Prior to the first examination, the adolescent should receive a thorough explanation and demonstration of what will be done and offered the opportunity to voice questions or concerns. Establishing a good rapport prior to the examination and maintaining eye contact and a professional but caring relationship during the examination are essential to the adolescent's psychological well-being.

CONFIDENTIALITY AND TRUST

Health care is traditionally provided in an environment of confidentiality and trust. But, when interacting with the adolescent, it is important to be aware of the unique issues of confidentiality and trust inherent in the client/provider relationship. Health issues related to sexuality and sexual activity raise unique dilemmas for the health care provider and can influence the provider's relationship with the client and thereby impact the quality of the care provided.

Most adolescents are minors, that is, under the age of 18. The power to consent to a minor's medical care has belonged traditonally to the parents or the parent's surrogate. The adolescent's status related to ability to seek and consent to health care is based either on the status of the minor or on the type of health care needed. Although there is variation among states, most states have laws that allow the adolescent the right to seek and consent to certain types of health care including the diagnosis and treatment of STDs, provision of contraception, and the diagnosis and treatment of pregnancy.[47] In addition, an individual under the age of 18 who has been declared an emancipated minor or meets the criteria for the mature minor rule may seek and consent to medical treatment. An emancipated minor is an individual who has attained a specific status based on marital status, parenthood or pregnancy, military service, or residency and financial independence.[48] Typically, the courts have considered these individuals emancipated from their parents. The status of emancipation, however, is rarely conferred by the court, proactively.[49] In fact, in most states, the right to seek emancipation of a minor belongs to the parent, not to the adolescent. Consequently, the designation of emancipation may need to be made by the health care provider within the context of the professional relationship. The mature minor doctrine states that there is "little likelihood that a practitioner will incur liability for failure to obtain parental consent in situations in which the minor is an older adolescent (typically at least age 15) who is capable of giving an informed consent and in which the care is not high risk, is for the minor's benefit, and is within the mainstream of established medical opinion."[48] Basically, the criteria for determining the adolescent's ability to consent is based in her ability not only to understand the risks, benefits, and alternatives but also to make a voluntary choice. These are the same criteria for informed consent with adult clients.

Issues of confidentiality should be discussed proactively with the adolescent and the parent. The nature of the adolescent's seeking health care, however, may not make these types of discussion realistic or desirable. Thus, the health care provider needs to be familiar with state statutes and needs to communicate his or her philosophy to the adolescent at the initiation of the client/provider relationship.

CONCLUSION

Unlike other cultures that celebrate the transition of adolescence, American culture views the adolescent period as a time of anxiety, awkwardness, and turmoil.[50] Although stereotypical descriptions predominate, adolescence is often a time of positive growth and development, a time for the development of healthy lifestyles, practices, and behaviors. The stage of adolescence includes a rapidly changing body and new expectations, norms, and social roles. Conceptualizations of adolescence need to focus on monitoring the physical changes as well as mastering the psychosocial tasks that allow advancement to higher levels of development. Health care providers must recognize that adolescents are "not just big children or small adults—they have unique problems that demand unique solutions."[51] A healthy adolescence equates with a successful transition manifested as physical well-being, coping, adaptation, and psychosocial growth. Working with adolescents offers the health care provider a unique opportunity for investing in the health and well-being of future generations.

REFERENCES

1. Hechinger, F. M. (1992). *Fateful choices: Healthy youth for the 21st century.* New York: Carnegie Foundation.
2. Great transitions: Preparing adolescents for a new century. (1995, October). *Concluding Report of the Carnegie Council on Adolescent Development.* New York: Carnegie Corporation of New York. October 1995.
3. Murray, R. B., & Zentner, J. P. (1996). *Health assessment promotion strategies through the life span.* (6th ed.). Stamford, CT: Appleton & Lange.
4. Oehninger, S., & Hodgen, G. (1993). Hypothalmic pituitary ovarian uterine axis. In L. Copeland (Ed.), *Textbook of gynecology.* (pp. 85–120) Philadelphia: W. B. Saunders.
5. Neinstein, L. S., & Kaufman, F. R. (1996). Normal physical growth and development. In L. S. Neinstein (Ed.), *Adolescent health care: A practical guide.* (3rd ed., pp. 3–39). Baltimore: Williams & Wilkins.
6. Polland, I. (1994). *A guide to reproduction.* (pp. 42–53) New York: Cambridge University Press.
7. Brook, C. G. D. (1993). Physical changes of adolescence. In C. G. D. Brook (Ed.), *The practice of medicine in adolescence.* (pp. 1–7) Boston: Little, Brown.
8. Albertsson-Wikland, K., Rosberg, S. Karlberg, J., & Groth, T. (1994). Analysis of the 24-hour growth hormone profiles in healthy boys and girls of normal stature: Relation to puberty. *Journal of Clinical Endocrinology and Metabolism, 78,* 1195–1201.
9. Sheets, E. E., & Goodman, H. M. (1995). The cervix. In K. J. Ryan, R. S. Berkowitz, & R. L. Barbiere, (Eds.), *Kistner's gynecology.* (6th ed.), pp. 103–137. St. Louis: Mosby.
10. Erikson, E. (1965). *Childhood and society.* New York: Norton.
11. Wadsworth, B. (1996). *Piaget's theory of cognitive and affective development* (5th ed.). New York: Longman.
12. Self-esteem from dating differs by gender. (1995). *The Menninger Letter, 3*(6), 3.
13. Moore, R. (1996). Overview of developmental and physical milestones and psychosocial issues. *Current practice issues in adolescent gynecology.* (pp. 4–7). Washington, DC: AWHONN and NANPRH.
14. Smith, S., & McClaugherty, L. O. (1993). Adolescent homosexuality: A primary care perspective. *American Family Physician, 48,* 33–36.
15. MacKenzie, R., Neinstein, L. S. (1996). Obesity. In L. S. Neinstein (Ed.), *Adolescent health care: A practical guide.* (3rd ed., pp. 547–563). Baltimore: Williams & Wilkins.
16. Edge, V., & Miller, M. (1994). *Women's health care.* St. Louis: Mosby.
17. Furniss, K. (1996). Common clinical problems and issues. *Current practice issues in adolescent gynecology* (pp. 8–14). Washington, DC: AWHONN and NANPRH.
18. Maxson, W. S., & Rosenwaks, Z. (1995). Dysmenorrhea and premenstrual syndrome. In K. J. Ryan, R. S. Berkowitz, & R. L. Barbiere (Eds.). *Kistner's Gynecology* (6th ed.), pp. 168–187. St. Louis: Mosby.
19. Hatcher, R. A., Trussell, J., & Stewart, F. (1994). Adolescent sexual behavior, pregnancy and childbearing. In *Contraceptive technology* (16th ed., pp. 571–600). New York: Irvington Publishers.

20. Centers for Disease Control and Prevention. (1994). Summary of notifiable diseases, United States. *1993 Morbidity and Mortality Weekly Report, 42*(53).

21. Millstein, S. G., Igra, V., & Gans, J. (1996). Delivery of STD/HIV preventive services to adolescents by primary care physicians. *Journal of Adolescent Health Care, 19,* 249–257.

22. Contraception and adolescents. (1995, July). *The Contraceptive Report,* 5–12.

23. Elster, A. B., & Kuzsets, N., (1993). *Guidelines for adolescent preventative services (GAPS).* Baltimore: Williams & Wilkins.

24. Alan Guttmacher Institute. (1994). *Sex and America's teenagers.* New York: Author.

25. Henshaw, S. (1993). *US teenage pregnancy statistics.* New York: AGI.

26. Capitulo, K. L., & Maffia, A. J. (1992). *Adolescent pregnancy.* New York: March of Dimes Birth Defect Foundation.

27. Butterworth, C. E., & Bendich, A. (1996). Folic acid and the prevention of birth defects. *Annual Review of Nutrition, 16,* 73–97.

28. Morris, D. L., Berenson, A. B., Lawson, J., & Wiemann, C. M. (1993). Comparison of adolescent pregnancy outcomes by prenatal care source. *Journal of Reproductive Medicine, 38*(5) 375–380.

29. Centers for Disease Control. (1995). State specific pregnancy and birth rates among teenagers. U.S., 1991–1992. *MMWR, 44,* 677–684.

30. Gidding, S. S. & Schydlower, M. (1994). Active and passive tobacco exposure: a serious pediatric health problem. *Pediatrics,* Nov. 94(5): 750–751.

31. Johnson, L. D., O'Mally, P. M., & Bachman, J. G. (1993 December 11). *Cigarette smoking among American teens rises again in 1995.* Ann Arbor, MI: News and Information Services of the University of Michigan.

32. Dappen, A., Schwartz, R. H., & O'Donnell, R. (1996). A survey of adolescent smoking patterns. *Journal of the American Board of Family Practice, 9*(1), 7–13.

33. Botvin, G. J., Goldberg, C. J., & Botvin, E. M. (1993). Smoking behavior of adolescents exposed to cigarette advertising. *Public Health Reports, 108,* 217.

34. Setterberg, S. R. (1992). Suicide behavior and suicide. In S. B. Friedman, M. Fisher, & S. K. Schonberg (Eds.), *Comprehensive adolescent health.* (pp. 862–866). St. Louis: Quality Medical Publishing.

35. Horton, J. A. (1995). Violence against women. In *The women's health data book: A profile of women's health in the United States* pp. 122–127). Washington, DC: Jacobson Institute.

36. Neinstein, L. S., Julian, M. A., & Shapario, J. (1996). Suicide. In L. S. Neinstein (Ed.), *Adolescent health care a practical guide.* (3rd ed., pp. 1116–1123). Baltimore: Williams & Wilkins.

37. Rosner, B., Prineas, R. J., & Loggie, J. M. H. (1993). Blood pressure nomograms for children and adolescents by height, sex and age in the United States. *Journal of Pediatrics, 123,* 871.

38. Greydanus, D., & Shearin, R. (1990). *Adolescent sexuality and gynecology* (pp. 245). Philadelphia: Lea & Febiger.

39. Speroff, L. & Darney, P. (1992). Oral contraception. In *A Clinical Guide for Contraception* (pp. 21–107). Baltimore: Williams and Wilkins.

40. AAP Committee of Adolescence. (1994). Sexual assault and the adolescent. *Pediatrics, 94,* 761.

41. Helton, A. (1986). Battering during pregnancy. *American Journal of Nursing, 86,* 910–913.

42. Devine, K. (1996). Communication, counseling and compliance issues. *Current practice issues in adolescent gynecology* (pp. 15–19). Washington, DC: AWHONN and NANPRH.

43. Schuster, M. A., Bell, R. M., Petersen, L. P. & Lanouse, D. E. (1996). Communications between adolescents and physicians about sexual behavior and risk prevention. *Archives of Pediatric Adolescent Medicine, 150,* 906–913.

44. U.S. Preventive Services Task Force. (1989). *Guide to clinical prevention: An assessment of the effectiveness of 169 interventions.* Baltimore: Williams & Wilkins.

45. Berry, P. L., Schubiner, H., & Giblin, P. T. (1990). Issues in adolescent gynecologic care. *Obstetrics and Gynecologic Clinics of North America, 17*(4), 837–848.

46. Rimasza, M. E. (1989). An illustrated guide to adolescent gyn. *Pediatric Clinics of North America, 36*(3), 639–662.

47. Johnson, K., & Moore, A.Y. (1990). *Improving health programs for low income youths.* Washington, DC: Children's Defense Fund, Adolescent Pregnancy Prevention Clearing House.

48. English, A. (1996). Understanding legal aspects of care. In L. S. Neinstein (Ed.), *Adolescent health care: A practical guide* (3rd ed., pp. 150–163). Baltimore: Williams & Wilkins.

49. Cohen, S. D. (1991). The evolving law of adolescent health care. *NAACOG's Clinical Issues in Perinatal and Women's Health Nursing, 2*(2), 201–208.

50. Brooks-Gunn, J., & Rieter, E. O. (1990). The roles of the pubertal process. In S. S. Feldman & G. R. Elliot (Eds.), *At the threshold: The developing adolescent.* Cambridge MA: Harvard University Press.

51. Shalala, D. E. (1996). I believe in angels. *Journal of Adolescent Health, 19,* 195.

CHAPTER 5

ASSESSING WOMEN'S HEALTH

Ellis Quinn Youngkin • Marcia Szmania Davis

Consider any in-teraction with a client a therapeutic in-tervention by permit-ting the free expression of issues and concerns.

Highlights

- Mortality, Morbidity, and Risk Factors
- Screening Methods
    - Health History
    - Special Assessment: Family, Nutrition, Stress/Risk, Fitness, Occupation, Sleep
    - Physical Examination
- Commonly Indicated Laboratory Tests
    - Papanicolaou Smear
    - Gonorrhea Culture
    - Chlamydia Trachomatis Tests
    - Wet Mounts
    - Urinalysis
    - Herpes Culture
    - Sensitivity, Specificity, and Predictive Value

► INTRODUCTION

Women's life span, opportunities and risks, and challenges and stresses are ever increasing. As perhaps the only person a woman sees for health care, the woman's health care provider must approach assessment holistically. Indeed, all factors impinging on the woman's health and well-being must be considered if significant omissions in detecting problems and offering care are to be avoided.

Pender, in discussing health and wellness, refers to Dunn's suggestion that optimum health, or high level wellness, only emanates from an environment that is favorable.[1] Thus, the provider must help the woman become more attuned to her body and its cues, and use the assessment period as an opportunity for teaching and counseling.

Healthy People 2000 has as its main goal helping Americans live longer, healthier lives.[2] One important focus for the provider is assessing the woman's risk factors and working with her to change her behaviors and lifestyle to more healthful ones.[3] Of interest are results of a study that examined the role of cognitive-perceptual factors (control over health, self-efficacy, and health status) in maintenance of health promoting behavior of over 1000 women.[4] The investigators found that cognitive-perceptual factors had only small effects on specific health promoting behaviors.

Some progress has been made to decrease deaths from heart disease, cancer, and stroke. According to Dr. J. Michael McGinnis of the U.S. Public Health Service, these diseases are moving toward the target goals for the year 2000, but some areas are worsening: obesity, homicide, teen pregnancy, pneumonia, and influenza.[5] The gap in health between the poor and uninsured and those with more resources continues to widen, especially among black Americans and Hispanic Americans who have less access to primary health care.

MORTALITY, MORBIDITY, AND RISK FACTORS IN AMERICAN WOMEN

LEADING CAUSES OF MORTALITY IN AMERICAN WOMEN

The average life expectancy for American women has increased from 77.6 years in 1979–1981 to 79.1 years in 1992.[6] The discrepancy between white and black American women, however, continues to be significant; 5.3 years in 1979–1981 rising to 5.9 years in 1992. The causes of death differ significantly for American women depending on age and race. Age groupings in this section are derived from statistical tables for mortality (see Tables 5–1, 5–2, and 5–3).[7,8] By 1992, infectious diseases as a whole ranked third as the leading cause of death across ages and races, following cardiovascular diseases and malignancies.[9] They were fifth in 1980, raising concerns relating to antibiotic resistance and the "potential volatility" of infectious diseases. Cancer deaths are reportedly down or declining, but the number of cases being diagnosed is up and people are living longer.[10] Better screening and diagnostic technologies are partially responsible for this trend. Smoking, excessive sun exposure, and AIDS have increased the numbers of cancers among women. Patterns were found to be similar between white and black Americans.

Adolescence to Young Adulthood (Ages 15 to 24). The number of young people in this country has increased since a decline from 1976 through 1991.[11] By 2020, 43 million teenagers, up from 35 million in 1992, will live in the United States. Adolescent and young adult women are at greatest risk for death from accidents and violence. Most unintentional injuries are from motor vehicle fatalities, and in adolescents, alcohol is a major contributing factor. Despite these grim findings, traffic deaths related to alcohol have decreased by one-third in the 15–24-year-old age group. Conversely, violence as

TABLE 5–1. SELECTED CAUSES OF MORTALITY FOR WOMEN BY AGE, 1992 (IN 1000s)

Age	Heart Disease	Cancer	Accidents	Cerebrovascular Diseases	COPD[a]	Pneumonia	Suicide	Liver Disease	DM[b]	Homicide and Legal Intervention
<15	0.5	0.7[z]	2.5	0.1[z]	[z]	0.4	0.1[z]	[z]	[z]	0.5
15–24	0.3	0.7	3.4	0.1	0.1	0.1	0.6	[z]	0.1	1.1
25–34	1.1	2.7	3.1	0.4	0.1	0.2	1.1	0.3	0.3	1.5
35–44	3.2	9.4	2.8	1.2	0.3	0.5	1.3	0.9	0.6	1.0
45–54	8.1	20.6	2.0	2.2	1.1	0.6	1.0	1.2	1.4	0.4
55–64	22.6	40.7	2.0	4.4	4.5	1.3	0.7	1.8	3.6	0.2
65–74	60.7	71.6	3.2	12.3	12.5	4.2	0.6	2.4	7.6	0.2
75–84	116.4	67.2	4.9	29.0	15.3	11.5	0.4	1.6	9.0	0.2
85–	147.0	32.7	5.2	37.3	7.5	21.4	0.1	0.5	5.8	0.1
Totals for women	360.2	245.7	28.9	87.1	41.5	40.3	6.0	8.8	28.4	5.4
Totals for men	357.5	274.8	57.9	56.6	50.5	35.5	24.5	16.5	21.7	20.1

[a]Chronic obstructive pulmonary diseases.
[b]Diabetes mellitus.
[z]Fewer than fifty in one or more age groups between birth and age 14.
Source: Reference 7.

a cause of death has increased, and homicide is the leading cause of death for black American females, ages 15–24, with rates 4 times that of white females. The other area where violent deaths has increased is in victim deaths from rape, robbery, and assault in the 12–19-year-old age group. Suicide, primarily by firearm, is third as a leading cause of death for young people ages 15–24. It is highest among Hispanic American youth and lowest among black Americans. Females are less likely to be successful. Deaths from human immunodeficiency virus (HIV) are rising rapidly; most are in men, but this, too, is changing rapidly (see Leading Causes of Mortality in American Women, Cancer).

Young Adulthood to Mid-Adulthood (Ages 25 to 44). Cancer (including HIV deaths), heart diseases, and suicide begin to increase as causes of death. Accidents and violence continue to be important causes, especially among black American women.

Mid-Adulthood to Older Adulthood (Ages 45 to 64). Heart diseases, cancer, cerebrovascular diseases (CVD), chronic obstructive pulmonary disease (COPD), chronic liver diseases/cirrhosis, and diabetes mellitus gain momentum as causes of death. Accidents, violence, and suicide decrease slightly but remain significant causes. Suicide is highest among white women in every age group

TABLE 5–2. ACCIDENTS AND VIOLENCE MORTALITY FOR WOMEN BY RACE, 1990–1992 (PER 100,000 POPULATION)

Cause of Death	White American	Black American
Motor vehicle accidents	10.2	8.8
All other accidents	12.4	12.7
Suicide	5.1	2.0
Homicide	2.8	13.1

Source: Reference 8.

TABLE 5–3. DEATHS RESULTING FROM ACCIDENTS AND VIOLENCE BY AGE GROUP, 1990–1992 (PER 100,000 POPULATION)

Age (in years)	White American	Black American
15–24	28.4	34.9
25–34	23.6	46.1
35–44	23.5	38.9
45–54	24.2	29.5
55–64	25.7	31.8
65–	78.6	72.6
65–74	38.7	43.9
75–84	83.9	89.5
85±	234.2	178.4

Source: Reference 8.

as compared with nonwhite women, peaking between ages 35 and 54. Liver disease peaks in mid- to older adulthood.

Maturity (Ages 65 and Older). Heart disease increases dramatically with age, as do cancer, CVD, COPD, pneumonia, and diabetes. Accidents again become a more prevalent cause, but suicides decrease. Falls are the main cause of injury resulting in death for women over 75, causing 47 percent of such deaths.[12] Falls occur significantly more often among elderly women than among elderly men.

Differences in Causes of Death for Women by Race. Compared with white women, black American women have a higher incidence of death from lung cancer, liver diseases, HIV infection, homicide and legal interventions, and diabetes mellitus (see Table 5–4 and Table 5–5).[13–16] Deaths from AIDS are significantly higher among African American and Hispanic youth.[11,17] Deaths from heart disease, cerebrovascular disease, all

cancers except respiratory cancer, COPD, pneumonia and influenzas, accidents and adverse effects, and suicides are higher among white women. Cancer is the leading cause of death for Asian and Pacific Islander women (see Table 5–6).[18] Heart diseases and malignant neoplasms are the leading killers of all women regardless of race. Although the risk of dying from pregnancy and childbirth-related causes is very low in the United States (i.e., 7.3 deaths per 100,000 live births in 1992), nonwhite women are at a greater risk of death, and black American women are at the greatest risk (i.e., 20.1 per 100,000 live births as compared with 4.7 for white women).[19] Pregnancy induced hypertension, hemorrhage, embolism, and ectopic pregnancy are the major causes of maternal death.[20]

Cancer. Lung cancer is the most preventable cancer but is the most common.[2] It rises in the 55 and over age group, and peaks at ages 75 to 84.[21] The incidence has increased since 1975, and is 12 percent for black women and 8 percent for white women.[2] Lung cancer became the leading cancer killer among white women in 1988, as women's smoking reached an all time high.[20] Smoking contributes to 25 percent of all cancer deaths in women. Whereas breast, colon and rectal, cervical and endometrial, and stomach cancer deaths have declined in women over the last 60 years, lung cancer deaths have continued to rise.[22] Digestive system, breast, genital, blood-related, urologic, and oral cancers rise steadily from age 45 to peak in the 85 and older age group.[21] Breast cancer is the leading cause of cancer deaths for women ages 35 to 54, and remains either the second or third cause of cancer deaths through old age. The death rate from HIV infection quadrupled between 1985 and 1994, and HIV related deaths became the sixth leading cause of death among American women 15 to 44 years old[23] (see Table 5–5). By the year 2000, it is anticipated that an equal number of men and women will be infected, and women represent the fastest growing group of new cases of AIDS in this country.[17] Transmission from injection of drugs was a more prevalent cause of infection early in the AIDS epidemic, but since 1992, heterosexual activity is the primary vehicle. As of 1990–1992, HIV

TABLE 5–4. DIFFERENCES IN DEATH RATES BY SELECTED CAUSE FOR ALL RACES, WHITE AMERICAN, AND BLACK AMERICAN WOMEN 1992 (PER 100,000 POPULATION)

Disease/Cause	All Races	White American	Black American
Heart diseases[13]	281.4	292.9	231.6
Cerebrovascular diseases[13]	56.4	70.3	57.8
Malignant neoplasms[13]	204.1	199.0	157.6
Respiratory cancer (1991)[14]	–	42.8	49.0
Breast cancer[14]	–	113.6	95.1
Chronic obstructive pulmonary disease[13]	36.0	35.8	13.7
Pneumonia/influenza[13]	29.7	33.6	19.5
Chronic liver disease and cirrhosis[13]	9.9	6.8	6.8
Accidents and adverse effects[13]	34.0	22.6	21.5
Motor vehicle accidents[15]	–	10.3	8.9
Suicide[13]	12.0	5.1	2.0
Homicide and legal intervention[13]	10.0	2.8	13.1
Diabetes mellitus[13]	19.6	20.7	32.3
Cancer of cervix[14]	–	7.5	12.9
Cancer of colon and rectum[14]	–	38.0	45.5
Cancer of uterus[14]	–	22.0	14.2
Human immunodeficiency virus (see Table 5–5)			

Source: References 13–15.

TABLE 5–5. DEATH RATES FOR HUMAN IMMUNODEFICIENCY VIRUS (HIV) INFECTION, ACCORDING TO SEX, DETAILED RACE, HISPANIC ORIGIN, AND AGE: UNITED STATES, 1987–1992 (PER 100,000 RESIDENT POPULATION)

Race and Sex	Age 25 to 44 Years		Age 45 to 64 Years	
	1987	*1990–1992*	*1987*	*1990–1992*
White male	19.2	39.1	9.9	21.1
Black male	60.2	119.6	27.3	70.6
Hispanic male	36.8	64.2	25.3	45.4
Asian/Pacific Islander male	4.1	8.9	*	6.3
American Indian/Alaskan Native male	*	11.7	*	5.9
Non-Hispanic white male	14.3	34.9	8.0	18.7
White female	1.2	3.0	0.5	1.2
Black female	11.6	28.5	2.6	10.9
Asian/Pacific Islander female	*	0.8	*	*
American Indian/Alaskan Native female	*	*	*	*
Hispanic female	4.9	10.6	*	5.4
Non-Hispanic white female	0.3	1.9	0.3	0.8

*Age-specific death rate based on fewer than 20 deaths.
Source: Reference 16.

infection caused deaths more frequently in black females, with the second highest rate in Hispanic females. Colorectal cancer is the third leading cause of cancer deaths in the United States but is declining, dropping from 25 deaths per 100,000 in 1950 to 15 in 1990.[24] The incidence is slightly higher among black women.

Heart Diseases. Heart diseases are the leading cause of death in women. All major causes of heart disease (ischemic, rheumatic, and hypertensive) rise continuously from middle age through old age, but ischemic heart disease is the dramatic killer.[25] In 1992, the total rate of death from heart disease for women in the United States was 275.8

TABLE 5–6. LEADING CAUSES OF DEATH BY RANK OF 1 THROUGH 10 IN AMERICAN FEMALES ACCORDING TO DETAILED RACE AND HISPANIC ORIGIN: UNITED STATES, 1992

Disease	White	Black	Indian/Alaskan	Asian/Pacific	Hispanic
Diseases of heart	1	1	1	2	1
Malignant neoplasms	2	2	2	1	2
Cerebrovascular	3	3	5	3	3
Unintentional injuries	6	5	3	4	5
Pneumonia/influenza	5	6	7	5	6
Diabetes mellitus	7	4	4	6	4
Atherosclerosis	8				
Chronic obstructive pulmonary disease	4	9	8	7	8
Perinatal conditions		7			7
Chronic liver disease			6		
Suicide				8	
Homicide/legal intervention		10			
HIV infection		8			10
Nephritis/nephrotic syndrome/nephrosis	9		9	10	
Septicemia	10				
Congenital anomalies			10	9	9

Source: Reference 18.

per 100,000 population. More than half of the nearly one million Americans who die annually from heart disease are women, and most are over 65. The National Institutes of Health (NIH) are now studying questions such as the relationships between diet, hormonal replacement therapy, exercise, and smoking cessation and the major causes of death and disability in women: cancer, cardiovascular disease, and osteoporosis. Smoking is the major risk factor for cardiovascular disease for women. As few as 4 or under cigarettes per day increases the risk of myocardial infarction by two times. Screening for and managing diabetes, hypertension, smoking, and cholesterol levels can decrease coronary heart disease risk significantly.[26]

LEADING CAUSES OF MORBIDITY IN AMERICAN WOMEN

Acute Conditions

For all of the following acute conditions except injuries, women have a higher incidence than do men.[27]

- Infective and parasitic diseases such as diarrhea are more common in children and adolescents. They become less frequent after age 18.
- The common cold and influenza are more common in women younger than 45.
- Digestive system conditions decline with age; the highest incidence is age 17 and under.
- Injuries occur most frequently during adolescence, young adulthood, and middle adulthood, declining from age 45 on.

Chronic Conditions

Heart diseases, hypertension, diabetes mellitus, and arthritis increase steadily in both sexes as they age. Women, however, have higher incidences of all of these conditions. Other chronic conditions more common in women than in men include constipation, indigestion, orthopedic impairments, cataracts, migraine, itching skin, corns/calluses/ingrown nails, dermatitis (eczema), hay fever, rhinitis without asthma, chronic bronchitis, asthma, hemorrhoids, and varicose veins.[28] Osteoporosis is considered one of three leading causes of disability in women

after age 45;[29] heart disease and cancer are the other two.

LEADING RISK FACTORS FOR WOMEN

An overall evaluation of risk factors should include assessment of the following behaviors.

Unsafe Lifestyle Behaviors

Such behaviors are related to personal choices and are amenable to change in most instances.

- **Cigarette smoking** is associated with lung cancer and other lung diseases, heart diseases, cerebrovascular diseases, peripheral vascular disease, cancers of the larynx, oral cavity, pharynx and esophagus, as well as with pancreatic, bladder, and peptic ulcer disease, deaths by fire, increased cataracts, lowered estrogen levels, early menopause, cervical cancer, rapid skin aging/wrinkling, and secondhand smoke risk.[2,30] One in six deaths in the United States is caused by cigarette smoking, even though the overall number of smokers has declined. Women have a 12 times higher risk of dying from lung cancer if they smoke than do lifetime nonsmokers.[2] Tobacco use generally begins before high school graduation and is highest in young people with lower self-esteem and low achievement in school.[11] Cigarette use has increased steadily since 1992 among adolescents. Females report slightly less smoking than do males; white youths report smoking five times more than black adolescents and two times more than Hispanic youths. Secondhand smoke, called environmental tobacco smoke (ETS), causes about 3000 cancer deaths annually, increases the risk of children's serious respiratory infections and middle ear infections, and is associated with coronary heart disease in nonsmokers.[30] A stronger association between Sudden Infant Death Syndrome and exposure to cigarette smoke is now evident. According to a 1995 study, nonsmokers' hearts are at greater risk from secondhand smoke than smokers' because the smokers' hearts have adapted to some extent to being overwhelmed with toxins, but the nonsmokers' hearts have not and small amounts of toxins can produce serious effects, that is, sticky platelets and decreased oxygen flow.[31] Assessment should include what the woman smokes, the number smoked per day, the number of years she has smoked, ill effects, and others in the household who smoke or are affected. Cigarette smoking in pregnancy is associated with prematurity, low birth weight, spontaneous abortion, and sudden infant death syndrome.[2]

- **Substance use/abuse** includes alcohol, nicotine, caffeine, cocaine, marijuana, and tranquilizers. Alcohol use is associated with cirrhosis, stroke, hypertension, accidents, increased risk of cancer, use of other addicting drugs, and psychosocial behavioral changes and their sequelae. Two-thirds of Americans drink alcohol occasionally, and most high school seniors report use at least once.[2] Dependence occurs in 7 percent of drinkers. Alcohol and drug abuse are associated with violent crime and sexually transmitted diseases. Deaths related to alcohol use in women are primarily from cancer, cardiovascular disease, digestive disorders, and unintentional and intentional injuries. Severe alcohol dependence is less of a problem causing morbidity and high costs than is problem drinking, defined as drinking more than limits considered safe and having one or more physical or social problems due to the alcohol.[32] The leading preventable cause of birth defects is fetal alcohol syndrome.[2] Nicotine, caffeine, cocaine, marijuana, and tranquilizers are each associated with health dangers (see Chapter 23). Damage to psychosocial relationships may be significant with substance use. Assessment includes the type of substance, amount used, years of use, unsafe associated behaviors, and effects. Though significant declines in reported 30-day prevalence of illicit drug use among high school seniors have occurred since 1979, increases in marijuana use among U.S. high school students occurred in 1993 and 1994.[11]
- **Overuse of any medication** may occur when clients fail to read warnings or are not cautioned about the excessive use of legal drugs, such as gastric mucosal irritation with nonsteroidal anti-inflammatory drugs (NSAID). Neurological abnormalities with excessive vitamin B_6 ingestion is another example.[33] Assess the type of drug, amount used, years of use, and effects.

- **Sedentary lifestyle and lack of exercise and personal fitness** are associated with coronary heart disease, hypertension, stroke, colon cancer, breast cancer, lung cancer, osteoporosis, noninsulin dependent diabetes, low back pain, obesity, depression, and anxiety.[34] Exercise increases endorphins and improves emotional health. Americans are among the most sedentary people in the world. The risk of coronary artery disease almost doubles in the sedentary person.[2] Those who exercise three or more times a week at a cardiovascular fitness level are less than 10 percent of the population; nearly one quarter of adults state they never relax by physical activity.
- **Nutritional excesses and deficits** are associated with cancer, cardiovascular disease, diabetes, eating disorders, obesity, malnutrition, and deficiency diseases. Coronary artery disease in women is highly associated with obesity.[35] Binging, purging, and anorexia are significantly more common in women than in men, occurring primarily in younger women.[36] Most (85 percent) diseases and illnesses occurring in the elderly are related to poor nutrition, and, therefore, potentially preventable.[37] Early and continued consumption of fruits and vegetables appears to be associated with cancer risk reduction, especially colorectal cancer.[38] The results of a 1995 survey of 3000 school children reported at the American Cancer Society, however, found that 24 percent of the children had eaten no fruit the prior day, and 25 percent had eaten no vegetable. Findings from the Nurses Study indicate that significant deaths are associated with being overweight.[39] Almost a third of the deaths from cancer were attributed to overweight. The study found that women of average weight by today's standards and those mildly overweight had death rates higher than lean women. The average American woman was found to be 5 feet 5 inches tall and weighed 150–160 pounds. This weight was found to be about 30 pounds too high and associated with a significant risk of cardiovascular and cancer deaths. More than one-fourth of Americans are overweight, especially minority and poor women.[2] Forty-four percent of African American women 20 years of age and over are obese.

- **Unsafe automobile driving,** inattention to precautions, and lapses in driving safety are associated with a high level of morbidity and mortality for women up to age 64, especially young women. Substance abuse, nonuse of protective devices (seatbelts), and reckless driving need to be assessed. Safety cautions should be integrated into the history routinely.[40]
- **Violence** encompasses homicide, suicide, sexual assault, physical abuse/battering, and emotional trauma (see Chapter 23). Women are more likely to be the victims of violence than its perpetrators.[20] They are injured most often by domestic violence, which occurs more than rape, muggings, and auto accidents combined. Assessment should include asking about dangerous, conflictual relationships and living conditions (e.g., violent families and neighborhoods). Sexual assault is a leading violent crime against women, and it is believed that most rapes are unreported.[41] Women who are young, single, students, African American, and unemployed are at greatest risk.[20] Spousal abuse is anticipated in 66 percent of all marriages.[42] African American women are at a fourfold greater risk of homicide, often from their partners, than Caucasian women are. Husbands or other intimate partners are the assailant in 35 percent or more of female homicides.[12] Although deaths from work related injuries constitute only about 6 percent, approximately 40 percent are from homicide. Estimates are that 20 percent or more visits by women to emergency rooms are due to assaults by partners or spouses. Pregnant women were found to have a one in six incidence of battering.[43] Elder abuse has become a serious problem for older women, with 3.2 percent of elderly adults experiencing either physical, psychological, or neglect abuse.[44]
- **Exposure to HIV, hepatitis, and sexually transmitted diseases (STDs)** may cause life threatening, incurable, or disabling conditions (see Chapter 11). Approximately 12 million new STD cases occur annually.[45] Sixty-six percent of all STDs are found in people 25 and under.[11] Women are likely to use pregnancy prevention but not STD prevention.[46] Assessment should include questions about the frequency of sexual contacts, the number of partners currently and in the past, the risk status of partners, forms of sexual expression, type of contraception and/or barrier/chemical methods of protection. Perception of risk should be assessed; it may be significantly different from real risk.
- **Lack of health-directed behaviors, or poor personal care,** is associated with a substandard health status and inadequate detection and prevention behaviors, such as immunization status, and use of contraception. Personal assessment should include breast self-exam, regular dental and eye exams, general screening physical and diagnostic exams including pelvic and rectal exams, Papanicolaou (Pap) smear and indicated cultures/tests, occult fecal blood testing, mammography, and vulvar self-exam. Demographic characteristics related to underuse of screening services in one study included such factors as being single, divorced or widowed; an educational level less than high school; older age (over 65); living in specific parts of the country, for example, women from the Northeast or South were less likely to have a clinical breast exam in the last year.[47] In one study of children to evaluate how lack of immunization history contributed to missed opportunities for immunizations, only 27 percent of patients had an immunization history taken during the initial visit, and 78 percent of caregivers brought no records with them.[48] No doubt this holds true for adults since many providers fail to ask about immunizations as a part of routine examinations.
- **Inadequate, excessive, or unusual sleep** is less a problem for women than for men. A sleep study found that women have better sleep quality than men, equal to a 10-year difference in age. This difference may be associated with women's longer life spans.[49] Sleep apnea occurs more often in men than women (affects 1 woman for every 10 men). The reason may be testosterone effects on the tongue (a muscle), making it heavier and more prone to fall back and block the airway during sleep. Also, progesterone may play a protective role in women.[49] It is important to note that after menopause, there are fewer sex differences related to sleep between men and women. Women present more often with the complaint of insomnia associated with depression, but this does not indicate a real difference between sexes in relation to

this problem since women tend to seek help more readily than do men. Evaluation should include breathing difficulties, snoring, smoking, neuroses, alcohol use, medication use, estrogen decline, time zone or job shift changes, sleepwalking, stress and depression, heavy exercise near bedtime, and environmental conditions for sleep. A sure clue that someone needs more sleep is that she dozes off during the day. People who are natural short sleepers do not need catch-up sleep or alarms. One serious concern with chronic insomnia is the increased likelihood of accidents secondary to fatigue.

Exposure to Environmental Hazards

Unsafe conditions may be found in the home or work environment.

- **Unsafe home environment** encompasses falls, exposure to chemical/toxic/radon hazards, fire, excessive heat or cold, unsanitary living conditions, unsafe drinking water, lack of running water, rodent or insect infestation, airborne pollutants, and infections among people living in crowded conditions. Tuberculosis, one example of a serious disease that proliferates in crowded conditions, is on the rise again because of new resistant strains of the causative organism and the deficient immunity of individuals with HIV infection. Another example is a study of children and fetuses exposed to home pesticides.[50] Children exposed in utero to hanging pest strips during the last three months of pregnancy had three times the increased risk of leukemia.
- **Unsafe occupational situations** are associated with life threatening, damaging, or debilitating conditions, such as asbestosis, lead poisoning, pesticide exposure, and radiation exposure. Illnesses and nonfatal injuries related to work seem to be on the increase, many in the 25- to 44-year-old age group.[2] Assessment should include the individual's type of work, work hazards and conditions, and effects. Biological, chemical, environmental-mechanical, physical, and psychosocial hazards should be assessed (see Screening Methods, Special Assessment Guides in this chapter and chapters 16 and 17 on pregnancy). Providers should be familiar with their local, state, and national resources such as the local poison control center hotline

or Occupational Safety and Health Administration (OSHA).

Negative Influences on Emotional Health

Such influences vary widely from family crises to unrealistic values of thinness.

- **Stress** is associated with a wide array of physical and emotional problems. American women are increasingly stressed with multiple roles and pressures, as well as fast-paced living. Assessment includes stressors related to work, home, family, and other relationships. One researcher, Lazarus, has more closely linked the effects of hassles (the little irritating or distressing occurrences that happen daily) rather than major life events to emotional health.[51] Stress can affect the person physically (reduced immune responses, increased risk of cardiovascular, reproductive, and gastrointestinal conditions) and mentally (post-traumatic stress syndrome, neuroses, and transient situational disturbances).
- **Family crises** mean increased physical and emotional risks for both the individual and the family. Assessment includes family health, values, health care beliefs, cultural influences, and coping abilities, as evidenced by past coping with crises, individual and family. Such crises include a wide array of problems such as death, serious illness, divorce, loss of a job, loss of a home, moving, or substance abuse of a member.
- **A poor or absent support system** is associated with feelings of loneliness, helplessness, hopelessness, and powerlessness. Social support appears to be related to better health and feelings of well-being.[1] Social networks are known to decrease health risks associated with occupational stress, cancer, and pregnancy.[52] Assessment of supports should include determining recent changes in life (e.g., marriage, divorce, birth, change of residence, change of job); distance from friends, relatives, cultural group, health resources; and access to support systems, such as church. Race and ethnic differences must be considered in evaluating women's support systems.[53]
- **Depression and other mood disorders** are common psychiatric illnesses in women[54] (see Chapter 23, Depression). A woman has a 20 percent

chance of developing depression in her lifetime. Rates of illness increase in adolescence, and are higher between ages 20 and 50. Depression is associated with suicide, a leading cause of death among women. In the United States, depression is significantly related to social, psychological, and physical loss. Typical signs and symptoms of depression such as eating or sleeping difficulties, unusual sadness, and suicidal thoughts must be assessed. Depression is more difficult to recognize in the elderly woman but should be considered as it frequently coexists with chronic illnesses and disabilities.[55]

- **Unrealistic values** of youth, beauty, and thinness lead to unhealthy, excessive concerns and behaviors related to appearance. These concerns may also indicate an inability to accept the aging process. Assessment includes appearance, age, weight, height, history of unusual or overuse of plastic/reparative surgery, diet and exercise history, any verbal and nonverbal cues, such as great concern with being overweight when in reality one is underweight (see Chapter 23, Eating Disorders). Much of the emphasis on attractiveness, weight loss, and fitness has come from the media, focusing on the positives of being thin to the extent that good nutrition and health may be jeopardized.[56] Adolescents and young adult women reap the fallout of this negative campaign to make money by the larger business world.

- **Lack of recreational and relaxation activities** can cause stress, overwork, anxiety, and in some instances depression. Assessment includes financial, social, physical, and psychological conditions and barriers. Relaxation takes planning and considered time to break from life's usual pressures and competitions.

Poverty, Insufficient Insurance, and Inadequate Material Resources

Women and children (including adolescents) are the fastest growing segment of those living in poverty. Being poor, as defined in the 1996 *Kids Count Data Book,* was a family of four with an annual income of $14,335.00 or less.[57] Being poor is no longer a problem only for welfare recipients. The consistent decrease in the value of low-skilled labor is inversely related to the in-

creasing number of children in working poor families, according to the survey's executive director. Two factors contribute to the working poor being more disadvantaged than welfare recipients: more working poor are without health insurance, and less time can be spent with children by the working poor. Poor people often delay seeking health care when ill, use fewer measures to prevent or alleviate illness, have less accurate information about health, and have fewer choices for access to health care. As significant changes in the welfare system occur, more consequences for the working poor will be seen.

As women age, a greater chance for poverty exists. "For virtually all of the chronic diseases that lead the Nation's list of killers, low income is a special risk factor" (p. 29).[2] A significant increase in the ranks of the uninsured had occurred among Hispanic Americans, especially those of Mexican descent from 1977 to 1992.[58] Findings from one large study indicated that Puerto Rican women had the highest percentage of insurance coverage, and women of Mexican and Cuban origin had the lowest.[59] Women below the poverty level had the least insurance coverage. African American and Hispanic women are affected adversely by the rising hospital employee cuts and the lower wages of employees in long-term care facilities.[60] Further cuts in Medicaid and Medicare will only lead to more job losses among minority women. Assessment of financial and material resource factors affecting women includes estimated income level, other sources of support, type of work and satisfaction, quality of nutrition and living conditions, untreated illnesses or conditions (acute and chronic), dental conditions untreated, disabilities, excessive sleep and sedentary living, depression and stresses associated with lifestyle, and inadequate self-concept and ability to change life. These latter areas provide real clues to the state of poverty. Choices for women are often limited because of family and child care needs.

Hereditary, Cultural, and Ethnic Influences

Family history and culture impact health.

- **Familial diseases** may be detected by assessing family history. Diabetes, breast cancer, colorectal cancer, ovarian cancer, diabetes, heart disease, asthma, and allergies are examples of disease risks inherited from family members. Significant health problems can be prevented or minimized by careful attention to risk factors and management of lifestyle, environmental and other conditions.

- **Race** is another consideration. According to *Healthy People 2000,* even though a disparate number of minority people die from disease—and much of this disparity can be attributed to socioeconomic factors—a part of the difference cannot be explained by poverty factors alone.[2] Race plays a role. Some diseases are more common among people of certain races; for example, osteoporosis is more prevalent in light- or yellow-skinned women; sickle cell disease is found in African Americans; and glucose-6-phosphate dehydrogenase (G-6-PD) deficiency occurs more often in people of Mediterranean descent. In many American Indian tribes, diabetes affects more than 20 percent of the members.
- **Ethnic, cultural, and religious influences** may be associated with unhealthy practices: eating uncooked meat, refusing to see a health care provider, lacking health directed behaviors, and lacking the understanding or education necessary for good health. As an example, Pender cites one study of a major source of saturated fat for different groups.[1] Hispanic and black children's intake of whole milk was significantly higher than that of white children based on the parents' beliefs that the whole milk was better for the children than lower fat or skim. In contrast, Asian Americans consume low fat-high carbohydrate diets, eating much healthier foods than Americans from European origins. Sensitivity to a client's culture, religion, and ethnic influences is essential in trying to assist her with any health behavior changes, for these variables strongly affect her health beliefs. The importance of gaining cultural competence to provide responsive access to women seeking primary health care is discussed in an article by Rorie, Paine, and Barger listed in the bibliography of this chapter. The authors point out the importance of addressing care issues from the context of the woman's background, religion, and sociocultural viewpoints.

Current or Past Medical Problems

Of particular concern are the risks of past and present problems, and the potential or real effects of current or past illness on new disease conditions. For example, recent research indicates a past history of smoking, even if the person no longer smokes, increases the risk of multiple myeloma and colon cancer. Multiple drug interactions may cause increased risks and confusing presentations. The use of multiple medications, seen most often in the elderly, is essential to assess as interactions may lead to serious consequences. Past pelvic inflammatory disease increases the risk of ectopic pregnancy or infertility.

SCREENING METHODS

HEALTH HISTORY[61–66]

Interview and Approach Considerations

Effective interviewing and interpersonal skills are required in order to gather accurate, useful data.

- Consider any interaction with a client a therapeutic intervention by permitting the free expression of issues and concerns. Treat the client with dignity and respect; be nonjudgmental, accepting, supportive, concerned, and an appropriate role model (e.g., do not smoke in a client's presence).
- Use clear language and terminology matched to the client's level of understanding, culture, and background. Consider the client's age, education, response to the interview, and ethical, cultural, and religious taboos. Avoid medical jargon and clarify by restating confusing information. Use an interpreter if necessary.
- Appropriate questioning technique includes using open questions early in the interview to facilitate broad information gathering and to assist with mental status and general survey assessment. Open questions draw forth an overview of the client's problems. Ask the client about her concerns. Avoid interrupting, which may cause valuable data to be lost. Use pointed, directive questions to obtain specific data. Avoid leading questions ("You've never had a sexually transmitted disease, have you?").

Phrase sensitive questions in a nonjudgmental manner ("How many partners do I need to notify about the risk of AIDS?").

- Be aware of nonverbal cues such as facial expressions, body movements, and signs of anxiety. The client may avoid making eye contact or answering questions. She may be reluctant to give information. Such cues may indicate fears or concerns.
- Help the woman understand the importance of telling you her concerns. If the client is able to talk freely, the interaction becomes healing, and there is the increased probability that something will be said that will help in understanding a problem or in management.[66]

Physical and psychological factors affect interaction.

- Provide a quiet, private place for the interview. Ideally, the interview should not take place in the examination room. Use measures, such as a sign on the door, to discourage others from walking in during the interview.
- Maintain the client's comfort. Permit her to remain dressed during the interview, and provide comfortable seating that will allow client and interviewer to be at the same eye level. Never obtain a history with the client in lithotomy position.
- Maintain a realistic time frame. Keep the interview focused to stay within a reasonable time limit, using more than one session if needed.

COMPONENTS OF HEALTH HISTORY

- **Demographic and biographical data, called identifying data (ID),** must be accurate. Record the client's full name; street and mailing addresses; telephone numbers for work, home, and contact persons; sex; age; birth date; Social Security number; city, county, state of birth; race, nationality, culture; marital status; dependents and persons living with client; years of formal education; religious preference; occupation; usual sources of medical care; and source and reliability of health information.
- **Record the chief complaint (CC) or reason for visit (RFV).** Use the client's own words in a brief statement and put into a time frame (e.g., "I've had chest pain for two days," or "I need a Pap test and checkup").
- **Probe the history of present illness (HPI) or current health status (CHS).** An introductory

statement for all women is essential: gravidity (G); parity (P); full-term or premature pregnancies; abortions (A), spontaneous and induced, with reasons and length of gestation; number of living children (LC); dates of last and previous normal menstrual periods based on first day of bleeding (LNMP, PNMP); and methods of contraception used by client and partner, for how long or when stopped. If the woman is older, include date of menopause and use of replacement hormone therapy.

Write the remainder of the paragraph as a narrative, giving the following:

- **Usual state of health.**
- **Clear, chronological development/analysis of complaints:** sequencing (starting with onset), causes or associated phenomena, factors worsening/lessening/relieving/aggravating, quality or character of complaint, quantity of problem, effect on activities, location, radiation, severity (on a scale of 1 to 10), timing, past occurrence, others with problem.
- **Relevant family history.**
- **Degree of disability.**
- **Significant negatives.**

If the visit is related to the menstrual cycle, a complete description of the menstrual cycles is needed, including characteristics before and after the use of hormonal or other contraception that may affect the cycles.

If the visit is for routine health maintenance, elicit information about the client's usual health, last exams or tests and their results, current medications, habits, and significant problems or negatives, such as diabetes mellitus or cardiac disease.

- **Assess and record the past medical history (PMH) or health status (PHS).**
  - *Childhood Diseases.* Measles, mumps, frequent infections, and so on.
  - *Immunizations and Screening Tests.* Dates of childhood immunizations: hepatitis B, diphtheria, pertussis, tetanus, Hemophilus influenza type B, measles, mumps, rubella, chickenpox, polio vaccines (types); dates of adult immunizations: tetanus toxoid, pneumococcus, influenza, hepatitis B, measles (those born after 1956), rubella (women without immunity), varicella; dates of other vaccinations: tuberculosis, meningococcus, smallpox, ty-

phoid, and other special vaccines for at-risk and older populations; screening tests (HIV, rubella, tuberculosis, sickle cell, G-6-PD). Urge importance of maintaining currency.[67,68] (See Table 5–7 for recommended routine adult immunizations. See Limited Bibliography at end of Chapter for more information.)[69]

- *Hospitalizations and Serious Illnesses.* Dates, places, health care providers, reasons, courses of recovery, sequelae.
- *Accidents and Injuries.* Type of injury, how it occurred, severity, treatment, where, by whom, sequelae.
- *Obstetric History.* All pregnancies, regardless of outcome; dates and types of deliveries, sex and weights of infants, lengths of gestations; antepartum, intrapartum, and postpartum complications.
- *Contraceptive History.* Types of contraceptives used by client or partner, length of use, complications, side effects, satisfaction with method.
- *Sexual History.* (See Chapter 6.) Assess safer sex methods used.
- *Allergies.* Specific allergens (food, environmental, medication), types of reactions, treatments, and results.
- *Medications.* Prescription, over-the-counter, herbal therapies, dosages, administration routes, frequencies, reasons for use, side effects. See Limited Bibliography at end of Chapter for more information on herbal therapies.
- *Habits.* Recreational or illicit drug use; tobacco, alcohol, caffeine use; type of substances, frequency, duration of use, effects, routes of administration, risk practices such as needle sharing.
- *Transfusions/Transplants.* Dates, reasons, exposure to HIV, hepatitis b and c.

- **Violence History.** Incidents of assault, incest, rape, other violence; injuries, treatment, counseling, sequelae.
- **Family history (FH)** includes hereditary, communicable, and environmental family diseases; causes of death of maternal and paternal grandparents, parents, siblings, children, partners, aunts, uncles, and cousins (if indicated). A genogram can be visually helpful (see Special Assessment Guides, Family Assessment). Note if family history is unknown or the client is adopted. Of particular importance is a family history of breast, colon, or ovarian cancer in mother or sister, congenital anomalies or retardation, multiple births, CVD, and anemia.

- **Psychosocial history taking (PSH) and personal history taking and assessment require sensitivity.**
  - *Nutrition.* (See Special Assessment Guides, Nutritional Assessment.)
  - *Family Relationships, Friendships, and Support Systems.* Significance and quality of relationships and interactions, areas of concern or conflict, verbal or physical abuse, living arrangements, availability of support systems, club and organization memberships, activities enjoyed with friends and relatives (see Special Assessment Guides, Family Assessment).
  - *Culture/Ethnicity.* Foods, religion, values, and beliefs affecting health.
  - *Occupation.* Full- or part-time employment, length of employment, type of work, hazards, stressors (see Special Assessment Guides, Occupational Assessment).
  - *Education.* Highest level obtained (formal and informal); client's feelings of satisfaction and how she learns best.
  - *Economic Status.* Adequacy of income for basic and recreational needs, monetary concerns, adequacy of insurance.
  - *Exercise and Activity.* Current levels and types of activity, length of time spent, frequency, tolerance, safety.
  - *Developmental Status.* Current level of task accomplishment according to developmental stage (see Chapters 3 and 4).
  - *Self-Concept.* Locus of control, positive and negative feelings about self, satisfaction with self, perceived strengths and weaknesses.
  - *Coping Mechanisms.* Stressors and usual methods of coping, perceived effectiveness (see Special Assessment Guides, Stress/Risk Assessment).
  - *Patterns and Maintenance of Health Care.* Types, sources, and frequency of health care visits; home/folk remedies; general experiences and attitudes about health and care.
  - *Sleep and Wakefulness.* Patterns, effects, problems, dreams, medication use to sleep or to stay awake (see Special Assessment Guides, Sleep Assessment).
  - *Recreation/Relaxation.* Hobbies and activities for fun or relaxation; associated patterns, roles, and relationships.

TABLE 5–7. ADULT AND ADOLESCENT IMMUNIZATIONS

Vaccine	Schedule/ Timing	Indications	Comments	Precaution/ Contraindications
Adult tetanus/diphtheria toxoid (Td)	First visit 1 IM dose Second visit 4 to 8 weeks after first dose Third visit 6 to 12 months after second dose Booster q 10 years through life	All unimmunized adults	1. Not contraindicated in pregnancy 2. Fully immunized women may not need further boosters > age 50	Neurologic or immediate hypersensitivity after prior dose; severe local reaction after prior dose
Polio vaccines Live oral polio virus (OPV)[a]	First dose at first visit Second dose in 2 months Third dose 6–12 months after second	1. Persons at risk for future exposure who previously received 1 or more doses of either oral or inactivated vaccine 2. Incomplete childhood series	1. Can give second dose in month if need to accelerate 2. Immunocompromised persons at higher risk for paralysis; rare in healthy persons; greatest risk for paralysis with first dose	1. Avoid in pregnancy unless immediate protection essential; then use OPV or E-IPV 2. Use E-IPV with immunocompromised persons 3. Do not give OPV to people with immunocompromised family members Hypersensitivity to streptomycin and neomycin (trace amounts are used in preparation of vaccine)
Enhanced-inactivated polio virus (E-IPV)[a]	First dose SC at first visit Second dose 1 to 2 months after first dose Third dose 8 to 14 months after first dose	1. **Preferred for primary adult vaccinations** 2. Unimmunized or partially immunized with compromised immunity 3. HIV infected—symptomatic or asymptomatic 4. Close contacts of immunodeficient individuals 5. Partially immunized or unimmunized in households where children receive OPV 6. Unimmunized at risk of exposure and has had primary series 7. Partially immunized with IVP or OPV at future risk of exposure 8. At future risk of exposure who have had primary series 9. Those refusing OPV 10. Those traveling outside U.S. 11. Incomplete childhood series	1. E-IPV means has enhanced potency and is equal to OPV in seroconversion rates; is available in U.S. 2. Preferred for primary adult vaccinations 3. For those adults who have completed primary vaccinations, booster can be either E-IPV or OPV	See OPV

TABLE 5–7. ADULT AND ADOLESCENT IMMUNIZATIONS (CONTINUED)

Vaccine	Schedule/ Timing	Indications	Comments	Precaution/ Contraindications
Measles vaccine	One dose SC; no boosters needed	1. Birthdate prior to 1957 gives immunity 2. No evidence of documented vaccination requires 2 doses 1 month apart 3. If person entering college, health care work, or traveling internationally, give revaccination. 4. Revaccinate if received killed vaccine between 1963 and 1967	1. Vaccine of choice is MMR 2. Is live virus vaccine	1. Pregnant women 2. Immunocompromised persons 3. History of anaphylactic reaction after ingesting egg or after receiving neomycin
Mumps vaccine	One dose SC; no boosters needed	1. Travelers without immunity 2. No documentation of disease or live vaccine 3. Elderly age no contraindication	1. Is live virus vaccine 2. MMR is vaccine of choice	1. Pregnant women 2. Immunocompromised persons 3. History of anaphylactic reaction after ingesting egg or after receiving neomycin
Rubella vaccine	One dose SC; no boosters needed	1. No documentation of live vaccine or immunity by lab test 2. Childbearing-age women 3. Employment in health care, colleges, military base 4. Travelers with susceptibility	1. Risk theoretically to fetus is considered negligible if given to mother in first trimester 2. If person also susceptible to measles and mumps, MMR is vaccine of choice	1. Pregnant women 2. Immunocompromised persons 3. History of anaphylactic reaction after receiving neomycin
MMR	First dose at first visit Second dose at 11–12 years after first visit If measles vaccine alone given and no past documentation, give 2 doses SC 1 month apart	1. Two doses needed if born >1957 2. Older people usually immune by contracting diseases 3. If entering college, immunize 4. No contraindication to vaccination if already immune	1. Susceptible postpartum women can receive vaccine even if breast-feeding 2. Revaccinate those vaccinated 1963–1967 with killed measles vaccine; also students entering college, health care workers, international travelers 3. Five to fifty-five percent have some local or systemic reaction	1. Do not administer to people with altered immunity except HIV-infected women who need measles protection (give MMR) 2. Contraindicated in pregnancy (live virus) 3. Postpartum women who received transfusion during peripartum—delay vaccine 3 months 4. History of anaphylactic reaction after ingesting egg or exposure to neomycin
Influenza (Whole or split-virus)	One dose (whole or split-virus) annually; generally in November, but may be offered as early as September	1. Healthy adults age 65± 2. Nursing home residents 3. Chronic care facility residents 4. All health care workers 5. Teens receiving long-term aspirin therapy	1. Provides protection against A&B strains 2. Does not cause the flu 3. May cause fever, malaise, myalgia 6–12 hours after given; lasts 1–2 days	1. Acute febrile illness (wait until all symptoms abate) 2. Known hypersensitivity to eggs

(Continued)

TABLE 5–7. ADULT AND ADOLESCENT IMMUNIZATIONS (CONTINUED)

Vaccine	Schedule/ Timing	Indications	Comments	Precaution/ Contraindications
Pneumococcal	One dose IM; another dose every 6 years may be considered	1. Adults age 65± 2. Immunocompetent adults with chronic disease 3. Immunocompromised adults 4. HIV-infected adults 5. Those living where increased risk of disease exists	1. Vaccinate high-risk women before or after pregnancy 2. Half experience injection site pain, erythema; 1% have fever, myalgias, severe local reaction	1. Contraindicated in pregnant women
Hepatitis B vaccine	First visit first dose Second dose in 4 weeks Third dose 5 months after second dose Screen with Hb_sAb before booster given; immunity lasts 7 years	1. All health care workers 2. All who are at increased risk occupationally, socially (includes family exposure)	1. Recombinant vaccine 2. Screening for susceptibility before vaccination variability cost effective 3. No therapeutic or adverse effects seen when given to HBV-infected persons	Not contraindicated in pregnancy
Varicella zoster vaccine (VZV)	Two doses 4–8 weeks apart	Age 12 months and older who have not had varicella	1. Live, attenuated vaccine 2. Herpes zoster risk ≤ natural disease 3. 25% have Erythema/soreness at injection site; 5%—rash	1. Avoid in immuno compromised, hypersensitive, or neomycin-allergic people 2. Avoid pregnancy for 1 month after vaccine 3. Nursing women at high risk for exposure may take

E-IVP—enhanced-potency inactivated poliovirus vaccine; IM—intramuscular; MMR—measles-mumps-rubella; SC-subcutaneous
ªFor detailed recommendations for poliomyelitis prevention, see Poliomyelitis Prevention in the United States: Introduction of a Sequential Vaccination Schedule of Inacti-vated Poliovirus Vaccine Followed by Oral Poliovirus Vaccine. (January 24, 1997). Morbidity and Morality Weekly Report. U.S. Department of Health and Human Services, PHS, CDC. Atlanta, GA.
Source: References 67, 68.

- *Living Environment.* Hazards (real or potential), level of comfort; privacy, space.
- *Religion.* Importance to client, source of strength or stress, level of involvement.
- *Daily Profile.* Description of a typical day for the client.

- **A review of systems (ROS)** includes a thorough past and present history of each system.

  - *General.* General health, fatigue, exercise tolerance, episodes of unusual weight/height loss or gain, malaise, ability to carry out activities of daily living (ADL).
  - *Skin, Hair, Nails.* Diseases; primary or secondary skin lesions, itching, flaking; changes in texture, moisture, color, skin temperature, amount of hair, care practices.

- *Head and Neck.* Injuries and their treatments, sequelae; headaches (type); range-of-motion limitations, pain, or stiffness; enlarged nodes; swelling.
- *Eyes.* Use of corrective lenses, reason for prescription, results of last exam and glaucoma test, diseases or infections, pain, itching, discharge, diplopia, cataracts, blurred vision, spots, halos, flashing lights, blind spots.
- *Ears.* Hearing acuity, test results and dates, use of aids and their effectiveness, diseases, pain, ringing, vertigo, infection, discharge, care habits.
- *Mouth, Teeth, and Throat.* Diseases; condition of teeth (loose, missing, caries), last exam and results, knowledge of routine care; sore throats, lesions, bleeding, hoarse-

ness, voice changes; chewing, swallowing, or taste problems.

- *Nose and Sinuses.* Diseases; problems with sense of smell; nosebleeds; allergies/seasonal problems, sneezing, congestion, drainage, pain; trauma; breathing difficulties; infections and their treatments.
- *Chest and Lungs.* Diseases; dyspnea, cough, hemoptysis, exertion breathing difficulty, wheezing, asthma, pneumonia, bronchitis, tuberculosis (TB), emphysema, orthopnea, night sweats, smoking; time of last chest x-ray, reason, and results; last TB test and results.
- *Cardiovascular.* Diseases; pain, cyanosis, palpitations, murmurs, bruits, irregular heart rate, mitral valve prolapse, hypertension, edema, varicosities, rheumatic fever; coldness, tingling, color changes, hair loss on extremities; recent cholesterol and lipid screening results.
- *Breasts and Axillae.* Diseases; pain, masses, changes related to menstrual cycle, discharge, color, characteristics; skin, vascular, temperature changes; breast self-exam (when, how); last provider exam; last mammogram results; breastfeeding history.
- *Gastrointestinal.* Diseases; abdominal pain, distention, masses, indigestion, food intolerances, belching, nausea, vomiting (character), reflux, jaundice, ascites, diarrhea, constipation, character of stools; hemorrhoids; use of antacids or laxatives; last hemoccult test, results.
- *Genitourinary*

  Reproductive. Onset of puberty, menarche (when, character, regularity of menses), current menstrual pattern (frequency, duration, flow amount); premenstrual syndrome (PMS); dysmenorrhea; tampon or pad use, size, correct use, number per day of flow, saturation; problems related to menses; use of medications or hormones, reasons, problems; last pelvic exam and Pap smear (if abnormal results, follow-up, sequelae); vaginitis, itching, discharge, lesions, diseases, abnormalities; sexually transmitted diseases (STDs), including pain, fever, chills; diethylstilbestrol (DES) exposure; fertility problems; sexual satisfaction, discomfort, problems. (Obstetric, sexual, contraceptive, and menopause history data may go here, or in HPI or CHS if it relates to the reason for visit; see Chapter 16 for further information about obstetric history.)

  Urinary. Character and regularity of urination/urine; diseases, infections (cystitis or pyelonephritis); dysuria, polyuria, oliguria, anuria, incontinence, hematuria, nocturia, urgency, stones, flank pain, fever, chills.
- *Musculoskeletal.* Diseases, fractures, or other injuries, cramping, pain, fasciculations, weakness/strength, range-of-motion/activities of daily living limitations, gait problems, joint complaints (swelling, redness, pain, deformity, crepitus); back discomfort, ache, or deformity; loss of height.
- *Neurological.* Diseases; fainting, loss of consciousness, seizures (and medication for them), sensory problems (numbness, tingling, paresthesia), motor problems (balance, gait, spasm, paralysis), cognitive problems (mood changes, memory loss, disorientation, loss of judgment, hallucinations); sleep disturbances.
- *Blood and Immune.* Diseases; anemias, bleeding tendencies, easy bruising, transfusions, allergies, treatments; unexplained infections or node enlargement; blood type.
- *Endocrine.* Diseases; unusual changes in weight, height, glove, or shoe size; increased thirst, urination, appetite; heat/cold intolerance; weakness/fatigue; changes in skin and hair (loss, excessive growth, hirsute, texture).

SPECIAL ASSESSMENT GUIDES

Family Assessment

Determine who lives in the family, their relationships, cultural origins, religious preferences, health practices; the role of each member (education, occupation), communication among members, material management (home, money), goals of the family, relaxation and recreational family activities; and strengths, weaknesses, conflicts, problems, past resolution methods.[61,70]

- **The McMaster Family Assessment Device (FAD)** looks at six family functioning areas, and assumes that some areas can be healthy functional areas while others are not.[70] It is a paper and pencil self-report 60-item tool that takes about 20 minutes to complete. Family members' scores can be compared. The overall measure of a family's functioning can be measured by the General Functioning Scale. Each of the six areas has optimal and unhealthy functioning well clarified. Problem solving, communication, roles, affective responsiveness, affective involvement, and behavior control are measured.[70]

- **"Family APGAR"** is one quick screening tool for identifying areas of family difficulty.[70] It uses five areas for scoring: *adaptation, partnership, growth, affection,* and *resolve.* Each category receives a score of 0 to 2 points. The provider asks the client to score 2 points for "almost always," 1 point for "some of the time," and 0 points for "hardly ever." The following statements are given to the client for scoring:

  - I am satisfied with the help that I receive from my family* when something is troubling me. (Adaptation)
  - I am satisfied with the way my family* discusses items of common interest and shares problem solving with me. (Partnership)
  - I find that my family* accepts my wishes to take on new activities or make changes in my lifestyle. (Growth)
  - I am satisfied with the way my family* expresses affection and responds to my feelings, such as anger, sorrow, and love. (Affection)
  - I am satisfied with the amount of time my family* and I spend together. (Resolve)

  A score of 0 to 3 is associated with a severely dysfunctional family; 4 to 6 with a moderately dysfunctional family; and 7 to 10 with a highly functional family.

  This tool is easy to use and focuses on perception of satisfaction.[70]

- **The *genogram* is** a family tree picture that contains a family's relationships, structure, health, and other important data over three generations.[70] It has been evolving since the 1970s. This visual picture may be very helpful in identifying tendencies of conditions within families and, thus, risk factors for individual clients. It is also helpful in providing the elderly client with a framework for looking at life events. Cultural differences are exhibited in genograms, as well as ways to compare heritages. Relationship and emotional behaviors can also be demonstrated with the genogram through use of a key that depicts such terms as "loving," "abusive," "domi-

---

*Substitute spouse, partner, significant other, parent, or children if necessary.

neering."[71] Standardization has not been accomplished yet, but the tool is useful nevertheless.

Nutritional Assessment

Appropriate nutrition with adequate exercise will ensure better health. Assess the client's 24-hour diet recall of food/drink intake for balance and adequacy of nutrients. For nonpregnant, nonlactating women, the table of governmental dietary guidelines gives the daily intake (the lesser amounts for less active or older women).[72] See Table 5–8 for examples of servings and foods from the food groups appropriate for the nonpregnant woman 25 and over.[73]

No more than 30 percent of calories should come from fat, and no more than 10 percent of fat should come from saturated fats (i.e., animal fat and tropical oils such as coconut or palm). Some women like to keep track of fat grams in the diet; active women who are not dieting should have about 1600 calories a day and about 44 grams of fat a day. Blood lipid levels should be maintained at healthful levels: total cholesterol under 200 mg/dL, HDL-cholesterol above 35 mg/dL (ideally for women above 50 mg/dL), and LDL cholesterol under 130mg/dL (optimum level equal to or under 100 mg/dL).[74] The triglyceride level is emerging as an independent risk factor for women; it should be under 250 mg/dL (optimum under 150 mg/dL).

Sugar and salt should be used in moderation. The maximum amount of salt daily in foods and added in cooking or at the table should be no more than 2400 mg. A variety of foods that provide the proper number of food group servings should be eaten daily. No more than one alcoholic drink (one ounce of distilled liquor, 8 ounces of wine, or the equivalent) per day is advised for a woman who drinks.

Eating adequate fruits and vegetables (5 servings a day) provides the body with antioxidants (3 or more of vegetables and 2 or more of fruits). Six or more servings of grains are needed daily. Fiber rich foods, such as apples, carrots, whole grains, bran, and legumes, are important for reducing risks of bowel cancer, diabetes, obesity, and decreasing serum cholesterol.[75] Adequate fiber intake (25–35 grams daily) is advised. Oat bran, kidney beans, and a pear are examples of 4 grams of soluble fiber per serving. Raisins,

TABLE 5–8. EXAMPLES OF FOODS GROUPS, FOODS, DAILY SERVINGS NEEDED AND SERVING SIZES FOR NONPREGNANT WOMEN 25 YEARS AND ABOVE

Food Group	Food Examples and Servings Sizes		Number Servings
Fruits/Vegetables			
High in Vitamin A	cantaloupe	1/4 medium	1
	tomato	2 medium	
	papaya	1/2 medium	
	apricot	3 medium	
	carrot, spinach, greens, sweet potato, winter squash	1/2 cup cooked or 1 cup raw	
	chili peppers	2 tbsp. raw/cooked	
High in Vitamin C	juices (orange, grapefruit)	6 ounces	1
	cantaloupe, papaya	1/4 medium	
	grapefruit	1/2 medium	
	orange, lemon, kiwi	1 medium	
	tomato	2 medium	
	broccoli, Brussel sprouts, strawberries, cauliflower, green pepper, cabbage	1/2 cup cooked or 1 cup raw	
Other	raisin	1/4 cup	3
	grapes/watermelon	1/2 cup	
	apple, banana, peach	1 medium	
	asparagus, green beans, potato, peas, yellow squash, corn	1/2 cup cooked or 1 cup raw	
	lettuce	1 cup raw	
Milk Products	milk, yogurt, custard	1 cup	2
	cheese	1-1/2 ounces	
	frozen yogurt, ice milk, ice cream	1-1/2 cups	
	cottage cheese	2 cups	
Breads/Cereals/Grains	bread	1 slice	5
	tortilla	1 small	
	cereal, cold	3/4 cup	
	cereal, hot	1/2 cup	
	macaroni/noodles/spaghetti, cooked	1/2 cup	
	rice, cooked	1/2 cup	
	hot dog/hamburger bun	1/2	
	biscuit, roll, muffin	1 small	
	pancake	1 medium	
	crackers	8	
Protein Foods	cooked dry beans/peas	1/2 cup	1/2
	peanut butter	2 tbsp.	
	tofu	3 ounces	
	nuts/seeds	1/4 cup	2
	meat/poultry/fish (serving size 2–3 ounces)	1 piece	
	eggs	1 substituted for 1 ounce meat/poultry/fish	
	canned tuna/fish	1/4 cup	3
Unsaturated Fats	avocado	1/8 medium	
	margarine, mayonnaise, vegetable oil	1 tsp	
	salad dressing—mayonnaise-based	2 tsp.	
	oil-based	1 tsp.	

Source: Adapted from Table 2.7 and Table 2.8 in reference 73.

prunes, and figs provide insoluble fiber that increases transit time and decreases constipation.

Megadoses of vitamins and minerals are not advised without provider knowledge and management. Folate 400 mcg daily is advised from foods or a multivitamin supplement to reduce the risk of neural tube defects in fetuses of childbearing age women.[75] By 1998, fortification will be added to most enriched breads, flours, and grain products. Calcium rich foods daily are advised, or calcium supplements, if such a diet is not adequate or not tolerated. Adolescents and younger women up to age 24 need 1200 mg/day.[73] Those 24 to 50 years (premenopausal) need 1000 mg daily. Women 50 to 64 years on hormone replacement therapy need 1000 mg a day; women 50 to 64 not on hormone replacement therapy and women 65 and over whether on or off HRT need 1500 mg daily.[76] Pregnant and nursing women need 1200–1500 mg daily. Foods high in calcium include dairy products, broccoli, kale, turnip greens, some legumes, canned fish, seeds, nuts and fortified products. Not all calcium supplements are as bioavailable as others. Calcium citrate is one of the better sources providing more bioavailable elemental calcium. Best absorption of supplements is in doses of 500 mg or less taken between meals. Calcium carbonate absorption is impaired without the presence of gastric acid, however, and so should be taken with foods promoting secretion of gastric acid. Calcium citrate is not dependent on gastric acid for absorption. Six to eight glasses of water are recommended daily for optimal body functioning.

Determine if the client eats breakfast; skips meals; uses vitamin and mineral supplements and types/amounts; wears dentures; eats snacks (how often and what); drinks caffeinated or carbonated beverages (what and how much); eats more beef than fish and poultry; consumes excessive fat, salt, sugar, or substitutes; eats alone or too quickly; chews adequately; uses alcohol, tobacco, or other substances or medications that could alter nutrient intake; is unable to tolerate some foods, eats charcoal grilled or fried foods; eats what someone else cooks; has wide weight fluctuations; abuses food when stressed; or diets constantly. Be sure that the client knows what is included in a balanced diet. For the elderly woman, it is important to assess for conditions that may

interfere with nutritional health. Ask about the effect on her diet of any illness, drug, or problem she may have such as tooth or mouth problems, if she has enough money for food, if she has someone to eat with or eats alone, how many meals she eats a day, unplanned weight loss, and how she shops and cooks for herself.[77] The Nursing Nutritional Screening Tool (NNST) is a quick and easy tool that may be used to identify women with actual or potential nutritional lacks.[78]

Vegetarians can get all the nutrients needed from a diet comprised mainly of plant foods, such as vegetables, grains, legumes, fruits, seeds and nuts, small amounts (3 servings per day) of low or nonfat dairy foods per day, and 3–4 egg yolks a week. Readers are referred to the January 1996 issue of the *Harvard Women's Health Watch* for a readable coverage of a vegetarian diet and nutrients requiring special attention, such as folate, calcium, vitamins B-12 and D, iron, and protein. Vegetarian diets are especially beneficial in providing fiber and antioxidants.

Correlate diet patterns with other history, physical examination, and diagnostic test findings; for example, high fat intake may be correlated with obesity and abnormal lipid levels. (See Chapter 17, for nutritional recommendations during pregnancy.) Data have shown that weight in the upper levels of normal and even moderate weight gains after age 18 increase a woman's risks of coronary heart disease.[79] Appropriate weight may be calculated roughly on the basis of the woman's height: 100 pounds for the first 5 feet and an additional 5 pounds for each additional inch.[80] If her body frame is large, add another 5 pounds; if small, subtract 5 pounds. Relative weight is another measure that may be helpful. A ratio that ideally is near 100 percent, relative weight can be calculated by dividing actual weight by ideal weight and multiplying by 100 (example: 64 inch woman weighs 155; relative weight = 129.2%). Other measures found valuable include the Body Mass Index (BMI) and Waist/Hip Ratio. BMI is calculated by dividing weight in kilograms by the square of the height in meters.[79]

The ideal BMI is 21 to 22; above 25, cardiovascular health risks rise.[39] As the amount of body fat increases and the amount of lean body mass decreases, the risks increase.[81] The waist to hip

TABLE 5–9. WEIGHTS AND HEIGHTS BASED ON BODY FRAME: WOMEN 25 YEARS AND OVER

| Height† | Weight in Pounds* | | | |
	Small Frame	Medium Frame	Large Frame	20% Overweight‡
4'9"	90–97	94–106	102–118	120
4'10"	92–100	97–109	106–121	124
4'11"	95–103	100–112	108–124	127
5'0"	98–106	103–116	111–127	131
5'1"	101–109	106–118	114–130	134
5'2"	104–112	109–122	117–134	139
5'3"	107–115	112–126	121–138	141
5'4"	110–119	116–131	125–142	148
5'5"	114–123	120–136	129–146	154
5'6"	118–127	124–139	133–150	158
5'7"	122–131	128–143	137–154	163
5'8"	126–136	132–147	141–159	167
5'9"	130–140	136–151	145–164	172
5'10"	134–144	140–155	149–169	177

*Without clothing
†Without shoes
‡20% over midpoint of medium-frame weight; not in original Metropolitan table
Adapted from: Metropolitan Life Insurance Company. New weight standards are for men and women. Stat Bull Metropol Life Insur Co. 1959;40:1–4 and Metropolitan height and weight tables. Stat Bull Metropol Life Insur Co. 1983;64:2–9. Reproduced by permission of the publisher; copyright © 1959 and 1983.
Reprinted with permission from April 1995 Nurse Practitioner 20(4), 66: Table 2 in Body Measurement.

ratio is calculated by dividing the waist measurement in inches by the hip measurement in inches. The optimal ratio should be 0.80 or under for women.[82] Any ratio above this optimum indicates a tendency for central obesity, a significant risk factor for heart disease (see Table 5–9 for desirable weights for women).[82] (See Chapter 17, Table 17–3, for weights at 120% and 135% of desirable midpoints.)

Stress/Risk Assessment

Assess the amount of healthy stress in the woman's life, and the amount of distress.[1] Distress is stress overload; therefore, look at factors such as financial problems; changing situations or relationships with family or significant others; and employment, unemployment, or underemployment problems or concerns (such as lack of control or input into the job situation). In addition, assess personal information (age, hereditary factors such as family history of depression, lifestyle, living conditions, habits), coping strategies, and social support. Stress and ineffective coping are associated with the development of illnesses, such as hypertension, coronary artery disease, headaches, back pain, and GI upsets; decreased immunity; mental health problems such as depression and substance abuse; and domestic violence, to name a few. A study to see if perceived family stress was predictive in forecasting health problems found that people reporting a high level of family stress had more severe illness follow-up visits, referrals, and hospitalizations over an 18-month period than low stress persons.[83] Research has also shown that the small stressors in life (daily hassles) can be important sources of stress, perhaps as much or more than major events.[84]

Helpful assessment tools for evaluating stress or anxiety are the Holmes and Rahe Life-Change Index, which measures the degree of change from major life events in one's life to predict the chance of illness;[85] the hassles and uplift scales;[84] and Speilberger's State-Trait Anxiety Inventory,[86] which measures the amount of anxiety a person feels at the time of testing. Signs of excessive stress (mood swings, disposition changes, physical signs and symptoms) must be correlated with other assessment findings (sleep, appearance, nutrition, relaxation, recreation, self-concept, social supports, use of medications/substances, or unusual behaviors).

Offering ways for managing stress to decrease the potential adverse effects becomes important as a routine part of women's health care in our society today. Using relaxation techniques is one effective way to inhibit the stress effects on the body. Domar and Dreher suggest minirelaxation techniques to use quickly and effectively in stressful situations.[87] These involve use of conscious abdominal breathing rather than chest breathing, which is associated with anxiety.

Fitness Assessment

Assess activities at work, home, or play for aerobic quality, stretching/flexibility movement, strength components, and sufficient intensity to meet therapeutic cardiovascular levels without compromising safety. Determine the duration of the exercise session, frequency per week, and the motivation of the client to exercise. To achieve a realistic assessment, evaluate fitness within a framework of lifestyle, diet, weight, stress, and substance use. *Healthy People 2000* goals aim for at least 30 percent of people over age 5 to exercise lightly to moderately each day for 30 minutes as a minimum.[2] Vigorous activity 3 times a week for 20 or more minutes is the goal for 20 percent of adults. Adolescents become more sedentary, especially females, indicating a need for early fitness habits in children.[1] The Centers for Disease Control and Prevention and the American College of Sports Medicine examined the research on recommended physical activity levels and concluded that every U.S. adult should "accumulate 30 minutes or more of moderate-intensity physical activity on most, preferably all, days of the week."[88] Previous recommendations had said that each person needed moderate- to high-intensity exercise 3 times a week for 20–60 minutes; however, the new recommendation is based on the findings that most health benefits can be attained with moderate-intensity exercise not necessarily found in a formal exercise program. Lifestyle exercise, those activities that cumulatively provide the person with moderate exercise during the day, should be assessed for adequacy in total amount (30 minutes) per day at less than 60 percent of maximum heart rate.[1]

Provide the woman with the benefits of exercise, such as the positive effects on blood pressure and cholesterol, the improved immunity effects, the decrease in body fat and improved glucose tolerance, the maintenance of bone density and increased lean muscle mass, and the improved self-concept.[1] A study of the effect of a single walking bout on a treadmill on serum lipids and lipoproteins in groups of premenopausal and postmenopausal women found that in the immediate postexercise period, even a single exercise event lowered the total cholesterol and the low density cholesterol (LDL-C) in the premenopausal women and lowered the LDL-C in the postmenopausal group.[89] The most favorable pattern of cholesterol and lipid changes in older women was produced by a combination of endurance exercise and hormone replacement therapy (HRT).[90] Over 11 months, total cholesterol, LDL-C, and high density lipoprotein cholesterol (HDL-C) all changed positively with the combined regimen. An accompanying editorial when this study was published warned that the safety of the HRT had not been addressed and was important.[91] A study of over 7000 women reported in the *Journal of the American Medical Association* found that women who were least fit had a 110 percent greater risk of death; women smokers had a 99 percent greater risk of death; nonsmoking women who were moderately fit had 55 percent lower all-cause risk of death than lower-fit women; and fitness appeared to offset some of the effects of smoking as well as impacts of hypertension and high cholesterol.[92]

For any exercise regimen, but especially for a moderate or higher intensity exercise program, teach the value of beginning slowly for short periods of time, then gradually building it, with emphasis on increasing tone, strengthening, reducing stress, enhancing flexibility and coordination, promoting relaxation, preventing injury, and improving self-concept. For a healthy woman who has no contraindications for exercise, advise building up to 20 to 40 minutes of aerobic activity, with a warm-up of 5 to 10 minutes before the more vigorous activity. Advise her to stretch after warming up and to cool down slowly for 5 to 10 minutes after exercising, monitoring her heartrate.

The intensity of exercise is aimed at safely improving cardiovascular function. The formula to determine approximate target heart rate zones for training, based on age, can be taught; however, referral to an exercise therapist may be necessary for a full assessment and program management. Recommended *target zones* (defined as 60 to 85 percent of the average maximum heart rate) for women, according to age and based on a resting heartrate of 80 are as follows:[93]

Age	Target Zone (heartbeats per minute)
20	120–170
25	117–166
30	114–162
35	111–157
40	108–153
45	105–149
50	102–144
55	99–140
60	96–136
65	93–132
70	90–123

Advise the client that for a conditioning response, the objective is to sustain the lower value of the target zone (60 percent) for 20 to 25 minutes. A good rule of thumb is that the client should be able to talk while in the target percentage range but probably not sing. An individual would have to be in peak fitness to sustain the upper end of the target zone for that extended time; it could cause exhaustion in the average person.[93] Activities that the usually sedentary individual can integrate into her life to provide short opportunities for moderate exercise include brisk walking, stair climbing, yard work, play with children, and gardening.[1] Suggestions include taking every opportunity to walk, such as changing channels by walking to the television, parking further from the destination, and taking the stairs instead of the elevator. Heel-to-toe walking is currently being touted as more fully beneficial than regular walking because it exercises all body parts—not just the heart, lungs, and legs—without stressing the joints.[94] A certain amount of practice is needed for this exercise for it to be useful and comfortable since it is more rhythmic and powerful than regular walking.

Occupational Assessment

Assess the type of work, amount, duration, physical labor involved, rest breaks, environmental risks, and stress overload. Problem areas include prolonged standing or sitting, heavy lifting, excessive noise, excessive heat or cold, exposure to toxins, exposure to chemicals or radiation, excessive hours on the job, boredom, low pay, low recognition, and little or no control over work. An area of increasing concern is environmental tobacco smoke exposure. A 39 percent excess risk of lung cancer was found with exposure in the workplace in a multicenter study that looked at lifetime lung cancer relative risk associated with environmental exposure.[95]

Be especially concerned about a pregnant woman (see Chapters 16 and 17); determine if she has been exposed to chemicals, anesthetic gases, radiation, or infections.[96] Consider the influence of multiple variables, such as secondhand smoke, stress, nutrition, lack of sleep, and exposure to hazardous materials. Estimates for the year 1984 were that occupational exposures caused about 125,000 illnesses, 5.3 million injuries, and 4000 to 12,000 deaths.[97] Three questions have been found to be essential for a simple occupational history: 1) What is your job like? Describe it; 2) Have you ever worked with any health hazard, such as asbestos, chemicals, noise, or repetitive motion?; and 3) Do you have any health problems that you believe may be related to your work or home? The chief complaint should always be examined for a relationship with the person's work or home activities or exposures. A more in-depth occupational history as presented in the reference by Twinings is needed if the simple history indicates problems.[97]

Sleep Assessment

Assess the sleep and rest patterns of the woman. Chronic sleep disorders cost Americans nearly $16 billion a year, and often this important aspect of living is never evaluated.[98] The stages of sleep consist of the following: Stage 1: NonRapid Eye Movement (NREM) sleep for a few minutes as the person moves in transitional sleep with dreamlike thoughts; Stage 2: NREM sleep that is deeper with fragmented thoughts for 15–20 minutes; Stages 3 and 4: Deeper NREM sleep stages (delta sleep) lasting 40–70 minutes; REM Stage: Follows the first four stages and is sleep (dream sleep) that can be considered as restorative, or as calisthenics for the brain. The cycles of sleep stages are repeated through the sleep period with increasingly lengthening REM stages until the person awakens. Many activities can interrupt the normal circadian rhythms, disrupting sleep, and causing distress. Lack of sufficient REM sleep affects memory and learning.

If the woman complains of awakening to go to the bathroom, look further as sleep apnea may be the cause.[99] Sleep apnea is either central or obstructive and affects 2 percent of women.[98] Cardiopulmonary altered function is common.[100] Loud snoring, especially with gasping/choking episodes, indicates apnea. Since obstructive problems decrease oxygen to the brain, the body nearly awakes as a warning. If this pattern is repeated multiple times a night, serious repercussions can occur and the woman needs to be seen by a specialist. A history of accidents on the job, sleeping on the job, and/or personality-cognitive changes should raise suspicions. A referral is also needed for women with narcolepsy (periods of sudden sleeping), which can lead to accidents.

Ask the following questions: Does it take you at least an hour to fall asleep? Do you wake up too early? Does your sleep partner complain that you are restless? Do you worry about getting enough sleep most nights? If you wake up in the night, can you go back to sleep? Do you use aids (pills or alcohol) to get to sleep? Do you feel exhausted from lack of sleep? Do you sleep in on days off or take daytime naps to make up for lack of sleep? Do you need caffeine to stay alert during the day? How much? Does your mind continue to work excessively during times when your body is resting? Five or more yes answers indicate problems.[101]

PHYSICAL EXAMINATION[61–65,102–103]

Overview

Accurate inspection, palpation, percussion, and auscultation are critical, as is the precise use of appropriate equipment. Understanding the findings is also essential.

- In preparation for the exam, explain all procedures to the client. Ensure privacy, draping, and comfort. Have all necessary equipment available and clean, and use good lighting. Ask the client to void before the exam. *Clean hands and the use of universal precautions are essential.*
- During the exam, give anticipatory advice and information; for example, teach abdominal breathing to help the client relax. Use the exam as an opportunity to teach. Be gentle, systematic, and sensitive. Avoid facial expressions or utterances indicating disgust. Provide tissues for the client after the pelvic exam. When finished, wash hands and allow the client to dress before reviewing findings.
- An abbreviated physical examination of a well woman, as done in some family planning clinics or private offices, includes assessment of blood pressure, height and weight, lymph nodes (head/neck, axillae, groin), thyroid, heart, lungs, breasts, abdomen, extremities, and genitourinary tracts and rectum.

General Survey

Obtain an overall first impression of the client. Obvious and more subtle clues are obtained primarily by sensory observation and listening with a "sixth sense."

- Note signs of respiratory, cardiac, and emotional distress, along with signs of pain.
- Assess levels of awareness and consciousness through levels of alertness, wakefulness, and appropriate timely response.
- Note the client's facial expression: its mobility, symmetry, and affect in response to questions.
- Observe the symmetry of gait and movements, and how coordinated the woman is when walking, sitting, and moving. Note any involuntary movements and her ability to move purposefully.
- Measure height and weight with clothes on and shoes off; compare findings to standardized charts. Consider racial effects: African Americans tend to be heavier and taller than Caucasians; Asians tend to be slighter and shorter than Caucasians. Consider age and gender effects: girls tend to reach peak height at puberty; older women tend to lose height after menopause.
- Note body type and posture, whether the woman is obese, slender, average, or stocky; her fat distribution and any deformities. Consider that an

older woman may develop a thoracic hump, especially if she is not on hormone replacement therapy. Observe her ability to stand and to sit straight.

- Note the client's speech, the pace at which she speaks, her ability to answer/speak spontaneously, clearly, logically, and with appropriate inflection.
- Observe personal hygiene, grooming, and dress.
- Evaluate the client's affect, manner, and orientation, including the cooperativeness, anxiety, manner toward others and examiner, and nonverbal clues.
- Body and breath odors may indicate problems: alcohol on the breath, urine on clothes, decaying teeth odor, acetone on the breath, halitosis.
- Determine vital signs, including accurate temperature, pulse rate, respiratory rate, and blood pressure. Use appropriate equipment and technique, such as a large cuff for obese clients and, if blood pressure is abnormal, checking both arms with client sitting and lying. Use a rectal thermometer if the client is not alert. Always recheck abnormal findings.
- Assess developmental changes of the breasts and reproductive system (sexual maturity). (See Physical Examination, Developmental Changes of the Breasts and the Reproductive System.)

Skin

Evaluate color, temperature, vascularity, turgor, moisture, texture, thickness, and primary and secondary lesions. Teach the client to examine moles for changes.

Hair

Note its color, texture, thickness, and distribution. Observe how the hair is cared for; observe the effects of dyes, permanent waves and other cosmetic changes; and check for nits and lice.

Nails

Observe for color, texture/consistency, care/cleanliness, clubbing, infection, damage/intactness, and smoothness.

Scalp, Head, Face

Note lesions, flaking, scaliness, abnormal contours, tenderness, lumps or masses, symmetry, and edema.

Eyes

Note symmetry, normal appearance, tenderness, lesions, and discharge. Assess intactness and abnormalities of eyes, eyebrows, eyelids, lens, cornea, conjunctiva, sclera, iris, and pupil. Test visual acuity, intact extraocular movements, accommodation and convergence, peripheral fields, and corneal light reflex. Do a fundoscopic.

Ears

Note symmetry, position, tenderness, masses, lesions, discharge, or normal appearance. Assess auditory acuity, internal canal, tympanic membrane, and external structures. If indicated, assess sensorineural/conduction loss.

Nose/Mucosa

Assess color, edema, discharge, lesions, bleeding, turbinates, and septum deviation.

Sinuses

Evaluate the frontal and maxillary sinuses for tenderness and swelling. Transillumination is done if indicated.

Lacrimal Glands and Sacs

Note swelling, tenderness, and punctual regurgitation.

Mouth, Teeth, Pharynx

Evaluate color, symmetry, texture, lesions, swelling, exudate, bleeding, tenderness, induration, lip moisture, buccal mucosa, gums, palate, ducts, tongue/papillae, pharynx, pillars, tonsils, sublingual area, and uvula. Note the number and condition of teeth.

Neck, Lymph Nodes, Thyroid, Trachea

Evaluate the range of motion, symmetry, pain, swelling, masses/nodules, lesions, enlarged nodes (mobility, size, shape, consistency, discreetness, tenderness), and tracheal position.

Thorax and Lungs

Evaluate the respiratory rate, rhythm, and effort; contour, symmetry, and shape of chest; bulges, retractions, deformities; tenderness, masses, lesions, thoracic expansion, tactile fremitus, and diaphragmatic excursion. Percussion and auscultation for adventitious sound are part of the examination.

Heart, Vessels

Assess chest symmetry, skin and mucous membrane color, pulsations, lifts, heaves, apical impulse, rate, rhythm, intensity, first heart sound (S_1), second heart sound (S_2), murmurs, and other extra sounds of the heart; amplitude, contour, rate, and rhythm of pulses; symmetry and pressure of jugular veins; color, temperature, hair pattern, and skin/vascular condition of extremities; Homan's sign.

Breasts, Areolae, Nipples and Axillae

Note sexual maturity, size, symmetry, dimpling, retractions, color, edema, thickening, vascular pattern, lesions/rashes/scaling, discharge, masses/nodules, rash, unusual pigmentation, abnormal lymph nodes. Teach breast self-exam.

Abdomen

Observe color of skin, lesions, contour, masses, distention, symmetry, vascularity, peristalsis, pulsations, and the umbilicus. Using percussion and/or palpation, assess pulsations, bowel sounds, bruits, ascites, organomegaly, and masses. Note inguinal node enlargement, tenderness/pain, rebound, and rigidity. Perform iliopsoas and obturator maneuvers with acute abdomen.

Musculoskeletal

Evaluate gait (stance, swing, abnormalities), joints and spine (limited range-of-motion, swelling, tenderness, warmth, redness, crepitation, scoliosis); note symmetry of structures, muscle strength, deformities, and abnormal condition of surrounding tissues.

Neurological/Psychological

Note mental status (mood, affect, appearance, posture, alertness/consciousness, orientation, facial expression, recent and remote memory, speech, abstract reasoning, judgment, and basic understanding). Test cranial nerves I through XII. Evaluate motor function (gait, posture, muscle tone, balance, muscle mass symmetry, muscle strength), coordination (rapid alternating movements, point-to-point testing), sensory (pain, temperature, light touch, vibration, position, stereognosis, graphesthesia, two point discrimination, extinction, point localization), and deep tendon reflexes (biceps, triceps, brachioradialis, patellar, plantar, Achilles, abdominal, clonus).

Case-finding instruments are valuable adjuncts in gathering data to diagnose major depression in primary care settings.[104] Several instruments such as the Beck Depression Inventory, the Center for Epidemiologic Studies Depression Screen, and the Zung Self-Assessment Depression Scale can be administered in 2–5 minutes, are easy in relation to literacy level, and are depression-specific. About 20 percent of depressed clients can be identified with use of a case-finding instrument, a decided improvement over the 50 percent missed if usual history and physical methods are used without a full diagnostic interview. Depression instruments should not be used to the exclusion of other instruments for case-finding additional disorders, however, such as anxiety or drug/alcohol abuse. Some instruments are multidimensional, such as the Primary Care Evaluation of Mental Disorders and the Symptom Driven Diagnostic System, and should be considered in gathering data. Additionally, specific examinations and tests are needed to rule out physical pathology of somatic complaints, such as chest pain in the woman with panic disorder or headache associated with depression.[105,106] The reader is referred to Chapter 23, Psychosocial Health Problems for more indepth assessment information.

Pelvic

Use gloves on both hands; maintain strict medical aseptic technique to prevent spread of organisms. Some clinicians recommend double gloves or special high-risk gloves if the HIV-AIDS/Hepatitis B status is known to be positive.

- *Inspect and palpate* femoral nodes, external genitalia and Bartholin glands, urethra, and Skene's (BUS) glands. This includes, in addition to the Bartholin glands and urethra, the mons pubis, labia minora and majora, clitoris, urethral meatus, and vaginal opening. Assess sexual maturity and check pubic hair for pattern/parasite. Note any swelling, enlargement, inflammation, lesions (e.g., excoriations, leukoplakia), pigmentation, discharge, relaxation/celes, and tenderness. Teach self-examination of the vulva.[107] The 2 minutes it takes to provide the woman with a "tour" of her genital area may save her life. The self-exam should be done monthly.
- *The vagina and cervix* are examined with a warmed speculum; lubricate with water only as lubricant may interfere with interpretation of cervical cytology.[102] The cervix may more readily come fully into view if the woman is asked to cough out loud 3 times with a hand covering the speculum and urethral openings.[108] Inspect the cervix and os: size, shape, color, lesions, discharge/bleeding, and position. Obtain the Pap smear and prepare cultures and wet prep specimens (see Overview of Commonly Indicated Laboratory Tests). Inspect the vagina for color, rugae, lesions (erosions, leukoplakia,

masses, ulcerations), inflammation, and discharge. With a cotton tipped applicator, gently remove any discharge that prevents adequate visualization of surfaces.
- *Assess the uterus and adnexa.* Lubricate index and middle gloved fingers; insert into vagina with other hand on abdomen above pubis. Note vaginal nodules, masses, or tenderness; note cervical size, consistency, nodules or masses, tenderness, pain with movement of the cervix, and closure of the os. Assess the position, size, shape, consistency, mobility, and tenderness of the uterus, adnexal organs, and any masses. Of interest is a paper published in Australia that the bimanual examination should not be performed routinely as a part of a well woman examination since, as a screening test, it does not fulfill appropriate levels of specificity, sensitivity and cost effectiveness.[109] Elimination of this part of the routine woman's health examination is not recommended by ACOG.
- *The rectovaginal area* is evaluated **after gloves are changed** and fingers lubricated again. Inspect the external anal area and palpate the sphincter, rectal walls, septum, posterior surface of the uterus, and palpable adnexal areas for tumors and tenderness. Test any stool on the gloved finger for blood. More colorectal carcinomas and polyps were found with Heme-Select and a combination of Hemoccult II Sensa plus HemeSelect than with Hemoccult II, the more widely used guaiac test for fecal occult blood.[110] Retroverted or retroflexed uteri are more accessible by rectal exam. Obese women may be evaluated more fully by the rectovaginal route.

Developmental Changes of the Breasts and the Reproductive System

- *Pubertal changes* include functional maturation of the reproductive organs. The breast bud (thelarche) is usually the first sign of puberty, followed soon afterward with the emergence of pubic hair. Axillary hair generally appears about 2 years after pubic hair begins; rarely does it precede pubic hair growth. Menarche (median age 12.8 years, range 9 to

15+ years) occurs after the peak of the growth spurt (median age 11.4 years, range 10–14 years). See Chapter 4 for more detail.

As the external genitalia develop into adult proportions, the clitoris becomes more erectile and the labia minora more vascular. The labia majora and mons pubis become more prominent at the same time as the breasts develop. The internal organs, including the uterus, ovaries, and fallopian tubes, increase in size and weight. The endometrial lining becomes thick in preparation for menarche, and vaginal secretions increase.[63,111]

■ *Tanner Staging.* This is widely used to assess adolescent pubertal development.[111,112] The sample used to develop these guidelines comprised white, middle-class English girls; therefore, modifications may be needed when applying the parameters to other groups.

- *Stage I (Prepubertal).* Breasts have elevated papilla only. No pubic hair present.
- *Stage II.* Breasts and papilla are elevated and appear as a small mound with enlarged areola diameter (median age 9.8 years, range <8 to 13 years). Sparse, long, pigmented hair develops chiefly along the labia majora (median age 10.5 years, range 8–13 years).
- *Stage III.* Further breast enlargement occurs without separation of breast and areola (median age 11.2 years). Dark, coarse, curled pubic hair is sparsely spread over mons (median age 11.4 years).
- *Stage IV.* Secondary mound of areola and papilla develop above the breast (median age 12.1 years). Adult-type pubic hair is abundant but limited to the mons pubis (median age 12 years).
- *Stage V (Final Adult Stage).* Recession of areola occurs (median age 14.6 years, range 12–18 years). Pubic hair is of adult type in both quantity and distribution (median age 13.7 years, range 12–18 years).
- *Although the normal time frame for sexual development varies greatly, deviations do occur.* Variations from normal development are identified by the terms *precocious* and *delayed.* The health care provider must be aware of these aberrations and must ensure that

complete family and medical histories are obtained (see Chapter 8).
- *Precocious Puberty.* Sexual development (see preceding discussion of Tanner staging) that occurs before age 8, or menarche before age 10.[113] This occurs rarely; it is usually due to early hypothalamic-pituitary-ovarian activation but requires evaluation.[111]
- *Delayed Puberty.* Menarche is absent at age 18, or breast budding is completely absent at age 13. This occurs rarely.[112,114]

■ The reproductive years (Tanner Stage V) involve additional changes, for example, cyclic changes in the size, nodularity, and tenderness of the breasts, related to hormonal changes in the menstrual cycle. These changes, along with an increase in total breast volume, occur maximally 3 to 4 days before the onset of menses and minimally in days 4 through 7 of the menstrual cycle. Structural changes also occur, unrelated to the cycle. Pubic hair may spread onto the inner aspect of the upper thighs. The labia majora increase in prominence; the labia minora and clitoris enlarge. Increased elasticity of vaginal tissue along with attainment of the mature vagina and ovarian size occurs.

■ Older women note profound breast and genitalia effects as ovulation and estrogen production decline. The perimenopause encompasses a period from about age 40 to 55. The average age of menopause is 51, with a normal range of 45 to 55.[111] Menopause before 40 is premature, and after 55, late. Ovulation usually continues until 1 to 2 years before menopause but declines in frequency from about age 40 until ending altogether.[111,115]

- *Breasts.* Breasts may begin to sag. Glandular tissue atrophies and is replaced by fat.
- *Hair Patterns.* Pubic hair turns gray and decreases in quantity. Axillary hair may also diminish. Hirsutism may develop, with coarse hair on the lip, chin, chest, abdomen, and back.
- *Genitalia and Reproductive Organs.* As estrogen levels decrease, the vulva appears atrophic and the labia and mons pubis flatten. Any lesion, especially in an older woman, may be cancerous and warrants evaluation.[103]

TABLE 5–10. GUIDELINES FOR SELECTED SCREENING EXAMINATIONS AND TESTS FOR WELL NONPREGNANT WOMEN

Exam/Test	18–39	40–59	60–74	75–
Physical examination including height/weight	q3y	q1y	q1y	q1y
Breast clinical examination	q1y	q1y	q1y	q1y
Pelvic and pap	q1y[a]	q1y	q1y	q1y
Rectal exam	q1y	q1y	q1y	q1y
Mammography	Baseline between age 35–40.	[b]	q1y or [c]	q1y or [c]
Hematocrit/hemoglobin	Baseline, q10y or [d]	q10y or [d]	q10y or [d]	q10y or [d]
Blood glucose	Baseline and [d]	q2y	q2y	q2y
Cholesterol, lipids	Baseline and q5y	q3–5y	q3–5y[g]	q3–5y[g]
Stool for occult blood	[d]	[d]	q1y	q1y
Protoscopy/sigmoidoscopy	[d]	q3–5y[e]	q3–5y	q3–5y
Blood pressure	q2y[f]	q2y[f]	q2y	q2y
Urinalysis	[d]	q5y	q5y	q1y
Dental	q1y	q1y	q1y	q1y
Eye exam and glaucoma test	Baseline then q3–5y or[d]	q2–4y or[d]	q1–2y or[d]	q1–2y or[d]
Hearing exam	Baseline @ 40	Repeat @ 50[h]	q1y[h]	q1y
Endometrial sampling	[d]	[d]	[d]	[d]
Tuberculosis	[d]	[d]	[d]	[d]
Chest x-ray	[d]	[d]	[d]	[d]
Thyroid testing(TSH)	[d]	Baseline	[d]	[d]

[a]If sexually active, begin earlier. STD screen advised for any client at high risk. *Women with hysterectomies for noncancer reasons do not need annual Pap smears.*
[b]General agreement exists among major national organizations setting standards for mammography, that women should have a mammogram every 1 year from age 40 to age 65.
[c]Mammograms are recommended q 2–3 years after age 65 by the American Geriatric Society.
[d]Indicated if risk factors present.
[e]After age 50. Should have 2 consecutive annual negative examinations before having q 3–5 years.
[f]Every year if blood pressure 130–139/85–89mm HG; if higher, repeat within 2 months.
[g]Total cholesterol (TCHO) screening optional after age 60. If TCHO 200–240 mg/dL, annual screening needed.
[h]Audiogram may be needed as the woman ages.
Source: References 116–123.

Gradually, the vaginal introitus constricts, the vagina becomes shorter and narrower, and the vaginal epithelium becomes thinner and less vascular, appearing pink, dry, and smooth with fewer rugae. The clitoris, cervix, and uterus become smaller. The uterus, about half the size of a woman's fist postmenopausally, may be difficult to palpate or may even prolapse, as the ligaments and connective tissue of the pelvis sometimes lose their elasticity and tone. The ovaries and fallopian tubes also atrophy. Many changes may be less drastic with hormone replacement therapy. If significant stenosis is present vaginally, a one finger bimanual examination is indicated. One third of pelvic masses in women over 50 are malignant.[103] Uterine fibroids occur in one in five menopausal women, especially in African American women. Any enlarged organ or mass must be evaluated by a gynecologist. The normal ovary in menopause is approximately $2cm \times 1.5cm \times 0.5cm$.

Guidelines for Routine Examinations and Screening Tests

After menarche until death, self-examination of the breasts, vulva, and skin is indicated for all women. Signs and symptoms of cancer should be taught (see Table 5–10).[116–123]

Guidelines for General Education and Anticipatory Guidance

Education and guidance in areas such as alcohol use, parenting, fitness, and immunizations are targeted for specific age groups (see Table 5–11). See Table 3–7 for indicated immunizations.

TABLE 5–11. ANTICIPATORY GUIDANCE TIME FRAME FOR SELECTED TOPICS BY AGE GROUP

Anticipatory Guidance	Ages 15–24	Ages 25–39	Ages 40–59	Ages 60–74	Ages 75–
Sun exposure	*	*	*	*	*
Smoking	*	*	*	*	*
Illicit drug use	*	*			
Alcohol use	*	*	*	*	*
Prescription/over-the-counter drug use	*	*	*	*	*
Nutrition	*	*	*	*	*
Driving accidents	*	*			*
Falls/other accidents				*	*
Family/marital/other relationships	*	*	*	*	*
Parenting	*	*	*	*	
School/work	*	*	*	*	
Retirement			*	*	*
Fitness	*	*	*	*	*
Stress	*	*	*	*	*
Sleep	*	*	*	*	*
Contraception	*	*	*		
Pregnancy	*	*	*		
Breast cancer	*	*	*	*	*
Loneliness/grief/loss			*	*	*
Menopause/climacteric/transitions		*	*	*	
Bowel/bladder problems			*	*	*
Self-care problems				*	*
Dental care	*	*	*	*	*
Sensory deficiency			*	*	*
Sexuality	*	*	*	*	*
Sexually transmitted disease/HIV risks	*	*	*		
Immunizations	*	*	*	*	*
Violence/abuse	*	*	*	*	*

Asterisk indicates that topic should be discussed.

OVERVIEW OF COMMONLY INDICATED LABORATORY TESTS

PAPANICOLAOU SMEAR

Purpose

The Papanicolaou (Pap) smear is a screening test for abnormal/atypical cells suggesting actual or preneoplastic cervical changes. Its primary use is in screening for cervical cancer. Cervical carcinoma is second only to breast cancer in the world as the most common malignancy.[124] New cases in the United States occur annually at a rate of 15,700, with 4,900 deaths each year, and it is particularly a disease of disadvantaged women. A National Institutes of Health (NIH) Consensus panel of experts found that women over 65, uninsured women, ethnic minorities, and poor and rural women have low screening rates and high cervical cancer rates. Additionally, about half the women diagnosed with cervical cancer have never had a Pap smear, and another 10 percent have not had one in 5 years.[124,125] The fact that cervical cancer is a major solid tumor that is virally induced in nearly all cases by human papillomavirus (HPV) DNA is unique.[124] Of the more than 70 types of HPV identified, 23 have been found to infect the cervix, half of these are associated with squamous intraepithelial lesions (SIL) or invasive cervical cancer, and the most common types (16, 18, 31, and 45) account for more than 80 percent of all invasive cancers of the cervix.[124]

Thirty-three percent of SIL lesions regress; 41 percent stay the same; and 25 percent become more advanced. Ten percent of these latter lesions become carcinoma in situ (CIS); one percent become invasive. Viral transmission is through sexual intercourse, with the prevalence decreasing with age. The peak incidence is between 22–25 years. Thus, a host immune response may occur, and this knowledge is fueling efforts to find preventive and curative vaccines.[124,126]

Because it has a long preclinical phase, squamous cervical cancer is ideal for screening.[124] The Pap smear definitely has reduced both morbidity and mortality. Additionally, the Pap smear can identify some infections of the cervix and vagina, but other more definitive tests are needed for diagnosis (see Chapter 11). Also, the Pap smear may be used to evaluate the hormonal status of squamous cells, but modern serum hormone levels are more precise.[127] Vaginal pool specimens are no longer considered useful. It is essential to know the reliability of the laboratory that reads the Pap smear; false negative reports may range from 6 to 50 percent.[128] The incidence of false negative reports declines with successive smears, so that the more negatives a person has, the more likely it is to be real. Also, false positives do occur, thus repeat Pap smears that are negative can be reassuring to clients.

Technique

To obtain the best possible specimen, be precise. It is essential to get samples from the transformation zone (the squamocolumnar junction), the usual site of abnormal changes (see Figure 5–1). Sampling error accounts for false negative smears as a major factor.[129] Be sure that the entire cervix is visible. Use the endocervical cytobrush instead of a cotton tipped applicator, and the plastic spatula instead of a wooden spatula; the cotton tipped applicator and wooden spatula may hold the best cells in porous material. The endocervical brush increases the endocervical cells obtained by seven-fold.[130] If a cotton tipped applicator must be used, wet in normal saline first so that the cells will be released from the fibers onto the slide. The brush may be used for the pregnant woman but warn her that spotting may occur; in fact, this is true for many nonpreg-

nant women. Do not use the long pointed end of the spatula in pregnancy. Be sure all slides are labeled correctly with name, date, source, and that the slides match the paperwork.

Steps in obtaining the Pap smear sample include the following:[129]

- Collect *before* the bimanual.
- *No* lubricant should be used on the speculum; will interfere with cytology. Water is acceptable.
- Collect the Pap smear *before* other tests, such as GC and chlamydia tests. This order of collection is clearly supported by ACOG; the rationale is to ensure the best sample with suspicious cells for the Pap smear.
- If a wet mount is to be done, collect the specimen from the vaginal fornices before the Pap or any test is done to avoid blood from the Pap.
- Remove large amounts of discharge from the portio of the cervix gently before taking smears.
- Do not take the sample if large amounts of menses are present; will obscure cytologic field.
- Obtain portio sample first with the spatula, then the endocervical brush sample since bleeding occurs frequently with the latter.
- Rotate the brush gently to minimize bleeding if possible.
- Apply smear material evenly on the slide without clumping and fix rapidly (within 10 seconds); drying will significantly alter the sample. If using one slide, material must be collected very quickly to prevent drying effects. Ideally, two slides are desirable.
- Be sure to rotate brush or paint cells with spatula onto a slide with slight pressure.
- The squamocolumnar junction may be out on the ectocervix. If so, use the more rounded end of the spatula to collect cells.
- If the newer, fan-type implement is used to collect the squamocolumnar junction specimen, rotate it several times in the os to get an adequate number of cells.

Interpretation of Results and Action

The Bethesda System is the test reporting system now being used nationwide.[131] Precise terminology

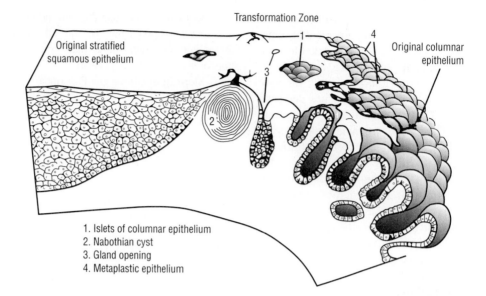

1. Islets of columnar epithelium
2. Nabothian cyst
3. Gland opening
4. Metaplastic epithelium

A

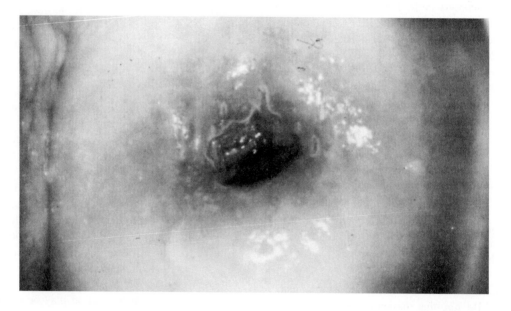

B

Figure 5–1. The transformation zone and the physiologic squamocolumnar junction. At birth, the squamocolumnar junction usually is located on the exocervix. Beginning in adolescence, it gradually migrates into the cervical canal as columnar epithelium, undergoes metaplasia, and matures into squamous epithelium. *A:* Schematic diagram. *B:* Colpophotograph of normal transformation zone. Note the squamocolumnar junction and gland openings. (Reproduced, with permission, from Burke L, Antonioli DA, Ducatman BS: *Colposcopy: Text and Atlas.* Appleton & Lange, 1991.)

tells the provider exactly what the findings are, eliminates traditional "class" groupings, includes a category "atypical squamous cells of undetermined significance" (ASCUS) to indicate the need for greater concern about atypia; includes HPV-associated changes with cervical intraepithelial neoplasia (CIN) 1 in a category called "low-grade squamous intraepithelial lesion" (LSIL); and places all the squamous cell carcinoma precursors (mild, moderate, severe dysplasia, and carcinoma

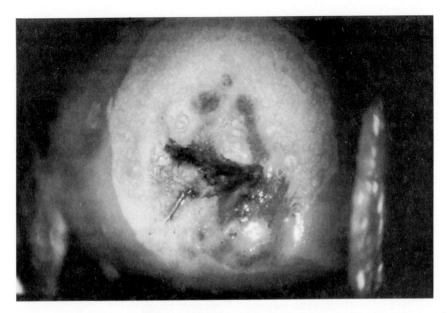

Figure 5–2. Colpophotograph after application of 3% acetic acid demonstrating acetowhitening and a mosaic vascular pattern. Biopsies revealed high-grade squamous intraepithelial lesions (HSIL). The broad area of dysplasia in this case is best treated with carbon dioxide laser vaporization rather than cryocautery. (Reproduced, with permission, from Burke L., Antonioli DA, Ducatman BS: *Colposcopy: Text and Atlas.* Appleton & Lange, 1991.)

in situ (CIS)) in the high-grade squamous intraepithelial lesion (HSIL) category (see Figures 5–2 and 5–3). Because the Pap smear does not yield a full thickness specimen, the entire thickness of the basement membrane cannot be examined with this method of testing. Thus, 25 to 77 percent of the women with atypia on Pap smear have been reported to have CIN that is not identified.[132] The guidelines in Table 5–12 are presented for interpretation and follow-up of report results.[124,129,133–137]

Pregnant women with atypia or dysplasia are referred for colposcopy. Generally, biopsy, diagnosis, and treatment are delayed until after pregnancy, unless a highly suspicious lesion is present.

Follow-Up after Treatment of Abnormal Pap Smear

Following treatment for an abnormal Pap smear, repeat Paps should be done every 4–6 months until one year of negative tests is obtained and annually thereafter as long as the results are normal.

It is important to wait at least 8 weeks between Paps or after treatment to allow for healing and more accurate results.[129] In one investigation of relevant probabilities, researchers studied the probability of invasive cervical cancer in women who had a repeat smear for ASCUS at 6 months versus those who were immediately referred for colposcopy and biopsy. They found that waiting to repeat the Pap smear was not likely to result in detectable increase in cancer.[138]

A National Cancer Institute (NCI) study is in progress currently to determine if women with mild cervical changes (ASCUS or LSIL) can safely wait longer before having colposcopy as well as to see which types of HPV infected cells will progress to HSIL versus reverting to normal. The use of automated, computerized systems, like PAPNET, as "double-checks" (see next section) will further increase numbers of women who must decide what to do after receiving a questionable Pap report. The NCI study results will provide more definitive guidance. See the Limited Bibliography for further references and issues related to the Pap smear.

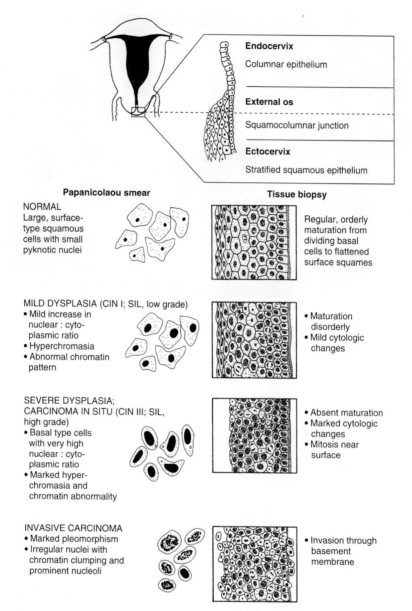

Figure 5–3. Squamous epithelial dysplasia and carcinoma of the cervix, showing criteria used to grade dysplasia. (Reproduced, with permission, from Chandrasoma P, Taylor CR: *Concise Pathology.* Appleton & Lange, 1991.)

Automated and Semiautomated Screening Tests

Concern over problems with the Pap test has led to development of automated and semiautomated cytologic screening systems.[139] Two such systems, PAPNET and NEOPATH, are being used as a back-up for the Pap smear evaluation by some laboratories. They utilize computers to recheck for abnormal cells and point them out. Both are FDA approved. The company marketing PAPNET claims it increases abnormal cell detection by up to 30 percent over regular Pap screening. Women can request one of these automated back-up tests but need to understand that an extra cost will be incurred. These tests are not yet available in all labs.

TABLE 5–12. PAP SMEAR REPORT RESULTS, INTERPRETATION, AND ACTION

Report Result	Interpretation	Action
Within normal limits (WNL); satisfactory for evaluation.	No abnormalities seen; specimen adequate.	Repeat in one year.
Within normal limits (WNL); satisfactory for evaluation, but limited by . . . (reason specified).	No abnormalities seen, but some problem exists such as insufficient endocervical or epithelial cells.	Repeat in one year if no known risks and 3 past Pap smears within normal limits. Consider repeating endocervical Pap at client's convenience if she is at high risk.
Unsatisfactory for evaluation.	No diagnosis is provided.	Repeat in 2–3 months.
Benign cellular changes: —Infection	Type of infection will be identified on the report. Make definitive diagnosis with appropriate test(s). Offer therapy.	Repeat in one year.
Reactive changes associated with the following: —Inflammation	Offer testing if not recently done; may be associated with infections such as gonorrhea or chlamydia; treat if indicated by follow-up.	Repeat 4–6 months; if repeat shows inflammation, refer for colposcopy. (Some institutions do not refer for colposcopy for inflammation only.)
—Atrophy with inflammation	Common in postmenopause. Offer hormone therapy.	Repeat Pap in 2–3 months.
—Intrauterine device	Normal finding in IUD users.	No therapy indicated; repeat Pap in one year.
Epithelial changes: —Atypical squamous cells of undetermined significance (ASCUS)	Will be qualified as favoring a reactive or premalignant/malignant process. ASCUS/premalignant is considered significant and if high risk factors present, refer for colposcopy and biopsy. High risk factors include HPV, HIV, smoking, multiple sexual partners.	If ASCUS/reactive, treat any specific infections and repeat in 3–6 months. Refer for colposcopy if 2 or more ASCUS reports within 18 months; biopsy suspicious lesions.
—Low-grade SIL	Includes HPV, mild dysplasia (i.e., koilocytes and CIN I). If woman unreliable or high risk, refer for colposcopy and biopsy initially.	If woman reliable and low risk, repeat Pap in 4–6 months. After 3 negative Paps, annual Paps indicated. Colposcopy indicated if abnormality persists. (Some institutions refer for colposcopy with an initial low-grade SIL.)
—High-grade SIL	Includes moderate and severe dysplasia (CIN II and III) and carcinoma in situ (CIS).	Refer for colposcopy and biopsy.
Glandular changes: —Endometrial cells in postmenopausal woman	May be benign; may be due to hyperplasia or malignancy.	Repeat Pap in 2–3 months; if same, refer for assessment of endocervical canal and endometrium.
—Atypical glandular cells of undetermined significance (AGCUS)	May be due to premalignant change.	Refer for endocervical canal/endometrial assessment.
—Adenocarcinoma	Specificity is high for endocervical or endometrial adenocarcinoma.	Refer to specialist for evaluation.

Source: References 124, 129, 133–138.

Other Screening Tests Being Studied

Several other screening tests are being studied. Please see the addendum at the end of this chapter for a brief summary of these tests.

GONORRHEA CULTURE

Purpose

A gonorrhea culture is done to diagnose *Neisseria gonorrhoeae* diplococci.

Technique

Obtain specimen for culture from each potential site (endocervix, urethra, Bartholin glands, Skene's ducts, rectum, pharynx, or conjunctivae) separately and label. For endocervical specimen (primary site in women; urethra secondary site),[140] gently remove excess mucus from the portio of the cervix. Insert sterile cotton tipped (some recommend synthetic tip over cotton) applicator 0.5 cm into os; rotate half turn; wait 10–30 seconds. Roll applicator onto Thayer-Martin (TM) medium in Z pattern, making slight impression in medium. Medium must be at room temperature. Place in carbon dioxide (CO_2) environment within 15 minutes. Keep bottles upright to prevent CO_2 from leaking out. Obtain GC sample after Pap smear if Pap is being taken.[129] Culture plates, if used, as well as TM medium should be brought to room temperature before inoculation. Most culture plates come with a carbon dioxide tablet that is placed in a well in the plate. The plate is sealed in a plastic bag to exclude oxygen.

Endocervical culture using selective media is the mainstay for diagnosis for women.[140] Sensitivity is about 80–90 percent. Gram-stained slides should be used only for immediate laboratory information with symptomatic women, but the culture should still be done. Gram-stained slides have 50–70 percent sensitivity and 97 percent specificity. Use of gram-stain allows more women to be treated during initial visit.

Direct fluorescent antibody tests are available and are sensitive and specific. Specimens are collected with a swab as with culture techniques. The same specimen may be tested for Chlamydia if need be. Results are available the same day.

Results

Positive test indicates need for treatment (see Chapter 11).

CHLAMYDIA TRACHOMATIS TESTS

Purpose

The tests are carried out to diagnose *Chlamydia trachomatis* intracellular parasite.

Technique

Definitive diagnosis is done by McCoy cell culture, but this is costly and requires substantial time. See Chapter 11, page 276 for directions. Several types of nonculture tests are available, including the following:

- *Enzyme-linked immunoassay (ELISA).* Insert a specially provided swab 0.5 cm into the cervical os; rotate vigorously; place in a tube with transport medium; and send for analysis by spectrophotometer. Has 90 percent sensitivity and 97 percent specificity with high risk populations.[140]
- *Monoclonal antibody test.* Insert an endocervical brush 0.5 cm into the cervical os; rotate vigorously; roll onto designated portion of specially provided slide and allow to dry; apply fixative and allow to dry; send for analysis. The slide is read by a medical technologist. Sensitivity in high risk populations is 89 percent; specificity 98 percent.[140] The sensitivity in low risk groups is 70 percent; specificity is 98 percent.
- *Amplified DNA diagnostic system.* Uses swab; uses highly sensitive ligase chain reaction technology.[141] Samples can be from urine or endocervix or urethra. Detected 30 percent more cases than culture in clinical studies. Results are possible in 3 hours. Tests for GC, TB, HPV, and pneumonia being developed for system.
- *Other.* A number of rapid tests are being marketed for office use. Check sensitivity and specificity for effective use with the population being screened.

Results

Positive report indicates need for treatment (see Chapter 11). Since available laboratory tests have a less than 100 percent sensitivity, false negative tests do occur. Similarly with specificity, false positive tests are possible.[140]

WET MOUNTS. NORMAL SALINE AND POTASSIUM HYDROXIDE

Purpose

Wet mounts are done to diagnose selected vaginal infections and to assist in determining causes of bleeding. A normal saline wet mount of vaginal secretions from a normal childbearing age non-pregnant woman shows lactobacilli and epithelial cells.

Technique

Wear gloves while handling specimens. Dip cotton swab into vaginal/cervical discharge; place in tube with 1 ml saline; mix; drop one drop on clean slide and cover with coverslip. Dip second swab into discharge; place in tube with 1 mL of 10 percent potassium hydroxide (KOH) and mix; drop one drop on clean slide or same slide at other end; cover. Blue or green food dye may be added to enhance visibility of organisms/cells. Evaluate with low and high power microscope objectives. The value of the specimen is proportional to the effectiveness of the collection techniques and the quality of the provider's interpretation. Vaginal/cervical discharge specimen may also be placed directly on a slide with a drop of solution, rather than placed in a tube, and covered with a coverslip for viewing. KOH is used to disrupt the epithelial cells (though not totally destroyed); gets rid of debris that may obscure hyphae and bacteria that are resistant to KOH and easily seen.[142]

Results

Clue cells indicate the occurrence of bacterial vaginosis (abundant coccoid bacilli and no white blood cells will be seen in fluid); spores and/or hyphae, leukocytes indicate fungal infection; motile protozoa, leukocytes indicate trichomoniasis vaginitis; leukocytosis (leukocytes in greater number than epithelial cells) indicates infections such as gonorrhea, chlamydia.[143,144] Excessive lactobacilli in epithelial cells indicate overgrowth and acidic vaginitis. Red blood cells indicate obvious or microscopic bleeding. (Because bleeding may be induced by examiner, wet mount specimens may be obtained before Pap and cultures; however, care must be taken not to take cells needed for Pap smear.) A greenish-yellow vaginal/cervical discharge on white background of cotton tipped swab indicates presence of bacterial infection. (See Chapter 11 for more details on STD and vaginitis diagnosis, as well as illustrations of findings microscopically, Figures 11–1, 11–2, 11–3, and 11–4.) Providers who use vaginal microscopy for diagnosis should gain depth in this area through special study.

Evaluating Vaginal pH

Purpose. A pH level of 3.8 to 4.2 is normal in the vagina and must be maintained to help keep the vaginal environment stable.[145] Lactobacillus acidophilus bacteria keep the vaginal ecosystem healthy by production of lactic acid that suppresses Gram-negative and Gram-positive anaerobes. Lactobacilli also produce toxic-to-anaerobes hydrogen peroxide. If the lactobacilli growth is suppressed, pH level rises, hydrogen ion concentration falls, and pathogen growth is favored. Testing pH level helps in determining imbalances.

Technique and Results

Special pH paper is placed on the lateral vaginal wall or in vaginal secretions. If the pH is >4.5, an increase in Gram-negative facultative anaerobes and Gram-positive and Gram-negative obligate anaerobes is the probable cause, as is seen with bacterial vaginosis.[145] Placing a drop of vaginal discharge in a drop of 10 percent potassium hydroxide (KOH) gives off a fishy odor as amines are released. This is called a positive whiff test and indicates possible clue cells or trichomonads.

URINALYSIS

Purpose

A urinalysis provides supportive data in diagnosing urinary complaints; however, it should not be used alone if results are negative but other findings indicate that a problem exists. A good portion of women with acute UTIs have as few as 100 colonies of causative bacteria.[146] Also, there may be up to 4 organisms causing the infection. Thus, the combination of symptoms, pyuria on urinalysis, and colony counts of at least 10^2 bacteria/mL on urine culture defines acute bladder infection currently.[147]

Technique

Instruct the client to wash her hands well and collect a midstream urine specimen. A clean-catch specimen is not necessary. Studies indicate that a midstream collection is adequate.[148] Use a tampon or cotton ball in the introitus during collection of urine if heavy vaginal discharge or bleeding is present. Test or culture the specimen within a few minutes, or refrigerate it with a tight cover and test within a few hours.

- If screening for nitrite and normal pH, a dipstick test is done on a first morning urine specimen. Keep dipsticks in cool, dark, tightly closed container. Assess glucose, ketones, blood, leukocytes, protein, and specific gravity.
- Microscopic examination should be done on centrifuged sediment, or a specimen may be sent out for analysis. Look for white blood cells (WBCs, or leukocytes) red blood cells (RBCs, or erythrocytes), crystals, bacteria, epithelial cells, and casts. Use low light to see casts better.
- Culture and sensitivity tests are indicated when the number of WBCs is greater than 5 per high power field or when Microstix indicates infection.

Results

All findings should be within normal limits (see standard laboratory testing text or manual).

HERPES CULTURE

Purpose

Culture is done to definitively diagnose herpes simplex genitalis. (See Chapter 11, pages 280 to 281 for more information.)

Technique

Wear goggles to protect eyes and cover unclothed skin with a mask, gloves, gown, and/or lab coat. Carefully puncture (unroof) intact vesicle with sterile tuberculin needle or rub open lesion vigorously (if vesicle already draining) with saline moistened Dacron tipped or cotton swab to get viral sample. Vesicular fluid is needed for testing; it is high in viral particles. Place specimen in culture medium immediately.[149] Do not swab to dry. If obtaining a cervical culture, the swab is inserted in the endocervix and rotated, then rubbed over the ectocervix. Refrigerate and transport within 12 hours or follow directions for transport and storage. Drainage from new lesions (those that have developed within 24 to 48 hours) can be applied to a glass slide and prepared as for Pap testing or other cytology staining for direct identification of multinucleated giant cells with intranuclear inclusions (called Tzanck smear). Culture is expensive and takes more time than Tzanck. The rapid monoclonal antibody test, employing immunoperoxidase staining or direct immunofluorescence cytology is inexpensive and is gaining popularity as the test of choice. Other methods include immunologic, electron microscope, and DNA hybridization.

Results

Positive growth of type 1 or type 2 herpes simplex virus (HSV) takes 2–3 days for results, but laboratories wait 7–14 days to be sure results are negative.[149] Identification of giant cells are highly reliable for diagnosis if seen on cytological examination.

SENSITIVITY, SPECIFICITY, AND PREDICTIVE VALUE OF TESTS[150]

Clinicians must understand the concepts of sensitivity, specificity, and predictive value to use and interpret test results effectively. The Bluestein and Archer reference is highly recommended to readers.

Sensitivity is the percentage of people who have a positive test who have the disease or condition. A sensitive test is used when the goal is to detect all people with the disease because undetection consequences can be disastrous. An example is the initial ELISA test for HIV antibodies. The test is to miss the lowest number of those exposed to the virus, though some nonexposed are expected to have a positive test.

Specificity is the percentage of people with no disease who have a negative test. It takes the number of people without disease and a negative test and divides it by the total number of nondiseased people. An example is the Western Blot test, which is very specific for HIV antibodies and is quite unlikely to be positive if HIV antibodies are absent.

Predictive value helps predict disease status. Positive predictive value (PV+) is the probability of disease if a test is positive, and negative predictive value (PV−) is the probability if the test is negative. The predictive value of a test utilizes disease prevalence in a particular site along with sensitivity and specificity. For example, a positive ELISA is more likely to be a false positive result in a setting where prevalence of disease is low.

Addendum on Other Cervical Screening Tests[151,152,153]

A test called ThinPrep 2000 by Cytyc is available. This test cleans the specimens for the Pap smear by filtering any blood, mucus, and debris before the cells are put on the slide. The specimen is collected by the provider and put into a preservative vial. The filtering process occurs at the laboratory by machine by the technician. Initial studies indicate less smudge on the slides than with the traditional Pap technique. The detection rate is the same. This method will be one used if automated slide review becomes a primary system of review.

A technique called cerviography in which high quality cervical photographs are taken may be useful for high risk populations who do not have colposcopy available to them, such as in remote areas of the country. This method has a high false positive rate, however, that may lead to unnecessary colposcopy.

Speculoscopy requires application of a dilute acetic acid solution to the cervix after the Pap smear is taken. The cervix is then viewed with a 5-power binocular or monocular magnification. This method is not a replacement for colposcopy, and is not approved as an adjunct to screening for cervical cancer at this time. The FDA has only approved it as safe, not for anything more.

REFERENCES

1. Pender, N. J. (1996). *Health promotion in nursing practice* (3rd. ed). Stamford, CT: Appleton & Lange.
2. *Healthy People 2000:* National health promotion and disease prevention objectives. (1990). Washington, DC: U.S. Public Health Service.
3. Burns, C. M. (1994). Toward Healthy People 2000: The role of the nurse practitioner and health promotion. *Journal of the American Academy of Nurse Practitioners, 6*(1), 29–35.
4. Bottorff, J. L., Johnson, J. L., Ratner, P. A., & Hayduk, L. A. (1996). The effects of cognitive-perceptual factors on health promotion behavior maintenance. *Nursing Research, 45*(1), 30–36.
5. Health results "not enough." (1995, April 12). *Richmond Times-Dispatch,* p. A10.
6. U.S. Bureau of the Census. (1995). Selected life table values: 1979 to 1992 (No. 115). *Statistical abstracts of the United States, 1995* (115th ed.). Washington, DC: U.S. Government Printing Office.
7. U.S. Bureau of the Census. (1995). Deaths, by selected cause and selected characteristics: 1992 (No. 126). *Statistical abstracts of the United States, 1995* (115th ed.). Washington, DC: U.S. Government Printing Office.
8. U.S. Bureau of the Census. (1995). Deaths from accidents and violence: 1990–1992 (No. 133). *Statistical abstracts of the United States, 1995* (115th ed.). Washington, DC: U.S. Government Printing Office.
9. Pinner, R. W., Teutsch, S. M., Simonsen, L., et al. (1996). Trends in infectious disease. *JAMA, 275*(3), 189–193.
10. Devesa, S., Blot, W., Stone, B., et al. (1995). Recent cancer trends in the United States. *JNCI, 87*(3), 175–182.
11. Sells, C. W., & Blum, R. W. (1996). Morbidity and mortality among U.S. adolescents: An overview of data and trends. *American Journal of Public Health, 86*(4), 513–519.
12. Schnitzer, P. G., & Runyan, C. W. (1995). Injuries to women in the United States: An Overview. *Women & Health, 23*(1), 9–27.
13. U.S. Bureau of the Census. (1995). Death rates by selected causes and age: 1980–1992. (No. 128). *Statistical abstracts of the United States, 1995* (115th ed.). Washington, DC: U.S. Government Printing Office.
14. National Center for Health Statistics. (1995). Age-adjusted cancer incidence rates for selected sites, according to sex and race: Selected geographical areas, selected years 1973–1991.

(No. 60). Health United States 1994, U.S. Department of Health and Human Services (DHHS Publication No. PHS 95-1232). Hyattsville, MD.

15. National Center for Health Statistics. (1995). Death rates for motor vehicle crashes, according to sex, detailed race, Hispanic origin, and age: United States, selected years 1950–1992 (No. 46). Health United States 1994, U.S. Department of Health and Human Services (DHHS Publication No. PHS 95-1232). Hyattsville, MD.

16. National Center for Health Statistics. (1995). Death rates for human immunodeficiency virus (HIV) infection, according to sex, detailed race, Hispanic origin, and age: United States, selected years 1987–1992 (No. 44). Health United States 1994, U.S. Department of Health and Human Services (DHHS Publication No. PHS 95-1232). Hyattsville, MD.

17. Bush, R. W. (1995). HIV infection. In D. Lemcke, J. Pattison, L. Marshall, & D. Cowliey (Eds.), *Primary care of women.* Norwalk, CT: Appleton & Lange.

18. National Center for Health Statistics. (1995). Leading causes of death and number of deaths, according to sex, detailed race, and Hispanic origin: United States, selected years 1980–1992 (No. 33). Health United States 1994, U.S. Department of Health and Human Services (DHHS Publication No. PHS 95-1232). Hyattsville, MD.

19. National Center for Health Statistics. (1995). Maternal morbidity rates for complications of pregnancy, childbirth, and the puerperium, according to race and age: United States, selected years 1950–1992 (No. 45). Health United States 1994, U.S. Department of Health and Human Services (DHHS Publication No. PHS 95-1232). Hyattsville, MD.

20. Horton, J. A. (1995). *The women's health data book: A profile of women's health in the United States.* (2nd Ed.). Washington, DC: Jacob's Institute for Women's Health.

21. U.S. Bureau of the Census. (1995). Death rates from cancer, by sex and age: 1970–1992 (No. 132). *Statistical abstracts of the United States, 1995* (115th ed.). Washington, DC: U.S. Government Printing Office.

22. Screening tests and cancer deaths. (1996). *Harvard Women's Health Watch, 3*(8), 7.

23. U.S. Bureau of the Census. (1995). Deaths by age and leading cause: 1992 (No. 127). *Statistical abstracts of the United States, 1995* (115th ed.). Washington, DC: U.S. Government Printing Office.

24. Colon cancer: Good news. 1994, September. *Harvard Women's Health Watch,* 7. Citing *The Journal National Cancer Institute,* July 6, 1994.

25. U.S. Bureau of the Census. (1995). Death rates from heart disease, by sex and age: 1970–1992 (No. 131). *Statistical abstracts of the United States, 1995* (115th ed.). Washington, DC: U.S. Government Printing Office.

26. Cardiovascular update for women, 1994, July 11. Issues in women's health, *ACOG News Release,* 1.

27. U.S. Bureau of the Census. (1995). Acute conditions by type: 1970–1993 (No. 214). *Statistical abstracts of the United States, 1995* (115th ed.). Washington, DC: U.S. Government Printing Office.

28. U.S. Bureau of the Census. (1995). Prevalence of selected reported chronic conditions, by age and sex: 1980–1993 (No. 215). *Statistical abstracts of the United States, 1995* (115th ed.). Washington, DC: U.S. Government Printing Office.

29. Healy, B. P. (1992). The women's health initiative. *Female Patient, 17,* 36–38.

30. Rigotti, N., & Polivogianis, L. (1995). In J. Carlson, S. Eisenstat, F. Frigoletto, & I. Schiff (Eds.), *Primary care of women.* St. Louis: Mosby.

31. Glantz, S., & Parmley, W. (1995). Passive smoking and heart disease: Mechanisms and risk. *JAMA, 273*(13), 1047–1053.

32. Kahan, M. (1996). Identifying and managing problem drinkers. *Canadian Family Physician, 42,* 661–671.

33. Schaumburg, H., Kaplan, J., Windebark, A., Vick, N., Rasmus, S., Pleasure, D., & Brown, M. (1983). Sensory neuropathy from pyridoxine abuse. *New England Journal of Nursing, 309,* 445–448.

34. Powell, K. E., Caspesen, C. J., Koplan, J. P., & Ford, E. S. (1989). Physical activity and chronic disease. *Am J Clin Nutrition.*

35. Manson, J. A., Stampfer, M. J., Willett, W.C., Rosner, B., Monson, R. R., Speizer, F. E., & Nennekens, C. H. (1990). A prospective study of obesity and risk of coronary heart disease in women. *New England Journal of Medicine, 322,* 882–889.

36. Eating disorders. (1994). In *Diagnostic and statistical manual of mental disorders* (4th ed.). Washington, DC: American Psychiatric Association.

37. Cope, K. A. (1994). Nutritional status: A basic "vital sign." *Home Health Care, 12*(2) 39–34.

38. Orndoff, B. (1995, March 29). Early diet linked to risk of cancer. *Richmond Times-Dispatch,* p. A9.

39. Manson, J. E., Willett, W. C., & Stampfer, M. J. (1995). Body weight and mortality among women. *NEJM, 333,* 677–685.

40. Lanman, G. (1995). Safety and accident prevention. In K. Carlson, S. Eisenstat, F. Frigoletto, & I. Schiff (Eds.), Primary care of women. St. Louis: Mosby.

41. Eisenstat, S. (1995). Domestic violence. In K. Carlson, S. Eisenstat, F. Frigoletto, & I. Schiff (Eds.), Primary care of women. St. Louis: Mosby.

42. McLeer, S., & Anwar, R. (1989). A study of battered women presenting in an emergency department. *AJ Public Health, 79,* 65–66.

43. McFarlane, J., Parker, B., Soeken, K., & Bullock, L. (1992). Assessing for abuse during pregnancy: Severity and frequency of injuries and associated entry into prenatal care. *JAMA, 267*(23), 3176–3178.

44. Sugg, N. (1995). Domestic Violence. In D. Lemcke, J. Pattison, L. Marshall, & A. Cowley (Eds.), *Primary care of women.* Norwalk, CT: Appleton & Lange.

45. Trends in STDs in the United States: Epidemiological synergy. (1994, May). In *Association of Preproductive Health Professionals Clinical Proceedings.* Washington, DC: ARHP.

46. Youngkin, E. (1995). Sexually transmitted diseases: Current and emerging concerns. *JOGNN, 24*(8), 743–758.

47. What's happening. (1996). Demographic predictors of clinical breast examination, mammography, and Pap test screening among older women. *J Am Ac NP, 8*(5), 231–236.

48. Watson, M. A., Feldman, K. W., Sugar, N. F., et al. (1996). Inadequate history as a barrier to immunization. *Arch Pediatric Adolescent Medicine, 150,* 135–139.

49. Ware, J. C., Director, Sleep Disorders Centre, Eastern Virginia Medical School and Sentera Norfolk General Hospital, Norfolk, VA. Telephone interview regarding differences in sleep patterns between sexes and relationship to longevity, November 24, 1993.

50. Leiss, J., & Savitz, D. (1995). Home pesticide use and childhood cancer. *Am J Public Health, 85*(2), 249–252.

51. Lazarus, R. S. (1981, July). Little hassles can be hazardous to health. *Psychology Today,* 59–62.

52. Auslander, G. K. (1988). Social networks and the functional health status of the poor: A secondary analysis of data from the national survey of personal health practices and consequences. *Journal of Community Health, 13,* 197–209.

53. Silverstein, M., & Waite, L. (1993). Are blacks more likely than whites to receive and provide social support in middle and old age? Yes, no, and maybe so. *J Gerontol, 48* (4), 5121–5222.

54. ACOG Technical Bulletin. (1992). *Depression in women* (No. 182). Washington, DC: ACOG.

55. NIH Consensus Development Conference. (1991). *Diagnosis and treatment of depression in later life 9*(3). Bethesda, MD: U.S. Department of HHS, PHS.

56. Guillen, E., & Barr, S. (1994). Nutrition, dieting, and fitness messages in a magazine for adolescent women, 1970–1990. *J Adolesc Health, 15,* 464–472.

57. Mason, J. (1996, June 3). Poverty more than welfare ill. *Richmond Times-Dispatch,* pp. B1, B5.

58. Berk, M. L., Albers, L. A., & Schur, C. L. (1996). The growth in the US uninsured population: Trends in Hispanic subgroups, 1977–1992. *AJPH, 86*(4), 572–576.

59. de la Torre, A., Friis, R., Hunter, H. R., and Garcia, L. (1996). The health insurance status of the US Latina women: A profile from the 1982–1984 HHANES. *AJPH, 86*(4), 533–537.

60. Himmelstein, D. U., Lewontin, J. P., & Woolhandler, S. (1996). Medical care employment in the United States, 1968–1993: The importance of health section jobs for African Americans and women. *AJPH, 86*(4), 525–528.

61. Morton, P. G. (1993). *Health assessment* (2nd ed.). Springhouse, PA: Springhouse.

62. Bates, B. (1995). *A guide to physical examination and history taking* (6th ed.). New York: Lippincott.

63. Seidel, H. M., Ball, J. W., Davis, J. E., & Benedict, G. W. (1995). *Mosby's guide to physical examination* (3rd ed.). St. Louis: Mosby Year Book.

64. Jarvis, C. (1996). *Physical examination and health assessment* (2nd ed.). Philadelphia: W.B. Saunders.

65. Eliopoulos, C. (1990). *Health assessment of the older adult* (2nd ed.). Redwood City, CA: Addison-Wesley Nursing.

66. Downs, H. (1996, June 30). The complete medical checkup: What you need to know. *Parade Magazine,* 4–5.

67. Johnson, C. (1996). Immunizations for adolescents and adults. In C. Johnson, B. Johnson, J. Murray, & B. Apgar (Eds.), *Women's health handbook.* Philadelphia: Hanley & Belfus; St. Louis: Mosby.

68. Gall, S. (1995). Making immunizations a priority for adults and adolescents. *Contemporary Nurse Practitioner, 1*(6), 17–27.

69. Vaccination against influenza in healthy adults. (1996). To the editor. *NEJM, 334*(6), 402–404.

70. Sawin, K., & Harrigan, M. (1995). *Measures of family functioning for research and practice.* New York: Springer Publishing.

71. Visscher, E., & Clore, E. (1992). The genogram: a strategy for assessment. *J Ped Health Care, 6*(6), 361–367.

72. U.S. Department of Agriculture. (August, 1992). *Food guide pyramid.* Pueblo, CO: Consumer Information Center, Department 159-Y.

73. Gutierrez, Y. (1994). *Nutrition in health mainte-nance and health promotion for primary care providers.* San Francisco: University of Califor-nia, School of Nursing.

74. Expert Panel on Detection, Evaluation, and Treatment of High Blood Cholesterol in Adults. (1993). Summary of the 2nd report of the Na-tional Cholesterol Education Program (NCEP) Expert Panel on detection, evaluation, and treat-ment of high blood cholesterol in adults. *JAMA, 269*(23), 3015–3023.

75. ACOG. (1996, May). FDA orders food fortifica-tion with folic acid. *ACOG Newsletter, 46*(5), 1–2.

76. *Optimal daily calcium intake.* (1994). National Institutes of Health Consensus Panel on Opti-mum Calcium Intake.

77. AAFP, ADA, & NCOA. (1994). *Incorporating nutrition screening and interventions into medical practice: A monograph for physicians.* Washing-ton, DC: The Nutrition Screening Initiative.

78. Phaneuf, C. (1996). Screening elders for nutri-tional deficits. *AJN, 96*(3), 58–60.

79. Willett, W., Manson, J., Stampfer, M., et al. (1995). Weight, weight change, and coronary heart disease in women. *JAMA, 273,* 461–465.

80. Star, W. L., Shannon, M. T., Samnors, L. N., Neeson, J. D., & Gutierrez, Y. (1992). *Ambula-tory obstetrics: Protocols for nurse practition-ers/nurse midwives.* San Francisco: University of California, School of Nursing.

81. Gerchufsky, M. (1996). How much is too much? Weighty questions. *ADVANCE for Nurse Practi-tioners, 4*(1), 17–19, 60.

82. Clinical guidelines. (1995). Body measurement. *NP, 20*(4), 65–66, 69.

83. Parkerson, G., Broadnead, W., & Tse, C. (1995). Perceived family stress as a predictor of health-related outcomes. *Archives of Family Medicine, 4,* 253–260.

84. Kanner, A., Cyne, J., Schaefer, C., & Lazarus, R. (1980). Comparison of two modes of stress man-agement: Daily hassles and uplifts versus major life events. *Journal of Behavioral Medicine, 4*(1), 1–35.

85. Holmes, T., & Rahe, R. (1967). The social read-justment rating scale. *Journal of Psychosomatic Research, 11,* 213.

86. Spielberger, C., Edwards, C., Lushene, R., et al. (1983). *Manual for state-trait anxiety inventory.* Palo Alto, CA: Consulting Psychologists Press, Inc.

87. Domar, A., & Dreher, H. (1996). *Healthy mind, healthy women: Using the mind-body connection to manage stress and take control of your health.* New York, NY: Henry Holt & Co.

88. Pate, R., Pratt, M., Blair, S., et al. (1995). Physi-cal activity and public health: A recommendation from the Centers for Disease Control and Pre-vention and the American College of Sports Medicine. *JAMA, 273*(5), 402–407.

89. Pronk, N., Crouse, S., O'Brien, B., & Rohack, J. (1995). Acute effects of walking on serum lipids and lipoproteins in women. *Journal of Sports Medicine and Physical Fitness, 35*(1), 50–57.

90. Binder, W., Birge, S., & Kohrt, W. (1996). Effects of endurance exercise and hormone replacement therapy on serum lipids in older women. *J Am Geriatr Soc, 44,* 231–236.

91. Grady, D. (1996). Exercise, hormone replace-ment therapy, and lipoprotein in women. *J Am Geriatr Soc, 44,* 331–332.

92. Blair, S., Kampert, J. Kohl II., H., et al. (1996). Influences of cardiopulmonary fitness and other precursors on cardiovascular disease and all-cause mortality in men and women. *JAMA, 276*(3), 205–210.

93. Dunn, M. M. (1987). Guidelines for an effective personal fitness prescription. *Nurse Practitioner, 12,* 9–10, 12, 14–16, 18, 23, 26.

94. Special Report. (1996, July). The best way to get fit after 40. *Prevention,* 65–73.

95. Fontham, E., Correa, P., Reynolds, P., et al. (1994). Environmental tobacco smoke and lung cancer in nonsmoking women. *JAMA, 27*(22), 1752–1759.

96. Keleher, K. C. (1991). Occupational health: How work environments can affect reproductive ca-pacity and outcome. *Nurse Practitioner, 16,* 23–37.

97. Twinings, S. (1995). The occupational and envi-ronmental health history: Guidelines for the pri-mary care nurse practitioner. *Nurse Practitioner Forum, 6*(2), 64–71.

98. Hahn, M. (1996). Search for Mr. Sandman. *AD-VANCE for Nurse Practitioners, 4*(5), 36–42.

99. Pressman, M., Figueroa, W., & Kendrick-Mohamed, J. (1996). A rarely recognized symp-tom of sleep apnea and other occult sleep disor-ders. *Archives of Internal Medicine, 156,* 545–550.

100. Strollo, P., & Rogers, R. (1996). Obstructive sleep apnea. *NEJM, 334*(2), 99–104.

101. Seaman, B. (1996, July/August). The scoop on sleep. *Modern Maturity,* 69–70.

102. Clinical guidelines. (1996). Adult cancer detec-tion screening by physical examination. *NP, 21*(3), 85–96.

103. Dumesic, D. (1996, January). Pelvic examina-tion: What to focus on in menopausal women. *Consultant,* 39–46.

104. Mulrow, C., Williams, Jr., J., Gerety, M., et al. (1995). Case-finding instrument for depression in primary care settings. *Ann Inter Med, 122,* 913–921.

105. Federici, C., & Tommasini, N. (1992). The assessment and management of panic disorder. *NP, 17*(3), 20, 22, 27–28, 31–32, 34.

106. Montano, C. B. (1994). Recognition and treatment of depression in a primary care setting. *J Clin Psychiatry, 55*(Supp. 12), 18–34.

107. STD Quarterly. (1995, June). Empower your patients by teaching genital self-exam. *Contraceptive Technology Update,* 73–74.

108. Clinical pearls. (1996, June). Easier cervical visualization. *Clinical Reviews, 49.*

109. Frover, S., & Quinn, M. (1995). Is there any value in bimanual pelvic examination as screening test? *Med J Australia, 162,* 408–410.

110. Allson, J., Tekawa, I., Ransom, M., & Adrain, A. (1996). A comparison of fecal occult-blood tests for colorectal-cancer screening. *NEJM, 334,* 155–159.

111. Speroff, L., Glass, R., & Kase, N. (1994). *Clinical gynecologic endocrinology and infertility* (5th ed.). Baltimore: Williams & Wilkins.

112. Murray, J. L. (1996). Preadolescent and adolescent health promotion and maintenance. In C. Johnson, B. Johnson, J. Murray, and B. Apgar (Eds.), *Women's health care handbook.* Philadelphia: Hanley & Belfus; St. Louis: Mosby.

113. Mattox, J. H. (1995). Disorders of menstruation. In V. Seltzer, & W. Pearse (Eds.), *Women's primary health care,* New York: McGraw-Hill, Inc.

114. Bates, G., & Blauer, K. (1995). Special needs of adolescents. In V. Seltzer, & W. Pearse (Eds.), *Women's primary health care.* New York: McGraw-Hill, Inc.

115. Varner, R., & Younger, J. (1995). Menopause. In V. Seltzer, & W. Pearse (Eds.), *Women's primary health care.* New York: McGraw-Hill, Inc.

116. *Preventive care guidelines for healthy women.* (1994). Clifton, NJ: Clinicians Publishing Group.

117. Clinical guidelines (1994). Mammography. *NP, 19*(11), 36–37.

118. ACOG Position on Mammography Screening. (1994, October 5). *ACOG News Release.* Washington, DC: Author.

119. What are the current recommendations for routine cancer screening in women? (1995). *AWHONN Voice, 3*(1), 6.

120. Dialogue. (1994). Colon cancer testing: What Kind? *University of California at Berkeley Wellness Letter, 10*(5), 5.

121. Speroff, L. (1992). *The routine gynecologic exam: How it changes as you age.* Published by Berlex Laboratories.

122. *Clinician's handbook of preventive services 1994.* Office of Disease Prevention and Health Promotion, Public Health Service, U.S. Department of Health and Human Services. Washington, DC: U.S. Government Printing Office.

123. Primary care preventive health care. (1992). *ACOG Final Task Report.* Washington, DC: ACOG.

124. National Institutes of Health Consensus Development Conference Statement: Cervical Cancer. (1996, April 1–3). Bethesda, MD.

125. Cervical cancer could be reduced through increased Pap testing. (1996). *ACOG Newsletter.* Washington, DC: *ACOG.*

126. Cervical cancer vaccine in trials. (1996, June 8), *The Pharmaceutical Journal, 256,* 781.

127. Pagana, K., & Pagana, T. (1995). *Mosby's diagnostic and laboratory test reference* (2nd ed.). St. Louis: Mosby.

128. Toffler, W. L., Pleudeman, C. K., Sinclair, A. E., Ireland, K. M., & Byrne, S. J. (1993). Comparative cytologic yield and quality of three Pap smear instruments. *Family Medicine, 25*(6), 403–407.

129. ACOG. (1993). Cervical cytology: Evaluation and management of abnormalities. *ACOG Technical Bulletin No. 183,* Washington, DC: ACOG.

130. Taylor, P. Jr., Andersen, W., Barber, S., et al. The screening Papanicolaou smear: Contribution of the endocervical brush. (1987). *Obstet Gynecol, 70,* 734–738.

131. Kurman, R. J., Malkasian, G. D., Sedlis, A., & Solomon, D. (1991). From Papanicolaou to Bethesda: The rationale for a new cervical cytologic classification. *Obstetrics & Gynecology, 77,* 779–781.

132. Soper, D. (1992, August 17). Presentation on Pap smears and HPV. Planned Parenthood of Richmond, VA.

133. Shingleton, H., Patrick, R., Johnston, W., & Smith, R. (1995). The current status of the Papanicolaou smear. *CA-A Cancer Journal for Clinicians, 45*(5), 315–319.

134. ACOG Criteria Set. (1995, April). *Ambulatory care criteria set: Atypical squamous cells of undetermined origin (ASCUS).* Washington, DC: ACOG.

135. ACOG Committee Opinion. (1995). *Absence of endocervical cells on a Pap test.* No. 153. Washington, DC: ACOG.

136. Classification and management of Pap smear results. (1994, October). Virginia League for Planned Parenthood Screening and Evaluation. Richmond, VA.

137. Nuovo, J., Melnikow, J., & Paliescheskey, M. (1995). Management of patients with atypical and low-grade Pap smear abnormalities. *Am Family Physician, 52*(8), 2243–2250.

138. Melnikow, J., Nuovo, J., & Paliescheskey, M. (1996). Management choices for Paps with "squamous atypia" on Papanicolaou smear. A toss up? *Medical Care, 34*(4), 336–347.

139. Slagel, D., Saleski, S., & Cohen, M. (1995). Efficacy of automated cytology screening. *Diag Cytopathol, 13*(1), 26–30.

140. ACOG Technical Bulletin. (1994). *Gonorrhea and chlamydial infections.* No. 190. Washington, DC: ACOG.

141. An amplified DNA diagnostic system for use with Chlamydia test. (1996). *Modern Medicine, 64,* 29.

142. Sommer, S. (1996, July). Consultation with Dr. Sommer, Associate Professor, Department of Medical Technology, Virginia Commonwealth University–Medical College of Virginia, Richmond, VA.

143. Freeman, S. (1995). Common genitourinary infections *JOGNN, 24*(8), 735–742.

144. Secor, M. (1994). Bacterial vaginosis: A common infection with serious sequelae. *ADVANCE for Nurse Practitioners, 2*(4), 11–16.

145. ACOG Technical Bulletin. (1996). *Vaginitis.* No. 226. Washington, DC: ACOG.

146. Barger, M., & Woolner, B. (1995). Primary care for women: Assessment and management of genitourinary tract disorders. *J Nurse, Midwifery, 40*(2), 231–245.

147. Elder, N. (1992). Acute urinary tract infection in women. *Postgrad Med, 92*(6), 159–166.

148. Leisure, M., Dudley, S., & Donowitz, L. (1993). Does a clean catch urine sample reduce bacterial contamination? *NEJM, 328*(4), 289–290.

149. Johnson, C. (1996). Genital herpes. In C. Johnson, B. Johnson, J. Murray, & B. Apgar (Eds.), *Women's health care handbook.* Philadelphia: Hanley & Belfus; St. Louis: Mosby.

150. Bluestein, D., & Archer, L. (1991). The sensitivity, specificity and predictive value of diagnostic information: A guide for clinicians. *NP, 16*(7), 39–45.

151. Two cervical cytologic tools approved. (1996). *ACOG Newsletter, 40*(8), 1,8,9.

152. Newest tools for cervical cytology and evaluation assessed. (1996). *ACOG Newsletter, 40*(8), 1,10.

153. Cervicography. (1993, April). ACOG Committee on Gynecologic Practice.

LIMITED BIBLIOGRAPHY

Centers for Disease Control and Prevention. (1996). Prevention of hepatitis A through active or passive immunization: Recommendations of the advising committee on immunization practices (ACIP). *MMWR, 45*(RR-15), 1–30.

Clinical Guidelines. (1997). Tetanus and diphtheria immunization/prophylaxis: Adults and older adults. *NP, 22*(3), 116–120.

Hefland, M., Marton, K. I., Simmer-Gembeck, M. J. et al. (1997). History of visible rectal bleeding in a primary care population. *JAMA, 277,* 44–48.

Korn, K. (1997). Computer comments: Today's health care news on the information superhighway. *JAANP, 9*(3), 141–142.

Leslie, M. & Mikanowicz, C. (1997). Assessment of body composition in the healthy adult. *JAANP, 9*(3), 123–127.

Mashburn, J. & Scharbo-DeHaan, M. (1997). A clinician's guide to Pap smear interpretation. *NP, 22*(4), 115–118, 124, 126–127, 130, 143.

McGill, H. C. Jr., McMahan, C. A., Malcom, G. T., et al. (1997). Effects of serum lipoproteins and smoking on atherosclerosis in young men and women. *Arterioscler Thromb Vasc Biol, 17,* 95–107.

Moser, D. K. (1997). Correcting misconceptions about women and heart disease. *AJN, 97*(4), 26–33.

Newman, A. B., Enright, P. L., Manolio, T. A., et al. (1997). Sleep disturbances, psychosocial correlates, and cardiovascular disease in 5201 older adults: The Cardiovascular Health Study. J *Am Geriatr Soc, 45,* 1–7.

Pursuing the Pap smear question. (1997, April). *Women's Health Watch, IV*(8), 1.

Ricchini, W. (1997). The antioxidant craze: Are vitamins the answer to good health? *Advance for Nurse Practitioners, 5*(4), 67–68.

Rorie, J. A., Paine, L. L., & Barger, M. K. (1996). Primary care of women: Cultural competence in primary care series. *J Nurse Midwifery, 41*(2), 92–100.

Youngkin, E. Q. & Israel, D. (1996). A review and critique of common herbal alternative therapies. *NP, 21*(10), 39–62.

CHAPTER 6

WOMEN
AND SEXUALITY

Catherine Ingram Fogel

Highlights

*P*athophysiological
causes of sexual
dysfunction are more
common than those that
are psychogenic; how-
ever, traumatic sexual
experiences, such as in-
cest and rape, may pre-
cipitate dysfunction.

- Dimensions of Sexuality
- Age Related Issues
- Illness Related Issues
- Sexual Problems and Dysfunction
- Sexual Health Care
- Sexual Assessment and History
- Interventions: PLISSIT Model

▶ INTRODUCTION

Sexuality is inextricably woven into the fabric of a woman's life and is an important aspect of her health. It is an integrated, unique expression of self that encompasses physiological and psychosocial processes inherent in sexual development, sexual response, sexual desire, view of self as a female including sexual orientation, and presentation of self to society as a woman.[1] Sexuality underlies much of who and what a person is, and it is an inherent, ever changing aspect of life from birth to death. It is expressed in different ways at different times—alone, with one partner, or with different partners.[2]

Although experts do not agree on a definition of sexual health or what constitutes normal sexual behavior, the World Health Organization definition provides a starting point: "Sexual health is the integration of somatic, emotional, intellectual, and social aspects of sexual beings in ways that are positively enriching and that enhance personality, communication and love."[3] Essential elements of this definition include a woman's capacity to live in a manner that is congruent with her personal and social ethic while enjoying and controlling sexual and reproductive behavior; the freedom from psychological factors such as guilt, anxiety, fear, shame, and misconceptions that impair sexual response and hurt sexual relationships; and the absence of disease, illness, organic disorders, or deficiencies that interfere with sexual function.[2] Integral to sexual health is an acceptance of one's self-concept, body image, sexual identity, and sexual orientation.

Sexual health is that emotional and physical state that allows enjoyment and the ability to respond to sexual feelings. In short, sexual health may be considered the physical and emotional state of well-being that enables us to enjoy and act on our sexual feelings.[4] Promoting sexual health is a legitimate role for health professionals and an essential nursing function. The nurse practitioner or other primary care provider can have a primary role in promoting and maintaining the sexual health of women.

Dimensions of sexuality

Sexuality is a broad concept that encompasses the dimensions of sexual desire, sexual response, view of self, sexual orientation, and presentation of self. Sexuality is a unique human quality that is an expression of a person's identity and a reflection of the basic need for emotional and physical closeness with another.[5] It is not limited by age, attractiveness, sexual orientation, or partner participation.[1]

SEXUAL DESIRE

Libido is the innate urge for sexual activity, produced by the activation of a specific system in the brain and experienced as a specific sensation that motivates a person to seek out or be receptive to sexual experience.[6] The amount of sexual desire experienced varies across a woman's life span and from woman to woman. Moreover, sexual desire is a response learned through feelings of pleasure, enjoyment, or dissatisfaction during sexual activity. Sexual desire derives from interest in sexual activity, preferred frequency of activity, and gender preference for a sexual partner.[1] Further, desire is influenced by one's health, past experiences, and/or cultural and environmental factors. Sexual desire has been incorporated into official diagnostic descriptions of the sexual response cycle[7] (see the following section for discussion).

SEXUAL RESPONSE CYCLE

The sexual response cycle may be divided into *capacity* (i.e., what a woman is able to experience) and *activity* (i.e., what she actually experiences). The two principal physiological responses to sexual stimulation are vasocongestion and myotonia. Vasocongestion corresponds to sexual excitement, as the tissues and blood vessels become engorged. Myotonia, an increase in muscle tension, peaks with orgasm.

Physiological Sexual Response Cycle (Masters and Johnson)

The most widely known approach for labeling and identifying the physiological response to sexual stimuli, this cycle has four phases: excitement, plateau, orgasm, and resolution.[8]

- *Excitement* is characterized by vaginal lubrication. This phase may develop from any bodily or psychic stimuli and may be interrupted, prolonged, or ended by distracting stimuli.
- *Plateau* is characterized by vaginal engorgement and clitoral retraction. This phase also may be interrupted by distracting stimuli.
- *Orgasm* is the peak of vasocongestion and myotonia released by involuntary climax.
- *Resolution* is characterized by bodily return to the preexcitement state. With adequate stimulation, a woman may again begin sexual response before complete resolution occurs.

Although these physiological changes are common to all women, not every woman experiences each response. Further, a woman may experience different aspects of response from cycle to cycle. And women experience the same sexual responses whether the stimulus is self-pleasuring, pleasuring from another women, from a man, or intercourse.[9]

Although the phases of sexual response are similar for men and women, three basic orgasmic patterns have been described for women and only one for men.[8,10] Further, women have the ability to experience multiple orgasms during a single sexual experience. Women experience single and multiple orgasms with sexual intercourse, masturbation, and petting.[10] Women have described three discrete stages in their orgasmic experiences: 1) intense clitoral awareness accompanied by a feeling of bearing down; 2) sensations of warmth that spread through the body; and 3) pelvic or uterine contractions followed by

pelvic throbbing.[5,8] Studies[11,12] suggest that women find orgasms occurring during masturbation to be more physically intense and more physically than psychologically satisfying than those associated with vaginal intercourse. Orgasms experienced during sexual intercourse have been reported to be more satisfying and less intense than those experienced during masturbation. All the women participating in these studies were orgasmic with masturbation, intercourse, and petting; however, the sexual orientation of the women was not reported or considered.

Questions have been raised about the existence of a Grafenberg or "G" spot and the occurrence of female ejaculation. Perry and Whipple[13] described the G-spot as a sexually sensitive area on the anterior wall of the vagina in the area of the urethra that responds to deep pressure and swells when stimulated. Additionally the release of vaginal fluid just prior to or during orgasm has been reported. Recent research documented that women do report having a fluid release at the moment of orgasm and awareness of a sensitive area in the vagina.[14] It is possible that this information could lead to more explicit anatomical information to assist women to more fully understand, explore, and enjoy their sexual responses.[5,15,16]

Women and men tend to report differences in body sensations of sexual pleasure. Women are more total body oriented for sexual touching and experience pleasurable, sexual sensations from their skin, whereas men are conditioned to be more genitally oriented. Women report high degrees of sensitivity from mouth or finger contact, whereas men commonly report intercourse to be the most pleasurable form of sexual stimulation.[8,17]

Recently, feminists have suggested that there is a need for an alternative to the prevailing genitocentric model of physiological arousal with orgasm as the only acceptable end response.[16] Chalker argues that a more inclusive model incorporating both biologic and psychosocial factors is necessary so that the element of consent is included.[15] Such models would place more emphasis on interaction between variations in an individual's emotional and spiritual dimensions, the sociocultural context in which sexual activity takes place, and the dynamics of relationships rather than solely on gender performance.[5,17]

American Psychiatric Association Sexual Response Cycle[7]

This well known approach that incorporates both biologic and psychological components is useful in categorizing sexual disorders.[7] It comprises four phases: appetitive, excitement, orgasm, and resolution.

- The *appetitive* phase is characterized by sexual fantasy and desire for sexual activity.
- *Excitement involves* pelvic vasocongestion with vaginal lubrication, swelling of external genitalia, narrowing of the lower third of the vagina, and lengthening of the upper two-thirds of the vagina, in addition to breast tumescence. Sensations of pleasure are experienced.
- *Orgasm* is the peaking of sexual pleasure followed by the release of sexual tension and rhythmic contractions of the perineal muscles, uterus, and in some women, the lower third of the vagina.
- *Resolution* is characterized by a sense of general relaxation and well-being.

VIEW OF SELF AS FEMALE

A woman's view of herself as female incorporates (a) concepts of gender identity (identification of self as female); (b) the sense of having characteristics customarily defined as female, masculine, or both; and (c) body image (a mental picture of one's body and its relationship to the environment).[1,19] Gender identity is influenced by biological sex although a person's gender identity is not necessarily consistent with her biological sex.[19]

PRESENTATION OF SELF AS A WOMAN

Gender role, or sex role, encompasses all attitudes and behaviors such as dress, hairstyle, speech pattern, and gait that are considered normal and appropriate for women in a specific culture.[19] These behaviors reflect a woman's internalization of sociocultural stereotypes and expectations of what a woman's behavior should be. Gender role proscriptions and expectations exert a strong influence on sexuality. Beliefs about females and males as well as assumptions about appropriate behaviors for each affect sexual behavior, patterns of communication, expectations of sexual rela-

tionships, and responses of others to an individual's sexuality.

SEXUAL LIFESTYLES

Sexual lifestyle provides the pattern and context for a woman's sexuality.[1] Several options exist.

- *Marriage with a Heterosexual Monogamous Partner.* The most frequently acknowledged pattern for women and the one that the majority of society assumes is most desirable.
- *Serial Heterosexual Monogamy.* An established pattern of having one monogamous relationship followed by another.
- *Nonmonogamous Heterosexual Marriage.* A married woman may participate in sexual activity with other individuals or couples—often called "swinging."
- *Heterosexual Coupling without Marriage.*
- *Single State.* Women with this lifestyle may be unmarried, divorced, or widowed. Society often considers this a transition phase.
- *Partnering with a Woman (Lesbianism).* Sexual and affectional preferences directed toward other women. A woman may be coupled or single with one or many sexual partners. The most typical pattern is serial monogamy.
- *Partnering with Either a Woman or a Man (Bisexuality).* Sexual and affectional preferences are directed toward persons of either sex. A woman may be married, have partners of both sexes serially or simultaneously, or have had lesbian relationships as well as sexual relationships with men in the past.
- *Celibacy.* Consciously chosen abstinence from sexual activity. A woman may view this lifestyle positively, as enabling her to focus all of her time and energy on other activities. Celibacy may also be nonvoluntary when a woman is between relationships.

FACTORS THAT AFFECT SEXUALITY

AGE RELATED ISSUES

Adolescence

The period between childhood and adulthood is a time of awareness and change in sexual feelings. The central issue in adolescent sexuality is defining sexuality through activities such as dating. During this time, one selects companions, tests ideas about oneself, and eventually experiences sexual pleasure. Adolescence is a time of developing a capacity for sexual intimacy, and sexual curiosity and experimentation are common.

In the United States, the mean age of first voluntary intercourse is 17.2 years for white women and 16.7 years for African American women;[20,21] 5 percent of white females and 12 percent of black females are sexually active before age 13.[22] Young women who initiate sexual activity early have greater numbers of sexual partners.[21] Teenagers often face peer pressure to become sexually active. For girls, a motivation to become sexually active may come from a desire for intimacy, not for the physical act of intercourse. Risks associated with early sexual activity include sexually transmitted diseases (STDs), including acquired immunodeficiency syndrome (AIDS), and pregnancy.

Reproductive Years

During the reproductive years, developmental tasks include achieving maturity in a sexual role and in the relationship tasks started in adolescence. Balancing career, children, and relationships is often of concern. For many, sexuality during pregnancy and the postpartum period also is of concern. During pregnancy, women often report diminished sexual desire and diminished frequency of intercourse. Fears about the effect of intercourse on the fetus and restrictions associated with high risk pregnancy may affect sexual activity and satisfaction during this period. Postpartally, women report declines in frequency of and desire for sexual activity and decreased sexual interest for up to six months following birth of the infant. Reasons for diminished sexual desire and activity are physical discomfort, lessened physical strength, dissatisfaction with appearance, and fatigue.[23,24] In addition, many lactating women experience a lack of sexual desire, primarily because of low estrogen levels. These women also may experience decreased vaginal secretions and therefore require some form of lubrication to prevent dyspareunia. Moreover,

struggling with infertility or repeated attempts to conceive can adversely affect sexual expression, activity, and desire.

Midlife

Sexuality during midlife is as varied as are women.[25,26] For some women sexual activity is very good, some say the best its ever been. Others report that sex is no longer the driving force in their lives. The physiological changes associated with menopause can affect sexual desire and expression. Physiological changes occur in the sexuality of women during midlife as a result of the climacteric or menopause. For some women, sleep disturbances associated with hot flushes and the resulting fatigue may adversely affect sexual desire. Vaginal dryness caused by decreasing estrogen levels may also diminish sexual activity. For some women, however, the lessened fear that they will become pregnant may increase sexual desire and lessen inhibitions.

Older Adulthood

Patterns of sexual behavior in old age are similar to patterns in midlife[27,28] (see Chapter 15). Further, although sexual frequency may decline, enjoyment of sexual activity sometimes increases with age.[19] One critical issue for women, however, is the availability of a partner. A second important factor is health with good health being positively related to sexual interest and activity.[29] Societal emphasis on youth, beauty, and slimness contributes to the expectation of asexuality in older women—a view that often becomes a self-fulfilling prophecy.

Physiological changes of aging (e.g., decreased estrogen supply, decreased tissue elasticity, thinning of vaginal tissues) may cause irritation or discomfort with penetration and may make women more susceptible to vaginitis. Loss of fatty tissue in the labia and mons pubis also may result in tenderness and easily damaged tissue or abrasions. Orgasms may decrease in intensity and may be painful for some. Breast size also decreases and breasts sag. These changes do not alter a woman's ability to respond sexually, but they may alter her view of her sexual self.

Physiological changes may require that the woman and her partners alter how they engage in sexual activity. A water-soluble lubricant may be used, foreplay increased, different positions used, and intercourse planned for when energy levels are highest.

Although sexual interest and activity may decrease somewhat, most older women do maintain sexual relationships if a partner is available. Older women with a partner may find that the opportunities for sexual expression in a relationship are increased in later years, as pressure from career, family, and achieving one's life goals may be reduced and more time is available for sharing with a partner.[19] Older women who become celibate due to lack of a partner retain their need for touch and closeness and should be encouraged to seek out opportunities for intimacy with another person.

ISSUES OF DISABILITY

The disabled are often perceived as asexual, by health care providers as well as by the public. Most disabled persons are not married.[2] How long a woman has had a disability may affect her sexuality: it has been suggested that women with an early onset of physical disability are less likely than those with a later onset to engage in various sexual activities.[30] In contrast, a recent study of women with spinal cord injury found that younger women were more likely to have had intercourse and that women injured at an earlier age were more likley to have resumed intercourse within 12 months after the injury.[31] An important issue is body image. The disabled woman may view her body as a problem and a source of anxiety rather than of pleasure (see Chapter 24).

THE WOMAN'S MOVEMENT

In the 1960s and 1970s, women began to redefine sexuality for themselves. New definitions recognized that sexuality is created by individuals, not anatomically prescribed. Women centered definitions of sexuality include the ideas of sensuality, closeness, mutuality, and relationships.[1]

SEXUAL CONCERNS OR PROBLEMS

ILLNESS RELATED ISSUES

Illness can affect sexuality in a number of ways. Chronic illness with its associated fatigue, pain, and stress affects sexual desire and arousal more often than it affects orgasm. For example, diabetic women report difficulties with vaginal lubrication, difficulties in reaching orgasm, and genital discomfort that negatively influences sexual functioning.[32] Also, they report that alterations in glucose levels and monilial infections interfere with sexual activity,[33] as well as more performance anxiety that interferes with sexual functioning and lower levels of sexual desire than do nondiabetic women.[33,34] Treatment of gynecological cancer has been associated with less frequent intercourse, sexual excitement, and arousal.[35,36] Women with endometrial cancer have emphasized the negative effect of symptoms (commonly vaginal bleeding) on sexual expression and that lethargy associated with treatment of the cancer adversely affected sexual functioning.[37] Results of studies on the effect of hysterectomy on sexuality vary widely and no longer document negative effects only.[38,39]

In our society where breasts are sexual, a woman with breast cancer may have sexuality concerns; greater sexuality problems may be experienced by women who dislike their breasts, have a negative self-image, have been sexually abused, lack a support system, or are uncomfortable discussing personal or sexual concerns.[2]

In addition, sexually transmitted diseases can have a tremendous impact on a woman's sexuality. Drastic changes may occur in her sexual behavior, including choice of partner, use of condoms, and specific sexual practices.

Medication, such as psychotropic drugs, can impair sexual response in women; the degree of impairment is dose related.[1]

Chemical dependency can have an adverse effect on sexuality. Issues such as incest and childhood sexual abuse experiences and violent relationships as adults are a concern for recovering chemically dependent women.[40] Women crack users report that crack is not an aphrodisiac as commonly supposed; rather, the drug has a negative impact on sexual feelings and functioning. In one study, almost half of the women reporting being orgasmic less than half the time or never.[41]

SEXUAL MYTHS

Sexual myths are common in every culture and society. These myths often interfere with women maximizing their full sexual potential and establishing fulfilling sexual relationships. The list of these myths is long.

- Women should satisfy men; women's needs are secondary. Related to this are the stereotypes that men are oversexed and women are undersexed and that women are recipients and men are initiators.
- Sexual pleasure is the responsibility of the partner. Related to this is the expectation that a partner should somehow sense what a woman's needs are.
- A great deal of stimulation is necessary to sexually arouse a woman; she becomes aroused more slowly than a man.
- Women who are raped asked for it; every woman wants to be raped; when a woman says no, she doesn't mean it.
- Little girls should not be told about sex, as that will put ideas in their heads.
- Women are not interested in sex; they are not capable of multiple orgasms.
- Women want sex only for procreative purposes.
- Women are so sexually aggressive they can never be satisfied.
- Sex is intercourse.
- A woman who initiates sex is immoral.
- A woman cannot enjoy sex unless she has an orgasm.
- There are absolute norms for sexual expression.
- Masturbation is dirty.
- Women can have an orgasm only with intercourse.

There are many sexual myths specific to the elderly.

- Old women do not have sexual desires.
- Old women are not able to make love, even if they want to.

- Old women are so frail that they might hurt themselves if they try to have sexual relations.
- Old women are physically unattractive and therefore sexually undesirable.
- Old women engaging in sexual activity is shameful.

LOSS OF A PARTNER

Women may define their identity through relationships, and thus the loss of a partner can be a loss of self. Furthermore, the stereotypical view of a widow is of a sad, grieving woman whose sexual life is over. A woman's sexuality after the loss of a partner may be influenced by her past extramarital sexual experiences, age, and sexual satisfaction in her marriage.[2,42,43] Remarriage is correlated with age; the older a woman, the less likely remarriage.

FAMILY INFLUENCE

Poor parent–child interactions contribute indirectly to sexual problems; such a child may have lower self-esteem or difficulty coping with intimacy.[44] In addition, less satisfactory relationships with fathers may contribute to orgasmic difficulties.[2] Restrictive family upbringing and the belief that expressions of intimacy or sexuality are shameful or taboo may affect a woman's later ability to express herself sexually. Sexual expression or enjoyment may be inhibited by messages that were taught within a restrictive family—messages such as "Sex is something to be endured" or "Women who enjoy sex are no good."

Incest contributes to sexual dysfunction particularly if its circumstances were associated with strong negative feelings, such as when threat or force was used, when the incest victim was an older child and more apt to have feelings of guilt, or when the incest was repeated over time.[44]

RELATIONSHIP ISSUES

Discord within a relationship may precipitate sexual dysfunction, so much so that many sex therapists believe that sexual dysfunction is a symptom of the underlying relationship problem. One or both partners may experience difficulty after the disclosure of sexual encounters out of their relationship. Communication problems are exacerbated by distrust, feelings of betrayal, and fear of disease. Sexual dysfunction in one's partner may precipitate dysfunction in the other. For example, premature ejaculation is often accompanied by female orgasmic difficulties and lack of desire.

SOCIOCULTURAL INFLUENCES

Religious and cultural beliefs may contribute to sexual concerns or problems. One such conviction is that using a contraceptive during the fertile period is amoral. In addition, attitudes and expectations exist regarding monogamy for males and females. Quite definitely, cultural practices that physically alter the anatomy of sexual response, such as a clitoridectomy, affect sexuality.

SEXUAL DYSFUNCTION

"Impaired, incomplete, or absent expressions of normally recurring human sexual desires and responses"[45] become dysfunctions only when there is subjective discomfort associated with them. It is not always easy to distinguish between aberrant or merely unconventional behaviors or between healthy and neurotic behaviors. Questions that the nurse practitioner might ask to assist in drawing these distinctions are the following:[5]

- How does the woman interpret the behavior?
- Does the behavior enhance or impoverish her sexual life and those with whom she has sexual relations?
- Does society in general tolerate the behavior?
- Is the behavior between two consenting adults?
- Does the behavior cause physical or psychological harm to a woman or her partner?
- Does the behavior involve coercion?

Several factors characterize sexual dysfunction.

- Dysfunction may occur in one or more phases of the sexual response cycle but is less common in the resolution phase.

- Dysfunction may occur during masturbation or, more commonly, during sexual activity with a partner.
- Dysfunction may be lifelong or develop after a period of normal responsiveness; it may occur once or recur.
- Most typically, dysfunction is seen among individuals in their late 20s or early 30s.

The prevalence of sexual dysfunctions in women is not precisely known, as epidemiological studies that include sexual dysfunction, especially in women, are rare. Additionally, clinicians often do not elicit the information when providing health care, and client discomfort in answering questions or reporting problems of a sexual nature contributes to underestimating the prevalence of sexual dysfunctions. It has been suggested that most individuals experience some degree of sexual difficulty at some point in their lives. For example, transient, delayed or absent sexual response might occur with illness or fatigue, when a woman is preoccupied with life demands or with certain medications, drugs, or alcohol. In contrast to popular belief, studies have shown that satisfaction with marriage does not imply adequate sexual functioning or satisfaction.[46]

CAUSES OF SEXUAL DYSFUNCTION

Pathophysiological causes of sexual dysfunction are more common than those that are psychogenic;[47] however, traumatic sexual experiences, such as incest and rape, may precipitate dysfunction. Other associated factors may be depression and life stress. Anxieties, including fear of partner rejection and fear of demand for performance, may also result in dysfunction.[6] An excessive need to please one's partner may cause sexual dysfunction. Poor communication between partners about sexual feelings, needs, and desires is common and can perpetuate an unsatisfying sexual pattern or escalate problems by limiting knowledge of each other or restricting standards of acceptable sexual behavior.

SEXUAL DYSFUNCTIONS IN WOMEN

Sexual dysfunctions commonly are categorized as disorders of desire, of arousal, or of orgasm.

TABLE 6–1. FEMALE SEXUAL DYSFUNCTIONS

Sexual Desire Disorders

Hyposexual Sexual Desire (HSD): Persistent absence or deficiency of sexual feelings, sexual fantasies, and the desire for sexual activity.
Sexual Aversion Disorder: Persistent or recurrent aversion to and avoidance of all or almost all genital contact with a sexual partner. More severe form of sexual inhibition.

Sexual Arousal Disorder

Partial or total lack of physical response indicated by lack of lubrication and vasocongestion of genitals. Persistent or total lack of a subjective sense of sexual excitement and pleasure during sexual activity.

Inhibited Female Orgasm

Persistent delay or absence of orgasm following a normal sexual excitement phase during sexual activity.

Sexual Pain Disorders

Dyspareunia: Recurrent genital pain before, during, or after vaginal intercourse.
Vaginismus: Recurrent involuntary spasm of the outer one-third of the vagina interfering with or preventing coitus.

Source: References 46, 48, 49.

Additionally, sexual pain disorders are considered in this classification (see Table 6–1). Sexual dysfunction also should be categorized as lifelong (has occurred throughout a woman's active sexual life) or acquired (there has been a time when a woman did not experience sexual dysfunction); and general (disorder occurs with all partners and in all situations) or situational (occurs only with certain partners or situations).[48] Dysfunctions may also be categorized as affecting one or both partners.[49]

Sexual Desire Disorders

Hyposexual Sexual Desire (HSD): Sexual desire depends on many things including inherent sexual drive, self-esteem, previous sexual satisfaction, an available partner, and a good relationship with one's partner in areas other than sex. HSD occurs when a woman lacks desire for sexual activity, sexual dreams or fantasies, or becomes frustrated if sexual activity does not occur. Sexual activity occurs infrequently or only in reluctant compliance with a partner's desire for activity.[46,48] It is a prevalent sexual

problem and one for which women most frequently seek assistance. Although the cause is unknown, the disorder is thought to be associated with depression, anxiety, and high levels of stress. Women with HSD may have deeper and more intense sexual anxieties, greater amounts of hostility and/or resentment in their relationships, and more tenacious defense mechanisms than do clients with arousal or orgasm phase difficulties.[49] Two common etiologies are trauma (sexual abuse, assault, or incest) or relationship issues that have created resentment and hostility.[49] Life events such as job loss or family trauma also may play a role. Psychological response to aging in a society that has strict cultural norms of female attractiveness may be a factor in some women. Physical factors also can be involved, particularly hormonal status, general health status, and use of recreational drugs and alcohol.

Desire disorders are difficult to diagnose, and a key issue is making a distinction between HSD as the primary diagnosis versus HSD as secondary to a psychiatric, medical, or other sexual dysfunction diagnosis.[49] Diagnosis is made more difficult because there are no norms for sexual desire across the life span and reasons for the development and maintenance of HSD are variable and imprecise.[46] Generalized life long hyposexual desire suggests a need for assessment for endocrine disorders, illness, and long-term medication use. Treatment depends on the extent of the dysfunction, taking into account factors that affect sexual functioning such as age, occupation, and the context of a woman's life. Underlying physical causes should be treated first as desire often returns when a woman's feelings of well-being are restored. Treatment of a primary sexual dysfunction such as dyspareunia or anorgasmia may also alleviate a lack of desire. Treatment is often difficult and frequently incorporates sensate focus and techniques to improve communication between partners.[1] It is essential that health care providers assisting women with HSD provide a supportive environment and frequent opportunities for expression of feelings. Often a client may require referral to a health care professional with advanced training in sexual counseling and therapy. This should not be done during a crisis period. If an underlying depression is suspected, the nurse practitioner should refer a client to a mental health provider for medication and/or psychotherapy. In some instances, referral for couple therapy will be appropriate.

Sexual Aversion Disorder. Extreme repulsion, loathing, and avoidance of almost all genital sexual contact with a partner is classified as sexual aversion disorder.[48] This disorder, which is far less common that HSD, may be the result of painful intercourse, feelings of guilt, or rape or other sexual trauma occurring in childhood or earlier in a woman's sexual life. Physical factors are not usually involved. These women, who experience intense irrational fear of sexual activity and a compelling desire to avoid sexual situations,[50] should be referred to a trained sex therapist for care. Therapy usually includes cognitive behavioral techniques, desensitization, and when relevant, working through issues of past abuse.

Sexual Arousal Disorder

Female sexual arousal disorder occurs in as many as one-third of all women.[48] The disorder is characterized by partial or complete failure to attain or maintain vaginal lubrication and swelling. Women also report a lack of sexual excitement or pleasure. A number of biological factors may cause insufficient vaginal lubrication, including medications such as antihistamines and anticholinergics or marijuana use prior to a sexual experience.[49] Postmenopausal women may experience lessened lubrication due to lowered estrogen levels. Chronic yeast infections, acute or chronic bacterial vaginosis or trichmoniasis also may be associated with inadequate lubrication. Once physical causes have been ruled out or treated, women with this disorder should be referred to a trained sex therapist for care.

Inhibited Female Orgasm

The inability to experience orgasm is defined as a disorder only if a woman reports receiving sufficient stimulation without orgasm. Women with this dysfunction do experience erotic feelings, genital swelling, and vaginal lubrication.

Rarely is primary (lifelong, generalized) orgasmic disorder caused by a physical factor, rather factors such as a restrictive home environment, negative cultural conditioning during childhood, unrealistic expectations about performance, current relationship issues, and lack of knowledge about female anatomy or the sexual response cycle are implicated. Physical causes of inhibited female orgasm include illnesses such as hypothyroidism and diabetes; vaginal damage such as episiotomy scars; any physical cause of dyspareunia; or endometriosis. Medications such as antihypertensives, central nervous system stimulants, serotonin-reuptake inhibitor or tricyclic antidepressants, and monoamine oxidase inhibitors also have been associated with inhibited orgasmic response.[48,51]

Women whose orgasmic difficulties have a physical basis should be treated for the underlying cause. Once physical causes have been corrected, the most common treatments for this problem are behavioral. For example, the woman is taught to experience orgasm through a series of exercises that increase her awareness of genital sensations and masturbatory techniques.[52] Once she has experienced an orgasm through self-stimulation, she is taught to transfer this knowledge to a partner experience. Women with a partner may be given specific couple exercises to practice. Women with an orgasmic dysfunction may also benefit from information about female anatomy and physiology and the differences between male and female response cycles.

Sexual Pain Disorders

Dyspareunia. Pain experienced in the labia, vagina, or pelvis during or after intercourse is called dyspareunia.[53] Pain may be experienced prior to, with penetration upon intromission, and/or with thrusting. Even when the actual pain is gone, the memory of the pain may persist and interfere with pleasure. Dyspareunia is both a symptom and a diagnosis.[48] All too often women do not seek care for this problem. The incidence of this problem is unknown; estimates of the prevalence in the general population are about 20 percent with a range of 4 percent to 40 percent. Some authorities suggest that as many as 60 percent of women experience dyspareunia at some

TABLE 6–2. POSSIBLE CAUSES OF DYSPAREUNIA

When Pain Occurs	Where Pain Occurs	Consider	Management
Precoital foreplay	External genitalia	Vulvovaginitis	Treat organism
		Inept male technique	Education & communication
		Vulvodynia	Treatment
		Arthritis in adjacent structures	Treatment
		Associated with abuse	Therapy (individual or group)
As penis enters	Introitus	Lack of lubrication	Education; water soluble lubricants
		Infection/vaginitis	Treatment
		Position/angle of penis	Education & communication
		Urethritis/cystitis	Treatment
		Scar tissue	Medical/surgical intervention
		Rigid hymen	Education; surgical intervention
		Postmenopausal changes	Education; HRT; water-soluble lubricant
Penis in midvagina	Vaginal canal & adjacent structures	Cystitis	Treatment
		Vaginitis	Treatment
		Postmenopausal changes	Education; HRT; water-soluble lubricant
		Scars	Medical/surgical
		Position of penis	Education
		Anorectal problems	Medical/surgical intervention
Deep penetration with thrusting	Lower back Lower abdomen Deep pelvis	Endometriosis	Medical (hormonal); surgical intervention
		PID-related	Medical/surgical treatment
		Position of penis	Education
		Arthritic/orthopedic problems	Medical/surgical interventions
		Post-trauma scars	Medical/surgical interventions
		Broad ligament varices	Medical/surgical interventions
During orgasm	Lower back Deep in pelvis Lower abdomen	Endometriosis	Medical (hormonal); surgical intervention
		Scars at vaginal vault or abdomen	Medical/surgical intervention
		Broad ligament varices	Medical/surgical intervention
Post coitus	Lower back Lower abdomen Deep in pelvis	Endometriosis	Medical (hormonal); surgical intervention
		Scars at vaginal vault or abdomen	Medical/surgical intervention
		Broad ligament varices	Medical/surgical intervention

Adapted from reference 49.

time in their lives.[53] Further, the incidence appears to be increasing; however, it is not clear if this is a result of the increasing incidence of sexually transmitted diseases, changes in sexual behavior, or women's increased willingness to talk about sexual matters.[54] As women age, they also report more dyspareunia associated with changes in the urogenital system.

Causes of dyspareunia are many and diverse (see Table 6–2 for etiology of dyspareunia). Physical causes are most common and numerous.[55] They include sexually transmitted disease, blad-der disease, diabetes, anatomic defects, and decreased estrogen due to aging. Mechanical causative factors may be excessive douching or the use of irritating soaps or sprays. Dyspareunia may also be caused by psychological factors related to family religious taboos or teachings that the vagina should not be touched; traumatic factors such as rape, incest, or previous painful intercourse; or other factors such as a lack of complete arousal and inadequate vaginal lubrication, personal problems, or negative feelings toward one's partner.[46,56,57]

Presentation of dyspareunia is diverse, necessitating a careful, logical sequence of history taking, physical examination, laboratory studies, and therapies.[54] In general, the history would include inquiring about the following:

- Sexual response cycle and any alterations in phases of sexual response cycle she has noticed.
- Attempts to conceive, previous high risk pregnancy, postpartal difficulties, contraceptive choices, and problems associated with them.
- Past and present illness, surgery, and medications.
- Client's self-concept and body image.
- Her view of herself as a sexual being and level of confidence in ability to function sexually.
- Past and current psychiatric problems or illness including anxiety and depression, and use of psychotrophic medications.
- Her satisfaction with current relationship.
- Any history of sexual abuse.
- Perceptions of sex appropriate roles for men and women in relationships; perception regarding her ability to fulfill these roles competently.
- Sources of sexual education, when received, and reactions to this information.
- A woman's religious affiliation and beliefs and ethnic and cultural belief system also should be noted.

The nurse practitioner should assess whether or not the information received was correct and accurate. A history that is specific for dyspareunia would include information about the pain: quality, quantity, location, duration, and aggravating/relieving factors. In addition, the nurse practitioner would obtain complete medical, surgical, obstetrical, gynecological, and contraceptive histories. Within this context, questions about previous vaginal or pelvic surgeries and pelvic trauma such as rape or sexual abuse should be asked. Finally, women are asked about medications, douching, and the use of perineal products such as sprays, deodorants, and minipads.

Physical examination is essential to determine the cause of dyspareunia. Possible components of the physical exam include vital signs, a general physical examination, and an abdominal examination. A pelvic exam always is performed. Special attention is paid to the external genitalia, observing for irritation, lesions, and discharge. During the bimanual examination, the nurse prac-

titioner would note any tenderness in the introitus, vagina, and pelvis and assess for unstretched or rigid hymen.[49] During the speculum examination, cultures, when indicated, are obtained.

The history and physical examination suggest which diagnostic tests are indicated. There are no tests specific to sexual assessment. Laboratory studies may be indicated when there is evidence of infection, for example, cultures for gonorrhea or chlamydia may be done when there is history of purulent discharge. If a woman complains of dyspareunia and a bladder infection is suspected, the nurse practitioner may elect to obtain a clean catch urine for culture and sensititivities.

Treatment for dyspareunia should address the specific cause of dyspareunia, for example, suggesting a water-soluble vaginal lubricant for the menopausal woman, treating the sexually transmitted disease, or providing information about techniques for sexual arousal. Further, the nurse practitioner may act as a consultant to mental health professionals who are referring a client with dyspareunia for a physical and gynecological examination.[49] (See Chapter 13, Common Gynecologic Pelvic Disorders for related information on dyspareunia.)

Vaginismus. This disorder involves the involuntary, spasmodic, sometimes painful contractions of the pubococcygeus and other muscles in the lower third of the vagina and the introitus.[46,48] The degree of vaginal spasm may range from partial (penetration is possible but painful) to complete (no penetration is possible).[49] Vaginismus can occur during any phase of the sexual response cycle when vaginal entry is attempted. Vaginismus can be associated with other sexual dysfunctions, including lack of desire, arousal, or orgasm.[48] Although rare, sex therapists believe vaginismus may be more common than is documented and women do not seek help for it.[1] Often a woman will not seek help until she experiences relationship difficulties or wishes to become pregnant.[46]

Causes of vaginismus are varied and include sexual trauma (rape, incest, or sexual abuse), phobia about sexual response or intercourse, strong conservative religious values in the woman's family of origin, dyspareunia, and hostile feelings toward one's sexual partner.[28,46] Further, repeated experiences with pain can establish a pain-fear-tension-pain syndrome that becomes self-maintaining. Generally, medical conditions are not a significant cause of vaginismus.[48]

When collecting a history from a woman who presents with symptoms suggestive of vaginismus, specific areas to assess include the degree of vaginal spasm she experiences, presence of desire, arousal, lubrication, and orgasm; history of previous pain related to penetration, fear of penetration or ripping; partner's sensitivity to pain; client's ability to communicate needs to partner; erectile difficulty in partner; use of lubricant; and attempts to penetrate virginal hymen. Vaginismus is diagnosed primarily by pelvic examination. It is important to remember that past or present pelvic exams may be connected to trauma. The nurse practitioner must discuss this possibility with a woman, and the two work together to make the exam as comfortable as possible. During the examination, the nurse practitioner should assess for involuntary contraction of vaginal muscles upon touching vulva or digitally entering vagina.

Treatment usually involves a desensitization process including insertion of progressively larger dilators into the vagina by the woman and/or her partner. At the same time, she is taught to relax vaginal muscles consciously. Often psychotherapy is needed. Treatment of this sexual dysfunction requires a health professional with advanced training in sexual therapy. Clients should be referred to such an individual.

Secondary/Other Sexual Dysfunctions

The majority of the sexual problems just reviewed (with the possible exception of dyspareunia) usually contain a psychological component or are solely caused by psychological factors, or cannot be accounted for by a general medical condition. There are sexual problems, however, that are the result of a medical condition such as a woman whose orgasm is inhibited by Cushing's disease or hypoparathyroidism. Further, a number of psychoactive drugs such as cocaine or alcohol may affect the sexual abilities of women.[48] Lack of sensation in the genital area may be a problem for women with neurologic disease or injury.[46]

SEXUAL HEALTH CARE ASSESSMENT AND HISTORY

In order to provide adequate sexual health care, nurse practitioners must be aware of their sexual biases, be comfortable with their sexuality, and have a genuine desire to help the client. MacLauren[5] suggests that health professionals can become aware of their personal attitudes and values about sex and sexuality by asking themselves the questions such as "My religious beliefs teach me that sex is . . ." and "In my culture, communicating my sexual needs to my partner is considered . . ." (see reference 5, page 109 for the complete list). When providing sexual health care, it is critical that assumptions not be made about a woman's sexual behavior, feelings, or attitudes. Health care providers should know how various health problems, diseases, and their treatment affect sexuality and sexual functioning.

Sexual assessment includes a physiological, psychological, and sociocultural evaluation. Data are gathered regarding the client's sexual response cycle and any alterations she has noted in its phases. The woman should be asked about attempts to conceive, any previous high risk pregnancy, postpartum difficulties, and contraceptive choices and any associated problems. In addition, data about past and present illness, surgery, and medications are obtained.

Components of psychological sexual assessment include the client's self-concept and body image; view of self as a sexual being and level of confidence in ability to function sexually; past and current psychiatric problems or illness including anxiety and depression; use of psychotropic medications; satisfaction with current relationship; and history of sexual abuse.

Sociocultural sexual assessment incorporates information about the client's perceptions of sex appropriate roles for men and women in relationships and her perception of her ability to fulfill those roles competently. Women should be asked about their sources of sexual education, when they received it, and their reactions to the information. The nurse practitioner/primary care provider should assess whether the information that the client received was correct and accurate. The woman's religious affiliation and beliefs and her ethnic and cultural belief system should be noted.

TECHNIQUES FOR TAKING A SEXUAL HISTORY

The health care provider should take responsibility for introducing the topic of sexual health problems. Choose a private location where the client is comfortable and assure her that the information will be held in strict confidence. It is essential that sufficient time be given to build trust and develop rapport before soliciting information that the client may consider highly personal or intimate. Several meetings may be needed to collect the history, especially if anxiety is high. Continually monitor your own responses to detect negative or embarrassed feelings that may easily be conveyed to the client. Usually you will obtain more information if you begin with open questions that will permit clients to tell their story on their own terms. Closed questions generally facilitate gathering specific information, such as medical history, menstrual history, and drug reactions.

From Simple to Complex

History taking should always begin with the least threatening material, for example, obstetric history or childhood sexual education, and progress to more sensitive topics, such as current sexual practices. A general guide is to begin with questions about the individual's sexual learning history, proceed to personal attitudes and beliefs about sexuality, and finally assess actual sexual behaviors. Explain to your clients the purpose of your questions. You can set limits on the length of responses if excessive or irrelevant information is offered or provide encouragement if progress is slow. Tell your clients if information becomes tangential.

Appropriate Terminology

Avoid using excessive medical terminology during an interview; in other words, make sure that both you and the client know the meaning of the terms used. Avoid euphemisms such as "slept with." Pose only one question at a time, and give the client sufficient time to answer it. Questions such as "How many times a week do you have sexual intercourse?" should not be asked because norms vary widely among individuals.

"Universalizing" or prefacing questions with phrases such as "Many people" or "The Kinsey Report shows" may make a client feel more comfortable when answering sensitive questions.

SEXUAL HISTORY FORMATS

A sexual history can be incorporated into a total health history (brief sexual history) or it can be more formal and inclusive (sexual problem history).

Brief Sexual History

When the sexual history is incorporated into the total health history, various formats can be used.

- Two questions that elicit sexual concerns are "Are you sexually active?" and "Are you having any sexual difficulties or problems at this time?"[58]
- The three question format is used to gather information about a client's usual sexual roles, views of self as a sexual being, and sexual functioning. These questions are "Has any [illness, pregnancy, surgery] interfered with your being a [mother, wife, partner]?" "Has any [surgery, medical treatment, illness] changed the way you feel about yourself as a woman?" and "Has any [surgery, disease, medication] altered your ability to function sexually?"[59]

Additional questions that could be asked in either of the above formats are "Is sex pleasurable for you?" (desire), "Are you having any difficulty with lubrication during sex?" (arousal), "Are you able to achieve orgasm?" (orgasm), and "Do you experience any pain or discomfort during sexual activity?" (pain). Two other categories that can be incorporated into assessment that relate specifically to sexual dysfunction are satisfaction: "Are you satisfied with your sexual relationship?" "Do you have other sexual complaints?"[60]

Other elements of a *routine* history are also significant for a sexual history. The woman's menstrual history is queried, including her age at menarche and the characteristics of her menstrual cycle (i.e., length, duration of flow, presence or absence of associated premenstrual symptoms, and ovulatory discomfort or dysmenorrhea). Ask your client about the presence of vaginal discharge, discomfort, or itching and about her preferred method of sanitary protection and level of satisfaction with that method. If the woman is beyond her childbearing years, ask when menopause occurred and whether she has experienced any difficulties with sexual functioning, such as vaginal dryness. If problems have occurred, ask her how she dealt with them.

Obstetric history data are significant and include the number of pregnancies, deliveries, and spontaneous and induced abortions. Note any difficulties the client has experienced conceiving and any history of infertility. Questions about her contraceptive history include the methods used, her satisfaction or dissatisfaction and confidence with each, and partner participation. Be sure to record any history of sexually transmitted disease, including pelvic inflammatory disease.

Obtain a brief description of the client's sexual response cycle. It is important to clarify the degree of lubrication that develops during sexual arousal or if pain occurs during sexual intercourse. Ask the client to describe briefly her present relationship and to rate it with respect to communication, affection, sexual needs met, and sexual communication.

Sexual Problem History

A sexual problem history is used to supplement a brief sexual history and is obtained within the context of sexual counseling and therapy. It is intended to collect information so that the provider can define the character, etiology, onset, severity, duration, and psychosocial effect of presenting sexual dysfunction. Formats may vary; however, certain commonalties should be explored.

- Description of the problem in the client's own words.
- Exploration of the onset and course of the problem.
- Determination of the client's assessment of the cause and persistence of the problem.
- A description of any past treatment and its results.
- The client's expectations of current therapy.[1]

An in-depth sexual history generally includes several factors.

- The nature of the presenting distress.
- Information about the client's present relationship, such as duration or other partners.
- Life cycle influences and events in childhood, adolescence, premarital adulthood, and marriage.
- The client's perception of self.
- The client's response to sensory stimuli.[61]

These histories can generate extensive information about experiences, feelings, sexual practices, and perceptions of self-concept. *History taking requires several hours of interviewing and is conducted only by health professionals with extensive training in sexual counseling or therapy.*

PHYSICAL EXAMINATION

A physical examination is done when indicated by history, presenting concern, treatment goals, or need for referral. Components might be determination of vital signs and a general physical examination, especially an abdominal and pelvic exam including external genitalia and internal genitalia (using a speculum and bimanual techniques).

DIAGNOSTIC TESTS/METHODS

Although no tests are specific to determine sexual assessment, laboratory studies may be indicated when infection is evident. For example, cultures may be done for gonorrhea or chlamydia if there is history of purulent discharge. If a woman complains of dyspareunia and a bladder infection is suspected, the nurse practitioner may elect to obtain a clean catch urine specimen for culture and sensitivity.

SEXUAL HEALTH INTERVENTIONS: PLISSIT MODEL

The PLISSIT model[62] is a schema for ordering levels of intervention for sexual problems and is the approach to sexual counseling most used by nurses. It incorporates four levels of counseling: permission, limited information, specific suggestions, and intensive therapy. As the complexity of intervention levels increases, more knowledge and skills are needed. All nurses should be able to provide permission and limited information related to many sexual concerns. Many nurses and all advanced nurse practitioners should also be able to intervene at the specific suggestion level. Intensive therapy, however, requires that nurses be specially trained in sexuality and sex therapy or that the client be referred to experts in sex therapy.

PERMISSION

The provider gives permission to the client to function sexually as she usually does and to accept herself and her desires. Reassurance is offered that such behaviors are normal. The health care professional may also encourage the woman to talk with her partner. It is important never to give permission for activities that are potentially harmful to a woman.

Permission giving involves answering questions about sexual fantasies, feelings, and dreams. Inquiring about the effect of developmental changes, illness, or lifestyle alterations may give a woman permission to be a sexual being. Permission giving is particularly useful for a client with a nursing diagnosis of anxiety related to sexual adequacy or of sexual dysfunction related to guilt over sexual enjoyment. Examples of interventions at this level include providing permission to be sexually aroused by normal feelings; to engage in safe activities that arouse sexual feelings, such as masturbation and fantasizing; and to have sexual intercourse as often as desired.

LIMITED INFORMATION

Provide the client with specific facts that are directly related to her area of sexual concern, making sure that the information is immediately relevant and limited in scope. Limited information helps to change potentially negative thoughts and attitudes about specific areas of sexuality and to refute sexual myths.

The purpose of providing limited information about sexual matters is to open the topic of sexual health for the client so that she, in turn, can discuss her concerns with the health care provider. This approach is particularly useful when the nursing diagnosis is knowledge deficit related to sexuality or anxiety related to sexual misinformation.

SPECIFIC SUGGESTIONS

The health care provider using the specific suggestions approach gives direct behavioral suggestions to relieve a sexual problem that is limited in scope or of brief duration. The client and the health care provider agree on specific goals, and the provider offers specific behavioral suggestions. These interventions are followed up after a brief period.

Numerous suggestions can be made, but they are always tailored to an individual's needs and particular situation. For example, a woman with a recent mastectomy might be counseled to use a side lying position for intercourse to avoid putting pressure on her wound. Or the health care provider might suggest that a postmenopausal woman who is experiencing vaginal dryness and dyspareunia use a water-soluble vaginal lubricant prior to penile penetration. Additional examples of specific suggestions include sensate focus exercises (mutual stimulation of erotic areas excluding the genitals); medication specific to the organism causing vaginal infection; and alternative ways of sexual pleasuring (oral-genital contact, mutual masturbation, cuddling, holding, massage).

Specific suggestions are used when the nursing diagnosis is sexual dysfunction related to pain with intercourse secondary to vaginal infection, or pain related to sexual position secondary to pregnancy, surgery, or other interfering factors.

INTENSIVE THERAPY

Intensive therapy is used when a client's problems are not relieved by interventions included in the first three levels (permission giving, limited information, and specific suggestions) or when the problems are personal and emotional difficulties that interfere with sexual expression. Intensive therapy is appropriate for women with a nursing diagnosis of sexual dysfunction related to inhibited female orgasm or to vaginismus. This level of intervention is the most complex and should be undertaken only by professionals with advanced training in sexual counseling and therapy. It is essential that nursing professionals recognize the limits of their own knowledge and refer the client appropriately.

REFERENCES

1. Fogel, C. I., & Lauver, D. (1990). *Sexual health promotion*. Philadelphia: Saunders.
2. Bernhard, L. (1995). Sexuality in women's lives. In C. I. Fogel & N. F. Woods (Eds.), *Women's health care*. Thousand Oaks, CA: Sage Publications.
3. World Health Organization. (1975). Education and treatment in human sexuality: The training of health professionals. Report of WHO meeting. *Technical Report Series, 572*.
4. Boston Women's Health Book Collective. (1992). *The new our bodies, ourselves*. New York: Simon & Schuster.
5. MacLauren, A. (1995). Comprehensive sexual assessment. *Journal of Nurse-Midwifery, 40*(2), 104–119.
6. Kaplan, H. (1979). *Disorders of sexual desire and other new concepts and techniques in sex therapy*. New York: Brunner/Mazel.
7. American Psychiatric Association. (1994). *Diagnostic and statistical manual of mental disorders, DSM-IV-R* (4th rev. ed.). Washington, DC: American Psychiatric Press.
8. Masters, W., & Johnson, V. (1966). *The human sexual response*. Boston: Little, Brown.
9. Woods, N. F. (1995). Women's bodies. In C. I. Fogel & N. F. Woods (Eds.), *Women's health care*. Thousand Oaks, CA: Sage Publications.
10. Zawid, C. S. (1994). *Sexual health; a nurse's guide*. Albany NY: Delmar Publishers Inc.
11. Darling, C. A., Davidson, J. K., & Jennings, D. A. (1991). The female sexual response revisited: understanding the multiorgasmic experience of women. *Archives of Sexual Behavior, 20*(6), 527–540.
12. Davidson, J. K. & Darling, C. A. (1989). Self-perceived differences in the female orgasmic response. *Family Practice Journal, 8*(2), 75–84.
13. Perry, J. D. & Whipple, B. (1981). Pelvic muscle strength of female ejaculators: Evidence in support of a new theory of orgasm. *Journal of Sex Research, 17*, 22–39.
14. Darling, C. A., Davidson, J. K. & Conway-Welch, C. (1990). Female ejaculation: Perceived origins, the Grafenberg spot/area, and sexual responsiveness. *Archives of Sexual Behavior, 19*(1), 29–47. 1990.
15. Chalker, R. (1994). Updating the model of female sexuality. *Siecus Report, 22*, 1–6.
16. Federation of Feminist Women's Health Centers. (1991). *A new view of a woman's body*. West Hollywood, CA: Feminist Health Press.
17. Hatcher, R. A., Trussel, J. Stewart F. et al. (1994). *Contraceptive technology*. (16th ed.). New York: Irvington Publishers Inc.
18. Tiefer, L. (1992). Feminism matters in sexology. In W. Bezemer, P. Cohen-Kettnis, K. Slob, & N. Van Scon-Schoones (Eds.), *Sex matters: Proceedings of the Tenth Congress of Sexology*. Amsterdam: Excepta Medica.
19. Alexander, L. L. & LaRosa, J. H. (1994). *New dimensions in women's health*. Boston: Jones and Barlett Publishers.
20. Wyatt, G. E. (1989). Reexamining factors predicting Afro-American and white American women's age at first coitus. *Archives of Sexual Behavior, 18*, 271–298.
21. Seidman, S. N., & Reider, R. O. (1994). A review of sexual behavior in the United States. *American Journal of Psychiatry, 151*(3), 330–341.
22. Coker A. L., et al. (1994). Correlates and consequences of early initiation of sexual intercourse. *Journal of School Health, 64*(9), 372–377.
23. Ellis, D. J., & Hewat, R. J. (1985). Mothers' postpartum perceptions of spousal relationships. *JOGNN, 14*(2), 140–146.
24. Fischman, S. H., Rankin, E. A., Soeken, K. L., & Lenz, E. R. (1986). Changes in sexual relationships in postpartum couples. *JOGNN, 15*(1), 58–63.
25. Taylor, D., & Sumral, A. C. (1993). *The time of our lives. Women write on sex after 40*. Freedom, CA: The Crossing Press.
26. Sang, B., Warshow, J., & Smith, A. J. (1991). *Lesbians at midlife: The creative transition*. Minneapolis: Spinsters Ink.
27. Steinke, E. E. (1988). Older adults' knowledge and attitudes about sexuality and aging. *IMAGE, 20*(2), 93–95.
28. Steinke, E. E. (1994). Knowledge and attitudes of older adults about sexuality in aging: a comparison of two studies. *Journal of Advanced Nursing, 19*, 477–485.
29. Johnson, B. K. (1996). Older adults and sexuality: A multidimensional perspective. *Journal of gerontological nursing, 22*(2), 6–15.
30. DeHaan, C. B., & Wallander, J. L. (1988). Self-concept, sexual knowledge and attitudes and parental support in the sexual adjustment of women with early- and late-onset physical disability. *Archives of Sexual Behavior, 13*, 233–245.

31. White, M. J., Rintala, D. H., Hart, K., & Fuhrer, M. J. (1994). A comparison of the sexual concerns of men and women with spinal cord injuries. *Rehabilitation Nursing Research, Summer, 1994,* 55–61.

32. Young, E. W., Koch, P. B., & Bailey, D. (1989). Research comparing the dyadic adjustment and sexual functioning concerns of diabetic and nondiabetic women. *Health Care for Women International, 10,* 377–394.

33. LeMone, P. (1993). Human sexuality in adults with insulin-dependent diabetes mellitus. *IMAGE, 25*(2), 101–105.

34. Watts, R. J. (1994). Sexual function of diabetic and nondiabetic African American women: A pilot study. *Journal of the National Black Nurses Association, 7*(1), 60–69.

35. Andersen, B. L., Anderson, B., & deProsse, C. (1989). Controlled prospective longitudinal study of women with cancer: I. Sexual functioning outcomes. *Journal of Consulting and Clinical Psychology, 57,* 683–691.

36. Schover, L. R., Fife, M., & Gershenson, D. M. (1989). Sexual dysfunction and treatment for early stage cervical cancer. *Cancer, 63,* 204–212.

37. Lamb, M. A., & Sheldon, T. A. (1994). The sexual adaptation of women treated for endometrial cancer. *Cancer Practice, 2*(2), 103–113.

38. Gath, D., Cooper, P., & Day, A. (1982). Hysterectomy and psychiatric disorder: I. Levels of psychiatric morbidity before and after hysterectomy. *British Journal of Psychiatry, 140,* 335–350.

39. Bernhard, L. A. (1992). Consequences of hysterectomy in the lives of women. *Health Care for Women International, 13,* 281–291.

40. Henderson, D. J., Boyd, C. J., & Whitmarsh, J. (1995). Women and illicit drugs: Sexuality and crack cocaine. *Health Care for Women International, 16,* 113–124.

41. Teets, J. M. (1990). What women talk about. Sexuality issues of chemically dependent women. *Journal of Psychosocial Nursing, 28*(12), 4–7.

42. Kansky, J. (1986). Sexuality of widows: A study of the sexual practices of widows during the first fourteen months of bereavement. *Journal of Sex and Marital Therapy, 12,* 307–321.

43. Malatesta, V. J., Chambless, D. L., Pollack, M., & Cantor, A. (1988). Widowhood, sexuality and aging: A life span analysis. *Journal of Sex and Marital Therapy, 14,* 49–62.

44. Sheaham, S. L. (1989). Identifying female sexual dysfunctions. *Nurse Practitioner, 14,* 25–26, 28, 30, 32, 34.

45. Renshaw, D. C. (1983). Recognition and treatment of sexual disorders. *Pennsylvania Medicine, 86,* 64–67.

46. Heiman, J. R. (1995). Evaluating sexual dysfunction. In D. P. Lemcke, J. Pattison, L. A. Marshall, & D. S. Cowley (Eds.), *Primary care of women.* Norwalk, CT: Appleton & Lange.

47. Field, M. (1990). In C. I. Fogel & D. Lauver (Eds.), *Sexual health promotion.* Philadelphia: Saunders.

48. Morrison, J. (1995). *DSM-IV made easy.* New York: The Guilford Press.

49. Ayers, A. (1995). Sexual dysfunction. *Women's primary health care. Protocols for practice.* Washington, DC: American Nurses Publishing.

50. Kaplan, H. S., & Klein, D. (1987). *Sexual aversion, sexual phobias, and panic disorder.* New York: Brunner/Mazel.

51. Seagraves, R. T. (1988). Psychiatric drugs and inhibited female orgasm. *Journal of Sex and Marital Therapy, 15,* 202–207.

52. Barbach, L. (1980). *Women discover orgasm.* New York: Free Press.

53. Glatt, A. E., Zinner, S. H., & McCormack, W. M. (1990). The prevalence of dyspareunia. *Obstetrics and Gynecology, 75,* 433–436.

54. Sarazin, S. K., & Seymour, S. F. (1991). Causes and treatment options for women with dyspareunia. *Nurse Practitioner, 16*(10), 30, 35–36, 38, 41.

55. Sandberg, G. & Quevillon, R. P. (1987). Dyspareunia: An integrated approach to assessment and diagnosis. The *Journal of Family Practice, 24*(1), 66–69.

56. Steege, J. F. & Ling, F. W. (1993). Dyspareunia. A special type of chronic pelvic pain. *Obstetrics and gynecology clinics of North America, 20*(4), 779–793.

57. Lazarus, A. A. (1989). Dyspareunia: A multimodel perspective. In S. R. Leiblum & R. C. Rosen (Eds.), *Principles and practices of sex therapy* (2nd ed.). New York: Guilford Press.

58. Bachman, G. A., Leiblum, S. R., & Grill, J. (1989). Brief sexual inquiry in gynecologic practice. *Obstetrics and Gynecology, 73,* 425–427.

59. Woods, N. F. (1984). *Human sexuality in health and illness* (3rd ed.). St. Louis: Mosby.

60. Heinman, J. R. (1994). Female sexual dysfunction: definitions, history-taking techniques, and workup. In C. Singer & W. J. Weiner (Eds.), *Sexual dysfunction: A neuro-medical approach.* Armonk, NY: Futura Publishing Co.

61. Masters, W., & Johnson, V. (1970). *Human sexual inadequacy.* Boston: Little, Brown.

62. Annon, J. S. (1974). *Behavioral treatment of sexual problems: Brief therapy.* New York: Harper & Row.

BIBLIOGRAPHY

Anderson, W. B. (1986). Use of a "permission giving" patient checklist in identification of social and sexual problems. *Henry Ford Hospital Medical Journal, 34,* 267–269.

Bernhard, L. A. (1993). Women's sexuality. In B. J. McElmurry & R. S. Parker (Eds.), *Annual review of women's health.* New York: National League for Nursing Press.

Chapman, J., & Sughrue, J. (1987). A model for sexual assessment and intervention. *Health Care for Women International, 8,* 87–99.

Collier, P. (1986). Education for sexual self-awareness. In V. J. Littlefield (Ed.), *Health education for women.* Norwalk, CT: Appleton-Century-Crofts.

Fogel, C. I. (1990). Sexual health promotion. In C. I. Fogel & D. Lauver (Eds.), *Sexual health promotion.* Philadelphia: Saunders.

Fogel, C. I., Forker, J., & Welch, M. B. (1990). Sexual health care. In C. I. Fogel & D. Lauver (Eds.), *Sexual health promotion.* Philadelphia: Saunders.

Fogel, C. I. & Rynerson, B. C. (1991). Sexuality concerns. In S. Cohen, C. Kenner, & A. Hollingsworth (Eds.), *Maternal, neonatal, and women's health nursing.* Springhouse, PA: Springhouse Corp.

Hunt, A. D., Litt, I. F., & Loebner, M. (1988). Obtaining a sexual history from adolescent girls. *Journal of Adolescent Health Care, 9,* 52–54.

MacElveen-Hoehn, P. (1985). Sexual assessment and counseling. *Seminars in Oncology Nursing, 1,* 69–75.

Morrison-Beedy, D., & Robbins, L. (1989). Sexual assessment and the aging female. *Nurse Practitioner, 14,* 35, 38–39, 42, 45.

Muscari, M. E. (1987). Obtaining the adolescent sexual history. *Pediatric Nursing, 13,* 307–310.

Sanderson, M. O. & Maddox, J. W. (1989). Guidelines for assessment and treatment of sexual dysfunction. *Obstetrics & Gynecology, 73,* 130–134.

CHAPTER 7

HEALTH NEEDS
OF LESBIANS

Ellis Quinn Youngkin • Marcia Szmania Davis • Catherine Ingram Fogel

*A*lthough the health care needs of lesbians are the same as those of all women in most instances, lesbians face additional unique health problems to which health care providers must attend.

Highlights

- Care Barriers for Lesbians
- Approach and Environment for Acceptance
- Assessing Coping Status
- Special Groups at Greater Risk
- Health Problems of Lesbians
- Desire to Parent
- Resources and Organizations

► INTRODUCTION

Women who form sexual and affectional relationships with women generally refer to themselves as lesbians.[1] Not all women who are partnered with women consider themselves lesbian. Rather, defining oneself as lesbian is a highly individualized choice and may be fluid over time.[1] The decision may be influenced by race/ethnicity, socioeconomic class, cultural values, psychological responses, age, or personal history.[1,2] Women who self-identify as lesbian may do so in their adolescence, as young adults, in middle age, or late in life. Their sexual behavior and preference may range from exclusively homosexual to bisexual to situationally heterosexual in response to economic considerations, cultural factors, or sexual desire.[3] As with all homosexuals, sexual preference is only one aspect of why a person considers her or himself same-sex identified.

Lesbians are as diverse as the population at large, crossing all age, occupation, ethnic/racial, religious, economic, and geographic boundaries. At least 1 in 10 women in the United States is lesbian,[4] although some suggest that this is an underestimation because many women never declare their sexual preference for fear of stigma.[5] One survey projected that 3.6 percent of U.S. women are lesbian,[6] while another offers an estimate of 2 percent to 10 percent.[3] Although the health care needs of lesbians are the same as those of all women in most instances, lesbians can experience some health problems with greater frequency than the average. Further, it is imperative that nurses caring for women be attuned to and respectful of this population and its healthcare needs and problems.

The increased number of articles discussing special needs and concerns of this population not only in the health professional literature but also in other disciplines and lay publications would seem to purport a mere tolerant attitude toward lesbians. Nevertheless, prejudice and ignorance remain, perpetuating bias and misinformation about this distinct cultural minority group.[6] Such bias is not limited to lay persons. A literature review of lesbian health care from 1970 to 1990 found that "prejudice is alive and well in present-day clinical practice and health care provider education. . . . This survey evidence suggests that lesbianism was still considered an affliction by many health care providers (p. 108)."[7] Knowing this prejudice exists often impedes lesbians from seeking care that may result in more debilitating, costlier medical problems. Providers can help to decrease barriers by acknowledging any internalized homophobia of their own and attempting to be as impartial as humanly possible to all their women clients.

The health care provider needs to understand first and foremost that, regardless of age, social status, education, and so on, every woman who becomes woman-identified and eventually self-identifies as a lesbian has generally gone through a period of "coming out"—realizing that her sexual and affectional preference is not of the societal norm. This can be a distressing period for the adolescent or the woman.[3] Because it requires a shift in core identity as well as a need to understand the pros and cons of disclosure, the person may need positive support and counseling. For the adolescent coping with developmental tasks as well as for the woman who finally begins to acknowledge that the heterosexual way of life is not fulfilling, it can be a time of great emotional distress, with greater risks of depression or suicide. Both families and health care providers need to consider questions about sexual identity as a reason for significant behavioral changes. Until the individual becomes comfortable with her choice, *every* "coming out" is a mine field: Will I be rejected, shunned, mocked? Can I live with that? Eventually, lesbians begin to understand that homophobia is the other person's problem. The hard part is knowing that the other's homophobia—internalized or externalized—can indeed affect the lesbian's life in very real and tangible ways.

Providing a safe, comfortable atmosphere, where truth can be told without repercussion, is the ideal. A client who allows a provider to know she is a lesbian has imparted a gift of self. That information should be handled gently and professionally.

CARE BARRIERS FOR LESBIANS

Lesbians experience the same barriers to care that other women do, such as having no transportation, child care, or leave time from work; inconvenient times/location of clinics/practices; inability to communicate due to language barriers or reading ability; physical barriers, or culture; "ism" barriers (race, sex, class, age, ability); putting others ahead of self for care; avoiding health screening as a way to deny problems or viewing it as a non-necessity; seeking care for serious problems only; history of abuse causing distancing from body; fear of procedures causing pain, embarrassment or fear of the unknown; fear of findings of tests; inability to pay; and/or lack of recommendation for a procedure by a health care provider.[1] In addition, lesbians may also face barriers that are particular to a gay identity/behavior (see Table 7–1).

Most lesbians (75 percent–94 percent) do have regular primary care providers, but more than half seek care only if they have a problem.[8] Of concern is the fact that care is often delayed. Stevens found in a narrative study of 45 lesbians in the San Francisco area that "noncare" was common.[9,10] "Noncare" was negative care, such as feeling a lack of respect, feeling not safe enough to continue with a particular provider, feeling generally poorly cared for. These results confirm prior studies' findings where providers' negative behaviors included such actions as clipped voice tones, constricted affect, roughness in handling, a hurried pace that frightened or humiliated or hurt, and false endearments.

TABLE 7–1. SPECIAL BARRIERS TO HEALTH CARE EXPERIENCED BY LESBIANS[1]

- Homophobia from the health care provider
- Internalized homophobia
- Lack of knowledge about special risks and screening needs of lesbians by lesbians themselves
- Incorrect knowledge about health care needs of lesbians by health care providers
- Belief (false) by lesbians and health care providers that lesbians are immune to STDs, cervical cancer, and HIV
- Preventive care sought less since lesbians need routine contraceptive and prenatal care less often
- Insurance lack and/or lack of access under partner's coverage
- Excluded or believe they are excluded from health promotion campaigns

Other reasons and examples of why lesbians may not seek health care, delay health care, or may not disclose their sexual orientation to health care providers include the following:[3,10–12]

- Prejudicial language. Examples are: When taking a history, do not ask any woman if she is married, ask who her support person is. Do not use the term "homosexual;" rather use "lesbian" which is thought to have a more positive connotation. Do not ask if she is "having intercourse;" ask if she is "sexually active." Better questions are "Are you single, partnered, or married?" "Who is in your immediate family?" If your client uses the term, lesbian, about herself and her family, she is probably relatively at ease with herself. The term, homosexual, generally refers to males in the gay culture.
- Negative behavior changes by the provider upon learning that the patient is lesbian. These can be avoiding touching her, superficial or condescending interaction with her, or outright hostility.
- Isolation from those they love—friends and relatives of choice—when in or visiting the hospital. The "traditional family" may be the only people allowed by the hospital staff to visit and support the client.
- Fear that coming out or disclosure, will lead to loss of confidentiality. If the client is "labeled" in the charts or records, it may become public knowledge, leading to personal-social-work losses.
- Fear of substandard care, or perhaps hurtful care.
- Fear after prior negative experiences.
- Lack of female provider (MD, NP, PA, CNM).

AN INCLUSIVE APPROACH AND ENVIRONMENT FOR ACCEPTANCE

Interview techniques and written materials that are inclusive in language allow a lesbian the freedom to respond with information that will be more helpful to the clinician.[1] Beginning with a reassuring statement to create a sensitive, nonjudgmental climate. The following suffices as an example:

> People are at risk for different diseases and need different tests depending on what activities they're engaging in now and in the past. I ask all my patients some personal questions about their sexual history to help me give you the best care tailored to your specific needs. Everything you tell me will be kept in confidence. (p. 6)[1]

In addition, a safe environment can be created that facilitates disclosure by using open body language, inviting the woman's partner or friend to participate if she wishes, assuring the confidentiality of medical documentation, and having a posted nondiscrimination policy and diversified reading materials prominently displayed in the waiting room.[1]

Too often, providers simply assume that the client is heterosexual.[8] The provider who asks a woman if she is sexually active, learns that she is and then immediately asks what form of contraception is being used, is both insensitive and judgmental.

Examples of questions that give the woman an opportunity to disclose her relationships include the following: "Are you in a committed relationship or partnership?" "Who are the support people in your life?" "Who is your immediate family?" "Who are the people important to you?" "Could you tell me about the people you live with?" "What is your relationship with the person(s) you live with?" "Are you in satisfying relationships with people important to you?" "Do you have any concerns you'd like to talk about?"[1,3]

Asking "Are you sexually active?" and receiving a "Yes" response should then lead to "Are you sexual with men . . . , women . . . , both . . . ?" Then, a further question is "Have your past partners been men, women, or both?"[1] Asking these questions in a matter of fact way allows the client to feel free to be truthful since the provider expects any of the answers. Questions about sexual relationships need to go further, however, than the sex of partner/s and the number of partners. The provider needs to determine if the relationship is a committed one—one where this partner is the most important support person for

the woman. This data is important for future reference in case of illness and hospitalization. Permission to chart the sexual orientation should be gained from the client before it is placed in the record.[5]

Additionally, the provider may need to ask if there is a need to discuss contraception, how the woman is protecting herself from sexually transmitted diseases (issues of safer sex), and if she has any other concerns to discuss.[1] Asking what the woman's major sources of stress, concern, and health risks and problems are is important.[1]

ASSESSING THE WOMAN'S COPING STATUS

To best meet the needs of the client, the provider must learn how the woman feels about herself, her level of self-esteem, and her ability to cope internally and externally with her identity.[11] How does she feel about being a lesbian? Does she share information about her sexual orientation with others and, if so, does she feel comfortable about this? How has she been and how is she treated by health care professionals? Has she been treated before by or know of health care providers who are open to caring for lesbians? What health needs and risks does she feel she has? Is she aware of support networks? The answers to these questions will allow the provider to give the client more information to help herself and to uncover areas for care.

Lesbians may, in fact, share little or nothing about their self-identification. By controlling this information, the client may believe her environment is safer.[13] She feels less likely to be mistreated, ignored, or misdiagnosed. This is seen as a survival method. Some women may increase their feelings of safety by bringing a friend who will be a witness if they are mistreated or be an advocate if needed. The provider needs to allow this type of support unless there is concern that the friend is abusive or coercive.

A lesbian—or any woman—who has been negatively sensitized from past experiences with the health care system[10,13] may act hostilely toward the provider from the outset, may be disruptive and dissonant. This kind of situation can make them feel more in control, believing that they will more likely receive needed care by using this behavior.

Lastly, a lesbian may be dealing with issues of self-worth and internalized homophobia. Some women may internalize societal self-hatred and have very poor self-esteem. This may be evidenced by depression, substance abuse, or negative behaviors.

SPECIAL GROUPS AT GREATER RISK

Children and Adolescents. Unless the young lesbian child or adolescent is lucky enough to be part of a family who is able to accept and support her in her development regardless of sexual orientation, she may be vulnerable to psychological trauma in her growth and development.[6] The usual message from families and adults who have contact with children today is still one that promotes the beliefs that lesbianism is a deviant, irreligious, and, perhaps, evil orientation. Thus, young girls who are battling inwardly with their same sex feelings and are being told outwardly that same sex feelings are wrong are subject to poor self-identity development, perhaps becoming runaways, homeless, isolated, depressed, or suicidal; furthermore, they may abuse substances, experience domestic violence, and fail in school or work.[14] These girls need positive lesbian role models and support in developing self-respect to help decrease the risks of these consequences. A number of larger cities have gay and lesbian adolescent social services organizations to which such clients can be referred. (See addresses for several such organizations at the end of the chapter.)

Older Lesbians. Nursing home personnel should be educated to understand the special needs of all clients, including lesbians. A clearinghouse of information on older lesbians is the National Association for Lesbian and Gay Gerontology in San Francisco. (Other resource centers for older lesbians are listed at the end of the chapter.) Older lesbians have a greater risk for unmet health needs because of their triple minority status: being old, being female, and being lesbian.[15] Additionally, older women may have been too afraid of negative consequences of affirming publicly their woman-identification and, thus, may never

have come out. Consequently, health care providers may not pick up on clues so that effective assistance can be offered to the older person, especially through support from the significant other.[13] Poverty and increasing health problems of aging add to the significant risks for lesbian elders. Health care providers will need to be particularly aware and sensitive to offer needed assistance.

Lesbians with Disabilities. See the special section on this topic provided in Chapter 24 on women with disabilities.

Racial and Ethnic Minority Lesbians. Not only do lesbians face unique challenges due to sexual orientation, but if they are members of a minority race/ethnic group, they face even greater risks of rejection based on racial or ethnic prejudices. Deevey states that "Lesbians of color report triple jeopardy because of their race, sexual orientation, and gender" (p. 197).[11]

HEALTH PROBLEMS OF LESBIANS

Lesbians seek health care for menstrual problems (painful or irregular periods), vaginal infections and sexually transmitted diseases (primarily vaginal infections and herpes), reproductive problems (pelvic pain, uterine infections, painful coitus or orgasms), urinary tract infections, musculoskeletal problems, and breast problems.[4] Many women never seek health interventions for these problems, except for musculoskeletal problems. Unique health concerns of lesbians that may go unaddressed if the provider assumes heterosexuality include appropriate screening for cancer, depression, substance abuse, STDs, HIV, as well as relationship issues, pregnancy, and parenting.[3,16]

In a study comparing lesbian and heterosexual women's lifestyles, Buenting (1992) found no difference between the groups on items of regular exercise, smoking cigarettes, social activities, community service, monthly self-breast exams, spiritual-religious activities, abstinence from alcohol, and drinking alcohol.[17] Lesbians had significantly higher mean scores, however, on use of recreational drugs, alternative diets, and meditation/relaxation techniques. Heterosexual women had significantly higher mean scores on regular Pap smears, use of prescribed medications, and fulfilling family obligations.

PHYSICAL HEALTH PROBLEMS

Menstrual Problems and Pelvic Pain. Dysmenorrhea, often severe, is a common complaint of lesbians (38–54 percent).[18] This complaint may never be acted upon because the woman is hesitant to seek care. Endometriosis is presumed to be high, based on the severe dysmenorrhea rate and the high rate of nulliparity. A reported higher rate of hysterectomy among lesbians than among heterosexual women may result from electing hysterectomies as definitive birth control.

Sexually Transmitted Diseases and Vaginal Infections. Rates of STDs are reported to be lower in lesbians than in heterosexual women or gay men.[3,8] Syphilis, gonorrhea, chlamydia, and herpes are reported as low in lesbians,[8] as well as hepatitis A, amebiasis, shigellosis and helminthism rates.[3] HPV rates have also been low in several studies.[8] Bacterial vaginosis, trichomonas, and vaginal candidiasis are the most common vaginal infections seen in lesbians, with some evidence of transmission between partners.[3]

One study of 503 lesbians found that STDs and vaginal complaints were the second most common reason for seeking health care.[4] Those who did not seek care were using herbal and other alternative therapies for self-care. Bisexual women are more likely to have a wider range of STDs or vaginitis than are lesbians who are exclusive with other exclusive women.[6] Thus, routine screening with this group of women for chlamydia, herpes, gonorrhea, trichomonas, and syphilis is not indicated. Women need to be reminded that oral sex can transmit some infections like herpes.

Although early studies of HIV in lesbians indicated that HIV infection was rare,[19,20] and many lesbian and bisexual women believed themselves to be at low risk, this may not be assumed today.[21] Although, to date, studies have not documented female-to-female transmission of HIV,[22] many women having sex with women engage in behaviors that place them at risk of HIV infection.[23] These behaviors include unprotected sex with men,

unprotected sex or sharing sex toys without protection, and injecting drug use.[22–25] Adolescent lesbians and bisexuals, like all adolescents, often "experiment" with sexual activities.[21] Thus, they may try heterosexual behaviors that put them at risk.

Women, in general, are at increased risk today for HIV infection; thus, safer sex information should be shared with lesbians.[5] Use of dental dams, latex gloves, and plastic kitchen wrap may offer some protection. More accurate information about increasing sexual safety and appropriate prevention rests in knowing the sexual preference of the client. It shows lack of awareness and insensitivity to ask every woman who walks in what kind of contraception she uses and to advise that her partner use condoms without knowing her sexual preference. Women who have male and female partners need to use condoms and spermicide with male partners, and other barriers with female partners. Avoidance of contact with blood and secretions/discharges of any partner is important protection from HIV infection.

Obesity. Herzog found that lesbians had a higher weight, preferred a higher ideal body weight, and were less concerned about thinness and appearance than were heterosexual women.[26] Lesbians are less likely to have eating disorders and to be concerned with body attractiveness.[27] Whether lesbians have a higher incidence of diseases attributable to obesity is unknown. Health care providers need to consider these general risks, however, in providing preventive care.

Cancer Risks. In a study of perceptions by sexual preference regarding cervical cancer, lesbians felt themselves less susceptible than heterosexuals despite the fact that 79 percent had had sexual intercourse with men.[28] Lesbians are likely to get Pap smears irregularly, regardless of sexual practices.[29] Reasons for not getting regular Pap smears include lack of health insurance, forgetting, misinformation about the need, lack of recommendation from health care providers, discomfort with the necessary exam, and history of past abuse. Many women are unaware of risk factors for cervical cancer.[28]

The actual rate of cervical dysplasia in lesbians is low, but since HPV can be transmitted by oral sex, cigarette smoking increases the risk of cervical cancer, and lesbians may have had at least one male partner in their lifetimes, it behooves health care providers to recommend yearly Paps for at risk women. Once any woman has had 3 negative Pap smears and has no risk factors for cervical cancer, Pap smears every several years may be considered.[6]

The incidence of breast cancer among lesbians is unknown, but there may be an increased rate secondary to lack of and delayed childbearing and increased alcohol exposure.[29] Additionally, if lesbians seek less health care or more irregular health care, they may be screened less often, and if they are separated from their families of origin because of their lifestyle, they may not be as aware of family disease risks. Lesbians do have a lower rate of performing breast self-examinations and having mammograms.[29]

Ovarian cancer risk may be higher in lesbians, although little data is available.[6] Any suppression of ovulation, such as full-term pregnancy, long-term use of oral contraceptives, or a history of tubal ligation, reduces the risk of ovarian cancer significantly. None of these is prevalent in the lesbian population as a whole. Similarly, lesbians as a group have a higher rate of a number of risk factors for endometrial cancer, including obesity, a high fat diet, and low parity, as well as a tendency to delay seeing a doctor about abnormal bleeding.[6] A high fat diet, high alcohol consumption, obesity, and a history of colon polyps are colon cancer risk factors found in lesbians.[6,30,31]

Heart Disease and Stroke. Those factors that may increase the risk of colon, breast, and endometrial cancer also may increase the lesbian's risk for heart disease and stroke. It is not known what the actual incidence among this group is for these diseases.

The glaring truth is that for all the cancer and cardiovascular risk factors, routine screening is one safeguard leading to early detection as well as to health promotion efforts that lesbians are less likely to have due to delayed care and irregular care. Both increase the risk of more serious disease.

MENTAL HEALTH ISSUES

Rates of depression among lesbians are similar to those among heterosexual women, but lesbians use counseling more, probably because it is stressful to live in a society where their identification is not readily accepted.[32] Saunders and Valente found a two and one-half times higher rate of suicide in a study of lesbians as compared with heterosexual women.[33] Adolescents seemed to be more at risk, accounting for half of the suicides among lesbians.[8] The leading cause of death of gay adolescents is suicide.[25] Suicide is the third leading cause of death of U.S. adolescents, and 30 percent of these are by gay adolescents. Information on other mental health problems on lesbians is limited.

If the provider assesses that depression is a health factor, it is appropriate to ask the client, in the course of narrowing down cause, if she has any problems relating to sexual orientation. Once disclosure has been made, the provider—who can comfortably do so—may then ask some or all of the following questions:

- How do you feel about your sexual orientation?
- When did you first come out to yourself?
- Have you been able to talk about this with your friends or family of origin? How did they respond?
- Have you been discriminated against or been victimized because of your orientation? By whom?
- Do you have a support system who you can turn to? Do you need information on how to find gay organizations in the area?

Providing the client with information about mental health professionals who routinely deal with these issues and/or support groups can be immensely helpful and affirming. Even in these so-called tolerant times, the client experiencing emotions toward someone of the same sex for the first time—or acknowledging it for the first time—may still think she's the only one on earth this has happened to. Being gay is a statement of selfhood and identity. Coming to terms with it can involve depression when too many forget that sexual identity is a spectrum and in fact seems to have a genetic basis.

Drinking alcohol has been reported as higher in lesbians, but the studies have been criticized as not being representative but being opportunistic.[3,8] Some studies have found higher rates of substance abuse, especially alcohol, among lesbians,[34–39] while others have not.[40,41] The criticism is that the data are biased since much of it was gathered in gay bars where there would be a higher number of women who drink. Newer studies show no greater abuse rates than nonlesbians have.

A substance abuse-identity development link may exist.[11] Alcohol abuse is estimated at 30 percent of lesbians as compared with 10 percent among the general population.[42,43] Additionally, alcohol use does not taper off as the young adult matures.[41] Some areas of the country have AA meetings that are specifically for women or lesbians or gays.

As with heterosexual relationships, lesbian relationships can be all encompassing to the point that the partners lose a sense of self.[44] Codependency (a pathologic and abnormal desire for closeness) may occur. Other relational conflicts occur as with any couple, but may be worsened by impinging issues related to being lesbians, such as not being able to wed, societal biases, or problems with self-concept.

Domestic violence in lesbian relationships does occur.[45,46] Eleven percent of lesbians reported being victims of domestic violence by their lesbian partners.[32] Violence seems to be related to alcohol use most commonly. Because there is a myth associated with lesbians that relationships are always loving and non-violent, however, battered lesbians rarely disclose their abuse or seek help.[5] Health care providers need to be aware that domestic violence is happening in this group of women. Support groups are available for assistance, including the Lesbian Caucus in Boston.

Other forms of violence are experienced by lesbians just as by heterosexual women. The special acts of violence born of hate, however, often unreported in years past, are being reported more often today. The National Gay and Lesbian Task Force hotline in Washington, DC (202-332-6483) offers a way for lesbians who have received violent threats to seek redress.

DESIRE TO PARENT

The needs of lesbians related to childbearing and child rearing have been in the public eye much of late. Health care providers must be aware that many lesbians and couples want to have children,[47] and should address this area in the history. Studies indicate that children raised in lesbian and gay families are like children from any other families developmentally, behaviorally, and otherwise.[5,48]

Artificial insemination is the usual choice to become pregnant of lesbian couples, and information about this process is often requested of the health care provider.[5] It is advisable for the sperm to come from a screened donor bank to decrease the possible risk of HIV. Adoption poses problems legally, especially if the legal parent dies or the couple separates. Seeking a male to have intercourse with for insemination purposes is another option for pregnancy. It is advisable for lesbians who wish to become pregnant to first consult a legal practitioner or call the Lesbian Mothers National Defense Fund in Seattle, WA (206-325-2643) for a list of attorneys who specialize in this field.[5]

Increased support may be needed when children from a previous heterosexual relationship or children from the lesbian relationship are involved in custody battles because of the client's sexual orientation. Other common fears relate to telling their children about their orientation and to interacting with the straight community—people in the schools, churches, and health care system.

Lesbians represent a large group of clients with unique medical, psychological, and social needs.[49] Often, providers remain unaware that a woman is lesbian and, therefore, unique and diverse needs may go unrecognized. The opportunity to provide optimal care is missed. Clinicians would benefit from further research on lesbian health issues in order to provide appropriate guidelines for care.[3]

LESBIAN HEALTH RESOURCES AND ORGANIZATIONS[1]

COMMUNITY SERVICES CENTERS

Lesbian and Gay Community Services Center
208 West 13th Street
New York, NY 10011
(212) 620–7310

**Los Angeles Lesbian and Gay Community
Services Center**
1625 Schrader Blvd.
Los Angeles, CA 90028–9998
(213) 993–7400

Gay and Lesbian Community Action Center
310 East 38th Street
Minneapolis, MN 55409
(612) 822–0127

YOUTH

**National Advocacy Coalition on Youth
and Sexual Orientation**
1025 Vermont Ave., N.W., Suite 200
Washington, DC 20005
(202) 783–4165

The Hetrick-Martin Institute
2 Astor Place
New York, NY 10003
(212) 674–2400

**Gay and Lesbian Adolescent Social Services
(GLASS)** .
650 N. Robertson Blvd. W.
Hollywood, CA 90069
(310) 358–8727

**Boston Alliance of Gay and Lesbian Youth
(BAGLY)**
P. O. Box 814
Boston, MA 02103
(800) 42–BAGLY (24-hour hotline)

Indianapolis Youth Group (IYG)
P. O. Box 20716
Indianapolis, IN 46220
(800) 347–TEEN (national peer help
line 7:00–11:45p.m., EST)

Out Youth Austin
2330 Guadalupe Street
Austin, TX 78705
(800) 96–YOUTH (peer hotline 5:30–9:30 P.M.,
EST)

National Runaway Switchboard
(800) 621–4000 (24-hour hotline)

ELDERS

**National Association for Lesbian and Gay
Gerontology (NALGG)**
1290 Sutter Street, Suite 8
San Francisco, CA 94109

Old Lesbians Organizing for Change (OLOC)
P. O. Box 980422
Houston, TX 77098

Senior Action in a Gay Environment (SAGE)
305 7th Ave.
New York, NY 10001
(212) 741–2247

Gay and Lesbian Outreach to Elders (GLOE)
1853 Market Street
San Francisco, CA 94103
(415) 626–7000

FAMILIES AND FRIENDS

**Parents and Friends of Lesbians
and Gays (P-FLAG)**
1011 14th Street NW, Suite 1030
Washington, DC 20005
(202) 638–4200

VIOLENCE

**New York City Gay and Lesbian
Anti-Violence Project**
647 Hudson Street
New York, NY 10014
(212) 807–0197 (24-hour hotline)
(212) 657–9465 (TDD)

**Tucson United Against Domestic
Violence/Brewster Center**
2711 E. Broadway
Tucson, AZ 85716

The Lesbian Caucus
107 South Street, Fifth Floor
Boston, MA 02111
(617) 426–8492

OTHER

**Sexuality Information and Education Council
of the United States (SIECUS)**
130 W. 42nd St., Suite 2500
New York, NY 10036
(212) 819–9770

National Women's Health Network
514 10th St. NW, Suite 400
Washington, DC 20004

REFERENCES

1. Rankow, L. (1995). Women's Health Issues: Planning for Diversity. Durham, N.C.: Duke University Medical Center.
2. Hollibaugh, A., Vazquez, C., & Plumb, M. (1993). *Lesbian health issues and recommendations.* Washington, DC: National Gay and Lesbian Task Force Policy Institute. Health Policy Project.
3. White, J. C., & Levinson, W. (1995). Lesbian health care: What a primary care physician needs to know. *West J Med, 162,* 463–466.
4. Trippet, S. E., & Bain, J. (1993). Physical health problems and concerns of lesbians. *Women & Health, 20*(2), 59–70.
5. Gentry, S. E. (1992). Caring for lesbians in a homophobic society. *Health Care for Women International, 13,* 173–180.
6. O'Hanlan, K. A. (1995). Lesbian health and homophobia: Perspectives for the treating obstetrician/gynecologist. *Curr Probl Obstet Gynecolog Fertil, 18*(4), 93–104.
7. Stevens, P. E. (1992). Lesbian health care research: A review of the literature from 1970–1990. *Health Care for Women International, 13,* 91–120.
8. Roberts, S. J., & Sorensen, L. (1995). Lesbian health care: A review and recommendations for health promotion in primary care settings. *NP, 20*(6), 42–47.
9. Stevens, P. E. (1994). Lesbians' health-related experiences of care and noncare. *Western J Nursing Research, 16*(6), 639–659.
10. Stevens, P. E. (1994). Protective strategies of lesbian clients in health care environments. *Research in Nursing & Health, 17,* 217–229.
11. Deevey, S. (1995). Lesbian health care. In C. I. Fogel, & N. F. Woods, (Eds.), *Women's health care: A comprehensive handbook.* Thousand Oaks, CA: Sage Publications.
12. Lucas, V. A. (1992). An investigation of the health care preferences of the lesbian population. *Health Care for Women International, 13,* 221–228.
13. Stevens, P. E. (1995). Structural and interpersonal impact of heterosexual assumptions on lesbian health care clients. *Nursing Research, 44*(1), 25–30.
14. American Academy of Pediatrics. (1993). Committee on Adolescence: homosexuality and adolescence. *Pediatrics, 92,* 631–634.
15. Deevey, S. (1990). Older lesbians: An invisible minority. *J Gerontological Nursing, 16*(5), 35–39.
16. Rankow, E. J. (1995). Lesbian health issues for the primary care provider. *J Fam Pract, 40*(5), 486–492.
17. Buenting, J. A. (1992). Health life-styles of lesbian and heterosexual women. *Health Care for Women International, 13,* 165–171.
18. Johnson, S. R., Smith, E. M., Guenther, S. M. (1987). Comparisons of gynecologic health care problems between lesbians and bisexual women: A survey of 2345 women. *J Reprod Med, 32,* 805–811.
19. Chu, S. Y., Buehler, J. W., Flemming, P. L., & Barkelman, R. L. (1990). Epidemiology of reported cases of AIDS in lesbians. United States 1980–1989. *AJPH, 80,* 1380–1381.
20. Petersen, L. R., Doll, L., & White, C. (1992). No evidence for female-to-female HIV transmission among 960,000 female blood donors. *J Acquir Immune Defic Syndr, 5,* 853–855.
21. Bevier, P. J., Chiasson, M. A., Heffernan, R. T., & Castro, K. G. (1995). Women at a sexually transmitted disease clinic who report same-sex contact: Their HIV seroprevalence and risk behaviors. *AJPH, 85*(10), 1366–1377.
22. Kennedy, M. B., Scarlett, M. I., Duerr, A. C., & Chu, S. Y. (1995). Assessing HIV risk among women who have sex with women: Scientific and communication issues. *JAMWA, 50*(3/4), 103–107.
23. Lemp, G. F., Jones, M., Kellogg, T. A., Nieri, G. N., Anderson, L., Withurn, D., & Katz, M. (1995). HIV seroprevalence and risk behaviors among lesbians and bisexual women in San Francisco and Berkley, California. *AJPH, 85,* 1549–1552.
24. Einhorn, L. & Pogar, M. (1994). HIV-risk behavior among lesbians and bisexual women. *AIDS Educ & Prevt, 6*(6), 514–523.
25. Nelson, J. A. (1997). Gay, lesbian, and bisexual adolescents: Providing esteem-enhancing care to a battered population. *NP, 22*(2), 94–109.
26. Herzog, D., Newman, K., Yeh, C., et al. (1992). Body image satisfaction in homosexual and heterosexual women. *Int J Eating Disorders, 11,* 391.
27. Siever, M. D. (1994). Sexual orientation and gender as factors in socioculturally acquired vulnerability to body dissatisfaction and eating disorders. *J Consult Clini Psychol, 62,* 252–260.
28. Price, J. H., Easton, A. N., Telljohann, S. K., & Wallace, P. B. (1996). Perceptions of cervical cancer and pap smear screening behavior by women's sexual orientation. *J Comm Health, 21*(2), 89–105.
29. Rankow, E. J. (1995). Breast and cervical cancer among lesbians. *WHI, 5*(3), 123–129.
30. Giovannucci, E., Stampfer, M. J., Colditz, G. A. et al. (1993). Folate, methionine, and alcohol intake and risk of colorectal adenoma. *J Natl Cancer Inst, 85,* 875–884.

31. Chute, C. G., Willett, W. C., Colditz, G. A. et al. (1991). A prospective study of body mass, height and smoking on the risk of colorectal cancer in women. *Cancer Causes Control, 2,* 117–124.

32. Bradford, J., Ryan, C., & Rothblum, E. (1994). National lesbian health care survey: Implications for mental health care. *J Consult Clin Psychol, 62*(2), 228–242.

33. Saunders, J. M., & Valente, S. M. (1987). Suicide risk among gay men and lesbians: A review. *Death Stud, 11*(1), 1–23.

34. Milman, D. H., & Su, E. H. (1973). Patterns of drug usage among university students. *J Am Coll Health Associ, 21,* 181–187.

35. Lewis, C. E., et al. (1982). Drinking patterns in homosexual and heterosexual women. *J Clin Psychiatry, 43*(7), 277–279.

36. Finnegan, D. G., & McNally, E. B. (1987). Dual identities: *Counseling chemically dependent gay men and lesbians.* Center City, MN: Hazelden.

37. Glaus, K. O. (1989). Alcoholism, chemical dependency, and the lesbian client. In E. D. Rothbaum & E. Cole (Eds.), *Loving boldly: Issues facing lesbians.* (pp. 131–144). New York: Harrington Park Press.

38. Kus, R. J. (1990). Alcoholism in the gay and lesbian communities. In R. J. Kus (Ed.), *Keys to caring: Assisting your lesbian and gay clients* (pp. 66–81). Boston: Alyson.

39. Nicoloff, L. K., & Stiglitz, E. A. (1987). Lesbian alcoholism: Etiology, treatment and recovery. In Boston Lesbian Psychologies Collective (Ed.), *Lesbian psychologies* (pp. 283–293). Urbana: University of Illinois Press.

40. Bloomfield, K. A. (1993). A comparison of alcohol consumption between lesbians and heterosexual women in an urban population. *Drg Alcohol Depend, 33,* 257–269.

41. McKirnan, D. J., & Peterson, P. C. (1989). Alcohol and drug abuse among homosexual men and women: Epidemiology and population characteristics. *Addictive Behaviors, 14,* 545–553.

42. Deevey, S., & Wall, L. J. (1992). How do lesbians develop serenity? *Health Care for Women International, 13*(2), 199–208.

43. Hall, J. M. (1990). Alcoholism and lesbians. Developmental, symbolic interactionism, and critical perspectives. *Health Care for Women International, 11*(1), 84–107.

44. McCandlish, B. M. (1981). Therapeutic issues with lesbian couples. *J Homosex, 7,* 71–78.

45. Morrow, J. (1994, April). Identifying and treating battered lesbians. *San Francisco Medicine,* 17–21.

46. Leeder, E. (1988). Enmeshed in pain: counseling lesbian battering couples. *Women and Therapy, 7,* 81–89.

47. Harvey, S. M., Carr, C., & Bernheine, S. (1989). Lesbian mothers: Health care experiences. *J Nurse-Midwifery, 34*(3), 115–119.

48. Laird, J. (1993). Lesbian and gay families. In F. Walsh (Ed.) *Normal family process* (pp. 282–328). New York: Guilford Press.

49. White, J. C., & Levinson, W. (1993). Primary care of lesbian patients. *J Gen Int Med, 8,* 41–47.

50. Gorham, M. (1997). Working toward recovery with the lesbian patient. *AJN, 97*(5), 69–70.

PROMOTION OF GYNECOLOGIC HEALTH CARE

CHAPTER 8

MENSTRUATION AND RELATED PROBLEMS AND CONCERNS

Sharon Baker

*M*ost women experience numerous changes in their menstrual cycle patterns during their reproductive life.

Highlights

- Myths
- Normal Onset and Occurrence
- Amenorrhea
- Dysfunctional Uterine Bleeding
- Dysmenorrhea
- Toxic Shock Syndrome
- Premenstrual Syndrome

▶ INTRODUCTION

Menstruation is a normal, cyclically recurring event for most women between the approximate ages of 12 and 50. Like childbirth, it usually occurs without major difficulties and is a universal event for most women. Unlike childbirth, however, menstruation has a very negative history. The menstruating woman has been thought to be possessed by evil spirits. Myths have portrayed the menses as a time of magic, danger, or even poison. Ancient physicians such as Pliny described how a menstruating woman could kill crops, drive animals mad, and even deter thieves. Aristotle wrote that the reflection of a menstruous woman in a mirror would bewitch the next person who looked into it.[1]

Historically, menstruation was viewed as a disease rather than a normal condition. Medical treatment during the second half of the 19th century rested on an explicit view of women as fragile and vulnerable, totally dominated by the cyclicity and disability of their reproductive system. This heritage has objectively and subjectively colored society's perceptions of the menstruating woman as weak, suffering, unstable, or physically unable to execute her normal duties competently. There is much argument in the literature about the effect of this conditioning on women's perceptions of menstrual symptoms and events. Feminist literature challenges much of the medical and psychiatric literature on menstrual cycle research as being biased and sexist.

The recent popularity of best sellers on the menstrual changes associated with menopause has opened the way for greater social awareness and knowledge of menstrual norms and changes, made the topic more acceptable for discussion, and continued to alter the attitudes of society toward menstruation. One can hope this trend will help to ameliorate the predominantly negative attitudes about menstruation that past studies have demonstrated. This is important since most women experience numerous changes in their menstrual cycle patterns during their reproductive life. In the United States, women aged 25–54 years make 2.9 million office visits annually for disorders of menstruation.[1] Adequate information about norms, comfort in discussing this body function, and access to reliable health care providers may decrease unnecessary visits, reduce embarrassment and anxiety about common problems, and encourage further studies on women's menstrual experiences.

ONSET OF NORMAL MENSES

Events preceding the first menses have a characteristic pattern. *Thelarche,* the development of breast buds; *adrenarche,* the appearance of pubic then axillary hair followed by the growth spurt; with culmination in *menarche.* See Chapter 4 and 5 for more details on these developmental milestones.

NORMAL OCCURRENCE OF MENSES

The menstrual cycle will be repeated 300–400 times in the life of the human female. Cycles vary in frequency from 21–40 days (regularity is normal), bleeding lasts 3–8 days, and blood loss averages 30 to 80 mL.[3,4] Small clots are normal; large clots indicate rapid bleeding and inability of fibrinogen to act in the uterus.

DESCRIPTIVE TERMS FOR MENSTRUAL ABNORMALITIES

- *Amenorrhea.* Absence of menses.
- *Oligomenorrhea.* Infrequently occurring menses at intervals greater than 35 days.
- *Polymenorrhea.* Menses at intervals of 21 days or fewer.
- *Hypermenorrhea/Menorrhagia.* Regularly occurring bleeding excessive in duration and flow (greater than 80mL/cycle or lasting longer than 7 days).
- *Metrorrhagia.* Bleeding occurring irregularly.
- *Menometrorrhagia.* Irregular, heavy bleeding.
- *Hypomenorrhea.* Regular bleeding in less than normal amount.
- *Intermenstrual Bleeding.* Bleeding at any time between otherwise normal menses.[3,5]

ABNORMALITIES RELATED TO THE MENSTRUAL CYCLE

AMENORRHEA

Amenorrhea is a symptom, not a diagnosis, and is categorized as primary or secondary. *Primary amenorrhea* is the absence of menses by age 16 whether or not normal growth and secondary sexual characteristics are present, or the absence of menses after age 14 when normal growth and signs of secondary sexual characteristics are present. *Secondary amenorrhea* is the absence of menses for 3 cycles or 6 months in women who have previously menstruated.[3,6,7]

Epidemiology

Etiology. Etiology includes pregnancy, lactation, and age appropriate menopause, which are by far the most likely causes of amenorrhea and are considered physiological. Among women of reproductive age, amenorrhea that is unrelated to pregnancy may signal stress or a life threatening disease. Causative factors include anatomic deviations, genetic factors, endocrine abnormalities or imbalances, defective enzyme systems, autoimmune diseases, tumors, eating disorders, excessive exercise, medications, or past surgery.[3]

Incidence. Secondary amenorrhea occurs in 1–3 percent of women. Incidence in subgroups such as college students and athletes are higher, 3–5 percent and 5–60 percent respectively. The prevalence of primary amenorrhea is 0.3 percent.[8]

Subjective Data

The etiology of amenorrhea is revealed in a woman's history most of the time. Questions about each of the following areas should be carefully posed.

- Menstrual history includes the following information: age of development of secondary sex characteristics and current status, absence of menarche or age it occurred, date of last menstrual period, symptoms associated with menses, interval between menses, duration and characteristics of flow.
- Past illnesses, hospitalizations, and surgeries should be noted. Chronic diseases such as childhood leukemia, thyroid or adrenal dysfunction, and renal or hepatic disease are recorded, along with a description of radiation therapy, chemotherapy, or surgery, particularly a dilation and curettage (D & C), which can affect the menstrual pattern.
- Obstetric history records the date and course of any pregnancy. Intrauterine or ectopic pregnancy, abortion, and type of delivery are also noted. Postpartum hemorrhage or infection could be a causative factor of amenorrhea.
- Prescription and over-the-counter drugs can affect menstrual function, and a history of oral contraceptives may alter usual patterns. Illicit drug use, smoking, and alcohol intake also can disturb normal cycles.
- Lifestyle evaluation includes eating patterns, weight loss or gain, critical level of body fat, exercise regimens, obesity, anorexia, bulimia, life stressors, and sexual behaviors, including contraception.
- History of present illness (HPI) is an assessment of bodily changes or abnormalities, such as nipple discharge, hirsutism, virilization, absence of menses alternating with heavy bleeding cycles, hot flashes, vaginal dryness, insomnia, headaches, or infertility.[3,8]

Objective Data

Physical Examination

- *General Appearance and Skin.* Observe carefully and note general body habitus, stage of development of secondary sexual characteristics (see Tanner stages, Chapter 5), amount and distribution of hair and fat, and presence of striae.
- *Vital Signs.* Gather baseline data, height, weight, and blood pressure and compare with norms.
- *Head and Eyes.* Perform a complete head-to-toe physical, including a visual field exam.[9]
- *Neck.* Examine thyroid for nodules or enlargement.
- *Breasts.* Observe breasts for discharge, then palpate for masses and attempt to express discharge.
- *Abdomen.* Palpate abdomen for masses or hernias.
- *Genitalia/Reproductive.* Examine genitalia for obstructive problems, such as imperforate hymen or vaginal septum. Observe the cervix for signs of pregnancy (bluish discoloration or softening). Palpate the uterus and adnexa for signs of pregnancy or tumor.[3,10]
- *Endocrine.* Assess for signs of androgen excess such as hirsutism, clitoromegaly, or acne. Evaluate hormonal status (estrogen and progesterone) by color of mucous membranes, presence or absence of rugae, amount and consistency of cervical mucus, and presence of ferning. Vaginal cells may be collected for maturation index.

In the normal woman of reproductive age, mucous membranes are pink and moist; rugae are present; and cervical mucus is clear and ferns if estrogen, without progesterone, is present.

Commonly Recommended Diagnostic Tests and Methods

- *A pregnancy test should always be done first* to rule out pregnancy or related complications: ectopic pregnancies, complete or incomplete abortions, or trophoblastic neoplasms. The serum beta human chorionic gonadotropin (β-hCG) test is most accurate, but expensive. Urine testing is usually adequate if the hCG level is not below 25 mIU/mL. [3,9]

- *Thyrotropin (TSH)* should be ordered after excluding pregnancy. It is relatively rare, but an easily treatable cause of amenorrhea.[3]
- The *prolactin (PRL)* test is the primary test for a pituitary tumor.[3,8] If galactorrhea is present, pituitary or central nervous system lesions are the second most common cause after drugs. Physician consultation is necessary for prolactin levels above 20ng/mL in order to rule out the presence of a pituitary tumor. The nurse practitioner can complete much of the workup if the consulting physician is agreeable. For prolactin above 20ng/mL, a coned-down lateral x-ray evaluation of the sella turcica is customary. If the prolactin level is greater than 100 ng/mL, or if the coned-down view is abnormal, a CT or MRI is necessary.[3,8] Physician management is essential.
- If tests for pregnancy, hypothyroidism, and pituitary tumor are negative, administer the *progesterone challenge test.* Progesterone in oil (200 mg I.M.) or orally active medroxyprogesterone acetate (10 mg daily for 5–10 days) is given to test for the presence of estrogen priming and the intactness of the outflow tract (uterus and vagina). If there is no galactorrhea and bleeding occurs in 2–7 days after concluding medication, anovulation is established as the diagnosis.[3,9]
- If no bleeding occurs with the progesterone challenge, administer 1.25 mg. of *conjugated estrogen* orally for 21 days to stimulate endometrial proliferation. *Add medroxyprogesterone acetate* 10 mg p.o. for the last 5 days of estrogen administration to achieve a withdrawal bleed. Bleeding after medications rules out defects of the outflow tract.[3,9]
- If no bleeding occurs after this regimen, *repeat medications to validate results.* Then, if no bleeding occurs, a diagnosis of defective uterus or outflow tract can be made. This is a relatively rare diagnosis with no history of infection or trauma in clients whose pelvic exam findings are normal.[3,8]
- If the history includes D & C or uterine infection, but no bleeding with an initial administration of estrogen and medroxyprogesterone or repeated regimen, *consult* with GYN physician to rule out Asherman's syndrome (intrauterine adhesions). The gynecologist may perform a

hysterosalpingogram or hysteroscopy to determine if uterine adhesions are causative.[8]

- If withdrawal bleeding occurs with the administration of estrogen and medroxyprogesterone, then the reason for the client's inability to produce adequate levels of estrogen must be determined. Consult with GYN or endocrine physician about evaluation of ovarian or adrenal factors that may be causative. Because estrogen/progesterone medications may affect endogenous gonadotropin levels, wait two weeks before initiating follow up testing.[3]

Ovarian Function Tests

- *Follicle-Stimulating Hormone (FSH).* A level greater than 30–50 mIU/mL indicates ovarian failure.[3,8]
- *Luteinizing Hormone (LH).* A normal LH level with a high FSH level indicates impending ovarian failure.
- *LH–FSH Ratio.* Higher than normal mean concentrations of LH with low or low-normal levels of FSH are present with persistent anovulation.[3]
- *Autoimmune Dysfunction.* Premature ovarian failure is associated with autoimmune diseases, particularly when ovarian failure and thyroid abnormalities occur together. Physician referral is recommended for further diagnostic workup of these two abnormal findings. Screening tests to rule out autoimmune dysfunction usually includes the following: sedimentation rate, antinuclear antibodies, complete blood cell (CBC) count with differential, rheumatoid factor, total serum protein, albumin-globulin ratio, and thyroid antibody studies (T4, calcium, phosphorous, and A.M. cortisol).[3,8]

Ovarian/Adrenal Function Tests

- *Total Testosterone.* Levels greater than 200 ng/dL suggest a tumor; the adrenal or ovarian source should be determined.[3]
- *Dehydroepiandrosterone Sulfate (DHEA-S).* A level greater than 400 µg/dL suggests an adrenal disorder or tumor.[7]
- *Cortisol Level.* Order this test if Cushing's stigmata are present in order to screen for adrenal hyperactivity.

Karyotype. Consult with physician about ordering this test if genetic or chromosomal abnormalities are suspected.[3,8]

CBC, Coagulation Profile, Serum Iron, or Ferritin. These tests may be ordered to rule out anemia or clotting disorders.[3]

Differential Medical Diagnoses

Pregnancy Related

- Pregnancy, lactation, or pregnancy complications such as ectopic pregnancy, missed abortion, postpartum hemorrhage, or trophoblastic neoplasm.

Hypothalamic-Pituitary-Ovarian (HPO) Axis Related

- Anovulation secondary to immature HPO axis, obesity, or polycystic ovaries.
- Premature ovarian failure secondary to genetic conditions, smoking, autoimmune diseases, chemotherapy, radiation, surgery, ovarian insensitivity to gonadotropins (Savage syndrome), or steroidogenic enzyme defect, 17 α-hydroxylase deficiency.
- Menopause secondary to age appropriate follicular depletion.
- Hyperprolactinemia secondary to pituitary tumor, stress, thyroid disorder, or drug induced.
- Inhibited gonadotropin-releasing hormone (GnRH) secondary to discontinuation of oral contraceptives, use of medications such as danazol or suppression of pulsatile GnRH secretion below its critical range secondary to anorexia or weight loss.

Obstructive Related

- Imperforate hymen.
- Transverse vaginal septum.
- Cervical stenosis following instrumentation or trauma.

Genetic/Chromosome Related

- Mayer-Rokintansky-Küster-Hauser syndrome (no apparent vagina).
- Testicular feminization (complete or incomplete).
- Gonadal dysgenesis (Turner's syndrome, Swyer's syndrome).

Autoimmune Disorders

Asherman's Syndrome
- See References [3,7,8,9,10]

Plan

Psychosocial Interventions. The health care provider must address the diverse causes of amenorrhea, the relationship to sexual identity, perception of normal menstrual function, possible infertility, tumor, or life threatening disease. Sensitive listening, interviewing, and individualized evaluation are essential. Always consider the possibility of pregnancy and related emergencies, despite the client's history or social situation. All patients diagnosed with ovarian failure prior to age 30 require physician referral for karyotype determination. These tests require sensitive explanations to avoid further emotional trauma.

Medication. The medication prescribed varies with the client situation. Combination oral contraceptives are superior to progesterone-only treatment in a sexually active, nonsmoking client who is younger than 35. Cyclic progesterone may be preferred when estrogen is contraindicated.

Medroxyprogesterone Acetate (MPA)
- Indications are to prevent endometrial hyperplasia by causing cyclic shedding in anovulatory clients who do not need contraception.[3,9]
- Administer 10 mg p.o. the first 10 to 14 days of each month or during cycle days 16 to 26.
- Side effects and adverse reactions most commonly reported include spotting, weight gain, fatigue, depression, or acne.
- Contraindications include pregnancy, thromboembolic disorders, liver dysfunction, known or suspected malignancy of breast or reproductive organs, undiagnosed vaginal bleeding, or missed abortion. The use of medroxyprogesterone acetate (MPA) as a diagnostic test for pregnancy is also contraindicated.
- Anticipated outcome on evaluation is that the client begins cyclic withdrawal spotting or bleeding 2–7 days after completing medication.
- Client teaching should include information about the possibility of bleeding being heavy when medication is completed. Emphasize the importance of taking the medication to prevent endometrial hyperplasia or cancer. Inform the client of side effects and tell her to report any abnormal bleeding or the absence of withdrawal bleeding. Stress the necessity of consistently using reliable birth control measures.

Low Dose Combination Oral Contraceptives
- Indications are to prevent endometrial hyperplasia *and* to provide contraception for clients with anovulatory cycles (first choice of therapy).
- Administer 21- or 28-day pack cyclic therapy.
- Side effects and adverse reactions most commonly reported include breast tenderness, weight gain, spotting, and scanty menses.
- Contraindications are pregnancy, undiagnosed vaginal bleeding, history of breast or reproductive tract cancer, history of thromboembolism, cerebrovascular or coronary heart disease, liver tumor or malignancy, or smoker older than 35.[11]
- Anticipated outcomes on evaluation are cyclic withdrawal bleeding, contraception, and absence of side effects of MPA.
- Client teaching and counseling should include information about how to take pills, manage missed pills, and recognize the danger signs (see Chapter 9). Instruct the client to chart dates of menses or spotting.

Hormone Replacement Therapy
- Indications are for hypoestrogenic states secondary to premature or physiological menopause, or in serious exercisers.
- Implications (see Chapter 9).

Other
- Other medication regimens should be managed by physician referral or with physician consultation, because of the complex etiology of amenorrhea.

Surgical Interventions. Endometrial biopsy—curette or flushing of endometrial cells for microscopic examination—may be done to evaluate the uterus for atrophy, phase of endometrium, or abnormalities, although the test is not commonly done unless prior tests and treatments yield no answer to the problem. Destroyed endometrium as a cause of secondary amenorrhea can be determined by hysterogram or hysteroscopy. It is an outpatient procedure. Client teaching and counseling include informing the client about the purpose of the biopsy, how the procedure is to be performed, relaxation techniques, follow-up, and the monetary cost.

Follow-Up. Once workup is completed, follow-up is done annually. Prior to refilling medications, evaluate the client's menstrual charts, the client's adherence to the medication schedule, the presence of danger signs or side effects, and the results of the Pap test and breast exam/mammography. Refer all clients with primary amenorrhea for physician evaluation. Reassure young amenorrheic teens and their parents; recommend watchful waiting if results of tests are normal. Refer all clients with secondary amenorrhea caused by central lesions, autoimmune diseases, psychiatric problems, or complex endocrine or metabolic diseases to a physician for evaluation and management.

DYSFUNCTIONAL UTERINE BLEEDING (DUB)

Dysfunctional uterine bleeding (DUB) is defined as excessive, prolonged, unpatterned bleeding from the endometrium in the absence of structural pelvic pathology and usually associated with anovulation.[5] DUB is not related to pregnancy, inflammation, genital tumor, or other anatomic uterine lesion.[3]

Epidemiology

Etiology. The etiology of DUB is usually hormonal disturbance with failure of ovarian follicular maturation resulting in lack of progesterone production, limitation of endometrial growth, and synchronous shedding. Chronic anovulation with continuous estrogen production increases endometrial vascularity and thickness without adequate stromal support for maintenance. Irregular spotting and episodes of profuse and usually painless bleeding result. An atrophic endometrium that bleeds irregularly may be formed by lack of estrogen due to menopause or formed pharmacologically through long-term use of low dose birth control pills. Excessive fibrinolytic activity and changes in prostaglandin also appear to be associated with DUB. Excessive use of acetylsalicylic acid (aspirin) may increase bleeding.[3,5]

Incidence. Incidence of dysfunctional uterine bleeding is primarily attributed to anovulation, and most commonly presents at the extreme ends of reproductive age.[11] One-half of all patients presenting with the problem are over 40, and about 20 percent are adolescents.[12] As much as 20 percent of adolescents with coagulopathies present with dysfunctional uterine bleeding.[3]

Subjective Data

A history of irregular menses is typically exhibited as episodes of heavy painless bleeding alternating with periods of amenorrhea. Subjective reports of excessive bleeding are frequently inaccurate. Factors indicating excessive blood loss include menses lasting longer than seven days, signs of volume depletion, or anemia. Dizziness, fainting, and orthostatic evaluation are important clues.[5]

Objective Data

Although no organic problems are associated with DUB, a complete physical examination, including pelvic and rectal exams, is performed to rule out neoplasia. Note passing tissue and test specimens if available and/or suspicious.

Diagnostic tests and methods include a CBC and Pap smear to rule out abnormalities. In a woman of reproductive age, particularly if unilateral abdominal pain is present, a serum β-hCG test and ultrasound should be done to rule out an ectopic pregnancy. Transvaginal ultrasound may be ordered to measure endometrial thickness. A patient or family history of bleeding disorders mandates coagulation studies. Severe DUB with anemia should be discussed with the physician and warrants coagulation studies. The initial coagulation screening should include platelet count, protime, partial thromboplastin time, and bleeding time.[5] Subclinical hypothyroidism has been implicated as causative of menorrhagia. A TSH assay is recommended.[5]

In-Office Endometrial Biopsy

- Evaluation of suspected uterine pathology is usually done by the physician, although some nurse practitioners perform endometrial biopsies. This diagnostic evaluation is done to determine the cytologic status of endometrial tissue. An in-office endometrial biopsy is recommended for patients at high risk for endometrial hyperplasia and cancer.[5] Age of the patient is not as important as duration of exposure to unopposed estrogen.[3,5]

- Test procedure involves helping the client to assume the lithotomy position. Then a small curette is passed through the cervix to the endometrial cavity in order to obtain a small amount of tissue for examination.

- Nursing implications and client teaching involve informing the client about the purpose of the test, obtaining her signature on the consent form, and explaining the cost of the procedures. Encourage relaxation breathing and convey the progression of each step to the client to alleviate her discomfort and anxiety. Spotting and cramping may occur up to 48 hours following biopsy. NSAIDS can be recommended if there are no contraindications.

Hysteroscopy

- *Hysteroscopy* is visualization of the endometrium through a scope to search for uterine fibroids, polyps, or structural abnormalities.[12] Observation and directed tissue sampling is replacing D & C as the diagnostic procedure of choice. (Minor treatments, such as polyp or septal removal, also can be done through the hysteroscope.)

- The procedure is done in the office or operating room. The hysteroscope is inserted when the cervix is dilated. The uterus is distended with dextran 70, carbon dioxide, or another distention medium to facilitate visualization of the endometrium.

- Nursing implications include teaching the client that some cramps and bleeding are expected following the procedure, and leakage of dextran 70 through the cervix and vagina can be messy. Carbon dioxide distention may cause cramps or shoulder pain. Pain medications should be provided. *Advise the client to report signs of infection, excessive bleeding, or pain— and to report any allergic response that occurs with dextran 70 at once.*

Dilation and Curettage (D & C)

- Dilation of the cervix and curettage (D & C) may be done for diagnostic evaluation. Endometrial D & C is recommended when medical regimens are ineffective, or if polyps, incomplete abortion, or neoplasia is suspected, or if a more complete biopsy sampling of the endometrium may be desired and hysteroscopy is unavailable.

- The procedure requires that the client be given local or general anesthesia and that specimens be sent to pathology.

- Nursing implications are to provide appropriate explanations of the procedure, anesthesia, cost, and risks. Postoperative instructions are given, advising the client to report signs of infection, excessive bleeding, and/or pain. Pain medication is also provided.

Differential Medical Diagnoses

Any early pregnancy disorder or ectopic pregnancy; fibroids/adenomyosis; endometrial polyps/carcinoma; endometriosis, coagulation defects (diagnosed in 20 percent of adolescents with DUB); ovarian abnormalities (polycystic ovaries, tumors); thyroid dysfunction; massive obesity; stress; drugs (anticoagulants, steroids, phenothiazides, digitalis, diet pills, anticholinergics).[3,5,10,11,12,13,14]

Plan

Psychosocial Interventions. Educate the client about normal menstrual cycles and possible reasons for her abnormal pattern. Be generous with reassurance. Menstrual calendars are helpful with instruction given about documenting any bleeding or spotting, days and dosages of medications, pad or tampon count, and associated symptoms of dysmenorrhea. By providing information about expected bleeding patterns on discontinuation of medications, you will help the client to avoid fears of recurrence or treatment failure. Because some medications are teratogenic, it is important to address birth control.

Medication

- A *low dose combination oral contraceptive (OC)* is the first choice of therapy for anovulatory bleeding in clients who need contraception.[3,5,12]

  - A requirement for beginning therapy is to rule out pregnancy prior to prescribing.

- Prescribe one 35 μg pill b.i.d. for 5 to 7 days.[3] Continue oral contraceptives in usual fashion for 3 to 6 months.
- Side effects and adverse reactions most commonly reported include breast tenderness, weight gain, spotting, and scanty menses.
- Contraindications are pregnancy, undiagnosed vaginal bleeding, history of breast or reproductive tract cancer, history of thromboembolism, cerebrovascular or coronary heart disease, liver tumor or malignancy, or smoker older than 35.[11]
- Anticipated outcome on evaluation is that bleeding will abate in 12–14 hours.
- *Client Teaching and Counseling.* If bleeding does not abate, consult a physician. If an anovulatory pattern returns after discontinuing OCs, then resume the low dose combination pills or progesterone therapy described below.

- *Medroxyprogesterone acetate (MPA)* is indicated for clients with anovulatory bleeding who do not need contraception.[3] If contraception is needed, barrier methods are advised with this treatment.

  - A requirement for beginning therapy is to rule out pregnancy.
  - Prescribe MPA 10 mg q.d. for 10–14 days for a medical D & C.

    Endometrial maturation and cyclic shedding can be maintained by prescribing 10 mg of progesterone on days 1 through 10–14 of each month, or cycle days 16–25.[3]
  - Side effects and adverse reactions most commonly reported include spotting, weight gain, fatigue, depression, or acne.
  - Contraindications include pregnancy, thromboembolic disorders, liver dysfunction, known or suspected malignancy of breast or reproductive organs, undiagnosed vaginal bleeding, or missed abortion. The use of medroxyprogesterone acetate (MPA) as a diagnostic test for pregnancy is also contraindicated.
  - Anticipated outcome on evaluation is that the first episode of bleeding after progesterone therapy will be heavy.
  - Client teaching should include information about the possibility of bleeding being heavy when medication is completed. Emphasize the importance of taking medication to pre-

vent endometrial hyperplasia or cancer. Inform the client of side effects and tell her to report any abnormal bleeding or the absence of withdrawal bleeding. Stress the necessity of consistently using reliable birth control measures.

- *Patients with severe anemia or life threatening bleeding require immediate physician management.* Intravenous fluids, blood replacement, and conjugated estrogen may be necessary.

  - Intravenous conjugated estrogen 25 mg q.4h. up to 3 doses until bleeding lessens. If bleeding initially is less, use 1.25 mg q.d. p.o. conjugated estrogen for 7–10 days. Follow either of these regimens with progestin treatment.[3,10]
  - Conjugated estrogens, 0.625–1.25 mg p.o. for days 1–25 of each month with MPA 10 mg p.o. days 12–25 of each month; or
  - Conjugated estrogens 1.25/day p.o. for 7–10 days.[3]

- *Prostaglandin synthetase inhibitors (PGSIs)* are a nonhormonal treatment of menorrhagia.

  - A requirement for beginning therapy is that pregnancy be ruled out. Prescribe mefenamic acid (Ponstel) 500 mg p.o. t.i.d. for 3 days *or* naproxen (Naprosyn) 500 mg p.o. b.i.d. *or* ibuprofen 400 mg every 6 hours. Instruct the client to take the medication with food.[5]
  - Side effects and adverse reactions include gastrointestinal upset, rash, and edema.
  - Contraindications include pregnancy, peptic ulcers, asthma, sensitivity to aspirin, and inflammatory bowel disease.
  - Anticipated outcome on evaluation is a 20–50 percent reduction in bleeding.[3]
  - Client teaching and counseling should include the precaution to take the medication with food. Instruct the client about the dosing regimen and the side effects of the drug.
  - GnRH agonist has been used in some women for short-term suppression of the hypothalamic pituitary axis to stop bleeding. This extreme measure is used if the woman cannot undergo D & C, or in transplant patients where the toxicity of immunosuppressive drugs makes the use of sex steroids less desirable. The expense and long-term side effects make this an unlikely choice for chronic therapy.[3,14]

Surgical Interventions

- Patients should be referred to a gynecologist if large structural lesions are noted on ultrasound or physical exam or if the patients are not responding to treatment. Diagnostic endometrial sampling, hysteroscopy, and occasionally D & C may be used. Myomectomy or removal of endometrial polyps may effectively control bleeding.[5]
- Hysterectomy is a radical procedure in which the uterus is removed. The surgery is reserved for perimenopausal women who fail to improve with hormonal therapy or for adolescents with severe blood dyscrasia.
- Endometrial ablation, an alternative to hysterectomy, is a technique to end bleeding difficulties by laser destruction, or excisional resection. Benefits include shorter surgical time and quicker recovery.[13] The uterus is not removed.

Explain all surgical procedures to the client carefully, including their purpose, risks, benefits, and cost. Before and after surgery, give instructions about pain medication, the expected postoperative course, and the follow-up schedule.

Follow-Up. Follow-up and referral may include iron therapy; 300 mg ferrous sulfate may be taken by mouth with orange juice 30 minutes after meals in addition to the therapy described above if the hemoglobin level is below 12 g. Anovulatory patterns tend to recur; therefore, clients should have a regular follow-up schedule and keep a menstrual and medication calendar. If more than a year elapses without a health care visit, notify the client. Cancer prevention should be a priority with this population.

DYSMENORRHEA

Dysmenorrhea is defined as abdominal pain, cramping or backache associated with menstrual bleeding. It is categorized as primary or secondary. Primary dysmenorrhea is usually without pelvic pathology; on the other hand, secondary dysmenorrhea is frequently accompanied by pelvic pathology.[15]

Epidemiology

Etiology. Primary dysmenorrhea occurs once ovulatory cycles are established and results from excessive prostaglandin release. Secondary dysmenorrhea is most frequently caused by endometriosis, adenomyosis, or pelvic infection.[15,16,17,18] Endometriosis is thought to affect 15 percent of American women.[16] Etiology may be obstructive defects, such as cervical stenosis, imperforate hymen, or müllerian defects, if pain begins at menarche rather than after a regular pattern of cycling is established.

Incidence. In cross-sectional surveys, 30–60 percent of women of reproductive age report experiencing menstrual pain, although the proportion of women who report severe pain sufficient to interfere with daily activity is considerably lower, ranging from 7–15 percent.[19]

Subjective Data

Primary dysmenorrhea. typically presents in ovulatory cycles 6–12 months following menarche, and is most commonly diagnosed in adolescents. Pain is suprapubic and described as "crampy"; it starts 12–24 hours before menses and is intermittent, except in severe cases. Pain is most severe during the first day of menses and disappears in 48–72 hours. The lower abdomen is most painful, but frequently pain extends to the back and thighs. Related molimina include fatigue, headaches, abdominal bloating, and occasionally nausea, vomiting, or light-headedness.[15]

Secondary dysmenorrhea typically presents in women with a history of painful menses that are increasingly intense or severe. It occurs most commonly in the third or fourth decades of life. Usually the location or duration of pain changes. Endometriosis presents in a variety of ways. Some women experience debilitating pain and cramping during menstruation; others experience no symptoms. The extent of disease and symptoms do not correlate. Associated symptoms are frequently dyspareunia, painful defecation, rectal pressure, heavy or irregular bleeding, urinary complaints, diarrhea and/or constipation during menstruation. Endometriosis has been diagnosed in 23–40 percent of infertile women.[16,20]

Objective Data

Physical Examination. A thorough pelvic exam is mandatory to establish a diagnosis. With primary dysmenorrhea, pelvic findings will be completely within normal limits. Secondary dysmenorrhea, however, may reveal an assortment of pelvic pathologies, depending on the etiology of the problem:

- Endometriosis may present with a normal pelvic exam, or the examination may reveal nodularity in the cul-de-sac, caused by implants, nonmobile ovaries or uterus due to adhesion formation, and possible enlarged ovaries secondary to endometrioma formation.[16]
- Adenomyosis will often present as an enlarged globular uterus, particularly in women who are in their 40s or 50s.
- Leiomyoma will present as an irregular or enlarged uterus and may be tender.
- Infection will present with discharge, adnexal tenderness, and/or uterine tenderness. Fever may be present.
- Pelvic inflammation is associated with pelvic tenderness, a history of dyspareunia, and bleeding between cycles.[18]

Diagnostic Tests and Methods

Variety of Tests
- Diagnostic evaluation to detect specific infection: gonorrhea, chlamydia, herpes; wet mounts for clue cells and/or white blood cells.
- Test procedure (see chapters 5 and 11).
- Nursing implications are to explain the purpose of the culture or test, the actual procedure, and the cost of specimen collection.

Ultrasound (Vaginal)
- Diagnostic evaluation to diagnose pelvic abnormalities: myomas, ovarian cysts, congenital malformations.
- Nursing implications are to explain the necessity of a full bladder for visualization and to teach the client about ultrasound, its purpose, and its cost.

Laparoscopy
- Diagnostic evaluation to stage and grade endometriosis if treatment fails or fertility workup is desired.

- The procedure is done with the client in lithotomy position in the operating room, using local or general anesthesia. An intrauterine manipulator is used to promote visibility. A small subumbilical incision is made and the laparoscope inserted to visualize the pelvic organs. Carbon dioxide or nitrous oxide is used to insufflate the pelvic region. Some surgery can be performed through the laparoscope.
- Nursing implications are to explain to the client the types of anesthesia, what the procedure entails, the risks, recovery, and the activity schedule that will follow surgery. Obtain the client's written consent for the laparoscopy, and prescribe pain medication p.r.n.[20]

Hysterosalpingogram, Hysteroscopy, or D & C. See Dysfunctional Uterine Bleeding (DUB), Objective Data.

Barium Enema
- Diagnostic evaluation done to rule out bowel pathology.
- Test procedure, generally outpatient, begins with barium enema followed by fluoroscopic and radiographic examination of the large intestine.
- Nursing implications and client teaching include explanations of preparation, procedure, follow-up, and test results.

Urinalysis
- Diagnostic evaluation done to rule out bladder pathology.
- Client teaching includes explanations of the procedure and its purpose, the cost, and the results.

Differential Medical Diagnoses

- Obstructive Defects. Cervical stenosis; imperforate hymen; congenital disorders of the müllerian tract.
- Endometriosis.
- Other Differential Diagnoses. Adenomyosis, pain secondary to an IUD, fibroids, endometrial polyps or carcinoma, pelvic inflammatory disease, urinary tract infection, infected rectal fissures, uterine malformations, ilioinguinal neuralgia, pelvic prolapse, pelvic tumors, pelvic congestion.[16,17,18]

Plan

Psychosocial Interventions. Helping the client to understand the normal events surrounding the menstrual cycle and the etiology of the dysmenorrhea is an important part of intervention. In addition, intervention is directed toward pain relief and coping strategies that will promote a productive lifestyle. Explaining the normal menstrual cycle will provide the client with the vocabulary to communicate more accurately about symptoms, and it will help to dispel myths. Give the client charts to record menses, onset of pain, timing of medication, relief afforded by the medication, and relationship of pain to basal body temperature. Charts are a teaching tool; they provide the client with a realistic picture of her pain and an objective record for modifying future therapy.

Carefully explain the nature and severity of the pathology associated with secondary dysmenorrhea. Discuss in detail the rationales for selecting particular tests, treatments, medications, or surgery; this will enhance client understanding and compliance. Be sure to address the impact that the disease and treatment will have on fertility.

Medication

Prostaglandin Synthetase Inhibitors (PGSIs)
- First choice of therapy for primary dysmenorrhea in clients not needing contraception. Administer these drugs to relieve pain. They prevent the synthesis of prostaglandins, thereby stopping uterine hypercontractility and ischemia and restoring normal function. Commonly prescribed inhibitors include ibuprofen (Motrin) 400 mg p.o. q. 4 hours; naproxen sodium (Napralan) 500 mg p.o., two tablets q.d., mefenamic acid (Ponstel) 500 mg p.o. stat., then 250 mg p.o. q. 6 hours.[3,17] Instruct the client to begin the medication at the onset of menstrual pain and to take the medication with food. Because the new PGSIs have a rapid onset of action, there is no need to begin treatment prior to menses.[16]
- Side effects and adverse reactions include gastrointestinal upset, rash, and edema.
- PGSIs may be teratogenic; therefore, they are contraindicated in pregnancy. Also, peptic ulcers, asthma, aspirin sensitivity, and inflammatory bowel disease are contraindications.

- Anticipated outcome on evaluation is relief of pain. The client should use one drug for a minimum of 2–4 cycles before evaluating effectiveness. If pain is not relieved, choose another PGSI, preferably from a different pharmacological group (e.g., naproxen sodium versus ibuprofen). If no relief occurs after another 2–4 months, initiate oral contraceptive therapy.
- Client teaching and counseling are the same as for DUB. Tell the client to take the medication with food. Give instructions about the dosing regimen and the side effects of the drug.

Low Dose Combination Oral Contraceptives
- Indication as first choice of therapy is for primary dysmenorrhea in clients who need contraception. Among women who have primary dysmenorrhea, 90 percent are relieved by using an oral contraceptive. Its use also can decrease the necessary dose of PGSI.
- Administer low dose combination oral contraceptives to reduce pain through the suppression of ovulation and endometrial proliferation. This reduces menstrual fluid volume and prostaglandin production to below normal.
- Side effects, adverse reactions, and contraindications are the same as for amenorrhea (see p. 144).
- Anticipated outcome on evaluation is relief of 90 percent of primary dysmenorrhea with oral contraceptives.
- Client teaching and counseling should include information about how to take pills, manage missed pills, and recognize the danger signs (see Chapter 9). Instruct the client to chart dates of menses or spotting.

Combined low dose oral contraceptives and PGSI treatment may be needed for some women. Failure of treatment warrants consideration of psychological factors or diagnostic laparoscopy.[3,17]

Surgical Interventions. One of several surgical procedures may be needed. Laparoscopy is recommended if medical treatment fails after a 6 to 12 month trial period. A D & C to correct cervical stenosis or to remove endometrial polyps is sometimes necessary. Uterosacral ligament division or a hysterectomy is considered a last resort therapy to relieve intractable pain.

Lifestyle Changes. Share information about lifestyle factors that can be initiated to restore some sense of control and alleviate the sense of frustration and victimization. For example, exercise increases endorphins, suppresses prostaglandin release, raises the estrone-estradiol ratio that decreases endometrial proliferation, and shunts blood away from the uterus; pelvic congestion and pain are thereby decreased. Menus can be planned to limit salty foods, increase fiber with fresh fruits and vegetables, and increase water to serve as a natural diuretic. Heating pads or warm baths decrease muscle spasms and may increase comfort. Relaxation techniques can supplement medication regimens and enhance the client's ability to deal with pain. Support groups may provide reassurance and alternative methods of pain relief such as massage and effleurage.

Follow-Up. Follow-up of clients with primary dysmenorrhea can be done on a regular gynecologic exam schedule, once a medical regimen has been found that relieves pain adequately and is well tolerated. Follow clients with secondary dysmenorrhea according to the diagnosis, the type of medication prescribed, and the need for investigative or therapeutic surgery. Because treatment of secondary dysmenorrhea is more varied and may involve infertility issues, much client education and reassurance is needed. Explain each procedure carefully, and allow adequate time for questioning.

TOXIC SHOCK SYNDROME (TSS)

Toxic shock syndrome (TSS) can be a potentially lethal disorder that affects many systems. It is caused in almost all cases by absorption of one or more toxins produced by colonized Staphylococcus aureus.[21,22,23] TSS requires immediate physician referral and hospitalization.

Epidemiology

Etiology. The etiology of TSS in the early 1980s shows that the overwhelming majority of cases occurred in association with menstruation. TSS not associated with menstruation now occurs as frequently. Initial studies found that significantly more women with menstrual TSS had used tampons than women in the control group; and women with TSS used tampons 24 hours per day during menstruation, significantly longer than did controls. Several mechanisms are *implicated* as causative, although no causation has been proved.

- Alterations in the normal vaginal flora.
- Mechanical blockage of menstrual fluids.
- Tampon contamination with *S. aureus.*
- Absorption of bacteriostatic cervical secretions.
- The superabsorbent or synthetic materials of which tampons are made.
- Damaged cervical and vaginal mucosa.
- Enhanced multiplication of the organism in the menstrual efflux.

Incidence. The incidence of TSS peaked in the late 70s and 80s, probably as a result of availability of super absorbent tampons. In 1980, approximately 95 percent of reported cases of TSS among women occurred during menstruation. By 1988, that rate dropped to 55 percent. The current overall rate of TSS is 1 to 3 per 100,000 per year. The overall fatality rate among persons with TSS has been 4 to 5 percent. TSS has been reported with prolonged tampon, contraceptive sponge or diaphragm use, after laser surgery for condylomata acuminatum, postpartum, and following nongynecologic surgery. It also has been isolated from many body tissues and reported in children and adult men.[21,22,23,24]

Incidence has decreased steadily as a result of education, altered patterns of tampon use, and removal of extremely high absorbency tampons from the market.[22]

Subjective Data

An abrupt onset of symptoms occurs, including high fever of about 104° F (40° C), chills, vomiting, watery diarrhea, myalgia, headaches, or abdominal pain in a previously healthy young woman during or shortly after menstruation. Other complaints include watery discharge, aching muscles, bloodshot eyes, sore throat, or dizziness.[22,23]

Objective Data

Physical Examination
- Multisystem involvement is typical; hemodynamic instability is prominent. Vital signs include

152 PROMOTION OF GYNECOLOGIC HEALTH CARE

a temperature of 102° F or higher; systolic blood pressure of less than 90 mm Hg. An orthostatic drop in pressure of 15 mm Hg or more may occur when moving from a lying to sitting position.

- The most characteristic symptom is a sunburn-like rash that develops within 24–48 hours of onset of symptoms and progresses to desquamation in 1–2 weeks. Palms and soles are particularly affected.
- Many clients have conjunctival hyperemia, oropharyngeal erythema, strawberry tongue, vaginal hyperemia.
- Nonspecific abdominal tenderness may be found.
- Neurological findings are general confusion and disorientation without focal neurological findings.
- Multisystemic involvement occurs. At least three organ systems must be involved, with no evidence of another cause.[21,22]

Diagnostic Tests and Methods
- CBC with Differential. A platelet count of 100,000/mm³ or less.
- Serum Electrolyte and Chemistry Determinations. Total bilirubin, SGOT, SGPT, and BUN or creatinine levels are twice the normal limit.
- Serology for syphilis, Rocky Mountain spotted fever, leptospirosis, and rubeola are negative.
- Cultures. Wound, throat, vagina, cervix, rectum, blood, urine, cerebrospinal fluid, and tampons, diaphragms, cervical caps or sponges removed. Usually negative for organisms other than *S. aureus.*

Differential Medical Diagnoses

Rocky Mountain spotted fever, leptospirosis, meningococcal meningitis, Kawasaki disease, scarlet fever, or septic shock; viral gastroenteritis or pelvic inflammatory disease.[22]

Plan

Psychosocial Interventions. Organize physician referral quickly. Most clients require intensive care in the hospital. Reassure that most clients suffer no apparent long-term effects. Inform that TSS can recur. Reoccurrence is reduced by taking antibiotics as prescribed and avoiding future tampon use.[22]

Medications

Antistaphylococcal Antibiotics
- Indications are to treat *Staphylococcus aureus* toxin.
- Beta-lactamase-resistant antibiotic therapy is used. Choices include methicillin, nafcillin, or oxacillin. For penicillin allergic patients, vancomycin, clindamycin, or genatmycin are alternatives.[22]
- Side effects and adverse reactions include acute or delayed allergic reaction to therapy, neurotoxicity, hepatotoxicity, or renal damage.
- Contraindications include hypersensitivity to penicillin. Use with caution in clients with significant allergies or asthma.[22,23]
- Anticipated outcome on evaluation is a decrease in the rate of menstrual TSS recurrence. No drug benefit has been proven for the acute illness.
- Client teaching and counseling should include information about bacteriologic studies that are done to determine causative organisms and susceptibility. With prolonged therapy, periodic assessment of renal, hepatic, and hematopoietic systems should be done. Blood cultures, white blood cell count, and differential cell counts should be obtained prior to therapy and continued at least weekly.

Intravenous Fluid Replacement. Aggressive intravenous fluid replacement is necessary when capillary leakage, fever, vomiting, and diarrhea cause volume depletion.

Follow-Up. Follow-up includes providing the client with information: inform her that subsequent attacks of TSS usually develop within 2–3 months, encourage compliance with antibiotics, and discourage tampon use. If tampons are continued, advise good handwashing with soap prior to insertion or removal of tampons and intermittent use with pads (e.g., tampons during the day and pads at night). Advise the client to be cautious when using a diaphragm or cervical cap and to adhere to the manufacturer's directions. *Advise her that if fever, vomiting, or diarrhea develops during a menstrual period, she must remove the tampon and seek medical care immediately.*[22,23,24,25]

PREMENSTRUAL SYNDROME (PMS)

Premenstrual syndrome (PMS) is a cyclic recurrence of a combination of distressing physical, psychological, and behavioral changes during the luteal phase of the menstrual cycle.[25,26] A range of over 150 symptoms is associated with the syndrome, and various techniques are used for diagnosis and treatment.

PMS is included as a provisional diagnosis in the *Diagnostic and Statistical Manual-IV*, in which it is termed premenstrual dysphoric disorder (PDD). For the diagnosis of PDD, 5 of 11 listed symptoms must be severe premenstrually with postmenstrual remission. The five symptoms must include at least one dysphoric symptom (irritability, mood swings, anxiety, or depression), and multiple physical symptoms are counted as one symptom. There is still considerable controversy about this attempt to systematize PMS symptomatology.[25,27] If PMS is a medical condition, the inclusion as a psychiatric diagnosis is questioned. Additionally, feminists note that other medical conditions cause behavioral changes, for example, thyroid abnormalities; yet they are not given a psychiatric label.[25]

Epidemiology

Etiology. The etiology of PMS is nebulous, and many theories abound. Epidemiologic studies of PMS have failed to show unequivocally an association between PMS and age, socioeconomic status, parity, diet, exercise, stress, menstrual cycle characteristics, or personality. Research is inconclusive because a universally agreed upon definition has not been used, timing of symptoms vary from study to study, severity of symptoms has not been quantified, or agreement about symptoms key to the diagnosis or number of symptoms necessary to be considered a syndrome have not been established. Sampling has been primarily with client populations, rather than a broader sampling of the community, and data collected retrospectively or prospectively have been compared. Feminist literature argues that PMS does not meet the usual criteria for definition as a disease, namely being "an aggregate of specific signs and symptoms" (p. 72).[25] They argue there is no empirical support for the accumulated list of treatments.

The medical literature considers PMS to be a complex disorder generally agreed to be linked to the cyclic activity of the hypothalamic-pituitary-ovarian axis; interactions between ovarian steroid hormones, endogenous opioid peptides, central neurotransmitters, prostaglandins, and peripheral autonomic and endocrine systems. Feminists maintain PMS is a socio-cultural phenomenon specific to Western cultures that work to maintain the status quo of acceptable feminine roles and behaviors. They point to historical similarities between "hysteria" and "PMS" in which uterine and neurological functions are "scientifically" reported to be related.[25]

They view the medical labels as potentially subjecting women to dangerous treatments, denial of insurance, and loss of custody of children in divorce cases. They point to past labels of hysteria with treatments of clitorectomy, ovariectomy, or seclusion, comparing them to present labels of PMS. Present treatments with hormones, or with potentially dangerous drugs such as lithium, as well as the stigma associated with a psychiatric diagnostic label are viewed as highly suspect. They point to the vast number of women that function very well premenstrually. The feminist construct views PMS as a "negotiated reality" between women and society (p. 82).[25] The complexity of multiple roles and societal expectations of women are noted to cause stress, fatigue, and irritability. Since these symptoms are trivialized, misunderstood, or ignored in Western society, PMS allows temporary expression of distress. Rather than being considered outside the boundaries of acceptable feminine behavior or expression with labels of inadequate or neurotic, PMS opens the door for seeking socially "legitimate" relief through medical solutions.[25]

The etiologies of PMS that have been proposed and debated include hormone imbalances, particularly an estrogen excess and a progesterone deficiency. More recently, the notion of estrogen deficiency at the time of symptoms, namely midcycle, and during the week of menses has been implicated. Comorbidity of PMS and depression has led to theories of serotonergic dysregulation in the pathogenesis of premenstrual dysphoria.[26] Other researchers challenge the results of treatment with serotonin reuptake inhibitors as only one of many pathways or neurotransmitters involved. The fluoxetine study reported improvement in 52 percent; and, therefore, a substantial 48 percent did not respond. Another explanation offered is that PDD is not a homogeneous entity, limited to the serotonin pathway alone. Enzyme deficiency, inborn error of metabolism, or triggering effect of the incoming wave of progesterone are initiating multiple changes at the central level.

Nutritional deficiencies have been proposed; the most popular theories describe a deficiency of B vitamins and/or magnesium.[1] Many endocrine imbalances are cited, including hypoglycemia, hyperprolactinemia, and hypothyroidism. Lifestyle factors have been cited as contributory if not causative; these include increased stress, decreased exercise, poor diet, and increased intake of caffeine, nicotine, alcohol, red meat, and salt. Also implicated are overgrowth of *Candida albicans,* amino acid deficiencies, hyperandrogenism, post-tubal ligation interruption in normal blood supply, sleep deprivation, and altered electroencephalogram (EEG) pattern.

Psychiatric hypotheses are that PMS is caused by negative "imprinting" regarding the menstrual cycle, denial of femininity, learned helplessness, attributing bad things in one's life to a physical event, dysfunctional family systems, and poor coping styles.[26,28]

Incidence. Because of numerous symptoms and diagnostic criteria, estimates of occurrence of PMS range from 5–97 percent of reproductive-age women.[25] At least 75 percent of women report minor or isolated PMS changes.[29] PDD differs from PMS in pattern, severity, and level of disability. Only 3–5 percent of women meet the criteria for PDD. The highest incidence of PMS is in the midreproductive years, as is the incidence of depression in women. The correlation of a history of depression is reported to occur in 30–75 percent of the PMS population as compared with 25 percent of the general population according to some authors.[1] If the requirements of the diagnosis include complete absence of symptoms postmenstrually, only 10–20 percent of women seeking treatment meet the criteria.[1]

Family history shows a significantly higher incidence of PMS in first degree relatives in some studies. This may reflect greater awareness, and less stringent criteria, however.[30]

Subjective Data

Typically, clients with PMS have a number of physical symptoms, for example, breast tenderness, fluid retention, abdominal bloating, increased appetite and weight gain, craving for salty or sweet foods—chocolate in particular—acne, fatigue, heart palpitations, dizziness, faintness, and/or headaches premenstrually. These symptoms may be stated as the chief complaint but are actually incidental when compared with the symptoms that are truly distressing the client. Usually, several of the following symptoms are present: mood swings, irritability, anxiety, hostility, depression, crying spells, thoughts of suicide, relationship conflict and fear of breakup, guilt over yelling at or battering children, feelings of inadequacy, increased or decreased libido, and inability to cope with the ever recurring symptoms.

Usually, clients delay treatment, deny the syndrome, make and cancel several appointments, and finally see a health care professional as a result of a recent crisis or threat from a significant other. The symptoms, usually present in the luteal phase, may present in one of four cyclic patterns.

- They appear at midcycle, disappear, and reappear the week prior to menstruation.
- They begin at midcycle with subtle changes that gradually escalate until menses.
- They appear the week prior to menses and intensify until menstruation ensues.
- They appear in the first or second luteal weeks and do not disappear until the end of menstruation.[31]

Objective Data

Although no specific physical findings or lab test can confirm PMS, a complete physical examination is required to rule out other causes of the signs and symptoms.[1]

Diagnostic tests and methods to rule out other illnesses may include a CBC, Pap smear, and urinalysis. Hormonal assays may be initiated to rule out menopause, hypothyroidism, hyperprolactinemia, hyperandrogynism, or hypoglycemia.

Differential Medical Diagnoses

Because of the nonspecific nature of PMS, many differential diagnoses emerge and need to be ruled out: cyclothymic disorder; dysfunctional marital situation; depression; bipolar depression type I or II; stress, "superwoman syndrome"; perimenopausal status; poor diet; endocrine abnormalities including hypoglycemia, diabetes, hypothyroidism, hyperprolactinemia, and hyperandrogynism; alcoholism; or drug addiction. Brain, breast, adrenal, or ovarian tumors should also be ruled out.

Plan

Psychosocial Interventions. Assure the client that her symptoms are real, that PMS exists and she is not "crazy." Acceptance and acknowledgment are therapeutic.

Briefly explain PMS. Provide the client with interesting, informative, and accurate articles and books on the topic.

Teach the client the basics of the menstrual cycle, and provide a menstrual symptoms chart for her to record and rate symptoms. This will enhance the client's awareness of her problem and the actual timing of PMS, and it will assist in planning and evaluating interventions. Symptoms should be prospectively charted for 2–3 months.

Focus on stresses contributing to PMS and ways to adjust lifestyle. Encourage the client to talk with family and friends about her needs and symptoms and to ask for nonthreatening types of support. Suggest assertiveness seminars or books about the subject. Role-play new strategies for dealing with troublesome situations that the client presented in her history. Teach her to schedule activities with PMS in mind, namely, not to overschedule when symptoms are worst. Encourage her to get adequate sleep, particularly during times of most severe symptoms.[28]

Lifestyle changes may include beginning a safe exercise program, preferably outdoors, to increase endorphin production, reduce stress, enhance cardiovascular health, and prevent osteoporosis. Encourage the client to exercise three to five times per week. Regular relaxation is effective in reducing symptoms.[27,28] Assist the client with planning a balanced diet that avoids salts, refined sugars, and includes a nutritious snack. Many symptoms can be relieved simply by eating a morning meal and avoiding self-induced hypoglycemia. Encourage the client to carry small, low calorie snacks in her purse for times when symptoms such as fatigue, difficulty concentrating, or irritability occur. Advise her to decrease caffeine intake gradually to avoid headaches with the goal of total elimination to reduce irritability and to enhance sleep. Recommend increasing water intake to achieve natural diuresis.

Give the client permission to set aside time for herself. Teach stress reduction techniques, for example, taking long baths and taking time for pleasurable activity, yoga, Lamaze, biofeedback, meditation, or visual imagery—or refer her to a specialist for instruction. Discuss the "superwoman syndrome" in which women try to excel in all areas of life in a perfectionistic way.[28] Suggest the book *Healing the Shame that Binds You* to help her gain insight into this problem.[28,29]

Dissuade client from blaming everything on PMS and perpetuating the role of victim. She *can* recognize and learn to cope with symptoms as do other chronic disease sufferers.[28] Encourage the client to approach her therapy a little at a time, to seek assistance, and to accept her mistakes. Discourage "all or nothing" thinking patterns.

Review a typical day's communication patterns, sources of conflict, and problematic lifestyle factors. With the client, select one or two realistic goals to begin to pursue right away; accomplishing even small changes enhances self-esteem and the desire to continue making changes. Discourage the client from making too many changes at once.

Stress the importance of *not* smoking because of the overall negative health consequences and toxicity to the ovaries. Encourage limited intake of alcohol or avoiding it, particularly high-sugar beverages such as wine, which may cause rebound hypoglycemia, headaches, palpitations, fatigue, and problems with mood.[28]

Encourage the client to evaluate her coping styles and discard unhealthy habits, such as alcohol consumption, drug abuse, and smoking, for more functional styles. Give the client permission to take care of herself.[32]

Provide information about assertiveness classes, support groups for PMS, Co-Dependency, Al-Anon, Alcoholics Anonymous, counselors, or psychiatrists.

Long-term pharmacological therapy may be needed; therefore, the client should be included in decisions regarding therapy so that concerns about cost and side effects are shared. Therapy should be individualized and tailored to troublesome symptoms determined from menstrual symptom diaries.

Medications. Part of the therapeutic effect from any drug used for PMS is due to the placebo effect.[1]

Selective Serotonin Reuptake Inhibitors (SSRIs). Indications for SSRIs are negative emotional symptoms. SSRIs are now frequently used as a first line drug therapy for PMS because of their apparent efficacy and tolerability. Emotional symptoms are decreased more than are physical symptoms, lending support to newer theories that altered serotonergic function is present in women with PMS. Fluoxetine has been shown to be superior to placebo in reducing symptoms. Long-term effectiveness is controversial. Reports vary from a drop in improvement from 55 percent to 37 percent after three cycles[33] to reports of study participants requesting prescriptions for fluoxetine after symptoms flared following discontinuation of the drug.[27,29]

Administer 20 mg of fluoxetine (Prozac) every A.M. Drug interactions with MAO inhibitors and tricyclics may occur. These agents, or combination with other SSRIs, should NOT be prescribed together.

Side effects of dizziness, nausea, headache, and insomnia are common, transient, and usually mild. In contrast to tricyclics, fluoxetine and other SSRIs do not have anticholinergic, hypotensive, or sedative effects. Dependency is not a concern, and they have no particular cardiovascular or serious toxic effects. Patients may have idiosyncratic responses to SSRIs, and their response should be monitored monthly for the first 3 months. If relief is not obtained, another agent should be chosen.

Advise clients about taking the medication appropriately and that beneficial effects are not immediate but may take as long as 2 weeks. In PMS, a positive clinical response has been noted to occur more immediately. At least one study suggests that a single dose of fluoxetine during the early luteal phase may be as effective as daily doses.[33] Pregnancy should be avoided while on these drugs, but increased teratogenicity has not been demonstrated.[1]

Advise clients of common side effects. Encourage them to give the medication at least a 2-week trial since most side effects are temporary. Elicit client's response to SSRI therapy, since the media has given a great deal of coverage to Prozac—both positive and negative. Advise clients that this therapy may well be long-term.

Vitamin and Mineral Supplements
- A good multivitamin supplement can be a benign beginning treatment while the client collects data for charts.
- Vitamins and minerals are commonly indicated for PMS therapy; however, there is no evidence that nutritional deficiencies cause PMS, and their use may be dangerous if taken in inappropriate amounts.
- Neurologic symptoms at pharmacologic doses, more than 500 mg daily of pyridoxine (vitamin B_6), have been shown to be directly related. In the absence of proven benefit pyridoxine is not recommended.[1]
- Overdosage of vitamin A must be avoided because research results have not been definitive on its use as a successful treatment. No more than the recommended daily allowance (5000 units) should be advised.
- Vitamin E, 400 units per day, has been associated with reduction of negative mood and food cravings, but it has not been shown to effectively reduce physical symptoms.[1]
- Calcium and magnesium have shown promise in recent studies but need further study.[26]

Prostaglandin Synthetase Inhibitors (PGSIs)
- Indications for these drugs include premenstrual headaches, tension, irritability, depression, abdominal pain, breast tenderness, abdominal bloating, and ankle edema. Affective and emotional symptoms are inconsistently improved, or NOT at all with PGSIs.[1]
- Side effects and contraindications are the same as for dysmenorrhea. Side effects and adverse reactions include gastrointestinal upset, rash,

and edema. PGSIs may be teratogenic; therefore, they are contraindicated in pregnancy. Also peptic ulcers, asthma, aspirin sensitivity, and inflammatory bowel disease are contraindications.

- Client teaching and counseling should begin with a discussion of the client's symptom records. It should include information about taking PGSIs with meals to avoid gastric upset or ulcer development. The medication should be initiated on the day of the luteal phase when symptoms and signs are perceived, as noted on a previous month's symptom record and limited to somatic symptoms.

Diuretics

- Have long been proposed to relieve weight gain and bloating premenstrually. Many types including thiazides, triamterene, and spironolactone have been evaluated. Weight gain and bloating may sometimes be improved with these agents, but diuretics may lead to hypotensive episodes and electrolyte abnormalities and are NOT recommended. If symptomatic relief is essential, or patient insistence intense, a potassium sparing diuretic, such as spironolactone, is recommended.[26]
- Administer spironolactone during the luteal phase (q.i.d. p.o. range daily for total does is 25–200 mg). The lowest effective dose is suggested.[34]
- Side effects include gynecomastia, GI upset, drowsiness, headache, rash, mental confusion, irregular menses or amenorrhea, and deepening of the voice.[34]
- Contraindications include anuria, acute renal insufficiency, significant renal impairment, and hyperkalemia.[34]
- Anticipated outcomes on evaluation are decreased bloating, feelings of fullness, and affective/physical symptoms associated with excessive fluid retention. The effects of spironolactone on behavioral symptoms are marginal.[26]
- Client teaching and counseling should make clear that potassium supplementation in the form of food or medication should NOT be taken with spironolactone. Furthermore, spironolactone should not be taken with other potassium-sparing diuretics. Follow clients

with fluid and electrolyte studies to avoid excessive potassium levels and resulting cardiac arrhythmias.[34] It is better to recommend increasing water intake and reducing sodium rather than to prescribe diuretics.

Oral Micronized Progesterone

- The indication for progesterone supplementation has been suggested since 1938 to relieve a wide variety of PMS symptoms. Controlled clinical trials have failed to demonstrate effectiveness superior to placebo. Natural progesterone appears benign and without major side effects, but long-term safety is NOT established, and progesterone therapy does not have FDA approval for PMS treatment.[1] Other therapies should be exhausted prior to prescribing progesterone.

Estradiol Therapy

- Indications for estradiol therapy are severe premenstrual headaches, insomnia, and depressive symptoms.[27]
- Ovarian steroid hormones can act directly on the nerve membrane, affecting its excitability, as well as acting on the vasomotor action of vessels. Cyclic symptoms are thought to be associated with low estradiol production particularly noted at midcycle or premenstrually. Occurrence of symptoms can be documented on patient symptom charts and compared with menstrual activities and estradiol levels. Estradiol levels are typically lowest the second day of the cycle.[35]
- Administer (apply) a 0.05 mg patch at the time during cycle when symptoms appear; remove it at the onset or completion of menses.
- Side effects and contraindications. Side effects of estrogen therapy include nausea, headache, breast tenderness and enlargement, fluid retention, cervical ectropion, and an increase in vaginal discharge. More severe adverse effects include thromboembolic development, cerebrovascular accident, pulmonary emboli, liver disease, uterine myoma growth, telangiectasia, hypertension, and myocardial infarction. Estrogen is contraindicated in pregnancy, cancer of the uterus or breast, in the presence of unusual/unexplained vaginal bleeding, endometriosis, or abnormal blood clotting. Women with hypertension, heart or kidney

disease, asthma, skin allergies, epilepsy, diabetes, migraine headache, or depression have a relative contraindication to estrogen use. Signs/symptoms of concern with estrogen therapy are severe headache, visual disturbance, dizziness, chest pain, shortness of breath, leg cramps, abdominal pain, and irregular bleeding. Estrogen patches may cause skin irritation, rash, or redness.
- Anticipated outcomes on evaluation are better sleep patterns and mood and fewer headaches.[34]
- Client teaching and counseling should help the client with her essential task of keeping accurate menstrual records and symptom charts. Pap tests and mammography must be current and normal.

Oral Contraceptives
- The indication for oral contraception is elimination of cyclic hormonal fluctuations. Both avoidance and the use of oral contraceptive pills have been recommended. Overall, the efficacy of OCs in the treatment of PMS has not been proven. OCs may be beneficial due to ovulation suppression, but this is not uniform to all pills. One study recently reported that OCs made premenstrual dysphoria worsen.[27] Depression may occur with OCs secondary to estrogen interference with the synthesis of tryptophan. This may be reversed with pyridoxine treatment.[26] Prescribe OCs only when all else fails and there are no contraindications.
- Administration, side effects, and contraindications. Administer oral contraceptives according to manufacturer's guidelines. (See Chapter 9 for detailed discussion of administration, side effects, and contraindications.) Side effects most commonly include breast tenderness, weight gain, spotting, and scanty menses. Contraindications are pregnancy, undiagnosed vaginal bleeding, history of breast or reproductive tract cancer, history of thromboembolism, cerebrovascular or coronary disease, liver tumor or malignancy, or smoker older than 35.[11]
- The anticipated outcome on evaluation is very limited. Little success occurs in reducing symptoms, and oral contraceptives may exacerbate depressive symptoms in some PMS sufferers.

- Client teaching and counseling. Advise regarding appropriate use of oral contraceptives (OC), danger signs, and side effects. Advise clients to record their response to OC therapy in order to decide whether the medication should be continued.

Anxiolytics
- The indication for anxiolytics is for the most troublesome emotional symptoms of PMS, notably anxiety, panic, irritability, and depression. Alprazolam administration can be limited to the luteal phase and has met with success in 37 percent of women in one study. Results are not uniform for all women with affective symptoms.[26]
- Administer alprazolam 0.25 or 0.5 mg p.o., b.i.d. or t.i.d. during the luteal phase. Prescribe in small amounts and evaluate patient response.
- Side effects include addiction potential, drowsiness, and if used with alcohol, a synergistic effect. Dependence has not been demonstrated in patients carefully diagnosed with PMS when dosage is limited to the luteal phase.[1]
- Contraindications include pregnancy, lactation, history of addiction, or acute narrow angle glaucoma. Alprazolam is used cautiously for clients with renal, hepatic, or pulmonary conditions.[34]
- The anticipated outcome on evaluation is that the therapy will allow temporary symptom reduction and enable the client to seek problem resolution through counseling or other therapies.
- Client teaching should encourage specialized counseling; therapists may be recommended. Discuss ways to reduce or cope with stress and discuss alternative PMS therapies that may be helpful.

Gonadotropin-Releasing Hormone Agonist (GnRH-a)
- Indications are extremely severe symptoms. GnRH agonists function by suppressing gonadotropin levels at the level of the pituitary and ultimately eliminating ovulation and sex steroid production.[1]
- *Administer with physician consultation only.* Requires daily subcutaneous injections (Lupron),

intramuscular injection (Depo Lupron), or intranasal sprays (Buserelin). Use of these agents without hormonal add back programs should not be longer than 6 consecutive months.[1]

- Side effects are menopause induced by complete ovulation cessation (see Chapter 15, Hypoestrogenic Changes, for effects of estrogen deficiency).
- The anticipated outcome is consistent elimination of menstrually related disorders through pharmacologic suppression of ovarian steroids. GnRH therapy is not successful in patients with concurrent major depression.[1]
- Client teaching and counseling require informed consent and in-depth education about the effects of this treatment. Although GnRH can reduce symptoms dramatically, hypoestrogenic effects, and risks of osteoporosis and cardiovascular disease need to be explained. If add back programs of estrogen and progesterone are used, these must be carefully explained to assure proper usage.[1,26]

Surgical Interventions. Oophorectomy is reserved for clients with the most severe cases of PMS and truly should be a last resort.[1] Frequently following surgery, clients who are placed on a hormone replacement regimen develop a chemically induced PMS; therefore, little is gained.

Hysterectomy has *no* place in the treatment of PMS and will not help the syndrome. Clients should be informed of this.

Follow-Up. Follow-up involves rescheduling the client in 1 or 2 months to evaluate her charts and progress and to arrive at a workable diagnosis and plan of care. The first few months involve intense examination of lifestyle, menstrual patterns, and coping strategies. Frequent visits provide time to review and provide more information, reinforce desired changes, give encouragement, assign reading, and discuss referrals. Results of initial lab work can be shared at this time, and continuation of symptom charting is stressed. As the client accrues knowledge and coping techniques and begins to see progress, her visits can be less frequent and shorter. The goal is to have yearly visits. An interdisciplinary team approach is useful in the management of PMS.[28]

NURSING DIAGNOSES

The following nursing diagnoses identified by the author are representative of those used in the health care plan of women with menstrual dysfunction; however, this is by no means an inclusive list:

- Activity limitation secondary to pain
- Anxiety
- Body image disturbance
- Discomfort
- Family coping ineffective
- Family processes altered
- Fatigue
- Fear
- Individual coping ineffective
- Infection, high risk
- Knowledge deficit concerning menstrual cycle and etiology of pain, alterations in menstrual cycle, and safe tampon use
- Nutrition altered: less than body requirements
- Powerlessness
- Role performance altered
- Self-esteem disturbance
- Social interaction impaired
- Tissue perfusion altered, cardiopulmonary and peripherally

REFERENCES

1. Barnhart, K., & Sondhemier, S. (1995). A clinician's guide to the premenstrual syndrome. *Medical Clinics of North America, 79*(6), 1457–1472.
2. Greydanus, D., & Shearin, R. (1990). *Adolescent sexuality and gynecology*. Philadelphia: Saunders.
3. Speroff, L., Glass, R., & Kase, N. (1994). *Clinical gynecologic endocrinology and infertility* (5th ed.). Baltimore: Williams & Wilkins.
4. Brown, J. S., & Crombleholme, W. R. (1993). *Handbook of gynecology and obstetrics*. Norwalk: Appleton & Lange.

5. Wathen, P., Henderson, M., & Witz, C. (1995). Abnormal uterine bleeding. *Medical Clinics of North America, 79*(2), 329–342.

6. Webb, T. (1995). Evaluation and Management of Amenorrhea. *ADVANCE for Nurse Practitioners, 3*(6), 28–30.

7. Warren, M. (1996) Evaluation of secondary amenorrhea. *Journal of Clinical Endocrinology & Metabolism, 81*(2), 437–442.

8. Kiningham, R., Apgar, B., & Schwenk, T. (1996). Evaluation of amenorrhea. *American Family Physician, 53*(4), 1185–1194.

9. Continuing education forum. (1995). Secondary amenorrhea. *Journal of the American Academy of Nurse Practitioners, 7*(9), 453–460.

10. Starr, W. L., Lommell, L. L., & Shannon, M. T. (1995). Abnormal uterine bleeding. *Women's Primary Care: Protocols for Practice.* Washington, DC: American Nurses Publishing.

11. Hatcher, R., Guest, F., Stewart, F., Steward, G., Trussell, J., Bowen, S., & Cates, W. (1992). *Contraceptive technology* (15th ed.). Atlanta: Printed Matter.

12. Jennings, J. C. (1995). Abnormal uterine bleeding. *Medical Clinics of North America, 79*(6): 1357–1376.

13. Dijhuizen, F., Brolmann, H., Potters, A., Bongers, M., & Heintz, A. (1996). The accuracy of transvaginal ultrasonography in the diagnosis of endometrial abnormalities. *Obstetrics & Gynecology, 87*(3), 345–349.

14. Rosenfeld, J. (1996). Treatment of menorrhagia due to dysfunctional uterine bleeding. *American Family Physician, 53*(1), 165–172.

15. Polaneczky, M., & Slap, G. (1992). Menstrual disorders in the adolescent: Dysmenorrhea & dysfunctional uterine bleeding. *Pediatrics in Review, 13*(3), 83–86.

16. Ziunuska, J. (1995). Endometriosis, an overview of diagnosis & treatment. *ADVANCE for Nurse Practitioners, 3*(1), 15–17.

17. Webb, T. (1996). Common menstrual disorders: Primary care management. *ADVANCE for Nurse Practitioners, 4*(1), 20–23.

18. Griffith, C. (1995). Pelvic inflammatory disease, an overview. *ADVANCE for Nurse Practitioners, 3*(8), 33–36.

19. Harlow, S., & Ephross, S. (1995). Epidemiology of menstruation and it's relevance to women's health. *Epidemiologic Reviews 17*(2), 265–286.

20. Garner, C. (1996). Coping with endometriosis. *Office Nurse, 9*(5), 14–20.

21. Centers for Disease Control. (1990). *Reduced incidence of menstrual toxic-shock syndrome—United States, 1980–1990* (DHHS Vol. 38, No. 25). Washington, DC: U.S. Government Printing Office.

22. Colbry, S. L. (1992). A review of toxic shock syndrome: The need for education still exists. *Nurse Practitioner, 17*(9) 39–46.

23. Creehan, P. (1995). Toxic shock syndrome: An opportunity for nursing intervention. *JOGNN, 24*(6), 557–560.

24. Sweet, R., & Gibbs, R. (1990). *Infectious diseases of the genital tract.* (2nd ed.). Baltimore: Williams & Wilkins.

25. Gurevich, M. (1995). Rethinking the label: Who benefits from the PMS construct? *Women and Health, 23*(2), 67–98.

26. ACOG Committee Opinion. (1995). Premenstrual syndrome. *International Journal of Gynecology & Obstetrics, 50,* 80–84.

27. Pearlstein, T. (1995). Hormones and depression: What are the facts about PMS, menopause, and hormone replacement therapy? *American Journal of Obstetrics and Gynecology, 173*(2), 646–653.

28. Warren, C., & Baker, S. (1992). Coping resources of women with premenstrual syndrome. *Archives of Psychiatric Nursing, 6*(1), 48–53.

29. van Leusden, H. A. (1995). Premenstrual syndrome no progesterone; Premenstrual dysphoric disorder no serotonin deficiency. *The Lancet, 346,* (8988), 1443–1444.

30. Chuong, C., & Burgos, D. M. (1995). Medical history in women with PMS. *Journal of Psychosomatic Obstetrics & Gynecology, 16*(1), 21–17.

31. Halbreich, U. (1995). Menstrually related disorders: What we do know, what we only believe that we know, and what we know that we do not know. *Critical Reviews in Neurobiology, 9*(2/3), 163–175.

32. Goodale, I., Domar, A., & Benson, H. (1990). Alleviation of premenstrual syndrome symptoms with the relaxation-response. *Obstetrics and Gynecology, 75,* 649–655.

33. Steiner, M., Steinberg, S., Stweart, D., Carter, D., Berger, C., Reid, R., Grover, D., & Streiner, D. (1995). Fluoxetine in the treatment of premenstrual dysphoria. *The New England Journal of Medicine, 332*(23), 1529–1534.

34. *Physicians' desk reference.* (1996). Oradell, NJ: Medical Economics.

35. Korhonen, S., Saarijavi, S., & Aito, M. (1995). Successful estradiol treatment of psychotic symptoms in the premenstrual phase: A case report. *ACTA Psychiatrica Scandinavica, 92*(1995), 237–238.

CONTROLLING FERTILITY

Kathryn A. Caufield

Highlights

- Historical and Political Perspectives
- Principles of Fertility Control
- Issues of Control, Safety, and Choice
- "Safer Sex"
- Evaluation of Clients
- Client Education, Informed Consent
- Combined Oral Contraceptives
- Progestin-Only Methods: Pills, Implants, Injections
- Postcoital Contraceptive Methods
- Male and Female Condoms
- Spermicides: Foams, Jellies, Creams, Suppositories, Vaginal Film
- Barrier Methods: Diaphragms, Cervical Caps
- Intrauterine Devices
- Sterilization
- Fertility Awareness Methods
- Withdrawal
- Lactational Amenorrhea Method
- Induced Abortion
- Outlook for Controlling Fertility: Men and Women

► INTRODUCTION

HISTORICAL AND POLITICAL PERSPECTIVES ON CONTRACEPTION

The desire of women and men to control their reproductive destinies has been evident since ancient times. Use of primitive barriers, spermicides, condoms, and withdrawal is documented in the writings of many ancient cultures. Until the mid-nineteenth century, however, few reliable methods to prevent or delay pregnancy were available. Herbal and chemical spermicides, condoms, and coitus interruptus (withdrawal) carried high risks of pregnancy; the latter two also depended on the cooperation of men.

Margaret Sanger (1883–1966), a nurse and feminist and the most important early leader of the U.S. family planning movement, introduced the diaphragm into the United States and fought for women's rights. She founded the American Birth Control League, which later became the Planned Parenthood Federation of America. A 1965 U.S. Supreme Court decision in the case of *Estelle T. Griswold and C. Lee Buxton v. State of Connecticut* declared birth control to be a basic right under the Bill of Rights. In the early 1960s, oral contraceptives and intrauterine devices (IUD) became available, beginning the "contraceptive revolution." In the late 1960s, New York, California and other states rewrote their abortion laws culminating in the 1973 U.S. Supreme Court decision of *Roe v. Wade,* which limited the circumstances under which "the right to privacy" could be restricted by local abortion laws. Abortion was thus legalized. The ability to control the timing and circumstances under which they would conceive and give birth bestowed on women a higher degree of personal control, more freedom of choice in many dimensions of their lives, and the self-determination to work toward equality.[1-6]

Not coincidentally, the women's movement gained momentum with the introduction of these more "modern" methods of birth control and the right to choose abortion. In turn, the women's movement provided the stimulus to limit family size and to move society toward acceptance of different roles for women. The availability of modern birth control methods has also dramatically reduced maternal and child mortality.

The national family planning program, Title X of the Public Health Service Act, was established by Congress in 1970. This program provides community based funding/support for comprehensive family planning services (not including abortion) and sexually transmitted disease (STD) care, free or at an affordable cost, based on income. In 1995, 5 million clients were served by the program nationwide.[7] Additionally, the United States provides support for numerous international family planning programs.

Large numbers of women continue to experience unplanned pregnancies, resulting in morbidity, mortality, and social distress. In fact, the United States is far behind other countries in varieties of birth control methods available. Numerous factors contribute to this phenomenon. Issues constraining contraceptive availability and research include product liability lawsuits; antifamily planning activism; pressure from well intended feminist, consumer, political, and religious groups; cautious and lengthy U.S. Food and Drug Administration (FDA) procedural requirements; too little knowledge about reproductive biology, and too little money.[3,6] Contraceptive technologies, however, are slowly but steadily evolving. Research and development underway in many parts of the world should eventually result in a wider array of contraceptive methods, offering advantages over some currently available contraceptive techniques and wider choices for consumers.

DEFINITION AND PURPOSE

Fertility control may be defined as follows.

1. Purposeful regulation of conception or childbirth.
2. Voluntary avoidance or delay of pregnancy or childbirth.
3. Use of devices, chemicals, abortion, or other techniques to prevent or terminate pregnancy.

Related terms often used interchangeably with fertility control include *birth control, family planning, contraception, pregnancy prevention,* and *planned parenthood.* The reasons for controlling fertility include personal convenience, economics, social values, and lifestyle.

Primary care clinicians are often the main source of accurate information and advice on responsible family planning practices for clients. Family planning services/programs should offer a variety of safe, effective, acceptable, affordable contraceptive methods to help women prevent unwanted pregnancies and STDs and to help them achieve their childbearing goals.[8]

SELECTING A METHOD OF CONTRACEPTION

A woman's reproductive life spans almost 40 years, and throughout those years, a variety of contraceptive methods may be used. Table 9–1 summarizes desirable method characteristics according to the stages of a woman's reproductive life. Women need assistance in reevaluating contraceptive choices as their needs change over time and in understanding and recognizing the many variables that can influence those choices. Many individual factors may enhance or impair contraceptive behavior and impact the selection of birth control methods.[8,9,10]

- Age and maturity.
- Stage of reproductive life (desire for future fertility).
- Marital status.

TABLE 9–1. STAGES OF REPRODUCTIVE LIFE AND CONTRACEPTIVE METHOD CHARACTERISTICS FOR A TYPICAL WOMAN IN THE U.S.

	Adolescents/Young Adults		Later Reproductive Years	
	Menarche to First Intercourse (ave. 4.9 yrs)	*First Intercourse to First Birth (ave. 8.6 yrs)*	*First Birth to Last Birth (ave. 4 yrs)*	*Last Birth to Menopause (ave. 18.4 yrs)*
Fertility Goals				
Births	Postpone	Postpone	Space	Stop
Ability to Have Children	Preserve	Preserve	Preserve	Irrelevant
Sexual Behavior				
# of Partners	None	Multiple?	One?	One?
Coital Frequency	Zero	Moderate to High	Moderate	Moderate to Low
Coital Predictability	Low	Moderate to High	High	High
Importance of Method Characteristics				
Pregnancy Prevention		High	Moderate	High
STD/PID Prevention[a]		High	Moderate	Low
Not Coitus Linked		High	High	Low
Reversibility		High	High	Low
Most Common Methods				
Most Common		Pill	Pill	Sterilization
Next Most Common		Condom	Condom	Pill, Condom

[a]STD = Sexually transmitted disease; PID = Pelvic inflammatory disease.
Source: Forrest, J. D. (1993). Timing of reproductive life stages. Obstet-Gynecology, 82*(1), 105–110. Adopted with permission from The American College of Obstetricians and Gynecologists.*

TABLE 9–2A. IMPORTANCE OF CHARACTERISTICS IMPACTING CONTRACEPTIVE SELECTION AND USE ACCORDING TO METHOD

Contraceptive Method	Cost	Ease of Use	Coitus Linked	Level of Convenience	Effectiveness	Systemic Effects	Level of Safety	Availability
Combined oral contraceptives	Mod	Great	No	High	High	Yes	High for nonsmokers	Wide
Progestin-only methods								
Progestin-only pills	Mod	Great	No	High	Mod	Yes	High	Wide
Implants	High	Great	No	High	High	Yes	Mod	Limited
Vaginal rings	Mod	Great	No	Mod to high	High	High	High	Limited
Injections	Mod	Great	No	High	High	Yes	High	Limited
Diaphragms	Mod to high	Mod	Yes	Mod	Mod	No	Mod to high	Mod
Cervical caps	Mod to high	Mod	Yes	Mod	Mod	No	Mod to high	Low
Postcoital methods	High	Difficult	No	Low	High	Yes	Mod	Limited
Male condoms	Low to mod	Mod	Yes	Mod to low	Mod	No	High	Wide
Female condoms	Mod	Mod	Yes	Low	Mod	No	High	Mod
Vaginal spermicides	Low to mod	Mod	Yes	Low	Mod	No	High	Wide
Intrauterine devices	High	Great	No	High	High	Some	Mod	Limited
Fertility awareness methods	Low	Difficult	Yes	Low	Low	No	Mod	Mod
Lactational amenorrhea method	Low	Mod	No	High	Mod	No	High	Wide
Withdrawal	None	Mod	Yes	Mod	Low	No	Mod	Wide
Female sterilization	High	Great	No	High	High	No	Mod	Mod
Male sterilization	Mod	Great	No	High	High	No	High	Mod

Note: Mod = moderate.
Source: References 6, 10, 12, 14, 16, 41.

- Cultural and religious beliefs.
- Health/medical history.
- Presence of physical or mental limitations.
- Motivation of the woman.
- Degree of cooperation of the male partner.
- Wishes and concerns of the partner.
- Degree of comfort with one's body and one's sexuality.
- Individual locus of control.
- Monogamous versus multiple sexual partners (risk of sexually transmitted diseases).
- Lactation status.
- Cost of methods.
- Previous experience with birth control methods (successes, failures, problems, side effects).
- Frequency of intercourse.
- Other patterns of sexual activity.
- Effectiveness of methods.
- Safety of methods.
- Access to health care.
- Noncontraceptive benefits.

- Short-term versus long-term contraceptive needs.
- Confidence in methods.
- Perceived convenience of methods.

Characteristics that may impact the selection and use of specific contraceptive methods are summarized in Tables 9–2A and 9–2B.

General Principles of Fertility Control[2,6,10]

- When the goal is to prevent pregnancy, any contraceptive method is better than none.
- *All* sexually active women of every age must have access to effective, confidential, and nonpunitive contraceptive services.
- Women need to know their options, the risks and benefits, and which methods may be contraindicated for them and why.
- Women are entitled to professional assistance when selecting a method that meets their own needs and circumstances.

TABLE 9–2B. IMPORTANCE OF CHARACTERISTICS IMPACTING CONTRACEPTIVE SELECTION AND USE ACCORDING TO METHOD

Contraceptive Method	Characteristics					
	Partner Involvement Required	Protection Against STDs/HIV	Prescription Required	Health Care System Contact Required	Return to Fertility After Discontinued Use	Can Be Used While Lactating
Combined oral contraceptives	None	None*	Yes	Yes	Delay—possibly 2–3 months	Not recommended
Progestin-only methods						
Progestin-only pills	None	None	Yes	Yes	Rapid	Yes
Implants	None	None	Yes	Yes	Delayed—possibly 2–3 months	Yes
Vaginal rings	None	None	Yes	Yes	Slight delay possible	Yes
Injections	None	None	Yes	Yes	Delayed, 6–12 months	Yes
Diaphragms	None	Mod	Yes	Yes	Immediate	Yes
Cervical caps	None	Mod	Yes	Yes	Immediate	Yes
Postcoital methods	None	None	Yes	Yes	Rapid	Not recommended
Male condoms	Yes	High	No	No	Immediate	Yes
Female condoms	Some	High	No	No	Immediate	Yes
Vaginal spermicides	None	Mod	No	No	Immediate	Yes
Intrauterine devices	None	None	Yes	Yes	Rapid	Yes
Fertility awareness methods	Yes	None	No	Yes for teaching	Immediate	Not reliable
Lactational amenorrhea method	No	No	No	No	Rapid	—
Withdrawal	Yes	Limited	No	No	Immediate	Yes
Female sterilization	None	None	No	Yes	Not applicable	Yes
Male sterilization	Yes	No	No	Yes	Not applicable	Yes

Note: STD = sexually transmitted disease; HIV = human immunodeficiency virus; Mod = moderate.
*Some protection against PID
Source: References 6, 10, 12, 14, 16, 41.

- Health professionals are obligated to educate clients, without undue bias, about the range of possible methods so that fully informed choices can be made.
- No birth control method is 100 percent effective in preventing pregnancy.
- Information and counseling about acquired immunodeficiency syndrome (AIDS) and human immunodeficiency virus (HIV) infection, sexually transmitted diseases (STDs), use of latex and non-allergenic protective condoms, and "safe sex" must be provided to individuals seeking family planning services.
- Responsibility for preventing pregnancy should ideally be shared by the man and the woman in a relationship.

ISSUES OF CONTROL, SAFETY, AND CHOICE

A "perfect" contraceptive would be 100 percent effective in preventing pregnancy, highly acceptable, free from health hazards and side effects not coitus related, low maintenance, and easily reversible. In addition, it would be relatively inexpensive and offer noncontraceptive benefits such as protection against sexually transmitted diseases (STDs). Currently, however, all available methods for controlling fertility carry some risks to users; therefore, disadvantages and risks must be carefully weighed against benefits. In assisting clients with contraceptive choices, it is often helpful to compare method risks with the

TABLE 9–3. SAFER SEX OPTIONS FOR PHYSICAL INTIMACY

Safe	Possibly Safe	Unsafe in the Absence of HIV Testing and Trust and Monogamy
Massage	Wet kissing with no broken skin, cracked lips, or damaged mouth tissue	Any vaginal or rectal intercourse without a latex or synthetic condom
Hugging		
Body rubbing	Vaginal or rectal intercourse using latex or synthetic condom correctly	Oral sex on a man without a latex or synthetic condom
Dry kissing		
Masturbation	Oral sex on a man using a latex or synthetic condom	Oral sex on a woman without a latex or synthetic barrier such as a female condom, dental dam, or modified male condom, especially if she is having her period or has a vaginal infection with discharge
Hand-to-genital touching (hand job) or mutual masturbation	Oral sex on a woman using a latex or synthetic barrier such as a female condom, dental dam, or modified male condom, especially if she does not have her period or a vaginal infection with discharge	
Erotic books and movies		
All sexual activities, when both partners are monogamous, trustworthy, and known by testing to be free of HIV		Semen in the mouth
		Oral-anal contact
	All sexual activities, when both partners are in a long-term monogamous relationship and trust each other	Sharing sex toys or douching equipment
		Blood contact of any kind, including menstrual blood, or any sex that causes tissue damage or bleeding

Source: Hatcher, R. A., Trussel, J., Stewart, F., Stewart, G., Kowal, D., Guest, F., Cates, W., Jr. & Policar, W. Contraceptive Technology *(16th ed.). (1994). Contraceptive Technology Communications, Inc. Used with permission.*

risks of full term delivery. In most cases, the risks associated with pregnancy and delivery are much greater than those associated with contraceptive use.

In an era when many women wish to delay pregnancy and simultaneously face many hazards to future fertility caused by STDs, choices are indeed difficult. Clients need assistance to select contraceptives that will protect them from both pregnancy and STDs. For young, healthy women, the combination of oral contraceptives and spermicidal condoms is a very sound choice; however, many options are presented in this chapter.[9,10]

CONTRACEPTION AND "SAFER SEX"

Responsibility for Prevention and Protection

When seeking birth control, both men and women bear responsibility. Today, the question of whether the method offers any protection against STDs must be added to other selection considerations such as convenience, effectiveness, failure rate, safety, and noncontraceptive benefits. Abstinence or sexual intercourse with

one mutually faithful, trustworthy, uninfected partner is the only totally effective prevention strategy against STDs. Individuals with multiple sexual partners must make difficult decisions about responsibility and consequences for actions, sexual expression, communication patterns with partners, and the long-term impact of these decisions.[10,11] All health care professionals must continue to do their part in providing individual and community education that is culturally and gender appropriate, geared toward safer sexual practices and reducing STD risk.

Safer Sex

When the HIV serostatus or STD status of a person is not certain, there is no such entity as "safe sex"; hence the term "safer sex." Though condoms are not 100 percent effective in preventing infections, male and/or female condoms are the best protection available at this time. Principal problems with male and/or female condom use are improper use, difficulty integrating use into sexual activity, and less often, condom breakage and slippage. Table 9–3 summarizes safer sex options.[10,12]

EVALUATION OF CLIENTS REQUESTING FERTILITY CONTROL

In many cases, women seeking care or advice about fertility control are in a state of physical wellness; however, they may or may not have been successful in their contraceptive efforts. Several examples of nursing diagnoses applied to clients seeking family planning services or using or attempting to use some method of birth control are listed in the Nursing Diagnoses box at the end of this chapter.[13]

Health care professionals must be aware that certain clients are at high risk for lack of contraceptive services: teenagers, low income women, and women in underserved areas. These women need services low in cost with convenient hours and accessible locations. Other groups with special family planning concerns include women with chronic illnesses, women who are physically or mentally handicapped, and women approaching midlife. All women need individualized plans of care, but these groups deserve special attention in order to meet their contraceptive needs fully (see chapters 4, 6, 15, and 20).

Initial Evaluation

A thorough initial assessment seeks data to identify risk factors and other influences on method selection (as discussed previously), and contraindications to certain methods. Subsequently, a database is established. During the initial evaluation a complete history is taken, including, but not limited to, the following.

- *Medical History.* Smoking, cardiovascular disease (CVD), thromboembolic disorder, reproductive tract cancer, breast cancer, diabetes mellitus (DM), frequent urinary tract infections (UTIs), etc.
- *Obstetric and Gynecologic History.* Menstrual, premenstrual syndrome (PMS), contraceptive, STDs, PID, vaginitis, and sexual.
- *Family History.* Especially cancer, CVD, DM, stroke, and other significant problems.
- *Review of Systems.*
- *Personal and Social Data.* Comfort with touching one's self, use of tampons and female hygiene products, desire or plans for children, and partner involvement.

Objective data are obtained from a complete screening physical examination with special attention to height, weight, blood pressure (BP), and examination of thyroid, breasts, abdomen, and pelvis (noting position of uterus and any anatomic variation), and extremities. Other components of physical examination may also require emphasis, depending on birth control methods being considered.

Diagnostic testing includes the following.

- Cervical cytology (Pap smear) essential.
- Wet mounts (saline and potassium hydroxide [KOH] highly recommended; others as indicated).
- Hematocrit.
- Urinalysis.
- STD (especially gonorrhea and chlamydia).

In addition, consider human papilloma virus (HPV) testing, such as polymerase chain reaction (PCR); and blood chemistries, especially lipid profile and blood glucose. In the presence of symptoms, all appropriate examinations/investigations should be carried out.

Subsequent Evaluations

All women who are sexually active or using a method of contraception that requires a prescription should be evaluated annually to evaluate new risk factors, contraindications, side effects, concerns, or new problems associated with the present birth control method and to identify any other reproductive problems.

Subjective data include a review of the client's history, any significant changes in her health status, and her method of birth control (including satisfaction with the method and any problems). Objective data include the client's weight and blood pressure, screening physical, breast, pelvic exam, and Pap smear. Other lab tests are performed as indicated (see previous information). Include a mammogram at the recommended intervals after age 35. (See Chapter 14.)

METHODS OF BIRTH CONTROL

Several birth control methods are currently available.

- Combined oral contraceptives (COCs—containing estrogen and progestin), also referred to as oral contraceptives (OCs), birth control pills (BCPs).
- Progestin-only methods (pills, implants, injections, vaginal rings).
- Postcoital methods (emergency contraception).
- Barriers (male and female condoms, sponges, diaphragms, cervical caps).
- Vaginal spermicides (creams, jellies, suppositories, films).
- Intrauterine devices (IUDs).
- Fertility awareness methods.
- Coitus interruptus (withdrawal).
- Lactational amenorrhea method.
- Sterilization.
- Abortion.

MANAGEMENT CONSIDERATIONS, GUIDELINES FOR CLIENT EDUCATION AND INFORMED CONSENT[1,10,14,15]

- The client must participate in choosing the birth control method; she must be an informed user.
- Always obtain informed consent, particularly for a client choosing an intrauterine device (IUD), implant, injection, or sterilization. *Informed consent* implies that client makes a knowledgeable, voluntary choice, receives complete counseling about the procedure and its consequences, and is free to change her mind prior to the procedure.
- When working with a client planning to use any birth control method, carefully screen for contraindications.
- Set aside time for teaching as a routine part of the clinic visit. During the initial visit, use counseling to help the client select a birth control method; then use additional counseling after the visit to teach specific information about the method chosen.
- *For certain methods (diaphragms, cervical caps, IUDs, implants, vaginal rings, sterilization), the health provider must receive formal education, training, and practice in fitting, insertion, and other technical aspects.*
- During the visit, the health professional is responsible for providing client education and the opportunity for practice and validation of skills pertaining to selected methods (as applicable).
- Make all presentations, counseling, and educational materials compatible with the language, culture, and education of the client.
- Be aware of local myths and misperceptions about particular methods. Address misconceptions sensitively but directly. For example, douching, or "washing" semen out of the woman's body, will not prevent sperm from entering the uterus. Indeed, douching could theoretically enhance the movement of sperm up the cervical canal by washing them deeper into the vagina toward the cervix or by washing away protective mucus.
- To prevent the omission of important information, use a standard teaching checklist outlining key information that the user should know.
- Instruct about female and male anatomy, using models and illustrations.
- Provide the client with method-specific teaching and counseling, using models, illustrations, and handouts to describe key information.

  - How the methods work.
  - Effectiveness of methods.
  - Advantages and disadvantages of methods.
  - Noncontraceptive benefits.
  - What to expect during the visit.
  - Recommendations concerning follow-up.
  - Descriptions of short- and long-term side effects that can occur, and how to deal with them.
  - Danger signs associated with the method selected.

- Explore factors that could place the client at risk for method failure (e.g., frequent intercourse, age, parity, previous failure of method, sexual or lifestyle patterns that make consistent use difficult). Counsel the client regarding these factors.
- If it is determined that the client is at risk for failure with her chosen method, recommend its use in combination with another method.

- Clients who choose a coitus associated method need accurate understanding of the timing of ovulation and awareness of days with high risk for conception. An additional method may be employed during high risk times.
- Provide both oral and written instructions. Instruct the client to read specific package literature and follow the instructions carefully.
- Inform the client that regardless of the method chosen, she must always keep a second birth control method available and be familiar with its use.
- Advise client to keep sufficient quantities of contraceptive products/supplies available at all times in a convenient location. Counsel her about the importance of budgeting her finances for the purchase of products and supplies and for annual exams.
- Teach the proper care and storage of contraceptive devices and supplies.
- For devices requiring insertion, instruct the client to wash her hands before and after insertion to minimize possible introduction of contaminants into the vagina; also instruct her to wash applicators with soap and water after each use.
- Ask the client to repeat important information.
- Inform all clients about the availability of postcoital protection (emergency contraception) in the event of method failure.

EFFECTIVENESS

In this chapter, the effectiveness of birth control methods is reported as estimated failure rates during the first year of use: among couples who used the method perfectly (i.e., correct use at every act of intercourse; lowest expected failure rate); and among typical users, including incorrect and inconsistent use as well as method failures. Table 9–4 shows these failure rates for each method discussed.[16]

COMBINED ORAL CONTRACEPTIVES

Birth control pills (BCPs) or oral contraceptives (OCs), also called "the Pill," have been available in the United States for over 35 years. It is estimated that about 60 million women worldwide

TABLE 9–4. PERCENTAGE OF WOMEN IN THE UNITED STATES EXPERIENCING A CONTRACEPTIVE FAILURE DURING THE FIRST YEAR OF TYPICAL USE AND THE FIRST YEAR OF PERFECT USE

Method	Percentage (%) of Women Experiencing an Accidental Pregnancy within the First Year of Use	
	Typical Use[1]	*Perfect Use*[2]
Chance	85	85
Spermicides	21	6
Periodic Abstinence	20	
Calendar		9
Ovulation Method		3
Sympto-Thermal		2
Post-Ovulation		1
Withdrawal	19	4
Cap		
Parous Women	36	26
Nulliparous Women	18	9
Sponge		
Parous Women	36	20
Nulliparous Women	18	9
Diaphragm	18	6
Condom		
Female (Reality)	21	5
Male	12	3
Pill	3	
Progestin Only		0.5
Combined		0.1
IUD		
Progesterone T	2.0	1.5
Copper T 380A	0.8	0.6
LNg20	0.1	0.1
Depo Provera	0.3	0.3
Norplant (6 Capsules)	0.09	0.09
Female Sterilization	0.4	0.4
Male Sterilization	0.15	0.10

Emergency Contraceptive Pills: Treatment initiated within 72 hours after unprotected intercourse reduces the risk of pregnancy by at least 75 percent.

Lactational Amenorrhea Method: LAM is a highly effective temporary method of contraception.

[1]Among typical couples who initiate use of a method (not necessarily for the first time), the percentage who experience an accidental pregnancy during the first year, if they do not stop use for any other reason.

[2]Among couples who initiate use of a method (not necessarily for the first time) and who use it perfectly (both consistently and correctly), the percentage who experienced an accidental pregnancy during the first year, if they do not stop use for any other reason.

Source: Hatcher, R. A., Trussel, J., Stewart, F., Stewart, G., Kowal, D., Guest, F., Cates, W., Jr. & Policar, W. Contraceptive Technology (16th ed.). (1994). Contraceptive Technology Communications, Inc. Used with permission.

and almost 20 million American women use OCs.[10] Pill use, its effectiveness, risks, benefits, and side effects have been well researched over the past 35 years. Low dosages of estrogen and progestin in today's pills make them very safe and effective for most women. Many noncontraceptive benefits have been identified.

Combined OCs contain two primary components, synthetic estrogen and progestin. The two estrogen compounds currently used in oral contraceptives in the United States are ethinyl estradiol or mestranol. Synthetic progestins are all derived from *19 nortestosterones*. OCs currently available in the United States contain one of several progestins. First generation progestins currently in use include norethindrone, norethindrone acetate, ethynodiol diacetate, norgestrel, and levonorgestrel. OCs containing norethynodrel are no longer marketed in this country.[6,10,14]

New generation progestins derived from levonorgestrel have been developed. These are gestodene, norgestimate, and desogestrel. Combined OCs containing desogestrel and norgestimate are now available in the United States. Gestodene is marketed in Europe and other countries. There appears to be little difference among these newer progestins with regard to clinical efficacy. These newer progestins are very potent in their ability to inhibit ovulation and to transform estrogen primed endometrium into secretory endometrium. Of the three newer agents, it appears that gestodene is most potent with regard to progestional activity. The three newer agents have little estrogenic effect and are weak anti-estrogens. They have far less androgenic activity in animal studies in vivo than older progestins.[17,18,19]

Several recent studies have shown a higher risk of venous thromboembolism (VTE) among women using two of these newer progestins, gestodene and desogestrel. As previously stated, of these two, only desogestrel is available in the United States and is contained in two currently marketed formulations, Desogen (Organon) and Ortho-Cept. The increase in risk of VTE is from 1 in 10,000 to 2 in 10,000 for the pills containing these progestins (pregnancy is associated with the greatest risk of VTE). This increased risk is

TABLE 9–5. RISK FACTORS FOR VENOUS THROMBOEMBOLISM (VTE)

1. Genetic predisposition[a]
2. Acquired predisposition (such as lupus, anticoagulant, malignancy)
3. Physiologic factors (such as dehydration)[b]
4. Mechanical factors (such as immobility or trauma)
5. Obesity (defined here as BMI of 30 or over)
6. Varicose veins (the data on the magnitude of risk attributable to varicose veins is conflicting. Extensive varicosities are likely to be a risk factor).

[a]Women with a family history of hereditary thrombophilia in a first degree relative should not be prescribed combined oral contraceptives unless thrombophilia has been ruled out.
[b]May be acute and/or temporary risk factors.
Source: Statement from the Clinical and Scientific Committee of the Faculty on Family Planning and Reproductive Health Care of the Royal College of Obstetricians and Gynecologists. (1995). Risk of venous thromboembolism and the combined oral contraceptive pill.

for VTE only and not for other cardiovascular events. In fact, recent studies have suggested a possible protective effect against myocardial infarction (MI) for women using OCs containing desogestrel and gestodene. More information regarding these findings will undoubtedly be forthcoming.[20–23] Family planning providers must be aware of the risk factors for VTE (Table 9–5).[24] Implications for practice, considering these studies, are included under Management Considerations later in this section.

Estrogen and progestin are combined in fixed dose pills (monophasic) or in variable amounts in relation to one another throughout the pill cycle, as in biphasic or triphasic preparations. Table 9–6 lists the types and dosages of OCs available in the United States and their comparable biologic activity.

Prescription

OCs are available in 21- or 28-day packs. Active pills are taken the first 21 days; 28-day preparations contain 7 "spacer" tablets that are inert (except for some Parke-Davis products that contain ferrous fumarate in the last 7 brown pills of the 28-day pack).

TABLE 9–6. ORAL CONTRACEPTIVE TYPES, DOSAGES, AND PHYSIOLOGICAL ACTIVITIES*

Oral Contraceptive	Progestational Activity	Androgenic Activity	Endometrial Activity
Low Dose Monophasics*			

Brevicon (Syntex) 21 or 28 day
  0.5 mg norethindrone
  0.035 mg ethinyl estradiol
	Low	Low	Intermediate

Demulen 1/35 (Searle) 21 or 28 day
  1 mg ethynodiol diacetate
  0.035 mg ethinyl estradiol
	Intermediate/High	Low	Low

Desogen (Organon) 28 day
  0.15 mg desogestrel
  0.03 mg ethinyl estradiol
	Intermediate/High	Low	Low/Intermediate

Genora 1/35 (Rugby) 28 day
  1 mg norethindrone
  0.035 mg ethinyl estradiol
	Intermediate	Low/Intermediate	Intermediate

Levlen (Berlex) 21 or 28 day
  0.15 mg levonorgestrel
  0.03 mg ethinyl estradiol
	Low/Intermediate	Intermediate	Intermediate

Loestrin 1/20 (Parke-Davis) 21 day
  1 mg norethindrone acetate
  0.02 mg ethinyl estradiol
	Intermediate	Intermediate/High	Low

Loestrin 1.5/30 (Parke-Davis) 21 day
  1.5 mg norethindrone acetate
  0.03 mg ethinyl estradiol
	Intermediate/High	Intermediate/High	Low

Loestrin Fe 1/20 (Parke-Davis) 28 day
  1 mg norethindrone acetate
  0.02 mg ethinyl estradiol
  7 pills 75 mg ferrous fumarate
	Intermediate	Intermediate/High	Low

Loestrin Fe 1.5/30 (Parke-Davis) 28 day
  1.5 mg norethindrone acetate
  0.03 mg ethinyl estradiol
  7 pills 75 mg ferrous fumarate
	Intermediate/High	Intermediate/High	Low

Lo-Ovral (Wyeth-Ayerst) 21 or 28 day
  0.3 mg norgestrel
  0.03 mg ethinyl estradiol
	Low/Intermediate	Intermediate	Low/Intermediate

Modicon (Ortho) 21 or 28 day
  0.5 mg norethindrone
  0.035 mg ethinyl estradiol
	Low	Low	Intermediate

Nelova 1/35E (Warner-Chilicott)
  1 mg norethindrone
  0.035 mg ethinyl estradiol
	Intermediate	Low/Intermediate	Intermediate

Nelova 0.5/35E (Warner-Chilicott)
  0.5 mg norethindrone
  0.035 mg ethinyl estradiol
	Low	Low	Intermediate

Nordette (Wyeth-Ayerst) 21 or 28 day
  0.15 mg levonorgestrel
  0.03 mg ethinyl estradiol
	Low/Intermediate	Intermediate	Intermediate

Norethin 1/35E (Schiapparelli Searle) 28 day
  1 mg norethindrone
  0.035 mg ethinyl estradiol
	Intermediate	Low/Intermediate	Intermediate

Norinyl 1+35 (Syntex) 21 or 28 day
  1 mg norethindrone
  0.035 mg ethinyl estradiol
	Intermediate	Low/Intermediate	Intermediate

(*Continued*)

TABLE 9–6. ORAL CONTRACEPTIVE TYPES, DOSAGES, AND PHYSIOLOGICAL ACTIVITIES (CONTINUED)

Oral Contraceptive	Progestational Activity	Androgenic Activity	Endometrial Activity
Ortho-Cept (Ortho) 21 or 28 day 0.15 mg desogestrel 0.03 mg ethinyl estradiol	Intermediate/High	Low	Intermediate
Ortho-Cyclen (Ortho) 21 or 28 day .25 mg norgestimate 0.035 mg ethinyl estradiol	Low	Low	Low/Intermediate
Ortho-Novum 1/35 (Ortho) 21 or 28 day 1 mg norethindrone 0.035 mg ethinyl estradiol	Intermediate	Low/Intermediate	Intermediate
Ovcon 35 (Mead Johnson) 21 or 28 day 0.4 mg norethindrone 0.035 mg ethinyl estradiol	Low	Low	Intermediate
Triphasics *			
Ortho-Novoum 7/7/7 (Ortho) 21 or 28 day 7 days: 0.5 mg norethindrone 0.035 mg ethinyl estradiol 7 days: 0.75 mg norethindrone 0.035 mg ethinyl estradiol 7 days: 1 mg norethindrone 0.035 mg ethinyl estradiol	Low/Intermediate	Low/Intermediate	Intermediate
Tri-Levlen (Berlex) 21 or 28 day 6 days: 0.05 mg levongorgestrel 0.03 mg ethinyl estradiol 5 days: 0.075 mg levonorgestrel 0.04 mg ethinyl estradiol 10 days: 0.125 mg levonorgestrel 0.03 mg ethinyl estradiol	Low	Low/Intermediate	Intermediate
Tri-Cyclen (Ortho) 21 or 28 day 7 days: 0.18 mg norgestimate 0.035 mg ethinyl estradiol 7 days: 0.215 mg norgestimate 0.035 mg ethinyl estradiol 7 days: 0.25 mg norgestimate 0.035 mg ethinyl estradiol	Low	Low	Low/Intermediate
Tri-Norinyl (Syntex) 21 or 28 day 7 days: 0.5 mg norethindrone 0.035 mg ethinyl estradiol 9 days: 1 mg norethindrone 0.035 mg ethinyl estradiol 5 days: 0.5 mg norethindrone 0.035 mg ethinyl estradiol	Low/Intermediate	Low/Intermediate	Intermediate
Triphasil (Wyeth-Ayerst) 21 or 28 day 6 days: 0.05 mg levonorgestrel 0.03 mg ethinyl estradiol 5 days: 0.075 mg levonorgestrel 0.04 mg ethinyl estradiol 10 days: 0.125 mg levonorgestrel 0.03 mg ethinyl estradiol	Low	Low/Intermediate	Intermediate
Biphasics			
Jenest (Organon) 28 day 7 days: 0.5 mg norethindrone 0.035 mg ethinyl estradiol 14 days: 1 mg norethindrone 0.035 mg ethinyl estradiol	Low/Intermediate	Low/Intermediate	Intermediate

TABLE 9–6. ORAL CONTRACEPTIVE TYPES, DOSAGES, AND PHYSIOLOGICAL ACTIVITIES (CONTINUED)

Oral Contraceptive	Progestational Activity	Androgenic Activity	Endometrial Activity

Ortho-Novum 10/11 (Ortho) 21 or 28 day
  10 days: 0.5 mg norethindrone
      0.035 mg ethinyl estradiol
  11 days: 1 mg norethindrone
      0.035 mg ethinyl estradiol
	Low/Intermediate	Low/Intermediate	Intermediate

Moderate Dose Monophasics			

Demulen 1/50 (Searle) 21 or 28 day
  1 mg ethynodiol diacetate
  0.050 mg ethinyl estradiol
	Intermediate/High	Low	Intermediate

Genora 1/50 (Rugby) 28 day
  1 mg norethindrone
  0.05 mg mestranol
	Intermediate	Low/Intermediate	Intermediate

Norethin 1/50M (Schiapparelli Searle) 28 day
  1 mg norethindrone
  0.05 mg mestranol
	Intermediate	Low/Intermediate	Intermediate

Norinyl 1+50 (Syntex) 21 or 28 day
  1 mg norethindrone
  0.05 mestranol
	Intermediate	Low/Intermediate	Intermediate

Norlestrin 1/50 (Parke-Davis) 21 day
  1 mg norethindrone acetate
  0.05 mg ethinyl estradiol
	Intermediate	Intermediate	Intermediate

Norlestrin FE 1/50 (Parke-Davis) 28 day
  1 mg norethindrone acetate
  0.05 mg ethinyl estradiol
  7 pills 75 mg ferrous fumerate
	Intermediate	Intermediate	Intermediate

Norlestrin 2.5/50 (Parke-Davis) 21 day
  2.5 mg norethindrone acetate
  0.05 mg ethinyl estradiol
	High	High	High

Norlestrin Fe 2.5/50 (Parke-Davis) 28 day
  2.5 mg norethindrone acetate
  0.05 mg ethinyl estradiol
  7 pills 75 mg ferrous fumerate
	High	High	High

Ortho-Novum 1/50 (Ortho) 21 or 28 day
  1 mg norethindrone
  0.05 mg mestranol
	Intermediate	Low/Intermediate	Intermediate

Ovcon 50 (Mead Johnson) 21 or 28 day
  1 mg norethindrone
  0.05 mg ethinyl estradiol
	Intermediate	Low/Intermediate	Intermediate

Ovral (Wyeth-Ayerst) 21 or 28 day
  0.5 mg norgtestrel
  0.05 mg ethinyl estradiol
	High	High	Intermediate/High

Progestin Only			
Micronor (Ortho) 28 day 0.35 mg norethindrone	Low	Low	Low
Nor-QD (Syntex) 42 day 0.35 mg norethindrone	Low	Low	Low
Ovrette (Wyeth-Ayerst) 28 day 0.075 mg norgestrel	Low	Low	Low

Source: Adapted from Dickey, R. P. Managing contraceptive pill patients (8th ed.). Durant, OK: Essential Medical Information Systems, Inc. 1994.

*Alesse (Wyeth-Ayerst) and Estrostep/Estrostep Fe (Park Davis) are newer oral contraceptives. See estimated activities page 222 in Addendum.

Mechanism of Action[6,10,14]

Pregnancy is prevented by several effects of estrogen and progestin.

- Gonadotropin-releasing hormone (GnRH) is suppressed, which in turn suppresses follicle-stimulating hormone (FSH) and luteinizing hormone (LH), inhibiting ovulation.
- Ovum/tubal transport is altered.
- Cervical mucus thickens, inhibiting sperm transport.
- Implantation is inhibited by suppression of the endometrium and alteration of uterine secretions.

Effectiveness

OCs are considered highly effective in preventing pregnancy (see Table 9–4). Failures are attributed to the following.

- Method failure, improper use, user error.
- Discontinuing the pill without immediate use of another method.
- Drug interactions.

Little difference exists in the failure rates among individual OCs.[10,14,16]

Advantages[10,14]

- High rate of effectiveness.
- Use not associated with the act of intercourse.
- Use controlled by the woman.
- Easy to use, convenient.
- Rapid reversal of effects after discontinuing use.
- Considered safe for most women throughout their reproductive life span when there are no contraindications.
- Multiple noncontraceptive benefits.

Noncontraceptive Benefits[6,10,14,25,26]

- *Improved Menstrual Characteristics.* OCs minimize dysmenorrhea and usually decrease the amount and duration of bleeding so that periods are regular and predictable. OCs relieve premenstrual syndrome (PMS) in some women, and they lower the incidence of iron deficiency anemia. They can be used to ameliorate amenorrhea and dysfunctional uterine bleeding.

- *Protection against Ovarian and Endometrial Cancer.* Compared with women who never used OCs, users have half the risk of developing these cancers. Protection is noted after a minimum of 12 months of use and persists long after pills are discontinued.
- *Lower Incidence of Ovarian Cysts.* Incidence is reduced by 90 percent, due to the suppression of ovulation.
- *Prevention of Ectopic Pregnancy.* Prevention occurs through the suppression of ovulation.
- *Lower Incidence of Endometriosis.* Incidence is reduced due to the suppression of endometrial growth. Also used in treatment.
- *Some Protection against Pelvic Inflammatory Disease (PID).* Incidence of PID is 20 to 50 percent lower among users of OCs than among those who use no contraceptive method. The greatest protection is against PID caused by gonorrhea.
- *Lower Incidence of Benign Breast Cysts and Fibroadenomas.* As a result, breast biopsy procedures are decreased.
- *Other Benefits.* OCs may reduce acne in some women; may reduce the incidence of rheumatoid arthritis; are used in treatment of hirsutism.

Disadvantages[10,14,25,26]

- Affects all body systems.
- User must remember to take pills daily.
- Some users experience undesirable side effects that cause discontinuance of pills.
- Should not be used while lactating.
- Provides no protection against HIV infection and other STDs.
- High cost for some women.
- For some women, slight delay in becoming pregnant after discontinuing (2 to 3 months).
- Prescription needed.
- Access to pharmacy needed.
- User must interact with medical system.
- OCs may interact with other drugs (see Table 9–7).
- Many possible side effects.

Side Effects and Complications

Side effects and complications are caused by systemic effects of OCs, and may be due to

TABLE 9–7. ORAL CONTRACEPTIVE INTERACTIONS WITH OTHER DRUGS

Effect	Substances	Comments
Drugs whose effects may be enhanced in combination with oral contraceptives.	Alcohol, tricyclic antidepressants,[a] some benzodiazepines (alprazolam, chlordiazepoxide, clorazepate, diazepam, flurazepam), β-blockers, corticosteroids, theophylline, Troleandomycin (Tao).[b]	Monitor blood levels when available and monitor affected body systems. Use these drugs with caution.
Drugs whose effects may be diminished in combination with oral contraceptives.	Acetaminophen,[b] oral anticoagulants, some benzodiazepines (lorazepam, oxazepam, temazepam), guanethidine,[a] oral hypoglycemic agents (chlorpropamide, glipizide, glyburide, tolazamide, tolbutamide), methyldopa.	Monitor physiological effect of drug, or use alternative drug, or use alternative contraceptive method.
Drugs that may diminish the effectiveness of oral contraceptives.	Any antibiotic (especially ampicillin, sulfonamides, tetracyclines), antacids, anticonvulsants (carbamazepine, ethosuximide, phenobarbital, phenytoin, primidone, valproic acid, valproate), barbiturates, griseofulvin, rifampin.	Could result in breakthrough bleeding or pregnancy. Use additional birth control method during drug use and for one cycle after drug discontinuation, or use alternative contraceptive method.

Note: Vitamin C, 1 g or more daily, may cause increased serum concentrations of estrogen and possibly increased adverse effects of estrogens.
[a]Clinical significance of this interaction is unknown.
[b]Increased risk of hepatotoxicity with simultaneous use.
Source: References 6, 10, 14, 15.

estrogenic, progestational, and/or androgenic activities, or their effects on serum lipoproteins. Pills with the lowest feasible biologic activity in each of these three areas should be chosen, because of potential long-term adverse effects on some body systems, particularly the cardiovascular system. Table 9–8 summarizes most common side effects of OCs based on their relation to excess or deficient hormone activity.

Managing Side Effects[10,14,17,27]

- Allow the client time to adjust to the pills (two or three packs).
- Determine that she is taking the pills correctly.
- Determine whether any symptom indicates the possible development of a serious health problem or OC-related complication (especially myocardial infarction, stroke, pulmonary embolism, thrombophlebitis, gallbladder or liver problems). Ask specific questions regarding early pill danger signs, remembering the acronym *ACHES*—severe *A*bdominal pain, severe *C*hest pain, severe *H*eadaches, *E*ye-visual changes, *S*hortness of breath. Other danger signs are severe leg pain, loss of coordination, speech problems, and depression.

- Determine which hormonal component of the OC is likely to be responsible for the symptom.
- Determine whether the side effect is due to an excess or deficiency of a hormonal component (see Table 9–8). If it is determined that the side effect is due to a deficiency or excess of a particular hormonal component, switch the client to a different OC product that has greater or lesser activity of the offending hormone (Table 9–6).

Table 9–9 lists common side effects, suggested hormone adjustments, and other management considerations. Table 9–6 includes hormonal activities of low and moderate dose OCs, and may be used when OC dosage and/or potency adjustments are indicated for management of specific side effects.

Effects of OCs on Blood Lipids

Use of OCs as a factor influencing blood lipoproteins has received a disproportionate amount of attention. No causal link between OC use and cardiovascular morbidity resulting from blood

TABLE 9–8 HORMONE CONTENT OF ORAL CONTRACEPTIVES AND RELATED SIDE EFFECTS

Estrogen Excess			Estrogen Deficiency
Reproductive System	*PMS-Type Symptoms*	*Cardiovascular System*	Absence of withdrawal bleeding
Hypermenorrhea, menorrhagia, and clotting	Nausea	Vascular headaches	Spotting and bleeding (day 1 to day 9, or continuously)
Cervical extrophy	Edema, leg cramps	Hypertension	Hypomenorrhea
Dysmenorrhea	Nonvascular headaches	Cerebrovascular accident	Nervousness
Breast enlargement and tenderness	Irritability	Deep vein thrombosis	Atrophic vaginitis
Mucorrhea	Bloating	Thromboembolic disorders	Vasomotor symptoms
Uterine fibroid growth	Dizziness, syncope	Telangiectasias	Pelvic relaxation
Enlargement of uterus	Cyclic weight gain		
Cystic breast changes	*Miscellaneous Symptoms*		
	Chloasma		
	Hayfever & allergic rhinitis		
	Urinary tract infection		
	Upper respiratory disorders		
	Epigastric distress		
Progestin Excess			**Progestin Deficiency**
Progestational	*Androgenic/Anabolic*	*Cardiovascular System*	Breakthrough bleeding and spotting during late cycle (days 10 to 21)
Reproduction Symptoms:	Increased libido	Hypertension	Delayed withdrawal bleeding
Post-pill amenorrhea	Acne	Dilation of leg veins	Dysmenorrhea
Libido decrease	Hirsutism	Lowered protective forms of high density lipoproteins (HDLs)	Menorrhagia and clotting
Light menses	Oil skin and scalp		
Cervicitis	Cholestatic jaundice		
Monilial vaginitis	Rash		
Miscellaneous Symptoms:	Pruritis		
Increased appetite	Edema		
Fatigue/weakness			
Depression, mood changes			
Noncyclic weight gain			

Source: References 6, 10,14.

lipid changes has been noted. Interest, however, has focused on lipoprotein changes that occur, because they are known indicators of increased risk for cardiovascular disease (CVD).

Studies show no increased risk of atherosclerosis in women who use or have used OCs. Recent data from the Nurses Health Study indicate no increased risk of coronary heart disease, stroke, or other heart disease among former OC users. Lipid values may indeed vary somewhat in OC users, but these variations tend to remain within the normal range and then return to normal during the pill free interval. This subtle impact is considered insignificant. The newer progestins demonstrate fewer atherogenic changes.[14,26,28–30]

OCs and Cardiovascular Disease

A dose-response relationship between the risk of arterial and venous thrombosis and the amount of estrogen in combined OCs has been established. Smoking and OC use increase the risk of serious cardiovascular side effects, including MI and stroke, this risk greatly increasing after age 35. Smokers over age 35 should be advised against using OCs. It should be noted that OCs containing 20 mcg. of estrogen have little or no effect on clotting parameters. These preparations should be considered for all smokers, for women over age 35, and for women with other CVD risk factors such as diabetes mellitus, focal migraine headaches and extreme obesity.[6,20,23,26,31,32]

TABLE 9–9. MANAGEMENT OF SIDE EFFECTS OF ORAL CONTRACEPTIVES

Sign, Symptom, Side Effect	Estrogen Adjustment	Progestin Adjustment	Comments and Other Considerations
Acne	Increase	*or* Decrease—less androgenic	Hygiene, diet, topical, antibiotic therapy
Amenorrhea or light menses	Increase	Decrease	Rule out pregnancy; change to pill with higher endometrial activity
Anemia	No change	No change or increase	Diet, iron supplements, evaluate anemia
Bloating, fluid retention	Decrease	No change	Consider minipill
Breakthrough bleeding, spotting	Early cycle (days 1 to 14) increase or give estrogen supplement	No change	Review history for misuse; check for infection, cervical changes, pregnancy
	Late cycle (days 15 to 21) No change	Increase or more biologically active	Change to pill with higher endometrial activity
Breast tenderness, fullness	Decrease	No change or decrease	Consider minipill; decrease sodium, caffeine intake; Vitamin E 400 IU b.i.d.
Breast or uterine cancer	Stop	Stop	Refer
Cervical eversion and increased mucus	Decrease	No change or decrease	Examine for infection
Chloasma	Decrease or stop	No change or less estrogenic	Consider minipill
Contact lens discomfort, refractive changes	Decrease or stop	No change	Consider minipill
Cyclic weight gain	Decrease	No change or decrease	
Decreased breast milk in nursing mothers	Stop	No change or decrease	Combined OCs not recommended—consider minipill
Decreased libido	Decrease or stop	Decrease or stop, or higher androgenic	Sexual counseling
Depression	Decrease or stop	Decrease or stop	Try vitamin B_6 20–25 mg per day; monitor closely
Diplopia, any loss of vision, papilledema	Stop	Stop	Evaluate
Diabetes, worsening of	Decrease or stop	Decrease or stop	Monitor closely
Dizziness	Decrease or stop	No change; or if hypoglycemia present, decrease	If hypoglycemia, eat regularly, and avoid simple carbohydrates
Dysmenorrhea	Decrease	Increase—higher progestational and androgenic	Rule out infection, other pathology
Gallbladder disease	Stop	Stop	Evaluate
Increased facial hair, hair changes, thinning scalp hair	Increase	Decrease—less androgenic	Rule out thyroid dysfunction
High-density lipoprotein (HDL) cholesterol, decrease	Decrease or stop	Decrease or stop	Triphasic pill or try pill with new generation progestin
Headache, migraine	Decrease or stop	Decrease or stop	Evaluate headaches, consult physician
Hypermenorrhea	Decrease	Increase—higher progestational and androgenic	Rule out pathology first; can combine estrogen with progestin/androgen change
Hypertension	Decrease or stop	Decrease or stop	Consider minipill, stop smoking, increase exercise, lose weight, reduce stress
Increased appetite	No change or decrease	Decrease—less androgenic	Dietary counseling
Increased growth of benign fibroid tumors	Decrease or stop	No change or decrease	Rule out malignancy

(Continued)

TABLE 9–9. MANAGEMENT OF SIDE EFFECTS OF ORAL CONTRACEPTIVES (CONTINUED)

Sign, Symptom, Side Effect	Estrogen Adjustment	Progestin Adjustment	Comments and Other Considerations
Liver disease, jaundice, or benign liver tumor	Stop	Stop	Evaluate
Myocardial infarction or stroke	Stop	Stop	Refer
Noncyclic weight gain	No change or decrease	Decrease—less androgenic	Avoid norgestrel and levonorgestrel
Nausea or vomiting	Decrease or change type	No change	Take after full meal; consider minipill
Nervousness	No change	Decrease or stop	Rule out hypoglycemia; try monophasic pill
Ovarian cysts	No change	Increase—moderate to high progestational activity	If on minipill, triphasic or very low dose OC, then switch to 35 μg dose monophasic or higher
Pelvic inflammatory disease (PID)	No change	No change	Evaluate and treat infection; monitor closely
Pulmonary embolism, thromboembolism, thrombophlebitis (or symptoms of)	Stop	Stop	Refer
Rheumatoid arthritis	No change	No change	Treat rheumatoid arthritis adequately
Thyroid function tests changes	No change	No change	Evaluate for thyroid dysfunction
Urinary tract infection	Decrease	No change	Treat infections
Vaginal dryness	Increase	Decrease	Use additional lubrication
Varicose veins	Decrease	No change	Consider minipill
Yeast infections	No change	Decrease	Hygiene measures, treat infection

Source: References 6, 10, 14, 15, 17, 27, 30.

Effects of OCs on Carbohydrate (CHO) Metabolism

Older high dose OCs were associated with slight increases in glucose levels, decreases in glucose tolerance and increases in plasma levels of insulin. Low dose OCs currently used, however, show minimal or no influences on CHO metabolism. The progestin component of the OC seems to have the greatest effect on CHO metabolism. For the non-diabetic OC user, the changes are so minimal as to be insignificant. No significant impact on glucose tolerance has been seen in women with risk factors for DM or with a history of gestational DM. In overtly diabetic women, low dose OCs may be given provided clients are followed closely. No progression or acceleration of diabetic retinopathy, nephropathy or cardiovascular complications has been attributed to use of the low dose OCs in diabetic women.[14,33–35]

Effects of OCs on the Risk of Breast Cancer

Whether a relationship exists between OC use and the development of breast cancer remains unclear and controversial. A few studies have suggested a link between the development of breast cancer at a relatively young age and long-term use of OCs; however, other studies refute these findings. Existing data suggest that the overall risk of breast cancer is not increased by the use of OCs. No increased breast cancer risk was noted for women older than 60 years who had used OCs. General conclusions are that the benefits of OCs greatly outweigh the risks for appropriately selected clients who are monitored regularly.[36–39]

Contraindications

Table 9–10 lists absolute and relative contraindications to the use of oral contraceptives.

TABLE 9–10. CONTRAINDICATIONS TO THE USE OF ORAL CONTRACEPTIVES

Absolute Contraindications (Refrain from prescribing OCs in presence of these conditions)

Thrombophlebitis or thromboembolic disorder

Family history of hereditary thrombophilia in a first degree relative

Cerebrovascular disease

Coronary artery or ischemic heart disease

Known or suspected breast cancer

Known or suspected estrogen-dependent neoplasia

Known or suspected pregnancy

Benign or malignant liver tumor

Current impaired liver function

Undiagnosed, abnormal vaginal bleeding

Relative Contraindications (Exercise caution if OC use is considered in presence of these conditions)

Vascular or migraine headaches, especially if they began or worsened with the use of combined oral contraceptives

Hypertension

Acute mononucleosis or recent hepatitis

Presence of factors predisposing to thromboembolic disorder, such as illness or surgery requiring immobilization, long leg cast, trauma to lower leg

Cardiac or renal dysfunction (or history of)

Diabetes mellitus

Obesity (of more than 20 percent of ideal body weight)

Varicose veins

Lactation

Age over 50

Age over 35 for a smoker (some providers feel that no heavy smoker should take birth control pills)

Psychic depression

History of myocardial infarction in an immediate family member before age 50 (especially a mother or a sister)

Hyperlipidemia

Active gallbladder disease

Sickle cell (SS) or sickle C disease

Completion of a term pregnancy within the past 10 to 14 days

Ulcerative colitis

Asthma

Source: References 6, 10, 14, 24, 30.

Management Considerations[6,10,14,40,41]

- All clients taking OCs should be advised to stop smoking. Nonsmoking, healthy women (without contraindications) older than 35 may take low dose OCs. Strongly consider a 20 mcg estrogen pill for these older women.
- Instruct that OCs do not protect against STDs, including HIV infection. If the client is not in a mutually monogamous relationship, advise that condoms with spermicide be used in addition to pills.
- Initial pill selection is based on individual client characteristics. New OC users should generally be started on the lowest dose that is still effective: a 35 µg (or less) pill. Since the introduction of triphasic preparations, many practitioners start new users on one of them. The lowest dose monophiasic combined OCs available, Loestrin 1/20 (Parke-Davis) or Alesse (Wyeth-Ayerst), should be considered for older women. Specific client characteristics that may influence initial OC selection include age, personal and family history, relative contraindications, menstrual patterns, and hormone sensitivity.

Because of the new and still controversial information regarding OCs containing desogestrel, it is prudent not to start new clients on these pills. For established users of OCs containing desogestrel, consider encouraging them to switch to other OCs until data are further clarified. If clients choose to remain on one of these preparations, fully inform them of the risk of VTE.[20–23] An informed consent document is advised.

New users should be reevaluated after 3 cycles of pill use to determine how they are adjusting. Instruct the client to contact the provider sooner if concerns arise. Early intervention and support when a client experiences bothersome side effects may prevent her from discontinuing the pill for nonmedical reasons.

- Instruct the client about how to take combined OCs. When first initiating pill use, one of the following methods is recommended.

  - Start pack on first Sunday after menses begins, regardless of whether bleeding is still present (preferred method). *or*
  - Start pack on first day of menstrual bleeding. *or*
  - Start pack on fifth day after menstrual bleeding begins.
  - Postpartum women (not lactating) may begin OCs at day 21 post-partum.
  - Postabortion or miscarriage may begin immediately (day 1 or 2).

Pill manufacturers often recommend specific routines for initiating use of their products. Instruct the client to swallow one pill daily, at the same time each day, until the pack is finished.

For second and subsequent packs:

- If using 28-day pack, begin new pack immediately. Do not skip any days.
- If using 21-day pack, stop pills for exactly 7 days, then start new pack.
- Periods may be very light while on pills. Even slight spotting or bleeding should be considered a period (as long as no pills were missed).

▪ Instruct the client to use a second birth control method, such as condoms or a diaphragm used with spermicide, until she completes the first 7 pills in the first pack. Another method is always kept on hand to use in case of missed pills, when taking another medication that might interfere with pill effectiveness (see Table 9–7), or when vomiting or diarrhea occurs.

▪ Missed pills are a common problem. Recent studies have shown that the most risky time to miss pills is at the beginning of the pack, right after the pill free interval (PFI), or during the third week of active pills, immediately prior to the start of the PFI. Preovulatory follicles may be present after 7 days without active pills. If the woman misses 1 or more pills close to the time of the PFI, thus extending the number of days without active pills to more than 7, she could ovulate and conceive. Missed pills during week 2 of the pack do not present a major concern. The following instructions apply if 1 or more pills are missed.

  - If 1 pill is missed, take the missed pill as soon as remembered and the next pill at the usual time. If the missed pill is taken more than 12 hours late, a backup contraceptive method must be used for the next 7 days.
  - If 2 or more pills are missed, take 2 as soon as remembered and discard the remainder of the missed pills. The next day's pill will be the one normally taken for that day, had no pills been forgotten. Spotting is very likely to occur. Again, use a backup method for the next 7 days.
  - If 1 or more pills are missed during week 3 of the pill pack, follow directions previously given, but skip the pill free interval (spacer pills) and go directly to the first pill in the new pack. Advise the woman that she may not have a period.

▪ If a period is missed and pills were taken correctly, the client should begin a new pack as usual. Pregnancy is unlikely. If two consecutive periods are missed and pills were taken correctly, a pregnancy test is done.

▪ If a period is missed and client missed one or more pills, pills are stopped; pregnancy test is done.

▪ If a decision is made to stop OCs and pregnancy is not desired, begin using another BC method immediately. If pregnancy is desired, use another method for two or three cycles after stopping pills.

▪ Birth control pills are considered medication. Always tell any health care provider when OCs are being taken.

▪ The client who seems to consistently miss pills should consider other methods of contraception

▪ Please refer to earlier section in this chapter, Management Considerations, Guidelines for Client Education and Informed Consent.

PROGESTIN-ONLY PILLS (POPS)

Referred to as "minipills," progestin-only pills (POPs) were introduced 10 years after combined oral contraceptives (COCs). POPs are taken daily with no pill-free interval. Although much less popular than COCs, POPs are well suited to women who want to take contraceptive pills but have contraindications to COCs (e.g., women with a history of thrombophlebitis, or who developed hypertension or severe headaches while taking COCs). Available POPs contain norethindrone or norgestrel; they contain a fixed dose of progestin in either 28- or 42-day packs (see Table 9–5).[6,10,14,25]

Mechanisms of Action

There are four mechanisms by which POPs may prevent pregnancy.[6,10,14]

▪ Ovulation is suppressed by inhibition of LH release from the anterior pituitary. Ovulation is inhibited in about 40 percent of cycles.

▪ Cervical mucus maintains a thick consistency, inhibiting sperm penetration.

▪ The endometrium becomes thin and atrophic.

- Tubal changes occur, including altered tubal transport, contractility, and histology.

Effectiveness

POPs are somewhat less effective than combined OCs (see Table 9–4). Efficacy increases significantly in women of older reproductive age and women who are lactating.[16]

Advantages[6,10,14,25,42]

- No estrogen related side effects.
- Overall safer than combined OCs (fewer and less serious complications).
- May be used by lactating women.
- May be used by clients with prior history of thrombophlebitis (no effect on blood clotting) or with history of other estrogen related contraindications to COC use.
- Minimal effect on carbohydrate metabolism; therefore, may be used (with caution) by diabetic women.
- Rapid reversal of effects after stopping.
- Several noncontraceptive benefits.

Noncontraceptive Benefits[6,10,14]

Most health benefits are similar to those of combined OCs. Because only a small number of women use POPs, large scale studies are not available. Menstrual cycle benefits include decreased cramping, lighter bleeding, shorter periods, decreased PMS-type symptoms, and lessened breast tenderness.

Disadvantages[6,10,14,42]

- Must be taken with meticulous accuracy; no more than 27 hours between pills.
- Less effective than combined OCs.
- May cause irregular bleeding with unpredictable patterns (may include spotting, breakthrough bleeding (BTB), amenorrhea, prolonged bleeding).
- No protection against HIV infection and other STDs.
- Interaction with other drugs can decrease effectiveness (see Table 9–7).
- Higher incidence of functional ovarian cysts.
- Higher incidence of ectopic pregnancy.

- Progestins may theoretically cause adverse effects on blood lipids by decreasing HDLs and increasing LDLs and triglycerides.
- Less widely available than combined OCs. Also refer to the section on combined OCs and to Tables 9–8 and 9–9 to evaluate and manage side effects.

Contraindications/Precautions

According to the FDA, progestin-only pills are required to carry the same contraindications as combined OCs, even though many of these contraindications are related to estrogen content (see Table 9–10). Several relative contraindications to POPs should be emphasized.

- History of functional ovarian cysts.
- History of ectopic pregnancy.
- Inability to take pills consistently.
- Undiagnosed abnormal vaginal bleeding during the preceding 3 months.
- Hyperlipidemia.

Management Considerations[6,10,14,41,42]

- All clients taking POPs should be advised to stop smoking. Nonsmoking, healthy women (without contraindications) older than 35 may take POPs. May also be used by women over 35 who smoke.
- Instruct that POPs do not protect against STDs, including HIV infection. If the client is not in a mutually monogamous relationship, advise that condoms with spermicide be used in addition to pills.
- If decision is made to stop POPs and pregnancy is not desired, begin using another BC method immediately. If pregnancy is desired, use another method for two or three cycles after stopping pills.
- Birth control pills are considered medication. Always tell any health care provider when POPs are being taken.
- When taking POPs, it is important to keep track of periods. Tell the client that if more than 45 days pass with no bleeding, a health care professional should be contacted for an examination and pregnancy test.
- Spotting or bleeding between periods is not unusual for a woman on the minipill, especially

during the first few months of use. Furthermore, some bleeding is very likely if one or more pills are missed. Heavy bleeding, pain, or fever is reported to the health care professional.

- *Initiating Use.* Pills are started on the first day of the period, or immediately after completing a 21-day pack of combined OC, or after the 21st pill of 28-day pack (placebo pills are discarded). A second birth control method is kept on hand to use for (a) the first 7 days on minipills, (b) times when pills are missed, (c) when on antibiotics, or (d) when experiencing diarrhea or vomiting.
- POPs may be started immediately following delivery, abortion, or miscarriage.
- One pill is swallowed daily until pack is finished; new pack is started the very next day—a day is never skipped. In addition, minipills must be taken at *exactly* the same time every day.
- When minipills are missed or forgotten, instruct the client as follows.
  - If pill is taken more than 3 hours late, use a backup birth control method for the next 48 hours.
  - If one pill is missed, take it as soon as remembered. Take the next pill at the regular time, even if this means taking two pills in 1 day. Use a backup method for the next 48 hours.
  - If two pills or more are missed in a row, there is good chance of pregnancy occurring. Take two pills as soon as remembered and two the next day. Start using a second method of birth control right away. If no period occurs in 4 to 6 weeks, a pregnancy test is needed.

OTHER PROGESTIN-ONLY CONTRACEPTIVES: IMPLANTS AND INJECTIONS

The newest methods available (and being tested) for controlling fertility are long acting progestin-only systems. These are ideal for women who desire long term, continuous contraception and who may desire future pregnancies. Norplant implants and depo-medroxyprogesterone acetate injections are discussed here.

Norplant

Approved for use in the United States in 1990 and marketed by Wyeth-Ayerst, Norplant is a timed-release implant of levonorgestrel. Once in place, it provides 5 years of continuous, highly effective contraception. The system consists of six Silastic capsules, each measuring 2.4×34 mm and containing 36 mg of levonorgestrel. Capsules are implanted in a fanlike pattern through a 3–5 mm incision, usually in the medial aspect of the upper arm (see Figure 9–1). The Norplant system releases 80 µg of levonorgestrel per day during the first few weeks after insertion, decreasing over the next 18 months to a constant rate of approximately 30 µg per day over a 5-year period.[6,10,14,43–46]

Depo-Provera Injections

Depo-Provera is an intramuscular (I.M.) injection of depo-medroxyprogesterone acetate (DMPA) that provides 3 months of protection. It was approved by the FDA for use as a contraceptive in the United States in 1992, after many years of controversy. The standard dosage is DMPA 150 mg I.M. every 90 days.[6,10,14,46–48]

Mechanisms of Action

Progestin-only systems vary in their delivery method, blood levels, and duration of action. The mechanisms of action by which pregnancy is prevented are the same, however.[6,10,14]

- Ovulation is suppressed by inhibition of LH release from the anterior pituitary. Ovulation is inhibited in about 40 percent of cycles.
- Cervical mucus maintains a thick consistency, inhibiting sperm penetration.
- The endometrium becomes thin and atrophic.
- Tubal changes occur, including altered tubal transport, contractility, and histology.

Effectiveness

Failure of long acting progestins is rare when they are properly administered and used no longer than the specified time limits. DMPA must be injected within the first 5 days of the menstrual cycle; implants are inserted within the first 7 days

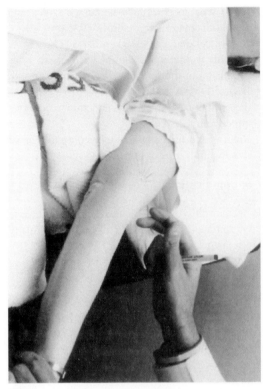

A

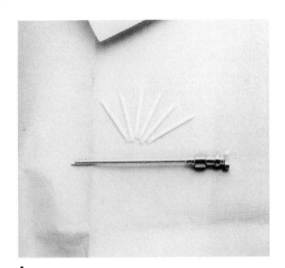

B

Figure 9–1. Norplant system: (A) components of system; (B) outline of pattern of insertion on the medial aspect of the upper arm. *(Reproduced, with permission, from Lemcke DP, Pattison J, Marshall LA, Cowley DS: Primary Care of Women. Appleton & Lange, 1995.)*

of onset of menses. *It must be determined that the woman is not pregnant.* These methods are considered highly effective (see Table 9–4).[16,44,46]

Advantages[6,10,43–48]

- Long duration of action.
- Highly effective.
- Relative low doses of hormone.
- Few systemic complications.
- Low ectopic pregnancy rates.
- Major complications are rare.
- Effects on blood lipids appear to be minimal.
- Estrogen free.
- Safe for women over 35.
- Use not associated with coitus.
- Very light menses or amenorrhea.
- May be used while lactating.
- May be used by smokers over 35.

- Receiving the DMPA injection early by a few days is not harmful. Grace period of 1 week if late receiving DMPA.
- Some noncontraceptive benefits.

Disadvantages[6,10,43–48]

- Most women experience some side effects; most are usually minor and related to menstrual irregularities. If bleeding is heavy, anemia may occur.
- Implants are very expensive.
- Implants may be slightly visible.
- Implants must be inserted and removed by a specially trained clinician.
- Removal of implants may be difficult.
- In rare instances infection can occur at the implant insertion site.

- If the woman is already depressed, signs and symptoms may increase on DMPA.
- No protection against HIV, other STDs.
- Possible weight gain, nausea, headaches.
- Expulsion of the implant system can occur.
- If first DMPA injection is given later than 5 days after onset of menses, injection may not be effective for 2 weeks.
- Return to fertility may be delayed up to 6 or 12 months after injection of DMPA.

Contraindications

Progestin-only methods must carry the same contraindications as COCs, even though many are related to estrogen content (see Table 9–10). Several relative contraindications to long acting progestin-only systems should be emphasized.

- Known pregnancy or suspected.
- History of undiagnosed abnormal vaginal bleeding during the 3 months prior to use of one of these methods.
- Acute liver disease.
- Jaundice.
- Significant concern about weight gain.
- For Depo-Provera injection; when rapid return to fertility is desired.[10,43–48]
- Hypercholesterolemia (DMPA).
- Current significant depression (DMPA).
- Women with existing or risk for bone density loss.

Management Considerations[10,43–48]

- The insertion and removal of implant systems must be done by a professional specifically trained in the proper techniques.
- Teaching and counseling must include information about how long the system is effective; what to expect regarding changes in bleeding patterns; and the importance of continuing annual gynecologic care (see Management Considerations, Guidelines for Client Information, and Informed Consent). Careful client selection, appropriate client education and supportive follow-up care can greatly enhance client satisfaction with these methods.
- Danger signs that indicate possible serious problems associated with use of the methods must be taught.

- Severe abdominal pain.
- Heavy vaginal bleeding.
- Frequent urination.
- Depression.
- Severe headache.
- Pus or bleeding at the insertion site.
- Excessive weight gain.
- Expulsion of the implant

- For prolonged and/or frequent bleeding (Norplant) obtain the following information: history of bleeding pattern, sexual activity pattern, intercurrent illness, unusual stressful events, medications, substance use/abuse.

  Examine for other causes of bleeding such as infection, genital lesions. Perform gonorrhea and chlamydia tests, saline and KOH preps.

  Treatment options:

1. Ibuprofen 800 mg. t.i.d. for 5 days.
2. Any currently available low dose OC (50 mcg. or less) for one cycle.
3. Levonorgestrel 37.5 mcg. b.i.d. for 20 days (Ovrette). *or*
   Megace 40 mg. daily for 30 days.
4. Ethinyl estradiol 20 or 50 mcg. for 10 days. If bleeding persists, continue for 20 days. *or* Premarin 0.625 mg. daily for 25 days.

For spotting/bleeding with DMPA, provide reassurance that by second or third injection she may be amenorrheic. If frequent or prolonged, work up as for Norplant outlined previously. Try treatment with one cycle of OCs.

- *Amenorrhea (Norplant or DMPA).* Provide reassurance. Obtain pregnancy test if client is worried or if insertion/injection not done at the recommended time (see previous information). No need to induce menses.
- *Norplant insertion and removal.* Remember the Norplant system that is carefully and properly inserted will be easier to remove. Most important is that all six capsules be at a uniform depth and uniform distance from the incision.

  Several techniques for removal have been developed (see Bibliography). When performing removal, allow 30 to 45 minutes for the procedure, make sure you and client are comfortable, have ample light and all equipment ready. Palpate all six capsules and mark their locations with a surgical marker. Perform preferred removal technique. Show client all capsules at completion of the removal. Note: Some communities have arranged that one or more providers become very proficient in Norplant removal and all removals are referred to them.[10,44–46]

POSTCOITAL CONTRACEPTIVE METHODS

Postcoital contraception, also called *emergency contraception* (BC), refers to intervention taken to prevent pregnancy after a single act of unprotected intercourse. Indications for use include sexual assault, condom breakage, dislodgement of a cervical cap, diaphragm or sponge, missed OC, or any unexpected event or emotion that leads to unprotected intercourse and the possibility of pregnancy. The treatment is indicated if the woman has had unprotected intercourse within the last 72 hours and does not wish to become pregnant. Care must be taken, however, that she is not already pregnant.

Emergency contraceptives available in the United States include oral contraceptive pills, progestin-only minipills and the postcoital insertion of a copper-T IUD. Danazol may also be used. Emergency contraception (EC) is underutilized in the United States primarily because women are not aware that it is available or they do not know how to obtain it.

In 1995, The Reproductive Health Technologies Project and Bridging the Gap Communications initiated the Emergency Contraceptive Hotline, a toll-free service that enables women to access information about emergency contraception and to obtain referrals to clinicians who provide emergency contraception. The service may be accessed 24 hours a day in English and Spanish. Access numbers are 1–800–584–9911, 1–888–NOT–2–LATE.[49–52]

Mechanisms of Action

Hormonal methods of EC work by disrupting ovarian hormone production, causing luteal phase dysfunction, asynchrony of endometrial development and disordered tubal transport. The copper IUD insertion alters the endometrium, producing an inflammatory response that makes the endometrium unsuitable for implantation; and interferes with fertilization and transport.[10,49]

Effectiveness

EC pills, including combined OC and minipills, reduce the chance of a pregnancy by 75 percent. This is not to say that 25 percent of women will become pregnant. Rather, if 100 women had unprotected intercourse once during the second or third week of their menstrual cycle, about eight would become pregnant. If those eight women had used EC pills, only two would have become pregnant. Danazol is somewhat less effective than the hormonal EC pills. Emergency insertion of a copper-T IUD is even more effective than pills.[49,53]

Emergency Contraceptive Pills

The combined oral contraceptive pills that have been studied and are now used for emergency contraception contain estrogen (ethinyl estradiol) and progestin (norgestrel or levonorgestrel). In the United States, these include Ovral, Lo/Ovral, Nordette, Levlen, Triphasil, Tri-levlen. The current treatment is one dose of the combined OC given as soon as possible after unprotected intercourse, but not later than 72 hours after, followed in 12 hours by a second dose. This method is referred to as the "Yuzpe" method. This is the most commonly used EC method, and almost all women can safely use it. Medical experts believe that even women who should not use estrogen on a continuous basis can usually use this method for one-time emergency contraception (see Table 9–11). Menses should begin in 2 to 3 weeks; if it does not, a pregnancy test should be performed. Nausea and vomiting are common with these pills. If vomiting occurs within 2 hours of taking a dose, that dose needs to be repeated. Extra pills should be dispensed in case this occurs. Antinausea medication may also be given. Also, teach pill danger signs (see *ACHES* page 175).[10,49–53]

Progestin-Only Pills

Progestin-only pills for EC require high doses. One regimen is to use 0.6 mg. of levonorgestrel within 12 hours of unprotected intercourse. No levonorgestrel-only tablet is available in the United States. Ovrette contains 0.075 mg. of norgestrel, which is equivalent to 0.0375 mg. of levonorgestrel. This would require a woman to take 16 Ovrette tablets. Another regimen is 0.75 mg. of levonorgestrel taken no more than 8 hours after intercourse and repeating the dose 24 hours later. This would require 20 Ovrette tablets for each of the two doses. One of these options might be helpful if a woman must avoid estrogen. Nausea and vomiting are less common (see Table 9–11).[10,49,50]

TABLE 9–11. EMERGENCY POSTCOITAL CONTRACEPTIVE OPTIONS

Method	Instructions
Combined Oral Contraceptives	
Ovral	Take 2 tablets within 72 hours of unprotected intercourse. Take 2 additional tablets 12 hours later.
Lo-Ovral Nordette Levlen Triphasil Tri-Levlen	Take 4 tablets within 72 hours of unprotected intercourse. Take 4 additional tablets 12 hours later. For Triphasil and Tri-Levlen, use yellow tablets only.
Progestin-Only pills	
Ovrette	Take 16 tablets within 12 hours of unprotected intercourse. *or* Take 20 tablets within 8 hours of unprotected intercourse. Take additional 20 tablets 24 hours later.
Danazol (synthetic androgen)	Take 400 mg within 72 hours of unprotected intercourse. Repeat 400 mg dose 12 hours later. Another Danazol regimen calls for a third 400 mg dose, 12 hours after the second dose.
IUD (copper containing such as CU T 380A)	Insert 5 to 7 days after unprotected intercourse. May be left in place for long-term contraception.

For all methods: Review contraindications. Evaluate for pregnancy if no menses by 3 weeks.

Source: References 10, 49, 51, 52.

Danazol

Danazol is a synthetic androgen often used in the treatment of endometriosis. Two regimens have been studied. In the first, Danazol 400 mg. is taken followed by the same dose 12 hours later. In the other regimen studied, a third dose is added, 12 hours after the second. Studies of efficacy have been inconsistent, but this method seems to be less effective than the Yuzpe method. Nausea and vomiting are less common.[10,49]

Postcoital IUD Insertion

Copper-containing IUDs can be inserted up to 7 days after unprotected intercourse to prevent implantation of a fertilized egg. This method prevents pregnancy 99 percent of the time when used postcoitally.[10] The same precautions and contraindications apply when an IUD is inserted for this purpose as when used for routine contraception (see Intrauterine Devices, later in this chapter). In addition, the copper-T IUD may be left in place to provide continuous effective contraception for up to 10 years.

Other Methods of EC

High dose oral estrogens in the forms of ethinyl estradiol (EE), diethylstilbestrol (DES), conjugated estrogen, or estrone have been used in the past for EC. These regimens were effective, but the incidence of side effects was high. Their use is no longer recommended.

The antiprogesterone drug, mifepristone (RU-486), is used in countries other than the United States as an emergency contraceptive. European studies have shown it to be highly effective when used within 3 days of unprotected intercourse. Mifepristone produces less nausea and vomiting than some other EC methods.[10,49-53]

THE MALE CONDOM

The male condom, also referred to as a rubber, prophylactic or skin, is a sheath that is worn over the erect penis to contain fluid from ejaculation. Most U.S. condoms are made from latex rubber. About 1 percent of condoms used in the United States are made of processed collagenous tissue from the intestinal caecum of lambs. Condoms are available in many colors, textures, sizes, shapes, and thicknesses. Clients must be sure to purchase condoms that are labeled for use as contraceptives/prophylactics and that bear a disease prevention claim. Novelty condoms do not prevent pregnancy or disease transmission. In 1994, the FDA approved Schmid Laboratories' Avanti brand polyurethane ("plastic") condom, even though limited testing had been performed. The public health need for a latex-free condom that would prevent pregnancy and disease prompted the FDA to approve the product. Clinical trials to evaluate efficacy are ongoing. Another nonlatex condom has been developed and is undergoing testing. It is not generally available as yet, but may be released soon. This is a latex-free natural rubber, nonallergenic product called the Tactylon condom. Tactylon is a synthetic thermoplastic elastomer, the same material used in the FDA approved nonallergenic examination gloves.[10,54–56]

Mechanism of Action

A *condom* is a mechanical barrier to prevent sperm from entering the vagina and cervix. Condoms prevent direct contact with semen, penile lesions, discharges, and infected secretions. Latex condoms prevent transmission of most sexually transmitted infections, including HIV. Spermicidal condoms have the additional action of nonoxynol-9 to immobilize and kill sperm after ejaculation and thus reduce the likelihood of transmitting STDs (see Spermicides, later in this chapter). Without condoms, infecting organisms can be physically transmitted into the uterus and tubes by sperm.

Effectiveness

Condoms are considered *moderately* effective at preventing accidental pregnancy (see Table 9–4). Failure to prevent pregnancy is most frequently attributed to inconsistent use. Condom breakage can occur, but this probably is not a major cause of accidental pregnancy. Effectiveness increases significantly, approaching the effectiveness of oral contraceptives or an IUD, when used concurrently with a vaginal spermicide.[10,16,54] Effective-

ness of the polyurethane and Tactylon condoms has not been determined.

Advantages[6,10,54]

- Available without a prescription or examination.
- Relatively inexpensive.
- Widely available.
- Physiologically safe.
- No adverse effect on fertility.
- Easily reversible contraception.
- Few side effects.
- Significant protection against most STDs and their consequences, including HIV disease.
- Possible protection against cancer of the cervix.
- Male participation in contraception is encouraged.
- Only reversible contraceptive available for use by men.
- May delay premature ejaculation in men for whom this is a concern.
- May be used during lactation.
- Lubricated condoms may reduce friction, preventing irritation to either partner.
- Postcoital drainage of semen from the vagina, which some women find objectionable, is eliminated.
- Allergic reactions are prevented for women who are sensitive to partner's semen.
- Polyurethane ("plastic") condom is stronger than latex and thinner. It may improve sensation and pleasure.
- Polyurethane condom can be safely used with oil based lubricants.

Disadvantages

- Fairly expensive for frequent use.
- Possible decreased sensation for man.
- Interferes with sexual spontaneity (requires forethought and preparedness).
- Necessity to interrupt foreplay to put condom on.
- "Skin" condoms made from animal membranes may not protect against some STDs, including HIV.
- Some women and men experience irritation with the use of particular lubricants or spermicides on condoms.
- Male partner may be unwilling to cooperate with condom use.

Contraindications

- Allergy of the man or woman to the latex in condoms. The incidence of latex allergy in our society is increasing, especially among individuals such as health care workers who have high environmental exposure to latex in the workplace. Individuals with latex allergies may use the nonallergenic, nonlatex condoms described earlier; or they may use a natural skin type condom over the latex condom (or under it, depending which partner has the allergy).[54,57]

Management Considerations[10,54–57]

The following instructions will be helpful to couples using condoms.

- Store condoms in a cool, dry place. Heat, even body heat, may weaken the rubber. Always keep the condom in its original package until use. Condoms should keep 5 years when properly stored. Consider using name brands; these may be of more reliable quality. Spermicidal condoms should be used.
- The condom is placed on the erect penis (either partner can do this) *before* the penis comes in contact with the woman's genital area.
- Roll the condom all the way down to the base of the penis.
- If the condom does not have a built-in reservoir, leave one-half inch of empty space at the end of it to collect ejaculate. This is accomplished by pinching the tip of the condom as it is rolled on. Leave no air in the tip; this could contribute to tearing.
- Be sure that the vagina and/or condom are well lubricated to prevent condom tearing. If additional lubrication is needed, use only water, saliva, water based jelly, or contraceptive foam, gel, or cream on latex condoms. Other products, especially petroleum based, will cause rapid deterioration and weakening of latex. Other vaginal products that cause latex condom weakening include miconazole nitrate (monistat), butoconazole nitrate (Femstat), estradiol (Estrace), and conjugated estrogen (Premarin) creams, Vagisil ointment, Rendell's Cone and Ovule Spermicide, and the sexual lubricant

called Elbow Grease. These lubricants do not affect the new polyurethane and Tactylon condoms.
- For added protection, use a second method of birth control (diaphragm, spermicidal foam, gel, film, suppository, or birth control pill).
- After intercourse, remove the condom immediately while the penis is still erect, holding on to the base of the condom to prevent spilling.
- Check the condom for tears, then throw it away. Use each condom only once. If tears are detected, immediately insert spermicidal gel or cream into the vagina.

FEMALE CONDOMS

The Reality female condom was approved by the FDA in 1993 for over-the-counter sale in the United States. The Reality Female Condom consists of a polyurethane sheath with an outer ring and inner ring (see Figure 9–2). Each condom is prelubricated with silicone, and a container of water based lubricant is supplied for those who prefer more lubrication. It is inserted vaginally, like a diaphragm and held in place by the pubic bone. The closed upper tip is anchored near the cervix by a flexible inner ring that holds the device in place, preventing expulsion. The condom covers the surfaces of the vaginal wall, allowing the penis to move freely inside the condom. An external ring at the outer opening of the pouch remains outside the vagina and partially covers the labia. It is used for one act of intercourse only; however, studies are underway to determine whether it may be used more than once. This would help to reduce cost. If used correctly with every sex act, the female condom also helps to prevent the spread of STD. This product is distributed by Wisconsin Pharmacal.[58–61]

Mechanism of Action

This device serves as a mechanical barrier to prevent sperm from entering the vagina or cervix. The polyurethane female condom also has the ability to prevent transmission of most STDs, including HIV.

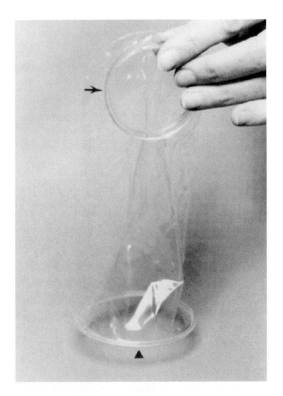

Figure 9–2. Female condom that shows the outer (arrowhead) and inner (arrow) rings. *(Reproduced, with permission, from Lemcke DP, Pattison J, Marshall LA, Cowley DS: Primary Care of Women. Appleton & Lange, 1995.)*

Effectiveness

The typical failure rate in U.S. studies was similar to that for diaphragm, sponge, and cervical cap during typical use. The female condom is impermeable to various STD organisms and HIV.[60,61] (See Table 9–4.)

Advantages[10,58–61]

- Use controlled by the woman.
- Available without a prescription or examination.
- Easily reversible.
- Considered medically safe.
- Little danger of systemic effects.
- May provide protection against STDs, cervical neoplasia.
- May be worn prior to intercourse.
- Not dependent on male arousal.

- May be used during lactation.
- May be removed immediately after intercourse.
- Provides improved sensation for man and woman and allows transfer of body heat.
- Eliminates postcoital drainage of semen.
- Prevents allergic reactions for women sensitive to partner's semen.

Disadvantages[10,58–61]

- Expensive for frequent use (about three times the price of the male condom).
- For single use only.
- Cumbersome; insertion of Reality can be difficult.
- Can slip or be pushed out of place.
- May make noise during use.
- Unsightly: Reality ring dangles outside the vagina.
- Breakage, tearing can occur (though rarely).

Contraindications

- Allergy of man or woman to polyurethane.
- Anatomic abnormalities that interfere with proper placement.
- Inability to master insertion technique.

Management Considerations[10,58–61]

The following instructions will be helpful to the client:

- Practice wearing and inserting the female condom before depending on it for protection.
- Be careful not to tear the condom with sharp objects such as rings or long fingernails.
- Extra spermicidal lubricant may be used if desired.
- Refer to the package inserts for detailed use and insertion instructions.
- After intercourse, remove the female condom carefully to avoid spilling semen.

SPERMICIDES

Spermicides are chemical substances that immobilize and kill sperm. Available in creams, foams, jellies, suppositories, and film, these products are inserted into the vagina prior to intercourse. When used alone, they are inserted vaginally near the cervix, forming a chemical barrier. Spermicides are also essential components of vaginal barrier methods of contraception (diaphragm, cervical cap, and sponge). Surfaces of male condoms may be coated with spermicide to enhance the effectiveness of this method as a contraceptive and as some protection against STDs.

When used alone, all spermicidal products provide protection for up to one hour and for one episode of intercourse only. Additional acts of intercourse, or intercourse occurring more than one hour after insertion, require repeated application of the product.[6,10,55]

Spermicide use reduces transmission of gonorrhea and chlamydia. Protection against HIV is undetermined. Developmental research is underway to discover new chemicals that have microbicidal properties with and/or without spermicidal activity. Chemical methods under study include a buffer gel that maintains a low vaginal pH and does not disturb the normal vaginal flora; sulfated polysaccharides designed to prevent adherence of HIV and chlamydia to cells in a woman's reproductive tract; N-docosanol, an antiviral product that works by inhibiting lipid-enveloped viruses; C31G, an amphoteric surfactant that disrupts cellular membranes but causes less irritation than nonoxynol-9; and squalamine, a steroid based compound that affects cell growth. Substances such as these would provide women with STD protection that would not necessarily require the cooperation of male partners.[62,63]

Foams, Jellies, Creams

These can be used alone or with a condom, diaphragm, or cervical cap. Foams are available in multidose aerosol containers or in small, single use, prefilled cartridges. Creams and jellies come in multidose tubes with reusable applicators. Some jellies are sold in single use packets.

Suppositories

Referred to as *spermicidal vaginal tablets,* the suppositories are a small ovoid shape. They can be used alone or with a condom but must be inserted 10 to 15 minutes before intercourse in order to melt and disperse the spermicide.

Vaginal Contraceptive Film (VCF)

VCF, which can be used alone or with a condom or diaphragm, is a paper-thin sheet of film containing nonoxynol-9, measuring 2×2 in. The sheet is inserted on or near the cervix (or inside a diaphragm) at least 5 minutes prior to intercourse in order to melt and disperse the spermicide.

New types of vaginal spermicide film are under development. One version, which incorporates benzalkonium chloride instead of nonoxynol-9 as the active agent, has undergone early clinical trials for safety. Other types, which are made of different materials than the film currently available, are being designed to dissolve more rapidly in the body but maintain their stability in tropical climates.

Advantage 24

Advantage 24 is a new nonoxynol-9 gel, which contains an agent that adheres to the vaginal surface, maintaining the spermicide's activity for up to 24 hours. The gel, which is used for one act of intercourse, will be marketed in the United States in 1997.[62,63]

Mechanism of Action

Spermicides contain a chemical that immobilizes and kills sperm (by destroying sperm cell membrane) and vehicle ingredients to keep the spermicide in place around the cervix. The active ingredient in most spermicidal products sold in the United States is nonoxynol-9. Octoxynol is the active agent in other products and is equally effective as a spermicide. In vitro studies of nonoxynol-9 show that it is lethal to organisms that cause trichomonas, gonorrhea, genital herpes, syphilis, and HIV/AIDS. Clinical studies have shown significant protection against gonorrhea and chlamydia for women who used nonoxynol-9 products alone or with a diaphragm when compared with women who used oral contraceptives or who were surgically sterilized. Studies in humans to determine if use of nonoxynol-9 decreases risk of HIV transmission have shown conflicting results.

When applying any of these findings, it is important to remember two points.

- The in vitro effect cannot be interpreted to mean absolute protection against transmission of these infections in humans.
- Gonorrhea, chlamydia, and HIV are intracellular organisms. An organism's location inside a cell could shield it from exposure to spermicide.

The presence of spermicide or even a physical barrier contraceptive does not preclude an organism's access to the body via open lesions or through areas beyond which barrier or spermicide is present, such as intracervical or endometrial areas.[10,62,63]

Effectiveness

Spermicides are moderately effective at preventing accidental pregnancy (see Table 9–4). Failures are most frequently attributed to inconsistent use. Proper use, including placement of the product deep inside the vagina against the cervix, is essential. Efficacy is much greater if used with a condom. Data are not available comparing the efficacies of various spermicidal products.[10,16]

Advantages[10,62,63]

- Widely available without a prescription or examination.
- Relatively inexpensive.
- Medically safe.
- Readily available as a backup method in a variety of circumstances:
  - In the event of condom rupture.
  - To augment other methods during midcycle, when the woman is most fertile.
  - When a woman begins using oral contraceptives.
  - When a woman taking oral contraceptives misses one or more pills.
- Can reduce STD transmission.
- Completely reversible.
- No effect on the return to fertility.
- Women can decide independently to use it.
- Can provide lubrication during intercourse.
- Can be used during lactation.
- Convenient, useful method of contraception after delivery and before the first postpartum visit, and when changing from one method to another.

Disadvantages[10,62,63]

- May interfere with sexual spontaneity (requires forethought and preparedness).
- Must be on hand at or near the time of intercourse.
- Suppositories and film require time to disperse before intercourse can take place.
- Perceived as messy by some individuals (drainage of the substance from the vagina occurs after intercourse).
- Incomplete dissolution of suppositories can cause an uncomfortable, gritty sensation for either partner, and may impair contraceptive effectiveness.
- Some users experience a warm sensation; some feel that the suppository "burns."
- For couples engaging in oral–genital sex, the taste of spermicides is unpleasant. Spermicide may be inserted after this activity, but before penis–vagina contact takes place.
- Skin irritation of the vulva or penis can result from frequent use of spermicides or from allergy or sensitivity to the spermicide or base ingredients. Another product may be tried.
- A few studies in the early 1980s reported possible adverse effects on the fetus if spermicide was used near or at the time of conception. Subsequent, more carefully designed and controlled studies failed to show adverse effects on the fetus.

Contraindications

- Allergy of either partner to spermicide or its other ingredients.
- Inability to "remember" to use the product associated with intercourse.
- Inability to learn the proper insertion technique.
- Anatomic abnormalities of the vagina that might interfere with the correct placement or retention of the spermicide.

Management Considerations[6,10,63]

The following instructions will be helpful to partners using a spermicide.

- The spermicide must be used every time intercourse occurs; must be in place prior to penis–vagina contact.

- Store spermicides in a cool, clean, and dry place.
- Wait the specified time after insertion so that the spermicide is adequately dispersed (for film and suppositories).
- One application is good for one hour after insertion and for one act of intercourse only. Additional application is needed if one hour has passed since insertion or before each additional act of intercourse.
- All spermicides must be left in place for at least 6 hours after the last act of intercourse. Do not douche or rinse the product out for at least six hours.
- Instructions for specific products include the following.
  - *Foam.* Shake vigorously at least 20 times before dispensing. Insert as for jelly or cream, below.
  - *Jelly or Cream.* Fill applicator by squeezing the tube from the bottom. Insert the applicator as far into the vagina as it will go comfortably. Holding the applicator in place, push the plunger to release the product.
  - *Suppository (Vaginal Tablet).* Remove the wrapper and insert as far as possible so that the tablet rests on or near cervix. Wait the specified time before intercourse.
  - *Film.* Fingers must be completely dry. Place one sheet of film on a fingertip and slide it along the back wall of the vagina as far as possible, so that the film rests on or near cervix. Wait at least 5 minutes before intercourse to allow dispersion.
- If burning or irritation occurs, stop use of the product. Changing brands or the form of spermicide may diminish reactions. If a reaction persists, discontinue use.

VAGINAL BARRIER METHODS: DIAPHRAGMS, CERVICAL CAPS, SPONGE

Diaphragm

A *diaphragm* is a dome-shaped cup made of latex rubber with a flexible-spring metal rim. It is inserted vaginally prior to intercourse, so that the posterior rim rests in the posterior fornix and the anterior rim fits snugly behind the pubic bone. Spermicidal cream, jelly, or film is applied inside the dome of the diaphragm and around the rim before insertion. Diaphragms are available in a range of sizes and four general styles. Specified sizes refer to millimeters in diameter across the rim, for example, 65 mm, 70 mm, 75 mm.

- *Coil Spring Rim.* This type has a sturdy rim with firm spring strength, which most women with average vaginal musculature and average pubic arch depth can use comfortably. The diaphragm folds flat for insertion and can be used with a plastic introducer. Specific products include Koromex diaphragm (latex), sizes 50–95; Ortho coil spring diaphragm (latex), sizes 50–95; Ramses flexible cushioned diaphragm (gum rubber), sizes 50–95.
- *Flat Spring Rim.* Having a thin, delicate rim with gentle spring strength, this type of diaphragm can be worn comfortably by nulliparous women with firm vaginal musculature or by women with a shallow notch behind the pubic bone. It folds flat for insertion and can be used with introducer. One example of this product is the Ortho-White diaphragm (latex), sizes 55–95.
- *Arcing Spring Rim.* The sturdy rim of this type of diaphragm imparts firm spring strength. Furthermore, the arcing rim facilitates insertion. Most women can use it comfortably, and it can be retained in the presence of cystocele and/or rectocele or relaxed vaginal muscle tone. Specific products include the Koroflex diaphragm (latex), sizes 60–95; Ortho All-Flex diaphragm (latex), sizes 55–95; Ramses Bendex diaphragm (gum rubber), sizes 65–95.
- *Wide-Seal Rim.* This type has a thin, flexible flange approximately 1.5 cm wide attached to the inner edge of the rim to keep spermicide in place inside the dome and to enhance the seal between the rim and the vaginal wall. It is made in two styles, arching and coil spring. Specific products include the Milex Wide-Seal arcing diaphragm (latex), sizes 60–95; Milex Wide-Seal Omniflex coil spring diaphragm (latex), sizes 60–95. Milex diaphragms are not available from pharmacies by prescription, but are only distributed to doctors and clinics by the manufacturer.[6,10,64]

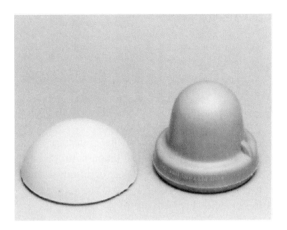

A

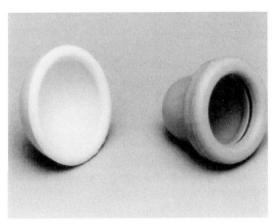

B

Figure 9–3. Prentif and Dumas cervical caps: (A) vaginal side; (B) cervical side. *(Reproduced, with permission, from Lemcke DP, Pattison J, Marshall LA, Cowley DS: Primary Care of Women. Appleton & Lange, 1995.)*

Vaginal Contraceptive Sponge

Manufacture of the *Today* vaginal contraceptive sponge has been discontinued. No other contraceptive sponges are available in the United States. Two other sponges are marketed in Canada and France.

Cervical Cap

The cervical cap is a soft, rubber, cup-shaped device, resembling a small diaphragm with a deep dome (much like a thimble). It fits over the cervix and is held in place by a seal that forms between its flexible rim and the outer surface of cervix. A small amount of spermicide is placed inside the cap, but not on the rim, which would interfere with the seal that needs to be formed.

The Prentif Cavity Rim Cervical Cap, the only cap currently approved by the FDA for general use in the United States, was first approved for general distribution in 1988 after several years of investigative testing. The Prentif cap is a soft, deep rubber cap with a firm, rounded rim (see Figure 9–3). A groove along the rim's inner circumference enhances the seal that forms between the inner rim and the surface of the cervix. Available in sizes 22–31 mm (inner rim diameter), it is manufactured in England and distributed in the United States by Cervical Cap Ltd., Los Gatos, California.

Other specific products (not generally available in the United States at this time) are the Dumas Cap and the Vimule Cap (see Figure 9–3).[6,10,65–68]

Mechanisms of Action

- The contraceptive effect of the diaphragm is related to the barrier effect, which prevents sperm entry into the cervix, and to the sperm-killing action of spermicide used with all diaphragms.
- Similar in action to the diaphragm, the cervical cap serves as a barrier to the cervix and holds spermicide within its dome.

Effectiveness

Contraceptive efficacy among these methods is comparable (see Table 9–4). Some cervical cap failures are attributed to cap dislodgement during intercourse and to deterioration of rubber after prolonged use.

Vaginal barrier methods depend largely on extremely conscientious use, although individual fertility characteristics are probably equally important. These methods must be used correctly and consistently. They are used with more success by women 30 years of age or older, who have intercourse fewer than four times weekly, and who may have slightly lower fertility than their younger counterparts. Many women who experience accidental pregnancy with these methods report misuse (including inconsistent use). Users must be highly motivated to prevent or delay pregnancy. The role of the clinician can be very significant in assisting women to use these products successfully.[10,16,64,66]

Advantages[10,64–68]

- Attractive method for women needing contraception on an irregular basis and whose sexual patterns are fairly predictable.
- Does not require partner involvement.
- Considered medically safe.
- Little danger of systemic effects.
- Easily reversible.
- Provides significant protection against STDs and PID.
- Can be used during lactation.
- Diaphragm may provide some protection against cervical neoplasia.

Disadvantages[10,64–68]

- Both the diaphragm and the cervical cap require accurate fitting by a professional clinician, often accompanied by lengthy office visit.
- Properly trained clinicians not widely available, especially for fitting the cervical cap.
- Costs related to use may be high (i.e., professional care, purchase of products).
- May interfere with sexual spontaneity if not readily available.
- Learning insertion and removal techniques may be difficult.
- Perceived as aesthetically objectionable or messy by some individuals.
- Latex, rubber, polyurethane, or spermicide could cause irritation or allergy in either partner.
- Foul odor or vaginal discharge may occur if the product is left in place more than a few days.
- Potential for vaginal trauma associated with difficult insertion or removal of the device.
- Increased risk of urinary tract infection (UTI) in diaphragm users (especially arcing spring).
- Potential for toxic shock syndrome (TSS).
- A few studies have reported Pap smear abnormalities with use of the cervical cap.

Contraindications

- Allergy to latex, rubber, polyurethane, or spermicide.
- Vaginal bleeding, even menses (because of possible risk of TSS).
- Delivery in prior 6 weeks or abortion in prior 2 weeks (for cap or sponge).
- Anatomic abnormalities that interfere with proper fitting of the cap or diaphragm.
- Inability to master insertion or removal techniques.
- Recurrent UTIs with use of the diaphragm.
- History of TSS.
- History of cervical malignancy or abnormal Pap that has not been evaluated (for cap).

Management Considerations

Fitting the Diaphragm. During the pelvic exam, check for a palpable pubic notch behind the symphysis pubis, as well as anatomic abnormalities. Estimate the diagonal length of the vaginal canal from the posterior vaginal fornix to the symphysis pubis, by inserting the middle and index fingers until the middle finger touches the posterior wall of the vagina. Use thumb of the same hand to mark the point that touches the symphysis pubis and withdraw fingers. Select a diaphragm with a diameter that equals the measurement from the tip of the middle finger to the point just in front of the thumb where symphysis pubis contact was made. Select the largest rim size that is comfortable for client. Insert the diaphragm and check its fit. The diaphragm should fit snugly between the posterior fornix and the symphysis pubis, touching lateral vaginal walls and covering the cervix. Check for displacement when the client bears down. Have her walk around the room, sit, and squat. Check again for displacement and client comfort. If the client feels the diaphragm while walking around, it may be too large. If it is easily displaced with a finger or with moving/walking, it can be displaced during intercourse. If in doubt about fit, try the next larger size. Two or three different sizes should be tried before a final decision is made. Instruct the client to practice removal and insertion three times, while you verify proper placement each time.[6,10,64]

Fitting the Cervical Cap. The client must be involved in the fitting process. During speculum examination, assist her to visualize her cervix. *Specific teaching sessions for health care professionals who will be fitting caps are strongly recommended.* Comprehensive training programs for prospective cap providers are available. Information on these programs may be obtained from the National Women's Health Network in Washington, DC.

During the pelvic exam, visualize the cervix to estimate cap size. The bimanual exam will determine the position and size of the cervix. The cervix must be fairly symmetrical, without excessive scarring or laceration that could interfere with complete contact between the cap rim and the cervix around its full circumference. The cervix also must be long enough to accommodate the depth of the cap. A cervix that is too flat cannot be fitted with the Prentif cap. Try two or more caps sizes to determine the best fit.

To insert the cap, pinch the sides of the cap together, compress the cap dome, insert into the vagina, and place over the cervix. As the dome is released, suction should form between the rim of the cap and the cervix. After inserting the cap, use one finger to feel around the entire circumference of the cap to be sure there are no gaps between the cap rim and the cervix. Probe the cap and cervix from various angles with a finger tip to be sure the cap is not easily dislodged. The cervix must be completely covered.

After a minute or two, check for evidence of suction by pinching the dome and tugging gently. The dome should feel collapsed (or dimpled) and the cap should resist the tug and not slide off easily. Finally, try to rotate the cap at the rim. If the cap rotates too easily or falls off, it is too large. If it does not rotate at all, it is too small and could cause trauma to the cervix. To remove the cap, press the index finger against the rim and tip the cap slightly to break the suction. Gently pull out the device. Instruct the client in proper insertion and removal techniques and have her practice three times during the visit, while you verify proper placement each time.[10,65–68]

Client Teaching and Counseling

A critical aspect of successful use of either the diaphragm or the cervical cap is that sufficient time be offered to the client for teaching and practice at the office visit. The following points should be part of client teaching.[6,10,64–68]

- Devices may be inserted immediately prior to intercourse; however, some experts recommend waiting 30 minutes after cervical cap insertion to be sure that the seal has formed between the rim and the cervix.
- Devices must be left in place for a minimum of 6 hours after the last act of intercourse.
- Diaphragm may not be reliable if coitus is to take place in water because spermicide could wash away.
- Do not use during menses (potential for TSS). Have an alternative method, such as condoms, available.
- The danger signs of TSS include sudden high fever, vomiting, diarrhea, dizziness, faintness, weakness, sore throat, aching muscles or joints, rash.
- The diaphragm or cap should be inspected prior to insertion for cracks, holes, tears, or drying of rubber or latex.
- After using a cap or diaphragm, wash the device with soap and water, dry thoroughly, and store in its container.
- Bring the cap or diaphragm to yearly gynecologic visit so that fit can be reevaluated.

Specific Instructions for Diaphragm Use

- Place approximately one tablespoon of spermicidal cream or jelly in the dome and around the rim of the diaphragm.
- Insert the diaphragm up to 6 hours prior to intercourse.
- The diaphragm must remain in place for 6 to 8 hours following each coitus. If coitus does not take place within 6 hours of insertion, remove the diaphragm and reapply spermicide. For subsequent acts of coitus, spermicide is added with an inserter, without removing diaphragm.

Specific Instructions for Cervical Cap Use

- To use a cervical cap, the woman should be at least 6 weeks postpartum or 2 weeks postabortion.
- Fill the dome of the cap to one-third with spermicidal cream or jelly. Do *not* apply spermicide

to the rim; this might interfere with the seal that must form around the cervix.

- Cap may be left in place up to 48 hours without regard to frequency of intercourse during that period. It is not necessary to insert additional spermicide.
- After inserting, check that the seal has formed around the cervix.

INTRAUTERINE DEVICES (IUDS)

Intrauterine devices (IUDs) are small objects, usually plastic, that are placed inside the uterus. They may contain substances such as copper or progesterone that enhance effectiveness. One or more strings are attached that protrude into the vagina so that the presence of the device can be checked by the user and removal facilitated. IUDs are packaged in individual sterile units that include the device, insertion barrel, and manufacturer literature.

Currently in the United States, two IUDs are available, the copper ParaGard-T-380A marketed by GynoPharma, and Progestasert, a progesterone-T device, available through Alza Corporation (see Figure 9–4). By 1986, most U.S. companies had voluntarily withdrawn IUDs from the American market, not for medical or scientific reasons, but, primarily because of decreased popularity, negative consumer perception, increasing litigation costs, and subsequent difficulty obtaining liability insurance.

The Dalkon Shield, associated with a high rate of pelvic infections and septic abortions, was removed from the U.S. market in 1975. The Lippes Loop was a popular IUD used in the

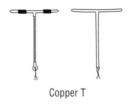

Copper T

Figure 9–4. Currently available IUDs: ParaGuard-T-380A (left) and Progestasert (right). *(Reproduced, with permission, from DeCherney AH and Pernoll ML: Current Obstetric & Gynecologic Diagnosis & Treatment, 8th Ed. Appleton & Lange, 1994.)*

1970s and early 1980s. The Lippes Loop was designed to be used indefinitely; consequently, some women still have these in place as they approach menopause.

Fears of side effects or complications continue to hamper widespread acceptance of IUDs among potential users, physicians, and other family planning providers. The modern IUDs, however, are safe, highly effective, and convenient for carefully screened potential users, and should be offered to appropriate clients, especially when hormonal contraceptive methods are contraindicated or not desired. In many countries of the world, IUDs are the most popular reversible method of birth control.[6,10]

Paragard-T-380A

Introduced in the United States in 1988, this is a T-shaped polyurethane device with barium sulphate added (for x-ray visibility). A very fine copper wire is wound around a vertical stem and crossbar. A white polyethylene string attached through a hole in the "T," creates a double string effect that, after insertion, protrudes into the vagina. ParaGard-T-380A is approved for 10 years of use.[10,69]

The Progesterone-T (Progestasert)

A T-shaped ethylene vinyl acetate copolymer; the vertical stem contains a reservoir holding 38 mg progesterone and barium sulphate in a silicone oil base. This IUD releases 65 μg progesterone per day. It may stay in place one year, then must be removed and/or replaced. Black double string is attached to the hole in the base of the "t," which after insertion, protrudes into the vagina.[10,70]

Mechanism of Action[6,10,71,72]

Precise mechanisms of IUD action are not fully understood. Theories are that IUDs affect fertilization, implantation, and the endometrium.

Fertilization. The IUD produces a foreign body reaction that is toxic to sperm or ova before fertilization occurs (fertilization is found to be rare in IUD users). It inhibits fertilization by increasing the speed of ovum transport through the fallopian tube, by immobilizing sperm, and by interfering with the migration of sperm from the vagina through the tubes.

Implantation. Interference with implantation is *not* the primary antifertility effect. Local foreign body inflammatory response and increased local production of prostaglandins prevent implantation and cause lysis and/or dislodgment of the blastocyte from the endometrium. The progestin-releasing IUD also interferes with the secretory (proliferative) maturation process of the endometrium.

Endometrium. Copper containing IUDs may also inhibit carbonic anhydrase and alkaline phosphatase activity, and interfere with estrogen uptake by uterine mucosa. Hormone releasing IUDs also produce an atrophic endometrium with long term use.

Effectiveness

IUDs are highly effective in preventing pregnancy, even more effective than OCs. Effectiveness is impacted by IUD characteristics, such as size, shape, expulsion rates, presence or copper or progesterone; and by user characteristics, such as age and parity. Also influential are medical variables, such as experience of the clinician inserting the device, the ease of insertion, placement of the device at the top of the fundus of the uterus, and likelihood that expulsion will be detected (see Table 9–4).[6,16,73]

Advantages[6,10,73,74]

- Once inserted, an IUD requires no continuing action, equipment, or motivation on the part of the user. Is immediately effective.
- Highly effective.
- Continuously effective.
- Very safe for carefully selected users.
- Allows for sexual spontaneity.
- Consider for women who have difficulty following directions or remembering to use a contraceptive or to take a pill every day.
- No messy substances needed.
- After initial cost little additional expense.

- Return to fertility not impaired.
- Progesterone-releasing IUD may decrease menstrual blood flow and dysmenorrhea.
- Can be used during lactation.

Disadvantages

Use of an IUD carries potential for some side effects and several serious complications; however, careful screening and counseling of potential users can prevent many of them. *If a contraindication to use arises, or when in doubt about the significance of a symptom or complaint, the recommended action is to remove the IUD immediately.* Always provide the client an alternate method of contraception. IUDs are best suited for parous women not desiring future pregnancy.

GynoPharma, the manufacturer of ParaGard-T-380A, distributes directly to physicians and clinics, provides detailed guidelines about who should use the product, and recommends it only for women who have had at least one child and are in a stable, monogamous relationship.[10,69,70]

- Insertion requires a skilled professional.
- May aggravate or initiate menstrual cramping.
- May increase bleeding patterns.
- User may experience pain or nausea during insertion.
- User may regularly check for presence of the IUD string.
- May increase the risk of pelvic infection, which could affect future fertility.
- Provides no protection against HIV or STDs.
- Device can be expelled without the user being aware.
- String may be felt by the partner.
- Progestasert lasts only one year; ParaGard-Cu T-380A for 10 years.
- User may neglect to see a health care professional for several years.

Contraindications[6,10,70–76]

Carefully screen potential IUD users for contraindications. Include general and focused histories, a physical examination, appropriate current lab work (CBC, Pap smear, STD testing) and other assessments as indicated.

Absolute Contraindications
(IUD Not Recommended)

- Current pelvic inflammatory disease (PID) or PID in past 3 months.
- Known or suspected pregnancy.

Strong Relative Contraindications
(Strongly Encourage Choice of Another
Contraceptive Method)

- History of ectopic pregnancy, especially if future pregnancy is desired.
- Undiagnosed, abnormal vaginal bleeding.
- Risk factors for PID: multiple sexual partners; past history of STD, especially gonorrhea or chlamydia; postpartum endometritis; infection following abortion in past 3 months; purulent cervicitis.
- Unresolved, abnormal Pap smear.
- Difficult access to medical care.
- Impaired ability (physical or mental) to check for IUD string.
- Known or suspected bleeding disorder.
- Valvular heart disease.
- Anatomic variations that make insertion or retention difficult (e.g., DES exposure, fibroids).
- Severe dysmenorrhea, heavy menses, endometriosis.
- Anemia.
- History of fainting or vasovagal response.
- Allergy to copper.
- History of impaired fertility (in a client desiring future pregnancy).

Managing Problems
and Complications[6,10,73–76]

- Spotting or bleeding may occur at the time of insertion or anytime after. Evaluate for anemia (though less likely with Progestasert), infection, pregnancy, other pathology. Treat according to findings. Remove IUD for severe anemia (Hgb < 9 gm), uterine infection.
- Cramping or pain also may occur at the time of insertion or at any time after. Giving a dose of a NSAID (assuming no allergy) prior to insertion is helpful. If these problems are severe, persistent or intolerable, remove the IUD. Partial expulsion of the IUD, uterine perforation, cervical or pelvic infection, and pregnancy (intrauterine or ectopic) must be ruled out.

- The IUD may be expulsed or partially expulsed. Most often, expulsion occurs during the first few weeks to months after insertion. Correct placement of the device high in the uterine fundus reduces the risk of expulsion. For partial expulsion, remove the IUD. In either case evaluate for uterine perforation, pregnancy, or infection. If no further problems are identified, another IUD may be inserted. A 5 to 7 day course of Doxycycline 100 mg. B.I.D. is recommended.
- The IUD can become embedded. If it cannot be removed after reasonable attempts, refer the client to a gynecologist.
- The IUD string may become lost. Attempt to determine whether the device has been partially or completely expulsed. Again, evaluate for uterine perforation, infection, pregnancy. If the IUD is determined to still be in place (this can be done with ultrasound), the strings are often in the cervical canal. Insertion of a Pap smear cytobrush into the endocervical canal and rotating it while withdrawing the brush will often extract the strings.
- Uterine perforation can occur. Perforation is most common during insertion, but can occur at any time. Suspect perforation if pain is present; if the string is no longer palpable; if the plastic of the device is felt or visible in the cervix. Ultrasound can help to confirm perforation. If perforation is suspected, refer the client to a gynecologist.
- Pregnancy, ectopic pregnancy (low incidence). There is an increased risk of septic abortion if pregnancy occurs. With delayed menses or suspected pregnancy, evaluate for pregnancy and infection. Ectopic pregnancy rates are higher among users of Progestasert than among users of copper IUD. Of users who become pregnant with IUD in place,

    - One-half will experience spontaneous abortion.
    - Twenty-five percent will abort if the IUD is removed early in pregnancy.
    - If the IUD is left in place, severe pelvic infection resulting in death could occur.
    - Five percent will have an ectopic pregnancy.

Inform the client of the above; assist her to determine whether to continue the pregnancy.

- Potential for increased risk of PID. Most reported cases of PID occur during the first 3 months after IUD insertion. This is believed to be due to introduction of bacteria into the uterus during the insertion procedure. Beyond 3 months postinsertion, when client selection procedures include diligent screening for women with risk factors for STDs and PID, the incidence of IUD related pelvic infection is low. *Appropriate* IUD users are at no greater risk of developing PID than non-users. PID is a serious complication that can be life threatening. Infection must be promptly and aggressively treated and the IUD removed. Providers and users of IUDs must be alert to the signs and symptoms suggestive of pelvic infection:

  - Fever of 101° F or higher.
  - Purulent discharge from the vagina/cervix.
  - Abdominal/pelvic pain.
  - Dyspareunia.
  - Cervicitis.
  - Suprapubic tenderness or guarding.
  - Pain with movement of the cervix on examination.
  - Tenderness on bimanual examination.
  - Adnexal tenderness or mass.

Management Considerations[10,73-76]

- Women planning to use an IUD must be carefully screened for contraindications. The ideal candidate for an IUD is a woman in a mutually monogamous relationship who has had at least one full term pregnancy. Give each IUD user an identification card with the name and a picture of the IUD, the day of insertion, and the recommended removal date printed on it.
- If the client is not accustomed to following a calendar, inform her about recommended dates for checkups and IUD removal.
- Samples of IUDs should be available so that the client can handle and examine them.
- Insertion may take place at any time during the menstrual cycle (insertion may be more comfortable at midcycle, when the cervix is softer) as long as it is certain that the client is not pregnant. Higher infection and expulsion rates are noted when IUDs are inserted during menses. The IUD may be inserted at 6 weeks postpartum. Studies conducted in other countries have found that an IUD may be safely inserted immediately after delivery of the placenta (within 10 minutes). Expulsion rates are only slightly higher than for some other types of insertions. IUDs may also be placed during cesarean section with even lower expulsion rates. High fundal placement and a provider trained in these specific postpartum insertion techniques are essential. Higher expulsion rates are associated with later postpartum IUD insertions (more than 10 minutes but fewer than 42 days after full term delivery).
- Insertions of IUDs require skill and experience on the part of the provider. Practicing insertions with a model and then several supervised insertions are strongly advised.
- IUD removal may take place at any time during the menstrual cycle, but may be easier at midcycle or at the time of menses.

Client Teaching and Counseling[10,76]

Several points are covered during client teaching and counseling.

- What to expect during and after IUD insertion.
- How and when to check for the IUD string (frequently during the first few months, then after each period or when abnormal cramping occurs).
- Signs of infection.
- Importance of keeping track of periods. Teach the client the IUD early danger signs, using *PAINS:*

  *P*eriod late, abnormal spotting or bleeding.
  *A*bdominal pain, pain with intercourse.
  *I*nfection exposure (especially gonorrhea), abnormal discharge.
  *N*ot feeling well, chills, fever.
  *S*tring missing, shorter, or longer.

VOLUNTARY STERILIZATION

Sterilization is the surgical interruption or closure of the pathways for sperm or ova, preventing fertilization. These methods are considered permanent means of contraception, although some surgical procedures to reverse both vasectomies and tubal ligations have been successful. Sterilization is the most popular method of contraception in the United States and worldwide.

Female Sterilization is accomplished by bilateral occlusion of the fallopian tubes, commonly referred to as bilateral tubal ligation (BTL). The fallopian tubes are ligated and cut, occluded with clips or rings, electrocoagulated or plugged to prevent the ovum from moving toward the uterus and joining with sperm. Sterilization is considered to be a safe operative procedure. A hysterectomy (removal of the uterus) accomplishes sterilization, but should *never* be performed solely for that purpose.[6,10,77,78]

Male Sterilization, or vasectomy, is an operative procedure that blocks the vas deferens to prevent the passage of sperm. Considered a simple procedure, it can be performed quickly, safely, and inexpensively in an office or clinic setting.[6,10,77,78]

Sterilization Techniques

Sterilization techniques may be performed using general or local anesthesia with sedation. Local anesthesia with light sedation has definite safety advantages over general anesthesia.

Suprapubic Minilaparotomy. Performed at 4 weeks or more postpartum or postabortion (when the uterus if fully involuted). Usually it is performed in lithotomy position. The procedure involves a small (2–5 cm) abdominal incision just above the pubic hairline. The uterus is elevated so that the uterus and tubes are close to the incision. The tubes are lifted, identified, and ligated by any of several occlusion techniques; the incision is sutured.[10,78]

Laparoscopy. A laparoscope consists of a viewing instrument, light source, and operating channel. *Single puncture technique* involves a small subumbilical incision. The abdomen is insufflated with a gaseous combination of nitrous oxide, carbon dioxide, and room air; the laparoscope is inserted, and the tubes are grasped and occluded through the operating channel of the instrument. With *double puncture technique,* a second tiny incision is made in the suprapubic region through which the operating channel is inserted and the procedure performed. Following bilateral tubal occlusion, the organs are inspected, the scope removed, gas gently expelled, and the incisions closed.[10,78]

Subumbilical Minilaparotomy. Most frequently used during the immediate postpartum/postabortion period, when the uterus and tubes remain high in the abdomen. A small (1.5–3.0 cm) incision is made just below the umbilicus. Oviducts are usually easily reached for the occlusion procedure. Lithotomy position is not needed, and organ manipulation and instrumentation are less extensive, facilitating a rapid recovery.[10,78]

Bilateral Tubal Ligation by Laparotomy. BTL using an abdominal incision greater than 5 cm, or vaginal access, or during cesarean section is associated with higher morbidity and complication rates. BTLs performed during cesarean section, however, are relatively common.

Nonsurgical Female Sterilization. Nonsurgical sterilization for women is being studied in several countries around the world. The method involves the use of *quinacrine hydrochloride,* a drug long used to prevent and treat malaria and other parasitic diseases. The quinacrine method of nonsurgical female sterilization involves transcervical uterine insertion of quinacrine pellets with a modified IUD inserter. This is done during the proliferative phase of the menstrual cycle. The drug causes inflammation and fibrosis in the proximal fallopian tube, leading to sterility. To date, more than 80,000 quinacrine pellet sterilizations have been performed worldwide. No deaths attributed to the use of the pellets have been reported. Experts conclude that further research is needed on toxicology, teratogenicity, and potential carcinogenicity of quinacrine. In the meantime, long-term follow-up studies on women who have already received the pellets are ongoing.[79,80]

Vasectomy (Male Sterilization). Each vas deferens is cut between two ligated sections, preventing sperm from mingling with ejaculate. Local anesthetic (e.g., 1 percent lidocaine without epinephrine) is injected into each side of the scrotum, where a small incision is made to isolate, occlude, and usually resect the vasa. Closure of the incision(s) requires one or two sutures. A no-scalpel technique for performing vasectomies is now widely used throughout the world and United States. This requires an instrument that "punctures" the scrotal skin and vas sheath. Once this is accomplished, the procedures to isolate, occlude, and resect are the same as for the scalpel technique. Little bleeding occurs, and no sutures are required. About 20 ejaculations are required for existing sperm in the vasa deferentia to be cleared.[10,78,81]

Effectiveness

Published in 1996, the U.S. Collaborative Review of Sterilization conducted by the Centers for Disease Control (CREST Study) assessed, over a 10-year period, the long-term risks and failure rates of female sterilization. Failure rates for BTL were found to be higher than previously believed. CREST reported an overall failure rate of 1.9 percent, which is more than double the usually reported failure rate of 0.4 percent. The 0.4 percent rate, however, reflects failures that occurred only during the first year after sterilization (Table 9–4), whereas CREST followed women for 10 years or longer.

The CREST study found that women sterilized at a young age had a higher risk of method failure; failure rates also varied by type of procedure. Unipolar coagulation, interval partial salpingectomy and postpartum partial salpingectomy all provided consistent protection over 10 years. On the other hand, silicone band application, spring clip application, and bipolar coagulation provided less protection, with failure rates increasing consistently and substantially over the 10-year period. In addition, a high percentage (33 percent) of pregnancies that occur following BTL run the risk of being ectopic. Any sterilized woman who suspects she might be pregnant should immediately contact her clinician because of the potential serious health risks involved.

Pregnancy rates following vasectomy (not including pregnancies resulting from intercourse before the reproductive tract was cleared of sperm) are less than 1 percent. Failures may result from errors in technique, such as failing to occlude the correct structure or spontaneous recanalization of the vas. Rarely, congenital duplication of the vas may be present and go unnoticed at the time of the procedure.

Advantages[6,10,77]

- One-time decision provides permanent sterility.
- Highly effective, convenient.

- Considered safe; low complication and morbidity rates.
- Following procedure and recovery, very few or no systemic or side effects occur.
- BTL has a protective effect against ovarian cancer.
- Partner cooperation not required.
- Short recovery time.
- Certain techniques can be performed immediately after childbirth or abortion.
- BTL immediately effective.
- Low long-term risks.
- Low long-term cost, covered by 85–90 percent of private insurance plans and Medicaid.
- Can be performed while lactating.
- Vasectomy is equally effective, simpler, safer, much less expensive than BTL.

Disadvantages[6,10,77,82–87]

- Carries risks inherent in any surgical procedure (infection, injury to other organs, hemorrhage, complications of anesthesia).
- Procedures are difficult to reverse.
- Initial cost may be high.
- Vasectomy is not immediately effective.
- Some states and third party payors require a waiting period between time of counseling/consent and actual procedure.
- Provides no protection against HIV or STDs.
- Some individuals may have regrets about having the procedure.
- Uterine perforation is possible.
- Some women report menstrual pattern changes, increased dysmenorrhea, PMS following BTL (research so far has been unable to support any pattern of identifiable changes).
- If BTL fails, high probability of ectopic pregnancy.
- Studies on the relationship between vasectomy and the development of prostate cancer remain inconsistent. In some recent studies, a weakly positive relationship has been found. Studies are continuing. Current recommendations state that vasectomy should continue to be offered and performed; vasectomy reversal is not warranted to prevent prostate cancer; prostate cancer screening should not be any different for men who have had a vasectomy than for men who have not.

- Vasectomy complications can occur (infection, bleeding, hematoma formation, congestive epididymitis, sperm granulation).

Contraindications

- Lack of adequately trained personnel to perform the procedure (especially important for laparoscopy techniques).
- Known or suspected pregnancy.
- Existing infection of the reproductive tract.
- Client ambivalence about sterilization.
- Serious uncontrolled health problems.

Management Considerations[82-89]

- A high skill level, involving special training and extensive practice, is needed to perform these procedures (especially for laparoscopy procedures).
- The client must provide informed consent prior to the procedure.
- When federal funds, and in some cases state funds, are used to reimburse for sterilization, the client must have signed informed consent at least 30 days prior to the procedure or before delivery or abortion, if sterilization is planned to immediately follow one of these procedures. The client must also be 21 years of age or older and mentally competent.
- Preoperative assessment includes history (with particular attention to the last menstrual period and most recent use of contraception, to be reasonably confident that the woman is not pregnant) and physical examination (with focus on position and mobility of uterus and detection of possible infection). Minimum lab requirements are hemoglobin and urinalysis.
- The client should have someone accompany her or him home following the procedure.
- The client should rest for a few days following the procedure.
- Sexual activity may be resumed after about one week for women and after 2 to 3 days for men.
- Men must be reminded that they are not sterile initially. Another method of contraception must be used for several weeks or for at least the next 20 ejaculations. Microscopic examination of semen is the best way to ascertain that sterility has been achieved.

Client Teaching and Counseling[78,88,89]

For several reasons, client teaching and counseling are especially important when an individual is considering sterilization. Sterilization is a surgical procedure, thus involving some risk; there are legal implications; and it is meant to be permanent. Postoperative regret about the sterilization decision is a serious concern. Indicators of future regret include young age (under age 34), having a BTL at the time of a cesarean section, change in marital status, decision was made during a time of crisis, children very young at the time of procedure. Reversal procedures often fail and are very costly. Documentation of adequate teaching/counseling is essential. In addition to the points in the counseling process that follow, also refer to the section at the beginning of this chapter on General Management Considerations, Client Education and Informed Consent.

- Assess client's interest in and readiness for sterilization.
- Emphasize permanence, discuss possibility of failure.
- Explain procedure using visual aids, discuss risks/benefits.
- Women who undergo sterilization are much less likely to use condoms or other barriers for prevention of STDs and HIV than are nonsterilized women. Men and women should be assessed and counseled about high risk sexual behaviors and how to adequately protect themselves and their partners.
- Have client read and sign informed consent form.
- Schedule appointment; provide copy of necessary forms.
- Discuss cost and payment.
- Provide pre- and postoperative instructions.
- Schedule postoperative follow-up visit.

FERTILITY AWARENESS METHODS

Fertility awareness methods, also referred to as menstrual cycle charting, natural family planning or periodic abstinence, involve making observations and charting of scientifically proven fertility signs that determine whether a woman is fertile on any given day. The three primary fertility signs are 1) waking temperature (basal body temperature), 2) cervical mucus/fluid, and 3) cervical position. These are normal physiological changes caused by hormonal fluctuations during the menstrual cycle that can be observed and charted so that fertile and infertile periods can be identified.[6,10,90]

Fertility awareness methods (FAM) are used in combination with coital abstinence or barrier methods during fertile days, when the desire is to prevent pregnancy. Fertility awareness also helps couple understand how to achieve pregnancy, detect probable pregnancy, detect impaired fertility, or manage PMS. The term *natural family planning* implies exclusive use of these methods and that absolute abstinence is maintained during the fertile phase.[10,90,91] The charting of observed changes is an important component for successful use of these methods. The techniques of FAM include basal body temperature method, cervical mucus/fluid (Billings or Ovulation) method, and symptothermal method. At least two of these techniques should be used simultaneously. Figure 9–5 is one example of a chart for recording fertility signs. Clients may design their own charts or adapt the one shown for their own use.

The calendar (rhythm) method is the original method based on periodic abstinence and is still widely used around the world. It is much less reliable than the newer methods listed previously, however, because it relies on a statistical prediction based on past cycles to predict fertility in future cycles. With newer, more effective and well researched methods available, the calendar (rhythm) method is no longer recommended.[6,10,90]

Modern fertility awareness methods are considered reliable and are acceptable to diverse population groups with varied religious and ethical beliefs and to couples who do not wish to use other methods for medical or personal reasons.[6,10,90]

Mechanism of Action

Pregnancy is prevented by avoidance of unprotected intercourse during times that a woman is determined to be fertile.

Calendar (Rhythm) Method.[10,90] This involves calculation of a woman's fertile period based on three assumptions:

- Ovulation occurs on the 14th day, plus or minus 2 days, prior to next menses.
- Sperm are viable for 3 days.
- The ovum is viable for 24 hours.

The client must chart the length of her menstrual cycles for a minimum of 8 months. The earliest day in the cycle she is likely to be fertile is determined by subtracting 18 days from the length of the shortest cycle occurring during that 8-month period. The latest day of potential fertility is obtained by subtracting 11 days from the longest cycle. These two numbers represent the beginning and end of the fertile period.

For example, if the client's shortest cycle was 27 days, subtract 18 from 27; on the 9th day (27 minus 18) the client must begin to abstain from sexual intercourse. If her longest cycle was 34 days, on the 23rd day (34 minus 11) abstinence may be ended. She must abstain from day 9 through day 23, a total of 14 days, during each cycle. This technique is most effective when menstrual cycles are regular. With less variable cycles, the period of required abstinence is shorter. The abstinent period cannot be less than 7 days.

As noted earlier, the calendar (rhythm) method is not based on tested scientific principles, relying on information from past cycles to predict fertile patterns in future cycles. Couples should instead be encouraged to utilize the more reliable methods to be discussed now.

Basal Body Temperature (BBT) Method.[6,10,90–93] Basal body temperature (waking temperature) refers to the lowest temperature reached by the body of a healthy person, taken upon wakening. Generally, a special BBT thermometer should be used (as opposed to a fever thermometer) because the temperatures are shown in increments of 0.1 degrees, and are easier to read and record. The temperature is taken daily after a minimum of 3 consecutive hours of sleep, before rising, eating, or drinking and is recorded on the chart (see Figure 9–5). The preovulatory temperatures are suppressed by estrogen, whereas postovulatory temperatures are increased by 0.4° to 0.8° F under the influence of heat inducing progesterone. Temperatures typically rise within a day or two *after* ovulation has occurred and remain elevated for 12 to 16 days, until menstruation

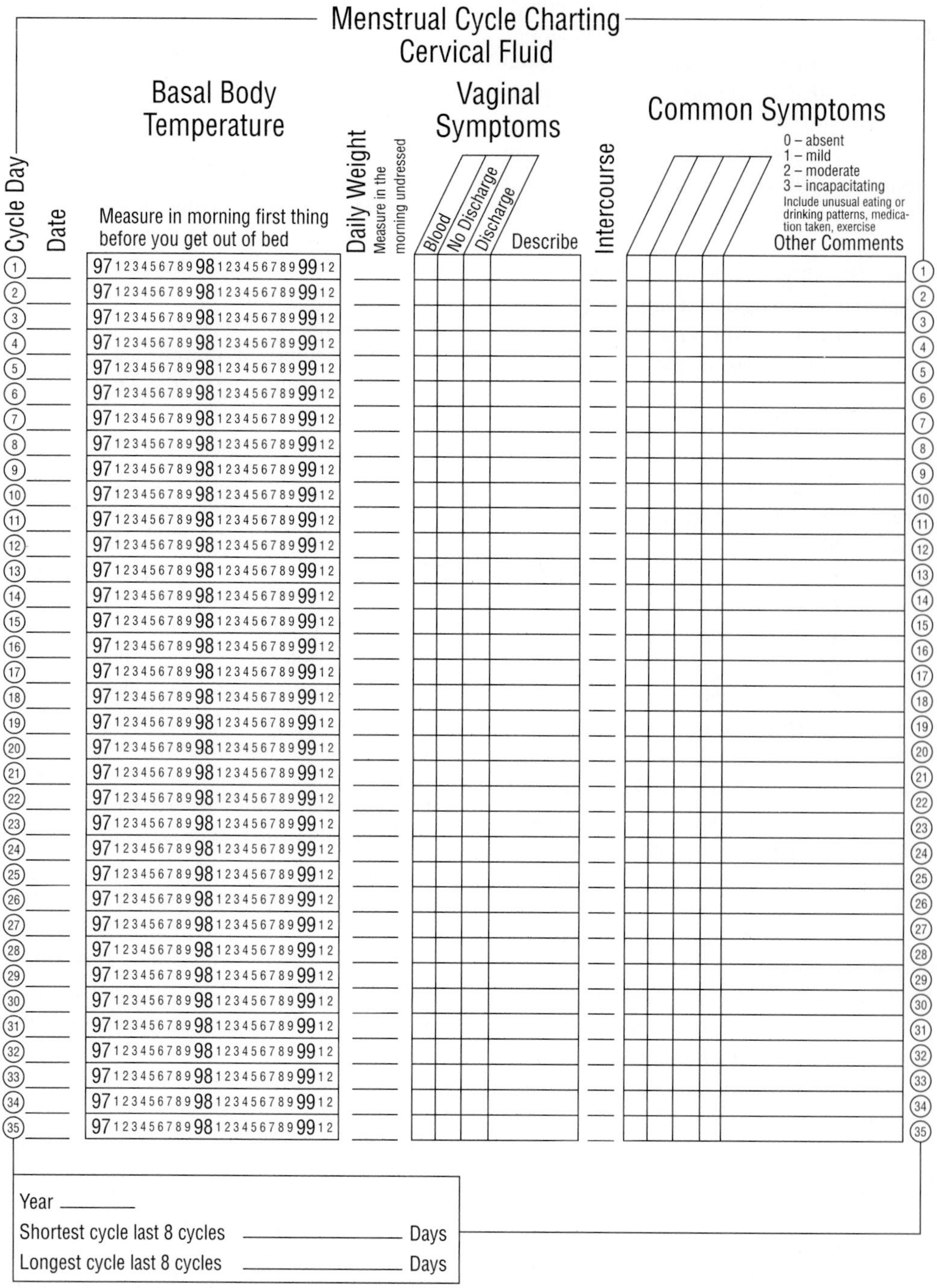

Menstrual Cycle Charting

Cervical Fluid

Cycle Day	Date	Basal Body Temperature — Measure in morning first thing before you get out of bed	Daily Weight — Measure in the morning undressed	Vaginal Symptoms: Blood	No Discharge	Discharge	Describe	Intercourse	Common Symptoms (0 – absent, 1 – mild, 2 – moderate, 3 – incapacitating)				Other Comments — Include unusual eating or drinking patterns, medication taken, exercise	
1		97 1 2 3 4 5 6 7 8 9 98 1 2 3 4 5 6 7 8 9 99 1 2												1
2		97 1 2 3 4 5 6 7 8 9 98 1 2 3 4 5 6 7 8 9 99 1 2												2
3		97 1 2 3 4 5 6 7 8 9 98 1 2 3 4 5 6 7 8 9 99 1 2												3
4		97 1 2 3 4 5 6 7 8 9 98 1 2 3 4 5 6 7 8 9 99 1 2												4
5		97 1 2 3 4 5 6 7 8 9 98 1 2 3 4 5 6 7 8 9 99 1 2												5
6		97 1 2 3 4 5 6 7 8 9 98 1 2 3 4 5 6 7 8 9 99 1 2												6
7		97 1 2 3 4 5 6 7 8 9 98 1 2 3 4 5 6 7 8 9 99 1 2												7
8		97 1 2 3 4 5 6 7 8 9 98 1 2 3 4 5 6 7 8 9 99 1 2												8
9		97 1 2 3 4 5 6 7 8 9 98 1 2 3 4 5 6 7 8 9 99 1 2												9
10		97 1 2 3 4 5 6 7 8 9 98 1 2 3 4 5 6 7 8 9 99 1 2												10
11		97 1 2 3 4 5 6 7 8 9 98 1 2 3 4 5 6 7 8 9 99 1 2												11
12		97 1 2 3 4 5 6 7 8 9 98 1 2 3 4 5 6 7 8 9 99 1 2												12
13		97 1 2 3 4 5 6 7 8 9 98 1 2 3 4 5 6 7 8 9 99 1 2												13
14		97 1 2 3 4 5 6 7 8 9 98 1 2 3 4 5 6 7 8 9 99 1 2												14
15		97 1 2 3 4 5 6 7 8 9 98 1 2 3 4 5 6 7 8 9 99 1 2												15
16		97 1 2 3 4 5 6 7 8 9 98 1 2 3 4 5 6 7 8 9 99 1 2												16
17		97 1 2 3 4 5 6 7 8 9 98 1 2 3 4 5 6 7 8 9 99 1 2												17
18		97 1 2 3 4 5 6 7 8 9 98 1 2 3 4 5 6 7 8 9 99 1 2												18
19		97 1 2 3 4 5 6 7 8 9 98 1 2 3 4 5 6 7 8 9 99 1 2												19
20		97 1 2 3 4 5 6 7 8 9 98 1 2 3 4 5 6 7 8 9 99 1 2												20
21		97 1 2 3 4 5 6 7 8 9 98 1 2 3 4 5 6 7 8 9 99 1 2												21
22		97 1 2 3 4 5 6 7 8 9 98 1 2 3 4 5 6 7 8 9 99 1 2												22
23		97 1 2 3 4 5 6 7 8 9 98 1 2 3 4 5 6 7 8 9 99 1 2												23
24		97 1 2 3 4 5 6 7 8 9 98 1 2 3 4 5 6 7 8 9 99 1 2												24
25		97 1 2 3 4 5 6 7 8 9 98 1 2 3 4 5 6 7 8 9 99 1 2												25
26		97 1 2 3 4 5 6 7 8 9 98 1 2 3 4 5 6 7 8 9 99 1 2												26
27		97 1 2 3 4 5 6 7 8 9 98 1 2 3 4 5 6 7 8 9 99 1 2												27
28		97 1 2 3 4 5 6 7 8 9 98 1 2 3 4 5 6 7 8 9 99 1 2												28
29		97 1 2 3 4 5 6 7 8 9 98 1 2 3 4 5 6 7 8 9 99 1 2												29
30		97 1 2 3 4 5 6 7 8 9 98 1 2 3 4 5 6 7 8 9 99 1 2												30
31		97 1 2 3 4 5 6 7 8 9 98 1 2 3 4 5 6 7 8 9 99 1 2												31
32		97 1 2 3 4 5 6 7 8 9 98 1 2 3 4 5 6 7 8 9 99 1 2												32
33		97 1 2 3 4 5 6 7 8 9 98 1 2 3 4 5 6 7 8 9 99 1 2												33
34		97 1 2 3 4 5 6 7 8 9 98 1 2 3 4 5 6 7 8 9 99 1 2												34
35		97 1 2 3 4 5 6 7 8 9 98 1 2 3 4 5 6 7 8 9 99 1 2												35

Year ________

Shortest cycle last 8 cycles ________________ Days

Longest cycle last 8 cycles ________________ Days

Figure 9–5. Chart for recording fertility signs. *(Reproduced, with permission, from Hatcher, R. et al.: Contraceptive Technology. 16th revised edition. New York: Irvington Publishers, Inc., 1994.)*

begins. If the woman were to become pregnant, the temperatures would remain elevated throughout the pregnancy. Some women experience a drop in BBT just prior to ovulation, but this is not a consistent occurrence. Based on the patterns observed, one should be able to predict the end of the fertile phase and the beginning of the safe, luteal phase of the cycle. If using BBT method alone, the client should avoid unprotected intercourse from the beginning of the menstrual cycle (or at least from day 4) until the BBT has been elevated for three days. Using other fertility awareness methods along with BBT should allow for shortening of the abstinent period.

It is important to know that numerous factors can delay or even prevent ovulation, thus prolonging the follicular (estrogenic) phase. These may include stress, travel, illness, medication, strenuous exercise, and sudden weight changes. Once ovulation occurs and the temperature rises, however, it is usually a standard 12 to 16 days until menses.

Cervical Mucus (Billings or Ovulation) Method.[10,90,93,94] This method assesses the character of cervical mucus. The mucus secreted by exocrine glands lining the cervical canal changes in character during the menstrual cycle in response to hormonal levels. The woman is taught to begin checking cervical mucus the first day the period is over and to check it prior to urinating about three times each day. She should first note whether there is a sensation of wetness or dryness in the vaginal area. Then the woman should obtain fluid from the vaginal opening and feel it with her fingers to note changes in the physical properties of the mucus. During a normal menstrual cycle, a woman experiences menses, then a few days of a dry sensation, then early mucus (may be milky white, translucent, yellow or clear, sticky at first and then smooth). As ovulation approaches, the mucus becomes more abundant, clear, slippery, and smooth. The mucus can be stretched between two fingers without breaking. This is called *spinnbarkeit* and closely resembles eggwhites. The vaginal sensation is one of lubrication, being wet and slippery. These characteristics correspond to the peak in estrogen occurring immediately prior to ovulation. This mucus is more permeable to sperm and can prolong the life of sperm. It is now known that sperm can live up to 5 days in the environment of wet quality cervical mucus. The *peak day* is the last day of eggwhite quality cervical mucus, or the lubricative vaginal sensation, or any midcycle spotting.

Before ovulation, the only days that are considered safe are those dry days in which there is no cervical fluid present. Postovulation, the woman is considered infertile the evening of the fourth consecutive day after the peak day. Charting must be done, noting observed cervical mucus characteristics.

Cervical position is an optional fertility sign that can be assessed to augment or confirm the changes in temperature and cervical mucus/fluid. The woman should insert one finger into the vagina and feel the conditions of the cervix, beginning when menses has ended. She palpates the cervix for height in the vagina (low, midway, high), softness (firm, medium, soft), openness (closed, partly open, open), and wetness (nothing, sticky, creamy, eggwhite). Near ovulation, the cervix feels high/deep in the vagina, soft, open, and wet. These observations should be noted on the chart, as well.[6,90]

Symptothermal Method. This method merely connotes that at least two indicators are being combined to identify the fertile period. The term *fertility awareness methods* also implies that more than one indicator is used. The symptothermal method usually combines the BBT and cervical mucus methods. It may also incorporate the changes in the cervix (position, texture, openness) described earlier, as well as secondary fertility signs that a woman might observe, such as breast tenderness, libido changes, midcycle pain, spotting, fluid retention, etc.

Effectiveness[6,10,16,90,95]

Fertility awareness methods are considered moderately effective for preventing pregnancy (see Table 9–4). Studies have concluded that when used perfectly, FAM is very effective in preventing pregnancy. It is extremely unforgiving, however, of imperfect use. Breaking the rules entails a 27 percent risk of pregnancy per cycle. Effectiveness would be increased if couples limited unprotected intercourse to the postovulatory period only. These techniques require high levels of commitment and participation by both partners. High motivation to prevent pregnancy and ability to learn the necessary concepts are needed. Failures are often related to poor understanding or improper teaching and poor use of methods. Some pregnancies result from couples having trouble coping with periods of abstinence. They may intentionally "break the rules" and take chances. Pregnancy must be an acceptable possible outcome of use of these methods.

Advantages[6,10,90–92]

- No damaging side effect.
- No interruption of normal body functions.
- No external or internal devices or chemicals.
- Acceptable to most religious groups.
- Low cost.
- Increases awareness of normal female body processes and fertility.
- Can facilitate diagnosis of gynecologic problems.
- Encourages communication between partners.
- The concepts and charting skills learned can also be applied to planning conception, diagnosis and treatment of fertility problems, and mapping symptoms of PMS.

Disadvantages[6,10,90–92]

- Low user effectiveness.
- Interferes with sexual spontaneity.
- Requires copious recordkeeping and intensive, ongoing teaching.
- Couples may have difficulty learning the techniques.
- Periodic abstinence is difficult for some couples.
- Is a less reliable method if infection is present.
- Is a less reliable method if menstrual periods are irregular.
- No identifiable BBT pattern is seen in some women's cycles, even when ovulating.
- Emotional and physiological stress, shift work, and travel can alter the timing of ovulation.
- No protection provided against HIV or STDs.
- Methods are unreliable during lactation and perimenopausal periods.

- If conception occurs, it may involve the fertilization of an "old" or overripe egg and an increased theoretical risk of fetal abnormalities. Convincing studies are unavailable either to support or negate this concern.

Contraindications[6,10]

There are no absolute contraindications to fertility awareness methods; however, if unplanned pregnancy would be unacceptable or inadvisable for a client or her family, for any reason, a more reliable contraceptive method should be considered. Relative contraindications include the following.

- Irregular menses.
- History of anovulatory cycles.
- Inability to keep careful records.
- Lack of partner cooperation.
- Frequent or persistent vaginal infections.

Management Considerations[6,10,90–92]

Clients must receive intensive and ongoing teaching by a trained fertility awareness counselor. They also will need assistance with interpreting charts. It is recommended that health care professionals be familiar with the available community resources for teaching these techniques and with the philosophy and teaching/learning resources used by the counselor. There should be a philosophical "match" between the needs and beliefs of the client and those of the counselor.

Teaching and counseling involves several aspects.

- Explanation of the normal menstrual cycle.
- Explanation of how the methods work.
- Selection of the methods.
- Techniques involved in the methods selected (e.g., how and when to take BBT, how to evaluate cervical mucus).
- Procedures for charting.
- How to determine fertile periods.
- Alternative sexual activity for fertile periods.

Some excellent references/resources are listed at the end of this chapter.

WITHDRAWAL (COITUS INTERRUPTUS)

Coitus interruptus, or withdrawal, involves the man removing his penis from the vagina before ejaculation so that ejaculation occurs away from the vagina and external genitalia. The man must rely on his own sensations to determine when he is about to ejaculate. Though not popular in the United States, withdrawal is one of the most common methods of preventing pregnancy in many countries and cultures of the world. Adolescents frequently use this method.[6,10,66]

Mechanism of Action[10]

Coitus interruptus prevents conception when sperm containing ejaculate is deposited away from the woman's genitalia, preventing contact between sperm and ovum. The man must interrupt intercourse and withdraw his penis from his partner's vagina before ejaculation occurs.

Effectiveness

Among typical users, about 19 percent experience method failure in the first year of use (see Table 9–4). Low success rates with this method may be due to the following:

- Presence of sperm in the preejaculate fluid that is emitted without sensation to the man.
- It is difficult for the man to predict when he will ejaculate.
- The required self-control is difficult to achieve.[10,16,96]

Advantages[6,10,96]

- Coitus interruptus involves no artificial devices or chemicals, costs nothing, is always available, and can be used during lactation.
- It is a backup method that is always available.

Disadvantages[6,10,96]

- High failure rate.
- Requires considerable self-control by the man.
- Can diminish enjoyment for the couple.
- Depends solely on the cooperation of the man.
- Puts the woman in a dependent role.
- Provides no protection against HIV or STDs.

- Sexual dysfunction and diminished pleasure could develop, as couples must remain alert, concentrate on timing, and interrupt the excitement or plateau phase of sexual response.

Contraindications

There are no absolute contraindications; however, if unplanned pregnancy is unacceptable or inadvisable, a more reliable method should be used. Relative contraindications include (a) questionable commitment of either partner to the method and (b) lack of effective communication between partners.

Management Considerations[10,96]

The method should be taught as part of contraceptive counseling, especially for those who tend to use this method (i.e, individuals inexperienced with contraceptive use or those who have exhausted all other contraceptive choices). Counseling and instruction should include several topics.

- Before intercourse, the man should urinate and wipe off any fluid on the tip of the penis; it may contain sperm. This is especially important if the couple intends to have more than one act of intercourse, because semen may be present in clear fluid at the tip of an erect penis.
- When a man feels impending ejaculation, he must immediately remove his penis from the vagina so that ejaculation occurs well away from the vagina.
- Condom use with this method would greatly increase its effectiveness and provide protection against HIV and other STDs.
- A supply of spermicide may be kept on hand in case withdrawal is not accomplished in time. An application could be inserted immediately, although this measure probably would not prevent some sperm from entering the uterus.
- Always advise clients about the availability of emergency contraception.

LACTATIONAL AMENORRHEA METHOD (LAM)

The Lactational Amenorrhea Method (LAM) is a highly effective temporary family planning method for breastfeeding women. LAM is based

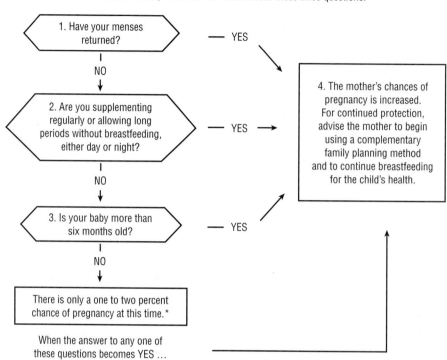

LAM: Lactational Amenorrhea Method
Ask the mother, or advise her to ask herself these three questions:

1. Have your menses returned? — YES

NO

2. Are you supplementing regularly or allowing long periods without breastfeeding, either day or night? — YES →

NO

3. Is your baby more than six months old? — YES

NO

4. The mother's chances of pregnancy is increased. For continued protection, advise the mother to begin using a complementary family planning method and to continue breastfeeding for the child's health.

There is only a one to two percent chance of pregnancy at this time.*

When the answer to any one of these questions becomes YES ...

*However, the mother may choose to use a complementary method at any time.

Figure 9–6. The Lactational Amenorrhea Method. *(Reproduced, with permission, from the Institute for Reproductive Health, Georgetown University, 1994.)*

on the utilization of lactational infertility for protection from pregnancy. LAM can provide women with natural protection against pregnancy for up to 6 months after a birth, and following the guidelines for this method encourages the timely introduction of complementary methods of birth control while breastfeeding continues beyond 6 months. Studies have shown that women who meet the three criteria for the method have a less than 2 percent pregnancy rate. The criteria include the following: 1) she is amenorrheic (no vaginal bleeding after 56 days postpartum); 2) she is fully or nearly fully breastfeeding (breastfeeding day and night, on demand. Intervals between feedings no more than 4 hours during the day and 6 hours at night; supplementation should not exceed 5 to 15 per-

cent of all feeding episodes, preferably less); 3) she is fewer than 6 months postpartum. LAM specifies that when any one of these conditions changes, the woman needs to begin to use a complementary family planning method if she desires to continue to have a low pregnancy risk (see Figure 9–6). LAM guidelines are considered extremely safe. Of the three criteria, the return of menses is the most important indication of the return of fertility.[97–100]

Mechanisms of Action

The physiology of LAM is based on the hypothalamic-pituitary-ovarian feedback system. The hypothalamus reacts to the suckling at the breast by reducing the pulsatile release of gonadotropin releasing hormone (GnRH). This, in turn, changes the pulsatile secretion of prolactin and the gonadotropin hormones, follicle stimulating hormone (FSH), and luteinizing hormone (LH). The result is decreased and disorganized follicular development.[97-100]

Effectiveness

Studies have demonstrated that women who met the LAM criteria had only a 1 to 2 percent chance of pregnancy during the first 6 months postpartum. The LAM method alone, by definition, cannot extend beyond 6 months. Research has emphasized the importance of full or nearly full breastfeeding patterns.[97-100]

Advantages[97-100]

- Highly effective (when used perfectly—see criteria).
- No supplies, low cost.
- Not coitus linked.
- Improved infant health through breastfeeding.
- Controlled by the woman.
- Gives women time to choose which complementary family planning method they will use.
- Acceptable to many religious groups.

Disadvantages[97-100]

- Temporary method, only effective in the postpartum months.
- If mother and baby are separated for extended periods, efficacy as a family planning method decreases.

Contraindications[97-100]

- Specific infant metabolic disorders.
- Maternal use of mood altering drugs.
- Maternal use of reserpine, ergotamine, anti metabolites, cyclosporine, cortisone, bromocriptine, radioactive drugs, lithium, anticoagulants.
- Maternal HIV infection/AIDS.
- Active tuberculosis.

Management Considerations[97-100]

In addition to teaching women the criteria for successful use of the Lactational Amenorrhea Method,

several points should be considered in client teaching and counseling.

- Emphasize that if there are disruptions in patterns of breastfeeding, resumption of ovulation and fertility cannot be accurately predicted. Woman can become pregnant while breastfeeding and before the first menstrual period occurs.
- Women who are uncertain about whether they can continue to meet the specified criteria for LAM, and wish to avoid the risk of pregnancy, should begin using a reliable method of birth control immediately. For some women, this may be at the time of the 6 week postpartum examination or even sooner.
- If the client wishes to rely on LAM for contraception, she must breastfeed her infant "on-demand" over each 24-hour period, with no formula or food supplementation. When the infant reaches 6 months or menses return, she must begin another method of birth control.
- Because U.S. women rarely adhere to such a rigorous breastfeeding pattern, most should be advised not to rely on lactation alone to prevent pregnancy. A complementary method is recommended.

DOUCHING

"Washing" semen out of the vagina through douching will not prevent sperm from entering the uterus. *Douching is not a reliable contraceptive,* because sperm enter the cervical canal too quickly, as soon as 15 seconds after ejaculation. In fact, douching could theoretically enhance movement of sperm up the cervical canal by washing it deeper into the vagina or by washing away protective mucus. Douching has also been associated with increased risk of pelvic infection and ectopic pregnancy.[10,101,102]

ELECTIVE TERMINATION OF PREGNANCY: INDUCED ABORTION

Induced abortions are voluntary interruptions of pregnancy and may be performed as elective or medically therapeutic procedures. Induced abortions involve the expulsion or extraction of the products of conception from the uterus by medical or surgical intervention before the embryo or fetus is capable of independent life. Abortion is the most common surgical procedure performed in the United States and may be the most common surgical procedure in the world. Excluding miscarriages, about 30 percent of all pregnancies in the United States end in abortions, with most abortions (90 percent) being performed during the first trimester of pregnancy.[6,10,103]

The 1973 U.S. Supreme Court decision *Roe v. Wade* allows women to choose to terminate pregnancy in the first trimester; after that point, individual state laws become effective. In recent years, several states have placed restrictions on access to abortion services in certain circumstances.[6,104]

Since abortion became widely available, controversy has been rampant in our society, and conflicts related to abortion rights will continue for years to come. It should be noted, however, that in a 1992 Gallop poll, only 14 percent of Americans surveyed believed that abortion should be illegal in all circumstances.[104] In order to provide health professionals with the information needed to counsel clients in a supportive manner, this section provides a discussion of the health needs of women seeking abortion services and a brief overview of abortion care.

Death as a result of legal induced abortion is unusual; in fact, maternal mortality associated with carrying a pregnancy to term is 16 times higher than the risk of death due to abortion. Risk of complications and death from induced abortion vary according to weeks of gestation, procedure used, and type of anesthesia. Later abortions and general anesthesia are more hazardous. Approximately 96 percent of first trimester abortions in the United States are performed by instrument evacuation, including vacuum aspiration and curettage. This is a very safe method of induced abortion. The number of American women reported as dying from abortion declined from nearly 300 deaths in 1961 (mostly illegal abortions), to only 6 in 1987, or 0.4 deaths for every 100,000 legal abortions. Major and minor complications associated with the procedures do occur. Major complications include retained tis-

sue, sepsis, uterine perforation, hemorrhage, incomplete abortion. Minor complications include mild infection, reaspiration (same day or later), cervical stenosis, cervical tear, underestimated gestation, convulsions/seizure. Major complications are 2.5 times higher for instillation methods than with instrument evacuation procedures in the second trimester. Use of general anesthesia during any abortion procedure carries a significantly higher risk of serious complications and death than use of local anesthesia.[6,105]

Risk of long-term complications after having one or more legal abortions is low. Subsequent problems with fertility, spontaneous abortion, premature delivery and low birth rate have not been found to be associated with first trimester abortions, or for later abortions when performed by skilled and well trained abortion providers. Concurrent abortion and sterilization procedures are not recommended due to higher rates of morbidity and mortality.[6,104,105]

CLIENT EVALUATION AND PREPARATION COUNSELING

Counseling can assist a woman in decision making and prepares her to give informed consent. When a woman finds out she is pregnant with an undesired conception, it is essential that she (and her partner or other supportive person, if appropriate) has the opportunity to discuss concerns and needs in a nonjudgmental atmosphere. Women seeking abortions may experience feelings of anxiety, conflict, isolation, or fear. If the abortion is sought because of a serious medical condition, loss or sadness may be prominent. Situations involving sexual abuse or rape will require referral for further counseling and support. Abortion counselors should convey the characteristics of empathy, warmth, and genuineness while helping women to resolve confusion, ambivalence, or guilt before the procedure is performed. Sensitivity to cultural differences among clients is essential. In addition, clients must be made to feel safe, considering today's volatile environment related to abortion.[6,10,104–106]

The client should be given the opportunity to discuss her current and future life situations, plans and expectations, and the possible impact of the pregnancy and/or abortion. For women who decide against abortion, referral should be made for prenatal care and information about adoption. The counselor must be able to provide other referrals that may be indicated such as social services, group or individual support, etc.[6,10,104–106]

It is the responsibility of the counselor to explain—in a kind thorough and objective manner—all aspects of the procedures, including options, risks, preparations for the procedures, techniques and their effects, pain management, and guidance in what to expect. Postabortion contraceptive options also need to be discussed.

History

The following historical data are needed.

- Menstrual history, especially last and previous menstrual periods.
- Contraceptive history and what methods the client wants to use in the future.
- Obstetric history.
- Reproductive system disease and/or prior surgery.
- Drug/anesthesia allergies.
- Other illnesses affecting health, past or present.
- Current medications.[10,105]

Physical and Reproductive Examination

The *physical exam* may be brief (heart, lungs, breasts, abdomen, vital signs); however, the *reproductive exam* should be thorough to estimate the size and position of the uterus, to estimate the state of the conceptus, and to determine any abnormality, such as a mass or anatomical variation.[10,105]

Diagnostic Tests

Several diagnostic tests may be done.

- *Pregnancy Test.* A urine test for first screening; if test is negative but pregnancy suspected, a sensitive serum test is done. A wait of 1 to 2 weeks may be needed for more definitive test results if the woman is 6 weeks or less from her last normal menstrual period.
- *Ultrasound Evaluation.* Done for accurate dating when a discrepancy exists between the size

of the uterus and gestational age. Ultrasound is routinely performed in the second trimester to ascertain accurate gestational age.
- *Hemoglobin/Hematocrit.*
- *Blood type.* Necessary to determine if a woman is Rh negative. Rh negative women will need to receive Rh(D) immunoglobulin (RhoGAM) after the procedure.
- *Vaginitis/STD Screening.* Chlamydia, gonorrhea, saline wet mount, and other if indicated.[10,104,105]

Reasons for Elective Termination

A woman may seek to terminate pregnancy for several reasons.

- *Elective Reasons* are unrelated to the health of the mother or the fetus, such as pregnancy due to rape or incest or the inability to afford the pregnancy.
- *Maternal indications* are reasons for which the mother's health would be jeopardized if the pregnancy were to continue, such as heart disease, severe depression, or cancer.
- *Fetal indications* most commonly are congenital defects, or exposure to a teratogenic agent.[104,106]

METHODS OF INDUCED ABORTION

Surgical Abortion Methods

Vacuum (suction) curettage is the most commonly used abortion procedure in the United States. It is an ambulatory care procedure and may be done through week 14 of gestation. The procedure is done under local anesthesia, a para-cervical block, and takes about 15 minutes. Prior to surgery, the cervix is dilated by osmotic dilators, which takes 4 or more hours. The products of conception are removed by suction evacuation, and completion confirmed by curettage.

Potential complications include incomplete abortion, cervical laceration, seizure, cardiac arrest, allergic reaction, uterine atony, uterine perforation, bleeding, and infection. Advantages of the procedure are that it costs less than procedures performed during later gestation and little time is lost from work. Private physician costs are generally higher. Dilation with a laminaria may be needed prior to the procedure, thus requiring an additional visit to the office.[6,10,104–106]

Other surgical methods include dilatation and curettage (D & C), though this is rarely used because of potential complications; dilatation and evacuation (D & E) is a commonly used procedure for second trimester abortions, after about 14 weeks. This involves dilatation of the cervix (to about 1.5 to 2 cm.) by various possible means, usually with a number of laminaria, and evacuation of the products of conception with specially designed forceps, followed by curettage, then suction. The D & E procedure is considered safer, faster, and less expensive for second trimester abortions than instillation methods (discussion to follow), and can be carried out under local anesthesia. Hysterotomy (essentially a cesarean section) is rarely performed due to high morbidity and mortality.[104–106]

Menstrual extraction is a term used to designate the performance of an early abortion before the diagnosis of pregnancy has been made by pregnancy test or examination. It is a simple procedure performed 5 to 6 weeks from the LMP, involving a suction device and a small cannula, accomplishing endometrial aspiration (if not pregnant) or an early abortion. It is not without risk, however, and because it is the general consensus of the medical community that potential risks outweigh the possible benefits, it is not recommended.[104–106]

Medical Abortion Methods

Substances used to induce medical abortion in the second trimester are prostaglandin E_2 suppositories, 12-methyl prostaglandin F_2 intramuscular injection, hypertonic saline intra-amniotic infusion, intra-amniotic prostaglandin infusion, or hypertonic urea intraamniotic infusion. These are generally referred to as instillation methods of induced abortion. Methods may be combined to ensure evacuation. To ease the procedure, dilation substances such as laminaria, or synthetic osmotic dilators, or prostaglandin suppositories to soften the cervix, are commonly used before the induction is

begun. It generally takes about 6 hours for a laminaria to dilate the cervix. To induce abortion, oxytocin may be given alone intravenously to cause uterine contractions, or it may be given in combination with other substances, such as saline. Infusions are inpatient or outpatient procedures; they become more expensive as a hospital stay lengthens. Costs for infusions averaged over $2000 in one report published in 1991.[107] Moreover, the psychological effects on the client may be traumatic.

The following two methods of medical abortion are carried out only in very early pregnancy. Women choose medical abortion in the first trimester for reasons of greater privacy and autonomy, less invasiveness and a more natural process than surgery.[108] The first to be discussed is the use of methotrexate (first developed as an antineoplastic agent), given intramuscularly at 50 mg. per square meter of body surface area, followed by the prostaglandin, misoprostol as an 800 microgram vaginal suppository or in oral form, 3 to 7 days later. Methotrexate induces abortion because of its toxicity to trophoblastic tissue and is most successful as an abortifacient when used at 8 or fewer weeks' gestation. When used in abortion, misoprostol, a prostaglandin, works by causing contractions of the uterus, helping to expel the uterine contents. If abortion does not occur within 7 to 10 days, a second dose of misoprostol is given. Side effects of methotrexate used in this way are minimal. Misoprostol side effects include diarrhea, nausea, vomiting. This method is 90 to 98 percent successful in accomplishing completed abortion. Incomplete abortions may require a surgical procedure to complete. Follow-up evaluation to be certain abortion is complete is important because of the potential teratogenicity of the drug, should the pregnancy continue. Use of methotrexate for the purpose of inducing abortion is not an FDA approved indication for this drug.[6,109–112]

A second method of medical induced first trimester abortion involves the use of mifepristone, also known as "the French abortion pill" or RU-486, followed by administration of the prostaglandin, misoprostol. Clinical trials of these drugs were conducted in the United States between 1994 and 1995. These trials were very successful and mifepristone has been recommended for FDA approval as an abortifacient.[113]

Mifepristone is a potent oral antiprogestogen. Mifepristone blocks the action of the natural hormone, progesterone, which prepares the lining of the uterus for the fertilized egg and then maintains the pregnancy. Without progesterone, the lining of the uterus softens, breaks down and bleeding begins. The pregnancy is thus interrupted in its early stages. The actions of misoprostol cause contractions of the uterus and expulsion of uterine contents.[114] The protocol for a mifepristone/misoprostol abortion, as used during the U.S. clinical trials, generally involves three visits. Following appropriate counseling and evaluation at the first visit, the woman swallows three tablets (200 mg each) of mifepristone and is observed for a period of time. At the second visit, 36 to 48 hours later, the woman is given two 200 microgram oral tablets of misoprostol and remains under supervision at the clinic for about 4 hours. Most women have the abortion during this 4-hour period, but it may occur in subsequent hours or days. The third visit is for follow-up evaluation and takes place 12 days after the second visit, to ensure that abortion is complete. If not complete, vacuum curettage is performed. Used in the first 9 weeks of pregnancy, this method is 95 percent effective. Five percent of women may require surgical completion of the abortion. No deaths or unexpected complications occurred during the U.S. trials. Side effects of the mifepristone are minimal, though some nausea, headache, weakness, and fatigue may occur. The misoprostol has possible side effects of cramping, abdominal pain, nausea, vomiting, diarrhea, uterine bleeding. Mifepristone is also being studied for use as an emergency contraceptive.[113–117]

COMPLICATIONS, SIGNS AND SYMPTOMS, AND PREVENTIVE MEASURES (see Table 9–12)

Postabortion Counseling

Clients who undergo vacuum aspiration or suction curettage need to expect menstrual cramping during and after the procedure and some vaginal bleeding that will taper over the next week. Clients undergoing a D & E in the second trimester can expect to enter the hospital, un-

dergo a 30-minutes procedure to place the laminaria, then allow about 6 hours or more for the laminaria's effect. Analgesia may be needed after the abortion for cramping and/or breast engorgement.

Infusions later in pregnancy require hospital stays of 1 to 3 days; severe cramping, necessitating analgesia, can be expected. Instruct all clients not to put anything in the vagina for 7 days after their procedure. They should expect to feel fatigue and breast tenderness for a few days and anticipate feelings of loss, sadness, or relief. Negative feelings are usually short-lived. A return visit should be scheduled for 2 to 4 weeks postoperatively.[104–107]

FUTURE METHODS OF FERTILITY CONTROL

Promising research is being conducted in many parts of the world to discover and test new technologies in contraception targeted for men and women. Methods being investigated for use by men, however, are most likely many years away.

MEN

- *Hormonal.* Administration of testosterone to men signals the pituitary to decrease the levels of testosterone needed for the testes to fully function, thus temporarily suppressing the production of sperm. An important finding from some early studies indicates that total suppression of sperm is not necessary to achieve highly effective contraception. Synthetic forms of testosterone are in varying stages of development, in the forms of injections, implants, transdermal patches or creams; alone or in combination with progestins such as DMPA or levonorgestrel, or in combination with luteinizing hormone releasing hormone (LHRH) antagonists.[118–120]
- *Vaccines.* Referred to as immunocontraception, vaccines would use the body's immune system to disable sperm. Vaccines under development are LHRH or FSH based, and would eliminate sperm production. Future vaccines will focus on interfering with highly specific aspects of spermatogenesis.[118–121]

TABLE 9–12. IMMEDIATE COMPLICATIONS OF INDUCED MEDICAL OR SURGICAL ABORTION, SIGNS AND SYMPTOMS, AND PREVENTIVE MEASURES

Complication	Signs and Symptoms	Preventive Measures
Excessive or prolonged bleeding	Occurs during or after procedure. Uterus may be atonic; bleeding may be from trauma (see below).	Local anesthesia, I.V. oxytocin or oral or I.M. ergot, uterine massage. Evacuation of placenta within hour of fetal expulsion. May require transfusion and ergotamine treatment if occurs.
Infection	Fever, chills, cramps, foul discharge, backache, abdominal pain, abdominal tenderness, muscle aches, tiredness.	Treatment of infections prior to procedure, complete evacuation of products of conception, antibiotic therapy prophylactically. Hospitalization may be indicated for adequate treatment if infection develops.
Intrauterine blood clots/retained products of conception (POC)	Occurs during first 5 days after abortion. Severe pain and cramps; uterus tense, tender, enlarged; no bleeding from cervix. May be accompanied by infection (endometritis). Seen with first trimester abortions.	Vacuum aspiration indicated; oral ergot may decrease occurrence of clots. Complete evacuation of uterus prevents retained POC.
Unsuccessful termination	Pregnancy signs/symptoms continue; products of conception not found.	Adequate uterine curettage.
Trauma to uterus (perforation) or to cervix (laceration)	Increased risks with younger woman, later gestation, prior delivery.	Preprocedure use of laminaria, osmotic dilators; safe, correct surgical procedure. Experienced practitioner.

Source: References 10, 104, 105, 106.

- *Sulfasalazine.* An ulcerative colitis drug, sulfasalazine causes decreased sperm counts and impairs sperm motility and function. The effects of this drug are quickly reversed.[121]

- *Occlusion of the Vas Deferens.* This is accomplished either by injection of a polymer or with flexible silicone plugs, producing a "reversible sterilization."[119,121,122]

- *Gossypol.* A natural substance found in cottonseed oil, gossypol suppresses sperm production, is reversible, and has no effect on androgens. Gossypol depletes potassium levels, however, and can lead to dangerous cardiac arrhythmias. Lower, safer doses are being investigated.[118,121]

- *Nifedipine.* Routinely used to treat hypertension, nifedipine appears to prevent sperm from fertilizing eggs by entering the membrane of the sperm and preventing it from discharging the enzymes needed to penetrate the protein coating of the egg. This is due to the blocking of calcium ion channels in the cell membrane. Dosage needs to be established.[121,123]

- *Mifepristone (RU-486) for Men.* Mifepristone and some of its chemical derivatives prevent calcium from penetrating sperm. Calcium is necessary for sperm motility and subsequent fertilization.[121,124]

WOMEN

- *Hormonal.* Newer long acting progestins are undergoing testing and in some cases are in use in countries other than the United States. They contain levonorgestrel, norethindrone, and other progestins, in the forms of removable and biodegradable implants, injections, and vaginal rings.[6,10,125]

  - *Removable implants.* Norplant II, an improved version of Norplant, contains two rods, is as effective and has similar duration of action as Norplant. Implanon is a one rod implant effective for 3 years. No incision is required for insertion; it is inserted under the skin, using a large needle. Contains etonogestrel.

  - *Biodegradable implants.* Eliminate need for surgical removal of implants. Annuelle consists of pellets the size of rice grains, containing norethindrone fused with cholesterol; effective for 2 years. Capronor contains levonorgestrel and is effective for up to two years.

- *Injectables.* A long acting ester, injectable levonorgestrel butanoate will be an alternative to DMPA. Injectables containing estrogen as well as a progestin are undergoing study. These are highly effective and minimize disruptions of bleeding patterns.
- *Vaginal Rings.* These may contain only progestin or a combination of estrogen and progestin. The combination ring would most likely be used 3 weeks on and 1 week off (like oral contraceptives) to allow for a withdrawal bleed.

- *Intrauterine devices.* The Levonorgestrel-20 (LNG-20) IUD is widely available throughout the world, though not in the United States. This device releases 20 mcg. of levonorgestrel into the uterine cavity daily, providing 7 years of highly effective contraception, light bleeding patterns, and decreased risk of ectopic pregnancy. The Nova-T is identical in size and shape to LNG-20, but contains copper rather than levonorgestrel.[6,10,126,127]

  An intracervical device is under investigation, a small plastic frame that is anchored to the inner wall of the cervix at about 1.5 cm. from the external os. Preliminary studies show high effectiveness, low expulsion rate, and the device is well tolerated by subjects.[128]

- *Barriers.* Efforts are underway to improve condoms, diaphragms, caps, and similar devices that provide physical barrier contraception, some of which can reduce exposure to STDs.[6,10,129,130]

  - *Female condoms.* New types of female condoms are being studied. The Bikini condom is worn like a panty. Another female condom product called Women's Choice is inserted with an applicator.
  - *Sponges.* Protectaid, available in Canada, is made of polyurethane and contains F-5 gel, a low dose combination of three spermicides (nonoxynol-9, benzalkonium chloride (BZK), and sodium cholate). A sponge containing BZK is available in Europe.
  - *Diaphragms.* Research is being conducted on the traditional diaphragms to make them easier and more appealing to use. These approaches include wearing the diaphragm for longer periods with and/or without spermi-

cide. A fit-free diaphragm is under development. A new type of diaphragm, made from silicone rather than latex, has been developed and is under study. This device is used without spermicide and worn continuously, removed only for washing. A disposable diaphragm that releases nonoxynol-9 is in early stages of development.
  - *Lea's Shield.* This is a one-size-fits-all cup shaped barrier that covers the cervix. It is made of silicone rubber and has a valve that allows draining of secretions and menstrual blood; it has a U-shaped loop for removal. It can be worn for 48 hours.[6,10,129,130]

- *Femcap.* This is a new type of cervical cap, made of silicone rubber, shaped like a hat with a wide upturned brim. It fits over the cervix, may be worn up to 48 hours, and may be effective without a spermicide.
- *Chemical barriers.* Research involving chemical barrier methods (spermicides) is examining these products for their ability to prevent the transmission of STDs, especially HIV, and ways to improve their ability to do so. Spermicides under study include nonoxynol-9, benzalkonium chloride, and menfegol. New delivery systems would enhance ease of use and would increase spreadability and cohesiveness to better protect against pathogens, including HIV, as well as sperm. These may be in the forms of new types of films, slow releasing pellets, gels, and a vaginal ring that would release spermicide for up to 30 days. Advantage 24 is a new spermicidal formulation that may be effective for 24 hours.[62,63,129,130]
- *Vaccines.* An antifertility vaccine is being studied that is directed against human chorionic gonadotropin (HCG). HCG is produced by the implanting embryo, and is essential for implantation and successful development of early pregnancy. Other vaccines are being developed that act against various targets in the body or at certain stages of embryonic growth. These include vaccines against FSH, LHRH, the zona pellucida, endometrial proteins, inactivation of the secretions of the blastocyte and other points in the processes of fertilization, postfertilization, and implantation.[131–133]

Nursing diagnoses

Nursing diagnoses reflecting actual or potential concerns or problems related to fertility control:[13]

- Powerlessness related to lack of knowledge about fertility control.
- Disturbed self-esteem related to past experience with contraceptive failure.
- Anxiety related to fear of pregnancy.
- Spiritual distress related to conflict between religious beliefs and desire to limit family size.
- Fear of unplanned pregnancy related to unprotected intercourse.
- Potential for sexual dysfunction related to fear of pregnancy.
- Potential for conflict in family (marital) processes related to disagreement about methods of birth control.
- Noncompliance with proper use of contraceptive method related to lack of understanding of instructions.
- Potential for guilt related to decision to terminate pregnancy.
- Others: Altered sexual patterns, ineffective individual coping, knowledge deficit, impaired social interaction, dysfunctional communication patterns (each requires a statement of etiology: related to . . .).

Nursing diagnoses reflecting functional health patterns for clients seeking family planning services or successfully using a selected birth control method:

- Positive self-concept related to successful efforts to control fertility.
- Positive health seeking behaviors (evidenced by timely request for fertility control counseling) related to adequate knowledge about contraception.
- Positive sexuality (reproductive) patterns related to successful achievement of desired family size.
- Effective individual coping related to confidence in sexual and reproductive choices.

REFERENCES

1. Fogel, C. I., & Woods, N. F. (1995). *Women's health care: A comprehensive handbook.* Thousand Oaks, CA: Sage Publications.
2. The Boston Women's Health Collective. (1992). *The new our bodies, ourselves.* New York: Simon and Schuster.
3. Potts, M. (1988). Birth control methods in the United States. *Family Planning Perspectives, 22,* 76–80.
4. Asbell, B. (1995). *The pill: A biography of the drug that changed the world.* New York: Random House.
5. Lynaugh, J. (1991). The death of Sadie Sachs. . . . Margaret Sanger. *Nursing Research, 40*(2), 124–25.
6. Speroff, L., & Darney, P. (1996). *A clinical guide for contraception* (2nd ed.). Baltimore: Williams and Wilkins.
7. National Family Planning and Reproductive Health Assoc. (1996). *Facts about the national family planning program, Title X of the Public Health Service Act.* Bulletin.
8. Barnett, B. (1995). Life stages affect method use. *Network: Family Health International, 15*(3), 14–17.
9. Forrest, J. D. (1993). Timing of reproductive life stages. *Obstet-Gynecology, 82*(1), 105–110.
10. Hatcher, R. A., Trussel, J., Stewart, F., Stewart, G., Kowal, D., Guest, F., Cates, W., Jr., & Policar, M. (1994). *Contraceptive technology* (16th rev. ed.). New York: Irvington Publishers, Inc.
11. Hearn, T. K. (1994). In the 1960s there was no free love—in the 1990s there is no safe sex. *Journal of American College Health, 42*(6), 298–302.
12. Nolte, S., Sohn, M. A., Koons, B. (1993). Prevention of HIV infection in women. *Journal of Obstetric, Gynecology, Neonatal Nursing, 22*(2), 128–134.
13. Carpenito, L. J. (1997). *Nursing diagnosis: Application to clinical practice* (7th ed.). Philadelphia: J. B. Lippincott Co.
14. Dickey, R. P. (1994). *Managing contraceptive pill patients* (8th ed.). Durant, OK: Essential Medical Information Systems, Inc.
15. Litchman, Ronnie, & Papera, Susan (1998). *Gynecology: Well-woman care.* Stamford, CT: Appleton & Lange.
16. Trussell, J., Hatcher, R. A., Cates, W., Jr., Stewart, F. H., & Kost, K. (1990). Contraceptive failure in the U.S. an update: *Studies in Family Planning, 21*(1), 51–54.

17. Blumenthal, Paul D., & Huggins, George R. (1992). A look at the new progestogen OCs. *Med. Aspects of Human Sexuality, 26*(1), 30–36.

18. Bringer, Jacques. (1992). Norgestimate: A clinical overview of a new progestin. *American Journal Ob-Gyn, 166* (6—Part 2), 1969–77.

19. Runnebaun, B., Grunwald, K., & Rabe, T. (1992). The efficacy and tolerability of norgestimate/ethinyl estradiol: Results of an open, multicenter study of 59,701 women. *American Journal Ob-Gyn, 166* (6—Part 2), 1963–68.

20. Jick, H., Jick, S. S., Gurewich, V., Myers, M. W., Vasilakis, C. (1995). Risk of idiopathic cardiovascular death and non-fatal venous thromboembolism in women using oral contraceptives with differing progestogen components. *Lancet, 346,* 1589–1593.

21. WHO Collaborative Study of CVD and Steroid Hormone Contraception. (1995). Venous thromboembolic disease and combined oral contraceptives: Results of international multicenter case-control study. *Lancet, 346,* 1575–82.

22. WHO Collaborative Study of CVD and Steroid Hormone Contraception. (1995). Effects of different progestogens in low estrogen OCs on venous thromboembolic disease. *Lancet, 3436,* 1592–88.

23. Lewis, M. A., Spitzer, W. O., & Heinemann, L. A. J. (1996). Third generation OCs and risk of myocardial infarction: An international case-control study. *British Medical Journal, 312,* 88–90.

24. Statement from the Clinical and Scientific Committee of the Faculty on Family Planning and Reproductive Health Care of the Royal College of Obstetricians and Gynecologists. (1995). *Risk of VTE and the combined oral contraceptive pill.*

25. Weisberg, E. (1995). Prescribing oral contraceptives. *Drugs, 49*(2), 224–231.

26. Staff. (1996). Metabolic effects of oral contraceptives. *The Contraceptive Report, 6*(6), 4–14.

27. Staff. (1992, Feb.). Maximizing oral contraceptive effectiveness: Changing perceptions. *ARHP Clinical Proceedings,* 1–15.

28. Simon, D., Sehan, C., Garnier, P., et al. (1990). Effects of oral contraceptives on carbohydrate and lipid metabolism in a healthy population: The Telacom Study. *American Journal Obstetrics-Gynecology, 163,* 382–387.

29. Colditz, G. A., & Nurses Health Study Research Group. (1994). Oral contraceptive use and mortality during 12 years of follow-up. The nurses health study. *Annals of Internal Medicine, 120,* 821–826.

30. Kraus, R. M., Burkman, R. T. (1992). The metabolic impact of oral contraceptives. *American Journal of Obstetrics-Gynecology, 167,* 1177–1183.

31. Barrett, D. H., Andra, R. F., Escobedo, L. G., Croft, J. B., Williamson, D. F., & Marks, J. S. (1994). Trends in oral contraceptive use and cigarette smoking. *Archives Family Medicine, 3,* 438–444.

32. Fruzzetti, F., Ricci, C., Fioretti, P. (1994). Haemostatic profile in smoking and non-smoking women taking low-dose OCs. *Contraception, 49,* 579–592.

33. Kjos, S. L., Shoupe, D., Douyan, S., Friedman, R. I., Bernstein, G. S., Mestman, J. H., & Mishall, D. R. (1990). Effects of low-dose oral contraceptive on carbohydrate and lipid metabolism in women with recent gestational diabetes: Results of a controlled, randomized prospective study. *American Journal of Obstetrics-Gynecology, 163,* 1822–1827.

34. Garg, S. K., Chase, H. P., Marshall, G., Hoops, S. L., Holmes, D. L., & Jackson, W. E. (1994). Oral contraceptives and renal and retinal complications in young women with IDDM. *JAMA, 271,* 1099–1102.

35. Peterson, K. R., Skouby, S. O., Sidelmann, J., Pedersen, L., & Jespersen, J. (1994). Effects of contraceptive steroids on cardiovascular risk factors in women with IDDM. *American Journal Obstetrics and Gynecology, 171,* 400–403.

36. Rookus, M. A., & Leeuwen, F. E., for the Netherlands OCs and Breast Cancer Study. (1994). Oral contraceptives and the risk of breast cancer in women aged 20–54. *Lancet, 344,* 844–851.

37. White, E., Malone, K. E., Weiss, N. S., Daling, J. R. (1994). Breast cancer among young U.S. women in relation to oral contraceptive use. *Journal National Cancer Institute, 86,* 505–514.

38. Brinton, L. A., Daling, J. R., Liff, J. M., Schoenberg, J. B., Malone, K. E., et al. (1995). Oral contraceptives and breast cancer risk among younger women. *Journal National Cancer Institute, 87,* 837–835.

39. LaVecchia, C., Negri, E., Franceschi, S., Talamini, R., Amadori, D., et al. (1995). Oral contraceptives and breast cancer: A cooperative Italian study. *International Journal Cancer, 60,* 163–167.

40. Letterie, G. S., & Chow, G. E. (1992). Effect of "missed pills" on oral contraceptive effectiveness. *Ob-Gyn, 79,* 979–982.

41. Szarewski, A., & Guillebaud, J. (1991). Contraception, current state of the art. *British Medical Journal, 302,* 23–25.

42. McCann, M. F., & Potter, L. S. (1994). Progestin-only oral contraceptives: A comprehensive review. *Contraception, 50* (Suppl.), S9–S195.

43. Darney, P. D. (1994). Hormonal implants: Contraception for a new century. *American Journal Ob-Gyn, 170,* 1536–1543.

44. Wehrle, K. E. (1994). The Norplant System: Easy to insert, easy to remove. *Nurse Practitioner, 19*(4), 47–54.

45. Archer, D. F. (1995). Management of bleeding in women using subdermal implants. *Contemporary Ob/Gyn,* Reprint.

46. Kaunitz, A. M. (1994). Long-acting injectable contraception with DMPA. *American Journal Ob-Gyn, 170*(5), 1543–1549.

47. Burkemaun, R. T. (1994). Non-contraceptive effects of hormonal contraceptives: Bone mass, STDs and PID, CVD, menstrual function and future fertility. *American Journal Ob-Gyn, 170*(5), 1569–1574.

48. Barnett, B. (1993). DMPA requires thorough counseling, other skills. *Network: Family Health International, 14*(1), 12–17.

49. Fahey, M. L. (1995). Pharmacologic update: Emergency post-coital therapies. *Journal of American Academy of Nurse Practitioners, 7*(10), 505–508.

50. Haspels, A. A. (1994). Emergency contraception: A review. *Contraception, 50*(2), 101–108.

51. Trussell, J., Ellerston, C., Rodriguez, G. (1996). The Yuzpe regimen of emergency contraception, how long after the morning after? *Ob-Gyn, 88*(1), 150–154.

52. Emergency contraceptive hotline fact sheet. (1997). Reproductive Health Technologies Project and Bridging the Gap Communications. Washington, DC.

53. Van Look, P. F., & Von Hertzen, H. (1993). Emergency contraception. *British Medical Bulletin, 49*(1), 158–170.

54. Gerchufsky, M. (1996). Ending condom confusion. *ADVANCE for Nurse Practitioners, 4*(6), 39–42, 60.

55. Gebbie, A. (1995). Barrier methods of contraception. *British Journal of Sexual Medicine,* 12–15.

56. Vinson, R. P., & Epperly, T. D. (1991). Counseling patients on proper use of condoms. *American Journal Family Practice, 43*(6), 2081–2085.

57. Gerchufsky, M. (1996). Issues and answers in latex sensitivity. *ADVANCE for Nurse Practitioners, 4*(6), 15–19.

58. Shiata, A. A., & Trussell, J. (1991). New female intravaginal barrier contraceptive device: Preliminary clinical trial. *Contraception, 44*(1), 11–19.

59. The Female Health Company. Division of Wisconsin Pharmacal. (1994). *Reality female condom: An alternative for women.* Chicago: Wisconsin Pharmacal.

60. Farr, G., Gabelnick, H., Sturgen, K., et al. (1994). Contraceptive efficacy and acceptability of the female condom. *American Journal Public Health, 84,* 1960–1964.

61. Staff. (1995). Contraceptive update: The female condom, controlled by women. *Network, Family Health International, 16*(1), 23–26.

62. Zekeng, L., Feldblum, P. J., Oliver, R. M., et al. (1993). Barrier Contraceptive use and HIV infection among high risk women in Cameroon. *AIDS, 7,* 725–731.

63. Barnett, B. (1996). Microbicide research aims to prevent STDs. *Network, Family Health International, 16*(3), 15–18.

64. Tagg, P. I. (1995). The diaphragm: Barrier contraception has a new social role. *Nurse Practitioner, 20*(12), 36–42.

65. Brokaw, A. K., Baker, N. N., & Harvey, S. L. (1988). Fitting the cervical cap. *Nurse Practitioner, 13*(7), 49–55.

66. Scott, P. M. (1996). How to fit a cervical cap. *JAAPA,* 83–88.

67. Rosenberg, M. J., Davidson, A. J., Chen, J. H., Judson, F. N., et al. (1992). Barrier contraception and STDs in women: A comparison of female-dependent methods and condoms. *American Journal Public Health, 82*(5), 669–674.

68. Chalker, R. (1987). *The complete cervical cap guide.* New York: Harper and Row.

69. GynoPharma. (1988). Paragard, CuT 380A. *Prescribing information.*

70. Alza Corporation. (1988). *Progestasert intrauterine progesterone contraceptive system.* Product information.

71. Ortiz, M. E., & Croxatto, H. B. (1987). The mode of action of IUDs. *Contraception, 36*(1), 37–53.

72. Siven, I. (1989). IUDs are contraceptives, not abortifacients: A comment on research and belief. *Studies in Family Planning, 20,* 355–359.

73. Sieven, I., Stern, J., Coutinho, E., Mattos, C. E. R., Diaz, S., et al. (1991). Prolonged intrauterine contraception: A seven-year randomized study of the levonorgestrel 20 mcg/day (L Ng20) and the Copper T 380A IUDs, *Contraception, 44*(5), 473–480.

74. Rivera, R., Farr, G., & Chi, I. (1993). *The copper IUD, safe and effective, the international experi-*

ence of Family Health International. Research Triangle Park, NC: Family Health International.

75. Farley, T. M., Rosenberg, M. S., Rowe, P. J., Chen, S. H., & Meirik, O. (1992). Intrauterine devices and PID: An international perspective. *Lancet, 339*(8796), 778–785.

76. Nelson, A. (1995, Oct.). Patient selection key to IUD success. *Contemporary Ob-Gyn,* Reprint.

77. Pollack, Amy. (1993). Male and female sterilization: Long term health consequences. *Outlook, 11*(1), 4–8.

78. Staff. (1996). Sterilization. *ACOG Technical Bulletin, 222,* 1–7.

79. Hieu, D. T., Tan, T. T., Tan, D. N., & Nguget, P. T. (1993). 31,781 cases of non-surgical female sterilization with quinacrine pellets in Vietnam. *Lancet, 342*(8865), 213–217.

80. Barnett, B. (1994). FHI's role in search for non-surgical sterilization. *Network: Family Health International, 14*(4), 26–29.

81. Staff. *No-scalpel vasectomy: An illustrated guide for surgeons.* NY: AVSC International.

82. Peterson, H. B. (1996). Update on female sterilization: Failure rates, counseling issues and post-sterilization regret. *The Contraceptive Report, 7*(3), 1–13.

83. Centers for Disease Control. (1992). Surgical sterilization among women and use of condoms, Baltimore, 1989–90. *MMWR, 41,* 568–575.

84. Hayes, R. B., Pattern, L. M., Greenberg, R., Schoeberg, J., Swanson, G. M., Liff, J., et al. (1993). Vasectomy and prostate cancer in U.S. blacks and whites. *American Journal of Epidemiology, 137,* 263–269.

85. Giovannuci, E., Ascherio, A., Rimm, E. B., Colditz, G. A., et al. (1993). A prospective cohort study of vasectomy and prostate cancer in U.S. men. *JAMA, 269,* 873–877.

86. Giovannucci, E., Tasteson, T. D., Speizer, F. E., et al. (1993). A retrospective cohort study of vasectomy and prostate cancer in U.S. men. *JAMA, 269,* 878–882.

87. Wilcox, L. S., Chu, S. U., Eaker, E. D., Zeger, S. L., & Peterson, H. B. (1991). Risk factors for regret after tubal sterilization: 5 years of follow-up in a prospective study. *Fertility-Sterilization, 55,* 927–933.

88. Peterson, H. B., Xia, Z., Hughes, J. M., Wilcox, L. S., Tyler, L. R., & Trussell, J. (1997). The risk of ectopic pregnancy after tubal sterilization. *New England Journal of Medicine, 336*(11), 762–767.

89. AVSC. (1992). *Family planning counseling: The international experience.* New York: Author.

90. Weschler, T. (1995). *Taking charge of your fertility: The definitive guide to natural birth control and pregnancy achievement.* New York: Harper Collins.

91. Kass-Annese, B., Danzer, H. (1992). *The fertility awareness handbook.* Alameda, CA: Hunter House.

92. Rodrigues-Garcia, R. (ed.). (1989). *Natural Family Planning: A good option.* Washington, DC: Institute for Reproductive Health, Georgetown University.

93. Labbok, M., & Queenan, J. (1989). The use of periodic abstinence for family planning. *Clinical Obstetrics and Gynecology, 32*(2), 387–402.

94. Katz, D. (1991). Human cervical mucus: Research update. *American Journal of Obstetrics and Gynecology, 165*(6–2), 1984–1986.

95. Trussell, J., & Grammer-Strawn, L. (1991). Further analysis of contraceptive failure of the ovulation method. *American Journal of Obstetrics-Gynecology, 165*(6–2), 2054–2059.

96. Lethbridge, D. J. (1991). Coitus interruptus: Considerations as a birth control method. *JOGN Nursing, 20*(1), 80–85.

97. Labbok, M. H., Perez, A., Valdes, V., Sevilla, F., et al. (1994). The Lactational Amenorrhea method (LAM): A postpartum introductory family planning method with policy and program implications. *Advances in Contraception, 10*(2), 93–109.

98. Labbok, M., & Queenan, J. (1992). Clinical study of the Lactational Amenorrhea Method for family planning. *The Lancet, 339,* 968–970.

99. Labbok, M., Cooney, K., & Cole, S. (1994). *Guidelines: Breastfeeding, family planning and the Lactational Amenorrhea Method.* Washington, DC: Institute for Reproductive Health.

100. Staff. (1996). *Are you offering your clients all the options?* Washington, DC: Institute for Reproductive Health.

101. Rosenberg, M. J., & Phillips, R. S. (1992). Does douching promote ascending infection? *Journal of Reproductive Medicine, 37*(11), 930–938.

102. Phillips, R. S., Tuomala, R. E., Feldblum, P. J., Schachter, J., Rosenberg, M. J., & Aronson, M. D. (1992). The effect of cigarette smoking, chlamydia trachamatis infection and vaginal douching in ectopic pregnancy. *Ob-Gyn, 79*(1), 85–90.

103. Gold, R. B. (1990). *Abortion and women's health: A turning point for America?* New York: Alan Guttmacher Institute.

104. Chalker, R., & Downer, C. (1992). *A woman's book of choices: Abortion, menstrual extraction,*

RU-486. New York, London: Four Walls Eight Windows.

105. Hern, W. (1990). *Abortion practice.* Philadelphia: J. B. Lippincott Co.

106. Hacker, N. F., & Moore, J. G. (1993). *Essentials of obstetrics and gynecology.* Philadelphia: Saunders.

107. Henshaw, S. K. (1991). The accessibility of abortion services in the United States. *Family Planning Perspectives, 20*(4), 169–176.

108. Winikoff, B. (1995). Acceptability of medical abortion in early pregnancy. *Family Planning Perspectives, 27*(4), 142–148, 185.

109. Wiebe, E. R. (1996). Abortion induced with methotrexate and misoprostol. *Canadian Medical Association Journal, 154*(2), 165–170.

110. Creinin, M. D., Vittinghoff, E., Galbraith, S., & Kaisle, C. (1995). A randomized trial comparing misoprostal three and seven days after methotrexate for early abortion. *American Journal of Obstetrics and Gynecology, 175*(5), 1578–1584.

111. Creinin, M. D., & Vittinghoff, E. (1994). Methotrexate and misoprostol alone for early abortion. A randomized controlled trial. *JAMA, 272*(15), 1190–1195.

112. Hausknecht, R. U. (1995). Methotrexate and misoprostol to terminate early pregnancy. *New England Journal of Medicine, 333*(9), 537–540.

113. Castle, M., Coeytaux, F. (1994). RU-486. Beyond the controversy: Implications for health care practice. *JAMWA. 49*(55), 154–164.

114. Brogden, R. N., Goa, K. L., & Faulds, D. (1993). Mifepristone. A review of its pharmacodynamic and pharmacokinetic properties and therapeutic potential. *Drugs, 45*(3), 384–409.

115. El-Refaey, H., Rajasekar, D., Abdalla, M., Caldar, L., & Templeton, A. Induction of abortion with mifepristone (RU-486) and oral or vaginal misoprostol. *New England Journal of Medicine, 332*(15), 983–987.

116. Weiss, B. D. (1993). RU-486. The progesterone antagonist. *Archives of Family Medicine, 2*(1), 63–69.

117. Baird, D. T. (1993). Clinical uses of mifepristone (RU-486). *Annals of Medicine, 25*(1), 65–69.

118. World Health Organization. *Special program of research development and research training in human reproduction.* (1994). Report of Task Force on methods for the regulation of male fertility.

119. Comhaire, F. H. (1994). Male contraception: Hormonal, mechanical and other. *Human Reproduction, 9*(4), 586–590.

120. World Health Organization Task Force on Methods for Regulation of Male Fertility. (1990). Contraceptive efficacy of testosterone-induced azoospermia in normal men. *Lancet, 336,* 955–959.

121. Finger, W. R. (1995). Future male methods may include injectables. *Network: Family Health Internations, 15*(3), 9–13.

122. Guha, S. K., Anand, S., Ansari, S., Farrog, A., & Sharma, D. N. (1990). Time controlled injectable occlusion of the vas deferens. *Contraception, 41*(3), 323–331.

123. Nowak, R. (1994). Antihypertension drug may double as male contraceptive. *Journal of NIH Research, 6,* 27–30.

124. Yang, J., Serres, C., Philibert, D., et al. (1994). Progesterone and RU-486: Opposing effects on human sperm. *Proc. National Academy of Science, 91,* 529–533.

125. Staff. (1995). One rod implant, easy to insert. *Network: Family Health International, 16*(1), 1.

126. Chi, I. (1993). The T Cu-380A (AG), ML Cu 375, and Nova-T IUDs and the IUD daily releasing 20 micrograms levonorgestrel-four pillars of IUD contraception for the nineties and beyond? *Contraception, 47,* 325.

127. Rybo, G., Anderson, K., & Odlind, V. (1993). Hormonal intrauterine devices. *Annals of Medicine, 25*(2), 143–147.

128. Van Os, W. A., deNooyer, C. C., Kivijarvi, A., & Nahmonovici, C. (1993). Intracervical anchoring: A new approach to intrauterine contraception. *Advances in Contraception, 9*(1), 65–69.

129. Barnett, Barbara. (1996). Developing new diaphragms, condoms and similar devices. *Network: Family Health International, 16*(3), 19.

130. Mauck, C. K., Cordero, M. Babelnick, H. L., et al. (1994). *Barrier contraceptives: current status and future prospects.* New York: Wiley-Liss.

131. Griffin, P. D. (1994). Immunization against HCG. *Human Reproduction, 9*(2), 267–272.

132. Bedford, J. M. (1994). The contraceptive potential of fertilization: A physiologic perspective. *Human Reproduction, 9*(5), 842–858.

133. Edwards, R. G. (1994). Implantation, interception and contraception. *Human Reproduction, 9*(6), 985–995.

BIBLIOGRAPHY

AVSC International. (1994). *No scalpel vasectomy: An illustrated guide for surgeons.* New York: AVSC.

Baylor College of Medicine. (1994). Inserting and removing levonorgestrel subdermal implants: An update. *Contraceptive Report, 5,* 4–12.

Darney, P. D. (1995). Contraceptive implants: Proper technique for rapid problem-free removal. *Women's Health Reports, 1,* 9–16.

Darney, P. D., Klaisle, C. M., & Walker, D. M. (1992). The pop-out method of Norplant removal. *Adv. Contraception, 8,* 188–189.

Guillebaud, J. (1994). *Contraception: Your questions answered.* Edinburgh: Churchill-Livingstone.

Hatcher, R. A., Trussel, J., Steward, F., Howells, S., Russell, C. R., & Kowal, D. (1995). *Emergency contraception: The nation's best kept secret.* Decatur, GA: Bridging the Gap Communications.

Klaisle, C., & Darney, P. D. (1995, March/April). A guide to removing contraceptive implants. *Contemp. NP,* 32–44.

Praptohardjo, U., & Wibowo, S. (1993). The "U" technique: A new method of Norplant removal. *Journal of Family Practice, 40,* 173–180.

Reynolds, R.D. (1995). The "Modified U" technique: A refined method of Norplant removal. *Journal of Family Practice, 40,* 173–180.

Sarma, S. P., & Hatcher, R. (1994). The Emory Method: A modified approach to Norplant implants removal. *Contraception, 49,* 551–556.

Shihata, A. A., Salzetti, R. G., Schnepper, F. W., et al. (1995). Innovative technique for Norplant implants removal. *Contraception, 51,* 83–85.

U.S. Preventive Services Taskforce. (1989). Adult counseling for STDs and HIV infection. In *Guide to clinical preventive services.* Baltimore: Williams and Wilkins.

U.S. Preventive Services Taskforce. (1989). Counseling to prevent unintended pregnancy. In *Guide to clinical preventive services.* Baltimore: Williams and Wilkins.

World Health Organization. (1990). *Norplant contraceptive subdermal implants: Managerial and technical guidelines.* Geneva, WHO.

ADDENDUM TO TABLE 9–6

Additions to Table 9–6 (pp. 171–173) have been added prior to press date.

ADDENDUM TO TABLE 9–6. ORAL CONTRACEPTIVE TYPES, DOSAGES, AND PHYSIOLOGICAL ACTIVITIES[a]

Oral Contraceptive	Progestational Activity	Androgenic Activity	Endometrial Activity
Low Dose Monophasics			

Alesse (Wyeth-Ayerst) 21 or 28 day
  0.10 mg levonorgestrel
  0.02 mg ethinyl estradiol
	Low	Low/Intermediate	Low

Triphasic			

Estrostep (Park-Davis) 21 day
  5 days: 1 mg norethindrone acetate
      0.02 mg ethinyl estradiol
  7 days: 1 mg norethindrone acetate
      0.03 mg ethinyl estradiol
  9 days: 1 mg norethindrone acetate
      0.035 mg ethinyl estradiol
	Intermediate	Intermediate	Low

Estrostep Fe (Park-Davis) 28 day
  5 days: 1 mg norethindrone acetate
      0.02 mg ethinyl estradiol
  7 days: 1 mg norethindrone acetate
      0.03 mg ethinyl estradiol
  9 days: 1 mg norethindrone acetate
      0.035 mg ethinyl estradiol
  7 days: 75 mg ferrous fumerate
	Intermediate	Intermediate	Low

[a]Physiological activities based upon author's interpretation of manufacturers' inserts and activities of similar oral contraceptive formulations in Table 9–6.

CHAPTER 10

INFERTILITY

Cathy A. James

The etiology of infertility can be identified in 85 to 90 percent of couples: 30 percent have male factor infertility, 35 percent have female factor infertility, and 20 percent have a combination of male and female factors.

Highlights

- History, Physical Examination, Diagnostic Studies
- Psychosocial Evaluation
- Female Infertility
    Hypothalamic Disorders
    Pituitary Disorders
    Adrenal Disorders
    Ovarian Disorders
    Uterine Disorders
    Pelvic Disorders
    Recurrent Pregnancy Loss
- Male Infertility
    Endocrine Disorders
    Varicocele
    Genetic Abnormalities, Acquired Obstruction
    Sperm Transport Dysfunction
- Combined Female and Male Factors
- Selected Infertility Treatments
    Ovulation Induction
    Artificial Insemination
    Assisted Reproductive Technologies
- Adoption, Surrogacy, Childfree Living
- Nursing Diagnoses

► INTRODUCTION

Infertility is the inability to conceive after a year of regular unprotected intercourse or to carry a pregnancy to a live birth. Primary infertility means that the couple has never conceived. Secondary infertility occurs when the couple has previously conceived, regardless of the pregnancy outcome.

Today, couples are more aware of specific causes of infertility and of the sophisticated treatments available. Consequently, they increasingly are seeking treatment, as infant adoption resources are becoming depleted. The number of available infertility services is increasing, as evidenced by increased membership in the American Society for Reproductive Medicine (formerly the American Fertility Society) and the creation of the subspecialty Reproductive Endocrinology by the American Board of Obstetrics and Gynecology. The National Certification Corporation for the Obstetric, Gynecologic, and Neonatal Nursing Specialties (NCC) offers certification for registered nurses in reproductive endocrinology/infertility. In many cases, however, health care insurance may not share the burden of treatment costs to diagnose or treat infertility.

Infertility is a widespread problem that often is initially identified in the obstetric/gynecologic, or less commonly, the urologic practice. It is imperative that the nurse practitioner recognize infertility and understand its causes and treatment options. Prevention of infertility is another piece that should be incorporated into the nurse practitioner's practice. Evaluation and treatment may be initiated in the general practice. The necessity of referral to a specialist is determined by the type of setting, credentials of staff, resources to treat, and efficacy of treatment, as well as the woman's age and diagnosis of woman.

The reproductive endocrinologist and nurse practitioner in the reproductive endocrinology/infertility practice collaborate as closely as they would in any medical setting. The health care provider's role is multifaceted: to diagnose and treat; to identify multiple impacts on the individual, couple, and significant others; to provide information, support, and counseling; and to refer to specialties of internal medicine, endocrinology, urology, psychiatry, and reproductive endocrinology. Other roles include research, community education, and advocacy.

Approximately 10 to 15 percent of couples in the United States experience infertility.[1] This is approximately 5 million couples, with 1.3 million seeking care for this problem.[2] Couples are postponing marriage and delaying childbearing to pursue advanced education and careers or to achieve financial stability. This delay may enhance factors related to infertility such as the effect of age on fecundity, increased risk of exposure to sexually transmitted diseases and increased risk of endometriosis with increased age.[3] In the 1980s and 1990s, one out of five American women had her first child after age 35. Yet, about one third of women who defer pregnancy until the mid-to-late 30s will have an infertility problem.[4]

CAUSATIVE FACTORS IN INFERTILITY

- *Aging.* Reduced frequency of intercourse, decline in ovarian and uterine function, decrease in oocyte quality, increase in aneuploidy and resulting spontaneous abortions, and increase in diseases of the reproductive tract, in particular endometriosis.[5]

- *Sexually Transmitted Diseases (STDs).* Leading to fallopian tube disease.
- *Exposure to Occupational Hazards.* Chemicals, radiation, noise.
- *Exposure to Environmental Hazards.* Heat, smoking, alcohol, drug abuse.

The cumulative effects of the choice to delay fertility—biologic factors, sexual practices, and exposure to environmental toxins—have resulted in an increase in infertility. The proportion of infertile couples has not changed, but there are more couples due to the aging of the baby boomers.[4]

INFERTILITY EVALUATION

Evaluation must be couple oriented, systematic, thorough, and completed within a reasonable time frame. The American Society for Reproductive Medicine (formerly the American Fertility Society) published Guidelines for the Provision of Infertility Services, which recognizes that many different health care providers, including nurse practitioners, provide care to couples experiencing infertility. As infertility treatments can range from basic to complex, three levels of care have been described.[6] Depending on the setting, protocols of practice in the state and the collaborative practice, the nurse practitioner may participate in the infertility evaluation, educate and support the couple, prescribe some initial interventions, and initiate referral to a specialist. Evaluation is recommended if a couple has not conceived after 1 year of attempting pregnancy or after 6 months if the woman is 35 or older.[5] The evaluation may begin sooner if other factors known to affect fertility exist or if the couple is very anxious.

The etiology of infertility can be identified in 90 percent of couples; 10–15 percent have unexplained infertility (no abnormality found). Thirty percent have male factor infertility, 35 percent have female factor infertility, and 20 percent have a combination of male and female factors.[4,7] Multiple factors of infertility become more difficult to overcome.

The essential data for a thorough evaluation are those gleaned from a history and physical examination of the couple (see Tables 10–1 through 10–5).

DIAGNOSTIC TESTS AND METHODS

Numbers 1 through 6 following are the steps of a routine assessment. The order in which they are performed depends on the client's history and age.

TABLE 10–1. FEMALE HISTORY: SUMMARY OF PERTINENT DATA

Age of client.

Menstrual history (age at menarche, length of cycle, duration of flow, amount of flow, dysmenorrhea. If amenorrhea present, duration).

Symptoms of ovulation (midcycle spotting, mittelschmerz, increased midcycle vaginal discharge, breast tenderness, mood swings, acne).

Gynecologic history (contraceptive history, especially IUDs and Depo-Provera; Pelvic Inflammatory Disease; sexually transmitted infection; diethylstilbestrol exposure; douching; D&C).

Obstetric history (previous pregnancies and outcomes, time taken to conceive).

Frequency of coitus, sexual practices, sexual dysfunction.

Medical history (galactorrhea, hirsutism, heat or cold intolerance).

Surgical history (cryotherapy, conization or loop electrosurgical excision procedure of cervix for abnormal Pap smear).

Social history (multiple partners, alcohol, tobacco or recreational drugs).

Family history (genetic or reproductive abnormalities).

Source: Adapted from Edwards, R. G., & Brody, S. A. (1995). Principles and practice of assisted human reproduction. Philadelphia: W.B. Saunders Company.

Basal Body Temperature (BBT) Chart

The BBT chart helps to determine the time of ovulation (after ovulation, a sustained temperature rise of 0.4–0.6° F occurs due to the influence of progesterone from the corpus luteum) and to plan and interpret fertility tests (see Chapter 9). A BBT thermometer or a digital thermometer should be used. The woman takes her temperature

TABLE 10–2. FEMALE PHYSICAL EXAM: SUMMARY OF PERTINENT DATA

Neurological symptoms (headache, visual field loss, papilledema, olfactory dysfunction).

Thyroid size, consistency, presence of nodules.

Breast development, lumps, galactorrhea.

Abdominal distention, tenderness.

Hair pattern over entire body. Tanner staging for pubic hair, male versus female pubic hair patterns.

External genitalia, normal Tanner staging, clitoromegaly.

Cervix: mucus correlated to cycle day, stenosis, pink, smooth, moist.

Uterus and ovaries, size, shape and consistency, mobility, tenderness.

Source: Adapted from Edwards, R. G., & Brody, S. A. (1995). Principles and practice of assisted human reproduction. Philadelphia: W.B. Saunders Company.

TABLE 10–3. MALE HISTORY: SUMMARY OF PERTINENT DATA

Duration of couple's infertility.

Previous paternities, including time to conceive.

General health, pubescence, disorders of the urogenital tract.

Frequency and timing of coitus, sexual practices.

Contraceptive methods (condoms, vasectomy).

Exposure to toxins, excessive warmth, or irradiation.

Drugs (chemotherapy, anabolic steroids, hypertensive medications, caffeine, nicotine, alcohol, recreational drugs).

Developmental characteristics, e.g., onset of secondary sex characteristics, descent of the testes, and abnormalities of general development. (This may indicate endocrinological causes of reproductive dysfunction.)

Histories of any sexually transmitted diseases, systemic febrile illnesses, or genital infections such as mumps, chickenpox, or other forms of orchitis.

Surgical history, e.g., inguinal herniorrhaphy, injuries to the vas or bladder neck, retroperitoneal node dissection, testicular cancer, or circumcision.

Testicular torsion or general trauma.

Gynecomastia or anosmia.

Source: Adapted from Edwards, R. G., & Brody, S. A. (1995). Principles and practice of assisted human reproduction. *Philadelphia: W.B. Saunders Company.*

TABLE 10–4. MALE PHYSICAL EXAM: SUMMARY OF PERTINENT DATA

State of virilization (hair pattern, body proportions, muscle development).

Neurological symptoms (libido, headache, visual symptoms, papilledema, olfactory dysfunction).

Thyroid size, consistency, presence of nodules.

Presence of gynecomastia and/or galactorrhea.

Penis, circumcised, Tanner staging.

Testicular location, size, volume, and consistency.

Presence of epididymis and vas deferens.

Varicocele.

Prostate size, consistency.

Source: Adapted from Sherins, R. J. (1995). How is male infertility defined? How is it diagnosed? Epidemiology, causes, work-up (history, physical, lab tests). In The American Society of Andrology, Handbook of Andrology. Lawrence, KS: Allen Press, Inc. Edwards, R. G., & Brody, S. A. (1995). Principles and practice of assisted human reproduction. *Philadelphia: W.B. Saunders Company.*

immediately upon waking in the morning. Three months or more of charts provide better prediction of ovulation. It must be emphasized that infections, travel, stress, and irregular sleep patterns may cause a 20–30 percent margin of error.[8]

Postcoital Test (PCT)

The PCT must be well timed: it is performed just before expected ovulation. BBT charts, urine or serum LH, or ultrasound monitoring may be used to predict ovulation based on timing of the LH surge.[9] The couple should refrain from intercourse during the 1 to 2 days before the test; then they should have intercourse without the use of lubricants (both surgilube and KY Jelly may immobilize sperm), 2 to 12 hours prior to the appointment. The woman may shower but should not take a tub bath or douche before the appointment. A sample of mucus is taken from the cervix and microscopically assessed for quality of mucus and number of motile sperm.

- A normal test, resulting from preovulatory estrogen levels, shows clear mucus; spinnbarkeit

(SPBK), the elasticity of cervical mucus, is approximately 10 cm. Ferning appears (on a dry slide), and 5 to 10 motile sperm per high power field (HPF) are seen. This test has become somewhat more objective by using the cervical mucus score (see Table 10–6).[10]

- An abnormal test may be due to improper timing. If that is the case, schedule a repeat in 2 days. If the PCT test is well timed, repeat it during the next cycle. Abnormality may be due to coital technique; ovulatory disorder; loss of endocervical secretory cells from cryotherapy, laser, loop electrosurgery excision procedure, or deep conization for treatment of cervical disease; sperm factors or the presence of antisperm antibodies.[9]

Semen Analysis (SA)

Early in a woman's evaluation, her partner, after 2–7 days of abstinence, collects a semen specimen by means of masturbation or, less commonly, by use of a special condom. The semen is deposited directly into a clean container and evaluated, within an hour of collection, microscopically on a dry slide or preferably in a Makler chamber. Semen analyses vary in different labs.

TABLE 10–5. COPING WITH INFERTILITY: INDIVIDUALS AND COUPLES

Coping with Infertility

Perception of problem, cause of infertility.

Knowledge of sexual function, anatomy, reproductive cycle.

Meaning of ability or inability to have a child (or another child).

Beliefs and values, motivations for pregnancy, responses of significant others to childbearing/child rearing.

Responses to Infertility

Stages of crisis/grief (shock or disbelief, anger, isolation, guilt, depression, grief, resolution).

Ability to identify and verbalize feelings; past experiences and effects on feelings, expectations of partner.

Affect on lives and relationship.

Affect on sexual relationship.

Significant others' awareness of infertility, responses to infertility/treatment.

Coping Strategies

Problem solving/decision making abilities.

Patterns of communication.

Use of support systems.

Ability to modify stressors in environment.

Source: Adapted from Menning, B. E. (1988). Infertility: A guide for the childless couple (2nd ed.). Englewood Cliffs, NJ: Prentice Hall Press.

- Normal semen analysis per the World Health Organization (WHO):[11]
  - *Volume.* 2 to 5 mL.
  - *Viscosity.* Liquefaction occurs in 1 hour.
  - *pH.* 7 to 8.
  - *Count.* Equal to or greater than 20 million per mL.
  - *Motility.* Equal to or greater than 50 percent.
  - *Quality of Motion (Forward Progression).* (How fast and how straight the sperm swims). Greater than 3 (on a 0–4 scale with 0 = no movement, to 4 = excellent forward progression).
  - *Morphology.* Greater than 30 percent normal oval heads, midpiece and tail.
  - *Kruger's Strict Criteria.* Greater than 14 percent normal forms. Kruger developed strict criteria for morphology, which have proven to be more predictive of fertilization in in vitro fertilization (IVF) cycles. This system identifies greater than 14 percent normal

TABLE 10–6. THE CERVICAL MUCUS SCORE

A. Volume

0: 0 mL
1: 0.1 mL
2: 0.2 mL
3: 0.3 mL or more

B. Consistency

0: Thick, highly "viscous," premenstrual mucus
1: Mucus of intermediate "viscosity"
2: Mildly "viscous" mucus
3: Watery, minimally "viscous," midcycle (preovulatory) mucus

C. Ferning

0: No crystallization
1: Atypical fern formation
2: Primary and secondary stem ferning
3: Tertiary and quaternary stem ferning

D. Spinnbarkeit

0: < 1 cm
1: 1–4 cm
2: 5–8 cm
3: 9 cm or more

E. Cellularity

0: > 20 WBCs per hpf
1: 11–20 WBCs per hpf
2: 1–10 WBCs per hpf
3: 0 WBCs
hpf—high power field

Source: Boyers, S. P. (1995). Evaluation and treatment of disorders of the cervix. In W. R. Keye, Jr., R. J. Chang, R. W. Rebar, & M. R. Soules (Eds.), Infertility: Evaluation and treatment. Philadelphia: W.B. Saunders Company. Used with permission.

forms as "normal," 4–14 percent as "good prognosis," and less than 4 percent as "poor prognosis."[12]
  - *White Blood Cell (WBC) Count.* Less than 1 million per mL.
- Abnormal semen analysis requires that the test be repeated in 4 to 6 weeks.
- If time is not critical, 3 months should be allowed to complete a sperm cycle if a viral illness, hot bath, or toxicants could have caused poor semen parameters.[5,13]
- Some studies suggest that ureaplasma attaches to sperm and reduces motility, so it is reasonable to obtain semen cultures if male factor infertility is present.[4] With positive ureaplasma/mycoplasma

semen culture, treatment of both partners is indicated: one coated 100-mg doxycycline hyclate pellet (Doryx) daily, p.o., for 30 days, beginning with the first day of the woman's full menstrual flow. It is necessary to prevent pregnancy by protected intercourse or abstinence during the cycle of treatment.

- Normal semen parameters indicate no further male evaluation is necessary unless infertility persists.[1]

Hysterosalpingogram (HSG)

An x-ray test is performed by the physician after menses but before ovulation. Radioactive dye is placed in the uterus to outline the uterine cavity and determine the patency of the fallopian tubes. Waterbased dye gives a better picture, but oil based can push mucus out the fallopian tubes, which may have been blocking them. Some physicians will use both to take advantage of the benefits of each type of dye. Cramping can be reduced by having the woman take 600–800 mg of ibuprofin 1 hour prior to the test. The client may have a paracervical block and/or be given a sedative, midazolam HCL/Roche (Versed), which will virtually eliminate discomfort. Advise the client that someone must accompany her home and that she should wear a sanitary pad for fluid leakage and spotting. Prophylactic antibiotic therapy is often given prior to HSG.

Endometrial Biopsy

The biopsy is performed late in the menstrual cycle, 2–3 days before expected menses. The nurse practitioner uses a Novak curette or pipelle to take a fundal sample of the endometrium[14] after making sure of a BBT rise (biphasic). It will document the probable occurrence of ovulation and the production of adequate luteal phase progesterone. Many health care providers perform an endometrial biopsy only after a negative pregnancy test. The risk of biopsy to an undetected pregnancy is small; however, some couples decide to have protected intercourse or to abstain during this cycle. Cramping during and shortly after the biopsy can be reduced by the client taking 600–800 mg of ibuprofin 1 hour prior to the test. Advise her

to wear a sanitary pad home because of the spotting that occurs (see Chapter 8).

- The endometrial tissue is assigned a cycle day based on histology findings.
- Test results are interpreted by the nurse practitioner only after the client has called with her menses, which becomes cycle day 28. The cycle day of the biopsy is determined by counting back from cycle day 28. The biopsy is normal, and thus no luteal phase deficiency, if the cycle days are ± 2 days. For example, an endometrial biopsy done on 5/1/97 is read as cycle day 25. Menses was three days later on 5/4/97, thus 5/3/97 is now classified as cycle day 28; 28 – 2 = cycle day 26 when the biopsy was done. The result reads 25, so this a normal test result.

Laparoscopy—Diagnostic or Therapeutic

The laparoscopy is performed early in the cycle, after menses, as outpatient surgery, usually under general anesthesia. It is recommended after other tests have been completed, unless the woman is experiencing severe pelvic pain. The laparoscope is inserted through the navel to visualize the pelvis. Laser or cautery can be used to treat endometriosis, pelvic adhesions or scarring, and some tubal diseases at the time of the diagnostic laparoscopy, thereby avoiding the need for major abdominal inpatient surgery. Usually the client can return home in several hours (see Chapter 13).

Hysteroscopy with Laparoscopy

The procedure is performed early during a woman's cycle, after menses, especially when uterine anomalies have been identified (abnormal HSG or ultrasound). Laparoscopy is performed in conjunction with hysteroscopy to delineate the external uterine contour, thus differentiating between a bicornate or septate uterus. The laser or cautery can be used at hysteroscopy to lyse adhesions, repair septa, or remove polyps or fibroids.

Additional Diagnostic Tests

A client's history may indicate the need for other tests. The history will determine how early in the workup these tests will be completed.

- A Papanicolaou (Pap) smear is done to rule out cervical cancer and inflammatory processes suggestive of infection. The procedure may suggest cervical stenosis (see Chapter 5).
- Chlamydia culture will rule out *Chlamydia trachomatis* infection (see Chapters 5 and 11).
- Serum progesterone will suggest the occurrence of ovulation but is not considered an absolute indicator of normal ovulation, as the client could have luteinized unruptured follicle syndrome.
- Serum prolactin test will rule out hyperprolactinemia (see Chapter 8).
- Serum thyroid stimulating hormone (TSH), triiodothyronine (T_3), thyroxine (T_4), and free T_4 tests will rule out hyperthyroid/hypothyroid disease including subclinical presentations.

PSYCHOSOCIAL ASPECTS OF INFERTILITY EVALUATION

Many couples take for granted that they are fertile and hence are not emotionally prepared for the psychological impact of a diagnosis of infertility. Pain and distress may be no less severe for couples who experience secondary infertility. A couple's ability to admit that they may have a fertility problem is an important first step, but they may also feel threatened as potential causes are identified and treatment recommended. Infertility is a couple's problem, not an individual's. Both partners need to be involved in diagnostic and treatment choices and to accompany each other to appointments when possible.

THE RESPONSES AND NEEDS OF PARTNERS

Crises of Infertility

Infertility threatens self-esteem, body image, masculinity/femininity, and sexual relations. It may not affect both partners at the same time or the same way. Table 10–7 lists some gender differences and the infertility experience.[15] Furthermore, one partner may not perceive the problem with the same emotional intensity or have the knowledge or energy to support the other partner. Prior coping strategies may be ineffective.[15]

TABLE 10–7. SOME GENDER DIFFERENCES AND THE INFERTILITY EXPERIENCE

Men

Expectations regarding fatherhood and family may be ambiguous.

Men often initially assume they are not the cause of the infertility.

In male factor infertility, men may experience strong guilt feelings, but are reluctant to express these feelings. They may undergo treatments or move forward with parenting alternatives prematurely.

Men often perceive their role as the optimist during the infertility crisis.

Workplace is seen by men as a distraction from the infertility crises.

Express anger and irritation toward medical personnel.

Women

See motherhood as primary goal of adulthood.

Women often initially assume they are the cause of the infertility.

In female factor infertility, women search endlessly for a cause and may reproach themselves for past "misdeeds."

Women become pessimistic regarding outcomes in an effort to protect themselves from disappointments.

Infertility often distracts women from efforts to be productive in the workplace.

Feel depressed and helpless.

Source: Applegarth, L. D. (1995). The psychological aspects of infertility. In W. R. Keye, Jr., R. J. Chang, R. W. Rebar, & M. R. Soules (Eds.), Infertility: Evaluation and treatment. Philadelphia: W.B. Saunders Company. Used with permission.

Emotional Responses

Shock and surprise are quickly replaced by denial (expressed as a need to try longer), which helps the couple to deal with intense feelings of loss. As denial subsides, anger emerges and intensifies as the couple loses privacy and undergoes invasive procedures. Often, significant others and health care professionals become targets for anger because the couple feels helpless and has experienced a loss of control. Anger displaced on the self becomes depression. Table 10–8 summarizes the common emotional responses to infertility.[15]

Support Systems

Partners may withdraw from each other and significant others in order to avoid uncomfortable sharing. It is often difficult for the couple to identify feelings, verbalize needs, and cope with multiple stressors. Significant persons may recognize the couple's needs but not know how to offer support. Ineffective communication results

TABLE 10–8. COMMON EMOTIONAL RESPONSES TO INFERTILITY (the manifestation of these responses may differ significantly between men and women)

Guilt
One or both partners assume blame for the infertility. Self-reproach increases and self-esteem decreases.

Depression
One or both partners develop a sense of hopelessness, loss and despair, tearfulness, fatigue, anxiety, sleep or eating disturbances, or an inability to concentrate. The onset of menses can often trigger a depression in many infertile couples.

Anger
The infertile couple often feels that life has treated them unfairly. They may feel out-of-control, resentful, and angry with others, including family, friends, and medical personnel.

Isolation
A sense of social separateness of feeling "left out" of the mainstream of life. Emotional and social isolation negatively impacts self-confidence and self-esteem.

Source: Applegarth, L. D. (1995). The psychological aspects of infertility. In W. R. Keye, Jr., R. J. Chang, R. W. Rebar, & M. R. Soules (Eds.), Infertility: Evaluation and treatment. Philadelphia: W. B. Saunders Company. Used with permission.

in increased stress, tension, guilt, and depression. It may even alter relationships and intensify marital dysfunction. If a couple has a child, they may have even less support in their quest to have another child because they "already have been blessed." When stepchildren are part of the family, the nonbiological parent may feel even more isolated and alone. Often, the partner who has experienced parenting does not have as much emotional energy invested in achieving a pregnancy.

Loss

Multiple losses, such as loss of control, loss of genetic continuity, loss of dream of jointly conceived children, loss of pregnancy and birth experience, and loss of opportunity to parent may accompany the infertility experience.[16] The couple needs to acknowledge these losses and to grieve in order to come to terms with the infertility.

Secondary Infertility

Couples who conceived previously with treatment soon remember the multiple impacts of infertility and experience hurt from the wounds that

they thought were healed. They also feel guilt because they want another child and feel pressured to conceive quickly using the same treatment as when they conceived previously.

PROFESSIONAL AND PSYCHOLOGICAL SUPPORT

The health care provider can assist the couple experiencing grief by giving accurate information; supporting or making referrals for individual, group, or sex therapy; and encouraging couples to use support services. Couples may contact the American Society for Reproductive Medicine (formerly the American Fertility Society) in Birmingham, Alabama, for information, or Resolve in Somerville, Massachusetts, to become involved in self-help groups on both a local and national level (see Resources). Couples may also need to be given permission to stop treatment.

The nurse practitioner can provide support and information to the couple to facilitate healthy adaptation/resolution. The many complex feelings associated with loss and infertility involve self-image, self-esteem, and sexuality. Past experiences and self-concept will affect the couple's understanding of problems and feelings and their problem solving or decision making abilities. Encourage clients to verbalize feelings and help them to strengthen their patterns of communication and support systems. The goal of intervention is to reduce stress, increase coping skills, and enable the couple to regain control and dignity. Referral to appropriate resources is often helpful. Resolution of infertility does not occur when a child is born or adopted, but rather when one no longer feels imperfect in relation to one's fertility, self-image, self-esteem, and sexuality. Couples who achieve a pregnancy after a history of infertility may either deny the pregnancy, thus not seek prenatal care in a timely fashion, or become hypervigilant regarding minor discomforts of pregnancy.[17] The nurse practitioner can help ease this transition by providing the couple with anticipatory guidance and by providing the obstetrician's office staff with the usual characteristics of such couples. Acknowledging and accepting differences between these couples and couples who have gotten pregnant in the usual manner are helpful to put the situation in perspective.

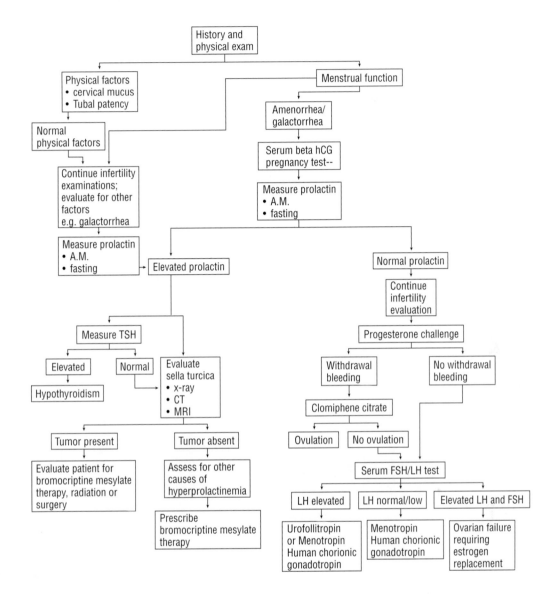

Figure 10–1. Suggested management guidelines: Diagnosis and treatment of the infertile female client. *(Used with the permission of Sandoz Pharmaceuticals Corporation.)*

FEMALE INFERTILITY: CAUSES, DIAGNOSES, AND INTERVENTIONS

Ovulatory disorders, which exist in 15 percent of infertile women,[4] may be related to hypothalamic, pituitary, adrenal, or ovarian dysfunction. Ovulation may occur infrequently (oligo-ovulation) or not at all (anovulation) (see Chapter 8).

Figure 10–1 outlines the diagnostic evaluation and treatment of the infertile female client. Table 10–9 describes specific treatment regimens for endocrine disorders and ovulation dysfunction. Drug dosages, common side effects, evaluation of the therapies, and continued treatment recommendations are included. Refer to *Drug Facts and Comparisons*[18] or other appropriate pharmacotherapeutic references for drug contraindications and a complete list of side effects.

TABLE 10–9. OVULATION INDUCTION[a]

Diagnosis	Drug/Action	Dose	Monitor	Side Effects	Continued Treatment
Increased DHEA-S (dehydroepiandrosterone sulfate).	Dexamethasone. Inhibits corticotropin release; decreases adrenal androgens.	0.5–0.75 mg p.o. q.h.s.	Serum cortisol. Basal body temperature (BBTs). Endometrial biopsy.	Rare. Decreases resistance to infection, response to medication. Masks symptoms of illness. (Wear ID bracelet.)	Anovulation: Clomiphene + dexamethasone
Increased PRL (prolactin).	Bromocriptine (dopamine agonist). Inhibits PRL production by pituitary. 90% attain normal PRL; 80% ovulate and conceive.	2.5–15 mg p.o. q.d. (Usual dose 2.5–7.5 mg.) Begin 1/2 tablet p.o. q.d.; add 1–2 tablets, p.o. q.d. over 2 weeks. Taper dose when discontinue.	PRL, 4 weeks after begin medication, then as necessary. Visual fields. BBTs. Endometrial biopsy.	Nausea (take with food/milk). Postural hypotension—causes dizziness. Careful operation of machinery. Headache.	Anovulation: Clomiphene + bromocriptine
Luteal phase defect.	Progesterone vaginal suppositories or progesterone capsules Enhances glandular development of endometrium. Conceive in 6–12 cycles.	Suppositories 25 mg b.i.d. 50 mg q.h.s. Capsules 100 mg p.o. t.i.d. Begin after BBT elevated for 2–3 days.	BBTs to assess change in luteal phase. Endometrial biopsy to determine endometrial response to treatment.	Delays onset of menses. Change in menstrual flow. Decrease in vaginal secretions. Vaginal irritation. Capsules may cause drowsiness; can take 1 in A.M. 2 in P.M.	No defect correction: Clomiphene
Oligo/anovulation. Polycystic ovarian syndrome (PCO). Normal PRL; increased LH; low to normal FSH.	Clomiphene citrate (CC) (antiestrogen). Binds to estrogen receptor sites. Prevents negative feedback of estrogen. Stimulates the pituitary. FSH rises; stimulates follicle development. 50–94% ovulate. 30–61% conceive. Conceive in 4–6 cycles. As indicated, use human chorionic gonadotropin hormone (Profasi, Pregnyl or APL) Finishes egg maturation. Triggers LH surge. Assists follicle rupture. Ovulation about 36 h after hCG.	50–200 mg p.o. Cycle days 5–9 (C$_{5–9}$). Start at 50-mg dose. In subsequent cycles increase dose by 50-mg increments if ovulation does not occur. Ovulation expected C$_{15–21}$. (Increased pregnancy rate occurs at lower doses.) Recommend 100 mg p.o. C$_{5–9}$ + ultrasound (U/S) C$_{15–17}$ and repeat p.r.n. until presence of 19–21 mm size follicle. Administer Profasi, Pregnyl, or APL 10,000 I.U. I.M.	BBTs to assess ovulation; pelvic or ultrasound exam (U/S) by C$_5$ to determine normal ovaries or presence of cyst. U/S monitoring of follicle development. Postcoital test (PCT) to check potential antiestrogen effects on cervical mucus. Intercourse midcycle week. Timed intercourse day of and next 2 days following administration of Profasi, Pregnyl or APL.	Mild headache, hot flashes, abdominal tenderness, bloating. With visual disturbances, stop clomiphene citrate. Multiple pregnancy rate (5%)—twins most often. Abdominal bloating, tenderness at injection site.	Clomiphene failure—no conception after 4–6 cycles. With anovulation or abnormal ovulation or abnormal cervical mucus, use: Gonadotropins Menotropin (Pergonal or Humegon): FSH/LH) or Urofollitropin (Metrodin or Fertinex: FSH).

232

Diagnosis	Treatment	Dose	Monitoring	Side Effects	Indications
Hypothalamic disorder. Hypogonadism.	*Priming Cycle* Medroxyprogesterone acetate (Provera) Conjugated estrogens, USP (Premarin) *and* Provera GnRH infusion pump: Factrel (subcutaneous)/Lutrepulse (I.V.) Directly stimulates hypothalamus— 90–95% ovulate, 30–35% conceive.[b] *Luteal Phase Support* Progesterone vaginal suppositories. (See Luteal Phase Defect.) *or* Profasi, Pregnyl, or APL. Enhances corpus luteum production of progesterone. (See Anovulation.)	10 mg p.o. × 10 days. *or* 1.25 mg p.o.—calendar days 1–25. 10 mg p.o. calendar days 14–25. Begin continuous infusion pump after menses. Subcutaneous 5–20 µg/dose. I.V. 2.5–5 µg/dose. Pulse q. 90 min. Ovulate within 3 weeks. See above. 1500–2500 I.U. I.M.× 3 doses.	Baseline serum estradiol (E_2)/FSH/LH. Repeat E_2 in 1 week of pump infusion and p.r.n. (Assesses biochemical activity of follicle—midcycle E_2 about 300 pg/mL.) Schedule ultrasound and repeat p.r.n. until follicle is about 20+ mm in size. BBTs. Use urine LH kit to detect LH surge to assist with timed intercourse. See Luteal Phase Defect. See Anovulation.	Provera: Spotting, headache, fluid retention, fatigue, depression. Premarin: Nausea, breast tenderness and fluid retention. GnRH infusion: Headache, hot flashes, abdominal discomfort, irritation at infusion site. Ovarian hyperstimulation. Treatment Expensive, multiple blood tests/office visits/adjustment to mechanics of pump. See Luteal Phase Defect. See Anovulation.	Anovulation or failure to conceive. Candidate for ovum donation IVF (does not respond well to gonadotropins).
Hypothalamic disorder (anorexia). Clomid failure.	Menotropin (Pergonal or Humegon) *or* Urofollitropin (Metrodin or Fertinex) Directly stimulates ovary. Increases FSH/LH 61–77% ovulate; 20–24% conceive in 6 cycles.[b] *and* Profasi, Pregnyl, or APL Day following last dose of gonadotropin. (See Anovulation.)	Begin cycle days 2–5 (C_{2-5}); 150 IU I.M. q.d. × 5 days, then vary pending E_2 and ultrasound results. May need 6–12 day course of daily injections. When appropriate E_2 levels and follicle size attained, administer hCG 5000–10,000 I.U. I.M.	Baseline; E_2 and U/S results serially p.r.n. (E_2 about 300 pg/mL per mature follicle 16–18 mm.) Urine LH kit to detect spontaneous LH surge. BBTs. PCT to determine adequacy of mucus. Timed intercourse (See Anovulation.)	Ovarian enlargement, abdominal bloating/ tenderness, fatigue, nausea, headache, diarrhea, weight gain; 6% of patients develop severe ovarian hyperstimulation syndrome, 20% have multiple gestation (twins). Irritation at injection sites. Painful/bruised arms due to blood tests.	Anovulation (poor responder): GnRH pump. Ovum donation/IVF. No conception: Assisted reproductive technologies (IVF/GIFT/ZIFT).

(Continued)

TABLE 10–9. OVULATION INDUCTION[a] (CONTINUED)

Diagnosis	Drug/Action	Dose	Monitor	Side Effects	Continued Treatment
	Luteal Phase Support Progesterone vaginal suppositories. (See Luteal Phase Defect.) *or* Profasi, Pregnyl or APL (See Luteal Phase Anovulation.)	See Luteal Phase Defect. 5000 I.U. I.M. × 1 dose (week after ovulatory dose). *or* 1500–2000 I.U. × 2–3 doses.	See Annovulation.	Treatment Expensive, inconvenient due to early A.M. lab and ultrasounds.	
Assisted reproductive technologies.	Leuprolide acetate (Lupron) (GnRH agonist) Suppresses pituitary production of FSH and LH. Helps control ovulation induction. *and* Metrodin or Fertinex/Pergonal, or Humegon.	See Figure 10–3. See Figure 10–3.	See Figure 10–3.	Mild headache, itching, redness, hive at injection site.	

Note: See Facts and Comparisons, 1996 for contraindications and complete list of side effects.

[a]Prior to induction, rule out pregnancy, complete infertility evaluation, including a semen analysis

[b]Difference in ovulation/and percent who conceive due to multiple factors of infertility.

Source: Adapted from Rivlin, M. (Ed.). (1990). Handbook of drug therapy in reproductive endocrinology and infertility. Boston: Little, Brown; and Ginsburg, J. (Ed.). (1996). Drug therapy in reproductive endocrinology. New York: Oxford University Press.

234

HYPOTHALAMIC DISORDERS

Hypothalamic Dysfunction

The dysfunction may result in multisystem disorders requiring that the client be referred to a reproductive endocrinologist. Hypothalamic problems that affect reproduction are diagnosed after pituitary abnormalities are excluded.

The exact cause of hypothalamic dysfunction is unknown; however, extreme weight loss, excessive exercise, and/or psychogenic stress that interfere with estrogen production do impact hypothalamic function. In addition, organic diseases, such as central nervous system and head trauma, can result in hypothalamic disorders. Hormone profiles reveal low serum estradiol (E_2 less than 35 pg/mL)[19] and low to normal levels of follicle stimulating hormone and luteinizing hormone.[20] Idiopathic dysfunction results in lowered gonadotropin releasing hormone (GnRH) production.

Subjective Data. Subjective data are obtained from an accurate menstrual history and determination of pubertal milestones. Inquire specifically about Crohn's disease, connective tissue disorders, hepatitis, galactorrhea, stress, adequacy of nutrition (take a dietary history to assess for eating disorders), exercise, and medications. Clients commonly report absent menses, monophasic basal body temperatures, history of excessive dieting or exercise, altered eating habits, and a stressful lifestyle.

Objective Data

■ *Physical Examination.* Includes assessment for low body weight, low fat, little breast tissue, normal secondary sexual characteristics, and hair patterns.
■ *Diagnostic Tests and Methods.* The following blood tests are used to diagnose hypothalamic dysfunction (see Appendix C for normal values). For each test, the results usually found with hypothalamic dysfunction are given:

  • *Pregnancy Test.* Negative; measure the β subunit of hCG with a lower sensitivity of 5 mIU/ml.[4] (Urine pregnancy tests have a lower sensitivity of 25 mIU and, therefore, are not as reliable as blood tests.)

  • *Serum Multiphasic Analysis-12 (SMA-12).* Results are evaluated for indications of systemic illnesses that could affect hypothalamic function; may be normal or abnormal.
  • *E_2.* Low.
  • *FSH/LH.* Low to normal.
  • *Thyroid Studies (TSH, T_3, T_4, free T_4).* May be abnormally high or low.
  • *Prolactin (PRL).* May be elevated; if so, complete pituitary workup is needed, including x-ray, computed tomography (CT) or magnetic resonance imaging (MRI) scan of the sella turcica to look for tumors. (Since thyroid releasing hormone can cause an increase in prolactin, as well as TSH, prolactin levels must be correlated with thyroid studies.)
  • *Gonadotropin Releasing Hormone (GnRH) Test.* Used to stimulate LH/FSH secretion. Two baseline blood samples are obtained at different intervals prior to I.V. infusion of 100 or 150 μg of GnRH. FSH/LH levels are obtained 30 and 60 minutes after infusion. In hypo-gonadal females, FSH response is greater than LH response. Exaggerated responses may suggest hypothyroidism.

Differential Medical Diagnoses. Anorexia nervosa, bulimia, psychiatric disorders, hyperprolactinemia, androgen excess, polycystic ovarian disease, central nervous system (CNS) infection (meningoencephalitis), neoplasms (craniopharyngioma), anosmia, congenital anomalies, drug ingestion (phenothiazines, oral contraceptives), idiopathic conditions.

Plan

■ Medical therapy as indicated.
■ Refer the client who desires fertility to a reproductive endocrinologist for continued evaluation and ovulation induction.
■ Psychosocial interventions are described on page 229–230. Counseling is related to the client's body image, ability to manage stress, and anxiety level.
■ Medication commonly includes monthly progesterone or cyclic oral estrogen/progesterone. Clomiphene, urofollitropin (Metrodin or Fertinex), menotropins (Pergonal or Humegon), or the GnRH pump are used to induce ovulation. Human chorionic gonadotropin (Profasi,

Pregnyl, or APL) I.M. and progesterone I.M. or vaginal suppositories may be administered to provide luteal phase support. For a description of the mechanism of action, usual dose, monitoring parameters, and side effects of these medications, see Hypothalamic Disorders; Hypogonadism, and Clomid Failure under *Diagnosis* in Table 10–9.

- *Medroxyprogesterone Acetate (Provera).* To induce cyclic menses or menses prior to ovulation induction, prescribe 10 mg p.o. for 10 days.
- *Conjugated Estrogens (Premarin).* When the client fails to have withdrawal bleeding after taking progesterone alone, prescribe conjugated estrogen (Premarin) 1.25 mg p.o. for calendar days 1 to 25 *with* Medroxyprogesterone acetate (Provera) 10 mg p.o. for days 14 to 25 to induce cyclic menses or menses prior to ovulation induction.

▪ Anticipated outcome on evaluation is cyclic menses, menses prior to ovulation induction, and normal ovulation induction.

▪ Teach the client the importance of drug compliance and the characteristics of the drug effects. The client should be provided with information regarding the benefits of adequate nutrition, and moderate versus excessive exercise. If hormonal replacement therapy is indicated, information regarding risks associated with decreased estrogen levels, such as osteoporosis and cardiovascular disease, should be addressed. Unopposed estrogen leads to endometrial hyperplasia increasing the client's risk of endometrial cancer. For the client desiring fertility, information regarding medications used for ovulation induction, risks of ovarian hyperstimulation syndrome, and the risks of multiple pregnancies should be supplied.

Follow-Up. Table 10–9 presents guidelines for monitoring and continuing treatment.

PITUITARY DISORDERS

Hyperprolactinemia is a common pituitary disorder; it requires extensive evaluation and referral. Hypogonadotropic hypogonadism and Sheehan's syndrome are rare causes of pituitary disorders.[4]

Hyperprolactinemia

Prolactin (PRL) levels are greater than 20 ng/mL. Elevated PRL interferes with GnRH release, which in turn results in lowered levels of FSH/LH. Elevated PRL may directly inhibit the gonads.[4]

Subjective Data. Take a complete history. Infertility; cyclic, irregular menses, or amenorrhea; spontaneous milky breast discharge; headache/visual field disturbances, and stress are commonly reported. Medications such as antipsychotics, antidepressants, clonidine, reserpine, metaclopramide, and cimetidine can cause an elevation in prolactin.[19]

Objective Data

▪ *Physical Examination.* This must include a thorough neurological exam. Note any milky breast discharge or abnormal neurological findings, especially visual field disturbances.
▪ *Diagnostic Tests and Methods.* The following are indicated:

- Pregnancy test.
- PRL level (must be elevated on more than one sample at least several days apart, before a breast exam, preferably fasting and prior to 11 A.M.).
- Slide of breast discharge to determine fat globules that would indicate milk.
- TSH and T_3, total T_4, free T_4 to rule out thyroid disease; (see Appendix C for normal values).
- X-ray, CT scan or MRI of the sella turcica to rule out pituitary adenoma.

Differential Medical Diagnoses. Galactorrhea, oligomenorrhea/amenorrhea, ovarian dysfunction (polycystic ovarian disease, luteal phase defect), hypothalamic lesions, pituitary lesions (tumors, acromegaly, Cushing's disease, empty sella syndrome), hypothyroidism, physiological conditions (pregnancy, breast stimulation), pharmacological effects (reserpine, cimetidine, tricyclic antidepressants, estrogens), idiopathic conditions.

Plan

▪ Refer the client who desires fertility to a reproductive endocrinologist for continued evaluation and ovulation induction.

- Refer the client to a neurologist, ophthalmologist, or surgeon as indicated.
- Psychosocial interventions are described on page 229–230. Provide the client with information, anticipatory guidance, stress management, and counseling for anxiety and body image disturbance.
- Medication as indicated:
  - *Bromocriptine.* Indicated for treatment of hyperprolactinemia. For administration and side effects, see Table 10–9. Anticipated outcomes on evaluation are normal PRL levels and thyroid function, decreased galactorrhea, and resumption of ovulatory menstrual cycles. Client teaching is related to drug characteristics (see Table 10–9).
  - *Levothyroxine Sodium.* Indicated for hypothyroid treatment among those few clients with galactorrhea and amenorrhea. The usual starting dose of 50 µg p.o. is taken daily with incremental increases of 25 µg every 2–3 weeks until a maintenance dosage of 100–200 µg daily is attained. The maintenance dosage is reflected by a normal metabolic state (TSH or T_3 levels) and should be achieved within the first month of therapy. Maintenance therapy is continued for an indefinite period. Anticipated outcomes on evaluation are normal prolactin levels, normal thyroid function, a decrease in galactorrhea, and resumption of cyclic menses. Client teaching is related to drug characteristics and the required follow-up evaluation.
  - *Bromocriptine with Clomiphene.* Indicated to induce normal ovulation; bromocriptine may correct hyperprolactinemia, but ovulation may not occur. Combined bromocriptine and clomiphene may be necessary to induce ovulation. For administration, side effects, and client teaching, see Table 10–9 and *Drug Facts and Comparisons*[18] or other appropriate pharmacotherapeutic references.
  - *Levothyroxine Sodium with Clomiphene.* Levothyroxine sodium therapy may correct hypothyroidism; however, ovulation may not occur. Levothyroxine sodium and clomiphene may be combined to induce normal ovulation. For administration, side effects, and client teaching, see *Drug Facts and Comparisons,*[18] or other appropriate pharmacotherapeutic references.

Hypogonadotropic Hypogonadism

The hypoestrogenic woman has a negative progesterone withdrawal (i.e., no menstrual bleeding after the administration of progesterone), normal or slightly lower than normal FSH/LH levels, and normal prolactin levels.[4] Amenorrhea can be caused by GnRH pulse suppression, which in turn inhibits pituitary function.

Subjective Data. Include reports of primary or secondary amenorrhea, vaginal dryness or perineal sensitivity, stress.

Objective Data. See Objective Data under Hypothalamic Disorders.

- A complete examination should be done. Assess for low body weight, low fat, little breast tissue, normal secondary sex characteristics, and hair patterns. The vagina is usually dry with decreased rugae, and the uterus is small. If the client has primary amenorrhea, assessing the patency of the cervix is included.
- Diagnostic tests for FSH/LH reveal normal/low normal values.

Differential Medical Diagnoses. Primary or secondary amenorrhea, anovulation, hyperprolactinemia, psychiatric disorder.

Plan
- Refer the client with primary amenorrhea (see Chapter 8).
- Medical therapy is indicated.
- Refer the client to a reproductive endocrinologist for evaluation and ovulation induction as indicated.
- Ovulation induction in clients with hypothalamic disorders is best managed with the GnRH pump, although clomiphene, menotropin, or urofollitropin are often used. Bromocriptine is used to treat hyperprolactinemia. If no ovulation results, then clomiphene is used. If this does not result in ovulation, menotropin or urofollitropin is used (see Table 10–9).

Androgen Excess

Adrenal gland or ovarian dysfunction may result in androgen excess. Androgen excess is a common cause of ovulatory dysfunction and may also be an indicator of adrenal or ovarian tumor.

Careful evaluation and referral are required. The three primary androgens in females are dehydroepiandrosterone sulfate (DHEA-S), androstenedione (A), and testosterone (T). Androgen excess interferes with feedback mechanisms and results in increased FSH/LH levels. Adrenal disorders result in the production of sex steroids which interact with GnRH, FSH/LH, and PRL.

Rapid progression of hirsutism, virilization, and changes in menstrual patterns are suggestive of a tumor. An adrenal tumor is suspected if serum DHEA-S levels are greater than 700 µg/dL.[21] Ovarian tumors are suspected if total female serum testosterone is greater than 200 µg/dL.[21]

Subjective Data. Reports a history of excessive body hair (fine to coarse), oily skin/acne, being overweight, and oligomenorrhea.

Objective Data
- *Physical Examination.* A complete physical exam is indicated. Assess the client's face, chin, and abdomen for male hair patterns (fine to coarse); note frontal balding, increased muscle mass, clitoral enlargement, decreased breast size, and voice changes. Assess for ovarian mass.
- *Diagnostic Tests.* Several are indicated:
  - *Testosterone.* Free. Normal is 100–200 pg/dL.[4]
  - *DHEA-S.* Normal is 80–350 µg/mL; normal ranges may decrease with age.[4]
  - *17-Hydroxyprogesterone (17 OHP).* Screens for androgen excess due to polycystic ovary syndrome (PCO), enzyme deficiency, or congenital adrenal hyperplasia (normal in follicular phase is 15–70 ng/dL; normal in luteal phase is 35–290 ng/dL). Significant elevation suggests adrenal hyperplasia.
  - *Dexamethasone Suppression.* Dexamethasone 1.0 mg is given orally at 11 P.M. Plasma cortisol is measured at 8 A.M.; if suppressed to less than 5 µg/mL, Cushing's disease is ruled out.[4]
  - *Corticotropin (ACTH) Stimulation Test.* At 8 A.M., an I.V. bolus of synthetic ACTH 0.25 mg is administered; blood samples for 17-OHP and cortisol are obtained prior to the bolus and at 60 minutes (normal random cortisol levels are 5–25 µg/dL; normal morning levels are 5–25 µg/dL; normal

evening levels are 2–12 µg/dL). Significant elevation suggests enzyme deficiency or adrenal hyperplasia.
- Additional testing is indicated: FSH/LH/E$_2$, PRL, TSH. A vaginal ultrasound may be recommended to rule out an ovarian mass or identify multiple follicular cysts.

Differential Medical Diagnoses. Ovarian disorders (polycystic ovary syndrome, hyperthecosis, androgen producing tumors, virilization of pregnancy). Adrenal disorders (congenital adrenal hyperplasia, androgen producing tumors, Cushing's disease, drug related, obesity, post menopause, incomplete testicular feminization, idiopathic conditions).

Plan
- Medical therapy as indicated.
- Refer the client to an endocrinologist and a surgeon as indicated.
- Refer the client to a reproductive endocrinologist for evaluation and management and possible ovulation induction.
- Psychosocial interventions include anticipatory guidance regarding treatment and medications. Offer the client support and referral to a psychologist or licensed counselor for self-esteem and body image disturbance. The client may need counseling to enhance her self-image (see Psychosocial Aspects of Infertility).
- *Medication.* For treatment of hirsutism and decrease of androgen production, medications may be used alone or in combination. Consider alternative or combination therapy if there is no clinical improvement in hirsutism after 3 to 6 months of treatment.

  - *Oral Contraceptives.* These are the standard drugs of choice. The usual dosage is ethinyl estradiol 35 µg, norethindrone 1.0 mg, or a similar formulation (see Chapter 9). Oral contraceptives work in two ways. The progestational agent interrupts the steady anovulation state, while the estrogen component increases sex hormone binding globulin levels, resulting in a greater androgen binding capacity and a decrease in free testosterone.[4]
  - *Spironolactone (Aldactone).* This aldosterone-antagonist diuretic is a potent antiandrogen that inhibits the ovarian and adrenal

biosyntheses of androgens, competes for the androgen receptor in hair follicles, and inhibits 5α-reductase activity in the skin, so there is clinical improvement in hirsutism.[4] The usual dosage, if used alone, is 50–200 mg p.o. daily.[21] Begin at 50 mg dose; may increase dose by 50 mg increments. Once a maximal effect has been seen, usually after 6 months, one can attempt to lower the dose to 25–50 mg qd for maintenance for 1–2 years. May split dose in morning and evening. Prior to initiating therapy, check serum electrolytes, blood urea nitrogen (BUN), and creatinine. Usual side effects include polyuria/polydipsia (during first few weeks of therapy), menstrual irregularities, and metrorrhagia. Contraindications include anuria, acute renal insufficiency, impaired renal function, and hyperkalemia. Avoid prescribing spironolactone to clients taking a potassium supplement, diuretic, or digoxin. Use care with clients taking antihypertensives. The drug is *not* recommended during pregnancy. The anticipated outcome on evaluation is a positive response from the use of spironolactone alone within 3 months of treatment, as evidenced by clinical improvement of hirsutism. Lab work to check serum electrolytes (especially potassium), BUN, creatinine, and androgen levels should be performed annually. Therapy should be discontinued after 1–2 years to observe the return of ovulatory cycles. Testosterone suppression may continue for 6 months to 2 years after discontinuing treatment. Client teaching is related to drug characteristics and the necessary follow-up evaluation.

- Spironolactone 100–150 mg p.o. daily *plus* contraceptive (ethinyl estradiol 35 μg and norethindrone 1.0 mg). Hirsutism is frequently treated by this combination of medications. Both drugs decrease androgens, and there is the added benefit of contraception.
- Spironolactone 100–150 mg p.o. daily *plus* dexamethasone 0.5 mg p.o. q.h.s.
- *Dexamethasone.* Usual dosage is 0.5 mg p.o. at bedtime. One should be certain of the diagnosis of androgen excess prior to initiating therapy, due to the significant side effects of this drug. Serum electrolytes and a complete blood count (CBC) should be performed. A usual side effect is decreased resistance to infection. Dexamethasone may complicate the detection and diagnosis of infection and may impair wound healing. Contraindications include drug hypersensitivity and systemic fungal infection; use with care during pregnancy or by clients with peptic ulcer disease, hypertension, renal insufficiency, osteoporosis, diverticulitis, hypothyroidism, and psychiatric disorders. Clients taking other medications should be carefully monitored. Maintenance therapy may be continued for 1 to 2 years. Lab work to assess serum electrolytes, CBC count, and androgen levels should be performed annually or sooner if signs of Cushingoid appearance, increased blood pressure, black tarry stools, bruising, or proximal muscle weakness occurs. Morning plasma cortisol levels should be monitored periodically. Reduce the dosage of dexamethasone if the morning basal cortisol level is less than 2.0 μg/dL.[4] When discontinuing the drug, the dosage must be tapered. Client teaching involves describing the drug side effects and the follow-up evaluation that is necessary.
- Dexamethasone 0.5 mg p.o. q.h.s. *plus* oral contraceptive (ethinyl estradiol 35 μg, norethindrone 1.0 mg). The dexamethasone will decrease adrenal androgens, while the estrogen and progestin in the oral contraceptives will feedback to the hypothalamus and pituitary to decrease LH secretion, which results in a decrease of ovarian androgens.
- Dexamethasone, along with clomiphene citrate (Clomid or Serephene), urofollitropin (Metrodin or Fertinex), or menotropin (Pergonal or Humegon) may be indicated for ovulation induction. For implications see Table 10–9 and other pharmacotherapeutic resources.

Follow-Up. Guidelines are presented in Table 10–9.

OVARIAN DISORDERS

Disorders that can cause infertility include polycystic ovary syndrome (PCO), premature ovarian failure (POF), gonadal dysgenesis, Turner's syndrome, luteinized unruptured follicle (LUF) syndrome, and luteal phase defect (LPD). Another rare disorder is resistant ovary syndrome.[4]

Polycystic Ovary Syndrome (PCO)

This syndrome results from a combination of androgen excess and anovulation. The symptoms begin during adolescence. LH levels are elevated; FSH levels are low or normal. Increased androgens and estrogen decrease FSH levels. Altered hormone levels interfere with GnRH secretion and follicle development.[4]

Subjective Data. Carefully record the client's family history of PCO, female obesity and/or hirsutism, and menstrual history. Ask the client about any use of danazol (Danocrine), progestins, glucocorticoids, anabolic steroids, phenytoin, or minoxidil. The client may reveal concern about a history of excessive body hair, oily skin or acne, being overweight, and having irregular menses.

Objective Data
- *Physical Examination.* A complete physical exam is indicated. Assess the client's face, chin, and abdomen for male hair patterns (fine to coarse); note frontal balding, increased muscle mass, clitoral enlargement, decreased breast size, and voice changes. Also note if obesity is present, and evaluate for ovarian mass.
- *Diagnostic Tests.* Several are indicated:
  - *FSH.* Low or normal.
  - *LH.* Elevated.
  - LH–FSH ratio greater than 3.
  - *Serum Testosterone and free Testosterone.* Mild to moderate elevation.
  - *DHEA-S.* Normal or elevated.
  - *17-Hydroxyprogesterone (17OHP).* Normal or mildly elevated.
  - *PRL.* Normal or mildly elevated.
  - *Basal Body Temperature (BBT).* For indication of ovulation and for scheduling endometrial biopsy, if client is ovulating at all.
  - *Endometrial Biopsy.* To diagnose hyperplasia and assess normal ovulation.
  - *Vaginal Ultrasound.* May be recommended to assess the ovaries (multiple cystic follicles present).

Differential Medical Diagnoses. Obesity, anovulation (amenorrhea, abnormal uterine bleeding), hyperprolactinemia, congenital adrenal hyperplasia (adult onset), adrenal/ovarian tumors, Cushing's disease, ovarian hyperthecosis, hilar cell hyperplasia, thyroid dysfunction, idiopathic hirsutism.

Plan
- Medical therapy as indicated.
- Refer the client to an endocrinologist or to a reproductive endocrinologist for evaluation and treatment.
- Psychosocial interventions include anticipatory guidance regarding treatment and medication. Offer the client support and referral to a counselor or psychologist for self-esteem and body image disturbance if indicated. (See section on Psychosocial Aspects of Infertility.)
- Review risks of endometrial cancer secondary to endometrial hyperplasia resulting from persistent anovulation.
- Prescribe appropriate medication for ovulation induction: clomiphene citrate, dexamethasone, urofollitropin (Metrodin or Fertinex), menotropin (Pergonal or Humegon) (see Table 10–9 and consult *Drug Facts and Comparisons*[18] or other appropriate pharmacotherapeutic reference). A recent study[22] has suggested that lowering the hyperinsulinemia in women with PCO with metformin lowered androgen levels. Some women spontaneously ovulated. More research is needed, but this may prove to be the treatment of choice for women with PCO in the future.
- Laparoscopy is indicated for clients who have an unsatisfactory response to ovulation induction. Laparoscopy permits laser or cautery drilling of multiple ovarian follicles, which decreases androgen production and results in short-term ovulation in the majority of clients. Laser or cautery drilling has replaced ovarian wedge resection that required laparotomy.[23]

Follow-Up. Guidelines are noted in Table 10–9.

Premature Ovarian Failure (POF)

In POF, failure of ovarian estrogen production results in elevated FSH levels (greater than 40 mIU/mL) on more than one serum sample.[20] The ovaries do not produce enough estrogen to inhibit hypothalamic release of GnRH. Continued release of GnRH results in elevated FSH/LH levels as ovulation ceases. Failure may occur at any age between menarche and 40 years and requires careful endocrine evaluation. POF can be caused by autoimmune disease.[4]

Subjective Data. These include amenorrhea, hot flashes/night sweats, vaginal dryness.

Objective Data. A complete physical examination is indicated; assess for signs of hypoestrogenicity (refer to Table 10–2). Several diagnostic tests are indicated.

- *Papanicolaou (Pap) Smear.* If a Maturation Index is done, a lack of superficial cells indicates decreased estrogen activity in the vaginal wall. (Often not done, as it is easy to obtain blood levels of estrogen).
- *FSH/LH.* Elevated (on more than one sample).
- *TSH, T_3, T_4, free T_4.* Rule out thyroid disease.
- *PRL.* Rule out hyperprolactinemia.

Additional tests to rule out autoimmune disorders include CBC with differential and sedimentation rate, total serum protein, albumin to globulin ratio, rheumatoid factor, antinuclear antibodies (ANA), antithyroid globulin, antimicrosomal antibodies, fasting blood sugar, A.M. cortisol, and serum calcium and phosphorus. If the woman is younger than 30 years, a karyotype is indicated (assessment of normal female versus presence of Y chromosome, which is associated with increased risk of malignant gonadal tumor).[4]

Differential Medical Diagnoses. Chromosome abnormality, autoimmune disease (polyendocrinopathy type I or II, myasthenia gravis, idiopathic thrombocytopenia purpura, hemolytic anemia), thyroid dysfunction (hypoparathyroidism, thyroiditis), adrenal insufficiency/failure, 17-hydroxylase deficiency, gonadal tumor.

Plan
- Medical therapy as indicated.
- Hormone replacement as necessary.
- Refer the client who desires fertility to a reproductive endocrinologist.
- Psychosocial interventions involve providing information and anticipatory guidance about the physical and emotional changes that accompany loss of ovarian function, including disturbances in body image, personal identity, self-esteem, the grief process, and sexual dysfunction. The client may need to be referred for individual/marital counseling and possible sex therapy. Review nutrition, including calcium and red meat intake, need for weight bearing exercise, as well as the risks of osteoporosis, cardiovascular disease, and endometrial cancer.
- Medication may include estrogen/progesterone replacement, lubricants, estradiol vaginal cream.
- In vitro fertilization (IVF) with donor oocyte/embryo transfer may be attempted.

Follow-Up. See Table 10–9 and *Drug Facts and Comparisons*[18] or other appropriate pharmacotherapeutic reference. An annual examination with Pap smear is necessary, as well as endometrial biopsy as indicated.

Gonadal Dysgenesis (Turner's Syndrome)

Gonadal Dysgenesis is a broad term for clients with female genitalia, normal müllerian structures and streak gonads.[4]

Dysgenesis results from the gonads undergoing partial or complete regression, which leads to abnormal sexual development.[24] Fibrous gonads caused by complete regression do not produce hormones. This syndrome is associated with a broad range of genetic patterns. Surprisingly, some women with pure gonadal dysgenesis have a normal XX chromosome pattern. A majority of clients with dysgenesis have only one X chromosome; others have multiple cell lines of varying sex chromosome composition (mosaicism).[4] Women with XY chromosome patterns (usually mosaic) are at risk for neoplastic changes in the gonads, thus requiring gonad removal.[4]

Turner's syndrome is a gonadal dysgenesis condition in which a woman has only one X chromosome, a structural abnormality in one X chromosome, or has mosaicism with an abnormal X. The fetus has a normal complement of ova at 20 weeks' gestation; however, they have totally or partially disappeared by birth. The ovaries appear as streak gonads. The incidence of Turner's syndrome is 1 in 2000–5000 liveborn girls.[4]

Subjective Data

- *Gonadal Dysgenesis.* Scant or absent pubic or axillary hair; primary or secondary amenorrhea, absent or arrested secondary sexual development.

Objective Data. A complete physical examination is necessary. (See Table 10–2.)

GONADAL DYSGENESIS CLIENTS MAY HAVE ANY OF THE FOLLOWING

- Normal height or short stature.
- Scant or absent pubic/axillary hair.
- Normal appearing female external genitalia.
- Normal or no breast development.
- Ambiguous genitalia (intra-abdominal testes often found in hernia), blind vaginal pouch, and absent or arrested secondary sex characteristics.
- May have no secondary sexual characteristics but normal appearing external female genitalia *or* ambiguous external genitalia.

TURNER'S SYNDROME CLIENTS CLASSICALLY HAVE THE FOLLOWING

- Short stature.
- Scant or absent pubic/axillary hair.
- Webbing of the neck.
- Broad shield-type chest with laterally placed nipples.
- Lack of breast development.
- Vagina and uterus present but infantile.
- Ovaries absent.
- Diagnostic Tests.
  - Karyotype—Abnormal chromosome pattern.
  - FSH/LH—Elevated.
  - Testosterone—Normal or Elevated.
  - Additional studies to detect cardiac malformations (coarctation of aorta) and renal abnormalities may be indicated in clients with Turner's syndrome.

Differential Medical Diagnoses. Turner's syndrome, testicular feminization, Swyer-James syndrome, coarctation of the aorta, kidney dysfunction.

Plan

- Refer the client to a reproductive endocrinologist and for genetic counseling.
- Medical therapy as indicated.
- During psychosocial interventions, information and anticipatory guidance are provided regarding physical differences and the emotional impacts of body stature, impaired sexual develop-

ment, and lack of reproductive capacity. Refer the client for individual/marital counseling and, possibly, sex therapy.
- Client teaching is related to estrogen deficiencies: review nutrition, exercise, hormone replacement and risks of osteoporosis, cardiovascular disease, glucose intolerance, and thyroid dysfunction.
- Medication in the management of Turner's syndrome includes oral cyclic administration of estrogen and progesterone. Oral contraceptives are not indicated for this client, as there are only streak gonads and the estrogen dose is not adequate to protect the bones and cardiovascular system.
- IVF with donor eggs is an option for the client with Turner's desiring fertility.

Luteinized Unruptured Follicle (LUF) Syndrome

Women with LUF Syndrome have regular cycles due to the luteinization of the granulosa cells, yet the follicle never ruptures to release the oocyte. There is controversy regarding this syndrome in terms of its impact on fertility. It has been shown that LUF may be quite sporadic. Dyssynchrony in the events controlling follicle rupture may result in LUF. It is reasonable to consider the syndrome as a possible cause of unexplained infertility.[4,25,26]

Subjective Data. Regular menses and biphasic BBTs are reported.

Objective Data. A complete examination is normal. The condition is diagnosed by monitoring BBT elevation, using a urine LH ovulation predictor kit, and serial ultrasound monitoring. Ultrasound is performed daily beginning with the LH surge and continued until after BBT elevation (2 to 4 days). Ultrasound demonstrates the continued presence of an echo-free dominant follicle for longer than 36 hours after the peak of the LH surge. (If echos are seen, ovulation has probably occurred and the follicle has filled with blood.) If LUF is identified, repeat testing in the subsequent cycle is indicated.

Differential Medical Diagnosis. Anovulation.

Plan. Provide the client with information and counseling related to ovulation induction, body image disturbance, and anxiety (see Psychosocial Aspects of Infertility).

Medication for ovulation induction is given in conjunction with ultrasound monitoring begun the day of the LH surge and continued daily until the follicle reaches 20 to 24 mm, as determined by ultrasound. Human chorionic gonadotropin (Profasi, Pregnyl, APL) 10,000 IU is then administered I.M. to trigger ovulation (see Table 10–9). Ovulation will occur within 36 hours. Intercourse is recommended the day human chorionic gonadotropin is administered and for the next 2 days. Ultrasound is performed 2 to 3 days post-hCG to assess follicular collapse.[5]

Follow-Up. Refer the client to a reproductive endocrinologist. Instruct her to telephone when menses begins or after BBT has been elevated for 14 days. Perform a pregnancy test or repeat ovulation induction if warranted.

Luteal Phase Defect (LPD)

An inadequate luteal phase occurs when progesterone secretion by the corpus luteum is decreased. Underlying causes of the defect may be abnormal secretion of FSH/LH, resulting in abnormal folliculogenesis, and a lack of normally responsive progesterone receptors in the endometrium. The condition is diagnosed after it has been detected in two cycles.[27] Luteal phase defect has been diagnosed in 3 to 4 percent of infertile women and 5 percent in women with a history of recurrent pregnancy loss.[4]

Subjective Data. Data reported may include a history of irregular (short) cycles and recurrent pregnancy loss.

Objective Data
- A complete physical examination is indicated to rule out other causes of irregular cycles or recurrent pregnancy loss.
- Diagnostic tests and methods are used to detect the defect:
  - BBT rise lasts fewer than 10 days; abnormal temperature curves are seen.
  - Endometrial biopsy is done to date the endometrium; biopsy is abnormal if the histology of the endometrium is 3 days or more out of phase. If the biopsy is abnormal, it is repeated before treatment is initiated.
  - Never treat LPD on the basis of only one abnormal biopsy. The second may be normal, in which case treatment is not necessary.
  - Normal serum progesterone levels are less than 3 ng/mL in the follicular phase; at least 6.5 ng/mL and preferably 10 ng/mL or more in the midluteal phase.[4]
  - Evaluate FSH/LH and prolactin to rule out other abnormalities.

Differential Medical Diagnoses. Mild hyperprolactinemia, abnormal FSH/LH production.

Plan
- Refer the client to a reproductive endocrinologist.
- Provide the client with information, support, anticipatory guidance, and counseling.
- Medication includes progesterone 50 mg vaginal suppositories, progesterone 50 mg capsules or progesterone 25 mg in oil IM to prolong the luteal phase. Bromocriptine may be indicated for mild hyperprolactinemia; clomiphene citrate if FSH/LH are abnormal. Urofollitropin (Methodin or Fertinex) or menotropin (Pergonal or Humegon) may also be used to treat abnormal folliculorgenesis (see Table 10–9).

Follow-Up. BBTs are indicated to monitor the client's cycle (see Table 10–9). Endometrial biopsy is indicated to assess efficacy of progesterone/ovulation induction treatment[27] and dosage is adjusted as needed. Ask the client to telephone with the beginning of menses; it is important to evaluate the characteristics of the cycle. A pelvic examination is done after a cycle of ovulation induction to assess ovarian size. Treatment in the subsequent cycle may be delayed if the ovaries remain enlarged. The dosage of medicine may be changed. If menses is late, perform pregnancy testing.

UTERINE DISORDERS

Uterine causes of infertility are classified in two groups: anatomic abnormality (congenital, diethylstilbestrol [DES] exposure, adhesions, infection, fibroids) and endometrial factor (luteal phase defect). Congenital anomalies result from

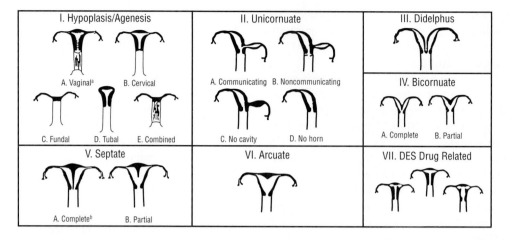

Figure 10–2. The American Society for Reproductive Medicine (formerly The American Fertility Society) classification of müllerian anomalies. [a]Uterus may be normal or take a variety of abnormal forms. [b]May have two distinct cervices. *(Adapted from The American Society for Reproductive Medicine (formerly The American Fertility Society) classifications of adnexal adhesion, distal tubal occlusion secondary to tubal ligation, tubal pregnancies, müllerian anomalies and intrauterine adhesions. Fertil Steril, 49: 6, 1988. Reproduced with permission of The American Society for Reproductive Medicine (formerly The American Fertility Society).)*

arrested uterine development, abnormal formation of the uterus, or incomplete fusion of the müllerian ducts.

Müllerian Anomalies

Such abnormalities may result from genetic patterns of inheritance or spontaneous mutations, such as trisomy 13 and 15, which would have been diagnosed as a neonate. Women who are presenting with a history of infertility or recurrent pregnancy loss may be found to have a subtle müllerian anomaly. Fortunately, uterine structural defects, except those caused by DES exposure, are often amenable to surgical correction (see Figure 10–2 and Table 10–10).

Subjective Data. May include a history of infertility and/or pregnancy loss, abnormal uterine bleeding, primary amenorrhea, dysmenorrhea, dyspareunia.

Objective Data
- A physical exam is indicated to assess for abnormal anatomic structures.
- Diagnostic tests and methods including ultrasound, hysterosalpingogram, and laparoscopy/hysteroscopy are used to detect structural abnormalities. Karyotype is performed to rule out chromosomal abnormalities. Cervical cultures may be indicated.

Differential Medical Diagnoses. Congenital anomalies, endometriosis, urinary tract anomalies, pelvic infection.

Plan
- Treat infections with appropriate antibiotic.
- Refer the client to a reproductive endocrinologist.
- Psychosocial interventions include providing information, anticipatory guidance, and support.
- If indicated, refer the client to a counselor for individual, group, or sex therapy.
- Pain management for dysmenorrhea includes acetaminophen and nonsteroidal anti-inflammatory agents.
- Laparoscopy/hysteroscopy (metroplasty) is done to correct vaginal and uterine abnormalities, to restore the uterine cavity or endometrium, and to provide some pain relief.

Follow-Up. Follow-up depends on the extent of the abnormalities and the procedures needed to correct them.

TABLE 10–10. CLASSIFICATION OF MÜLLERIAN ANOMALIES

Hypoplasia or Agenesis Malformations: Abnormal development of the caudal portion of the uterovaginal primordium. Malformations range from a transverse membrane in the vagina, to vaginal atresia with normal or abnormal uterine shapes, to hypoplasia of the endometrium, to segmental agenesis of the fallopian tubes. Infertility may be the presenting symptom. Obstetrical (OB) complications depend on the anomaly.

Unicornate Uterus: Unilateral abnormality caused by arrested development of one müllerian duct. If implantation occurs in a rudimentary horn pregnancy wastage or tubal pregnancy can be the result. OB complications include malpresentations, intrauterine growth retardation, premature labor and incompetent cervix.

Uterus Didelphus: The müllerian ducts never fused, so there are two uteri, two cervices, and possibly two vaginas. Outflow from one uterus may be obstructed and cause symptoms. OB complications include malpresentations and premature labor.

Bicornuate Uterus: Partial lack of fusion of the two müllerian ducts produces a single cervix with a varying degree of separation in the two horns. OB complications include early abortions, preterm labor and breech presentations.

Septate Uterus: Lack of resorption of the midline septum between the two müllerian ducts resulting in defects varying from a slight midline septum to a septum dividing the uterus and vagina. OB complications depend on the severity of the defect, but can include recurrent pregnancy loss, preterm labor and breech presentations.

Arcuate Uterus: A mild form of Septate Uterus (heart-shaped cavity) not associated with pregnancy loss.

Diethylstilbestrol (DES) Related Anomaly: Due to in utero DES exposure. T-shaped uterus, small cavity, constriction rings may present in any combination. Cervical defects include anterior cervical ridge, a cervical collar, a hypoplastic cervix, or a pseudopolyp. All may lead to an incompetent cervix.

Source: Adapted from Speroff, L., Glass, R. H., & Kase, N. G. (1994). Clinical gynecologic endocrinology and infertility *(5th ed.). Baltimore: Williams and Wilkins; and Sims, J. A. & Gibbons, W. E. (1996).* Treatment of human infertility: The cervical and uterine factors, *in E. Y. Adashi, J. A. Rock, & Z. Rosenwaks. (Eds.),* Reproductive endocrinology, surgery and technology. *Philadelphia: Lippincott-Raven.*

DES (Diethylstilbestrol) Exposure

Exposure of the female fetus to diethylstilbestrol is associated with uterine cavity abnormalities, including T-shaped uteri, hypoplastic cavities, intrauterine adhesions, and cervical stenosis. In addition, DES exposure in utero is linked with ectopic pregnancy, pregnancy loss, and preterm birth.[4] Later cellular abnormalities (adenosis) in vaginal or ectocervical epithelium are associated with DES exposure during fetal life, resulting in susceptibility to carcinogenic effects of endogenous estrogens (clear cell adenocarcinomas). (See DES Exposure, Chapter 13.)

DES was synthesized in 1938 and used by several million women from 1948–1971 to prevent pregnancy loss, toxemia, stillbirth, and preterm labor.[28] Research has documented an increased occurrence of clear cell adenocarcinoma in DES exposed women between 14 and 22 years of age, with a peak incidence at age 19. It is unknown whether female offspring of DES exposed offspring will also sustain structural defects.[29]

Subjective Data. Data reveal a history of maternal DES treatment and a client history of menstrual abnormalities, miscarriage, lower fertility rate, ectopic pregnancy, premature delivery, incompetent cervix, or abnormal Pap smears.

Objective Data. A complete physical examination is indicated to detect abnormalities of anatomic structure. DES exposed women need to begin having pelvic examinations soon after the onset of menses and to have them at least annually. Common abnormalities include vaginal adenosis (ridge, septum, malformation), cervical adenosis (collar, hood, polyp, malformation, stenosis), and müllerian anomalies.

Diagnostic tests and methods include a Pap smear of the cervix to screen for squamous cell carcinoma, and a colposcopy and biopsy of abnormal vaginal and cervical tissue. Other methods may be indicated to evaluate anatomic abnormalities (ultrasound, hysterosalpingogram, laparoscopy/hysteroscopy).

Differential Medical Diagnoses. Congenital anomalies, chromosomal abnormalities.

Plan. Psychosocial interventions include providing information, anticipatory guidance, and support. No medication is recommended. No treatment is indicated unless complications—such as abnormal Pap smears, pregnancy complications, or infertility arise.

Follow-Up. Referrals for individual, group, or sex therapy may be indicated; or an infertility specialist may be indicated if the client is unable to become pregnant or has a history of pregnancy loss. Careful follow-up for clear cell adenocarcinoma and squamous cell carcinoma is required; immediate referral is made if suspicious findings occur.

Intrauterine Adhesions (Asherman's Syndrome)

The syndrome results from damage to the endometrium after excessive curettage, cesarean birth, metroplasty, myomectomy, as well as from infections.[28] It interferes with fertility by disrupting sperm migration, mechanically obstructing tubal ostia, and impeding blastocyst implantation. Pregnancy loss may result from decreased size of the uterine cavity or inadequate endometrium.[4]

Subjective Data. The client may report a history of menstrual abnormalities (scant flow, secondary amenorrhea, dysmenorrhea), or normal menses, dyspareunia, uterine infection, pregnancy losses, surgical procedures.

Objective Data
- A complete physical examination is indicated. Often, findings are normal. Assess for cervical stenosis; cervical discharge; signs of cervical, vaginal or uterine infection; and abnormal uterine contour, firmness, immobility, tenderness.
- Diagnostic tests and methods include endometrial biopsy to diagnose tuberculosis of the endometrium; hysterosalpingogram to determine abnormalities in uterine contour; laparoscopy and hysteroscopy (when indicated). Repeat hysterosalpingogram may be indicated after surgical correction if conception does not occur. (An endometrial biopsy may diagnose fibrosis, but a normal result does not rule out fibrosis in another area of the uterus.)

Differential Medical Diagnoses. Amenorrhea, dysmenorrhea, cervical stenosis.

Plan
- Provide the client with information, anticipatory guidance, and support.
- Medication may include cyclic high dose estrogen/progesterone replacement to help restore normal endometrium after surgical correction (see Table 10–9). Postoperative pain is usually managed with acetaminophen or nonsteroidal anti-inflammatory agents.
- Laparoscopy and hysteroscopy may be indicated for lysis of adhesions and cervical dilation.
- Following lysis of adhesions, an IUD or pediatric foley inflated with 3 ml fluid left in for 7 days may be used to keep the uterine sides from adhering to each other.[4]

Follow-Up. Refer the client to a reproductive endocrinologist and for counseling. Repeat procedures to lyse adhesions are indicated if normal menses is not established.

Endometritis

Endometritis is an endometrial inflammation due to infection caused by pathogens. It may result from ascending vaginal organisms, use of an intrauterine device (IUD), endometrial trauma, or as a secondary infection associated with cancer. Common pathogens include aerobic/anaerobic bacteria, mycoplasma, chlamydia, gonorrhea, viruses, toxoplasmas, parasites, and rarely mycobacterium tuberculosis. Treatment is controversial when no pathogen is identified because resolution may occur spontaneously. Infertility may be associated with an unfavorable endometrial environment that results from infection and interferes with blastocyst implantation.[14]

Tuberculosis (TB) endometritis is rare. Infertility occurs due to extensive tubal scarring and uterine adhesions. Diagnosis is made by curettage and culture of the premenstrual endometrium. Antituberculosis medications are used until repeat curettage is normal.

Subjective Data. The client may report uterine tenderness, dyspareunia, dysmenorrhea, and an abnormal vaginal discharge. She may also report a history of D & C or trauma to cervix (decreasing secretion of cervical mucus).[14] Infertility may be the only sign of chronic endometritis.

Objective Data. Physical examination will reveal tenderness or bimanual examination, especially if it is acute endometritis. If discharge is unusually foul and client is elderly, suspect cancer.

Diagnosis of chronic endometritis is accomplished by follicular phase endometrial biopsy with culture, as well as histologic evaluation of the biopsy tissue.[14] (See Pelvic Inflammatory Disease in Chapter 13 for tests to diagnose acute infection.)

Differential Medical Diagnoses. Urinary tract infection (UTI), acute pyelonephritis, appendicitis, pelvic abscess, thromboembolism, gastrointestinal disease, endometriosis, uterine adhesions.

Plan

- Psychosocial interventions include teaching the client about the causes, treatment, prevention, and effects of infection. Provide support and counseling, and encourage support from significant others.
- Medication specific to the identified organism is prescribed for recurrent endometrial/pelvic infections because the inflammation, abnormal endometrium, and adhesion formation associated with infection decrease fertility (see Chapter 11).
- Endometrial biopsy (follicular phase) is indicated after antibiotic treatment to determine resolution of endometritis.
- Pain management is often indicated.

Follow-Up. Refer the client to a reproductive endocrinologist for continued evaluation and infertility treatment. Diagnostic evaluation and treatment will be affected by the history of recurrent infection and the degree of pelvic and tubal pathology.

- Other interventions that may be indicated are hysterosalpingogram, laparoscopy, laparoscopy/hysteroscopy, and laparotomy for lysis of adhesions and tubal repair. After tubal repair, clients are at risk for ectopic pregnancy. IVF may be necessary if other corrective therapies cannot restore normal tubal function. A client with the diagnosis of TB endometritis who wishes to become pregnant will probably require IVF, unless the endometrium is atrophic, in which case there is no further treatment available.[30]

Leiomyomas (Fibroids)

These tumors, of smooth muscle origin, arise from the myometrium. They may enlarge during pregnancy or when exogenous estrogen is given because of an increase in estrogen receptor levels in the fibroid. Distortion of the pelvic and uterine cavities may interfere with fertility, preventing conception or maintenance of pregnancy.[28] Therapeutic intervention is determined by the size and location of the fibroid and the desire for fertility. Fibroid tumors occur more frequently during the fourth and fifth decade of life. They are more prevalent among African American women.[31] (Chapter 13 has more information related to leiomyomas.)

Subjective Data. The client may report pain, especially dysmenorrhea or dyspareunia; increased, prolonged, or irregular menstrual flow.[32] Small fibroids may be asymptomatic.

Objective Data. A complete physical exam may reveal an enlarged, irregularly shaped, firm uterus.

- Diagnostic tests and methods may include ultrasound and hysterosalpingogram to access the uterine cavity.

Plan

- Refer the client to a gynecologist.
- *Preoperative Medication.* Surgery may be necessary for a successful pregnancy. Use of Depot Lupron (leuprolide acetate) or other GnRH analogue preoperatively may be indicated with large tumors to impose anovulation and thereby decrease tumor size, the risk of hemorrhage, and trauma to the uterus. Medications such as leuprolide acetate suppress the growth of the fibroid tumor, but as it causes a medical menopause, the risk of osteoporosis increases, and consequently cannot be given on a long-term basis. When the drug is stopped, the tumor starts to grow again, so usually Lupron is used on a short-term (3–6 month) basis to shrink the tumor prior to surgery.
  - Common transient side effects include hot flashes, night sweats, breakthrough bleeding, vaginal dryness.
  - Protected intercourse is indicated during entire course of therapy.
- Laparotomy is required to remove large fibroids; small fibroids may be removed with laparoscopy/hysteroscopy.
- Pain (dysmenorrhea) management includes acetaminophen and nonsteroidal anti-inflammatory agents.

Cervical Factor

Abnormalities in cervical mucus or in mucus-spermatozoa interactions have been identified in 5 to 15 percent of infertile couples.[33] Adequate cervical mucus is critical to sperm transport and storage. Midcycle mucus increases in quantity and quality (clear, thin) with increased levels of estrogen. Abnormalities may result from female or male causes. Poor timing of the postcoital test gives a false result of mucus abnormality.

Female causes include ovulatory disorders, severe dyspareunia, previous cervical surgery or infection, DES exposure, anatomic abnormalities (polyps, severe stenosis), drugs clomiphene), use of lubricants and douches, and the presence of antisperm antibodies. Male causes include retrograde ejaculation, hypospadias, semen abnormalities, antisperm antibodies and impotence from performing on demand.[10]

Subjective Data. May reveal a history of infertility, as well as cervical mucus that is clear and thin, thick and sticky, or absent.

Objective Data. A physical examination is indicated, focusing on cervical discharge and moisture (as related to cycle day), as well as cervical appearance (pink, smooth).

- *Diagnostic Tests and Methods:*
  - *Basal Body Temperatures (BBTs).* Sometimes used with a urinary LH predictor kit, BBTs help to schedule the postcoital test appropriately and interpret the test results.
  - *Postcoital Test (PCT).* (See PCT, page 226.) Two days of abstinence prior to the PCT is encouraged.
  - *Postinsemination Test (PIT).* The PIT is performed after a second abnormal PCT. (See PCT, page 226.) The client's partner must collect a semen specimen in a sterile container. Semen is placed in the cervical canal with a catheter. Cervical insemination is performed in the office and an endocervical mucus sample is obtained 2 to 4 hours later.
  - *Semen Analysis (SA).* (See SA, page 226.)
  - *Female/Male Antisperm Antibodies Test.* (Discussed later in this chapter.)

Differential Medical Diagnoses. Ovulatory disorder, cervicitis, cervical anatomic abnormality (polyps, stenosis, surgery, DES exposure), semen

abnormalities, female/male antisperm antibodies, sexual dysfunction.

Plan
- Psychosocial interventions include providing information and support, counseling the client regarding causes of infertility, the diagnostic testing, and treatment.
- Elimination of alcohol and tobacco use due to their negative effect on cervical mucus production.[8]
- *Medications:*
  - *Antibiotic Therapy.* Indicated for cervicitis (see Chapter 11).
  - *Conjugated Equine Estrogen.* Premarin 0.3 mg p.o. is given daily, beginning cycle day 6 and continuing until the day of urine LH surge. (Start and stop dates of medication vary depending on day of ovulation; the client may take the medication for 6 to 12 days.) Low dose estrogen may improve the quality of the cervical mucus but may also delay ovulation. The PCT must be repeated on the day of the urine LH surge. If the PCT result is normal while the client is taking conjugated estrogen, continue treatment for approximately 6 to 9 cycles. If the PCT result is abnormal, discontinue conjugated estrogen and treat with intrauterine insemination (IUI).
- Inseminations are performed to place sperm as close to the egg as possible. (See discussion of Selected Infertility Treatments.)

Follow-Up. Referral for more extensive counseling and therapy may be indicated.

PELVIC DISORDERS

Sequelae of pelvic inflammatory disease, postoperative adhesions, and endometriosis are involved in the pathogenesis of impaired fertility.

Pelvic Inflammatory Disease (PID)

Every year, one million women are treated for PID; ectopic rates have quadrupled.[34] Westrom's classic study demonstrated that the incidence of tubal occlusion after one episode is

11.4 percent, after two episodes, 23.1 percent, and after three or more episodes, 54.3 percent.[35] Early diagnosis of acute PID and aggressive antimicrobial treatment decreases the chances of resulting sequelae.[36] Tubal pathology is one of the most common causes of infertility in women. Sexually transmitted diseases caused by *Neisseria gonorrhoeae* and *Chlamydia trachomatis* are the major source of tubal disease. Tubal repair may be accomplished by laser or cutting laparoscopy or laparotomy (salpingostomy, fimbrioplasty, reanastomosis). The success of tubal repair depends on the extent of disease and, due to the delicate microsurgery involved, the skill of the surgeon. Further fertility treatment if repair is unsuccessful may include IVF. A repeat surgery usually does not result in functional tubes (see Uterine Disorders; Endometritis; and Chapter 13).

Pelvic Adhesions

Pelvic adhesions that interfere with pickup/transport of the oocyte are a major cause of infertility in women. Meticulous surgical technique, minimal tissue handling, stringent hemostasis, constant irrigation, avoidance of abrasion between raw surfaces (adhesion barriers), and microsurgery using unipolar fine wire cautery or the laser will reduce adhesions formation and preserve fertility (laparoscopy/laparotomy).[37] Other causes of pelvic adhesions include infections with gonorrhea, chlamydia, toxoplasmas, parasites, and aerobic/anaerobic bacteria.

Subjective Data. The client may report a history of chronic pelvic pain, dyspareunia, menstrual disorders, pelvic surgery. In half of the cases, a history of infertility with no history of antecedent disease is the presentation.

Objective Data. An examination is indicated. Tenderness and a fixed uterus on bimanual examination are common. Diagnostic methods are a hysterosalpingogram, and a laparoscopy to diagnose and treat pelvic pathology.

Differential Medical Diagnoses. Chronic salpingitis, residual inflammatory disease, tubal blockage, PID.

Plan
- Psychosocial interventions include providing information and support. Refer, if necessary, for counseling (individual, group, sex therapy). Relaxation techniques, biofeedback, and pain management may also be indicated.
- Antibiotic and pain therapy may be used prior to invasive procedures.
- Other possible interventions include laser or cautery laparoscopy for lysis of adhesions; tubal repair (salpingostomy, neosalpingostomy, fimbrioplasty) as indicated; laparotomy to treat severe pelvic disease (adhesion lysis; microscopic tubal or cornual reanastomosis); in vitro fertilization if indicated.
- Refer the client to a reproductive endocrinologist.

Endometriosis[37a]

Endometriosis, a major cause of infertility, is a condition in which endometrial tissue, glands and stroma, are located outside of the uterine cavity. The tissue responds to cyclic hormones like the endometrial lining, but may be out of phase with it (see Chapter 13). Fertility is impaired by mechanical factors interfering with ovum pickup and tubal transport; by ovulatory dysfunction, and by interference with sperm function, fertilization and implantation.[38] Treatment depends on the severity of symptoms and the desire for fertility. Infertility management may include both laparoscopy and medical management with GnRH agonists. In mild cases, conservative management (doing nothing), or laser or cautery laparoscopy may be the only treatment needed. Moderate disease may be treated with medication such as Depot Lupron and nafarelin acetate or danazol for 6 months. These medications suppress estrogen and progesterone production so that atrophy of the endometrial implants occurs. Symptoms often return after the medications are stopped. Severe cases, however, may also require either preoperative or postoperative danazol, Depot Lupron, or nafarelin acetate (Synarel).[33] Further infertility treatment may include stimulated ovulation induction IUI or IVF/GIFT/ZIFT.

Recurrent Pregnancy Loss

The most common obstetrical complication is spontaneous abortion, which is seen in 15–20 percent of all clinically recognized pregnancies. *Recurrent abortion* is defined as three or more consecutive spontaneous pregnancy losses prior to 20 weeks' gestation. This is discouraging for both the couple and the provider. The good news is that almost 70 percent of women will eventually achieve a live birth in subsequent pregnancies without treatment. Treatment is designed to decrease the risk of subsequent pregnancy losses.[39]

Evaluation of a couple experiencing recurrent abortion should begin after three pregnancy losses, or after two if the woman is over 35 years of age. Pregnancy loss may be caused by anatomic, endocrine, genetic, or immunologic variations; infection; chronic illness; or environmental toxins.

Subjective Data. The client may report a history of recurrent abortion.

Objective Data. A complete physical examination is indicated. During the pelvic examination, special attention is given to detecting anatomic abnormalities, such as fibroids or a soft cervix. Diagnostic tests include PRL; TSH, T_3, T_4, free T_4; systemic lupus screen; lupus anticoagulant; anticardiolipin antibodies; karyotype (both partners); chlamydia, ureaplasma, and mycoplasma cultures; endometrial biopsy; hysterosalpingography; ultrasound; laparoscopy/hysteroscopy.[39]

Differential Medical Diagnoses
- *Anatomic Abnormalities (Uterus).* Müllerian defects, fibroids, septum defects, Asherman's syndrome, incompetent cervix.
- *Endocrine Abnormalities.* Thyroid (hypothyroid), hyperprolactinemia, ovulatory dysfunction/LPD.
- *Infection.* Chlamydia, TORCH (T, toxoplasmosis; O, other infections (varicella, listeria, syphilis); R, rubella; C, cytomegalovirus; H, herpes simplex virus), ureaplasma/mycoplasma.
- *Chronic Illness.* Wilson's disease, heart/renal disease, blood dyscrasias.
- *Genetic Abnormality.* Aneuploidy of products of conception; balanced translocation, sex chromosome mosaicism, chromosome inversions and ring chromosomes of the couple.[4]
- *Immunologic Disorders.* Systemic lupus erythematosus (SLE), parental histocompatibilities.

- *Environmental Toxins.* Radiation, chemotherapy/drugs, smoking, ethyl alcohol abuse, caffeine.

Plan
- Provide the client with information and psychological support; be available for questions and listening. Evaluate the client's stage of crisis and grief, communication patterns, relationships, coping abilities, and use of support systems.
- Collaborate with medical (reproductive endocrinology) and mental health specialists.
- Medication or surgery is determined by the cause of the recurrent pregnancy loss.[4,39]

Follow-Up. As appropriate, provide information about Compassionate Friends (see Resources), a support group for individuals and families who have lost pregnancies or children.

MALE INFERTILITY: CAUSES, DIAGNOSES, AND INTERVENTIONS

Male factor infertility is found alone in approximately 30 percent of cases, and is involved in another 20 percent where there is also a female problem. Thus, male factor is implicated in 50 percent of infertile cases.[40] Male factor infertility may result from a variety of causes, such as endocrine disorders, varicocele, antisperm antibodies, occupational and environmental practices, and sexual dysfunction. Evaluation of a man's fertility should be coordinated with the evaluation of the woman's. Evaluation may be initiated in the general practice or gynecology office. Referral is made to a urologist when semen abnormalities are identified. Frequently, medical therapies are unsuccessful, but surgery has often been successful in treating post-testicular and ductal disorders.

Subjective Data. A detailed history is essential to identify factors that may affect sperm production (see Table 10–3). For normal spermatogenesis, a delicate balance must exist between the neuroendocrine system and testes.[4,5,40]

Objective Data
- A thorough physical examination (see Table 10–4) and Doppler evaluation are indicated when sperm parameters are abnormal.

- Diagnostic tests begin with a semen analysis (performed twice) (see SA under Infertility Evaluation).

Semen culture is obtained if there are five or more white blood cells per high power field or if agglutination of sperm indicates a need for culture and for antisperm antibody testing. Other tests may include TSH, T_3, T_4, free T_4; FSH (normal is 5–25 mIU/ml); LH (normal is 6–26 mIU/ml); testosterone (normal is 250–1200 ng/dL); PRL; CT Scan/MRI of sella turcica; karyotyping. Tests that are rarely used today include bovine mucus penetration (because the results would not change the clinical management, which is washed IUI), and the sperm penetration assay (because it does not predict the ability of sperm to bind to or penetrate a human zona pellucida).[40]

CAUSES OF MALE INFERTILITY

Endocrine Disorders

Such disorders constitute rare causes of male infertility, and as such endocrine evaluation is indicated when sperm concentration is very low or if there is a clinical suspicion.[40] Measurement of TSH, T_3, T_4, free T_4, FSH/LH, PRL, and testosterone may identify abnormalities.[4] Some specific endocrine problems with usual test results are the following.

- Germ cell aplasia; elevated FSH/LH.
- Testicular failure: elevated FSH/LH.
- Pituitary adenoma/impotence: elevated PRL.
- Thyroid dysfunction: elevated or low TSH, T_3, T_4, free T_4.
- Hypogonadotropic hypogonadism (Kallmann's syndrome): low FSH/LH, testosterone.[41]

Varicocele

This varicosity of the internal spermatic vein is usually on the left side and found in both fertile and infertile men. It impairs infertility by raising testicular temperature, thus killing sperm. Surgical correction is beneficial in some cases.[4]

Disorders of Sperm Transport

Sperm transport can be caused by congenital disorders, such as absence of major portions of the epididymis, vas deferens and seminal vesicles in males with cystic fibrosis, or acquired disorders due to infections, surgery, or trauma. Such conditions may be surgically corrected.

Functional obstruction occurs in clients with spinal cord injuries, diabetic males with autonomic neuropathy, and with medications such as tranquilizers, antidepressants, and antihypertensives.

Sperm Transport Dysfunction

Clients with hypospadias, retrograde ejaculation, or sexual dysfunction are unable to deliver sperm to cervical mucus. Sperm collection by means of masturbation for cervical insemination may be indicated. Sperm may also be retrieved from alkalinized urine and prepared for intrauterine insemination in the client with retrograde ejaculation.

Interventions

- *Medications:*
  - Clomiphene citrate (Clomid or Serephene) 25 mg, p.o. days 1–25 of the calendar for 6–9 months, to increase sperm count; *or*
  - Human chorionic gonadotropin (Profasi, Pregnyl or APL) 2000–2500 IU, I.M. Three times per week for 8–10 weeks, to increase sperm motility; *or*
  - Menotropin (Pergonal or Humegon) 25–75 IU, I.M. Three times per week *plus* human chorionic gonadotropin (Profasi, Pregnyl or APL) 2000–2500 IU I.M. Three times per week for 8–10 weeks, to increase spermatogenesis; *or*
  - GnRH Pump, pulsation q. 2 hours, long-term therapy to provide normal gonadotropin pulsation to increase spermatogenesis (see Table 10–9).

- Surgery (varicocelectomy, removal of obstruction, vasectomy reversal).
- Artificial insemination—husband (AIH-cervix).
- Artificial insemination—donor (AID-cervix).
- Stimulated ovulation induction IUI—husband or donor.
- Electroejaculation.
- IVF/ZIFT/GIFT
- Intracytoplasmic sperm injection (ICSI) where one sperm is injected directly into the oocyte.

- *Psychosocial support must be* assessed, as self-esteem issues are often dramatic when the diagnosis of male infertility is made. Referral may be indicated for counseling.[42]

COMBINED FACTORS OF MALE AND FEMALE INFERTILITY

Combined factors of male and female infertility may be more difficult to overcome. It is critically important to assess each partner's fertility status before the other undergoes corrective surgery. For example, in vitro fertilization (IVF) may be indicated instead of surgical intervention for couples with tubal pathology and a severe male factor. Individual and couple factors determine the choice of therapy. To maximize chances of conception, evaluation and intervention are coordinated, for example, using varicocele repair and endometriosis surgery.[40]

UNEXPLAINED INFERTILITY

For 5 percent of infertile couples, no specific cause of infertility can be identified by any of the standard tests.[33] Some couples with unexplained infertility will conceive at an unpredictable time, but many will not. They have multiple needs; although they have the biologic potential to conceive, efforts have been unsuccessful, resulting in frustration for the couple, and there is nothing identified to treat.

Subjective Data. The couple reports a history of infertility.

Objective Data. A complete infertility evaluation is performed resulting in normal findings.

Differential Medical Diagnoses. Luteinized unruptured follicle (LUF) syndrome, immunologic factor; female/male antisperm antibody.

Plan
- Refer the couple to a reproductive endocrinologist.
- Psychosocial interventions include providing information and, as treatment becomes more complex, using a variety of educational strategies, such as written information, videotape, demonstration, and individual and group sessions. It is important to be available to answer questions and provide psychosocial support for the individual and couple. Explore all treatment options and allow the couple to regain control by decision making.
- Medication. Stimulation ovulation induction intrauterine insemination (IUI) is accomplished with clomiphene and menotropin, or urofollitropin, and human chorionic gonadotropin. (See Table 10–9 and Female Infertility: Causes, Diagnoses, and Interventions.)
- IVF/GIFT/ZIFT.
- Referral may be made for the individual or couple for counseling for psychological support.

FEMALE AND MALE ANTISPERM ANTIBODIES

Antisperm antibodies can be found in either partner. The exact cause of female antisperm antibody formation is unknown; an increased incidence of male antisperm antibodies has been noted if they have breaches of the blood-testis barrier (i.e., congenital absence of the vas or epididymis, vasectomy, local inflammation or infection).[5] Antibodies have been found in serum, cervical mucus, seminal plasma, directly on the sperm surface, and in the reproductive tracts of fertile and infertile couples. Antibodies decrease sperm motility, transport, and ability to penetrate the egg.[5] Couples with unexplained infertility should have antibody screening performed. Antibodies are thought to result in 10 percent of unexplained infertility in men.[5]

Subjective Data. Clients may report a history of infertility, genital tract infections, surgery, trauma. A man may have cryptorchidism, varicocele, or vasectomy reversal.

Objective Data. A complete physical examination of the female is indicated. Diagnostic tests and methods include antisperm/antibody testing and semen analysis.

Antisperm/antibody testing is recommended with a history of vasectomy reversal, unexplained infertility, and two abnormal postcoital tests (PCTs) (normal cervical mucus with no sperm; with poorly motile, shaking, or clumping sperm; and a history of normal semen analysis). Testing of both partners is recommended. The antisperm-antibody screen is performed on serum for the woman (indirect immunobead) and semen (direct immunobead) samples. The level of serum antibodies does not correlate to the semen level, and only the semen level impacts fertility in the male.

Immunobead binding determines the presence and location of antibodies. It is used to identify the percentage of sperm coated with antibodies, the area of sperm surface bound to antibodies (head, neck, tail), and type of antibody present (IgG, IgM, IgA). The type of antibody present affects sperm function. The more sperm that are bound and the greater the sperm surface area involved, the greater the risk of impaired fertility.[4] A test result is considered positive if there is binding to more than 40 percent of motile sperm (tail tip binding is not clinically significant).[43]

When semen analyses in the past have been normal, suspect antisperm antibody if "clumping," agglutination of sperm, or decreased motility is seen in the current specimen.

Differential Medical Diagnosis. Unexplained infertility.

Plan

- Refer the couple to a reproductive endocrinologist.
- Psychosocial interventions include providing information and support.
- Treatment indicated for female antisperm antibodies is stimulated ovulation induction IUI (see Table 10–9). In the past, oral steroids were used to decrease antibody titers for male and female antisperm antibodies. The risks and benefits of oral steroids must be balanced because of the large therapeutic dosage required and the increased side effects (see Table 10–9).[4]
- Stimulated ovulation induction IUI involves the development and ovulation of multiple eggs coupled with timed inseminations. This results in the presence of more than one oocyte (egg) available for sperm penetration. IUI shortens the distance that sperm must travel to reach oocytes and helps to prevent the loss of sperm motility due to antibody binding. A male with positive antibodies should collect the semen specimen in a container with medium. The specimen should be prepared (washed) immediately to decrease agglutination.
- IVF, GIFT, ZIFT (see Infertility Treatment).
- Condom use by the male for 6 months was once thought to decrease cervical mucus antibody titers; however, it has limited effectiveness, delays conception, and has been abandoned.
- Refer the clients for counseling (individual, group, sex therapy).

SELECTED INFERTILITY TREATMENTS

OVULATION INDUCTION

This therapy may be used alone (timed intercourse) or in combination with inseminations or assisted reproductive technologies. See Table 10–9 for drugs used, mechanism of action, dose, monitoring and side effects. Table 10–11 depicts five different ovulation induction drug regimens. These regimens are merely guides. Ovarian response to hMG or uFSH determines dose and duration of therapy. Often a practice uses two or three of these regimens, changing only if the woman's ovaries fail to respond.

There is controversy in the field regarding the taking of fertility drugs and the risk of ovarian cancer. Whittemore and colleagues[44] in November 1992 published the findings of a meta-analysis of twelve studies in the *American Journal of Epidemiology*. There were some flaws in the study, including only three studies having information on fertility drugs, so the numbers were small. The study showed that if the infertile woman becomes pregnant, her risk of ovarian cancer did not increase.

Another study published in 1994 by Rossing and co-workers[45] found a possible link between the use of clomiphene citrate for 12 or more cycles and ovarian cancer. Today's standard of care with close monitoring makes it highly unusual for a client to have more than 6 cycles of clomiphene before the recommendation is made to change therapies. To add more confusion, Rossing and colleagues[46] in 1996 published an article that stated the use of clomiphene may reduce the risk of *cervical* neoplasia. Also in 1996, Shushan and others[47] concluded that human menopausal gonadotropin may increase the risk of epithelial ovarian cancer. Mosgaard and co-workers, in a case-control study from Denmark published in 1997, reported that treatment with clomiphene, hMG or hCG did not increase the risk of ovarian

TABLE 10–11. OVARIAN STIMULATION PROTOCOLS

	Luteal Phase (begins with ovulation)								Follicular Phase (begins day one of menses)												
										menses											
Days of menstrual cycle	21	22	23	24	25	26	27	28	1	2	3	4	5	6	7	8	9	10	11	12

Drug

CC — CC (days 3–8)

hMG/uFSH — hMG and/or uFSH (days 3–9), hCG

GnRHa / hMG/uFSH (long protocol) — GnRHa (days 22–8); hMG and/or uFSH (days 5–11); hCG

GnRHa / hMG/uFSH (short protocol OR Flare) — GnRHa (days 3–8); hMG and/or uFSH (days 4–10); hCG

GnRHa / hMG/uFSH (ultra short protocol) — GnRHa (days 3–5); hMG and/or uFSH (days 4–10); hCG

CC = clomiphene citrate; GnRHa = Lupron; hMG = Pergonal or Humegon; hCG = Profasi, Pregnyl or APL; uFSH = highly purified FSH, Fertinex. Luteal phase support could be with progesterone or hCG. (See Table 10–9.)

cancer, regardless of pregnancy, when compared to nontreated infertile women.[48]

We do not know the answer to this question. In the first 5 years of data collection in the NIH supported "Health Surveillance of Women Treated for Infertility by In Vitro Fertilization," no cases of ovarian cancer were reported among approximately 3100 women.[49] This study has been stopped. As this is an important question to answer, the National Institute of Health is funding a retrospective study of cancer patients and is trying to determine if they took fertility drugs. In a prospective study, women, after taking fertility drugs 10 years ago, will be followed to determine the incidence of cancer. Rossing is the primary investigator in both studies (Personal communication with Dr. Robert Spirtas, of the National Institute of Child Health and Human Development). Clients should be made aware of the potential ramifications of ovulation induction. Since parity is a protective factor, if the client gets pregnant, all risks may be negated and may provide protection. Each client must balance the risks, benefits, and her own needs to make a decision.

ARTIFICIAL INSEMINATION

Husband or donor sperm may be used for intracervical or intrauterine insemination (IUI). Indications for intracervical insemination (ICI) include hypospadias, impotence, vaginismus, dyspareunia or donor sperm.[50] Establish a rationale for insemination that identifies male and/or female factors of infertility necessitating the consideration of artificial insemination (see Table 10–12). Insemination enables sperm to be deposited closer to the oocyte, which may improve the chances of conception. Therapeutic insemination provides hope of parenthood for many single women and infertile couples; however, it raises many physical, psychological, ethical, legal, religious, and financial concerns.

Procedures

- *Artificial Insemination—Husband (AIH).* Requires a fresh specimen for cervical insemination. The partner may assist with insemination. Cervical insemination has a role when due to

TABLE 10–12. INDICATIONS FOR IUI

I. Normal Semen Analysis
A. Anatomic male causes
  1. Retrograde ejaculation
    a. Surgery
    b. Trauma
    c. Systemic disease
    d. Medications
B. Female causes
  1. Cervical stenosis (conization, cauterization, diethylstilbestrol exposure)
  2. Deficiencies in cervical mucus
  3. Defects in sperm transport or survival
C. Coital dysfunction
  1. Impotence
  2. Premature ejaculation
  3. Vaginismus
D. Unexplained infertility

II. Abnormal Semen Analysis
A. Oligospermia
B. Asthenospermia
C. Volume disorders
D. Immune mediated disorders
E. Multiple male factor disorders

III. Frozen Sperm
A. Husband (sperm stored prior to vasectomy, chemotherapy, or radiation)
B. Donor (azoospermia, genetic disease, Rh incompatibility, single woman)

Source: Byrd, W. (1995). Sperm preparation and homologous insemination. In W. R. Keye, Jr., R. J. Chang, R. W. Rebar, & M. R. Soules (Eds.), Infertility: Evaluation and treatment. Philadelphia: W.B. Saunders Company. Used with permission and adapted from Garner, C. (1995). Infertility. In C. I. Fogel, & N. F. Woods (Eds.), Women's health care: A comprehensive handbook. Thousand Oaks, CA: Sage Publications, Inc.

physical or psychological factors, sperm cannot be deposited in the vagina by intercourse. Otherwise, IUI is the procedure of choice.

- *Therapeutic Donor Insemination (TDI).* Must be performed according to The American Society for Reproductive Medicine (formerly The American Fertility Society) Guidelines for Gamete Donation: 1993.[50] Consent forms are signed and donors selected. Female evaluation includes current history and physical examination, including Pap smear, chlamydia and gonorrhea cultures, rubella titer, cytomegalovirus (CMV) titer, serologic test for syphilis, hepatitis profile, and human immunodeficiency virus (HIV) test. Both partners have blood type and Rh determinations in donor matching. The female may have an antisperm antibody screen as indicated. Donors are extensively screened, with cryopreserved specimens stored for at least 6 months, and donors are rescreened for HIV prior to release for use. Laboratory tests include serologic tests for syphilis, hepatitis profile, CMV titer, HIV test, and chlamydia and gonorrhea cultures. Specimens are thawed approximately 20 minutes prior to use. The partner may assist with insemination. Some couples request that the partner's sperm be mixed with the donor sperm.

- *Intrauterine Insemination (IUI).* Performed using washed partner's specimen or thawed, cryopreserved donor specimen. The sperm is separated from the seminal fluid to prevent the proteins, prostaglandins, and bacteria in semen from being deposited in the uterus.[4]

Timing of insemination is determined by using basal body temperature (BBT) readings and urine luteinizing hormone (LH) ovulation predictor kits or ultrasounds for follicular growth and serum LH monitoring. Cervical insemination is performed the day of the LH surge and may be repeated the next day if the BBT is not elevated. Unstimulated IUI is performed the day after the LH surge. Stimulated ovulation induction IUIs are performed approximately 18 and 40 hours after ovulation is induced by administration of human chorionic gonadotropin (Profasi, Pregnyl or APL).

If conception with AIH cervical insemination (fresh specimen) does not occur within 6 cycles, then treatment proceeds to unstimulated IUI for 3 to 4 cycles, then to stimulated ovulation induction IUI for 4 cycles.

With TDI utilizing thawed specimens, conception should occur no later than 12 cycles. Attempt 3 cycles of cervical insemination; then proceed to unstimulated IUI for 3 to 6 cycles; then proceed to stimulated ovulation induction IUI cycles. If conception does not occur after 4 stimulated IUI cycles, assisted reproductive technologies are recommended. If the woman is older, it is reasonable to move more quickly to stimulated IUI. Due to the expense of donor sperm, many health care providers start with IUI cycles.

ASSISTED REPRODUCTIVE TECHNOLOGIES

When other treatment options have been exhausted or when other therapies have a poor prognosis, assisted reproductive technologies are used. Options include in vitro fertilization (IVF); gamete intrafallopian transfer (GIFT); zygote intrafallopian transfer (ZIFT); embryo cryopreservation, assisted hatching, and intracytoplasmic sperm injection. Assisted reproductive technologies may include the use of donor gametes. The therapy recommended will be determined by the couple's diagnosis and age (see Table 10–13 and Figure 10–3).

Success Rates

Success rates are variable. Overall, a clinical pregnancy rate of 26.3 percent per retrieval with IVF embryo transfer; and 36.3 percent with GIFT retrieval was reported for 1994.[52] *Clinical pregnancy* is defined by rising beta human chorionic gonadotropin (β-hCG) titers and the presence of a gestational sac in the uterine cavity, detected by ultrasound monitoring. Multiple gestation and spontaneous abortion may both occur.

Treatment Consideration

Couples must consider the treatment prognosis and their desire for a biologic child. Grief over the loss of a potential unborn child may be intensified as a couple undergoes treatment. The complex stressors and impacts of infertility may heighten the couple's feelings of loss of control. Additional stressors may include physical, emotional, social, family, religious, ethical, legal, and financial issues. Treatment choice is often dictated by finances and insurance coverage. Both couples and individuals may benefit from counseling, referral, stress management, and assistance with resolving grief.[15]

Lesbian couples have the same stressors and decision making problems as straight couples, plus they have co-parenting and adoption-by-partner concerns (see Chapter 23). Single women are opting for infertility treatment, as it has become more acceptable for single women to keep their babies. It is imperative for the nurse practitioner to discuss social support with the client.

Treatment Selection

The specific criteria, as well as risks and benefits of each treatment need to be carefully weighed before one is selected. Information about clinics in the United States may be obtained from the American Society for Reproductive Medicine (formerly the American Fertility Society), Birmingham, Alabama, and from Resolve, Somerville, Massachusetts (see Resources).

Stress Management

Intensive treatment involving rigorous scheduling and invasive procedures is stressful. During the seemingly long interval between the transfer and pregnancy testing, clients may experience symptoms of pregnancy due to hormone stimulation. Couples may be ambivalent and fearful about the outcome or may feel isolated from the IVF team when daily visits stop.[15]

A positive pregnancy test means heightened anxiety for the couple. Although it is joyous news, the couple fears "something will happen." It is difficult to enjoy pregnancy because of past disappointments.[42]

Failure to conceive is devastating physically, emotionally, and financially. These couples experience tremendous personal loss; they may apologize for "letting the IVF team down." Guilt and self-doubt are often expressed. Ambivalence regarding starting a new cycle can add to the stress.[16]

Follow-Up. Maintain the health of the individuals and the couple to enable them to cope and eventually resolve their infertility. Education, support, counseling, and referral are part of the intervention.

ALTERNATIVES TO PREGNANCY

ADOPTION

The hardest part of adoption is the gradual process of deciding to adopt and how to proceed. During infertility treatment, guide the couple toward adoption resources if they are interested. They may, however, perceive adoption as "giving up on their bodies," and fear that this choice will affect their response to treatment and chance of

TABLE 10–13. SUMMARY OF PROCEDURE AND INDICATIONS FOR ASSISTED REPRODUCTIVE TECHNOLOGIES

In Vitro Fertilization (IVF)

Procedure:
Oocytes are fertilized in the laboratory.
Resulting embryos are transferred to the uterus.

Indications:
Tubal factor.
Male factor.
Immunological infertility.
Endometriosis.
Unexplained infertility.

Gamete Intrafallopian Transfer (GIFT)**

Procedure:
Gametes (oocytes and sperm) are transferred to the fallopian tubes.

Indications:
Male infertility (if fertilization has been or will be proven in same cycle by IVF).
Immunological infertility.
Endometriosis.
Unexplained infertility.

Zygote Intrafallopian Transfer (ZIFT)**

Procedure:
Oocytes are fertilized in the laboratory.
Resulting zygotes or fertilized oocytes are transferred to the fallopian tubes.

Indications:
Same as for GIFT.

Intracytoplasmic Sperm Injection (ICSI)

Procedure:
One sperm is injected directly into the cytoplasm of the oocyte.

Indications:
Male factor infertility.

Assisted Hatching

Procedure:
A hole is made in the zona pellucida with a microinjection needle, laser or acidic Tyrode's solution to enhance embryo hatching.

Indications:
Failed IVF cycle.
Woman 35 years or older.
Frozen embryos.

Donor Oocytes

Procedure:
Oocytes are retrieved from a donor and transferred to a recipient in an IVF, GIFT, or ZIFT cycle.

Indications:
Premature ovarian failure.
Loss of gonadal function due to surgery, radiation or chemotherapy.
Congenital absence of ovaries.
Genetic disorder carrier (X-linked or autosomally dominant).
Repeated, unexplained pregnancy loss.
Poor response to gonadotropins.

Gestational Carrier

Procedure:
Oocytes are fertilized in the laboratory.
Resulting embryos are transferred to the uterus of another woman, who will carry the pregnancy.

Indications:
Uterine absence or anomaly (congenital, distortion of cavity).
Medical contraindication to pregnancy.

Embryo Cryopreservation

Procedure:
Freeze extra embryos from an IVF, GIFT or ZIFT cycle.

Indications:
To allow for a subsequent attempt at pregnancy without ovarian stimulation or retrieval.

**Absolute contraindication for GIFT or ZIFT is not having an open fallopian tube.
Source: Adapted from Broer, K. H., & Turanli, I. (Eds.). (1996). New trends in reproductive medicine. Berlin, Germany: Springer.

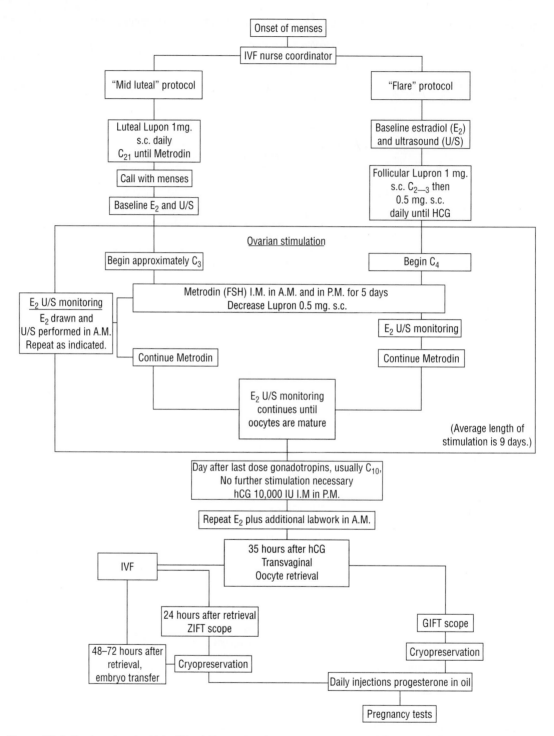

Figure 10–3. Treatment cycle. *Note:* Stimulation protocols vary among programs. Cycles may be canceled at different stages depending on treatment response. *(Source: Medical College of Virginia In Vitro Fertilization Program.)*

conceiving. Some couples feel that they can cope only with the stresses of infertility and not with adoption stresses at the same time. Moreover, adoption does not resolve the couple's feelings about infertility, and they must resolve them, with the support of each other, significant others, and professionals.[53]

A couple's concerns relate to their lack of prenatal control and their ability to love and bond to a child not biologically related. In addition, they may have fears related to their parenting abilities. They wonder, too, how they will manage with psychological, financial, and legal issues, and how they will cope with the potential special needs of an adopted child. The couple must deal with the responses of significant others to adoption, as well as with societal responses.[42]

Options for adoption are by means of a private arrangement (parental placement) or through an agency or international organization. Many adoption agencies insisted that all infertility treatment be complete and neither partner is over 40 years old. Waiting lists may be years long. The adoptive child may have special needs or be an older child. The processes can be complicated, time consuming, and costly. The couple may feel that again they have lost control.[53]

SURROGACY

Traditionally, surrogacy meant that a woman was inseminated with the rearing father's sperm, and at time of delivery, relinquished her rights to the child. Utilizing ART technologies, the surrogate no longer has to donate any genetic material. She can be simply the gestational carrier for an embryo created with donor gametes or gametes from the rearing parents. Surrogacy may also imply a kind of adoption, as the child may or may not have a biologic connection with his or her parents. Couples considering surrogacy need information, support, counseling and legal service.

Social and Ethical Concerns

The potential negative effects of surrogacy on the child, the donor, and their families are the focus of concern. Extensive screening must be completed on both donor and recipient, as both parties must be physically and emotionally healthy. Appropriate precautions during pregnancy must be outlined and maintained.[54]

Secrecy versus open conception is a controversial topic. The impact on the child's self-identity is unknown. Secrecy may be regarded as damaging to the child's trusting relationship with his or her parents. Yet, for the child to learn of others' disapproval and that the "mother" was paid to conceive, gestate, and give the child away is considered destructive. Questions arise regarding trauma to donors (bonding in utero and loss of a child) and their families (loss of a sibling). Recipients undergo stress while waiting for the child to be born, fearing the unknown, the loss of a child, or the inability to bond. The long-term effects of contact between surrogates and recipients and the potential for shared parenting may create conflict and stress.[54]

Payment for surrogacy is taboo, and illegal in some states; it is unacceptable to "sell babies" or to discriminate against those who would choose surrogacy if they could afford this option. It is feared that incest may result if surrogacy becomes more widespread. Legal controversy concerns the rights and responsibilities of donor and recipient, breech of contract, and payment for services. Legislation is needed to regulate but not eliminate surrogacy.[54]

CHILDFREE LIVING

Infertile couples have many difficult decisions to make: how great is their motivation for parenthood? their energy and resources to continue treatment? the value of continuing treatment? Choosing to remain without children is painful, and the couple must come to terms with the loss.[16] The decision is made gradually, and it is a mutual decision. It requires close personal examination and intense communication by the couple.

Finally, the couple feels relieved that their family is complete without children. They no longer feel pressured to "perform on demand," put their "lives on hold," or conform to medical therapies. They are able to regain privacy, control their lives, and focus their energies on themselves, each other, their relationship, and future life goals.[55]

The decision to remain childfree is not easily understood by others. Couples who have resolved their infertility and professionals who work with infertile men and women can help others understand the impact of infertility and the process that occurred in deciding not to have children. Others should be helped to understand that this choice is a positive solution.[42]

NURSING DIAGNOSES

The following nursing diagnoses are representative of those used in the health care plan of women and their partners with an infertility problem. The list, however, is by no means inclusive.

- Anxiety.
- Body image disturbance.
- Comfort, altered.
- Coping ineffective, individual.
- Family coping: potential for growth.
- Grieving.
- Health seeking behaviors.
- Hopelessness.
- Impaired adjustment.
- Nutrition, less or more than body requirements, altered.
- Pain.
- Personal identity disturbance.
- Powerlessness.
- Role performance, altered.
- Role relationship disturbance.
- Self-concept disturbance.
- Self-esteem disturbance.
- Sexual dysfunction.
- Sexuality, reproductive disturbance.
- Skin integrity, risk for impaired.
- Social isolation.
- Spiritual distress.

RESOURCES

Adoptive Families of America
2309 Como Avenue
St. Paul, Minnesota 55108
Phone: (800) 372–3300
Fax: (612) 645–0055
Web Site at http://www.adoptivefam.org

Network of families built by or interested in adoption. Goals are education, support and advocacy. Bimonthly magazine available.

The American Society for Reproductive Medicine
1209 Montgomery Highway
Birmingham, Alabama 35216–2809
Phone: (205) 978–5000
Fax: (205) 978–5005
Web Site at http://www.asrm.com

Patient education booklets, fact sheets, guidelines available. Nurses' Professional Group of ASRM has developed protocols and procedures to provide nursing care.

The Compassionate Friends
P.O. Box 3696
Oak Brook, IL 60522-3696
Phone: (630) 990–0010
Fax: (630) 990–0246
Web Site at http://pages.prodigy.com/CA/lycq97a/lycq97tcf.html

National self-help group to provide support to families who have experienced the death of a child. National newsletter for parents and grandparents and a newsletter for siblings are available. National and regional conferences are held annually.

Resolve, Inc.
1310 Broadway
Somerville, MA 02144–1731
Helpline: (617) 623–0744

National lay organization with local chapters dedicated to providing education, support, and advocacy for couples experiencing infertility. Newsletter and fact sheets available.

Serono Symposia, Inc.
100 Longwater Circle
Norwell, MA 02061
Phone: (617) 982–9000 *or* (800) 283–8088
Fax: (617) 982–9481
Web Site at http://www.springer-ny.com/serosym

Has free patient education booklets on various infertility topics. Sponsors professional and lay symposia to provide education in the field of reproductive medicine. Syllabi from various symposia are available free of charge to nonparticipants of the symposia.

REFERENCES

1. The American College of Obstetricians and Gynecologists. (1996). *Guidelines for women's health care* (pp. 121–127). Washington, DC: Author.
2. Stephen, E. H. (1996). Projections of impaired fecundity among women in the United States: 1995–2020. *Fertil Steril, 66,* 205–209.
3. Kessel, B. (1995). Reproductive cycles in women: quality of life impact. In B. P. Sachs, R. Bears, & E. Papiernik (Eds.), *Reproductive health care for women and babies* (pp. 18–39). New York: Oxford University Press.
4. Speroff, L., Glass, R. H., & Kase, N. G. (1994). *Clinical gynecologic endocrinology and infertility* (5th ed.). Baltimore: Williams & Wilkins.
5. Edwards, R.G., & Brody, S. A. (1995). *Principles and practice of assisted human reproduction.* Philadelphia: W.B. Saunders Company.
6. American Society for Reproductive Medicine (formerly The American Fertility Society). (1996). *Guidelines for the provision of infertility services.* Birmingham, Alabama: Author.
7. Aiken, R. D. (1995). Male infertility: Prognostic value of old and new tests. *Assisted Reproductive Reviews, 5,* 26–27.
8. Broer, K. H., & Turanli, I. (Eds.). (1996). *New trends in reproductive medicine.* Berlin, Germany: Springer.
9. Hall, L.-L., & Rice, V. M. (1995). Ovulation predictors and postcoital testing. In W. R. Meyer. (Ed.), *Infertility and Reproductive Medicine Clinics of North America, 6,* 179–197. Philadelphia: W. B. Saunders Company.
10. Boyers, S. P. (1995). Evaluation and treatment of disorders of the cervix. In W. R. Keye, Jr., R. J. Chang, R. W. Rebar, & M. R. Soules (Eds.), *Infertility: Evaluation and treatment* (pp. 195–229). Philadelphia: W.B. Saunders.
11. World Health Organization. (1992). *Laboratory manual for the examination of human semen and sperm-cervical mucus interaction.* Cambridge: Cambridge University Press.
12. Kruger, T. F., Acosta, A. A., Simmons, K. F., Swanson, R. J., Matta, J. F., & Oehninger, S. (1988). Predictive value of abnormal sperm morphology in in vitro fertilization. *Fertil Steril, 49,* 112–117.
13. Sherins, R. J. (1995). How is male infertility defined? How is it diagnosed? Epidemiology, causes, work-up (history, physical, lab tests). In *The American Society of Andrology, Handbook of Andrology* (pp. 48–51). Lawrence, KS: Allen Press, Inc.
14. Winkel, C. A. (1995). Lesions affecting the uterine cavity. In W. R. Keye, Jr., R. J. Chang, R. W. Rebar, & M. R. Soules (Eds.), *Infertility: Evaluation and treatment* (pp. 425–443). Philadelphia: W.B. Saunders Company.
15. Applegarth, L. D. (1995). The psychological aspects of infertility. In W. R. Keye, Jr., R. J. Chang, R. W. Rebar, & M. R. Soules (Eds.), *Infertility: Evaluation and treatment* (pp. 25–41). Philadelphia: W.B. Saunders Company.
16. Johnston, P. I. (1995). Infertility: A patient's perspective. In W. R. Keye, Jr., R. J. Chang, R. W. Rebar, & M. R. Soules (Eds.), *Infertility: Evaluation and treatment* (pp. 19–24). Philadelphia: W.B. Saunders Company.
17. Burns, L. H. (1996). Pregnancy after infertility. In A. M. Braverman (Ed.), *Infertility and Reproductive Medicine Clinics of North America, 7,* 503–520. Philadelphia: W.B. Saunders Company.
18. *Drug facts and comparisons.* (1997 ed.). St. Louis: Facts and Comparisons.
19. Liu, J. H. (1995). Hypothalamic-pituitary disorders. In W. R. Keye, Jr., R. J. Chang, R. W. Rebar, & M. R. Soules (Eds.), *Infertility: Evaluation and treatment.* Philadelphia: W.B. Saunders Company.
20. Zuckerman, A. L. (1995). Amenorrhea: Diagnosis, evaluation, and treatment. In W. R. Meyer (Ed.), *Infertility and Reproductive Medicine Clinics of North America, 6*(1), 25–36. Philadelphia: W.B. Saunders Company.
21. Levy, M. J. (1995). Hirsutism. In W. R. Meyer (Ed.), *Infertility and Reproductive Medicine Clinics of North America, 6*(1), 215–227. Philadelphia: W.B. Saunders Company.
22. Nestler, J. E., & Jakubowicz, D. J. (1996). Decreases in ovarian cytochrome P450c17 α activity and serum free testosterone after reduction of insulin secretion in polycystic ovary syndrome. *N Engl J Med., 335,* 617–623.

23. Lobo, R. A. (1995). Chronic anovulation and polycystic ovary syndrome: treatment for infertility. In W. R. Keye, Jr., R. J. Chang, R. W. Rebar, & M. R. Soules (Eds.), *Infertility: Evaluation and treatment* (pp. 168–177). Philadelphia: W.B. Saunders.

24. Ostrer, H. (1996). Sex determination. In E. Y. Adashi, J. A. Rock, & Z. Rosenwaks (Eds.), *Reproductive endocrinology, surgery, and technology* (pp. 41–58). Philadelphia: Lippincott-Raven.

25. Yee, B., Rosen, G. F., & Cassidenti, D. L. (1995). *Transvaginal sonography in infertility.* Philadelphia: Lippincott-Raven.

26. Schenken, R. S. (1996). Treatment of human infertility: The special case of endometriosis. In E. Y. Adashi, J. A. Rock, & Z. Rosenwaks (Eds.), *Reproductive endocrinology, surgery, and technology* (pp. 2121–2139). Philadelphia: Lippincott-Raven.

27. Castelbaum, A. J., Lessey, B. A. (1995). Insights into the evaluation of the luteal phase. In W. R. Meyer (Ed.), *Infertility and Reproductive Medicine Clinics of North America, 6*(1), 199–213. Philadelphia: W.B. Saunders Company.

28. Sims, J. A., & Gibbons, W. E. (1996). Treatment of human infertility: The cervical and uterine factors. In E. Y. Adashi, J. A. Rock, & Z. Rosenwaks (Eds.), *Reproductive endocrinology, surgery, and technology* (pp. 2141–2169). Philadelphia: Lippincott-Raven.

29. Rock, J. A., & Markham, S. M. (1995). Developmental anomalies of the reproductive tract. In W. R. Keye, Jr., R. J. Chang, R. W. Rebar, & M. R. Soules (Eds.), *Infertility: Evaluation and treatment* (pp. 387–411). Philadelphia: W.B. Saunders.

30. Marcus, S. F., Rizk, B., Fountain, S., & Brinsden, P. (1994). Tuberculous infertility and in vitro fertilization. *Am J Obstet Gynecol., 171,* 1593–1596.

31. Verkauf, B. S. (1995). The myomatous uterus and reproductive failure: Diagnostic aids for planning therapy. In W. R. Meyer (Ed.), *Infertility and Reproductive Medicine Clinics of North America, 6*(1), 103–134. Philadelphia: W.B. Saunders Company.

32. Lowdermilk, D. L. (1995). Reproductive Surgery. In C. I. Fogel, & N. F. Woods (Eds.), *Women's health care: A comprehensive handbook* (pp. 629–650). Thousand Oaks, CA: Sage Publications.

33. Garner, C. (1995). Infertility. In C. I. Fogel, & N. F. Woods (Eds.), *Women's health care: A comprehensive handbook* (pp. 611–628). Thousand Oaks, CA: Sage Publications, Inc.

34. Lewis, J. A., & Bernstein, J. (1996). *Women's health: A relational perspective across the life cycle.* Boston: Jones and Bartlett Publishers.

35. Westrom, L. (1980). Incidence, prevalence, and trends of acute pelvic inflammatory disease and its consequences in industrialized countries. *AM J Obstet Gynecol, 138*(7), 880–892.

36. Rogers, S. F. (1995). Pelvic inflammatory disease: Effects on future fertility. In W. R. Meyer (Ed.), *Infertility and Reproductive Medicine Clinics of North America, 6*(1), 95–101. Philadelphia: W.B. Saunders Company.

37. Strickler, R. C. (1995). Factors influencing fertility. In W. R. Keye, Jr., R. J. Chang, R. W. Rebar, & M. R. Soules (Eds.), *Infertility: Evaluation and treatment* (pp. 8–18). Philadelphia: W.B. Saunders Company.

37a. Readers are encouraged to review the revised classification of endometriosis appearing in the May 1997 issue of *Fertility and Sterility* (Volume 67, No. 5, pages 817–821). This revised classification provides a standardized form for recording pathologic findings and assigning scalar values to disease status in order to better predict the probability of pregnancy following treatment.

38. Halme, J., & Sahakian, V. (1995). Endometriosis: Pathophysiology and presentation. In W. R. Keye, Jr., R. J. Chang, R. W. Rebar, & M. R. Soules (Eds.), *Infertility: Evaluation and treatment* (pp. 496–508). Philadelphia: W.B. Saunders Company.

39. Scott, J. R., & Branch, D. W. (1995). Evaluation and treatment of recurrent miscarriages. In W. R. Keye, Jr., R. J. Chang, R. W. Rebar, & M. R. Soules (Eds.), *Infertility: Evaluation and treatment* (pp. 230–248). Philadelphia: W.B. Saunders Company.

40. Shaban, S. F. (1995). Male factor infertility. In W. R. Meyer (Ed.), *Infertility and Reproductive Medicine Clinics of North America, 6*(1), 134–256. Philadelphia: W.B. Saunders Company.

41. Matsumoto, A. M. (1995). Pathophysiology of male infertility. In W. R. Keye, Jr., R. J. Chang, R. W. Rebar, & M. R. Soules (Eds.), *Infertility: Evaluation and treatment* (pp. 555–579). Philadelphia: W.B. Saunders Company.

42. Read, J. (1995). *Counselling for fertility problems.* London: Sage Publications.

43. de Kretser, D. M., & Baker, H. W. (1996). Human infertility: The male factor. In E. Y. Adashi, J. A. Rock, & Z. Rosenwaks (Eds.), *Reproductive endocrinology, surgery, and technology* (pp. 2031–2061). Philadelphia: Lippincott-Raven.

44. Whittemore, A. S., Harris, R., Itnyre, J., Halpern, J., & The Collaborative Ovarian Cancer Group.

(1992). Characteristics relating to ovarian cancer risk: Collaborative analysis of 12 US case-control studies. *American Journal of Epidemiology, 136,* 1175–1220.

45. Rossing, M. A., Daling, J. R., Weiss, N. S., Moore, D. E., & Self, S. G. (1994). Ovarian tumors in a cohort of infertile women. *N Engl J Med., 331,* 771–776.

46. Rossing, M. A., Daling, J. R., Weiss, N. S., Moore, D. E., & Self, S. G. (1996). In situ and invasive cervical carcinoma in a cohort of infertile women. *Fertil Steril, 65,* 19–22.

47. Shushan, A., Paltiel, O., Iscovich, J., Elchalal, U., Peretz, T., & Schenker, J. G. (1996). Human menopausal gonadotropin and the risk of epithelial ovarian cancer. *Fertil Steril, 65,* 13–18.

48. Mosgaard, B. J., Lidegaard, Ø., Kjaer, S. K., Schou, G., Andersen, A. N. (1997). Infertility, fertility drugs and invasive ovarian cancer: a case-control study. *Fertil Steril, 67*(6), 1005–1012.

49. Marrs, R. P., & Hartz, S. C. (1993). *Comments on the possible association between ovulation inducing agents and ovarian cancer.* Statement from The American Fertility Society to its Members, January 1993.

50. Byrd, W. (1995). Sperm preparation and homologous insemination. In W. R. Keye, Jr., R. J. Chang, R. W. Rebar, & M. R. Soules (Eds.), *Infertility: Evaluation and treatment* (pp. 696–711). Philadelphia: W.B. Saunders Company.

51. The American Fertility Society. (1993). Guidelines for gamete donation: 1993. *Fertil Steril, 59* (Suppl. 1), 1S–7S.

52. The Society for Assisted Reproductive Technology and The American Society for Reproductive Medicine. (1996). Assisted Reproductive Technology in the United States and Canada: 1994 Results generated from The American Society for Reproductive Medicine/Society for Assisted Reproductive Technology Registry. *Fertil Steril, 66,* 697–708.

53. Johnston, P. (1992). *Adopting after infertility.* Indianapolis, IN: Perspective Press.

54. Robertson, J. A. (1994). *Children of choice: Freedom and the new reproductive technologies.* Princeton, NJ: Princeton University Press.

55. Carter, J., & Carter, M. (1989). *Sweet grapes: How to stop being infertile and start living again.* Indianapolis, IN: Perspective Press.

CHAPTER 11

VAGINITIS AND SEXUALLY TRANSMITTED DISEASES

Susan D. Schaffer

---

*R*esearch supports the protective benefits of latex condoms against HIV, HSV, genital ulcers, gonorrhea, chlamydia, cytomegalovirus, and hepatitis B virus.[1,2]

Highlights

- The Centers for Disease Control
- Vaginitis
    - Bacterial Vaginosis
    - Candida Albicans
    - Cytolytic Vaginosis
    - Trichomoniasis
- Cervicitis
    - Chlamydia Trachomatis
    - Gonorrhea
    - Mucopurulent Cervicitis
- Ulcerative Genital Infections
    - Herpes Simplex Virus
    - Syphilis
    - Chancroid
    - Granuloma Inguinale
    - Lymphogranuloma Venereum
- Epidermal Diseases
    - Human Papillomavirus
    - Molluscum Contagiosum
    - Pediculosis Pubis
- Hepatitis B

▶ INTRODUCTION

Vaginitis and sexually transmitted diseases (STDs) are frequently occurring problems among women. These conditions occur most often during the reproductive years; in fact, many reach their peak incidence during adolescence and young adulthood. Sexual activity and direct intimate contact are responsible for STD transmission in most cases. It is well known that women who are frequently sexually active with multiple partners are at greater risk for STDs than women who are sexually inactive or those with stable, mutually monogamous partners. Nevertheless, broad assumptions about women with STDs are inappropriate.

Billions of dollars are expended annually in the United States to diagnose and treat STDs. Many STDs are uncomplicated (e.g., trichomonas); on the other hand, many have serious long-term health consequences (e.g., chlamydia), and some may be life threatening (e.g., hepatitis B). Prevention should be the primary focus when dealing with all STDs. The effectiveness of latex condoms in reducing the risk of AIDS has had a spillover effect in reducing the risk of other STDs. Similarly, the introduction of universal precautions for health care professionals, a di-

rect result of the human immunodeficiency virus (HIV) epidemic, has made the workplace safer against the transmission of all bloodborne infections.

Women with vaginitis and/or sexually transmitted diseases are represented in every socioeconomic class, culture, age group, and workplace. Their story is often one of fear, anxiety, frustration, anger, shame, and guilt. Often, it is also an untold story. A health care provider giving primary care to women must be able to offer treatment, education, and counseling. Complete, accurate information conveyed in an open, professional manner is essential. Information rapidly changes and requires constant updating. In providing care, sensitivity and kindness are essential. The emotional impact that a sexually transmitted disease has on a client is intense; there is no place for judgmental attitudes. Table 11–1 provides an overview of general information that should be provided to women with vaginitis or a sexually transmitted disease.

Note: Revised Centers for Disease Control sexually transmitted diseases guidelines are due to be released Fall, 1997 as this book goes to press.

SEXUALLY TRANSMITTED DISEASES AND THE CENTERS FOR DISEASE CONTROL

Some STDs, but not all, are reportable by state agencies to the Centers for Disease Control (CDC) in Atlanta, Georgia. The CDC is part of the U.S. Public Health Service and charged with, among other functions, assisting states to identify and control certain diseases. The actual mandate to report specific diseases comes from individual states through their legislative bodies. The CDC can recommend which diseases should be reported; however, the final decision rests with the states. The following STDs are reportable by states to the CDC: AIDS, gonorrhea, hepatitis B, and syphilis.

In addition, some states also require the reporting of HIV infection, Herpes Simplex, nonspecific urethritis, and chlamydia trachomatis.[3]

Three factors are considered in determining which diseases should be reported.

ABILITY TO TEST. If no reasonable test for a condition is readily available (e.g., herpes), then that disease is unlikely to become reportable.

ABILITY TO CURE. Especially important to report are readily curable diseases (e.g., gonorrhea) in order to control epidemics.

PUBLIC AWARENESS. Diseases that gain widespread public attention and represent a public health threat (e.g., AIDS) are usually reportable.

TABLE 11–1. GENERAL INFORMATION NEEDED IN THE CARE OF WOMEN WITH VAGINITIS AND SEXUALLY TRANSMITTED DISEASES (STDS)

Provide both written information and verbal explanations to the client.

Disease Process	Etiology, incubation, risk factors, diagnosis, management, follow-up.
Treatments	Medications and their side effects; signs of allergic response; discomfort; time commitments; simultaneous partner treatment; the need to keep appointments for treatment and thereby control growth and spread of lesions and worsening of disease and symptoms; avoidance of douching and tampon use (unless medically directed) until healing is complete.
Transmission	A description of all possible modes; the need to suspend genital and oral sexual relations, foreign body insertion, and manual manipulation until healing is complete; use of lubricated latex condoms until partners are examined and determined disease-free; the dangers of multiple partners and the principles of "safer sex."
Comfort Measures	Sitz baths and oral analgesics may help some conditions.
Hygiene	The importance of cleanliness and dryness to enhance healing. Use of a hair dryer on low setting to aid drying. Avoidance of powders, douches (especially perfumed or deodorized), perfumed sprays. Discussion of secondary infection and how it may occur. Wearing clean cotton underwear, loose clothing and fabrics that "breathe"; washing hands thoroughly before and after touching genitalia; not wearing underwear more than one day; not wearing anyone else's underwear; not allowing anyone other than oneself to wear one's underwear or tight fitting trousers; changing out of moist clothing as soon as possible.
Other Prevention	Decreasing smoking in infection with human papillomavirus (HPV); self-monitoring of the vulva (HPV); client examination of partner and asking about past exposure; empowerment of client (through role playing) to be motivated and skillful in talking about sensitive issues with her partner; caution in new sexual liaisons; avoidance of alcohol and drugs that limit inhibitions; an agreement ("contract") with her partner that they have a mutually monogamous relationship; for their mutual safety, an agreement between the two partners in the relationship to tell each other if either one has sexual relations with someone else.

Source: Bennett, M. (1994). Vaginitis and Sexually Transmitted Diseases in Youngkin, E. & Davis, M. Women's Health: A Primary Care Clinical Guide. (1st Ed.) Norwalk, CT: Appleton & Lange.

In addition to compiling STD statistics, the CDC recommends treatment for individual diseases. Approximately every 4–5 years, it publishes STD treatment guidelines. The most recent of these guidelines, published in 1993, are used throughout this chapter when discussing medication, although some newer research based recommendations are also included. *Readers should compare the newest CDC guidelines with those provided in this chapter when they are published.*

The remainder of this chapter is organized according to clinical syndromes. This facilitates clinical decision making when the clinician is faced with vaginitis or a possible STD. First, the clinician must determine the type of clinical syndrome based on presenting symptoms. Then the possible causes of that syndrome can be considered. Although HIV infection is primarily sexually transmitted, it is discussed in a separate chapter due to the complex psychosocial and medical manage-

ment required by persons with this infection (see Chapter 12).

VAGINITIS

Vaginitis occurs when the vaginal ecosystem has been disturbed, either by the introduction of an organism, or by a disturbance that allows the pathogens normally residing in this environment to proliferate. Factors that may alter the vaginal ecosystem include antibiotics, hormones, contraceptive preparations (oral and topical), douches, vaginal medication, sexual intercourse, STDs, stress, and changes in sexual partners.[4] The hallmarks of vaginitis are excessive or malodorous vaginal discharge, pruritus or irritation, and sometimes external dysuria. Diagnosis of vaginitis is made by close inspection of the external genitalia, determination of the pH of the vaginal discharge (normally 3.8–4.2) and microscopic examination of the discharge.

BACTERIAL VAGINOSIS (BV)

Bacterial infections of the vagina have been known by various names such as Gardnerella vaginalis, hemophilus vaginalis, nonspecific vaginitis, and bacterial vaginitis. *Bacterial vaginosis* is currently preferred because it highlights the polymicrobial nature of the infection and the frequent absence of inflammatory cells.[5]

BV is the most prevalent form of vaginitis among childbearing women. It is a syndrome in which normal H_2O_2 producing Lactobacilli in the vagina are replaced with high concentrations of anaerobic bacteria (e.g., Gardnerella vaginalis, Mobiluncus species, Mycoplasma hominis and Bacteroides.[4,5] Research suggests that BV is associated with preterm labor, chorioamnionitis, postpartum endometritis, and PID.[6]

Epidemiology

Etiology/Risk Factors. Antibiotics, douching, or intercourse may raise the normally acidic vaginal pH, altering the hydrogen ion concentration and favoring increased growth of pathologic anaerobic bacteria.[4] Although women who have never been sexually active are rarely affected, BV is not considered to be exclusively an STD.[6] However, women with recurrent BV should be assessed for other sexually transmitted infections, particularly gonorrhea and chlamydia.[6]

Transmission. Research suggests a nonsexual mode of transmission, although BV occurs almost exclusively in sexually active women.[7] The treatment of male partners does not reduce the risk of recurrence. Since BV associated bacteria can be recovered from the urethra of male partners, some investigators recommend that a couple abstain from intercourse or that condoms be used during treatment.[4]

Incidence. BV has been found in 10–25 percent of patients in general gynecology clinics and in up to 64 percent of patients visiting STD clinics.[8,9,10]

Subjective Data

Clients with BV may be asymptomatic or may have malodorous vaginal discharge. Often, clients report foul odor after intercourse. Symptoms such

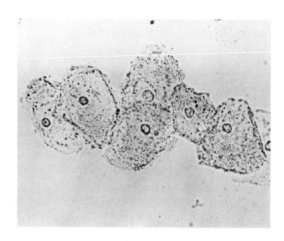

Figure 11–1. Saline wet mount of clue cells from Gardnerella vaginalis infection. Note the absence of inflammatory cells. *(Reproduced with permission, from DeCherney, A. H., & Pernoll, M. L.:* Current Obstetric & Gynecologic Diagnosis & Treatment, *8th Ed. Appleton & Lange, 1994.)*

as pruritus, abdominal pain, dyspareunia, and dysuria do not reliably correlate with BV.

Objective Data

Physical Examination. Clinical diagnosis of BV requires that three of the following four criteria be met: thin, dark or dull gray homogeneous malodorous adherent vaginal discharge, pH level above 4.5, positive whiff test, and/or presence of clue cells on wet-mount microscopic examination. Cultures are not recommended.[4]

Diagnostic Tests and Methods
- *Saline Wet Mount.* Diagnostic evaluation for clue cells: characteristic epithelial cells with bacteria adherent to the cell wall, giving it a stippled, granular appearance (see Figure 11-1). Cell margins become blurred, and few white blood cells are noted.

  The test procedure is to mix a sample of vaginal secretions (obtained from the vaginal pool or posterior blade of the speculum) with normal saline, place on a slide, and cover with a coverslip. Examine microscopically under low and high power. Explain the procedure to the client. Advise her that an immediate diagnosis is possible.
- *"Whiff" Test.* Diagnostic evaluation for a "fishy" amine odor. The test procedure is to mix

vaginal secretions with 10 percent potassium hydroxide (KOH); the characteristic odor is readily emitted. Advise the client of the test purpose.

- *Vaginal pH.* Diagnostic evaluation for acidity of vaginal secretions. In BV, pH is greater than or equal to 4.5, but this is not specific for BV alone. The test procedure is to dip appropriate pH paper (pH range 4.0 to 6.0) into vaginal secretions and observe the color change. The sample may be obtained by swabbing the lateral and posterior fornix and applying directly to pH paper, or by dipping pH paper into the posterior blade of the speculum after removal from the vagina. Advise the client of the purpose of the test.

Differential Medical Diagnoses

Trichomonas vaginitis, foreign body vaginitis, monilia.

Plan

Psychosocial Interventions. Because the etiology of BV is uncertain and changing, a client's confusion is understandable. Counsel clients about what is currently known and what is being suggested. If BV is related to an organism that is sexually transmitted is unknown, male partners need not be treated. Routine treatment is recommended for asymptomatic women, particularly those who are planning pregnancy or at high risk for pregnancy. Recurrence rates are high. Over-the-counter remedies such as lactobacillus products are not therapeutic.

Medication

Metronidazole Oral Tablets/
Metronidazole Vaginal Gel

- *Indications.* Oral metronidazole is recommended treatment for BV in females (including the second trimester of pregnancy) and males. Vaginal gel has demonstrated efficacy in female patients.[10]
- *Administration.* Oral tablets: 500 mg b.i.d. for 7 days or 2 g single dose stat.[6] The single dose regimen may enhance compliance but is slightly less effective (69 percent) and may cause more GI upset.[11] Vaginal gel 0.75 percent: one applicator full intravaginally q.d. or b.i.d. for 5 days.

- *Side Effects and Adverse Reactions.* All alcohol products must be avoided with any metronidazole regimen because profuse nausea and vomiting (disulfiram reaction) may occur. Transient nausea and a metallic taste have also been reported. Because metronidazole has a broad antimicrobial spectrum, normal vaginal flora may be suppressed with subsequent monilial infection. Vaginal gel: vaginal candidiasis, occasional genitourinary-perineal itching, irritation, swelling; gastrointestinal complaints.
- *Contraindications.* Known allergy to metronidazole. Do not use during the first trimester of pregnancy.
- *Anticipated Outcomes on Evaluation.* Symptoms clear rapidly after treatment. A test for cure is not routinely indicated.
- *Client Teaching and Counseling.* Stress the need to avoid alcohol. If symptoms return, re-examination is indicated. Treatment of the sexual partner with recurrent infection is recommended. Sexual abstinence or use of condoms during treatment is recommended. Advise the client about side effects.

Clindamycin

- *Indications.* Alternative treatment of BV; may be useful in recurrent cases and during the first trimester of pregnancy.
- *Administration.* Two percent clindamycin cream intravaginally daily (usually at bedtime) for 7 days.[4,6] Clindamycin may be used orally 300 mg b.i.d. for 7 days,[5] but severe side effects are more common with this regimen.
- *Side Effects and Adverse Reactions.* Colitis, may be severe (more common with oral form). Vaginitis from *Candida albicans* is more common with clindamycin use.
- *Contraindications.* Known sensitivity to clindamycin. Do not use condom or diaphragm within 72 hours. Vaginal cream not recommended in pregnancy due to possible preterm birth association.
- *Anticipated Outcome on Evaluation.* Symptoms resolve rapidly. Test for cure is not necessary.
- *Client Teaching and Counseling.* The regimen of medication must be completed.
- *Follow-Up and Referral.* No follow-up is necessary.

CANDIDIASIS

About 30 percent of women with a healthy vaginal environment harbor Candida, usually Candida albicans. An upset in the homeostatic balance in the vagina leads to an overgrowth of this organism and symptoms of infection. These changes may be phenotypic changes in the organism or changes in the vaginal environment.[4] Vulvovaginal candidiasis (VVC) is a common, irritating, and recurrent cause of vaginitis that is not generally sexually transmitted. Predisposing factors include antibiotic use, obesity, diabetes, HIV infection (or other immunosuppressive conditions), and pregnancy. Other names for the condition are monilia and yeast infection.

Epidemiology

C. albicans is a fungal species that is responsible for 75–85 percent of infections. C. tropicalis and C. glabrata are responsible for the remainder of infections.[4,12] As many as 75 percent of women will experience at least one episode of VVC during their lifetime; 40–50 percent of women will experience two or more infections.[13] The organism gains access to the vaginal mucosa primarily from the perianal area.

C. albicans can be transmitted from infected mother to newborn at delivery. Neonates develop an oral infection known as thrush.

Subjective Data

VVC presents with vaginal itching, burning, and irritation. Dysuria (burning when urine hits the involved tissue) is common. Vaginal discharge, which may be scanty or profuse, is white and thick. Symptoms frequently worsen prior to menses. Most clients report an acute onset of symptoms that rapidly clear with treatment. A small subset of women experience persistent chronic infection that does not respond well to classic treatment.

Objective Data

Physical Examination. The vulva may be red and inflamed and edematous or appear normal. Excoriations may be present. Typically, a white dis-

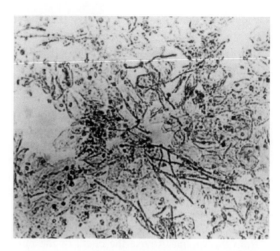

Figure 11–2. Saline wet mount demonstrating Candida albicans. *(Reproduced with permission, from DeCherney, A. H., & Pernoll, M. L.* Current Obstetric & Gynecologic Diagnosis & Treatment, *8th Ed. Appleton & Lange, 1994.)*

charge with the consistency of cottage cheese is adherent to the vaginal mucosa, which may also be inflamed and edematous. Odor is absent and the pH is normal.

Diagnostic Tests and Methods. Microscopic examination of vaginal solution diluted with saline (wet mount) or 10 percent KOH preparations will demonstrate hyphal forms or budding yeast cells in 50–70 percent of infected women (see Figures 11–2 and 11–3). The test procedure involves mixing a sample of vaginal secretions with saline, covering with coverslip, and viewing under microscope. A wet mount prepared with 10 percent potassium hydroxide will obliterate cellular material so that yeasts may be seen more easily.

Some cases of VVC are not detected in a wet mount because there are relatively few organisms or because of poor smear technique. Additionally, nonalbicans species tend not to form pseudohyphae.[4]

Focus client teaching on explaining that immediate diagnosis is possible.

- *Vaginal Culture.* Although routine culture is not cost effective, cultures may be helpful in recurrent VVC. Cultures are prepared by placing

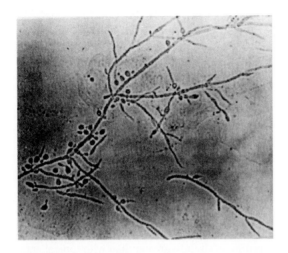

Figure 11–3. KOH preparation showing branched and budding Candida albicans. *(Reproduced with permission, from DeCherney, A. H., & Pernoll, M. L.* Current Obstetric & Gynecologic Diagnosis & Treatment, *8th Ed. Appleton & Lange, 1994.)*

a sample of vaginal secretions on Nickerson's medium or Sabouraud's agar. Accurate culture is only possible using the appropriate medium. Advise the client that the yeast culture is the most sensitive test but results take up to 72 hours to obtain.

Differential Medical Diagnoses

Bacterial vaginosis, trichomonas, allergic contact dermatitis, pediculosis pubis, cytolytic vaginosis.

Plan

Psychosocial Interventions. Advise the client that infection is not sexually transmitted and treatment of her partner is unnecessary unless pruritic balanitis is present in her partner. Rigorous, immediate treatment in pregnancy is recommended to avoid neonatal thrush. Women with chronic moniliasis need intensive counseling to cope with discomfort and long-term medication regimens. Often chronic infection leads to chronic dyspareunia, which can stress relationships. Advise clients to wear cotton underwear, avoid tight fitting nylons and slacks, wipe the perineum from front to back, and use mild soaps. Douching

should be avoided. **Clients should be advised that topical vaginal creams or ointments formulated with petrolatum will weaken latex; latex condoms and diaphragms may not be reliable if used during treatment.**

Medication. Uncomplicated, acute VVC can now be effectively treated with a wide variety of products, including a recently FDA approved single dose oral agent. Treatment length can vary from a single dose to a 7-day therapy regimen; however, uncomplicated, mild, nonrecurrent VVC may be most likely to respond to single dose therapy.[14] Most C. albicans species are susceptible to over-the-counter preparations; however, nonalbicans species may require prescription antifungal agents. The more commonly prescribed medications are discussed here.

MICONAZOLE (MONISTAT). 2 percent cream, 100 mg vaginal suppository, 200 mg vaginal suppository. Available over the counter.

- *Indications.* Acute and chronic infections. Safe during pregnancy.
- *Administration.* One applicator of cream in vagina q.h.s. for 7 nights, *or* one 100 mg vaginal suppository q.h.s. for 7 nights, *or* one 200 mg suppository q.h.s. for 3 nights. Clients who are diagnosed soon after the onset of symptoms may be treated with a 3-day regimen. Those with longstanding symptoms should use a 7-day treatment.[4,6]
- *Side Effects and Adverse Reactions.* Few reactions are reported. Occasional burning after application may occur.
- *Contraindications.* Known hypersensitivity to miconazole.
- *Anticipated Outcomes on Evaluation.* Symptoms will rapidly resolve. Routine test for cure (wet mount) is not recommended for acute infection but is advised with chronic recurrent vaginitis.
- *Client Teaching and Counseling.* Advise the client that medication is to be completed as prescribed. Symptoms often will abate before medication is finished, but it must be completed to avoid recurrence. Cream or suppositories should be inserted immediately before retiring or lying down. Some may leak out on arising.

Panty liners are helpful during the daytime to prevent moist underwear. Avoid tampon use with cream or suppository because tampons absorb medication, interfering with delivery of the therapeutic dose.

CLOTRIMAZOLE (GYNE-LOTRIMIN, MYCELEX). 1 percent cream, 100 mg vaginal tablet (over the counter). 500 mg vaginal tablet.[4]

- *Indications.* Acute and chronic infections. Safe during pregnancy.
- *Administration.* One applicator of cream in vagina q.h.s. for 7 to 14 nights, *or* 1 vaginal tablet q.h.s. for 7 nights, *or* 2 vaginal tablets q.h.s. for 3 nights, *or* 1 single 500 mg vaginal suppository once.[4,6]
- *Side Effects and Adverse Reactions.* Same as miconazole/clotrimazole.
- *Contraindications.* Known hypersensitivity to miconazole.
- *Anticipated Outcomes on Evaluation.* Symptoms will rapidly resolve. Routine test for cure (wet mount) is not recommended for acute infection but is advised with chronic recurrent vaginitis.
- *Client Teaching and Counseling.* Advise the client that medication is to be completed as prescribed. Symptoms often will abate before medication is finished, but it must be completed to avoid recurrence. Cream or suppositories should be inserted immediately before retiring or lying down. Some may leak out on arising. Panty liners are helpful during the daytime to prevent moist underwear. Avoid tampon use with cream or suppository because tampons absorb medication, interfering with delivery of the therapeutic doses.

TERCONAZOLE (TERAZOL). 0.4 or 0.8 percent vaginal cream; 80 mg vaginal suppository.

- *Indications.* Acute infection; suspected C. tropicalis and C. glabrata may respond better to terconazole than to miconazole or clotrimazole.
- *Administration.* One applicator of 0.4 percent cream intravaginally q.h.s. for 7 days; or 1 application of 0.8 percent cream intravaginally q.h.s. for 3 days; or 1 vaginal suppository q.h.s. for 3 days.[4,6]
- *Side Effects and Adverse Reactions.* Same as miconazole.

- *Contraindications.* Same as miconazole.
- *Anticipated Outcomes on Evaluation.* Same as miconazole.
- *Client Teaching and Counseling.* Same as miconazole.

FLUCONAZOLE (DIFLUCAN). 150 mg oral tablet.

- *Indications.* Acute infection with Candida (not recommended for non-Candidal species) for clients who prefer not to use topical vaginal medications. Not recommended in pregnancy (pregnancy category C).
- *Administration.* One 150 mg oral tablet.
- *Side Effects and Adverse Reactions.* Side effect profile is slightly greater than with topical antifungals (26 percent versus 16 percent).[14] Most common side effects include headache, nausea, and abdominal pain. Skin rashes have been reported. Hepatic toxicity has been associated with Fluconazole (not dose related).[14]
- *Contraindications.* Hypersensitivity to Fluconazole. There is no information related to cross hypersensitivity between Fluconazole and other azoles.
- *Drug Interactions.* Clinically significant hypoglycemia may be precipitated by the use of Diflucan with oral hypoglycemic agents. Prothrombin time may be increased in patients receiving Fluconazole with coumarin-type anticoagulants. Diflucan increases the plasma levels of Dilantin, cyclosporin, and theophylline. Rifampin enhances the metabolism of Fluconazole (may require increased dose of Diflucan when given with Rifampin). Fluconazole may inhibit the metabolism of ethinyl estradiol and levonorgestrel. The clinical significance of these effects is unknown. Although no interaction has been observed between Fluconazole and terfenadine, patients receiving these drugs concurrently should be monitored for cardiac dysrhythmias.[14]
- *Anticipated Outcomes on Evaluation.* Symptoms will improve.
- *Client Teaching and Counseling.* Client should be advised of possible drug interactions.

KETOCONAZOLE (NIZORAL). 200 mg oral tablet.

- *Indications.* Effective for acute infection but very expensive and not FDA approved for this use. Should be reserved for long-term suppression of chronic infection with *C. albicans* (resistance, however, has been associated with chronic use).

- *Administration.* Acute infection: one tablet p.o. b.i.d. for 5 days. Suppressive therapy: 1/2 tablet to one tablet p.o daily for 6 months.[4]
- *Side Effects and Adverse Reactions.* Liver toxicity has been reported; therefore, liver function studies should be obtained with long-term therapy. GI irritation, fever, chills, and hormonal effects have also been reported.
- *Contraindications.* Known sensitivity to ketoconazole.
- *Anticipated Outcomes on Evaluation.* Symptoms will improve.
- *Client Teaching and Counseling.* Once long-term therapy is completed, rebound infection may result. Oral absorption may be impaired by antacids, cimetadine, or rifampin.

OTHER MEDICATIONS. Other intravaginal formulations that may be used include butoconazole 2 percent cream q.d. for 3 days or tioconazole 6.5 percent ointment once intravaginally in one single dose (now available over-the-counter).[4,6]

Nontraditional Interventions. Boric acid 600 mgs in size 0 gelatin capsules inserted into the vagina nightly for 14 days has been reported to be effective for resistant infections.[4] Boric acid has not gained widespread acceptance, perhaps because so many other preparations are readily available. The use of intravaginal yogurt has not been scientifically studied, and reports of its efficacy are only anecdotal; however, a recent study compared the rates of infection among women who ate yogurt containing *Lactobacillus acidophilus* for 6 months and women who did not. The yogurt group had significantly fewer infections.[15]

Follow-Up and Referral

Clients with simple, acute candidiasis do not require a follow-up visit. Those with chronic infection must be seen 1 to 2 weeks after treatment. A test for cure, preferably via culture, should be done.

CYTOLYTIC VAGINOSIS

Although not well studied, this condition is increasingly recognized as a cause of recurring (cyclic) vaginitis. It is frequently confused with vulvovaginal candidiasis since the symptoms are similar. Formerly known as Doderlein's cytolysis, it is diagnosed by excluding other common causes of vaginitis and identifying increased numbers of lactobacillus on a wet mount along with cytolysis of the vaginal epithelium (cell membranes of epithelial cells are dissolved, leaving bare nuclei).[16] A similar condition also recurring during the second half of the menstrual cycle and characterized by increased numbers of long anaerobic lactobacilli but without cytolysis of the vaginal epithelium has also been described.[17]

Epidemiology

Cytolytic vaginosis is not sexually transmitted but is believed to be caused by an overgrowth of lactobacilli and possibly other nonpathogenic bacteria. The cause of this overgrowth is unknown. Symptoms may increase during the second half of the menstrual cycle and decrease with onset of menses.[17]

Subjective Data

Symptoms include increased vaginal discharge, dyspareunia, vulvar pruritus, and dysuria. There are no systemic symptoms.

Objective Data

Physical Examination. Physical examination is unremarkable except for the presence of frothy or thick white discharge and a pH level between 3.5 and 4.5.

Diagnostic Tests and Methods. Diagnosis is made on the basis of a wet mount examination. Diagnostic criteria are 1) absence of trichomonas, clue cells, and Candida 2) few leukocytes, 3) increased lactobacilli,[16,17] and 4) cytolysis of vaginal epithelial cells.[16]

Differential Medical Diagnosis

Trichomonas, vulvovaginal candidiasis, bacterial vaginosis.

Plan

Psychosocial Intervention. Assure the client that her symptoms are not evidence of sexually transmitted infection and have no known sequela. The client should stop antifungal medications, stop tampons, and stop douches except as recommended. Baking soda baths (2 tablespoons of baking soda in 2 inches of warm bath water) may be soothing. Conservative vulvar care may be beneficial (avoiding soap, wearing white cotton underwear, applying petroleum jelly or pure mineral oil to pruritic areas b.i.d.).[18]

Medication. Two treatments have been described for Cytolytic vaginosis. One treatment increases the pH of the vagina using sodium bicarbonate douches. The client should mix 30–60 grams of sodium bicarbonate to one liter of warm water and douche with the solution two to three times a week, then weekly as needed. The patient can be advised to begin treatment during the second half of her menstrual cycle if she experiences recurrent luteal symptoms.[16] Partner treatment is not indicated. Follow-up examination is not required.

Another approach directed toward eradication of the overgrowth of lactobacilli is to use Augmentin 500 mg p.o. t.i.d. for 7 days.[17] A concurrent antifungal agent may be beneficial.[18]

TRICHOMONIASIS

In this common form of vaginitis, women may be markedly symptomatic or asymptomatic. Men are asymptomatic carriers. Although this infection is localized, there is increased incidence of premature delivery and postpartum endometritis in women infected with Trichomonas vaginalis.[13]

Epidemiology

Trichomonas vaginalis, a flagellated, anaerobic protozoan, is the causative organism. Sexual contact is the primary means of transmission. Although nonsexual transmission via fomites is theoretically possible, clinically it is rare. The organism lives in the vagina, urethra, Bartholin's and Skene's glands in women and in the urethra and prostate gland of men. It is transmitted during vaginal-penile intercourse, and transmission rates are high. There is no finite incubation period. Trichomoniasis occurs in approximately 3 million women annually,[19] and is responsible for one

fourth of vulvovaginitis complaints.[4] Prevalence is highest in STD clinics and lowest in the private sector. Use of oral contraceptives and barrier methods decreases prevalence.[19]

Subjective Data

Foul-smelling, yellow-green, frothy vaginal discharge may be profuse or scanty. Vaginal odor is the primary presenting symptom. Infrequently, women report dyspareunia and dysuria. Rarely, men have symptoms of urethritis or prostatitis.

Objective Data

Physical Examination. Infection is often detected on routine examination in the absence of subjective complaints. In addition to discharge as previously described, physical examination reveals vulvar erythema and edema and occasionally petechial lesions on the cervix (sometimes called "strawberry cervix"). The pH will be elevated. Signs and symptoms alone are insufficient to make the diagnosis.

Diagnostic Tests and Methods. A culture is the most sensitive and specific diagnostic method, but it is expensive and not widely available. Wet mount using saline is the most clinically useful test. Diagnosis is made when a motile flagellated trichomonad is visualized (see Figure 11–4). In addition, an increased number of white blood cells may be evident in the wet mount. Pap smear results often include reporting of trichomonads, but the sensitivity of the method is low (65 percent).

Differential Medical Diagnoses

Bacterial vaginosis, candidiasis, foreign body vaginitis, cytolytic vaginosis.

Plan

Psychosocial Interventions. The client may experience anxiety and fear with the knowledge that trichomoniasis is sexually transmitted. Reassure her that the infection is curable. Pregnant clients must wait until the second trimester for treatment. Counseling should include the need to treat male partners.

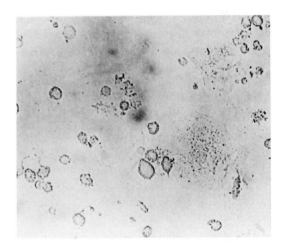

Figure 11–4. Saline wet mount with motile trichomonads in the center. *(Reproduced with permission, from DeCherney, A. H., & Pernoll, M. L.* Current Obstetric & Gynecologic Diagnosis & Treatment, *8th Ed. Appleton & Lange, 1994.)*

Medication

METRONIDAZOLE

- *Indications.* Symptomatic and asymptomatic clients and partners; it is the drug of choice for *Trichomonas* infection.
- *Administration.* Metronidazole 2 g p.o., in a single dose for both partners. If treatment fails, clients should be retreated with metronidazole 500 mg b.i.d. for 7 days. Another alternative is 2 g p.o., daily for 3 to 5 days.[6]
- *Side Effects and Adverse Reactions.* Occur with the use of alcohol when taking metronidazole; vomiting and flushing may result. Transient nausea and a metallic taste have also been reported. Because metronidazole has a broad antimicrobial spectrum, normal vaginal flora may be suppressed with subsequent candidal infection.
- *Contraindications.* Known allergy to metronidazole. Do not use during the first trimester of pregnancy.
- *Anticipated Outcomes on Evaluation.* Symptoms clear rapidly after treatment. A test for cure is not routinely indicated.
- *Client Teaching and Counseling.* Stress the need to avoid alcohol 24 hours before and 48 hours after treatment. If symptoms return, reexamination is indicated. Routine treatment of the

sexual partner is recommended, and the client should be sexually abstinent or use condoms until her partner is treated.

CERVICITIS

Although many sexually transmitted pathogens may gain entry through the vagina, vulva, or cervix, infections characterized by cervicitis primarily use the cervix as a portal of entry. Thus, barrier methods such as condoms and diaphragms are particularly effective in the prevention of cervicitis. Clinical syndromes characterized by cervicitis are considered when mucoid or purulent discharge is observed in the cervical os. Women with cervicitis may have vaginal discharge and dysuria, although many women with cervicitis (perhaps most) are asymptomatic.

CHLAMYDIA TRACHOMATIS INFECTIONS

Chlamydia trachomatis is the most common STD in Western countries, with more than 4 million estimated new cases each year.[20] Men and women may be asymptomatic or symptomatic. Men primarily develop urethritis. In women, chlamydia is associated with cervicitis, acute urethral syndrome, salpingitis, pelvic inflammatory disease, infertility, and perihepatitis. Some women with apparently uncomplicated cervical infection have been shown to have subclinical upper reproductive tract infection.[21] All women with chlamydia should be tested for gonorrhea before treatment is begun.[22]

Newborns delivered to infected mothers may develop conjunctivitis or pneumonitis. In the adult population worldwide, chlamydia is the etiologic agent of trachoma, the leading cause of preventable blindness. Trachoma is not endemic to the United States, however.

Epidemiology

Chlamydia trachomatis is an obligate intracellular parasite that displays some bacterial properties and some viral properties. Unable to produce its own energy, it depends on the host for survival. Risk factors parallel those of gonorrhea. Transmission may be sexual, requiring direct contact with an infected individual; or it may be congenital, acquired at birth when delivery occurs through an infected birth canal. Transplacental transmission does not occur. The incubation period is 10 to 30 days.

The infection is particularly prevalent among adolescents and young adults, so testing sexually active adolescent women should be routine during gynecologic examination. Women using oral contraceptives have been found to be at increased risk for Chlamydia, possibly because oral contraceptive induced ectopy exposes more susceptible cells to infection.[23]

Chlamydial infection is not reportable to the CDC, but the infection is reportable in some states. Incidence ranges from 3 to 5 percent among asymptomatic women and 20 percent among women attending STD clinics.

Subjective Data

Women may be asymptomatic. Subjective symptoms are similar to those seen with gonorrhea and relate to the site of infection. They include vaginal discharge, pelvic pain (dull or severe), fever, dysuria (frequency and urgency). Men may report a penile discharge and burning with urination.

Objective Data

Physical Examination. Because the majority of women with chlamydial infection are asymptomatic, the physical examination may reveal nothing abnormal. The cervix, however, may show mucopurulent discharge, hypertrophic ectopy, and friability. There may be mild to severe adnexal tenderness and/or cervical motion tenderness.

Diagnostic Tests and Methods.[23a,b] A wet mount of the discharge may show numerous white blood cells but also may be negative in the presence of infection. Urine culture may be sterile in the presence of urinary symptoms.

CULTURE. Diagnostic evaluation for symptomatic or asymptomatic chlamydial infection. A culture is the "gold standard" for identification of infection, but is expensive, requires special transport and storage, and requires 3–9 days for results.

The test procedure involves collection of a sample that contains many epithelial cells. This is essential. Cleanse the ectocervix of excessive secretions. Insert a cytologic brush or sterile Dacron tipped swab 1 to 2 cm into the endocervix. Rotate it and withdraw it. Place the swab in transport media. Refrigerate and transport the swab on ice to a laboratory within 24 hours. Explain to the client the minor discomfort that may occur with endocervical sampling.

ANTIGEN DETECTION TESTS. Diagnostic evaluation for symptomatic or asymptomatic infection. These nonculture, rapid detection methods use enzyme linked immunoassay (e.g., Chlamydiazyme) or direct immunofluorescent staining (e.g., Microtrak). These indirect tests have sensitivity and specificity of about 75–90 percent and 95 percent respectively.[23]

First, obtain an adequate sample, as noted previously for culture. Many commercial kits are available. Follow the manufacturer's directions exactly. Prepare the client for the minor discomfort that may occur with sampling. Advise her that results are available in 1 to 2 days, depending on the method used and laboratory access.

The direct smear is best suited to labs that handle a small number of samples. It requires a high quality fluorescent microscope and a well trained technician, and it is labor intensive. The enzyme linked immunoassay is better suited to labs that run a large number of samples. They are automated and labor saving. Both are good for screening high risk populations. If the availability of chlamydial testing is limited, priority should be given to screening adolescents, high risk pregnant women, and those with multiple sexual partners.

PAPANICOLAOU (PAP) SMEAR. Diagnostic evaluation is nonspecific for chlamydia but may show a characteristic inflammatory pattern that suggests the need for definitive testing. For test procedure and nursing implications/client teaching, see chapters 5 and 13.

Differential Medical Diagnoses

Gonorrhea, mucopurulent cervicitis, salpingitis, pelvic inflammatory disease.

Plan

Psychosocial Interventions. Encourage clients to have chlamydia screening if they are in a risk group. Those with multiple partners or a new sexual partner are especially at risk. Partners of individuals diagnosed with chlamydia should be tested and treated; if testing is unavailable, the partners should be treated presumptively. High risk pregnant women need screening and treatment to prevent congenital transmission. Individuals with chlamydia should be tested for other STDs because of the high rate of concurrent disease.

Medication

DOXYCYCLINE

- *Indications.* Treatment of uncomplicated urethral, endocervical, and rectal infections in women and men.
- *Administration.* Doxycycline 100 mg p.o., b.i.d. for 7 days.[6]
- *Side Effects and Adverse Reactions.* Gastrointestinal (GI) upset, rash, photosensitivity. Overgrowth of vaginal candida.
- *Contraindications.* Known pregnancy, sensitivity to tetracyclines. Not for use in children.
- *Anticipated Outcomes on Evaluation.* Antimicrobial resistance to this treatment has not been observed. Provided that treatment is completed, test for cure is not recommended.
- *Client Teaching and Counseling.* Instruct the client that all medication must be taken. Use of antacids must be avoided during treatment. Partners should be treated concurrently and should abstain from intercourse until the treatment is completed.

ERYTHROMYCIN

- *Indications.* Chlamydial infection during pregnancy.
- *Administration.* 500 mg p.o., q.i.d. for 7 days.[6]
- *Side Effects and Adverse Reactions.* Gastrointestinal distress.
- *Contraindications.* Sensitivity to erythromycin.
- *Anticipated Outcomes on Evaluation.* Because experience in treating with erythromycin is limited, a test for cure 3 weeks after completion of medication is recommended. Retesting with the DNA probe should be done at 6 weeks because of increased false positive results at 3 weeks.[22]
- *Follow-Up and Referral.* Necessary only if the client was nonresponsive to the medication.

AZITHROMYCIN

- *Indications.* Treatment of uncomplicated urethral, endocervical, and rectal infections in women and men. Useful if compliance may be a problem. Expense must be considered.
- *Administration.* 1 gm once p.o.[4,21]
- *Side Effects and Adverse Reactions.* GI side effects, photosensitivity, and overgrowth of vaginal candida are common; hepatic changes (cholestatic jaundice), renal changes, headache, dizziness, rash, and angioedema are less common. Caution should be used in patients with impaired hepatic function. Although *not* reported with Azithromycin, the following reactions/interactions have been observed with other macrolides: ventricular arrthymias, increased serum levels of theophylline, increased anticoagulant effects with coumarins, elevated digoxin levels, elevated ergot levels, increased pharmacologic effect of Trizolam, and elevated levels of Dilantin, carbamazepine, cyclosporine, and hexobarbital. Because of the long half-life of azithromycin, allergic reactions may be persistent and should be carefully monitored.
- *Contraindications.* Sensitivity to macrolides. May be used in pregnancy although experience is limited.[25]
- *Anticipated Outcomes on Evaluation.* Test of cure unnecessary.

OTHER MEDICATIONS. Ofloxacin 300 mg p.o., b.i.d. for 7 days has been recommended by the CDC, but is expensive and cannot be used in pregnancy or with adolescents age 17 years and under. A recent meta-analysis found that Amoxicillin 500 mgs t.i.d. for 7 days is more effective than erythromycin in the treatment of antenatal chlamydia infection and has better compliance.[26]

GONORRHEA

Gonorrhea is a classic bacterial STD that can be symptomatic or asymptomatic in both men and women. In women, gonorrhea primarily infects the cervix and fallopian tubes and is a leading cause of PID. Rectal transmission is common with anal intercourse, and pharyngeal transmission with oral sex is possible but rare. Gonorrhea (GC) can be transmitted during birth and cause conjunctivitis and blindness in neonates. Other rare manifestations of gonorrhea include arthritis, meningitis, perihepatitis, and disseminated gonococcal infection. In pregnancy, gonorrhea has been associated with chorioamnionitis, premature labor, premature rupture of membranes, and postpartum endometritis.

Epidemiology

More than 1.3 million new cases of gonorrhea are reported each year in the United States.[27] The causative agent is *Neisseria gonorrhoeae,* a gram-negative intracellular diplococcus. Risk factors include low socioeconomic status, urban residency, non-married status, and multiple sexual partners. Infection rates in African Americans and Latins are greater than those in whites. Women who use oral contraceptives have a higher rate of gonorrhea; women who use spermicides have lower rates.[28] Often, gonorrhea and chlamydia coexist.[6]

Direct sexual contact with mucosal surfaces of an infected individual is required for the transmission of gonorrhea. Although the organism has been recovered from inanimate objects artificially inoculated with the bacteria, there is no evidence that natural transmission occurs this way. The incubation period is 3 to 7 days.

Subjective Data

Among women, asymptomatic infection can be present in the urethra, endocervix, rectum, or pharynx. Symptoms may include vaginal discharge, pelvic pain, fever, menstrual irregularities, and dysuria.

Objective Data

Physical Examination. The examination may be normal. Some women exhibit mucopurulent cervicitis, erythema, and friability of the endocervix. Bartholin's abscess is infrequent. Other infections, among them chlamydia, trichomonas, monilia, and herpes, are frequently seen with gonorrhea and may confound the clinical picture.

Diagnostic Tests and Methods. Although gram stains showing intracellular gram-negative diplococci are reliable in males with gonorrhea, gram stains are not reliable in females.

CULTURE USING MODIFIED THAYER MARTIN MEDIUM. (See Chapter 5, page 96.)

CULTURE USING TRANSGROW MEDIUM. (See Chapter 5, page 96.)

DIRECT FLUORESCENT ANTIBODY TEST. (See Chapter 5, page 96.)

Differential Medical Diagnoses

Chlamydia trachomatis infection, mucopurulent cervicitis.

Plan

Psychosocial Interventions. Advise the client that persons with untreated gonorrhea risk the development of PID and subsequent infertility. Sexual partners must be treated concurrently and abstain from intercourse during their treatment. With appropriate treatment gonorrhea is curable. Clients must be checked for other STDs before treatment, especially Chlamydia and syphilis, as multiple infections are common. Pregnant clients should be screened at the first prenatal visit, and those at high risk should be rescreened late in the third trimester.

Medication

CEFTRIAXONE
- *Indications.* This is the treatment of choice for uncomplicated urethral, endocervical, and rectal infection.
- *Administration.* Ceftriaxone 125 mg I.M. once.[6] Ceftriaxone is the most effective drug for pharyngeal infection and anal infection in males. All persons diagnosed with gonorrhea should also be treated for presumptive Chlamydia with Doxycycline 100 mgs. b.i.d. for 7 days or 1 gram of Azithromycin orally.[6] For pregnant clients, Doxycycline may not be used but, Azithromycin 1 gram orally, Amoxicillin 500 mgs. t.i.d. for 7 days or erythromycin 500 mg p.o., q.i.d. for 7 days may be given for Chlamydia coverage.
- *Side Effects and Adverse Reactions.* Although usually well tolerated, ceftriaxone has occasionally been associated with pain at injection site, diarrhea, rash, and headache. See discussions of Chlamydia for more information about drugs for concurrent treatment of chlamydia.
- *Contraindications.* Known sensitivity to cephalosporins. Ceftriaxone should be used with caution in clients sensitive to penicillin.

- *Anticipated Outcomes on Evaluation.* Treatment failure is rare. Test for cure with this regimen is not essential.
- *Client Teaching and Counseling.* Advise the client to complete all oral medication and report any drug intolerance. If symptoms recur, retesting is needed. Stress the need for the partner's treatment.

OTHER MEDICATIONS. Other recommended regimens for uncomplicated gonococcal infections among adolescents and adults include cefixime 400 mg p.o. in a single dose *or* Ciprofloxacin 500 mg p.o. in a single dose *or* Ofloxacin 400 mg p.o. in a single dose.[6] Pregnant women may not take Ciprofloxin or Ofloxacin. Pregnant women allergic to Cephalosporins antibiotics may be treated with Spectinomycin 2 grams IM (not effective for pharyngeal gonorrhea).[6] All of these drugs must also be given concurrently with an antibiotic that will cover Chlamydia.

Recommended treatment schedules for special circumstances and complications are available from the CDC.[6]

MUCOPURULENT CERVICITIS (MPC)

Chlamydia trachomatis and gonorrhea are the most common etiologic agents in women who have mucopurulent cervical discharge. In about a third of women with mucopurulent discharge, however, the diagnosis cannot be established.[29] In men with nongonococcal urethritis (NGU), Ureaplasma urealyticum causes 20–40 percent of cases.[6] Since mucopurulent cervicitis is the biologic equivalent of NGU,[29] Ureaplasma (or the related species Mycoplasma hominis) are reasonable diagnoses of exclusion in women with MPC. Although these ubiquitous organisms have been found in the absence of disease, their association with infertility, spontaneous abortion, salpingitis and possibly pelvic abscess makes their pathogenic potential clear.[30]

Epidemiology

Ureaplasma urealyticum and Mycoplasma hominis are bacterial organisms that are sexually transmitted in adults. Colonization in infants may occur through an infected birth canal, although

disease rarely results and colonization does not persist. The incidence of genital mycoplasma infections is unknown, but it is believed to be common. Infection is more common among low socioeconomic groups and minorities.

Subjective Data

May be asymptomatic or may present with dysuria, vaginal discharge, abnormal vaginal bleeding and/or abdominal pain. Mycoplasma/ureaplasma infection may also be suspected in women who present with infertility or recurrent miscarriages.

Objective Data

Physical Examination. Mucopurulent cervicitis is characterized by a yellow endocervical exudate visible in the endocervical canal or in an endocervical swab specimen (the yellow color of the exudate is apparent when contrasted with the white swab).

Diagnostic Tests and Methods. Tests for Chlamydia, gonorrhea will be negative. Wet prep will contain many white blood cells, but no Candida or Trichomonads.

CULTURE. MPC may be treated empirically by many clinicians; however, confirmation of the diagnosis may be made by vaginal culture. Culture is particularly important when the client has infertility or recurrent miscarriage. The test procedure is to do a vaginal culture, which is better than an endocervical culture. An adequate sample from the vagina is necessary to enhance the yield. Obtain the specimens, place them immediately in medium, and transport them to the lab as soon as possible. Keep specimens refrigerated. Mycoplasma culture facilities are not widely available. Explain the procedure to the client.

Differential Medical Diagnoses

Chlamydia trachomatis, gonorrhea.

Plan

Psychosocial Interventions. Explain to the client the widespread, nonspecific nature of genital mycoplasmas and the difficulty in establishing a definitive diagnosis. Partners should be treated empirically.

Medication. Medications effective for Chlamydia are also effective for MPC.

Doxycycline 100 mgs b.i.d. for 7 days (see Chlamydia treatment for prescribing details).

Azithromycin 1 gram orally as a single dose (some ureaplasma strains are resistant to Doxycycline).[31] May be used in pregnancy (see Chlamydia treatment for prescribing cautions).

Ofloxacin 500 mg b.i.d. for 7 days (expensive, but also effective for resistant strains).[31] Not in pregnancy or with adolescents under age 18.

ULCERATIVE GENITAL INFECTIONS

In the United States, most genital ulcers are caused by herpes simplex infections. Diagnosis based on history and physical alone, however, is often inaccurate.[21] All persons with suspected genital herpes infection should also be tested for syphilis. Since syphilis management is very complex, clinicians unfamiliar with diagnostic and treatment protocols should seek consultation for questions related to diagnostic and treatment strategies. Consultation is also recommended if one of the rare bacterial ulcerative diseases is suspected.

HERPES SIMPLEX VIRUS (HSV)

No cure is known for this acute, recurring viral disease. Characteristic painful lesions can occur in the mouth and genitalia of men and women, although virtually any skin or mucous membrane is vulnerable. Neonates who contract the virus congenitally develop infection of the central nervous system (CNS) and eyes. Significant perinatal morbidity and mortality are associated with congenital herpes simplex.[32] Persons who are immunosuppressed are at risk for disseminated HSV, which often presents as meningitis/ encephalitis. Once it enters the body, the herpes virus never leaves, although clinical manifestations disappear as the virus becomes dormant (it is believed in neural ganglia). When recurrence is triggered, the virus travels from nerve roots to the skin surface, where lesions develop. Triggers for reactivation are multifactorial; some triggers re-

ported by women are stress, overexertion, and sexual intercourse.[22] Many clients with HSV infection are asymptomatic.

Epidemiology

Herpes simplex virus type 1 (HSV-1) primarily produces oral lesions, and herpes simplex virus type 2 (HSV-2) primarily produces genital lesions. Differentiation of the two types is academic because they are transmitted identically, their symptomatology is the same, and the procedures for diagnosis and treatment are the same.

Herpes simplex virus is transmitted primarily by direct contact with an infected individual who is shedding the virus. On the basis of serologic studies, approximately 30 million persons in the United States may have genital HSV infection.[6] Approximately 32 percent of the U.S. population was reported to have acquired HSV-2 by the early 1990s.[33] Kissing, sexual contact, and vaginal delivery are means of transmission. Prolonged asymptomatic shedding follows in 20 percent of primary type 2 infections and appears to be responsible for transmission. Primary herpes in pregnancy may be passed to the neonate transplacentally or at birth. Autoinoculation is possible.

The transmission rate of primary HSV in pregnancy may be as high as 50 percent, whereas neonatal transmission of recurrent HSV is estimated to be only 3 to 5 percent. The incubation period of HSV is 7 to 10 days.

Subjective Data

Primary herpes is a systemic disease characterized by multiple painful vesicular lesions, fever, chills, malaise, and severe dysuria if the lesions are genital. Symptoms peak 4 to 5 days after onset and may last 2 to 3 weeks. *Recurrent herpes,* on the other hand, is a localized disease characterized by typical HSV lesions at the site of initial viral entry. Recurrent herpes lesions usually are fewer, are less painful, and resolve more rapidly than primary herpes lesions. Recurrent HSV lasts an average of 5 to 7 days, preceded by a prodromal symptom—frequently a burning, itching or swelling sensation. Lesions will appear within 24 hours of prodrome.

Objective Data

Physical Examination. Characteristic lesions are visible on the vulva and/or cervix. They are vesicular, usually multiple, and exquisitely painful to touch. The vesicles will open and weep and finally crust over, dry, and disappear without scar formation. Clients with primary HSV may have low grade fever and tender lymphadenopathy.

Diagnostic Tests and Methods

VIRAL CULTURE. Diagnostic evaluation for primary and recurrent HSV infections, which are often diagnosed by clinical signs and symptoms. The culture yield is best if the specimen is taken during the vesicular stage of disease; viral isolation is markedly reduced as lesions resolve. In primary episodes, viral shedding is prolonged and HSV more easily isolated.

Advise the client that obtaining the culture will be painful because vigorous sampling is essential to collect adequate cells. (see Chapter 5, page 98 for test details).

SEROLOGIC TESTING FOR HSV ANTIBODIES. Diagnostic evaluation may be accomplished by antibody testing to document past infection with HSV-1 and HSV-2. In addition, it may be useful to differentiate seronegative individuals from seropositive individuals and asymptomatic carriers. Many widely used serological assays, however, do not differentiate HSV-1 and HSV-2 antibodies. Furthermore, serological testing is not always reliable. Hence, it should be used with caution.

Differential Medical Diagnoses

Primary syphilis, mucocutaneous manifestations of Crohn's disease, Behçet's syndrome, chancroid, lymphogranuloma venereum (LGV).

Plan

Psychosocial Interventions. Clients diagnosed with herpes require extensive counseling to understand the complex nature of the disease and its ramifications. Support groups may be helpful. Advise clients to abstain from intercourse during the prodrome and when lesions are present in any stage. Consistent condom use may reduce transmission rates. In addition, clients must know to wash their hands after touching lesions to avoid autoinoculation. Risk of acquiring HIV may be enhanced while genital lesions are present. Clients with a history of genital HSV should know to advise their care provider of this history if they become pregnant.

There is no evidence that HSV causes cervical cancer. Earlier suspicions that implicated it as an etiologic agent of cervical malignancy have been laid to rest.[32] Annual Pap smears are recommended for women with HSV infection since persons with one STD are at risk for the acquisition of other sexually transmitted infections.

Clients with genital HSV, both primary and recurrent, will benefit from such comfort measures as nonconstricting clothes, lukewarm sitz baths, and air drying of lesions with a hand held hair dryer on medium setting. Clients with severe dysuria may benefit by urinating in water. Extremes of temperature such as ice packs or heating pads should be avoided, as should steroid creams, anesthetic sprays, and any type of lotion or gel (e.g., petroleum jelly).

Management of HSV in Pregnancy. Pregnant women should be asked whether they or their partners have had genital herpes lesions. Suspicious or recurrent lesions should be cultured to document HSV. Women with documented primary HSV during pregnancy should be cultured near time of delivery to document viral shedding; positive cultures or visible lesions at time of delivery are indications for cesarean delivery in this subgroup.[34] Routine screening cultures in women with a history of recurrent HSV, however, have not been shown to predict women who will be shedding virus at delivery.[34] Women with a history of recurrent HSV should be examined carefully at onset of labor for evidence of signs, symptoms, or prodrome. If no lesions are evident during labor, an HSV culture should be performed and vaginal delivery should proceed.[35]

Medication

ACYCLOVIR (ZOVIRAX)
- *Indications.* Primary herpes infection and severe recurrent disease. Clients with frequent recurrences (more than six per year) may benefit from daily suppressive therapy. After 1 year of therapy, medication may be stopped and the

client evaluated for recurrences. The safety and effectiveness for up to 3 years of acyclovir use have been documented.

- *Administration.* For primary HSV: 200 mg p.o., 5 times daily for 7 to 10 days or until symptoms resolve. For recurrent HSV: 200 mg p.o., 5 times daily for 5 days, *or* 800 mg p.o., 2 times daily for 5 days. Daily suppression: 200 mg p.o., 2 to 5 times daily. Dosage may be individualized.[6]
- *Side Effects and Adverse Reactions.* These are minimal, even with long-term use. Nausea, vomiting, and headache have been reported, however. Clients on long-term suppression can expect a rebound recurrence when therapy is stopped.
- *Contraindications.* Known hypersensitivity to acyclovir.
- *Anticipated Outcomes on Evaluation.* Accelerated healing and shortened course of the disease.
- *Client Teaching and Counseling.* Advise the client that short courses of acyclovir neither eradicate HSV nor have an impact on the subsequent risk and frequency of recurrences. Daily suppressive therapy reduces the frequency and severity of recurrences, but this effect does not persist after medication is discontinued.[32] Topical therapy with acyclovir ointment is substantially less effective than oral medications.[32] Safe use during pregnancy has *not* been established; however, treatment of pregnant women with primary infection has been recommended by some authorities to prevent severe disease in the mother.[34] Advise the client not to exceed recommended doses and not to share acyclovir with others.[6]

OTHER MEDICATIONS. Famciclovir tablets (Famvir) are approved for the management of recurrent genital herpes in immunocompetent adults. The recommended dose for this indication is 125 mg b.i.d. for 5 days, initiated at the first sign of symptom of recurrence.[36] Side effects and activity are similar to acyclovir. Clinical trials with immunocompromised clients are underway.

Valacyclovir HCL caplets (Valtrex) are also approved for the management of recurrent genital herpes in immunocompetent adults. Recommended dose is 500 mgs b.i.d. for 5 days initiated at first sign of recurrence.[37] Side effects and activity are similar to acyclovir.

SYPHILIS

Syphilis is a complex sexually transmitted disease that can lead to serious systemic illness and even death if untreated. Infection manifests in distinct stages with diverse clinical manifestations. Its natural history begins with *primary syphilis,* which is characterized by a chancre at the site of bacterial entry. *Secondary syphilis* is recognized by flulike symptoms and a maculopapular rash of the palms and soles. Following secondary syphilis, *latency* occurs. Ultimately *tertiary (late) syphilis* occurs, characterized by irreversible cardiovascular, neurologic, dermatologic, or bony disease. Accelerated clinical courses of syphilis have been described in persons infected with HIV.[38]

Clients with any STD or genital ulcer should be evaluated for syphilis. All pregnant women should have a nontreponemal serologic test for syphilis at the first prenatal visit. Women suspected of being at risk for syphilis should have the test repeated during the third trimester and at delivery.[38] Clients who have been exposed to syphilis within the preceding 3 months may be infected but sero-negative and thus should be treated for early syphilis.[38]

Epidemiology

Treponema pallidum, a bacterium in the spirochete family, is the causative organism. Direct sexual contact (or less frequently blood contact) with an infected individual transmits the disease. The risk of developing syphilis after one unprotected contact is up to 50 percent.[38] Because the initial anorectal or vaginal chancres are not likely to be noticed, syphilis is infrequently diagnosed in the primary stage among women or homosexuals. Males, however, notice penile chancres 40 percent of the time.[39] Transplacental transmission of an infected mother to her fetus is also possible and results in about 60 percent fetal loss; up to half of surviving infants have stigmata.[39] Longstanding untreated disease is less contagious than the primary or secondary stage. The incubation period is from 10 to 90 days (3 weeks average).

Before penicillin, syphilis affected upwards of 25 percent of the population. Widespread use of antibiotics dramatically decreased incidence.

Since 1958, however, there has been no net progress against syphilis in the United States.[40] In 1990, more than 50,000 cases were reported in the United States, the highest incidence since 1949. Rates are highest among young adult African Americans in urban areas, and in the southern states. A substantial portion of the current syphilis epidemic is directly attributable to crack cocaine use which is accompanied by an increase in the exchange of sex for money and drugs.[40]

Subjective Data

- *Primary Syphilis.* Client is an asymptomatic contact or may report a lesion.
- *Secondary Syphilis.* Low grade fever, headache, sore throat, rash on the palms and soles.
- *Tertiary Syphilis.* Cardiovascular symptoms (chest pain, cough), neurological symptoms (headache, irritability, impaired balance, memory loss, tremor) skeletal (arthritis, myalgia, myositis), or skin (multiple nodules or ulcers).
- *Congenital Syphilis.* See Objective Data.

Objective Data

Physical Examination

- *Primary Syphilis.* Classic chancre is a painless, rounded, indurated ulcer with serous exudate (see Figure 11–5). It may be genital or extragenital. Usually a single chancre occurs, but multiple chancres may be present. An extragenital chancre is likely to be atypical in appearance. Lymphadenopathy, which may accompany the chancre, will resolve spontaneously in 3 to 6 weeks. Must be distinguished from genital herpes, chancroid, lymphogranuloma, or neoplasm.
- *Secondary Syphilis.* Classic maculopapular rash that gradually covers the body, including the palms and the soles. Less common signs include patchy alopecia, generalized nontender lymphadenopathy, mucosal ulcers, and condyloma lata (flat broad wartlike papules on warm, moist skin surfaces). Spontaneous healing of all secondary manifestations occurs. Must be distinguished from infectious exanthems, pityriasis rosea, and drug eruptions.
- *Tertiary Syphilis.* Manifestations are dependent on whether the client has neurosyphilis,

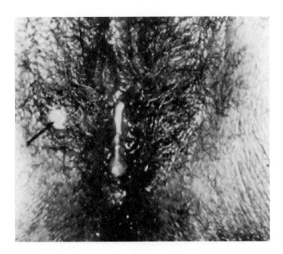

Figure 11–5. Chancre of primary syphilis (arrow). *(Reproduced with permission, from DeCherney, A. H., & Pernoll, M. L. Current Obstetric & Gynecologic Diagnosis & Treatment, 8th Ed. Appleton & Lange, 1994.)*

cardiovascular syphilis, or other expressions of the disease. Aortic diastolic murmur, aneurysms, and congestive failure characterize cardiovascular syphilis; meningeal irritation, unequal reflexes, irregular pupils with poor light response, wide based gait, and personality deterioration characterize neurosyphilis. Must be distinguished from neoplasms of the skin, liver, stomach or brain; other forms of meningitis, and primary neurologic lesions.

- *Congenital Syphilis.* Premature birth, intrauterine growth retardation, mucocutaneous lesions, snuffles (serous nasal discharge), hepatosplenomegaly, condyloma lata, skeletal lesions, CNS involvement, ocular lesions, and others.

Diagnostic Tests and Methods. Diagnosis is largely dependent on microscopic examination of primary and secondary lesion tissue and serology during latency and late infection. Direct darkfield microscopic examination requires considerable expertise and is unavailable in most offices. However, an immunofluorescent staining technique is available for demonstrating *T. pallidum* in fluid taken from suspicious lesions, spread on slides, fixed appropriately and mailed to a reference lab.

DIRECT MICROSCOPIC EXAMINATION. Diagnostic evaluation for definitive identification of *T. pallidum* is possible when lesions (e.g., chancre, rash) are present. If antibiotics have been taken, the test is not useful.

The test procedure is first to cleanse the lesion with sterile saline. Then gently abrade to produce oozing of serous fluid. Avoid active bleeding. Collect serous fluid on a slide and fix as directed by the laboratory. Advise the client that the testing procedure is not uncomfortable, but results will have to be obtained from the laboratory.

SEROLOGICAL TESTS, NONTREPONEMAL. Diagnostic evaluation for antilipid antibodies produced by the host exposed to *T. pallidum*. Examples are Venereal Disease Research Laboratory (VDRL) and Rapid Plasma Reagent (RPR). Used for syphilis screening and follow-up after treatment. Twenty-five percent of patients with syphilis develop negative nontreponemal tests in late latent disease; however, treponemal tests will still be positive.[39]

The test procedure is to collect a blood sample in a dry tube without anticoagulant. Advise the client that venipuncture is required. Results are reported as either reactive (positive) or nonreactive (negative). *Reactive results* are quantitated in the form of a titer. The false positive rate is 1 to 2 percent in the general population, higher in low risk groups. False positive reactions are encountered in connective tissue diseases, mononucleosis, febrile diseases, intravenous drug use, old age, and pregnancy.[38] False negative results may occur when high antibody levels are present. If syphilis is strongly suspected and the nontreponemal test is negative, the laboratory should be instructed to dilute the specimen to detect a positive reaction.

All reactive results require confirmation by the treponemal test (description follows). Tests become reactive 14 days after the chancre appears. If results are equivocal, repeat testing is indicated. A rising titer is evidence of primary syphilis. If syphilis is suspected and the initial nontreponemal test is nonreactive, repeat in 1 week, 1 month, and 3 months. *Nonreactive results* after 3 months exclude the diagnosis of syphilis.

SEROLOGICAL TESTS, TREPONEMAL. Diagnostic evaluation to detect *T. pallidum* specific antibodies. This test is designed to confirm the diagnosis of a re-

active nontreponemal test. One example is fluorescent treponemal antibody absorption (FTA-ABS). The test procedure is to collect a blood sample in a dry tube without anticoagulant.

A venipuncture is required. The treponemal test should only be used *after* the nontreponemal test is reactive—never as the initial screen. It is also used if symptoms of tertiary syphilis are present. The results are reported as reactive or nonreactive. Once reactive, the client usually may remain so for life, even with adequate treatment. The false positive rate is 1 percent. Final decisions about the significance of serologic tests results must be based on a total clinical appraisal of risks.[38]

Plan

Psychosocial Interventions. Extensive counseling and support are needed. Explain the complex nature of the disease and its ramifications. Case finding and treatment of sexual partners are essential to epidemic control but difficult when the relationship is associated with crack or cocaine use. The need must be stressed for follow-up testing to ensure adequate treatment. Explain the meaning of test results, especially rising or falling titers and persistent reactive results. Clients with serological evidence of syphilis in any stage are best treated by practitioners experienced in the management of this complex disease. Suggest HIV counseling and testing.

Medication. Penicillin is the treatment of choice for all clients with syphilis and the only proven therapy for syphilis during pregnancy and for congenital syphilis. Current dual-drug therapy for gonorrhea will probably cure incubating syphilis.[38] Penicillin prevents congenital syphilis in 90 percent of cases, even when given late in pregnancy.[38]

BENZATHINE PENICILLIN G

- *Indications.* Primary and secondary syphilis and early latent syphilis of less than 1 year's duration.
- *Administration.* 2.4 million units I.M. in one dose. Clients with syphilis of greater than a year's duration (latent or tertiary stages) require weekly treatment with 2.4 million units of Benzathine Penicillin G for 3 weeks. Neurosyphilis

(diagnosed by lumbar puncture) requires intravenous treatment.[7]

- *Side Effects and Adverse Reactions.* Penicillin adverse effects include wheezing, weakness, abdominal pain, nausea or vomiting, diarrhea, rash, fever, increased thirst, and seizures. In addition, Jarisch-Herxheimer reaction, an acute febrile illness with headache and flulike symptoms, may occur a few hours after antibiotic administration. It is probably due to treponemal lysis and subsides within 24 hours.[38] It may be severe.
- *Contraindications.* A known sensitivity to penicillin.
- *Anticipated Outcomes on Evaluation.* Clients treated for syphilis must be followed with a nontreponemal test at 3 and 6 months. Titers should fall fourfold by 6 months in those treated for primary and secondary syphilis, indicating adequate therapy. In patients with early latent syphilis, a fourfold drop may take 12–24 months. Titers may be expected to become negative in 72 percent of those treated for primary syphilis and 50 percent of those with secondary syphilis after 3 years.[38]
- *Client Teaching and Counseling.* Provide the client with information about the possibility of the Jarisch-Herxheimer reaction and its treatment: rest, fluids, and antipyretics. Stress the importance of follow-up testing. Clients allergic to penicillin may be treated with doxycycline/tetracycline/erythromycin/Ceftriaxone (not single dose). Specific protocols are recommended by the Centers for Disease Control (CDC).[76]

CHANCROID

Chancroid is a sexually transmitted disease characterized by painful genital ulceration. Lesions are usually confined to the genitals and accompanied by inguinal lymphadenopathy. Systemic illness does not occur. Although more common in Africa, the West Indies and Asia, it is endemic in many parts of the United States.[41] Ten percent of patients with chancroid have co-infection with herpes simplex virus and/or syphilis. An increased rate of HIV infection has also been associated with chancroid.[41]

Epidemiology

Haemophilus ducreyi, a gram negative bacillus, is the causative agent. The incubation period is 3–5 days. The condition occurs most commonly in uncircumcised males; incidence among women is low. Transmission is by direct contact with an infected individual. Fomite transmission does not occur.

Subjective Data

The initial lesion is a vesicopapule that breaks down to form a painful soft ulcer. Multiple lesions may develop, spread by auto-inoculation. These may rupture spontaneously. Fever, malaise, and chills may also develop. Women may have nonspecific symptoms such as dysuria, vaginal discharge, and dyspareunia or they may be asymptomatic.

Objective Data

Physical Examination. A characteristic ulcerative lesion is seen on the genitalia with a necrotic base and surrounding erythema. In over 50 percent of the cases, a bubo will be present (a greatly enlarged, inflamed lymph node). This unilateral inguinal adenitis is tender and the overlying skin is inflamed. Buboes may spontaneously rupture. One or two lesions are the norm, although more may occur.

Diagnostic Tests and Methods

CULTURE OF ULCERS. Diagnostic evaluation to isolate *H. ducreyi.* The test procedure is to swab the base of the ulcerative lesion with a cotton or calcium alginate swab. Transport the specimen to a laboratory within 4 hours (refrigerate the swab if transportation time is longer). Do not culture a bubo unless it has ruptured; unruptured bubos are usually sterile.

The laboratory must be informed that chancroid is suspected. The organism is best cultured on chocolate agar with 1 percent Isovitalex and vancomycin 3 mg/ml.[24] Explain to the client that a culture is the best test. (A gram stain may be inaccurate, and newer enzyme immunoassay tests are still being developed.) Culture results take up to 1 week.

Differential Medical Diagnoses

Genital herpes, syphilis, granuloma inguinale.

Plan

Psychosocial Interventions. Chancroid may increase the risk of HIV infection. Advise the client that her sexual partners within the past 10 days need examination and treatment. Symptoms improve within 3 days; ulcers heal within 7 days. Bubos resolve more slowly and may require aspiration.

Medication

AZITHROMYCIN

- *Indications.* Suspected or culture proven chancroid. A presumptive diagnosis is made if the clinical picture is clear. Single dose facilitates compliance; however, treatment failures have been reported with single dose Azithromycin in HIV positive clients.[42]
- *Administration.* One gram orally as a single dose.[21,24]
- *Side Effects and Adverse Reactions.* Gastrointestinal distress, rare angioedema and cholestatic jaundice. Caution should be used in patients with impaired hepatic function. See also side effects listed under Chlamydia.
- *Contraindications.* Known hypersensitivity to any macrolide drug.
- *Anticipated Outcomes on Evaluation.* Ulcerative lesions resolve.
- *Client Teaching and Counseling.* Azithromycin must be taken 1 hour before or 2 hours after a meal. It should not be taken with food. If no improvement occurs within 2–3 days, diagnosis must be reconsidered. Infection with other STDs, including HIV, may also exist. Partners should be treated.

CEFTRIAXONE

- *Indications.* Suspected or culture proven chancroid. A presumptive diagnosis is made if the clinical picture is clear. Single dose facilitates compliance.
- *Administration.* 250 mg I.M.[6]
- *Side Effects and Adverse Reactions.* Although usually well tolerated, ceftriaxone is occasionally associated with pain at the injection site, diarrhea, rash, and headache.

- *Contraindications.* Known sensitivity to cephalosporins. Use with caution for clients sensitive to penicillin.
- *Anticipated Outcomes on Evaluation.* Treatment failure is rare. Test for cure with this regimen is not essential.
- *Client Teaching and Counseling.* Stress the need for the client's partner to be treated.

ERYTHROMYCIN

- *Indications.* Suspected or culture proven chancroid. A presumptive diagnosis is made if the clinical picture is clear.
- *Administration.* 500 mg p.o., q.i.d. for 7 days.[6]
- *Side Effects and Adverse Reactions.* Gastrointestinal distress. (See Azithromycin under Chlamydia treatment for drug reactions/interactions that have been reported with macrolides.)
- *Contraindications.* Known hypersensitivity to erythromycin. Concomitant use of terfenadine (Seldane) or ketaconazole (Nizoral).
- *Anticipated Outcomes on Evaluation.* Ulcerative lesions resolve.
- *Client Teaching and Counseling.* Advise the client to complete the entire course of medication. If no improvement occurs within 7 days, diagnosis must be reconsidered. Infection with other STDs, including HIV, may also exist, so screening for other infections is recommended. Partners should be treated.

OTHER MEDICATIONS. Two other possible alternatives are amoxicillin 500 mg plus clavulanic acid 125 mg p.o., t.i.d. for 7 days or ciprofloxacin 500 mg p.o., b.i.d. for 3 days.[24] With the exception of ciprofloxacin, which is contraindicated for pregnant and lactating women and children under 17, all of the regimens just listed may be used in pregnancy.

Follow-Up/Referral

Only if nonresponsive to drug treatment.

GRANULOMA INGUINALE

A chronic, progressive bacterial infection of the genitals, Granuloma inguinale presents with large, unsightly ulcers of the genitalia, inguinal region, and anus. Other names for the condition are donovanosis and granuloma venereum. Since other sexually transmitted diseases frequently co-exist, cultures for these and a serological test for syphilis must be performed.

Epidemiology

Calymmatobacterium granulomatis, a gram negative bacterium, is the causative agent. Anal intercourse, often associated with homosexuality, is a particular risk factor. Transmission is by sexual or nonsexual trauma to infected sites, primarily the anus and penis. The disease is mildly contagious; repeated exposures are needed in order for clinical manifestations to develop. The incubation period is 7 days to 12 weeks.[24]

Rarely reported in the United States, granuloma inguinale is epidemic in parts of Australia and common in India and many tropical and subtropical environments. Donovan bodies (bacteria encapsulated in mononuclear leukocytes) are found in tissue scrapings that are stained with Wright's stain.

Subjective Data

The disorder often begins as a papule, which then ulcerates leaving a beefy-red, relatively painless granular area with clean sharp rolled edges (see Figure 11–6). The ulcer is persistent, and satellite ulcers may unite to form a large ulcer. Inguinal swelling is common, with late formation of painful abscesses (buboes). Superinfection of the ulcer with spirochete-fusiform organisms is common; the ulcer then becomes purulent, painful, and foul smelling. Rarely, granuloma inguinale presents with granulomatous cervical lesions which must be distinguished from carcinoma.[41]

Objective Data

Physical Examination. An examination reveals the characteristic lesions, as noted previously.

Diagnostic Tests and Methods. Wright's or Giemsa Stain. Diagnostic evaluation for pathognomonic Donovan bodies (common name for causative organism). The test procedure is to crush/smear a clean piece of granulation tissue on a slide. Air dry, then stain using appropriate Wright's or Giemsa staining technique. Explain to the client that the test procedure is simple and

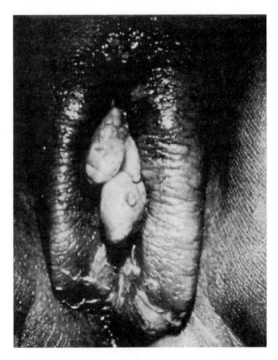

Figure 11–6. Granuloma inguinale. *(Reproduced with permission, from DeCherney, A. H., & Pernoll, M. L. Current Obstetric & Gynecologic Diagnosis & Treatment, 8th Ed. Appleton & Lange, 1994.)*

reliable. Must be done by a laboratory familiar with these techniques.

Differential Medical Diagnoses

Chancroid, carcinoma, syphilis, amebiasis.

Plan

Medication. A variety of antibiotics are useful. The first line treatment is Doxycycline.

DOXYCYCLINE
- *Indications.* Positive diagnosis of Granuloma inguinale.
- *Administration.* Doxycycline 100 mgs b.i.d. for 1–4 weeks until lesions have healed.[42]
- *Side Effects and Adverse Reactions.* GI upset, rash, photosensitivity. Overgrowth of vaginal candida.
- *Contraindications.* Pregnancy; allergy to tetracyclines.

- *Anticipated Outcomes on Evaluation.* Lesions will heal and Donovan bodies will disappear from the smears.
- *Client Teaching and Counseling.* Advise the client that compliance with treatment is critical. Medication must be continued until all lesions are healed. This may take up to 4 weeks. Discontinuing therapy early results in high recurrence rates.

OTHER MEDICATIONS. Trimethoprim 80 mg/sulfamethoxazole 400 mg (Bactrim) tablets b.i.d. for 14 days or until lesions have healed.[42] Erythromycin 500 mg q.i.d. for at least 4 weeks may be used in pregnancy.[41]

Follow-Up and Referral

The client should be seen 1 to 2 months after the initial diagnosis to ensure resolution. Partners must be treated.

LYMPHOGRANULOMA VENEREUM (LGV)

This chronic bacterial STD initially presents as a vesiculopustular eruption that may go unnoticed. After the genital lesion disappears, the infection spreads to lymph channels and lymph nodes of the genital and rectal areas (in women the genital lymph drainage is to the perirectal glands). This secondary invasion is characterized by painful ulceration, lymphedema and draining abscesses (buboes) (see Figure 11–7). Early anorectal manifestations are proctitis with tenesmus and bloody purulent discharge; late rectal manifestations include inflammation, scarring, and stricture of rectal and vaginal tissue. Systemic symptoms (fever, headache, abdominal pain, chills, and arthralgias) may develop.

Epidemiology

The causative organisms are *Chlamydia trachomatis serovars:* L1, L2, and L3. In the United States, LGV is more common in urban settings, and in the Southeastern United States.[41] Men with the disease outnumber women by 5 to 1. The incubation period is 3 to 12 days or longer.

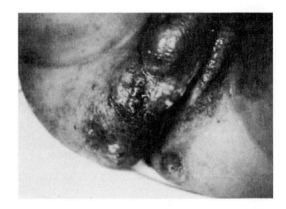

Figure 11–7. Lymphogranuloma venereum. Note involvement of perineum and spread over buttocks. *(Reproduced with permission, from DeCherney, A. H., & Pernoll, M. L.* Current Obstetric & Gynecologic Diagnosis & Treatment, *8th Ed. Appleton & Lange, 1994.)*

Subjective Data

LGV contacts are initially asymptomatic, or may report genital ulcers and painful groin nodes or abscesses. A wide variety of nonspecific symptoms may be present.

Objective Data

Physical Examination. Tender inguinal lymphadenopathy is the most common sign. A spectrum of other clinical symptoms may occur, including papules, ulcers, cervicitis, proctitis, bubo formation (tender abscesses), and genital edema. A hard cutaneous induration may also be present.

Diagnostic Tests and Methods. Serological tests using fixation, neutralizing antibody, or immunofluorescents are available. Because LGV is so rare in the United States, specific information should be obtained from the local laboratory when testing is required.

Differential Medical Diagnoses

Chancroid, genital herpes, syphilis. Lymph node involvement must be distinguished from that due to tularemia, tuberculosis, or neoplasm. Rectal strictures must be distinguished from neoplasm and ulcerative colitis.

Plan

Psychosocial Interventions. Prevention is critical. When LGV is diagnosed, all sexual contacts must be identified and treated to eliminate a reservoir of continued transmission.[6] Surgical excision of lesions may be necessary after infection has been halted.

Medication. *Clients should be referred to an infectious disease specialist if LGV is suspected.* Antibiotic therapy is indicated, and adequate treatment and follow-up are essential.

DOXYCYCLINE

- *Administration.* Doxycycline 100 mg p.o., b.i.d. for 21 days.[6]
- *Side Effects and Contraindications.* The same as those discussed in the section on tetracycline therapy for granuloma inguinale.
- *Anticipated Outcomes on Evaluation.* Resolution of symptoms. Relapse is common.
- *Client Teaching and Counseling.* Assist the client to complete the medication regimen, which is difficult because it lasts 21 days.

OTHER MEDICATIONS. Alternative treatment regimens include erythromycin 500 mg p.o., q.i.d. for 21 days (may be used in pregnancy) *or* sulfisoxazole 500 mg p.o., q.i.d. for 21 days.[6,42]

EPIDERMAL DISEASES

Clinical syndromes with epidermal manifestations vary in seriousness, persistence and treatment approaches. Human papillomavirus infections are unique in that different viral types have different clinical manifestations.

HUMAN PAPILLOMAVIRUS (HPV) INFECTION

About one third of the sexually active population in the United States is thought to be infected with one or more of the human papillomaviruses, making this infection the most common viral sexually transmitted infection.[43] The outcome of exposure to these viruses depends on multiple factors including HPV type, type of skin infected, host immunity, and smoking status.[44] Of particular concern is the strong association between HPV infection, progressive cervical neoplasia, and carcinoma.[45] HPV infections are differentiated from HPV associated carcinoma in this chapter, however, since it appears that other factors are necessary for malignant transformation.[44,46]

It is speculated that HPV infection may persist in a dormant (latent) state throughout the lifetime of most infected persons, with intermittent subclinical or clinical evidence of infection.[47] Individuals with evidence of HPV in one genital site have a significant risk of other HPV manifestations in another genital site (vulva, vagina, cervix, urethra, perianal skin, and rectum).[48] Unlike the treatment goal for bacterial sexually transmitted infections, the goal of HPV treatment is to remove obvious lesions and prevent the progression of neoplasias, not to eradicate HPV.

HPV infections are classified as clinical, subclinical, or latent. Clinical lesions can be identified without the aid of magnification and are typically called condyloma acuminata. Subclinical lesions are identified as whitened areas visible after application of 5 percent acetic acid and inspection under magnification. Subclinical infection of the cervix is generally diagnosed by typical changes (koilocytosis or neoplasias) diagnosed by Papanicolaou smear.[21] Latent infections have no visible lesions and are evident only by DNA hybridization tests for HPV.[48] The clinical implications of latent infection continue to be explored, but routine use of DNA hybridization tests is not currently recommended.[48]

Epidemiology

Human papillomavirus (HPV) is a slow growing DNA virus of the papovavirus family; more than 60 strains are identified, 20 of which have been associated with genital tract infections.[49] Condyloma acuminata and low grade neoplasias are usually associated with human papilloma types 6 and 11. Other HPV types in the anogenital area (16, 18, 31, 33, and 35) are strongly associated with higher grades of genital dysplasia and carcinoma.[21,46] More than one type may be present at one time.

HPV is most commonly spread by means of sexual or other intimate contact. The organism may have limited survival on fomites, but non-sexual transmission is rare and difficult to document. Autoinoculation and mother-child transfer at birth can occur. The incubation period is 3 weeks to 8 months or longer. There is an initial proliferative period in which the virus replicates uncontrolled by immunologic response. During this proliferative period, a large number of virions are produced that infect adjacent tissue.[44]

Subjective Data

Clinical HPV lesions are papular lesions with a warty, granular surface. They are usually painless; however, malodorous vaginal discharge, pain and burning with urination, pruritus, and bleeding during and after coitus may occur. The lack of visible lesions or complaints is not uncommon, however. A woman may have a history of an infected partner but have no evidence of infection. Lesions may grow so large in pregnancy as to affect urination, defecation, mobility, and descent of the fetus, although rarely is cesarean delivery necessitated.[48]

Objective Data

Physical Examination. Genitalia/reproductive tract shows one or more soft, pale, pink or flesh-colored, dry, irregular lesions on the external genitalia, perineum, or anus. The lesions, 1 mm or larger, may be flat, papular, or pedunculated papules on the vulva, introitus, vagina, cervix, perineum, urethra, and/or anus. Small condylomata should not be confused with vulval vestibular papillae that are normally located on the epithelium of both labia minora. In true condyloma acuminata, multiple papilla converge toward a single base, whereas each papillae has its own base in normal vulvar tissue.[50] Examination of the vulva after topical application of 3–5 percent acetic acid may assist in identification of subclinical lesions. These will be slightly elevated, well demarcated, and aceto-white. Candidiasis, folliculitis, contact dermatitis, and psoriasis may also turn white, however, with acetic acid application.[50] Large lesions may be cauliflower-like in appearance, exist in coalesced clusters, and be friable. Areas most often traumatized during coitus are common sites for HPV infection.

Diagnostic Tests and Methods

PAP SMEAR (CYTOLOGY). It is imperative that women with vulvar HPV or partners with HPV have a cervical examination with a Papanicolaou smear. The application of 3–5 percent acetic acid to the cervix may identify areas of acetowhitening that can be targeted by the Pap smear. This screening evaluation will identify koilocytosis, dyskaryosis, keratinizing atypia, or dysplasia on traditional reports, or squamous intraepithelial lesions on Bethesda System reports. A Pap smear is a screening test and not diagnostic since the sample can miss the lesion. The severity of any cervical lesion reported on a Pap smear can be determined best by colposcopically directed cervical biopsy. (See chapters 5 and 13 for Pap smear techniques and management of abnormal Pap smears.) It is important to note that any grossly visible suspicious cervical lesion requires biopsy, regardless of the Pap smear findings.

COLPOSCOPY WITH DIRECTED BIOPSY (HISTOLOGY). Diagnostic evaluation for subclinical lesions, dysplasia, and malignancy, performed by trained, experienced colposcopist using colposcope. The procedure provides a magnified view of direct biopsy sites. An abnormal Pap report, cervical lesions, or extensive external lesions warrant referral for colposcopy and biopsy. Endocervical curettage should not be performed if the client is pregnant.

The test procedure includes the application of 3 to 5 percent acetic acid to the tissue of the vulva or cervix. After several seconds, abnormal areas turn white. The tissue is then examined under magnification with the colposcope. Directed biopsy is done on the most abnormal sites (e.g., acetowhite with punctuation and mosaic pattern).

Explain the procedure to the client: no anesthesia required; lithotomy position; instrument introduced through wide speculum opening; uncomfortable stinging from acetic acid; pinching, cramping sensation when tissue is removed. Tell the client that no excessive bleeding should occur, although a blood tinged discharge may continue for 2 to 3 days; no coitus, douching, tampon use, or putting other objects in the vagina for 3 days.

DNA Typing (Nucleic Acid Hybridization Tests). Diagnostic evaluation to determine the specific HPV strain; may be useful to identify latent infection. The test procedure includes the use of Virapap and ViraType HPV detection kits, which are commercially available but limited in the number of HPV strains they are able to detect. Other DNA probes are being researched. Obtaining an adequate sample is critical; the cytologic brush method appears to be most effective.

Explain to the client that HPV typing may identify particularly virulent strains of the virus. Explain the procedure and that its cost may be high. In addition, results take a long time and false negatives do occur. (DNA typing is not considered cost effective for mass screening.)

Differential Medical Diagnoses

Condyloma lata, molluscum contagiosum; carcinoma; concomitant sexually transmitted diseases.

Plan

Considerable disagreement exists regarding protocols and recommendations for diagnosis and treatment. There is no consensus on treatment for male partners of women infected with HPV, and there is disagreement on the effectiveness of condoms in preventing transmission or recurrence of HPV.[51] Although 53 percent of male sexual partners of women with CIN have HPV lesions themselves, and wives of men whose first wives died of cervical cancer are at greater risk for cervical cancer,[51] studies have found no difference in recurrence rates of genital warts in women whose male partners were or were not treated for HPV lesions.[50] Recurrence rates of 25–50 percent are believed to be an evolution from latent to active infection at different sites or reexposure of the healing treated area to the woman's colonized adjacent tissue.[51]

Although treatment of subclinical lesions in monogamous sexual partners may not be justified, treatment of subclinical lesions and condom use is likely to prevent the spread of HPV to other partners. Condom use during treatment of clinical or subclinical warts may also reduce viral spread in partners who may not yet be infected.

Psychosocial Interventions. Implications for counseling include relationship dissatisfaction, depression, and fear related to the seriousness of the diagnosis (dysplasia or cancer). Referral may be indicated. Discuss treatment options with the client (and partner, if appropriate); fully involve her in the therapy plans.

Emotionally, HPV infection may affect self-esteem, body image, feelings (shame, guilt, or blame), satisfaction with intimate relationships, and overall mental health.[21] Anxiety associated with knowing one has a potentially malignant disease and lack of a definitive cure may necessitate referral for psychological counseling and support. Partners may also be involved in counseling. A client's concerns may relate to sharing with future partners the fact that she has the disease. Through education about HPV, anxiety may be reduced. Involvement in controlling decisions empowers the client by decreasing her dependency.[52]

Medication. Drug therapies may be alternated or combined in some arrangement, such as TCA and liquid nitrogen on alternating weeks. With any topical application, an alternative treatment should be tried if lesions have not resolved in four to five treatments. Clients should be referred for biopsy of any nonresponsive or atypical lesions.

Trichloracetic Acid (TCA). 80 to 90 percent.
- *Indications.* To reduce the size of external genital and vaginal lesions, therefore, viral shedding.
- *Administration.* Apply TCA solution sparingly to lesions, using a cotton swab and avoiding the surrounding tissue. Calcium alginate swabs may be preferred since they are smaller and decrease damage to surrounding tissue. Treated areas will turn white. A mixture of baking soda and water may be applied to neutralize the acid after application or to prevent damage from solution inadvertently applied to normal skin. A burning sensation occurs for several minutes following application but may be avoided by pretreatment spraying of topical anesthetic.[44] Applications are repeated once weekly; may be repeated twice weekly if the client can tolerate it.
- *Side Effects and Adverse Reactions.* Burning sensation on application should resolve quickly. There may be erythema, tenderness, swelling,

and sloughing of tissue in the area for a few days after application. No systemic effects.

- *Contraindications.* TCA is contraindicated with severely irritated tissues. The medication has been used safely in pregnancy.
- *Anticipated Outcomes on Evaluation.* Lesions will become smaller and finally disappear after a few applications. If no visible improvement occurs after three treatments, use another method. If lesions persist or are multiple or internal, refer the client to a gynecologist.
- *Client Teaching and Counseling.* Tell the client that it is not necessary to wash off the acid. Persistent leukorrhea, increased pain, and redness may indicate infection. Spotting or bleeding may occur if the healing tissue is jarred. In addition, lidocaine (Xylocaine) ointment may be given, or warm sitz baths and a baking soda/water mixture may soothe.

LIQUID NITROGEN CRYOTHERAPY

- *Indications.* External warts. For internal lesions, the client is referred to a gynecologist.
- *Administration.* Application may be accomplished with a finely twisted cotton tip, or the wooden end of a cotton tipped applicator, or a special applicator jet. The lesion will turn white. May be followed by application of podophyllin or TCA.
- *Side Effects and Adverse Reactions.* The same as for TCA and podophyllin.
- *Contraindications.* None.
- *Anticipated Outcomes on Evaluation.* The lesions will disappear after 1–4 weekly treatments.
- *Client Teaching and Counseling.* Inform the client that the application of the drug may burn. For the discomfort, the same teaching and counseling as used for application of TCA or podophyllin are appropriate.

PODOFILOX. 0.5 percent. Podofilox 0.5 percent, a self-treatment, may be prescribed. Unlike podophyllin, this is a stable, purified product that does not need to be washed off.[21] Advise the client to apply it twice a day (only to the warts) for 3 days with a cotton swab followed by 4 days of no therapy. The treatment may be repeated for a total of 4 cycles. The health care provider must teach wart identification, proper medicine appli-

cation, and avoidance of getting any solution on other areas. The total treatment area should be 10^2 cm or less. No more than 0.5 mL of solution should be used daily. It is not used in pregnancy.[6]

PODOPHYLLIN. 10 to 25 percent in tincture of benzoin compound.

- *Indications.* For external lesions only. Because of potential toxicity and variations in potency of this natural plant extract, podophyllin is not recommended as a first line treatment.
- *Administration.* Compound is applied to the lesion using a cotton swab and avoiding normal tissue. Unaffected areas may be protected by applying petroleum or lubricant jelly to them. Podophyllin must be washed off 4 hours after application. Applications are repeated weekly; more frequent use may result in burning.
- *Side Effects and Adverse Reactions.* Erythema, burning, swelling, tissue damage. Lesions may become tender several days after treatment.
- *Contraindications.* Pregnancy or presence of large warts. Absorption may cause toxicity.
- *Anticipated Outcomes on Evaluation.* The same as for trichloracetic acid (TCA), discussed previously. Do not exceed four applications if no significant improvement results.
- *Client Teaching and Counseling.* Provide the client with information about the signs of toxicity: nausea, vomiting, lethargy, coma, paralysis. Repeated use may be carcinogenic. Instruct the client to wash off podophyllin 4 hours after application with mild soap and water, sooner if irritation causes discomfort.

Surgery and Other Interventions. Indications are internal lesions, large lesions, or external lesions unresponsive to prior therapy. The client is referred to a trained, experienced specialist.

LASER CARBON DIOXIDE VAPORIZATION. This outpatient procedure is done with the client under general or regional anesthesia or heavy sedation. A laser beam vaporizes large areas of lesions without scarring. Small lesions are done under local anesthesia. During the procedure, warmth and menstrual-like cramps are felt. Pain after treatment is mild to moderate; profuse, watery discharge occurs for up to 2 weeks. Healing takes 3 to 4 weeks. The secondary infection rate is higher with large treatment areas.

ELECTRODIATHERMY LOOP EXCISION PROCEDURE (LEEP). Leep is increasingly popular as an office procedure for cervical lesions when the entire lesion and entire transformation zone can be visualized by colposcopy, there is no evidence of endocervical involvement, and there is no evidence of invasive disease.[54] Leep procedures result in less thermal damage compared to cryotherapy and also provide a specimen for histology.[53]

CRYOSURGERY (NITROUS OXIDE). Cryosurgery is performed as an office procedure for cervical disease (dysplasia). Lesions treated by cryosurgery must meet the same criteria as those treated by LEEP. Nitrous oxide is the freezing agent of choice. The cryoprobe is applied to the cervix using a 3–5–3 minute technique. Mild to moderate cramping during the procedure usually subsides once freezing is complete. A profuse, watery, foul smelling vaginal discharge continues for 2 to 3 weeks. Nothing is to be put into the vagina for 3 weeks. The client may shower or bathe in a clean tub.

SURGICAL EXCISION. Performed on an outpatient or inpatient basis, depending on the extent of disease and the location of lesions. Healing varies with the degree of trauma but generally takes 2 to 3 weeks for smaller lesions.

INTERFERON. Interferon is an antiviral agent thought to reduce human papillomavirus (HPV) lesions by improving the immune system. It is injected directly into lesions three times per week for 1 month. Useful for recalcitrant cases or immunosuppressed clients.[44] This expensive treatment is available primarily in medical centers. Side effects include fever, flulike symptoms, and malaise.

5-FLUOROURACIL. 5 percent cream (Efudex).
- *Indications.* Used by specialists to treat widespread papillary vaginal lesions. Flat, keratinized lesions in the vagina do not respond as well as do papillary lesions. It is a cytotoxic agent and not useful for external warts, because side effects are too severe. Because of variable response, treatment must be individualized to prevent chronic vaginal ulcerations.
- *Administration.* Treatment protocols vary widely. *Initial treatment:* 2 grams of a 5 percent cream inserted deep in the vagina at bedtime once a week. Monitor weekly for side effects.[44]

- *Side Effects and Adverse Reactions.* Denuding, chemical vaginitis, adenosis, and vulvar vestibulitis.[50]
- *Contraindications.* Pregnancy: During pregnancy the drug is teratogenic. No systemic toxicity is usual.
- *Anticipated Outcomes on Evaluation.* Vaginal warts will disappear and the Pap smear return to normal. The client should be reevaluated in 3 months.
- *Client Teaching and Counseling.* Include information about inflammation, discharge, and local discomfort caused by 5-fluorouracil. Severe pain and burning are *not* usual. A vaginal tampon may be inserted after application to reduce irritation to other tissues. Effective contraception is essential since this medication is teratogenic (some clinicians will not use in patients who are capable of becoming pregnant).

Long Term Follow-Up

Women with any history of HPV infection should be evaluated with biannual Pap smears for the first 2 years after treatment and annually thereafter.[46] Self-examination of external genitalia is recommended on a regular basis.

Future Directions for HPV Research

The firmly established causal relationship between HPV infection and neoplasia makes vaccine strategies appropriate as prophylactic and therapeutic approaches. Research in these areas is currently underway.[46]

MOLLUSCUM CONTAGIOSUM

This benign, viral, papular infection occurs on the abdomen, thighs, and genitals of adults and on the face, trunk, and extremities of children. Molluscum are common in persons infected with HIV and are difficult to eradicate in these persons. The infection is generally minor and self-limited. Another name for the condition is seed wart.

Epidemiology

Molluscum contagiosum virus (*MCV*), a member of the pox virus family, is the causative organism.[35]

In adults, transmission is primarily sexual; in children, it is nonsexual and via fomites. Autoinoculation may also occur. The incubation period ranges from 1 week to 6 months (2 to 3 month average). The exact incidence is unknown but is thought to be low.

Subjective Data

The client is generally asymptomatic, and diagnosis is often made when treatment is sought for some other reason.

Objective Data

Physical Examination. A firm, smooth, waxy nontender dome shaped papule with a central umbilication is seen (may be single or multiple). Lesions contain a caseous material. Principal sites of involvement include face, upper thighs, lower abdomen, and genitals.[54]

Diagnostic Tests and Methods. Diagnosis is made upon sight of a characteristic lesion. Biopsy reveals molluscum bodies.

Differential Medical Diagnoses

Genital warts, genital herpes, dermatologic folliculitis, lichen planus, basal cell epithelioma.

Plan

Psychosocial Interventions. Reassure the client that MCV is benign, self-limiting, and grows slowly. Clients with multiple or persistent lesions, however, should be questioned about risk factors for HIV. Many cases spontaneously resolve over a few months. Bacterial superinfection may require a systemic antibiotic, but such a condition is rare. Clients should avoid sharing razors. Advocate good handwashing.

Surgical Interventions. Unroofing the lesion with a fine gauge needle to remove the central core is effective and practical if there are only a few lesions. Multiple lesions have been successfully treated using cryotherapy with liquid nitrogen; direct destruction is achieved. Electrosurgery with a fine needle may be used.[54]

PEDICULOSIS PUBIS

A species of human lice causes this common sexually transmitted disease. Another name for this condition is pubic lice or crabs. Body and head lice also occur in humans but do not infect the pubic area. Pubic lice, however, have been found in axillae, beards, eyebrows, and eyelashes.

Epidemiology

Phthirius pubis is the crab louse. It requires human blood to survive. Off the host, pubic lice will die within 24 hours. Sexual or other direct contact must occur for transmission. Some cases of fomite transmission have been documented.[54] The examination table and toilet used by the client will need to be washed with an appropriate disinfectant, or the rooms may be closed for the life span of the lice (24 hours) if this is feasible. Young adults (15–25 years old) have the highest incidence of pubic lice; prevalence declines after age 35.

Subjective Data

Itching is the primary symptom. It leads to scratching, erythema, and skin irritation. The client may be asymptomatic. Some clients report small dark red or black "dots" (excrement of the pubic lice) in their underwear.

Objective Data

Physical Examination. Adult lice may be viewed moving along pubic hairs. Eggs (nits) appear as minute white dots adherent to pubic hair. Occasionally small scabs (crab bites) are noted on underlying skin.

Diagnostic Tests and Methods. Characteristic lice and nits may be observed; microscopic examination confirms.

Differential Medical Diagnoses

If small white flakes are noted in the pubic hair, seborrheic dermatitis must be considered.

Plan

Psychosocial Interventions. Assist the client to deal with the anxiety and embarrassment that diagnosis causes. Tell her that pubic lice are usually curable and have no long-term consequences. In addition, advise her that contacts need to be checked and treated if they are infected. Clothing and household items require disinfection. Washable items may be laundered in hot water or dry cleaned. Nonwashable items can be treated with products that contain pyrethrin (Black Flag or Raid). These products should be used only on inanimate objects.

Medication. A variety of prescription and over-the-counter medications are available. Ideally, medication should be lethal to both adult lice and eggs, however, there is some indication that head lice are developing resistance to usual treatments and this may be seen in the future with pubic lice.

PERMETHRIN. 1 percent liquid (Nix).
- *Indications.* For treatment of pubic lice and eggs.[54] This is an over-the-counter preparation.
- *Administration.* Application is as a shampoo or liquid. Manufacturer's directions for application must be followed exactly. Repeat application is usually unnecessary but may be done 7 to 10 days after initial treatment. Do not exceed two applications within 24 hours.
- *Side Effects and Adverse Reactions.* Minimal but minor skin irritation may occur. Avoid contact with mucous membranes. May be used during pregnancy.
- *Contraindications.* Sensitivity to ragweed: for these individuals the solutions should be used with caution.
- *Anticipated Outcomes on Evaluation.* Destruction of pubic lice and eggs. Reexamination is needed 1 week after initial treatment to confirm positive outcome.
- *Client Teaching and Counseling.* Encourage the client to follow the directions exactly. Instruct her in the use of the fine-tooth comb usually provided with the medication; dead nits are combed out of the pubic hair.

LINDANE. 1 percent (Kwell).
- *Indications.* This prescription solution is used in the treatment of pubic lice. It kills both adult lice and eggs.
- *Administration.* Application is as a shampoo. Apply exactly according to the manufacturer's directions. One application is usually adequate, but the treatment may be repeated in 7 days.

- *Side Effects and Adverse Reactions.* May include skin irritation, but it is usually minor. Lindane permeates human skin and has potential central nervous system (CNS) toxicity. Care must be taken to avoid contact with the eyes.
- *Contraindications.* Known seizure disorders and known sensitivity to lindane. Do not use during pregnancy and lactation or on infants/children.
- *Anticipated Outcomes on Evaluation.* The same as that achieved with the use of permethrins.
- *Client Teaching and Counseling.* Clients who telephone to say they have pubic lice can be believed and given treatment over the telephone. No office visit is needed to confirm the diagnosis.

OTHER MEDICATIONS. Lindane pyrethrins (RID) and Crotamiton (Eurax) are also effective.[41]

HEPATITIS B

Hepatitis B, or serum hepatitis, is a viral inflammation of the liver that results in a broad spectrum of disease from mild illness to chronic carrier state with possible cirrhosis, liver cancer, and death secondary to liver failure. Most infected persons never become jaundiced; their illness is mistaken for a nonspecific viral syndrome unless liver biochemical tests are ordered.

Women infected with hepatitis B may transmit the virus to their neonates at the time of delivery; the risk of chronic infection in the infant is as high as 90 percent.[47] Testing for hepatitis B is indicated for persons who are jaundiced, who have elevated liver transaminases (ALT and AST), or who are sexual partners of a person diagnosed with hepatitis B. Persons with presumptive hepatitis B should also be tested for hepatitis A, hepatitis C, and hepatitis D. Hepatitis D is caused by a defective RNA virus that requires coinfection with hepatitis B. Further information about hepatitis A and C is beyond the scope of this chapter since their transmission is not primarily sexual.[55]

Epidemiology

Hepatitis B virus (HBV) is the causative organism. Those at special risk include intravenous drug users, heterosexuals and homosexuals with multiple partners, sexual partners of HBV carriers, infants of HBV infected mothers, health workers who have contact with blood, and people born in areas where HBV is endemic. Hepatitis B may occasionally be transmitted to household contacts. Hepatitis B may be transmitted parenterally, sexually, or perinatally. The incubation period ranges from 4 weeks to 6 months (average is 12 weeks).[56] One percent to 2 percent of persons with hepatitis B become chronic carriers, remain capable of transmitting the virus, and may progress to cirrhosis or liver failure.

Although up to 300,000 cases and 350 deaths due to fulminant disease have been reported each year in the United States,[6] cases are expected to drop with routine immunization of health care workers and infants. The majority of current cases in the United States are adults.

Subjective Data

Many persons have asymptomatic infection and develop lifelong immunity. The symptoms, which may be mild or severe, include fatigue, loss of appetite, dark urine, light colored bowel movements, nausea/vomiting, diarrhea, malaise, and myalgias. The onset of symptoms is usually gradual, and resolution is slow.

Objective Data

Physical Examination. Examination may reveal jaundice, low grade fever, or the only sign may be mild right upper quadrant pain.

Diagnostic Tests and Methods. Initial diagnostic workup for acute hepatitis should include a urinalysis (for bilirubin), a check of serum transaminases (ALT and AST), hepatitis B surface antigen (HBsAG), antibody to hepatitis B core antibody (Anti-HBc IgM), antibody to hepatitis A (Anti-HAV IgM), and antibody to hepatitis C (Anti-HCV). Antibody to hepatitis D (anti-HDV) should be measured in all persons diagnosed with acute hepatitis B. If hepatitis B is diagnosed, prothrombin time and serum albumin should be measured.[57] The test procedure is to obtain a blood sample. Advise the client that blood testing is highly accurate and can determine active infection.

Differential Medical Diagnoses

Hepatitis A, C, and D.

Plan

Medical Management. Nonphenothiazine antiemetics (such as Tigan suppositories 200 mgs t.i.d.) should be used to control nausea and vomiting since phenothiazines may cause cholestatic jaundice.[57] Clients should be followed weekly in the acute phase to monitor symptom management.

Prothrombin time, serum bilirubin, and aminotransferases should be rechecked weekly if there is suspicion of worsening. At 3 months, transaminases should be repeated along with serum bilirubin and prothrombin time. HBsAG should be rechecked to determine antigen status. If symptoms and laboratory evidence of activity persist after 3 months, evaluations should be repeated monthly. If antigen persists 6 months after acute infection, referral for liver biopsy should be considered.[57]

Psychosocial Interventions. Advise the client that there is no specific treatment for hepatitis B. Rest and nutritious diet are important. Alcohol should be restricted, but oral contraceptives need not be stopped.[57] Activity restrictions are based on how the individual feels. Sexual partners and household contacts should be vaccinated. In addition to vaccination, general counseling to prevent transmission of HBV includes information about using latex condoms, and not sharing needles, razors, or toothbrushes.

Medication

HEPATITIS B IMMUNE GLOBULIN (HBIG)

- *Indications.* Sexual contacts of clients with acute HBV, those who have sexual contact with HBV carriers, nonimmunized health care workers with needlesticks from patients with hepatitis B, and newborns of mothers with HBV. HBIG should be followed by HBV immunization.
- *Administration.* Intramuscular injection, 0.06 mL/kg. In neonates, 0.5 cc I.M. at birth.
- *Side Effects and Adverse Reactions.* Minimal, local irritation at the injection site.
- *Contraindications.* None known.

- *Anticipated Outcomes on Evaluation.* Highly effective, immediate immunity, although temporary.
- *Client Teaching and Counseling.* HBIG should be given within 14 days of HBV exposure.[6] Three dose immunization with hepatitis B vaccine should follow.

HEPATITIS B VACCINATION

- *Indications.* Persons with multiple sexual partners, homosexual/bisexual men, illicit intravenous drug users, prison inmates and other institutionalized individuals, prostitutes, health care workers with exposure to blood products, infants of HBV infected mothers, clients attending STD clinics, and household or sexual contacts of HBV carriers. Universal vaccination of newborns is now recommended.[7]
- *Administration.* Requires three intramuscular injections: an initial injection, another 1 month later, and the third at 6 months. The deltoid muscle should be used. May give first dose concurrently with HBIG.
- *Side Effects and Adverse Reactions.* Minimal, local soreness at injection site.
- *Contraindications.* None.
- *Anticipated Outcomes on Evaluation.* Active immunity to HBV, lasting 5 years or longer. Postvaccination testing to confirm immunity is not routinely recommended.
- *Client Teaching and Counseling.* Educate the client that prevaccination HBV testing is recommended only for very high risk groups where the presence of HBV antibodies would negate the necessity of vaccination. The cost effectiveness of such testing in moderate risk groups must be considered. HBsAg positive individuals who receive the vaccine are unharmed.

NURSING DIAGNOSES

The following nursing diagnoses are representative of those used in the health care plan of women with general vaginitis and sexually transmitted diseases. The list, however, is by no means inclusive.

- Anxiety.
- Body image disturbance.
- Disruption in skin integrity.

- Discomfort.
- Fatigue.
- Fear.
- Grieving, anticipatory.
- Infection, high risk for.
- Knowledge deficit.
- Lowered self-esteem.
- Pain.
- Sexual dysfunction.
- Sexuality pattern, altered.
- Skin integrity, impaired.
- Social interaction, impaired.
- Social isolation.

REFERENCES

1. American College of Obstetricians and Gynecologists (ACOG). (1995). Condom availability for adolescents. *ACOG Committee Opinion, 154.* Washington, DC: Author.
2. Update: Barrier protection against HIV infection and other sexually transmitted diseases. (1993). *Morbidity and Mortality Weekly Report, 42*(30), 589–597.
3. Schaffer, S. D., Garzon, L. S., Heroux, D. L., & Korniewicz, D. M. (1996). *Pocket guide to infection prevention and safe practice.* Baltimore: Mosby-Year Book, Inc.
4. American College of Obstetricians and Gynecologists (ACOG). (1996). Vaginitis. *ACOG Technical Bulletin, 221,* 1–9.
5. Faro, S. (1993). Review of vaginitis. *Infectious Diseases in Obstetrics and Gynecology, 1,* 153–161.
6. Morbidity and Mortality Weekly Report. (1993, September 24). *1993 Sexually Transmitted Diseases Treatment Guidelines* Vol. 42, No. RR-14, Atlanta, GA: U.S. Department of Health and Human Services, PHS, Centers for Disease Control and Prevention.
7. Eschenbach, D. A., et al. (1987). Diagnosis and clinical manifestations of bacterial vaginosis. *American Journal of Obstetrics and Gynecology, 158,* 819–828.
8. Embree, J., Caliando, J. J., & McCormack, W. M. (1984). Nonspecific vaginitis among women attending a sexually transmitted diseases clinic. *Sexually Transmitted Diseases, 11,* 81–84.

9. Hallen, A., Pahlson, D., & Forsum, U. (1987). Bacterial vaginosis in women attending STD clinics: Diagnostic criteria and prevalence of Mobiluncus spp. *Genitourinary Medicine, 63,* 386–389.

10. Livengood, C. H., et al. (1994). Bacterial vaginosis: Efficacy and safety of intravaginal metronidazole treatment. *American Journal of Obstetrics and Gynecology, 170,* 759–764.

11. Lugo-Miro, V. I., Green, M., & Mazur, L. (1992). Comparison of different metronidazole therapeutic regimens for bacterial vaginosis. A meta-analysis. *JAMA, 268,* 92–95.

12. Carcio, H. A., & Secor, M. C. (1992). Vulvovaginal candidiasis: A current update. *Nurse practitioner Forum, 3*(3), 135–144.

13. Freeman, Sarah B. (1995). Common genitourinary infections. *JOGNN, 24*(8), 735–742.

14. Pfizer Incorporated. (1995). *Diflucan brief summary for vaginal candidiasis.* Author.

15. Hilton, E., Isenberg, H., Alperstein, P., France, K., Borenstein, M., et al. (1992). Ingestion of yogurt containing lactobacillus acidophilus as prophylaxis for candidal vaginitis. *Annals of Internal Medicine, 116,* 353–357.

16. Cibley, L. J., & Cibley, L. J. (1991). Cytolytic vaginosis. *American Journal of Obstetrics and Gynecology, 165,* 1245–1249.

17. Horowitz, B. J. (1994). Vaginal lactobacillosis. *American Journal of Obstetrics and Gynecology, 170,* 857–861.

18. Cecor, R. M. (1996, March 15). *Cyclic vulvovaginitis: Diagnostic and management challenges.* Presented at Contraceptive Technology Conference.

19. Moulton, A. W., & Montgomery, K. M. (1995). Approach to the patient with a vaginal discharge. In A. H. Goroll, L. A. May, & A. G. Mulley. *Primary care medicine: Office evaluation and management of the adult patient* (3rd ed.). Philadelphia: J. B. Lippincott.

20. Randall, J. (1993). New tools ready for chlamydia diagnosis, treatment, but teens need education most. *JAMA, 269,* 2716–2717.

21. Krieger, J. N. (1995). New sexually transmitted diseases treatment guidelines. *The Journal of Urology, 154,* 209–213.

22. Youngkin, E. Q. (1995). Sexually transmitted diseases: Current and emerging concerns. *JOGNN, 24*(8), 743–758.

23. Cottingham, J., & Hunter, D. (1992). Chlamydia trachomatis and oral contraceptive use: A quantitative review. *Genitourinary Medicine, 68,* 209–216.

23a. The Ligase Chain Reaction (LCR) Amplification Assay was introduced in February, 1997, by the Clinical Microbiology Laboratory. This is a nucleic acid amplification assay for use in diagnosing Chlamydia trachomatis and Neisseria gonorrhea, and is considered more sensitive than any other method in use today, including culture, antigen detection by EIA, or nucleic acid detection by DNA probe hybridization. Specificity of the LCR is superior to non-culture tests. One single specimen is used for this test.[58] Either a urogenital swab or first voided urine specimen may be used.

23b. The DNA probe remains positive for 30 days. This may be confusing if a test-of-cure is done before 30 days because the DNA material that remains, even though dead, will yield a positive test. Use clinical parameters to determine if infection is still present such as lack of signs or symptoms of infection.

24. Chambers, H. F. (1996). Infectious diseases: Bacterial and chlamydial. In L. M. Tierney, S. J. McPhee, & M. A. Papadakis. *Current medical diagnosis & treatment. (36th ed.)* Stamford, CT: Appleton & Lange.

25. Bush, M. R., & Rosa, C. (1994). Azithromycin and erythromycin in the treatment of cervical chlamydial infection during pregnancy. *Obstetrics & Gynecology, 84,* 61–63.

26. Turrentine, M. A., & Newton, E. R. (1995). Amoxicillin or erythromycin for the treatment of antenatal chlamydial infection: A meta-analysis. *Obstetrics & Gynecology, 86*(6), 1021–1025.

27. Hatcher, R. A., et al. (1994). *Contraceptive technology* (16th ed.). New York: Irvington Publishers.

28. Trends in STDs in the United States: Epidemiological synergy (1994, May). In *Association of Reproductive Health Professionals Clinical Proceedings* (p. 3). Washington DC: ARHP.

29. Ingalls, R. R., & Rice, P. A. (1996). Sexually transmitted diseases. In J. Noble (Ed.), *Textbook of primary care medicine* (2nd ed.). Baltimore: Mosby-Year Book Inc.

30. Curry, S. L., & Barclay, D. L. (1994). Benign disorders of the vulva and vagina. In A. H. DeCherney, & M. L. Pernoll (Eds.). *Current obstetric and gynecologic diagnosis & treatment.* Norwalk, CT: Appleton & Lange.

31. Goodson, J. D. (1995). Approach to the male patient with urethritis. In A. H. Goroll, L. A. May, & A. G. Mulley. (Eds.). *Primary care medicine: Office evaluation and management of the adult patient* (3rd ed.). Philadelphia: J. B. Lippincott.

32. Galpin, J. E. (1995). Management of cutaneous and genital herpes simplex. In A. H. Goroll, L. A. May, & A. G. Mulley (Eds.), *Primary care medi-*

cine: Office evaluation and management of the adult patient. (3d ed.). Philadelphia: J. B. Lippincott.

33. Swanson, J., Dibble, S., & Chenitz, C. (1995). Clinical features and psychosocial factors in young adults with genital herpes. *Image: Journal of Nursing Scholarship, 27*(1), 16–22.

34. Eisenstat, S. A. (1995). Infectious exposure and immunization during pregnancy. In K. J. Carlson, S. A. Eisenstat, F. D. Frigoletto, & I. Schiff (Eds.), *Primary care of women.* Baltimore: Mosby.

35. Apgar, B. S. (1996). Pregnancy. In C. A. Johnson, B. E. Johnson, J. L. Murray, & B. S. Apgar (Eds.), *Women's health care handbook.* Baltimore: Mosby.

36. Famiciclovir gains genital herpes indication. (1996). *The Female Patient, 21,* 13.

37. Product Information. (1995, December). Valtrex. Glaxo Wellcome.

38. Jacobs, R. A. (1996). Infectious diseases: Spirochetal. In L. M. Tierney, S. J. McPhee, & M. A. Papadakis (Eds.), *Current medical diagnosis & treatment.* (35th ed.). Stamford, CT: Appleton & Lange.

39. Simon, H. B. (1995). Management of syphilis and other venereal diseases. In A. H. Goroll, L. A. May, & A. G. Mulley. (Eds.), *Primary care medicine: Office evaluation and management of the adult patient* (3rd ed.). Philadelphia: J. B. Lippincott.

40. Nakashima, A. K., et al. (1996). Epidemiology of syphilis in the United States, 1941–1993. *Sexually Transmitted Diseases, 23*(1), 16–23.

41. Ramin, S. M., Wendel, G. D. & Hemsell, D. L. (1994). Sexually transmitted diseases and pelvic infections. In A. H. DeCherney, & M. L. Pernoll (Eds.), *Current obstetric and gynecologic diagnosis & treatment.* Norwalk: CT: Appleton & Lange.

42. Sanford, J. P., Gilbert, D. N., & Sande, M. A. (1996). *Sanford guide to antimicrobial therapy* (26th ed.). Vienna, VA: Antimicrobial Therapy, Inc.

43. Heaton, C. L. (1995). Clinical manifestations and modern management of condylomata acuminata: A dermatologic perspective. *American Journal of Obstetrics and Gynecology, 172*(4), 1344–1349.

44. Hatch, K. D. (1995). Clinical appearance and treatment strategies for human papillomavirus: A gynecologic perspective. *American Journal of Obstetrics and Gynecology, 172*(4), 1340–1343.

45. Koutsky, L. A., et al. (1992). A cohort study of the risks of cervical intraepithelial neoplasia grade 2 or 3 in relation to papillomavirus infec-

tion. *New England Journal of Medicine, 327,* 1272–1278.

46. National Institutes of Health. (1996). Consensus development conference statement: Cervical cancer. Author.

47. Soper, D. E. (1995). Sexually transmitted diseases & pelvic inflammatory disease. In D. P. Lemche, J. Pattison, L. A. Marshall, & D. S. Cowley (Eds.), *Primary care of women.* Norwalk: CT: Appleton & Lange.

48. American College of Obstetricians and Gynecologists (ACOG). (1994). Genital human papillomavirus infections. *ACOG Technical Bulletin, 194,* 1–7.

49. Lorincz, A. T., et al. (1992). Human papillomavirus infection of the cervix: Relative risk association of 15 common anogenital types. *Obstetrics & Gynecology, 79,* 328–337.

50. Ferenczy, A. (1995). Epidemiology and clinical pathophysiology of condylomata acuminata. *American Journal of Obstetrics and Gynecology, 172*(4), 1331–1339.

51. Keller, M. L. (1995). Genital human papillomavirus infection: Common but not trivial. *Health Care for Women International, 16,* 351–363.

52. Enterline, J., & Leonardo, J. (1989). Condyloma acuminata. *Nurse Practitioner, 14,* 8–16.

53. Cannistra, S. A. & Nilof, J. M. (1996). Cancer of the uterine cervix. *The New England Journal of Medicine, 334*(16), 1030–1038.

54. Berger, T. G., Goldstein, S. M., & Odom, R. B. (1997). Skin & appendages. In L. M. Tierney, S. J. McPhee, & M. A. Papadakis (Eds.), *Current medical diagnosis & treatment.* (35th ed.). Stamford, CT: Appleton & Lange.

55. Friedman, L. S. (1996). Liver, biliary tract, & pancreas. In L. M. Tierney, S. J. McPhee, & M. A. Papadakis (Eds.), *Current medical diagnosis & treatment.* (35th ed.). Stamford, CT: Appleton & Lange.

56. Dienstag, J. L. (1995). Prevention of viral hepatitis. In A. H. Goroll, L. A. May, & A. G. Mulley (Eds.), *Primary care medicine: Office evaluation and management of the adult patient* (3rd ed.). Philadelphia: J. B. Lippincott.

57. Dienstag, J. L. (1995). Management of hepatitis. In A. H. Goroll, L. A. May, & A. G. Mulley (Eds.), *Primary care medicine: Office evaluation and management of the adult patient* (3rd ed.). Philadelphia: J. B. Lippincott.

58. New clinical testing. (April, 1997). *The Pathology Scope.* Richmond, VA: School of Medicine, Medical College of Virginia–Virginia Commonwealth University, *3*(1), 1.

CHAPTER 12

WOMEN
AND HIV

Susan D. Schaffer

*A*IDS requires us
to reconsider our
basic assumptions and
to question received
wisdom in the form of
convenient categoriza-
tions. One such simpli-
fication treats health
and human rights as
distinct and separate—
and often conflicting—
concerns. . . .[1]

Highlights

- Epidemiology of HIV
    Viral Life Cycle
    Incidence
    Transmission
    Risk Factors
- Diagnostic Testing
    Pre- and Post-Test Counseling
- Initial Evaluation of the Woman with HIV
    Subjective
    Objective
- Management of Early HIV Infection
    Self-Care Strategies
    Immunizations
    Gynecological Care
    Contraception
    M. Tuberculosis Prevention
    Monitoring Immune Status
- Management of Late HIV Infection
    Antiretroviral Therapy
    Pneumocystis Carinii Prophylaxis
    Mycobacterium Avium Complex
    Cytomegalovirus Infection

► INTRODUCTION

Acquired Immune Deficiency Syndrome (AIDS), first identified in 1981, is a viral infection caused by the Human Immunodeficiency Virus (HIV). The spectrum of HIV disease ranges from asymptomatic to full blown infection that is almost universally fatal through a loss of cell mediated immune function and the depletion of T4 lymphocytes.[2] Humoral immunity (circulating antibodies carried by immunoglobulins) is also affected, but this mechanism of action is not well understood.[3] This deterioration of the immune system confers susceptibility to rare opportunistic infections and malignant tumors. These phenomena, along with dementia and a wasting syndrome, signal the end stage of HIV infection (AIDS).[2] HIV infection has a profound effect on women both as an illness and as a social and economic challenge. HIV affects women's care taking role in the family; women must deal with their own life threatening illness while they also deal with the impact of disease on their families. Women who become pregnant while HIV infected or who contemplate pregnancy while infected need information on risks to the fetus as well as information on caring for themselves. The stigma attached to HIV/AIDS can subject women to discrimination, job loss, social rejection, and other violations of their rights.[4] Although primarily sexually transmitted, AIDS is covered in a separate chapter from other sexually transmitted infections because of the devastating effect AIDS has on infected women and their families and because of the complex psychosocial and medical management that is required to delay the effects and to promote a high quality of life in infected women.

Since there is no cure for HIV infection, primary prevention remains the most important strategy for primary care providers. Recent advances in the use of antiviral agents (particularly during pregnancy) and in the strategic use of antibiotics and antivirals to prevent debilitating opportunistic infection, however, highlight the importance of early diagnosis. Women with HIV infection require the ongoing provider relationship that is the hallmark of primary care. Primary care providers should perform periodic physical examinations, monitor prognostic markers (CD4+ counts and viral load tests), prescribe initial antiviral and prophylactic therapy, initiate diagnostic evaluation and therapy for HIV related complications, provide supportive counseling, and offer assistance with pain control and durable power of attorney.[5] Specialists should be consulted for patients unable to tolerate standard antiviral drugs and for patients with complicated opportunistic infections.[3] Strategies to combat HIV infection depend on understanding the epidemiology of the virus.

EPIDEMIOLOGY OF HIV

VIRAL LIFE CYCLE

T lymphocytes play a central part in the immune system by destroying infected cells and helping B cells make antibodies. T4 helper cells (CD4+ cells) are specialized T lymphocytes that do little to repel intruding substances themselves but instead become activated to alert B cells, killer cells, and phagocytes to the presence of a bacterial, fungal, or viral antigens. When the HIV virus is introduced into the bloodstream, the virus joins the host T4 cell's DNA and awaits activation of the cell. Only after the HIV infected T4 cells are activated by some non-HIV antigen do the T4 cells manufacture HIV viral RNA strands, replicating the virus and destroying themselves in the process.[6] With ongoing destruction and replacement of the T4 cells, the body gradually loses its ability to mount an immune response. Minimizing T4 cell activation in HIV infected persons by controlling other infections may thus be one key to delaying progression of the infection.[2,6]

INCIDENCE

As of mid-1995, about 20 million people were HIV infected worldwide; 36 percent were women.[2] By the end of the 20th century there will be as many women as men with AIDS.[7] In the United States, HIV infection first appeared in homosexual and bisexual men; however, 18 percent (14,302) of persons with AIDS in 1994 were women, up from 7 percent (534) in 1985.[8] In 1994, 60 percent of all new female HIV infections in the United States occurred in women by age 20.[9] More than three-fourths (77 percent) of cases among women occurred among blacks and Hispanics; however, race and ethnicity are not risk factors but serve as markers of socioeconomic status and access to medical care.[10]

During 1995, vaginal intercourse replaced parenteral drug use as the leading cause of acquisition of HIV in women.[11] For infants and young children, perinatally acquired HIV is already among the ten leading causes of death, and is likely to be among the five leading causes of death within the next several years.[2]

TRANSMISSION

Three main routes of HIV transmission have been documented: 1) sexual contact with infected body fluids; 2) contact with infected blood or blood products via transfusion, organ transplants, shared needles, or accidental needlestick injury (health care workers); and 3) transmission from an infected woman to her infant prenatally, at birth, or during breast feeding. Current use of third generation antibody screening for donated blood has all but eliminated the risk of transfusion associated HIV transmission. (One case of HIV transmission is currently expected for every 450,000 to 660,000 donations of screened blood.[12]) Transmission via casual contacts, fomites, and insect bites does not occur. Transmission via artificial insemination is possible; however, current safeguards make this unlikely. Oral transmission of HIV has been demonstrated in a simian model, making oral-genital contact a

likely route of transmission for humans.[13] Receptive anal intercourse is especially risky because traumatic lacerations of the delicate rectal mucosa provide direct bloodstream access for the HIV virus.

Women are at far greater risk of contracting HIV during heterosexual intercourse than are men for several reasons. First, semen has greater quantities of lymphocytes that may be infected than does vaginal fluid.[2] Seminal fluid has also been postulated to have an immunosuppressive effect upon mucosa that facilitates the absorption of HIV.[14] Women have a larger mucosal surface area available for HIV penetration (vagina and cervix), but the only exposed mucosal surface in men is the urethra. Vaginal mucosa can suffer microscopic abrasions during intercourse, increasing susceptibility to HIV penetration. Finally, there are currently more HIV infected men than women in the United States.[2]

RISK FACTORS

HIV infected individuals may be asymptomatic or relatively asymptomatic for 10 years or longer, but with current advances in treatment, diagnosis while asymptomatic provides optimal opportunities to slow disease progression. Testing for antibodies to HIV is an important first step in establishing a diagnosis. Based on a recent study documenting the efficacy of zidovudine (ZDV) therapy in reducing the perinatal transmission of HIV,[15] the Centers for Disease Control and Prevention (CDC) has published guidelines urging routine counseling and voluntary testing for all pregnant women in the United States.[16] Recommendations for testing of nonpregnant women should be based on risk behaviors and/or symptoms that include the following.

Risk Behaviors (since 1978). Anal sexual activity, injection drug use, frequent casual intercourse, intercourse with commercial sex workers, previous treatment for sexually transmitted infections (human papilloma virus, herpes simplex, gonorrhea, syphilis, Chlamydia), blood transfusions before 1985, or sexual activity with partners having any of these characteristics.

Symptoms. Unexplained fever or weight loss, severe fatigue, recurrent vaginal candidiasis, oral thrush, dysphagia, shingles, swollen glands, diarrhea, and other nonspecific but persistent symptoms.

Signs. Signs that should alert practitioners to possible HIV infection include persistent or recurrent vaginal candidiasis, weight loss, enlarged lymph nodes and/or tonsillar enlargement, oral candidiasis or oral hairy leukoplakia of the tongue, skin lesions such as Kaposi's Sarcoma, varicella-zoster, psoriasis, or seborrheic dermatitis. Persistent or recurrent genital herpes simplex infection, recurrent cervical neoplasia (despite treatment), and nonspecific genital ulcers may suggest HIV infection. Recurrent (nonpneumocystis) pneumonias, recurrent or particularly severe pelvic inflammatory disease (PID), and persistent urinary tract infections unresponsive to standard treatments may also be markers for early HIV infection. Hepatosplenomegaly and/or mental status changes may also be suspicious.

DIAGNOSTIC TESTING

Except for blood donors, newborns, military recruits, and immigrants, HIV testing must be performed only with voluntary informed consent.[17] Although HIV antibodies have been found as early as 1 week after exposure, 50 percent of exposed persons seroconvert within 3 months, and 90 percent within 6 months.[2] The enzyme linked immunosorbent assay (ELISA) test detects antibody to HIV antigens and is used as an initial screening test for HIV. The ELISA test is usually performed on venous blood obtained through venipuncture. As with all blood collection, gloves should be worn. In an effort to support testing in persons who have shunned blood tests, the Food and Drug Administration (FDA) approved an antibody test in 1996 that uses a treated cotton pad to scrape a tissue sample from between the gum and cheek.[18]

If the ELISA is positive, it is repeated by the reference lab before results are reported. People may test false positive for the ELISA if they have underlying liver disease, have received a blood transfusion or gamma globulin within 6 weeks of the test, have had several children, have had rheumatological diseases, are injection drug users, or have received vaccines for influenza or hepatitis B.[19,20] The confirmatory Western blot test, however, will almost always be negative in these cases.[2] Combined ELISA and Western blot tests, if repeatedly run, have a better than 99 percent overall accuracy rate.[21]

In addition to these antibody tests, quantification of viral burden in persons known to be HIV infected can be performed by polymerase chain reaction (PCR), nucleic acid sequence-based amplification, or branched chain DNA signal amplification. These methods quantify single strands of HIV RNA in plasma.[22]

PRE- AND POST-TEST COUNSELING

Counseling both before and after HIV testing has become a standard of practice.[23] This counseling has been shown to provide reassurance and motivation to modify lifestyle as well as reduction of anxiety and depression.[24] It is recommended that all women being tested for HIV receive extensive pretest counseling about viral transmission, implications for pregnancy, modes and prevention of transmission, personal risk, possibility of positive test results, and available support mechanisms. It is generally preferable for all HIV test results to be presented in person, although a home HIV test has recently been approved that will provide results over the phone.[25]

Persons testing negative for HIV can probably be reassured that they are virus free if it has been 6 months since their last possible exposure to HIV. Persons testing negative should be counseled about primary prevention strategies, however, and should be encouraged to have the test repeated if they have had more recent possible exposure.

Women testing (repeatedly) positive for HIV require extensive counseling. Disclosure should consider social, cultural, and psychologic characteristics of the person tested. Immediate interventions should include assessing the woman for the potential for violence to herself or others, ensuring access to a comprehensive medical evaluation, scheduling the next appointment, prevention of further HIV transmission, assessing the availability of key support persons and providing information on local and national sources of support. Referral should be made for any services not available on site.[5]

Later counseling should also include the natural history of HIV infection and available treatments.[26] Disclosure of HIV status to sexual and needle sharing partners by the woman should be encouraged so they can be tested. At the same time providers must be aware of the potential for domestic violence that may be triggered by this disclosure. Women should be advised that discrimination based on HIV status or AIDS regarding matters of employment, housing, state programs or public accommodations is illegal.[4] It should also be recommended that children born after acquisition of maternal infection be tested.

HIV infected pregnant women should additionally be advised of the risk for perinatal HIV transmission (25–30 percent), ways to reduce this risk (including not breastfeeding), and the prognosis for infants who become infected.[5] They should be given information concerning zidovudine (ZVD) therapy to reduce the risk for perinatal transmission. One study, for example, documented reduction of risk from 25 percent to 8 percent with use of oral ZVD taken prenatally for 6 months, intravenously during labor, and then taken orally by infants for 6 weeks.[15] Information about ZVD treatment should include addressing the potential benefit and short-term safety of zidovudine and the uncertainties regarding risks of therapy and effectiveness in women with clinical characteristics unlike those of study participants. A woman's decision not to accept zidovudine treatment should not result in punitive action or denial of care.

INITIAL EVALUATION OF THE WOMAN WITH HIV

SUBJECTIVE DATA

The medical history for all HIV infected women should include the following: sexual and drug use history, and history of exposure to bacterial, viral, parasitic, and fungal infections such as tuberculosis, syphilis, herpes simplex and other STDs, or giardia lamblia. Immunization history should be determined as well as the presence of household pets (cat litter boxes transmit Toxoplasmosis, and reptiles transmit salmonella). A social history should include family system history, occupational history, socioeconomic needs (insurance, disability benefits, etc.), and psychiatric history (medications and potential for suicide).

OBJECTIVE DATA

A complete physical examination should be done including weight and nutritional status, blood pressure and temperature, oral cavity and tongue, skin and nails (lesions and clubbing), fundoscopic exam (for exudates associated with CMV retinitis), ears, nose, and sinuses, neurological status (including mental status, cranial nerves, reflexes, gait, and fine motor skills), lymph nodes, heart and lungs, extremities, (muscle mass, myositis), and abdominal exam (hepatomegaly, splenomegaly, or tenderness). A breast exam and complete vaginal and perirectal exam should also be done.[27]

Recommended baseline labs include a lymphocyte panel (CD4+ count and percent), viral load determination, CBC with differential and platelets, chemistry panel including liver functions, hepatitis B panel, serological test for syphilis, urinalysis, and PPD. Simultaneous administration of two additional antigens (tetanus and candida) to test for anergy has been recommended by the Early HIV Infection Guidelines Panel,[5] but not by the USPHS/IDSA Working Group.[26] A Pap smear, specimens for gonorrhea and chlamydia, and wet mounts for bacterial vaginosis, trichomonas, white blood cells, and Candida should be obtained. Some authorities recommend a baseline chest x-ray and determination of antibodies to Toxoplasma gondii.[27] Since many HIV related infections are reactivation illnesses, tuberculin testing, syphilis serologic tests, and toxoplasma antibody status in particular can guide the practitioner diagnostically when an acute illness occurs.[10]

Management of Early HIV Infection

It has been demonstrated that HIV infected persons who are followed in a comprehensive program of care survive longer than those who present for care only according to their symptoms.[28] The establishment of trust in a nonjudgmental care provider and sufficient time to express concerns are crucial. Care providers for HIV infected women should refer them for comprehensive case management services if they are unable to provide such services.[5] Advance directives regarding life sustaining treatments, durable power of attorney for health care, and guardianship of dependent children should be addressed when rapport allows.[10]

The CD4+ lymphocyte count is currently the best documented test for monitoring immune function in persons with HIV infection. Plasma viral load as measured by RNA amplification, however, has been shown to be a better predictor of regression to AIDS and death than the number of CD4+ cells.[29] Measuring viral load (viremia) is also useful as a gauge of antiviral efficacy.[22,30] Guidelines for directing therapy according to these measures are expected to evolve as use of RNA amplification becomes widespread.

Women with asymptomatic HIV infection should be followed by a primary care provider every 3–6 months as long as their CD4+ counts remain normal.[27] In addition to measuring CD4+ counts, each visit should include monitoring for mental disorders, alcohol and drug abuse, measurement of weight and temperature, neurological status (including mental status and mood), abdominal examination, assessment of lymph nodes, and assessment of skin, oral cavity, and retina for characteristic lesions.[27] Although the USPHS recommends annual Pap smears after two normal smears 6 months apart, other authorities recommend Pap smears every 6 months for HIV infected women, particularly when CD4+ counts drop below normal.[31] Rescreening for sexually transmitted infection should be based on individual risk assessments. Additional strategies for ongoing care of HIV infected women follow.

SELF-CARE STRATEGIES

Management of early HIV infection requires extensive teaching in health maintenance and in the avoidance of infectious disease risks. Latex condoms (or latex dental dams) should be encouraged for all vaginal, oral, and anal intercourse for the protection of HIV infected persons and their partners (see section on Contraception). Smoking cessation decreases the risk of oral candidiasis, hairy leukoplakia, and bacteria pneumonia.[32] Women who are abusing drugs or alcohol should be referred to treatment programs. HIV infected persons experience several unique oral conditions, including frequent oral lesions and rapidly progressive periodontal disease and should receive twice yearly dental prophylaxis.

HIV infected persons should avoid pet reptiles who may carry salmonella; they should avoid young animals with diarrhea who may carry enteric pathogens, and they should avoid contact with cat feces that may be infected with Toxoplasma gondii. Since Toxoplasma may be present in soil, hands should be washed after gardening, and raw fruits and vegetables should be washed before eating. Poultry and meats should be well cooked (> 165 degrees), and uncooked meats should not come into contact with foods that will be eaten raw.[5]

HIV infected persons should be counseled about avoidance of Cryptosporidium (transmitted through contact with stools of infected adults and diaper age children), contact with infected animals, contact with contaminated drinking water, and contact with contaminated lake and river water. Using drinking water purified through reverse osmosis or through distillation may be considered by HIV infected persons whose municipal water supply is known to be contaminated by Cryptosporidium.[5]

IMMUNIZATIONS

Although live vaccines (except measles-mumps-rubella) are contraindicated in persons with HIV, pneumococcal vaccine, hepatitis B vaccine (in susceptible persons) and annual influenza vaccines have been recommended by the U. S. Public Health Service for prevention of infection in HIV infected persons and have become the standard of care.[5] Despite these guidelines, evidence is emerging that vaccination may stimulate HIV replication (at least temporarily) by activating CD4+ lymphocytes.[6,33] Although the clinical implications of this temporary increase in viral burden are unknown, this finding may stir new debate about the risks and benefits of routine vaccination. It is likely that pneumococcal vaccine (given once after HIV diagnosis) should continue to be offered routinely since HIV infected persons are at high risk for invasive and recurrent pneumococcal disease and since an adequate antibody response to the vaccine has been demonstrated in persons with low CD4+ counts. The benefit of annual influenza vaccine may be marginal, however, since an increased risk from influenza has not been demonstrated in HIV infected persons and since persons with low CD4+ counts demonstrate suboptimal antibody formation.[33,34]

GYNECOLOGIC CARE

Cervical dysplasia, vaginal candidiasis, and pelvic inflammatory disease are more common in HIV infected women, and tend to follow more aggressive courses. Since coexistent cervical intraepithelial neoplasia (CIN) is more prevalent in HIV infected women who have atypia of any type on a Pap smear, referral for colposcopy and biopsy is recommended for HIV infected women with atypia or any grade of CIN.[3,31,35] Evaluation of the anal canal with cytology and anoscopy has also been recommended for HIV positive women with high grade HPV lesions.[31]

Vaginal candidiasis, although not life threatening, is not a trivial condition in HIV infected women. Severe pruritus and excoriation can be disabling. Extension of candida to vulvae and thighs is common. Symptoms can often be controlled with topical antifungals, but oral fluconazole (100–200 mg daily for 10–14 days) or oral ketoconazole (200 mg daily for 10–14 days) may be necessary. It is not recommended that oral antifungals be given prophylactically because development of imidazole resistance is likely.[3]

Although the bacteriology remains the same, PID is more common in HIV infected women and is often more severe. Accordingly, inpatient management should be considered.[3]

Genital herpes simplex infections occur more frequently, tend to be more severe, and are more likely to disseminate in immunocompromised hosts. Because of the risk of progressive disease, all herpes simplex attacks should be treated with acyclovir 200 mg orally five times a day. Chronic acyclovir administration (400 mg orally b.i.d.) may be considered for women with a history of recurrent herpes infection; acyclovir resistance among herpes strains cultured from HIV patients is a possibility.[3] Valacyclovir (Valtrex) and famciclovir (Famvir) are alternative therapies.[36,37]

CONTRACEPTION

For HIV positive women, serostatus has been documented as only one of many factors that influence reproductive decision making.[36] Providers should advise about relative risks and therapeutic options and dangers and refrain from directive counseling where moral judgment is involved. The decision to initiate a pregnancy or to continue a pregnancy must remain a choice of the woman and her partner.[23]

Consistent use of latex condoms provides protection against most sexually transmitted infections (including HIV) as well as pregnancy. Condoms should be strongly recommended for consistent use by HIV positive women in addition to other contraceptive methods that may be selected. Condoms are helpful in protecting uninfected partners and also protect HIV infected women from increased HIV viral load and new viral strains from HIV positive partners. Polyurethane male condoms or polyurethane female condoms may be recommended for persons who are allergic to latex as laboratory evidence has documented their impermeability to HIV.[36]

Vaginal spermicides (nonoxynol-9) used with latex condoms enhance prevention of pregnancy as well as STDs such as gonorrhea and chlamydia. Nonoxynol-9 has also been shown to exert anti-HIV activity in vitro. The utility of nonoxynol-9 as protection against HIV transmission has been questioned, however, following a study demonstrating increased genital ulcers and increased acquisition of HIV infection in third world prostitutes who used contraceptive sponges.[37] Until this finding is better understood, the benefits of nonoxynol-9 as an adjunct to condoms is questionable in women infected with HIV.

Intrauterine devices are not recommended for use in HIV positive women since an impaired immune response and increased PID risk are strong relative contraindications.[38] Diaphragms and cervical caps have been associated with microabrasions and they leave most of the woman's vaginal vault unprotected. They also require use of vaginal spermicides such as nonoxynol-9. These problems make these methods less desirable for HIV infected women; they should be used only when no other contraceptive option is available.[36] To enhance prevention of pregnancy and STDs, these cervical barrier methods should be combined with use of a latex condom by the woman's partner.[36]

There is currently no documentation that the use of combined oral contraceptives by HIV positive women contributes to the progression of their immune disease; however, there is a possibility of interaction between oral contraceptives and some of the drugs used for HIV treatment.[36] Because of the association between estrogen levels, cervical ectopy, and subsequent increased cervical secretions, there is also a theoretical concern about increased risk of HIV transmission to an infected woman's sexual partner.[36]

Hormonal contraception containing only progestin (injections, pills, or subdermal implants) avoids possible estrogen related problems, but one simian study has shown increased risk of simian HIV in monkeys given progestin implants.[39] Nine other studies of human Norplant use, however, have failed to show an association between progestin and HIV.[40] Until further studies clarify these complex issues, highly efficient hormonal contraception—with careful explanation of risks and benefits—should be provided to HIV infected women who want it.

M. TUBERCULOSIS PREVENTION

Since immunosuppression caused by HIV can cause rapid progression of M. tuberculosis infection to an active state, PPD positive persons with negative x-rays should receive isoniazid (INH) therapy, usually 300 mg. p.o. daily for 12 months.[5] The addition of 50–100 mgs. of pyroxidine (B6) p.o. daily will prevent peripheral neuritis. Since INH is hepatotoxic, persons taking it should be monitored monthly for the development of adverse effects such as nausea, anorexia, fever, rash, visual problems, or jaundice. Monthly hepatic enzymes should be monitored in those over age 35. INH should be avoided in pregnant women (preventive therapy should be deferred until after delivery). A PPD reaction of 5 mm or greater is considered positive in a person with HIV infection.[5] Women should be assessed for health and social conditions (alcoholism, mental illness, or failure to keep appointments) that may affect their ability to complete a course of INH treatment. Case management and directly observed therapy should be used when needed to ensure successful completion of INH treatment.[5]

Women presenting with weight loss, hemoptysis, night sweats, or fever should receive an immediate chest x-ray and a sputum smear should be examined. Those who are coughing with symptoms of TB should be placed on respiratory isolation until active TB has been ruled out. Active tuberculosis or infection with possibly drug resistant organisms should be managed by an infectious disease specialist.

Monitoring Immune Status

The assessment of immune status is a key element in the ongoing management of early HIV infection. Measurement of plasma viral load should be used with physical findings and CD4+ cell counts to stage patients and to determine appropriate time for initiating antiretroviral therapy and prophylaxis for p carinii pneumonia and other opportunistic infections. CD4+ cells should be measured every 6 months when the count is greater than 600, and every 3 months when the CD4+ count is between 200 and 600 cells per microliter[5] (589–1505 is normal).[41] Persons with CD4+

counts lower than 200 should be monitored according to their symptoms.

MANAGEMENT OF LATE HIV INFECTION (AIDS)

Although recurrent vaginal candidiasis, pulmonary tuberculosis, bacterial pneumonia, and persistent generalized lymphadenopathy may occur during early HIV infection,[42] most of the conditions associated with AIDS occur when the CD4+ count falls below 500 cells per microliter. According to the CDC,[43] HIV infection is termed AIDS with the diagnosis of one of the conditions listed in the 1993 Expanded Surveillance case definition for AIDS (see Table 12–1). The distinction between HIV infection and AIDS is important for reporting purposes in some states (see Table 12–2). Persons with AIDS should be managed in conjunction with an infectious disease specialist, and may also require referral to oncology or other sub-specialty care.

ANTIRETROVIRAL THERAPY[43a]

Although available research data do not define optimal timing for initiation of antiretroviral agents or a single first-line antiretroviral regimen

TABLE 12–1. 1993 EXPANDED SURVEILLANCE CASE DEFINITION FOR AIDS

HIV Seropositivity *and* CD4+ Count < 200/mm³ *or* One or More of the Following Conditions:

Candidiasis of bronchi, trachea, esophagus, or lungs, invasive cervical cancer, extrapulmonary Coccidioidomycosis (disseminated or extrapulmonary), Cryptococcosis, Cryptosporidiosis, Cytomegalovirus (CMV) disease (other than spleen, liver, and nodes), or CMV retinitis, Encephalopathy, Herpes Simplex virus (chronic ulcers, esophagitis, or bronchitis), Histoplasmosis, Isosporiasis, Kaposi's Sarcoma, Lymphoma (Burkitt's, immunoblastic, or primary), mycobacterium tuberculosis (any site) Mycobacterium avium complex, Mycoplasma kansasii or other species (disseminated or extrapulmonary), pneumocystis carinii pneumonia, any recurrent pneumonia, progressive multifocal leukoencephalopathy, salmonella septicemia (recurrent), Toxoplasmosis of brain, or wasting syndrome due to HIV.

Source: Centers for Disease Control (1993). Revised classification system for HIV infection and expanded surveillance case definition for AIDS among adolescents and adults. MMWR 41, 1–19.

TABLE 12–2. REPORTING REQUIREMENTS FOR HIV INFECTION*

By Name	Anonymous	Not Required
Alabama	Georgia	Alaska
Arizona	Iowa	California
Arkansas	Kansas	Connecticut
Colorado	Kentucky	Delaware
Idaho	Maine	Florida
Illinois	Montana	Hawaii
Indiana	New Hampshire	Louisiana
Michigan	Oregon	Maryland #
Minnesota	Rhode Island	Massachusetts
Mississippi	Texas	Nebraska
Missouri		New Mexico
Nevada		New York
New Jersey		Pennsylvania
North Carolina		Vermont
South Dakota		Washington #
Tennessee		District of Columbia
Utah		
Virginia		
West Virginia		
Wisconsin		
Wyoming		

*Current as of March 3, 1993. *ALL* states require reporting of AIDS cases by name at the state/local level.
Requires reports of symptomatic HIV infection by name.
Source: Early HIV Infection Guideline Panel (1994). American Family Physician 49, 801–814.

for any given indication, rational treatment decisions can be made on the basis of available data.[44] Clinical trial data support the initiation of therapy in patients with CD4+ counts below 0.500×10^9/L. Some clinicians prefer to wait until the CD4+ count drops to 200–300, weighing likely benefits against substantial toxicities and quality of life considerations.[45] Starting antiretroviral treatment with CD4+ counts between 0.300×10^9 and 0.500×10^9 is recommended for asymptomatic patients with more than 30,000–50,000 HIV RNA copies/ml. or for those with rapidly declining CD4+ counts (a greater than 0.300×10^9 decline over 12–18 months) based on risk of rapid progression.[44] Antiretroviral treatment should be initiated in all persons with symptomatic HIV disease irregardless of laboratory parameters.[44]

Combinations of nucleoside analogues have proved significantly better than monotherapies.[44] Treatments with the most demonstrated benefits are zidovudine/didanosine (ZVD/ddi) and zidovudine/zalcitabine (ZVD/ddC).[44] Didanosine monotherapy is a reasonable option for those who cannot tolerate zidovudine. Newly approved protease inhibitors could be added to these regimens for symptomatic patients, patients with lower or falling CD4+ counts, and those with high plasma HIV RNA levels.[44] Studies using two nucleoside analogues plus a protease inhibitor have demonstrated reductions in HIV RNA to below detectable levels in a majority of patients after 24–48 weeks of treatment.[46] The clinical value of using three drug combination regimens to maximally suppress viral replication is controversial. It remains to be seen whether plasma viral suppression can be sustained and whether viral replication is also suppressed in the lymph nodes and central nervous system.[47]

The most frequently used dose of zidovudine is 200 mgs p.o. t.i.d.[45] Common adverse effects of ZDV include granulocytopenia, anemia, nausea, headache, confusion, myositis, hepatitis, seizures, and nail discoloration.[5] The CBC with differential should be monitored during therapy at two weeks, at one month, and if the value is stable, every three months thereafter. If the hemoglobin drops between 9.5–10.5 or the absolute neutrophil count (ANC) drops between 1000–1500, the CBC should be monitored every two weeks; if one hemoglobin drops between 8–9.4 or the ANC below 750–999, the CBC should be monitored every week.[45] Anemia or neutropenia below these levels require cessation of ZDV therapy until blood levels improve.[27]

Didanosine (ddi) is dosed 200 mgs p.o. b.i.d. This agent also has serious adverse effects, notably pancreatitis, liver failure, and peripheral neuropathy.[44] Didanosine must be dosed one hour before or two hours after meals. Concurrent use of alcohol is contraindicated.

Zalcitabine is dosed 0.005–0.01 mg/kg orally every 8 hours. Although it is not associated with hematologic side effects, it may cause peripheral neuropathy and rare pancreatitis.

Of the available protease inhibitors, indinavir demonstrates the best bioavailability and the fewest adverse effects.[44] Toxic effects include benign hyperbilirubinemia and a 3 percent to 4 percent rate of nephrolithiasis.[44] To prevent nephrolithiasis, patients should try to drink large amounts of water (1.5 liters) throughout the day.[47]

Similar to all protease inhibitors, serious complications may result from concurrent administration of indinavir and agents that interact with the hepatic cytochrome P450 3A4 system such as rifampin, rifabutin, terfenadine, astemizole, cisapride, trizoloam, and midazolam.[47] The bioavailability of indinavir is reduced by food, so it should be taken one hour before or two hours after meals (or with a low fat, low protein meal if this enhances compliance). The usual dose of indinavir is 800 mgs. every 8 hours (not three times per day) to maintain constant blood levels.[47] The development of viral resistance is a significant barrier to the long term use of protease inhibitors. To minimize resistance, protease inhibitors should not be used as monotherapy and they should always be started and continued at optimal therapeutic doses.[47] Although unanswered questions about long term benefits remain, combination antiretroviral drug therapies are an important development in long-term treatment of HIV infection that should be closely watched by those caring for HIV infected persons.

PNEUMOCYSTIS CARINII PROPHYLAXIS

Pneumocystis carinii pneumonia (PCP) is the most common opportunistic infection in persons with AIDS. Prophylaxis with the preferred agent trimethoprim/sulfamethoxazole (TMP/SMX), one double strength tablet daily, not only prevents this common infection but also prolongs life.[45] PCP prophylaxis is recommended for adults and adolescents with a CD4+ count below 200 mm/l[3], a prior episode of PCP, oral candidiasis, or unexplained fever lasting 2 weeks or more.[26] PCP prophylaxis should continue for the life of the woman. Because of the importance of TMP/SMX, attempts should be made to continue it even in those who develop the fever and skin rash typical of an allergic reaction, although care must be taken to ensure that life threatening allergic symptoms do not develop. Women can be referred to an allergist for desensitization, or the dose may be reduced to a daily single strength tablet or a double strength tablet 3 times a week.[45]

For those unable to tolerate TMP/SMX, Dapsone 50 mg p.o. b.i.d. or 100 mg daily, Dapsone 50 mg p.o. daily with pyrimethamine 50 mg p.o./week and leucovorin 25 mg p.o./week, or aerosolized pentamidine 300 mg monthly, (administered by the Respirgard II nebulizer) are alternatives.[45] When TMP/SMX is used, it is necessary to monitor for anemia, neutropenia, and agranulocytosis.[26] Severe dermatologic reactions such as Stevens-Johnson syndrome, erythema nodosum, erythema multiforme, or epidermal necrolysis are possible with TMX/SMX and Dapsone.[26] With the exception of pentamidine, agents recommended for prevention of PCP will also prevent toxoplasmosis encephalitis in persons who have a positive titer.[45]

MYCOBACTERIUM AVIUM COMPLEX

Mycobacterium avium complex (MAC) typically occurs at CD4+ counts below $75/mm^3$.[45] Drugs for disseminated MAC prophylaxis are generally started at CD4+ counts of 75 for those with previous infections and at CD4+ counts of 50 for those without previous infections. Rifabutin 300 mg daily of 150 mg b.i.d. (taken with food), or Clarithromycin 500 mg b.i.d. or azithromycin 500 mg 3 times a week are currently approved for this use.[45]

CYTOMEGALOVIRUS INFECTION

Cytomegalovirus (CMV) retinitis is a common opportunistic infection associated with visual loss in HIV infected persons. Ganciclovir may be used to delay onset of CMV disease in those with CD4+ counts < 50.[45] Those with visual symptoms suggestive of CMV retinitis should be referred to an opthamologist for confirmation of diagnosis.[5]

REFERENCES

1. Mann, J. (1994). In A. Kurth (Ed.), *Until the cure: Caring for women with HIV* (p. xi). New Haven, CT: Yale University Press.
2. Stine, G. J. (1996). *Acquired immune deficiency syndrome: Biological, medical, social, and legal issues* (2nd ed.). Englewood Cliffs, NJ: Prentice Hall.
3. Hollander, H., & Katz, M. H. (1996). HIV infection. In L. M. Tierney, S. J. McPhee, and M. A. Papadakis (Eds.), *Current medical diagnosis & treatment.* Stamford, CT: Appleton & Lange.
4. Kurth, A. (1994). An overview of women and HIV disease. In A. Kurth (Ed.), *Until the cure: Caring for women with HIV.* New Haven, CT: Yale University Press.
5. Centers for Disease Control and Prevention. (1995). USPHS/IDSA guidelines for the prevention of opportunistic infections in persons infected with human immunodeficiency virus: A summary. *MMWR, 44*(RR–8), 1–34.
6. Stanley, S. K., et al. (1996). Effect of immunization with a common recall antigen on viral expression in patients infected with human immunodeficiency virus type 1. *The New England Journal of Medicine, 334*(19), 1222–1229.
7. Centers for Disease Control and Prevention. (1991a, September). *HIV/AIDS Surveillance Report.*
8. Update: AIDS among women—United States, 1994. *MMWR, 44,* 81–84.
9. Cotton, P. (1994). U. S. sticks head in sand on AIDS prevention. *JAMA, 272,* 756–757.
10. Bush, R. W. (1995). HIV infection. In D. P. Lemcke, J. Pattison, L. A. Marshall, & D. S. Cowley (Eds.), *Primary care of women.* Norwalk, CT: Appleton & Lange.
11. Simpson, M. (1996). HIV/AIDS update 1996. *Practical Reviews in Internal Medicine, 31*(1A & B), 1–2.
12. Lackritz, E. M., et al. (1995). Estimated risk of transmission of the human immunodeficiency virus by screened blood in the United States. *The New England Journal of Medicine, 333,* 1721–1725.
13. HIV data raise concern on oral-sex risk. (1996). *Science 272,* 142.
14. Brown, R. K. (1987, Nov.). AIDS: A perspective. *Am. Chem. Prod. Rev.,* 44–47.
15. Connor, E. M., et al. (1994). Reduction of maternal-infant transmission of human immunodeficiency virus with zidovudine treatment. *The New England Journal of Medicine, 331,* 1173–1180.
16. Centers for Disease Control and Prevention. (1994). Recommendations of the U. S. Public Health Service Task Force on the use of zidovudine to reduce perinatal transmission of human immunodeficiency virus. *MMWR, 43,* 1–15.
17. Minkoff, H., & Willoughby, A. (1995). Pediatric HIV disease, zidovudine in pregnancy, and unblinding heelstick surveys: Reframing the debate on prenatal HIV testing. *JAMA, 274*(14), 1165–1168.
18. FDA approves 2 tests dealing with AIDS virus. (1996, June 4). *Virginian Pilot,* p. C1.
19. Fang, C. T., et al. (1989). HIV testing and patient counseling. *Patient Care, 23,* 19–44.
20. MacKenzie, W. R., et al. (1992). Multiple false positive serologic tests for HIV, HTLV-1 and hepatitis C following influenza vaccination, 1991. *JAMA, 268,* 1015–1017.
21. Testing for antibodies to HIV-2 in the United States. *MMWR, 41,* 1–9.

22. Murphy, R. L. (1996). Advances in antiretroviral therapy and viral load monitoring. *Special Report: XI International Conference on AIDS.* Cedar Knolls, NJ: World Medical Communication Organization.

23. Rojansky, N., & Schenker, J. G. (1995). Ethical aspects of assisted reproduction in AIDS patients. *Journal of Assisted Reproduction in AIDS Patients, 12*(8), 537–541.

24. Faden, R. R., et al. (1991). HIV infection, pregnant women, and newborns: A policy proposal for information and testing. In R. R. Faden, G. Geller, & M. Powers (Eds.), *AIDS, women, and the next generation.* New York: Oxford University Press.

25. Scripps Howard News Service. (1996, May 15). Home HIV-test kit gets FDA approval. *Richmond Times-Dispatch,* p. A9.

26. Early HIV Infection Guideline Panel. (1994). Managing early HIV infection. *American Family Physician, 49*(4), 801–814.

27. Young, M. (1994). In A. Kurth (Ed.), *Until the cure: Caring for women with HIV.* New Haven, CT: Yale University Press.

28. Laraque, F., et al. (1996). Effect of comprehensive intervention program on survival of patients with human immunodeficiency virus infection. *Archives of Internal Medicine, 156,* 169–175.

29. Mellors, J. W., et al. (1996). Prognosis in HIV infection predicted by the quantity of virus in plasma. *Science, 272,* 1167–1170.

30. Ho, D. (1996). Viral counts count in HIV infection. *Science, 272,* 1124–1125.

31. Palefsky, J. (1995). Human papillomavirus-associated malignancies in HIV-positive men and women. *Current Opinion in Oncology, 7,* 437–441.

32. *Infectious Disease Alert.* (1995, March). Abstract No. 16. 91.

33. Singer, M., & Sax, P. (1996). Routine immunization in HIV: Helpful or harmful? *AIDS Clinical Care, 8*(2), 11–15.

34. Kroon, F. P., van Dissel, J. T., de Jong, J. C. & van Furth, R. (1994). Antibody response to influenza, tetanus, and pneumococcal vaccines in HIV-seropositive individuals in relation to the number of CD4+ lymphocytes. *AIDS, 8*(4), 469–476.

35. Wright, T., Jr., et al. (1994). Cervical intraepithelial neoplasia in women infected with human immunodeficiency virus: Prevalence, risk factors, and validity of Papanicolaou smears. New York Cervical Disease Study. *Obstetrics and Gynecology, 84,* 591–597.

36. Hutchison, M., & Shannon, M. (1994). In A. Kurth (Ed.), *Until the cure: Caring for women with HIV.* New Haven, CT: Yale University Press.

37. Kreiss, J., et al. (1992). Efficacy of nonoxyl-9 contraceptive sponge use in preventing heterosexual acquisition of HIV in Nairobi prostitutes. *JAMA, 268*(4), 477–482.

38. Hatcher, R. A., et al. (1994). Intrauterine devices. In R. A. Hatcher, et al. (Eds.), *Contraceptive Technology* (16th ed.). New York: Irvington Publishers Inc.

39. Cohen, J. (1996). Monkey study promps high level public health response. *Science, 272,* 805.

40. Monkey study prompts high-level public health response. (1996, May 10). *Science 272,* 805.

41. Fischbach, F. (1996). *A manual of laboratory and diagnostic tests.* (5th ed.). New York: Lippincott.

42. Godofsky E. W., et al. (1996). Primary care of the HIV-infected patient. In J. Noble (Ed.) *Textbook of primary care medicine,* (2nd ed.). Baltimore: Mosby.

43. Centers for Disease Control. (1993). Revised classification system for HIV infection and expanded surveillance case definition for AIDS among adolescents and adults. *MMWR, 41,* 1–19.

43a. Readers are advised to consult the Consensus Statement on antiretroviral therapy for HIV infection in 1997 from the International AIDS Society—USA Panel reported in the June 25, 1997 issue of the *Journal of the American Medical Association* (Volume 277, No. 24, pages 1962–1969). This is an updated panel recommendation based on new clinical and basic science study results, as well as expert opinions. Earlier initiation of more aggressive therapy is supported. Use of plasma viral load as a crucial element of clinical management for evaluating prognosis and therapy effectiveness is discussed. Therapy regimens will continue to evolve as more new data emerges.

44. Carpenter, C. C. J., Fischl, M. A., Hammer, S. M., Hirsch, M. S., et al. (1996). Antiretroviral therapy for HIV infection in 1996: Recommendations of an international panel. *JAMA, 276,* 146–154.

45. Cotton, D. J., Horowita, H. W., & Powderly, W. G. (1996, March). Keeping HIV patients healthy. *Contemporary OB/GYN,* 89–114.

46. Murphy, R. L. (1996). Changing the paradigm: Emerging strategies in the treatment of HIV disease. *Special report: XI International Conference on AIDS.* Cedar Knolls, NJ: World Medical Communication Organization.

47. Deeks, S. G., Smith, M., Holodniy, M., & Kahn, J. O. (1997). HIV-1 protease inhibitors: A review for clinicians. *JAMA, 277,* 145–153.

CHAPTER 13

COMMON GYNECOLOGIC PELVIC DISORDERS

Donna E. Forrest

*F*rustrating for all health care providers is the client who presents with chronic pelvic pain, because in most cases, a specific etiology cannot be determined and care is very difficult.

Highlights

- Endometriosis
- Adenomyosis
- Pelvic Inflammatory Disease
- Adnexal Masses: Functional, Inflammatory, Metaplastic, and Neoplastic Ovarian Tumors
- Dyspareunia
- Nonmalignant Disorders of the Vulva
- Leiomyomas
- Pelvic Relaxation Syndrome
- Chronic Pelvic Pain
- Cervicitis
- Bartholin's Gland Duct Cysts and Bartholinitis
- Cervical Polyps
- Cancers: Cervical, Uterine, Ovarian, and Vulvar
- Diethylstilbestrol Exposure

► INTRODUCTION

The health care provider needs to be familiar with the diagnosis, management, and follow-up of the more common gynecologic pelvic disorders encountered in practice, and must recognize when a client should be referred for further evaluation and management. With the changing health care climate where managed care and cost effectiveness are major influences, the practitioner must use sound clinical judgment in gathering pertinent history and physical examination data, selecting cost efficient diagnostic tests, and implementing medical, nursing, and adjunct therapies. The population of older women is growing rapidly in the United States and quality of life issues are most important and should always be in the forefront of the provider's mind. The provider should be more knowledgeable about those disorders more common in older women, such as genital prolapse, and the importance of screening for gynecologic cancers.

The evaluation of any complaint of pelvic symptoms begins with a thorough client history that includes the following:

- The onset and description of the pelvic symptoms and any associated abdominal symptoms.
- A description of the character, nature, location, and timing of any pain.
- A detailed menstrual and sexual history.
- A history of previous related surgeries or hospitalizations.
- An obstetric history.
- A thorough psychosocial history.

Frustrating for all health care providers, including the gynecologist, is the client who presents with chronic pelvic pain, because in most cases, a specific etiology cannot be determined and care is very difficult. For these clients, a thorough history, physical examination, and diagnostic evaluation are critical. Consultation with a gynecologist is necessary, and in most situations, consultation with a psychotherapist is beneficial.

Although a goal is to prevent unnecessary medical and surgical intervention, the fact remains that surgical intervention often is necessary to evaluate and manage pelvic disorders. The health care provider has a responsibility to the client to review alternative therapies, to evaluate the severity of her symptoms and their impact on her lifestyle, to discuss the potential benefits of proposed surgery, and to assist the client in seeking consultation with a qualified, reputable surgeon.

In many clinical situations, the provider will find him or herself in a unique position to thoroughly evaluate a chronic or ongoing problem. In the evaluation, management, and follow-up of nonmalignant vulvar disorders, especially vulvodynia, the provider's most important role is to obtain a complete history, to offer emotional support, and to evaluate therapy.

This section cannot completely address all pelvic/gynecologic disorders. It is intended to be a clinical guideline for current evaluation and management of common, more frequently seen problems. The provider should always be aware of when to seek consultation and/or when to refer. It goes without saying that the provider should stay abreast of ever changing developments in gynecologic health care as she or he continues to gain clinical experience.

ENDOMETRIOSIS[1a]

Endometriosis is the presence of endometrial tissue, composed of glands and stroma, at sites outside the endometrial cavity. The most common sites include the ovary, anterior and posterior cul-de-sac, uterosacral ligaments, posterior uterus and posterior broad ligaments;[1] however, endometrial implants can occur in any organ. Endometrial tissue responds cyclically to estrogen by swelling and producing local inflammation. The severity of pain appears unrelated to the extent of the disease so that clients with small implants of endometriosis may experience the severest pain. The condition commonly occurs in women in their twenties and thirties; it does not occur before menarche or after menopause. Endometriosis is a major cause of infertility.[1,2]

EPIDEMIOLOGY

A specific etiology for endometriosis is unknown, although several theories have been put forth. Many researchers conclude that endometriosis develops as a result of a combination of factors. Modern explanations of the pathogenesis of endometriosis include the following:

- Sampson's theory of retrograde menstruation describes menstrual or endometrial tissue flowing backward through the fallopian tubes and into the abdominal cavity.
- Lymphatic spread theory describes endometrial tissue spreading to distant sites through the lymphatic system.
- Coelomic metaplasia theory describes the metaplasia of peritoneal mesothelial cells into endometrial epithelium under some unidentified influence, such as repeated inflammation.
- Müllerian cell theory suggests that remnant müllerian cells remain in the pelvic tissue during the development of the müllerian system and later, perhaps under the influence of estrogen, develop into endometrial glands and stroma.
- Recent research suggests that immunologic and genetic factors may have a role in the initiation and progression of endometriosis.[1,2]

Endometriosis is found equally among caucasian and African Americans, but has a slightly higher prevalence in Asian women.[3] It occurs across all socioeconomic groups. It is more likely to occur and progress in women with early menarche, longer cycle length (greater than 30 days), years of menstruation uninterrupted by pregnancy, and positive family history. It is found more frequently in women who have used an IUD for 2 or more years and less commonly in oral contraceptive users. The risk of endometriosis decreases as parity increases.[3]

Endometriosis occurs in 5–10 percent of women of reproductive age.[1-3] The actual prevalence is difficult to determine because of the difficulty of diagnosis. Two to 4 million women in the United States report symptoms of endometriosis, and it is the primary cause of infertility in 30–40 percent of infertile women.[4] About 4 in 1000 women aged 15–64 are hospitalized annually with endometriosis.[2,3]

SUBJECTIVE DATA

Dysmenorrhea, pelvic pain, dyspareunia, intermenstrual bleeding, and infertility are the most commonly reported symptoms. The client may also complain of perimenstrual back pain, dyschezia, abdominal pain, urinary symptoms, and/or rectal pain or bleeding. Reported symptoms may be cyclical or constant.[1,2,5,6] Because of the strong association of sexual abuse with reported pelvic pain, all clients should be screened for the possibility of past or present physical or emotional abuse.[1]

OBJECTIVE DATA

Physical Examination

The genitalia and reproductive tract may appear completely normal if lesions are small and few. In more advanced disease, a speculum exam reveals cervical displacement of 1 cm or more to the left or right of the midline; bimanual exam tenderness and nodularity of the uterosacral ligaments and posterior cul-de-sac are detected. Clinical examination during menstruation may better enable the practitioner to identify tender nodules of endometriosis.[6] Also seen are fixed retroversion of the uterus and adnexal masses that vary in size, shape, and consistency and may be asymmetric, fixed, cystic, or indurated.[1,2,5]

If the history and physical exam suggest endometriosis, especially in the presence of pain and history of infertility, refer the client for gynecologic consultation.

Diagnostic Tests and Methods

CA-125 Assay. Serum cancer antigen is a cell surface antigen found on certain cells derived from embryonic coelomic epithelium.[5] These tissues include the epithelium of the endocervix, endometrium, fallopian tubes, mesothelial lining of the peritoneum, pleura, pericardium and fetal müllerian ducts. Used mainly as a marker of response to treatment of ovarian epithelial neoplasms, CA-125 levels are elevated in clients with endometriosis. Levels correlate with severity of the disease and response to treatment.[2] Because elevation of Ca-125 levels occurs in several gynecologic and nongynecologic conditions, it is not useful in the diagnosis of endometriosis. Current research suggests that CA-125 may be useful in differentiating endometriotic ovarian cysts from functional ovarian cysts, predicting severe disease in clients with suspected endometriosis, and monitoring response to therapy.[5] One promising clinical application for diagnostic use of CA-125 is predicting which clients with endometriosis are more likely to conceive following surgical treatment. This remains under investigation.[5]

The test procedure is to obtain a blood sample and send it to a laboratory with experience in analyzing CA-125.

Tell the client that the assay is very expensive and will most likely not be covered by her insurance. Providing such information will facilitate decisions related to the necessity of the assay. In addition, consult with the physician ordering the assay to ascertain his specific plans for utilizing the test. Assist and educate the client as to its role in her overall plan of care. This assay should be used only in consultation with a physician.

Diagnostic Laparoscopy. Diagnostic evaluation through direct visualization of endometriosis. Procedure of choice for definitive diagnosis of endometriosis.[1] Positive findings include "powder burns" (flat, brownish discolorations of the peritoneal surface due to adherent endometrial

implants), "mulberry spots" (raised, bluish implants of endometriosis), and adhesions.[2] Gynecologic surgeons employ the American Fertility Society's classification system as a means of communicating and documenting their findings. This assists the practitioner in understanding the severity and extent of disease, as well as choice of treatment in an individual client.[2,6]

The test procedure requires that the client be referred to a gynecologic surgeon with special training and experience using the laparoscope. Laparoscopy is usually performed as an outpatient procedure, with the client under general anesthesia. The laparoscope is inserted through a small incision just above the navel after the abdomen has been inflated with carbon dioxide gas. The surgeon is able to visualize the pelvic organs directly.

Explain the procedure to the client in detail. In addition, discuss the risks. Complications, which are rare, may include bleeding or injuries to nearby organs. Anesthesia complications are rare. Discuss the recovery process. Usually, the client may return home the same day. Common discomforts are neck and shoulder pain from the gas used to inflate the abdomen, mild nausea, pelvic discomfort at the incision site, mild cramps, and mild vaginal discharge. Instruct the client that she may shower or bathe in 24 hours and return to normal activities as soon as she feels able. Review the signs and symptoms of infection and explain how to keep the incision site clean and dry. To reinforce this discussion, provide the client with written information about the procedure and recovery.

DIFFERENTIAL MEDICAL DIAGNOSES

Chronic pelvic inflammatory disease (PID), recurrent acute salpingitis, hemorrhagic corpus luteum benign or malignant ovarian neoplasm, ectopic pregnancy, adenomyosis.[6]

PLAN

Management of the client with endometriosis should be determined by one or more of the following factors:

- Severity of symptoms.
- Desire for fertility.
- Degree of disease.
- Client's therapeutic goals.

Medical management should be considered initially in clients with mild to moderate symptoms who wish to maintain their fertility potential. Conservative surgery is indicated when medical therapy fails, but fertility is still desired. Medical therapy and conservative surgery can be combined. Those clients who have severe endometriosis with debilitating pain should be counseled to complete their childbearing. Total abdominal hysterectomy and bilateral salpingo-oophorectomy represent definitive treatment of endometriosis.

There are a variety of therapeutic options. Assist the client in determining her desired therapeutic outcome. Monitor side effects of medications and response to therapy. Provide education and emotional support.

Psychosocial Interventions

Encourage active participation by the client and her significant other in treatment decisions. Assess the client's lifestyle and future plans, such as childbearing, marriage, education, and career. Discuss the impact of the disease on her life and which treatment option will best suit her lifestyle. Assess the client for depression, which can be initiated or worsened by chronic pain. Many of the hormonal therapies have side effects such as depression, loss of libido, and/or mood swings. Inform the client of these potential side effects. Sexual therapy should be offered if the disease has significantly impacted sexual relations.[7]

Medication

The goal of medication is to interrupt cycles of stimulation and bleeding. The various medications are comparable in their ability to provide relief from dysmenorrhea, dyspareunia, and pelvic pain associated with endometriosis. They are not of proven value in improving fertility.[2] The basis for medical management of endometriosis is to create states of pseudopregnancy, pseudomenopause or chronic anovulation.

None of the following medications is indicated over any of the others.[2] Recent studies demonstrated that Danazol and Naferelin were equally effective in relieving dysmenorrhea, dyspareunia, and pelvic pain in clients with endometriosis.[8] GnRH analogs continue to be ex-

pensive. All have side effects that may be poorly tolerated by the client. Recurrence of endometriosis is common after completion of medical therapies at rates from 20–50 percent.[9]

Progestogens
- *Indications.* Suppression of the cyclic hormonal response of endometrial implants, and resorption of tissue. Indicated in mild to moderate endometriosis. Progestogens are better tolerated than combination oral contraceptives, having fewer estrogen related side effects and are less costly than Danazol and GnRH analogs, making them a better initial choice of therapy.
- *Administration.* Medroxyprogesterone acetate (Depo-Provera), 100 mg I.M. every 2 weeks for 4 doses, followed by 200 mg I.M. monthly for 4 additional months, or MPA (Provera), 30 mg p.o. every day for 6 months.
- *Side Effects and Adverse Reactions.* Breakthrough bleeding, depression, delayed fertility, headache, dizziness, weight gain, nausea, fluid retention, breast tenderness.
- *Contraindications.* Traditionally, contraindications for progestin-only medication have been the same as those for combination oral contraceptives (see Contraindications for Oral Contraceptives, Chapter 8). Progestin-only is also contraindicated for women with undiagnosed abnormal genital bleeding. A relative contraindication is for women who desire fertility immediately after completing therapy.
- *Anticipated Outcomes on Evaluation.* The relief of pain and the resorption of endometrial implants.
- *Client Teaching and Counseling.* Review with the client the instructions for selected regimens, their possible side effects, and the danger signs (see Combined Oral Contraceptives).[1,2]

Danazol
- *Indications.* Mild to moderate endometriosis in women who desire fertility but not in the immediate future. Traditionally the medication of choice, Danazol is now considered no more effective than the other available therapies.[2]
- *Administration.* An 800 mg dose is given as two 200 mg tablets p.o. twice daily for 6 to 9 months beginning on the fifth day of menses. Newer studies suggest lower doses may be

effective for less severe disease. Therefore, an option is to start at 400 mg daily given as one 200 mg tablet twice daily. If no relief occurs within 6 weeks, increase the dosage.

- *Side Effects and Adverse Reactions.* Possible weight gain, fluid retention, fatigue, decreased breast size, acne, oily skin, hirsutism, atrophic vaginitis, hot flushes, muscle cramps, emotional lability, voice changes, spotting, and/or decreased HDL cholesterol.
- *Contraindications.* A history of liver disease, hypertension, hyperlipidemia, congestive heart failure, or renal impairment, or pregnancy.
- *Anticipated Outcomes on Evaluation.* The relief of pain, resorption of endometrial implants, return to fertility, and pregnancy if desired; few side effects.
- *Client Teaching and Counseling.* Tell the client about the high cost of Danazol therapy and the length of treatment. Review the side effects, and stress the importance of following the administration regimen correctly. Barrier contraception is recommended during therapy with Danazol and during the first menstrual cycle after treatment.

Combined Oral Contraceptives (OCs)

- *Indications.* Suppression of the cyclic hormonal response of endometrial implants and eventual resorption of the tissue. Oral contraceptives (OCs) induce a "pseudopregnancy." The combination of estrogen and progestin causes endometrial tissue to become decidual and necrotic, leading to resorption. The therapy may be useful for mild to moderate endometriosis associated with clinical symptoms of pain or infertility.
- *Administration.* One pill p.o. daily, of a low dose, monophasic, taken continuously for 6 to 12 months. If breakthrough bleeding occurs, add conjugated estrogen, 1.25 mg per day for 1 week. Alternatively, the OC dosage may be increased to two tablets or more per day if breakthrough bleeding occurs.
- *Side Effects and Adverse Reactions.* Possible weight gain, breast pain and tenderness, abdominal bloating, nausea, increased appetite, breast secretion, superficial vein varicosities, and increased risk of deep vein thrombosis.

TABLE 13–1. GnRH-ANALOGUE THERAPY FOR ENDOMETRIOSIS

Drug	Dosage	Route
Lupron (Leuprolide acetate)	3.75 mg. IM q 28–33 days	IM sustained release depot
Synarel (Nafarelin acetate)	400–800 mcg. (1–2 sprays b.i.d.)	Nasal spray
Zoladex (Goserelin acetate)	3.36 mg. implant abdomen q 28 days	Subcutaneous sustained release

Source: References 2, 9, 10. Adapted from Winkel, Postgraduate Medicine, 1994.

- *Contraindication.* In addition to those usually listed for OCs, other contraindications are known or suspected pregnancy, history of thromboembolic disease, and liver disease (see Chapter 9 and the current *Physicians' Desk Reference*).
- *Anticipated Outcomes on Evaluation.* The relief of pain, resorption of endometrial implants, return to fertility, and pregnancy if desired.
- *Client Teaching and Counseling.* Review with the client the instructions for taking OCs continuously, stressing the importance of not skipping pills. Warn her of the possible side effects and danger signs, for example, abdominal pain, severe headache, and leg pain. Explain the purpose of the therapy.[1]

Gonadotropin-Releasing Hormone Analogues (GnRH-a)

- *Indications.* Suppression of endometriosis by creating a pseudomenopause.
- *Administration.* See Table 13–1, GnRH-Analogue Therapy for Endometriosis.[10]
- *Side Effects and Adverse Reactions.* Hot flushes, vaginal dryness, mood swings, depression, weight gain, decreased breast size, decreased libido, fatigue, and insomnia. In addition, GnRH-a may interfere with calcium and bone metabolism.
- *Contradictions.* Known or suspected pregnancy, hypersensitivity to GnRH, undiagnosed abnormal vaginal bleeding, breastfeeding.
- *Anticipated Outcomes on Evaluation.* The relief of pain, resorption of endometrial implants, return to fertility, and pregnancy if desired; few side effects.

- *Client Teaching and Counseling.* Provide instructions for the drug's proper administration, and tell the client that the therapy is costly and will continue for 6 months. Review the side effects. A calcium supplement may be necessary: 1000–1500 mg q.d. Barrier contraception is recommended during therapy and for the first menstrual cycle.[2]

Surgical Interventions

Conservative Surgery. One surgical option is to destroy and dissect endometriomas and endometriotic implants while preserving reproductive function. The procedure may be performed by a specially trained gynecologic surgeon directly after laparoscopic diagnosis, while the client is still under anesthesia. Conservative methods include fulguration, excision and resection, and/or laser vaporization. Conservative surgery is indicated for adnexal masses, symptoms unresponsive to medical therapy, severe endometriosis in a client who desires future fertility, and concomitant conditions such as leiomyomas or adhesions. Some women have been treated with presacral neurectomy and uterosacral ligament ablation for pain if they wish to preserve fertility.[11]

The possible adverse effects are few: a reaction to anesthesia, incisional infection, bleeding, or injury to nearby organs. The anticipated outcomes on evaluation are the relief of pain and return to fertility.

When explaining the procedure to the client, point out that conservative surgery is not curative. Review the postoperative instructions, addressing the client's return to activity, resumption of sexual relations, and signs and symptoms of infection.

Definitive Surgery. Abdominal hysterectomy, with or without bilateral salpingo-oophorectomy, is indicated for clients with severe disease. These are women who either have completed their families or have no desire for future fertility, or whose disease has not responded to medical therapy or conservative surgery, or whose disease involves other organs, such as the bowel or bladder. Referral is made to a board certified gynecologic surgeon. The procedure, performed under general anesthesia, involves removal of the uterus through an abdominal incision. The ovaries and fallopian tubes may or may not be removed; among the determining factors are the age of the client and the extent of endometriosis.

There are possible adverse effects, namely, bleeding, infection, wound infection, or damage to nearby organs. The anticipated outcome on evaluation is complete resolution of the disease, including relief of dysmenorrhea, dyspareunia, dyschezia, and/or dysuria.[5]

Prepare the client by giving her a thorough explanation of the anatomy and physiology, surgical procedure, and risks and benefits. Reassure her that femininity remains unchanged by the surgery. Hormonal replacement therapy may be needed. Full recovery usually takes about 6 weeks. Review the postoperative instructions, including topics such as the return of activity, the expectation that vaginal bleeding will change to clear discharge, signs of infection, return to sexual activity, and dietary needs.

FOLLOW-UP AND REFERRAL

Endometriosis tends to recur at a rate of 5 to 20 percent per year when definitive surgery is not performed.[2] Appropriate follow-up intervals depend on the choice of therapy and the client's needs. An initial evaluation, made after 6 months of therapy, should report the incidence, severity, and cyclicity of pain, dysmenorrhea, and dyspareunia. Review the side effects and their impact on the client. Inquire about the issue of pregnancy and provide emotional support and encouragement.

ADENOMYOSIS

Adenomyosis occurs when the endometrial glands and stroma within the endometrium grow into the myometrium. The cause is believed to be disruption of the uterine wall during pregnancy, labor, and postpartum involution. It occurs in 5–70 percent of multiparous women in their 30s, 40s, and 50s, but it does not occur in postmenopausal women.[11,12] It is difficult to diagnose and is most commonly identified posthysterectomy.

SUBJECTIVE DATA

Clients are often asymptomatic but may report severe dysmenorrhea and abnormal uterine bleeding.[12]

OBJECTIVE DATA

Physical Examination

Bimanual examination of the genitalia and reproductive organs may reveal a large, symmetrical uterus.[12]

Diagnostic Tests and Methods

Endometrial Biopsy. Diagnostic evaluation of any abnormal bleeding; requires referral to a gynecologist. Explain the procedure to the client. The test is performed with a biopsy curette, or a suction catheter, or other instrument passed through the cervical canal into the uterus. The client will be an outpatient, and, generally, no anesthesia will be necessary. Obtain the client's menstrual history. Explain that she may return to normal activities immediately.

Ultrasound. Diagnostic evaluation to rule out leiomyomas or other tumors. Transvaginal ultrasound in the hands of a skilled technician can identify the irregular hyperechogenic outlines in the myometrium.[13] The procedure should be performed by a trained professional with expertise in obstetrics and gynecology. The method, performed abdominally or vaginally, employs sound waves to provide detailed images of the pelvic structures.

Explain the procedure to the client and assure her that it is painless. In the *abdominal method,* the lower abdomen is covered with a water soluble gel, a probe is moved slowly across the abdomen, and images are projected onto a video display monitor. In the *vaginal method,* a probe with ultrasound gel is inserted into the vagina. The client remains awake. In order to obtain clearer images, a client may be required to undergo a 24-hour bowel preparation (i.e., laxative, enema, clear liquid diet).

Magnetic Resonance Imaging (MRI). An accurate non surgical diagnostic test for adenomyosis, it is indicated preoperatively in symptomatic women who wish to maintain their fertility and who are considering conservative surgery for removal of the adenomyomas. Its usefulness is limited by its cost, and its clinical necessity is best determined by the gynecologic surgeon.[14]

DIFFERENTIAL MEDICAL DIAGNOSES

Leiomyomas, endometriosis.

PLAN

Psychosocial Interventions

Discuss the condition with the client and determine the impact of her symptoms. The severity of symptoms will determine therapy, which should be described to the client. Reassure her if necessary.

Medication

No specific medications are given for treatment or resolution of adenomyosis. If symptoms are mild, however, palliative management with nonsteroidal anti-inflammatory drugs (NSAIDs) is helpful (see Chronic Pelvic Pain). Most recently, GnRH-analogues have proven to effectively reduce symptoms[12] (see Table 13–1).

Surgical Interventions

Hysterectomy is indicated for severe, symptomatic adenomyosis, including severe dysmenorrhea, menorrhagia, or enlarged uterus. (For procedure, see Definitive Surgery, under Endometriosis.)[11]

FOLLOW-UP AND REFERRAL

If medical therapy is the initial treatment of choice, then the client is evaluated in 3 to 6 months. Increasing pain or bleeding may necessitate referral to a gynecologic surgeon for possible hysterectomy. Sarcoma can be a complication.

PELVIC INFLAMMATORY DISEASE (PID)

In pelvic inflammatory disease (PID), infection and inflammation develop in the pelvic organs—namely the uterus, fallopian tubes, and ovaries. Most often, the condition is localized in the tubes;

however, it may occur anywhere in the upper genital tract. Complications include ectopic pregnancy, pelvic abscess, infertility, recurrent or chronic episodes of the disease, chronic abdominal pain, pelvic adhesions, premature hysterectomy, and depression. Because of the seriousness of the potential complications of PID, accurate diagnosis is imperative.[15]

EPIDEMIOLOGY

Neisseria gonorrhoeae and Chlamydia trachomatis are the two major causative organisms; however, PID is usually a mixed infection caused by both aerobic and anaerobic organisms. Recent studies demonstrate the presence of bacterial vaginosis in cases of confirmed PID. It is suggested that BV may facilitate the ascent of gonorrhoeae or C. trachomatis.[16,17,18] Adolescents and young women are three times more likely to develop the infection. Nonwhite women are higher risk. Other risk factors include multiple sex partners (greater than two in the previous 30–60 days considered a major risk factor); a history of PID or sexually transmitted disease (STD); intercourse with a partner who has untreated urethritis; recent intrauterine device (IUD) insertion; and nulliparity. Additional risk factors include douching, cigarette smoking, and sex with menses.[18] PID is more likely to occur during the first 5 days of the menstrual cycle.

The causative organisms are transmitted through sexual intercourse with an infected partner. One million new episodes are diagnosed annually in the United States, requiring 300,000 hospitalizations.[16]

SUBJECTIVE DATA

Because of a wide variety of presenting signs and symptoms in clients with PID, clinical diagnosis can be difficult. A client may report one or all of the following symptoms: pain and tenderness of the lower abdomen, fever, chills, nausea, vomiting, increased vaginal discharge, symptoms of urinary tract infection (UTI), and irregular bleeding. The severity symptoms may be mild or severe. Recently, experts agree that many cases of PID have gone undiagnosed. The term "silent PID" refers to such clients.[19] Abdominal pain is usually present. If Fitz-Hugh-Curtis syndrome is present, upper abdominal pain will occur due to liver capsule inflammation. A client may also report experiencing any of the aforementioned risk factors. Consultation with a gynecologist is advised due to the seriousness of this condition. The Centers for Disease Control's (CDC) minimum criteria for empiric treatment of PID include all of the following:

- Lower abdominal tenderness.
- Adnexal tenderness.
- Cervical motion tenderness.[20]

OBJECTIVE DATA

Physical Examination

Determination of vital signs may show an elevated body temperature. The abdomen may be distended with rebound tenderness, guarding and hypoactive bowel sounds. The genital and reproductive exam is positive for cervical motion tenderness (pain upon movement of the cervix), purulent cervical discharge, uterine tenderness, adnexal pain and fullness, or the presence of an adnexal mass. CDC routine criteria for diagnosing PID include the following:

- Oral temperature > 38.3° C.
- Abnormal cervical or vaginal discharge.
- Elevated erythrocyte sedimentation rate.
- Laboratory documentation of cervical infection with N. gonorrhoeae or C. trachomatis.[20]

Diagnostic Tests and Methods

Complete Blood Count (CBC) and Erythrocyte Sedimentation Rate (ESR). Diagnostic evaluation to detect any inflammatory process. The white blood cell (WBC) count is above 10,000 and erythrocyte sedimentation rate (ESR) is elevated in PID. A venous blood sample is obtained according to laboratory protocol after the procedure and its purpose have been explained to the client.

Pregnancy Test. Diagnostic evaluation (urine or blood level of human chorionic gonadotropin [hCG]) for unsuspected intrauterine pregnancy or suspected ectopic pregnancy. A urine pregnancy test is done, or if ectopic pregnancy is suspected, blood quantitative radioimmunoassay of hCG.

Explain the procedure to the client and determine her last normal menstrual period. If the client is pregnant, ultrasound should be ordered to rule out ectopic pregnancy or missed abortion. Whether a treatment regimen is contraindicated during pregnancy must be determined.

C-Reactive Protein. Diagnostic evaluation to detect inflammation; the test is highly sensitive for detecting PID. A venous blood sample is obtained according to laboratory protocol after the procedure and its purpose have been explained to the client.

Vaginal Smears/Cervical Cultures. Diagnostic evaluation to detect the causative organisms of infection. Wet mount with saline can detect bacterial vaginosis or trichomoniasis. Cervical tests will detect *N. gonorrhoeae* and *C. trachomatis*. PID is usually due to polymicrobial, ascending infection (see Chapter 11 for the test procedures).

Ultrasound. Diagnostic evaluation to identify fluid in the cul-de-sac, distended tubes, masses or a pelvic abscess, and to rule out intrauterine and ectopic pregnancy (see Adenomyosis for a description of the test procedure).

Laparoscopy. Diagnostic evaluation to identify fluid in the cul-de-sac, distended tubes, masses or pelvic abscess.[14] Indicated if the diagnosis is uncertain, if the client fails to respond to therapy, or if symptoms recur soon after adequate therapy.[16] It may also reveal tubal occlusion and tubal factor infertility associated with PID.[21]

DIFFERENTIAL MEDICAL DIAGNOSES

Ectopic pregnancy, appendicitis, ruptured corpus luteum cyst, septic abortion, torsion of an adnexal mass, pyelonephritis, degeneration of a leiomyoma, endometriosis, endometritis, ulcerative colitis.[16]

PLAN

Psychosocial Interventions

Thoroughly discuss with the client the disease, its implications, and risk factors. If possible, the client's partner should participate. Review the serious sequelae that may occur if the disease is not treated or if the client does not comply with treatment. Refer partners for evaluation and treatment of any sexually transmitted disease that is diagnosed. Discuss the use of condoms, especially if the client has multiple sexual partners. Provide emotional support. Stress the importance of follow-up care and evaluation.[21,22]

Medication

The client is treated on an ambulatory basis or admitted for hospitalization, and the medication regimen is determined by this choice.

Ambulatory Medication. This regimen is followed when a client with PID can be managed safely on an outpatient basis at home and is based upon the 1993 CDC guidelines.[20] *Newer guidelines anticipated by early 1998 should be reviewed for any changes.*

Regimen A:

Cefoxitin 2 grams plus probenecid, 1 gram orally in a single dose, concurrently

or

Ceftriaxone 250 mg I.M.

plus

Doxycycline 100 mg orally b.i.d. for 14 days.

Regimen B:

Ofloxacin 400 mg. orally b.i.d. for 14 days

plus

either Clindamycin 450 mg. orally q.i.d.

or

Metronidiazole 500 mg. orally b.i.d. for 14 days.

Stress to the client the importance of taking the complete medication prescription to help prevent complications; review all medication related instructions. *Convey the importance of returning for a follow-up evaluation 48 to 72 hours after the medication is started and again in 7 to 10 days.* Instruct the client that if symptoms worsen during outpatient treatment, she must call the health professional immediately because hospitalization will probably be necessary. Oflaxacin should not be used in adolescents. It is deposited in the cartilage of young women. It is also contraindicated if pregnancy is diagnosed or suspected.

The following factors will contribute to the decision to refer a client to a physician for hospital admission and care.

- Questionable diagnosis.
- Possible ectopic pregnancy or appendicitis.
- Suspected pelvic abscess.
- Severe illness (nausea, vomiting, fever greater or equal to 30.0° C, severe pain, dehydration).
- Pregnancy.
- Inability to tolerate or follow an outpatient regiment.
- Lack of response to outpatient treatment after 48 to 72 hours.
- Prepubertal client or adolescent.
- Inability of the client to seek follow-up evaluation in 48 to 72 hours.
- Presence of HIV infection.[20]

In-Hospital Medication
Regimen A:[20]

Cefoxitin 2 grams I.V. every 6 hours

or

Cefotetan 2 grams I.V. every 12 hours

plus

Doxycycline 100 mg I.V. or orally every 12 hours.

(This regimen should be continued for at least 48 hours after the client demonstrates substantial clinical improvement, after which doxycycline 100 mg orally b.i.d. should be continued for a total of 14 days.)

Regimen B:[20]

Clindamycin 900 mg I.V. every 8 hours

plus

Gentamicin loading dose I.V. or I.M. (2 mg/kg of body weight), followed by a maintenance dose of (1.5 mg/kg) every 8 hours.

(This regimen should be continued for at least 48 hours after the client demonstrates substantial clinical improvement, then followed with doxycycline 100 mg orally b.i.d. or clindamycin 450 mg orally q.i.d. to complete a total of 14 days of therapy.)

Explain to the client the necessity of hospitalization. Make sure that the client understands all discharge instructions and the need to return for evaluation after discharge.

Side Effects and Adverse Reactions
- *Cefoxitan, Cefotetan, Ceftriaxone (Cephalosporins).* Few; most serious is pseudomembranous colitis.
- *Doxycycline.* Gastrointestinal (GI) distress, fetal teeth discoloration if given during pregnancy, photosensitivity.
- *Gentamicin.* Nephrotoxicity, ototoxicity.
- *Clindamycin.* Diarrhea, pseudomembranous enterocolitis.

Contraindications
- *Cefoxitin, Cefotetan, Ceftriaxone (Cephalosporins).* Known allergy to cephalosporins.
- *Doxycycline.* Pregnancy or hypersensivity to tetracyclines.
- *Gentamicin.* Hypersensitivity to aminoglycosides.
- *Clindamycin.* Hypersensitivity to aminoglycosides.

Anticipated outcomes on evaluation are the resolution of symptoms of pelvic inflammatory disease and the prevention of serous sequelae.

Surgical Interventions

Conservative Surgery. This involves removal of grossly abnormal tissue only. The uterus and at least one ovary are preserved to allow for possible later in vitro fertilization. Conservative surgery is indicated when the hospitalized client with acute PID or a pelvic mass does not respond after 72 hours of appropriate therapy or when a ruptured tubovarian abscess is suspected.[16,23] An experienced gynecologic surgeon should perform the surgery. Preservation of reproductive capability.

The potential adverse effects are few: the usual potential anesthesia complications and the risk of excessive bleeding or postoperative infection. The anticipated outcomes on evaluation are the resolution of pelvic infection with the preservation of reproductive capability.

Explain the procedure to the client and inform her that it will be carried out using general anesthesia. Informed consent forms must be signed. Provide postoperative instructions regarding the return to activity, signs and symptoms of infection, and return to sexual activity.[16,23]

Colpotomy. Colpotomy permits drainage of abscesses located in Douglas' cul-de-sac. It is performed transvaginally by an experienced gynecologic surgeon using direct ultrasonographic or radiographic guidance.

The possible adverse effects include the usual anesthesia complications and the risk of excessive bleeding or postoperative complications. The anticipated outcomes on evaluation are the resolution of the pelvic abscess and the prevention of chronic pelvic infection and chronic pelvic pain.

Explain the procedure to the client and inform her that it will be carried out using general anesthesia. Informed consent forms must be signed. Provide postoperative instructions regarding the return to activity, signs and symptoms of infection, and return to sexual activity.[23]

Unilateral/Bilateral Salpingo-Oophorectomy. One or both fallopian tubes and ovaries are removed, depending on the location and extent of a tubo-ovarian abscess. Indications for the surgery are extensive involvement of the tubes or ovaries by the inflammatory process, including scarring and abscess.

The possible adverse effects are few; the most severe is loss of reproductive capability with a bilateral salpingo-oophorectomy. The usual potential for anesthesia complications and postoperative infection also exists. The anticipated outcomes on evaluation are the complete resolution of infection and symptoms and the prevention of chronic pelvic pain and chronic pelvic infections.

Discuss with the client the impact of the surgery on her reproductive function. Provide emotional support, and refer the client for counseling if her reproductive function is lost.

FOLLOW-UP AND REFERRAL

Any woman with PID who is being treated on an outpatient basis should be seen again in 48–72 hours after therapy is initiated. Marked improvement in symptoms should be exhibited by then. If no or less improvement than is deemed acceptable has occurred, the client must be referred to a specialist or hospitalized. If ambulatory care is progressing acceptably, reevaluate again in 1 week. If tenderness or any mass persists, refer immediately to a specialist. Advise immediate treatment for any sexual partner who has not received evaluation and treatment.

ADNEXAL MASSES (OVARIAN TUMORS)

The word *adnexal* pertains to the appendages of the uterus: the ovaries, fallopian tubes, and ligaments of the uterus. The adnexal masses discussed here are ovarian tumors.

CATEGORIES OF OVARIAN TUMORS

Four major categories of ovarian tumors have been identified: functional, inflammatory, metaplastic, and neoplastic.[24]

Functional Ovarian Tumors

- *Follicular cyst* is caused by the failure of the ovarian follicle to rupture in the course of follicular development and ovulation. The cyst formed is lined by one or more layers of granulosa cells, is thin walled, and usually 5–6 cm. or less in diameter.[25]
- *Lutein cyst* forms when the corpus luteum becomes cystic or hemorrhagic and fails to degenerate after 14 days.
- *Theca-lutein cyst* development is accompanied by abnormally high blood levels of human chorionic gonadotropin (hCG). The cyst occurs in clients with hydatiform mole, or with choriocarcinoma, or who are undergoing ovulation induction with gonadotropins or clomiphene.
- *Polycystic ovary syndrome* (Stein-Leventhal syndrome) is characterized by the presence of multiple inactive follicle cysts within the ovary. The syndrome is associated with androgen excess and chronic anovulation.[24]

Inflammatory Ovarian Tumors

- *Salpingo-oophoritis* is inflammation of a fallopian tube and ovary. (Salpingo-oophorectomy is discussed in the preceding section on Pelvic Inflammatory disease.)

- *Tubo-ovarian abscess* is the tumor that develops in direct response to acute or chronic salpingo-oophoritis.

Metaplastic Ovarian Tumor

Endometriosis is the presence of endometrial tissue, composed of glands and stroma, at sites outside the endometrial cavity (see Endometriosis, page 315).

Neoplastic Ovarian Tumors

- *Epithelial tumors,* the most common type of tumor, include serous tumors, mucinous tumors, and endometrioid tumors. Epithelial tumors are derived from mesothelial cells lining the peritoneal cavity. They have the highest potential for malignancy.
- *Stromal tumors* are derived from the sex cords and specialized stroma of developing gonads. They include fibromas, granulosa-theca cell tumors, and Sertoli-Leydig cell tumors.
- *Germ cell tumor* is a benign cystic teratoma or dermoid cyst, derived from early embryonic germ cells. It may contain calcifications; the majority are benign.[25,26]

EPIDEMIOLOGY

The etiology of adnexal masses is unclear. It is known, however, that the risk of ovarian malignancy increases significantly with age. Benign cystic teratoma (germ cell tumor) is the most common *ovarian* neoplasm; epithelial neoplasm is the most common *malignant* neoplasm. Stromal neoplasms, on the other hand, are uncommon. During the reproductive years, 70 percent of all noninflammatory tumors are functional; 20 percent are neoplastic; 10 percent are endometriomas. After menopause, half of all ovarian tumors are malignant; however, before puberty, only 10 percent are malignant.[24–27]

SUBJECTIVE DATA

- *Functional Ovarian Tumors.* A follicular cyst is usually asymptomatic but can cause minor lower abdominal discomfort, pelvic pain, or dyspareunia. A lutein cyst causes pain or signs of peritoneal irritation, delayed menses. The rupture of a cyst may produce acute lower abdominal pain and tenderness.
- *Inflammatory Ovarian Tumors.* A client may report symptoms that are similar to those of pelvic inflammatory disease (discussed earlier in this chapter): pain and tenderness of the lower abdomen, fever, chills, nausea, vomiting, increased vaginal discharge, irregular bleeding patterns.
- *Metaplastic Ovarian Tumors.* A client may report symptoms that are similar to those of endometriosis (discussed earlier in this chapter): dysmenorrhea, dyspareunia, perimenstrual back pain, infertility, dyschezia, abdominal pain, irregular bleeding.
- *Neoplastic Ovarian Tumors.* Subjective data are nonspecific. The client may be asymptomatic unless torsion or rupture occurs. Abdominal enlargement or bloating may occur, usually later in the tumor development. With rupture or torsion of the tumor, mild, intermittent pelvic pain or severe pelvic pain may be reported, as well as peritoneal irritation.

OBJECTIVE DATA

Physical Examination

Physical examination, including bimanual gynecologic exam, is done to detect the following.

- Functional ovarian tumor is 4 to 8 cm, noted on bimanual examination. It regresses following the next menstrual cycle, is mobile, unilateral, and may be tender.
- Inflammatory ovarian tumor (see Pelvic Inflammatory Disease).
- Metaplastic ovarian tumor (see Endometriosis).
- Neoplastic ovarian tumor may be palpable by an abdominal exam; percussion may reveal dullness anteriorly with tympany toward the flanks as a result of bowel displacement. Bimanual exam is usually positive for an adnexal mass.

The bimanual pelvic examination should include a rectovaginal examination. Palpate the uterus, adnexae and cervix; repeat with rectovaginal exam. Rectovaginal exam allows detection of lateral and posterior masses. Uterus should be midline. Cervical motion tenderness indicates inflammation versus cyst or tumor. Benign masses are generally cystic, smooth, less than 8 cm. and mobile.[25]

Diagnostic Tests and Methods

In some situations, it may be appropriate to begin an initial diagnostic workup, the description of which follows; however, *if the client is premenarcheal or postmenopausal and a palpable adnexal mass is discovered, then refer her immediately to a gynecologist for further evaluation and management.*[27]

Pregnancy Test. Diagnostic evaluation to rule out pregnancy (uterine enlargement may be mistaken for an adnexal mass) and ectopic pregnancy. A urine or blood sample is obtained and measured for quantitative human chorionic gonadotropin (hCG).

Explain the procedure to the client and determine her last normal menstrual period.

Pelvic Ultrasound. Diagnostic evaluation to confirm the suspicion of an adnexal mass, especially in an obese client or uncooperative client. With ultrasound it is possible to exclude intrauterine or extrauterine pregnancy, distinguish between solid or cystic masses, or identify calcification associated with a teratoma. Ultrasound is also helpful in measuring the mass.[14] Explain to the client the various aspects of the ultrasound procedure (see Adenomyosis).

Intravenous Pyelogram. Diagnostic evaluation to determine the size of the mass by evaluating ureteral displacement and distortion of the bladder contour. Kidney position and function and ureteral obstruction are also evaluated, especially before diagnostic laparoscopy.

It is necessary to evacuate the bowels using bisacodyl suppositories the night before the pyelogram. On the day of the test, a contrast dye is infused intravenously, and x-rays are taken at set intervals. The dye is traced through the glomeruli, renal tubules, renal pelvis, ureters, and bladder.

Before beginning, ask the client if she is allergic to iodine. Explain the procedure. Tell client to expect flushing of her face, a feeling of warmth, and a salty taste.

Laparotomy/Laparoscopy. Diagnostic evaluation of any adnexal mass larger than 8 cm. or any adnexal mass in a premenarcheal or postmenopausal client. (See Endometriosis for the test procedure.) These procedures make it possible to distinguish between a uterine myoma, hydrosalpinx, and an ovarian tumor. Functional cysts and benign neoplasms, however, cannot be differentiated.[27]

DIFFERENTIAL MEDICAL DIAGNOSES

Pelvic inflammatory disease (PID), endometriosis, uterine leiomyomas, nongynecologic masses (e.g., neoplastic colon mass), pelvic kidney, pregnancy. If rupture or torsion of the mass occurs and pain is present, rule out ectopic pregnancy and acute PID.

PLAN

If the mass is smaller than 8 cm, unilateral, mobile, smooth, and suspected to be a functional ovarian cyst, then wait and reevaluate the mass after the next menstrual period. If the mass does not meet these criteria or if it does not regress after the next menstrual period, then the health care provider must consult with a gynecologist and refer the client for further evaluation and management. In addition, refer all premenarcheal and postmenopausal clients with a palpable adnexal mass immediately.

Psychosocial Interventions

The client will experience major fear and anxiety with any suspicion of malignancy. Therefore, it is particularly important to provide support, encouragement, and reassurance during any period of observation or evaluation. Stress the importance of compliance with diagnostic testing requirements and of keeping scheduled appointments. Make certain that she understands that early diagnosis and treatment provide the best prognosis.

Medication

An oral contraceptive (OC) is indicated in the management of a functional ovarian cyst. By suppressing gonadotropin levels, the OC increases resolution of the cyst.[6]

Details about OC administration, side effects, and contraindications are discussed in Chapter 9. The anticipated outcome on evaluation is complete resolution of the adnexal mass (functional cyst).

Provide the client with detailed instructions about taking OCs; stress the importance of not skipping any pills. Warn her that pregnancy is possible during the first cycle of pills, and urge use of a barrier method of contraception; and emphasize the importance of returning for the follow-up visit immediately after the first menstrual cycle.

Surgical Interventions

Surgical exploration and management of adnexal masses is headed by a board-certified surgeon specializing in gynecology. The surgical procedure varies with the type of ovarian tumor, but the health care provider should be aware of the possibilities in order to provide counseling and support to the client. Definitive treatment will depend on the client's age and her desire for reproductive capability.

Epithelial ovarian neoplasms may be managed with unilateral salpingo-oophorectomy, including appendectomy. If the client is older than 40, then total abdominal hysterectomy and bilateral salpingo-oophorectomy may be indicated. On the other hand, if the client is young and nulliparous and the ovarian neoplasm is unilocular with no excrescences within the cyst, an ovarian cystectomy that preserves the ovary is performed.[27]

Stromal neoplasma may be managed with unilateral salpingo-oophorectomy and appendectomy. If the client is older than 40, then a total abdominal hysterectomy and bilateral salpingo-oophorectomy may be indicated.[27]

Germ cell tumors are managed with an ovarian cystectomy if future childbearing is desired. If it is not desired, then total abdominal hysterectomy and bilateral salpingo-oophorectomy are indicated.[27]

FOLLOW-UP AND REFERRAL

If a functional ovarian mass is suspected, follow-up examination should occur in 4 to 6 weeks, or immediately after the next menstrual period. If the mass persists, referral to a gynecologist for further evaluation and management is necessary.

Dyspareunia

Dyspareunia or painful coitus, occurs either on intromission (entry) or on deep penetration of the penis. Pain results from any number of factors, such as infection, inflammation, anatomic abnormalities, pelvic pathology, atrophy or failure of lubrication, or psychological conflicts.[28]

EPIDEMIOLOGY

Introital pain may be caused by vulvovaginitis (recurrent and chronic), vulvar vestibulitis (see section on Vulvar Disorders), urethritis/urethral syndrome, interstitial cystitis, cervicitis, lack of lubrication, or levator spasm. Pain on deep penetration may be caused by uterine retroversion, pelvic relaxation, endometriosis, adhesions, adenomyosis, pelvic congestion syndrome or lack of vaginal expansion due to insufficient arousal.[28]

Risk factors for dyspareunia include menopause, psychological factors (including restrictive sexual attitudes), relationship difficulties and history of sexual trauma, history of sexually transmitted disease (STD), recurrent infection (candidiasis), and poor hygiene.[29]

The incidence is unclear because clients tend not to report dyspareunia to health professionals. Of the reported cases, the most common cause is vulvo/vaginitis infection. In one 1990 study of 313 women, over 60 percent had experienced dyspareunia at some point in their lives. The average age of women in this study was the early 30s.[30]

SUBJECTIVE DATA

A client's history is crucial to determining the etiology of dyspareunia. One problem, such as vaginitis, may cause another problem, such as anxiety or fear about pain with intercourse, thus altering sexual response, decreasing lubrication, and increasing pain.[28] Pain may occur on intromission or on deep penetration; it may occur after long pain free intervals or with first intercourse. Vaginal discharge or irritation may be present. There may be a history of chronic pelvic pain.

Relationship difficulties may be reported. The client may have been unable to use tampons previously or may have had difficult pelvic exams. Menopausal symptoms may be beginning.[28,31]

OBJECTIVE DATA

Physical Examination

Examination includes the genitalia and reproductive tract. The vulvar/vaginal mucosa may reveal irritation, inflammation, lesions, discharge, atrophy, hymenal remnants, Bartholin's cyst/abscess or vestibulitis (focal irritation/inflammation of the vestibular glands, see section on Vulvar Disorders). Involuntary contractions of the perineal muscles (vaginismus) may occur during a speculum or digital exam, prohibiting examination. In this situation, proceed carefully and allow the client control during pelvic exam. Bimanual exam may reveal uterine prolapse, pelvic mass, nodularity of endometriosis, cervical motion tenderness of pelvic inflammatory disease, or loss of pelvic support (cystocele, rectocele).[31]

Diagnostic Tests and Methods

Select tests discriminately as indicated by the findings of the history and physical examination. Review previous test results in order to avoid unnecessary and repetitive diagnostic testing.

Complete Blood Count (CBC) and Erythrocyte Sedimentation Rate (ESR). Diagnostic evaluation to detect any inflammatory process (see Pelvic Inflammatory Disease for test procedure). The white blood cell (WBC) count and ESR are elevated in pelvic inflammatory disease.

Urinalysis. Diagnostic evaluation to identify any urinary tract conditions that might be a source of pain. White blood cells, bacteria, or red blood cells in the urine may indicate chronic or recurrent urinary tract infection (UTI).

To enhance test accuracy, explain to the client how to obtain a clean catch urine sample in a sterile container.

Pregnancy Test (Urine or Blood Level of beta hCG). Diagnostic evaluation to detect unsuspected intrauterine pregnancy or suspected ectopic pregnancy (see Pelvic Inflammatory Disease for procedure).

Vaginal Smears/Cervical Cultures. Diagnostic evaluation to determine whether infection is present. Wet mount with normal saline is used to detect bacterial vaginosis or trichomoniasis; potassium hydroxide (IOH) preparation is used to detect candidiasis; and cervical tests can detect *N. gonorrhoeae* and *C. trachomatis* (see Chapter 11 for the test procedures).

Ultrasound. Diagnostic evaluation using ultrasound may be useful if a bimanual exam is difficult, as with clients who are obese or unable to tolerate the exam. The procedure is most useful in diagnosing acute pelvic pain conditions, such as ruptured ovarian cyst, adnexal masses, or ectopic pregnancy; it should not be performed in clients with a clearly negative pelvic examination (see Adenomyosis for the test procedure).[14]

Diagnostic Laparoscopy. Diagnostic evaluation is accomplished by directly visualizing the pelvic pathology that may be causing dyspareunia (see Endometriosis for the test procedure).

DIFFERENTIAL MEDICAL DIAGNOSES

Vulvovaginitis, atrophic vulvovaginitis, vulvar vestibulitis, urethritis, urethral syndrome, cystitis, cervicitis, muscle spasm, hymenal strands, scar tissue, episiotomy, vaginismus, pelvic relaxation, uterine prolapse, PID, endometriosis, adenomyosis, adhesions, pelvic masses, Bartholin's cyst. Consider possible contributing psychological factors, such as previous sexual trauma, conflictual relationships, stress, or restrictive sexual attitudes. Also consider inappropriate sexual technique, including lack of foreplay, or low estrogen in the oral contraceptive.[28,29,31]

PLAN

The management of dyspareunia depends on the symptoms and etiology.

Psychosocial Interventions

Refer the client for psychotherapy if her history reveals the possibility of a psychological component to the dyspareunia or if significant discord is present in the couple's relationship. Select a therapist with special training in sexual problems. Discuss fully with the client the findings of the physical examination and diagnostic testing, and include her partner whenever possible. Address and discuss all client fears, concerns, and anxieties. Sexual attitudes may need to be addressed.[28,29,31]

Medication

The etiology of the dyspareunia determines whether medication is prescribed.

- *Vaginitis/Sexually Transmitted Disease.* See Chapter 11.
- *Atrophic Vaginitis.*
  - Hormonal replacement therapy (HRT) (see Chapter 15). HRT may be the treatment of choice for perimenopausal or menopausal women with atrophic vaginitis. Estrogen revitalizes atrophic tissues.
  - A water based lubricant (K-Y jelly or Replens) available over the counter or vegetable oil or shortening is indicated for poor vaginal lubrication. The lubricant may be administered prior to or during intercourse to improve vaginal lubrication and enhance foreplay. Do not use latex contraceptives with vegetable based lubricants.[28] Vaginal suppositories may be inserted three times weekly, without regard to intercourse. Instructing the client in the use of a lubricant is important.
  - Anticipated outcomes on evaluation are improved vaginal lubrication and relief of dyspareunia secondary to vaginal dryness. Local allergic irritation is a potential adverse reaction, however, that would contraindicate lubricant use.
- *Pelvic Inflammatory Disease, Endometriosis, Adnexal Mass, and Leiomyoma.* Medications for these causes of dyspareunia are described in other sections of this chapter.

Surgical Intervention

The cause of dyspareunia determines whether surgery is necessary. In cases where surgical evaluation is needed, referral should be made to a board-certified gynecologist. For descriptions of specific surgical interventions, see the appropriate section in this chapter: Endometriosis, Pelvic Inflammatory Disease, Adnexal Masses, Leiomyomas, or Pelvic Relaxation Syndrome. Other surgical interventions would depend on the specific cause, such as marsupialization of a Bartholin's cyst.

Progressive Dilation and Muscle Awareness Exercise

This procedure, with appropriate counseling, is indicated for clients with vaginismus, an anatomically narrow introitus, hymenal remnants or scar tissue, or psychogenic factors.

Begin by reviewing the anatomy and physiology of the sexual organs and sexual response, stressing the normalcy of vulvar tissue. Using a mirror, have the client become familiar with her genitalia. Instruct the client on how to perform Kegel's exercises to increase her awareness of the muscles involved. Involve the client's partner whenever possible.

For progressive dilation, the client or health care provider inserts progressively larger objects into the vagina, beginning with a single finger, then a medium Pederson's speculum, two fingers, and finally a medium Graves' speculum. Measured vaginal dilators are also available. Allow the client to stop at any point that pain occurs. Have her bear down on insertion and use water-soluble lubricant to alleviate discomfort.

Progressive digital dilation may be practiced by the client at home in order to familiarize her with her tissue, sensitization, and muscular control.[31] The partner is gradually included in a "bridge-over" manner.[28] Cross-wise intercourse position is suggested to provide the woman with more control over entry and penetration depth.[28]

FOLLOW-UP AND REFERRAL

As with the entire evaluation and plan of care for clients with dyspareunia, follow-up will depend on the cause and the therapy selected. Follow-up evaluation is important, especially when dyspareunia is multifactorial. Stress to the client the importance of keeping follow-up appointments. Reassess the client frequently to determine whether psychological intervention is needed.

NONMALIGNANT DISORDERS OF THE VULVA

The client who presents with vulvar symptoms requires conscientious evaluation by the primary care provider/nurse practitioner. Knowledge of the more common nonmalignant disorders of the vulva is important in deciding whether to initiate careful medical therapy or to refer for further evaluation and management, including biopsy and/or surgical therapy. In this section, the more common vulvar conditions are presented. The clinician will most often find her or himself confronted with the client complaining of vulvar burning, itching, and pain. For this reason, vulvar pain/discomfort/irritation will be the primary focus. It is helpful for the practitioner to have available for reference a comprehensive textbook of genital dermatology and/or vulvar disorders such as Lynch and Edwards' *Genital Dermatology* (Churchill Livingstone, Inc., 1994).

Most clients who present with either recurrent pain, itching, burning, or irritation are frustrated, desperate for relief, and have previously used a variety of antifungal and/or steroid creams. Many will have already seen a variety of health care providers without resolution of symptoms. Psychological distress, depression, and anxiety may be present as either a risk factor for the current problem or as a result of the chronic discomfort.

The practitioner is in a unique position to obtain a comprehensive, detailed history related to the problem, to identify possible causative factors, to initiate and evaluate therapy, and to provide emotional support. The more experience the clinician gains, the better she or he is able to evaluate and manage vulvar problems. It is most critical to recognize the need for referral to a knowledgeable specialist when necessary.

VULVODYNIA

The International Society for the Study of Vulvar Disease (ISSVD) defines *vulvodynia* as chronic vulvar discomfort characterized by the client's complaint of burning, stinging, irritation, and/or rawness.[32] Vulvodynia, "burning vulva syndrome" or "vulvar pain syndrome," all terms for the same entity, includes subsets of vulvar disorders. These disorders include the following:[33]

- *Vulvar vestibulitis.* Episodic or continuous stinging or burning accompanied by hyperemia and point tenderness of the vestibule and characterized by dyspareunia.
- *Cyclic vulvovaginitis.* Cyclic burning and/or itching centered around the menses and/or just after intercourse.
- *Vulvar dermatoses.* Characterized by noncyclic pruritus, scratching, dyspareunia and changes in the epithelium, such as in Lichen sclerosus.
- *Vulvar dysesthesia.* Also known as idiopathic vulvodynia, this condition consists of constant severe burning pain of the vulva in the absence of visible pathology.

EPIDEMIOLOGY

The vulvar pain syndrome was recognized and described as early as 1889 by Dr. A. J. C. Skene in his *Treastise on the Diseases of Women.* Many theories exist as to the etiology for vulvodynia. It has been proposed that the syndrome may be precipitated by candidiasis infection, Human Papilloma virus (HPV), oxalate crystalluria (elevated urinary levels of calcium oxalate), contact dermatitis, allergic response, sexual dysfunction, emotional stress, or hormonal reactions. None of these hypotheses has been proven in the literature and, therefore, a specific etiology is unknown.[32] Most experts agree that the etiology is most likely multifactorial with both pathophysiologic and psychological components.

The exact incidence of vulvodynia is unknown due to the difficulty in making a diagnosis, but current estimates are about 15 percent in the general gynecologic population.[34]

The client with vulvodynia will usually be white and nulliparous with a wide age range. Mean age range is about 32. The client will most likely have been to multiple clinicians for the condition. Research has shown a high incidence of sexual abuse. The client may have a history of allergies to various substances and/or repeated candida infections. There may be a higher incidence of depression. Sexual history reveals a limited number of sexual partners with a low incidence of history of STDs.

SUBJECTIVE DATA

Pain is often acute in onset and is described as "burning, stinging, irritation, or rawness." Onset may be associated with recent episodes of vaginitis. Dyspareunia interferes with sexual function. Pain can be mild to severe, interfering with normal activities, and may be continuous or episodic.

Previous treatments have provided either partial or no relief. Clients will report having seen many different clinicians and will generally express frustration and anxiety.

The practitioner can play a major role in evaluating vulvodynia by obtaining a complete history. A comprehensive history for evaluating vulvodynia should include *all* of the following information:

- Description of the client's major symptoms including the duration, quality, cyclicity, and any aggravating or soothing factors.
- Any precipitating event that correlated to the onset of symptoms.
- Complete sexual history including any current or past history of abuse, number of partners, past history of STDs.
- Hygiene habits including use of powders, types of soaps, overbathing, scrubbing, or excessive douching, feminine hygiene sprays.
- Use of personal products such as dryer sheets, types of tampons, chronic use of minipads, contraceptive gels, foams, or suppositories, use of condoms, lubricants.
- Exercise habits such as biking, aerobics, swimming, running, and intensity and frequency of workout sessions.
- Relationship of vulvar symptoms to urinary symptoms.
- History of musculoskeletal trauma, back pain or congenital skeletal abnormalities.
- List of previous treatments used, results of any previous cultures or other diagnostic testing and response to treatments.
- Psychological history including history of traumatic events, marital stress, history of chronic pain, history of depression or anxiety disorder.[33,34,35]

OBJECTIVE DATA

Physical Examination

Initial inspection of the vulva generally fails to reveal any obvious abnormality. Closer exam may reveal hyperemia, fine linear excoriations, and/or thickening, atrophy, or whitening of the epithelium in vulvar dermatoses. The vulvar vestibulum consists of the area between the labia minora and hymenal ring, extending upward to the frenulum of the clitoris and posteriorly from the fourchette to the vaginal introitus. The vulvar vestibulum includes the urethra, Skene's glands, Bartholin's glands, and the minor vestibular glands.

Micropapillations are a normal finding of the vulva. Frequently misdiagnosed as HPV, these normal anatomical findings are 1–3 mm symmetric papillae that may cover most of the mucosal surface of the labia minora. HPV is more patchy.[36,37]

The Q-tip test is essential for assessing vulvar vestibulitis. This test consists of touching the vestibulum lightly with a moist cotton tipped swab. Ask the client to respond by rating the amount of discomfort she experiences in each area of the vestibulum. Clients with vulvar vestibulities will experience marked pain at 5 and 7 o'clock between the introitus and posterior fourchette.[34,36,37]

Although vaginal exam is usually unremarkable in the client with vulvodynia, obtain vaginal secretions for saline and KOH wet mounts. Inspect the vagina for any abnormalities. Use of a Pederson speculum is essential to minimize discomfort.[34]

Screen for any musculoskeletal abnormalities including asymmetry of the spine.

Diagnostic Tests and Methods

Wet Mount and Cultures. Indicated for making a differential diagnosis and for determining any precipitating etiology(ies). Examination of vaginal secretions should include a pH determination and careful microscopic exam for the presence of hyphae, clue cells, trichomonas, lactobacilli, an/or WBCs. The practitioner whenever possible should examine his or her own microscopic slides. Cultures for candidiasis, chlamydia, gonorrhea may be necessary.

- *Vulvar Biopsy.* Indicated for any diagnostically questionable areas or for any suspicion of vulvar intraepithelial neoplasia. Not usually helpful in differentiating vestibulitis. The following are suggested indications for vulvar biopsy.
- Lesions surrounded by either thickened skin or color changes.
- Slightly raised, red or pigmented lesions.
- Lesions presumed to be genital warts, which do not respond to therapy.
- Chronic dermatoses that do not respond to therapy.
- Any suspicious lesion for neoplasia.[37,38]

Unless the practitioner has specialized training in vulvar biopsy, referral should be made to either a dermatologist or gynecologist for the procedure. Under local anesthesia, the lesion is biopsied using one of these techniques. The shave biopsy is indicated when the lesion is superficial. A #15 scalpel blade is used to remove a sample of skin well under the lesion but not through to fat. Sutures are not used. Monsel's solution or silver nitrate is used for controlling any bleeding. The punch biopsy is indicated for an ulcer or inflammatory skin condition and removes epidermis, dermis, and some fat. A special punch instrument such as a Keyes biopsy is used, and simple sutures may be necessary.

The biopsy procedure is rapid and can be performed in the office setting, and adverse reactions are rare. Explain to the client the purpose of the procedure and how it will be done. Reassure the client that adverse effects are unusual; rarely, women experience scarring, infection, soreness, bleeding, or bruising. Tissue is sent to a pathologist for diagnostic evaluation.[36]

Acetowhitening/Colposcopy of the Vulva. Application of acetic acid solution with the use of a specialized microscopic instrument called a colposcope is indicated for directed biopsy and when there is a history of HPV. Colposcopy should also be performed of the vagina and cervix if HPV is found on the vulva. Typically, acetowhite lesions that are diffuse and flat are a result of chronic trauma or inflammation, and those that are raised are typical of HPV infection.

Unless the practitioner has specialized formal training, certification, and experience with colposcopy, referral should be made to the gynecologist for colposcopy.

Caution should be exercised in the diagnosis of HPV. Current research and expert opinion demonstrate that HPV has been overdiagnosed as a cause for vulvodynia and, therefore, unnecessary treatment has occurred, many times worsening the client's symptoms.[37,38]

DIFFERENTIAL MEDICAL DIAGNOSES

Lichen sclerosus, Lichen planus, contact dermatitis, candidiasis, postmenopausal atrophic vaginitis, Human Papillomavirus infection, Herpes simplex infection, pudendal neuralgia, overuse of topical steroids, erythema multiform, Bechet's disease, Reiter's disease, pellagra.[34,37,38]

PLAN

Psychosocial Interventions

The most important intervention in caring for the client with vulvodynia is to validate her feelings. Acknowledge that her pain is real and encourage her to become a partner in her care. Explain the multifactorial nature of the problem and that currently, there is no single known etiology for the condition. Suggest the use of a journal for recording exacerbations and possible related events, foods eaten, stressful events, etc. Request that she not self-medicate and initially, that she be seen for office evaluation during acute episodes. This allows the practitioner to differentiate obvious causes that may confuse the clinical picture such as trichomoniasis, candidiasis, bacterial vaginosis, or urinary tract infection. Include the partner on all discussions to increase his understanding.[39]

Refer for psychiatric evaluation and intervention if there are clinical signs of depression and/or history of sexual abuse. Refer couples for sexual therapy when indicated.[39]

Medication[32,33,36,39,40]

Before initiating medical therapy stop all current topical vulvar medications and review proper vulvar hygiene including the use of cotton underwear, avoidance of constrictive clothing that promotes heat and chafing (pantyhose, jeans, spandex shorts, tights, etc.), use of unscented, hypoallergenic products, avoidance of chemical allergens (hygiene sprays, perfumes, talcum pow-

TABLE 13–2. EVALUATION AND MANAGEMENT OF COMMON VULVAR DISORDERS

	Diagnostic Characteristics			
Disorder	*Subjective*	*Objective*	*Medical Therapy*	*Adjunct Therapy*
Vulvar Vestibulitis	Burning, stinging, irritation, rawness, entry dyspareunia	Positive Q-tip test, hyperemia	Topical anesthetics: *2–5 percent topical Xylocaine, *alpha-Interferon injections, °Calcium citrate*	Low-oxalate diet; *vestibulectomy
Dysesthetic Vulvodynia	Constant, severe, burning pain, most common in perimenopausal or menopausal women	Little or no objective findings	Tricyclic antidepressants: *Amitriptyline, 10–75 mg daily*	Psychological counseling; physical therapy; biofeedback
Cyclic Vulvovaginitis	Itching, burning, cyclic, often related to the menses; irritation following coitus; frequent use of antibiotics	Erythema, edema of the vulva with fissure, pustules, scaling, +KOH or yeast culture	Suppressive therapy; 4–6 mos. oral antifungals (*ketodonazole, Diflucan*)	
Lichen Sclerosus	Pruritus, pain, or may be asymptomatic	Well demarcated white plaques of thin, fragile skin; agglutination of labia in advanced cases; may be sores, excoriations	Medium-potent topical steroid, ointment based (*triamcinolone*) or *testosterone cream,* b.i.d. for 4–6 mos., then, twice/wk	Monitor annually for malignancy; biopsy as indicated; sleep aides when itching or pain is severe

*Requires physician consultation/referral.
°Theoretical.
Source: References 32–40.

ders, shaving lotions), and use of vaginal lubricants that are nonirritating. Most experts in the area of vulvar disorders recommend the use of Crisco or other vegetable oil as a lubricant for use during intercourse (Do not use latex contraceptives with vegetable lubricants). One may also use Vitamin E skin oil.[32,33]

Because medical therapy is specific to each subset of vulvodynia, Table 13–2 will be utilized to provide descriptions of the various diagnostic subsets, identifying characteristics and commonly accepted medical therapies. Table 13–3 describes common differential diagnoses, characteristics and treatment.

Medium-Potency Topical Steroids (examples: triamcinolone acetonide 0.1 percent, hydrocortisone valerate 0.2 percent, betamethasone valerate 0.1 percent)
- *Indications.* Prompt improvement of symptoms of Lichen sclerosus; fast becoming first-line treatment.[34,35]
- *Administration.* Apply thinly b.i.d. to t.i.d.; prescribe in small tubes without refills, ointment base more soothing.

- *Side-Effects and Adverse Reactions.* Super-infection, atrophy, steroid dermatitis, and striae.
- *Contraindications.* Allergy to topical steroids.
- *Anticipated Outcomes on Evaluation.* Relief of symptoms and improvement of the disease process. Noticeable healing of skin, lessening of white lesions.
- *Client Teaching and Counseling.* Instruct to apply creams sparingly, in a thin layer and only as often as prescribed. Review the risks of atrophy of the normal skin with overuse.

High-Potency Topical Steroid, Clobetasol Propionate (Temovate)
- *Indications.* Improvement of symptoms quickly in more severe, long standing cases of Lichen sclerosus.
- *Administration.* Apply thinly once or twice daily to affected area for about 12 weeks.
- *Side Effects, Adverse Reactions, Contraindications, Anticipated Outcomes on Evaluation, Client Teaching.* The same as associated with medium-potency topical steroids.

TABLE 13–3. COMMON NONMALIGNANT VULVAR DISORDERS: DIFFERENTIAL DIAGNOSES

	Diagnostic Characteristics			
Disorder	*Subjective*	*Objective*	*Medical Therapy*	*Adjunct Therapy*
Contact/Allergic Dermatitis	Pruritis, burning, stinging; begins 1–2 days after exposure to an irritating agent	Hyperemic, may be vesicular, marked edema, scaling, linear plaques, papules, fissuring, lichenification	Wet prep to r/o yeast; possible biopsy if hx. unclear; low or midpotency steroids; night-time sedation w/antihistamine or tricyclic antidepressant	Avoid all irritants
Seborrheic Dermatitis	More common in men than women; more common in AIDS pts	Erythematous, poorly margined plaques; yellow scale w/greasy texture; lesions occur more in scalp, ears, central face; more severe cases affect genitalia	1 percent hydrocortisone cream; severe cases: oral prednisone, 40 mg 5–10 days	Good hygiene
Hidradenitis	Occurs primarily in the axilla, anogenital areas; occurs after puberty, ages 20–40; higher incidence in African Americans	Red papules, multiform, enlarge to be nodular or cystic; resembles furuncles; draining, scarring, edema may occur; regional lymphadenopathy present	*Tetracycline 500 mg* b.i.d. for several mos; *oral contraceptives* at 50 mcg	Refer for surgery w/severe cases
Furunculosis	Presence of painful boils; fever, malaise may be present	Eythematous nodules that drain	*Dicloxacillin, Cephalexin, Erythromycin*	
Epidermal Cysts	Asymptomatic	White or yellow nodule, firm nontender, varies in size 1mm–several cms.; located near hair follicles		I & D
Lichen Planus	Pain, itching purulent, painful irritating discharge	Well circumscribed flat-topped papules; shiny surface, white, fernlike lesions; ulcers/erosions may be present; may be lesions in the mouth; may be increased vaginal discharge; Vaginal pH > 5.0	Mid- to high-potency topical steroid, b.i.d.	Vulvar biopsy

Source: Reference 36.

Testosterone Propionate 2 Percent

- *Indications.* Most often used treatment for Lichen sclerosus. Recent research findings, however, indicate that testosterone may have little place in current treatment of Lichen sclerosus.[36]
- *Administration.* Must be made up by the pharmacist of 2 percent testosterone propriate in petrolatum. Should be replaced every 6 months. Apply to affected area twice a day for 4 to 6 months. When improvement occurs, taper to twice/week.
- *Side Effects and Adverse Reactions.* Clitoral hypertrophy, increased libido, hirsutism, deepening of the voice. The most common side effect is local irritation and flare up of itching and irritation.
- *Contraindications.* Should not be used in children.

- *Expected Outcomes on Evaluation.* Relief of symptoms. There is generally no improvement in the appearance of the skin.
- *Client Teaching and Counseling.* Discuss possible side effects and advise the client to report changes as soon as possible.

Amitriptyline

- *Indications.* Treatment of essential vulvodynia.
- *Administration.* Initiate at the lowest dose of 10 to 25 mg p.o. in early evening. Gradually increase until relief of symptoms up to 75 mg. Continue at least 2 months.
- *Side Effects and Adverse Reactions.* Drowsiness, dry mouth, weight gain, tinnitus, palpitations, constipation, loss of balance (especially in the elderly).
- *Contraindications.* Previous hypersensitivity. Should not be given concurrently with monoamine oxidase inhibitors.
- *Expected Outcomes on Evaluation.* Relief of symptoms of burning, pain, and irritation.
- *Client Education and Counseling.* Reassure the client that mitriptyline is commonly used to manage pain syndromes because of its effect on cutaneous nerves and not because they are "crazy" or that the problem is psychosomatic.[40] Discuss common side effects. Advise the client that she will begin with the lowest dosage and will increase the dose by 10 mg every 1 to 2 weeks until relief is achieved. If she has difficulty arising in the morning, she may take it at dinnertime.

Antifungals. See Chapter 4.

Topical Anesthetics (Xylocaine Jelly 2 percent or Ointment 5 percent)

- *Indications.* Relief of symptoms of vulvar vestibulitis, may be prescribed for use during sexual activity. First line therapy for management of vulvar vestibulitis.[33,36,39]
- *Administration.* Apply first in the office setting with a cotton swab to check for burning and local irritation. Then, the client may apply the gel or ointment 15 minutes before anticipated coital activity.
- *Side Effects and Adverse Reactions.* Local irritation.
- *Contraindications.* Should not be used in clients with allergy to benzocaines.

- *Expected Outcomes on Evaluation.* Relief of symptoms, decrease in dyspareunia.
- *Client Teaching and Counseling.* Instruct in proper application. Advise clients to avoid activities that might irritate the affected tissues. Add other lubricants during intercourse.

Interferon

- *Indications.* Last line therapy for vulvar vestibulitis recommended in conjunction with physician consultation.[33,36]
- *Administration.* Local injections of 1 million units (0.2 ml) intradermally in the vestibule around the circumference on Monday, Wednesday, and Friday for 4 weeks for a total of 12 injections.
- *Side Effects and Adverse Reactions.* Myalgias, headache, fever and other flulike symptoms; develop about 4 hours after injection.
- *Contraindications.* Hypersensitivity.
- *Expected Outcomes on Evaluation.* Decrease in symptoms of pain and burning and dyspareunia.
- *Client Teaching and Counseling.* Take 650 mg of acetaminophen prior to the injection and every 4–6 hours afterward until flulike symptoms resolve. Document thorough informed consent.

Surgical Intervention

Vestibulectomy. Excision of the vestibule to include the hymenal ring. The vagina is undermined and advanced to cover the area. This procedure is indicated when pain and discomfort are severe and interfere with normal daily living and when conservative measures fail. Success rates are reported at 60–90 percent. Adverse outcomes include the potential risks involved with anesthesia; postoperative pain and possible scarring. The anticipated outcomes on evaluation are the complete relief of symptoms with return to normal sexual function.

Discuss with the client the potential risks and the benefits of the surgery. Warn that pain may continue long-term following the surgery. Explain the procedure using anatomical models. The procedure should only be performed by an experienced gynecologic surgeon.

Dietary Interventions

Low-Oxalate Diet. One theory concerning vulvar pain proposes that clients have an elevated urinary level of calcium oxalate, an end product of metabolism. Therefore, it may be beneficial to provide the client with a list of foods that may represent possible dietary irritants and advise her to avoid or limit these particular foods. The following foods are considered to increase calcium oxalate:

- *Beverages.* All teas, coffee, cocoa, and most wines.
- *Fruits and Vegetables.* Beans, beets, berries, celery, cranberries, cranberry juice, eggplant, green peppers, lima beans, plums, prunes, rhubarb, spinach, summer squash, sweet potatoes, tomatoes, vegetable soup, Vitamin C supplement > 250 mg/day.
- *Spices and Condiments.* Black pepper, chiles, dill, mustard, soy sauce, vinegar.
- *Other.* Chocolate, fruit cake, nuts, peanut butter, tofu, wheat germ.

Although a 24-hour urine test for calcium oxalate may help confirm this theory and/or be used to evaluate dietary changes, it is often expensive and may not be covered by insurance. This therapy is best used empirically. Have the client keep a food recall diary and symptom record.

Alternative Therapies

As with any chronic pain syndrome, clients may benefit from biofeedback, massage, acupuncture, acupressure and/or hypnotism. Support the client in pursuing these avenues and evaluate for relief of symptoms.

FOLLOW-UP AND REFERRAL

Continuing, consistent follow-up is extremely important in managing vulvar pain syndromes. Careful observation for visible improvement or worsening of vulvar tissue is crucial. Offer continued emotional support. Clients may need to be seen biweekly when initiating therapy, monthly during active medical therapy, and perhaps every 1 to 2 months as improvement occurs.

If improvement does not occur or if the clinician is unsure of the diagnosis, referral to a specialist with knowledge of vulvar disorders is mandatory. Always be aware of the indications for vulvar biopsy (discussed earlier in this section) and refer when indicated. Refer for psychological evaluation and counseling when signs of depression are apparent, when sexual dysfunction is present, or in light of a history of sexual/physical abuse.

LEIOMYOMAS

Leiomyomas are benign smooth muscle tumors of the uterus, commonly called "fibroids." They are classified according to their location within the uterus.

- *Submucous,* protruding into the uterine cavity. Most commonly symptomatic, leading reason for hysterectomy.[21]
- *Intramural,* within the myometrial wall.
- *Subserous,* growing toward the serous surface of the uterus.
- *Intraligamentous,* located in the cervix or in between the folds of the broad ligament.

Leiomyomas are estrogen dependent; they rarely occur before menarche or after menopause. Although leiomyomas may grow larger during pregnancy, most do not. If growth occurs, it is usually during the first trimester. Most regress in size after pregnancy.[2] Rarely malignant, leiomyomas may be small and asymptomatic or may grow very large and extend up into the abdomen. They are the most common indication for hysterectomy and account for an undetermined amount of major and minor conservative surgical procedures, outpatient consultations, and disabilities.[2]

ETIOLOGY/EPIDEMIOLOGY

Leiomyomas develop from a single neoplastic smooth muscle cell. Cytogenetic analyses demonstrate abnormalities in chromosomal patterns, but it is still unclear what factors are responsible for the initial neoplastic transformation.[41] Growth of uterine leiomyomata is influenced by steroid hormones including estrogen and progesterone.[2,42]

This condition occurs in 25 percent of women of reproductive age with a 3–9 times higher incidence in African American women.[2,41,42] Increased risk is also associated with women who are nulliparous, over age 35, obese, sedentary, or who are nonsmokers. It is no longer accepted that oral contraceptives increase the risk for leiomyomas.[2]

SUBJECTIVE DATA

The majority of clients with uterine leiomyomas are asymptomatic. Symptoms increase as the tumors grow. The most common symptom is menorrhagia, occurring in 10–40 percent of women with leiomyomas.[43] Other symptoms include pelvic pressure, bloating, pelvic congestion, a feeling of heaviness, urinary frequency, urgency, and/or incontinence, dysmenorrhea, and, less commonly pain.[2] Clients may report infertility. Pregnant women complain more frequently of pain due to "red" degeneration of the leiomyoma. Loss of blood supply to the leiomyoma causes degeneration leading to acute, self-limited pain.[2,42]

OBJECTIVE DATA

Physical Examination

An abdominal exam may reveal a large mass if the leiomyoma has grown larger than a 12–14 week pregnant uterus. The absence of ascites and presence of rebound tenderness and normal bowel sounds should be noted.

The genitalia and reproductive tract are also examined. Examine cervix for any extraneous tissue or distortion and examine any bleeding or discharge. Prior to the pelvic exam, ask the client to empty her bladder so that the examiner avoids confusing the tumor with the bladder. A pelvic exam may reveal an enlarged uterus that is firm and irregular but not tender. Usually palpated at midline, a leiomyoma may feel very firm or soft and cystic. If it is situated laterally, it may be mistaken for an adnexal mass. If the mass moves with the cervix, then it is likely to be a leiomyoma. Size should be described in terms of gestational size.[4,44]

Diagnostic Tests and Methods

Hemoglobin or Hematocrit. Diagnostic evaluation to determine whether the client is anemic, especially if she has experienced menometrorrhagia.[2,43] May usually be obtained by fingerstick and performed via traditional centrifuge or newer instant analyses.

Urinalysis. Diagnostic evaluation to identify urinary tract conditions that might account for any urinary tract symptoms. White blood cells, bacteria, or red blood cells in the urine may indicate chronic or recurrent urinary tract infection (UTI). Hematuria may indicate the presence of renal stone or a tumor of the urinary tract. Further diagnostic testing may be indicated, specifically cystoscopy or intravenous pyelogram.

Explain to the client how to obtain a clean catch urine sample.

Pregnancy Test (Urine or Blood Level of β-hCG). Diagnostic evaluation for unsuspected intrauterine pregnancy (see Pelvic Inflammatory Disease for procedure).

Stool Guiac (Colocare or Hemoccult). Diagnostic evaluation to detect gastrointestinal (GI) pathology that may be the source of a palpable abdominal mass, for example, an inflammatory diverticulum or an intestinal mass. A stool found to be positive for occult blood suggests GI polyps or malignancy, but that result alone is insufficient for a definitive diagnosis. If the test is positive, or if the client's history and physical exam are suggestive, then refer her for gastroenterology consultation and further diagnostic testing, such as upper GI series, barium enema, sigmoidoscopy, and/or colonoscopy.

With the Colocare method, the client floats a special card in the toilet after a bowel movement. A specific color change represents a positive result. The test should be repeated for three bowel movements at home. Alternatively, the older guaiac test (Hemoccult) requires the client to smear a stool sample onto a card and return the card to the health care professional, who subsequently applies solution to it; bluish discoloration represents a positive result. This test also should be repeated three times.

Provide instructions that will prepare the client for the test. Tell her that for 2 days before the test and during the testing period she is not to eat red or rare meats and is not to take vitamin C supplements, laxatives, or medications such as aspirin, corticosteroids, reserpine, indomethacin, or phenylbutazone. A high fiber diet is advised.

Ultrasound. Diagnostic evaluation to identify the leiomyoma and confirm its location. Should identify the uterine volume, number of fibroids, location relative to the endometrial stripe, evaluation of adnexa, and a cursory scan of the kidneys.[43] Ultrasound helps to distinguish between uterine leiomyoma and an adnexal mass, and helps in assessing obese clients or others for whom the exam is not well tolerated (see Adenomyosis for the test procedure).

Barium Enema. See Adnexal Masses.

Intravenous Pyelogram. See Adnexal Masses.

Diagnostic Hysteroscopy. Hysteroscopy employs the use of endoscopic equipment to view the uterine cavity. It enables direct examination of the endocervical canal and lower uterine segment.

The most common indications for hysteroscopy are evaluation of abnormal uterine bleeding and direct observation of uterine fibroids, polyps, adhesions, and location of IUDs. It enables the provider to identify the exact presence, location, size, and number of fibroids and is helpful in treatment planning.

Contraindications to the procedure include a recent or present episode of salpingitis or diagnosed cervical or uterine malignancy. The procedure should be performed with careful consideration in women who are bleeding heavily, pregnant, or have cardiovascular or systemic disease.

Risks are infrequent and include possible cervical trauma, uterine perforation, and infection.

Prior to the procedure, the client is placed in the dorsal lithotomy position and the cervix is cleansed with provodone iodine solution. Paracervical anesthesia may be employed. A light source, camera, carbon dioxide and saline lines are connected, and the hysteroscope is introduced through the cervical canal. The procedure in experienced hands takes about 10 minutes.

Counsel the client that she may expect shoulder pain as a result of the CO_2 gas escaping into the abdomen and mild tolerable cramping. She will rest about 10 minutes following the procedure and may return home afterward. Advise her to expect possible shoulder pain, cramping, and mild spotting to continue for the next 1–3 days. She should abstain from intercourse, douching or use of tampons for 2 weeks and call if she experiences heavy bleeding, abdominal pain, discharge with odor or fever.[45,46]

DIFFERENTIAL MEDICAL DIAGNOSES

Ovarian neoplasm, tubo-ovarian inflammatory mass, diverticular inflammatory mass, pregnancy, ectopic pregnancy, adenomyosis, pelvic kidney, malignancy, interstitial cystitis, irritable bowel syndrome, obstipation.[43]

PLAN

Psychosocial Interventions

Provide the client with explanations and printed information about leiomyomas (fibroids). Reassure her that leiomyomas occur commonly, that they are rarely malignant, and that if she is asymptomatic or if symptoms are mild, treatment will be unnecessary. Assess her future reproductive plans and the extent of her symptoms. Stress the importance of regular monitoring and follow-up examinations.

If the client is or becomes pregnant, provide reassurance and support. Reassure her that in most pregnancies, fibroids do not grow enough to cause complication. Advise the client of the signs and symptoms of preterm labor later in the pregnancy.

Medical Management

Expectant Management. Fifty percent of clients with leiomyomata are asymptomatic. In these clients, reassure that no further intervention is necessary. Indications for the treatment of fibroids include menorrhagia, pelvic pressure or pain, infertility or habitual abortion, and compromise of adjacent organs.[43]

Medication

The goal of medical therapy is to reduce the symptoms and myoma size.

NSAIDS

- *Indications.* To relieve discomfort and to decrease menorrhagia. Studies show a reduction in menorrhagia by 30–50 percent with the use of NSAIDs initiated 102 days prior to the expected menses.[44]
- *Administration.* Several types of NSAIDs are available, and their dosages vary. The most widely accepted and least expensive are the following:
  - Ibuprofen 600 mg, p.o., q.i.d.
  - Naproxen sodium (Naprosyn, Anaprox, Aleve), 550 mg, p.o., b.i.d.
- *Side Effects and Adverse Reactions.* Most often reported is GI irritation. Advise taking with food or after meals.
- *Contraindications.* Previous allergy to NSAIDs and a history of ulcer disease.

Oral Iron Preparation

- *Indications.* The client who is experiencing significant menorrhagia or metrorrhagia and whose hemoglobin and hematocrit are falling below normal levels.
- *Administration.* Select one of many commercially available preparations. Begin with one tablet (300 mg ferrous sulfate or the equivalent) daily; increase to two daily if hemoglobin falls below 10.0 g/dL. Follow with reticulocyte counts to monitor response to the therapy.
- *Side Effects and Adverse Reactions.* Constipation and other gastrointestinal symptoms, such as indigestion, nausea, loss of appetite.
- *Contraindication.* Known allergy to oral iron preparations.
- *Anticipated Outcome or Evaluation.* Anemia secondary to menometrorrhagia is prevented.
- *Client Teaching and Counseling.* Provide information about foods that are rich in iron (leafy green vegetables, enriched flour products, raisins, prunes, dried apricots). Instruct the client that for better absorption of the iron, she should take the preparation with a citrus juice and avoid eating or drinking dairy products for 1 hour before and 1 hour after.

Gonadotropin Releasing Hormone Agonist (GnRHa) (Leuprorelin, Nafarelin, Goserelin).

GnRH analogues bind to GnRH receptors resulting in a decrease in LH and FSH, which produces a hypoestrogenic effect.

- *Indications.* To suppress the growth of leiomyomas and promote possible shrinkage. GnRH-a are useful for reducing the size of the leiomyoma prior to surgery; it may permit vaginal hysterectomy rather than abdominal hysterectomy. It also may prevent the need for surgery in the perimenopausal client.
- *Administration. Leuprorelin (Lupron),* 0.5 mg s.c., q.d. for 8–12 weeks *or* 3.75–7.5 mg Depot Luporn once every 28 days. *Nafarelin (Synarel),* one spray (200 mg/spray) into one nostril q.a.m. and one spray into the other nostril q.h.s. 8–12 weeks. *Goserelin (Zoladex)* consists of a small biodegradable cylinder which is inserted subcutaneously monthly.
- *Side Effects and Adverse Reactions.* Hot flashes (75 percent of clients report hot flashes), vaginal dryness, mood swings, depression, weight gain, reduced breast size, decreased libido, fatigue, insomnia, headache, joint and muscle stiffness, and irregular vaginal bleeding.[5]
- *Contraindications.* Known or suspected pregnancy, hypersensitivity to GnRH agonists, undiagnosed abnormal vaginal bleeding, breastfeeding.
- *Anticipated Outcomes on Evaluation.* A reduction in uterine and leiomyoma size.
- *Client Teaching and Counseling.* Instruct the client about proper drug administration and inform her that the GnRH agonists are very expensive. The length of therapy (8–12 weeks) needs to be discussed. Review the side effects and the possible need for calcium carbonate supplementation. Barrier contraception is recommended during therapy and for the first menstrual cycle. Explain that it is likely that within 6 months following treatment the leiomyomas will recur.

Add-Back Therapy. Although still currently under continuing investigation, the results of add-back therapy look promising. Because of concerns about bone loss associated with GnRH agonists and because of the hypoestrogenic symptoms that are poorly tolerated by many patients, the addition of estrogen/progesterone therapy to the GnRH-a regimen is being advocated.[2,43] The practitioner should be aware of this trend so that she may better counsel her clients.

Surgery

Myomectomy. This procedure entails the abdominal removal of leiomyomata indicated when the client is symptomatic, the uterus is greater than 12 weeks' size, and conservation of fertility is desired.[21,41] The leiomyoma(s) appears to be either interfering with fertility or causing pregnancy loss.

Refer the client to a board-certified gynecologist. The size and location of the leiomyomas will determine the site of abdominal incision. Some surgeons are skilled at removing small myomas through the laparoscope or hysteroscope. Smaller tumors may be destroyed with the laser. The goal of surgery is to remove all leiomyomas, relieve symptoms, and increase fertility. Adverse effects may develop as a result of a difficult, demanding procedure with the potential for increased blood loss, increased operating time, increased postoperative risks of infection, ileus, anemia, and increased pain. Among women who undergo myomectomy, 27 percent must have repeated surgery due to recurrence.[41] Most myomectomy clients who subsequently become pregnant will require delivery by cesarean section.

Discuss the difficult surgery and its potential complications with the client. Inform her about the high rate of myoma recurrence and the possible later need for a hysterectomy. Warn her not to attempt pregnancy until 4 to 6 months after the procedure. Review the postoperative/discharge instruction.[47]

Hysterectomy. This procedure is definitive treatment, indicated when the fibroids become palpable abdominally and are a concern to the client or when menorrhagia occurs or worsens, placing the client at risk for anemia.[42] In addition, hysterectomy may be done to resolve any of the following: pelvic pain and secondary dysmenorrhea, urinary symptoms, or uterine growth after menopause. The surgery is indicated if the client has completed childbearing or if the health care provider is unable to evaluate the adnexa because the uterus has become an abdominal organ. The route of hysterectomy depends on the size of the leiomyoma; if less than 12 weeks' size, vaginal hysterectomy is possible.

Surgery should accomplish complete relief of symptoms. Few adverse effects occur; however, bleeding, infection, and damage to nearby organs are possible. After the surgery, the client is at risk for depression, sexual dysfunction, and cardiovascular disease without hormone replacement therapy.

Client teaching and counseling include discussion of the alternatives to hysterectomy, especially if there is indecision regarding future childbearing. Provide the client with a thorough explanation of hysterectomy, including descriptions of anatomy, physiology, and the surgical procedure, its risks and benefits. Reassure the client that femininity remains unchanged. Hormonal replacement therapy may need to be initiated if salpingo-oophorectomy is done. Full recovery usually occurs within 6 weeks. Review the postoperative instructions, including the return to activity, expectation that vaginal bleeding will change to clear discharge, signs of infection, resumption of sexual activity when bleeding ceases (usually in about 14 days), and dietary counseling (including information about preventing constipation and weight gain).[21]

FOLLOW-UP AND REFERRAL

For the client who is asymptomatic or has mild symptoms, the treatment of choice is expectant management.[21,42,44] During pregnancy, rest and analgesics are appropriate if pain is present. Stress the importance of keeping appointments for close follow-up. If expectant management, medical therapy, or myomectomy is chosen as a treatment option, the client should be reexamined at 3- to 6-month intervals. It is generally accepted that cancer does not develop from leiomyomata. The client may be monitored without risk of the development of cancer. Rapid increase in uterine size raises the question of malignancy.[2,21] Uterine size and the leiomyoma should be evaluated carefully by pelvic exam and, if necessary, ultrasound should be used. Discuss with the client any new or worsening symptomology. Alter the plan of care as necessary. Monitor hemoglobin and hematocrit frequently if menorrhagia or metrorrhagia is present. Refer for physician consultation if there is rapid increase in size, increase in menorrhagia or development, or increase in pain/pressure.

Pelvic relaxation syndrome

Pelvic relaxation syndrome is the failure of the pelvic musculature to maintain support and position of the pelvic organs. When supporting pelvic ligaments, muscles, and fascia can no longer withstand constant increased intra-abdominal pressure, such as that which occurs with obstetric damage, chronic coughing or straining, surgery, or aging, the vaginal wall weakens, descends, and the pelvic organs protrude into the vaginal canal. Five major types of genital prolapse may occur; cystocele, urethrocele, rectocele, enterocele, and uterine prolapse.[48] The vagina can also prolapse to or beyond the introitus but this generally occurs only when the uterus has been removed.

Types of Genital Prolapse
- *Cystocele.* Prolapse of the posterior bladder wall through the anterior vaginal wall.
- *Urethrocele.* Bulging of the urethra through the anterior vaginal wall; usually not a single entity, occurs with cystocele.
- *Rectocele.* Bulging of the bowel through the posterior vaginal wall; involves loss of support of the fascia and levator ani muscles.
- *Enterocele.* Bulging of the bowel through the posterior cul-de-sac and vaginal wall; may be part of a high rectocele.
- *Uterine Prolapse.* Descent of the uterus through the pelvic floor and into the vaginal canal. (See Figure 13–1.)

The extent of genital organ prolapse is described in terms of degree: first degree, prolapse of an organ into the vaginal canal; second degree, presence of an organ at the hymenal ring; third degree, presence of an organ beyond the hymenal ring; and fourth degree, organ is fully outside the hymenal ring.[49]

EPIDEMIOLOGY
- Weakening of the pelvic support through the stretching and trauma of childbirth.
- Increased intra-abdominal pressure secondary to chronic respiratory problems, heavy lifting, ascites, obesity, and habitual straining due to constipation.
- Normal downward pressure because the human posture is erect.
- Atrophy of the supporting tissues with aging, especially after menopause.
- Congenital weakness.

Risk factors include obesity, caucasian race, multiparity, and menopause with lack of estrogen replacement.[24]

Pelvic relaxation occurs with increasing frequency during the postreproductive years; in fact, the majority of parous women show some evidence of pelvic relaxation. Approximately 10–15 percent will require surgery.[24]

There are 6 million women in the United States over the age of 75. With the increase in the aging population, quality of life concerns are increasingly important when caring for this group of women. Factors related to prolapse of the pelvic organs will take a greater portion of the practitioner's time.[48]

SUBJECTIVE DATA

Clients frequently state, "Something feels as if it is falling out." Other symptoms include backache, pelvic pressure or heaviness; bearing-down sensation; urinary frequency, urgency, or incontinence; dyspareunia; discomfort walking or sitting; difficult defecation; or protrusion of an organ through the introitus.[24,50]

OBJECTIVE DATA

Physical Examination

Physical examination, including complete gynecologic inspection, is the most important step in diagnosing pelvic relaxation. It should include an overall assessment of the client's general physical health, including measurement of blood pressure, weight, and height in stocking feet. Note at each annual exam, any possible changes indicating osteoporosis and vertebral compression. Include auscultation of heart and lungs. Note the client's posture and presence and width of abdominal wall striae. This is indicative of the client's elastic index. The greater the striae, the less elasticity and the higher the risk of prolapse.[48]

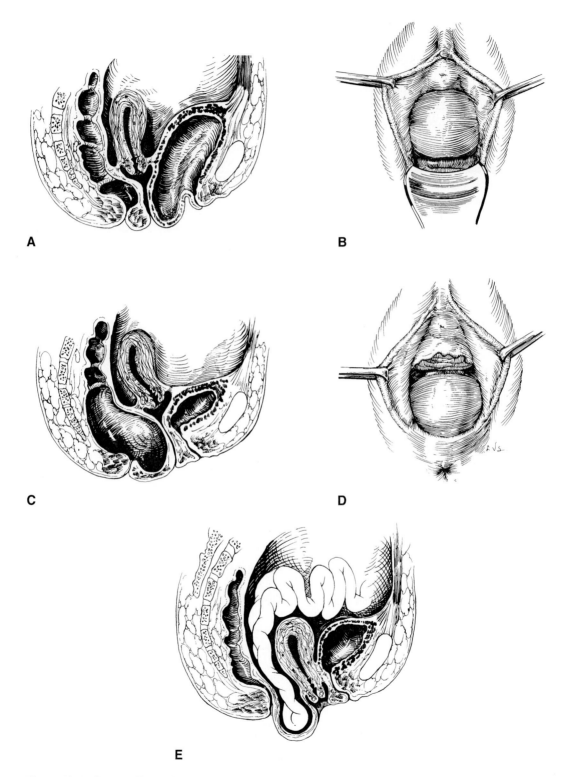

Figure 13–1. Common Types of Pelvic Floor Relaxation. Diagrammatic representation of cystocele (A & B), rectocele (C & D), and enterocele and prolapsed uterus (E). *(Source: DeCherney, A. H. & Pernoll, M. L. (1994).* Current Obstetric & Gynecologic Diagnostics & Treatment. *Norwalk, CT: Appleton & Lange.)*

During the physical examination, the practitioner should be assessing for any of the common complications of prolapse, such as mucosal hypertrophy, irritative bleeding, chronic excoriation, ulceration, and urinary retention.[50]

Examine the external genitalia for atrophy and any obvious protrusion of the uterus, bladder, urethra, or vaginal wall. Use lithotomy position and Sim's speculum (Graves' speculum may be used if the anterior blade is removed). Ask the client to perform the Valsalva maneuver; note which organ prolapses first and the degree to which it occurs.

Systematically examine the anterior and posterior walls of the vagina. Ask the client to contract the pubococcygeal muscles (Kegel's exercise); with two fingers in the vagina, note the strength and symmetry of the contraction. Note any ulcerations of the cervix and uterus if third degree prolapse is present. Note bladder leakage during the exam.

Perform a rectal exam; observe any bleeding, and determine muscle tone and the presence of any rectocele. The client should also be asked to stand and be assessed for prolapse of the vaginal walls or uterus.

The Q-tip test is used by some to assess the degree of descent of the bladder neck. A sterile lubricated tip applicator is placed in the urethra of the urethrovesical junction. It should be at zero degrees in the dorsal-lithotomy position and should only change minimally when the client is asked to strain. If the support of the bladder neck is lax, the applicator will move upward > than 30 degrees.[49,50] A 1993 research study by Caputo and colleagues found that this test is unreliable and not a good assessment of urethral support defects.[51]

Since genital organ prolapse can cause urinary symptoms, such as incontinence or retention, bladder function must be assessed.[50] Determine postvoid residual with catheterization. Retention is present if residual is more than 60 to 100 mL. The client should be referred for further urodynamic evaluation and testing if she is older than 65, has indications for surgery, has had previous unsuccessful anti-incontinence surgery, has serious medical problems, has possible intrinsic sphincter damage or other unexplained urinary symptoms.[50]

DIFFERENTIAL MEDICAL DIAGNOSES

Pelvic or abdominal tumors, tumors of the rectovaginal septum, cervical hypertrophy, Gartner's cyst, urethral diverticulum.

PLAN

Psychosocial Interventions

Describe the normal anatomy and the etiologies for pelvic prolapse to the client. Determine the impact of the prolapse on the client's daily functioning and ask whether she has future reproductive desires. Reassure the client that she can achieve relief of symptoms, restoration or partial restoration of anatomy, and return to normal functioning.

Medication

Estrogen Replacement Therapy. Indicated to improve tone and vascularity of the supporting tissue in perimenopausal and menopausal women.

Nonnarcotic Analgesics. Indicated for temporary relief of associated discomfort, especially back pain. The desired outcome of treatment is partial or complete pain relief. Over-the-counter analgesics, such as acetaminophen, should be tried first, but more potent nonsteroidal anti-inflammatory drugs (NSAIDs) may be needed.

- *Administration.* Continuous use is most effective. Several types of NSAIDs are available, and their dosages vary.
  - Ibuprofen (Motrin), 400–800 mg. p.o. q.i.d.
  - Naproxen (Naprosyn, Anaprox, Aleve), 200 mg. p.o. t.i.d. to 550 mg. p.o. b.i.d.
  - Ketoprofen (Orudis), 50–100 mg. p.o. b.i.d.

Newly available NSAIDs enter the market continually. It is imperative that the clinician remains current on the dosages, benefits, risks and side effects. It is probably best to select one or two which are inexpensive, low in side effects, and simple to dose and to use these interchangeably.

- *Side Effects and Adverse Reactions.* Most often reported is GI irritation. If GI irritation occurs, sucralfate (a GI antiulcerative) may be added to the regimen. Sucralfate dosage is one 1 g tablet p.o. 1 hour before or 2 hours after meals and at bedtime.

- *Contraindications.* Previous allergy to NSAIDs and a history of ulcer disease.
- *Client Teaching and Counseling.* Stress the need to follow the NSAID regimen carefully and to take the drug with food. Counsel the client to report immediately any signs of indigestion, epigastric pain, or hematochezia.

Dietary Interventions

Dietary habits can exacerbate the prolapse by causing constipation and consequently chronic straining. Dietary modifications will help to establish regular bowel movements without discomfort and eliminate excessive gas or bloating.

Teach the client about increasing dietary fiber and fluids to prevent constipation. Explain how constipation can contribute to straining and pelvic prolapse. Provide the client with instruction, materials, and support.[24,48]

Respiratory Interventions

Correction or improvement of respiratory problems that cause chronic cough will decrease intra-abdominal pressure and thereby prevent worsening of pelvic prolapse. Intervention is indicated for clients who smoke, have asthma, or have chronic bronchitis. Anticipated outcomes on evaluation are that the client has stopped smoking, coughs less, and has less shortness of breath.

Counseling of a client who is not receiving care for a respiratory problem should include referral for evaluation and management. Encourage her to follow prescribed regimens, to stop smoking, and, if possible, to join a support group. Discuss with the client how reducing respiratory symptoms will help improve the symptoms of prolapse and prevent them from worsening.[48] Reinforce the discussion by providing written information.

Surgery

Surgical treatment of genital organ prolapse is designed to correct specific defects, with the goals being restoration of normal anatomy and preservation of function. Procedures that are frequently done include the following.[49]

- Anterior colporrhaphy (plication of the pubocervical fascia) to correct cystocele/urethrocele.
- Posterior colporrhaphy (midline approximation of the endopelvic fascia and perineal muscles) to correct rectocele/enterocele.
- Enterocele repair (approximation of the uterosacral ligaments and levator ani muscles after reduction of the bowel).
- Manchester operation (involves anterior colporrhaphy, posterior colporrhaphy, amputation of the cervix, and suturing of the cardinal ligaments in front of the stump) to preserve, support, and antevert the uterus.
- Vaginal hysterectomy, done for any degree of uterine prolapse.
- Le-Fort's partial colpocleisis (suturing of the anterior and posterior vaginal walls so that the uterus is supported above), performed in elderly clients with substantial prolapse.

Indications for surgery are when childbearing is completed and/or symptoms begin to interfere with the client's daily living patterns and do not respond to nonsurgical treatment. The procedure chosen depends on the type and severity of pelvic prolapse. The client is referred to a board-certified gynecologic surgeon for evaluation.

Potential adverse effects depend on the surgical procedure performed. For example, with preservation of the uterus and closure of the vaginal canal, abnormal uterine bleeding could occur undetected. Coitus is also affected. A major adverse effect is recurrence of the prolapse; other effects include urinary retention, chronic urinary tract infection (UTI), incontinence, and difficult defecation.

Anticipated outcomes on evaluation are a return to optimal function; cessation or significantly fewer and less severe symptoms; normal patterns of elimination; and prevention of prolapse of other organs and of recurrence of the prolapse that was repaired.

Provide in-depth discussions of the procedure to be performed, emphasizing anatomy and postoperative instructions. Allow the client to express her fears and anxieties. Stress that femininity will be preserved; however, discuss how sexual function may be altered.[52]

Pessaries[50,52]

A *pessary* is a hard rubber or plastic ring used to maintain the normal position of the uterus or bladder by exerting pressure and providing support. It is placed in the vagina behind the pubic arch and the posterior fornix. An indication for pessary use is uterine prolapse or cystocele especially among elderly clients for whom surgery is contraindicated.

The best type of pessary depends on the individual client's anatomy and symptoms. Clients with uterine prolapse without incontinence require only a space occupying type (doughnut, inflatable). Clients with urinary incontinence benefit from a Smith-Hodge pessary.

Types of pessaries include the following:

- Smith-Hodge pessaries elevate the bladder neck and support it in a retropubic position.
- Ring pessaries are similar to diaphragms and are easily accepted by most clients. Inserted similarly to a diaphragm.
- Cube pessaries remain in place by adhering to the vaginal side walls. The incidence of mucosal inflammation and ulceration is high with this type, especially in the presence of atrophic vaginitis.
- Gellhorn pessaries are the best choice for large prolapse of the anterior vaginal wall.
- Inflatable pessaries are inserted and then inflated with a bulb.
- Doughnut pessaries are indicated for severe prolapse, may be difficult for the elderly client to insert and remove (see Figure 13–2).

Select the largest pessary that can be comfortably admitted through the vaginal orifice. Vaginal estrogen should be used twice weekly (1 gram). The most common recommendations for pessary care include removing the pessary twice weekly and cleansing with soap and water; using lubrication upon insertion, and having regular follow-up exams every 6 to 12 months after an initial period of adjustment.

Adverse effects include chronic vaginal infection and UTI. Vaginal erosion may occur. Anticipated outcomes on evaluation are that the uterus and bladder are supported, symptoms are decreased, and no interference occurs with intercourse. Client teaching must include instruction for removing and cleaning the pessary. Review the untoward symptoms/signs associated with pessary use; leukorrhea; vaginal burning or itching; loss of pessary; urinary retention; frequency, urgency, and dysuria. Instruct the client to report any symptoms.

Kegel's Exercises

The exercises strengthen pelvic muscles, which prevents further prolapse. They can be performed at any time and are very easy to learn. They have no adverse effect. If the prolapse extends to or beyond the vaginal introitus, however, Kegel exercises are no longer useful.[50]

Help the client to identify the pubococcygeus muscle by having her stop and start her urinary flow. Have her tighten the muscle for a count of 3, then relax it. The client should repeat the exercise 10 times. Then instruct the client to contract and relax the muscle rapidly 10 times. In addition, have her try to bring up the entire pelvic floor and bear down 10 times. This movement may be repeated 5 times daily.

Lifestyle Changes

Several changes in lifestyle may help to prevent pelvic relaxation. For example, the client should attempt to achieve her ideal weight; wear a girdle or abdominal support best; avoid or reduce heavy lifting; avoid high impact aerobics and jogging, and quit smoking.

FOLLOW-UP AND REFERRAL

Emphasize to all clients that worsening or recurrence of any symptoms should be reported immediately. If nonsurgical therapies are employed, regular follow-up visits at least every 6 months are necessary to assess the degree of prolapse and any worsening symptomatology. If a pessary is used, the client should be seen every 2 to 6 months to remove the device for inspection and cleaning. After surgery, the client should be seen at least annually to assess any recurrent prolapse.

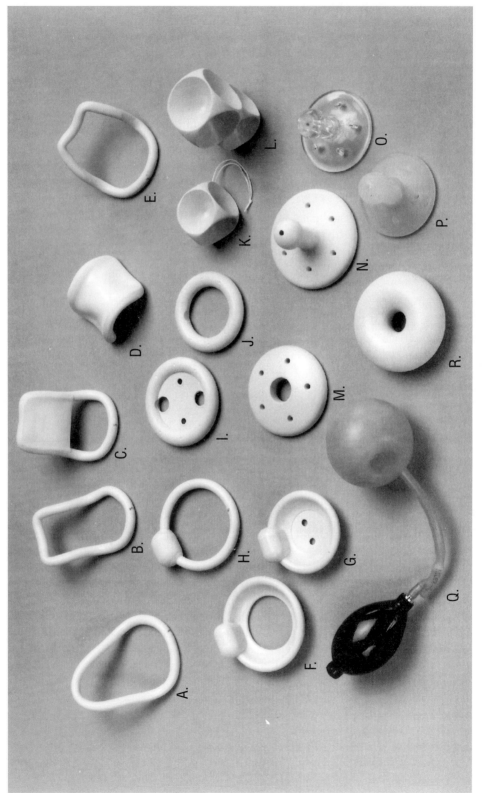

Figure 13–2. Types of Pessaries. A. Smith (Silicone)-(Folding); B. Hodge without Support (Silicone)-(Folding); C. Hodge with Support (Silicone)-(Folding); D. Gehrung with Support (Silicone)-(Folding); E. Risser (Silicone)-(Folding); F. Incontinence Dish without Support (Silicone)-(Folding); G. Incontinence Dish with Support (Silicone)-(Folding); H. Incontinence Ring (Silicone)-(Folding); I. Ring without Support (Silicone)-(Folding); J. Ring with Support (Silicone)-(Folding); K. Cube (Silicone)-(Flexible); L. Tandem-Cube (Silicone)-(Flexible); M. Shaatz (Silicone)-(Folding); N. Gellhorn (Silicone)-(Flexible)-(Multi-Drain); O. Gellhorn (Acrylic)-(Rigid)-(Multi-Drain); P. Gellhorn (95% Rigid Silicone)-(Multi-Drain); Q. Inflatoball (Latex); R. Donut (Silicone).

CHRONIC PELVIC PAIN

Chronic pain persists for longer than 6 months and significantly impacts a woman's daily functioning and relationships. It can be *episodic* (i.e., cyclic, recurrent pain that is interspersed with pain free intervals) or *continuous* (i.e., noncyclic pain). Chronic pelvic pain frustrates both the client and her health care providers. Many times an etiology for chronic pain cannot be found or treatment of the presumed etiology fails; hence, pain becomes the illness.

EPIDEMIOLOGY

One third of clients with chronic pelvic pain have no obvious pelvic pathology.[53] Since the 1920s researchers have attempted to discover etiologies for chronic pelvic pain syndrome. At various times, different theories gained popularity, but the studies on which they were based were problematic (e.g., small samples, observer bias). Among the more popular theories that lack definite diagnostic criteria and management protocol are Allen-Masters Syndrome (universal joint syndrome), pelvic congestion syndrome, and retrodisplacement of the uterus.[54] The more common etiologies of chronic pelvic pain are as follows.

- *Episodic.* Dyspareunia, midcycle pelvic pain (mittelschmerz), dysmenorrhea.
- *Continuous.* Endometriosis, adenomyosis, chronic salpingitis, adhesions, loss of pelvic support.

In clients under 30, the cause of pelvic pain is more likely to be endometriosis or chronic pelvic inflammatory disease. In clients who are older, the causes are more likely to be one of the following: leiomyoma; adenomyosis; pelvic relaxation.[53]

Risk factors include the following:

- History of childhood or adult sexual abuse or trauma.
- Previous pelvic surgery.
- Personal or family history of depression.
- History of other chronic pain syndromes.
- History of alcohol and drug abuse.
- Tendency toward somatization.
- Dysfunctional family and marital relationships.[53]

Chronic pelvic pain comprises up to 10 percent of outpatient gynecologic visits and is the reason for 20 percent of laparoscopies and 12 percent of hysterectomies. Approximately 75,000 hysterectomies are performed annually because of chronic pelvic pain. Recent cost estimates are 2.8 billion dollars annually for physician and mental health visits. Additionally, women who report chronic pelvic pain admit to significantly poorer general health.[53]

SUBJECTIVE DATA

The major goals in the evaluation of chronic pelvic pain are as follows:

- To identify any treatable sources of pain, either gyn or nongyn.
- To rule out any potentially life threatening pathologies.
- To identify associated problems such as depression.

Because the evaluation of chronic pelvic pain can be complicated, a consistent approach to history taking and physical examination is essential.[55] Inquiry about the presence of pelvic pain should be a routine part of health care for women.[56]

The history should include these essential components:

- Detailed description of the onset, location, nature, character, and timing of the pain.
- Description of any associated symptoms such as nausea, vomiting, fever, urinary symptoms, constipation, diarrhea, bloating, vaginal discharge, dyspareunia.
- Detailed menstrual history including last menstrual period, bleeding patterns, dysmenorrhea, menarche, menopause.
- Reproductive history including pregnancies, births, miscarriages, elective terminations, ectopics, infertility.
- Sexual history including the number of sex partners, use of contraception, history of PID, STDs.
- Psychosocial history with careful attention to any past or present physical or sexual abuse; how the pain has impacted the client's lifestyle (work, sick days, relationships, normal activities, recreation).

- Past medical history and review of systems is pertinent to establishing differential diagnoses and should include past surgeries, previous therapies for the pain, use of pain medications, other providers seen, history of gastrointestinal problems, genitourinary problems, and musculoskeletal problems.

The client may report pain duration of 6 months or longer; incomplete relief by most previous treatments, including surgery and nonnarcotic analgesics; significantly impaired functioning at home or work; signs of depression such as early morning awakening, weight loss, and anorexia; pain out of proportion to pathology; and altered family roles. The client may also have a history of childhood abuse, incest, rape or other sexual trauma, substance abuse, or current sexual dysfunction. A client usually reports previous consultation with one or more health care providers and dissatisfaction with their management of her condition.[56]

OBJECTIVE DATA

Physical Examination

Perform a systematic physical examination of the abdominal, pelvic, and rectal areas, focusing on the location and intensity of the pain. Attempt to reproduce the pain. The use of relaxation/breathing techniques will facilitate examination for both client and health professional.[57,58] *Check the client's vital signs; fever indicates an acute process.*

Note the client's general appearance, demeanor, and gait; these may suggest the severity of pain and possible neuromuscular etiology. Vomiting may indicate an acute process.

Abdominal symptoms of a more acute process are rebound tenderness (peritoneal irritation) and decreased abdominal pain on palpation with tension of the rectus muscles. Ask the client to perform a straight leg raise; with the client's legs slightly raised and rectus muscles taut, pain on deep palpation will decrease if it is of pelvic origin and increase if it is of abdominal wall or myofascial origin. Inspect and note any well healed scars. Palpate scars for incisional hernias, and palpate for any unsuspected masses. To help identify femoral or inguinal hernias, palpate the groin while the client performs the Valsalva maneuver.

During the speculum exam, note any cervicitis, which may be a source of parametrial irritation. With bimanual/rectal exam, a tender pelvic or adnexal mass, abnormal bleeding, tender uterine fundus, or cervical motion tenderness may indicate an acute process, such as pelvic inflammatory disease (PID), ectopic pregnancy, or a ruptured ovarian cyst.

Nonmobility of the uterus may indicate the presence of pelvic adhesions. Note existence of any adnexal mass, fullness, or tenderness. Cul-de-sac nodularities are palpable with endometriosis. Identify any areas that reproduce deep dyspareunia.

Palpate the coccyx, both internally and externally, for tenderness of coccydynia.

Musculoskeletal exam should be performed. View the spine while client is sitting, standing and walking. Observe gait, leg length, and range of motion. Have the client bend at the waist to assess for scoliosis.[57–59]

Diagnostic Tests and Methods

Diagnostic tests should be selected discriminately as indicated by the findings of the history and physical examination. Review previous test results in order to avoid unnecessary and repetitive diagnostic testing.

Complete Blood Count (CBC) and Erythrocyte Sedimentation Rate (ESR). See Pelvic Inflammatory Disease.

Urinalysis. Diagnostic evaluation to identify any urinary tract conditions that might represent the source of pain. White blood cells, bacteria, or red blood cells may indicate either chronic or recurrent urinary tract infections (UTI). Hematuria may indicate renal stones or a tumor of the urinary tract. Further diagnostic testing, specifically cystoscopy or intravenous pyelogram, may be indicated.

Teach the client how to obtain a clean catch urine sample in a sterile container.

Pregnancy Test (Urine or Blood Level of hCG). See Pelvic Inflammatory Disease.

Vaginal Smears/Cervical Cultures. Diagnostic evaluation to detect existing pelvic infection as the etiology of acute or chronic pelvic pain. Wet mount with saline can detect bacterial vaginosis or trichomoniasis. Cervical tests can detect *N. gonorrhoeae* and *C. trachomatis* (see Chapter 11 for the test procedures).

Stool Guaiac (Colocare or Hemoccult). Diagnostic evaluation to detect gastrointestinal (GI) pathology as a possible source of pain (see Leiomyomas for the test procedure). The stool may be positive for occult blood in cases of ulcerative colitis, irritable bowel syndrome, GI polyps, or malignancy, although this test is not definitive. If the result is positive or if history and physical exam suggest, then refer the client for gastroenterology consultation and further diagnostic testing, such as upper GI series, barium enema, sigmoidoscopy, and/or colonoscopy.

Ultrasound. Diagnostic evaluation to identify and locate potential causes of pelvic pain (see Adenomyosis for the test procedure).

Laparoscopy. Diagnostic evaluation accomplished by direct visualization, performed when pelvic pathology is not detectable by pelvic exam or other diagnostic testing (see Endometriosis for the test procedure). Laparoscopy is useful in the diagnosis of acute or chronic salpingitis, ectopic pregnancy, hydrosalpinx, endometriosis, ovarian tumors and cysts, torsion, appendicitis, and adhesions. Clients may experience less anxiety about their symptoms when no serous pathology is found.[60] Researchers have been unable to demonstrate a direct correlation between laparoscopic findings and the severity of pelvic pain.[61]

DIFFERENTIAL MEDICAL DIAGNOSES

The evaluation of pelvic pain must differentiate between acute and chronic etiologies and gynecologic and nongynecologic. Table 13–4 summarizes common causes of pelvic pain.

Common medical conditions that are not gynecologic but may present as chronic pelvic pain include GI conditions, such as irritable bowel syndrome, ulcerative colitis, and diverticulosis; urinary tract disease; and neuromuscular/musculoskeletal disorders, such as disc problems.[57]

TABLE 13–4. COMMON CAUSES OF ACUTE AND CHRONIC PELVIC PAIN

Common GYN Causes of Acute Pelvic Pain	Common GYN Causes of Chronic Pelvic Pain
Ectopic pregnancy	Endometriosis
Salpingitis	Adenomyosis
Abortion	Uterine fibroids
Ruptured ovarian cyst	Chronic salpingitis
Adnexal torsion	Adhesions
Endometriosis	Dysmenorrhea
Menstruation	Dyspareunia
Ovulation pain	Pelvic relaxation
	Psychopathology/Enigmatic (30–50 percent)

Common NonGYN Causes of Acute Pelvic Pain	Common NonGYN Causes of Chronic Pelvic Pain
Appendicitis	Chronic appendicitis
Cystitis	Irritable bowel syndrome
Diverticulitis	Ulcerative colitis
Ureteral calculus	Diverticulosis
Gastroenteritis/Spastic colon	Urinary tract disease
Trauma	Neuromuscular disorders

Source: References 11, 57.

PLAN

Specific management of a client with chronic pelvic pain depends on the pain's etiology. Therefore, careful physical, psychosocial, and diagnostic evaluations represent the most important steps in providing care for these clients. Many clients, however, either fail to respond to therapy or do not demonstrate any known pathology.

The goal of care is to alleviate pain so that the client is able to maintain optimal daily functioning. The emotional, psychological, and physical aspects of the pain should be managed simultaneously.

Psychosocial Interventions

Listen carefully and demonstrate an attitude of caring and concern. Validate the fact that the client's symptoms are real. If she has one or more of the following indications, the refer her for skilled psychological evaluation and therapy.

- No apparent etiology for pain found during a thorough evaluation, including diagnostic laparoscopy.
- History of psychosexual trauma.

- History of consultation and therapy for multiple unrelated somatic symptoms.
- Symptoms of depression.

Review all findings with the client and involve her in decisions about care. If appropriate, involve the client's partner in planning care. Set realistic goals for evaluating therapy, stressing that a "cure" may not be possible. Refer the client for sexual counseling and therapy if indicated. Encourage her to keep a diary of the timing, location, and severity of the pain and the significant circumstance surrounding it.[55]

Medication

The goal of treatment with medication is to ameliorate pain, not eliminate it. Long-term narcotic use has been proved ineffective in the management of chronic pelvic pain and may lead to abuse and dependency behaviors.[55,57]

Nonsteroidal Anti-Inflammatory Drugs (NSAIDs). See section on Pelvic Organ Prolapse.

Antidepressants. Antidepressants are used to enhance the effectiveness of NSAIDs, manage simultaneous depression, and improve sleep patterns. Many different types are available, with varying side effects and actions. Tricyclic antidepressants have been most commonly used in the past. The Serotonin-reuptake inhibitors, for example, *Prozac* and *Zoloft* are increasingly used. See Chapter 23, Tables 23–1 and 23–2 for a comprehensive list with side effects and dosages.

The anticipated outcomes on evaluation are perception of decreased pain and less interference with the activities of daily living. Instruct the client to monitor her response to the drug and its side effects. Help ensure that the client takes the proper dose and understands the possible side effects.

Oral Contraceptives. Indicated for the management of cyclic, chronic pain, specifically that associated with dysmenorrhea, mild endometriosis, and recurrent functional ovarian cysts (see Endometriosis and Chapter 8, Dysmenorrhea).

GnRH Analogues. Indicated for the management of chronic pain associated with endometriosis and/or uterine fibroids (see sections on Endometriosis and Leiomyomas).

Dietary Interventions

Modifications in diet may be indicated when the client is experiencing constipation, bloating, edema, excessive fatigue, irritability, or lethargy, or is overweight. Dietary habits may contribute to the pain pattern, although not directly cause it.

Anticipated outcomes on evaluation are regular bowel movements without discomfort; decreased gas, bloating, and edema; improved energy level and stability of mood; and attainment and maintenance of ideal body weight.

Provide the client with information about the need for a high fiber diet and increased fluids to prevent constipation; explain how constipation can contribute to the pain pattern. In addition, less sodium, caffeine, and carbonated beverages reduce edema and abdominal bloating. Discuss with the client alternative cooking and seasoning methods, explain pertinent information on food labels, and suggest alternatives to soft drinks, coffee, and tea in order to limit intake of caffeine and carbonated beverages. Instruction may also include information about achieving stable blood sugar levels and weight loss by reducing refined carbohydrates and sugar in the diet and by eating low fat foods with fewer calories. Reinforce the information with printed materials.

Surgical Interventions

Laparoscopy. Indications are for the therapeutic as well as diagnostic purposes. Therapeutically, laparoscopy may be used for lysis of pelvic adhesions and ablation of endometrial implants.

Hysterectomy. This type of surgery is indicated when a known pathology is suspected to represent the source of pain, for example, leiomyomas, endometriosis, chronic PID, adenomyosis, or suspected malignancy. Pain that does not have a known or suspected etiology is not an indication for a hysterectomy; however, chronic pelvic pain is listed as the indication for 10 to 15 percent of the hysterectomies performed in the United States.[58] In a recent study, hysterectomy proved effective in ameliorating pain; however, 25 percent of the hysterectomy clients reported persistent pain one year after surgery.[61]

Alternative Interventions

Other interventions for the management of chronic pelvic pain include biofeedback, stress management techniques, self-hypnosis, relaxation therapy, transcutaneous nerve stimulation (TNS), trigger-point injections, spinal anesthesia, and nerve blocks. For many of these alternative interventions, referral to a chronic pelvic pain clinic is recommended.[55,57]

FOLLOW-UP AND REFERRAL

Regularly scheduled client appointments are crucial to the management of chronic pelvic pain. Visits are scheduled at intervals unrelated to specific pain episodes. Maintain consistent communication with the client, coordinate results of other providers' evaluations and therapies, and review this information with the client.[57]

CERVICITIS

Cervicitis is inflammation or ectopy of the cervix as evidenced by visual presence of yellow endocervical exudate, quantification of leukocytes in cervical exudate or histologic examination of the cervix. Cervical ectopy (ectopia, ectropion, eversion, erosion) refers to the extension of the columnar epithelium from the endocervix outward over the ectocervix, joining the squamous epithelium at the transformation zone, or squamocolumnar junction. Cervical ectopy without the presence of infection is a normal finding in most female adolescents and in women on oral contraceptives.[62]

EPIDEMIOLOGY

C. trachomatis is the most common organism infecting the cervix, present in over 66 percent of women seen at STD clinics.[49] *N. gonorrhoeae* is the next common organism, occurring along with *C. trachomatis* about 40 percent of the time.[63] Herpes simplex virus (HSV) and human papillomavirus are also common causes of cervicitis, with HPV playing a significant role in the development of cervical cancer.[49,63]

Acute or chronic infectious cervicitis is one of the most common gynecologic disorders affecting more than 50 percent of all women at some time during their adult life. Risk factors for the increased incidence of cervicitis include young age, early age of first intercourse, the presence of *C. trachomatis;* use of oral contraceptives, and sexual contact with men who have nongonococcal urethritis.

SUBJECTIVE DATA

Clients report purulent discharge, postcoital or postdouche vaginal spotting or bleeding.

OBJECTIVE DATA

Physical Examination

Red, edematous, often friable cervix, with the presence of tenacious, yellowish-white discharge. With trichomoniasis, the characteristic "strawberry" cervix is seen with grayish-green discharge.

Diagnostic Tests and Methods

Wet Mount. Microscopic examination of vaginal and cervical discharge for leukocytes, trichomoniasis, candida. See Chapter 5 on Assessment and Chapter 11 on Vaginitis and STDs.

Cultures. Obtain specific cultures for *C. trachomatis, N. gonorrhoeae, Herpes.* See Chapter 5 on Assessment and Chapter 11 on Vaginitis and STDs.

Pap Smear. Indicated to rule out early cervical neoplasia. See Chapter 5 on Assessment and this chapter on Screening for Gynecologic Cancers.

Colposcopy. Indicated if Pap smear shows atypia after repeated dysplasia or if cervicitis is persistent and/or unresponsive to medical therapy. If the practitioner has experience with colposcopic examination, he or she may proceed with evaluation, including biopsy. Otherwise, refer to a gynecologist.

DIFFERENTIAL MEDICAL DIAGNOSES

Ovulation (mucus of ovulation is clear with scant leukocytes); pelvic abscess or mass above the cervix; early neoplasia; syphilis; chronic granulomatous ulcerations of tuberculosis and granuloma inguinale.[63]

PLAN

Psychosocial

Discuss the disease process with the client, reviewing the anatomy and physiology of the vagina, cervix, and uterus. If there is abnormal bleeding, show the client where the bleeding is originating on the cervix, and reassure her that this does not represent an *abnormal period*. Discuss the purpose and importance of the Pap smear in the evaluation of cervicitis. Review the common causes of cervicitis and discuss how high risk sexual behaviors can contribute to the transmission of infection. Encourage the use of condoms. Provide the client with written information. Include the partner when possible and encourage him to be evaluated for the presence of any sexually transmitted diseases.

Medication

Antibiotic therapy should be based upon the specific etiology. See Chapter 11 for specific treatments. Discuss with the client the importance of taking prescribed medications correctly and of completing therapy.

Surgery

Surgical measures in the treatment of cervicitis are indicated for chronic cervicitis that is unresponsive to medical therapy and especially when accompanied by ectopy. Before any procedure is begun, colposcopic examination and biopsy, if indicated, should be performed to rule out cervical neoplasia. Common methods include the following:

- *Cryosurgery.* Destroys tissue by freezing with liquid CO_2, nitrogen, freon, or nitrous oxide. A probe is placed directly on the cervical os. Advantages include lack of discomfort, less postoperative bleeding, and less incidence of cervical stenosis. Adverse effects include heavy vaginal discharge for 2–3 weeks after the procedure.

- *Electrocauterization/Loop electrosurgical excision procedure (LEEP).* Employs the use of heat using a thin wire to incise and destroy diseased tissue. Advantages include good control of tissue destruction, and ability to perform in the office without the use of anesthesia. Adverse effects include postoperative bleeding and cervical stenosis.

- *Laser.* Use of directed laser to destroy diseased tissue. Advantages include lack of sloughing of tissue and no resulting leukorrhea, lack of scarring, and control of degree of cellular destruction.[63]

Outcomes on evaluation include destruction of infected tissues with subsequent healing by fibroplastic proliferation and reepitheliazation. Counsel the client about the procedure to be utilized and possible adverse effects. Explain that complete healing may take up to 6 weeks.

FOLLOW-UP AND REFERRAL

Complications of untreated cervicitis include leukorrhea, cervical stenosis, salpingitis, chronic infection of the urinary tract, and chronic cervicitis. Once treatment is initiated, have the client return in 2 weeks, and 4 to 8 weeks thereafter until resolved. Refer for further evaluation if the cervicitis does not resolve or if Pap smear reveals cervical intraepithelial neoplasia.

Bartholin's Gland Duct Cysts and Bartholinitis

The Bartholin's glands are two pea-sized glands located bilaterally beneath the vaginal vestibule. They are considered major mucous secreting glands, helping to lubricate the vestibule.[36]

A Bartholin's gland duct cyst results from obstruction of the gland leading to dilatation of the duct. Bartholinitis is the inflammation of one or both of the Bartholin's glands.[63]

EPIDEMIOLOGY

Obstruction of the duct may occur as a result of infection, inspissated mucous, or trauma. Secondary infection is commonly caused by

N. gonorrhoeae, staphylococcus, streptococcus, escherichia coli, trichomoniasis and bacteroides. Gonococcus is implicated about 20–30 percent of the time.[49]

Approximately 2 percent of adult women develop Bartholinitis.[64]

SUBJECTIVE DATA

May be asymptomatic; however, when size increases, inflammation develops, and clients report unilateral swelling of the labia; extreme tenderness, pain, and throbbing; dyspareunia; and pain when walking or sitting. The client may have a history of recurrent abscess.

OBJECTIVE DATA

Examination of the genitalia/reproductive tract may reveal erythema, acute tenderness, edema, a fluctuant mass located laterally to the vestibule, purulent drainage, tender and enlarged inguinal nodes.[64]

A culture and sensitivity test is done to identify the source of infection, especially with recurrent infection. Drainage from the gland is collected on a sterile swab. If gonorrhea is suspected, Thayer-Martin medium may be used for the culture. Explain the procedure to the client.[49]

DIFFERENTIAL MEDICAL DIAGNOSES

Inclusion cyst, sebaceous cyst, primary cancer of Bartholin's gland or duct (especially among women older than 40), secondary metastatic malignancy, lipoma, fibroma, hernia, hydrocele.[64]

PLAN

Psychosocial Interventions

Describe for the client how the infection occurs, and explain the treatment in detail. Allow time for questions and concerns to be expressed.

Medication

Broad Spectrum Antibiotics (Erythromycin, Doxycycline, Cephalosporins). Indicated when gonorrhea is suspected or identified (see Chapter 11). Administer erythromycin, 250 mg. p.o., q.i.d.

for 10 days; or doxycycline, 100 mg. p.o., b.i.d. for 10 days; or cephalexin, 250 mg. p.o., q.i.d. for 10 days.

A side effect is GI upset: contraindications include previous sensitivity to any of the aforementioned antibiotics. Doxycycline/tetracycline is contraindicated during pregnancy.

Anticipated outcomes on evaluation are relief of symptoms and resolution of infection/abscess. Instruct the client to take the medication with food (meal or snack) but not with milk, to complete the entire course of medication, and if taking doxycycline, to stay out of the sun or use sunscreen.

Analgesics. Used to relieve pain.

Surgical Interventions

Incision and Drainage/Insertion of Word Catheter. This procedure is done by a gynecologist in cases of abscess formation and when response to antibiotic therapy is inadequate. If a practitioner has specialized skills training and experience, he or she may place a word catheter. The procedure involves cleansing the area with povidone iodine (Betadine) and using local anesthetic, such as lidocaine (1 percent). A small incision is made approximately at the opening of the duct, and as much purulent drainage as possible is expressed. The cavity is explored for other pockets of infection. Finally, a word catheter (a bulb-tipped inflatable catheter that remains in the cyst) is inserted and 2 to 4 mL of sterile water is injected to hold the catheter in place for 4 to 6 weeks. The plugged end of the catheter is tucked into the vagina.

An adverse effect of overinflation of the bulb is pressure necrosis of the cyst wall with chronic defect.

The anticipated outcome on evaluation is complete resolution of the abscess and infection.

Provide the client with instructions to follow during the 4 to 6 weeks that the catheter is in place. The catheter is checked weekly and deflated as the abscess becomes smaller and drainage slows. The client may take sitz baths and warm soaks for comfort. Sexual intercourse is permitted as soon as tenderness subsides; care must be taken not to dislodge the catheter.[64]

Marsupialization. Creation of a pouch is performed in cases of recurrent abscess formation. Referral is made to a gynecologic surgeon, who performs the procedure on an outpatient basis using local, regional, or general anesthesia. After an incision is made over the cyst, exploration and drainage is performed if necessary, and the wall of the cyst is everted and fixed to the surrounding skin. Adverse effects, although rare, may include postoperative infection and pain.

The anticipated outcomes on evaluation are permanent drainage and no further cyst/abscess recurrences.[49,63]

Alternative Intervention

Rest, heat, and sitz baths may also be used to treat bartholinitis.

FOLLOW-UP AND REFERRAL

Follow-up for conservative treatment (antibiotics, rest, heat) should occur 7 to 10 days after the treatment is begun. Swelling, pain, erythema, and tenderness or throbbing should be resolved or resolving. If a word catheter is inserted, follow up weekly. A 4 to 6 week follow-up is appropriate for marsupialization.[64]

CERVICAL POLYPS

Cervical polyps are benign, pedunculated growths of varying size that extend from the ectocervix or endocervical canal. Polyps may occur singularly or they may be multiple.[63]

EPIDEMIOLOGY

The etiology is unknown. Polyps are believed to result from chronic inflammation, however; they may be associated with hyperestrogen states; and they are found commonly with endometrial hyperplasia. Polyps are most common among multiparous women in their thirties and forties.

Cervical polyps are the most common benign neoplastic growths of the cervix and occur in 4 percent of all gynecologic clients.[64]

SUBJECTIVE DATA

The client is usually asymptomatic, although thick leukorrhea, postcoital bleeding, intermenstrual bleeding, menorrhagia, postmenopausal bleeding, or mucopurulent or blood tinged vaginal discharge may occur.[63]

OBJECTIVE DATA

Physical Examination

Single or multiple pear shaped growths may protrude from the cervix into the vaginal canal. They are usually smooth, soft, reddish purple to cherry red, and readily bleed when touched. They may be small or very large.

Diagnostic Tests and Methods

Pathology. A diagnostic microscopic evaluation of all polyps should be done by a pathologist; diagnosis is confirmed during evaluation. This requires collection of a specimen to be labeled and sent in preservative medium to a pathology laboratory. (See Surgical Interventions, following, for a description of the procedure.)

Explain the procedure to the client and tell her when she can expect test results. Reassure her that the majority of polyps are benign.

Papanicolaou (Pap) Smear. See Chapter 5.

DIFFERENTIAL MEDICAL DIAGNOSES

Endometrial polyps, small prolapsed myomas, cervical malignancy.[64]

PLAN

Psychosocial Interventions

Explain to the client what polyps are and that they are usually benign; encourage her to express her concerns.

Surgical Interventions

Cervical polyps should be removed and sent to a pathology laboratory. The procedure can be performed in an office without anesthesia by any appropriately trained health care provider. Paint the cervix with povidone-iodine (Betadine); using ring forceps, grasp and twist the polyp at the base. Apply silver nitrate or Monsel's solution to the site of removal to control bleeding. Excessive bleeding is a potential adverse effect.

Client teaching includes the need for pelvic rest for 24 hours to ensure that bleeding does not occur at the removal site. If excessive bleeding or excessive vaginal discharge does occur, the client must return for evaluation and possible endometrial sampling.

Treatment of Vaginal Infections

Accompanying vaginal infections must be treated appropriately (see Chapter 11).

FOLLOW-UP AND REFERRAL

Regular Pap smears and gynecologic exams are important, and this needs to be stressed to the client.

GYNECOLOGIC CANCERS: SCREENING AND REFERRAL

CIN AND CERVICAL CANCER

Invasive carcinoma of the cervix is decreasing in incidence in the United States due to the effectiveness of Pap smear screening programs and early treatment.[65] There has been an increase, however, in the prevalence of dysplasia and preinvasive lesions.[66] It is important that the practitioner be aware of the most common risk factors for CIN and cervical cancer, currently recommended screening protocols, and appropriate follow-up.

Cervical intrapepithelial neoplasia (CIN) is defined as "the spectrum of intraepithelial changes beginning as with a well-differentiated neoplasm, traditionally classified as mild dysplasia, and ending with invasive carcinoma" (p. 347).[66]

Cervical cancer (CIS) occurs when malignant cells penetrate the underlying basement membrane of the epithelium and infiltrate the stroma, now considered invasive cervical cancer.

Epidemiology

In 1995, there were 15,800 cases of invasive cervical cancer in the United States with 4800 deaths.[65] Recent data reveal that the incidence of cervical cancer in the United States is about 8–9 percent, with higher rates reported in Native Americans, Hispanics, African Americans, and Filipinos.[66] The lowest rates occur in Japanese women.[66] African American women have about twice the age adjusted incidence rate per 100,000 women compared with white women.[66,67] Cervical cancer is the third most common cancer among women in the United States and is the second most common worldwide.[65,66]

Human papillomavirus infection is highly prevalent, detected in one-third of American female college students and is associated with cervical cancer. HPV types 16 and 18 are the most prevalent types.

Risk Factors
- Early age at first intercourse.
- Multiple sexual partners.
- First child prior to age 20.
- Lower socioeconomic status.
- History of sexually transmitted diseases (STDs, especially HPV).
- Exposure to diethylstilbestrol (DES) in utero.
- Cigarette smoking.[65–67]

Screening. Screening for cervical cancer is very effective because of the presence of a precursor lesion, cervical intraepithelial neoplasm (CIN). The goal of screening is to identify the precursor lesions at an early stage before progression to malignancy. Fortunately, these precursor lesions appear to have a long latent phase in most cases.[67]

Screening is performed using the Pap smear (see Chapter 5). Along with the spatula, the Cytobrush or the Cytopick is now recommended to obtain better endocervical samples in nonpregnant women.[68]

Most recently, several new methods of cervical cancer screening are appearing including the following:

- Automated slide thin-layer preparation. The collection instrument is rinsed in a vial of liquid preservative, which is sent to the laboratory. Slides are then prepared with automated equipment. The major advantage is that specimen quality is improved.

- Automated readers. An automated microscope conveys a picture to a computer where it is analyzed. May be used as a quality control method.
- Denvu. Uses colposcopy to obtain a digital image of a section of the cervix, which is then computer analyzed. Advantages are that the slides can be sent by modem for consultations, made into slides, or compared with later images.
- Cervicography. Photographs of the cervix are obtained and enlarged, allowing physicians to read results as in reading x-rays. Disadvantage is that it may miss low grade lesions.

Although none of these techniques is currently accepted as standard of care, they are under development and may be employed in the future.[69]

The American College of Obstetricians and Gynecologists and the American Cancer Society recommend that annual screening commence when women become sexually active or reach the age of 18 years. If three or more consecutive annual examinations have been normal in a low risk client, then Pap tests may be performed less frequently at the practitioner's discretion. It is appropriate to continue to perform annual Pap tests in women considered to be at high risk for cervical cancer on the basis of the known risk factors.[65]

Management of Abnormal Results. Management of abnormal Pap results remains somewhat controversial with varying opinions on how to follow low grade abnormalities such as atypical squamous cells of undetermined significance (*ascus*). Using the Bethesda system, the currently accepted method of reporting Pap smear results (see Chapter 5), the following are commonly accepted guidelines.[70]

- With normal findings, repeat screening every year (see ACOG and American Cancer Society guidelines above).
- Inflammatory changes, atypia, or ASCUS. Reevaluate for evidence of a specific infecting organism (e.g., Chlamydia trachomatis, Neisseria gonorrhoeae, Candida albicans, Trichomonas vaginalis) or bacterial vaginosis, and appropriate treatment should be started. Repeat

the Pap smear 2 to 3 months after treatment. If still abnormal, refer.
- CIN of any grade (*mild, moderate, or severe dysplasia*). Refer for colposcopic examination and biopsy. CIN 1 is equated with the low grade squamous intraepithelial lesion (SIL); CIN 2 and 3 with high grade SIL (Bethesda System).

Treatment Modalities. The practitioner should be aware of current treatment modalities for CIN:

- *Cryosurgery.* Destroys tissue by freezing with liquid CO_2, nitrogen, freon, or nitrous oxide. A probe is placed directly on the cervical os. Studies show a 90 percent cure rate. Advantages include lack of discomfort, less postoperative bleeding, and less incidence of cervical stenosis. Adverse effects include heavy vaginal discharge for 2–3 weeks after the procedure.
- *Loop Electrosurgical Excision Procedure (LEEP).* Employs the use of heat using a thin wire to incise and destroy diseased tissue. Studies show a 95 percent cure rate, slightly better than the rate of cryosurgery or laser. Advantages include good control of tissue destruction and ability to perform in the office without the use of anesthesia. Adverse effects include postoperative bleeding and cervical stenosis.[71] LEEP can also be used to both biopsy and treat within the same procedure. This should only be performed, however, when results are unequivocal intraepithelial lesions.[71]
- *Laser.* Use of directed laser to destroy diseased tissue. Advantages include lack of sloughing of tissue and no resulting leukorrhea; lack of scarring and control of degree of cellular destruction.[63,66]
- *Cone Biopsies.* Removal of a cone shaped section of cervical tissue, including a portion of the endocervix indicated in higher grade or invasive lesions. Can be performed using LEEP, laser, or *cold knife conization.*

Prevention and Education
- Encourage clients to recognize their personal risk factors and to obtain annual screening.
- Encourage prevention of STDs and reduction of risk factors.
- Advocate postponing sexual activity when counseling adolescents.

- Encourage the use of barrier methods of contraception.
- Encourage smoking cessation.

UTERINE CANCER

Endometrial or uterine cancer is the most common gynecologic malignancy.[72] It may occur with exposure of the endometrium to high levels of exogenous and/or endogenous estrogen.

Epidemiology

In 1995, an estimated 32,800 new cases of cancer of the corpus uteri were found, causing about 5900 women to die. It is the eighth most common malignancy in women worldwide, and the fourth most common in the United States. Its incident rate in the United States is about 20 percent. It occurs more frequently in caucasian and Hawaiian women, moderately in African Americans, Japanese, and Chinese women, and less frequently in Filipino, Korean, and Native American women. It has one of the highest survival rates of all cancers.[72]

Risk Factors
- Unopposed estrogen replacement.
- Obesity.
- Nulliparity or low parity.
- History of diabetes.
- History of hypertension.
- Menopause.
- Chronic anovulation.

Screening. The incidence of uterine cancer in women younger than 40 is low; hence routine screening of these women is not recommended. Screening of all women over age 40 is neither practical nor cost effective. The criteria used in performing endometrial sampling include the following:

- Any unexplained peri- or postmenopausal bleeding.
- Premenopausal clients with polycystic ovarian syndrome.
- Premenopausal clients taking unopposed exogenous estrogen.
- Obese, nulliparous clients with diabetes or hypertension.
- Tamoxifen therapy (baseline, then annually).[67,72]

Techniques for endometrial sampling vary. Screening is performed by an experienced gynecologist, usually in an office without anesthesia. Fractional dilation and curettage (D & C) in a hospital may be required in some circumstances.

The most commonly used and easiest technique is the pipelle biopsy. It can be performed by the nurse practitioner if he or she has experience and training in the appropriate setting. It employs the use of a slender suction catheter to obtain a small amount of tissue for pathology.[73]

Transvaginal ultrasonography for measuring the endometrial lining is a new method that is showing promise in detecting possible endometrial hyperplasia. If the endometrial lining measures less than 4 mm, then the client is at lower risk.[14,73]

Follow-Up and Referral

Any high risk client (see criteria for endometrial sampling) should be followed with regular biopsies. Positive findings warrant immediate referral to an experienced gynecologist.

Prevention and Education. Prevention should be aimed at weight management and control of obesity, the use of a progestin in hormone replacement therapy, and the early evaluation of any abnormal bleeding.[67]

OVARIAN CANCER

Epidemiology

Ovarian cancer is the seventh most common cancer in women worldwide, the second most common gynecologic cancer, and the leading cause of death from gynecologic malignancies. There were an estimated 26,600 cases of ovarian cancer in the United States with 14,500 women dying from the disease. Ovarian cancer has the highest incidence in developed countries and the lowest incidence in developing countries.[74] It has a higher incidence among caucasians and Hawaiian women, moderate risk in African American, Hispanic, and Asian women, and the lowest incidence among Native American women.

Risk Factors
- Age greater than 45.
- Postmenopause.

- Periods of prolonged ovulation without pregnancy.
- Mother or sister with ovarian cancer, colon, or breast cancer.
- Father or brother with colon cancer.
- Caucasian.
- High fat diet.
- Possibly, use of fertility drugs.[67,75]

Screening. No effective method of mass screening has yet been developed. Publicity has increased the public's awareness of the difficulty of early detection. Clients may ask about routine ultrasound and CA-125, although neither method is currently recommended for routine screening due to expense and poor sensitivity and reliability. It may be used in women with a first degree relative with ovarian cancer or with a combination of the above risk factors.[75] An annual bimanual examination is currently recommended. Symptoms of ovarian cancer are not specific, i.e., abdominal fullness and bloating, pain, or intestinal complaints.[67,74]

Follow-Up and Referral

Any postmenopausal client with a palpable ovary or mass should be referred for laparoscopic evaluation. Any woman who has completed childbearing and who has a first degree relative with ovarian cancer should be considered for a prophylactic bilateral oophorectomy.[74]

Prevention and Education. Pregnancy and oral contraceptives both lower the total number of ovulatory cycles in a woman's lifetime and decrease the risk of ovarian cancer. Discuss the known risk factors with the client. Emphasize the lack of good screening methods and encourage compliance with the annual gynecologic exam. Maintain a healthy weight and low fat diet.

VULVAR INTRAEPITHELIAL NEOPLASIA AND VULVAR CANCER

Vulvar intraepithelial neoplasia (VIN) is a cancer precursor that is often associated with human papillomavirus.[76] It is classified just as cervical intraepithelial neoplasia as VIN 1-3, based upon the grade of undifferentiated cells. Invasive vulvar cancer is the presence of a lesion that breaks through the basement membrane.[77] Although the

incidence of vulvar cancer has remained stable over the past several years, the incidence of VIN is increasing.[76]

Epidemiology

The incidence of VIN in the United States has increased from 1.2 to 2.1 per 100,000 women in the last 20 years.[77] It has increased significantly in caucasian women under age 35 years. Vulvar cancer is responsible for 1 percent of all malignancies in women and 3–5 percent of all female genital cancers.

Vulvar cancer is predominately found in older women, increasing to more than 50 percent of cases in women age 70 years and older.[77]

Risk Factors
- Young age at first intercourse.
- Lifetime history of multiple sexual partners.
- History of sexually transmitted disease.[78]
- Smoking.
- Infrequent Pap smears.
- HPV infection.[77]

Screening. The diagnosis of vulvar carcinoma is almost always delayed because symptoms are similar to other conditions. Vulvar pruritis is the most consistent complaint, and women will self-treat with over-the-counter vaginal preparations.

Simple inspection of the vulva with biopsy of suspicious lesions is the only available screening method. Careful inspection of the vulva should be an essential part of any physical examination, especially in high-risk clients.[76] Physical examination may reveal some of the various lesions.

Paget disease presents with extreme pruritis and soreness, usually of long duration. Red or bright pink, desquamated, eczematoid areas among scattered, raised, white patches of hyperkeratosis. The borders are well-demarcated and raised.

Basal cell carcinoma is very rare and is associated with a long history of pruritis. The carcinoma occurs over the anterior two-thirds of the labia majora, with slightly elevated margins.

Verrucous carcinoma appears as condyloma, but does not respond to treatment. Invasive squamous cell carcinoma occurs when a woman is in her 60s and 70s. It presents with ulceration, friability, or induration of surrounding tissues.

A melanoma of the vulva involves the labia minora and clitoris. It is a darkly pigmented lesion, rare among African American women. Any recent growths, changes in appearance of existing moles, or bleeding of growths should be investigated. Sarcoma occurs in women of all ages. The vulvar sarcoma is a rapidly expanding, painful mass.

Follow-Up and Referral

Any client with a persistent lesion of the vulva should be referred to a gynecologist for colposcopy, biopsy, and further evaluation and treatment.[67]

Prevention and Education. Teach clients self-examination and advise them to seek evaluation of any persistent itching or unusual lesions. Encourage smoking cessation. Advise clients to avoid constricting undergarments and perfumes and dyes in the vulvar region. Advocate condom use and prevention of STDs. Perform or refer for biopsy for any suspicious lesions.[77]

DIETHYLSTILBESTROL (DES) EXPOSURE

DES was used extensively in the United States during the 1940s and early 1950s to treat pregnancy complications, including bleeding, premature labor, diabetes, and preeclampsia.[11] Although studies during the late 1950s proved its ineffectiveness, DES use continued through 1971. An estimated 5 to 10 million were prescribed DES during pregnancy or were exposed to the drug in utero.[79]

DES Exposure Sequelae

Women exposed to DES may exhibit one or more of the following sequelae:

- Structural changes including transverse vaginal and cervical ridges (cocks combs, collars, and pseudopolyps), abnormally shaped uterine cavity, uterine hypoplasia.
- Vaginal adenosis with columnar epithelium on or beneath the vaginal muscosa; it is self-limiting and gradually disappears.
- Clear-cell adenocarcinoma of the cervix or vagina (incidence rises at age 15 and median age at diagnosis is 19 years).

- Increased incidences of spontaneous abortion, ectopic pregnancy, premature cervical dilation, and premature rupture of membranes.
- Increased incidence of breast cancer.

Risk. Women who were born in the United States between 1945 and 1971 to mothers who had complicated pregnancies and received DES.[11]

Screening. All women born between 1940 and 1971 should be questioned about possible exposure to DES. If history suggests exposure, the following screening techniques may be employed.

- An initial examination is recommended following menarche or at age 14 if no menarche; routine examination is every 6 to 12 months thereafter and includes inspection, palpation, and cytology.
- Cytology requires vaginal scrapings taken from all four quadrants of the fornix and fixed on slides for cytological review.[80]
- Careful inspection of the cervix and vagina using one-half strength Lugol's solution and palpation of the entire vaginal wall.[80]
- Colposcopy is performed by an experienced colposcopist if the Pap smear is abnormal. Appropriate biopsies are done for evaluation.
- DES daughters should be followed as high risk obstetric patients because of the increased risk of spontaneous abortion, ectopic pregnancy, early cervical effacement, and premature labor.

Follow-Up and Referral

Any abnormal cytology or undiagnosed lesion requires referral to a gynecologist.

Provide the client with information about DES and its possible effects. Stress the importance of having a regular examination and cytology. Allow time for the client to express her concerns. In addition, stress that DES exposure is not known to interfere with fertility, although there may be some risk of premature delivery. Practitioners are encouraged to refer women with known in utero exposure to centers that have focused on the follow-up, treatment and education of these women. There are no known contraindications to oral contraceptive use.

Third generation DES exposed women are now being studied for any possible long-term effects of exposure.[80]

Nursing diagnoses

The following nursing diagnoses are representative of those used in the health care plan of women with gynecologic pelvic disorders. The list, however, is by no means inclusive.

- Activity intolerance, potential for.
- Altered patterns of urination.
- Altered patterns of sexuality.
- Altered family processes.
- Altered comfort; pain, chronic pain.
- Altered bowel elimination; dyschezia, constipation.
- Altered role performance.
- Anxiety.
- Disturbance in self-concept, self-esteem, body image.
- Fear.
- Hopelessness.
- Hyperthermia.
- Impaired mobility.
- Incontinence.
- Ineffective coping; family, individual.
- Knowledge deficit concerning sexual function, technique, etiology of pain.
- Post-trauma response.
- Potential for infection.
- Potential for decreased tissue perfusion secondary to anemia.
- Potential activity intolerance.
- Potential fluid volume deficit.
- Powerlessness.
- Rape trauma syndrome.
- Sensory alterations.
- Sexual dysfunction or altered sexual patterns.
- Sleep pattern disturbance.
- Social isolation.

REFERENCES

1a. Readers are encouraged to review the revised classification of endometriosis appearing in the May 1997 issue of *Fertility and Sterility* (Volume 67, No. 5, pages 817–821). This revised classification provides a standardized form for recording pathologic findings and assigning scalar values to disease status in order to better predict the probability of pregnancy following treatment.

1. Lu, P. Y., & Org, S. J. (1995). Endometriosis: Current management. *Mayo Clinic Proceedings, 70,* 453–463.

2. Speroff, L., Glass, R. H., & Kase, N. G. (1994). *Clinical gynecologic endocrinology and infertility* (5th ed.). Baltimore: Williams and Wilkins.

3. Sangai-Haghpeykar, H., & Poindexter, A. N. (1995). Epidemiology of endometriosis among parous women. *Obstetrics and Gynecology, 85,* 983–992.

4. Pittaway, D. E. (1996). Management options for infertile patients with endometriosis. *Contemporary OB-GYN, 5,* 27–50.

5. Keltz, M. D., & Olive, D. L. (1993). Diagnostic and therapeutic options in endometriosis. *Hospital Practice, 10,* 15–31.

6. Koninckx, P. R., Meuleman, C., Oosterlynck, D., et al. (1996). Diagnosis of deep endometriosis by clinical examination during menstruation and plasma CA-125 concentration. *Fertility and Sterility, 65,* 280–287.

7. Waller, K. G., & Shaw, R. W. (1995). Endometriosis, pelvic pain, and psychological functioning. *Fertility and Sterility, 63,* 796–800.

8. Adamson, G. D. Kwei, L., & Edgren, R. A. (1994). Pain of endometriosis; Effects of Nafarelin and Danazol therapy. *International Journal of Fertility, 39,* 215–217.

9. Carter, J. E., & Trotter, P. P. (1995). GnRH analogs in the treatment of endometriosis, clinical and economical considerations. *The Female Patient, 20,* 13–18.

10. Winkel, C. A. (1994). Gonadotropin-releasing hormone agonists; Current uses for these increasingly important drugs. *Postgraduate Medicine, 95,* 111–118.

11. Seltzer, V. L., & Pearse, W. H. (1995). *Women's primary health care.* New York: McGraw-Hill.

12. Siegler, A. M., & Camilien, L. (1994). Adenomyosis. *The Journal of Reproductive Medicine, 39,* 841–853.

13. American College of Obstetricians and Gynecologists. (1993). Gynecologic ultrasonography. *ACOG Technical Bulletin,* No. 215.

14. Arnold, L. L., Ascher, S. M., Schruefer, J. J., et al. (1995). The nonsurgical diagnosis of adenomyosis. *Obstetrics and Gynecology, 86,* 461–465.

15. Peipert, J. F., Boardman, L., Hogan, J. W., et al. (1996). Laboratory evaluation of acute upper genital tract infection. *Obstetrics and Gynecology, 87,* 730–736.

16. Sweet, R. L. (1996). *Pelvic inflammatory disease.* Presentation at the 20th annual Post-Graduate Seminar, University of Pennsylvania. Philadelphia, PA.

17. Soper, D. E., Brockwell, N. J., Dalton, H. P., & Johnson, D. (1994). Observations concerning the microbial etiology of acute salpingitis. *American Journal of Obstetrics and Gynecology, 170,* 1008–1017.

18. Joessens, M. R., Schachter, J., & Sweet, R. L. (1994). Risk factors associated with pelvic inflammatory disease of differing microbial etiology. *Obstetrics and Gynecology, 83,* 989–997.

19. Wolner-Hanssen, P. (1995). Silent pelvic inflammatory disease, is it overstated? *Obstetrics and Gynecology, 86,* 321–325.

20. Centers for Disease Control and Prevention. (1993). Sexually transmitted diseases treatment guidelines. *MMWR, 42* (no. RR-14).

21. ACOG. (1996). *Guidelines for women's health care.* Washington, DC: Author.

22. Jossens, M. O., Eskenazi, B., Schachter, J., & Sweet, R. L. (1995, May–June). Risk factors for pelvic inflammatory disease: A case control study. *Sexually Transmitted Diseases,* 239–247.

23. Apuzzio, J. J., & Pelosi, M. A. (1989). The "new" salpingitis: Subtle symptoms, aggressive management. *Female Patient, 14,* 25–66.

24. Hacker, N. F., & Moore, J. G. (1992). *Essential of obstetrics and gynecology* (2nd ed.). Philadelphia: Saunders.

25. Barber, H. R. K., Creasman, W. T., & Knapp, R. C. (1993). A rational approach to ovarian masses. *Patient Care, 12,* 50–72.

26. Curtin, J. P. (1994). Management of the adnexal mass. Gynecologic Oncology. 55: 542–546.

27. American College of Obstetricians and Gynecologists. (1993). Disorders of the Ovaries. Precis V., 255–260.

28. Steege, J. (1995). Chronic pelvic pain and dyspareunia. In Seltzer, V. and Pearse, W., Women's Primary Health Care. New York: McGraw-Hill.

29. American College of Obstetricians and Gynecologists. (1993). Sexuality and Sexual Dysfunction. Precis V. 97–103.

30. Glatt, A. E., Zinner, S. H., & McCormack, W. M. (1990). The prevalence of dyspareunia. *Obstetrics and Gynecology, 75,* 433–436.

31. Steege, J. F., & Ling, F. W. (1993). Dyspareunia, a special type of chronic pelvic pain. *Obstetrics and Gynecology Clinics of North America, 20,* 779–793.

32. Baggish, M. S., & Miklos, J. R. (1995). Vulvar pain syndrome: A review. *Obstetrical and Gynecological Survey, 50,* 618–627.

33. Spadt, S. K. (1995). Suffering in silence: Managing vulvar pain patients. *Contemporary Nurse Practitioner, 1,* 32–38.

34. Paavonen, J. (1995). Diagnosis and treatment of vulvodynia. *Annals of Medicine, 27,* 175–181.

35. Paavonen, J. (1995). Vulvodynia—A complex syndrome of vulvar pain. *Acta Obstetriciaa et Gynecologica Scandinavica, 74,* 243–247.

36. Lynch, P. J., & Edwards, L. (1994). *Genital dermatology.* New York: Churchill Livingstone, Inc.

37. Apgar, B. S., & Cox, J. T. (1996). Differentiating normal and abnormal findings of the vulva. *American Family Physician, 53,* 1171–1180.

38. McKay, M. (1992). Vulvodynia: Diagnostic patterns. *Dermatologic Clinics, 10,* 423–433.

39. Clarke-Secor, R. M., & Fertitta, L. (1992). Vulvar vestibulitis syndrome. *Nurse Practitioner Forum, 3,* 161–168.

40. McKay, M. (1993). Dyesthetic ("essential") vulvodynia, treatment with amitriptyline. *Journal of Reproductive Medicine, 38,* 9–13.

41. Greenberg, M. D., & Kazamel, T. I. G. (1995). Medical and socioeconomic impact of uterine fibroids. *Obstetric and Gynecology Clinics of North America, 22,* 625–636.

42. ACOG. (1994). Uterine Leiomyomata. *ACOG Technical Bulletin* (No. 192). Author.

43. Hutchins, F. L. (1995). Uterine fibroids, diagnosis and indications for treatment. *Obstetric and Gynecologic Clinics of North America, 22,* 659–665.

44. Davis, K. M., & Schlaff, W. D. (1995). Medical management of uterine fibromyomata. *Obstetric and Gynecologic Clinics of North America, 22,* 727–738.

45. Prather, C. (1995). Hysteroscopy: The nurses' role in office hysteroscopy. *JOGNN, 24,* 813–816.

46. Siegler, A. M. (1995). Office hysteroscopy. *Obstetric and Gynecologic Clinics of North America, 22,* 457–471.

47. Hutchins, F. L. (1995). Abdominal myomectomy as a treatment for symptomatic uterine fibroids. *Obstetric and Gynecologic Clinics of North America, 22,* 781–789.

48. American College of Obstetricians and Gynecologists. (1993). Anatomic support defects and dysfunction. *Precis V,* 230–234.

49. Ryan, K. J., Berkowitz, R. S., & Barbieri, R. L. (1995). *Kistner's gynecology.* St. Louis: Mosby.

50. Davila, G. W. (1996). Vaginal prolapse, management with nonsurgical techniques. *Postgraduate Medicine, 99,* 171–185.

51. Caputo, R. M., & Benson, J. T. (1993). The Q-tip test and urethrovesical junction mobility. *Obstetrics and Gynecology, 82,* 892–896.

52. Weber, A. M., Walters, M. D., Schover, L. R., et al. (1995). Sexual function in women with uterovaginal prolapse and urinary incontinence. *Obstetrics and Gynecology, 85,* 483–487.

53. Mathias, S. D., Kupperman, M., Liberman, R. F., et al. (1996). Chronic pelvic pain: Prevailing health-related quality of life, and economic correlates. *Obstetrics and Gynecology, 87,* 321–327.

54. Stenchever, M. A. (1990). Symptomatic retrodisplacement, pelvic congestion, universal joint, and peritoneal defects: Fact or fiction? *Clinical Obstetrics and Gynecology, 33,* 161–176.

55. Milburn, A., Reiter, R. C., & Rhomberg, A. T. (1993). Multidisciplinary approach to chronic pelvic pain. *Obstetrics and Gynecology Clinics of North America, 20,* 643–661.

56. Jamieson, D. J., & Steege, J. F. (1996). The prevalence of dysmenorrhea, dyspareunia, pelvic pain and irritable bowel syndrome in primary care practices. *Obstetrics and Gynecology, 87,* 55–58.

57. American College of Obstetricians and Gynecologists. (1996). Chronic pelvic pain. *ACOG Technical Bulletin* (No. 223). Author.

58. Reiter, R. C. (1990). A profile of women with chronic pelvic pain. *Clinical Obstetric and Gynecology, 33,* 130–136.

59. Baker, P. K. (1993). Musculoskeletal origins of chronic pelvic pain. *Obstetric and Gynecology Clinics of North America, 20,* 719–742.

60. Lipscomb, G. H., & Ling, F. W. (1993). Relationship of pelvic infection and chronic pelvic pain. *Obstetrics and Gynecology Clinics of North America, 20,* 643–661.

61. Hillis, S. D., Marchbanks, R. A., & Peterson, H. B. (1995). The effectiveness for hysterectomy for chronic pelvic pain. *Obstetrics and Gynecology, 86,* 941–945.

62. Critchlow, C. W., Wolner-Hanssen, P., Eschenbach, D. A., et al. (1995). Determinants of cervical ectopia and of cervicitis: Age, oral contraception, specific cervical infection, smoking, and douching. *American Journal of Obstetrics and Gynecology, 173,* 534–543.

63. DeCherney, A. H., & Pernoll, M. L. *Current obstetric and gynecologic diagnosis and treatment.* Norwalk: CT: Appleton & Lange.

64. American College of Obstetricians and Gynecologists. (1993). Bartholin duct cyst and abscess. *Precis V,* 227–228.

65. Cannistra, S. A., & Niloff, J. M. (1996). Cancer of the uterine cervix. *The New England Journal of Medicine, 334,* 1030–1038.

66. Morris, M., Tortolero-Luna, G., Malpica, A., et al. (1996). Cervical intraepithelial neoplasia and cervical cancer. *Obstetrics and Gynecology Clinics of North America, 23,* 347–410.

67. Huff, B. C. (1996). Prevention, screening and early detection of gynecologic cancers. *Voice (AWHONN), 4, 1,* 11–12.

68. Shingleton, H. M., Roman, L. P., Johnston, W. W., & Smith, R. A. (1995). The current of status of the Papanicolaou smear. *CA-A Cancer Journal for Clinicians, 45,* 305–320.

69. McNeil, C. (1995). Novel technologies for cervical cancer screening seen on the horizon. *Journal of the National Cancer Institute, 87,* 789–790.

70. Nuovo, J., Melnikow, J., & Paliescheskey, M. (1995). Management of patients with atypical and low-grade Pap smear abnormalities. *American Family Physician, 52,* 2243–2250.

71. Ferenczy, A., Choukroun, D., & Arseneau, J. (1996). Loop electrosurgical excision procedure for squamous intraepithelial lesions of the cervix: Advantages and potential pitfalls. *Obstetrics and Gynecology, 87,* 332–337.

72. Burke, T. W., Tortolero-Luna, G., Malpica, A., et al. (1996). Endometrial hyperplasia and endometrial cancer. *Obstetrics and Gynecology Clinics of North America, 23,* 411–456.

73. Patsner, B. (1993, March). Screening for gynecologic malignancies in primary care: Uterine cancer. *Emergency Medicine,* 157–161.

74. Gershenson, D. M. (1996). Ovarian intraepithelial neoplasia and ovarian cancer. *Obstetrics and Gynecology Clinics of North America, 23,* 475–543.

75. Piver, M. S. (1993, March). Screening for gynecologic malignancies in primary care: Ovarian cancer. *Emergency Medicine,* 141–148.

76. Hording, U., Junge, J., Hemming, P., et al. (1995). Vulvar intraepithelial neoplasia III: A viral disease of undetermined progressive potential. *Gynecologic Oncology, 56,* 276–279.

77. Edwards, C. L., Tortolero-Luna, G., Linares, A. C., et al. (1996). Vulvar intraepithelial neoplasia and vulvar cancer. *Obstetrics and Gynecology Clinics of North America, 23,* 295–345.

78. Trimble, C. L., Hildesheim, A., Brinton, L., et al. (1996). Heterogeneous etiology of squamous carcinoma of the vulva. *Obstetrics and Gynecology, 87,* 59–64.

79. Guiste, R. M., Iwamoto, K., & Hatch, E. E. (1995). Diethylstilbestrol revisited: A review of the long-term health effects. *Annals of Internal Medicine, 122,* 778–788.

80. Wilcox, A. J., Umbach, D. M., Hornsby, P. P., et al. (1995). Age at menarche among diethylstilbestrol granddaughters. *American Journal of Obstetrics and Gynecology, 173,* 835–836.

CHAPTER 14

BREAST HEALTH

Lynette Galloway Branch

*T*horough breast assessment, including history taking for risk factors and education regarding BSE, should be standard protocol for the health provider during a client's annual exam.

Highlights

- Breast Examination: Professional, Self-Exam, and Mammography
- Benign Breast Disorders
    Fibrocystic Changes
    Fibroadenoma
    Nipple Discharge
- Malignant Neoplasms
- Breast Reconstruction
    Tissue Transfer
    Augmentation Mammoplasty
    Mastopexy
    Breast Reduction

▶ INTRODUCTION

The female breast is closely linked with womanhood in the American culture. The more amply endowed the female bosom, the "sexier" and more womanly one is perceived. Although the primary function of the breasts is lactation, breasts are perceived as erotic. They are attractive and alluring to men and a source of sensual pleasure for women as well. Thus, the loss or injury of these important anatomic structures is potentially psychologically devastating to both sexes.

For women in their childbearing years, breast injury or loss threatens the ability to nourish and nurture offspring by means of breastfeeding. This intimate, interactional process may be perceived as the ultimate way of connecting and communicating with a newborn. Middle-age women, who have begun to observe the effects of aging on their bodies, may perceive breast loss or injury as an additional change to their once youthful appearing bodies. Elderly women, who are living longer, desire to maintain their fitness, which entails keeping their bodies healthy and intact. Hence, maintaining breast health is conducive to maintaining optimal physical and psychological health.

Concerns about breasts and breast symptoms are among the most common complaints of women who seek medical attention. Although most concerns have no disease or have benign changes as their underlying condition, the fear of cancer causes great anxiety and stress for most women who have any breast symptoms. This anxiety is indeed warranted since breast cancer now occurs in one of every eight women and is the second most common occurring cancer in women.[1]

Since concerns about breast health are common in primary care settings and since the primary care provider is most often the first point of contact in today's health delivery system, it is important that health care providers have substantial knowledge about breast related disorders and diseases. A basic understanding of the most severe form of breast disease—cancer—is paramount so that immediate referral can be made and mortality reduced.

BREAST EXAMINATION AND ASSESSMENT

Breast examination has a pivotal role in the early detection of breast cancer and diseases. This examination may be carried out by a health professional, the client herself, or by means of mammography. Breast self-examination (BSE) is practiced today by many women. In fact, it has been found that breast cancer patients who regularly perform this examination present to their health care providers with smaller lesions.[2] Yet, many more women fail to carry out this valuable monthly exercise. Why is not clear. It is speculated, however, that motivating factors are health beliefs, fear and anxiety of discovering a lump, hence, a cancer; lack of knowledge or self-confidence regarding the technique of BSE; denial; discomfort with body manipulation; lack of perceived susceptibility to or risk of breast cancer; lack of perceived benefits; and apathy.[3] If this 10-minute routine is not incorporated into a woman's lifestyle, breast cancer may not be detected early and the risk of death due to breast cancer may increase. Table 14–1 indicates the American Cancer Society's recommended examination schedule to detect breast cancer in asymptomatic women.[1]

In 1993 the National Cancer Institute (NCI) decided that they would not recommend universal mammography screening for women at age 40.[4] At that time, the organization felt that there was no clear scientific evidence to indicate that women in their 40s, who underwent regular screening mammograms, had a reduced risk of dying from breast cancer.

**TABLE 14–1. RECOMMENDED BREAST CANCER
SCREENING FOR ASSYMPTOMATIC WOMEN**

Age	Recommendation
20–39	Monthly breast self-exam, clinical breast exam every 3 years
40–49	Monthly breast self-exam, annual clinical breast exam, mammography every 1–2 years
50 and over	Monthly breast self-exam, annual clinical breast exam, annual mammography

Source: American Cancer Society (1996). Breast cancer facts and figures. *Atlanta, GA: American Cancer Society.*

In March, 1997, the National Cancer Institute changed its position on mammography screening. The NCI adopted the recommendations of the Breast Cancer Advisory Board, a presidentially appointed committee, that advises and consults with the director of the NCI with respect to National Cancer Institute activities and policies.[4] In response to research that revealed that regular mammography screening of women in their 40s reduced deaths from breast cancer by approximately 17 percent, the National Cancer Advisory Board recommended the following screening guidelines:[4]

- Mammography screening every 1 to 2 years for women between the ages of 40 and 49 who are at average risk for breast cancer;
- Women at higher risk for breast cancer should seek medical advice about beginning mammography before age 40.

MAMMOGRAPHY SCREENING AND COSTS

Although the American Cancer Society and the National Cancer Institute provide mammography screening guidelines, the health care provider should consider several issues when a screening mammogram is recommended. Currently, 40 states require that third party payers cover all or part of the cost of a screening mammogram for women in their 40s.[4] An additional four states have pending legislation.

Medicare covers one screening mammogram every two years for its beneficiaries who are in their 40s and every year for women in their 40s with a personal family history of breast cancer.[4] Some women who are medicare recipients may

find funding the cost of a mammogram during the year that the mammogram is not covered by medicare prohibitive. This is especially true for women who do not have secondary health insurance coverage. Thus, the health care provider may find it expedient to recommend screening through agencies in their communities that offer free or discounted mammography during the year that medicare does not provide coverage. If no such agency exists, screening mammography may be recommended every two years and a diagnostic mammogram recommended when abnormalities are found.

TECHNIQUE FOR BREAST SELF-EXAMINATION (BSE)

BSE follows a specific technique (see Figure 14–1).[5] The exam should be done each month, after the menstrual period; day 4, 5, 6, or 7 is optimal. Menopausal and pregnant women should perform the exam on the first day of each month. For menstruating women, a note placed on a box of feminine hygiene pads or tampons, or on a personal calendar may serve as a reminder to perform BSE.

The Sensor Pad, designed to help women to examine their breasts has been approved by the Food and Drug Administration. This pad has 2 layers, is 10 inches in diameter and is filled with a small amount of silicon lubricant. The silicon lubricant is designed to help the fingers to glide easily over the breasts as they do when the breasts are lathered with soap.[6] This pad, used after instruction, not only may help to detect breast lumps but may also serve as a reminder to perform breast exam. Currently, the pad is available by prescription for patients who are interested. Patients who are not interested in using the pad or who find the cost of the pad prohibitive can be encouraged to examine their breasts while bathing.

Breast self-examination proceeds in the following manner:

1. While standing in front of a mirror, observe both breasts for symmetry, dimpling, scaling, redness, bruising, and nipple irritation, discharge, or retraction (Figure 14–1A).
2. Continue observations with hands elevated above the head (Figure 14–1B).

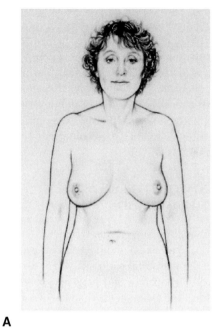

A

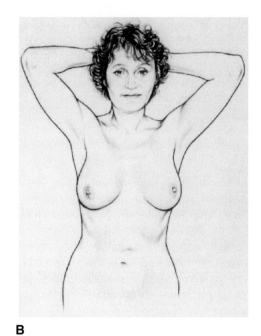

B

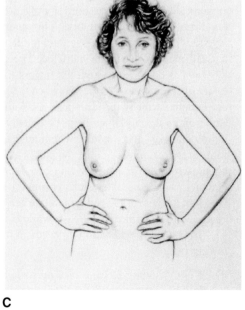

C

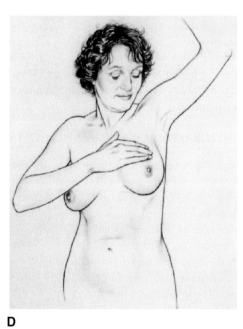

D

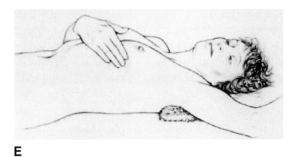

E

Figure 14–1. Breast self-examination (BSE) (perform procedure each month). See pages 282–283. *(From National Cancer Institute (March, 1984). Breast Exams—What You Should Know. (NIH pub. no. 84-2000.) Bethesda, MD: National Institutes of Health.)*

3. Continue observations with hands placed firmly on the hips, and body bowed slightly forward (Figures 14–1C).

4. Place one arm above the head and palpate the breast closest to that arm for lumps, masses, and tenderness. Use the fingers (not fingertips) of the opposite hand to glide over the breast in a circular fashion, starting in the upper outer quadrant of the breast and continuing until the entire breast, including the areola and nipple, has been examined (Figure 14–1D).

   Observe the nipple for discharge during this examination. Next, thoroughly palpate the axillary region for enlarged or tender nodes. Repeat the procedure for the other breast. (*Note:* Right hand examines the left breast, and left hand examines the right breast.)

5. Finally, lie supine with a pillow or towel behind the chest wall of one breast; examine the breast as in step 4 (Figure 14–1E). Move the pillow or towel to the opposite side and repeat the procedure for the other breast.

BREAST ASSESSMENT BY THE HEALTH CARE PROVIDER

Thorough breast assessment, including history taking for risk factors and education regarding BSE, should be standard protocol for the health provider during a client's annual exam.

History

Obtain the client's history and her family history of breast disease, breast symptoms and breast cancer. Special attention should be given to breast diseases in the maternal family, especially the mother, siblings or daughter, since breast cancer in a first degree relative increases the client's risk of cancer.[1,5] Also inquire about the client's menstrual and reproductive history, including information about menarche, onset of menopause, number of pregnancies and deliveries and age at both, as well as lactation or breast-feeding history. Ask the client about her current medication usage—specifically, psychotropic drugs, antihypertensives, hormonal therapy (estrogen, progesterone), and oral contraceptives, which could induce breast changes. Also inquire about her dietary habits, including caffeine intake, and frequency of BSE, clinical examination and mammography.

Breast Examination

The health care provider should devote ample time to examining the breasts, teaching the proper technique for BSE, and encouraging monthly BSE. The client should be provided the opportunity and encouraged to demonstrate BSE. Breast models that allow clients to practice on normal and abnormal breasts often help to increase client confidence in BSE. The breast exam by the health care provider should be systematic:[5]

1. Observe the client while she is sitting with her hands resting in her lap, with hands overhead and chest wall forward, and with her hands placed firmly on her hips (which contracts the pectoral muscles). Observe the breasts for dimpling, retraction, color changes, skin

thickening, spontaneous nipple discharge, and asymmetry. (*Note:* Some asymmetry is normal, i.e., one breast may be slightly larger or smaller than the other. It is important to ask the client if the asymmetry had been previously observed.)

2. If the client has large, pendulous breasts, ask her to lean over while placing her hands on your shoulders. In this position, observe the breasts for symmetry, retraction, and dimpling.
3. Allow the client's arm to rest diagonally on your arm (positioned from the client's right to your right) as you palpate the axillary nodes. Repeat this procedure for the opposite axilla. Then palpate the supraclavicular and infraclavicular lymph nodes. If the breasts are pendulous, palpate them while the client is seated.
4. Ask the client to lie supine and extend the arm on the side of the breast to be examined overhead. Place a pillow beneath the same shoulder.
5. Then palpate the client's breast from the upper outer quadrant to the nipple in a circular fashion, taking care to cover each breast quadrant. Give careful attention to the Tail of Spence.
6. Observe the nipple for discharge.
7. Perform steps 3 through 6 on the opposite breast.

Benign Breast Conditions

Benign breast conditions account for most breast symptoms and complaints seen in the primary care setting.[7] Frequently, a significant amount of time must be spent reassuring the client that the lesion is indeed benign, thus patience and support are essential.

FIBROCYSTIC CHANGES

Fibrocystic changes of the breast are the most frequently encountered benign breast condition.[8] The term includes a broad grouping of lesions including cystic mastitis, ductal hyperplasia, large and small cyst formation, apocrine metaplasia and sclerosing adenosis.[8,9] Breast thickness,

lumpiness and/or palpable nodularity is present. Pain is almost always present and is the most common sign and symptom of fibrocystic change.[9] Sometimes fibrocystic changes will mask atypia and proliferative changes that are frequently a precursor to cancer.[9]

Epidemiology

Several theories exist regarding the etiology of fibrocystic breast changes. The development of mastalgia and tender nodularity is thought to represent a physiological response to hormonal outflow.[8] It is thought that an imbalance between estrogen and progestin produces excessive ductal stimulation and proliferation, which produces these symptoms. Pain is also thought to be due to stromal edema. Nodularity and tenderness may be physiological and due to hormone stimulation, or they may be secondary to estrogen excess. Another theory is that the breast tissue becomes extra sensitive to estrogen and proliferates.[7–9]

Hyperprolactinemia has been considered a cause of fibrocystic changes. Prolactin levels are elevated in one-third of women with fibrocystic breast changes.[8] The hyperprolactinemia is thought to be related to the increased levels of estrogen noticed in some patients. It has not been found to be a consistent causative factor in fibrocystic changes of the breasts; thus, it does not apply to all cases.

The incidence of fibrocystic changes is greatest in women 20 to 50 years of age who are in their reproductive or premenopausal years.[9] The frequency of the condition increases with age occurring in approximately 10 percent of women younger than 21 years of age, 25 percent of menstruating women and 50 percent of perimenopausal women.[8]

The incidence and variability of the lesions suggest that fibrocystic changes should not be considered a disease process.[8] It is suggested that fibrocystic changes occur in three clinical stages that overlap:[9]

1. Mazoplasia, the first stage, occurs in women who are in their twenties. The pain is found most often in the upper outer breast quadrants. The most tender area is the indurated axillary Tail of Spence.

2. The second clinical stage, adenosis, generally occurs in women in their thirties. Multiple breast nodules, which may be 2 to 10 mm in size, occur with premenstrual breast pain and tenderness. Marked proliferation and hyperplasia of ducts and alveolar cells occur.

3. In the third stage, the cystic phase, solitary or multiple cysts may occur. Lumps are tender, slightly mobile, and fairly well delineated. There may be point tenderness with palpation when a cyst increases in size. This stage occurs mostly in women in their forties.

Subjective Data

The client reports bilateral or unilateral breast pain and tenderness (the symptom is usually bilateral).[7,8] The pain is cyclic and frequently begins 7 to 14 days prior to the menses and resolves sometime after the onset of menses.[10] Sometimes, however, pain is present at all times. Breast lumpiness and nodularity is also noted and may be localized, especially in the upper outer quadrants of the breasts.[7,8] The client may also report that the breasts are engorged and occasionally a spontaneous nipple discharge is seen.[7]

Objective Data

Physical Examination. Examination of the breasts reveals thickening and lumpiness (usually bilateral), which is palpated primarily in the outer quadrants. Usually no discharge from the nipples is seen; however, some clear discharge may be expressed or may occur without manipulation.[8] Lymphatic examination reveals tender palpable axillary lymph nodes among 20 percent of clients. No clavicular nodal enlargement is palpable. In older or postmenopausal women, a ridge of nodularity may be found along the inframammary margin, particularly in the lower quadrant of the breast.

Diagnostic Tests and Methods

MAMMOGRAPHY. Mammography remains the best breast imaging modality available today.[11] It is performed to identify and characterize a breast mass and to detect an early malignancy. Mammography can detect lesions before they become clinically evident,[12] sometimes by as many as 2 to

4 years.[13] The test procedure involves taking radiographic pictures of the bare breasts while they are compressed between two plastic plates. Generally two views of the compressed breasts are taken; however, other images may be taken during diagnostic studies to help to predict the origin of a lesion.[13] Most women find the 10-minute procedure temporarily uncomfortable but not painful. To decrease discomfort, advise routine mammography for the week after menses. Mammography in clients younger than 35 years of age is controversial and is usually not recommended because breast tissue in this population is dense. Although a mammograph may detect cancer in younger women, it should not be a standard method of evaluation. Also a woman should be advised that 10 percent of breast cancers can be missed by mammography.[12]

Inform the client that the tenderness that may be caused by breast compression may be relieved by acetaminophen, ibuprofen, or aspirin. To decrease discomfort, the procedure may be scheduled for a time of the menstrual cycle when breasts are less tender. Deodorant and powder can cause shadows to appear on the x-rays, making them more difficult to read;[14] therefore, they should be removed with soap and water before x-ray or they should be avoided on the day of the exam.

Help the client to choose a mammography facility that is accredited by the American College of Radiology (ACR) and ascertain that machines are designed specifically for mammography. Try to ensure that the mammogram is performed by a registered technologist and that the radiologist is trained to read mammography.[15] The radiology facility may not reveal the results of the x-ray to the client; therefore, it is important that a follow-up visit be scheduled as soon as possible to discuss the mammography findings.

ULTRASOUND. Sonography is a useful problem-solving tool and is an excellent adjunct to mammography for breast evaluation. The procedure helps to differentiate a cystic mass from a solid one.[12,13,16] Ultrasound is usually performed after mammography in the patient older than 30 years of age and may be the only modality employed in women younger than age 30.[16] Images of the breasts are produced via sound waves that travel through a gel medium that is applied to the breasts.

Explain the procedure to the client and offer support. The test must be performed by a qualified radiologist. It is not contraindicated in pregnancy.

Differential Medical Diagnoses

Malignant breast mass; physiological nodularity (when nodularity varies with the menstrual cycle). Pain may be due to cervical (neck) radiculopathy, costochondritis, respiratory infection, rib fracture, peptic ulcer disease, or hiatal hernia.[10]

Plan

Psychosocial Intervention. Spend significant time performing a thorough breast exam that might assure the client that her complaint is taken seriously. If symptoms are minimal, i.e., occurring two to three days prior to menses, reassurance may be sufficient.[8] Focus on helping to alleviate anxiety by informing the client of the frequency and generally benign nature of the breast changes. Have literature available that provides information in a simplistic manner. Also provide reference books for those who might be interested.

Medication

ORAL CONTRACEPTIVES (OCs)
- *Indications.* Oral contraceptives prevent or slow the development of new fibrocystic changes and minimize symptoms of existing changes.[8] Symptoms are suppressed in 88 percent of clients with fibrocystic changes.[8] An OC tends to be very helpful when pain is cyclic[10] and is especially appropriate if the client needs a birth control method and OC use is not contraindicated. The effectiveness of oral contraceptives is based on the reduction of ovarian estradiol production and on the modulation of breast estrogen receptors by progestin.[8]
- *Administration.* Low dose estrogen (e.g., ethinyl estradiol, 0.02 mg) and relatively high dose progesterone (e.g., norethindrone, 1.0 mg) pill daily for 3–6 months or longer. Frequently, symptoms improve drastically after 1 year and maximally after 2 years.[8] If contraception is needed, 0.030 to 0.035 mg of ethinyl estradiol with progestin is used.

- *Side Effects and Adverse Reactions.* Possible water retention, weight gain, hypertension, cardiovascular changes, and breakthrough bleeding (see Chapter 9).
- *Contraindications.* See Chapter 9.
- *Anticipated Outcomes on Evaluation.* A decrease in symptoms associated with fibrocystic changes. If improvement is noted, oral contraceptives are continued. Symptoms will probably recur when therapy is discontinued.
- *Client Teaching and Counseling.* Explain to the client that her menstrual cycle may change and that breakthrough bleeding is possible when the pill is not taken as prescribed. Counsel her about the side effects and danger signs associated with pill use (see Chapter 9). Caution the client about expecting immediate results; some breast symptoms may improve immediately; however, more severe symptoms require more time. Have the client keep a record of the effectiveness (or lack of) of the medication. Daily recording of symptoms may be extremely beneficial immediately after initiating OCs. Advise the client that symptoms may return when therapy is discontinued. The wearing of a supportive brassiere is essential.

DANAZOL
- *Indications.* Danazol, a steroid, reduces pain, tenderness and nodularity caused by fibrocystic changes. It is the primary drug of preference for the treatment of severe symptomatology of fibrocystic changes[9] and is the only FDA approved pharmaceutical treatment for mastalgia.[10] Danazol creates a postmenopausal hormonal environment that reduces estrogen production and concentration in breast tissue, thereby reducing symptoms.[8] It should be noted that as Danazol reduces the nodularity of small fibrocystic lesions, large cysts may appear to be more prominent and may require aspiration.[8,9]
- *Administration.* Usual dose of Danazol is 100 mg to 400 mg per day in divided doses.[8–10] Start with Danazol 200 mg per day beginning on menstrual cycle day two.[2] If response is obtained the dosage may be decreased to 100 mg per day for 2 months.[10] If symptomatic relief is maintained, the dosage may be reduced to 25 mg to 100 mg per day. Therapy should begin during menstruation or after a negative preg-

nancy test. Three to 4 months may pass before improvement in symptoms is observed;[8] however, breast pain and tenderness may be significantly relieved in the first month and eliminated in 2 to 3 months.[17] The elimination of nodularity usually requires 4 to 6 months of uninterrupted therapy.[17]

- *Side Effects and Adverse Reactions.* Weight gain, menstrual irregularity (including amenorrhea), acne, increased cholesterol levels, decreased breast size, oily skin, growth of facial hair, hair loss, deepening voice (which may continue after therapy is terminated), sore throat, hoarseness, liver dysfunction, nervousness, depression, vaginitis.[8–10,17]

- *Contraindications.* Undiagnosed abnormal genital bleeding; markedly impaired hepatic, renal, or cardiac function; pregnancy; breastfeeding; and clients whose symptoms occur only during the premenstrual period or who experience mild fibrocystic changes.

- *Anticipated Outcomes on Evaluation.* A decrease in breast tenderness and nodularity, and a decrease in the size of the breast cyst(s) if present.

- *Client Teaching and Counseling.* Advise the client that improvement normally occurs within the first month of therapy but may require 4 to 6 months. Also inform her that 50 percent to 65 percent of clients notice the return of some symptoms when Danazol is discontinued.[8,17] High cholesterol foods should be decreased in the diet, and a lipid profile and liver function tests should be drawn 3 months after therapy is initiated. The wearing of a supportive brassiere should be encouraged. A daily diary reflecting the effectiveness of Danazol therapy should be maintained throughout the use of the drug.

TAMOXIFEN

- *Indications.* Tamoxifen, known more for its use in breast cancer, reduces pain, tenderness, and nodularity caused by fibrocystic changes. It is an estrogen agonist that binds to the estrogen receptor and competes with estradiol for receptors of estrogen located in the breasts, thus, decreasing pain. Reduction of symptoms, especially pain, is improved in 65 to 75 percent of patients.[7–9]

- *Administration.* Tamoxifen 10 mg per day will normally decrease symptoms after 2 to 3 months.[8]

- *Side Effects.* Nausea, vomiting, vaginal discharge, vaginal bleeding, malaise, urticaria, alopecia, weight gain, depression and hot flashes may occur.[10,17] An increased risk for endometrial cancer also exists.[17-20]

- *Contraindications.* Pregnancy.

- *Anticipated Outcomes.* A decrease in breast tenderness and nodularity.

- *Client Teaching.* After assuring that the client is not pregnant by performing a serum pregnancy test, advise the client to avoid pregnancy by consistent use of a barrier method of contraception. Also inform her that breast tenderness may actually increase during the first 1 to 4 weeks of therapy but should resolve after that time.[8] Discuss all possible side effects of Tamoxifen. Strongly encourage regular Pap smears and endometrial surveillance (see Figure 14–2). Discuss risk of endometrial cancer. As with other therapies, use of a supportive brassiere should be advocated and a daily diary of breast symptoms should be maintained.

BROMOCRIPTINE

- *Indications.* This dopamine receptor agonist may reduce the pain and nodularity of fibrocystic changes. Because of the possible role of prolactin in the cause of breast pain, bromocriptine is used to decrease serum prolactin levels.[10] Its use, though controversial, has been found to reduce pain and nodularity in some patients.[8,10] Bromocriptine should not be used frequently and should be restricted to very select patients who may not have had success with other therapies.[8]

- *Administration.* Bromocriptine is given at 5 mg per day in two divided doses throughout therapy.[9] Doses may start at 1.25 mg at bedtime, increasing by 1.25 mg every 3 to 4 days until the aforementioned dosage is reached.[10]

- *Side Effects and Adverse Reactions.* Nausea, vomiting, alopecia, dizziness, edema, headache, and abdominal cramping.[8,10,17] Side effects are experienced in 70 percent of patients.[21]

- *Contraindications.* Clients receiving diuretics and antihypertensives as well as those who are sensitive to ergot alkaloids.

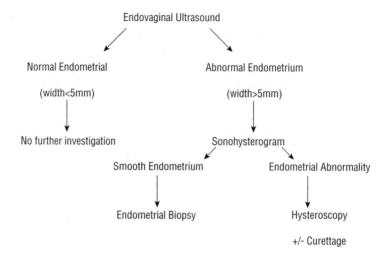

Figure 14–2. Algorithm for Endometrial Surveillance with Tamoxifen. *(Reproduced with permission from Odom LD: Endometrial surveillance in tamoxifen-treated patients. Contemporary OB/GYN 1966; 133–134, 139–140, 142 passim.)*

- *Anticipated Outcomes on Evaluation.* A decrease in pain and breast nodularity.
- *Client Teaching and Counseling.* Inform the client of the possible side effects of this drug. Advise the client to avoid pregnancy through the consistent use of a barrier form of birth control. Encourage the client to wear a supportive brassiere. A daily record of symptoms should be maintained throughout therapy.

Dietary Intervention

CAFFEINE. Consumption should be reduced, as this may alleviate breast tenderness and reduce nodularity. This treatment, the effectiveness of which is controversial,[8] may be tried in conjunction with other treatment modalities. Other nonprescriptive or lifestyle interventions that may help reduce fibrocystic discomfort include low salt diet, warm compresses, a supportive brassiere (even for sleep), and mild analgesics. The anticipated outcomes on evaluation by the client include decreased breast pain, tenderness, and nodularity.

Advise the client to decrease her intake of coffee, tea, cola drinks, chocolate, and drugs containing caffeine. Explain that 3 to 6 months may be required for symptoms to improve. Encourage perseverance, as many clients find it difficult to eliminate such foods as cola, coffee, and chocolate from their diet. Caffeine should be gradually reduced to prevent withdrawal symptoms.

VITAMIN E (EFFECTIVENESS CONTROVERSIAL)
- *Indications.* Vitamin E (alphatocopherol) often decreases pain and tenderness associated with fibrocystic change. It also decreases the proliferation of breast tissue. Even though the use of Vitamin E is controversial, it has been proven effective in relieving the symptoms of fibrocystic changes in some women, with its effectiveness thought to be due to altered lipid metabolism.[9]
- *Administration.* Oral Vitamin E, 150 to 600 IU daily.
- *Side Effects and Adverse Reactions.* Vitamin E's fat solubility and slow excretion may cause it to build up to a toxic level. Blood vessels may become constricted; therefore, the vitamin should be used cautiously in individuals with hypertension, diabetes mellitus, or cardiovascular disease.
- *Contraindications.* Hypertension, diabetes mellitus, or cardiovascular disease.
- *Anticipated Outcomes on Evaluation.* Decrease in pain, lumpiness, and thickness.
- *Client Teaching and Counseling.* Explain that Vitamin E is given on a trial basis and should be discontinued in 2–3 months if no improvement occurs. Caution the client about the dangers of overusing this fat soluble vitamin since vitamin toxicity may result.

EVENING PRIMROSE OIL

- *Indications.* This homeopathic herb is frequently used in Britain as an initial attempt to control cyclic breast pain.[10] Its effectiveness is variable.[22,23,24] The exact mechanism of action of evening primrose oil is unknown; however, it has been found to normalize the ratio of essential fatty acids to saturated fatty acids in some women with cyclic mastalgia.[10] Primrose oil may be especially useful in young women who require long-term treatment as well as those who desire to avoid hormonal manipulation.[10]
- *Administration.* Two 500 mg capsules should be taken 3 times per day for a minimum of 3 to 4 months.[10]
- *Side Effects and Adverse Reactions.* Side effects are few and usually include bloating and nausea.
- *Contraindications.* None, however, conflicting reports regarding its efficacy require that the provider be familiar with this herb. In addition, herbal medications are not regulated by the Food and Drug Administration, and some products advertised as evening primrose oil may contain other ingredients that may result in little if any effectiveness.[25]
- *Anticipated Outcome.* Reduction of breast pain.
- *Client Teaching and Counseling.* Inform the client that a minimum trial of 3 to 4 months may be required to determine the effectiveness of this therapy. Also describe that side effects are possible with this oil. Advise her that primrose oil may be purchased in health food stores and that no prescription is required.

Alternative Therapy. Hypnosis. Although the response is unpredictable, hypnotherapy may be tried[10] and has been found to be effective in some clients who have been unresponsive to other therapies.[26]

Surgical Intervention

PROPHYLACTIC BILATERAL TOTAL MASTECTOMY (SEE BREAST CANCER). Indications for the surgery are to decrease the likelihood of developing cancer in clients who have a strong family history of cancer[27] or who have progressive fibrocystic disease with atypia.[8] The procedure is usually considered too aggressive an approach in treating precancerous changes or as a request from patients who are tired of the pain caused by fibrocystic changes. All breast tissue is removed, including the nipple-areolar complex and some axillary nodes. A subcutaneous mastectomy in which the nipple remains attached to the skin envelope and the nipple-areola complex remains intact may be performed. Possible adverse effects include mild lymphedema, disfigurement, and anesthesia reactions.

The anticipated outcomes on evaluation include decreased anxiety related to developing cancer. Survivability may improve in high risk clients. High risk clients who undergo bilateral total mastectomy have a 2.5 to 5 percent chance of developing invasive cancer and a 5 to 10 percent chance of developing cancer in situ.[8]

When counseling the client, carefully convey the risks and advantages of the voluntary procedure. Advise the client that breast cancer may not be prevented, even if mastectomy is performed; however, the risk should be decreased. Cancer may develop in subcutaneous tissue that may be left after surgery.[27] Suggest that testing for the BRCA1 gene be done (see Breast Cancer). Professional counseling is strongly advised prior to this extreme surgery. The client should be advised to include significant others of choice in the decision-making process. Refer the client to at least three qualified surgeons for their opinions about the surgery.

Follow-Up

Clients who receive oral contraceptives for fibrocystic breast changes should have a physical examination and evaluation every 3 months for the first 6 months of therapy, followed by a breast exam 6 months later. Clinical breast exam should take place annually thereafter (see Chapter 9).

Clients who receive Danazol will require a lipid profile and liver function tests after 3 months of therapy as well as at the termination of therapy. Normally symptoms associated with fibrocystic breast changes resolve in 3 to 6 months, and Danazol can be terminated.

Bromocriptine should be used infrequently and clients who receive bromocriptine should be followed monthly.

Clients who have surgery should be followed per the recommendations of the surgeon.

Advise all clients to try caffeine reduction for 3 to 6 months to ascertain if pain and nodularity decrease. Continue reduced intake indefinitely if improvements are noticed.

Evening primrose oil may be tried by all clients as well. The oil may be used indefinitely if effective. Remember to caution about the variability of its effectiveness and preparation.

It is important that the health care provider exhibit openness to alternative therapies for those clients who choose such methods as hypnosis. A follow-up should be planned 4 to 6 weeks after the initiation of hypnotherapy to assess its effectiveness. All clients should be reminded to wear well fitted supportive brassieres and to continue to practice monthly BSE.

FIBROADENOMA

A fibroadenoma is the most common benign solid breast tumor.[7,28] It is a discrete, smooth, solid, firm, or rubbery, well defined mobile mass that is usually painless.[29] It may be stony hard when calcified.[7] The mass is usually found unilaterally as a single breast mass but may be multiple and bilateral.

Epidemiology

A fibroadenoma is thought to be a hormonally induced change in breast tissue.[30] The mass, considered a disorder of normal breast development—not a neoplasm—presumably arises from the lobules and terminal ducts of the breast.[29] It is basically an overgrowth of elements thought to be found in these ducts and is composed of stromal and epithelial cells.[30] Usually a mass will grow to 2 to 4 cm in diameter and remain that size.[7] A small number, however, grow to be larger than 5 cm; these are called giant fibroadenoma.[30] A fibroadenoma is usually hormonally responsive and may increase in size toward the end of each menstrual cycle.[7] The risk of a clinical fibroadenoma being a neoplasm is virtually confined to women over 35 years of age. It does not undergo malignant change and any cancers that are reported are thought to be chance occurrences.[29]

The occurrence of a unilateral discrete breast mass is most common after puberty and before age 30.[30] Peak incidence is between ages 20 and 30.[29] Often a mass may be detected in postmenopausal women, but it is most likely in these cases that the fibroadenoma developed prior to menopause and became clinically apparent during the involution of surrounding breast tissue.[7] Growth of these tumors often occurs during pregnancy[31] and sometimes the growth during pregnancy may be rapid because of the excess hormone levels associated with pregnancy. Though a fibroadenoma is normally a single, unilateral lesion, it may be multiple and found in both breasts. The risk of developing fibroadenoma is *not* increased by age, weight, parity, age at first pregnancy, socioeconomic status, or a family history of breast cancer.

Subjective Data

The client reports a "seed-like" or "marble-like," discrete, mobile, painless lump in one breast. Less often, she will find a lump in both breasts. It may be observed in any area of the breast, but is most frequently found in the upper outer quadrant. No nipple discharge or retraction, dimpling, or other breast symptoms are reported.

Objective Data

Physical Examination. A physical examination of the breasts reveals a firm, well delineated, freely mobile, nontender mass, best palpated with the client in the dorsal recumbent position with hand behind her head. Usually the mass is palpable unilaterally, but it also may be bilateral.

Diagnostic Tests and Methods

FINE-NEEDLE ASPIRATION. Diagnostic evaluation using fine needle aspiration is done to identify a solid tumor, cyst, or malignancy. The procedure should be done by a trained health care provider, usually an obstetrics/gynecology specialist or a surgeon. The test procedure involves first cleaning the breast with an antiseptic solution (usually isopropyl alcohol). Then the mass is stabilized between the fingers of one hand and compressed downward. It should be pushed up and over a rib and stabilized.[32] A 22 gauge needle is inserted into the mass.[33] A finer gauge needle may be chosen, but withdrawal of fluid and tissue will occur more slowly, which may result in more anxiety for the patient.[33] As the needle is moved around in the mass, suction is applied to remove the contents. The needle is gently withdrawn, and pressure is applied to the puncture site. Tissue from a fibroadenoma tends to stick to the needle so that it must be forcefully withdrawn.[32] The specimen should then be placed on a clean glass slide and gently spread at a 10 degree angle. Fix the slide with alcohol. Prepare a second slide and allow it to air dry. Send both slides to a cytology lab. If straw colored fluid is withdrawn, the diagnosis is usually benign; in this case the fluid may be discarded. If, however, there is doubt, send the remaining fluid to the lab in a sterile glass tube. Absence of fluid may indicate a solid mass, which is suspicious of malignancy, necessitating open biopsy.

Fine needle aspiration is cytologically diagnostic if there are abundant sheets of benign ductal epithelial cells, benign stroma and abundant bipolar, bare, benign nuclei.[28]

Provide the client with an explanation of fine needle aspiration and a rationale for it. If referral is necessary, allow the client to participate in the selection of the care provider. If the client wishes to have the mass removed, refer her to a surgeon. Encourage her to continue BSE.

MAMMOGRAPHY. (See benign breast conditions, fibrocystic changes.) A mammogram may be used to evaluate any mass. Fibroadenoma are most common in young adult women who have dense breast tissue, however, fibroadenoma may not be visualized accurately via mammography in this age group. Mammography usually shows a circumscribed mass with clear borders and intermediate density. A well defined mass may show a halo effect from compression of the surrounding breast tissue.[28]

ULTRASOUND. (See benign breast conditions, fibrocystic changes.) Sonography will differentiate a cystic mass from a solid mass. A fibroadenoma is shown as a circumscribed or lobulated mass with distinct borders and moderate internal echoes.[28] The well differentiated, low-level echoes are homogeneous throughout.[28]

Differential Medical Diagnosis

Breast macrocyst, cystosarcoma phyllodes, tubular adenoma, and mucinous carcinoma.

Plan

Psychological Interventions. Psychological interventions include helping the client to alleviate anxiety by informing her of the usual benign status of this mass. In addition, literature should be provided about common benign breast lesions. Assure her that a fibroadenoma should not impair her ability to breastfeed in the future.

Medication is not indicated.

Surgical Intervention

EXCISIONAL (OPEN) BIOPSY. This procedure is done to remove and diagnose a breast lesion. It is performed especially if the lesion persists after repeated aspiration;[33] when a suspicious mass persists beyond menses; if the fluid in a cyst is bloody; if nipple discharge is serous or serosanguineous with no mass but a trigger point is present; or, when a suspicious mammogram occurs without clinical findings. It has also been advised that these lesions be removed before a client decides to become pregnant (even in adolescence) since pregnancy frequently causes the lesions to grow.[31] The lesion may later infarct causing significant increase in size and pain. Removal of a larger lesion causes more unsightly cosmetic changes.

The fibroadenoma is surgically excised under local anesthesia, and adhesive strips are used to close the excision. Adverse effects are virtually nonexistent. The client, however, may react to the local anesthesia, and bleeding and infection is possible with virtually any surgical procedure.

The anticipated outcomes on evaluation include reduced anxiety because the lesion has been removed. Greater accuracy is achieved in diagnosis because the lesion is sent to a pathology lab.

Explain to the client that the surgery may be done in an ambulatory setting under local anesthesia. A small dressing will be required. The pain is usually mild, but over the counter analgesics may be used if needed. Time lost from work is usually minimal. No heavy lifting or strenuous work should be done until the site is healed.

Conservative Treatment. Since fibroadenoma do not undergo malignant change, nonsurgical management may be considered in women who are younger than 30 years of age.[29] This conservative treatment may take place only after a confident diagnosis of fibroadenoma is made via clinical examination, cytologic evaluation, and breast imaging.[29,34] Women should be advised to be reevaluated in 6 months, perform monthly BSE, and return annually for a clinical breast exam. The client should be encouraged to return if she has any anxiety regarding the presence of the lesion or if the fibroadenoma increases in size.[29]

Follow-Up

After fine needle aspiration and surgery, follow-up should be done at the physician's discretion, but usually in 2 to 4 weeks. Routine clinical breast exams should be done every year by a health professional, and breast self-examination (BSE) should be carried out monthly.

NIPPLE DISCHARGE

Fluid emission from the mammary nipple is a common complaint by women seen by health care providers. Nipple discharge is commonly treated in patients in the office or clinic because many types of discharge can be treated medically and do not require surgery.[7] Nipple discharge is more commonly associated with benign rather than malignant conditions,[7,35] however, persistent nipple discharge is attributed to cancer in 4 percent to 21 percent of cases.[35] Discharge may be caused by factors outside the breasts, primarily neuroendocrine or drug induced; by pathology of the ductal system; or by disease of the nipple.[31,36]

At least seven types of nipple discharge have been identified: serous (yellow), serosanguineous, bloody, clear (watery), milky, purulent, and multicolored.[7,35]

NIPPLE DISCHARGE CAUSED BY FACTORS OUTSIDE THE BREASTS

Galactorrhea

Galactorrhea is a spontaneous milky nipple discharge that is nonpuerperal or unrelated to lactation.[21] It is usually bilateral, comes from multiple ducts, and is most often found in women of childbearing age.[30] The condition is most commonly observed after pregnancy and may last as long as 2 years.[7]

Epidemiology. The etiology of galactorrhea may involve medications. For example, it can be induced by oral contraceptives (OCs), antihypertensive medications (e.g., reserpine, methyldopa and verapamil), or psychotropic medications (e.g., imipramine).[35] Estrogen in oral contraceptives causes an increase in prolactin producing cells of the pituitary.[21] Oral contraceptives also stimulate the breasts and prepare them for lactation; estrogen stimulates the ductal system while progesterone stimulates the alveolar system.[21] Antihypertensive medications like reserpine and methyldopa inhibit the synthesis of dopamine while opiates suppress dopamine and stimulate prolactin release, thereby causing hyperprolactinemia.[21] Galactorrhea can also be due to Forbes-Albright Syndrome, hypothyroidism, chest lesions, renal disease, nonpituitary prolactin producing tumors (such as of the lung or kidney), and dysfunction of the hypothalamus and pituitary tumors.[21] In addition, prolonged stimulation of the nipples and breasts can substantially increase prolactin to high levels and cause galactorrhea. Galactorrhea is often associated with menstrual abnormalities. Details about the incidence of galactorrhea are unknown.

Subjective Data. The client reports an unelicited milky white discharge from both nipples and says that she is not pregnant or lactating. She also indicates that she neither has experienced trauma nor has pain. She may, however, acknowledge amenorrhea or irregular menses. Visual complaints of spots, whiteness, glowing, or progressive blurring may be given by a client suspected of having a pituitary tumor.

Objective Data

PHYSICAL EXAMINATION. Physical examination of the breasts reveals a milky nipple discharge that occurs spontaneously and with manual stimulation. It is not expressed from any particular areolar quadrant or duct. No redness or tenderness is visible. Fundoscopic examination of the eye may be normal.

DIAGNOSTIC TESTS AND METHODS

PREGNANCY TEST. The absence of a pregnancy should be confirmed by performing a pregnancy test. A sensitive urine or blood pregnancy test that measures human chorionic gonadotropin should be performed in the office or sent to a laboratory.

SERUM PROLACTIN TEST. This diagnostic evaluation is performed to identify elevated prolactin, which may be indicative of a pituitary tumor or thyroid disorder. Values greater than 20 ng/mL are considered abnormal. A level of 20–100 ng/mL usually represents a tumor or functional hyperprolactenemia.[21] A level between 100 and 200 ng/mL is very suggestive of a tumor. When values of 200 to 300 ng/mL are found, a tumor is present 90 percent of the time. Values greater than 300 ng/mL are essentially diagnostic of a prolactin secreting tumor.[21] If the blood level is elevated, the test may be repeated to ensure accuracy.

The test procedure is to draw 3 to 5 mL of blood in a red-top tube and send it to a lab for evaluation. Use universal precautions when performing venipuncture.

Explain to the client the rationale for the laboratory test and help to allay her anxiety about the diagnosis.

THYROID FUNCTION TEST. This diagnostic test may identify an elevated level of thyrotropin (TSH), which may be indicative of thyroid disease (hypothyroidism). Thyroid-stimulating hormone releasing hormone of the hypothalamus that releases TSH also releases prolactin. If primary hypothyroidism is present, the thyrotropin-releasing hormone increases, which releases TSH and prolactin causing galactorrhea. Hypothyroidism is the etiology of hyperprolactenemia in 5–10 percent of cases.[21] This test should also be done if the serum prolactin test results show an elevated prolactin level.

The test procedure is to draw 5 mL of blood in a red-top tube and send it to a lab for evaluation. Use universal precautions when drawing blood.

Explain the rationale for the laboratory test and help to allay any anxiety.

SERUM CREATININE/BLOOD UREA NITROGEN. This diagnostic test identifies abnormality in renal function and should be done to rule out a kidney disorder.

Blood (5 mL) should be collected in a red-top tube and sent to the laboratory for evaluation. Universal precautions should be observed.

Rationale for the test should be provided the patient. An expected date that the test results will be available should be indicated.

COMPUTED AXIAL TOMOGRAPHIC SCAN (CT) SCAN OF THE PITUITARY FOSSA. A CT Scan is done to identify pituitary tumors and is performed if the client has hyperprolactinemia, specifically, a prolactin level greater than 60 ng/mL.[21]

The test procedure involves the use of narrow x-ray beams to reveal the differences in radiation absorption among different kinds of tissue. Intravenous dye (usually Renografin) is used to enhance the x-ray contrast of vascular lesions. Axial tomography scans 1 mm slices of the pituitary gland and hypothalamus in the coronal plane after 200 cc of iodinated contrast medium is administered. The coronal plane is selected because prolactinomas are usually located in the lateral wing of the anterior pituitary.[21]

Explain to the client the rationale for the test and refer her for financial screening if the test is not covered by medical insurance. Determine if the client is allergic to dyes. Support the client and help to allay any anxiety. Explain that the test is painless, but the client may be required to remain still for long periods during testing.

MAGNETIC RESONANCE IMAGING (MRI). This test, like the CT scan, will diagnose a pituitary tumor; however, MRI can provide resolution to 1 mm without radiation. Hydrogen nuclei in static magnetic fields, exposed to radiowaves of specific frequency, resonate and depict tissue hydrogen density.[21] This test should also be performed if the prolactin level is elevated.

Explain the test to the client and provide literature if possible. Advise of the expense of testing and suggest financial screening at the local imaging center if available. Inform the client that she may have to remain immobile for a long period of time during the test.

VISUAL FIELDS MEASUREMENT. This diagnostic evaluation is performed to determine visual field defects caused by a pituitary tumor or mass. It is performed if the CT scan result is abnormal or if the client has visual complaints. Referral to an ophthalmologist is warranted for precise testing to evaluate peripheral vision; gross screening and a fundoscopic exam should be performed by the primary care provider.

Explain the reason for referral and the rationale for the exam. Involve the client in the selection of an ophthalmologist.

CHEST RADIOGRAPH (X-RAY). Radiology of the chest identifies anomalies and lesions of the chest cavity, including the lungs and ribs. Frequently, a cardiac silhouette can also be visualized.

Radiation is used in this brief examination that normally takes fewer than 5 minutes.

Although most clients are familiar with this exam an explanation should be offered. Provide test results as soon as possible.

MAMMOGRAPHY. (See benign breast disorders, fibrocystic changes.)

Differential Medical Diagnoses. Drug induced galactorrhea, pituitary tumor, prolactinoma, hypothyroidism, chest lesion, renal disease, nonpituitary prolactin producing tumor, and Forbes-Albright Syndrome.

Plan

PSYCHOSOCIAL INTERVENTIONS. Help to allay the client's anxiety through teaching and providing literature about galactorrhea. Assure the client that galactorrhea is rarely associated with breast cancer.[35] Encourage significant persons in the client's life to be supportive. Discuss sexuality and body image issues as appropriate. (*Note:* Close consultation with the physician is essential while managing a client with galactorrhea.)

MEDICATION

BROMOCRIPTINE

- *Indications.* Bromocriptine is the drug of choice in the treatment of galactorrhea.[21] This most effective treatment is a dopamine agonist that inhibits the secretion of prolactin. It activates dopamine receptors, acting like long acting dopamine. It is used to lower prolactin levels, end galactorrhea, and restore the menses to normal if they have been irregular. Bromocriptine may even be used when a tumor is identified, since surgery frequently yields fair to poor results.[21] It may be used successfully when a microadenoma (less than 1 cm) or macroadenoma (greater than 1 cm) is identified since it

often causes shrinkage or necrosis of parts of the tumor.

- *Administration.* Start with 1.5–2.5 mg of bromocriptine daily, with the evening meal, for 1 week. The dosage is then increased to 1.25–2.25 mg twice daily. If necessary, doses of 1.25–2.25 mg three times a day may be prescribed.[21] Bromocriptine may also be given vaginally and is as effective as the oral dose when administered by this route. There are practically no gastrointestinal effects when used intravaginally because the metabolism is slower and the liver is bypassed. The daily dosage is a 2.5 mg tablet placed in the fornix of the vagina daily.[21]
- *Side Effects and Adverse Reactions.* Nausea, vomiting, dizziness, fatigue, headache, abdominal cramps, diarrhea, constipation, nasal congestion, and drowsiness.[8,10,17,21] Side effects are experienced by 70 percent of patients.[21]
- *Contraindications.* Clients receiving antihypertensives, diuretics and those who are sensitive to ergot alkaloids.
- *Anticipated Outcome on Evaluation.* Cessation of nipple discharge.
- *Client Teaching and Counseling.* Advise the client to practice safe, effective birth control (barrier method) to avoid pregnancy while taking bromocriptine and to notify her care provider of any side effects.

SURGICAL INTERVENTION

TRANSSPHENOIDAL EXCISION OF PITUITARY TUMOR. The purpose of this surgery is to remove the causative pathology and consequently abate the symptom. The tumor is excised through the nasal cavity. Tumor recurrence is possible.[21] Results with surgery depend on the tumor size and prolactin level. If a microadenoma is present and the prolactin level is less than 200 ng/mL, the cure rate is 80 percent and the mortality risk and risk for diabetes insipidus is negligible.[21] When a macroadenoma is present and the prolactin level is greater than 200 ng/mL, the cure rate is 40 percent, the mortality rate 0.5 percent, and the risk for diabetes insipidus 20 percent.[21]

The anticipated outcome on evaluation is cessation of nipple discharge without other adverse health conditions.

Refer the client to a qualified surgeon, encouraging client participation in the selection of a surgeon.

Follow-Up. Consultation with a physician is strongly recommended. If the galactorrhea is being managed with bromocriptine, the client should be evaluated every month. The medication may be discontinued if the symptom resolves in 2 to 3 months; thereafter, the client may be evaluated in 6 months and yearly. If, however, the symptom does not abate in 2 to 3 months, bromocriptine may be continued and the client evaluated 1 month later. If at that time galactorrhea is unresolved, the client should be referred to a physician or managed with frequent consultation with a physician. Bromocriptine should be discontinued temporarily every 2 years and a prolactin level should be measured 6 weeks later.

If hypothyroidism is the cause of galactorrhea, then the disorder may be managed with thyroid hormone. The client may be referred to an internist or endocrinologist for management if desired. Evaluate the client every 6 months once hypothyroidism is stabilized.

If the prolactin level is increased, no microadenoma exists, the client does not desire pregnancy and has adequate estrogen levels, treatment may consist of observation only with a CT scan or MRI every 2 years.[21]

If surgery is required for tumor removal, then follow-up is per the surgeon's recommendations.

NIPPLE DISCHARGE CAUSED BY DUCTAL SYSTEM DISORDERS

Intraductal Papilloma

The intraductal papilloma is a small, usually nonpalpable, benign tumor located in the mammary duct that produces a spontaneous serous or sero-sanguineous nipple discharge.[24,37] The tumor is usually solitary and affects only one duct, but occasionally it affects multiple ducts (see Figure 14–3).

Epidemiology. It is thought that intraductal papilloma is caused by a proliferation and overgrowth of ductal epithelial tissue. On rare occasions the papilloma may be intracystic rather than intraductal; however, in these cases, discharge will occur

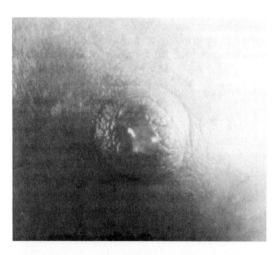

Figure 14–3. *Single duct nipple discharge.* Whether the discharge is clear or contains blood is not as useful a diagnostic sign as is often quoted. It is more important to discover whether a palpable or mammagraphic abnormality is present.

If cytology of the discharge is carried out and obvious cancer cells are found, clearly an underlying breast cancer is indicated. However, suspicious cells found in nipple discharge are often merely degenerate duct cells.

only if the cyst communes with a duct. Although a papilloma is usually millimeters in size and nonpalpable, it can grow large enough to obstruct the duct and thereby become palpable. A nodule is usually located close to the areola.[24,30]

Multiple papilloma may exist, especially in younger women, and are frequently bilateral and located in the periphery of the breasts.[7,28] Multiple lesions are a substantial risk for papillary carcinoma.[7,28]

Intraductal papilloma occurs most frequently among women in their late menstrual years.[28] Usually the tumor occurs just prior to menopause, but it may occur at any time from adolescence to old age.

Subjective Data. The client reports yellow or bloody discharge on her clothing. The discharge may occur spontaneously or with nipple stimulation. If the papilloma is large, the client may be able to observe a nonpainful, mobile mass usually in the areola. On rare occasions, the client may be able only to palpate the mass. She may complain of an associated feeling of fullness or pain beneath the areola.

Objective Data

PHYSICAL EXAMINATION. A physical examination of the breasts reveals serous or sero-sanguineous discharge, which is expressed manually from the affected duct when the nipple is systematically massaged in quadrants. The tumor, if palpable, may be a 1 to 3 cm mass, soft and poorly delineated and felt in the nipple area.[28] When multiple lesions are present, they are normally palpated in the periphery.[7] Occasionally, skin dimpling is observed.

DIAGNOSTIC TESTS AND METHODS

TEST FOR OCCULT BLOOD IN BREAST FLUIDS. This diagnostic evaluation identifies the presence of blood in nipple discharge. The procedure involves placing a small amount of nipple discharge on the designated area of a Hemoccult™ card (front side). Use a gloved finger to transfer the specimen from the nipple (use universal precautions). Apply 2 drops of developer on the designated area on the reverse side of the card. Blue coloration indicates the presence of blood.

Explain the purpose of the test to the client.

CYTOLOGY OF BREAST FLUID (PAPANICOLAOU SMEAR). Cytologic evaluation screens for cancerous cells. Cytology is obligatory for any blood stained breast discharge.[38] Usually, on microscopic examination, an intraductal papilloma shows scattered macrophages and tight clusters of epithelial cells with minimal atypia.[30] Test results should be treated with caution, because negative results are not diagnostic of intraductal papilloma since false negative results may occur.[36]

The test procedure requires that a drop of breast fluid be expressed onto a clean glass slide. The glass slide is held at the opening of the duct and the nipple discharge is expressed directly from the nipple onto the slide.[36] Then fix the slide with alcohol immediately, label it to indicate which breast the sample was taken from, and send it to a lab. Immediate fixing is vital to avoid any drying artifact. A small specimen bottle of alcohol preservative works well because the patient may hold the bottle while the nipple discharge is obtained or the bottle may be placed close to the procedure site.

Because the discharge is more cellular in the last drops of secretions, it is recommended that 4–6 slides be obtained.[36]

Explain the procedure and its purpose to the client; caution that the results are inconclusive.

MAMMOGRAPHY. (See benign breast conditions, fibrocystic changes.) Mammography may reveal dilated ducts near the nipple. When a mass is seen, borders are usually obscured by overlying glandular tissue. Benign appearing calcifications may be present.[28]

ULTRASOUND. (See benign breast conditions, fibrocystic changes.) Sonogram may reveal dilated ducts, but rarely identifies a lesion. Low level of internal echoes are present when lesions are seen.[28]

DUCTOGRAPHY (CONTROVERSIAL). This diagnostic evaluation to identify, by means of radiography, the ductal orifice that drains the pathological ductal system is not commonly performed. The test offers better visualization of small intraductal papillomas.[35] Ductography will not differentiate benign lesions from malignant lesions; thus, surgery will ultimately be required.[35] The test is considered unnecessary by some because the affected ductal quadrant can be identified by manual examination of the nipple and surgery is required whether or not this radiological procedure is done. Some specialists, however, find the test valuable for a more precise diagnosis; however, it may best be reserved for preoperative evaluation.[28]

The test procedure requires introducing radiographic dye through a cannulated duct, followed by x-rays.[35,36]

Discuss the pros and cons of this procedure with the client and assist her in choosing a qualified radiologist.

Differential Medical Diagnoses. Intraductal carcinoma, multiple papillomatosis.

Plan

PSYCHOSOCIAL INTERVENTIONS. Counsel the client regarding the benign etiology of this diagnosis. Encourage her to verbalize her feelings and emotions. Discuss sexuality issues as appropriate.

MEDICATION. Not given for intraductal papilloma.

SURGICAL INTERVENTION

WEDGE EXCISION. Wedge excision of the affected duct is the removal of the pathological ductal system and papilloma. This is the only method of differentiating this benign lesion from papillary carcinoma.[28] Also, the nipple discharge will continue if the diseased duct is not removed. Local anesthesia is used. The excised papilloma and duct are sent to a pathology lab to rule out cancer.

Adverse effects may include a reaction to the anesthetic or possibly infection. The anticipated outcomes on evaluation include cessation of the discharge. In addition, anxiety is relieved if pathology results show a benign lesion.

Client counseling includes information that the procedure can be performed in an outpatient surgical setting under local or general anesthesia. Tell the client that usually only a small areolar incision is required; thus, major alteration in the cosmetics of the breast is averted. Only a small surgical dressing is necessary. More extensive surgery is required if the lesion is hard to access. Referral to a surgeon who specializes in the treatment of the breast is required; and client participation in the selection of a surgeon is appropriate.

Encourage the client to follow through with recommendations since surgery is the only method to determine if cancer is present. Advise the client to continue with annual breast exams performed by the health care provider and monthly breast self-examination (BSE).

Duct Ectasia

Duct ectasia is dilation and inflammation of the major mammary ducts, resulting in noncyclic breast pain and pasty nipple discharge that may be straw-colored, cream-colored, green, brown, yellow, gray, or reddish-brown.[35]

Epidemiology. The etiology of duct ectasia is unclear; however, several theories exist. Endocrine induced relaxation/hypertrophy of the muscle of the duct wall has been suggested.[39] Another theory is that the duct wall is destroyed by inflammation caused by bacterial infection or autoimmunity.[39] Mammary ducts are also thought to become distended with cellular debris and pressure, sometimes caused by nipple inversion, which causes a subareolar duct obstruction.[39] Lymphocytes and plasma cells accumulate around the duct wall. Longstanding inflammation results in loss of elasticity and weakening of the

cell wall so that it sags or dilates.[40] Subsequently, secretion within the duct becomes thick and static and the duct wall becomes fibrotic and scarred.[40] Sometimes long linear calcifications may develop within the lumen and are sometimes associated with obliteration of the lumen.[40]

The median age for the appearance of duct ectasia is 43 years, and it occurs frequently in women between 37 and 53 years of age.[35] It tends to affect perimenopausal women in their fifties and usually occurs with a history of nipple discharge upon manipulation.[35] Clients are usually parous and have lactated but may have experienced difficult lactation because of inverted nipples.

Subjective Data. Clients report a bilateral, pasty discharge that may be green, cream, brown, or straw-colored. In addition, dull nipple pain, a "drawing" sensation, subareolar swelling, and burning and nipple itching frequently occur.[7] When the condition is advanced, the client may report an inflammatory breast mass and nipple retractions.[7]

Objective Data

PHYSICAL EXAMINATION. Physical examination of the breasts may reveal subareolar redness and swelling. Tortuous tubular swellings are frequently palpated beneath the areola.[7] Nipple retraction and dimpling may also be present. There is often mild to moderate tenderness on palpation. Nipple discharge, manually expressed, is green, brown, straw-colored, or cream-colored with the consistency of toothpaste. Discharge is usually observed from one ductal quadrant of the nipple when the breast is palpated in a systematic fashion. In advanced cases, a round, firm, and somewhat fixed tumor may be palpable. Also in advanced cases, axillary lymphadenopathy is observed.

DIAGNOSTIC TESTS AND METHODS

TEST FOR OCCULT BLOOD IN BREAST FLUID. (See benign breast conditions, intraductal papilloma, page 380.) In addition to testing for the presence of blood by using a Hemocult™ card, placing a sample of the nipple discharge on a small white gauze pad will frequently reveal the presence of blood in the nipple discharge. The color of the stain usually reflects the true color of the discharge.[7]

MAMMOGRAPHY. (Performed most often for clients with a palpable mass; see benign breast conditions, fibrocystic breast changes, page 369.) Mammography may show tubular dilated ducts radiating from the nipple. An abundance of dense tissue may also appear behind the nipple.[28]

ULTRASOUND. (See benign breast conditions, fibrocystic changes, page 369.) Well differentiated dilated ducts may be visualized when viewed longitudinally, and lesions that appear to be cysts may be observed when viewed cross sectionally.[28]

CYTOLOGY. (See benign breast conditions, intraductal papilloma, page 380.) Cytologic exam normally shows acellular material with debris and desquamated epithelium.

DUCTOGRAPHY. (See benign breast conditions, intraductal papilloma, page 380.)

Differential Medical Diagnoses. Intraductal carcinoma.

Plan

PSYCHOSOCIAL INTERVENTIONS. Provide information on the benign status of the disease to help alleviate the client's anxiety. Use the opportunity to promote breast self-examination (BSE). Encourage support by significant others in the client's life and encourage the client to express her feelings and emotions. Discuss sexuality issues if problematic and refer the client for professional counseling if indicated.

SURGICAL INTERVENTION

WEDGE EXCISION. The affected duct, including any mass that is present, is surgically removed by wedge excision and sent to pathology for evaluation. This is the only procedure that may eliminate the symptom.[28]

Follow-Up. Some health care providers believe that this nipple discharge is self-limiting and does not require surgery.[36] Thus, the client should be encouraged to clean nipples daily with a betadine solution or hexachlorophene for 2 to 5 minutes.[36] If a mass is present or an abscess occurs, it is recommended that wedge excision be performed.[36] If surgery is performed, follow-up care is directed by the surgeon. If symptoms recur, an ice pack may be used for inflammation and nonsteroidal anti-inflammatory drugs (NSAIDs) may be used for pain until a health care provider can be consulted. The usual routine of clinical breast exam should be carried out by the primary care provider, and monthly BSE is done by the client.

Galactocele

A galactocele is a discrete, milk filled, cystic or firm mass in the breast of a lactating or recently lactating woman. It may or may not be painful.

Epidemiology. The galactocele is thought to arise from dilation and obstruction of the lactiferous duct with retained milk and desquamated epithelial cells.[7,31] It is most often found in the upper quadrants beyond the areolar border and may be singular or multiple.[7]

Subjective Data. The client may report a lump, knot, or cyst in her breast that may or may not be painful. Usually no bloody or purulent nipple discharge is reported but occasionally pain may be described. She may note that the lesion was discovered after lactation was terminated.[28]

Objective Data

PHYSICAL EXAMINATION. Physical examination usually reveals a visible, palpable, firm, round mass in one or both breasts. Milk may be manually expressed from the nipple and pain may be elicited upon palpation.

FINE NEEDLE ASPIRATION. (See benign breast conditions, fibroadenoma.) This test is performed to identify and eradicate the lesion (see page 374 for the procedure). If the fluid is milky, it may be discarded and cytology is not required; however, if doubt exists, the fluid may be sent for cytologic examination. Most often, no further treatment is needed if the mass disappears with aspiration, as aspiration is often curative.[7,28] If the fluid is other than milky or if the galactocele does not disappear with aspiration, an excisional biopsy is indicated.

MAMMOGRAPHY. (Described on page 369.) The mammogram usually reveals a well circumscribed radiolucent mass with clean margins.[28]

ULTRASOUND. (See page 369.) Sonography frequently shows a hypoechoic, well delineated mass with variable shadowing and some compressibility.[28]

Differential Medical Diagnosis. Microcyst, fibroadenoma.

Plan

PSYCHOSOCIAL INTERVENTIONS. Once a definitive diagnosis is made, reassure the client that galactocele is a benign condition that rarely interferes with current or future lactation. In addition, discuss issues related to self-concept or sexuality. Encourage the client to express her feelings and concerns. If necessary, refer her to a breastfeeding support group, for example, La Leche League.

SURGICAL INTERVENTION

EXCISION OF THE AFFECTED DUCT. This surgery, though rarely needed,[31] is indicated if the lesion recurs frequently. An incision is made in the quadrant of the areola where the affected duct is located. The duct is then removed and sent to a pathology lab. (More often than surgery, a repeat aspiration is needed.)[31]

Adverse effects, or complications of surgery, may include infection and a possible reaction to the local anesthetic. The anticipated outcome on evaluation is total obliteration of the mass.

Help the client to choose a surgeon with expertise in this type of breast surgery. In addition, explain that the procedure is most often performed in ambulatory surgery under local anesthesia. Inform the client that a periareolar incision is usually made and only a small bandage is required. A minor cosmetic change may result. Mild to moderate pain is associated with the procedure, but there are virtually no complications.

Follow-up visits should be made to the surgeon as directed. Routine breast exams should be continued by the health care provider and a monthly BSE is advocated for the client during and following lactation.

MALIGNANT BREAST NEOPLASMS (BREAST CANCER)

Breast cancer, an overgrowth of neoplastic cells of the breast, is a life threatening, and when diagnosed, a life altering disease. Now that women are living longer, the threat of breast cancer is increasing.

Epidemiology

The precise etiology of breast cancer is unknown; however, the disease is thought to develop in response to a number of related factors: increasing age, positive family history, previous breast cancer, late menopause, hormonal factors, and nulliparity.[14,41] Increased fat intake, once thought to have a positive association with the incidence of breast cancer, has now been found to have no positive association with this disease.[42,43,44] No reduction of risk was found even when dietary fat intake was reduced to less than 20 percent of the total caloric intake.[43]

Breast cancer accounts for one out of every three cancer diagnoses in the United States.[1] It occurs second only to skin cancer in American women; in fact, it is estimated that one out of every eight women in the United States will develop breast cancer.[1] Approximately 44,300 deaths from breast cancer and the diagnosis of approximately 184,300 new cases among American women were estimated for 1996.[1] Only lung cancer causes more deaths in women than breast cancer.[1]

Breast cancer is rare among young women, accounting for one case in every 100,000 women between the ages of 20–24.[1] The incidence rises to 25.2 cases per 100,000 for women ages 30–34; 125.4 cases per 100,000 for women ages 40–44, and 232.7 cases in women 50–54 years of age.[45] Thus, the incidence of breast cancer increases with age and approximately 77 percent of women newly diagnosed with breast cancer each year are over the age of 50.[1] Unfortunately, breast cancer is the leading cause of death for women between the ages of 45 and 50.[2]

Caucasian women are more likely to develop breast cancer than African American women, with a rate of 113.1 per 100,000 women.[45] The rate for African American women is 101.0 cases per 100,000 women.[45] For all women younger than 45 years of age, African American women are more likely to develop cancer, and among all women African American women are more likely to die of breast cancer than caucasian women.[1,45] It is proposed that breast cancer in African American women may be diagnosed at later stages, may be more estrogen-receptor negative, and may be more difficult to treat.[1] Limited access to health care as well as socioeconomic and cultural factors may contribute to the late diagnosis of breast cancer and mortality associated with breast cancer in African American women.[1,41]

Hispanic women who were diagnosed with breast cancer in California between 1988 and 1992 had an incidence of 69 per 100,000 women and a mortality rate of 18 per 100,000 women.[46] Rates varied among Asian women in California during the same period of time (Korean 23.3/100,000; Southeast Asian 31.8/100,000; Chinese 52.1/100,000; Japanese 74.0/100,000; Filipino 73.8/100,000). Mortality rates ranged from 7 per 100,000 among Korean women to 14 per 100,000 for Filipino and Japanese women.[46]

Breast cancer is two to three times more likely to develop in women whose mothers or sisters have had breast cancer,[1,47] and its incidence is higher among nulliparous women and women whose first full-term pregnancy occurred after age 30.[47] There is a four fold increased risk of breast cancer in the daughters of premenopausal women with breast cancer, but there is no increased risk in daughters of women who developed breast cancer after menopause. If a mother or sister has premenopausal unilateral breast cancer, the likelihood of a woman developing breast cancer is 10 to 30 percent.[48] Women whose mothers or sisters have bilateral premenopausal breast cancer have a 40 to 50 percent likelihood of developing the disease.[48]

Hormone replacement therapy (HRT) might provide a modest risk of breast cancer.[49] The risk increases with 5 or more years of HRT and is greatest for women between the ages of 60 to 64. There are estimates of a 1.3 to 2 fold increase in breast cancer in those using HRT, depending on duration of use, age, alcohol consumption, and use of concomitant progestins.[50,51]

There are other studies that have found no risk or a decreased risk of breast cancer with the use of hormone replacement therapy.[52,53] The data has lead to confusion regarding the relationship between hormone replacement therapy and breast cancer. It is noted, however, that the lack of uniformity and consistency in study results indicates that if there is an impact of hormone replacement therapy on breast cancer, it is likely a small one.[52]

It is believed that bone mass may be the key to determining the body's cumulative exposure to estrogen, thereby, being a predictor of risk of breast cancer.[54] A recent report has linked high bone density with an increased risk of breast cancer in postmenopausal woman.[54] Women with the highest bone mass were found to be at much greater risk of postmenopausal breast cancer than those with lower bone mass. This maybe important information for future treatment with hormone replacement therapy and in screening for breast cancer in African American females.

Nulliparity has also been associated with increases in breast cancer as well as late age of first full term pregnancy.[1,41] It is thought that a woman giving birth before age 20 has half the risk of developing breast cancer as a woman giving birth after age 30.[41] Some studies have shown a slightly increased risk of breast cancer among women with a history of pregnancy termination, which occurred spontaneously or via elective abortion.[55-59] Recently, studies have shown no relationship.[60]

A history of contralateral breast cancer is one of the strongest single risk factors for the development of a secondary primary breast cancer.[12] A history of endometrial, ovarian, or colon cancer has also been linked to an increased risk of breast cancer.[49]

BRCA1/BRCA2 Genes. The BRCA1 Gene, a tumor suppressor gene, was isolated in the latter half of 1994.[61] It has been localized or mapped to chromosome 17q12-21 by genetic linkages to families with many cases of breast cancer.[48,62] A woman with this gene who has multiple relatives with early onset breast cancer may have a breast cancer risk of 95 percent.[48] Mutations of this gene account for disease in 80 to 90 percent of families with breast and ovarian cancer, and there are now more than 80 mutations of the BRCA1 gene.[63,64]

The BRCA1 gene has been found in women with no first degree family history of breast or ovarian cancer. Eighty percent of those women have a risk of getting the disease.[65]

It has been estimated that 1 in 100 women of Ashkenazi Jewish origin carries the 185 del AG frame shift mutation of the BRCA1 gene, making them more at risk for breast cancer.[66] Jewish women, in whom breast cancer has been diagnosed prior to age 40, have a 20 percent chance of having the 185 del ag mutation regardless of family history of breast cancer.[67] Though found primarily in Ashkenazi Jewish women, Jewish researchers recently found a woman of non-Ashkenazi origin with the mutation.[68] Hence, many physicians now suggest that all women of Jewish ancestry, who have an increased risk of breast cancer, be tested for the mutation.[68]

It is also suspected that genetic susceptibility to breast cancer in high-risk African American women under age 60 can be explained by the BRCA1 gene.[69]

Carriers of the BRCA1 gene or its mutation face difficult and uncertain choices about medical or surgical options to reduce the risk for breast cancer.[70] Controversy exists regarding whether new findings related to the BRCA1 gene are justification for increased genetic screening, though women with the gene are at increased risk of getting breast cancer.[71] Testing for the BRCA1 Gene is available.[69]

A second gene, called BRCA2, has been mapped to a specific region on chromosome 13.[48] Breast cancer survival is worse in patients with the BRCA2 breast cancer gene as these tumors are usually more aggressive.[72] Research continues that investigates both of these genes.[73,74]

Tumor Marker CA27.29. In 1996, the Food and Drug Administration approved the first blood test for breast cancer recurrence.[75] The test measures CA27.29, a tumor marker found in the blood of patients with breast cancer and other types of cancer. Normally, as breast cancer progresses, the level of CA27.29 antigen in the blood rises. The new test is not intended as the sole basis for the diagnosis of cancer, which can be made only after the results are verified by other procedures such as biopsy; however, it provides health care providers with an additional tool to help detect the recurrence of breast cancer in the earliest stages.[75]

Her-2/neu Oncogene

Her-2/neu is an oncogene whose proteins are often elevated in tumors of patients with metastases.[1] Overexpression of her-2/neu in breast carcinomas correlates with poor prognosis, though strength as a prognostic indicator varies.[76] The overexpression of this gene may have prognostic significance with respect to local relapse in the conservatively treated breast.[77]

Profile of Specific Malignant Tumors[30,37,40,78,79]

Invasive Ductal Carcinoma. Represents about 80 percent of all breast cancers. It can spread rapidly to axillary and other lymph nodes even while small. Breast hardness, dimpling, and nipple retraction develops. Lesions appear more lobulated as they enlarge. This most common type of breast cancer starts in the ducts, breaks through the duct wall, and invades fatty breast tissue.

Medullary Carcinoma. Represents 5 percent of breast cancers and is most often found among women younger than 50 years. It is a rounded, somewhat soft tumor that characteristically grows rapidly. In this infiltrating breast cancer, the tumor appears well defined with obvious boundaries between the tumor and normal tissue. Necrosis in this lesion is common, which may result in liquefaction and cyst formation. There is a better than average prognosis since it is slow to metastasize. Signs include a large palpable tumor that is fixed to the chest wall or skin and ulceration.

Comedocarcinoma. This cancer originates in the lining of the mammary duct, and as it grows, fills the duct. Cancer cells undergo necrosis and slough into the lumen of the duct, forming a large quantity of necrotic debris. The tumor is sometimes large but is not likely to spread beyond the breast or into the skin. The prognosis is usually good.

Mucinous Carcinoma. A ductal cancer that accounts for about 2 percent of breast cancers. Usually it grows slowly and rarely spreads to the nodes. There is characteristically an abundance of extracellular mucin around the tumor cell that is produced by the cancer cells. Mucinous carcinoma may have sharp borders and may be confused with a fibroadenoma. It usually presents as a mass but may be accompanied by nipple discharge, fixation, and skin ulceration. Less often, it is associated with metastasis; thus, prognosis is usually good.

Tubular Ductal Carcinoma. This is the best differentiated of the ductal carcinomas and the type with the best prognosis. It is an invasive cancer whose cells are arranged in regular, well defined tubules typically lined by one epithelial layer and accompanied by fibrous stroma. Axillary metastases are uncommon. The presenting symptom, a palpable mass, is occasionally accompanied by skin retraction or fixation. The prognosis is better than for invasive carcinoma.

Invasive Lobular Carcinoma. This cancer arises in the milk producing lobules of the breasts, then breaks through the lobular wall. It then spreads invasively elsewhere throughout the breasts. It usually presents as a nondescript skin thickening. Axillary node involvement is common, and this cancer usually metastasizes to sites in the lung, breast, and liver. The presenting tumor is frequently located in the upper, outer breast quadrant. Skin retraction and fixation accompany large lesions. The prognosis is poor.

Paget's Disease. A cancer of the nipple that is almost always associated with an underlying intraductal carcinoma and frequently with a long history of eczema of the nipple. Itching, burning, oozing, erythema, crusting or bleeding of the nipple and areola occur. There is frequently a unilateral lesion (see Figure 14–4).

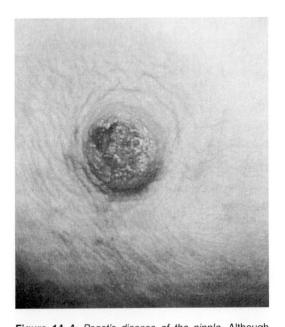

Figure 14–4. *Paget's disease of the nipple.* Although there is only a small area of excoriation, biopsy showed this to be Paget's disease of the nipple. Any area of eczematous change of the nipple should be biopsied. Paget's disease of the nipple may heal between episodes of excoriation and a recent history of excoriation is also an indication for biopsy.

Subjective Data (see prior descriptions)

A client may report one or more of the following conditions.

- A fixed, poorly defined lump or mass may be noted in one breast. Rarely is it painful. The lump is usually located in the upper, outer quadrant of the breast. (*Note:* A lump can be palpated when it reaches a size of approximately 1 cm; it has possibly been present for 7 to 8 years when palpable at that size.)
- Spontaneous nipple discharge that is clear, yellow, or bloody may appear unilaterally.
- Persistent nipple irritation is reported.
- Dimpling or redness of the skin, nipple retraction, change in breast contour, inflammation, swelling and peau d'orange skin (advanced malignancy) may occur. (These are characteristics of what is called inflammatory breast cancer, which is not a distinct cancer, but represents an extension of the tumor into the intradermal lymphatics.)
- Axillary adenopathy, or supraclavicular/ intraclavicular adenopathy (advanced malignancy) is described.

Objective Data

Physical Examination. Physical examination should be performed in a slow and meticulous manner. Examination of the breast requires observation for and palpation of the subjective symptoms. Peau d'orange skin of the breast may also be observed, and in advanced malignancies, a mass fixed to the chest wall may be palpated.

Careful lymphatic palpation is performed to determine supraclavicular, infraclavicular, and axillary nodal involvement.

Diagnostic Tests and Methods

MAMMOGRAPHY. (See benign breast conditions, fibrocystic breast changes, page 369.)

ULTRASOUND. (See benign breast conditions, fibrocystic breast changes, page 369.)

FINE NEEDLE ASPIRATION. (See benign breast conditions, fibroadema, page 374.) The procedure for fine needle aspiration is altered for a solid mass in that several passes are made through the mass while aspirating.[33] The aspiration continues until aspirate is visualized in the hub of the needle. Aspiration is then stopped and the needle is removed cleanly. The specimen should be sent to the lab preserved in isopropyl alcohol.

STEREOTACTIC CORE BIOPSY. This computerized mammographic biopsy yields highly accurate results.[80] When done well it has a 98 percent sensitivity, which is similar to that of needle localized excisional biopsy.[81] Computerized mammography triangulates the location of the breast lesion to within 1 mm. The lesion is then sampled using a 14 gauge needle and the sample is sent to the lab for histologic diagnosis.[80] This procedure can be done with a local anesthetic, may be painful, and normally causes little or no scarring of the breast. The client can usually resume routine activities in 24 hours.

NEEDLE LOCALIZATION BIOPSY. This is a very significant methodology to use with lesions that are detected by mammography but are not palpable.[14,33] Mammography is used to provide guidance for surgical biopsy of the lesion,[33] in fact, the mammographer's goal is to place the needle close to the lesion so that the surgeon can maximize the size of the biopsy.[16]

A thin guide wire is placed through a percutaneous needle. The wire has a hooked tip that is anchored within the lesion.[33] Mediolateral and craniocaudal views are obtained with the needle and wire in place. Dye may be injected near the lesion as an alternative to the needle, or both may be used.[33] A more precise identification of the lesion is provided with needle localization, and less normal tissue is removed with the biopsy. Less than 5 percent of needle localized biopsies do not contain the lesion.

Local anesthesia is often used and the procedure can be performed on the client as an outpatient. If the lesion is close to the chest wall or deeply situated in large breasts, a more than allowable dose of local anesthetic may be required. General anesthesia may be best suited in these cases.[33]

EXCISIONAL BIOPSY. (See benign breast conditions/fibroadenoma breast changes, page 375.) This diagnostic procedure is usually the standard for breast cancer diagnosis.[48] This technique usually reveals one cancer for every three or four benign findings. Excisional biopsy is optimal for removing small lesions of the breast since the entire mass is often removed with this technique.[14] The procedure requires cleansing the breast with an antiseptic solution. The mass is then surgically excised under local anesthesia, and the biopsied lesion is sent to the pathology lab. When a deeper lesion is present, a combination of intravenous and local anesthetic is very effective.[48] The incision is sutured or held together with adhesive strips.

Explain the procedure to the client and refer her to a qualified surgeon. The client should participate in selecting the surgeon. Review the possible complications of the procedure: hematoma, stitch abscess, malignant tumor remaining partially intact, reaction to local anesthetic, and infection. Provide client support.

INCISIONAL BIOPSY. This procedure is usually performed for diagnostic purposes,[14] particularly in a minimally suspicious lesion or in a large surgically unresectable lesion, to obtain tissue for hormone receptor analysis.[33] This diagnostic evaluation is done to determine quickly, prior to surgical intervention, whether a tumor is malignant. The decision to use this form of biopsy depends on the size and location of the lesion and the degree of clinical suspicion.[33] It can confirm the diagnosis of advanced cancer.

The procedure requires skin preparation with an antiseptic solution. Under local anesthesia, a small wedge of tissue is excised with sharp dissection from the diseased area. The incision is then closed. Adhesive strips may be used to close the wound. The specimen is submitted to the pathology lab for histologic evaluation.

Explain the procedure to the client and be supportive. Teach her about possible complications: bleeding, infection, reaction to local anesthetic. In explaining, reinforce for the client that only a small wedge of the lesion will be taken and that the remaining, possibly malignant, tumor will be left intact. Referral to a qualified surgeon is required. Encourage the client to participate in selecting a surgeon.

HORMONE RECEPTOR ASSAYS. This procedure is done to determine a tumor's dependency on female hormone.[37] The assay predicts metastatic disease response to hormone manipulation.[27] If the estrogen receptor (ER) is negative, the client is less likely to benefit from hormonal therapy.[12,14] In contrast, if the estrogen receptor is positive, the client is likely to respond to hormonal therapy. Positive ER levels are those greater than or equal to 10 fm/mg protein. Negative levels are those less than 10 fm/mg protein.

The tumor is excised, put in a sterile container, and immediately chilled. If necessary, the specimen can be frozen and stored until it is sent to a lab for analysis. The procedure is done under local anesthesia.

Explain the procedure to the client and provide support. Also explain the possible complications: bleeding, infection, and reaction to local anesthetic. Referral to a qualified surgeon is required; encourage the client to participate in the selection of a surgeon.

Differential Medical Diagnoses

Fibroadenoma, intraductal papilloma, eczema.

Plan

Psychosocial Interventions. Help the client to cope with her fear, anxiety, and impaired self-image, if present, and encourage family support. Referral to a support group, for example, Reach to Recovery, or to a counselor or minister may be appropriate. Remember to provide culturally sensitive counseling. (The client's family usually needs support as well and an appropriate referral should be made.) A cooperative/interactive team approach with this client is vital.

If surgery is performed, explain to the client that the absence of breasts or breast function may not decrease her female sexual response. Orgasm should still be possible, if not directly tied to nipple manipulation and stimulation, since clitoral function is primary to the female sexual response and is still possible.[3] Also, advise the client and her family that the diagnosis of cancer neither equates to imminent death, decrease in attractiveness, nor diminished sexual appetite.[3] Assure her that past misdeeds, family sins, nor improper health caused her to develop breast cancer; however, be mindful that women of some cultures may continue to hold this belief.

Medication

ADJUVANT THERAPY. Adjuvant therapy, usually chemotherapy or hormonal therapy postsurgery, is most often a preventative measure but actually represents an attempt to ablate micrometastatic disease that may lead to tumor recurrence.[82] Patients are treated with potentially dangerous drugs in hopes of this long-term benefit. Adjuvant systemic therapy had been generally reserved for patients with positive lymph nodes; however, many node negative patients were offered this treatment during the National Surgical Adjuvant Breast and Bowel Project (NSABP), which began in 1992.[12] The current recommendations for adjuvant chemotherapy and hormonal therapy in breast cancer are the following:[12]

- Treat menopausal patients with positive lymph nodes with adjuvant combination therapy;
- Consider chemotherapy for premenopausal patients with negative axillary nodes but with other high risk features (e.g., large tumors, high grade tumors, high levels of epidermal growth factor);
- Treat menopausal patients who have negative lymph nodes and positive hormone receptor levels with adjuvant tamoxifen (Those with positive nodes may receive either cytoxic or hormonal therapy); and
- Consider adjuvant chemotherapy for post menopausal patients who have negative hormone receptor levels.

Adjuvant systemic therapy is not currently recommended for small nonpalpable tumors, those that cannot be quantitatively tested for hormone receptor, or those with favorable DNA studies and negative axillary lymph nodes.[49] The use of adjuvant therapy must also be evaluated in terms of the emotional effect on the quality of life and the toxicity of the drug.[82]

CHEMOTHERAPY. Any of 50 or more chemotherapy agents may be used; however, a combination of cyclophosphamide, methotrexate and fluorouracil(CMF) is most commonly used.[20,82] Usually a combination of two to five drugs is used, though a single drug is sometimes very effective. For example, Doxorubicin (Adriamycin) is the most active single agent used in the treatment of metastatic breast cancer.[20] Doxorubicin, though more toxic, may be used for a shorter period of time than the 3 to 8 months usually allotted for CMF therapy.[20] Women with ten or more positive nodes are often referred for high dose chemotherapy.[20]

In patients with localized inoperable or marginally operable breast cancer, cytotoxic drugs have been used to downstage the patient to a more operable state.[82]

- *Administration.* Administration of the therapy depends on the agent, disease stage, (which is used to determine the extent of local, regional or distant cancer involvement; see Table 14–2, and the site of metastasis if present. It is given intravenously, orally, or possibly intrathecally.
- *Side Effects.* Side effects include nausea, vomiting, alopecia, stomatitis, leukopenia, destruction of healthy cells, cardiotoxicity, early menopause, and infertility.[14,19,17,73]
- *Anticipated Outcomes on Evaluation.* Regression in the dissemination of cancer, ablation of micrometastatic disease, and improvement in survivability.
- *Client Teaching and Counseling.* Refer the client to a qualified oncologist for treatment, and advise her to consult with more than one. Provide literature about chemotherapeutic drugs. Discuss possible adverse reactions to the drugs and other possible drug effects on body image, self-perception, or self-esteem. Inform the client that medications may be prescribed to treat some symptoms and that a cap is available to help reduce hair loss. Refer her to a local support group such as Reach to Recovery.

HORMONAL THERAPY

- *Indications.* Hormone therapy is given to promote tumor regression and to delay recurrence, post-mastectomy, among women who have cancer that is sensitive to estrogen.[14] The basis of the therapy is to block or counter the effect of estrogen. Tamoxifen, a widely used antiestrogenic agent, is indicated when the cancerous tumor shows estrogen receptors.[20] Tamoxifen is often used in women with 1 to 3 positive nodes and those who are considered at low risk. It may decrease the incidence of cancer in the contralateral breast.[82] It has been used exten-

TABLE 14–2. STAGING OF BREAST CANCER

Stage	Characteristics
0	The earliest type of breast cancer, the disease is in situ.
I	The tumor is less than 1 inch in diameter and has not spread beyond the breast.
II	The tumor is about 1 to 2 inches in diameter and/or has spread to axillary lymph nodes.
III	The tumor is about 2 inches or larger and may have spread to the axillary nodes and/or to other lymph nodes, or to other tissues near the breast.
IV	The cancer has metastasized to other body organs.

Source: American Cancer Society (1995). Breast cancer dictionary. Atlanta, GA: American Cancer Society. American.

Cancer Society (1995). For women facing breast cancer. Atlanta, GA: American Cancer Society.

sively in the National Surgical Adjuvant Breast and Bowel Project (NSABP), which began in 1992. Most oncologists prescribe tamoxifen therapy for 5 years, though the duration of therapy is controversial.[20]

- *Administration.* Tamoxifen, one to two 10-mg tablets, p.o., b.i.d.
- *Side Effects and Adverse Reactions.* Hot flashes, nausea, depression, vomiting, vaginal bleeding and discharge, unintended pregnancy, menstrual irregularities, and bone pain. More serious side effects are endometrial cancer, liver cancer, thromboembolitic disease, and retinopathy.[14,17,82]
- *Contraindications.* None are known.
- *Anticipated Outcomes on Evaluation.* Tumor regression and increased likelihood of survival. An additional benefit of reduction in cardiovascular death is anticipated because tamoxifen lowers the cholesterol level. This effect occurs within the first 3 to 6 months and is sustained during the treatment.
- *Client Teaching and Counseling.* Refer the client to a qualified oncologist; the client should consult with more than one oncologist. Inform the client that therapy is most effective in cancers sensitive to estrogen. Discuss the side effects/risk factors in detail. Discuss data related to the tamoxifen trials. Advise endometrial evaluation to rule out cancer, and recommend close follow-up with the oncologist.

Radiation Therapy. Radiation therapy is used to treat early stage breast cancer. It is generally used in combination with breast conservation surgery to destroy or suppress cells that are not removed by surgery[14] and offers a small but important survival advantage.[83] The use of radiation following chemotherapy in women at substantial risk for metastasis is said to improve control of distant disease and survival without compromising the control of local disease.[84] Chemotherapy followed by radiation therapy is currently being used more often to treat early stage breast cancer.

External radiation (x-rays) is directed to the breast and possibly the axillary lymph nodes. Sometimes a booster or concentrated dose of radiation is given in the area where cancer is located.[14] Radiation may be administered by electron beam or internal radioactive implant.

- *Adverse Effects.* Fatigue, temporary discoloration of the skin, itching or peeling, leukopenia, retraction of the breast, breast fibrosis, cancer secondary to radiation therapy, and pleural effusion.[14]
- *Anticipated Outcomes on Evaluation.* Eradication of the pathology, maintenance of breast integrity, and improved chances for survival.
- *Client Teaching and Counseling.* Provide the client with information about the course of radiation therapy: Noting that it usually requires 5 to 6 weeks and daily trips to the treatment site, where a qualified radiologist administers therapy. Advise the client that she may feel fatigued and that the skin directly exposed to radiation may look or feel as though it has been sunburned.[14] Assure her that the skin should return to normal in 1 or more months after therapy has been completed and that the use of a sunscreen and protective clothing should help to prevent further irritation. Refer the client to a support group, such as Reach to Recovery. Discuss the need for annual mammography.

Surgical Interventions.*[14,37,48,85]* Surgery for breast cancer involves removal of the tumor, with or without complete mastectomy or axillary node dissection and subsequent breast reconstruction if desired.[85] The surgery performed fits in one of two groups; partial mastectomy, which usually conserves the breast, or complete mastectomy, which removes the breast.

Several factors are important in determining whether breast conservation therapy should be used: size, location, invasiveness and histopathology of the tumor, risk for tumor recurrence, as well as the client's age and attitude regarding the surgery. Patients with tumors measuring up to 4 cm. are normally considered candidates; however, when the tumor is 3 cm or more in size it may be difficult to obtain the desired cosmetic result or to clearly define the tumor margins. In addition, removal of a tumor that is large in relationship to the breast size may produce an undesired cosmetic outcome. It may also be difficult to obtain a good cosmetic result when multiple tumors are present.

Lesions that are removed from the periphery of the breast normally provide a more aesthetically pleasing outcome than tumors that are removed from central locations that include the nipple-areola complex. This should not necessarily deter breast conservation therapy if the client chooses it with full knowledge of the potential cosmetic impairment.

Breast conservation therapy may be performed in invasive and noninvasive cancer and will normally be followed by radiation in invasive disease. Radiation may or may not be used in noninvasive disease.

The specific type of breast cancer is not usually considered a strong determinant of the feasibility of breast conservation surgery. In the presence of invasive lobular cancer, with its wide diffuse and vague margins, complete mastectomy might provide a safer choice for the patient.

There is no age limit for breast conservation surgery; however, breast cancer may recur after lumpectomy, and young women who may live longer can be more at risk for cancer recurrence.[86] Because of this, breast conservation surgery may not be favored in women younger than 40 years of age.

Clients who have anxiety regarding cancer recurrence following breast conservation surgery may choose to have a complete mastectomy. On the other hand, some clients are more concerned about their physical appearance and may consider breast conservation surgery the only desired option.

Patients who choose breast conservation therapy must have access to a radiation facility and must be followed closely. They must clearly understand that cancer recurrence is a possibility.

PARTIAL MASTECTOMY

LUMPECTOMY OR SEGMENTAL MASTECTOMY.
Lumpectomy, which has best results when used on small lesions, involves the gross removal of the tumor and a wedge of surrounding normal breast tissue in node negative cancers. Usually axillary lymph nodes are removed. If nodes are not removed, undetected microscopic nodal involvement may be left in place, necessitating later surgery or resulting in disease recurrence. Radiation often follows and adjuvant therapy may be administered. Infection postsurgery may occur.

This procedure may be cosmetically unappealing for women with small breasts if a large portion of breast is removed.

The anticipated outcomes on evaluation are removal of pathology, preservation of the breast, and improved chances for survival. Client teaching includes clearly explaining the surgery and referral to a qualified surgeon. The client should be advised that a greater risk of cancer recurrence exists, especially if nodes are not evaluated.

COMPLETE MASTECTOMY

TOTAL MASTECTOMY.
This surgery is indicated for women with carcinoma in situ (ductal or lobular) with no suspicious axillary involvement or in women whose tumor recurred after partial mastectomy and axillary dissection. The surgery involves removal of the breast and pectoralis major muscle fascia.

Adverse effects may arise if the axillary chain is left intact and not evaluated for cancer. Nodal involvement may be microscopic and nonpalpable. If cancer is later detected in the lymph chain, further surgery, radiation, or other adjuvant therapy may be required. Postoperative infection is possible.

The anticipated outcomes on evaluation are removal of the pathology and improved survival.

In client teaching, contrast and compare total and modified radical mastectomy. Include a discussion of reconstructive surgery. Inform the client that breast prostheses are available. Radiation therapy will frequently be recommended and requires discussion. Refer the client to a support group such as Reach to Recovery for preoperative and postoperative support. Reinforce the practice of BSE.

MODIFIED RADICAL MASTECTOMY.
Modified radical mastectomy is indicated when tumors are not large or bulky, when axillary adenopathy is not bulky, and when interpectoral nodes are not grossly involved. The surgery involves removal of the breast, axillary nodes, and, often, the pectoralis minor. Adverse effects include lymphedema, infection, and hematoma.

The anticipated outcomes on evaluation are removal of the pathology and improved chances of survival.

Provide the client with information about the procedure (e.g, surgeon qualifications, anesthesia, and possible complications of surgery). Referral to physical and occupational therapy is imperative. Counsel the client about breast reconstruction and inform her that breast prostheses are available. Refer her to a support group for preoperative and postoperative support. In addition, a professional counselor may be needed. A team approach is necessary for the client's rehabilitation. Reinforce the practice of BSE.

RADICAL MASTECTOMY.
Radical mastectomy is indicated for the removal of cancers with large bulky tumors involving the pectoralis major or fascia, bulky axillary lymph involvement, or grossly involved interpectoral nodes. With improvements in early detection, radical mastectomy is done less frequently. The surgery involves removal of the breast, pectoralis major and pectoralis minor muscles, skin overlying the tumor, and all axillary nodes. Adverse effects include extensive scarring, hollow chest, lymphedema, infection, skin necrosis, and disfigurement. Breast reconstruction is difficult if possible at all.

The anticipated outcomes on evaluation are the removal of the pathology and improved chances for survival.

Center client teaching on the procedure and its possible adverse effects. Hospitalization and general anesthesia are required. In addition to a qualified surgeon, a physical and/or occupational therapist will be needed. A team approach is preferable for rehabilitation. Discuss

TABLE 14–3. RECOMMENDED FOLLOW-UP SCHEDULE FOR BREAST CANCER PATIENTS

Examination	Mastectomy	Breast Conserving	Advanced Disease
H&P	Every 3 mos. X 1 year, Every 6 mos thereafter	Every 3 mos. X 3–5 yrs, Every 6 mos. thereafter	Every 3 mos.
Mammography	Annually	Yearly contralateral every 6mos Ipsilateral until stable, then yearly	Annually
Lab analysis (CBC)	Annually	Annually	Every 3–6 mos
Chest XRAY	Annually	Annually	Every 3–6 mos or as symptons arise
Bone Scans	For symptoms only	For symptoms only	For symptoms only
Liver Scans	For symptoms only	For symptoms only	For symptoms only

Adapted with permission from Pace, B. W.; Tinker, M. D.: Follow-up of patients with breast cancer. Clinical Obstet Gynecol 1994; 37(4)998–1002.

the difficulty of breast reconstruction, and inform the client that breast prostheses are available. A visit by a specialist in fitting breast forms or foundations may be arranged. The management of lymphedema and other side effects must also be taught, and exercises to reduce lymphedema or arm stiffness should begin 24 hours after surgery. Encourage ROM exercises and encourage the client to avoid restrictive clothing such as tight sleeves. The client should also avoid underarm creams, depilatories, and deodorants. Reinforce the importance of BSE and refer the client to a support group such as Reach to Recovery for preoperative and postoperative support. If indicated, suggest professional counseling.

AUTOLOGOUS BONE MARROW TRANSPLANT.[37,87] Transplanted bone marrow is indicated for the treatment of extremely aggressive breast cancer or cancers that have metastasized. Bone marrow is withdrawn from the client to protect it. It is cleaned, treated and stored. Extremely high doses of chemotherapy are then administered to the client to destroy cancerous cells. Bone marrow is also destroyed, which robs the body of its natural ability to fight infection. Next, the bone marrow is reinjected or transplanted after chemotherapeutic agents have been absorbed. Adverse effects include nausea, vomiting, alopecia, leukopenia, and fatigue. The anticipated outcome on evaluation is regression of the spread of cancer and improved survivability. Clients who are in complete or partial remission prior to transplantation often have a higher response rate.[87]

Advise the client that several weeks of hospitalization will be required. A hospital with the facilities and staff capable of performing transplant will need to be selected. Advise the client that most insurance companies do not cover the cost of this high risk therapy.

Follow-Up (see Table 14–3)

The follow-up of clients who have had chemotherapy is variable, and depends on their response to the drugs and on the oncologist's recommendations. Clients may receive tamoxifen for 2 to 5 years, with follow-up every 6 months or per the oncologists's preference.

Clients who receive tamoxifen should have a physical examination every 3 to 4 months for the first 5 years with a CBC twice yearly and a chest x-ray and mammogram annually. Endometrial evaluation should be performed routinely (see Figure 14–2).

Breast conservation clients who are asymptomatic are often requested to have mammography every 6 months for the first 2 to 3 years after radiation therapy.[88]

Clients who undergo a mastectomy are evaluated postoperatively at the discretion of the surgeon. Complications, if encountered, may require more frequent evaluation or may necessitate rehospitalization. Clients undergoing autologous bone marrow transplants are followed closely by the oncologist and may require weekly visits after leaving the hospital.

BREAST RECONSTRUCTION

Breast reconstruction, a voluntary procedure, is available to many women who have undergone mastectomy. In addition to being an option following mastectomy, breast reconstruction and augmentation may also be chosen for cosmetic reasons that are unrelated to cancer surgery.[3,89]

The process of breast reconstruction surgery changed dramatically in 1992 when the Food and Drug Administration (FDA) restricted the use of silicone implants, the most common breast implant used in the United States.[90,91] Silicone breast implants had been used for reconstruction and cosmetic enhancement of the breasts since the early 1960s.[92] Multiple complaints of rheumatic conditions, including fibromyalgia, systemic lupus erythematosus, polymyositis and Raynaud's phenomenon were reported and associated with silicone implants, which caused the utilization of this long used implant to cease.[91] Though the use of these implants was terminated in strictly cosmetic surgeries, the FDA later (1992) approved the use of silicone implants in patients undergoing breast reconstruction surgery, following mastectomy, who were involved in clinical trials. This ruling stands today. Saline breast implants are now the only implant available for elective cosmetic breast augmentation that is unrelated to breast cancer.

Some studies show that patients with silicone breast implants are no more likely to get symptoms of connective tissue diseases than are other patients.[93,94] Still, in 1994 a settlement fund was established by Dow Corning and other manufacturers of silicone gel implants that provided more than 4.2 billion dollars to pay compensation for recipients of these implants who had experienced certain rheumatologic and/or neurologic conditions.[91]

A new implant consisting of a silicone elastomer bag filled with soybean oil is currently being investigated.[90]

TISSUE TRANSFER (TRAM): RECTUS ABDOMINIS MYOCUTANEOUS FLAP[37,48]

Tissue transfer is recommended when the client chooses to have breast reconstruction while avoiding the possible side effects of breast implants. It offers the potential for soft, naturally appearing breast mounds without the associated risks of implanting foreign/manufactured materials.[95] A similar procedure, the latissimus dorsi musculocutaneous flap, may be performed as well when the client has small or moderate sized breasts and does not desire breast implants.[96]

The rectus abdominis muscle is transferred from the abdomen via a tunnel under the skin and extended through a new incision in the breast area. The flap is sutured into position and, along with fat, is contoured to form a breast. Sufficient abdominal girth is required to perform the procedure, which can be very painful and may require 6 to 8 weeks for recuperation. Untoward responses to anesthesia and postoperative infection and bleeding are possible. Initially, sensitivity in the reconstructed breast(s) may be decreased; however, it may later return.[97]

The anticipated outcome on evaluation is a favorable body image.

Explain to the client that the recovery period required is often long and that appropriate pain management will be necessary. Inform her that tissue transfer is not recommended for women who smoke or who have chronic disease. In addition, further surgery will be necessary for nipple formation.

AUGMENTATION MAMMOPLASTY (BREAST ENLARGEMENT)

Augmentation mammoplasty is performed to improve the cosmetic appearance of the breast by increasing its size. Many women choose to undergo this procedure to attain a well proportioned figure[98] or a figure that complies with their and/or society's ideal. When this procedure is performed following mastectomy, it is given the term reconstructive breast surgery.

The surgical procedure involves placing an implant behind the breast through an inframammary, periareolar, or transaxillary incision.[98] The inframammary placement is preferred by some surgeons because it allows complete visualization of the pockets, which enhances symmetry and allows better hemostasis prior to placement of the implants.[98]

Periareolar incisions introduce the implant in a submuscular or subglandular position. This

TABLE 14–4. GRADING OF A CAPSULAR CONTRACTION

Grade	Features
Grade 1	The augmented breast is as soft as an unoperated breast; no palpable firmness.
Grade 2	The breast has minimal firmness; is less soft; the implant can be palpated with no visible abnormalities.
Grade 3	The breast is moderately firm; the implant is easily palpated; implant or distortion caused by it is visible.
Grade 4	Severe contracture with tender, painful, cold breast; marked di'stortion exists.

Source: Howrigan, P. J. (1994). Reduction and augmentation mammoplasty. Obstet Clin North Am. 21:539–549.
Baker, J. T. Jr. (1978). Augmentation mammoplasty. In Ownsley, J. Q. (Ed) Symposium in aesthetic surgery of the breast. St. Louis, MO: Mosby.

may produce a less noticeable scar, but the technique has increased risk of contamination by bacteria contained in the milk ducts.[98] The procedure also has a greater chance of interfering with (decreasing) nipple sensation.

The transaxillary approach produces a remote scar that is well hidden in the axilla.[98,99] Pockets are dissected deep into the pectoralis major muscle, providing less exposure of implants to bacteria from ducts. Care must be given to attain symmetry.

A smooth surfaced silicone elastomer bag filled with silicone gel has historically been the most prevalently used implant.[90] Though it may still be used during breast reconstruction postmastectomy, the saline implant consisting of an elastomer shell filled with saline is now used for all other breast augmentation surgeries.[90]

A common complication of silicone gel and saline implants is the formation of a fibrous capsule or capsular contracture around the implant, which causes a firm rigidity of the breast.[90,100] This fibrous capsule forms as a part of the body's normal response to a foreign body.[90] The capsule may contract and become constrictive. This converts the normally disc shaped implants to appear as a sphere. Some cases may cause disfigurement. Grading of the capsular contracture occurs during physical examination[101] (see Table 14–4).

Treatment of capsular contracture is normally considered ineffective since it probably will recur,[100] however, some surgeons recommend the use of steroids to reduce the formation of scar tissue.[98] Placing steroids in the pocket or instilling them into the implants has been suggested. Placing steroids in the pocket can cause thinning of the skin and subcutaneous tissues at the lower border of the pocket during the postoperative period.[98] Steroid placement in the implant may reduce capsular contracture in the early postoperative period.[98]

Implant rupture may occur spontaneously or after trauma and may cause nodules, decreased breast size, asymmetry, and pain.[90]

Possible side effects of breast enlargement surgery are delayed wound healing, infection, hematoma, changes in breast/nipple sensation, galactorrhea or galactocele, wrinkling, shifting and extrusion of the implant, asymmetry, and dissatisfaction with cosmetic results.[98,100] Untoward reactions to general anesthesia may occur. Wound infection occurs in 2 to 3 percent of cases.[98] Deflamation, rippling, wrinkling, sloshing, and encapsulation diminish client's satisfaction with saline implants.[102]

Breastfeeding with the presence of breast implants should be possible and should not present problems for the nursing infants or mothers.[91] One study, however, revealed esophageal motility disturbances in infants nursed by mothers with breast implants.[103] This symptom is consistent with that sometimes seen in scleroderma.

Screening for breast cancer and for implant integrity may be difficult. Breast implants obscure breast tissue. Mammography, the most common method used to image breasts with implants has two major limitations: (a) it is unable to display the entire implant, leaving the posterior one-third or one-fourth excluded, and (b) it relies primarily on an evaluation of the morphology of the implant.[104] As a result, ruptures that occur around the deep margins of an implant may be missed, and the use of mammography in the diagnosis of an intracapsular rupture is very constricted.[90]

Ultrasound is a very useful tool for the evaluation of the integrity of implants. There is no ionizing radiation, the interior of the implant can be visualized and areas that are difficult or impossible to image with mammography can be seen.[90] The disadvantages of using sonography are that it is very time consuming and requires a highly skilled operator who will scan the breasts meticulously.

Magnetic resonance imaging (MRI) offers an excellent option in the evaluation of the breasts with implants. Its major advantage is its ability to distinguish silicone from normal tissues within the breast.[90] Intracapsular ruptures can be diagnosed. The disadvantage is the cost of the test, especially for women who lack insurance coverage. Also many, if not most, insurances might refuse to cover the cost of this test because it is not routinely used.

The anticipated outcomes upon completion of breast augmentation surgery are improved self-esteem and a favorable body image.

Inform the client of the controversies surrounding breast implants and the possible complications of implants and augmentation surgery. Discuss the possibility of decreased sexual pleasure associated with nipple numbness and breast firmness. Clients with a history of or a propensity for keloid formation (common among African Americans) should consider the possibility of unsightly keloid scarring. Encourage the client to continue BSE and provide her with the instruction she needs (see Figure 14–1). Inform her about the American Cancer Society guidelines for mammography screening. Discuss the difficulties associated with imaging breast tissue when breast implants are present, and help the client to find a mammography facility that uses specialized techniques for women with breast implants.

MASTOPEXY (CORRECTION OF PTOSIS)

Mastopexy is performed to improve the appearance of sagging breasts, which may be caused by gravity, hormone regression (postpartum, menopausal) or weight loss. Surgical resection of the breasts is done, with elevation of the breast mount, areola, and nipple to a new (usually higher) location.

Markings for breast location following surgery are performed with the client in an upright position, and new sites for the nipple-areola complex are chosen.[98] Placement of the nipple-areola complex that is considered aesthetically most attractive is 21cms. from the sternal notch and 21cms. from the midclavicular line.[105]

General anesthesia is used, and infection, hematoma, nipple numbness (usually temporary), asymmetry, and scarring of the breast may develop postoperatively. A reaction to the anesthesia is possible.

The anticipated outcomes on evaluation are a favorable body image and improved self-esteem.

Encourage the client to weigh very carefully the risks and advantages of the procedure. Clients with a history of or a propensity to develop keloids (particularly common in African Americans) should consider possible formation of unsightly keloid scarring. Inform the client that breast ptosis may recur and that sensation in the breast and nipple may be lost, which may decrease sexual gratification. If desired by the client, include significant others in decision making and advise them to seek the opinions of at least two surgeons. Encourage BSE and mammography if age appropriate.

BREAST REDUCTION

The goal of breast reduction surgery is to alleviate the physical symptoms associated with large breasts and to create a breast size and shape that is appropriate for the client's age, body habitus or desire.[98] Breast reduction surgery is performed to reduce breast size and relieve back and shoulder pain caused by heavy pendulous breasts.[106] Many women with large breasts or macromastia complain of neck strain, occipital headache, shoulder pain, disfigurement caused by brassiere straps that burrow into the skin, low back pain, anterior chest discomfort, and paresthesia of the little fingers.[98,106] Often clients with macromastia find participation in exercise and sports activities difficult because of discomfort or self-consciousness.[98] Frequently, unsolicited sexual advances occur, which might be troubling for young adolescents and women who are establishing a sexual identity.[98]

Reduction surgery, which makes breasts smaller, helps to relieve these symptoms and may resolve them totally (scarring and deep shoulder grooves caused by brassiere straps may not resolve). Neck and back pain are relieved in 85 to 95 percent of patients.[98] Smaller breasts may also help those who feel embarrassed about their large breasts to improve their self-image and self-esteem.

During breast reduction surgery, the breasts are surgically restructured and made smaller. Preoperative markings are performed as with mastopexy. In some cases the nipple-areola complex requires resection as a full thickness skin graft and is transplanted to the appropriate position on the breast mound. This often occurs when very large resections of tissue are necessary (greater than 1500 to 2000 gms.); when pronounced ptosis occurs; when it is necessary to limit anesthesia time; and in clients with previous surgery that may result in a compromise of the viability of the nipple-areola complex.[98] The grafted nipple-areola complex will not have normal sensation and may have irregular pigmentation.[98]

The potential adverse effects and complications are asymmetry, infection, hematoma, nipple numbness, extensive scarring, necrosis of the skin flap or nipple-areola complex, and nipple inversion.[98,106]

The anticipated outcomes on evaluation are reduced back and shoulder pain, reduced pressure on skin and irritation from brassiere straps, and improved self-esteem. Some patients find the surgery to be an incentive for total body weight reduction.[106]

Encourage the client to weigh the advantages and risks of this elective surgical procedure. Clients with a history of or propensity to develop keloid (common among African Americans) should consider the possibility of extensive and unsightly keloid scarring. Include significant others of the client's choosing in decision making. Discuss the possible relationship between nipple numbness and decreased sexual gratification. Encourage BSE and mammography if appropriate. Advise the client to seek the opinions of at least two surgeons. Inform her that the procedure generally is covered by insurance because it is not performed for cosmetic reasons alone. The client, however, should consult with her insurance company.

Follow-Up

Clients should follow the postoperative care guidelines provided by the surgeon. Immediate evaluation is especially important if signs or symptoms of infection occur in a client who has had the TRAM flap procedure, because abdominal and chest wounds are present. When possible, refer the client to women who have had breast reconstruction and augmentation surgery who are willing to discuss their experiences.

Routine screening mammography should be continued, and annual clinician exam as well as monthly BSE should continue. Mammography should not be performed sooner than 6 months after surgery has been completed.

NURSING DIAGNOSES

The following nursing diagnoses are representative of those used in the health care plan of women with breast problems. The list, however, is by no means inclusive.

- Altered role performance.
- Anticipatory grieving.
- Anxiety.
- Body image disturbance.
- Denial.
- Dysfunctional grieving.
- Fear.
- Grief.
- High risk for infection.
- Hopelessness.
- Impaired skin integrity.
- Ineffective breastfeeding.
- Ineffective individual or family coping.
- Knowledge deficit.
- Low self-esteem.
- Pain.
- Powerlessness.
- Sexual dysfunction.
- Situational low self-esteem.
- Sleep pattern disturbance.
- Spiritual distress.

REFERENCES

1. American Cancer Society. (1996). *Breast cancer facts and figures.* Atlanta, GA: Author.
2. Henderson, C. (1995). Breast cancer. In G. P. Murphey, W. L. Lawrence, R. E. Lenhard, (Eds.). *Clinical Oncology.* Atlanta, GA: American Cancer Society.
3. Small, E. C. (1994). Psycho-sexual issues. *Obstet Gynecol Clin North Am, 21,* 773–780.
4. National Cancer Institute. *Cancer facts.* March 26, 1997, pp. 1–7.
5. Lawrence, H. C. (1994). History, physical examination, and education in breast self-examination. *Clin Obstet Gynecol, 37,* 881–886.
6. Mechcatie, E. (1996, February 15). Self-exam aid approved for prescription only. *Internal Medicine New.* p. 32.
7. Isaacs, J. H. (1994). Benign tumors of the breast. *Obstet Gynecol Clin North Am, 21,* 487–497.
8. Drukker, B. H. (1994). Fibrocystic changes of the breast. *Clin Obstet Gynecol, 37,* 903–915.
9. Fiorica, J. V. (1994). Fibrocystic changes. *Obstet Gynecol Clin North Am, 21,* 445–452.
10. BeLieu, R. M. (1994). Mastodynia. *Obstet Gynecol Clin North Am, 21,* 461–477.
11. Jackson, V. P. (1995). Management of solid breast nodules: What is the role of sonography? *Radiology, 196,* 14–15.
12. Bell, M. C., & Partridge, E. E. (1995, Dec.). Early breast carcinoma: Risk factors, screening, and treatment. Dec. *Contemp OB/GYN,* 31–32, 36, 40 passim.
13. Schilling, K., & Love, N. (1995). Screening and diagnostic breast imaging procedures. *Postgrad Med,* 44–46, 51, 56 passim.
14. American Cancer Society. (1995). *For women facing breast cancer.* Atlanta, GA: Author.
15. Schapira, D. V., & Levine, R. B. (1996). Breast cancer screening and compliance and evaluation of lesions. *Med Clin North Am, 80,* 15–26.
16. Xenophon, L. (1994). Imaging techniques for breast disease. *Clin Obstet Gynecol, 37,* 933–943.
17. Medical Economics Data Production Company. (1996). *Physicians' desk reference.* (1996). Montvale, NJ: Author.
18. Fisher, B., Constantino, J., Redmond, C., et al. (1994). Endometrial cancer in tamoxifen-treated breast cancer patients. Findings from the national surgical adjuvant breast and bowel project (NSABP) B-14. *J Natl Cancer Inst, 86,* 527.
19. Odom, L. D. (1996). Endometrial surveillance in tamoxifen-treated patients. *Contemp Obstet Gynecol,* 133–134, 139–140, 142 passim.
20. Berkowitz, L. D., & Love, N. (1995). Adjuvant systemic therapy for breast cancer. *Postgrad Med, 98,* 85–86, 88, 91 passim.
21. Benjamin, F. (1994). Normal lactation and galactorrhea. *Clin Obstet Gynecol, 37,* 887–897.
22. Gateley, C., Miers, M., Mansel, R., & Hughes, L. (1992). Drug treatments for mastalagia: 17 years experience in the Cardiff Mastalgia Clinic. *J of Social Medicine, 85,* 12–5.
23. Wetzig, N. (1994). Mastalgia: A 3 year Australian study. *Aust N Z J Surg, 64,* 329–331.
24. McFayden, I., Forrest, A., Chetty, V., & Raab, G. (1992). Cyclical breast pain—Some observations and difficulties in treatment. *Br J Clin Pract, 46,* 161–164.
25. Tyler, V. (1993). *The honest herbal: A sensible guide to the use of herbs and related remedies.* New York: Pharmaceutical Products Press.
26. Serewel, A., Haggie, J., & Cade, D. (1990). A randomized trial of medroxyprogesterone acetate in mastalgia. *Ann R Coll Surg Engl, 72,* 273
27. Lopez, M. J., & Porter, K. A. (1996). The current role of prophylactic mastectomy. *Surg Clin North Am, 76,* 231–242.
28. Hindle, W. H. (1994). Other benign breast problems. *Clin Obstet Gynecol, 37,* 916–924.
29. Carty, N. J., Carter, C., Rubin, C., et al. (1995). Management of fibroadenoma of the breast. *Ann R Coll Surg Engl, 77,* 127–130.
30. Bradley, A. L., & Sharp, K. W. (1995). Breast disease. *Med Clin North Am, 79,* 1443–1455.
31. Scott-Conner, C. E. H., & Schorr, S. J. (1995). The diagnosis and management of breast problems during pregnancy and lactation. *Am J Surg, 170,* 401–405.
32. Hindle, W. H. (1994). The diagnostic evaluation. *Obstet Gynecol Clin North Am, 21,* 499–517.
33. Chalas, E., & Valea, F. (1994). The gynecologist and surgical procedures for breast disease. *Clin Obstet Gynecol, 37,* 948–953.
34. Dixon, J., Dobie, V., Lamb, J., Walsh, J., & Chetty, U. (1996). Assessment of the acceptability of conservative management of fibroadenoma of the breast. *Br J Surg, 83,* 264–265.
35. Fiorica, J. V. (1994). Nipple discharge. *Obstet Clin North Am, 21,* 453–460.
36. Isaacs, J. H. (1994). Other nipple disharge. *Clin Obstet Gynecol, 37,* 898–902.
37. American Cancer Society. (1995). *Breast cancer dictionary.* Atlanta, GA: Author.
38. Webb, A. J. (1995). Mammary duct ectasia-periductal mastitis complex. *Br J Surg, 82,* 1300–1302.

39. Hughes, L. E. (1991). Non-lactational inflammation and duct-ectasia. *Br. Med Bulletin, 47,* 272–283.

40. Sewell, C. W. (1995). Pathology and benign and malignant breast disorders. *Rad Clin North Am, 33,* 1067–1080.

41. Nichols, D. H. (1994). The epidemiologic characteristics of breast cancer. *Clin Obstet Gynecol, 37,* 925–932.

42. Hunter, D. J., Spiegelman, D., Hans-Olov, A., et al. (1996). Cohort studies of fat intake and the risk of breast cancer—A pooled analysis. *New Engl J Med, 334,* 356–361.

43. Pooled analysis dispels link between fat and breast cancer. (1996). *ACOG Newsletter.*

44. National Institute of Child Health and Human Development. (1996). Reduction of dietary fat and breast cancer prevention. *Research reports.* Bethesda, MD: Author.

45. Kosary, C. L., Ries, L. A. G., Miller, B. A., et al. (1995). *Seer cancer statistics review, 1973–1992.* Bethesda, MD: Natl Cancer Inst.

46. Perkins, C. L., Morris, C. R., Wright, W. E., & Young, J. L. (1995). *Cancer incidence and mortality in California by detailed race/ethnicity, 1988–1992.* Sacramento, CA: California Department of Health Services.

47. Crowe, J. P. (1996). An update on breast cancer: Evolving treatments and persistent questions. *Cleveland J of Medicine, 63,* 48–56.

48. Guilano, A. E. (1994). Breast diseases. In J. S. Berek, N. F. Hacker, (Eds.). *Practical gynecologic oncology.* Baltimore, MD: Williams & Wilkins.

49. Colditz, G. A., Hankinson, S. E., Junter, D. J., et al. (1995). The use of estrogens and progestins and the risk of breast cancer in postmenopausal women. *N Engl J Med, 332,* 1589–1593.

50. Hulka, B. S., Liu, E. T., & Lininger, R. A. (1994). Steroid hormones and risk of breast cancer. *Cancer, 74*(Suppl 3), 1111–1124.

51. Isaacs, C., & Swain, S. (1994). Hormone replacement therapy in women with a history of breast carcinoma. *Hem Onc Clin North Am,* 179–195.

52. Speroff, L. (1996). Postmenopausal hormone therapy and breast cancer. *Obstet and Gynecol., 87,* (2 supp) 44s–54s.

53. Theriault, R. (1996). Hormone replacement therapy and breast cancer: An overview. *Br. J. Obstet and Gynecol, 103* (13 supp) 87–91.

54. Zhang, Y., Kiel, D., Kreger, B., et al. (1997). Bone mass and the risk of breast cancer among postmenopausal women. *New Eng J. Medicine, 336,* 611–617.

55. Newcomb, P. A., Storer, B. E., Lognecker, M. P., et al. (1996). Pregnancy termination in relation to risk of breast cancer. *JAMA, 275,* 283–287.

56. Daling, J. R., Malone, K. E., Voight, L. F., et al. (1994). Risk of breast cancer among young women: Relationship to induced abortion. *J Natl Cancer Inst, 86,* 1584–1592.

57. Andrieu, N., Duffy, S. W., Rohan, T. E., et al. (1995). Familial risk, abortion and their interactive effect on the risk of breast cancer: A combined analysis of six case control studies. *Br. J Cancer, 72,* 744–751.

58. Andrieu, N., Clavel, F., Gourard, B., et al. (1994). Familial risk of breast cancer and abortion. *Cancer Detect Prev, 18,* 51–55.

59. Lipworth, L., Katsouyanni, K., Ekbon, A., et al. (1995). Abortion and the risk of breast cancer: A case-control study in Greece. *Int J Cancer, 61,* 181–184.

60. Melbye, M., Wohlfahrt, J., Olsen, J., et al. (1997). Induced abortion and the risk of breast cancer. *N Engl J Med, 336,* 81–85.

61. Weber, B. L., Abel, K. J., Brody, L. C., et al. (1994). Familial breast cancer: approaching the isolation of a susceptibility gene. *Cancer, 74,* 1013–1020.

62. Wooster, R., & Stratton, M. R. (1995). Breast cancer susceptibility: A complex disease unravels. *Trends Genet, 11,* 3–5.

63. Miki, Y., Swensen, J., Shattuck-Eidens, D., et al. (1994). A strong candidate for the 17q-linked breast and ovarian cancer susceptibility gene BRCA1. *Science, 266,* 66–77.

64. Futreal, P. A., Liu, Q., Shattuck-Eidens, D., et al. (1994). BRCA1 mutations in primary breast and ovarian carcinoma. *Science, 266,* 120–122.

65. Langston, A. A., Malone, K. E., Thompson, J. D., et al. (1996). BRCA1 mutations in the population-based sample of young women with cancer. *N Engl J Med, 334,* 137–142.

66. Strueing, J. P., Abeleovich, D., Peretz, T., et al. (1995). The carrier frequency of the BRCA1 185 del AG mutation is approximately one percent in Ashkenazi Jewish individuals. *Nat Genet, 11,* 193–200.

67. Huber, D. A., Garber, J. E., & Finkelstein, D. (1996). Letter to the editor. *N Engl J Med, 334,* 1199–1200.

68. Sher, C. M., Sharabani-Gargir, L., & Shohat, M. (1996). Letter to the editor. *N Engl J Med, 334,* 1199.

69. Gao, Q., Neuhausen, S., Cummings, S., Luce, M., & Olopade, O. (1997). Recurrent germ-line BRCA1 mutations in extended African American

families with early-onset breast cancer. *Am J Human Genet, 60,* 1233–1236.

70. Hoskins, K. F., Stopher, J. E., Calzone, K. A., et al. (1995). Assessment and counseling for women with a family history of breast cancer: A guide for clinicians. *JAMA, 273,* 577–585.

71. Goldman, E. L. (1996, February 15). BRCA1 findings shouldn't change screening. *Internal Medicine News,* p. 36.

72. Jancin, B. (1996, February 15). BRCA2 tumors more agressive, survival poorer. *Internal Medicine News,* p. 36.

73. Weber, B. (1996). Familial breast cancer. *Recent Results Cancer Res, 140,* 5–16.

74. Berman, D., Costalas, J., Schultz, D., Grana, G., Daly, M., & Godwin, A. (1996). A common mutation in BRCA2 that predisposes to a variety of cancers is found in both Jewish Ashkenazi and non-Jewish individuals. *Cancer Res, 56,* 3409–3414.

75. Department of Health and Human Services. (1996). FDA approves first blood test for breast cancer recurrence. *FDA Medical Bulletin, 26,* 2.

76. DiGiovanna, M., Carter, D., Flynn, S., & Stern, D. (1996). Functional assay for Her-2/neu demonstrates active signaling in a minority of Her-2/neu-overexpressing invasive human breast tumors. *Br J Cancer, 74,* 802–806.

77. Haffty, B., Brown, F., Carter, D., & Flynn, S. (1996). Evaluation of Her-2 neu oncoprotein expression as a prognostic indicator of local recurrence in conservatively treated breast cancer: A case control study. *Int J Radiat Oncol Biol Phys, 35,* 751–757.

78. Yuan, J. M., Wang, Q. S., Ross, R. K., et al. (1995). Diet and breast cancer in Shanghai and Tianjin, China. *Br J Cancer, 71,* 1353–1358.

79. Jamali, F. R., Ricci, A., & Deckers, P. J. (1996). Paget's disease of the nipple-areola complex. *Surg Clin North Am, 76,* 365–381.

80. Schilling, K., & Love, N. (1995). Screening and diagnostic breast imaging procedures. A look at lesions through a radiologist's eyes. *Postgrad Med, 94,* 44–46, 51, 56 passim.

81. Parker, S. H., Burbank, F., Jackman, R.J., et al. (1994). Percutaneous larger-core breast biopsy: A multi-institutional study. *Radiology, 193,* 359–364.

82. Budman, D. R., & Citron, M. L. (1994). Adjuvant therapy for breast cancer. *Clin Obstet Gynecol, 37,* 978–987.

83. Levitt, S., Aeppli, D., & Nierengarten, M. (1996). The impact of radiation on early breast carcinoma survival. A Bayesian analysis. *Cancer, 78,* 1035–1042

84. Thurlimann, B., & Senn, H. (1996). Editorial. Changing approach to early breast cancer. *N Engl J Med, 34,* 1397–1398.

85. Porterfield, L. A., & Love, N. (1995). Local regional therapy for primary breast tumors. *Postgrad Med, 98,* 65–68, 73, 77 passim.

86. Neff, P., Bear, H., Pierce, C., et al. (1996). Long term results of breast conservation therapy for breast cancer. *Ann Surg, 233,* 709–716.

87. Saez, R., Selby, G., Slease, R., et al. (1994). Autologous bone marrow transplantation for metastatic breast cancer. *J Okla State Med Assoc, 87,* 405–410

88. Pace, B. W., & Tinker, M. A. (1994). Follow-up of patients with breast cancer. *Clin Obstet Gynecol, 37,* 998–1002.

89. Allen, M., & Oberle, K. (1996). Augmentation mammoplasty: A complex choice. *Health Care for Women International, 17,* 81–90.

90. Reynolds, H. E. (1995). Evaluation of the augmented breast. *Rad Clin North Am, 33,* 1131–1145.

91. Stracner, J., & Bohan, A. (1995). Silicone breast implants. Understanding the current controversies. *Clinician Reviews, 5,* 55–57, 59–60, 62, passim.

92. Cronin, T. D., & Gerrow, F. J. (1964). Augmentation mammoplasty: A new "natural feel" prosthesis. Transactions at the third international congress of plastic surgery. Amsterdam. *Excerpta Medica Foundation,* 41–49.

93. Gabriel, S. E., O'Fallon, W. M., Kurland, L., et al. (1994). Risk of connective tissue diseases and other disorders after breast implantation. *N Engl J Med, 330,* 1697–1702.

94. Goldman, J. A., Greenblatt, J., Joines, R., et al. (1995). Breast implants, rheumatoid arthritis, connective tissue diseases in a clinical practice. *J Clin Epidemiology, 48,* 571–582.

95. Harden, J., & Girard, N. (1994). Breast reconstruction using an innovative flap procedure. *AORN J, 60,* 184–192.

96. Germann, G., & Steinau, H. (1996). Breast reconstruction with the extended latissimus dorsi flap. *Plast Reconstr Surg, 97,* 519–526.

97. Liew, S., & Pennington, D. (1996). Sensory recovery following free TRAM flap breast reconstruction. *Br J Plast Surg, 49,* 210–213.

98. Howrigan, P. J. (1994). Reduction and augmentation mammoplasty. *Obstet Clin North Am, 21,* 539–549.

99. Troilius, C. (1995). Total muscle coverage of a breast implant is possible through the transaxillary approach. *Plastr Reconstr Surg, 95,* 509–512.

CHAPTER 15

THE CLIMACTERIC, MENOPAUSE, AND THE PROCESS OF AGING

Valerie T. Cotter

*W*omen today can expect to live one-third of their lives after their reproductive years.

Highlights

- Physiology of Menopause
- Physical Changes of Aging: Body Systems
- Sexuality and Aging
- Hypoestrogenic Changes
    Vasomotor
    Vaginal
    Urinary
    Menstrual
- Alterations in Mood
- Cognitive Function/Memory Loss/Alzheimer's Disease
- Sleep Disorders
- Hormone Replacement Therapy
    Counseling, Assessment
    Treatment Considerations: Preparations, Contraindications, Follow-Up
- Midlife and Late Life Education, Evaluation, Screening
- Osteoporosis
- Hirsutism/Virilism
- Nonreproductive Health Concerns
    Insurance and Income
    Social Support
    Elder Mistreatment
    Chronic Illness
    Functional Status
    Depression and Suicide Risk
    Polypharmacy
    Injury Prevention
    Access to Care

► INTRODUCTION

In 1900, the average life expectancy was 48.7 years for white American women and 33.5 years for African American women. By 1991, however, average life expectancy was higher for women (79 years) than for men (72 years) generally. Today, a woman in the United States who reaches age 65 can expect to live to be 82.[1]

The elderly population has grown substantially in this century and will continue to grow into the 21st century. In 1900, the elderly comprised only 1 in every 25 Americans (3.1 million) and made up 1 in 18 (33.2 million) in 1994.[1] According to the Census Bureau's projections, the elderly population will more than double between now and the year 2050, to 80 million.[1] The elderly population is becoming more racially and ethnically diverse. In 1994, 1 in 10 elderly were a race other than white. In 2050, this proportion will rise to 2 in 10, and the proportion of elderly who are Hispanic is expected to climb from 4 percent to 16 percent.[1]

Only recently, then, has society been faced with the issues of aging beyond menopause. Research is now focusing on factors that positively impact physical and psychological aging. Women today can expect to live one-third of their lives after their reproductive years, or one-half of their adult life,[2] and preventive health care and healthy lifestyle habits can greatly improve the quality of life in those later years.

As women age they face numerous transitions that require adaptation. During the middle years, the 20-year span of time between 50 and 70, a woman refines and integrates the emotional growth that she underwent during the previous 20 or so years and assumes primary responsibility for the continued survival and enhancement of the nation.[3] During late adulthood, the years between 70 and death, a woman experiences a continuing process of maturation and assumes responsibility for sharing the

wisdom of age, reviewing life, and putting affairs in order.[3]

Developmental Tasks for Age 50–70 Years[3]

- Maintaining flexible views in occupational, civic, political, religious, and social positions.
- Keeping current on relevant scientific, political, and cultural changes.
- Developing mutually supportive (interdependent) relationships with grown offspring and other members of the younger generation.
- Reevaluating and enhancing the relationship with spouse or most significant other or adjusting to her/his loss.
- Helping aged parents or other relatives progress through the last stage of life.
- Deriving satisfaction from increased availability of leisure time.
- Preparing for retirement and planning another career when feasible.
- Adapting self and behavior to signals of accelerated aging processes.

Developmental Tasks of Late Adulthood[3]

- Pursuing a second or third career, new interest, hobbies, and/or community activities that fulfill some untapped inner resource or otherwise enhance the self-image and maintain worth in society.
- Learning new skills that are well removed from prior learnings or at least do not produce cognitive dissonance with prior learnings.
- Sharing wisdom accrued from the past with individuals, groups, communities, and nations.
- Evaluating the totality of past life and putting successes and failures into perspective.
- Progressing through the stages of grief, death, and dying with significant others and with oneself.

The Climacteric and Menopause

Menopause as defined by the World Health Organization is the permanent cessation of menstruation resulting from loss of ovarian follicular activity and 12 months of amenorrhea at the time of midlife.[4] It is possible to induce menopause surgically by bilateral oophorectomy. *The climacteric or perimenopause* refers to the 2 to 8 years prior to the menopause, and to the subsequent 1 year of amenorrhea following menopause.[4] The Greek *climacteric* means "rungs on a ladder"—a rather appropriate and positive way to view maturation. The postmenopause is defined as the time after the menopause, including the year of amenorrhea.[4]

The average age of menopause in the United States is 50 years. Despite consistent lowering of the age of puberty, the age of natural menopause has remained consistent.[5] Ovarian failure prior to 30 is premature and requires chromosomal analysis to rule out gonadal dysgenesis. Menopause between ages 31 and 40 is considered early and, because of the increased incidence of autoimmune disorders, requires referral for medical endocrine evaluation. Menopause after age 40 is considered normal. The only consistent predisposing factor for earlier menopause, typically 1–2 years earlier, is cigarette smoking. Another factor that has been suggested is shorter menstrual cycles, fewer than 26 days.[6] Nulliparity and oral contraceptive use have been associated with later onset of menopause.[7,8]

THE PHYSIOLOGY OF MENOPAUSE

Menopause results from a series of changes initiated in the ovary. General atresia of ovarian follicles begins with the onset of puberty and becomes more significant after age 35 when the ovary contains fewer follicles that are responsive to FSH. Eventually the atresia leads to a decline in ovarian production of estrogen and progesterone.

Loss of Estrogen Feedback

In the normal menstrual cycle, rising levels of FSH stimulate the developing dominant follicle to secrete increasing amounts of estradiol. The increasing level of estradiol as well as inhibin from the granulosa cells exert a negative feedback on the hypothalamus and result in decreasing FSH. After menopause, there is an increase in FSH because of the reduction in pituitary gonadotropin inhibition of estrogen and progesterone. This change in ovarian steroid production is often gradual, resulting in anovulatory bleeding patterns. Eventually, the ovaries are completely unable to respond to FSH and LH, and the level of gonadotropin hyperactivity stabilizes. Gonadotropin levels never return to premenopausal levels.[9]

Diagnosis of Menopause

- If on no hormonal medication (e.g., HRT, ERT, oral contraceptives), a rise in FSH 30mIU/ml is diagnostic.
- If on combined oral contraceptives: beginning at age 50, do annual FSH on day 5, 6, or 7 of placebo-pill week; FSH will rise during this week if woman is menopausal. By mid-50s, test not necessary; assumption is that menopause has occurred.
- If on progestin-only contraception or therapy, FSH levels are not affected and can be measured at anytime.[10]

Postmenopausal Estrogen Sources

The major source of estradiol prior to menopause is the ovarian follicle. Estradiol is produced cyclically, and the ovary accounts for over 90 percent of total body production. Relatively constant production of estrone by adrenal glandular secretion and peripheral conversion of androstenedione, the major circulating androgen in women, also occur. Postmenopause, little estradiol is produced in the ovarian follicles. Ovarian stroma, under stimulation by LH, continues to produce androstenedione and testosterone, which along with androstenedione produced by adrenal glands, are converted to estrone in peripheral adipose tissue. Thus, the body weight of the woman contributes to her overall postmenopausal level of circulating estrogen. Initially, both the ovary and the adrenal glands are major sources of androstenedione. With advanced age, however, the ovarian stroma ceases production of androstenedione and is unable to maintain sufficient estrone production. Specific target deficiencies may then be noted. The degree of deficiency will vary with the individual woman. During the climacteric, ovarian secretion of androgens decreases markedly; androgens, especially testosterone, may play a role in the maintenance of sexual desire, normal affect, and normal cognition[11] (see Hirsutism).

THE PHYSICAL CHANGES OF AGING

The changes that occur as a woman ages are the culmination of heredity, the effects of living and lifestyle, and hormonal changes.

DERMAL CHANGES

With aging, the skin undergoes progressive changes: the epidermis becomes thinner and flatter; the density of scalp and body hair follicles decreases; and the sebaceous glands and sweat glands have reduced function and become less responsive to stimuli.[12] The dermis becomes less elastic, collagen is lost, and a wrinkling of the epidermis results. Decreases in resilience, protection, and moisture occur. The incidence of skin cancer increases markedly after age 50. Hair grays as functioning melanocytes in hair decrease.[12]

SENSORY CHANGES

Visual disorders (i.e., decreased visual acuity, visual field narrowing, increased light percep-

tion threshold, decreased depth perception), increase with age. Nearly 13 percent of older adults age 65 or older and 28 percent of those over 85 years of age have some degree of visual impairment.[13] Visual disorders frequently lead to motor vehicle accidents, injurious falls, and functional decline.

Presbycusis, the bilateral hearing loss associated with advanced age gradually occurs after age 50 and is characterized by a decreased sensitivity to high frequency tones.

CARDIOVASCULAR CHANGES

Cardiovascular disease (CVD) is the leading cause of morbidity and mortality in postmenopausal women in the United States. Nearly half of postmenopausal women will develop coronary heart disease (CHD) in their lifetime, 30 percent will die from CHD, and 20 percent will have a stroke.[14,15,16] The efficiency and muscle contractility of the heart decrease with aging, causing reduced cardiac output. This decreased output is tolerable under normal conditions, but with hemodynamic stresses or acute illness, the heart is less able to adapt.[17]

The changes in lipid components that accompany postmenopausal estrogen deficiency (see Table 15–1) favor the slow formation of atherosclerosis.[18] These changes are compounded by elevated blood pressure, smoking, obesity, and heredity. The usual postmenopausal lipid changes are as follows.[18]

Decreased catabolism in low density lipoproteins (LDL).
Decreased production of high density lipoproteins (HDL).
A gradual increase in total cholesterol (TCHO) and triglyceride levels.

PULMONARY CHANGES

Lung expansion decreases gradually with aging, as the thorax becomes more rigid and tissues less elastic. Reductions occur in pulmonary reserve and in vital capacity, and there is a decline over time in arterial oxygen concentration.[19] The elderly are able to compensate for age associated changes in the pulmonary system; however, they are vulnerable to acute respiratory infections.

TABLE 15–1. LABORATORY VALUES WITH OLDER ADULTS

Test	Unchanged/Same as Younger Reference	Decrease with Older Subjects	Increase with Older Subjects
CBC			
RBC	unchanged	or slight decrease	
Hgb	unchanged	or slight decrease	
Hct	unchanged	or slight decrease	
RBC indices	unchanged		
WBC count	unchanged		
Differential			
Basophils	unchanged		
Eosinophils	unchanged		
Myelocytes	unchanged		
Bands	unchanged		
Monocytes	unchanged		
Lymphocytes	unchanged	or slight decrease	
Platelets	unchanged		
ESR			slight increase
B_{12}		decrease	
Folate/folic acid		decrease	
TIBC/transferrin	unchanged		
Serum Fe	unchanged		
Blood chemistry electrolytes			
Na	unchanged	or slight decrease	
K	unchanged		or slight increase
Cl	unchanged		
Ca	unchanged	or slight decrease	
P	unchanged		
Mg		decrease	
Glucose			
FBS	unchanged		or slight increase
PPBS			increase
OGTT			increase
HgA_{1c}			increase
End products of metabolism			
BUN	unchanged		or slight increase
Creatinine	unchanged		or slight increase
Creatinine clearance		decrease	
Bilirubin	unchanged		
Uric acid			slight increase
Liver function tests			
ALAT (SGPT)	unchanged		
AST (SGOT)	unchanged		
LDH	unchanged		or slight increase
Alkaline phosphatase			gradual increase
Total protein	unchanged	or slight decrease	
Albumin		decrease	
Globulin	unchanged		
Lipoproteins			gradual increase
Total cholesterol			gradual increase
LDL			increase

(*Continued*)

TABLE 15–1. LABORATORY VALUES WITH OLDER ADULTS (CONTINUED)

Test	Unchanged/Same as Younger Reference	Decrease with Older Subjects	Increase with Older Subjects
HDL	unchanged	or slight decrease in women	or slight increase in men
Triglycerides			increase
Thyroid function tests			
T$_4$	unchanged	or slight decrease	
T$_3$		decrease	
TSH			slight increase

Source: Reprinted by permission of the publisher from Interpretation of Laboratory Values in Older Adults, by K. D. Melillo, in Nurse Practitioner *18(7) 59–67. Copyright 1993 by Elsevier Science Publishing Co., Inc.*

GASTROINTESTINAL (GI) CHANGES

The GI system can handle food that is chewed properly, albeit more sluggishly with aging. For proper chewing, gums and teeth must be in good condition. Estrogen deficiency can cause atrophic changes in the gums and influence mastication, as can poor dental hygiene and gum disease. Generally, the amount of hydrochloric acid in the stomach decreases with age, as does pepsin. Peristaltic action and emptying times decrease, and absorption of certain substances, such as the B vitamins, iron, and calcium, is affected.

REPRODUCTIVE CHANGES

- *Vulva.* With the loss of estrogen, the vulva undergoes atrophy, and subcutaneous tissues diminish.[20] The labia majora become small and the labia minora almost nonexistent.

  The skin becomes thinner, and pubic hair loss is progressive. Dystrophies and pruritus are more frequent.
- *Vagina.* Epithelial maturation decreases. The failure to produce glycogen containing superficial cells causes an increase in the vaginal pH, which may predispose the woman to vaginitis or leukorrhea.[20] The vagina becomes shortened, thinned, and narrowed, with obliteration of the vaginal fornices and eventual loss of vaginal rugae. Sebaceous gland secretions decrease and the vagina loses most of its lubricating ability, especially in response to sexual stimulation. Changes may be prevented or slowed by the continuation of regular intercourse.

Over time, the uterus decreases in size and the endometrium atrophies; however, the endometrium continues to respond to hormonal stimulation.[21] The cervix pales and shrinks with loss of the fornices so that the external os is nearly flush with the vaginal wall. The endocervix becomes atrophic and the cervical canal stenotic. The ovaries and fallopian tubes atrophy and are usually not palpable on examination; in fact, any adnexal mass in a woman over 50 is considered malignant until proven otherwise.[22]

- *Pelvic Floor.* The muscular tissue loses tone after menopause, causing increases in uterine prolapse, cystocele, and rectocele.[23] This loss of tone may be heightened by past pregnancy and vaginal delivery.
- *Breast.* Breast size tends to diminish as glandular breast tissue decreases and is replaced by fat; the breasts often hang lower on the chest.[24]

URINARY CHANGES

Urinary tract changes are secondary to estrogen deficiency, aging, and past trauma from childbearing. The distal portion of the urethra shortens, thins and the opening shifts closer to the introitus. Bladder capacity decreases and the bladder and urethral tissue lose tone. With age, there is an increase in uninhibited bladder contractions and postvoid residual volume.[25] Renal clearance diminishes, but the kidneys are able to maintain a proper fluid balance in the body, unless concurrent disease or severe stressors are imposed.

ENDOCRINE CHANGES

- *Thyroid.* Irregularity and nodularity of the thyroid increase with age.[12] Thyroid function appears to remain stable after menopause, although hyperthyroidism and hypothyroidism are more common in women, in general, and in the elderly.[13] See Table 15–1 for normal changes in thyroid values with aging.
- *Pituitary.* Adequate hormonal secretion continues despite decreased pituitary size.

MUSCULOSKELETAL CHANGES

Muscle tone is related to exercise. In the sedentary woman, normal tone and strength diminish. Atrophy occurs more rapidly with aging if muscles are not used (see Osteoporosis). The proportion of fat and water change with aging: fat increases and water decreases.

NEUROLOGICAL CHANGES

Forgetfulness is not uncommon and may be related to neuron loss that begins when a woman is in her 20s. Some brain and spinal cord efficiency is lost, which is evident, for example, in slowed pupillary response. Sleep may be more easily disrupted. The incidence of Alzheimer's disease increases with age. The third leading cause of death in the United States is cerebrovascular accident (CVA). The principal risk factors are age, hypertension, smoking, coronary artery disease, and diabetes.

SEXUALITY AND AGING

Sexuality continues as an important component of a woman's life until her death. It represents a need to be accepted, a need for intimacy and companionship. Sexuality is influenced by many factors. Although most older adults continue to be sexually active, physical changes associated with aging, illness, and opportunity have major influence on the frequency and satisfaction of sexual behaviors. Physical changes in women that may have a negative impact on sexuality include the following:[26]

- Thinning of vaginal walls.
- Vaginal lubrication volume smaller and occurs after several minutes of stimulation.
- Increased time to reach orgasm.
- Shorter duration of orgasm.
- Decreased strength of orgasmic contractions.
- Decrease in clitoral hood/body.
- Loss of elasticity, length, and width of vagina.
- Decreased strength of orgasmic contractions.

Changes caused by hormonal deficiency may be lessened with estrogen or testosterone therapy. Other factors that affect sexuality, either positively or negatively, include longer life span; issues surrounding aging, such as physical and social losses and transitions; an increase in chronic illness; body image changes; effects of medications on libido; more time for intimacy; and freedom from worry about contraception/pregnancy. Sexuality is seldom considered in the counseling of midlife and aging women, yet women in this age group have a variety of concerns and information needs. Women need information about sexually transmitted diseases and "safer sex." Whether single or married, women may desire information about common sexuality concerns, such as masturbation. They may also want information about male sexuality and aging, and may need help adapting sexual practices to accommodate physical and emotional changes. It is estimated that 10 percent of older adults are homosexual.[27] Sensitivity to the needs and concerns of lesbian couples should be the same as for any other couple.

HYPOESTROGENIC CHANGES

The loss of estradiol with decreasing ovarian function results in a host of changes among postmenopausal women. The incidence and severity of complaints vary greatly, but most frequently, they involve vasomotor instability, vaginal and urinary tract changes, headaches, insomnia and menstrual irregularity. Research suggests that the vasomotor instability and genitourinary changes are clearly related to the physiologic changes of menopause, but the impact of psychological, social, and cultural factors on other associated symptoms is less clear.[28,29]

VASOMOTOR INSTABILITY

Vasomotor instability, better known as hot flashes or flushes, coincides with a surge of LH and is followed by a measurable increase in body surface heat and a fall in core temperature. The hot flash is an intense feeling of heat that begins in the upper chest or neck and proceeds up the face and head. It typically lasts for 5 to 12 minutes and concludes with profuse perspiration. Hot flashes tend to increase at night. They can occur in the premenopause, but more frequently in postmenopause, lasting in most women for 1 to 2 years, but in some (25–50 percent) for longer than 5 years.[9]

Epidemiology

Hot flashes and flushes are the most consistently reported symptom of the menopause. As many as 72 percent of women experience hot flushes in the perimenopausal years; however, only 25–30 percent of menopausal women seek medical attention.[30] The symptoms of vasomotor instability are greater in the first 2 years after menopause;[31] their severity varies with the individual.

Subjective Data

Evaluate the client's menstrual history for changes suggestive of perimenopause, such as decreasing or increasing intervals between menses and dysfunctional/anovulatory bleeding patterns. The client will report episodes of feeling extreme warmth rising from the chest up to the face and head, followed by perspiration and sometimes chills. If these vasomotor symptoms occur at night, they disrupt sleep—causing insomnia, exhaustion, and irritability. Flushes can occur frequently during a 24-hour period; hence the client may report the need to change clothing and bed linens often.

Objective Data

Physical Examination. Findings are frequently absent, but may include vasodilation of peripheral blood vessels in the skin coupled with mild increase in pulse, but without alteration in blood pressure; increased digital temperature; and decreased intracore temperature with chills.

Diagnostic Tests and Methods

- *Serum FSH Level.* A level greater than 30 IU/L is diagnostic of menopause;[10] FSH is less reliable during the perimenopause when there are irregular bursts of follicular function alternating with no ovarian response.
- *Client Diary of Episodes.* Confirms oral history.

Differential Medical Diagnoses

Hypothalamic/pituitary tumor, infection (viral illness, tuberculosis, systemic infection with fever, human immunodeficiency virus [HIV] infection), alcoholism, thyroid disease.

Plan

Psychosocial Interventions. Reassure the client that vasomotor instability is normal during the perimenopause. In addition, explain the physiology of menopause. Offer adaptive measures as follows.

- Adjust the room temperature; leave a window open; use a portable fan to accommodate an office environment.
- Wear clothing in layers for ease of removal; wear more cotton.
- Try stress management techniques such as relaxation exercises, meditation, and yoga.

Medication. Hormone Replacement Therapy (HRT) or Estrogen Replacement Therapy (ERT) are effective in greater than 90 percent of women. Adjust the dosage to accommodate client symptoms. (See Hormone Replacement Therapy, later in this chapter, for a complete description of administration, side effects, contraindications, evaluation outcomes, and teaching/counseling.)

Alternative Therapies. Alternative therapy is indicated if HRT or ERT is contraindicated. The following drugs may be offered to decrease vasomotor instability.

- *Medroxyprogesterone Acetate (MPA).* Prescribe 10 to 20 mg q.d. Side effects include weight gain, depression, and breast tenderness. MPA treatment is moderately effective (see Hormone

Replacement Therapy for more information about MPA).

- *Clonidine.* Transdermal clonidine can be applied in a 100-ug dose once weekly. Side effects include severe hypotensive episodes, dizziness, nausea, and mood swings.[32] Treatment is moderately effective.
- *Vitamin B Complex.* 1–2 daily after meals aids in detoxification and elimination of FSH and LH by the liver.[20] Possibly effective.
- *Vitamin E.* Prescribe 100 IU daily, increasing over weeks or a few months to 600 IU, until relief of symptoms.[20] Possibly effective.
- *Other Interventions.* Advise the client to limit her caffeine and alcohol intake and not to smoke. Drinking 8 to 10 glasses of water daily is also advised; drinking cold water at the beginning of a flush may help to alleviate the discomfort. Hot drinks and foods should be avoided. Separate bed sheets and blankets can be used, then taken off without disturbing the bed partner. Regular exercise every day may improve sleep; however, heavy exercise must be avoided immediately before bedtime.
- *Herbal Therapies.* Many herbal therapies are available that promise relief of symptoms. Advise caution in use as FDA approval is very limited for these substances and no standardization exists at present.[101,102] (The reader is referred to Youngkin, E. and Israel, D. in the references for an in-depth review.)

Follow-Up

Call the client to evaluate the effectiveness of therapy in relieving the signs and symptoms of perimenopause. (See Hormone Replacement Therapy for follow-up related to that therapy.) If therapy is ineffective, suggest referral to a gynecologist.

VAGINAL CHANGES

The vagina, composed of thick tissue with accordionlike folds (rugae) during the childbearing years, thins dramatically in the absence of estrogen. This process predisposes the woman to vaginal infection, trauma, and pain.

Epidemiology

Decreased estrogen, whether because of natural or surgical menopause, contributes to vaginal atrophy. Vaginal changes including vaginal wall friability, increase in pH, irritation, susceptibility to infection, dyspareunia, and related loss of sexual desire are common among postmenopausal women and often occur during perimenopause.

Subjective Data

A menstrual history will reveal symptoms of vaginal change, possibly including vaginal dryness, loss of lubrication with intercourse, pain or soreness with penile thrusting during intercourse, unusual vaginal discharge, infection, and postcoital bleeding.

Objective Data

Physical Examination. Findings include thinning and paleness of vaginal epithelia, bloody vaginal discharge, brittle pubic hair, disappearance of rugae, and infection.

Diagnostic Tests and Methods

SERUM FSH. A level of greater than 30 mIU per mL is diagnostic of menopause; FSH is less reliable during the perimenopause when there are irregular bursts of follicular function alternating with no ovarian response.

PAPANICOLAOU (PAP) SMEAR. Maturation index for indication of estrogen deficiency (test is optional, not as diagnostic as FSH level is). Over 50 percent parabasal cells equates with a marked estrogen decline.

GONORRHEA CULTURE, WET MOUNT, AND CHLAMYDIA TEST. Performed if appropriate.

Differential Medical Diagnoses

Vaginitis and sexually transmitted diseases (bacterial, viral, fungal infection), leukoplakia, lichen sclerosis, malignancy, postmenopausal uterine bleeding, diabetes mellitus.

Plan

Psychosocial Interventions. Teach the client about the normal physiological changes of menopause, aging, and sexuality that may occur.

Medication. *Estrogen* cream (Premarin Vaginal Cream) is indicated to reverse vaginal atrophic changes (see Hormone Replacement Therapy for a general description of hormone use).

Apply 1 g estrogen cream or the equivalent intravaginally daily, for 2–4 weeks; then decrease to 1 g, 2–3 times weekly when symptom relief is achieved. Then decrease to one application per week or eliminate altogether based on symptoms. Vaginal absorption into the bloodstream is very efficient; therefore, the client is at risk for endometrial hyperplasia due to unopposed estrogen stimulation of the endometrium. Medroxyprogesterone acetate (Provera), 10 mg for 10–12 days every 3 months, is recommended if the uterus is intact.[9] Oral hormone replacement therapy (HRT) is described later in this chapter.

Other Interventions. Treat any vaginal infection as indicated, and educate the client about "safer sex" (see chapters 9 and 11). Teach her Kegel's exercises, as these may help with arousal (see Chapter 21, Urinary Incontinence, Pelvic Muscle Exercises, for more detail). Offer the client suggestions or readings on sexual pleasuring to increase arousal (see Chapter 6). Advise her to use a water soluble vaginal lubricant with intercourse to prevent trauma from penile thrusting and alleviate the discomfort of friction (lubricants will not reverse epithelial changes). Lubricant jellies, creams, and suppositories are available over the counter (without prescription). Vegetable oils or lotions without perfume may be suggested. Advise the client to wash her hands thoroughly before and after applying any vaginal lubricant.

Lᴜʙʀɪɴ Vᴀɢɪɴᴀʟ Sᴜᴘᴘᴏsɪᴛᴏʀɪᴇs. Insert one suppository 5 to 20 minutes prior to intercourse as needed.

K-Y Jᴇʟʟʏ. Apply as needed.

Rᴇᴘʟᴇɴs Vᴀɢɪɴᴀʟ Sᴜᴘᴘᴏsɪᴛᴏʀɪᴇs ᴏʀ Cʀᴇᴀᴍ. Insert cream or suppository 5 to 20 minutes prior to intercourse. May be used as needed.

Asᴛʀᴏɢʟɪᴅᴇ. Apply intravaginally as needed.

Follow-Up

Advise the client to return to the health care provider if no relief occurs. Referral for sexual therapy may be indicated if the problem seems unrelated to physical changes in the vagina.

URINARY TRACT CHANGES

Urgency, nocturia, increased incidence of urinary tract infection, and incontinence are common among postmenopausal women and often occur during the perimenopause. The urethra and bladder have large numbers of estrogen receptors and subsequently atrophy during menopause. Detrusor instability (urge incontinence) and/or urethral sphincter incompetence (stress incontinence) are the most common causes of urinary incontinence in women over age 60. These conditions are influenced not only by hypoestrogenism but also by age, medications, endocrine disorders, pelvic floor denervation, prolapse, excessive weight, and smoking.[33] (See Chapter 21, Urinary Incontinence.)

MENSTRUAL IRREGULARITY

As the number of ovarian follicles capable of producing estrogen decreases, a woman experiences irregularities of the menstrual cycle. Ideally her periods are shorter and less frequent, but often they are a mix of heavy, longer bleeding episodes that are closer together due to anovulation. With anovulation, the epithelium builds from unopposed estrogen stimulation with no progesterone to transpose it to a secretory state. Although irregular bleeding is common, endometrial cancer must be ruled out. If an episode of bleeding occurs more often than 21 days, lasts longer than 8 days, is very heavy, or occurs after a 6-month interval of amenorrhea, or if the bleeding occurs in an irregular pattern, then evaluation must be done for endometrial hyperplasia.[34]

Subjective Data

The client's history indicates a change in the regularity of cycles and characteristics of menses (waxing and waning menses) or the absence of menses, and, often, other symptoms of hypoestrogenism.

Objective Data

Physical Examination. The physical and pelvic exam should be normal, and may or may not reveal changes suggestive of approaching menopause (see Chapter 8 for causes of abnormal menstrual bleeding and physical findings).

Diagnostic Tests and Methods. A pregnancy test must be used to rule out pregnancy as a cause of the bleeding. A serum FSH level of greater than 30 IU/L is diagnostic of menopause; FSH reachs a maximal level 1 to 3 years after menopause, then declines gradually.[9] Endometrial abnormalities (hyperplasia and carcinoma) may be ruled out with an endometrial biopsy. If anemia is suspected, a hemoglobin and hematocrit may be done.

Differential Medical Diagnoses

Pregnancy, spontaneous abortion, anovulation, hyperplasia, carcinoma, infection, abnormalities of the uterus such as fibroids or polyps, endometriosis, adenomyosis, injury, ovarian abnormalities such as tumors or cysts.

Plan

Psychosocial Interventions. Reassure the client that bodily changes are normal; explain the physiology of menopause; and educate regarding methods of treatment, if indicated.

Medication. For the perimenopausal women who is ovulating, recommended treatment is low dose oral contraceptives or continuous progestin, either oral or depot. For the perimenopausal woman with anovulatory cycles, estrogen with cyclic progestin is the treatment of choice, unless amenorrhea is desired, then continuous progestin or DMPA is recommended.[35]

Endometrial Biopsy. Office based endometrial biopsy has replaced dilation and curettage (D & C) as the method of choice for diagnosing endometrial abnormalities; it offers 90 percent accuracy in detecting hyperplasia and cancer.[22]

Follow-Up

Refer the client to a gynecologist for evaluation of suspected abnormalities, especially carcinoma. Any bleeding that does not respond to therapy also requires that the client be referred. Any postmenopausal woman who bleeds requires referral to rule out pelvic cancer, unless on HRT and the bleeding pattern is consistent for the therapy.

ALTERATIONS IN MOOD

A significant number of women report that changes in mood and concentration, irritability, nervousness, and depression occur during midlife. The relationships between hormonal changes and anxiety and depression in the perimenopausal woman remain to be clarified, however. Both the central and peripheral nervous systems contain 17 b-estradiol sensitive cells, and even the brain responds to withdrawal or absence of ovarian steroids. Estrogen influences the concentrations and availability of neurotransmitters, including serotonin, in the brain. Research has shown that estrogen increases the degradation of monoamine oxidase, the enzyme that catabolizes serotonin, regulates the amount of free tryptophan, the precursor for serotonin, and enhances the transport of serotonin.[36] Very few clinical correlations are available.

EPIDEMIOLOGY

No single cause for mood alterations has been identified. Hormonal deficiency may play a role, but consideration must be given to other factors in the client's life, such as aging and how she feels about it. American society reveres youth, and the reality of lost youth and changes in body image may upset some women. Other major life changes that are common for a woman of perimenopausal and menopausal age include one's children leaving home; death or disability of a spouse or partner; helping aging parents; realization that one may not have achieved all of one's life goals, loss of child-bearing capacity; and concerns about retirement and finances. Psychologic symptoms, including loss of concentration, loss of memory, mood changes, depression, and loss of sexual desire not related to vaginal changes, have been attributed to menopause.[2] Many of these symptoms may be interrelated to the physical symptoms of menopause, such as hot flashes causing insomnia, leading to loss of concentration from loss of sleep. The interrelationships among hormone levels, affective symptoms, and lifestyle factors, need further examination.

SUBJECTIVE DATA

The client's history may reveal periods of crying, anger, sadness, irritability, depression, anxiety attacks, family members' reports of mood swings, and expressions of suicide. If a psychological disorder is suspected, a referral to a mental health professional is indicated.

OBJECTIVE DATA

Physical Examination

Findings on physical examination may include decreased affect, lethargy, inappropriate responses, and crying. A complete examination is indicated to rule out systemic diseases, drug use, or other conditions that could affect physiological function and cause symptoms.

Diagnostic Tests and Methods

General diagnostic tests, such as complete blood cell (CBC) count, thyroid studies, FSH/LH, urinalysis, and blood chemistry analysis are indicated to determine normal baselines and deviations. Drug testing may also be indicated. Other tests that may be done are psychological scales and questionnaires, such as CAGE and MAST alcoholism questionnaires,[37,38] and Zung, Beck, or Geriatric Depression scales.[39–41]

DIFFERENTIAL MEDICAL DIAGNOSES

Depression, anxiety disorders, neurological impairment, sexual dysfunction, psychiatric disorder.

PLAN

Psychosocial Interventions

Refer the client for psychological evaluation as appropriate; protect if the client is suicidal.

Life transitions, grief work, and affective and physical changes associated with perimenopausal transitions may require individual or group therapy and support. Educational programs focused on midlife and menopause that emphasize accurate information, positive attitudes, and connection with other women may reassure the client.

Medication

Hormone replacement therapy (discussed later in this chapter). Although women seek hormone therapy to help with their mood, concentration, or depressive symptoms, current research does not justify the use of HRT for these symptoms without other indications for use.[2] (See antianxiety and antidepressant therapy in Chapter 23 or other reference texts.)

Exercise

Advise the client to engage in regular aerobic exercise and resistance training to improve muscle strength, unless contraindicated. Exercise may improve the client's psychological outlook and reduce mood swings.

Balanced Diet

Advise the client to maintain a nutritionally balanced diet and to avoid simple carbohydrates, which can induce hypoglycemic reactions.

Stress Reduction Techniques

Relaxation exercises, yoga, meditation, and regular physical exercise may reduce stress.

FOLLOW-UP

If the client does not respond to lifestyle changes and/or medication therapy, she should be referred to an appropriate mental health professional for additional treatment.

COGNITIVE FUNCTION/ MEMORY LOSS/ALZHEIMER'S DISEASE

Cognition emcompasses the entire range of human intellectual functions, including learning and memory. Whether or not cognitive decline is related to advancing age or changes in sex hormones remains controversial. Estrogen may enhance or preserve cognitive functions of the brain.[36]

There is convincing evidence that estrogen influences neuroanatomical structures and neuro-chemical mechanisms known to be important for memory. Studies on healthy middle-aged and older postmenopausal women that have investigated the association between estrogen and memory support the hypothesis that estrogen helps to maintain aspects of verbal memory, and has no effect, or possibly even a negative influence, on spatial memory.[36] A recent study demonstrated that postmenopausal women who took estrogen longer than 1 year (average 13.6 years) had a significantly reduced risk of developing Alzheimer's disease (5.8 percent estrogen users vs. 16.3 percent nonusers) and the age of onset was significantly delayed.[42] Initiating HRT as a preventive measure for Alzheimer's disease may prove to be of value, although the research data is just beginning to come in. The risk of Alzheimer's disease is said to be reduced by half in women who use estrogen therapy postmenopausally.[103]

SUBJECTIVE DATA

The client, or significant other, may report signs and symptoms of declining mental functioning, e.g., forgetfulness, decreased concentration and attention, getting lost in familiar environments, and expressive or receptive language impairment.

OBJECTIVE DATA

A comprehensive history and physical examination, review of prescribed and over-the-counter medications are done to rule out reversible and potentially treatable causes of cognitive impairment. Screening for cognitive impairment can be done with instruments such as the Mini Mental Status Examination (MMSE),[43] or Short Portable Mental Status Questionnaire (SPMSQ).[44]

Diagnostic Tests

CBC, thyroid profile, B12 and folate levels, RPR, urinalysis, blood chemistry analysis, and EKG. CT or MRI of the brain is usually indicated.

DIFFERENTIAL MEDICAL DIAGNOSES

Benign senescent forgetfulness, multi-infarct dementia, Alzheimer's disease, alcohol dementia, depression, delirium, toxic effects of medications, malignancy, infection, thyroid disorders.

PLAN

Psychosocial Interventions

Depending upon the duration and severity of cognitive impairment, refer the client for consultation with a neurologist, neuropsychologist, mental health professional or other primary care provider for further evaluation. If symptoms are mild and complete evaluation, including cognitive screening, is normal, reevaluate in 6 to 12 months, and reassure the client about benign senescent forgetfulness. Individual and group therapy may be considered.

SLEEP DISORDERS

With aging, sleep stages 3 (early phase of deep sleep) and 4 (deep sleep and relaxation) decrease and brief arousals become more frequent.[12] Alterations in sleep patterns may be the result of hot flushes and night sweats. The need for overall sleep diminishes slightly with age; the average adult needs 5 to 7 hours of sleep each day.

EPIDEMIOLOGY

Any number of factors may contribute to sleep disturbances in addition to estrogen decline: lack of exercise, excessive napping during the day, stress, depression, anxiety, illness, restless sleep partner, uncomfortable sleeping accommodations, excessive activity prior to bedtime, and stimulant drugs. Sleep disorders are common among the general population and increase in the perimenopausal and postmenopausal years. The exact incidence is unknown.

SUBJECTIVE DATA

The client reports signs and symptoms of menopause, as well as irritability, interrupted sleep, and feelings of tiredness.

OBJECTIVE DATA

Findings on physical examination include lethargy, dark circles under the eyes, and possible altered response time. Diagnostic tests are used to rule out other diseases that cause lethargy, fatigue, and insomnia, such as anemia, sleep apnea, or hypothyroidism. Be sure that obstructive sleep apnea, associated with significant daytime sleepiness and increased motorvehicle accidents, is not a factor. This condition is a risk factor for cardiovascular death.[45]

DIFFERENTIAL MEDICAL DIAGNOSES

Neurological disorders, psychological disturbances.

PLAN

Reassure and educate the client about causes and remedies of sleep disorders. Referral to a sleep therapy specialist may be indicated. Consult current pharmacological therapy references for information on sedatives and sleeping medications, but only after giving nonpharmacological interventions a fair trial of several months.

Nonpharmacological Interventions

Evaluate naps. Encourage 10 to 30 minute naps during the daytime if the client is severely sleep deprived. If napping is interfering with night sleep, however, urge decreasing naps if possible.

- *Avoid caffeine.* Foods and beverages containing caffeine should be decreased or eliminated, especially after 5 P.M. Evaluate prescription and over-the-counter medications that might contain caffeine, for example, some cold remedies.

- *Limit alcohol intake.* Alcohol consumption should be less than 4 oz. per day or, preferably, eliminated altogether.
- *Avoid smoking.* Encourage the client to stop smoking. Offer literature and referral to a group for support.
- *Exercise before or in the early evening.* Exercising should occur no later than 7 P.M. (Aerobic exercise in late evening increases wakefulness.)
- *Arrange for a comfortable sleep environment.* Make suggestions concerning mattress comfort, soundproofing or earplugs, room darkening, sleeping clothes, room temperature, elimination of distractions.
- *Arrange quiet activity prior to bedtime.* Reading or listening to soothing music or environmental sounds may encourage sleep.
- *Avoid sleeping medications.* If the client is unable to sleep, advise her to get up and read or watch television, then try again in 30 to 60 minutes. Learning relaxation techniques, such as slow breathing from the diaphragm or playing mental games, and using them at bedtime may be beneficial. By setting aside a time to review concerns and activities of the day and coming up with solutions to problems before going to bed, the client may succeed in separating worries from the act of going to bed. (The bed should not be used as an office.) Taking warm baths, drinking milk (but not too much), and eating light (nonsugar) snacks before bedtime may also be helpful.

FOLLOW-UP

The client may require referral to a sleep disorder program.

HORMONE REPLACEMENT THERAPY (HRT)

Women now have the option, unless medically contraindicated, of hormone replacement therapy (HRT)(estrogen and progestin therapy) during the perimenopause and after. The concerns related to an increased risk of endometrial cancer, which peaked during the 1970s, have been tempered by the realization that the addition of a progestin to estrogen replacement therapy (ERT)(unopposed estrogen) offers significant protection against progressive hyperplasia. This benefit of the progestin, however, must be weighed against its possible negative effects, such as symptoms similar to premenstrual syndrome (PMS), attenuation of HDL-cholesterol, or breast pathology. Thus, the decision to use HRT must be made by the informed client. In the past, many women chose HRT to help relieve menopausal symptoms, but as more information regarding hormones is reported in the professional literature and popular media, the likelihood is that hormone use to prevent risks of cardiovascular disease, osteoporosis, and Alzheimer's disease will continue to rise. Researchers studying participants in the Nurses' Health Study reported that current hormone users had a 37% lower risk of mortality from all causes after adjustment for a number of risk factors such as cigarette smoking than nonusers, particularly for death due to coronary heart disease. However, the benefits declined after 10 years or more of current hormone use, due to an increased risk of breast cancer mortality by 43% after 10 years of use.[104] Short-term use was associated with a decreased risk of death from breast cancer.

CLIENT EDUCATION AND COUNSELING

The health care provider must provide the client with accurate, current information about the probable benefits and possible adverse effects of HRT. The following factors have consistently demonstrated improved compliance: patient education, patient involvement in decision making and treatment monitoring, simplification of the treatment regimen, and reduction of side effects caused by medications.[46] Generally, the following areas are included in discussion with the client.

Signs and Symptoms of Hypoestrogenism. Estrogen taken orally, transdermally, or vaginally is effective in relieving vasomotor and urogenital symptoms(dyspareunia, dysuria, incontinence, and urinary tract infections).[47] The dosage is individualized for relief of physical and subjective symptoms of anxiety or distress.

OSTEOPOROSIS. Bone loss begins in the third or fourth decade of a woman's life, and accelerates rapidly because of estrogen deficiency in the first postmenopausal decade. The standard of care for preventing and treating postmenopausal bone loss is ERT and should be considered for all women without contraindications.[48] (Osteoporosis is discussed more fully later in this chapter.)

ENDOMETRIAL CANCER. Both continuous and cyclic regimens of progestins prevent estrogen induced endometrial hyperplasia.[49] The addition of a progestin, recommended for the client who still has a uterus, does not detract from the favorable estrogen effects on bone density, or most other hypoestrogen complaints.

LIPID CHANGES. Although estrogen alone positively impacts lipid fractions by lowering LDL and raising HDL, conflicting studies exist on the impact of estrogen-progestin combination on the lipid profile. Progestins, especially those that closely resemble androgens, attenuate the HDL cholesterol elevating properties of estrogens.[50] Because HRT is usually given in combination with progestin, the data concerning the cardioprotective effects are important. In several long term studies,[51,52] HDL cholesterol levels did not differ significantly between those receiving either estrogen or combined HRT therapy. The results of large prospective, placebo controlled trials, the Heart Estrogen Replacement Study and the Women's Health Initiative, will not be available for years.

BREAST CANCER. Study results are mixed on the relationship of postmenopausal hormone therapy on breast cancer. Although approximately 40 observational studies have been done to date, there is no uniformity or consistency in the studies, nor are there any results of a randomized clinical trial.[53] A small, but significant, increase in breast cancer is probably associated with long-term hormone therapy. In a risk/benefit analysis, however, coronary heart disease (CHD) is more common than breast cancer after the menopause. Both estrogen and estrogen-progestin therapy are predicted to prolong life expectancy (> 2 year average) for most women, even if the risk of breast cancer is increased up to 50 percent.[54] Dosages of estrogen known to protect against osteoporosis and cardiovascular disease (0.625 mg conjugated estrogens and 1.0 mg estradiol) are presently not associated with any clear-cut increased risk of breast cancer, nor is adding a progestin.[53]

BLOOD PRESSURE. In the PEPI trial, no significant effects on blood pressure were noted with either estrogen alone or in combination with a progestin.[50]

STROKE. Recent studies suggest no significant effect of estrogen use on risk of stroke.[2]

CARDIOVASCULAR DISEASE. Many studies have indicated that HRT reduces cardiovascular mortality by about 50 percent;[55] estrogen-progestin therapy and unopposed estrogen were each associated with significant and comparable reductions in risk of CHD compared with women who did not use hormones.[56,57] HRT may also have direct beneficial effects on the arterial wall, vascular smooth muscle, blood flow, and platelet aggregation, as well as favorable effects on body fat distribution.[18,55,58] Variations in dosages, types of estrogen, and modes of delivery produce somewhat different results. Oral ERT increases HDL and triglycerides, lowers LDL and total cholesterol; transdermal ERT alters HDL, LDL, and total cholesterol levels like oral ERT, but to a lesser extent, and lowers triglycerides.[59] (Oral and transdermal ERTs are discussed later in this chapter.) Efforts to prevent or slow the progression of cardiovascular disease in women should also focus on the woman's total cardiovascular risk profile. This includes exercise, weight control, diet, cholesterol control, blood pressure control, and smoking cessation.

GALLBLADDER DISEASE. Estrogen may increase the risk of gallbladder disease.[2] Estrogen may increase the risk of gallstones in obese women and women with a personal or family history of the condition. The primary cause of gallstones in women is obesity; cholesterol gallstones occur when cholesterol in the bile exceeds the normal range and precipitates out. The precipitate creates seeds, or crystals, that form stones. In women who are not obese, gallstones are caused by a reduced rate of production of bile salts and other substances. In evaluating each client, family history, current risk factors, and the need for preventive health measures are assessed.

MOOD AND SLEEP. Many women report improved overall psychological well-being while taking estrogen, although studies are inconclusive.[60]

RHEUMATOID ARTHRITIS. There is no apparent effect of ERT or HRT on rheumatoid arthritis.[2,31]

GLUCOSE TOLERANCE. The use of estrogen and medroxyprogesterone acetate (MPA) is not associated with impaired glucose tolerance.[2]

BLEEDING PATTERNS. Therapy with cyclic progestin with an estrogen produces menstrual-like vaginal bleeding and spotting in many women. For some, this is an unacceptable side effect. Continuous combined regimens of estrogen and progestin reduce the incidence of unwanted bleeding. Continuous dosage regimens (conjugated estrogen [CE] 0.625 g/medroxyprogesterone [MPA] 2.5 mg and CE 0.625 mg/MPA 5.0 mg) produce amenorrhea in 61.4 percent and 72.8 percent, respectively and sequential regimens (CE 0.625 mg/MPA 5.0 mg cycle days 15–28 and CE 0.625 mg/MPA 10 mg cycle days 15–28) produce regular withdrawal bleeding or spotting 81.3 percent and 77 percent, respectively.[61]

REQUIRED ASSESSMENT BEFORE INITIATING HRT

Take a complete client history with special emphasis on symptoms of hypoestrogenism, and note any family history of osteoporosis, heart disease, or hypertension. During the required complete physical examination, note signs of hypo-estrogenism in the presence or absence of menses.

Diagnostic Tests and Methods

Complete evaluation per midlife and late life protocol includes determination of baseline values for common tests. The basic testing/evaluations done initially include cholesterol and lipid profile, urinalysis, complete blood count, blood chemistry profile, a screen for colorectal cancer, cervical screening, and mammogram. Time intervals for testing are provided in the subsequent section on Midlife and Late-life Women's Health Care Program.

- Serum FSH level may be indicated, but a 1 year period of amenorrhea is also diagnostic of ovarian failure.
- Bone density evaluation may be indicated if the reason for initiating therapy is to prevent or inhibit osteoporosis.

- Endometrial biopsy is indicated if dysfunctional bleeding is present or if the client is at high risk for endometrial cancer (obese, family history of endometrial or breast cancer, long history of amenorrhea or oligomenorrhea during the reproductive years).
- A menstrual diary and an accurate record of other bleeding episodes over several months may provide insights for diagnosis and treatment. The diary may also be helpful after HRT is begun.

Ovarian/pelvic ultrasound is indicated if the ovaries are nonpalpable due to obesity, or if there is a suspected enlarged ovary or pelvic mass, or if there is a family history of ovarian cancer.

TREATMENT CONSIDERATIONS

Hormone dosages, preparations, and schedules are individualized according to symptoms and client choice. In general, there are three protocols for administering hormone therapy: (1) estrogen only, (2) estrogen with addition of cyclic progestins, and (3) continuous estrogen with the addition of continuous progestins. Table 15–2 lists some of the more widely used preparations of estrogen, progestin, and testosterone and their dosages.

Absolute Contraindications to Estrogen Use

- Known or suspected cancer of the breast (undiagnosed breast mass).
- Known or suspected estrogen dependent neoplasia.
- Undiagnosed, abnormal genital bleeding.
- Active thrombophlebitis or thromboembolic disorders. (A history of thrombotic disease is not a contraindication, but an indication to use transdermal, rather than oral, estrogen.)[62]
- Consult with a physician in treating the client with such a history.
- Pregnancy.
- Impaired liver function may require a transdermal route, as may migraine headaches.[62]
- Both conditions warrant physician consult, as differing dosages and routes may be needed.

TABLE 15–2. HORMONE REPLACEMENT REGIMENS

Cyclic Treatment Regimens
(Estrogens daily, progestin on days 1–12 of the month, or estrogen on days 1–25 and progestins on days 14–25)

Estrogens (dose in mg)	
conjugated estrogens	0.625, 1.25
estropipate	0.625, 1.25
micronized estradiol	1.0, 2.0
estradiol valerate	1.0, 2.0
Progestins (dose in mg)	
medroxyprogesterone acetate	5.0, 10.0
norethindrone	2.5, 5.0
norethindrone acetate	5.0, 10.0

Continuous Treatment Regimens
(Estrogen and progestin daily)

Estrogens (dose in mg)	
conjugated estrogens	0.625
estropipate	0.625
micronized estradiol	2.0
Progestins (dose in mg)	
medroxyprogesterone acetate	2.5, 5
norethindrone	0.35, 2.1
norethindrone acetate	1.0

Combination Therapy (dose in mg)

Premphase
  conjugated estrogens .625 for 28 days 1st and 2nd blister card
  & MPA 5 for 14 days 2nd blister card
Prempro
  conjugated estrogens .625 & MPA 2.5 1 tab daily

Estrogen & Testosterone Daily Regimens

esterified estrogen 1.25 & methyltestosterone 2.5
esterified estrogen 0.625 & methyltestosterone 1.25
conjugated estrogen 0.625 & methyltestosterone 5.0
conjugated estrogen 1.25 & methyltestosterone 10.0

Transdermal Estradiol Patches (dose in mg/day)

Climara	0.05, 0.1 applied weekly
Estraderm	0.05, 0.1 applied biweekly
Vivelle	0.375, 0.05, 0.075, 0.1

Vaginal Estrogen Creams (daily, cyclically, or as directed)

conjugated estrogen	0.625 mg/g
estradiol	0.01 percent
estropipate	1.5 mg/g

Adapted from LeBoeuf, F. J. & Carter, S. G. (1996). Discomforts of the Perimenopause. JOGNN, 25(2), 173–180.

Absolute Contraindications to Progestin Use

- Active thrombophlebitis or thromboembolic disorders.
- Liver dysfunction or disease.
- Known or suspected cancer of the breast.
- Undiagnosed abnormal vaginal bleeding.
- Pregnancy.

Breast Cancer and Hormone Replacement Therapy

Evidence is conflicting at this time about the effect of estrogen and the risk of breast cancer, although some studies suggest that a slightly increased risk of breast cancer is associated with prolonged estrogen use (over 5 to 15 years) and older age.[63,64] There is no longer the need to administer estrogen cyclically in order to minimize the risk, and the addition of progestin does not seem to increase the risk of breast cancer, although long-term data on combined estrogen and progestin are limited.[53,64]

FOLLOW-UP EVALUATION AND HORMONE REPLACEMENT THERAPY

Follow-up assessment on an annual basis for all clients on HRT should include the following: interim history, complete medical examination, including breast and pelvic examinations, mammography, and Papanicolaou smear, if indicated. Endometrial evaluation is indicated for clients on ERT without progestin, and those with prolonged bleeding (> 10 days), or persistent, irregular bleeding. Office based endometrial biopsy is the standard method of evaluation; transvaginal ultrasound may be used as an initial test to determine which clients need biopsy, or dilation and curettage may be necessary when office based biopsy is not possible and endometrial thickness is greater than 4 mm. Routine endometrial evaluation at onset of HRT or while on HRT is not recommended.[65]

POSTMENOPAUSAL HORMONE REPLACEMENT THERAPY

Hormone replacement therapy (estrogen, progestin, and/or testosterone) is given orally, trans-dermally, and vaginally. Oral estrogens include natural, conjugated, and synthetic estrogens. Natural estrogens, such as micronized estradiol (Estrace) and estropipate (Ogen), are converted in the liver to estrone, which becomes the primary circulating estrogen. Oral estrogens all have a reduction in bioavailability because of the first-pass effect through the liver, and less potency than transdermal delivery because they have to pass through the gastrointestinal tract.[55] For osteoporosis, oral and epidermally applied estrogen are effective for prevention and inhibition of bone loss with doses 1 to 2 mg of 17B-estradiol or 0.625 mg of conjugated estrogen daily.[48] The most commonly used progestin is medroxyprogesterone acetate (Provera). Norethindrone is also frequently used. The most commonly used testosterone is methyltestosterone. Side effects of the hormonal components are estrogen or progestin or androgen related. Estrogen related side effects include breast tenderness, nausea (usually subsides in 3 to 6 months), and headaches. Progestin related side effects include nausea, acne, headaches, and PMS-like symptoms, such as irritability. Androgen related side effects include acne and hirsutism.

Oral Regimens

Cyclic Estrogen/Progestin Therapy. Start with continuous daily conjugated estrogens (Premarin) 0.625 mg, or an equivalent. If hypoestrogenic symptoms persist after 30 days of Premarin, increase the daily dosage incrementally to 0.9 mg or 1.25 mg. If the client has an intact uterus, add medroxyprogesterone acetate (Provera) 5–10 mg daily, on days 1 to 12 or days 13 to 25 of the month. It is well established that 10 mg daily for 12 days is protective against endometrial cancer;[66] however, the side effects of progestin at this dosage may not be acceptable to the client. Equivalent dosages of other progestins may be tried. Some clinicians reduce the Provera to 5 mg and carefully observe the effects, as this dosage may not offer the endometrial protection of 10 mg. Prolonged withdrawal bleeding more than 10 days may indicate the need for endometrial biopsy. If bleeding begins before day 10 of the progestin administration and is cyclic, increase dosage or duration of progestin to see if this regulates the bleeding pattern. If not, a biopsy is indicated.[62]

ADVANTAGES. Cyclic therapy is effective for relief of hypoestrogenic symptoms and prevention of osteoporosis.

DISADVANTAGES. Withdrawal bleeding after the progestin is stopped may lead to decreased client compliance; however, dosing every 3 months may be less problematic (10 mg per day for 12 to 14 days). Whether this type of regimen protects the endometrium is unproved by research at this time.

Continuous Daily Estrogen/Progestin Therapy. Start with conjugated estrogens (Premarin) 0.625 mg, once a day, or an equivalent. If the uterus is intact, continuous medroxyprogesterone acetate (Provera) 2.5 mg is added daily. If hypoestrogenic symptoms persist after 30 days of Premarin, increase the dosage incrementally to 0.9 mg or 1.25 mg daily. If Premarin is increased, also increase Provera to 5 to 10 mg daily.

Two combination packs are currently available: 1) conjugated estrogens 0.625 mg for full 28-day cycle plus MPA 5 mg given on days 15 through 28 (Premphase) and 2) conjugated estrogens 0.625 mg plus MPA 2.5 mg given daily (Prempro).

ADVANTAGES. No cyclic bleeding occurs with the continuous therapy, and therapy is effective in preventing osteoporosis.

DISADVANTAGES. The client may have acyclic bleeding during the first few months; this usually resolves by 6 months. The client may find the unpredictable bleeding pattern unacceptable; if so, switch to the cyclic option, and convert to the continuous method some years later. Prolonged and persistent bleeding requires biopsy. Also, once amenorrhea is established, if bleeding occurs, biopsy is indicated.[62]

The most exhaustive data on efficacy have been collected on Premarin, but Table 15–2 also lists substitutes. *Generic estrogens are not recommended because of quality control issues.*

Transdermal Estrogen

Transdermal estradiol, Estraderm and Climara, deliver human 17-beta estradiol directly to the bloodstream, bypassing the liver. Both patches are available in 0.05 mg/day and 1.0 mg/day; estraderm is replaced biweekly, and Climara re-

placed weekly. If hypoestrogenic symptoms persist after 30 days, increase the dosage to 0.1 mg. If the uterus is intact, add medroxyprogesterone acetate (Provera) 10 mg or progestin equivalent for 12 days per month or Provera 2.5 mg continuously as presented previously in the continuous daily estrogen/progestin therapy discussion.

ADVANTAGES. Among the advantages of transdermal estrogen are prompt relief of hypoestrogenic symptoms and delivery of natural 17b-estradiol directly to target cells. Continuous levels are delivered without fluctuation. Improved compliance is noted among women who do not desire oral medication. Short-term data suggest that the patch is equal to oral estrogens in the prevention of osteoporosis. The patch does not significantly affect clotting factors or any other liver functions, as if taken orally.[59]

DISADVANTAGES. Skin irritation from the patch may occur; however, preventive measures can be taken.

- Make sure that the application area is clean, dry, and free of oil, powder, perfume, and soap.
- Leave the system open to the air (with protective covering off) for 10 to 15 minutes prior to application to allow some of the alcohol to evaporate.
- Rotate the patch with each change. Apply to upper outer quadrants of buttocks (less sensitive). Do not use on breasts.

Lipid profile data in transdermal estrogen use are inclusive; to date, they have less effect on lipids and are of undetermined benefit against heart disease.[59]

Transvaginal Estrogen

Vaginal application of estrogen is absorbed and enters the systemic circulation, achieving 25 percent of the serum level of an equal oral dose.[67] It exerts a potent local effect, however, enhancing revascularization of the vaginal epithelium. Vaginal administration of estrogen is indicated for the treatment of atrophic vaginitis. One applicator of estrogen cream inserted twice weekly usually is adequate to relieve symptoms. Most of the side effects seen with oral estrogen can be experienced with vaginal estrogen.

Testosterone Therapy

Esterified estrogens with methyltestosterone (Estratest tablets) or conjugated estrogens (Premarin) with methyltestosterone may be used when a client's primary complaint is loss of libido, in the absence of other medical and psychosocial factors. (Progestins must be added if the client has an intact uterus.)

ADVANTAGES. Improvement in libido with some women; prevention of osteoporosis, relief of hypoestrogenic symptoms.

DISADVANTAGES. Androgenic side effects: acne, hirsutism, clitoromegaly.

Side effects are infrequent and dose-related and usually resolve after discontinuation of therapy. Lipid profile data for testosterone therapy are inclusive; in women with a low HDL cholesterol level, documented atherosclerotic cardiovascular disease, or a strong family history of cardiovascular disease, it is best to avoid estrogen-androgen products.[68]

PERIMENOPAUSAL HORMONE REPLACEMENT THERAPY

Clients who are still ovulating may need contraception as they approach menopause, yet have indications for supplemental estrogen therapy as their estrogen level declines. The points to consider in continuing or initiating low dose contraceptive therapy are many.

- Estrogen may be necessary as the aging ovary begins to secrete lower levels of estradiol several years prior to the last menstrual period. The client may have some beginning signs or symptoms of deficiency but continue to have regular menses. *Reference point:* Postmenopausal estrogens are about 1 percent as potent as ethinyl estradiol. Thus, 10 μg of ethinyl estradiol (EE) is about equivalent to 1 mg of conjugated estrogen. Knowing when to change from oral contraception to postmenopausal hormone therapy is important. It is necessary to change because even with the lowest estrogen dose oral contraceptive available, the estrogen dose is four-fold greater than the standard postmenopausal dose, and with increasing age, the dose related risks with estrogen become significant.[9]

- Control of irregular or breakthrough bleeding may be required. The bleeding may occur because of inadequate production of luteal phase hormone or because of an estradiol peak without subsequent ovulation.
- HRT does not provide contraception. Elective abortion is highest among women under age 25 (58 percent); 1.5 percent of elective abortions are in women over age 40.[69] Postmenopausal estrogens will not provide contraception, although they will ameliorate symptoms.
- No data suggest an increased risk of heart disease. Studies indicate no increased risk in women over age 35 using low dose ethinyl estradiol (less than 35 μg) oral contraceptives, provided they do not smoke.[70]
- Oral contraceptive (OC) users are at decreased risk to develop endometrial and ovarian cancer.[70]
- Data from formal studies regarding the effect of OCs on cervical neoplasia lack consistency.[70] OC users are likely to be sexually active, often not using a barrier method, a risk factor for cervical cancer.
- Studies on the use of oral contraceptives do not demonstrate an increased risk of breast cancer, nor any protection against it.[9]
- The incidence of fibroids is 30 percent lower among OC users.[70]
- Pelvic inflammatory disease (PID) and ectopic pregnancy are less common among OC users.[70]

Therapy options to regulate anovulatory cycles for perimenopausal women include oral contraceptives containing less than 35 μg of estrogen or low dose progestational treatment. These may be used if no contraindications exist. Low dose oral conjugated estrogen (0.3–0.625 mg Premarin) or an estrogen patch are options if contraception is not an issue. Progestin is added when the uterus is intact. Management includes annual screening exams—Pap smear, colorectal cancer screen, and FSH level evaluation. Begin annual FSH evaluation when the client is 50 years old: when the FSH level exceeds 30 IU/L on days 5 to 7 of a pill free week, switch the client to ERT/HRT.[9] (See subsequent section on the Midlife Women's Health Care Program for other tests/diagnostic methods that may be indicated based on age and assessment findings.) Allay the fears of older clients about the increased risks of heart disease and stroke. Communicate to the client the contraindications to OC use: smoking, hypertension, diabetes, thromboembolic disorders, impaired liver function, and known or suspected estrogen dependent neoplasm (see Chapter 9).

OPTIONS AFTER HYSTERECTOMY/ OOPHORECTOMY

Posthysterectomy (without Oophorectomy)

Hysterectomy promotes earlier ovarian failure; the surgery itself may compromise blood supply to the ovaries, and the uterus contributes hormonally to ovarian function.[71] Monitor the client for hypoestrogenic symptoms. Measure the FSH level every 1 to 2 years.

Postoophorectomy

An abrupt, drastic fall in estradiol occurs following oophorectomy (no gradual adaptation is possible, as with natural menopause). The symptoms are often severe, particularly hot flushes and intestinal symptoms. Surgical menopause is a predisposing factor to osteoporosis, and it is known that bone is maintained by ERT.[2] ERT is generally begun immediately postoperatively; high doses, such as 1.25 mg of Premarin, may be needed for up to a year postoperatively.

INITIATING HORMONE REPLACEMENT THERAPY AND FOLLOW-UP

Provide the client with written and oral information about HRT. Explain the risks and benefits as they apply to the client's own situation. Request that the client keep a menstrual calendar; educate her concerning what constitutes abnormal bleeding. Advise the client to telephone the health care provider immediately if she experiences any of the following:

- Unexpected bleeding.
- Abdominal pains, bloating.
- An increase in headaches.
- Symptoms not relieved or that increase.
- Visual disturbances.
- Shortness of breath or chest pain.
- Calf pain.

Obtaining written consent for HRT from the client is optional, but advised because consumers continue to be confused about estrogen and its risks and benefits.

Adequate follow-up is critical in maximizing compliance, to evaluate the response to medications, and side effects. A reasonable approach is to call the client in a month, and schedule a 2–3 month visit after therapy is initiated. Clients should be encouraged to call with questions or concerns at any time. Stress to the client that even if she experiences no problems, annual exams, routine tests, and communication are important.

CHANGING DOSAGE OR DISCONTINUATION OF THERAPY

Adjustment of ERT dosage may be needed to provide symptom relief. The dosage is increased gradually to find the minimum level needed for symptom relief. After 6 months of adequate relief at a dosage higher than 0.625 mg Premarin or equivalent, gradually decrease doses to 0.625 mg (see Table 15–2). (*Example:* 1.25 mg for 3 weeks, 0.9 mg for 1 week; if tolerated, 1.25 mg for 2 weeks, 0.9 mg for 1 week; 1.25 mg for 1 week, 0.9 mg for 1 week; stabilize at 0.9 mg for 2 weeks, then 0.9 mg for 3 weeks, 6.25 mg for 1 week, and so on.)

Hormone replacement therapy (HRT) should be discontinued gradually. (*Example:* 7 tablets per week for 1 month; 6 tablets per week for 1 month; 5 tablets per week for 1 month, and so on until zero.)

WOMEN'S MIDLIFE AND LATE LIFE HEALTH CARE PROGRAM

Comprehensive health care, which includes traditional medical care, as well as health promotion and disease prevention, should be individualized for each client. The plan of care focuses on the existing health problems and projected long-range health outcomes, and each client's preferences concerning the risks and benefits of preventive measures. Emphasis is on health education, appropriate screenings for early detection of disease, and discussion of positive health behaviors. A holistic health care program includes education and appropriate evaluation and testing.

EDUCATION

Many women lack knowledge of the emotional, sexual, social, and medical aspects of the perimenopausal and postmenopausal phases of life; hence, client education must be comprehensive. Approximately half of all deaths occuring in the United States in 1990 may be attributed to factors such as tobacco, alcohol, and illicit drug use, diet and activity patterns, motor vehicles, and sexual behavior, and are potentially preventable by changes in personal health practices.[72]

Anatomy and Physiology. Explain the changes expected with the perimenopausal transition and postmenopausal period, including the most common signs and symptoms and usual nonmedical and medical methods of management.

Nutrition and Dental Health. Dietary excess and imbalance is associated with diseases such as breast and colon cancer, stroke, coronary heart disease, hypertension, and osteoporosis. Explain the dietary need to decrease fat, especially saturated fats (Table 15–3); increase complex carbohydrates and fiber; have a moderate protein intake; and increase dietary calcium or add a calcium supplement. Counsel clients to visit a dental care provider on a regular basis, floss daily, and brush their teeth daily with a fluoride containing toothpaste.

Exercise/Obesity. Thirty-three point five percent of white women, and 49.6 percent of black women are at least 20 percent above their ideal weight according to the National Health and Nutrition Examination Survey III.[73] The risk of CHD is three times higher among obese women than women at their ideal weight.[74] Physical inactivity is also related to an increased risk of CHD. Research has shown a 60 percent–75 percent lower risk of CHD in physically active women.[75] Encourage weightbearing, aerobic, flexibility, and joint mobility activities (Table 15–4). Adults should be encouraged to increase activity gradually, with the goal of at least 30 minutes daily of physical activity of moderate intensity, (e.g., brisk walking, stair climbing); more strenuous activities such as slow jogging, cycling, field and court games, and swimming.[76]

Smoking, Alcohol, and Drug Use. Communicate the need to stop all untoward substance use. Refer the client to a smoking cessation program, Alcoholics Anonymous, or drug treatment program as appropriate. Stress the need for caution with prescription drug use also (see Chapter 23 and Nonreproductive Health Concerns of Aging Women, end of Chapter 15).

Relaxation and Stress Reduction. Emphasize the need for awareness of one's stress level and the contributing factors. Promote the use of relaxation techniques and behavior modification, rather than alcohol or drugs.

Contraception. Give information about effective, safe birth control methods if the client desires protection during the transition before menopause (see Chapter 9).

Hormone Replacement Therapy. Tell the client about the risks, benefits, and side effects of HRT. Provide written information.

Sexuality. Discuss how the transition to menopause will affect sexuality, particularly the frequent vaginal changes and ways to counter them satisfactorily (e.g., lubrication and Kegel's exercises). Assessing sexual function and counseling clients to prevent sexually transmitted diseases and HIV should be a routine part of the evaluation, regardless of age.

Accident Prevention. Counsel all clients to use auto safety belts, wear bicycle helmets, and refrain from driving while under the influence of alcohol or other drugs (see Accident Prevention, in Nonreproductive Health Concerns of Aging Women).

PERIODIC EVALUATION AND TESTING

Preventive services for the early detection of disease have been associated with reductions in morbidity and mortality. Periodic health evaluation and selected screening tests are recommended based on effectiveness of the specific test, age, and other individual risk factors of the client. A comprehensive health history that

TABLE 15–3. EXAMPLES OF FOODS TO CHOOSE OR DECREASE FOR THE STEP I AND STEP II DIETS*

Food Group	Choose	Decrease
Lean Meat, Poultry, and Fish ≤ 5–6 oz. per day	Beef, pork, lamb—lean cuts well trimmed before cooking Poultry without skin Fish, shellfish Processed meat—prepared from lean meat, e.g., lean ham, lean frankfurters, lean meat with soy protein or carrageenan	Beef, pork, lamb—regular ground beef, fatty cuts, spare ribs, organ meats Poultry with skin, fried chicken Fried fish, fried shellfish Regular luncheon meat, e.g., bologna, salami, sausage, frankfurters
Eggs ≤ 4 yolks per week, Step I ≤ 2 yolks per week, Step II	Egg whites (two whites can be substituted for one whole egg in recipes) cholesterol free egg substitute	Egg yolks (if more than four per week on Step I or if more than two per week on Step II); includes eggs used in cooking and baking
Low Fat Dairy Products 2–3 servings per day	Milk—skim, 1/2%, or 1% fat (fluid, powdered, evaporated), buttermilk Yogurt—nonfat or low fat yogurt or yogurt beverages Cheese—low fat natural or processed cheese Low fat or nonfat varieties, e.g.: cottage cheese—low fat, nonfat, or dry curd (0 to 20% fat) Frozen dairy dessert—ice milk, frozen yogurt, (low fat or nonfat) Low fat coffee creamer Low fat or nonfat sour cream	Whole milk (fluid, evaporated, condensed), 2% fat milk (lowfat milk), imitation milk Whole milk yogurt, whole milk yogurt beverages Regular cheeses (American, blue, Brie, cheddar, Colby, Edam, Monterey Jack, whole-milk mozzarella, Parmesan, Swiss), cream cheese, Neufchatel cheese Cottage cheese (4% fat) Ice cream Cream, half & half, whipping cream, nondairy creamer, whipped topping, sour cream
Fats and Oils ≤ 6–8 teaspoons per day	Unsaturated oils—safflower, sunflower, corn, soybean, cottonseed, canola, olive, peanut Margarine—made from unsaturated oils listed above, light or diet margarine, especially soft or liquid forms Salad dressings—made with unsaturated oils listed above, low fat or fat free Seeds or nuts—peanut butter, other nut butters Cocoa powder	Coconut oil, palm kernel oil, palm oil Butter, lard, shortening, bacon fat, hard margarine Dressings made with egg yolk, cheese, sour cream, whole milk Coconut Milk chocolate
Breads and Cereals 6 or more servings per day	Breads—whole-grain bread, English muffins, bagels, buns, corn or flour tortilla Cereals—oat, wheat, corn, multigrain, Pasta Rice Dry beans and peas Crackers, low fat—animal-type, graham, soda crackers, breadsticks, melba toast Homemade baked goods using unsaturated oil, skim or 1% milk, and egg substitute—quick breads, biscuits, cornbread muffins, bran muffins, pancakes, waffles	Bread in which eggs, fat, and/or butter are a major ingredient; croissants Most granolas High fat crackers Commercial baked pastries, muffins, biscuits
Soups	Reduced or low fat and reduced sodium varieties, e.g., chicken or beef noodle, minestrone, tomato, vegetable, potato, reduced fat soups made with skim milk	Soup containing whole milk, cream, meat fat, poultry fat, or poultry skin
Vegetables 3–5 servings per day	Fresh, frozen, or canned, without added fat or sauce	Vegetables fried or prepared with butter, cheese, or cream sauce
Fruits 2–4 servings per day	Fruit—fresh, frozen, canned, or dried Fruit juice—fresh, frozen, or canned	Fried fruit or fruit served with butter or cream sauce

*Careful selection of processed foods is necessary to stay within the sodium < 2,400 mg guideline.

(Continued)

TABLE 15–3. EXAMPLES OF FOODS TO CHOOSE OR DECREASE FOR THE STEP I AND STEP II DIETS* (CONTINUED)

Food Group	Choose	Decrease
Sweets and Modified Fat Desserts	Beverages—fruit-flavored drinks, lemonade, fruit punch	
	Sweets—sugar, syrup, honey, jam, preserves, candy made without fat (candy corn, gumdrops, hard candy), fruit-flavored gelatin	Candy made with milk chocolate, coconut oil, palm kernel oil, palm oil
	Frozen desserts—low fat and nonfat yogurt, ice milk, sherbet, sorbet, fruit ice, popsicles	Ice cream and frozen treats made with ice cream
	Cookies, cake, pie, pudding—prepared with egg whites, egg substitute, skim milk or 1% milk, and unsaturated oil or margarine; ginger snaps; fig and other fruit bar cookies, fat free cookies; angel food cake	Commercial baked pies, cakes, doughnuts, high-fat cookies, cream pies

Source: Expert Panel. (1993). Second Report of the Expert Panel on Detection, Evaluation, and Treatment of High Blood Cholesteral in Adults. NIH Publication No. 93–3095.

specifically addresses midlife or late life issues is invaluable. A complete physical examination, also necessary, includes height, weight, integumentary, oral cavity, thyroid, cardiovascular and thoracic systems, breasts (including instruction in breast self-examination [BSE]), abdomen, extremities, and pelvic and rectal components.

Diagnostic Tests and Methods

Cholesterol and/or Lipid Profile. (See Chapter 5 for general screening guidelines.) If no prior testing has been done, obtain baseline data in early adulthood or when HRT is initiated. Draw a lipid profile if cholesterol is over 240 mg/dL, or if the total cholesterol is 200 mg/dL or above and the client has 2 or more CHD risk factors, or if the client has an HDL-cholesterol less than 35mg/dL;[13] if normal, repeat every 5 years to age 64, and then every 3 to 5 years thereafter.[13] If cholesterol is 200 mg/dL or above, advise a low cholesterol, low fat, high fiber diet and regular exercise for 3 months and then repeat the test. If cholesterol is still elevated, referral to a primary care provider is appropriate.

Dipstick Urinalysis. For preventive care perform yearly, as appropriate in all women.

Hemoglobin Levels. Routine screening for anemia is not recommended.[13] For women with a history of excessive menstrual flow, and for women 65 years of age or older, hemoglobin levels should be measured as part of routine preventive care.[13]

Blood Chemistry Profile. All major U.S. authorities do not recommend multiple blood chemistry screens for asymptomatic normal risk individuals.[13]

Colorectal Cancer Screening. For women at normal risk, begin annual screening with a digital rectal exam, at age 40, annual fecal occult blood testing beginning at age 50, and sigmoidoscopy every 3 to 5 years beginning at age 50.[13] For women at an increased risk of colorectal cancer, more frequent screening is recommended. What constitutes increased risk and the frequency of screening differs among authorities.

Cervical Screening. Annual Pap smear and pelvic exam are recommended for all women age 18 and older. If a client has three or more consecutive normal Pap smears, then the test may be done less frequently, at the discretion of the client and health care professional.[13] Annual pelvic exams are warranted however, to evaluate other areas, for example, the ovaries. If the client has had a hysterectomy for benign disease, then repeat the Pap smear 1 year after surgery; if negative, then every 2 years. If the cervix was not removed, or if the client has ever had an abnormal Pap, then continue Pap smears annually.

Ovarian Cancer Screening. Bimanual pelvic examination is of unknown sensitivity in detecting

TABLE 15–4. EXERCISES FOR MIDLIFE WOMEN

Run in place, or around a room. (This is just as beneficial as running, or jogging, outdoors.)

Lie on your back, knees slightly bent. Catch your feet securely under a bed, couch, cabinet, or heavy chair. Clasp your hands behind your head. Rise to a sitting position, then return to a reclining position.

Lie flat, with knees slightly bent and arms at your sides. Raise your left leg straight up. Lower it. Repeat with your right leg.

Repeat the exercise above, but when leg is raised, swing it slowly to one side and back up, then lower it to the floor.

Stand, placing your hands flat against each other as if in prayer. Push them together as hard as you can.

Lie down, knees flexed, soles on the floor. Extend your left leg as far as you can, pointing your toe. Return to a flexed position, then relax it. Repeat with your right leg.

Kneel and put hands on floor. Raise your back the way a cat stretches, then lower your abdomen in a reverse movement. Repeat several times.

Sit on the floor cross-legged. Reach as high as you can with your right hand, then with your left hand. Repeat. Do the same thing, reaching forward with each hand.

Stand on your tiptoes. Rock back and forth from heels to toes.

Stand straight. Keeping your knees slightly bent, bend to touch the floor with your fingertips.

Stand straight. Reach for the ceiling with both hands.

Note: These exercises emphasize strength and stretching, and they are suitable for women who have not been very active.
Source: Fogel, C. I. (1991) Nutrition and health patterns in midlife women. *In C. H. Garner (Ed.),* NAACOG's Clinical Issues in Perinatal and Women's Health Nursing: Mid-Life Women's Health 2(4), 523. Used with permission.

ovarian cancer; small, early stage ovarian tumors are often not detected by palpation.[72] Routine screening by transvaginal ultrasound or serum tumor markers is not recommended in asymptomatic women.[72] The NIH Consensus Conference concluded that women with hereditary cancer syndrome should undergo annual pelvic examinations, CA-125 measurements, and transvaginal ultrasound until childbearing is completed or at age 35, and then undergo prophylactic bilateral oophorectomy.[77]

Endometrial Cancer Screening. Routine screening is neither cost effective nor warranted.[9] A biopsy is indicated if abnormal uterine bleeding occurs.

Lung Cancer Screening. No suitable techniques are available, although some clinicians support annual chest x-rays for women 50 years and older who smoke more than a pack of cigarettes daily.

All major U.S. authorities do not routinely recommend chest x-rays for asymptomatic normal risk individuals.[13] Advise the client to stop smoking, because of the increased risks of breast disease, hypertension, osteoporosis, cervical cancer, early menopause, and lung cancer.

Breast Cancer Screening. Teaching and reinforcing BSE, and encouraging an annual exam by a health care provider are important. A baseline mammogram is needed between ages 35 and 40 years, every 1 to 2 years from ages 40 to 49, and annually after age 50.[13] The American Geriatrics Society recommends that women over 65 years receive mammograms at least every 2 or 3 years until at least 85 years of age.[13] Recommendations vary for women at increased risk of breast cancer (see Chapter 14).

Skin Cancer Screening. Skin cancer is the most common type of cancer in the United States and is virtually 100 percent curable if diagnosed and excised early.[13] Skin examination should be performed for clients with a family or personal history of skin cancer, increased exposure to sunlight, or clinical evidence of precursor lesions (e.g., dysplatic nevi, congenital nevi).[13]

Cardiovascular Screening. All major United States authorities do not recommend routine screening electrocardiograms (ECGs) for asymptomatic, normal risk individuals.[13] The risk of cardiovascular disease does increase with age, however, and the health professional may want to consider more regular ECG use in the later decades of a client's life.

Hearing Examinations. Hearing screening is not necessary for asymptomatic women under age 65, except for those exposed regularly to excessive noise, but women 65 years and older should be evaluated for hearing loss.[13] An otoscopic exam and audiometric testing are practical methods to evaluate hearing loss.

Vision Screening. A comprehensive eye examination, including visual acuity and glaucoma screening by an opthalmologist, should be done every 3 to 5 years in African Americans age 20 to 39 years, and regardless of race, every 2 to 4 years age at 40 to 64 years, and every 1 to 2 years beginning at age 65.[13]

Immunizations. Updated diphtheria and tetanus immunizations are needed every 10 years. Annual influenza immunization beginning at age 65 and Pneumovax (pneumonia vaccine) at age 65 are recommended.[13] Hepatitis B Virus (HBV) immunization is recommended in women at increased risk for HBV infection: high occupational risk, heterosexual women who have had more than one partner in the previous 6 months and/or those with a recent episode of a sexually transmitted disease, international travelers in areas with high HBV infection, hemophiliacs, hemodialysis clients, and injection drug users.[13]

Bone Density Screening. Routine screening in asymptomatic women is not currently recommended due to the costs and inconvenience, but may be useful for identifying women at high risk of osteoporosis or fracture who might not otherwise consider preventive treatment (see Osteoporosis). Bone density measurement is more reliable than clinical assessment, and may help the client and primary care provider make more informed decisions about the potential benefits and risks of therapies such as estrogen.[72]

- Dual photon absorptiometry (DPA) uses the radioisotope gadolinium to project gamma rays through the body. They are measured by computer to calculate the quantity of minerals present.
- QCT densitometry—modified quantitative computerized tomography of the lumbar spine—calculates bone mass. This method is more costly and uses a higher dosage of radiation.
- Dual-energy x-ray absorptiometry (DEXA), or dual x-ray absorptiometry (DXA), is widely used in the clinical setting and is safe, accurate, and precise, with shorter examination times (5–10 vs. 20–40 minutes) than DPA.[72] This measure is being used more than DPA or QCT as it is less expensive and can be done rapidly.
- Single photon absorptiometry (SPA) measures the density of cortical bone of the distal radius or calcaneus. SPA is accurate, less expensive, and predictive for future risk of nonspine fracture.

Diabetic Screening. Fasting plasma glucose level should be periodically measured in women who are at high risk due to a personal history of gestational diabetes, a family history of diabetes, or marked obesity[13] (see Chapter 21).

Endometrial Biopsy

- *With Hormone Replacement Therapy.* Routine screening for endometrial hyperplasia or cancer is not recommended for clients on HRT; however if taking unopposed estrogen (ERT), endometrial biopsy at onset of treatment and then yearly is recommended.[65] (See also DUB, which follows.)
- *With Dysfunctional Uterine Bleeding (DUB).* DUB is defined as any bleeding that occurs a year or more after a previous episode of perimenopausal bleeding (single episodes of spotting or blood tinged discharge are significant), heavy or frequent bleeding episodes, or bleeding at inappropriate times with hormone replacement therapy (HRT). Initially, the health are provider must rule out endometrial carcinoma; refer the client to a gynecologist for evaluation (see Chapter 8).

Blood Pressure Screening. Elevated blood pressure puts clients at risk for coronary artery disease, peripheral vascular disease, stroke, renal disease, and retinopathy. Blood pressure should be measured as part of the periodic evaluation, which should occur annually or as appropriate.[13]

Thyroid Dysfunction. Hypothyroidism and hyperthyroidism are more common in women, older adults, and clients with a family history of thyroid disease. Thyroid malignancy occurs twice as frequently in women as in men. Thyroid palpation should be part of the periodic examination for all women over age 18, and thyroid stimulating hormone (TSH) levels should be obtained every 3 to 5 years for all women aged 65 and older and for younger women with an autoimmune condition or strong family history of thyroid disease.[13]

OSTEOPOROSIS

Osteoporosis is a condition characterized by low bone mass, deterioration of bone tissue leading to bone fragility, and consequent susceptibility to fracture. Bone mass peaks at age 30, and as much as 50 percent of the bone that women lose during their life span is lost before menopause.[78] At menopause, the rate of bone loss accelerates and is most significant in the first postmenopausal decade.[79] The greatest loss occurs in the femoral neck and lumbar vertebrae comprised of trabecular bone, which is subject to future fracture. A long, silent, asymptomatic period (10 to 20 years postmenopause) is typical. Osteoporosis related fractures commonly involve the proximal femur (hip), vertebral body, and distal forearm, of these sites, the proximal femur has the greatest effect on morbidity and mortality.

Osteoporosis and related skeletal fractures result in enmorous economic costs, considerable disability, and premature death. The perimenopausal and postmenopausal woman requires knowledge of the epidemiology, risk factors, screening tests, and treatment regimens for osteoporosis.

EPIDEMIOLOGY

Osteoporotic fractures in aging women are a major public health problem. In the United States, approximately 150,000–250,000 hip fractures occur annually in women over age 65, with 15 to 25 percent needing long-term home nursing care. Five percent to 20 percent of hip fracture victims will die within 1 year of fracture, and more than 50 percent of survivors will be incapacitated, many of them permanently.[48] Estimates for vertebral fracture approach 650,000 cases per year, with a prevalence of 40 percent by age 80. There is good evidence that oral estrogen can reduce the rate of bone loss and improve bone mineral density in postmenopausal women. Greater benefit is achieved with current use, long-term use (> 5 years), and therapy begun close to menopause. Since bone loss resumes after estrogen is discontinued, hormones may need to be taken indefinitely to provide maximal protection after age 75, when the risk of fracture is greatest.[81] Women should be aware of the value of HRT in preventing osteoporosis to enhance long-term compliance.

SUBJECTIVE DATA

The client may report some of the risk factors listed in Table 15–5; these risk factors can help

TABLE 15–5. RISK FACTORS FOR LOW BONE MASS

Age

Caucasian or Asian race

Sedentary lifestyle

Smoking

Low body weight

Family history of osteoporosis

Excessive alcohol intake

Prolonged calcium deficient diet

Nulliparity

Long-term use of certain medications (e.g., glucocorticoids, phenytoin, excessive thyroxine)

Estrogen deficient states

AACE. (1996) AACE Clinical Practice Guideline for Prevention and Treatment of Postmenopausal Osteoporosis. Endocrine Practice, 2(2), 157–171.

identify clients who are susceptible to fracture and to develop an osteoporosis prevention program, but fail to identify a substantial proportion of clients with low bone mass.[79] The medical evaluation includes a family and a medical history. Medications or coexisting diseases that cause or aggravate bone loss need to be eliminated or appropriately treated.

OBJECTIVE DATA

Physical Examination

A complete physical and gynecologic examination is indicated. Findings may include spinal injuries or other adverse effects such as loss of height and "dowager's hump" (curvature of the cervical and upper thoracic spine). Maintain a careful record of the client's height in centimeters, in order to detect any decrease.

Diagnostic Tests and Methods

Bone Mineral Density Measurements. Currently DXA, the preferred method for baseline and follow-up measurements, should be done for the following:[79] 1) for risk assessment in perimenopausal or postmenopausal women who are concerned about osteoporosis and willing to accept interventions, 2) in women with x-ray findings that suggest osteoporosis, 3) in women beginning or receiving long-term glucocorticoid therapy, 4) for periomenopausal or postmenopausal women with asymptomatic primary hyperparathyroidism in whom evidence of skeletal loss would result in parathyroidectomy, and 5) in women undergoing treatment for osteoporosis, as a tool for monitoring the therapeutic response.

Laboratory Tests. CBC, serum chemistry, urinalysis. Additional tests may be indicated if secondary causes for bone loss are suspected.

DIFFERENTIAL MEDICAL DIAGNOSES

Multiple myeloma, Cushing's syndrome, hyperparathyroidism, glucocorticoid use, thyrotoxicosis.

PLAN

Psychosocial Interventions

Discuss with the client the importance of preventing or inhibiting further bone loss during the perimenopausal and postmenopausal years. Stress diet, exercise, health, and medication regimens. Advise the client to eliminate or decrease her alcohol intake, and to improve ERT effectiveness, eliminate smoking.

MEDICATION

Therapies approved by the FDA for osteoporosis prevention and treatment include estrogen (with or without MPA), alendronate, and calcitonin. Calcium and vitamin D supplementation do not require FDA approval and are recommended. Sodium Fluoride stimulates bone formation but has not been approved by the FDA for these indications.

Estrogen Replacement Therapy (ERT). ERT is the most significant therapy for the prevention and treatment of postmenopausal osteoporosis. Therapy should begin at the time of menopause or oophorectomy, although can be initiated any time after menopause.[79] Evidence suggests that most women taking estrogen therapy for 7 to 10 years or longer have a 50 percent or greater reduction in the incidence of osteoporotic fractures.[82,83] For the prevention and treatment of osteoporosis, continuous daily estrogen doses

of 0.625 mg Premarin or the equivalent are recommended.

Calcium. By itself, calcium does not significantly influence bone resorption;[84] however, adequate intake is necessary for a positive calcium balance. A negative balance pulls calcium stores from the bone. Calcium and vitamin D supplementation can be administered to most women for a lifetime.

- *Dietary Calcium.* Optimal dietary calcium comes from dairy products and tofu (bean curd), derived from soy bean milk. Factors that interfere with absorption include being older than 35, taking aluminum containing antacids, consuming caffeine, and a high protein diet. Generally, about 500 mg of calcium can be gained through the diet (see Table 15–6, Calcium Content of Various Calcium Rich Foods).
- *Calcium and Vitamin D Supplements.* The recommended daily calcium intake for white women 65 years or younger is 1000 mg per day if taking ERT/HRT and 1500 mg per day if not taking ERT/HRT, and 1500 mg per day for all women older than 65 years.[79] Requirements may differ in other ethnic groups and in persons with lower protein intakes and small skeletal size.[48] When dietary intake is insufficient, a supplement is indicated. Products with calcium carbonate, for example Tums, provide the most calcium for the money. To minimize gastrointestinal side effects and enhance absorption, clients should take calcium with meals and with a bedtime snack. Calcium supplementation is contraindicated in women who have a history of renal stones. Hypercalciuria is unusual at dosages of < 1.5 gm/day.

Alendronate Sodium. An aminobisphosphonate, which inhibits osteoclast activity and bone resorption, is approved by the FDA for treatment of osteoporosis in postmenopausal women. Treatment with alendronate for 3 years has been shown to increase bone mineral density of the vertebrae, femoral neck, and femoral trochanter in postmenopausal women with osteoporosis with mean percentile increases of 7 to 10, 5 to 6, and 7 to 8, respectively.[85] The client should be instructed to take alendronate in the morning at

TABLE 15–6. CALCIUM CONTENT OF VARIOUS CALCIUM RICH FOODS

Food	Serving Size	Calcium per Serving (mg)*
Dairy products:		
Milk†	1 cup	290–300
Swiss cheese	1 oz (slice)	250–270
Yogurt	1 cup	240–400
American cheese	1 oz (slice)	165–200
Ice cream or frozen dessert	1/2 cup	90–100
Cottage cheese	1/2 cup	80–100
Parmesan cheese	1 Tb	70
Powdered nonfat milk	1 tsp	50
Other:		
Sardines in oil (with bones)	3 oz	370
Canned salmon (with bones)	3 oz	170–210
Broccoli	1 cup	160–180
Soybean curd (tofu)	4 oz	145–155
Turnip greens	1/2 cup, cooked	100–125
Kale	1/2 cup, cooked	90–100
Corn bread	2 1/2-inch square	80–90
Egg	1 medium	55
Calcium fortified food		
(bread, cereal, fruit juices)‡	1 serving	160

*A simple formula for calculating dietary calcium assigns 300 mg for the dairy free diet, 300 mg for each serving of a dairy product (cup or slice), and 160 mg for each serving of calcium fortified food.
†All milks (skim, 1%, 2%, and whole) have the same calcium content.
‡Breads and cereals, unless fortified with calcium, are relatively low sources of calcium but still contribute substantially to calcium intake because these foods constitute such a large part of the diet.
Source: From AACA. (1996). AACE clinical practice guidelines for the prevention and treatment of postmenoposal osteoporosis. Endocrine Practice, 2(2), 157–171.

least 30 minutes before the first food, beverage, or medication of the day, swallow whole with 6–8 oz. of water, and avoid recumbancy for at least 30 minutes after taking the dose. The drug should be stopped if symptoms of esophageal disease (e.g., heartburn, difficulty swallowing) develop.

Calcitonin. May be used with hormone replacement therapy to decrease bone resorption. Calcitonin may produce an analgesic effect and is useful in the immediate postfracture phase. It is an alternative to ERT and biphosphonate therapy for postmenopausal women who cannot or will not take ERT or a biphosphonate. The recommended dosage is 50 units subcutaneously 3 times per week (may be increased to 100 units) or 200 units intranasally daily.

Fluoride. A slow release form of sodium fluoride has received a preliminary recommendation by an FDA advisory committee and will likely receive final approval shortly.[79] Fluoride stimulates bone formation through a direct effect on osteoblasts.

Weightbearing Exercise

Weightbearing, muscle strengthening exercise stimulates new bone formation and maintains the mineral content of the bone. There is evidence of a protective effect of past physical activity and of moderate levels of recent physical activity on the risk of hip fracture in postmenopausal women.[86] For clients with established osteoporosis, referral to physical therapy can help prevent falls and develop a program for decreasing kyphotic posture and improving overall muscle strength.

FOLLOW-UP

Consultation with or referral to a gynecologic and/or orthopedic specialist or osteoporosis center is indicated for progressing disease.

Preventive measures in childbearing clients include adequate dietary or supplemental calcium, weightbearing exercise several times per week, and evaluation for estrogen deficiency during periods of amenorrhea longer than 6 months, particularly during adolescence.

Hirsutism/Virilism

Hirsutism (increased hair in unusual amounts and places) is one sign of benign hyperandrogynism (the appearance of testosterone stimulated characteristics). The signs include excess facial and abdominal hair of a coarse nature and oily skin or acne. Hirsutism often causes extreme distress in women. The more severe states of virilization (clitoromegaly, deepening of the voice, balding, and changes in body habitus) are rare and usually secondary to adrenal hyperplasia or androgen producing tumors.[9]

EPIDEMIOLOGY

Androgens enter the blood from the adrenal glands, ovaries, and peripheral sites, such as the liver, spleen, and adipose tissue. Benign rises in androstenedione and testosterone levels are caused by ovarian stromal hyperplasia that sometimes develops under the influence of high luteinizing hormone (LH) levels. Testosterone levels, however, decrease in all women between the fourth and fifth postmenopausal year. Hirsutism is usually associated with persistent anovulation. Estrogen-androgen combination therapy for treatment of menopausal women may produce masculinizing side effects. Side effects are usually dose dependent but can develop even with low dose methyltestosterone.

SUBJECTIVE DATA

The client may report an increase in facial, areolar, abdominal, and chest hair, and acne.

OBJECTIVE DATA

During the physical examination, note any increase in facial, upper abdomen, chest, and upper back and shoulder hair. Virilization is suggestive by temporal and vertical scalp hair loss, deep voice, acne, increase in muscle mass, and clitoromegaly. On pelvic examination, palpate for the presence of bilaterally enlarged ovaries (Ovaries should not be palpable in postmenopausal women).

Diagnostic tests include serum testosterone level to rule out ovarian and adrenal tumors, and dehydroepiandrosterone sulfate (DHAS) level and 17-hydroxyprogesterone (17-OHP) to rule out adrenal tumor. If either serum testosterone or DHAS is elevated, refer the client immediately to a gynecologist to rule out an androgen-producing tumor.

DIFFERENTIAL MEDICAL DIAGNOSES

Ovarian or adrenal androgen producing tumors, Cushing's syndrome, drugs such as anabolic steroids and androgenic progestogens, and polycystic ovary disease.

PLAN

Approaches to the management of hirsutism are based on the underlying pathophysiology. They include the following: reassurance that the increased hair growth is not abnormal and that it may abate as testosterone levels decrease in a few years, suggestions for its removal (e.g., electrolysis), medications to suppress ovarian and adrenal androgen overproduction, and curative treatment of underlying diseases, such as Cushing's syndrome or ovarian tumors. Spironolactone (aldosterone antagonist) 25 mg q.i.d. *or* 50 mg b.i.d. may help to decrease androgen production and block the effect of testosterone on hair follicles. Cimetidine, generally used to treat ulcers and excess gastric acid, may also provide an antiandrogenic effect. Dexamethasone (corticosteroid) 1.0 mg q.h.s. has been used to suppress adrenal hyperfunction, but this drug can cause osteoporosis and suppression of the hypothalamic-pituitary-adrenal axis, so it should be used with caution. Consult a current pharmacotherapeutics reference before prescribing drugs to treat hirsutism, and confer with a gynecologist who specializes in endocrinology.

FOLLOW-UP

Immediate referral to a gynecologic specialist is required whenever androgen producing tumors are suspected.

NONREPRODUCTIVE HEALTH CONCERNS OF AGING WOMEN

More women are taking a proactive role in health maintenance and the prevention of disease. Preventive health care is a major area that the health care provider must focus on with women, especially as they age. The menopause provides a unique opportunity for the provider to assist the woman in maintaining ongoing cost effective health care that includes appropriate referrals if necessary. Many risk factors can be modified by adapting positive health measures, such as not smoking, eating a low fat, low cholesterol diet (Table 15–3), and exercising (Table 15–4). The aging process, however, is affected by biologic, social, economic, and psychological influences. Assessment of all these factors is critical to the development of an effective health care strategy for older women. Certain areas posing more serious problems for the aging woman that may negatively affect her health include the following.

HEALTH CARE INSURANCE AND INCOME

Ninety-nine percent of Americans over age 65 have private or government health insurance coverage.[87] Women who have lost spouses through death, divorce, or separation are more likely to have only public health care coverage or no insurance. Making co-payments, payment for services not covered by Medicare, or payment of insurance deductible is often a hardship for elderly women. Medicare and Medicaid managed care plans are increasing in numbers to help meet the economic challenge of caring for older adults and controlling costs. Elderly women who live alone or who are of ethnic minority tend to be poorer than elderly men. Social Security benefits are the largest single source of income for elderly people. The median yearly income for older women in 1992 was $8189 and was $14,548 for older men.[1] Income disparities persist among various elderly subgroups: white elderly men median income, $15,276; elderly black women, $6220; and elderly hispanic women, $5968.[1] White women are more likely to have private insurance than nonwhite women. Women are more likely to have health insurance than men are, except in the 45- to 64-year-old group. Research shows that if people cannot pay, they are unable to get needed health care, which clearly affects their health status and longevity.[88] Out-of-pocket costs of health care, including medications, often increase with acute and chronic illness as the woman ages; and if a choice among rent, food, and medicine confronts the elderly woman, she may forgo her medication. More serious illness is a likely consequence. It is essential that the health care provider be aware of resources in her/his locale to use for referral that can aid the woman in maintaining her finances in health or illness. The Area Agency on Aging(AAA) is a good resource and available in every county in the United States.

SOCIAL SUPPORT

With a life expectancy of over 75 years, most American women will live half of their adult lives after their last child has left home. Nearly one-quarter of women over age 70 have no surviving children.[88] Approximately 32 percent of women age 65 to 74 live alone; 57 percent of women over age 85 live alone.[1] Only 41 percent of elderly women are married, compared with 75 percent of elderly men.[1] Since the proportion of women to men increases after age 65, the likelihood of finding male partners is decreased. Thus, while most elderly men have a spouse for assistance, most elderly women do not. The lack of social support can be a source of serious concern and increasing health risks in the elderly. The health care provider must be sensitive to the social living conditions of the woman, and work with her to find ways to enhance her support systems.

ELDER MISTREATMENT

Elder mistreatment, including physical abuse, psychological abuse, financial abuse, and neglect, has reached alarming proportions in the United States.[89] In assessing the older woman, the health care provider should always evaluate for signs of actual abuse or neglect. Dependency and increasing longevity put the elderly woman at risk for abuse and neglect. Although about 4 percent of elderly Americans are victims of abuse yearly, it is likely to be underreported.[90] Detection of mistreatment is often difficult and, if suspected, requires more substantial assessment. Assisting the woman to seek appropriate avenues for support, as well as reporting suspected abuse, are inherent in providing holistic health care.

CHRONIC ILLNESS

Chronic illnesses increase in women over age 60; women are likely to have three or more chronic conditions.[88] As a result of aging and chronic illness, the client may experience limitations in functional capacities for managing daily living. A small minority, approximately 5 percent of elderly, have physical and health changes that significantly affect activities of daily living and impact upon independent living.[91]

Common Chronic Problems
- Visual and hearing impairments.
- Arthritis.
- Hypertension.
- Heart disease.
- Diabetes.
- Orthopedic problems.
- Chronic respiratory disease.

Heart disease, cancer, and stroke continue to be the leading causes of death among older women.[31]

FUNCTIONAL STATUS

The primary goal of health promotion and disease prevention in the elderly is to promote independent functioning as long as possible. All elderly clients should be asked about the level of independence in carrying out basic activities of daily living (ADL) including bathing, grooming, dressing, toileting, transferring, eating, and walking and instrumental activities of daily living (IADL). The IADLs, including meal preparation, shopping, housework, telephoning, money management, and medication management, are critical to maintaining independence in the community. Functional changes can be a warning sign of a beginning pathological process[92] such as drug toxicities, early dementia, or acute illness.

DEPRESSION AND SUICIDE RISK

As well as assessing for physical changes, the provider must be alert to depressive symptoms in the aging woman. Depression is one of the most common emotional problems affecting older adults. Community based surveys of older adults estimate that prevalence rates of significant depressive symptoms are higher compared to major depression (4 to 8 percent vs. 1 to 2 percent). Depression is associated with physical illness and disability at all ages, and older persons are at greater risk of concurrent depression and disability than younger adults.[93] In the United States, persons age 65 and older have the highest suicide rate of any age group; the ratio of completed to attempted suicides rises from about 1 in 200 among young adult women to 1 in 4 among elderly persons of both genders.[94] Of all the risk factors for completed suicide, the most common is a single episode of major affective illness occurring at the time of suicide.[95]

Risk Factors for Depression
- Unrecognized or untreated affective disorders.
- Physical illness.
- Losses and changes in older age (decreases in physical vigor, mental agility, income, relocation, social roles).
- Bereavement.
- Isolation.
- Prior depressive episode.

Depressed older women may present with multiple somatic complaints (e.g., insomnia, fatigue, constipation, anorexia) or with a lack of interest in self-care or a functional decline. The elderly seldom complain of a depressed mood or seek care for emotional symptoms.[96] A detailed history and mental status examination can help to distinguish the thinking and behavioral changes associated with depression from those of dementia. Pseudodementia (depression manifesting as cognitive impairment) is an important consideration in the differential diagnosis of older adults with cognitive impairment. Early and aggressive detection and treatment of depression among the elderly is critical because prognosis is good and it may be a life saving treatment. Referral for psychiatric consultation is recommended.

POLYPHARMACY

The elderly consume 25 percent to 30 percent of all prescription drugs in the United States, and 30 percent of those over 65 years take eight or more prescription drugs daily.[97] This does not account for the over-the-counter medications. The elderly are at significantly high risk of drug-drug interactions, drug toxicity, and adverse drug reactions. Drug therapy may also play a role in accidents and injuries. Review of current prescription and nonprescription drug use should be done at each periodic health visit. Additionally, interactions with foods must be considered.

INJURY PREVENTION

Falls

Falls are the leading cause of nonfatal injuries and unintentional injury deaths among Americans 65 years and older in the United States.[98,99] Approximately 30 percent of community dwelling elderly fall one or more times each year; in residential institutions, the proportion is higher, about 40–50 percent.[100] Frail elderly persons, with the following multiple intrinsic risk factors are at high risk: postural instability, gait disturbances, decreased muscle strength and proprioception, poor vision, cognitive impairment, multiple medications, and use of psychoactive and antihypertensive drugs. Extrinsic or environmental risk factors include stairs, cluttered furniture, slippery surfaces, inadequate lighting, incorrect footwear, and absence of assistive devices in the bathroom. Periodic fall assessment and education are recommended with elderly clients to prevent injuries.

Fires/Burns

Fires and burns are also leading causes of death in older adults. Older persons may be at increased risk of dying in residential fires because of impaired vision, hearing, mobility, or mental status. Cigarette smoking is a leading cause for burn injuries and deaths among the elderly; scald burns primarily involve hot tap water, food, and drinks. Measures to promote safety in the home are important, such as installing and maintaining effective smoke detectors, removal of hazardous heaters, and setting household water heaters at or below 120° F.

LIMITED ACCESS TO CARE

Decreasing vision and other physical impairments may limit an older woman's driving ability and access to care. Alternative transportation may create a financial burden, particularly if multiple health services at multiple sites are needed.

There may be a shortage of health care providers who are trained and interested in holistic care of perimenopausal and postmenopausal women, or who will accept Medicare and Medicaid. When family members and other caretakers are lacking, elders become dependent on the health care system, particularly nursing homes. But for the women of midlife who are the caretakers for elderly parents, stress is increased during the perimenopausal transition. Women's health care providers must emphasize preventive measures and appropriate use of early detection in order to address the problems of morbidity and chronic illness in the elderly. Health and social services for older women are often interdependent, providing a comprehensive, holistic approach.

REFERENCES

1. Bureau of the Census. (1995). *Statistical brief: Sixty-five plus in the United States.* Washington, DC: U.S. Department of Commerce.
2. Lichtman, R. (1996). Perimenopausal and postmenopausal hormone replacement therapy: Part 1. An update of the literature on benefits and risks. *Journal of Nurse-Midwifery, 41*(1), 3–28.
3. Stevenson, J. S. (1977). *Issues and crises during middlescence.* New York: Appleton-Century-Crofts.

4. World Health Organization. (1981). Research on the menopause. *WHO Technical Report Series* (No. 670). Geneva, Switzerland.

5. McKinley, W. M., Brambilla, D. J., & Posner, J. G. (1992). The normal menopausal transition. *Maturitas, 14,* 102.

6. Whelan, E. A., Sandler, D. P., McConnaughey, D. R., et al. (1990). Menstrual and reproductive characteristics and age at natural menopause. *Am J Epidemiol, 131,* 625–632.

7. Stanford, J. L., Hartge, P., Brinton, L. A., et al. (1987). Factors influencing the age at natural menopause. *J Chronic Dis, 40,* 995–1002.

8. VanKeep, P. A., Brand, P. C., & Lehert, P. (1979). Factors affecting the age at menopause. *J Biosoc Sci,* (Suppl. 6), 37–55.

9. Speroff, L., Glass, R. H., & Kase, N. G. (1994). *Clinical gynecologic endocrinology and infertility* (5th ed). Baltimore: Williams & Wilkins.

10. Johnson, C. A. (1996). Menopausal symptoms. In C. A. Johnson, B. E. Johnson, J. L. Murray, B. S. Apgar, (Eds.), *Women's health care handbook.* Philadelphia: Hanley & Belfus, Inc. and St. Louis: Mosby.

11. Udoff, L. C., & Adashi, E. Y. (1996, May). Androgens: The other class of female hormones. In a special report: Optimizing hormone replacement therapy. *Postgraduate Medicine,* 5–9.

12. Fretwell, M. D. (1993). Aging changes in structure and function. In D. L. Carnevali, & M. Patrick (Eds.), *Nursing management for the elderly* (3rd ed.). Philadelphia: J. B. Lippincott Co.

13. U.S. Public Health Service. (1994). *The clinician's handbook of preventive services: Put prevention into practice.* Alexandria, VA: International Medical Publishing, Inc.

14. Kuhn, F.E., & Rackley, C.E. (1993). Coronary artery disease in women: Risk factors, evaluation, treatment and prevention. *Arch Intern Med, 153,* 2626–2636.

15. Cummings, S. R., Black, D. M., & Rubin, S. M. (1989). Lifetime risks of hip, Colles' or vertebral fracture and coronary heart disease among white postmenopausal women. *Arch Intern Med, 149,* 2445–2448.

16. Grady, D, Rubin, S. M., Petitti, D. B., et al. (1992). Hormone therapy to prevent disease and prolong life in postmenopausal women. *Ann Intern Med, 117,* 1016–1037.

17. Wei, J. Y. (1992). Age and the cardiovascular system. *New Engl J Med, 327*(4), 1735–1739.

18. Wild, R. A. (1996). Estrogen: Effects on the cardiovascular tree. *Obstet Gynecol, 87*(2), 27S–35S.

19. Blair, K. A. (1990). Aging: Physiological aspects and clinical implications. *Nurse Practitioner, 15(2),* 14–28.

20. LeBoeuf, F. J., & Carter, S. G. (1996). Discomforts of the perimenopause. *JOGNN, 25,* 173–180.

21. Eliopoulos, C. (1993). *Gerontological nursing* (3rd ed.). Philadelphia: J. B. Lippincott Co.

22. Dumesic, D. A. (1996, Jan). Pelvic examination: What to focus on in menopausal women. *Consultant,* 39–46.

23. Morrison-Beedy, D., & Robbins, L. (1989). Sexual assessment and the aging female. *Nurse Practitioner, 14*(12), 37–43.

24. Bates, B. (1995). *A guide to physical examination and history taking.* (6th ed.). Philadelphia: J. B. Lippincott.

25. Berry, L. (1993). Incontinence and urinary problems. In D. Carnevali, & M. Patrick (Eds.), *Nursing management for the elderly* (3rd ed.). Philadelphia: J. B. Lippincott Co.

26. Glickstein, J. K. (Ed.). (1991). Sexuality and aging. *Focus on Geriatric Care & Rehabilitation, 4*(7), 1–8.

27. Patrick, M. (1993). Challenges of daily living and development in later life stages. In D. L. Carnevali, & M. Patrick, (Eds.), *Nursing management for the elderly* (3rd ed.). Philadelphia: J. B. Lippincott Co.

28. Hote, A. (1992). Influence of natural menopause on health complaints: A prospective study of healthy Norwegian women. *Maturitas, 14,* 157–160.

29. Kaufert, P. A. (1994). A health and social profile of the menopausal woman. *Exp. Gerontol, 29,* 343–350.

30. Bosarge, P. (1995). Hormone therapy: The woman's decision. *Contemporary Nurse Practitioner* (Suppl. 1), 3–10.

31. Sowers, R. & LaPietra, M. T. (1995). Menopause: Its epidemiology and potential association with chronic diseases. *Epidemiologic Reviews, 17*(2), 287–302.

32. Goldberg, R. M., Loprinzi, C. L., O'Fallen, J. R., et al. (1994). Transdermal clonidine for ameliorating tamoxifen-induced hot flashes. *J Clin Oncol, 12,* 155.

33. Fantyl, J. A., Cardozo, L., McClish, D. K., & the Hormones and Urogenital Therapy Committee. (1994). Estrogen therapy in the management of urinary incontinence in postmenopausal women: A meta-analysis. First report of the Hormones and Urogenital Therapy Committee. *Obstet Gynecol, 83,* 12–18.

34. Hammond, C. B. (1996). Menopause and hormone replacement therapy: An overview. *Obstetrics and Gynecology, 87,* (Suppl. 2), 2–19.

35. Hormonal therapy during the perimenopausal period. (July, 1993) *ARHP Clinical Proceedings,* 15–16.

36. Sherwin, B. B. (1996). Hormones, mood, and cognitive functioning in postmenopausal women. *Obstetrics & Gynecology, 87,* 20S–26S.

37. Mayfield, D., McLeod, G., & Hall, P. (1984). The CAGE questionnaire. *American Journal of Psychiatry, 131,* 1121.

38. Selzer, M. L. (1980). The Michigan Alcoholism Screening Test (MAST). *American Journal of Psychology,* (revised) *25*(3), 176–181, 197.

39. Zung, W. W. K. (1965). A self-rating depression scale. *Arch Gen Psychiatry,* 12, 63–70.

40. Beck, A. P., Rial, W. Y., & Rickels, K. (1974). Short form of depression inventory: Cross validation. *Psychol Rep, 34,* 1184–1186.

41. Yesavage, J. A., & Brink, T. L. (1983). Development and validation of Geriatric Depression Scale: A preliminary report. *Journal of Psychiatric Research, 17,* 41.

42. Tang, M. X., Jacobs, D., Stern, Y., Marder, K., Schofield, P., Gurland, B., Andrews, H., & Mayeux, R. (1996). Effect of oestrogen during menopause on risk and age at onset of Alzheimer's disease. *Lancet, 348,* 429–432.

43. Folstein, M. F., Folstein, S. E., & McHugh, P. R. (1975). Mini-mental state : A practical method for grading the cognitive state of patients for the clinician. *J Psychiatr Res, 12,* 189–198.

44. Pfeiffer, E. (1975). A short portable mental status questionnaire for the assessment of organic brain deficit in elderly patients. *Journal of the American Geriatric Society, 23,* 433–441.

45. Dantzker, D. R., & Multz, A. S. (1995). Pulmonary disorders. In V. L. Seltzer, & W. H. Pearse (Eds.), *Women's primary health care.* New York: McGraw-Hill.

46. Wheeler, J. L. (1996, May). Compliance with hormone replacement therapy: Strategies for improvement. In A Special Report: Optimizing hormone replacement therapy. *Postgraduate Medicine,* 14–18.

47. Report of the U.S. Preventive Services Task Force. (1996). Postmenopausal hormone prophylaxis. In *Guide to clinical preventive services* (2nd ed.) Baltimore, MD: Williams & Wilkins.

48. Consensus Development Conference: Diagnosis, prophylaxis, and treatment of osteoporosis. (1993). *Am J Med, 94,* 646–650.

49. Grady, D., Gebretsadik, T., Kerlikowske, K., Ernster, V., & Petitti, D. (1995). Hormone replacement therapy and endometrial cancer risk: A meta-analysis. *Obstetrics & Gynecology, 85,* 304–313.

50. The Writing Group for the PEPI Trial. (1995). Effects of estrogen or estrogen/progestin regimens on heart disease risk factors in postmenopausal women. *JAMA, 273,* 199–208.

51. Barrett-Conner, E., Wingard, D. L., & Criqui, M. H. (1989). Postmenopausal estrogen use and heart disease risk factors in the 1980s. Rancho Bernardo, California revisited. *JAMA, 267,* 2095–2100.

52. Nabulsi, A. A., Folsom, A. R., White, A., et al. (1993). Association of hormone replacement therapy with various cardiovascular risk factors in postmenopausal women. *N Engl J Med, 328,* 1069–1075.

53. Speroff, L. (1996). Postmenopausal hormone therapy and breast cancer. *Obstetrics & Gynecology, 87,* 44S–54S.

54. Gorsky, R. D., Koplan, J. P., Peterson, H. B., et al. (1994). Relative risks and benefits of long-term estrogen replacement therapy: A decision analysis. *Obstetrics & Gynecology, 83,* 161–166.

55. Sullivan, J. M., & Fowlkes, L. P. (1996). The clinical aspects of estrogen and the cardiovascular system. *Obstetrics & Gynecology, 87,* 36S–43S.

56. Psaty, B. M., Heckbert, S. R., Atkins, D. et al. (1994). The risk of myocardial infarction associated with the combined use of estrogens and progestins in postmenopausal women. *N Engl J Med, 328,* 1069–1075.

57. Falkeborn, M., Persson, I., Adami, H. O., et al. (1992). The risk of acute myocardial infarction after oestrogen and oestrogen-progestogen replacement. *Br J Obstet Gynecol, 99,* 821–828.

58. Kritz-Silverstein, D., & Barrett-Connor, E. (1996). Long-term postmenopausal hormone use, obesity, and fat distribution in older women. *JAMA, 275,* 46–49.

59. Nachtigall, L. E. (1995). Emerging delivery systems for estrogen replacement: Aspects of transdermal and oral delivery. *Am J Obstet Gynecol, 173,* 993–997.

60. Pearce, J., Hawton, K., & Blake, F. (1995). Psychological and sexual symptoms associated with the menopause and the effects of hormone replacement therapy. *British Journal of Psychiatry, 167,* 163–173.

61. Archer, D. F., Pickar, J. H., & Bottiglioni, F., for the Menopause Study Group. (1994). Bleeding patterns in postmenopausal women taking continuous combined or sequential regimens of

conjugated estrogens with medroxyprogesterone acetate. *Obstetrics & Gynecology, 83,* 686–692.

62. Lemcke, D., Marshall, L., & Pattison, J. (1995). Menopause and hormone replacement therapy. In D. Lemcke, J. Pattison, L. Marshall, & D. Cowley, (Eds.), *Primary care of women.* Norwalk CT: Appleton & Lange.

63. Dupont, W., Page, D. (1991). Menopausal estrogen replacement therapy and breast cancer. *Arch Intern Med, 151,* 67–72.

64. Colditz, G., Hankinson, S., Hunter, D., et al. (1995). The use of estrogens and progestins and the risk of breast cancer in postmenopausal women. *N Engl J Med, 332,* 1589–1593.

65. American College of Physicians. (1992). Guidelines for counseling postmenopausal women about preventive hormone therapy. *Ann Int Med, 117,* 1038–1041.

66. Williams, D. B. & Moley, K. H. (1994). Progestin replacement in the menopause: Effects on the endometrium and serum lipids. *Curr Opin Obstet Gynecol, 6,* 284–292.

67. Gasbarro, R. (1996, May). Managing hormone replacement therapy. *American Druggist, 40*–47.

68. Timmons, M. C. (1996, May). Estrogen-androgen therapy for postmenopausal women-safety and adverse effects. In a special report: Optimizing hormone replacement therapy. *Postgraduate Medicine, 10*–13.

69. Dept. for Economic & Social Information & Policy Analysis Population Division. (1995). *Abortion policies: A global review* (Vol. 3). New York: United Nations.

70. Hatcher, R. A., Trussell, J., Stewart, G. K., et al. (1994). *Contraceptive technology* (16th ed.). New York: Irvington Pub, Inc.

71. Grodstein, F., & Stampfer, M. J. (1996). Cardiovascular disease & impact of sex steroid replacement. In E. Y. Adashi, J. A. Rock, & Z. Rosenwalls, (Eds.), *Reproductive endocrinology, surgery, and technology* (Vol. 2). Philadelphia: Lippincott-Raven Pub.

72. Report of the U.S. Preventive Services Task Force. (1996). *Guide to clinical preventive services* (2nd. ed.). Baltimore, MD: Williams & Wilkins.

73. Dept. of Health and Human Services. (1990). National Health and Nutrition Examination Survey III Data Collection Forms. Hyattsville, MD.

74. Stampfer, M. J., Colditz, G. A., Willett, W. C., et al. (1991). Postmenopausal estrogen therapy and cardiovascular disease: Ten-year follow-up from the Nurses' Health Study. *N Engl J Med, 325*(26), 1758.

75. American Heart Association. (1995). Heart and stroke facts: 1995 statistical supplement. *Dallas,* 1–23.

76. WHO/FIMS Committee on Physical Activity for Health. (1995) Exercise for health. *Bulletin of the World Health Organization, 73*(2), 135–136.

77. National Institutes of Health. (1994, April 5–7). Ovarian cancer: Screening, treatment, and follow-up. National Institutes of Health Consensus Conference Statement.

78. Northrup, C. (1994). Menopause. In C. Northrup (Ed.), *Women's bodies, women's wisdom.* New York: Bantam.

79. AACE. (1996). AACE clinical practice guidelines for the prevention and treatment of postmenopausal osteoporosis. *Endocrine Practice, 2*(2), 157–171.

80. Nussbaum, S. R. (1995). Screening for osteoporosis. In A. H. Gorroll, L. A. May, & A. G. Mulley (Eds.), *Primary care medicine: Office evaluation and management of the adult patient* (3rd ed.). Philadelphia: J. B. Lippincott Co.

81. Ettinger, B., & Grady, D. (1993). The waning effect of postmenopausal estrogen therapy on osteoporosis. *N Engl J Med, 329,* 1192–1193.

82. World Health Organization. (1994). Assessment of fracture risk and its application to screening postmenopausal osteoporosis: Report of a WHO study group. *Technical Report Series 843.*

83. Consensus Development Conference. (1991). Prophylaxis and treatment of osteoporosis. *Am J Med, 90,* 107–110.

84. Haines, C. J., Chung, T. K., Leung, P. C., Hsu, S. Y. C., & Leung, D. H. Y (1995). Calcium supplementation and bone mineral density in postmenopausal women using estrogen replacement therapy. *Bone, 16,* 529–531.

85. Liberman, U., Weiss, S., Broll, J., et al. for the Alendronate Phase III Osteoporosis Treatment Study Group. (1995). Effect of oral alendronate on bone mineral density and the incidence of fractures in postmenopausal osteoporosis. *N Engl J Med, 333,* 1437–1443.

86. Jaglal, S. B., Kreiger, N., & Darlington, G. (1993). Past and recent physical activity and risk of hip fracture. *Am J Epidemiol, 138,* 107–118.

87. U.S. Dept. of Commerce. (1995). *Statistical abstract of the U.S.* (115 ed.). Washington, DC: Bureau of Census.

88. Horton, J. A. (1995). *The women's health data book: A profile of women's health in the United States.* Washington, DC: Jacobs Institute of Women's Health, Elsevier.

89. Fulmer, T., & Ashley, J. (1989). Clinical indicators of elder neglect. *Applied Nursing Research, 2*(4), 161–167.

90. Capezuti, E. (1989). Preventing elder abuse and neglect. In R. Lavizzo-Mourey, et al. (Eds.), *Practicing prevention for the elderly.* Philadelphia: Hanley & Belfus.

91. Enloe, C. (1993). Managing daily living with diminishing resources and losses. In D. Carnevali, & M. Patrick (Eds.), *Nursing management for the elderly* (3rd ed.). Philadelphia: J. B. Lippincott Co.

92. Calvani, D., & Douris, K. (1991). Functional assessment: A holistic approach to rehabilitation of the geriatric client. *Rehabilitation Nursing, 16*(6), 330–335.

93. Kurlowicz, L. (1993). Social factors and depression in late life. *Archives of Psychiatric Nursing, 7*(1), 30–36.

94. Conwell, Y. (1995). Suicide among elderly persons. *Psychiatric Services, 46*(6), 563–564.

95. Conwell, Y. (1994). Suicide in the elderly. In L. S. Schneider, C. F. Reynolds III, B. D. Lebowitz, et al. (Eds.), *Diagnosis and treatment of depression in late-life.* Washington, DC: American Psychiatric Press.

96. Martin, L. M., Fleming, K. C., & Evans, J. M. (1995). Recognition and management of anxiety and depression in elderly patients. *Mayo Clin Proc, 70,* 999–1006.

97. Kotthoff-Burrell, E. (1992). Health promotion and disease prevention for the older adult: An overview of the current recommendations and a practical application. *Nurse Practitioner Forum, 3*(4), 195–209.

98. National Safety Council. (1992). *Accident facts.* Chicago: National Safety Council.

99. Rice, D. P., MacKenzie, E. J., et al. (1989). *Cost of injury in the United States: A report to Congress 1989.* Baltimore: Johns Hopkins Univ.

100. Grisso, J. A., Capezuti, E., & Schwartz, A. (1996). Falls as risk factors for fractures. In R. Marcus, D. Feldman, & J. Kelsey (Eds.), *Osteoporosis.* New York: Academic Press.

101. Youngkin, E. & Israel, D. (1996). A review and critique of common herbal alternative therapies. *The Nurse Practitioner, 21*(10), 39–62.

102. Israel, D. & Youngkin, E. Q. (1997). Herbal therapies for perimenopausal and menopausal complaints. *Pharmacotherapy, 17*(5), 970–984.

103. Associated Press. (June 19, 1997). 2 studies energize estrogen debate. *Richmond Times Dispatch,* A1–A2.

104. Grodstein, F., Stampfer, M., Colditz, G., Willett, W., et al. (1997). Postmenopausal hormone therapy and mortality. *NEJM, 336*(25), 1769–1775.

PROMOTION OF WOMEN'S HEALTH CARE DURING PREGNANCY

CHAPTER 16

ASSESSING HEALTH DURING PREGNANCY

Cynthia W. Bailey

A National Institutes of Health and Human Services expert panel . . . recommended that prenatal care begin prior to conception, preferably within 1 year of a planned pregnancy.

Highlights

- Barriers to Prenatal Care
- Preconception Counseling, Assessment
- Presumptive, Probable, and Positive Signs and Symptoms
- Sexuality During Pregnancy
- Initial Prenatal Visit, Subsequent Visits
- Progressing Physical Changes
- Commonly Recommended Tests
- Risk Assessment
    Genetic and Preterm Assessments
    Attachment
    Environmental, Occupational Hazards
- Psychosocial Assessment
    Domestic Violence
- Nutrition
- Major Theories of Maternal Role Development
- Preparation for Childbirth: Counseling and Classes
- Adolescent Pregnancy
- Delayed Pregnancy
- Nontraditional Families
- Substance Abuse Screening

► INTRODUCTION

Prior to the early 1900s few women received prenatal care or evaluation. The advent of consistent and comprehensive prenatal care, begun in early pregnancy, has markedly decreased both maternal and infant morbidity and mortality in the United States. Today prenatal care encompasses risk assessment, social services, client education, and medical care. Ideally this care should begin prior to conception.[1]

Despite advances in prenatal care, several barriers to initiating care exist.[1,2]

BARRIERS TO PRENATAL CARE

- *Unrecognized Pregnancy.* Pregnancy may go unrecognized because of lack of knowledge about the signs and symptoms of pregnancy, limited body awareness, a history of irregular menses, or obesity.
- *Denied Pregnancy.* Pregnancy may be denied, particularly if unplanned, because of the woman's ambivalence regarding motherhood.
- *Limited Finances.* Financial constraints or limited health insurance may discourage a woman from securing prenatal care.
- *Inaccessibility of the Health Care System.* An inconvenient location of the health care facility, lack of transportation, lack of provider availability, or fear of the health care system may make it difficult for a woman to obtain prenatal care.

Today many women have jobs outside the home both for financial reasons and for professional accomplishment. In two income families, partners share childrearing responsibilities, and the male partner is expected to be active in the care and nurturing of offspring. Our concept of *family* has expanded to include nontraditional households, such as same sex relationships, single parent families, and cohabitation.

The advent of consumerism in health care also has influenced our concept of pregnancy.[2] Current biostatistics indicate that the typical American couple will have one or two children. Many women/couples make a conscientious effort to have a healthy pregnancy, and therefore couples with the availability of modern medical technology have greater expectations for a healthy pregnancy and infant. Ultimately, this raises legal and ethical demands on health care providers, particularly in obstetrics and gynecology.[3]

Clients as consumers have come to expect an optimal outcome in pregnancy, and preconception counseling has become common. Throughout pregnancy, women may question the safety of various activities and the effects of substances on the developing fetus. Women and their partners are also increasingly included in the decision making process, and frequently they participate in community prenatal classes. All of these changes make for a different experience of pregnancy and parenthood for today's women.

PLANNING FOR A HEALTHY PREGNANCY

PRECONCEPTION COUNSELING

Interest in preconception education and counseling began in the 1980s in the United States. In evaluating new information and reconsidering older data, many health care providers became convinced that pregnancy may be too late for expectant parents to correct unhealthy habits. A National Institutes of Health and Human Services expert panel reviewed the factors that contribute to good pregnancy outcomes for women and infants, and subsequently recommended that prenatal care begin prior to conception, preferably within 1 year of a planned pregnancy.[2] The status of a woman's health can influence not only her ability to conceive, but also her ability to maintain the pregnancy.[4]

At the time of conception, a woman should be in an optimal state of emotional and physical health. Health educators and health care providers have concluded that this directly improves pregnancy outcomes.[1] The goal of preconception care and counseling is to maximize the health of the woman and the health of her potential infant.[1] Ideally, preconception counseling is accompanied by a complete physical and psychosocial evaluation. Prior to conception, prospective parents have an opportunity to make informed decisions and ultimately to make lifestyle adjustments to maximize their chances of a successful outcome in pregnancy.[5]

Teaching/Learning Methods

A healthy lifestyle can be promoted through individual teaching during routine examinations, community adult health education programs, or traditional classes with content directed toward prospective parents. Although current studies do not demonstrate that preconception education directly influences perinatal outcomes, new information can be acquired that enhances a positive perinatal outcome.[5] Demonstrated statistical changes in the ultimate outcome for pregnancy may not be available for several generations of infants, thus long term goals such as parental behavior changes and improved health status in someday parents needs to be the guiding philosophy for marketing these classes.[3]

Reva Rubin investigated the relationship between social support and pregnancy outcomes and found that the mother's ability to identify with the developing fetus fostered attachment to the child. Hence, the quality of the social support given to a woman during pregnancy correlates positively with maternal-fetal attachment.[3] In addition, enhancing a parent's knowledge about fetal growth and development promotes intrauterine bonding and subsequent parenting skills. These concepts reinforce the importance of programs directed toward preconception health promotion.[6]

Nonpregnant persons may not feel compelled to attend preparation classes; therefore, tools must convey the importance of preconception education and the potential for improved perinatal outcomes. Information should focus strongly on maternal and fetal health, timing of pregnancy, and how these factors influence the overall life plan.[4] The normal physiological changes associated with pregnancy and their affect on the woman's body and self-image, and legal/ethical issues, such as genetic and diagnostic testing, are other subjects that need to be covered in these classes. Moreover, pertinent information about community agencies and family services should be provided for those in need of follow-up support.[7]

PRECONCEPTION ASSESSMENT DATA

Preconception care and counseling are valuable in identifying risks in the client's medical history and current health status, and their potential impact on a pregnancy. Assessment includes history taking and a physical examination, often augmented by laboratory/diagnostic testing.[8]

Subjective Data

During the evaluation, obtain a detailed medical, social, reproductive, and family history. By identifying problems early, it is sometimes possible to resolve them prior to conception and ultimately improve perinatal outcome.[5]

A comprehensive screening tool, such as the Preconceptional Health Assessment (see Figure 16–1) can facilitate risk assessment with prospective parents.[5] This appraisal includes a checklist that assesses the health status of the prospective mother. Through it, information specific to the client's family, medical, reproductive, and drug histories can be obtained. Nutrition and lifestyle choices also can be evaluated.

In addition, it is important to assess human immunodeficiency virus (HIV) risk factors. These factors include history of homosexual activity, intravenous drug use, multiple sexual contacts, blood or blood product transfusion, or close contact with bodily fluids.

Objective Data

Physical Examination. A complete physical examination is needed, with special emphasis on the systems identified during the risk appraisal. A

PRECONCEPTIONAL HEALTH ASSESSMENT

What is your main interest in seeking preconceptional counseling?

_____

_____

_____

    So that we can address your specific interests and concerns, we ask that you complete the following questionnaire. You may use the back of the form to provide additional information when necessary.

Place an X next to any item that applies to you.

SOCIAL HISTORY

Do you

_____ drink beer, wine, or hard liquor

_____ smoke cigarettes or use any other tobacco products

_____ use marijuana, cocaine, or any recreational drugs

_____ use lead or chemicals at home or at work.
If yes, list the specific chemicals if you know what they are:

_____

_____

_____ work with radiation

_____ participate in an exercise program

Are you

_____ 34 years of age or older

NUTRITION HISTORY

On the back of this sheet, list by meal everything you ate and drank yesterday, including the approximate amount; indicate snacks separately.

Do you

_____ practice vegetarianism

_____ eat unusual substances, such as laundry starch or clay

_____ have a history of bulimia or anorexia

_____ follow a special diet
If yes, describe:

_____

_____

_____ supplement your diet with vitamins
If yes, list vitamins and dosages:

_____

Figure 16–1. Preconceptional health assessment. *(Source: Reprinted with permission from the authors. Cefalo R.C., & Moos M.K. (1995) Preconceptual health care: A practical guide (2nd ed.). St. Louis, Missouri: Mosby-Year Book.)*

_____ take medications, including oral contraceptives

_____ have an intolerance for milk

MEDICAL HISTORY

Do you now have or have you ever had

_____ diabetes

_____ thyroid disease

_____ phenylketonuria (PKU)

_____ asthma

_____ heart disease

_____ high blood pressure

_____ deep venous thrombosis (blood clots)

_____ kidney disease

_____ systemic lupus erythematosus (SLE)

_____ epilepsy

_____ sickle cell disease

_____ cancer

_____ other health problems that require medical or surgical care
If yes, describe:

_____

_____

INFECTIOUS DISEASE HISTORY

Do you or your partner have a history of

_____ recurrent genital infections

_____ herpes simplex

_____ *Chlamydia* infection

_____ human papillomavirus (genital warts)

_____ gonorrhea

_____ syphilis

_____ viral hepatitis or high-risk behavior, including use of intravenous street drugs, intimate bisexual/homosexual contact, or multiple sexual partners

_____ acquired immunodeficiency syndrome (AIDS) or high-risk behavior, including use of intravenous street drugs, intimate bisexual/homosexual contact, or multiple sexual partners

_____ occupational exposure to the blood or bodily secretions of others

_____ blood transfusions

(Continued)

Do you

_____ own or work with cats

_____ have documented immunity to rubella

MEDICATION HISTORY

Do you

_____ routinely or occasionally take prescribed medications
If yes, list names and dosages:

_____

_____

_____ routinely or occasionally take over-the-counter medications
If yes, list names and dosages:

_____

_____

REPRODUCTIVE HISTORY

Do you have a history of

_____ uterine or cervical abnormalities

_____ two or more pregnancies that ended between 14 and 28 weeks of gestation

_____ one or more fetal deaths

_____ one or more infants who weighed less than 5½ lbs. at birth

_____ one or more infants who were admitted to a neonatal intensive care unit

_____ one or more infants with a birth defect

FAMILY HISTORY

Do you, your partner, or members of either of your families, including children, have

_____ hemophilia

_____ thalassemia

_____ Tay-Sachs disease

_____ sickle cell disease or trait

_____ phenylketonuria (PKU)

_____ cystic fibrosis

_____ a birth defect

_____ mental retardation

_____ Are you and your partner related outside of marriage (such as cousins)?

_____ Do you and your partner have the same ethnic or racial background, such as Ashkenazic Jewish, Mediterranean, or black?

Figure 16–1. Preconceptional health assessment. (Continued)

thorough pelvic examination should also be performed, including a Papanicolaou (Pap) smear, cultures for gonorrhea and chlamydia, and a wet smear evaluation.[5,8]

Diagnostic Tests and Methods. These include rubella titer and antibody screen, serology for syphilis, complete blood cell (CBC) count with indices, blood type/Rh, random blood sugar, and urinalysis.[5] Hemoglobin electrophoresis may be performed if sickle cell or thalassemia status is of concern. If positive, test the father for these traits also. Refer for genetic testing if both display traits. Screening for viral disease, such as HIV, hepatitis, cytomegalovirus (CMV), or toxoplasmosis, can be offered.[5] Encourage testing father for syphilis, HIV, hepatitis and type/Rh.

Provide instruction in basal body temperature (BBT) assessment, charting, and timing of intercourse to interested couples (see Chapter 10). Also review menstruation and fertility awareness methods to enhance possibility of conception (see Chapter 8).

CLIENT EDUCATION AND COUNSELING

Preconception counseling and intervention for the client and her partner should focus on the following areas.[8]

- ***Menstrual Cycles.*** Advise the client to keep an accurate record of her menstrual cycles in order to help establish gestational dating.
- ***Adequate Exercise and Nutrition.*** A vitamin/mineral supplement is often recommended to increase maternal nutrition stores. In September 1992, the U.S. Public Health Service Centers for Disease Control announced new recommendations regarding folic acid supplementation in the periconceptional period. These advise all women of childbearing age to consume 0.4 mg of folic acid per day for the purpose of reducing the risk of a neural-tube-defect affected pregnancy. Women with a history of an affected pregnancy are at particular risk in each subsequent pregnancy, and thus may also benefit from supplementation during the periconceptional period.[9] Folic acid supplementation is contraindicated in those women with pernicious anemia.[5] Food sources of folic acid include broccoli, leafy green vegetables, eggs, and orange juice. Encourage overweight or underweight clients to attain an ideal weight prior to conception. Obesity increases the risk of perinatal mortality and morbidity. It may contribute to the development of hypertension and diabetes in pregnancy.[1] Recent studies suggest that obesity increases the risk of neural tube defect regardless of folic acid intake.[10,11] Low pregravid weight increases the risk of premature birth and intrauterine growth retardation.[12] Beginning an exercise program prior to pregnancy will hopefully improve cardiovascular status and impart a feeling of overall well-being into the pregnancy as well. Exercise may also help the overweight woman attain close to ideal and ideal weight.
- ***Avoidance of Teratogens.*** Warn the client that potential teratogens can be related to occupation and lifestyle, for example, cleaning solutions, hair colors/perms, photography solutions, radiation, aromatic hydrocarbons, and chemicals used in processing food and textiles.
- ***Affirmation of Pregnancy Decision.*** Stress that the couple needs time to affirm the decision to attempt pregnancy.
- ***Readiness for Parenthood.*** Assess the couple's social, financial, and psychological readiness for pregnancy and commitment to parenthood.
- ***Identification of Unhealthy Behaviors.*** Assist the couple to identify and alter unhealthy behaviors, such as smoking, alcohol consumption, and drug use (i.e., prescription, over-the-counter, and illegal drugs).
- ***Treatment of Jeopardizing Conditions.*** Ensure that medical conditions, i.e., hypertension, diabetes, hepatitis, sexually transmitted diseases, which may jeopardize the pregnancy outcome are evaluated. Refer the couple to a specialist as needed.
- ***Identify Genetic Risk.*** When risks are identified, refer the couple for genetic counseling and laboratory testing to determine carrier status (see Figure 16–2).
- ***Effective Professional Relationship.*** To encourage the client's early entry into prenatal care, initiate and nurture a positive professional relationship.
- ***Preconception Classes.*** Where appropriate, refer the couple to community adult educational resources for preconception classes (e.g., March of Dimes).

Name _____   Patient # _____   Date _____

1. Will you be 35 years or older when the baby is due?   Yes ____   No ____
2. Have you, the baby's father, or anyone in either of your families ever had any of the following disorders?
   - Down syndrome (mongolism)   Yes ____   No ____
   - Other chromosomal abnormality   Yes ____   No ____
   - Neural tube defect, spina bifida (meningomyelocele or open spine), anencephaly   Yes ____   No ____
   - Hemophilia   Yes ____   No ____
   - Muscular dystrophy   Yes ____   No ____
   - Cystic fibrosis   Yes ____   No ____
   If yes, indicate the relationship of the affected person to you or to the baby's father: _____
3. Do you or the baby's father have a birth defect?   Yes ____   No ____
   If yes, who has the defect and what is it?_____
4. In any previous marriages, have you or the baby's father had a child, born dead or alive
   with a birth defect not listed in question 2 above?   Yes ____   No ____
   If yes, what was the defect and who had it? _____
5. Do you or the baby's father have any close relatives with mental retardation?   Yes ____   No ____
   If yes, indicate the relationship of the affected person to you or to the baby's father: _____
   Indicate the cause, if known: _____
6. Do you, the baby's father, or a close relative in either of your families have a birth defect,
   any familial disorder, or a chromosomal abnormality not listed above?   Yes ____   No ____
   If yes, indicate the condition and the relationship of the affected person to you or to the
   baby's father: _____
   _____
7. In any previous marriages, have you or the baby's father had a stillborn child or three or more first
   trimester spontaneous pregnancy losses?   Yes ____   No ____
   Have either of you had a chromosomal study?   Yes ____   No ____
   If yes, indicate who and the results: _____
   _____
8. If you or the baby's father is of Jewish ancestry, have either of you been screened for
   Tay-sachs disease?   Yes ____   No ____
   If yes, indicate who and the results: _____
   _____
9. If you or the baby's father is black, have either of you been screened for sickle cell trait?   Yes ____   No ____
   If yes, indicate who and the results: _____
   _____
10. If you or the baby's father is of Italian, Greek, or Mediterranean background, have either of
    you been tested for ß-thalassemia?   Yes ____   No ____
    If yes, indicate who and the results: _____
    _____
11. If you or the baby's father is of Philipine or Southeast Asian ancestry, have either of you been
    tested for α-thalassemia?   Yes ____   No ____
    If yes, indicate who and the results: _____
    _____
12. Excluding iron and vitamins, have you taken any medications or recreational drugs since
    being pregnant or since your last menstrual period? (Include nonprescription drugs.)   Yes ____   No ____
    If yes, give name of medication and time taken during pregnancy: _____
    _____

Note: Any patient replying "YES" to questions should be offered appropriate counseling. If the patient declines further counseling or testing, this should be noted in the chart. Given that genetics is a field in a state of flux, alterations or updates to this form will be required periodically.

Figure 16–2. Sample prenatal genetic screen. *(Source: Reference 25.)*

- *Laboratory Tests.* Order all appropriate laboratory tests, evaluate the results, and discuss the findings and their implications with the client.
- *Appropriate Vaccinations.* If the client is not immune to rubella, administer the vaccine and advise the client to wait 3 months before attempting conception. Also vaccinate for tetanus, hepatitis, and varicella when indicated.
- *Special Dietary Needs.* If the client has special dietary needs (e.g., vegetarian, cultural, overweight, underweight), refer her to a dietician. Use of megavitamin/mineral supplements are to be avoided. Assess for eating disorders, pica. Economic constraints may negatively affect dietary intake.

ASSESSMENT DURING PREGNANCY

Well woman's health care during pregnancy begins with a complete history and thorough physical examination during the initial visit. The initial visit is the ideal time to screen for particular risk factors suggesting preterm delivery or other poor outcomes (see Risk Assessment, later in this chapter). Since many women continue to experience unintended pregnancy, however, routine exams are also ideal for screening and education.

Encourage the client to seek prenatal care early in pregnancy.

The health care provider and the client establish the foundation of a trusting relationship by jointly developing a plan of care for the pregnancy. This plan is tailored to the client's lifestyle preferences as much as possible and focuses primarily on education for overall wellness during pregnancy. The ultimate goal is early detection and prevention of potential problems in the pregnancy.

Return office visits include physical evaluation of the client and her fetus, client education, and the continuation of a holistic approach to pregnancy care. (Nursing diagnoses that might be established during this period are listed at the end of this chapter.)

SIGNS AND SYMPTOMS OF PREGNANCY

Signs and symptoms that may be reported by the pregnant client are traditionally categorized into three groups, defined as follows and summarized in Table 16–1.

- *Presumptive.* Signs or symptoms frequently reported with pregnancy, although not conclusive for pregnancy.
- *Probable.* Signs or symptoms that are more reliable indicators of pregnancy, often noted on the physical examination or with laboratory testing.

TABLE 16–1. SIGNS AND SYMPTOMS OF PREGNANCY

Presumptive	Probable	Positive
Amenorrhea.	Abdominal enlargement.	Auscultation of fetal heart sounds.
Breast tenderness and enlargement.	Ballottement.	Palpation of fetal movements.
Chadwick's sign.	Braxton-Hicks contractions.	Radiological and/or ultrasonic verification of gestation.
Fatigue.	Goodell's sign.	
Hyperpigmentation.	Hegar's sign.	
Chloasma.	Palpation of fetal contours.	
Linea nigra.	Positive pregnancy test.	
Fetal movements (quickening).	Uterine enlargement.	
Urinary frequency.		
Nausea/vomiting.		

Source: Adapted from reference 13.

- *Positive.* Signs or symptoms noted when absolute confirmation of pregnancy is made.

Although these signs and symptoms assist in confirming pregnancy, they *cannot* enable the health care provider to differentiate an intrauterine pregnancy from an ectopic pregnancy.

OVERVIEW OF INITIAL PRENATAL VISIT

During the initial visit, the health care provider performs a complete assessment and counsels the client about risk factors and prenatal care. Several components are included.[14,15]

- *Confirmation of Pregnancy.* Perform a beta-human chorionic gonadotropin (β-hCG) urine test if seen prior to FHT's, ultrasound; if negative, retest using a radioimmunoassay (RIA) β-hCG serum test (see Table 16–5 on page 454).
- *History.* Obtain a complete medical, psychosocial, family, and reproductive history (see Chapter 5). Several areas require more in-depth evaluation during pregnancy. Information obtained may help date the pregnancy.[13]
  - Menstrual history—last normal menses.
  - Contraceptive history—last time used, dates of unprotected intercourse.
  - Gynecologic history.
  - Sexual history—high-risk behavior.
  - Surgical history.
- *Physical Examination.* (See Chapter 5.) Assess the client's vital signs and perform a complete head-to-toe examination with particular attention to the pelvic evaluation. Establish the client's baseline cervical status and perform clinical pelvimetry if it is part of the protocol in a particular setting. The normal pregnant cervix is usually 3–4 cm long, closed, firm in texture and usually mid to posterior in position. Testing the adequacy of the pelvis, if unproven by previous vaginal delivery, includes measurement of the diagonal conjugate from the posterior inferior edge of the symphysis pubis to the sacral promontory (normally 12.5 cm or greater), which estimates the inlet; the transverse diameter of the midpelvis includes evaluation of the ischial spines (sharp or blunt and degree of prominence) and of the antero-posterior diameter by the shape of the sacrum

(curved or flat). The ischial tuberosities should be 8 cm or more apart.[15]
- *Laboratory Tests.* Perform routine laboratory tests (Table 16–2) and additional testing as needed (Table 16–3).
- *Risk Assessment.* Refer the client for thorough risk assessment as indicated (see pages 458–460).
- *Prenatal Educational Materials.* Provide and review information about prenatal classes, nu-

---

TABLE 16–2. ROUTINE TESTS TO BE PERFORMED ON ALL PREGNANCY CLIENTS[a]

ABO blood group/Rh factor identification/Antibody screen.

Complete blood cell count with indices (Hb, Hct, MCV, MCH, MCHC).

Rubella titer.

Syphilis screening/VDRL, RPR.

Hepatitis screening.

Urinalysis.

Chlamydia screening.

Gonorrhea screening.

Group Beta strep screening.

Pap smear.

[a]Values may vary according to the laboratory used.

Note: Hb = hemoglobin; Hct = hematocrit; MCV = mean corpuscular volume; MCH = mean corpuscular hemoglobin; MCHC = mean corpuscular hemoglobin concentration; VDRL = Venereal Disease Research Laboratories test; RPR = rapid plasma reagin; HIV = human immunodeficiency virus.
Source: References 14, 15, 18.

TABLE 16–3. ADDITIONAL TESTS PERFORMED ON THE BASIS OF THE PREGNANT CLIENT'S HISTORY[a]

α-fetoprotein/triple screen.

Antibody screening.

Blood chemistry.

Cytomegalovirus titer.

Fifth disease titer.

Glucose tolerance tests.

Hemoglobin A1C.

Hemoglobin electrophoresis.

Herpes culture.

HIV screening.

Serum iron studies.

Toxoplasmosis titer.

Thyroid studies.

Urine culture.

Tuberculin skin test.

[a]Values may vary according to the laboratory used.
Source: References 14, 15, 18.

trition, exercise, teratogens, sexuality, and choices in infant feeding.

- *Sexuality During Pregnancy.* See discussion that follows.
- *Schedule Follow-Up Visits.* Discuss the importance of continued prenatal care and work out a schedule for follow-up visits.

SEXUALITY DURING PREGNANCY

Physiological Changes

Table 16–4 gives a summary of physiological changes that may enhance pleasure or diminish a woman's sexual response during pregnancy. Second trimester changes, such as increased pelvic congestion and vaginal lubrication, may enhance sexual enjoyment. Opportunities arise to review the physiological changes that influence sexuality both during the initial prenatal visit and during subsequent visits.

Psychosocial Changes

Pregnancy is often a time of profound emotional and developmental upheaval and can present a developmental crisis for both partners. Some couples experience increased intimacy and closeness from the bond pregnancy creates. Sexuality during pregnancy can be affected directly. The health care provider's role involves providing anticipatory guidance through sexuality education and assessment, both at the initial prenatal evaluation and during subsequent visits. Several concerns are often reported.[16,17]

- Fear of causing miscarriage or harm to the developing fetus.
- Need for modifications in positioning for coitus with advancing gestation.

- Fluctuating libido by both partners and the resulting effect on sexual desire and contact.
- The woman's perceived loss of attractiveness to her sexual partner, body image changes.
- Misinformation and misconception regarding sexuality, safety; the impact of religious taboos.
- A declining desire for intimacy as the woman withdraws or focuses on infant preparation.

Guidelines for Intervention

Take a sexual history early in the pregnancy to establish baseline information, e.g., frequency, monogamy, risk factors, about both partners. Knowledge of sexual activity since last normal menses may help with dating the pregnancy. To the extent that medical findings allow, give permission for the couple to be sexually active during and after pregnancy.

Contraindications to Sexual Intercourse

The following conditions may preclude sexual relations during a portion of the pregnancy.[16,17,18]

- History of repeated miscarriage.
- History of cervical incompetence, without cerclage.
- Current possibility of threatened abortion.
- Placenta previa.
- Undiagnosed vaginal bleeding.
- Premature rupture of membranes, preterm labor.
- Severe vulvar varicosities.

SUBSEQUENT PRENATAL VISITS

At each subsequent prenatal visit, measure the client's weight and blood pressure; assess for quickening/fetal movement; evaluate the client's

TABLE 16–4. PHYSIOLOGICAL CHANGES IN PREGNANCY THAT INFLUENCE SEXUALITY

First Trimester	Second Trimester	Third Trimester
Fatigue and lethargy.	Increased pelvic congestion.	Physical discomfort, backache.
Nausea and vomiting.	Increased vaginal moisture.	Increasing uterine irritability.
Breast tenderness.		Excessive pelvic congestion.
Abdominal bloating.		Vulvar/femoral varicosities.
Increased urination.		

Source: References 13, 16, 17.

urine for blood, protein, ketones, nitrites, and glucose; determine fundal height; and assess fetal heart tones. Also at each visit, evaluate any client complaints and answer questions appropriately. Review appropriate nutrition and use of prenatal vitamin/mineral supplements. Leopold's maneuvers should be performed weekly after 35 weeks to determine fetal presentation and position.[1,15] Include the partner when possible in auscultation of fetal heart tones and palpation of fundal height changes. Share positive aspects of the exam, e.g., normal heart tones, good growth. Review with the couple the common discomforts of pregnancy and how they may influence sexuality. Encourage the partner's participation in the labor and delivery process to improve his ability to empathize during the postpartum period. As appropriate, offer the couple suggestions about sexual frequency, foreplay, and alternate forms of intimacy. As the pregnancy advances, offer advice on coital positioning.

Weeks 12 to 16

Review laboratory findings with the client and her partner. If appropriate order genetic testing, such as amniocentesis or α-fetoprotein serum. Screen the father of the baby for sickle cell (hemoglobin electrophoresis) disease, blood type/Rh as indicated.

Weeks 16 to 20

Assess for fetal movements (quickening). Ultrasound evaluation may be performed to confirm gestational age and assess fetal well-being. Encourage the couple to enroll in prenatal classes.

Weeks 24 to 28

If Rh negative, reevaluate the antibody screen titer. Perform glucose screening for gestational diabetes. Administer RhoGAM immune globulin as indicated. Reactions to RhoGAM [$Rh_o(D)$ immune globulin] are infrequent, mild, and primarily at the injection site. An occasional person may react more strongly. A few women may experience a slight temperature elevation. Retest hemoglobin and hematocrit. Evaluate the client for risk of preterm labor and perform a cervical assessment including cervical position, consistency, length and dilation.

Weeks 28 to 32

Offer the client counseling regarding the choice of health care provider for the infant. Assess the client's breasts and discuss preparation for breastfeeding. Discuss the importance of daily fetal movement as an indicator of fetal well-being.

Weeks 32 to 34

Reassess the client for risk of preterm labor; assess the cervix as indicated.

Weeks 34 to 36

Review with the client the signs and symptoms of labor; provide a handout listing them. Obtain a vaginal/anorectal culture for GBS (group Beta strep).[19] According to setting protocol, begin weekly cervical cultures for active HSV (herpes simplex virus) in those with positive history. Retest for chlamydia and gonorrhea in those with infections earlier in pregnancy.

Weeks 36 to 40

Assess fetal position and presentation. Review and negotiate the client's birth expectations. Forward a copy of the client's prenatal records to the hospital labor area for future reference. Document the client's final choice of a pediatrician. Initiate fetal surveillance as indicated. A cervical examination may be performed per the protocol of the institution. Review client desires for postpartal contraception. Reinforce preparation for breastfeeding. Arrange for infant car seat.

Week 40 and Beyond

Prepare the client for postdate pregnancy protocol. Perform a cervical assessment. Institute fetal surveillance, such as ultrasound, nonstress testing, and biweekly office visits. Check via ultrasound for AFV (amniotic fluid volume).

PROGRESSING PHYSICAL CHANGE

Several changes commonly occur during pregnancy.[1]

- *Skin.* Increased vascularity; increased pigmentation of face (chloasma), areola, abdomen (linea nigra), and genitalia; striae of breasts and abdomen.

- *Head.* Mild changes in scalp; excessive oiliness or dryness.
- *Eyes.* Vessel dilation in the sclera.
- *Mouth.* Edematous, friable gums.
- *Chest/Cardiovascular.* Increased respiratory effort and rate; progressive elevation of the diaphragm; hand/pedal edema by third trimester.
- *Breasts.* Increased fullness, tenderness, and enlargement; and excretion of colostrum are common by the third trimester.
- *Heart.* Exaggerated heart sounds, particularly functional murmurs in systole.
- *Abdomen.* Distention secondary to flatus and increased uterine size; diminished bowel sounds as peristaltic movements are slowed; enlarging uterus, which displaces abdominal organs.
- *Genitalia/Reproductive*
  - *External.* Increased pigmentation; pubic hair may lengthen. Near term, pelvic congestion and overall swelling of labia majora are common; vulvar varicosities may be noted.
  - *Vagina.* Increased pelvic congestion and hypertrophy; rugation of vaginal mucosa is prominent.
  - *Cervix.* Positive Chadwick's sign (bluish/purple color) is noted; may soften, dilate, and efface close to term. Positive Goodell's sign (softening with growth of cervical glands) may be noted.
  - *Uterus.* Positive Hegar's sign (softening of the lower uterine segment) often present by 6 weeks' gestation. At 12 weeks' gestation the fundus is noted at the symphysis pubis; at 16 weeks' gestation the fundus is midway between the symphysis and the umbilicus. Uterine enlargement occurs in linear fashion (1 cm per week). The uterine fundus can be palpated at the umbilicus at approximately 20 weeks and measures 20 cm. By the 36th week the fundus is just below the ensiform cartilage and measures approximately 36 cm; the fundal height drops slightly near term (lightening). Measurement may then no longer correspond with week of gestation. The uterus maintains a globular/ovoid shape throughout pregnancy.
  - *Adnexa.* Discomfort may be noted with exam due to stretching of the round ligaments throughout pregnancy. The ovaries are not palpable once the uterus fills the pelvic cavity at 12 to 14 weeks' gestation.
  - *Urinary.* The bladder may be palpable; frequency and incontinence are common, particularly with multiparity.
  - *Rectal.* Increased vascular congestion with resulting hemorrhoids is often noted.
- *Musculoskeletal.* Increased relaxation of pelvic structures; lordosis; sciatica and discomfort at the symphysis pubis are common. Pain from round ligament syndrome often noted at sulcus of thighs.
- *Endocrine.* May have mildly enlarged thyroid; however, diffusely enlarged thyroid nodularity or increased firmness is abnormal.

DIAGNOSTIC TESTS AND METHODS

To assess the development of the fetus and the well-being of the mother, the health care provider may use a variety of invasive and noninvasive tests.

Pregnancy Tests[18,20]

It is important to diagnose pregnancy as early as possible to maximize the benefits from health care and minimize risks to the developing fetus. (See Table 16–5 for a description of pregnancy tests.)

Human chorionic gonadotropin (hCG) is detected in pregnancy at about the time of implantation. Levels in normal pregnancy usually double every 48 to 72 hours; by the first missed period, serum values reach 50 to 250 mIU per mL. Levels peak at approximately 60 to 70 days postfertilization, then decrease to plateau at 100 to 130 days of pregnancy. Tests vary in sensitivity, specificity, and accuracy—influenced by the length of gestation, concentration of specimen, proteins or blood present, and some drugs. Human chorionic gonadotropin is composed of alpha and beta subunits. The alpha subunit of hCG reacts with the alpha subunits of luteinizing hormone (LH), follicle stimulating hormone (FSH), and thyrotropin (TSH) due to similar molecular structure. Tests that are specific for

TABLE 16–5. PREGNANCY TESTS

Type	Specimen Source	Sensitivity (mIU/mL)	Example	Comments
Beta Subunit Radioimmunoassay (RIA).	Serum	5	Used mainly in hospitals and large outpatient laboratories.	Radioisotopes. *Uses:* Quantifies ß-hCG. Serial measurements useful in determination of pregnancy viability, trophoblastic disease, ectopic pregnancy. *Specificity:* For ß-hCG. No cross-reaction with LH, FSH, TSH. *Reliable:* 7 days postconception. *Time:* 1 to 2 hours, usually run in batches.
Enzyme-liked immunosorbent assay (ELISA); immunometric test.	Serum urine	25–100	Clearview hCG (Wampole), Icon II hCG (Wampole), Precise (Becton-Dickinson). Quick Vue (Quick 1). Testpack Plus hCG (Abbot).	Monoclonal antibodies; enzyme coupling. *Uses:* Serum tests quantify ß-hCG and hCG. Same as RIA if ß-hCG specific; urine tests qualify ß-hCG. *Specificity:* No cross-reaction with LH FSH, TSH if ß-hCG specific. *Reliable:* 7 to 10 days postconception. *Time:* 1–7 minutes.
Agglutination inhibition tests.	Urine	150–2500	Pregnospia (Organon, UCG-Beta Slide (Wampole), ß-hCG (Ortho), Pregnosticon (Organon).	Agglutination of coated latex particles and hCG antibodies. Positive if no agglutination occurs. *Uses:* Qualifies pregnancy. *Specificity:* Varies; if ß-hCG specific, no cross-reaction to LH, FSH, TSH. Sensitivity set at higher levels to decrease cross-reaction in test to whole hCG molecule. *Reliable:* 14 to 21 days postconception. *Test:* 2 minutes.

Source: References 18, 20.

beta subunit are more accurate; serum tests are generally more sensitive and specific than urine tests.

Quantitative, serial measurements of serum *beta-human chorionic gonadotropin* (β-hCG) are valuable in documenting the viability of the gestation. Serum and urine tests specific for β-hCG have accuracy rates of 99 percent, with few false positives. With urine testing, early gestational age and decreased specimen concentration may yield false negatives (Table 16–5).

Technological advances in *ultrasonic imaging* (see Chapter 19) have enabled accurate evaluation or monitoring of several aspects of pregnancy.[1]

- Early identification of intrauterine pregnancy, ectopic, and/or multiple pregnancy.
- Demonstration of growth and viability of the embryo.
- Identification and evaluation of uterine, fetal, and placental anomalies.
- Serial measurements to evaluate fetal growth.
- Evaluation of amniotic fluid levels.
- Biophysical profile to evaluate fetal well-being in later stages of pregnancy. Commonly recommended tests are described in Tables 16–6 and 16–7.[1,14,18,19,21,22]

TABLE 16–6. LABORATORY AND DIAGNOSTIC TESTS OFTEN PERFORMED DURING PREGNANCY

Test	Nonpregnant Values	Pregnant Values	Implications for Mother/Fetus
Cervix-Vagina			
Chlamydia	Negative	Negative	Culture remains gold standard for diagnosis; neonatal infection; implicated preterm labor.
Gonorrhea	Negative	Negative	Culture remains gold standard for diagnosis; neonatal infection; implicated in preterm labor, spontaneous abortion, ectopic pregnancy, chorioamnionitis, IUGR.
Group beta strep	Negative	Negative	May be considered normal vaginal flora in a client who is not pregnant, however, neonatal infection can be fatal; implicated in preterm labor, chorioamnionitis, UTI, endomyometritis.
Herpes simplex genitalis	Negative	Negative	Neonatal infection can be fatal. Implicated in preterm labor and spontaneous abortions. Primary infection third trimester carries higher fetal/neonatal risk.
Listeria	Negative	Negative	Strong association with intrauterine fetal demise (IUFD); preterm delivery and chorioamnionitis. Congenital defects not widely noted. Found in unpasteurized dairy products.
Mycoplasma	Negative	Negative	May be considered normal vaginal flora in a client who is not pregnant; however, implicated in spontaneous abortions; controversial rare cause of anencephaly, stillbirth.
Bacterial vaginosis	Negative	Negative	Condition marked by shift in normal vaginal flora from predominence of lactobacilli to anaerobes. Implicated in PROM, preterm birth, endometritis.
Trichomonas	Negative	Negative	Controversial cause of LBW, PROM.
Serology			
Antibody screen	Negative	Negative	Positive screen indicates sensitization; done at initial and 28th week visits, and after maternal fetal blood exchange in Rh-negative woman.
Cytomegalovirus	Negative	Stable titer	Majority demonstrate immunity; maternal immunity does not prevent congenital infection; primary infection is more severe for fetus; cytomegalic inclusion disease is evident in 5–10 percent of those affected; overall fetal morbidity, cost factors, predictability of occurrence/recurrence limit use of this testing.
Hepatitis	Negative	Negative	If positive screen in HB_sAg or HB_eAg, IgM titer to assess active, chronic, convalescent states; the presence of anti-HB_c IgG indicates previous infection; anti-HB_s is positive only in those with successful vaccination; transplacental transmission is rare; neonatal infection can occur. Screen for HCV is those at risk.
Rubella	Immunity greater than 1:10	Stable titer	If nonimmune, vaccinate postpartum, compatible with breastfeeding. No evidence amassed of adverse consequence noted in infants or pregnancies inadvertantly vaccinated first trimester. Infection during first trimester associated with high rates of spontaneous abortion and congenital malformation.
Syphilis	Nonreactive	Nonreactive	If reactive, perform FTA-ABS test or MHA-TP to confirm presence of *Treponema pallidum* organism; if woman is untreated, approximately 25 percent of offspring die in utero, 25 percent perinatally/neonatally, 40 percent develop syphilis; long-term sequelae beginning in newborn.

(Continued)

TABLE 16–6. LABORATORY AND DIAGNOSTIC TESTS OFTEN PERFORMED DURING PREGNANCY (CONTINUED)

Test	Nonpregnant Values	Pregnant Values	Implications for Mother/Fetus
Serology (cont.)			
Toxoplasmosis (IgG titer	Negative	Stable titer	If positive, repeat titer in 2 weeks: An 8-fold increase in IgG, or positive IgM titer, indicates active infection; more virulent if new infection during first trimester, but less frequent; less than 10 percent of infants infected third trimester display disease; for woman with risk of exposure to seropositive cats or uncooked meat and eggs.
HIV (ELISA)	Nonreactive	Nonreactive	Immunofloresence, Western Blot confirm diagnosis; mandatory in many states to offer testing; recent studies indicate AZT given in pregnancy to infected woman reduces vertical transmission to fetus; virus can be transmitted via breast milk to neonate. False negative confirmed by polymerase chain reaction (PCR) testing.
Type/Rh	A+ A– B+ B– O+ O– AB+ AB–		If Rh negative, screen for antibodies; ABO incompatibility usually result of O woman carrying an A or B fetus; degree of hemolysis is usually mild.
Fifth disease (erythema infectiosum) IgM titer	Immune	Stable titer	Human parvovirus B19; controversial rare cause of fetal aplastic anemia and nonimmune hydrops; 50 percent of women are immune. Follow exposed, at risk women who are IgM positive, IgG negative, for perinatal sequelae.
Hematology			
Red blood cell count	3.5–5.5/mm^3	Increases 20 percent by term	Stable during pregnancy.
White blood cell count	4.5–11/mm^3	5–12/mm^3; may increase	Values of up to 25 mm^3 have been noted during labor.
Hematocrit	37–47/percent	28.6–38.4 percent	Decreased values reflect overall 50 percent increase in plasma volume—physiological anemia.
Hemoglobin	12–16 g/dL	11–16 g/dL	Increased oxygen carrying capacity of red blood cells compensates for volume expansion.
Platelets	250,000–500,000/mm^3		May decrease with severe preeclampsia. Rule out immune thrombocytopenic purpura (ITP).
Hemoglobin A1c	4.0–8.2 percent	6.5 percent	Measure of long term glucose control in identified gestational diabetic; changes are seen in 3–5 weeks after optimal diet and insulin control; not accurate in diabetics with chronic renal failure or disease that impairs erythrocytes.
Hemoglobin electrophoresis	HgbA1 96–98.5 percent; HgbA2 1.5–4.0 percent; HgbF 0–2.0 percent	Same	Detects amounts of hemoglobin normally found and presence of HgbS HgbC; diagnosis of trait and disease is dependent on percentage of types to HgbA; screen all African American, Mediterranean, Asian women; occasionally noted in white population.
Blood Chemistry			
Alkaline phosphatase (Total)	12–63 IU/L	May double	Elevated in liver conditions; increases due to placental involvement; in diseases involving connective tissue.
Blood urea nitrogen (BUN)	10–15 mg/dL	8–10 mg/dL	Pregnant values are lower due to increased glomerular filtration rate. In pregnancy induced hypertension (PIH), values increase to nonpregnant levels due to pathological arterial spasm and vasoconstriction.

TABLE 16–6. LABORATORY AND DIAGNOSTIC TESTS OFTEN PERFORMED DURING PREGNANCY (CONTINUED)

Test	Nonpregnant Values	Pregnant Values	Implications for Mother/Fetus
Blood Chemistry (cont.)			
Cholesterol	130–200 mg/dL	243–305 mg/dL	Accurate levels not reflected in pregnancy.
Creatinine	0.8 mg/dL	0.5–0.7 mg/dL	Pregnant values are lower due to increased glomerular filtration rate. In PIH, values increase to nonpregnant levels due to pathological arterial spasm and vasoconstriction.
Iron—serum	60–160 µg/dL	Decrease	Iron demands increase during pregnancy.
Lactate dehydrogenase (LDH)	30–200 IU/L		Elevated in various conditions, especially those with tissue destruction, hypoxia, or an inflammatory process; seen in heparin therapy.
Serum alanine aminotransferase (ALT, SGPT)	3–35 IU/L		Used primarily to monitor the liver; may increase in severe preeclampsia.
Serum aspartate aminotransferase (AST, SGOT)	5–40 IU/L	May decrease	Elevated in conditions where cardiac or hepatic damage occurs; also elevated post IM injections; may also be depressed in diabetic ketoacidosis (DKA) and beriberi.
Thyroid panel: triiodothyronine (T_3)	24–35 percent	Decrease	Due to increase of thyroid binding globulins by estrogen.
Thyroxine (T_4)	5.3–14.5 µg/dL	Increase	Basal metabolic rate increases by 25 percent; increased thyroid binding globulins.
Thyrotropin (TSH)	0.5–10 µU/mL		Most sensitive indicator for hypothyroid/hyperthyroid states in pregnancy.
Total iron binding capacity (TIBC)	250–460 µg/dL	Increase	Estrogen increases ability for iron to bind to transferrin, which regulates transport in the body.
Uric Acid	4.2–6.0 mg/dL	3.0–4.2 mg/dL	Pregnant values are lower due to increased glomerular filtration rate. In PIH, values increase to nonpregnant levels due to pathological arterial spasm and vasoconstriction.
Urinalysis			
Albumin	Negative	Less than 100 mg/24 h	Elevations seen in preeclampsia and urinary tract infections.
Chloride	170–250 mEg/24 h	Slight increase	Due to increased glomerular filtration rate.
Creatinine	1.0–1.8 g/24 h	Elevated	Due to increased glomerular filtration rate.
Glucose	120 g/24 h	Elevated	Due to decrease renal threshold and increased glomerular filtration rate.
Ketones	Negative	Same	Presence may indicate dehydration; starvation states; ketoacidosis in insulin-dependent diabetic strenuous exercise.
White blood cells	Less than 1–3 per high power field	Same	Often vaginal contamination, urinary tract infection if other indicators.
Red blood cells	Less than 2–3 per high power field	Same	May be due to violent exercise, kidney trauma, systemic or renal disease.
Bacteria	Greater than 100,000 colonies/mL	Greater than 10,000 colonies/mL	Infection if same species.
Nitrites	Negative	Negative	Some bacteria convert urine nitrates into nitrites in the bladder. Positive indicates infection. Urine must be retained in the bladder several hours for conversion to occur. Gram positive cocci do not produce nitrites, E. coli may.

Note: HCV = hepatitis C virus; IUGR = intrauterine growth retardation; UTI = urinary tract infection; PROM = premature rupture of membranes; LBW = low birth weight; HB_sAg = hepatitis B surface antigen; HB_cAg = hepatitis B core antigen; IG = immunoglobulin; FTA-ABS = fluorescent treponemal antibody absorption; MHA-TP = micro-hemagglutination assay for antibody to *Treponema pallidium*; PCR = polymerase chain reaction.
Source: References 1, 14, 18, 19, 21, 22.

TABLE 16–7. ADDITIONAL TESTS OFTEN CARRIED OUT DURING PREGNANCY

Test	Values	Significance	Implications
Maternal serum α-fetoprotein (MSAFP)	Less than 0.4 MOM (multiples of the mean	At risk for aneuploidy Down syndrome, trisomy 18	Relative to maternal weight, age, race, gestational dating, diabetic status, singleton vs. multiple gestation. A triple screen aids in the detection of chromosomal abnormalities in low MSAFP. BHCG and unconjugated estriol measurements viewed in relation to MSAFP value increase sensitivity of test.
	0.4–2.5 MOM	Normal range is 85 to 95 percent	Margin of error is 5–15 percent.
	Greater than 2.5 MOM	At risk for neural tube defect, Turners syndrome, abdominal wall defect, esophageal atresia. May indicate risk for PTB, IUGR, pregnancy loss.	All abnormal values should be evaluated selectively by ultrasound, fetal scan, and amniocentesis; identified strong family/maternal history of neural tube defect.
Fasting blood sugar (FBS)	70–105 mg/dL	≥ 105 mg/dL elevated	Not valuable in healthy pregnancy.
1-hour glucose tolerance test (GTT)	135–140 mg/dL	≥ 140 mg/dL elevated	Suspicious for diagnosis of gestation diabetes. Screening done at 24–28 weeks' gestation; screen earlier if H/O[a] 4000-g infant, history of gestational diabetes, or previous fetal death. Repeat 24–28 weeks if initial screen normal.
3-hour GTT			Diagnostic of gestational diabetes.
FBS	70–105 mg/dL	≥ 105 mg/dL elevated	Requires fasting 8 hours prior to testing. Carbohydrate loading of 200–300 gram/day for 3 days prior to testing increases sensitivity of test.
1 h	120–190 mg/dL	≥ 190 mg/dL elevated	Elevated FBS is indicator of probable need for insulin therapy.
2 h	120–165 mg/dL	≥ 165 mg/dL elevated	Criterion: Requires treatment if 2 of the 4 values are elevated.
3 h	70–145 mg/dL	≥ 145 mg/dL elevated	

[a]H/O = history of; PTB = preterm birth; IUGR = intrauterine growth retardation; BHCG = beta human chorionic gonadotropin
Source: References 1, 18, 21, 22, 23.

ASSESSMENT OF COMMON CONCERNS

The pregnant client may report common concerns in a multitude of areas. These concerns are mainly physical (see Chapter 17) and may include nausea and vomiting, fatigue, backache, constipation, and edema. Psychological/developmental concerns (see Chapter 17) may include changes in libido, emotional lability, and nightmares.

RISK ASSESSMENT

Assessment of a maternity client for risk factors encompasses physical, historical, and psychosocial aspects. The client at risk is identified, evaluated, and observed, with special consideration given to the course and outcome of pregnancy.

Screening is done to detect genetic defects, to determine the risk of preterm labor and delivery, and to assess parental-fetal attachment and hazards in the environment and workplace. Screening should ideally be done at the initial visit, during each remaining trimester, and whenever necessary.

Genetic Screening

The purpose of genetic screening is to identify those at risk for an inherited or acquired defect and to identify unrecognized defects in healthy individuals.[18] Genetic defects account for most of all first trimester spontaneous abortion. It is estimated that 3 to 5 percent of infants in the United States have recognizable defects present at birth. Up to 15 percent of all live births will reveal defects when assessed 5–10 years after delivery.[15,18] Approximately one-third of children in pediatric hospitals are treated for conditions that have a genetic component.[24] Approximately 25 percent of birth defects are attributed to genetic factors, 15 percent to environmental factors, 30 percent to a combination of these—leaving 30 percent unaccountable. It is estimated that 50 percent of spontaneous abortions and 5 to 7 percent of intrauterine fetal deaths are caused by chromosomal abnormalities.[18,24] Clients with potential risks (Figure 16–2) should receive further counseling, testing, education, and guidance in decision making.[24,25]

Tools for the Detection and Diagnosis of Genetic Defects (Also See Chapter 19)

- *Family Pedigree.* A graphic record of family medical history may reveal an inheritance pattern and help to identify whether further laboratory testing and clinical evaluation are needed.[24]
- *Alpha-fetoprotein.* Levels of a α-fetoprotein circulating in maternal serum or amniotic fluid are evaluated in relation to gestational age, maternal age, weight, race, presence of diabetes, or previous history of neural tube defects. Increased levels may indicate neural tube defect (NTD), Turners syndrome, oomphalocele, tetralogy of fallot. Decreased levels may indicate Down Syndrome, trisomy 18. In decreased levels, a triple serum of MSAFP, BHCG, and unconjugated estriol increases sensitivity of testing.[23]
- *Amniocentesis.* Fluid aspirated from the amniotic sac has multiple test applications such as chromosome analysis, karyotype, α-fetoprotein, deoxyribonucleic acid (DNA) markers, viral studies, biochemical linkage assays, and inborn errors of metabolism.[24]
- *Chorionic Villus Sampling.* Transcervical aspiration of chorionic villi permits results for the same test as does amniocentesis, with the exception of α-fetoprotein results.[24]
- *Fetal Blood Sampling.* Improvements in ultrasound technology allow for percutaneous umbilical blood sampling (PUBS) of the fetus. Used to diagnose hemophilia A, various immunologic diseases in which fetal blood not contaminated with amniotic fluid is needed.[26]

- *Fetal Skin Sampling.* Ultrasound guided biopsy of fetal skin. Used to diagnose rare dermatologic disorders such as epidermolysis bullosa and ichthyosis.[26]
- *Fetal Muscle Biopsy.* Ultrasound guided biopsy of fetal muscle tissue. Used to diagnose/exclude certain forms of muscle dystrophy.[26]
- *Level 2 Ultrasound/Fetal Scan.* Indirect visualization of the fetus enables evaluation of overt, structural changes; it is usually performed in a tertiary setting.[24]
- *Fetoscopy.* Direct visualization of the fetus and placenta allows for tissue sampling or limited interventions with the fetus in life threatening situations. Fetoscopy is rarely used since the advent of recombinant DNA techniques and amniocentesis. The risk of miscarriage with fetoscopy is 3 to 5 percent higher than with amniocentesis or chorionic villus sampling.[1,15]

Preterm Labor Screening

The demographic, historical, and psychosocial factors associated with increased incidence of preterm labor and delivery are assessed with preterm screening. *Preterm labor* is the presence of regular uterine contractions causing cervical dilation and effacement prior to 37 completed weeks' gestation and after 20 completed weeks. The etiology of preterm labor is unknown. Current estimates are that preterm labor occurs in 8–17 percent of women.[15] Perinatal morbidity/mortality increase as length of gestation decreases. Even with the most advanced technology, outcomes are poor for gestations of fewer than 26 weeks. Long-term sequelae such as chronic respiratory and neurological handicaps, blindness, learning disabilities, and financial strain are often reported.[18,26] Parental emotional and financial strain may be significant.

The incidence of preterm labor and delivery may be reduced by early identification of risk factors, continuous assessment of physical changes, education, and treatment that reduces controllable risk factors. A screening tool is illustrated in Table 16–8.[26] If one or more major factors, or two or more minor factors, are present, the client is identified as belonging to a high risk group. (For further information on diagnosis and treatment, see Chapter 18.)

TABLE 16–8. MAJOR AND MINOR RISK FACTORS IN THE PREDICTION OF SPONTANEOUS PRETERM LABOR

Major	Minor
Multiple gestation.	Febrile illness.
Diethylstilbestrol (DES) exposure.	Bleeding after 12 weeks' gestation.
Hydramnios.	History of pylonephritis.
Uterine anomaly	Cigarette smoking—more than 10 per day.
Cervic dilated more than 1 cm at 32 weeks' gestation.	Second trimester abortion.
2 second-trimester abortions.	More than 2 first-trimester abortions.
Previous preterm delivery.	
Previous preterm labor.	
Abdominal surgery during pregnancy.	
History of cone biopsy.	
Cervical shortening of less than 1 cm at 32 weeks' gestation.	
Uterine irritability.	
Cocaine abuse.	

Note: Presence of one or more major factors and/or two or more minor factors places client in high risk group.
Source: Reference 26. Printed with permission.

Assessment of Parental-Fetal Attachment

Assessing parental-fetal attachment may help to identify a family at risk for maladaptive behaviors in relation to the developmental tasks of pregnancy. The major developmental task for the family is achieving a strong sense of self (differentiation), while maintaining psychological and physical closeness (attachment). Another task is establishing a safe environment for the family unit.[27]

Major risk factors for maladaptive behaviors are unintended pregnancy, marital discord or family violence, sexually transmitted disease, limited finances, substance abuse, positive HIV status, and adolescence. Other risk factors include poor social support system and educational background, adverse pregnancy outcome, or conditions that interfere with the ability to reason effectively.[18,27,28] *All* women have the potential for maladaptive behaviors during pregnancy; therefore, interventions are directed toward reducing the effect of situations that lead to maladjustment.

Family assessment tools may provide a means for identifying women at risk for less than optimal maternal-fetal and maternal-infant attachment.[27] These tools can be found in listed reference.

- *The Family Environment Scale* uses self-reporting to assess the internal family milieu.
- *The Card Sort Procedure* measures how family members relate to one another through a group problem-solving task.
- *The Support System Questionnaire* assesses the support system within the family, assesses outside influences on the family, and identifies family members at perinatal risk.

Assessment of Environmental and Occupational Hazards

The environmental and occupational factors that place mother and fetus at risk for injury or death need to be identified. Women of childbearing age comprise a significant proportion of the U.S. work force. Women are exposed to chemicals and infectious agents, demanding labor, and often less than ideal working conditions. Assessment should be made of the possible exposure to teratogens, physical demands of employment, and the workplace environment.[18,29,30,31]

Teratogens are substances or disorders with the potential to alter the fetus permanently in form or function.[31] Strongly suspected teratogens include various drugs, chemicals, infectious agents, heavy metals such as lead, and selected maternal disorders. Often the effect is dose related; the effect is greatest during fetal organogenesis (see Chapter 17).

Physically intensive employment increases the likelihood of low birthweight and preterm labor and delivery. Standing for long periods; increased pulling, pushing, or lifting of more than 10–25 pounds; and decreased rest periods also increase these risks.[18,29] The physical setting needs to be assessed for risks of falling or being crushed; exposure to temperature extremes; and exposure to teratogens such as radiation, chemicals, or infectious agents.[32]

Recommended favorable working conditions for pregnant women include:

- Work only 8-hour shifts: no more than 48 hours per week, ideally less than 40 hours per week.
- Limit hours of work to between 6 A.M. and midnight.

- Take at least two 10-minute rest periods and one nutrition break per shift, with adequate rest facilities available.
- Avoid occupations that involve heavy lifting, hard physical labor, continuous standing, or constant moving about.
- Do not work in places where a good sense of balance is required for job safety, or where there is exposure to toxic substances.
- Be aware that substances permissible by state codes for a nonpregnant individual may be *unsafe* for a pregnant woman and a developing fetus. The Occupational Safety and Health Administration (OSHA) can answer questions about specific substances and situations (see Chapter 17).

PSYCHOSOCIAL ASSESSMENT AND INTERVENTIONS[33]

During the first trimester, assess the meaning of pregnancy to the client and the positive, negative, or ambivalent feelings she may have, particularly if her pregnancy is unplanned. Explore her feelings about this pregnancy, her economic concerns, and her level of anxiety. Validate the pregnancy with and help her to identify her support systems. Suggest childbirth education classes; begin anticipatory guidance counseling (see Chapter 17).

During the second trimester, assess the client's adaptation to pregnancy and to the body changes she has experienced. Explain how fetal growth/development and the client's own body/emotional changes will facilitate adaptation.

During the third trimester, determine how well the client is prepared for birth, delivery, and the physical needs of a newborn including infant feeding and child care needs. Explore her expectations about labor, birth, and the newborn—and her fears concerning motherhood, pain of labor, loss of control, and harm to herself or the fetus. Begin planning for postpartal contraception.

Domestic Violence[34,35]

Throughout pregnancy, assess for subtle and overt signs of physical, sexual and emotional abuse. The five questions Abuse Assessment Screen (Figure 16–3) may help to identify abused clients.

The incidence of abuse is high but often goes unreported. It is estimated that abuse occurs in 1 out of 6 pregnancies, often occurring/escalating initially during pregnancy. The risk/incidence of abuse increases in the presence of alcohol and substance abuse.

Abused women are less likely to seek prenatal care or follow medical advice. Abuse places the mother and fetus at risk for perinatal complications, injury, homicide, and suicide.

DIETARY ASSESSMENT1[1,12]

A well-balanced diet is essential to optimal nutrition for maternal well-being and fetal growth (see also Chapter 17). Requirements during pregnancy include daily servings of dairy products, meat products, fruits/vegetables, and grains/bread. Routine dietary supplements also are required during pregnancy. Mega vitamin/mineral supplements are to be avoided.

It is always desirable that maternal weight gain and fetal growth be adequate; that appropriate weight be achieved by the neonate, depending on gestation age; that labor and delivery do not occur preterm; and that the mother be normotensive with stable hemoglobin. However, inadequate nutrition may place the client at risk for having a low birthweight infant, preterm labor, pregnancy induced hypertension, and anemia with resulting sequelae.[1,12]

PREPARATION FOR SURGICAL INTERVENTION

Complications related to fetal distress and failure for labor to progress at delivery are the primary reasons for surgical intervention. Surgical options include cesarean section, episiotomy, and forceps birth.[15,18] Maternal medical conditions unrelated to pregnancy, such as appendicitis, also may necessitate surgery. Counsel clients at risk about the reasons for an episiotomy at delivery and the care involved; and discuss cesarean birth with clients whose medical conditions predispose them to this type of delivery. For those needing forceps delivery, instruction is given at the time of delivery. *Providing in-depth education concerning surgical intervention to clients not at risk may add to their anxiety level.*

1. Have you **ever** been emotionally or physically abused by your partner or someone important to you?

    YES ☐ NO ☐

2. **WITHIN THE LAST YEAR,**

    have you been hit, slapped, kicked, or otherwise physically hurt by someone?   YES ☐ NO ☐

    If YES, by whom?_____ Total number of times_____

3. Since you've been pregnant, were you hit, slapped, kicked, or otherwise

    physically hurt by someone?   YES ☐ NO ☐

    If YES, by whom?_____ Total number of times_____

MARK THE AREA OF INJURY ON THE BODY MAP. SCORE EACH INCIDENT ACCORDING TO THE FOLLOWING SCALE:

SCORE

1= Threats of abuse including use
   of a weapon

2= Slapping, pushing; no
   injuries and/or lasting pain

3= Punching, kicking, bruises,
   cuts and/or continuing pain

4= Beating up, severe
   contusions,
   burns, broken bones

5= Head injury, internal injury,
   permanent injury

6= Use of weapon; wound from
   weapon

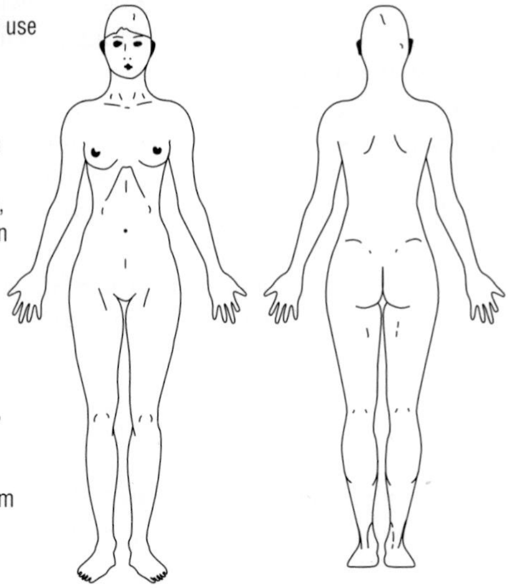

If any of the descriptions for the higher number apply, use the higher number.

4. **WITHIN THE LAST YEAR,**

    has anyone forced you to have sexual activities?   YES ☐ NO ☐

    If YES, who? _____ Total number of times _____

5. Are you afraid of your partner or anyone you listed above?   YES ☐ NO ☐

Developed by the Nursing Research Consortium on Violence and Abuse. Readers are encouraged to reproduce and use this assessment tool.

Figure 16–3. Abuse assessment screen. *(Source: Reprinted with permission from author, Barbara Parker, RN, Ph.D., professor University of Virginia, School of Nursing, Charlottesville, Virginia.)*

Cesarean Birth[18,26]

Any condition that prevents the safe passage of the fetus through the birth canal or that seriously compromises maternal-fetal well-being may be an indication for cesarean birth. Examples include breech and transverse presentations, maternal-fetal hemorrhage, fetal distress, active genital herpes infection, severely impaired maternal cardiac status, cephalopelvic disproportion, placenta previa, and placental abruption.

Implications. It is estimated that 1 out of 5 deliveries in the United States is by cesarean birth. Statistics vary regionally. Several factors may explain the increase that has occurred.

- Reduced parity with greater numbers of nulliparous women.
- Electronic fetal monitoring (EFM), which facilitates detection of fetal distress.
- Repeat cesarean deliveries, usually with prior classical incision.
- Fewer forceps deliveries.
- More advanced-age pregnancies.
- Greater threat and incidence of legal malpractice suits.

Surgery is done under regional or general anesthesia with combination cold-knife, electrocautery techniques. Vaginal birth after cesarean birth (VBAC) is common today, as most surgeons employ a low transverse uterine incision to deliver the infant. The vertical, or classical, incision requires cesarean birth for subsequent births, as the uterus is more likely to rupture during active labor.

Side Effects and Adverse Reactions. The side effects of a cesarean birth are related to infection, hemorrhage, embolus, injury to proximal organs, and anesthesia. Studies in maternal mortality statistics vary, with approximately 5–40 per 100,000 cesarean births. Select studies show substantially lower rates of maternal mortality related to the cesarean section itself.

Contraindications. Vaginal delivery is preferred in cases of maternal coagulopathies, or when the fetus has died or is too premature to survive outside the uterus.

Counseling. Inform the client about the procedure and its rationale, anesthesia, recovery, and post-operative care. Explain how the surgery will affect the newborn, breastfeeding, and activities of daily living. Also explain that signs of infection/complication will be monitored.

THE DEVELOPMENTAL STAGES OF PREGNANCY

Maternal role attainment is not an inevitable, instinctive event initiated by the act of birth; instead it is an active process requiring personal motivation. It is believed that the "roots" of this role develop during childhood. During pregnancy a woman actively works on assuming the behaviors she believes encompass the "ideal" mother.[27,36,37]

MAJOR THEORIES OF MATERNAL ROLE DEVELOPMENT

Two leading theorists in maternal role development are Reva Rubin and Regina Lederman.

Reva Rubin's contributions to maternity nursing provide valuable insights into the biopsychosocial experience of childbearing. Rubin developed a framework for the process of maternal role assumption in 1967, although she published from 1961 to 1984. Her early publications "Basic Maternal Behaviors" and "Maternal Touch" are considered classics in maternity nursing.[36]

Rubin's writings include concepts about body image, self-esteem, and thought process during pregnancy, as well as assumption of the maternal role prior to and after delivery.[36] Without the desire for children, there is no active motivation to assume a maternal role. Rubin identified maternal tasks and behaviors normally seen during the antepartum and postpartum periods. Assessment of those behaviors can be used to evaluate the mother's progress toward assumption of a maternal role (see Table 16–9).[27,36,37] Rubin concluded that if the mother perceived a threat to her pregnancy, such as HIV infection or miscarriage, then she was less likely to bond with her infant and therefore was at risk for poor attachment.

When Rubin made her initial observations of maternal behaviors, strong consumer participation in childbirth education and health care was in its infancy. Today, childbearing couples have the

TABLE 16–9. REVA RUBIN THEORY: THE ANTEPARTUM PHASE

Trimester	Maternal Task/Behavior	Nursing Significance
First	"Who me?" "Pregnant?" "Now?"	Question of identity—conception thought to be a surprise—resulting ambivalence related to the reality of pregnancy. Incorporation of concept of fetus into self. Acceptance of pregnancy/fetus by self and significant others.
Second	Seeking safe passage for self and child. Ensuring the acceptance of the child fetus. Protective behaviors by the mother for the child.	Acceptance of growing fetus by self, others. Willingness to "house" fetus even with body/role/ego changes. Passage of socially accepted values, behaviors, attitudes, skills from mother to child.
Third	Mother's binding-in to her unknown child. Learning to give of self.	"Binding-in" developed from initial maternal-fetal bonds to adult-child companionship. These bonds include fetal movements, maternal anatomic changes. Nurturant behaviors given from mother to child.

Source: References 27, 36, 37.

option of knowing the gender of their fetus, see their fetus through the technology of ultrasound, and are more knowledgeable and less passive than parents of previous generations. Ultimately, some of Rubin's observations may have less relevance for contemporary women, but they are a timeless framework for family-centered maternity care. Using Reva Rubin's three postpartum developmental phases, a mother's progress during the postpartum period may be assessed. (The three phases and their characteristic behaviors are described in Table 16–10.)[27,36,38]

Regina Lederman views maternal role assumption as identification with motherhood; namely, as part of the larger process of psychosocial development in pregnancy that includes taking the developmental step from being a woman without child to being a woman with child.[39] This process is a progressive change in thinking for the mother, away from concerns about self and more toward concern for the mother-infant unit. Two important factors come into play to achieve this goal: motivation and the degree of preparation for the mothering role.

According to Lederman, motivation for motherhood is reflected by the degree to which one expresses the interest and the ability to nurture and empathize with a child. This encompasses the perception of motherhood as a life fulfilling event.[39] The woman's motivation for pregnancy is questioned if her thoughts toward the child (fetus) are infrequent, aversive, avoided or denied, or if the woman desires the pregnancy but not the child.

Preparation for motherhood involves acquiring the ability to see oneself as a mother.[39] This is

TABLE 16–10. REVA RUBIN THEORY: THE POSTPARTUM PHASE

Phase	Behaviors
Taking in	Passive, receptive, dependent infant mode; sleep, food are paramount. Often thought to be a process of regeneration. Mother spends time claiming her infant, bringing the infant into her social fabric. Mother begins with initial touching activities: first fingertips then to whole-hand touching within days 1 to 5 postdelivery.
Taking hold	Increased autonomy, independence usually begin on third day postpartum. Characterized by accomplishing what *must* be done over the next 2 to 3 weeks of the postpartum period. Mother demonstrates mastery of her own body's functioning, readiness to master some of her many tasks of motherhood.
Letting go	Starts during second and third weeks postdelivery. Mother begins to separate herself from the symbiotic relationship she and her infant enjoyed during pregnancy/delivery. Prior to this point, guilt was predominate feeling for the mother when separated from her infant.

Source: References 27, 36, 38.

accomplished through *fantasizing/dreaming,* which is an arena for rehearsing motherhood skills. The woman relies on her life experiences of being nurtured, and on her ability to identify with other women in their positive role as mothers. According to Lederman, all women bring conflicts to a pregnancy. But if the conflicts are not resolved through preparation and bargaining during pregnancy, then the woman may find the motherhood role unrewarding, thereby increasing her feelings of inadequacy.

Lederman describes a woman's relationship with her own mother as the final aspect of maternal role development. The availability of the client's own mother, her acceptance of that pregnancy, her respect for the daughter's autonomy, and her willingness to share her previous childbearing/childrearing experiences all impact the outcome of preparation.[39]

Rubin's and Lederman's frameworks are generally considered compatible, although they use different names for similar concepts. Absence of these processes or inability to pass through them satisfactorily may impede the progress of maternal role development.[27,36,38] This recognition is fundamental for nursing assessment during pregnancy and the postpartum period.

Implications of Rubin's and Lederman's Theories

- Identify whether the client is at higher risk for maladaptation at initial and ongoing prenatal visits.
- Monitor the client's progress by observing for expected role behaviors.
- When maladaptive behaviors are identified, refer the client for appropriate counseling.

Preparation for Childbirth: Counseling and Classes

The prospect of having a problem-free pregnancy and healthy baby is aided by early and complete prenatal education. Maternal expectations of labor and delivery based on prenatal experience/knowledge are predictive of postpartum maternal-infant attachment. The primary goal of childbirth education classes is to reduce the fear-pain-tension cycle and make the childbirth experience a positive one—and thereby facilitate maternal-infant attachment.[14]

Prior to the 19th century, childbirth was a social event, centered in the home with family members and friends. That changed, but by the 1960s women began to question the extensive procedures and strong medications often used for hospital managed labor and delivery. Women began to change the rigid structure of medical practice.

Society was finally ready for the 1944 classic by Grantley Dick-Read, *Childbirth without Fear,* which espoused that the pain of labor could be eliminated by reducing the fear, apprehension, and tension associated with childbirth. The underlying principle behind childbirth education is that the woman can use skills and intellect to control her body during childbirth.[14,39]

STRATEGIES FOR PREPARATION[13,14,33]

In *childbirth preparation classes,* accurate information is provided about the physiological and psychological adaptations that occur during parturition. Only information pertinent to managing labor and delivery process is included. In *prenatal parenting classes,* on the other hand, discussions may include a variety of topics surrounding parenting. In addition, comprehensive formats may be presented as refresher courses. How many clients pursue some form of prenatal education with their first baby is not known.

The education may be sought in a traditional classroom, from a resource book at the library, or from group sessions organized by local health departments. Programs are also offered by hospitals, community agencies and groups, or individuals qualified to teach childbirth education. The participation of health care providers and obstetric staff nurses as educators is desirable to ensure continuity of care and consistency of childbirth preparation instruction (see Table 16–11). To help ensure that a client is adequately prepared for childbirth, the health care provider may implement various strategies.

- During the initial prenatal evaluation, encourage enrollment in a prenatal class.
- Provide the client with resources according to her assessed knowledge level and financial ability.

TABLE 16–11. SUBJECTS COMMONLY COVERED IN PRENATAL CLASSES

Anatomy and physiology of reproduction.

Physiological and psychological changes during pregnancy.

Sexuality during pregnancy.

Nutritional needs.

Teratogens and their impact on the fetus.

Danger signs in pregnancy.

Fetal growth and development.

Role of the father and siblings.

Prenatal exercise.

Signs and stages of labor.

Preparation for labor and delivery.

Cesarean delivery.

Postpartum support groups/parenting skills.

Infant care.

Infant safety/first aid/cardiopulmonary resuscitation (CPR).

Postpartum family planning

Source: References 14, 33, 39.

- Provide prenatal counseling on an individual basis during ongoing prenatal visits.
- Supply pertinent pamphlets regarding pregnancy concerns throughout antepartum care.
- Act as role model and client advocate to encourage the client's educational responsibility.
- Periodically evaluate the client's knowledge deficits and intervene when appropriate.

CHILDBIRTH METHODS

Some couples will need help choosing birth preparation classes; they may be confronted with many alternatives. Childbirth education classes, such as Bradley (partner coached) and Lamaze (psychoprophylactic) techniques serve the dual purpose of explaining the birth process and dispelling fears concerning labor and delivery.[14,34]

The Lamaze Method

Classes in the Lamaze method or "prepared childbirth classes" are the most popular. This method uses techniques that focus the mother's attention on breathing and relaxation exercises as well as massage.[14,34] Consequently, the perception of pain is lessened, as is the amount of medication needed for pain relief. The father's presence and active support during the birthing process can heighten the sense of family at the moment of birth, thereby increasing the perception of a positive birthing experience. Partner or coach involvement is a fundamental cornerstone of both methods.

The Bradley Method

The primary goal of the Bradley method is a completely unmedicated labor and delivery. The training techniques are directed toward the coach, not the mother. The coach is educated in massage/comfort techniques to use during labor and delivery.

Other Options

The Read method, or "natural" childbirth, is also based on relaxation and breathing technique; the Wright method, based on psychoprophylaxis but with less active breathing than that in the Lamaze method, is also called "new childbirth." Sheila Kitzinger's psychosexual method includes chest breathing and simultaneous abdominal release. Yoga and hypnosis are other techniques that are used.

In counseling the client regarding the many approaches to childbirth education, it is paramount to consider her readiness to learn, knowledge base, attitudes and fears about pregnancy, and the support systems available to her. It is an ongoing process, begun at the initial prenatal evaluation.

ADOLESCENT PREGNANCY

Adolescent pregnancy is usually defined as pregnancy occurring between the age of menarche and 19 years of age, but it also can be viewed in relation to emotional maturity and financial independence. Most adolescent pregnancy is unintended. Often adolescent mothers and their babies form a nontraditional family (nontraditional families are discussed later in this chapter). Perinatal/maternal morbidity is significantly higher in pregnancies of adolescent mothers, which is in part due to incomplete maternal growth and the increased psychological needs of adolescent women. "Magical" thinking, feelings of invincibility, and limited abstract thought processes contribute significantly to the incidence of unintended pregnancy.[18,28,33,40]

FACTS ABOUT ADOLESCENT PREGNANCY[18,28,33,40]

- Adolescent pregnancy can be related to cultural norms, peer interaction, immature cognitive abilities, psychological needs, increasing societal acceptance, unprotected coitus, birth control failure or misuse.
- It is estimated that 23 percent of females are sexually active by age 15; 71.4 percent by age 19.
- Less than 40 percent of sexually active adolescents attempt some form of birth control; use is often sporadic.
- Adolescents are typically sexually active for 6 to 12 months prior to seeking birth control services or choosing a method of contraception.
- Among 15- to 19-year-old sexually active women, 1 of 10 will become pregnant during a calendar year; among that group (estimated at 1 million), 39 percent will end their pregnancies in abortion. A significant number will conceive again shortly thereafter.
- Many young women deny signs and symptoms of pregnancy, feel embarrassed to admit their inability to use birth control, or feel embarrassed to use birth control.
- One in three pregnant adolescents will drop out of high school.
- Pregnant adolescents are less likely to seek early, regular prenatal care.
- As they age, women who give birth during adolescence have approximately half of the median family income noted in those who have their first child mid-twenties and older.
- One out of 5 pregnant adolescents experiences emotional, sexual, or physical abuse.

OBJECTIVE DATA

A physical exam will reveal changes similar to those seen during an adult physical exam, particularly during the breast, abdominal, and pelvic evaluations. Evaluate Tanner staging (see Chapter 5), as young adolescents may be physically immature, which would significantly impact growth and development in pregnancy. A final area of evaluation would be for evidence of eating disorders, substance abuse, or depression.[18,28]

DIFFERENTIAL MEDICAL DIAGNOSIS

Ectopic pregnancy, endometrial regression, polycystic ovary disease, immature hypothalamic-pituitary-gonadal axis with primary amenorrhea, secondary amenorrhea, pseudocyesis, anorexia/eating disorders, ovarian tumors.[1,14]

NURSING DIAGNOSES

Potential nursing diagnoses include those related to adult pregnancy (see list at the end of the chapter) as well as high risk for altered parenting.

PLAN

Pregnant adolescents, especially those younger than 16 years, are at risk for having low-birth-weight infants and preterm births. Moreover, they are at increased risk for cesarean births. Cephalopelvic disproportion may result from immature skeletal development of the pelvis. It remains the primary goal of the health care provider to promote the best possible pregnancy outcome through client evaluation and education. Therefore, focus education on general health maintenance and how pregnancy needs will change health status. The cognitive abilities of adolescents vary, however, as do their abilities to assimilate information. Foster behaviors that will promote independence in adolescent development.[28,40]

Encourage the client to maintain peer interactions and continue to meet educational needs. Help her to clarify the father's role, make use of family support systems, and set realistic goals. Assess the client's cognitive abilities (e.g., concrete versus abstract). Encourage behaviors that foster parenting skills such as attending classes for this, and demonstration of what has been learned. Be aware of the increased rate of suicide among adolescents, the risk of substance abuse, and the need to promote a nonjudgmental atmosphere in which the client may express views about the pregnancy.

Health care providers need to assess their own value system, particularly to avoid stereotyping. The foundation for a trusting relationship is based on mutual acceptance, caring, and a nonjudgmental approach. Assisting the client to achieve the developmental tasks of adolescence, such as financial, emotional, and physical independence, is the underlying task for the health provider.[28,40] Remember that despite increasing public awareness and concern, adolescents continue to need support from the community in the areas of wellness, education, finance, and family planning.

MEDICATION

Stress the importance of *no* medication use without the consent of a health care provider.

DIET

The adolescent diet is notoriously inadequate. Because of the increased risk for inadequate nutrition, it is imperative to stress normal, adequate nutrition and the value of daily prenatal vitamins and iron supplementation. Educate the client on what constitutes appropriate nutritional choices. Changing body image and the increased demands of fetal growth and development place adolescent mothers at further risk for eating disorders. Careful periodic assessment during prenatal care will aid the health care provider in early detection of inadequate nutrition.

Adolescent dietary needs include 38–50 kcal/per kg of body weight, and 1.5–1.7 grams of protein per kilogram of body weight per day is recommended. A 25- to 30-pound weight gain depending on prepregnant weight is recommended.[28,33] Encourage a balanced diet from the food pyramid, and limit nonnutritional foods or snacks. Instruction in good nutrition is related to maternal/fetal growth needs and should reinforce the need for adherence on the part of the adolescent mother.

SMOKING

Although the harmful effects of smoking cigarettes are well documented, adolescents continue to smoke at alarming rates; adolescent females smoke more than adolescent males. Cigarette smoking is highly correlated to early sexual activity; it is often seen as a display of "adult" behavior, rebellion, or peer pressure.[26,40]

Smoking increases the risk of spontaneous abortion, preterm labor and birth, hypertension, placenta previa/abruptio, low birthweight infants, perinatal death, Sudden Infant Death Syndrome (SIDS), and long term developmental delays in offspring.[15,28] Direct counseling strategies toward decreasing or cessation of smoking and investigating support groups for that purpose. Education must be appropriate for the client's knowledge level and address both the immediate and long term impact of tobacco on the client and her offspring. Another strategy to help a client stop smoking is to encourage other outlets, such as chewing gum, sugarless candy, handiwork, and exercise.

SELF-CARE

Emphasize proper hygiene techniques. Advise the client to avoid contact sports but maintain physical activity by walking, swimming, and participating in prenatal exercise classes. Stress the importance of not consuming chemical substances during pregnancy without knowledge or direction of a health care provider.

EDUCATION

Encourage the client to remain in school during pregnancy or to obtain her general equivalency diploma. Home tutoring and schools for pregnant adolescents are also viable options, although peer interaction is decreased.

FINANCES

Financial concerns are heightened if education is interrupted as a result of pregnancy. Three areas of assessment may be helpful: insurance coverage; government assistance through such programs as Women/Infant/Children (WIC) or Aid to Dependent Children (ADC); job benefits (if employed).

FAMILY PLANNING

Frequent conception is common with adolescent mothers; as many as 40 to 50 percent conceive again within 24 months. Discuss motivation, maturity, and physical and financial practicality of contraceptive methods. Advise the client to choose a reliable method prior to completion of pregnancy. Explore the client's options for contraception, sexual responsibility, and risk behaviors for sexually transmitted disease.

FOLLOW-UP

Adolescent mothers are at higher risk for inflicting child abuse, being victims of domestic violence, conceiving frequently, contracting sexually transmitted disease (including HIV), having education disrupted, and having maladaptive peer interaction. Evaluate such situations when they become evident and initiate intervention in areas of greatest concern.

DELAYED PREGNANCY

Any woman who completes her pregnancy on or after her 35th birthday is referred to as a mother of advanced maternal age.[1] Extensive literature in medicine and genetics has debated whether any significant risks are associated with childbearing after age 35. These risks generally stem from pre-existing medical conditions, infertility, chromosomal abnormalities, or nutritional deficits.[41] With proper control of underlying medical conditions, most women can have successful pregnancy outcomes. The highest absolute risk and sharpest rise in maternal mortality, however, occurs after the age of 40. Older gravidas are more likely to experience gestational diabetes, preeclampsia, placenta previa, pulmonary embolus and exacerbation of underlying medical conditions. The woman over 40 is at increased risk for cesarean and operative vaginal delivery, as well as ectopic pregnancy, spontaneous abortion, multiple gestation, preterm labor, abnormal labor patterns, and neonatal intensive care unit admissions.[41,42]

Women may delay childbearing for medical or economic reasons, or because of career or personal relationship choices. By postponing childbearing, women have increased their life experiences and psychological stability.[43] This may better equip them to rear children. A major influence on a woman's parenting behavior is the type and number of roles she has undertaken in life. Taking on multiple roles is thought to be either self-enhancing (promoting self-esteem and personal fulfillment) or personally divisive (increasing stress and anxiety).[43] Older mothers may particularly cherish the ability to have children, and if these mothers have higher salaries they may be better able to provide for their children financially.[43] Society encourages increased paternal involvement; consequently, the financial and emotional needs of parenting are shared more by both partners. Furthermore, postponing parenthood or choosing not to have children has gained acceptance, as well as delaying subsequent pregnancies.

Delayed parenting is probably influenced to the greatest degree by the increasing availability of effective contraception. Advances in contraceptive techniques have enabled greater freedom to time the birth of the first child. An additional reason for delayed childbearing may be the steady increase in late or second marriages. Moreover, for women who previously suffered from infertility, the prospect of bearing a child has improved with advances in reproductive technology.

HISTORY AND PHYSICAL EXAMINATION

For women whose pregnancy occurs later in life, the history and physical examination are the same as for other pregnant clients. Devote particular attention to nutritional and immunization status; reproductive, medical, occupational, and social histories; chemical substance use; and genetic concerns. Offer the client referral for genetic counseling and a review of available genetic testing. Identify any occupational hazards.

DIAGNOSTIC TESTS AND METHODS

The minimum standard tests are needed; medical conditions may require additional individual assessment. The American College of Obstetricians and Gynecologists (ACOG) recommends genetic testing for all women who are 35 years of age or older at the time of delivery. If the client elects genetic testing after counseling has been completed, scheduling for amniocentesis or chorionic villus sampling follows.

PLAN

Initiate discussions of pregnancy and encourage the client's questions. Several subjects may require review and counseling.[43]

- Normal physiology of pregnancy.
- Pertinent medical history findings.
- Genetic concerns and the testing available.
- Occupational hazards; exposure to teratogens.
- Nutrition and weight control.
- Warning signs in pregnancy; client do's and don'ts.
- Substance use/abuse.
- Exercise, travel, and leisure activities.
- Sexuality.

Make referrals where appropriate and encourage the client to explore educational resources within the community (e.g., prenatal classes). Tailor follow-up visits to pertinent medical findings and individual needs.

NONTRADITIONAL FAMILIES

The American family has made several remarkable changes in the past 25 years. Today's American families include the "typical" nuclear family and nontraditional families, including one parent households, same sex parents, single-by-choice parents, unmarried heterosexual couples living together, and those choosing to remain childfree. These patterns are the result of profound social and demographic changes in the United States and are becoming increasingly accepted. The contraceptive revolution of the 1960s greatly influenced family structure by changing the role of women. Selective fertility has played a fundamental role in economic shifts within households.

THE RISKS

Increased stress and maladaptive behaviors are reported among many nontraditional families. For health care providers, particular attention to the client's lifestyle choices may help in identifying her particular needs prior to pregnancy. Often women in nontraditional families have greater financial, education, and legal concerns. They may make many requests of their health care provider

or they may feel reluctant to share their private lives. As always, the establishment of a trusting relationship is vital for both health care provider and client.

Though all behaviors cross boundaries, a higher incidence of the following maladaptive behaviors has been reported among some nontraditional mothers.[34,40,44,45]

- Suicide (adolescents).
- Alcoholism/chemical abuse (lesbians, adolescents).
- Greater dependency on welfare monies (adolescents).
- Domestic violence (nontraditional families).
- Higher incidence of noncompliance with health care advice due to mistrust of "the system" (lesbians, adolescents).

HISTORY AND PHYSICAL EXAMINATION

History taking during the initial workup is important in identifying nontraditional family units. Several areas need to be explored.

- Sexual preference/practices.
- Legal status of relationship (i.e., paternity).
- Length of relationship and overall support systems for pregnancy.
- Employment setting, income, and how loss of income would impact pregnancy.
- Social ramifications of role modeling as a parent in a nontraditional household.
- Dietary practices (provide nutritional counseling and referral where appropriate).[23,45]

During the initial prenatal examination, carefully observe for signals of physical or chemical abuse (e.g., bruises, unusual marks, history of numerous bone fractures or excessive "accidents"). Women in nontraditional lifestyles may be at risk for maladaptive behaviors.

DIFFERENTIAL MEDICAL DIAGNOSES

Intrauterine pregnancy, substance abuse, dysfunctional adolescence, battering.[1,45]

PLAN

Counseling, support, anticipatory guidance, and education are among the psychosocial interventions.[14,15,44]

- Counsel the client about feelings of anger, hostility, fear, anxiety, aversion, and ambivalence throughout the pregnancy.
- Provide a calm, supportive, nonjudgmental environment for improved communication.
- Give anticipatory guidance regarding common stressors of pregnancy, both physical and emotional.
- Counsel about general wellness issues such as hygiene and breast self-exam (BSE), anatomy and physiology, and prevention of sexually transmitted diseases and HIV infection.
- Provide resource/referral information when domestic violence or substance abuse is a potential or identified risk, or when financial concerns are great.

FOLLOW-UP

Periodically throughout pregnancy and postpartum, reevaluate the client for continued risk. In addition, periodically evaluate the strength of the client's support systems.

SUBSTANCE ABUSE SCREENING IN PREGNANCY*

Screening is done to detect the use or misuse of any substance known or suspected to exert a deleterious effect on the client or her fetus.[46] The effects of specific drugs are difficult to assign, because often multiple drugs are used and nutritional status is poor. The use of multiple drugs is associated with intrauterine growth retardation (IUGR) and increased anomalies. Factors that may impact a drug's effects are duration of use, dosage, timing in gestation, and use of other drugs.[46,47] Ideally, counseling a client concerning substance abuse begins prior to conception. Open discussions may make a client aware of the need to prevent pregnancy and to obtain counseling if necessary. Clients who use substances only occasionally need to be aware of the potential teratogenic effect of one exposure.

Ascertain whether the mother and fetus have been exposed to harmful substances, assess the mother's need for counseling, and design intervention that targets and eliminates the abuse and decreases potential harm to mother and fetus. Being nonjudgmental is a key to success; a client is more apt to trust and reveal patterns of abuse if the health provider does not display dismay or disgust.

Initially the goal of the health care provider is to prevent complications of pregnancy and in utero exposure, thereby minimizing permanent sequelae. Behavioral problems, learning disabilities, and physical anomalies may be present in the newborn. If multigenerational drug use is to be prevented, a link in the chain of addiction must be broken. Getting the client into treatment may help to identify her needs as an individual, teach her how to cope with the stresses that lead to drug use, and perhaps introduce skills for coping and potential parenting. In turn, these measures may enhance parent-child bonding and reduce the incidence of emotional, physical, or sexual abuse and neglect, which are often a common experience among children of substance abusers.[31,48,49]

It is important to stop drug abuse during pregnancy to prevent the potential for parents to give their infant or child drugs in food or a bottle as a means of consoling, or for a mother to breast-feed her infant while continuing to use illicit drugs. Accidental ingestion of drugs may occur if drugs are in the house. Current studies do not suggest that drug or alcohol use by the father of the baby influences the outcome of the pregnancy. Concern over chromosomal damage caused by hallucinogens and cannabinoids is also unwarranted. Drug use by the father, however, may be indicative of other factors that adversely affect outcomes.[46]

SCREENING QUESTIONS

The questions below may aid the health care provider evaluate a client who is at risk for substance abuse during pregnancy. Using accepting terminology may encourage honest answers without fear of reproach. Some clients may be offended by assumption of use, however, in terms such as "How often do you use."

1. Have you ever used recreational drugs? If so, what, when, and how much?

*The author wishes to acknowledge the contributions of Marion Fuqua, RNC, MS, OGNP to this section.

2. Have you ever taken a prescription drug other than as intended? If so, what, when, and how much?
3. Have you used any legal or recreational drugs during this pregnancy? What, when, and how much?
4. How often do you drink alcohol? What, when, how much?
5. How often do you smoke cigarettes? How many per day?
6. What are your feelings about drug use during pregnancy?

ASSESSMENT

The following overview briefly describes only a few side effects of specific drug use. Further reading is encouraged concerning other substances and sequelae documented in research.

Smoking

Smoking increases the risk of spontaneous abortion, preterm labor and delivery, maternal hypertension, placenta previa, abruptio placenta, low birthweight infant, perinatal death, and possibly long term developmental delays in offspring.[15,18,28,50,51] The perinatal death rate among infants of smoking mothers is 20–35 percent higher.[15] Central apnea, intrauterine growth retardation, and increased incidence of childhood respiratory infections have been noted.[52] Nicotine reduces fetal blood flow, and this may be related to the transient decrease in fetal movement associated with maternal smoking. There is an association between maternal smoking and increased risk of congenital urinary tract anomalies.[53] Alcohol and smoking combined increases the risk for adverse perinatal outcomes. They both are frequently associated with use of other chemicals in pregnancy.[15] Prenatal exposure and passive exposure after birth may be a risk factor for sudden infant death syndrome (SIDS).[54]

In counseling a client, present measures to decrease smoking cues and behaviors; provide information about support groups for smoking cessation; stress the immediate and long term impact of tobacco use on her and her fetus; encourage her to seek appropriate outlets to replace smoking, such as chewing gum, eating sugarless candy, doing handiwork or exercise. Use of nicotine gum is contraindicated in pregnancy. The adverse effects of smoking appear to be dose related. The pregnant client who smokes 20 or more cigarettes per day may benefit from a nicotine transdermal patch. Circulating levels of nicotine from smoking cigarettes would be reduced as would exposure to other toxins found in cigarettes such as carbon monoxide.[51]

Counsel the patient that smoking cessation may decrease the risk of infant and fetal mortality by 10 to 50 percent. The greatest impact is seen if cessation occurs in the first trimester.[51]

Cocaine

Decreased plasma cholinesterase activity in the pregnant woman, fetus, and newborn increases the risk of cocaine toxicity. Cocaine use produces vasoconstriction, tachycardia, and hypertension in both the mother and fetus.[15,31] Uteroplacental insufficiency may result secondary to reduced uterine blood flow and placental perfusion. Studies suggest that perinatal cocaine use increases the risk for spontaneous abortion, preterm labor with rupture of membranes and delivery, intrauterine growth retardation, intrauterine fetal distress and demise, seizures, withdrawal, cerebral infarcts, and complications of the neonatal course. Cocaine may increase the risk of placental abruption, uterine rupture, SIDS, and congenital anomalies.[15,26,31,46]

Alcohol

Excessive alcohol use remains a major public health issue in the United States. Underreporting of alcohol intake makes it difficult to estimate the rate of alcohol use in pregnancy.[31] Maternal-fetal effects of alcohol usage appear to be dose related. Fetal alcohol syndrome (FAS) is generally thought to occur in infants born to women who consume six standard drinks per day and is estimated to occur in 1–2/1000 live births. Characteristics of FAS include craniofacial dysmorphia, intrauterine growth retardation, microcephaly, and congenital anomalies such as limb abnormalities and cardiac defects. Long-term sequelae include postnatal growth retardation, attention deficits, delayed reaction time, and poor scholastic performance. FAS is the most common cause of mental retardation in the United States.

Other adverse outcomes of alcohol usage in pregnancy include intrauterine fetal demise and an increased rate of spontaneous abortion.[15,31,46] Fetal alcohol effects (FAE) are less severe and are noted in those consuming two to six standard drinks per day. Though some studies failed to demonstrate adverse consequences with fewer than two standard drinks per day, no known safe threshold for alcohol consumption exists. Alcohol and smoking combined have an additive risk for adverse perinatal outcomes.[46]

LSD

Usage of lysergic acid diethylamide in pregnancy is not known to increase perinatal morbidity or mortality. Long-term effects on development, however, are not known.[15,26]

Opiates/Narcotics

Opiates such as heroin may induce intense addiction in both mother and neonate. Neonatal withdrawal occurs in up to 95 percent of neonates exposed in utero.[15]

An increased incidence of sudden infant death syndrome (SIDS) has been found among these infants.[15] Intrauterine growth retardation, increased fetal distress, and persistently small fetal head circumference have also been noted.[48,52]

Though not teratogenic alone, opiates may become so when "cut" with other substances. Reported complications in addicts also include preeclampsia, premature rupture of membranes, placental abruption, and meconium staining.[47,48] When compared with drug free children, opiate exposed children had deficits ranging from poor motor performance to hyperactivity and impulsiveness.[49]

A woman's withdrawal from opiates has been associated with fetal demise.[48] Methadone substitution has been successful during pregnancy but must be used in a closely supervised treatment program.[48] Narcotic antagonists, such as Narcan® (Naloxone), Nubaine® (Nalbuphine) and Stadol® (Butorphanol) (frequently given in labor), can pre-

cipitate withdrawal symptoms. Narcan® may be used to reverse narcotic overdose.[15]

Methamphetamines

Methamphetamines produce some of the same effects as cocaine, such as increased risk for abruption, hemorrhage, preterm labor, eclampsia, increased perinatal mortality, fetal distress, and intrauterine growth retardation. Evidence exists that exposure may also increase the incidence of cerebral hemorrhage, infarction, or cavitation. Use of methamphetamines does not increase risk of congenital defects.[46,47]

Marijuana

In the general population, marijuana is the most frequently used illicit drug. Fetal levels are several times lower than maternal. Use of marijuana is highly correlated with use of alcohol and cigarettes. Usage may lead to preterm delivery and intrauterine growth retardation, however marijuana is not considered teratogenic.[15]

Organic Solvents/Aromatic Hydrocarbons

Organic solvents/aromatic hydrocarbons (AHC) are present in paints, glue, enamel, varnish, lacquer, and resins. They are easily absorbed through the skin, lungs, gastrointestinal tract, and easily cross the placenta. Exposure may occur in the workplace or be recreational ("huffing" or "sniffing"). Toluene is the most popular AHC for this purpose. Usage during pregnancy may lead to intrauterine growth retardation, microcephaly, hydrocephaly, limb anomalies, and craniofacial dysmorphia similar to FAS. Toluene exposure places the mother and fetus at risk for hyperchloremic metabolic acidosis.[15,46,55]

Physical Examination

The physical examination of a woman abusing a chemical substance may reveal fresh needle or track marks, a dazed appearance, inappropriate behavior or affect, extreme agitation or stupor, frequent conjunctivitis, tremors, flecks of paint around the mouth and nose, fetal/maternal tachycardia, or poor maternal weight gain (or weight loss) not attributed to underlying maternal disease. (See chapters 18 and 23 for evaluation, diagnosis, and treatment.)

Plan

Client counseling must continue into the postpartum period. During that time, her problem may worsen if the infant is not feeding, sleeping only for short intervals, crying shrilly, difficult to console, and avoiding eye contact. For some women addicts, fear of legal action may deter them from getting any form of prenatal care, and they may choose to forgo hospital delivery. Recidivism is high.[15,46,56]

A drug screen should be done to identify all drugs that a client is using since multiple drug usage is common. Assist the client to enroll in a drug rehabilitation program that offers her ease of accessibility and provides optimum social support. (Be aware that resources for treating pregnant substance abusers are often limited and have long waiting lists.) Management includes dietary counseling, ideally by a nutritionist. The client should be seen perhaps every one to two weeks and begin non-stress tests by 30 weeks' gestation. Serial ultrasounds are indicated to assess fetal growth patterns and placental health.

Constant encouragement and motivation are required to reinforce the need for compliance. Be honest about drug effects, but do not humiliate the client. Be open and direct with questions while being supportive of her efforts. Some women do not see their infant as part of themselves, nor do they care to. Most, however, genuinely do not want to harm their child. Consequently, those who can only focus on the present may benefit from counseling on the immediate effects of substance use on both mother and baby. Discussion of long-term effects may heighten compliance and promote a sense of maternal responsibility for the fetus and infant. The mother may consider her own needs first when she is making a decision about continuing to use drugs.[56] Most importantly, clients need to understand and value consistent prenatal care.

NURSING DIAGNOSES

The following nursing diagnoses are representative of those used in the health care plan of some pregnant women. This list, however, is by no means inclusive.[57]

- Activity intolerance.
- Anxiety.
- Body image disturbance.
- Constipation.
- Decisional conflict.
- Denial, ineffective.
- Family coping compromised, disabling, ineffective.
- Family processes altered.
- Family coping, potential for growth.
- Fatigue.
- Fear.
- Grieving, anticipatory.
- Health seeking behaviors.
- Hopelessness.
- Incontinence.
- Individual coping ineffective.
- Knowledge deficit.
- Noncompliance.
- Nutrition altered, less or more than body requirements.
- Parenting role conflict.
- Parenting altered.
- Personal identity disturbance.
- Physical mobility impairment.
- Powerlessness.
- Protection altered.
- Role performance altered.
- Self-esteem disturbance.
- Sexual performance altered.
- Sleep pattern disturbance.
- Social interaction impaired.
- Social isolation.
- Stress.
- Violence, high risk for, self-directed or directed at others.

REFERENCES

1. Scott, J., DiSaio, P., Hammond, C., & Spellacy, W. (1994). *Danforth's obstetrics and gynecology* (2nd ed.). Philadelphia: Lippincott.
2. Maloni, J. et al. (1996). Transforming prenatal care: Reflections on the past and present with implications for the future. *Journal of Obstetric, Gynecologic and Neonatal Nursing, 25,* 17–23.
3. Bushy, A. (1992). Preconception health promotion: Another approach to improve pregnancy outcomes. *Public Health Nursing, 9,* 10–14.
4. Cefalo, R., & Moos, M. K. (1995). Preconceptional health care: A practical guide (2nd ed.). St. Louis: Mosby.
5. ACOG Committee. (1995). *ACOG technical bulletin: Preconceptional care* (No. 205). Washington, DC: American College of Obstetrics and Gynecology.
6. Davis, M., & Akridge, K. (1987). The effects of promoting intrauterine attachment in primiparas on post delivery attachment. *Journal of Obstetric, Gynecologic and Neonatal Nursing, 16,* 430–437.
7. Bushy, A., & Graner, R. (1990). Preconceptional education: A program of community health nurses. *Family and Community Health, 13,* 82–84.
8. Swan, L., & Apgar, B. (1995). Preconceptual obstetric risk assessment and health promotion. *American Family Physician, 51,* 1875–1885.
9. Murphy, P. (1992). Periconceptional supplementation with folic acid: Does it prevent neural tube defects? *Journal of Nurse Midwifery, 37,* 25–32.
10. Werler, M., et al. (1996). Prepregnant weight in relation to risk of neural tube defects. *Journal of the American Medical Association, 275,* 1089–1092.
11. Shaw, M., et al. (1996). Risk of neural tube defect-affected pregnancies among obese women. *Journal of the American Medical Association, 275,* 1093–1096.
12. Luke, B., et al. (1993). *Clinical maternal-fetal nutrition.* Boston: Little, Brown.
13. Pillitteri, Adele. (1995). Maternal and child health nursing (2nd ed.). Philadelphia: J. B. Lippincott.
14. American College of Obstetrics and Gynecology. (1992). *Guidelines for perinatal care.* Washington, DC: Author.
15. Niswander, K. (1994). *Manual of obstetrics: Diagnosis and therapy* (4th ed.). Boston: Little, Brown.
16. Zalar, M. (1976). Sexual counseling for pregnant couples. *Maternal Child Nursing, 2,* 176–181.
17. Mims, F., & Swenson, M. (1980). *Sexuality: A nursing perspective.* New York: McGraw-Hill.
18. Cunningham, G., MacDonald, P., & Gant, N. (1993). *Williams obstetrics* (19th ed.). Norwalk, CT: Appleton & Lange.
19. Mead, P., & Larsen, J. (1996). Guidelines for preventing perinatal GBS infection. *Contemporary OB/GYN, 41,* 83–94.
20. Hatcher, R., Stewart, F., Trussell, J., Kowal, D., Guest, F., Stewart, G., & Cates, W. (1994–1996). *Contraceptive technology* (16th ed.). New York: Irvington.
21. Gomella, L., (1993). *Clinicians pocket reference* (7th ed.). Norwalk, CT: Appleton & Lange.
22. Chernecky, C., Krech, R., & Berger, B. (1993). *Laboratory tests and diagnostic procedures.* Philadelphia: W. B. Saunders.
23. Mishell, R., & Brenner, P. (1994). *Management of common problems in obstetrics and gynecology* (3rd ed.). Boston: Blackwell.
24. Mange, E., & Mange, A. (1994). *Basic human genetics.* Sunderland: Sinauer Associates Inc.
25. Simpson, J. (1987). *ACOG technical bulletin: Antenatal diagnosis of genetic disorder* (No. 108). Washington, DC: American College of Obstetrics and Gynecology.
26. Creasy, R., & Resnick, R. (1994). *Maternal-fetal medicine: Principles and practice* (3rd ed.). Philadelphia: Saunders.
27. Sherwen, L. (1987). *Psychosocial dimensions of the pregnant family.* New York: Springer.
28. Goldstein, P., (1990). *ACOG technical bulletin: Adolescent obstetric-gynecologic client* (No. 145). Washington, DC: American College of Obstetrics and Gynecology.
29. Keleher, K. (1991). Occupational health: How work environments can affect reproductive capacity and outcome. *Nurse Practitioner, 16,* 23–37.
30. Keleher, K. (1995). Environmental assessment of the home, community, and workplace. *Journal of Nurse-Midwifery, 40,* 88–96.
31. Paul, M. (1993). *Occupational and environmental reproductive hazards.* Baltimore: Williams & Wilkins.
32. Jones, J. M., Cox, A. R., Levy, E. Y., & Thompson, C. E. (1984). *Women's health management: Guidelines for nurse practitioners.* Englewood Cliffs, NJ: Prentice Hall.
33. Sherwen, L., et al. (1995). *Nursing care of the childbearing family* (2nd ed.). Norwalk, CT: Appleton & Lange.
34. McFarlane, J., & Parker, B. (1994). Preventing abuse during pregnancy: An assessment and intervention protocol. *Maternal Child Nursing, 19,* 321–324.
35. Mayer, L. (1995). The severely abused woman in obstetric and gynecologic care—Guidelines for recognition and management. *Journal of Reproductive Medicine, 40,* 13–18.

36. Gay, J., Edgil, A., & Douglas, A. (1988). Reva Rubin revisited. *Journal of Obstetric Gynecologic and Neonatal Nursing, 17,* 394–399.

37. Rubin, R. (1984). *Maternal identity and the maternal experience.* New York: Springer.

38. Ament, L. (1990). Maternal task of the puerperium reidentified. *Journal of Obstetric Gynecologic and Neonatal Nursing, 19,* 330–335.

39. Lederman, R. (1996). *Psychosocial adaptation in pregnancy* (2nd ed.). Englewood Cliffs, NJ: Prentice Hall.

40. Jannke, S. (1996). Teen pregnancy. *Childbirth Educator* (2nd quarter), 14–16, 37.

41. O'Reilly-Green, C., & Cohen, W. (1993). Pregnancy in women aged 40 and older. *Obstetrics and Gynecology, 87,* 917–922.

42. Bianco, A., et. al. (1996). Pregnancy outcome at age 40 and older. *Obstetrics and Gynecology, 87,* 917–922.

43. Harker, L., & Thorpe, K. (1992). The last egg in the basket? Elderly primiparity: A review of findings. *Birth, 19,* 23–29.

44. Carr, P., et al. (1995). *The medical care of women.* Philadelphia: W. B. Saunders Company.

45. Ziedenstein, L. (1990). Gynecological and childbearing needs of lesbians. *Journal of Nurse Midwifery, 35,* 10–18.

46. Koren, G. (1994). *Maternal-fetal toxicology* (2nd ed.). New York: Marcel Dekker.

47. Gilstrap, L., & Little, B. (1992). *Drugs and pregnancy.* New York: Elsevier.

48. Siney, C. (1995). *Pregnant drug addict.* Cheshire: Books for Midwives Press.

49. Bays, J. (1990). Substance abuse and child abuse. *Pediatric Clinics of North America, 37,* 881–891.

50. ACOG Committee. (1993). *ACOG technical bulletin: Smoking and reproductive health* (No. 180). Washington, DC: American College of Obstetrics and Gynecology.

51. Zagon, I., & Slotkin, T. (1992). *Maternal substance abuse and the developing nervous system.* San Diego, CA: Academic Press Inc.

52. De-Kyn, Li., et al. (1996). Maternal smoking during pregnancy and the risk of congenital urinary tract anomalies. *American Journal of Public Health, 86,* 249–252.

53. Stewart, D., & Streiner, D. (1995). Cigarette smoking during pregnancy. *Canadian Journal of Psychiatry, 40,* 603–607.

54. Blair, P., et al. (1996). Smoking and sudden infant death syndrome. *British Medical Journal, 313,* 180–181.

55. Arnold, G., et al. (1994). Toluene embryopathy: Clinical delineation and developmental follow-up. *Pediatrics, 93,* 216–220.

56. Poland, M., et al. (1993). Punishing pregnant users: Enhancing the flight from care. *Drug and Alcohol Dependency, 31,* 199–203.

57. Carpenito, L. J. (1991). *Handbook of nursing diagnosis* (4th ed.). Philadelphia: Lippincott Company.

CHAPTER 17

PROMOTING A HEALTHY PREGNANCY

Maryellen C. Remich

The issues of concern to pregnant women involve safety, comfort, and uncertainty about what to expect during pregnancy, labor, and delivery.

Highlights

- Nutrition and Weight Gain
- Immunization
- Common Complaints
- Anticipatory Guidance
    - Chemical Use, Radiation
    - The Workplace
    - Sexual Activity
    - Exercise
    - Dental Care, Bathing
    - Travel
    - Accidents, Blows to the Abdomen
    - Infant Care
    - Sibling Rivalry
    - Family Planning
- Danger Signs: First, Second, and Third Trimesters
- Initial Assessment in Labor

▶ INTRODUCTION

The ultimate goal of pregnancy is the birth of a healthy infant into a healthy and nurturing family who can provide for his or her physical, psychological, emotional, and spiritual needs. During pregnancy, many normal physiological changes lead to discomfort or concern for the mother. Health care providers must differentiate between normal and pathological changes, educate clients about changes, and help them to recognize and respond appropriately to signs of pathology and labor. In addition, health care providers need to individualize client education about prenatal nutrition and weight gain.

NUTRITION AND WEIGHT GAIN

Good nutrition before and during pregnancy decreases the risks of significant infant health problems, such as premature birth, low birthweight, malformations, and inadequate cell development. Pregnant women with poor dietary habits are at increased risk for anemia, preeclampsia, obesity, and osteoporosis with associated morbidity and mortality. Women who are underweight or who gain little weight during pregnancy are more likely to have a small-for-gestational-age infant.[1] Women who are obese or whose weight gain is excessive are at risk for having an infant with a neural tube defect,[2,3] hypertension, and diabetes. Ideally, issues of nutrition and weight gain should be addressed during preconception counseling (see Chapter 16). Because most women are highly motivated to eat properly during pregnancy, the nutrition instruction that they receive during pregnancy could result in positive and sustained dietary changes for the entire family.

SUBJECTIVE DATA

Several points are assessed during the first prenatal interview and reassessed as necessary at subsequent visits.

- Nutrition knowledge.
- A recall of the client's diet, ideally 7-day, though 24-hour is often more attainable.
- Food storage and preparation capacities.

- Portion of income spent for food.
- Food buying practices.
- Cultural and religious preferences.
- Food aversions or allergies (e.g., lactose intolerance).
- Meanings attached to eating (e.g., celebration).
- Prepregnancy weight; and body mass index (see Figure 17–1).
- Activity level and any change since pregnancy.
- Lactation during or just prior to pregnancy.
- Reproductive age (number of years menstruating).
- Gravity and parity (two or more pregnancies within 2 years or five or more total deliveries increase risk of perinatal and maternal health problems, e.g., anemia).
- Megavitamin or supplemental vitamin use.
- Nicotine, alcohol, or drug use.
- Psychosocial disorders (e.g., depression, bulimia) that may affect food intake.
- Discomforts from pregnancy (e.g., dyspepsia) that may affect food intake.
- Complications during past pregnancies (e.g., small-for-gestational-age neonate, preterm delivery, perinatal loss, gestational diabetes).[4]
- Maternal nutritional risk factor (see Table 17–1).

OBJECTIVE DATA

Physical Examination

Table 17–2 describes clinical signs that may indicate nutritional deficiency and require additional workup.

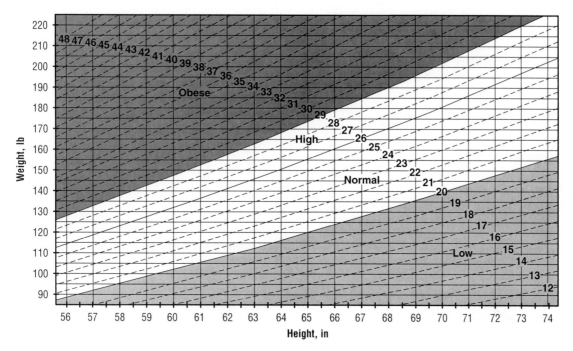

Figure 17–1. Chart for Estimating Body Mass Index (MBI) Category and BMI. To find BMI category (e.g., obese), find the point where the woman's height and weight intersect. To estimate BMI, read the bold number on the dashed line that is closest to this point. *(Source: Courtesy of the Food and Nutrition Board, Institute of Medicine. Copyright 1992 by the National Academy of Sciences, Washington, DC.)*

Abnormal weight gain patterns (see Figure 17–2), an increase in blood pressure, and non-dependent edema are additional signs that may appear in late pregnancy, indicating nutritional risk (e.g., intrauterine growth retardation, pregnancy induced hypertension, macrosomia).[4]

Diagnostic Tests and Methods

- Complete blood cell count (CBC) to screen for anemia
- One-hour 50-g Glucola to rule out gestational diabetes
- Urine dipstick to detect proteinuria (suggestive of pregnancy induced hypertension), glycosuria (suggestive of gestational diabetes), and ketonuria (suggestive of hyperemesis gravidarum)
- Other less commonly used laboratory assays available to diagnose other nutritional deficiencies (normal values in pregnancy differ from nonpregnant values) (see Chapter 16).[4]

DIFFERENTIAL MEDICAL DIAGNOSES

Normal nutrition in pregnancy, ruling out overweight or underweight; anemia; gestational diabetes; drug, alcohol, or nicotine abuse; eating disorders; problems affecting nutrition (e.g., cultural, economic, psychosocial); and complications of pregnancy requiring dietary intervention.

PLAN

Psychosocial Interventions

Encourage the client to verbalize any physical and psychosocial problems and explore interventions with her. Interventions for the normal physiological changes that may interfere with a woman's ability to eat an adequate diet are described later in the chapter (see Common Complaints).

TABLE 17–1. MATERNAL NUTRITIONAL RISK FACTORS*

Anthropometric

Moderately Overweight

Greater than 120% of desirable pregravid weight for height

BMI of greater than 26.0 to 29.0

Very Overweight

Greater than 135% of desirable pregravid weight for height

BMI of greater than 29.0

Underweight

Less than 90% of desirable pregravid weight for height

BMI less than 19.8

Inadequate Weight Gain (During Pregnancy)

During trimesters 2 and 3:
    Less than 1 lb (0.5 kg) per month for very overweight women
    Less than 2 lbs (1 kg) per month for all other women

Excessive Weight Gain (During Pregnancy)

More than 6.5 lbs (3 kg) per month

Biochemical (Laboratory)

Anemia

Nonpregnant, 12 through 14 years old:
    Hb below 11.8 g/dL (or 118 g/L)
    Hct below 35.5 vol % (or 0.35)

Nonpregnant, 15 years or older:
    Hb below 12.0 g/dL (or 120 g/L)
    Hct below 36.0 vol % (or 0.36)

Pregnant, weeks 1–13:
    Hb below 11.0 (or 110 g/L)
    Hct below 33.0 (or 0.33)

Pregnant, weeks 14–28:
    Hb below 10.5 (or 105 g/L)
    Hct below 32.0 (or 0.32)

Pregnant, weeks 29+:
    Hb below 11.0 (or 110 g/L)
    Hct below 33.0 (or 0.33)

Hypovolemia
(Inadequate Plasma Volume Expansion During Pregnancy)

Between 24 and 34 weeks:
    Hb above 13.9 g/dL (or 139 g/L)
    Hct above 41.9 vol % (or 0.419)

Abnormal Glucose Levels

1-hour glucose loading test:
    venous plasma glucose above 140 g/dL (7.8 mmol/L) one hour after 50-gm oral glucose load

3-hour 100-gm oral glucose tolerance test—two or more of the following venous plasma concentrations must be met or exceeded:
    fasting, 105 mg/dL (5.8 mmol/L)
    1-hour, 190 mg/dL (10.6 mmol/L)
    2-hour, 165 mg/dL (9.2 mmol/L)
    3-hour, 145 mg/dL (8.1 mmol/L)

Clinical (Physical/Medical/Obstetrical)

Previous Obstetrical Complications

Hyperemesis gravidarum

Gestational diabetes

Preeclampsia

Anemia

Preterm labor

Inadequate weight gain

Neonatal death (death within first 28 days after birth)

Stillbirth (greater than 20 weeks gestation)

Fetal loss (less than 20 weeks gestation)

Premature delivery (less than 37 weeks gestation)

Low-birth-weight infant (less than 2,500 g)

Small-for-gestational-age infant

High-birth-weight infant (more than 4,000 g)

Congenital anomaly

Postpartum hemorrhage

Adolescence

Less than 18 years at last menstrual period

Less than reproductive biologic year 3 (biologic age = chronologic age minus menarcheal age)

High Parity

5 or more previous deliveries at greater than 20 weeks gestation

Short Interpregnancy Interval

12 months or less between delivery (or termination of pregnancy) and conception

Breast-Feeding

Breast-feeding during current pregnancy

Inadequate milk supply

TABLE 17–1. MATERNAL NUTRITIONAL RISK FACTORS* (CONTINUED)

Clinical (Physical/Medical/Obstetrical) (cont.)

Current Medical/Obstetrical Complications

Diabetes (insulin-dependent, non-insulin-dependent, or gestational)

Hypertension (chronic or associated with preeclampsia)

Chronic renal disease

Chronic liver disease

Cancer

Cardiopulmonary disease:

Functional heart disease (N.Y. Heart Assoc. Class 2 or higher)
Organic disease (e.g., tuberculosis, pneumonia)
Asthma requiring treatment

Thyroid disease

Gastrointestinal disease (including parasites, malabsorption more severe than lactase deficiency)

Use of prescribed drugs known to affect or suspected of affecting the fetus (e.g., Dilantin or phenobarbital for epilepsy)

Multiple pregnancy

Intrauterine growth retardation

Severe infection (e.g., pyelonephritis, hepatitis, toxoplasmosis, listeriosis, HIV positive)

Venereal disease (positive VDRL, genital herpes, chlamydia, trichomoniasis)

Anesthesia/surgery/trauma shortly before or during the perinatal period

Systemic evidence of nutritional deficiency

Socioeconomic

Low Income

Eligible for local, state, or federal assistance programs

Substance Abuse

Alcohol

Average daily intake of more than 1 oz absolute alcohol
(1 oz absolute alcohol = 2 mixed drinks or 2 cans beer or
2 6-oz glasses wine)
Binge drinking

Cigarettes:

More than 10 cigarettes/day

Recreational/street drugs:

Use of narcotics, cocaine, hallucinogens, marijuana, amphetamines, and/or other recreational/street drugs

Over-the-counter (OTC) medications and herbal remedies:

Chronic use of laxatives, antacids or other OTC drugs known to affect nutritional status
Use of herbal remedies known or suspected to cause toxic side effects

Vitamin and mineral supplements:

Excessive use of nutrient supplements (over toxicity limits):

Vitamin A   > 8,000 IU daily
Vitamin D   > 400 IU daily
Vitamin C   > 2,000 mg daily
Vitamin B-6 > 100 mg daily
Iodine   > 11 mg daily

Substance Abuse (cont.)

Caffeine:

Excessive intake of caffeine (more than 300 mg/day). This amount of caffeine is found in about 3 cups coffee, 4 cups tea, or 6 cans of cola.

Pica

Eating of nonfood substances

Psychological Problems

Depression influencing appetite or eating

Current or past history of eating disorders (e.g., anorexia nervosa, bulimia)

Mental retardation

Mental Illness

Dietary

Poor Diet/Inappropriate Food Consumption

Less than minimum recommended servings for each food group in the Daily Food Guide for Women

Excessive intake of fat, sugar, or salt

*Broader and more inclusive definitions for these risk factors are appropriate to determine eligibility for public health programs such as WIC, as they identify individuals who may be predisposed to poor nutritional status and will benefit from nutritional education.
Source: California Department of Health Services. (1990). Nutrition during pregnancy and the postpartum period: A manual for health care professionals. *Sacramento, CA: Author*

TABLE 17–2. SELECTED CLINICAL SIGNS FOR NUTRITIONAL EVALUATION

Body Area	Clinical Signs	Possible Nutritional Implications
Hair	Dull, dry, sparse, shedding, or lightening of normal color.	Protein-calorie malnutrition. (May also be due to hypothyroidism.)
Face	General lightening of skin color.	Protein-calorie malnutrition.
	Scaling with dry, greasy, gray or yellowish threadlike material around nostrils; also on bridge of nose, eyebrows, and back of ears. Sebaceous gland ducts plugged.	Riboflavin, niacin, or pyridoxine deficiency. (May also be due to poor hygiene.)
Eyes	Pale conjunctivae.	Iron, folate, or B-12 deficiency.
	Redness of membranes; redness and fissuring of eyelid corners.	Riboflavin and niacin deficiency.
	Dryness of membranes; dullness of cornea.	Vitamin A deficiency.
Lips	Cracks, redness, and flaking at corners of the mouth. Scars at corners of the mouth. Important only if bilateral.	Riboflavin, niacin, iron, and pyridoxine deficiency. (Also results from poor dentures, herpes, and syphilis.)
	Vertical cracks on lips, usually in center of the lower lip. Lips are red, swollen, and inner mucosa appears to extend out onto the lip. May be ulcerated.	Riboflavin and niacin deficiency. (May also occur from environmental exposure.)
Tongue	Pale.	Iron deficiency.
	Purplish red (magenta).	Riboflavin deficiency.
	Taste buds are atrophied. Tongue appears smooth, pale, and slick (even when slightly scraped).	Folate, niacin, riboflavin, iron, or B-12 deficiency. (May also occur in nonnutritional anemia.)
	Tongue is beefy, red, painful, and taste buds are atrophied. Usually hypersensitivity, burning, and even taste changes, especially when eating. Oral mucosa may also be red and swollen.	Niacin, folate, riboflavin, iron, B-12, pyridoxine, and tryptophan deficiency.
Teeth	Carious or missing.	Excessive intake of carbohydrate (sucrose) or alcohol, poor hygiene, or multiple nutrient inadequacies (e.g., calcium).
	Mottled enamel.	Fluorine excess.
Gums	Swollen, bleeding.	Vitamin C deficiency. (May also be caused by chronic overdoses of hydantoinates [e.g., Dilantin], poor hygiene, and lymphoma.)
Glands	Thyroid enlargement (goiter).	Iodine inadequacy or toxicity. (May also be caused by cysts, tumors, and hyperthyroidism.)
Skin	Dry, flaking, or scaly; skin feels like sandpaper.	Vitamin A or essential fatty acid deficiency. (Also occurs with fungus infection, syphilis, etc.)
	Petechiae (small purple spots or hemorrhages under the skin).	Vitamin C and vitamin K deficiency. (Also occurs in hematological disorders, trauma, liver disease, and anticoagulant overdose.)
	Poor turgor or tone; pressure sores.	Multiple nutrient inadequacies, especially of protein and vitamin C.
	Xanthomas (fat deposits under the skin, around joints, and under the eyes).	Increased serum levels of LDLs or VLDLs with resultant hyperlipo-proteinemia.
Nails	Brittle, ridged, or spoonshaped.	Iron deficiency. (May also occur in thalassemia.)
Abdomen	Edematous.	Protein-calorie malnutrition.
Extremities	Muscle wasting.	Protein-calorie malnutrition.
	Edematous.	Protein-calorie malnutrition.
Nervous System	Listless and apathetic.	Protein deficiency.
	Mental irritability and confusion.	Protein deficiency.
	Sensory loss.	Thiamin deficiency.

TABLE 17–2. SELECTED CLINICAL SIGNS FOR NUTRITIONAL EVALUATION (CONTINUED)

Body Area	Clinical Signs	Possible Nutritional Implications
Nervous System (cont.)	Motor weakness (inability to squat and then stand three to four times in a row).	Thiamin deficiency.
	Loss of vibratory sense (significant only if bilateral).	Thiamin and B-12 deficiency. (Consider other cause of peripheral neuropathy.)
	Loss of ankle and knee jerks (significant only if absolute and bilateral).	Thiamin and B-12 deficiency. (Consider other cause of peripheral neuropathy.)
	Calf tenderness (significant only if bilateral).	Thiamin deficiency. (Consider deep vein thrombosis and other causes of peripheral neuropathy.)

Source: California Department of Health Services. (1990). Nutrition during pregnancy and the postpartum period: A manual for health care professionals. Sacramento, CA: Author.

Dietary Interventions

Ask the client to recall her diet during the previous 24 hours, though a week is ideal; assess its adequacy (see Table 17–3). Assuming the client's dietary intake was adequate before conception and her weight is within a normal range, protein intake should increase by 10 g per day and total kilocalories (kcal) by 200 to 300. Normal weight gain is 25 to 35 pounds (see Figure 17–2).[4,5] Educate the client about the dietary adjustments needed to supply nutrients, taking into account the client's cultural, religious, and personal preferences, as well as lifestyle, food preferences, intolerances, and aversions.

High or low activity levels require adjustment of calorie and protein intake. To calculate energy needs, the client 19–24 years old should consume 23.3 kcal/kg. The 25–50 year old should consume 21.9 kcal/kg. These numbers are then multiplied by 1.3 for very light activity, 1.5 for light activity, 1.6 for moderate activity, 1.9 for heavy activity, or 2.2 for exceptionally heavy activity. Add 300 kcal m the second and third trimester.[4] Encourage an ideal weight gain pattern.

Inadequate calcium intake has been implicated in pregnancy induced hypertension along with thiamine, B_6, B_{12}, magnesium, and sodium.[5,6] Advise clients with lower than optimal intake of calcium to increase their dietary calcium with dairy products, green leafy vegetables, tofu, canned salmon, egg yolks, whole grains, legumes, and nuts. Juices and bread with calcium supplementation have recently become available. In one study, the calcium in the juices was shown to have good bioavailability.[7] A calcium supplement may be necessary. Clients with lactose intolerance may benefit from taking lactase supplements (e.g., Lactaid), eating lactose-reduced dairy products (yogurt, cheese, milk, or cottage cheese), or eating dairy products in small quantities.

Vegetarians choose this lifestyle for cultural, religious, personal or philosophic reasons. Types of vegetarians' diets vary: excluding all animal food sources, including milk, eggs, fish, and/or poultry, fruit as a main dietary staple, or macrobiotics who eat mainly cereals. In most cases, with the help of a registered dietician, these clients can plan a diet that meets their pregnancy needs. These clients are particularly advised to use a prenatal vitamin and mineral supplement.[4]

If the client's body weight at conception is above or below her normal range, counsel her to adjust her caloric intake appropriately. Figure 17–1 shows the desirable weight range (normal), weights that are low, weights that are high, and weights that are obese. Recommended weight gain is 28 to 40 pounds if low, 25 to 35 pounds if normal weight, 15–25 pounds if high weight, and 15 pounds if obese (Figures 17–1 and 17–2).[5]

Adolescents have nutritional needs not only of the pregnancy but also of their own growth. Pregnant teens, 11–14 years old, need 28.5 kcal/kg. This should be multiplied by 1.3 for very light physical activity, 1.5 for light, 1.6 for moderate, 1.9 for heavy, and 2.2 for exceptionally heavy activity. Protein needs are calculated by multiplying 1 g/kg and adding 10 gms. If this number is less than 60, use 60 gms; 1.2 gms of calcium is recommended. Teens aged 15–18

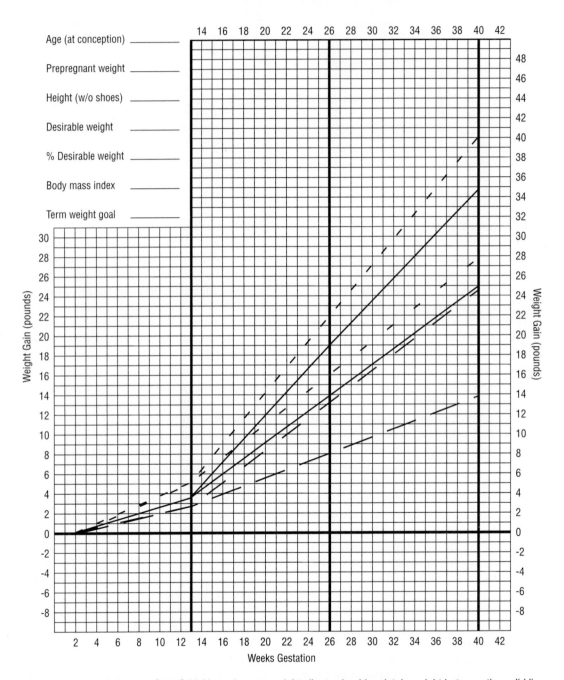

Figure 17–2. Prenatal Weight-Gain Grid. Normal to overweight clients should maintain weight between the solid lines, underweight clients between the short dashed lines, and overweight clients between the long dashed lines. Young adolescents, African American women, and smokers should strive for gains at the upper end of the recommended ranges. Short women (<62 inches) should strive for gains at the lower end of the range *(Source: Adapted with permission from Nutrition during pregnancy, copyright 1990 by the National Academy of Sciences. Courtesy of the National Academy Press, Washington, DC.)*

require 24.9 kcal/kg, multiplying by the same factors for activity. Protein needs are 0.8 gm/kg plus 10 grams or 60 grams, whichever is more; 1.2 gms of calcium is recommended, 300 kcal are added to all diets in the second and third trimester.[4]

For clients with multiple gestations, data indicate that a weight gain of 35 to 45 pounds is ideal.[1] Although recommendations for calorie, protein, or calcium intake are lacking, prudence suggests that increases in these nutrients are needed.

For the client with five or more pregnancies or with pregnancies that are closely spaced, emphasize optimal nutrition in all areas but particularly protein, calcium, iron, and folic acid.

Risk factors for anemia include menorrhagia, vegetarian diet (particularly with the exclusion of eggs), diets lacking red meat or low in vitamin C, multiple gestation, more than three blood donations per year, and chronic aspirin use. In pregnancy, anemia is present with a hemoglobin of less than 11.0 g/dL in the first and third trimester and 10.5 g/dL in the second trimester.[8] Encourage a diet that includes foods high in iron (e.g., liver, lean red meats, oysters, dark green vegetables, peas, iron-fortified cereals, dried beans, and blackstrap molasses). Iron supplementation is recommended.

If the client has been diagnosed with hyperemesis gravidarum, optimal nutrition is essential for the remainder of pregnancy. Weight gains in the second and third trimesters have the greatest impact on fetal growth.[9] In one study, impaired fetal growth was reported if more than 8 pounds of prepregnant weight was lost.[9]

Recent research has revealed several areas of interest when counseling a pregnant client on nutrition. Prepregnant obesity may be related to an increased risk of neural tube defects and possibly other significant defects of the central nervous system, great vessels, ventral wall or intestines.[2,3] Folic acid may reduce the incidence of neural tube defects in at risk clients if supplemented from 1 month preconceptually to 3 months of gestation. Supplementation for normal risk clients continues to be researched.[10] For clients at risk for pregnancy induced hypertension, calcium supplementation has shown significant reduction of blood pressure but whether it reduces morbidity is not yet clear.[6] Supplementation with 25 mg of zinc was shown to increase both birth weight and head circumference in clients with low plasma zinc concentrations early in pregnancy.[11] Vitamin A supplementation was shown to be teratogenic in doses of 10,000 or above. Beta-carotene, the natural precursor found in food, was not shown to produce birth defects.[12,13]

Medication

Prenatal Vitamin/Mineral Supplements. Although needed only by those whose diet is inadequate or otherwise at nutritional risk, supplements are usually prescribed for all pregnant women.

- *Administration.* One tablet by mouth each day. The supplement should contain at least 30 mg elemental iron, 15 mg zinc, 2 mg copper, 250 mg calcium (*not* in the form of calcium phosphate), 2 mg vitamin B_6, 300 μg of folate (most supplements contain 0.8 to 1.0 mg folic acid), 50 mg vitamin C and 5 μg (200 I.U.) of vitamin D.[4]
- *Side Effects and Adverse Reactions.* Gastric upset, constipation, diarrhea.
- *Contraindications.* None are known.
- *Anticipated Outcomes on Evaluation.* The client's hemoglobin level is within normal range, and neither the client nor the infant develops pathology related to vitamin or mineral deficiencies.
- *Client Teaching and Counseling.* Inform the client of the need for a healthy, balanced diet even when taking a prenatal supplement. To maximize the absorption of iron in the supplement, the tablet should be taken when the stomach is empty, with a drink high in vitamin C content, not with coffee, tea, or milk.[9] The client should discontinue other vitamin supplementation.

Iron Supplementation. If the client is not anemic, a supplement of 30 mg elemental iron is recommended during the second and third trimesters, usually supplied in the prenatal vitamin. If the client is anemic, supplementation of 60 to 120 elemental mg iron is recommended.[4,8,9]

- *Administration.* Thirty mg of elemental iron twice a day, as 150 mg ferrous sulfate, 300 ferrous gluconate, or 100 mg ferrous fulmate.[8]
- *Side Effects and Adverse Reactions.* Gastric upset, constipation, diarrhea.

TABLE 17–3. DAILY FOOD GUIDE FOR WOMEN

Food Group	One Serving Equals	Recommended Minimum Servings		
		Nonpregnant/ Nonlactating		Pregnant/ Lactating
		11–24 yrs.	25+ yrs.	
Protein Foods Provide protein, iron, zinc, and B vitamins for growth of muscles, bone, blood, and nerves. Vegetable protein provides fiber to prevent constipation	Animal Protein 1 oz cooked chicken or turkey 1 oz cooked lean beef, lamb, or pork 1 oz or ¼ cup fish or other seafood 1 egg 2 fish sticks or hot dogs 2 slices luncheon meat Vegetable Protein ½ cup cooked dry beans, lentils, or split peas 3 oz tofu 1 oz or ¼ cup peanuts, pumpkin, or sunflower seeds 1½ oz or ⅓ cup other nuts 2 tbsp peanut butter	5 A half serving of vegetable protein daily	5 A half serving of vegetable protein daily	7 One serving of vegetable protein daily
Milk Products Provide protein and calcium to build strong bones, teeth, healthy nerves and muscles, and promote normal blood clotting.	8 oz milk 8 oz yogurt 1 cup milk shake 1½ cups cream soup (made with milk) 1½ oz or ⅓ cup grated cheese (like cheddar, monterey, mozzarella, or swiss) 1½–2 slices presliced American cheese 4 tbsp parmesan cheese 2 cups cottage cheese 1 cup pudding 1 cup custard or flan 1½ cups ice milk, ice cream, or frozen yogurt	3	2	3
Breads, Cereals, Grains Provide carbohydrates and B vitamins for energy and healthy nerves. Also provide iron for healthy blood. Whole grains provide fiber to prevent constipation.	1 slice bread 1 dinner roll ½ bun or bagel ½ English muffin or pita 1 small tortilla ¾ cup dry cereal ½ cup granola ½ cup cooked cereal ½ cup rice ½ cup noodles or spaghetti ¼ cup wheat germ 1 4-in pancake or waffle 1 small muffin 8 medium crackers 4 graham cracker squares 3 cups popcorn	7 Four servings of whole-grain products daily	6 Four servings of whole-grain products daily	7 Four servings of whole-grain products daily
Vitamin C-Rich Fruits and Vegetables Provide vitamin C to prevent infection and to promote healing and iron absorption. Also provide fiber to prevent constipation.	6 oz orange, grapefruit, or fruit juice enriched with vitamin C 6 oz tomato juice or vegetable juice cocktail 1 orange, kiwi, mango ½ grapefruit, cantaloupe ½ cup papaya 2 tangerines ½ cup strawberries ½ cup cooked or 1 cup raw cabbage ½ cup broccoli, Brussels sprouts, or cauliflower ½ cup snow peas, sweet peppers, or tomato puree 2 tomatoes	1	1	1

Food Group / Description	Serving Examples			
Vitamin A-Rich Fruits and Vegetables Provide beta-carotene and vitamin A to prevent infection and to promote wound healing and night vision. Also provide fiber to prevent constipation.	6 oz apricot nectar or vegetable juice cocktail 3 raw or 1/4 cup dried apricots 1/4 cantaloupe or mango 1 small or 1/2 cup sliced carrots 2 tomatoes	1/2 cup cooked or 1 cup raw spinach 1/2 cup cooked greens (beet, chard, collards, dandelion, kale, mustard) 1/2 cup pumpkin, sweet potato, winter squash, or yams	1	1	1
Other Fruits and Vegetables Provide carbohydrates for energy and fiber to prevent constipation.	6 oz fruit juice (if not listed above) 1 medium or 1/2 cup sliced fruit (apple, banana, peach, pear) 1/2 cup berries (other than strawberries) 1/2 cup cherries or grapes 1/2 cup pineapple 1/2 cup watermelon	1/4 cup dried fruit 1/2 cup sliced vegetable (asparagus, beets, green beans, celery, corn, eggplant, mushrooms, onion, peas, potato, summer squash, zucchini) 1/2 artichoke 1 cup lettuce	3	3	3
Unsaturated Fats Provide vitamine E to protect tissue.	1/8 med. avocado 1 tsp margarine 1 tsp mayonnaise 1 tsp vegetable oil	2 tsp salad dressing (mayonnaise-based) 1 tbsp salad dressing (oil based)	3	3	3

Source: California Department of Health Services. (1990). Nutrition during pregnancy and the postpartum period: A manual for health care professionals. Sacramento, CA: Author.

- *Contraindications.* Some hemoglobinopathies (e.g., β-thalassemia without a dietary deficiency in iron; see Chapter 18).[4]
- *Anticipated Outcomes on Evaluation.* Hemoglobin levels above 11.0 g/dL in the first and third trimester and 10.5 g/dL in the second trimester.[8] Recheck hemoglobin level after 6 weeks. If the hemoglobin rises, continue for 2–4 months, or until reaches 12.0 g/dL. A maintenance dose of 30 mg elemental iron should be continued for 6 months.[8]
- *Client Teaching and Counseling.* Advise the client to take the iron supplement on an empty stomach, separate from the prenatal vitamin, and with liquids containing vitamin C (e.g., orange, cranberry or tomato juice), not with milk, tea, or coffee. The addition of 15 mg of zinc and 2 mg copper is recommended because high levels of iron interfere with absorption of those minerals.[8,9]

Calcium Supplement. A calcium supplement may be recommended. Women younger than 25 years whose calcium intake is less than 600 mg receive 600 mg of supplemental calcium per day.[9] Ten μg (400 I.U.) of vitamin D is recommended if the client does not use dairy products.[4]

- *Administration.* The concentration of elemental calcium varies among common calcium supplements: calcium carbonate supplies 40 percent elemental calcium; calcium citrate supplies 24 percent; calcium lactate supplies 14 percent; and calcium gluconate supplies 9 percent. Because calcium phosphate is poorly absorbed and interferes with iron absorption, it is not recommended.[5] Other calcium sources (e.g., dolomite, oyster shell calcium) are not recommended. Calcium will be better absorbed if given in divided doses.
- *Side Effects and Adverse Reactions.* Increased intestinal gas.
- *Contraindications.* History of kidney stones.
- *Anticipated Outcome on Evaluation.* Neither the client nor the infant develops pathology related to inadequate calcium intake.
- *Client Teaching and Counseling.* Advise the client to split the calcium supplement into 250- to 300-mg doses and take with a light meal or snack to enhance absorption. Calcium should not be taken at same time as an iron supplement.[9]

FOLLOW-UP

Weight gain should be assessed at each visit. The gain should be steady and in the parameters described (see Figure 17–2). Maternal weight is gained primarily in the first half of the pregnancy. Fetal weight gain is primarily in the third trimester. Each client's weight gain should be evaluated with that knowledge. Abnormal weight gains should be evaluated by ruling out pregnancy induced hypertension and by assessing diet quality, activity levels, food preferences and intolerance, and socioeconomic and psychologic factors. Refer to a dietitian any client at nutritional risk (see Tables 17–1 and 17–2) with a drug or alcohol abuse problem, a chronic medical problem that requires a therapeutic diet, gestational diabetes, or a vegetarian diet. If psychosocial problems are affecting the client's diet or appetite, refer her to a mental health care provider. If the client has inadequate financial resources, refer her to a social workers for advice about government and private programs (e.g., Women, Infants, and Children [WIC]).[9]

IMMUNIZATION

BEFORE PREGNANCY

Clients should have all childhood immunizations before conception to protect the fetus from an illness that could produce congenital anomalies and from the theoretical risk of exposure to immunizations. The health care provider should be aware of changes in the measles, mumps, and rubella (MMR) immunization schedule, which may require that the client receive an additional MMR immunization. Diphtheria/tetanus boosters are required every 10 years. Varicella vaccination is now available.[14] These issues should be addressed at the preconception checkup (see Table 17–4).

DURING PREGNANCY

Rubella

Despite large-scale immunization of preschool-age children, a resurgence of rubella and congen-

TABLE 17–4. VACCINATION DURING PREGNANCY

	Vaccine	Indications for Vaccination During Pregnancy
Live virus vaccine		
Measles	Live-attenuated	Contraindicated.
Mumps		
Rubella		
Yellow fever	Live-attenuated	Contraindicated except if exposure to yellow fever virus is unavoidable.
Poliomyelitis	Trivalent live-attenuated (OPV)	Persons at substantial risk of exposure to polio.
Inactivated virus vaccines		
Hepatitis B	Recombinant produced, purified hepatitis B surface antigen	Pregnancy is not a contraindication.
Influenza	Inactivated type A and type B virus vaccines	Usually recommended only for patients with serious underlying disease. Consult health authorities for current recommendations.
Japanese Encephalitis	Killed virus	Should reflect actual risks of disease and probable benefits of vaccine.
Poliomyelitis	Killed virus (IPV)	OPV preferred when immediate protection of pregnant females is needed; however, IPV is alternative if complete vaccination series can be administered before exposure.
Rabies	Killed virus	Substantial risk of exposure.
	Rabies IG	
Live bacterial vaccines		
Typhoid (Ty21a)	Live bacterial	Should reflect actual risks of disease and probable benefits of vaccine.
Inactivated bacterial vaccines		
Cholera	Killed bacterial	Should reflect actual risks of disease and probable benefits of vaccine.
Typhoid		
Plague	Killed bacterial	Selective vaccination of exposed persons.
Meningococcal	Polysaccharide	Only in unusual outbreak situations.
Pneumococcal	Polysaccharide	Only for high-risk persons.
Haemophilus b conjugate	Polysaccharide-protein	Only for high-risk persons.
Toxoids		
Tetanus-diphtheria (Td)	Combined tetanus-diphtheria toxoids, adult formulation	Lack of primary series, or no booster within past 10 years.
Immune globulins, pooled or hyperimmune	Immune globulin or specific globulin preparations	Exposure or anticipated unavoidable exposure to measles, hepatitis A, hepatitis B, rabies, or tetanus.

Source: Health Information for International Travel. (1994, June). CDC, HHS Pub No 94–8280. U.S. Dept. of Health and Human Services. Division of Quarantine, Atlanta, GA 30333.

ital rubella syndrome occurred between 1988 and 1990. Among women of reproductive age, 6 to 11 percent remain seronegative. The risk of congenital rubella syndrome is related to the gestational age of the fetus at the time of maternal infection. One study showed a fetal infection rate of 90 percent before 11 weeks, 33 percent at 11 to 12 weeks, 11 percent at 13 to 14 weeks, 24 percent at 15 to 16 weeks, and 0 percent after 16 weeks.[15]

Administering serum immunoglobulin to a pregnant client with rubella reduces her symptoms but does not alter the risk or severity of congenital rubella syndrome in the fetus.[15] The theoretical risk of congenital rubella syndrome from immunization just prior to pregnancy or during the first trimester is as high as 1.7 percent, but the observed risk is 0 percent.[16]

If the client has a positive serological test, then there is no risk to the fetus if she is exposed to rubella. *All prenatal clients should be tested.* If seronegative, they should be cautioned to avoid anyone with a rash or viral illness.

All nonimmune clients should be immunized postpartum. Breastfeeding is not a contraindication. If Rho(D) immune globulin (human) (RhoGAM) is given seroconversion should be checked at the postpartum visit. Theoretically, RhoGAM could block antibody development.[15]

All preschool children should be immunized even if a pregnant woman is in the household. Furthermore, all nonpregnant persons of unknown immunity status should be immunized, particularly health care providers. Because of theoretical risk, women of childbearing age should not become pregnant for 3 months following immunization.[16]

Hepatitis B Virus

Infection with hepatitis B virus (HBV) carries significant sequelae if the client becomes a chronic carrier. Infection can lead to chronic hepatitis, cirrhosis, or primary hepatocellular carcinoma. Infants whose mothers test positive for hepatitis B surface antigen (HBsAg) may become infected and are at 25 percent risk for the same serious sequelae. Certain populations are at high risk for HBV infection, but limiting screening to persons in those groups results in failure to identify 50 percent of women who are HBV carriers.[17]

All clients should be screened for HBsAg prenatally or, if not then, when they are admitted to the hospital. If HBsAg is positive, further testing of the client, her children, and her sexual partner is advised. The pediatrician should be advised of the mother's positive status and is responsible for appropriate care of the infant.

If a client is HBsAg and HBsAb (antibody to HBsAg) negative and at risk for infection, immunization is encouraged as pregnancy is not a contraindication.[17] Groups at risk include women of Asian, Pacific Island, or Eskimo descent, no matter where they were born; women born in Haiti or sub-Saharan Africa; women with work histories in public safety or health care (especially those exposed to blood); women who live with HBV carriers or hemodialysis clients; or women who have a history of intravenous drug use or sexual partners who have used intravenous drugs. Others at risk are women with a history of acute or chronic liver disease, women who work or live in institutions for the mentally disabled, women who have been rejected as a blood donor, women with a history of blood transfusion, or women with multiple sexually transmitted disease (STD) episodes, multiple sexual partners, or whose partner has multiple sexual partners.[17]

Other Immunizations

Other immunizations (e.g., influenza) are usually not indicated during pregnancy. The decision to immunize should be made only after the risk of disease has been weighed against the risk of vaccination and after several factors have been taken into account.

Determination of susceptibility should include a history of prior illness, previous vaccinations, and, most important, serological tests. Other information is helpful, but *only serological tests can prove immunity.* The Centers for Disease Control (CDC) have developed definitions of susceptibility, which may be obtained through the Immunization Practices Advisory Committee.

Risk of exposure is reduced by avoiding travel to endemic areas, practicing appropriate hygiene, and avoiding infected persons. This strategy is preferred to immunization.

Pregnancy may alter the rate of maternal complications in some diseases and cause special health problems.

In general, live vaccines are to be avoided; killed vaccines are safer (see Table 17–4).[16]

New Vaccines

Varicella-zoster immunoglobulin is recommended for susceptible, exposed pregnant women within 96 hours of exposure. The varicella vaccination is available for nonimmune clients. It is not recommended during pregnancy and clients should avoid pregnancy for 3 months after vaccination.[14]

COMMON COMPLAINTS

Many symptoms that are frequently reported to health care providers are most often attributable to pregnancy but must be evaluated to rule out other pathology.

FIRST TRIMESTER

Nausea and Vomiting

Etiology. Physiological changes that cause nausea and vomiting during pregnancy are unknown; however, unusually high levels of estrogen and progesterone and the introduction of human chorionic gonadotropin (hCG) have been studied.[18] Smooth muscle relaxation in the gastrointestinal (GI) tract causing delayed emptying of the stomach has been implicated. Decreased hydrochloric acid and pepsis secretion, fatigue of early pregnancy, emotional factors, and dietary factors, including vitamin B_6 deficiency have been explored.[4] Multiple gestation and molar pregnancies are associated with higher incidences of nausea and vomiting. Sixty to eighty percent of Western women experience nausea and vomiting, but women in other cultures experience those symptoms less frequently.[4,19] They generally last 14 to 17 weeks into pregnancy and are usually associated with a positive pregnancy outcome.

Subjective Data. Nausea and/or vomiting are reported by the client between the 4th and 16th weeks of pregnancy. It may or may not be limited to certain times of the day.[20] The client may have had nausea while taking oral contraceptives. The history should *not* include fever, lethargy, muscle aches, abdominal pain, cramping, diarrhea, jaundice, dark urine, changes in the shape or color of bowel movements, vaginal bleeding, head injury, headache, projectile vomiting, vomiting blood, excessive thirst, neurological signs, ataxia, chest pain, ear pain or ringing, or psychosocial distress, as these symptoms/signs indicate other conditions that may require medical or other appropriate follow-up.[21]

Objective Data. Physical examination and vital signs are within normal limits. Thyroid dysfunction has been associated with hyperemesis. The thyroid should be normal size.[18] Significant negatives include the absence of signs of dehydration and vaginal bleeding. A hydatidiform gestation may present with hyperemesis and possible prolonged vaginal spotting. Multiple pregnancies often cause severe nausea and/or vomiting.[18]

Uterine size should be appropriate for dates. Fetal heart tones should be audible at 12 weeks' gestation.

Weight loss, dehydration, and ketosis suggest hyperemesis gravidarum.[18]

Urine ketone and specific gravity tests are used to rule out dehydration.

Differential Medical Diagnoses. Nausea and vomiting related to pregnancy ruling out hyperemesis gravidarum, multiple gestation, hydatidiform gestation, gastroenteritis, cholecystitis, hepatitis, inner ear infection, sinusitis, hiatal hernia, diabetes, thyroid dysfunction, increased intracranial pressure, migraine headache, pica, food poisoning, vitamin deficiencies, emotional problems, eating disorders, myocardial infarction.[21]

Plan

PSYCHOSOCIAL INTERVENTIONS. Explain to the client that nausea and vomiting usually are limited to the first trimester and are usually related to positive pregnancy outcomes. Advise her to notify the health care provider if any symptoms rules out during history taking occur in the future.

MEDICATION

- Vitamin B_6 Supplement
  - *Indications.* Nausea and vomiting in pregnancy.
  - *Administration.* Vitamin B_6 25 mg p.o. t.i.d. × 3 days.
  - *Side Effects and Adverse Reactions.* None are known.
  - *Contraindications.* None are known.
  - *Anticipated Outcome on Evaluation.* Decreased nausea and vomiting.
  - *Client Teaching and Counseling.* This therapy works best with severe, not mild or moderate nausea and vomiting.[22] Instruct the client not to exceed 100 mg per day as toxicity may result.[18]

- Phosphorated Carbohydrate Solution (Emetrol)
  - *Indications.* To reduce smooth muscle contractions of hyperactive gastric muscles.

- *Administration.* Emetrol 1 to 2 tablespoons. Repeat every 15 minutes up to 5 times until nausea and vomiting are relieved.
- *Side Effects and Adverse Reactions.* None are known.
- *Contraindications.* Diabetes or hereditary fructose intolerance.
- *Anticipated Outcome on Evaluation.* Decreased nausea and vomiting.
- *Client Teaching and Counseling.* Instruct the client never to dilute this medication[23] or drink fluids of any kind immediately before or after taking a dose.

LIFESTYLE CHANGES

- Ask the client to keep a diary listing when and for how long nausea and vomiting occur and what activities, associated factors, or foods trigger or improve symptoms. Interventions suggested by this diary are most likely to succeed.
- Advise the client to rest when the nausea occurs, avoid stress, avoid sights and smells that trigger nausea, refrain from wearing clothing that is tight and constricting about the abdomen, and reduce work loads. Support and assistance from the client's partner may also improve symptoms.
- Suggest hypnosis, acupressure (e.g., Seabands), cold compresses to the throat, or acupuncture as a possible intervention. To reduce the risk of human immunodeficiency virus (HIV) or hepatitis B infection, acupuncture should be performed only by a specially trained physician.
- Describe relaxation techniques that may help: progressive relaxation (systematic tensing and relaxing of muscle groups), autogenic training (using suggestions such as "My right arm is heavy"), meditation (repeating a sound or gazing at an object while clearing the mind of all distractions), visual imagery (visualizing self in a relaxing place), and touching/massage.

DIETARY INTERVENTIONS

- Symptoms may be relieved by eating small, frequent meals that do not allow the stomach to become too empty or full, including high-carbohydrate or high-protein, easily digested meals and snacks, sipping carbonated drinks, including foods that tend to neutralize stomach acid (e.g., apples, milk, bread, potatoes, calcium carbonate tablets), eating crackers on arising, drinking fluids between meals instead of with meals, and avoiding foods that may irritate the stomach (e.g., spicy or fatty foods).[18] Lemonade and potato chips have more nutrients and may be more effective than soda and crackers.[19]
- Sit upright after eating.[18]
- If a vitamin/mineral supplement is causing nausea, it may be discontinued until the client is less nauseated, often after about 14 to 16 weeks of pregnancy. A balanced diet would provide all necessary vitamins and minerals, except iron needed in the second and third trimester (see Nutrition and Weight Gain).
- Remind the client of the need for adequate hydration (6 to 8 glasses per day). Sipping lukewarm fluids every 5 minutes is tolerated better than drinking an entire glass of fluid at one time.
- Ginger root tea and capsules have been studied but their safety during pregnancy has not been established.[19]

Follow-Up. Refer to a physician any client who is unable to hold down liquids for more than 12 hours, who loses 5 pounds or more, or who has ketonuria or any symptoms of pathology.

Constipation

Etiology. Large amounts of circulating progesterone cause decreased contractility of the GI tract, resulting in slow movement of chyme and increased water reabsorption from the bowel. The large bowel is also mechanically compressed by the enlarging uterus, most noticeably in the first and third trimesters. The client may have changed her food and fluid intake or exercise level in response to nausea and vomiting, fatigue, culturally prescribed expectations of pregnant women, or medically prescribed treatment. Prenatal vitamins with iron or calcium can also be constipating.[4,19,20]

Subjective Data. The client may report abdominal cramping, flatulence, or increasing difficulty with bowel movements or intervals between them. Stools may be small, hard, round, and dark. Often the client has a history of constipation before pregnancy. Her diet may be low in bulk and fluids, and she may rarely exercise. The client may have taken antacids, calcium, iron supplements, anticholinergics, tricyclic antidepressants, or codeine medications; these can constipate. The history should *not* include change in stool (i.e., color, shape, or pattern), diarrhea, abdominal pain, fever, anorexia, periumbilical pain, rectal bleeding, emotional distress, or excessive laxative use for weight control (purging), as these symptoms/signs may indicate other conditions requiring medical or other appropriate follow-up.[21]

Objective Data. Physical examination and vital signs are within normal limits, although hyperactive bowel sounds, constipated stool in the rectum, a sausage-shaped mass in the lower left quadrant that disappears after bowel movements, hemorrhoids, or hemorrhoidal tags may be revealed.

The *stool for occult blood* test is used to detect the presence of blood in the stool. A stool sample is collected during a digital rectal examination. The stool is applied to the card provided, and a drop of developer is placed on the card. If the card turns bright blue, blood is present.

Client teaching in preparation for the test includes diet information. For the most accurate results, the client should eliminate meats, fish, poultry, and green leafy vegetables for 3 days prior to the test. Aspirin should not be consumed during that same 3-day period. Hemorrhoids, anal fissures, and vaginal bleeding may also result in positive readings.

Differential Medical Diagnosis. Constipation related to pregnancy ruling out preterm labor, pica irritable bowel syndrome, appendicitis, intestinal obstruction, fecal impaction, chronic laxative use, use of medications known to cause constipation (e.g., codeine), or anal pain.[21]

Plan

PSYCHOSOCIAL INTERVENTIONS. Explain to the client how pregnancy exacerbates the symptoms of constipation and that symptoms should improve after delivery. Advise her to notify the health care provider if any symptoms ruled out during history-taking occur in the future.

MEDICATION. Advise the client to avoid mineral oil, as it will decrease the absorption of fat-soluble vitamins. Cathartics are contraindicated in pregnancy but particularly if the client is at risk for preterm labor.[4]

Review with client what other medication (e.g., codeine, iron) she is taking to determine whether constipation is a side effect—then help her to reduce their use if possible.

- Bulk-forming, nonnutritive laxatives (e.g., Metamucil, Fibercon)
  - *Indications.* Constipation caused by low dietary bulk.
  - *Administration.* Available in tablets or granules. Take per package instructions.
  - *Side Effects and Adverse Reactions.* If taken without adequate fluids, may swell in throat or esophagus, causing choking.
  - *Contraindications.* Fecal impaction or intestinal obstruction.
  - *Anticipated Outcome on Evaluation.* Softer stools with decreased constipation.
  - *Client Teaching and Counseling.* Instruct the client to drink 8 oz of water or more with each dose. Do not use if having difficulty breathing or swallowing, chest pain or vomiting. If these occur advise to seek immediate medical attention. She may need to continue treatment for 2 to 3 days before maximum effect is noted.[23]

- Docusate sodium (e.g., Colace, Ex-Lax Stool Softener), a stool softener.
  - *Indications.* Can be used to prevent constipation.
  - *Administration.* 50 to 200 mg per day.
  - *Side Effects and Adverse Reactions.* Bitter taste, throat irritation, nausea.
  - *Contraindications.* Sensitivity to docusate sodium.
  - *Anticipated Outcome on Evaluation.* Formation of softer, less constipating stools in 1–3 days.
  - *Client Teaching and Counseling.* Though listed as a category C drug, docusate sodium has not been associated with congenital defects. Instruct the client to take docusate sodium with milk or juice to mask its bitter taste.[23] Hypomagnesiumenia in one neonate was noted with chronic use of doses of 150–250 mg. Advise the client against this type of use.[24]

LIFESTYLE CHANGES. Encourage the client to exercise regularly (according to ACOG guidelines), to establish a time of day to defecate, to avoid prolonged attempts to defecate, and to elevate her feet on a stool while defecating to avoid straining.

DIETARY INTERVENTIONS. Advise the client to eat foods high in bulk (e.g., fresh fruits and vegetables, whole-grain breads and cereals) and to drink fluids (6 to 8 glasses of water per day above that drunk with meals) and to drink warm fluids on arising to stimulate bowel motility. Explain that if she takes her vitamin/mineral supplement every second or third day or changes to a supplement without iron and calcium temporarily, then constipation may be less of a problem. If any foods or juices (e.g., bran, prune juice) have helped the client in the past, encourage their use.

Follow-Up. If prenatal vitamins or iron are discontinued, monitor the client for anemia. If purging or psychosocial stress is causing constipation, refer the client to a mental health care provider. If symptoms of a pathological condition develop, refer the client to a physician.

Hemorrhoids

Etiology. Hemorrhoids occur when the vascular submucosa in the rectoanal canal bulges and becomes congested with varicosities. They become significant only when they become symptomatic. Hemorrhoids are exacerbated during pregnancy by increased intravascular pressure in veins below the uterus, constipation, and straining at stool.[4,25]

Subjective Data. The client may report a history of constipation, hemorrhoids before pregnancy, multiparity, increased age, or a family history of hemorrhoids. She may notice swelling, fullness, or a lump at her anus; bright red, painless bleeding on the stool surface during defecation; or increased mucus with defecation. If an anal fissure develops, defecation is often painful.

Objective Data. Physical examination and vital signs may be within normal limits, or hemorrhoids may be visible externally or palpated internally. Anal fissures or hemorrhoidal tags may be noted. Thrombosed hemorrhoids are a painful, shiny, bluish or purple clot-containing mass near the anus.

Diagnostic tests and methods include evaluation of the *hemoglobin level* in the blood. The hemoglobin level may be decreased if bleeding is extensive or prolonged.

Stool for occult blood is the other diagnostic tool (see Constipation).

Differential Medical Diagnosis. Hemorrhoids exacerbated by pregnancy; rule out abscessed or thrombosed hemorrhoids, cancerous lesions, idiopathic pruritus ani, condyloma acuminata, all of which may require more extensive medical referral and intervention.[21]

Plan

PSYCHOSOCIAL INTERVENTIONS. Explain to the client the underlying changes that created or exacerbated the hemorrhoids, and assure her that the condition will improve or resolve after pregnancy. Encourage her to contact a health care provider if any symptoms occur in the future.

MEDICATION

- Topical Anesthetics (e.g., Preparation H, Anusol)
  - *Indications.* To shrink the swelling of hemorrhoids and reduce itching.
  - *Administration.* Free application of cream, as needed, to hemorrhoids up to three to five times per day: in the morning, at night, and after each bowel movement. If a suppository is used, insert it into the rectum after cleaning and drying the anal area, six times per day as needed after bowel movements.
  - *Side Effects and Adverse Reactions.* Occasional burning of irritated tissues.
  - *Contraindications.* Client sensitivity to components of the medication. Heart disease, thyroid disease, and diabetes are contraindications to suppository use.
  - *Anticipated Outcomes on Evaluation.* Decreased swelling, pain, or itching of hemorrhoids.
  - *Client Teaching and Counseling.* Instruct the client in cream or suppository use. With the suppository, remove the foil wrapper before insertion. If soft, hold under cold water (in foil) for 2–3 minutes. With the cream, use a dispensing cap: Attach the cap to the tube and fill it by squeezing the tube. Lubricate the tip, gently insert it into the anus, and squeeze the tube to deliver cream into the rectum. Clean the cap with soap and water after use.[23]

LIFESTYLE CHANGES. Advise the client to try to avoid constipation by following the measures described in the preceding section (see Constipation). Encourage her to use warm or cool sitz baths (Epsom salts may be added), witch hazel pads (e.g., Tucks), and ice packs or cold compresses to reduce the size of the hemorrhoids. Furthermore, advise her to avoid straining by elevating her feet on a stool while attempting to defecate. Applying petroleum jelly around the anus before defecating will help reduce pain and bleeding.

Advise the client to sleep and rest on her side. Moreover, Kegel's exercises will improve circulation. To learn the feel of tightening the pubococcygeal (Kegel) muscles, first have the client sit on the commode and start and stop her urine flow. Next, insert a clean finger into the vagina and tighten the muscles. To do the exercise, squeeze and tighten 3 seconds each 10 times. Next, squeeze and tighten as fast as possible 10–25 times. Pretend to suck water into the vagina and hold for 3 seconds 10 times. Push out as if having a bowel movement with vaginal muscles holding for 3 seconds 10 times. Repeat the entire series 3 times a day.[4] Self-digital replacement of hemorrhoids if possible and careful perineal cleansing habits are also helpful.

Refer the client to a physician if she has symptoms of thrombosed hemorrhoids, does not respond to interventions, or has symptoms of other pathology.

Flatulence

Etiology. The physiological changes that result in constipation also may result in increased flatulence.[4]

Subjective Data. A client may report increased passage of rectal gas, abdominal bloating, epigastric pain, constipation, or belching, but not abdominal pain, use of food or medications that cause gas, change in bowels, greasy bowel movements, anxiety or depression.[21]

Objective Data. Often, hyperactive bowel sounds or abdominal distention is detected on physical exam.

Differential Medical Diagnoses. Flatulence; rule out irritable bowel syndrome, lactose or food intolerance, medication side effects, hyperventilation.[21]

Plan

PSYCHOSOCIAL INTERVENTIONS. Reassure the client that increased flatulence is related to pregnancy and should resolve afterward.

LIFESTYLE CHANGES. Teach the client measures to avoid constipation. Help her to recognize the symptoms of hyperventilation or air swallowing in order to alleviate flatulence. The client may find that she is breathing fast, sighing, or feeling the need for frequent deep breaths. She may feel tingling in her fingers, toes, or lips, dizziness, or confusion. Rebreathing air that is exhaled into a paper bag or cupped hands may help decrease symptoms. Because stress often causes hyperventilation, becoming aware of areas in her life that cause stress may be helpful for the client. Avoiding gum chewing, large meals, and smoking also will reduce flatulence.

DIETARY INTERVENTIONS. Advise the client to limit gas-forming foods (e.g., carbonated beverages, cruciferous vegetables, baking soda, cheese, beans, bananas, peanuts, calcium carbonate supplements). Pasta, corn, and whole grains when cooked, refrigerated or frozen, then reheated form gas producing substances. Each cooling and reheating makes them more potent.[26]

Follow-Up. Refer her to a mental health care provider if symptoms of psychosocial stress are evident.

Fatigue

Etiology. Fatigue during pregnancy occurs primarily during the first and third trimesters (the highest energy levels often occur during the second trimester). First-trimester fatigue may be caused by physical changes (e.g., increased oxygen consumption, progesterone and relaxin levels, and fetal demands) and psychosocial changes (e.g., reexamination of roles). Mood swings and depression may also cause insomnia.[25] Third-trimester fatigue is usually caused by sleep disturbances that result from increased weight, physical discomforts, and decreased exercise. Fatigue, in particular, can be a symptom in most pathological problems—emotional, physical, or dietary.[4]

Subjective Data. The client may report fatigue despite normal amounts of sleep or insomnia due to difficulty in getting comfortable, fetal movements, urinary frequency, vivid dreams, increased stress, or emotional problems. Her family or work situation may not allow her to rest during the day. The history should *not* include depression, anxiety, difficulty with concentration, anorexia, anemia, exercise intolerance, chest pain or discomfort, change in bowel habits, flulike symptoms, sore throat, coughing, or dyspnea, or other symptoms/signs indicating other conditions requiring medical or other appropriate follow-up.[21]

Objective Data. The physical examination and vital signs are within normal limits.

A *complete blood count* (CBC) is used to evaluate the client for signs of anemia, infection, or blood dyscrasias. The procedure involves venipuncture and withdrawal of blood which is sent to laboratory for evaluation. The client may apply pressure to the venipuncture site until bleeding stops. Hematoma formation at the site is common and will resolve.

Differential Medical Diagnosis. Fatigue due to pregnancy ruling out other pathological states.

Plan

PSYCHOSOCIAL INTERVENTIONS. Explain to the client that increased fatigue is expected in the first trimester and insomnia is common in the third. Encourage her to contact the health care provider if she develops other symptoms.

Encourage verbalization of psychosocial problems and explore appropriate interventions. Encourage the client to accept offers of help. Advise the client to avoid, if possible, major life stresses (e.g., moving) during pregnancy.

MEDICATION. Supplemental iron may be appropriate if anemic. No sleeping medications are prescribed.

LIFESTYLE CHANGES. Encourage adequate sleep and rest periods; help the client to arrange work, child care, and other activities to permit additional rest.

Encourage good posture, wearing of lowheeled shoes, and pelvic rock exercises to ease backaches. Pelvic rock exercises are taught to the client by having her stand against a wall,

bend knees slightly, and insert her hand behind the small of her back. Move the pelvis to roll her uterus up toward her chest and push her buttocks toward the floor. This should push her hand against the wall. Encourage her to do this while standing, walking, and sitting.

Suggest ways to increase comfort and reduce insomnia (e.g., placing pillows behind her back, raising the head of the bed up on blocks).

Establishing a regular sleep time and routine may induce sleep.

Demonstrate exercises that consume less energy (isometric instead of aerobic exercises). Have the client avoid exercise during the 2 hours prior to sleep.

Recommend exercise for sedentary clients (see Exercise, later in chapter).

Relaxation techniques may help.

Measures to reduce leg cramps may decrease their occurrence (see Leg/Muscle Cramps).

DIETARY INTERVENTIONS. Correct nutritional inadequacies, paying attention to total nutrient intake and distribution of those nutrients throughout the day (see Nutrition).[4] Advise client to avoid caffeine after midday and heavy meals at the end of the day. Suggest that warm milk may induce sleep. Encourage higher fluid intake earlier in the day, decreasing in the evening.

Follow-Up. Refer the client to a physician if symptoms of pathology are evident. When severe psychosocial stress, anxiety, or depression are noted, referral to a mental health care provider is appropriate.

Urinary Frequency or Incontinence

Etiology. A physiologic change during the first trimester that causes urinary difficulty is the enlargement of the uterus. which compresses the bladder. In the second trimester, however, as the uterus becomes an abdominal organ, these symptoms improve. In the third trimester, fetal presenting parts often compress the bladder.[20] This, in addition to hyperplasia and hyperemia of the pelvic organs and increased kidney output, leads to urinary frequency and incontinence.[4]

Subjective Data. The client may report increased urination, nocturia, or involuntary loss of urine. The history should *not* include back pain, fever, flulike symptoms, hematuria, dysuria, urgency, dark, cloudy or blood urine, dribbling, suprapubic pain, polyuria, polydipsia, polyphagia, history of perineal or abdominal trauma, as these symptoms/signs indicate other conditions requiring more thorough followup and possible medical referral.[21] She may report use of alcohol or caffeine.

To differentiate urine loss from rupture of membranes (ROM), know that ROM may be described as fluid from her vagina that cannot be controlled with Kegel exercises or as fluid that does not smell of urine and that may increase while she is lying down, gush at first when she stands, then decrease after standing.

Objective Data. Physical examination and vital signs are within normal limits. The costal vertebral angle and suprapubic area are not tender. Vaginal exam does not reveal pooling of amniotic fluid but may reveal a cystocele. Abdominal exam does not reveal contractions or uterine irritability.

Urinalysis and culture and sensitivity tests are used to detect urinary tract infection, renal and metabolic diseases. The test procedure first involves obtaining the best specimen. Instruct the client to wash her hands, then separate her labia. Provide three cleansing wipes and have her wipe from front to back once with each wipe, on the right side, then the left side, and then the middle. She should start to urinate in the commode, then catch a small amount of urine midstream in a sterile cup, and finish urinating in the commode. She should replace the lid on the cup tightly without touching the inside or top edge. Client teaching should stress that failing to follow this procedure jeopardizes the accuracy of the test.

The urine can be poured over a urine dipstick. Presence of nitrites, or 3–4 plus protein, suggests a urinary tract infection, plus glucose suggests ruling out diabetes (see Chapter 21).

The *nitrazine test* discriminates between vaginal discharge and amniotic fluid. Use of a sterile technique reduces the possibility of introducing infection if the membranes have ruptured. A sterile cotton tipped applicator is used to remove discharge from the vaginal pool. It is placed on nitrazine paper and the color change is compared with the chart. If the pH is 3.5 to 5, the fluid is normal vaginal discharge. If the pH is 7, the

discharge may be amniotic fluid, Note that blood and vaginal discharge associated with certain vaginal infections (e.g., bacterial vaginosis and trichomonas vaginitis) may give a higher than normal pH reading.

The *fern test* also discriminates between vaginal discharge and amniotic fluid. Again, a sterile speculum is used. The sample of vaginal discharge is placed on a clean slide and allowed to dry. Amniotic fluid forms a fernlike pattern under microscopic examination. Inform the client that the nitrazine and fern tests are the best way to discriminate between vaginal discharge and amniotic fluid. Differentiation is important because premature rupture of membranes can cause amniotitis or preterm labor. The practitioner may also look for fluid leaking from the cervix, which may not necessarily be amniotic fluid, but would certainly raise suspicion.

A screening 50-g glucola test that is negative (see Chapter 16) reduces the likelihood of diabetes.

Differential Medical Diagnosis. Urinary frequency/incontinence due to pregnancy ruling out urinary tract infection, pyelonephritis, kidney stone, stress urinary incontinence, gestational diabetes, preexisting diabetes mellitus, hypokalemia, and spontaneous rupture of membranes.[21]

Plan

PSYCHOSOCIAL INTERVENTIONS. Show the client diagrams of female anatomy. Often when a client can view the anatomical changes that occur during pregnancy, she understands the reason for urinary frequency and incontinence. Reassure her that these symptoms should improve after delivery. Advise the client to notify the health care provider if any symptoms ruled out during history taking occur in the future.

LIFESTYLE CHANGES. Resting and sleeping in the lateral recumbent position enhance kidney function. Kegel exercises increase perineal muscle tone.

DIETARY INTERVENTIONS. Advise the client to maintain an adequate fluid intake (6 to 8 glasses of water) to decrease the incidence of urinary tract infections. Water intake should decrease 2 to 3 hours before bedtime. In addition, advise the client to discontinue drinking beverages that contain alcohol or caffeine.

Follow-Up. A client with urinary tract infection (UTI) must be treated appropriately. Refer clients with symptoms of pathology, such as frequently repeated UTIs, to a urologist.

Varicosities of Vulva and Legs

Etiology. Physiologic changes during pregnancy that exacerbate varicosities are the increased venous stasis caused by the pressure of the gravid uterus and the vasodilation resulting from hormonal changes.[4,20] Women who develop varicosities often have a genetic predisposition, are inactive, obese, and have poor muscle tone. Prolonged standing or sitting aggravates the condition.

Subjective Data. The client may report aching, throbbing, swelling, or heaviness in the legs or vulvar area. The client may also report multiparity, prolonged standing or sitting, or decreased activity. She may note increased symptoms as she becomes older. A family history of varicosities may be reported. The history should *not* include clotting; swelling, redness, or tenderness; or a white, cold, numb leg, as these symptoms/signs indicate other conditions requiring immediate medical follow-up.

Objective Data. Diagnostic tests are not necessary. Physical examination and vital signs are within normal limits. Knotted, twisted, and swollen veins, however, are visible in the legs or vulva with possible edema below the varicosities. Peripheral pulses are normal. Significant negatives include no inflammation over the varicosities: no firm, cordlike feel: no dependent cyanosis: no positive Homan's sign; no deep pain on palpation; no distention of veins on the dorsal side of the foot after it is elevated 45 degrees; no positive Louvel's sign (pain in calf with coughing or sneezing that decreases with compression above varicosities); and no restlessness, fever, or tachycardia.[4]

Differential Medical Diagnosis. Varicosities of legs and/or vulva exacerbated by pregnancy ruling out venous thrombosis, thrombophlebitis, phlebothrombosis, edema from pregnancy-induced hypertension, and physiologic edema of pregnancy.

Plan

PSYCHOLOGICAL INTERVENTIONS. Explain to the client the reasons for the varicosities and inform her that the varicosities will not resolve until after delivery. Advise the client to notify the health care provider if any symptoms ruled out during the history taking occur in the future.

Any surgical intervention would be delayed until after delivery or, optimally, until after childbearing is complete.

LIFESTYLE CHANGES. Some lifestyle changes may help to relieve discomfort. Teach the client proper application of support hose and compression stockings: Have her lie flat and raise her legs to drain the veins. While her legs are elevated, have her roll the stockings on. Advise the client to do this before she rises in the morning and to leave the stockings on until she goes to bed at night.

Instruct the client to avoid crossing her legs and not to wear knee-high stockings or a constrictive band around the legs.[20]

Because orthostatic hypotension is common, tell the client to change position gradually when rising to avoid dizziness.

Explain the importance of elevating the legs above the level of the heart at least twice a day. Advise the client to wear comfortable shoes, to avoid prolonged standing or sitting, altering position frequently.

Instruct the client in the use of perineal pads with a sanitary belt or maternity girdle to compress vulvar varicosities.

Explain to the client the need to avoid leg or vulvar injury, as hemorrhage may result.

DIETARY INTERVENTIONS. Warn the client to avoid excess weight gain during pregnancy, and encourage weight loss during the postpartum period.

Follow-Up. Refer a client with symptoms of pathology to a physician.

Headache

Etiology. Physiologic changes during pregnancy that cause headaches include increased circulatory volume, vasodilation caused by high levels of circulating progesterone, tissue edema resulting from vascular congestion, stress, fatigue, and low blood sugar. Other causes include muscle spasm, allergens, hyperventilation or noxious fumes. Headaches not caused by pathology are very common in pregnancy. Women who had headaches prior to pregnancy improve 60 percent of the time, worsen 13 percent of the time, and remain unchanged 27 percent of the time. Headache can be a symptom of serious illness, which must be ruled out.[4,19]

Subjective Data. Focus on the nature, frequency, intensity, location, an description of the pain; factors that trigger, worsen, or alleviate it; and changes that have occurred during pregnancy in the quality of the headaches. The client may report a past or family history of headaches or increased stress. The history should *not* include injury to the head, neck, or back; nausea, vomiting, fever; migraine aura; occupational exposure to chemicals; consumption of alcohol, chocolate or aged cheese; unbalanced intake of calories; fatigue, as these symptoms/signs may indicate other conditions requiring medical or other appropriate follow-up. Pathology may also be present if there is a history of facial edema; changes in the level of consciousness; memory changes; depression, anxiety, motor, visual, or sensory changes; nausea; vomiting; stiff neck; fever; ear or eye pain; rhinitis; flulike symptoms; injury; or prodomata (i.e., visual, auditory, or sensory changes preceding a headache).[21]

Objective Data. Physical examination and vital signs, particularly blood pressure, weight gain pattern, ophthalmoscopic examination, and ear, nose, throat, neurological, musculoskeletal, and upper respiratory exams, are within normal limits.

A *urine dipstick test* that is negative for protein and ketones reduces the possibility of pregnancy-induced hypertension and dehydration from vomiting.

The *serum glucose test* (to rule out hypoglycemia) procedure begins with venipuncture; blood is withdrawn into a tube containing chemicals that stabilize the glucose. The tube is sent to a laboratory. Another method involves performing a fingerstick to withdraw a drop of blood that is then placed on a reagent strip. The strip is then analyzed in a machine or read against a scale (least accurate method).

Teach the client that a hematoma is common at the venipuncture site and will resolve. Tenderness at the fingerstick is common. Accurate interpretation of the results depends on obtaining an accurate history of food intake during the time preceding the test. This test is other performed after the client fasts or ingests a measured amount of glucose.

A complete blood count is another diagnostic test used (see Fatigue).

Differential Medical Diagnosis. Benign vascular headache of pregnancy ruling out pregnancy induced hypertension; upper respiratory sinus or dental infection; fever; cardiovascular disease; hypertensive crisis; cervical arthritis; muscle tension headache; cerebral mass or hemorrhage; central nervous system infections; hypoglycemia; migraine or cluster headache.[21]

Plan

PSYCHOSOCIAL INTERVENTIONS. Explain to the client the physiologic changes that are causing the headache and that it may improve in the second trimester. Advise the client to notify the health care provider if any symptoms ruled out during the history taking occur in the future.

Ask the client to keep a diary of activities, foods, and environmental stimuli that occur around the time of the headache. This may reveal triggering factors.

Teach the client symptoms of pregnancy induced hypertension (headache that is different in nature, visual changes, photophobia, confusion, swelling in the face or hands, severe swelling in the feet, epigastric pain) and encourage immediate contact with a physician.

MEDICATION. Acetaminophen is indicated for headache and other pain.

- *Administration.* 325 to 650 mg every 4 hours as needed for pain.
- *Side Effects and Adverse Reactions.* None are known.
- *Contraindication.* Sensitivity to acetaminophen; consuming 3 or more alcoholic drinks a day; history of liver damage.
- *Anticipated Outcome on Evaluation.* Reduced headache pain.

- *Client Counseling.* Instruct the client to notify the health care provider if headache pain continues. Overdose of acetaminophen requires prompt attention. It has been associated with liver damage.[23] Advise against chronic use.[24]

LIFESTYLE CHANGES. Advise the client to avoid activities and situations that may trigger headaches (stress, smoking, smoke filled rooms, blinking lights, sleeping late). Advise her to reduce stress as much as possible, get adequate sleep, have her neck and shoulders massaged with heat or coolness applied.

Encourage the client to practice relaxation techniques (see Nausea and Vomiting).

DIETARY INTERVENTIONS. Advise the client to eat a regular, balanced diet and to avoid intake of food that triggers headaches (e.g., caffeine, chocolate, nitrites, hard aged cheese, alcohol—especially red wine).

Refer the client to a physician if the headache is severe, does not respond to interventions, requires strong pain killers, or demonstrates other signs of pregnancy induced hypertension, pathology, or eye strain. If signs of severe psychosocial stress are present, refer the client to a mental health care provider. Referral to a pain center may help severe headache that is not due to pathology.

Breast Pain, Enlargement, and Changes in Pigmentation

Etiology. Physiologic changes that underlie these complaints are the increased levels of estrogen and progesterone, which cause the fat layer of breasts to thicken and the numbers and development of milk ducts and glands to increase. As a result, the breasts, especially the area round the areola, increase in size, weight, and tenderness, and bluish veins appear on the chest. The nipples become erect, melatonin causes the areolae to darken, the Montgomery tubercles enlarge, and there is a slight colostrum discharge.[4,19,20]

Subjective Data. The client may report increasing tenderness, weight, and size of the breasts, darkening of the areolae, leakage of colostrum from the nipples. The client should *not* report pain and redness localized in one area of the breast, fever, flulike symptoms, injury, masses, dimples,

bloody discharge, changes in skin texture, or changes in breast or nipple size, shape, symmetry, as these symptoms/signs may indicate other conditions requiring medical follow-up.[4,21] Some medications are known to cause galactorrhea.

Objective Data. No diagnostic tests are necessary. Physical examination and vital signs are within normal limits. Areas of induration, inflammation, or heat; masses; skin dimpling; skin changes; enlarged nodes; or unilateral or bloody nipple discharge should not be present.

Differential Medical Diagnosis. Breast tenderness, enlargement, and pigment changes due to pregnancy ruling out mastitis, fibrocystic breast tissue, breast injury, and breast cancer.[21]

Plan

PSYCHOSOCIAL INTERVENTIONS. Explain to the client the reasons for the breast changes. Inform her that pain often improves in the second trimester but the other changes will remain until after lactation ends. Advise the client to notify the health care provider if any symptoms ruled out during the history taking occur in the future.

LIFESTYLE CHANGES. Advise the client to examine her breasts in the same way as before pregnancy, except that no special time of month is indicated. If instruction is necessary, provide it (see Chapter 14).

In addition, the client may need to constantly wear a supportive bra. Correct fit is important as breast size changes in pregnancy. She may find wearing a bra while sleeping more comfortable.

DIETARY INTERVENTIONS. Advise the client to avoid the use of caffeine.

Follow-Up. Clients with symptoms of mastitis must be treated appropriately (see Chapter 14). Refer the client with symptoms of pathology to a physician.

Menstrual-like Cramping

Etiology. The physiologic changes underlying the sensation of cramping may be the increased vascular congestion in the pelvis, the pressure exerted by the presenting fetal part, or stretching of the round ligaments.[25] Many women report such cramping during the first 1 or 2 months of pregnancy and again at the end of pregnancy.

Subjective Data. The client reports sensations similar to those she experienced just prior to her menses, before she was pregnant. The client should *not,* however, report severe cramping, unilateral or suprapubic abdominal pain, contractions, vaginal bleeding, rupture of membranes, bowel or urinary tract symptoms (see Urinary Frequency or Incontinence and Constipation), as these symptoms/signs may indicate other conditions which may require medical follow-up.[21]

Objective Data. Physical examination and vital signs are within normal limits. There is no vaginal bleeding, cervical dilatation, adnexal masses, tenderness, or vaginal pooling of amniotic fluid. Uterine size equals dates. There is no suprapubic tenderness.

Serum β *Human chorionic gonadotropin-quantitative* (hCG) is evaluated to identify and monitor pregnancy and to diagnose certain pregnancy related complications (e.g., abortion, ectopic pregnancy, hydatidiform gestation). A blood sample is withdrawn by venipuncture and sent to a laboratory. In normal pregnancies, the hCG level is expected to double every other day. A deviation could indicate a complication of pregnancy and requires further testing.

Nitrazine and *fern tests* and *urinalysis and culture and sensitivity* may also be indicated (see Urinary Frequency and Incontinence).

Differential Medical Diagnosis. Normal menstrual-like cramping in pelvis ruling out ectopic pregnancy, abortion, premature labor, gastroenteritus, other bowel disorders, and urinary tract infection.[21]

Plan

PSYCHOSOCIAL INTERVENTIONS. Explain to the client the physiologic changes that underlie the sensations. In addition, inform the client that no signs of imminent abortion or labor exist and that the sensations should decrease in the second trimester but may return again in the third. Advise the client to notify the health care provider if any symptoms ruled out during the history-taking occur in the future.

Follow-Up. Refer the client with symptoms of pathology to a physician.

SECOND TRIMESTER

Backache

Etiology. Physiologic change underlying a backache is the shift in the center of gravity caused by the enlarging uterus. Muscle strain results. In addition, a high level of circulating progesterone softens cartilage and loosens once stable joints, thereby increasing discomfort. Upper back pain can also be caused by increased breast size.[4,19] Night backache may result from pressure on the lower back from venous stasis and the gravid uterus.[19] One author, Ostgaard (1994), distinguished between lumbar-type backache and sciatica, both well known, and posterior pelvic pain. Posterior pelvic pain is distal and lateral to the lumbar sacral spine and may radiate to the posterior thigh to below the knee.[27]

Subjective Data. The client reports dull, aching pain in the upper or lower back that increases as the day goes on. Ask the client to describe the location, nature, and duration of the pain, exacerbating and relieving factors, the changes in pain that occur with movement. She may wear improperly fitting or high-heeled shoes. The client may have gained excessive weight, report being obese before pregnancy, must stand or sit for long time periods or be fatigued. She may be large busted and/or wear an improperly fitting or poorly supporting bra. Many clients lift heavy objects by bending from the waist rather than bending the knees; low back muscles are strained as a result of this movement. Ostgaard (1994) defined posterior pelvic pain as time and weight-bearing related pain deep in the gluteals, stabbing with possible radiation down the thigh to the knee but not beyond. Turning in bed often causes the pain.[27] There should be *no* history of back injury or other problems, surgery, or symptoms of urinary tract infection, vaginal infection, ruptured membranes, uterine contractions, pain or numbness in buttocks, legs or hips, or neurologic deficit.[21]

Objective Data. No diagnostic tests are done. Physical examination and vital signs are within normal limits; however, lordosis, abnormal gait,

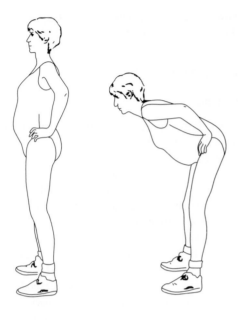

Upper Body Bends

This exercise strengthens the muscles of your back and torso.

- Stand with your legs apart, knees bent slightly, with your hands on your hips.
- Bend forward slowly, keeping your upper back straight. You should feel a slight pull along your upper thigh.
- Repeat 10 times.

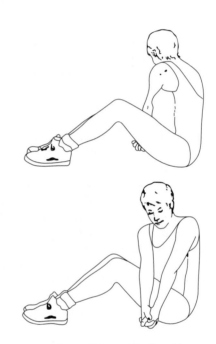

Diagonal Curl

This exercise strengthens the muscles of your back, hips, and abdomen. If you have not already been exercising regularly, skip this exercise.

- Sit on the floor with your knees bent, feet on the floor, and hands clasped in front of you.
- Twist your upper torso to the left until your hands touch the floor.
- Do the same movement to the right.
- Repeat on both sides 5 times.

Figure 17–3. A Healthy Back. Exercises that strengthen and stretch muscles to support the back and legs, promote good posture, help ease back pain, and prepare for labor and delivery. *(Source: American College of Obstetricians and Gynecologists, Planning for pregnancy, birth and beyond, Second Edition. Washington, D.C., ACOG © 1995.)* Reprinted with permission.

or tenderness along paraspinous muscles may be revealed. The posterior pelvic pain provocation test, described by Ostgaard, recreates the specific pain. While the client is supine, the knee on the affected side is bent vertically, the other leg remains straight, and the health care provider pushes straight down on the knee toward the pelvis while stabilizing the pelvis.[27] Significant negatives include no costal vertebral angle tenderness; no pain with straight-leg raises; normal patellar, deep tendon, and plantar reflexes; and a normal neurologic exam. No uri-

nary tract symptoms (see Urinary Frequency and Incontinence), no abnormal vaginal discharge (see Leukorrhea), and no uterine contractions are detected.

Differential Medical Diagnoses. Backache or posterior pelvic pain related to pregnancy ruling out uterine contractions, genital infections, urinary tract infections, kidney stone, pancreatitis, ulcer, fracture, sciatica, herniated disk, vertebral tumor, osteomyelitis, arthritis, ankylosing spondylitis, muscle sprain, or strain.[21]

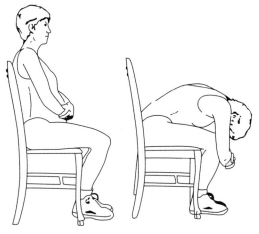

Forward Bend

This exercise stretches and strengthens the muscles of your back.

- Sit on a chair in a comfortable position. Keep your arms relaxed.
- Bend forward slowly, with your arms in front and hanging down.
- If you feel any discomfort or pressure on your abdomen, do not push any further.
- Hold this position for a count of 5, then get up slowly without arching your back.
- Repeat 5 times.

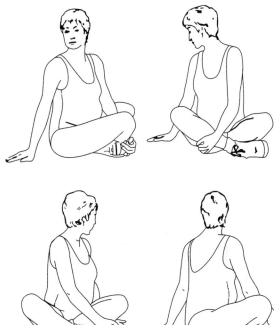

Trunk Twist

This exercise stretches the muscles of your back, spine, and upper torso.

- Sit on the floor with your legs crossed, with your left hand holding your left foot and your right hand on the floor at your side for support.
- Slowly twist your upper torso to the right.
- Do the same movement to the left, after switching your hands (right hand holding right foot and left hand supporting you).
- Repeat on both sides 5–10 times.

Figure 17–3. (Continued)

Plan

PSYCHOSOCIAL INTERVENTIONS. Explain to the client the changes underlying the backache, and inform her that it should decrease or resolve after pregnancy. Advise the client to notify the health care provider if any symptoms ruled out during the history taking occur in the future.

MEDICATION. Acetaminophen (see Headache).

LIFESTYLE CHANGES. Instruct client in the pelvic tilt exercise (see Fatigue). Proper body mechanics, particularly when lifting require her to keep her back straight when lifting and to bend her knees, keeping the object close to her body;[20] if she must hold her breath to lift an object, it is too heavy. Advise her to avoid excessive twisting, bending, and stretching. Back rubs may help.[19]

Inform the client that an exercise program encourages general fitness.

Exercises for the back may help back pain but not posterior pelvic pain (see Figure 17–3).

Advise the client, when standing for long periods, to rest one foot on a low stool, and when

Backward Stretch

This exercise stretches and strengthens the muscles of your back, pelvis, and thighs.

- Kneel on hands and knees, with your knees 8–10 inches apart and your arms straight (hands under your shoulders).
- Curl backward slowly, tucking your head toward your knees and keeping your arms extended.
- Hold this position for a count of 5, then come back up to all fours slowly.
- Repeat 5 times.

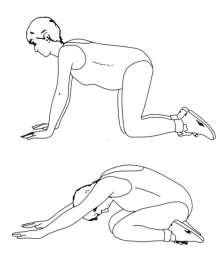

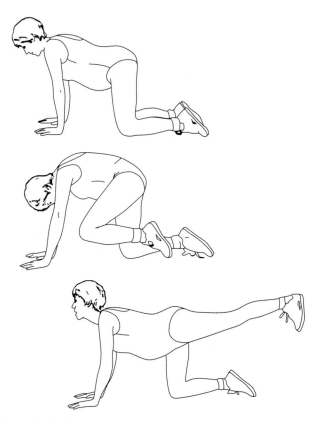

Leg Lift Crawl

This exercise strengthens the muscles of your back and abdomen.

- Kneel on hands and knees, with your weight distributed evenly and your arms straight (hands under your shoulders).
- Lift your left knee and bring it toward your elbow.
- Straighten your leg without locking your knee.
- Extend your leg up and back.
- Do this exercise to a count of 5. Move slowly; don't fling your leg back or arch your back.
- Repeat on both sides 5–10 times.

Figure 17–3. (Continued)

sitting for long periods, to rest her feet on a low stool, to raise her knees above the waist, and to sit with her back firmly against the back of the chair.[20] While driving, she should sit straight and position the seat so that her knees are slightly bent when using the pedals.

Advise the client to avoid excessive walking or standing. A nonelastic sacroiliac belt offers some relief from pain while walking to clients with posterior pelvic pain.[27]

Inform the client that a firm, supportive mattress may be helpful. Advise her to assume a lateral recumbent position while sleeping, with pillows supporting the back and legs; sleeping in this position promotes comfort. Some clients sleep better on the couch.

Rocking Back Arch

This exercise stretches and strengthens the muscles of your back, hips, and abdomen.

- Kneel on hands and knees, with your weight distributed evenly and your back straight.
- Rock back and forth, to a count of 5.
- Return to the original position and curl your back upward as much as you can.
- Repeat 5–10 times.

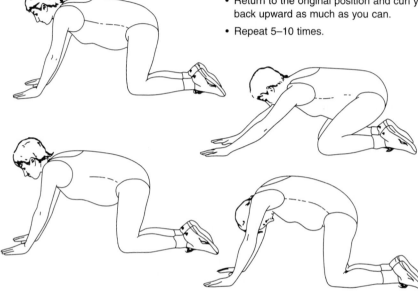

Back Press

This exercise strengthens the muscles of your back, torso, and upper body and promotes good posture.

- Stand with your feet 10–12 inches away from a wall and your back against it.
- Press the lower part of your back against the wall.
- Hold this position for a count of 10, then release.
- Repeat 10 times.

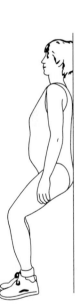

Figure 17–3. (Continued)

Advise the client with upper back pain to wear a good, supportive bra, and the client with lower back pain, to wear a maternity support girdle.

Warm tub baths may be soothing. Advise the client to be careful when rising from the tub, as she may experience dizziness; she should have someone's help or hold on to some other support. Do not recommend tub baths for clients in whom rupture of membranes is suspected.

Inform the client that massage and relaxation techniques, as well as use of a heating pad for short periods, but not during sleep (to avoid a burn), may promote comfort.

DIETARY INTERVENTIONS. Advise the client to avoid gaining excessive weight.

Follow-Up. If severe pain does not respond to intervention, refer the client to a physical therapist. Refer any client who requires strong pain medication or who has symptoms of pathology to a physician.

Syncope

Etiology. The physiologic changes underlying syncope (feeling dizzy or faint) are related to pooling of blood in the lower extremities, expansion of blood volume, and compression of the vena cava and lungs by the gravid uterus.[25] True vertigo is often described as the room spinning or disorientation in relation to space. Syncope is also caused by nausea and vomiting, low blood sugar, substance abuse, hyperventilation, postural hypotension, and illness.

Subjective Data. The client reports lightheadedness or dizziness that lasts a minute or less when she is standing, lying on her back, or changing position. She may report low or sporadic intake of calories. There should be *no* history of loss of consciousness; use of medications; exposure to toxic agents; substance abuse; sinus or ear problems, numbness or tingling in the digits or around the mouth; nausea or vomiting; melena; heart palpitations; shortness of breath; double vision; loss of strength or sensation; incoordination; or anxiety or depression, as these symptoms/signs may indicate other conditions that may require medical or other appropriate follow-up.[21]

Objective Data. Physical examination and vital signs are within normal limits. *Hemoglobin* tests may reveal anemia.

Differential Medical Diagnosis. Syncope related to the hemodynamic changes in pregnancy ruling out orthostatic hypotension, compression of vena cava, hyperventilation, anemia, hypoglycemia, dehydration, substance abuse, exposure to a toxic agent, psychosocial stress, or central nervous system, cardiac, respiratory, endocrine, eye, ear, or sinus pathology.

Plan

Psychosocial Interventions. Explain to the client the physiologic changes causing syncope. Advise the client to notify the health care provider if any symptoms ruled out during the history taking occur in the future.

Advise the client to avoid stressful situations. Teach her to recognize hyperventilation. Encourage her to verbalize problems and explore appropriate responses.

Lifestyle Changes. Advise the client to rest in the lateral recumbent position; to change position gradually, holding on to something when rising; or to lower her head below the level of the heart if feeling faint.

To reduce blood pooling in the extremities, instruct the client to apply compression stockings before getting out of bed and to perform leg pumping exercises (flexing and extending the ankle several times).

If being in a crowd induces symptoms, advise the client to move to an open window or go outside and loosen or remove layers of clothing.

Dietary Interventions. Advise the client to eat regularly throughout the day. Assess her diet for adequate calorie and fluid intake and distribution.

Follow-Up. Refer a client with symptoms of pathology to a physician.

Leukorrhea

Etiology. The physiologic changes underlying leukorrhea arise from the high levels of estrogen that cause increased vascularity and hypertrophy of cervical glands as well as vaginal cells. As a consequence, leukorrhea production increases; the discharge is white or yellow, thin, and more acidic than normal vaginal discharge.[4]

Subjective Data. The client reports increased vaginal discharge. She should *not*, however, report green, watery, bloody, itchy, or irritating discharge that smells foul or fishy; fever; flulike symptoms; abdominal pain: bleeding after intercourse; dysuria or dyspareunia.[21] Ask the client if she has multiple or new sexual partners, has recently resumed sexual activity or douching, has had abnormal Pap smears in the past, or has recently used antibiotics.

Objective Data. Physical examination and vital signs are within normal limits: however, the pelvic exam may show increased but normal-appearing vaginal discharge.

A *normal saline and potassium hydroxide test* (wet mount) is used to determine whether candida, trichomonads, clue cells, white or red blood cells, or bacteria are present in the vaginal discharge. A Q-tip is used to obtain some vaginal, not cervical, discharge which is placed on two clean, dry microscope slides. A drop of normal saline is placed on one and a drop of potassium hydroxide on the other. Coverslips are used and the specimens are examined under the microscope. Candida, trichomonads, clue cells, and abnormal numbers of coccal bacteria, red cells, and white blood cells all indicate a vaginal infection.

A *Papanicolaou smear* is done to detect changes in the cervical or endocervical cells that could indicate dysplasia, carcinoma, or human papillomavirus. Signs of vaginal infection or herpes simplex may also be noted.

Both tests are speculum exams; that is, cervical and endocervical cells are collected using a wooden or preferably plastic spatula and cytobrush (though during pregnancy, a Q-tip is preferred to reduce cervical bleeding from the collection procedure), placed on a microscope slide, sprayed with a fixative, and sent to a pathology laboratory for examination.

Inform the client that the Pap smear is a screening test used to determine which clients require additional testing. Advise the client that she should not douche, use vaginal medications, or have intercourse for 24 hours before the test. The procedure may cause slight spotting up to 24 hours afterward.

The *nitrazine* and *fern tests* are also used (see Urinary Frequency and Incontinence).

Differential Medical Diagnoses. Physiologic leukorrhea of pregnancy ruling out ruptured membranes, vaginitis, cervicitis, urinary tract infection, condyloma acuminatum, genital herpes, sexually transmitted diseases, and cervical dysplasia or neoplasia.[21]

Plan

PSYCHOSOCIAL INTERVENTIONS. Reassure the client that increased leukorrhea is normal and will decrease postpartum. Advise the client to notify the health care provider if any symptoms ruled out during the history taking occur in the future.

LIFESTYLE CHANGES. Advise the client to keep the vulva clean and dry; to avoid pantyhose and other tight or layered clothing; to wear cotton underwear and a nightgown without underwear at night; and if using panty liners to use unscented/nondeodorant ones, changing them frequently. Also, advise her to avoid douching and tampon use unless otherwise instructed by the health care provider. Feminine sprays, powders, etc. should not be used.

DIETARY INTERVENTIONS. Some clients have recurrent monilia during pregnancy. Instruct these clients to avoid large amounts of simple sugar in their diets. If an antibiotic has been prescribed, advise the client to eat yogurt containing active cultures (aspartame sweetened yogurt unless the client has phenylketonuria or sensitivity to aspartame) to reduce the risk of candida infection. Inform the client that adding lactobacillus, in tablet or granular form, to food may also help; it may be purchased at a pharmacy, where it is kept refrigerated.

Follow-Up. Refer all clients with abnormal Pap smears or symptoms of pathology for appropriate follow-up. Clients with symptoms of vaginitis require appropriate treatment (see Chapter 11).

Epistaxis and Epulis

Etiology. The physiologic change underlying epistaxis and epulis is the high level of circulating estrogen. The nasal mucosa and gums become hypertrophic and hyperemic and, as a result, bleed more easily.[4]

Subjective Data. The client reports that her nose or gums bleed easily, but she is able to control a nosebleed within 15 minutes. Nosebleeds are usually preceded by blowing the nose, picking at the nose, or overexertion. Gums bleed after teeth brushing or flossing, but the bleeding stops quickly. The client reports continuing her dental care during pregnancy. She has no history of hypertension, bleeding problems, sinus symptoms, upper respiratory infection, swollen glands, fever, trauma, cocaine or chronic nasal spray use.[21] She may report a history of nasal stuffiness, postnasal drip, or hay fever.

Objective Data. Physical examination and vital signs, particularly blood pressure, are within normal limits. The nasal mucosa may be swollen and dull red or pink, and clotted blood may be observed. Increased vascularization may be evident as may postnasal drip. The gums may show evidence of trauma caused by a toothbrush or floss, and may look swollen and inflamed. Nasal polyps, growths, and evidence of cocaine use should not be observed. A *complete blood count* is the diagnostic test performed (see Fatigue).

Differential Medical Diagnoses. Epistaxis and/or epulis of pregnancy ruling out sinusitis, upper respiratory infection, polyps, or ulcerative disease of the nasal mucosa, hypertension, anemia, bleeding disorders, cocaine or chronic nasal spray use, gingivitis; or other dental disease.[21]

Plan

PSYCHOSOCIAL INTERVENTIONS. Explain to the client the underlying physiologic changes that cause the problem and inform her that the condition should resolve after pregnancy. Advise the client to notify the health care provider if any symptoms ruled out during the history taking occur in the future.

LIFESTYLE CHANGES. Advise the client, when nosebleeds occur, to loosen clothing around the neck, sit with her head tilted forward, pinch her nostrils for 10 to 15 minutes, and apply ice packs to her nose. Light packing of the nose with sterile gauze may help. Inform her that applying petroleum jelly to the nostrils will lubricate and protect the mucosa. Advise the client to avoid overheated air, excessive exertion, and nasal sprays. Cool mist vaporizer may help humidify the air. Do not use if allergic to molds or mildew.

Inform the client that the reduced air pressure at high altitudes may precipitate nosebleeds. Instruct the client to blow her nose gently, one nostril at a time and not to pick at her nose.

Advise clients with epulis to practice good oral hygiene, using a soft toothbrush and flossing regularly and gently. Instruct clients that warm saline mouthwashes relieve discomfort. Regular dental care is advised. Dental x-rays while shielding the abdomen and use of local anesthesia are safe.[20]

DIETARY INTERVENTIONS. Advise the client to maintain a healthy diet; to avoid decay causing sugary, starchy food; and to cut food that is difficult to chew into small pieces to reduce gum trauma.

Follow-Up. Refer clients with gum and tooth disease to a dentist. Clients whose nose bleeds cannot be controlled within 15 minutes or who have high blood pressure or symptoms of pathology should be referred to a physician.

Muscle Cramps in the Calf, Thigh, or Buttocks

Etiology. The physiologic change underlying muscle cramps in pregnancy is uncertain. An imbalance in the phosphorus/calcium ratio has been postulated, but a correlation with calcium intake has not been established. Cramps occur primarily in the second and third trimesters and could be related to the pressure of the gravid uterus on pelvic nerves and blood vessels.[19]

Subjective Data. The client reports calf, thigh, or buttocks cramps that occur mostly at night or in the early morning. She may report a similar history with previous pregnancies, excessive exercise or walking, wearing of high-heeled or poorly supporting shoes, or consumption of foods very high or low in calcium. There should be *no* history of deep-vein thromboembolytic disease, recent trauma or surgery, inability to walk, lower back pain, or arthritis.[21]

Objective Data. Physical examination and vital signs, particularly Homan's sign, and pulses are within normal limits. No redness, tenderness, heat, swelling, coldness, numbness, or whiteness appears in a calf or leg.[19]

Diagnostic tests are not done unless pathology is suspected.

Differential Medical Diagnoses. Calf, thigh, or buttocks cramps, ruling out thromboembolytic disease, varicosities, dehydration, arthritis, sciatica, and nerve root compression.[21]

Plan

PSYCHOSOCIAL INTERVENTIONS. Explain to the client the physiologic changes that could possibly cause muscle cramping and inform her that the condition should improve after delivery. Advise the client to notify the health care provider if any symptoms ruled out during the history-taking occur in the future.

LIFESTYLE CHANGES. Advise the client to avoid stretching her legs, pointing toes, walking excessively, and lying on her back, and to wear low-heeled shoes.

Instruct the client in calf stretching: Have the client stand 3 ft from a wall and lean toward it to rest the lower arms against the wall, keeping her heels on the floor. Advise her that performing this exercise 10 to 12 times before going to bed may reduce cramping.[19]

DIETARY INTERVENTIONS. Correct excessive or inadequate intake of dairy and calcium products.

Follow-Up. Refer a client with symptoms of pathology to the physician.

Ligament Pain

Etiology. The physiologic change underlying ligament pain is the growth of the uterus, which causes ligaments in the pelvis to stretch.[4,20] The round ligaments attach to the uterus at the top of the fundus, extend anteriorly and inferiorly to the oviducts, through the inguinal canal, and attach at the labia majora. Other ligaments attach at the upper fundus, extend bilaterally to the upper labia majora and from the posterior cervix to the sacrum.[19]

Subjective Data. Usually in the second trimester, the client reports sharp or dull pain on either or both sides of the uterus. The pain often starts or worsens with twisting, stretching, or quick movements. The client, however, does *not* report contractions, constipation, diarrhea, vomiting, vomiting blood, tarry or bloody stools, low-grade fever, anorexia, periumbilical pain, right lower abdominal flank pain, urinary tract infection symptoms, a tender lump in the groin that tends to worsen the longer she stands, or one-sided constant pain that increases (if the pregnancy is less than 14 to 16 weeks). These symptoms may indicate problems other than ligament pain, and require further evaluation.[21]

Objective Data. Physical examination and vital signs are within normal limits. Tenderness at the supravaginal insertion site or laterally to the uterus may occur on pelvic exam. Significant negatives include no contractions, cervical dilatation, effacement or softening, rupture of membranes, adnexal or abdominal masses, hernias, hyperactive or underactive bowel sounds, rebound tenderness, or tenderness on abdominal palpation other than along the affected ligament.

Differential Medical Diagnoses. Stretching of ligaments ruling out preterm labor, ectopic pregnancy, rupture of an ovarian cyst, constipation, intestinal obstruction, ulcer, diverticulitis, gastroenteritis, appendicitis; ureteral stone, and inguinal hernia.[21]

Plan

PSYCHOSOCIAL INTERVENTIONS. Explain to the client the underlying physiologic change causing the pain and inform her that the pain will resolve after pregnancy. Advise the client to notify the health care provider if any symptoms ruled out during history taking occur in the future.

LIFESTYLE CHANGES. Advise the client to avoid sudden, twisting or stretching movements. Inform her that getting out of bed by turning onto her side and pushing up with her arm will reduce abdominal muscle and back strain.

Fingertip massage warm bath, or heat to the affected area may provide relief. Heating pads should not be used during sleep to avoid burns. Advise her to avoid excessive exercise, standing, or walking. Frequent, short rest periods during the day may help.

Follow-Up. Refer clients with symptoms of pathology to a physician.

Excessive Salivation and Bad Taste in Mouth

Etiology. The etiology of oral changes is not known. It is theorized that because swallowing saliva increases nausea, clients are reluctant to swallow, which results in their perception of more saliva.[4,19]

Subjective Data. The client reports increased salivation or a bitter taste in her mouth. She does *not* report a sore throat, fever, flulike symptoms, heat, pain or lesions in the mouth, bad breath, upper abdominal pain, bloating, lethargy, dental problems, or pica. In addition, the client practices good dental hygiene and does not have symptoms of a psychiatric disorder.

Objective Data. No diagnostic tests are necessary. Physical examination and vital signs, particularly the condition of the mouth and teeth, are within normal limits. Occasionally, perioral irritation, red-coated tongue, swollen glands, drooling, or salivation interfering with speech may occur.

Differential Medical Diagnoses. Excessive salivation related to pregnancy ruling out stomatitis, tonsillitis, pharyngitis, gastric, hepatic or pancreatic disorders, dental problems, and pica.[21]

Plan

PSYCHOSOCIAL INTERVENTIONS. Reassure the client that the complaint is related to pregnancy and that the condition should resolve after the pregnancy. Also, inform the client that her breath does not smell unpleasant. Advise the client to notify the health care provider if any symptoms ruled out during the history taking occur in the future.

LIFESTYLE CHANGES. Advise the client to maintain good oral hygiene.

DIETARY INTERVENTIONS: Advise the client to avoid excessive starch intake and to maintain a good diet and adequate hydration. Inform her that sucking hard candy or breath mints or chewing gum may improve the taste in her mouth.

Follow-Up. Refer a client with symptoms of pathology to a physician. Refer a client with symptoms of dental disease to a dentist.

Discomfort in the Upper Extremities

Etiology. Postural changes caused by the enlarging breasts may cause a flexion of the neck and slumping shoulders. This plus the retention of fluids can cause aching, numbness, and weakness of the upper extremities. Carpal tunnel syndrome results from swelling in the wrists, causing numbness, tingling, weakness, and pain in the first through third digits.[25]

Subjective Data. The client may report pain, numbness, weakness, or tingling in the upper arms or hands. She does not report cardiac symptoms; chest pain, palpitations, air hunger, sweating, nausea and/or vomiting, symptoms of hyperventilation; numbness around mouth with nausea or sweating, loss of sensation in the extremities, loss of ability to grip, history of trauma to neck, shoulder, arm or wrist, recent chest trauma or surgery, psoriasis, or arthritis.[21] She may report a past history of carpal tunnel syndrome.

Objective Data. The fingers may exhibit decreased sensation during neurological testing.

The hands may be edematous. Pain produced by forced flexion at wrist or tapping on the carpal tunnel indicates carpal tunnel syndrome. Otherwise the physical examination and vital signs are within normal limits.[21]

Differential Medical Diagnoses. Pain, numbness, tingling, or weakness in the upper extremities ruling out carpal tunnel syndrome, trauma, infection, arthritis, cervical neck injury or disease, nerve damage in the hands, cardiac problems or psychosocial problems causing hyperventilation.

Plan

PSYCHOSOCIAL INTERVENTIONS. Assure the client that the discomfort is related to pregnancy and will resolve after the pregnancy is over.

LIFESTYLE CHANGES. Wearing a wrist splint especially to bed at night to prevent sleeping on flexed wrists. During the day, if the hands are affected, raise hands above the head and pump the fists. At night, put the hands over the side of the bed and shake vigorously. Acupuncture is sometimes helpful.[25] Avoid aggravating movements, especially fine motor movements (e.g., typing, writing).

DIETARY INTERVENTIONS. See Edema for interventions to reduce swelling.

Follow-Up. Refer any client with symptoms of pathology to a physician. Any client with recurrent hyperventilation should be referred for counseling.

Pica and Changes in Taste and Smell

Etiology. The physiologic change underlying pica (i.e., eating nonnutritive substances) is unknown. It occurs in all cultures but in some, for example, among African American women in the southeastern United States, it is very common. Many clients notice a change in their senses of taste and smell but do not report pica.[4]

Subjective Data. The client reports changes in her senses of taste and smell. Common changes include those in the taste of coffee, tobacco, alcohol, milk, eggs, and red meats. The client may report cravings for nonfood items (pica) or state that eating specific items is important for a healthy pregnancy, delivery, and baby and not eating them may cause harm or birthmarks.

Pica may lead to constipation, bowel obstruction or perforation, parotid gland obstruction, anemia, lead intoxication, or parasitic infection.[4,9]

Clients may also report financial problems affecting the food budget.

Objective Data. Physical examination, particularly of the abdomen and mouth, and vital signs are within normal limits.

Diagnostic tests include the *urine dipstick,* which if negative for ketones rules out ketonuria, and a *complete blood count.*

Differential Medical Diagnoses. Changes in taste and smell related to pregnancy ruling out pica. If pica is diagnosed, rule out anemia, ketonuria, obstruction, parasitic intestinal problems, poor nutrition, and lead poisoning.

Plan

PSYCHOSOCIAL INTERVENTIONS. Reassure the client that the changes in taste and smell should resolve after the pregnancy and may improve as pregnancy advances. While respecting cultural variations, explain that eating nonfood items (e.g., starch) may hurt rather than protect the mother or fetus. Advise the client to notify the health care provider if any symptoms ruled out during the history taking occur in the future.

DIETARY INTERVENTIONS. Evaluate the client's diet to determine its adequacy. If pica is diagnosed, explain the need to maintain a healthy diet and that problems could occur if the craved substance either is substituting for nutritious food or is harmful to the mother or fetus.

Follow-Up. Refer a client with symptoms of pathology to a physician or a client eating an inadequate diet to a dietitian. A client without adequate financial resources may be referred to a social worker.

THIRD TRIMESTER

Braxton-Hicks Contractions

Etiology. In early gestation, the uterus begins painless, irregular contractions known as Braxton-Hicks contractions. No cervical dilatation occurs. The contractions are thought to arise from stretching of the myometrium and increase the tone of uterine muscles in preparation for labor.[4]

Subjective Data. The client may report a sudden tightening or pressure in the uterus, without the sensation of building, that lasts from 30 seconds to 2 minutes. The contractions may decrease with position change or emptying of the bladder. The client does *not* report regular contractions, vaginal bleeding, bloody show, leaking or rupture of membranes, symptoms of urinary tract infection, constipation, diarrhea, fever, flulike symptoms, or cramping, as these symptoms/signs may indicate other conditions requiring medical follow-up Increased vaginal discharge may signal cervical dilatation.[4]

Objective Data. Physical examination and vital signs are within normal limits. The pelvic exam, particularly cervical dilatation, effacement, and station, is within normal limits. No bleeding from the cervical os or pooling of amniotic fluid is evident. The abdominal exam does not reveal regular contractions, rigid, tender uterus, or suprapubic tenderness. Bowel sounds are normal. The fetus should be normally active.

Differential Medical Diagnoses. Braxton-Hicks contractions ruling out preterm labor, premature rupture of membranes, urinary tract infection, pyelonephritis, gastroenteritis, constipation, and normal fetal activity.

Plan

PSYCHOSOCIAL INTERVENTIONS. Reassure the client that Braxton-Hicks contractions are normal. Teach the client to differentiate between Braxton-Hicks and labor contractions. Labor contractions grow longer, stronger, and closer together and occur at regular intervals. Often, activity strengthens labor contractions, but decreases Braxton-Hicks contractions. Labor is differentiated from Braxton-Hicks contractions by the presence of cervical changes.

Advise the client to notify the health care provider if any symptoms ruled out during the history taking occur in the future.

LIFESTYLE CHANGES. Advise the client to empty her bladder frequently, though she must stay well hydrated. Inform her that resting in a lateral recumbent position, walking, or exercising lightly may relieve contractions.

As Lamaze breathing eases the discomfort of contractions, teach the client to breathe slowly and deeply at about half her normal rate. Make sure that she is inhaling and exhaling approximately equal amounts of air. Advise the client to contact the health care provider if contractions become strong or different in character from previous contractions.

Follow-Up. Refer a client with possible preterm labor, premature rupture of membranes, or symptoms of pathology to a physician.

Dyspnea

Etiology. The physiologic change underlying dyspnea is the enlarging uterus, which presses up against the abdominal organs and diaphragm, preventing full expansion of the lungs. The woman has an increased awareness of the need to breathe. Dyspnea can be aggravated by the pressure of the gravid uterus against the vena cava, reducing venous return to the heart.[4]

Subjective Data. The client reports shortness of breath, which may or may not be associated with exercise, dizziness, or lightheadedness. There should be *no* history of headache, sore throat, coughing, flulike symptoms, fever, night sweats, wheezing, chest pain, indigestion, or exercise intolerance with vomiting, sweating, hyperventilation, or anxiety. Neither does the client smoke or have a history of respiratory or cardiac problems.[21]

Objective Data. Diagnostic tests are not necessary. Physical examination, particularly of the upper respiratory tract, heart, lungs, and vital signs are within normal limits.

Differential Medical Diagnosis. Dyspnea related to pregnancy ruling out upper respiratory infection pulmonary or cardiac problems, and anemia.[21]

Plan

PSYCHOSOCIAL INTERVENTIONS. Reassure the client that her dyspnea is related to normal physiologic changes of pregnancy and that it will improve when the fetus drops into the pelvis. Inform her that it is not an indication that she or the fetus is receiving insufficient air. Advise the client to notify the health care provider if any symptoms ruled out during history-taking occur in the future.

LIFESTYLE CHANGES. Advise the client to avoid exercise that precipitates dyspnea, to rest after exercise, and to avoid overheating and very warm environments. Instruct her not to wear restrictive clothing. Inform the client that sitting up very straight or elevating her head with pillows may help relieve dyspnea, as may lying in the lateral recumbent position, which displaces the uterus off the vena cava.

Follow-Up. Refer a client with symptoms of pathology to a physician.

Edema

Etiology. The physiologic change underlying edema is increased capillary permeability caused by elevated hormone levels. Sodium and water are retained. Thirst increases. Plasma osmolarity is lowered and the osmoreceptors for vasopressin are suppressed. Edema occurs most often in dependent areas. Moreover, the pressure of the gravid uterus slows down venous return to the heart. Consequently, more fluid passes into intracellular spaces.[4]

Subjective Data. The client reports mild edema in her hands and feet that worsens as the day progresses. Warm weather or prolonged sitting and standing may increase edema; it should improve by morning, however. Ask the client if she wears constrictive bands on her legs. Question her about her diet; a diet deficient in protein, calories or fluids or high in sodium, fat, or sugar may increase edema.

The client does *not* report numbness, loss of sensation or muscle strength in the fingers of either or both hands. Edema is not generalized and improves after a night's sleep. There is *no* report or evidence of facial edema, edema in one extremity, especially one leg, confusion, headache, flashing lights, fatigue, nausea, vomiting, dyspnea, hives, upper abdominal pain, decreased fetal movement, decreased urine output, or rapid weight gain (i.e., more than 2 pounds per week).[4,21]

Objective Data. Physical examination, particularly of the heart, lungs, extremities, and abdomen, and vital signs are within normal limits. It is important to rule out pregnancy-induced hypertension.[4] By definition, pregnancy induced hypertension occurs after 20 weeks of pregnancy except with a hydatidiform gestation. Hypertension before this time is considered preexisting, undiagnosed hypertension. The client's systolic blood pressure has not risen 30 mm Hg, or her diastolic 15 mm Hg, above the baseline reading taken in the first trimester. The client's weight gain pattern is less than 2 pounds per week in the third trimester, 1 pound per week in the second trimester. Edema of the extremities is 0 (no swelling) to +1 (after pressing skin for 5 seconds, the indentation is slight and the contour normal). Deep tendon reflexes are also normal. Jaundice, upper abdominal pain, or headache are not noted.[4]

The *urine dipstick for protein* should be negative or show only a trace.[4]

Differential Medical Diagnoses. Physiologic edema of pregnancy ruling out pregnancy induced hypertension, chronic hypertension, HELLP (i.e., hemolysis, elevated liver enzymes and low platelet count) syndrome, renal or liver disease, varicosities, local trauma or infection to extremities, allergic reaction, carpal tunnel syndrome, and congestive heart failure.[21]

Plan

PSYCHOSOCIAL INTERVENTIONS. Reassure the client that edema in pregnancy is normal and will resolve after pregnancy. Advise the client to notify the health care provider if any symptoms ruled out during the history taking occur in the future.

LIFESTYLE CHANGES. Advise the client to lie in a lateral recumbent position for 1 to 2 hours twice a day and to sleep in that position at night. Also advise her to avoid long periods of sitting or standing. If a client must sit for extended periods, she should also stand—preferably walk—10 minutes every 1 to 2 hours, or vice versa.

Instruct the client not to wear constrictive bands on the legs and arms; however, she should wear maternity support pantyhose.

Inform the client that raising arms and legs above the level of the heart for short periods and pumping hands and feet may decrease edema. Advise her not to curl her hands under her head or pillow at night if they are swollen or numb. Use of wrists supports would decrease swelling and numbness. Regular aerobic exercise may improve blood flow to legs.[19]

DIETARY INTERVENTIONS. Advise the client to eat adequate protein and calories, drink 6 to 8 glasses of water a day (reducing fluids does not reduce edema), and avoid high intake of sugar and fats (they can cause water retention). Sodium intake should be moderate; a low intake may be detrimental to the pregnancy and a high intake may increase water retention.

Follow-Up. Refer a client with symptoms of pregnancy induced hypertension or with symptoms of pathology to the physician. A dietitian may assist with special dietary needs.

Dyspepsia

Etiology. The physiologic changes underlying dyspepsia are the increase in levels of circulating progesterone that causes decreased gastrointestinal peristalsis and the relaxation of the hiatal sphincter. In addition, the pressure of the gravid uterus against the intestines and stomach increases the reflux of gastric contents into the esophagus.[4,20]

Subjective Data. The client reports heartburn and bloating. The client may be under stress, depressed, swallowing air, or overweight. The client does *not* report chest pain; shortness of breath; exercise intolerance; palpitations; sweating; anxiety; upper abdominal pain, especially after heavy, fatty, or spicy meals; fatty, foul-smelling stools; nausea, diarrhea, constipation, or vomiting; fever, or flulike symptoms, as these symptoms/signs may indicate other conditions requiring medical follow-up.[21]

Objective Data. No diagnostic tests are necessary. Physical examination, particularly of the heart and abdomen, and vital signs are within normal limits.

Differential Medical Diagnoses. Dyspepsia related to pregnancy ruling out cardiac, gallbladder, reflux, ulcer, irritable bowel syndrome, epigastric, or pancreatic disease, gastroenteritis, and a hiatal hernia.[21]

Plan

PSYCHOSOCIAL INTERVENTIONS. Reassure the client that dyspepsia is related to pregnancy and should improve or disappear after pregnancy. Advise the client to notify the health care provider if any symptoms ruled out during history taking occur in the future.

Calcium carbonate is indicated for hyperacidity. One to two tablets are recommended every hour, as needed (see Nutrition section). Abdominal bloating may occur in some clients. Inform the client that calcium carbonate is an additional source of calcium.[23]

LIFESTYLE CHANGES. Advise the client not to lie down, bend, or stoop for 2 hours after eating. Inform her that for sleeping, the head of the bed can be elevated 6 inches. Instruct the client not to wear restrictive clothing around the abdomen or waist.

Teach the client to recognize her hyperventilation and swallowing of air, which may aggravate dyspepsia.

Advise the client to stop smoking.

DIETARY INTERVENTIONS. Advise the client to avoid hot, spicy, fatty, gas-forming foods; coffee; alcohol; and gum chewing. Instruct her to eat small, frequent meals and to chew slowly and thoroughly. Inform her that sipping water, milk, hot tea, or a tablespoonful of heavy cream, yogurt, or half-and-half may help dyspepsia.

Advise the client to avoid excessive weight gain.

Follow-Up. Refer any client with symptoms of pathology to a physician.

Joint Pain/Ache

Etiology. The physiologic changes underlying joint discomfort are hormonal. Hormone changes, primarily increased relaxin, increased the mobility of the sacroiliac, sacrococcygeal, and pubic joints, which, in turn, slightly increases the size of the pelvis in preparation for delivery. The increased mobility of the joint is often painful.[4,19]

Subjective Data. The client reports pain in the pelvis or hip joints. Pain often increases after fetal engagement. The client does *not* report contractions, symptoms of urinary tract infection, or transient pain, swelling, stiffness, or redness in the joints with fever, abnormally cold and/or white digits and other flulike symptoms, as these symptoms/signs indicate other conditions requiring medical follow-up.[21] There is no history of tick bites or being in a wooded area where ticks could bite.

Objective Data. Physical examination and vital signs, particularly the joints and musculoskeletal system, are within normal limits; however, tenderness may be noted when palpating the symphysis pubis. There are no signs of labor.

Differential Medical Diagnoses. Joint pain ruling out urinary tract infection, contractions, Lyme's disease, or other rheumatic or joint diseases.[21]

Plan

PSYCHOSOCIAL INTERVENTIONS. Reassure the client that the discomfort is limited to pregnancy. Advise her to notify the health care provider if any symptoms ruled out during the history taking occur in the future.

MEDICATION. Acetaminophen may be taken.

LIFESTYLE CHANGES. Advise the client to avoid excessive walking, high-heeled shoes, jarring movements, high-impact activities, or other movements that can cause pain. Inform her that she may apply a heating pad or warm moist heat to the painful area for 15 to 20 minutes and that good posture is helpful. Instruct the client that she may place pillows between the thighs and underneath her abdomen to support and align the back while sleeping.

Follow-Up. Refer any client with symptoms of pathology to a physician.

Emotional Lability/Anxiety/Depression

Etiology. The physiologic change underlying lability is the constant rising and falling of hormonal levels during pregnancy. Progesterone has a depressant effect on the central nervous system. Fears about personal and fetal vulnerability, increased responsibility, new and changing roles often produce anxiety.[4,19,20]

Subjective Data. The client may report emotional instability, mood swings, feeling blue, depressed, or frequent crying. She may have sleep disturbances. She has adequate support systems and denies fatigue and physical or psychosocial problems.

Objective Data. Physical examination and vital signs are within normal limits with a normal affect and weight gain pattern.

Differential Medical Diagnoses. Emotional lability or anxiety from pregnancy ruling out fatigue and physical or emotional disorders (e.g., depression).

Plan

PSYCHOSOCIAL INTERVENTIONS. Psychosocial interventions should be considered.

- Reassure the client that mood swings are common and should improve after the postpartum period (see Chapter 20).
- Explain the normal introversion that occurs in pregnancy and its role in mood swings.
- Assess the adequacy of the client's support systems, including support and communication between partners. Encourage her to discuss her feelings with a trusted person.
- Teach the client communication techniques. Use of "I" statements, describe the feelings of the speaker without transferring blame to or labeling the feelings of the listener (e.g., "I am embarrassed by your behavior" rather than "You embarrassed me with that behavior"). Encourage both the client and her significant other to observe the accompanying body language ("I'm OK" while crying indicates that the speaker may not be OK). Encourage clarification and guard against not fully listening to the speaker but instead formulating a response while listening. Instruct the client to use reflective responses for clarification (i.e., they reword and reflect what the listener has said). Advise her to use silence to encourage the speaker to continue or clarify his or her thoughts.
- Encourage the client to participate in pleasurable activities and to take time for rest, sleep, exercise, and grooming.
- Encourage the client to express her concerns, listening in a nonjudgmental environment. Explore ideas and solutions for problems.
- A birth plan may help the client to express her fears surrounding labor and delivery and to construct a method of coping with them.
- All explanations to the client should be clear, concise, simple, and honest as she may have difficulty concentrating.
- Address all the physical discomforts experienced by the client to enhance her ability to rest.[19]
- Encourage socialization.

DIETARY INTERVENTIONS. Assess the adequacy of the client's diet and that caloric intake is spread throughout the day.

Follow Up. Refer a client with symptoms of mental illness to a mental health care provider. Couples may also need specialized interventions.

Altered Body Image

Etiology. The physiologic changes underlying body image alterations result from hormonal fluctuations and the growing uterus. Chloasma, uneven brown patches across the nose or cheeks and around the eyes, can appear lighter on black or brown skin. The areolae, vulva, and upper, inner thighs darken. The normally vertical, pale line that stretches from the umbilicus to the mons darkens (linea nigra). Some women experience acne as a result of increased levels of circulating progesterone, whereas others note improvement. Striae are stretch marks on the skin. Mild pruritus from dryness, as well as stretching, is frequent. Some clients develop spider nevi and palmar erythema. Breasts enlarge in preparation for lactation. The abdomen enlarges with the growing fetus.[4,20]

Subjective Data. The client may report any of the previously described changes. Severe, generalized itching; jaundice; upper abdominal pain; bloating; malaise; constipation; diarrhea; change in stool color or shape; and severe psychosocial stress are *not* reported.

Objective Data

- Physical examination and vital signs are within normal limits.
- A *bile acid* (*cholyglycine*) *test* is done with severe abdominal pruritus to determine the level of bile acids in the serum. A venipuncture is performed and blood withdrawn for laboratory evaluation. The client must be instructed to fast for 8 hours before the test. The bile acid level is significantly elevated in pruritus gravidarum.

Differential Medical Diagnoses. Changes in skin, breasts, and/or abdomen ruling out liver disease, pruritis gravidarum, scabies, and dermatologic or emotional problems.

Plan

PSYCHOSOCIAL INTERVENTIONS. Psychosocial interventions are predominantly to encourage verbalization of concerns.

- Reassure the client that changes are due to pregnancy and will either fade (e.g., striae) or gradually disappear (e.g., nipple darkening, linea nigra) after delivery.

- Encourage the client to verbalize her concerns, including her perception of her partner's reaction to the pregnancy and body changes. Encourage her to communicate with her partner. (See Emotional liability.)

LIFESTYLE CHANGES. Lifestyle changes may improve body image.

- If acne is a problem, advise the client to wash her face carefully, to use a topical astringent, to avoid wearing makeup that clogs pores, and to apply a strong sunblock when in the sun (a strong sunblock may minimize chloasma).
- Moisturizing lotions may reduce itching, but will not help striae.
- Advise the client to avoid irritating soaps (e.g., those with fragrance, antibacterial properties, or deodorants), long, hot showers, and other drying agents.
- Encourage regular exercise to control weight gain if no contraindications to exercise exist.
- Encourage the client to consider breastfeeding, emphasizing that it will induce faster involution of the uterus and easier postpartum weight loss.

DIETARY INTERVENTIONS. Advise the client to maintain a well-balanced diet (see Nutrition) with adequate fluids, which may help reduce acne breakouts and minimize unnecessary weight gain.

Follow-Up. Refer a client with symptoms of pathology to the physician. A client with severe relationship or psychosocial stress may be referred to a mental health care provider.

ANTICIPATORY GUIDANCE DURING PREGNANCY

The issues of concern to pregnant women involve safety, comfort, and uncertainty about what to expect during pregnancy, labor, and delivery.

CHEMICAL USE AND SAFETY

Tobacco

Smoking is related to bleeding, preterm rupture of membranes, abruptio placenta, placenta previa, spontaneous abortion, premature birth, low birthweight, Sudden Infant Death Syndrome

(SIDS), lags in developmental milestones, and low IQ in the child. The adverse effects of smoking increase with the number of cigarettes smoked each day and with the years that the client has smoked. Recent research demonstrates increased rates of SIDS with prenatal and postnatal exposure that is dose related. A slight decrease in fetal birthweight with second-hand smoke exposure has been demonstrated. Encourage the client and all household members to stop smoking.[20,28,29,30,31] Refer to a smoking cessation clinic. Transdermal patch may be considered if client cannot stop smoking otherwise and smokes more than one pack per day. Although exposing the fetus to nicotine, it eliminates the many other toxins in smoke including carbon monoxide. Risks vs. benefits must be explained, particularly that of smoking while using the patch. A non-nicotine, pill form, alternative is bupropion hydrochloride (zyban) which has an FDA Pregnancy Category B designation (see Chapter 23). Clinical experience is limited with pregnant and lactating women, therefore risk and benefits of use must be weighed carefully.[24]

Alcohol

Alcohol use can cause low birthweight, fetal alcohol syndrome (intrauterine growth retardation, malformations, characteristic facial features, behavior and learning problems), and fetal alcohol effects (learning and behavior disabilities only).[32] (See Table 17–5.) Studies are not conclusive, but as little as 1 oz of alcohol per day (e.g., one beer or glass of wine or one shot of liquor) has been implicated.[32] Currently, the best advice for a pregnant woman is complete abstinence from alcohol.

- If the client is concerned about alcohol she consumed after her last menstrual period but before she knew she was pregnant, explain that all studies showing deleterious effects were done with women who consumed alcohol throughout pregnancy, though effects are worse with drinking in the third trimester.[32] This information may be reassuring.
- Refer a client to a mental health care provider or Alcoholics Anonymous if needed.
- If the client stops drinking alcohol before the last trimester, her chances of having abnormal neonate are significantly decreased.[32]

TABLE 17–5. KNOWN TERATOGENS THAT CAUSE HUMAN MALFORMATIONS

Teratogen	Classification	Effects of Embryo/Fetus
Drugs		
Testosterone	Male hormone	May cause virilization of female fetus; ambiguous genitalia with hypertrophy of clitoris and fusion of labia
Estrogens diethylstilbestrol (DES), stilbestrol	Female hormone	Cause a variety of genital malformations in female fetuses and some possible changes in males. Genital cancer may occur in female offspring of mothers who took DES during their pregnancy
Cyclophosphamide (Cytoxan, Endoxana)	Antineoplast and immunosuppressant (folic acid antagonist)	Blocks synthesis of DNA, RNA, and protein. During first trimester of pregnancy, it is used only when potential benefits to mother outweigh hazards to fetus because it causes many major congenital deformities
Busulfan (Myleran)	Antineoplast (tumor-inhibiting)	May cause skeletal deformities, corneal opacities, cleft palate, hypoplasia of organs, and stunted growth
Methotrexate (Amethopterin, Mexate)	Antineoplast	Multiple skeletal deformities of face, skull, limbs, and vertebral column
Aminopterin	Antineoplast	May result in death of conceptus during embryonic period. Multiple skeletal and other congenital malformations may occur if fetus survives
Phenytoin (Dilantin)	Anticonvulsant	Causes fetal hydantoin syndrome: IUGR, mental retardation, microcephaly, inner epicanthic folds, ptosis of the eyelids, depressed nasal bridge, phalangeal hypoplasia
Warfarin (Coumadin)	Anticoagulant	Nasal hypoplasia, mental retardation, microcephaly, optic atrophy, chondroplasia punctata
Lithium carbonate (Cibalith, Eskalith, Lithane, Lithobid)	Psychotropic drug (used to control manic episodes of manic-depressive psychosis)	May cause a variety of malformations, particularly involving heart and great vessels
Thalidomide	Antiemetic in early pregnancy (no longer available)	Absence of one or more limbs, meromelia and other limb deformities; and malformations of heart, gastrointestinal system, and external ear
Alcohol	Drug	Fetal alcohol syndrome: IUGR, mental retardation, microcephaly, ocular anomalies, joint abnormalities, short palpebral fissures
Isotretinoin (Accutain)	Antiacne agent	Causes a wide range of anomalies (CNS, CV, craniofacial defects, thymus gland abnormalities and microcephaly, hydrocephaly) and blindness
Ribavinin (Virazole)	Antiviral	Malformation of skull, palate, eye, jaw and GI tract
Tetracycline	Antibiotic (Antiinfective)	Hypoplastic tooth enamel; bone and tooth anomalies
Maternal Disease		
Herpesvirus	Infection	Microcephaly, microphthalmia, retinal dysplasia, mental retardation
Rubella virus (German measles)	Infection	Cataracts, cardiac malformations, deafness, glaucoma, chorioretinitis
Cytomegalovirus	Infection	Abortion during embryonic period, IUGR, microphthalmia, chorioretinitis, blindness, microcephaly, mental retardation, deafness, cerebral palsy, cerebral calcifications, hepatosplenomegaly (enlargement of liver and spleen)
Toxoplasma gondii (contracted by eating raw or poorly cooked meat; infects cats; causes toxoplasmosis)	Protozoan infection (intracellular parasite)	Oocyst of contaminated cat crosses human placenta, causing microcephaly, microphthalmia, hydrocephaly
Treponema pallidum (causes syphilis)	Spirochete infection	Hydrocephaly, deafness, mental retardation, Hutchinson's teeth, saddle nose, poorly developed maxilla

(Continued)

TABLE 17–5. KNOWN TERATOGENS THAT CAUSE HUMAN MALFORMATIONS (CONTINUED)

Teratogen	Classification	Effects of Embryo/Fetus
Maternal Disease (cont.)		
Syphilis	Infection	Deformed nails; osteochondritis at joints of extremities; abnormal epiphyses
Varicella zoster (chickenpox)	Infection	Skin and muscle defects; limb abnormalities; eye anomalies
Diabetes mellitus	Carbohydrate intolerance	CNS and cardiac defects
Phenylketonuria	Inborn error in metabolism	Microcephaly; mental retardation
Chemical Agents		
Lead	Heavy metal	CNS anomalies; mental retardation
Methyl mercury	Metal compound	CNS anomalies; microcephaly blindness
Radiation		
High-level radiation therapy, radio-iodine, atomic weapons	Radiation	Microcephaly, mental retardation, skeletal deformities

Source: May, K. A., & Mahlmeister, L. (1994). Maternal and neonatal nursing: Family-centered care (3rd ed.). Philadelphia: Lippincott. Reprinted with permission.

Artificial Sweeteners

Aspartame (Nutrasweet) has not been shown to cause harmful effects when used in moderation. This sweetener is composed of two naturally occurring amino acids, phenylalanine and aspartic acid. Clients with phenylketonuria, though, are not able to use it. Saccharin is not advised as a slight increase in cancer in the offspring has been shown in animal studies.[25]

Caffeine

Though caffeine has not been shown to be teratogenic, it may increase risk of spontaneous abortion. It is a diuretic, often displaces more nutritious food choices, can exacerbate mood swings, disturb rest, and cause fetal or newborn heartbeat irregularities.[25]

Inform the client of caffeine sources: coffee, tea, chocolate, some sodas, and some over-the-counter pain and cold medications. Explain the physical effects of caffeine withdrawal (e.g., lethargy, irritability, headache) and their usual duration (3 to 4 days). Mixing decaffeinated and caffeinated products in increasing ratios to wean from caffeine use may reduce these effects.

Illegal Drugs

The risks of using illegal drugs are fetal addiction, prematurity, low birthweight, placental abruption, stillbirth, and hepatitis B and HIV infection.[32] Advise clients to stop using drugs. Refer clients using illegal drugs to a drug detoxification center specializing in the needs of pregnant women or to a mental health care provider whose expertise is drug abuse (see Chapter 18).

Over-the-Counter Medications

Health care providers do recommend some over-the-counter medications for minor complaints, such as headaches. Some medications (e.g., pseudoephedrine) can restrict blood flow through the placenta. Ventral wall defects have also been associated with pseudoephedrine use in the first trimester.[32] Advise the client not to take any medication without first consulting a health care provider. Also advise her that megadoses of vitamins (e.g., vitamins A and D) could harm both her and the fetus;[25] she should take only a vitamin/mineral supplement advised by a health care provider.

Prescription Drugs

Some prescription drugs are harmful to the fetus. Advise the client to report all medications she is taking to her health care provider for evaluation (see Table 17–5).

Environmental Exposure

The client can be exposed to various chemicals in her work setting, home, or other environments.

Ideally, the client should avoid exposure to chemicals, particularly during the first trimester in which organogenesis occurs. To reduce exposure when using chemicals (e.g., household cleaning items), the client should ensure that work areas are well ventilated and wear protective gloves. Advise the client to avoid inhaling chemical fumes, particularly from paint or turpentine, and to wash off any chemicals on the skin immediately. Also advise her if she is in doubt about the toxicity of a chemical to which she has been exposed, she should notify a health care provider or go to an emergency room.

Knowledge about teratogens is growing. To obtain the most current information, several hotlines are available.

- Reproductive Toxicology Center (1–202–293–5137), Columbia Women's Hospital, Washington DC. Information to professionals via online computer, FAX, or written request. A subscription service.
- National Pesticides Telecommunications Network (1–800–858–7378).
- A Material Safety Data Sheet (MSDS) is required to be available wherever chemicals are used in the workplace. Pregnancy issues are addressed.

Lead Poisoning

Lead poisoning can be a problem for clients who live in homes built before 1980. It can cause mental retardation and central nervous system anomalies in the fetus,[4,33] as well as in children and adults. Lead-base paint on walls, plastic miniblinds, or lead pipes can be a source of lead contamination. Inhabitants of these homes should run cold water for consumption for five minutes before drinking. Advise clients who are planning home improvements during their pregnancy to check the house for lead first. Stay away from the construction. Instruct clients to wash fruits and vegetables well to remove lead residue and to remove food from cans before storage, as the solder used to seam cans may contain lead that could leach into food. (This effect could also be caused by drinking liquids stored in lead crystal or eating off lead-paint glazed dishes, usually old, handmade, or imported.) Hobbies of creating pottery with lead glaze or leaded glass work or occupations in lead smelting, printing, battery manufac-

turing, paint manufacturing, toll booth attendants or clients who work on heavily traveled roads or tunnels could have high blood lead levels.[25,34]

THE WORKPLACE

In general, healthy women may work until delivery if they have an uncomplicated pregnancy and work at jobs where the potential hazard is no greater than that of normal community life.[34] Because of risk to the fetus in the first trimester, encourage clients to inform their employers of the pregnancy as early as possible.

Modifications

Some modifications may be needed in employment.

- The client should not work longer than 8 hours per day and 48 hours per week.
- The client should take two 10-minute breaks and one meal break each 8-hour shift.
- The client should have a place to rest on her side and should be able to elevate her legs and use the restroom.
- A client who must either sit or stand excessively should be allowed a short time every 1 to 2 hours to sit or walk, whichever is different from her work routine. Standing over 4 hours a day increases risk of preterm labor in some studies.[34,35]
- The client should avoid exhaustion, discomfort, extreme temperatures, smoking areas, noxious odors, chemical fumes, continuous loud noises, activities that require good balance, and potential trauma to the abdomen.[34,36]
- If the job is strenuous, reduce heavy work or exercise, and increase rest times while at home. Be sure the calorie intake meets the increased energy needs.[25]
- Clients with strenuous jobs should avoid hard physical labor,[35,37] stop or reduce work 2 to 4 weeks before the expected date of delivery, and limit lifting to 25 pounds and use proper lifting technique.[25]
- Clients have certain rights that are protected by law. The Pregnancy Discrimination Act requires the employer to treat pregnancy as any other disability would be treated. The Occupational Safety and Health Administration ensures that

employers either provide a workplace free of hazards likely to cause death or serious harm or provide information about dangerous chemicals or substances. The Family and Medical Leave Act requires employers of more than 50 persons to give 12 weeks of unpaid leave with birth, adoption or foster care of a child, care of a spouse, child, parent with a serious health condition, or if unable to perform the job because of any disability including pregnancy. Vacation and sick pay must be given if earned, and health benefits cannot be changed. The same or equal job must be available upon return to work.[20]

- Health care workers exposed to chemotherapy agents or ionizing radiation should avoid exposure.[34] Child care workers need to use gloves, and careful hand washing after exposure to childrens' body fluids (e.g. changing diapers) to avoid cytomegalovirus infection (see Cytomegalovirus).
- Handling cats and raw meat increases risk of exposure to toxoplasmosis. Clients employed in animal care and meat preparation should wear gloves and wash hands carefully after exposure (see Toxoplasmosis).

Variables

Several variables interact to determine the extent of workplace hazard, particularly in relationship to teratogen exposure: the type of hazard (see Table 17–5); duration and level of exposure; the method of exposure (i.e., inhalation or ingestion); and/or the health and genetic makeup of the client (e.g., lead or benzene exposure induces or exacerbates anemia); and the genetic makeup of the fetus.[32,36]

Factors That Prohibit Work

Several physical conditions may make work impossible: incompetent cervix, history of fetal loss, cervical cerclage, heart disease classification greater than II (no symptoms at rest but minor limitations of physical activity due to fatigue, palpitations, or dyspnea),[4] uterine abnormalities, Marfan's syndrome, hemoglobinopathies, hypertension, retinopathy greater

than stage 1, severe anemia, herpes genitalis if the pain is severe, diabetes, renal disease, severe disorders requiring medication, asthma, and disk or back problems.[37]

The Occupational Safety and Health Administration is a federal agency that determines and enforces standards regarding workplace safety.

CONTACT WITH DISEASE

Ideally, clients should avoid persons with disease. In addition, immunizations should be up-to-date prior to pregnancy. The client should also be assessed for susceptibility to hepatitis B, rubella, toxoplasmosis, cytomegalovirus, and varicella–oster before pregnancy or early in the prenatal period (see Chapter 16).

Toxoplasmosis

Advise clients to avoid *Toxoplasma* infection by not handling raw meat or gardening without gloves and avoiding outdoor sandboxes and litter boxes. If the client must change a cat's litter, she should wear gloves. Afterward, hands are washed well.[32]

Cytomegalovirus

Twenty-five to 60 percent of all preschoolers carry cytomegalovirus, which can be excreted for quite a long time from the saliva, urine, and feces. It is not very contagious. Clients who care for preschoolers are advised to use careful hand washing technique when handling diapers or any body fluids. Many child care sites require their employees to use disposable gloves. Avoid contact with saliva (e.g., kissing or sharing food) with preschoolers, particularly in a child care setting. Cytomegalovirus[20,25] can also be transmitted by sexual intercourse.

Fifth's Disease

Clients are advised to avoid exposure to children with undiagnosed rashes. Fifth's disease can, though rarely, cause fetal hydrops in a client who contracts the disease while pregnant.[20,25]

Varicella Zoster

Chickenpox can rarely affect the fetus if the client becomes infected during the first half of the pregnancy. Adults, particularly if pregnant, are at much greater risk of developing severe complications. If infected close to term, the greatest danger lies in the newborn developing the disease before the mother has developed antibodies and transferred them to the fetus transplacentally. Any client without a history of chickenpox exposure is advised to avoid exposure. Immunization prior to pregnancy may be advised. If it occurs, immunity can be tested and immune globulin is advised within 96 hours of exposure. She should contact her health care provider immediately.[20,25]

Mumps

If contracted during pregnancy, mumps can cause uterine contractions leading to miscarriage or preterm labor. If not immune or vaccinated, the client should avoid exposure.[20,25]

Measles

Rubeola is not linked to fetal defects but may cause miscarriage or preterm labor. Infection close to term could result in the fetus developing the disease without sufficient antibodies to protect it. Avoidance of exposure is advised and contacting the health care provider immediately upon exposure is recommended as an immune gamma globulin is available.[20,25]

Lyme Disease

Lyme Disease can be transmitted to the fetus through the placenta and is suspected to cause heart defects. Advise avoidance of exposure by wearing long pants tucked into boots and long sleeves in grassy or wooded areas. Insect repellant can be applied to the clothes but not directly to the skin. A skin check for ticks is recommended after potential exposure. Contact a health care provider with suspected exposure.[20,25]

Rubella

German measles can cause significant harm to the fetus if the client contracts it in the first half of her pregnancy. All clients should be tested prenatally and, ideally, preconceptionally. If nonimmune, advise the client to avoid exposure to anyone with an undiagnosed rash. If exposed contact the health care provider immediately. Nonimmune clients should be vaccinated immediately postpartum (see Immunizations).[20,25]

Listeriosis

Listeriosis is caused by bacteria infecting milk, cheese, raw vegetables, and shellfish. If contracted early in the pregnancy, miscarriage is more likely. Babies infected at birth can have feeding and breathing problems, which may not develop until they are several weeks old. The symptoms are flulike. Advise clients to contact their health care provider if flulike symptoms occur.[20]

Tuberculosis

The incidence of tuberculosis is rising. If client is exposed, a skin test or chest x-ray is advised. Refer to a physician if she tests positive. She can be treated during pregnancy. The newborn can be exposed at birth. Advise contact with the health care provider if exposure is suspected.[4,20]

Sexually Transmitted Diseases

Sexually transmitted diseases (STDs) pose a health threat to the fetus. Assess the client for a history of STDs; ask about the number of sexual partners she has and her use of condoms. Advise her to use condoms if she has multiple partners or a new partner, if she is unsure of her partner's sexual or drug use history, or if her partner has multiple sexual partners.

Educate clients to recognize symptoms of infection and if exposed to high-risk sexual partners to contact a health care provider as soon as possible (see Chapter 11).

SEXUAL ACTIVITY

Many fluctuating factors—physical, hormonal, and psychosocial—influence sexual desire and sexual response throughout pregnancy.

Normal Sexual Activity

Normal sexual activity is permissible, unless history of miscarriage exists, bleeding occurs, preterm labor is a risk, infection develops, intercourse is painful, placenta previa exists, or membranes rupture or are suspected of rupturing.

Assure the couple that the fetus will not be injured by intercourse nor is the fetus able to understand what is happening.

Encourage the couple to experiment with positions that may be more comfortable (e.g., woman on top, side lying).[4,25]

Inform couples that uterine contractions may occur with orgasm. This is safe if the client is not at risk for preterm labor.[25]

Communication

A couple may require help adjusting to changes brought about by pregnancy. Some women have increased sexual desire, some less. The woman, though, often has an increased need for closeness during pregnancy. She should communicate this to her partner, stressing that she is not rejecting him. Emphasize to the couple that closeness and cuddling need not always culminate in intercourse. A mental health care provider may be consulted if necessary.

Alternative Forms of Sexual Expression

Cunnilingus is safe if the partner does not blow air into the vagina. Air embolisms are more likely.[25] Condoms are advised with anal sex. Advise changing the condom if vaginal intercourse is then desired. If intercourse is prohibited, specify what is meant: orgasm, vaginal penetration, or unprotected penetration. Other forms of sexual expression (e.g., cuddling, kissing, masturbation) may be advised.

EXERCISE

Regular exercise during pregnancy increases a client's sense of well-being, improves sleep, helps to control weight gain, tone muscles, and, after delivery, hastens recovery.

General Guidelines

A client who was physically active before conception should be able to engage in the same activities throughout pregnancy. You may need to advise clients not to take up new activities or sports if this activity requires balance because their sense of balance is decreased and their joints are looser, which increases the risk of injury.

Many exercise programs for pregnant women exist but because exercise specialists are not regulated, advise clients to consult their health care provider and to check the credentials of the instructor.

- The client should exercise three to four times per week, not sporadically.
- The client should drink water before, during, and after exercise to replace what is lost during exercise. Eat a light snack before exercising rather than exercising on an empty stomach.[25] Be sure calorie intake includes exercise expenditure.
- The client should not exercise in hot, humid conditions or when feeling ill.
- The client should make a 5- to 10-minute warmup of stretching exercises routine. Exertion should be moderate, stopping if fatigued, breathless, profusely sweating, or unable to converse. After a 5- to 10-minute cooldown period of stretching, the heart rate should be under 100 beats per minute. The length and intensity of the program are built gradually, though often must decrease in the third trimester.
- The client should exercise on a floor that absorbs impact (e.g., rug-covered or wooden floor). The client should wear clothes that are loose or stretch and a well-fitting support bra. Sneakers are supportive and absorb impact. Deep knee bends should be avoided as should pointing toes, full situps, double leg raises, and straight toe touches; these exercises may injure joints or cause cramps.
- To avoid dizziness, the client should rise slowly following exercise.
- The client should avoid high-impact exercises (jumping, jerking, rapid direction changes), exercises that may force air into the vagina (upside-down bicycles), exercises that stretch the adductor muscles of the legs (putting soles of feet together and pushing down or bouncing

legs), exercises that require uncomfortable positions, and exercises that exaggerate the normal curvature of the spine.[25]

- After the first trimester, the client should not lie on her back for more than a few minutes at a time.
- Weight lifting exercise may be continued if started preconceptually, without increasing the weight. Use of circuit machines or spotter is advised.
- The client should modify the exercise program as the physical load of pregnancy increases.
- The client should stop exercising and contact a health care provider if any of the following occur: pain, bleeding, suspected membrane rupture, dizziness that does not resolve quickly after rising, shortness of breath (unable to talk comfortably), palpitations, faintness, tachycardia, back pain, pelvic pain or pressure, or difficulty walking.[20,25,38]

Prohibited Sports

Advise the client not to participate in snow or water skiing, surfing, diving, scuba diving, ice or roller skating, sprinting, or any sport performed where oxygen deprivation (e.g., mountain sickness) or abdominal trauma are possible because they pose a risk of serious injury to mother and fetus.[25,38]

Pregnancy Complications

Several complications of pregnancy may prohibit exercise. These include premature labor (current or past pregnancies), placental abruption or previa, threatened abortion, a history of three or more spontaneous abortions, incompetent cervix, intrauterine growth retardation, history of stillbirth, small for gestational age, client is underweight or has inadequate weight gain, and medical diseases. Clients at risk should speak with a physician. Toning and stretching exercises, however, reduce the complications of bedrest.[25,38]

SAUNAS, HOT TUBS, WHIRLPOOLS, TANNING BEDS

Advise clients not to use such equipment. The high water temperature (higher than 100° F) could raise body temperature 1.5 to 2° F above normal, which is not considered safe. In addition, because blood is shunted to the skin in the sauna or whirlpool, the heart has difficulty maintaining circulation. Syncope could result.[25,32] Tanning is not advised due to risk of serious sunburn, dehydration, and skin cancer.

RADIATION EXPOSURE

Ionizing Radiation (X-Ray, Radiation Therapy)

Dosage of ionizing radiation greater than 5 rad over an entire pregnancy may harm the fetus. The greatest risk is between 8–15 weeks of gestation. Total exposure during a barium enema series is 2–4 rad. Several guidelines are suggested that pertain to exposure to diagnostic x-rays.[39]

- Avoid unnecessary x-rays, wait until after 15 weeks, use ultrasound or magnetic resonance imaging (MRI). With all testing, weigh risk vs. benefits, waiting if possible.[39]
- Advise the client to inform anyone ordering or taking an x-ray that she is pregnant, to insist on lead shielding of the abdomen, and to use low exposure techniques if possible.
- Advise the client to follow exactly the directions of the technician to avoid having to retake x-rays.
- Advise a regularly inspected facility staffed with certified technicians and supervised by a radiologist.
- Advise the client that if x-rays are necessary, fetal risk is low, particularly as the pregnancy advances.[39]

Nonionizing Radiation

Emissions from video display terminals, televisions, and microwave ovens are very low. Although studies are not conclusive, the fetus does not appear to be at risk.[40]

Ultrasound

The use of ultrasound, high-frequency sound waves, poses no risk to the fetus, according to several studies.[39,40]

Nuclear Medicine

Radioscope procedures generally expose the client to very low radiation doses. Several types are available. Consultation with a radiologist is advised. Radioactive isotopes of iodine are contraindicated.[39]

DENTAL CARE

Regular dental care is important during pregnancy. The dentist must be told of the pregnancy and x-rays performed only if necessary, with an abdominal shield. Local anesthesia is usually safe.[20]

TRAVEL

Generally, travel is best undertaken during the second trimester when risk of complications is low and the client is feeling her best.[4,20]

General Guidelines

- The client should check with her health care provider prior to traveling. Travel may be contraindicated with certain complications: risk for preterm labor, repeated spontaneous abortions, pregnancy induced hypertension, bleeding, intrauterine growth retardation, or a medical condition, e.g., cardiac disease.
- If planning to fly, the client should check with the airline about regulations is concerning pregnancy. Pregnant women should not fly in unpressurized planes.
- The client should walk for 5 to 10 minutes every 1 to 2 hours while traveling. If driving, she should plan to make stops; if flying or traveling by train or bus, she should arrange for an aisle seat.
- To exercise while seated, take a deep breath, extend lower legs, flex feet, wiggle toes, and contract abdominal and buttocks muscles. With swollen hands, stretch above head and open and close fists.[25]
- The client should drink adequate fluids and urinate every 2 hours to increase comfort. Light snacks may help reduce nausea.
- The client should not take medication for motion sickness or constipation without first consulting a health care provider.

- The client should be provided with names of obstetricians in the area to which she will be traveling and given a copy of her prenatal record in case of unexpected complications.[25]
- Travel to high altitudes or where additional immunization is required should be avoided.[4,20]

Foreign Travel Guidelines

- Immunizations required for travel should be received at least 3 months before conception.
- Use of chloroquine during pregnancy (to prevent malaria) is safe. Advise the client to start the medication 2 weeks before traveling to the risk area. Covering exposed skin, mosquito netting, and spraying bug repellents on clothing reduce chance of being bitten. In some areas (East Africa, Thailand), the strains of malaria are resistant to chloroquine; no other safe medications are available. Because malaria during pregnancy carries increased risk to the mother and fetus, travel to these destinations should be postponed until after delivery.[20]
- In areas where water has been known to be contaminated, clients should avoid drinking it, as well as eating raw fruits and vegetables and using ice made from contaminated water or glasses washed in it. Water purification tablets containing iodine are not safe for pregnant women. She should drink only boiled or bottled water, soft drinks, or bottled fruit juices. Advise the client which medications and antibiotics to use if she should develop nausea, vomiting, or diarrhea and prescribe them for her if necessary.
- All meat should be thoroughly cooked.[20]
- The American College of Obstetricians and Gynecologists publishes a directory of board-certified obstetricians practicing in foreign countries.

Seat Belts

Advise the client to use shoulder and lap belts when traveling in a car. Correct positioning of a seat belt requires that the lap portion be placed below the abdomen, across the upper thighs. The shoulder belt should rest between the breasts. Both belts should be worn snugly. If only the lap belt is available, it is used alone. Studies show that in most accidents the fetus recovers quickly from any damage caused by a seat belt, but not from impact against the dash or steering wheel.[4,20,25]

CHILDBIRTH PREPARATION

Although all pregnant women do not have the same goals for their labor and delivery experience, most clients in their first pregnancy benefit from prepared childbirth classes. A birthing partner assists the client during her labor and delivery. The partner may be her husband, the baby's father, a friend, her parent, a sibling, or a paid birthing attendant.

Three Philosophies

- Grantly Dick-Read uses education and relaxation techniques to reduce the fear–tension–pain cycle.[25]
- Bradley teaches nutrition, exercise to prepare muscles, relaxation techniques, and inward focusing with deep abdominal breathing to achieve labor and delivery without medication.[25]
- Lamaze uses relaxation techniques, contrived breathing techniques, outward focusing, and conditioned response to reduce the need for medication.[25]

Shared Concepts

Some classes adapt parts of the three philosophies. The best classes usually comprise five to six couples, employ varied media to present materials, permit discussion, and ultimately prepare the client and her partner for many different experiences during labor and delivery, including use of pain medication.[25]

VIVID DREAMS AND FANTASIES

Vivid dreams and fantasies are common, healthy, and normal during pregnancy. Most commonly, pregnant women dream or imagine they are unprepared, being attacked, hurt or trapped, have forgotten something, or of becoming physically unattractive. In addition, fantasies and dreams may focus on sex, death and resurrection, delivery at home, and the physical appearance of baby.[25] Recurrent themes may indicate an area of concern for the client.

Assess the need for intervention. Reassure the client that she is not mentally ill, that she will not be a bad mother, and that the dreams do not predict the future.

CONCERN FOR BABY

Reassure the client that her concern about whether the baby will be normal is not unusual. The many tests that are available to diagnose problems prenatally may be discussed, if appropriate. If her concern seems excessive, refer the client for counseling.

ACCIDENTS OR BLOWS TO THE ABDOMEN

Reassure the client that the amniotic fluid and abdominal structure protect the fetus, although a very serious blow to the abdomen could cause injury (e.g., hitting the steering wheel during an auto accident). Recommend that she contact a health care provider if an abdominal blow should occur, particularly if there is vaginal bleeding or fluid, abdominal pain, uterine contractions, or fewer or no fetal movements.[25] Abusive relationships may intensify during pregnancy. If a woman is in a potentially abusive relationship, abuse may begin once she is pregnant. Refer her to a mental health care provider if abuse is suspected (see Chapter 23).

FETAL HICCUPS

Hiccups are common and do not harm the fetus.

BATHING

Advise the client that she may take tub baths if ruptured membranes are not suspected and if she takes safety precautions in case she experiences syncope. Late in pregnancy, a woman may need help rising out of a low tub.

INFANT SAFETY SEATS

By state law in many cases, most hospitals do not discharge infants unless the parents' car is equipped with an infant safety seat. These seats can be rented or purchased, and sometimes are available from charitable organizations and government social service offices. Hospitals, car dealers, baby stores, and consumer safety councils have the information.

FEEDING METHOD

Whether to breastfeed or bottle feed is a woman's personal choice, although breast milk is the ideal infant food.

Advantages of Breastfeeding

Breast milk is ideally suited for the newborn and changes as the infant grows, adjusting to fulfill his or her nutritional needs, particularly advantageous for a premature baby.[4] The milk is digestible, economical, and always ready. Breastfeeding encourages bonding between mother and child, speeds up uterine involution, suppresses ovulation (although not a reliable method of birth control), and helps weight loss. The sucking motion of nursing helps to develop the infant's jaws, teeth, and palate. Antibodies in breast milk provide protection against disease and reduce the development of allergies.[4] Any adverse reaction to breast milk is usually related to the mother's diet, and removing the offending food often solves the problem. Special techniques and equipment help mother and baby to have a successful nursing experience in unusual or difficult situations (e.g., mouth deformities, Down's syndrome, twins or multiples, mastectomy, breast surgery or congenitally absent breast tissue). Many mothers successfully continue nursing after returning to work by pumping and storing milk.[4,20]

Disadvantages of Breastfeeding

Breast discomfort, sore or leaking nipples, increased incidence of mastitis, engorgement, less personal time than if bottle feeding, vaginal dryness and decreased libido are often cited as disadvantages.

Breastfeeding Contraindications

Breastfeeding is prohibited in the face of serious illness, very low maternal weight, certain infections (e.g., active, untreated tuberculosis, HIV disease or AIDS, hepatitis B, herpes lesion on the aerola). Breastfeeding is also contraindicated if the mother is taking certain medications or abusing drugs or if the infant has certain metabolic disorders (e.g., phenylketonuria).[25]

Preparation for Breastfeeding

Educating a mother about breastfeeding will increase the likelihood of a successful breastfeeding experience. Encourage the client to attend a class (e.g., those offered by La Leche League), to read a good reference book about lactation, and to find a support person (a woman who had a successful nursing experience).

Nipple preparation is unnecessary unless nipples are inverted and do not become erect when stimulated. Assess for this by placing the forefinger and thumb above and below the areola, compressing behind the nipple. It should become erect and protrude. If it flattens or inverts, advise the client to wear breast shells during the last 2 months of pregnancy.[4] They are worn inside the bra with the nipples centered in the hole and a plastic dome fitted over it. The client should begin wearing the breast shells 1 hour a day for 1 week, and increase wearing time 1 hour each day until she is wearing the shells 8 hours a day. The client should maintain this schedule until after delivery, and then wear the shells 24 hours a day until the baby latches on easily when they are not used.

The nipples should not be rubbed roughly with a towel or rolled. No drying agents (e.g., alcohol, witch hazel, or soap) should be applied.

Advantages of Bottle Feeding

The client can return to work more easily, go on a strict reducing diet, and have others share in the baby's feeding.

Preparation for Bottle Feeding

If the client has chosen bottle feeding, emphasize that infant formula is recommended for the entire first year. Many formulas are available, for example, modified cow's milk and soy-based formulas with varied levels of iron and calories. Formulas are also designed for infants with special dietary needs. The pediatrician will advise the mother about the best formula for her baby. Formulas can be purchased in various forms: concentrated (need to be diluted with equal amounts of water);

powdered (to be mixed with water); ready to use (poured directly into bottles); and prepackaged (ready to use in disposable bottles). Advise the client to follow directions carefully and never over- or underdilute the formula.

If a clean water source is available, bottles and nipples need only be cleaned carefully with soap and water and stored away from sources of contamination.

Infants should always be held during feedings. The bonding that occurs while an infant is held is essential to her or his emotional growth. The bottle should not be propped up against the infant. Propping can cause a newborn to aspirate formula. An older baby who lies down with a propped bottle is more likely to develop otitis media. Falling asleep with a bottle contributes to early dental caries.[4]

CIRCUMCISION

The decision to circumcise is up to the parents. The procedure is usually performed before discharge from the hospital.

Proponents argue that circumcision prevents urinary tract infection (rare) and infection around the penis. Cleanliness and personal, religious, or cultural preference are the most common reasons for circumcision.

Opponents argue that circumcision may cause injury, infection, and pain (local anesthesia is available). It is not medically indicated in normal circumstances and routine circumcision is not advised by the American Academy of Pediatrics.

SIBLING RIVALRY

Many parents need reassurance that sibling rivalry is normal.

Techniques to Minimize Rivalry

Parents can use the following techniques to minimize rivalry.

- Enroll the older child(ren) in sibling classes.
- Encourage the older child(ren) to verbalize his or her emotions and acknowledge the emotions.
- Role play with a doll safe handling of a newborn.
- Expect and tolerate some regression.

- If the older child(ren) is to be moved from a crib to a bed or into another room to accommodate the baby, do so before the baby is born, preferably 2 to 3 months before.
- If the older child(ren) desires, buy a gift that she or he can give to the new infant. Be sure that the gift is safe for an infant and request that it be placed in the bassinette (purchase an item that can be cleaned or sterilized). The older child(ren) can then identify the infant in the nursery.
- The first time the child(ren) comes to visit, have the infant in the bassinette. Give the older child(ren) individual attention until he or she expresses an interest in the infant.
- It may also help to have a gift from the infant to the older child(ren).
- Encourage grandparents and visitors to pay attention first to the older child(ren) and to have her or him introduce the baby.
- Find time every day to be alone with the older child(ren).

GRANDPARENTING

The grandparents of the newborn must go through developmental changes, which can either result in a closer, supportive relationship with their children or widen the communication gap. Much new information about pregnancy, feeding—particularly breast feeding—and child rearing has emerged. The grandparents may or may not desire to be active participants in the newborn's life. Role changes must occur, adult children now being considered equals. New parents lack confidence in their parenting skills, wanting their parents' support without criticism. Grandparents have life experiences, traditions, knowledge, time, and often money the new parents don't have. They can provide stability and unconditional love to the older siblings. Grandparents, not infrequently, have taken the parenting role when the parent is unable or unwilling to do so.

Assess the communication skills, role expectations, and support skills of the parents and grandparents. Encourage the grandparents to learn about new parenting, feeding and child rearing skills their children may use. Teach good communication skills. Encourage attendance at grandparenting classes if available.[4]

FAMILY PLANNING

Encourage the client to begin thinking about family planning methods before delivery.

Spacing Births

Ideally, women should space births at least 2 years apart to allow their bodies to recover and replace reserves.

Lactational Amenorrhea Method

The lactational amenorrhea method of birth control is believed to carry a 2 percent risk of pregnancy if the client is 6 months or fewer postpartum, fully or nearly fully breastfeeding (at least 15 feedings lasting at least 10 minutes each), and amenorrheic. If any of these criteria are not met, a complimentary form of birth control should be used.[41]

Oral Contraceptives

Progestin only oral contraceptives are very effective when used during breastfeeding, and some progestins may increase milk supply. Combination oral contraceptives are not contraindicated while nursing but often reduce milk supply. For this reason, they are not prescribed until at least 6 weeks postpartum. The World Health Organization does not recommend combination oral contraceptives as a first choice while lactating.[41]

Depo-Provera

Depo-Provera has shown no effect on lactation in many studies.[41]

Subdermal Implants

Subdermal implants (Norplant) do not effect lactation and may be inserted immediately postpartum, though the Food and Drug Administration suggests inserting 6 weeks postpartum.[41]

Barrier Methods

Foam, suppositories, and lubricated condoms are recommended if a client has intercourse. They also counteract the normal vaginal dryness that occurs postpartum and with breastfeeding.[41]

Condoms are always recommended to reduce STD exposure risk, as well as to provide for contraception.

Diaphragm and Cervical Cap

If the client used a diaphragm or cervical cap prior to conception and wants to use it again, it must be refitted.[41]

Intrauterine Devices

Intrauterine devices (IUDs) are usually inserted 6 weeks postpartum or after a menstrual period. In some settings, an IUD is inserted immediately after delivery.[41]

Ovulation and Sympto-Thermal Methods

If these methods are desired, refer the client and her sexual partner to classes. Advise them that the first ovulation following pregnancy can occur at any time; they should wait until after the first menses to use this method.[41]

Sterilization

If a client desires sterilization, the procedure may be done on the first postpartum day, during a cesarean birth, or after her postpartum visit. Anesthetic agents may sedate the infant temporarily if nursing.[41]

Vasectomy

If the woman's partner decides to have a vasectomy, the procedure can be done at any time. Both partners, however, must be aware that a man is not sterile until his sperm count is zero. A second sperm count to confirm is recommended.[4]

DANGER SIGNS AND SYMPTOMS

Potential problems in pregnancy may be indicated by the development of particular signs. Should she recognize such a sign, the client should contact the health care provider as soon as possible.

FIRST TRIMESTER

Signs in the first trimester including spotting or bleeding; cramping; painful urination; severe vomiting and/or diarrhea; fever higher than 100° F; low abdominal pain located on either side or in the middle; lightheadedness; and dizziness, particularly if accompanied by shoulder pain.

SECOND TRIMESTER

Signs in the second trimester include all those noted for the first trimester plus regular uterine contractions; pain in one leg or calf, often increased with foot flexion and redness, heat, and tenderness, or coldness, numbness, and whiteness; symptoms of vaginal infection or sexually transmitted disease; sudden gush of fluid that cannot be controlled by Kegel exercises; absence of fetal movement for more than 24 hours after quickening; a sudden weight gain; periorbital or facial swelling; or severe upper abdominal pain or headache with visual changes and/or photophobia.

THIRD TRIMESTER

Signs in the third trimester (after 26 weeks) include all those noted for the first and second trimesters plus a decrease in the daily fetal movement indexes (see Chapter 19). If movement is insufficient, she should contact the health care provider immediately.[4]

INITIAL ASSESSMENT IN LABOR

PRELABOR

The prelabor stage can begin 1 month to 1 hour before labor begins. It is a period of cervical softening, effacement, and descent of the presenting part into the pelvis. Dilatation of the cervix can also occur during this time.

Subjective Data

Lightening, dropping, or engagement occurs when the presenting part descends into the pelvis. The client notes easier breathing but increased pelvic pressure, cramping, low back pain, and more frequent urination. Among primiparas, lightening can occur 2 to 4 weeks before labor and, among multiparas, during labor. Either increasing (nesting) or decreasing energy levels are noted. Vaginal discharge increases and thickens. The client may notice loss of the mucous plug (a thick red or brown plug) and/or bloody show (a pink tinged mucous discharge. Braxton-Hicks contractions may increase and become more intense. They are irregular, feel high and in front, occur suddenly without buildup, and decrease after urinating or changing position.

Labor contractions are felt in the back, legs, or lower abdomen, and frequently are accompanied by menstrual-like or gastrointestinal cramping sensations. With walking or over time, they grow longer, stronger, regular, and close together.

Diarrhea sometimes occurs.[25]

Objective Data

Physical examination reveals a weight loss of 1 to 2 pounds since the last visit. Softening of the cervix, effacement, and possibly some dilatation occur; dilatation is occasionally as much as 4 cm. The cervix moves more anterior. With descent of the presenting part into the pelvis, the fundal measurement may decrease and presenting part may palpate vaginally.

DECISION TO GO TO HOSPITAL OR BIRTHING CENTER

Subjective Data

Usually, when contractions are 3 to 5 if a primipara or 5 to 8 minutes apart if a multipara with the characteristics of true labor, the client should go to the hospital/birthing center. Each client, though, should be individually assessed based on her pregnancy risk and the distance the client lives from the hospital. Also, if the client was scheduled for a cesarean section, has a history of precipitous labor, or has a high-risk pregnancy, she may need to go to the hospital/birthing center earlier.

Signs indicating a client should be in the hospital as soon as possible include a significant decrease in fetal movement; menstrual-like bleeding; constant, severe contractions without relief;

and rupture or suspected rupture of membranes. If the umbilical cord is in the vagina (see Chapter 18) the client should call an ambulance and assume a knee-chest position.

Objective Data

If the cervix is dilated 4 cm or greater, if amniotic fluid is present in the vagina, if the presenting part is not vertex and the client is having contractions (see Chapter 18), and if the uterus is hard and tender without relaxation, the client should be in the hospital.

Palpation of the umbilical cord during a pelvic exam signals a life threatening emergency. The health care provider should attempt to push the presenting part back into the uterus while the physician is contacted immediately (see Chapter 18).

NURSING DIAGNOSES

The following nursing diagnoses identified by the author are representative of those used in a health care plan for pregnant women; however, these diagnoses by no means constitute an inclusive list.

- Activity intolerance related to syncope.
- Anxiety related to dyspnea in pregnancy.
- Body image disturbance related to changes in the skin and figure.
- Bowel elimination altered related to flatulence, constipation.
- Comfort and nutrition altered related to dyspepsia, potential for less or more nutrition than body requirements.
- Comfort altered with sleep pattern disturbance related to backache or calf, buttocks, or thigh cramps.
- Comfort altered and verbal communication impaired.
- Comfort altered related to Braxton-Hicks contractions; increased vaginal discharge; breast tenderness, enlargement, and pigmentation change; menstrual-like sensations in pelvis; increased salivation/bitter taste and/or speech difficulties.

- Coping ineffective, individual and/or family, related to emotional lability.
- Mobility impaired related to joint discomfort in pregnancy.
- Nutrition altered, potential for more or less than body requirements related to changes in taste and smell, pica, or nausea/vomiting.
- Sleep pattern disturbance related to insomnia or increased sleep needs during pregnancy.
- Tissue perfusion altered related to edema.
- Tissue integrity, altered oral and nasal mucous membranes related to epistaxis and/or epulis.
- Urinary elimination, altered patterns related to urinary frequency and/or incontinence.

REFERENCES

1. American College of Obstetricians and Gynecologists. (1993, April). Nutrition during pregnancy. *Technical Bulletin, 179.* Author.
2. Werler, M., Louik, C., Shapiro, S., & Mitchell, A. (1996, April 10). Prepregnant weight in relation to risk of neural tube defects. *Journal of the American Medical Association, 275*(14), 1089–1092.
3. Shaw, G., Velie, E., & Schaffer, D. (1996, April 10). Risk of neural tube defect—Affected pregnancies among obese women. *Journal of the American Medical Association, 275*(14), 1093–1096.
4. May, K., & Mahlmeister, L. (1994). *Maternal and neonatal nursing: Family-centered care* (3rd ed.). Philadelphia, Lippincott.
5. Giotta, M. (1993, March). Nutrition during pregnancy: Reducing obstetric risk. *Journal of Perinatal and Neonatal Nursing, 6*(4), 1–12.
6. Bucher, H., Guyatt, G., Cook, R., Hatala, R., Cook, D., Lang, J., & Hunt, D. (1996, April 10). Effects of calcium supplementation on pregnancy-induced hypertension and preeclampsia: A meta-analysis of randomized clinical trials. *Journal of the American Medical Association, 275*(14), 1113–1117.
7. Smith, K., Heaney, R., Flora, L., & Hinders, S. (1987). Calcium absorption from a new calcium delivery system. *Calcified Tissue International,* 351–352.

8. Neibyl, J. (1996, March). Iron therapy in pregnancy. *Contemporary OB/GYN,* 146–150.

9. National Academy of Sciences. (1990). *Nutrition during pregnancy.* Washington, DC: National Academy Press.

10. American College of Obstetricians and Gynecologists. (1993, March). Folic acid for the prevention of recurrent neural tube defects. *ACOG Committee Opinion, 120.* Author.

11. Goldenberg, R., Tamura, T., Neggers, Y., Cooper, R., Johnston, K., DuBard, M., & Hauth, J. (1995, Aug. 8). The effects of zinc supplementation on pregnancy outcome. *Journal of the American Medical Association, 274*(6), 463–468.

12. American College of Obstetricians and Gynecologist (1995, Sept.). Vitamin A supplementation during pregnancy. *ACOG Committee Opinion, 157.* Author.

13. Rothman, K., Moore, L., Singer, M., Nguyen, U., Mannino, S., & Milunsky, A. (1995, Nov. 23). Teratogenicity of high vitamin A supplementation. *The New England Journal of Medicine, 333*(21), 1369–1373.

14. Greco, H. (1995). Prevention of chickenpox in reproductive age women. *Primary Care Update for Obstetricians and Gynecologists, 2*(6), 221–223.

15. American College of Obstetricians and Gynecologists. (1992, Aug.). Rubella and pregnancy. *ACOG Technical Bulletin, 171.* Author.

16. U.S. Department of Health and Human Services: Public Health Service. (1994, January 28). General recommendations on immunization: Recommendations of the Advisory Committee on Immunization Practices. *Centers for Disease Control and Prevention:* Author.

17. American College of Obstetricians and Gynecologists. (1990, Jan.). Guidelines for hepatitis B screening and vaccination during pregnancy. *ACOG Committee Opinion, Committee on Obstetrics 78, Maternal and Fetal Medicine.* Author.

18. Newman, V., Fullerton, J., & Anderson, P. (1993, Nov./Dec.). Clinical advances in the management of severe nausea and vomiting during pregnancy. *Journal of Obstetrical, Gynecologic and Neonatal Nursing, 22*(6), 483–490.

19. Davis, D. (1996, Jan.). The discomforts of pregnancy. *Journal of Obstetrical, Gynecologic and Neonatal Nursing, 25*(1), 73–81.

20. Holzman, G., & Rinehart, R. (Eds.). (1995). *Planning for pregnancy, birth and beyond* (2nd ed.). Washington, DC: American College of Obstetricians and Gynecologists.

21. Wasson, J., Walsh, B., Tompkins, R., Sox, H., & Pantell, R. (1992). *The common symptom guide* (3rd ed.). New York: McGraw-Hill.

22. Sakakian, V., Rouse, D., Sipes, S., Rose, N., & Niebyl, J. (1991, July). Vitamin B$_6$ is effective therapy for nausea and vomiting of pregnancy: A randomized double-blind study placebo-controlled study. *Obstetrics and Gynecology, 78*(1), 33–36.

23. *Physicians' desk reference for nonprescriptive drugs.* (16th ed.). (1995). Montvale, NJ: Medical Economics Data.

24. Briggs, G., Freeman, R., & Yaffer, S. (1994). *Drugs in pregnancy and lactation* (4th ed.). Baltimore: Williams & Wilkins.

25. Eisenberg, A., Murkoff, H., & Hathaway, S. (1991). *What to expect when you are expecting* (2nd ed.). New York: Workman Publishing.

26. Kotz, D. (1996, Aug.). The hidden causes of gas pain. *Good Housekeeping, 222*(8), 130.

27. Ostgaard, H., Zetherstrom, G., Roos-Hansson, E., & Svanberg, B. (1994, Nov.). Reduction of back and posterior pelvic pain in pregnancy. *Spine, 19*(8), 894–900.

28. Dominquez-Rojas, V., Juanes-Pardo, J., Ortega-Molina, P., & Gordillo-Florencio, E. (1994). Spontaneous abortion abortion in a hospital population: Are tobacco and coffee intake risk factors? *European Journal of Epidemiology, 10,* 665–668.

29. American College of Obstetricians and Gynecologists. (1993, May). Smoking and reproductive health. *ACOG Technical Bulletin,* 180. Author.

30. Blair, P., Fleming, P. J., Bensley, D., Smith, I., Bacon, C., Taylor, E., Berry, J., Golding, J., & Tripp, J. (1996). Smoking and the sudden infant death syndrome: Results from 1993–5 case-control study for confidential inquiry into stillbirths and deaths in infancy. *British Medical Journal, 313,* 195–198.

31. Eskenazi, B., & Christianson, R., (1995, Mar.). Passive and active maternal smoking as measured by serum cotinine: The effect on birthweight. *American Journal of Public Health, 5*(3), 395–398.

32. Conover, E. (1994, July–Aug.). Hazardous exposure during pregnancy. *Journal of Obstetrical, Gynecologic and Neonatal Nursing, 23*(6), 524–531.

33. Barker, P., & Lewis, D. (1990). The management of lead exposure in pediatric populations. *Nurse Practitioner, 15*(12), 8–16.

34. American College of Obstetricians and Gynecologists. (1992, Sept.). Working during your pregnancy. *ACOG Patient Education.* Author.

35. Ahlorg, G. (1995, Aug.). Physical work load and pregnancy outcome. *Journal of Environmental Medicine, 37*(8), 941–943.

CHAPTER 18

COMPLICATIONS OF PREGNANCY

Joan Corder-Mabe

*T*he advanced prac-
tice role in high risk
care includes several
functions: assessment,
anticipating concerns,
education, advocating
for the client, and
counseling.

Highlights

- Infections
    - Hepatitis
    - Rubella
    - Varicella-Zoster
    - Cytomegalovirus
    - Parvovirus B19
    - Toxoplasmosis
    - HIV/AIDS
    - Sexually Transmitted Diseases Affecting Pregnancy
    - Pyelonephritis
    - Intra-amniotic and Amniotic Infections
- Bleeding
    - Spontaneous Abortion
    - Ectopic Pregnancy
    - Gestational Trophoblastic Disease
    - Placenta Previa
    - Abruptio Placenta
- Anemias
    - Iron and Folate Deficiency Anemias
    - Thalassemia
    - Sickle Cell Anemia
- Pregnancy Induced Hypertension
- Diabetes
- Preterm Labor and Birth
- Substance Abuse
- Multiple Gestation

► INTRODUCTION

A high risk pregnancy is one in which a condition exists that jeopardizes the health of the mother, her fetus, or both. The condition may be pre-existing or may have occurred solely because of the pregnancy. Between 1900 and 1980, the maternal mortality rate was drastically reduced. Since the 1980s, the rate of decline has slowed. In 1992, of the over 4 million live births in the United States, there were over 300 maternal deaths; approximately 7.7 per 100,000 women died annually.[1] Yet one statistic raises much concern and many questions: the maternal mortality rate among African American women and women of color is more than four times that of white women.[2,3] Older women are also at increased risk.[4,5]

Prenatal care has long been known to influence perinatal outcome because it allows timely and appropriate intervention to prevent or lessen the impact of untoward occurrences. Even though more women are receiving prenatal care in the first trimester, in 1993 21 percent of pregnant women had little or no prenatal care. The early receipt of prenatal care varies substantially among racial and ethnic groups.[1,3] Lack of or late prenatal care is associated with low birth weight infants who are at increased risk of neonatal mortality. The reasons that women frequently give for not seeking prenatal care are lack of money, no transportation, and not being aware of their pregnancy. Moreover, increased stress levels and inadequate support systems have been associated with complications of pregnancy. Is it the lack of prenatal care or the social and behavioral factors associated with inadequate care that contribute to the increased maternal and fetal morbidity and mortality?

Infant mortality is frequently used as a benchmark of the health status of nations and/or communities. In the United States, the infant mortality has gradually declined in the past 20 years, mostly due to increased technology of caring for the sick neonate. The black infant mortality rate was 2.4 times the white infant mortality rate in 1992, a ratio that has persisted for several years. In 1992 and 1993, the United States ranked twenty-second among industrialized nations. Even with all of our advances and increased resources spent for maternal and child health care, the United States has steadily fallen behind other nations. Birth weight is the single most important predictor of infant survival. In the United States, most infant deaths are associated with low birth weight. As with infant mortality rates, racial disparities persist in low birth weight categories, with black infants being much more likely than white infants to be of low birth weight.[6]

Optimal perinatal health care involves effective systems to assess all obstetrical clients for risk factors and to identify those women who are at risk. Appropriate interventions and procedures must then be implemented to minimize perinatal mortality or morbidity. Many perinatal centers have established antenatal care units to provide this specialized medical and nursing care. Home care programs have also been developed that provide cost effective, personal care to high risk pregnant women in surroundings that are familiar to them. Much needs to be learned about the effectiveness and efficiency of these strategies.[7]

The advanced practice role in high risk care includes several functions: assessment, anticipating concerns, education, advocating for the client, and counseling. The practitioner assesses the physical and emotional health of the woman; assists the family to activate their own strengths and develop strategies to deal with stressors of high risk pregnancy; anticipates the needs and concerns the family may have and assists them to make appropriate plans to meet their needs; edu-cates the woman and her family about all aspects of the treatment and care so that they can actively participate in the management; advocates for the woman and assists her to communicate and interact with the health care system; and counsels the client throughout her pregnancy.

Even with comprehensive, high quality prenatal care, many of the conditions discussed in this chapter will continue to occur with less than optimal outcome. The goal of care at all times is the best possible outcome for the woman and her family; the ultimate goal is a healthy mother with a healthy infant.

INFECTIONS

HEPATITIS

Hepatitis is an acute, systemic, viral infection and the most frequent cause of jaundice during pregnancy. It occurs as hepatitis A (HAV); hepatitis B (HBV); non-A, non-B [includes hepatitis C (HCV) and hepatitis E (HEV)] hepatitis; and delta hepatitis. Hepatitis A is an RNA virus formerly known as infectious hepatitis, because it causes an acute, mild, self-limiting hepatitis without major risk to health. Liver enzymes are temporarily affected and the woman does not become a carrier. Hepatitis B, formerly known as serum hepatitis, is a DNA virus that causes an acute, more severe infection. Forty to forty-five percent of all cases of hepatitis are caused by the hepatitis B virus.[8] Among its sequelae are chronic hepatitis, cirrhosis, and hepatocellular cancer. Pregnancy does not affect the severity or outcome of the disease. Non-A, non-B hepatitis is a viral syndrome that behaves much like hepatitis A and is transmitted either by parenteral (hepatitis C) or enteric (hepatitis E) routes.[8] It does not, however, have markers for hepatitis A or hepatitis B. Delta hepatitis is a hybrid particle with a delta core and a hepatitis B surface antigen coat. It can only occur with hepatitis B. Transmission is similar to hepatitis B. Generally a coexisting infection is not more virulent except in homosexuals and parenteral drug abusers when fatality can approach 5 to 10 percent. Hepatitis B vaccination seems reasonable to prevent delta hepatitis in the mother and therefore neonatal infection.

Epidemiology

Hepatitis A: HAV infection is acquired primarily by the fecal-oral route by either person-to-person contact or ingestion of contaminated food, particularly milk and shellfish, or polluted water. High risk populations are American Indians, Alaskan Natives, and those women living in western states. The rates are highest in children and employees in day care centers.[9]

Hepatitis B: Traditionally, risk populations for hepatitis B were defined by ethnic origin and historical data. Asians, Pacific Island residents, Eskimos, and certain African peoples are at increased risk. Hepatitis B virus (HBV) is transmitted through contaminated blood and blood products and through sexual intercourse. Skin punctures with contaminated needles, syringes, or medical instruments can also transmit the virus. Perinatal transmission does occur. The fetus is not at risk for the disease until it comes in contact with contaminated blood at delivery.

Incidence reports reveal that the hepatitis B carrier state affects 5 percent of the world population, with a higher percentage in tropical areas and Southeast Asia.

Hepatitis C: Risk factors for obstetric population include women with sexually transmitted diseases such as HIV and hepatitis B, multiple sexual partners, history of blood transfusions, and history of intravenous drug use.

Hepatitis D: Occurring as co-infection with hepatitis B, it has the same transmission and risks.[8] Perinatal transmission has been reported, but immunoprophylaxis for hepatitis B has been effective in preventing neonatal infection.[8]

Hepatitis E: Although rare in the United States, hepatitis E is endemic in developing countries and is transmitted by fecal/oral route.[8] Risk to obstetric population involves women who travel to developing countries. Once the pregnant woman recovers from the acute phase of infection, perinatal transmission does not occur.

Subjective Data

Hepatitis A produces flulike symptoms with malaise, fatigue, anorexia, nausea, pruritus, fever, and upper right quadrant pain. Symptoms of hepatitis B are similar to those of hepatitis A but with less fever and skin involvement. The older the woman is, the more severe her symptoms. Infection may be inapparent to the woman or the provider. Most clients with hepatitis C, D, or E are asymptomatic or have general flulike symptoms similar to hepatitis A.

Objective Data

Physical examination may reveal a normal general appearance. Jaundice of the skin, sclera, or nail beds may be present.

Hepatitis A: Serological testing to detect IgM antibody is done to confirm acute infection; becomes detectable 5–10 days after exposure and can remain positive for up to 6 months.

Hepatitis B: The immunoglobulin M antibody response occurs 3 to 4 weeks after exposure to the virus and before elevation of liver enzymes. When the IgM level is elevated in the absence of IgG elevation, then acute infection is suspected. The level of IgM usually returns to normal in 8 weeks. Explain to the client that the test will differentiate acute infection from chronic disease.

The immunoglobulin G antibody response occurs about 2 weeks after the IgM response begins. The level of IgG increases rapidly and slowly returns to normal. The IgG level may remain elevated for years. When the IgG is elevated in the absence of IgM elevation, chronic disease is suspected.

Hepatitis B virus antigens and antibodies are identified in a laboratory screening. The testing for HBsAg should be included in the initial prenatal assessment for all clients and repeated later in pregnancy for women in high risk groups.[8,10,11]

HBV, also called the Dane particle, consists of an inner core and an outer surface capsule. Laboratory screening is used to identify the presence of hepatitis B surface antigen in the blood, as well as antibodies to the virus surface or core. The hepatitis B surface antigen (HBsAg) screening test is most commonly performed, as a rise in HBsAg appears at the onset of clinical symptoms and generally indicates active infection. If HBsAg persists in the blood, the client is identified as a carrier. The hepatitis B surface antibody (HBsAb) appears 4 weeks after the surface antigen and indicates immunity. Elevation of hepatitis B core antibody (HBcAb) occurs in the period between disappearance of HbsAg and appearance of HBsAb. HBcAb is the only marker in this period that indicates a recent hepatitis infection.

Prepare the client for repeat testing, as HBV screening tests may also be used to monitor the progression of infection.

Serum levels of glutamic-pyruvic transaminase (SGPT) and serum glutamic-oxaloacetic transaminase (SGOT), cellular enzymes found in the liver, are evaluated to determine liver damage. When liver damage occurs, increased amounts of these enzymes are released into the bloodstream.

As these enzymes are evaluated as part of a complete panel of blood work, usually following a positive screening for HBV or clinical signs of illness, inform the client that enzyme levels will be retested to monitor the severity and progression of disease.

Hepatitis C: Confirmed by the identification of anti-C antibody performed with an enzyme immunoassay (EIA). Testing for hepatitis C is not widely available or recommended at present.[10]

Hepatitis D: For acute infection, serologic test will have positive antigen and positive IgM antibody.[8]

Hepatitis E: Confirmation done through electron microscopy of stool sample; fluorescent antibody blocking assay and Western blot assay are also available.[8]

Differential Medical Diagnoses

Fatty liver disease, pregnancy induced hypertension with HELLP (hemolysis, elevated liver enzymes, and low platelets) syndrome, secondary syphilis, drug induced hepatitis.

Plan

Psychosocial Interventions. Reassure the client that the fetus is at minimal risk. Family members should be encouraged to assist with household and child care duties to allow the client to rest.

Medication. *Hepatitis A:* Immune globulin (gamma globulin) or immune-specific globulin (ISG) is indicated for any pregnant woman exposed to HAV to provide passive immunity through injected antibodies. All household contacts should also receive gamma globulin. Gamma globulin is given intramuscularly. Immune globulin intravenous (IGIV) is available to provide passive immunity.

Hepatitis B: Immune globulin (HBIG) contains a high titer of hepatitis B surface antigen (HBsAg), which provides passive immunity to hepatitis B. Pregnant women with definite exposure to HBV should receive HBIG as soon as possible after contact and again 30 days later. Any household or sexual contact should be tested and, if negative, receive immunoprophylaxis with HBIG. Those individuals should also receive the vaccination series. The newborn of a woman positive for HBV should be given HBIG within 12 hours of delivery. If a woman is suspected of having an acute infection during pregnancy, serial HBsAg tests are done. Disappearance of HBsAg indicates that the fetus is no longer at risk. Close contacts of women with HBV should also receive HBIG, if not already immunized.

Hepatitis B vaccine is indicated for the newborn of a woman who has tested positive for HBsAg to stimulate the newborn's active immunity. It should be given as soon as possible after birth up to 7 days of life, and again at 30 and 60 days. The Centers for Disease Control and Prevention (CDC) recommend routine vaccination of all newborns.[10] Dosage recommendations depend upon the status of the mother. The vaccination is not contraindicated during pregnancy. Recombivax HB and Energix-B are the two approved products for hepatitis B vaccination.[11]

Hepatitis C, D, and E: No current licensed vaccine for use with hepatitis C or D infection.[10,12]

Hygienic Measures. All caregivers, whether health care providers or family members, should use universal precautions at all times.[12] Stress to the client and her family that hepatitis A, C, D, and E are highly contagious. Explain the mode of transmission in the instruction and advise family and friends concerning good hand washing and hygiene.

Diet. Recommend a bland diet with additional fluids, depending on the extent of a client's nausea and vomiting. Intravenous fluid hydration may become necessary.

Breastfeeding. Infants who have received prophylaxis at birth and are currently on the immunization schedule should continue breastfeeding.

Follow-Up

Frankly discuss and assess possible drug use, as hepatitis is frequently associated with substance abuse. In addition, as hepatitis is sexually transmitted, recommend the use of condoms throughout the remainder of the pregnancy, and arrange to repeat screening tests for sexually transmitted diseases, especially human immunodeficiency virus (HIV) infection.

RUBELLA

Commonly called German measles or 3-day measles, rubella is an acute, mild, contagious disease caused by the rubella virus.

Epidemiology

The etiology and risk factors of rubella are important in relation to pregnancy because of the potential teratogenic effects of the virus on the fetus, particularly in the first trimester. When infection occurs in the first 4 weeks of conception, 50 percent of fetuses have signs of rubella infection; in the second 4-week interval following conception, 25 percent of fetuses will be affected; in the third month, 10 percent of fetuses will be affected; and beyond the first trimester only 1 percent of fetuses will be infected.[8] The disease occurs worldwide, more frequently in springtime, and is more likely among adolescents and young adults.

Transmission occurs by direct contact with urine, stool, or nasopharyngeal secretions with an incubation period of 2–3 weeks. Infected individuals can transmit the infection for several days without experiencing the characteristic symptoms or rash. The disease is transmitted to the fetus through transplacental infestation.

The low incidence of rubella and related congenital anomalies is attributed to the availability of rubella vaccine since 1969. It is estimated that 5 to 15 percent of women of childbearing age are susceptible to rubella.

Subjective Data

The client reports a nonpruritic rash, fever, and a feeling of general malaise. She has no history of the disease or vaccination.

Objective Data

Postauricular and occipital lymphadenopathy is present early in process. Fever may range from 99.5–101.7° F, and conjunctival erythema (mild conjunctivitis) may be noted. The characteristic maculopapular rash starts on the face, spreads to the trunk, and disappears by the third day.

The diagnostic test used is hemagglutination inhibition (HI). A serum sample is obtained and sent for laboratory evaluation. Antibodies are usually not present in the serum until after the rash has developed. When confirmation of rubella infection is important, as it is in pregnancy, an HI antibody titer is drawn immediately after exposure to the virus and repeated in 2 to 3 weeks. An initial titer of 1:8 indicates absence of previous rubella infection. A fourfold rise in antibody titer in 2 to 3 weeks indicates infection. Prepare the client for repeat testing.

When rubella affects the fetus, it is termed *rubella syndrome;* defects of the eyes (cataracts, retinopathy, glaucoma), ears (degenerative changes in inner ear, hearing loss), and heart (patent ductus arteriosus, pulmonary artery stenosis) may result. Also associated with the syndrome are decreased head circumference, mental retardation, and poor childhood growth and language and motor development. Seizures related to encephalitis from central nervous system damage also may occur.

Differential Medical Diagnoses

Rubeola, scarlet fever, drug reaction.

Plan

Ideally, all women have been vaccinated and have adequate immunity; however, it is recommended that all women be screened during the initial prenatal visit. Assessment of rubella status should be included in a preconception visit. If negative, vaccination should be done a minimum of 3 months prior to conception. Counsel clients who do not have adequate immunity to avoid situations where they may come in contact with infected persons. Vaccination is recommended during the immediate postpartum period. Breastfeeding is not a contraindication to vaccination.[8]

If active disease occurs during the first trimester, counsel the client concerning the risks to her fetus. Support her decision to continue or terminate the pregnancy.

VARICELLA-ZOSTER (CHICKENPOX)

Varicella-zoster is a highly contagious infection caused by a virus of the same name (varicella-zoster virus or VZV).[13] Varicella is a member of the herpes virus family and, like herpes, varicella can lay dormant in the dorsal root ganglia and reactivate later. Less than 10 percent of occurrences are in individuals over 10 years of age. It is a common benign childhood disease that can be more serious in adulthood. In pregnant women, the severity of the disease may be further increased, particularly if there is pulmonary involvement. Once an individual is infected, immunity is usually lifelong. Therefore, varicella is rare in pregnancy; 95 percent of pregnant women have antibodies to VZV. Immunization is available and may be used prior to conception if indicated.

Epidemiology

Pregnant women are at risk for developing varicella when they come in close physical contact with children who have active infection. (Most adults have had chickenpox.) The virus is transmitted through direct contact with respiratory tract secretions with an incubation period of 10–14 days. Individuals are infectious the 24 hours prior to the rash until all cutaneous lesions have crusted. Complications of varicella infection in children are rare, but encephalitis and pneumonia are life threatening complications that occur in adult infection.[8,14]

The major consequence of varicella in pregnancy is infection in the neonate. Ten to 20 percent of infants of mothers who had acute varicella infection during pregnancy develop varicella through dissemination of the virus across the placenta. Neonatal signs appear within 5–10 days postdelivery. The symptoms are variable including nothing but scattered skin lesions to more generalized rash with visceral infection and possible pneumonia. Prior to treatment with acyclovir, neonatal mortality was 20–30 percent.[8] Infection during the first half of pregnancy is associated with low birth weight, limb hypoplasia, microcephaly, chorioretinitis, and cataracts.[13]

Subjective Data

The client reports fever, malaise, and a generalized pruritic rash predominantly on the trunk. Usually, her history reveals exposure during the previous 2 weeks.

Objective Data

Physical examination of the client reveals a characteristic rash. Fluid from the vesicles may be examined for diagnosis and several antibody tests performed.

Diagnosis of varicella is usually made by clinical exam alone.[8,14] Physical examination shows a maculopapular rash on the trunk. The rash quickly progresses to vesicles that erupt and then crust over. New vesicles form daily for 2–3 days. Consequently, a mixture of red papules, vesicles, and scabs appears at one time. Fever of 101 to 103° F may be present. Prenatal infection can lead to varicella embryopathy or varicella in the newborn. Congenital anomalies associated with varicella are limb atrophy, microencephaly, cortical atrophy, motor and sensory manifestations, and eye problems such as cataracts, chorioretinitis, microphthalmia, and Horner's syndrome.

Diagnostic methods include clinical evaluation of the virus isolated from vesicular fluid. Several antibody tests are also used to detect infection: complement fixation (CF), radioimmunoassay (RIA), latex agglutination (LA), enzyme-linked immunosorbent assay (ELISA), fluorescent antibody against membrane antigen (FAMA), and immune adherence hemagglutina-

tion (IAHA). None of these tests is in widespread use for screening at this time, but the two most useful are the FAMA and ELISA.

Medical Differential Diagnoses

Rubella, rubeola.

Plan

Psychosocial Interventions. Focus on identifying women who are at risk prior to or shortly after exposure to the virus. Counsel any woman who has been exposed and has not previously had the infection to be tested for VZV antibody.

The primary care provider must educate all pregnant women to avoid situations where they may come in contact with varicella.[14] When infection does occur, women require instructions on how to avoid spread of infection and how to relieve the discomforts of skin eruptions.

Medication. Medication is given for symptomatic relief of pruritic; acetaminophen is given to control fever. For severe varicella infection in pregnancy involving pneumonia and high fever, intravenous acyclovir may be recommended. The safety of systemic acyclovir therapy among pregnant women has not been established.[13]

Varicella zoster immune globulin (VZIG) is administered as soon as possible after a woman who has not had varicella infection or who has not been previously immunized is exposed to the virus. A newborn whose mother had an onset of varicella 5 days before or 2 days after delivery should receive VZIG.[8,13]

Immunization. Women of reproductive age should be assessed for varicella immunity prior to pregnancy and offered the vaccine, Varivax. The vaccine is administered in two subcutaneous doses, 4 to 8 weeks apart. Pregnancy should be avoided for a minimum of 3 months following the last vaccination. Effects of the varicella virus on the fetus are unknown; therefore, pregnant women should not be vaccinated.[15] If a pregnant woman is vaccinated, she should be advised of the potential effects on the fetus. Because the risks are small, the decision to terminate a pregnancy should not be based on whether vaccine was administered during pregnancy.

Breastfeeding. Most live viruses are not secreted in breast milk. Whether attenuated varicella vaccine is excreted in breast milk or causes infection is not known. Attenuated rubella vaccine has been detected in breast milk but only produces asymptomatic infection in the nursing infant. Therefore, varicella virus vaccine may also be considered for a nursing mother.[8,13]

Other Interventions. Institute measures to prevent the spread of infection. Isolate the client until the rash has disappeared, which is usually about 7 days. Take respiratory and skin precautions if the client is in labor and in the hospital. Following delivery, she should be isolated with her neonate in a private room.

CYTOMEGALOVIRUS

Cytomegalovirus (CMV) is a DNA virus that is widely spread throughout the human population.[16] Congenital infection is different from perinatal infection. Congenital CMV infections, especially those that occur in the first 20 weeks of gestation, are associated with symptomatic disease at birth and possible long-term problems of mental retardation, microencephaly, intracranial calcification, chorioretinitis, hearing loss, or cerebral palsy. The most common cause of hearing loss in children is perinatal CMV.[8] Acute congenital effects of the neonate include hepatosplenomegaly, thrombocytopenia, hepatitis with jaundice, and/or anemia.

Epidemiology

The etiology of congenital disease involves in utero infection. Congenital CMV infection results from hepatogenous dissemination of virus across the placenta secondary to primary maternal CMV infection. In women, the likelihood of seropositivity has been correlated with low socioeconomic status, older age, multigravidity, large number of sexual partners, and a first pregnancy before age 15. Women who fit these criteria are at most risk for primary CMV infection. Perinatal CMV is acquired through intrapartum exposure to secretions or postpartum exposure to CMV in breast milk or blood transfusions.

Pregnant women acquire active disease mostly from sexual contact, blood transfusions, and contact with children in daycare centers. Reactivation of previous infection can also occur and cause congenital CMV. Incidence reports reveal that congenital CMV occurs among 0.5 to 2.9 percent of all infants. In women who acquire primary disease during pregnancy, 40–50 percent of those infants will be affected.[8]

Subjective Data

Most women with primary infections are asymptomatic. Women may, however, report flulike symptoms, including myalgia, chills, and malaise.

Objective Data

Lymphadenopathy and hepatosplenomegaly may be present.[8] Blood work demonstrates leukocytosis and lymphocytosis; liver function tests are elevated. Diagnosis is most often made by means of antibody tests, including hemagglutination inhibition, ELISA, and fluorescent antibody. A positive CMV-specific IgM test confirms that infection occurred during the previous 60 days. A fourfold rise in IgG antibody titer indicates recent infection.[16] Other laboratory findings will include atypical lymphocytes on differential WBC, low platelet count, and elevated serum transaminase concentrations.[8]

Differential Medical Diagnoses

Mononucleosis, HIV disease.

Plan

No therapy prevents or treats CMV infection. Screening for CMV using cervical cultures or blood tests are not recommended. Women with documented infection may elect termination of their pregnancy, depending on the gestational age. Discuss the risks and be sensitive to the client's concerns and anxiety.

Teaching all pregnant women about good hygiene and handwashing helps decrease the spread of disease. Advise pregnant women to avoid exposure to individuals with CMV infection (e.g., persons with AIDS). Explain that CMV is sexually transmitted and advise the use of condoms and limiting sexual partners as strategies that reduce the transmission of the infection.

ERYTHEMA INFECTIOSUM (FIFTH DISEASE)

This type of virus (parvovirus B19) usually does not cause infection in humans. When, however, acute infection does occur during pregnancy, particularly before 18 weeks of gestation, fetal infection and stillbirth are possible.

Epidemiology

The prevalence of infection among pregnant women and fetuses is not known. Among adults, 30 percent are carriers of antibodies for parvovirus. Infection is spread transplacentally, by oropharyngeal route in casual contact, and through infected blood components. Estimating risk is impossible because studies are limited. Erythema infectiosum is a self-limiting disease and complete recovery usually occurs.[8]

The most significant effect of human parvovirus on the fetus is the occurrence of fetal hydrops. The hydrops develops as a result from the aplastic anemia secondary to the viral infection, and subsequent congestive heart failure. The incidence of hydrops is varied from 0–38 percent, with most researchers reporting 5–15 percent.[8]

Subjective Data

A client may report a facial rash and sometimes arthritic pain of the hands, wrists, and knees.

Objective Data

The most characteristic sign of parvovirus B19 infection is the "slapped-face" rash, a macular rash that may also be found on the trunk. The rash may subside only to return in response to stress, exercise, sunlight, or bathing.[8]

Viral infection of the bone marrow causes destruction of red blood cell precursors so blood work reveals a transient aplastic crisis. The crisis usually happens only in women who have an underlying hemoglobinopathy. IgG shows a 30 per-

cent rise with acute infection.[8,16,17] The serum maternal α-fetoprotein is also elevated. When there is a history of parvovirus B19 in the first trimester, a level II sonogram is ordered between 20 and 22 weeks to evaluate fetal structures and to detect the presence of hydrops. If there are not signs of hydrops, no further testing is necessary.[8] With hydrops, fetal edema and ascites are observed.[17] There have been reports of subsequent sonograms that revealed resolution of previously detected hydrops.[18]

Medical Differential Diagnoses

Rubella, rubeola, roseola, scarlet fever.

Plan

Sonography. A Level II sonogram should be done in any woman with suspicion of parvovirus infection. Serial sonograms should be ordered after acute infection to monitor for the occurrence of hydrops. With the sonographic findings that have reported resolution of hydrops associated with Fifth disease, prognosis may not be as grave as earlier thought.[8,18] The health care provider should share what information is available and be sensitive to the client's concerns.

TOXOPLASMOSIS

Toxoplasmosis is a common infectious disease caused by the intracellular protozoan parasite *Toxoplasma gondii.*[14] Primary infection during pregnancy is associated with stillbirth or congenital infection. Symptoms usually appear at birth. About 10 percent of infected infants manifest severe disease characterized by chorioretinitis, cyanosis, pneumonia, hepatosplenomegaly, jaundice, and thrombocytopenia purpura. Infants who survive sustain some permanent neurological damage.

Epidemiology

Risk factors for maternal infection include eating raw or undercooked meats and living in rural areas.

Usual transmission is through ingestion of tissue cysts in contaminated meat or through contact with oocytes in feces of infected cats or farm animals, or eating unwashed fruit, berries or vegetables with contagious oocytes on their surface. During acute primary maternal infection, the fetus is transplacentally infected about 40 percent of the time. Any history of maternal infection affords permanent immunity. Spontaneous abortion, stillbirth, or severe congenital infection occurs in 10 to 15 percent of pregnancies complicated with toxoplasmosis. Congenital infection is more likely to occur when maternal infection occurs in the third trimester.

Women who are positive for HIV or who are on immunosuppressive therapy following transplantation will be more susceptible to toxoplasmosis.

The overall incidence is 0.25 to 1.0 per 1000 live births. About 30 percent of the U.S. population has been infected with toxoplasma organism.[14]

Subjective Data

Although most women are asymptomatic, the client may report fatigue, fever, rash, depression, malaise, headache, and sore throat. Infection occurs 1 to 2 weeks after exposure, and the client may remain symptomatic for as long as several months.

Objective Data

Physical examination reveals lymph node enlargement, particularly in the posterior cervical chain.

Diagnosis is made by means of serial toxoplasma antibody tests (two or more) done 3 weeks apart. The second sample shows significantly higher levels of antibodies if active infection is present. An indirect fluorescent antibody test of 1:512 or greater correlates with active infection. Recently, testing for toxoplasma DNA in amniotic fluid has been used to determine presence of fetal infection.[14]

Some countries screen all pregnant women for toxoplasmosis during the initial prenatal visit. That is not currently an acceptable approach in this country.

Differential Medical Diagnosis

Infectious mononucleosis.

Plan

Psychosocial Interventions. Educate prenatal clients about the risk of toxoplasmosis and discuss prevention. Advise pregnant women to avoid handling cat litter, to wear gloves when gardening, to always wash their hands well after handling cats, and to avoid eating undercooked or raw meats. Prevention of disease is the key to management.

If primary infection occurs in the first trimester, discuss the option of terminating the pregnancy with the client and her family.

Medication. Medications include pyrimethamine and sulfonamides, but pyrimethamine is not recommended in the first trimester because of possible teratogenicity.[8] Some success may occur in treating maternal toxoplasmosis if the drugs are administered throughout pregnancy. Although the treatment reduces the severity of maternal toxoplasmosis, it is not currently standard therapy.

An investigational drug, Spiramycin, may be used to prevent placental transmission of the parasite in the first trimester.[14] It is being used in France with success but is not a common practice in the United States.[8]

A newborn whose mother was treated antenatally for toxoplasmosis should be treated prophylactically with a combination of pyrimethamine and sulfadiazine (antimalarial drug). An infant with symptoms or an asymptomatic infant with positive cerebrospinal fluid should also be treated.

HUMAN IMMUNODEFICIENCY VIRUS (HIV)*

Human Immunodeficiency Virus (HIV) attacks the T4 cells, decreases the CD-4 cell count and disables the immune system. As the CD-4 cell count decreases, immune system dysfunction occurs. Organs such as the kidney and liver can suffer tissue damage before major system dysfunction is apparent. The condition progresses to a severe immunosuppressed state termed Acquired Immunodeficiency Syndrome (AIDS). Recent reports indicate that pregnancy does not accelerate the progression of HIV to AIDS and/or death.[8,19]

---

*Refer to Chapter 12 for a more complete discussion of HIV/AIDS.

The CDC definition of AIDS is an HIV-infected person with a specific opportunistic infection or a CD-4 count less than 200 mm.

Epidemiology

The disease was not recognized until the early 1980s and there is no reliable data collection system for the number of HIV-positive individuals. Historically, HIV/AIDS was a disease of homosexual males. Now, the incidence of HIV/AIDS has increased in women. In 1995, of the 73,380 AIDS cases reported, women accounted for 13,764 (19 percent). HIV infection is the third leading cause of death among all U.S. women aged 25–44 years and the leading cause of death among black women in this age group.[20] Most of the women affected by HIV have male partners who use injectable drugs or who are bisexual men. Women who use drugs themselves or are prostitutes are more likely to be HIV affected. Unfortunately, the mortality rate for people with AIDS is 90 percent.

An estimated 7000 infants are born to HIV infected women in the United States each year.[20] Most cases of infant HIV infection are due to perinatal transmission. The chances of a woman having an infant who has HIV infection varies from 5 to 60 percent with an average of 20 to 30 percent. The large variance reported in transmission statistics relates to advances in treatment being developed over the short time that women are beginning to be represented in the HIV positive population. Using prenatal drug treatment may be able to decrease vertical transmission from 30 percent to 8 percent. Vertical transmission is affected by the viral load of the mother, status of the maternal immune system, route of delivery, general health of the fetus, presence of maternal infection, and exposure to genital secretions. The greater the viral load of the mother the more likely that vertical transmission of the virus will occur.[21,22] Women with AIDS and the suppressed immune system are more likely to transmit the virus to the fetus. A first twin during vaginal delivery also has increased risk to contract the virus because of its longer exposure to cervical/vaginal secretions. Any delivery complication such as forceps delivery, lacerations, or episiotomy add to fetal risk for the same reason.

Placental vasculitis (chorioamnionitis) facilitates the spread of the virus.[8]

Most HIV infections in the United States are HIV-1, but HIV-2 is endemic in other countries such as Africa.

Another rare HIV-1 group O has been reported. Because this group is not detected by the standard HIV testing, there is concern that undetected transmission of HIV is occurring.[20]

HIV infection is acquired by sexual contact, exposure to blood or bodily fluids, vertical transmission to the fetus, and perinatal exposure at delivery and by breastfeeding. Historically, HIV/AIDS was associated with the male homosexual community and intravenous drug abusers. The prevalence of HIV infection and AIDS is now increasing more rapidly among women than among men.[20,23] Most women with AIDS have acquired the disease through heterosexual contact, and a majority of those women are mothers. Pregnancy rates among women infected with HIV remain high.[24] The implications to discuss this disease in women's and infants' health are obvious.

The relationship between pregnancy and HIV infection is difficult to separate because so many of the women with HIV/AIDs have other risks associated with complications of pregnancy. Many of these women affected by HIV also have problems with drug addiction, access to prenatal care, adequate nutrition, poverty, and increased incidence of sexually transmitted diseases. Considering these factors, women affected by HIV also have increased risk for preterm delivery, premature rupture of membranes, intrauterine growth retardation, postpartum endometritis, and increased perinatal mortality.[8]

Risk of acquiring HIV through heterosexual contact is greater for women because semen has high concentration of the virus, and coitus causes more breaks in the vaginal lining as compared to the penile skin. The presence of other genital infections increases those chances.

Subjective Data

Most people remain asymptomatic after exposure to the virus. Within the first few months of being infected, many persons experience an acute viral infection similar to mononucleosis with complaints such as weight loss, fever, night sweats, pharyngitis, rash, and lymphadenopathy. These symptoms resolve within a few weeks and are frequently not perceived by the client as significant.

The woman may experience several episodes of discrete illnesses such as weight loss or an infection that have a definitive beginning and end. Once the symptoms subside, the woman returns to a prediagnosis level of function. At some point, these illnesses become chronic and, even though controlled, are not cured. Usually, at this time the woman is on prophylaxis drug therapy. The symptoms experienced at this point are varied and reflect which organ systems are most affected by the virus. Common symptoms include dyspnea and fatigue, decreased muscle strength, cramping pain in the extremities, nausea and vomiting, and recurrent vaginal yeast infections.[25] Because these are also common complaints associated with pregnancy, identifying onset of illness may be difficult.

Objective Data

The enzyme linked immunosorbent assay (ELISA) detects antibodies to the virus that develop within 12 weeks of exposure. It is the screening test for exposure to HIV and, if reactive on two separate tests, is followed by the Western blot assay. The Western blot is the confirmatory diagnostic test.

With advancing technology, ways of assessing the status of the immune system and level of invasion of the virus are being developed. Monitoring of CD-4 cell count assesses a person's status as to the invasion of the virus, and RNA levels or viral load assessments are used as a staging indicator of the disease. (Refer to Chapter 12 for more detailed information on screening and monitoring status of HIV.)

Differential Medical Diagnosis

Refer to Chapter 12.

Plan

Prevention. Major media campaigns have educated citizens on the need to protect themselves from the spread of HIV. "Safer sex" has become the focus of many national and local campaigns including advice to reduce the number of sexual partners, avoid partners with high risk histories (multiple partners, homosexual relations, intravenous drug users), and use latex condoms, preferably with Nonoxynol 9, during all sexual encounters. Abstinence based educational campaigns have also emerged.

In February 1994, the National Institutes of Health announced findings of a study sponsored by the Pediatric Clinical Trials Group (ACTG), which found that administering Zidovudine (ZDV) during pregnancy, labor and delivery, and during the neonatal period reduced perinatal transmission of HIV by two-thirds. Women with advanced HIV disease or previous antiretroviral therapy were not included in this study. The ACTG, warning that the study had limitations, recommended the development of national policies and protocols for the counseling and screening of all pregnant women. Since then, much effort by governmental agencies, professional groups, and concerned citizens has occurred to educate women about this potential preventive strategy.[26,27,28,29,30]

Numerous reports indicate that women know about HIV and its transmission. There are only a few studies that specifically report the knowledge, attitudes, and practices of pregnant women.[31] The problem now is that many pregnant women particularly minority and women of other cultures, may have inadequate knowledge about the treatment and perinatal transmission of HIV/AIDS.[31] In the past, education programs targeted homosexual males and intravenous drug users. Because women constitute the fastest growing population affected by HIV/AIDS, educational programs designed for minority and women of other cultures are necessary to be effective in reducing the incidence of HIV.[31,32,33]

PRENATAL SCREENING. Initially, selected testing based upon assessment of risk behaviors in pregnant women was standard, but it was later discovered that significant numbers of women who tested HIV positive had not given any history of risk behaviors.[20,29] Some groups, including the American Medical Association, have proposed national policies to mandate testing for all pregnant women. So far, most groups feel that mandatory testing would deter many of the affected women from seeking prenatal care and have proposed mandatory counseling and informed consent for testing.[25,29,34] The prenatal counseling recommendation is to discuss with the pregnant woman how HIV is acquired, strategies to reduce transmission, perinatal transmission and strategies to prevent transmission to the fetus. Pharmaceutical treatment should be offered. At present, federal funds to states for HIV programs include stipulations encouraging statewide systems to promote interview screening of all pregnant women for HIV. As knowledge is gained in the prevention of perinatal transmission and treatment of HIV/AIDS, recommendations about prenatal screening may change.

Women who are seropositive for HIV should be counseled about the risk of perinatal transmission and potential for obstetric complications. A discussion of the options on continuing the pregnancy is appropriate.

PRENATAL CARE. Women affected by HIV warrant comprehensive prenatal care that can be provided by the local obstetrical care delivery system. Community based care with appropriate consultation and guidance from the appropriate referral center is preferred. The usual screening tests done in normal pregnancy should also be done with emphasis on sexually transmitted diseases. Screening for gonorrhea, chlamydia, herpes, hepatitis B,C, and D, and syphilis are particularly important. Testing for antibody to CMV and toxoplasmosis is also recommended.[8] If not routinely done for the normal pregnant women in the prenatal setting, a tuberculin skin test with follow-up chest x-ray as indicated for the woman who is HIV positive. Vaccinations for hepatitis B, pneumococcal infection, hemophilus B influenza and viral influenza should be done to offer protection for opportunistic infections. Close scrutiny and follow-up of suspicious Pap smear results are prudent because of the increased risk of cervical changes associated with HIV.

NEWBORN SCREENING. Many states anonymously test all newborns for HIV in order to assess the prevalence of the virus. Some states have taken efforts to make these records available to women or to pediatricians as deemed necessary.[29,34] Prior to the ACTG 076 protocol, some professionals were calling for mandatory newborn screening. At present, mandatory screening of newborns is not occurring in any states.

Medication. Nucleoside analog reverse transcriptase inhibitors, non-nucleoside reverse transcriptase inhibitors, and protease inhibitors are available and are being used in the treatment of persons positive for HIV. Much research continues as to when treatment is initiated, which drugs to choose, and in what combination. Over time, resistance to the drugs occurs and, therefore, it is not clearly known when changes to other drugs are most advantageous. The nucleoside analog reverse transcriptase inhibitors inhibit the binding site of the reverse transcriptase enzyme, the key enzyme in transforming viral RNA to DNA. They do not kill the virus but inhibit viral replication.[35] Azidothymidine (AZT), the most popular, remains the initial therapy is most cases. The non-nucleoside reverse transcriptase inhibitors (NNRTIS) alter the shape of the active site on the binding site of the reverse transcriptase enzyme. These drugs are only available in clinical trials at present.[35] The protease inhibitors work by inhibiting the HIV protease enzyme, a necessary enzyme for formation of the protein capsule surrounding the viral RNA in mature viruses.[35,36] Treatment with protease has reduced HIV replication and increased CD-4 cell counts better than the other categories of drugs.[37] The use of these drugs during pregnancy is being investigated and usage varies by geographical areas. At present no clear recommendations are in place.

AVAILABLE ANTIRETROVIRAL DRUGS
Nucleoside Analog Reverse Transcriptase Inhibitors
Azidothymidine(AZT)—Retrovir, Zidovudine
Didanosine (ddI)—Videx
Zalcitabine (ddC)—Hivid
Stavudine (d4T)—Zerit
Lamivudine (3TC)—Epivir

Non-Nucleoside Reverse Transcriptase Inhibitors (NNRTIS)
Delavirdine—Rescriptor
Nevirapine—Viramune

Protease Inhibitors
Saquinavir—Invirase
Indinavir—Crixivan
Ritonavir—Norvir

The protocol for the prevention of perinatal transmission of HIV includes the following:

- Zidovudine 500 mg per day beginning in the second or third trimester.
- Zidovudine IV 2 mg/kg loading dose followed by 1 mg/kg per hour during labor.
- Zidovudine 2 mg/kg per day for the infant during the first 6 weeks of life.[21,23]

Since the release of the protocol, there are reports of the relationship of the maternal viral load to success of treatment with ZDV.[21] ZDV has a protective effect prenatally but may not be as effective late in the third trimester or intrapartally if the viral load is increasing or is high at that time of administration.[21] The major sign of toxicity is bone marrow suppression, so hematocrit, white cell count, and platelet count should be done periodically.[8] Those women on Zidovudine during pregnancy should also be monitored by a monthly complete blood cell count and liver function tests. Trimethoprim-sulfamethoxazole is the drug of choice for prophylaxis for pneumonia carinii infection, a common opportunistic infection associated with AIDS. This regimen also provides protection against toxoplasmic encephalitis.[8] The CD-4 and T-lymphocyte count should be monitored each trimester to determine need for initiation of prophylaxis for opportunistic infections.

Physical Concerns. Fatigue or decreased physical endurance has been identified by HIV positive clients and their caregivers as a major health care problem.[38] Exercise has been proposed as a strategy to increase endurance and improve mental outlook. Direct positive effect on the immune system has been theorized but as yet has not been demonstrated.[38] Effects of exercise including prenatal exercises and prepared childbirth have not been studied for their effects on the HIV positive pregnant woman.

Psychosocial Issues. The issues of women who are positive for HIV are complex and difficult. Women are more likely to be involved in full-time caregiving roles, are more likely to be in poverty and be less able to access health care.[23,24] Even when the diagnosis of HIV positive is made, the women is usually not symptomatic and, therefore, is likely to react with denial. Because of this denial, discussions about planning for the future, accepting preventive treatment for perinatal transmission, and reducing the transmission of HIV to present partners is difficult. Previous experience and general mental health will attribute to the women's ability to cope with the disease and/or the pregnancy. With the emphasis on prenatal screening, many of these women are having to deal with an initial diagnosis of a fatal disease as well with stressors of a pregnancy. Those women who abuse drugs are even more difficult to help because of the nature of their lifestyle, which is usually disorganized and without adequate family or community support. A discussion about the option of termination of the pregnancy may be appropriate.

Women who have progressed to AIDS face a daily risk of developing an opportunistic infection, are challenged dealing with normal activities of daily living with compromised energy level and decreased physical endurance, overwhelmed by financial burdens of medical and drug therapies and emotional responses to a life threatening condition as well as concern regarding who will care for their infants if they becomes ill. A home care model with the appropriate supportive care including nutritional services, counseling, nursing, homemaker and spiritual care is the most effective, client oriented and cost effective approach.[25,39] Case management involves being able to identify the strengths of the woman and develop a plan of care that provides comprehensive care while maintaining the woman's independence as long as possible.

As the disease progresses and the woman's coping with the stresses of the illness and its treatment, the woman affected by HIV is at increased risk for clinical depression and suicide.[25] The applicability of this observation to pregnant and postpartum women is unknown.

Many community based, multicultural organizations have developed programs throughout the country to address the various issues regarding HIV/AIDS. Many communities have AIDS service directories, volunteer organizations and academically based and/or federally funded projects to assist HIV affected women access resources. The national AIDS hotline 1–800–342–AIDS is an excellent source of information for clients and providers.

Education/Counseling. The HIV positive pregnant woman will need education concerning infection control issues at home, safer sex precautions, stages of the HIV disease, and treatment modalities at these various stages. She will need information about the preventive drug therapies for her unborn child. Much national attention supported with federal funds has been spent to disseminate the prevention of HIV message.

Health care provider attitudes and fears may compromise care given to HIV affected women. It has been reported that professionals with negative attitudes about the HIV affected person reflect that anxiety and concern about contracting the disease through exposure to that person. Rejection and avoidance have been documented.[40,41] Education about HIV has been shown to reduce the fear and resentment toward HIV affected persons and has been associated with less rejection and avoidance behavior.[31,40] Nationally supported educational programs have been established but programs to address specific issues regarding HIV and pregnant women are needed.

Delivery. Some reports suggest that cesarean birth may decrease the risk of HIV transmission.[28] It has been shown that the risk of HIV transmission increases when the fetal membranes have been ruptured more than 4 hours before delivery, which may attribute to lower transmission rates in cesarean births.[42] For that reason, fetal membranes should remain intact until delivery.[8] Studies are being conducted in Europe, but, at present in the United States, the recommendation is to offer intrapartum zidovudine therapy and plan for vaginal delivery.[28] Efforts to reduce instrumentation such as avoiding use of episiotomy, fetal scalp electrodes and scalp pH are necessary to decrease the newborn's exposure to maternal vaginal secretions and blood.

Breastfeeding. Even though there have been only a few cases of transmission of HIV to an infant through breastfeeding, the Public Health Service recommends women who are HIV positive avoid breastfeeding.[25,43] In addition, the Committee on Pediatric AIDS recommends women with known risks for HIV be counseled specifically regarding the appropriateness of breastfeeding.[43]

Postpartum Contraception. In some groups, rates of pregnancy in HIV affected women are high. Reasons women continue to be at risk for pregnancy are complex and multifactorial. Reasons include denial of illness and its meaning, positive secondary gains related to the pregnancy, perception of the low risk of transmission to the child, ethical and cultural beliefs about contraception and conception, lack of access to health care including family planning services, or the inability to negotiate with partner for safer sex practices including pregnancy prevention practices.[24,25] For the woman who is also abusing drugs, pregnancy may be a low priority issue for her. Intrauterine devices (IUD) are usually not advised in these women because of the risk of pelvic infection. All other methods are viable options with emphasis that latex condoms should be used in addition to reduce transmission to the partner. Surgical sterilization may be desired and should be discussed. Contraceptive services including sterilization should be available and affordable.[24,25] Important to any discussion of contraception regarding HIV affected women is sensitivity to the woman's choice. The provider's responsibility is to ensure the client makes an informed decision based upon current knowledge. Even though effective contraception seems to be logical for the provider, directive counseling on contraception, especially sterilization, is inappropriate.[44]

Legal Issues. Because of the previous documented discrimination that has occurred in HIV positive persons, maintaining confidentiality is critical to the woman and her family. Legal issues regarding a positive HIV include insurance coverage, job security, documentation policies, state testing and reporting protocols, and guardianship of surviving children. The provider must maintain current knowledge of local laws and policies that affect the health care of the HIV affected woman and her newborn. Referral to community legal services is appropriate.

SEXUALLY TRANSMITTED DISEASES AFFECTING PREGNANCY

Many sexually transmitted infections, including HIV, are known to have fatal or severely debilitating effects on the fetus. Table 18–1 summarizes

TABLE 18–1. SEXUALLY TRANSMITTED DISEASES AFFECTING PREGNANCY

Organism	Incidence in Pregnancy	Affect on Pregnancy	Medications	Other Concerns
Herpes simplex virus	About 10% of all pregnant women have incidence of primary or recurrent herpes in pregnancy. Perinatal transmission occurs 1 in 2,000 to 1 in 10,000 live births. There is a 60% infant mortality rate associated with infants affected by genital herpes and about 50% of the surviving infants suffer serious neurological damage.	The same painful vesicular lesions appear as in the nonpregnant client. Not all infants born through an infected birth canal become infected, in fact, most infected infants are not born to women with a history of herpes genitalis. Perinatal transmission is more likely if the initial infection is near the time of delivery. Infants manifest HSV in localized form by lesions on the skin, eyes or oral cavity. In more severe, systemic forms shown by lethargy, poor feeding, fever, irritability, convulsions, jaundice, apnea, shock and possible death.	Oral and topical Acyclovir have been used. Usual regimen is 200 mg orally 5 times day for 7–10 days until lesions resolve. Hospitalization for intravenous administration of Acyclovir has been used to decrease chances of infant becoming infected or treat life-threatening maternal infections including encephalitis, pneumonitis, or hepatitis. Prophylactic administration of Acyclovir intrapartially for women with a history of HSV is NOT recommended. The safety of Acyclovir is not established.	Instructions for the client include symptomatic relief measures as nonpregnant women. Cool perineal compressors, sitz baths, loose fitting clothes help to alleviate pain. Cesarean delivery is not necessary for every client with a history of herpes; only recommended when active lesions are present. Infants born through an HSV infected birth canal should be monitored carefully for neonatal complications.
Syphilis (Treponema pallidum)	40–50% of infants of infected mothers contract congenital syphilis	Syphilis unaltered by course of pregnancy. Chancre often unnoticed and/or internal and not diagnosed during pregnancy. Treponemas cross placenta at all stages of pregnancy but fetal involvement rare prior to 18 weeks of gestation. Maternal infection increases risk of endarteritis, stromal hyperplasia, and immature villi. Increased risk of premature labor and birth. Congenital syphilis signs and symptoms; hepatosplenomegaly, osteochondritis, jaundice, rhinitis, anemia, lymphadenopathy, nervous system involvement.	Benzathine penicillin G 2.4 million units IM. No known alternative to penicillin treatment in pregnancy. Treat pregnant women with penicillin after desensitization. Some experts recommend a second dose 1 week after initial treatment when woman in third trimester. Erythromycin should not be used because it cannot be relied upon to cure an infected fetus. Erythromycin estolate should NOT be given in pregnancy because of possible hepatotoxicity.	All pregnant woman should be screened in early pregnancy. Serologic test should be reported in third trimester in populations with high incidence or women at high-risk. Infant diagnosed with congenital syphilis should be placed in isolation until treatment administered All women infected with syphilis should be tested for HIV. Any woman who delivers a stillborn infant after 20 weeks gestation should be tested for syphilis. No infant should leave the hospital without documentation of results of maternal syphilis test

Disease	Epidemiology	Clinical	Treatment	Comments
Gonorrhea (Neissaeria gonorrhea)	Estimated 1 million cases a year in the U.S.	85% of infected women have no symptoms Ophthalium neonatorum: results from delivery through infected birth canal.	Ceftriaxone, 125 mg IM in a single dose or cefixime, 400 mg po in a single dose followed by presumptive treatment for chlamydia. Erythromycin base or stearate 500 mg po qid x 7 days or Erythromycin ethyisuccinate 800 mg po qid x 7 days Pregnant women who cannot tolerate a cephalosporin should receive Spectinomycin 2 gm IM (single-dose)	Gonorrhea screening should be done at initial prenatal visit and repeated in the third trimester. Test of cure not recommended when using drug of choice. Test for syphilis with positive gonorrhea. All states have mandated prophylaxis in the first hour of life. Newborn prophylaxis: Tetracycline or erythromycin ointments, silver nitrade ophthalmic drops and Penicillin GM have all been used as prophylaxis. Partners must be treated. Avoid coitus until both partners are cured.
C Trachomatic (Chlamydial cervicitis)	Most common STD. Occurs in 5 percent of pregnant women with a range of 3–37 percent.	Frequently the woman is asymptomatic. It is a common cause of mucopurulent cervicitis. Chlamydial infection during pregnancy is associated with prematurity and stillbirth. Urinary tract infection caused by Chlamydia untreated may progress to pyelonephritis. Infants born vaginally to infected women have a 10–20 percent chance of acquiring conjunctivitis. The newborn may also develop a pneumonia type of infection with congestion, wheezing and cough up to 12 weeks of age. It may also cause a middle ear infection in the infant.	Tetracycline is drug of choice but contraindicated in pregnancy. Erythromycin 500 mg qid for 7 days. (See Gonorrhea above.)	Treatment is essential for the sexual partner. Encouragement of abstinence during treatment is important to prevent reinfection. Treatment prior to delivery will eradicate maternal cervical chlamydial infection and prevent vertical transmission to the newborn. Many states mandate the use of erythromycin topical eye ointment within the first one hour of birth to prevent both gonorrhea and chlamydial infection.
Trichomonas	Occurs in 20–30% of all pregnant women	No untoward effects on pregnancy documented. Recent reports suggest association between any prenatal vaginal infections and preterm delivery.	Metronidazole 2 g initial treatment. Metromidazole 500 mg BID x 7 days. Metromidazole not recommended in first trimester because safety of drug not established	Partners need treatment. Instruct client to avoid sexual intercourse until she and her partner have completed therapy.

MMWR: (1993). Sexually Transmitted Diseases Treatment and Guidelines: Supplement Vol 42, RR–14. U.S. Department Health and Human Services. Center for Disease Control. Atlanta, Georgia.

the infections most commonly faced by providers in prenatal care. For early treatment and prevention of vertical transmission, screening for many sexually transmitted diseases is done at the initial prenatal visit. Refer to Chapter 11 for a more detailed discussion of these diseases and their impact on women's health (see Table 18–1).

PYELONEPHRITIS

Acute pyelonephritis in pregnancy is a common renal disorder defined as the presence of actively multiplying bacteria in the upper urinary tract. It usually, although not always, follows a previous asymptomatic bacteriuria (ASB). Escherichia coli (E.coli) is the most common organism for ASB.

Epidemiology

In normal pregnancy, the ureters become dilated and compressed secondary to the influence of progesterone and compression of the gravid uterus. In addition, the renal plasma flow increases about 35 percent during pregnancy. The glomerular filtration rate (GFR) rises 50 percent after the first trimester and remains elevated through delivery. This increased ratio of the glomerular filtration ratio leads to an increase in electrolytes, glucose, and other filtered substances reaching the renal tubules. Reabsorption of sodium usually is maintained, but glucose reabsorption does not increase proportionately. Glucosuria during pregnancy is not unusual and contributes to an environment conducive to bacterial growth. Increase in the GFR accelerates the excretion of creatinine, urea, and uric acid, which manifest in a fall in the blood urea nitrogen (BUN) and serum creatinine values. Secondary to pressure from the gravid uterus, the bladder loses muscle tone, becomes more easily distended, and predisposes to lower urinary tract infection. All of these factors contribute to the incidence of urinary tract infections in pregnancy.

Acute pyelonephritis occurs in up to 2 percent of all pregnancies and is the most common nonobstetrical reason for antepartum admissions.[8] Ascension of bacteria to the kidney will lead to pyelonephritis. Effects on the mother include bacterial endotoxemia leading to endo-toxin shock and acute renal dysfunction leading to acute renal failure. Pyelonephritis in pregnancy has been associated with small-for-gestational-age babies and premature delivery.[8] Pyelonephritis occurs more frequently in women affected by sickle cell anemia and diabetes.[8]

Subjective Data

Maternal symptoms include fever, shaking chills, malaise, flank pain, nausea and vomiting, headache, increased urinary frequency, and dysuria. Symptoms of mild cough to severe respiratory distress syndrome are present when severe cases lead to pulmonary dysfunction.

Objective Data

Traditionally, all pregnant women are screened by urine culture on the initial prenatal visit and monitored throughout pregnancy with a dipstick method for presence of nitrites.[45,46] Recently, efforts are being made to develop less costly alternatives methods using rapid enzymatic screens.[46]

For the symptomatic woman, a urine culture is necessary. Bacteriuria, with pyuria and white blood cell casts will be present in urine examination. A count of 1–2 bacteria per high power field in spun urine or more than 20 bacteria in the sediment of a centrifuged specimen of urine collected by bladder catheterization is diagnostic. Hematuria may be present. Urine culture is necessary for diagnosis and determination of causative agent. Determining the causative agent is important in monitoring recurring episodes. Also, if the causative organism is Group Beta Streptococcus, intrapartum chemoprophylaxis is recommended to reduce neonatal Group Beta Streptococcal Disease.

Differential Medical Diagnoses

Acute cystitis, urinary calculi, glomerulonephritis.

Plan

Prevention. The incidence of pyelonephritis can be significantly reduced by screening and treating asymptomatic bacteriuria during prenatal visits. Clean catch urine cultures are recommended at the initial prenatal visit for all pregnant women. If on the client's initial prenatal visit, urine culture reveals > 100,000 organisms per millimeter, the client should be treated regardless of the presence of symptoms. For those women treated for bacteriuria during pregnancy, prophylaxis antibiotic maintenance may be ordered by some providers throughout the remainder of the pregnancy. Close monitoring and urine screening for all pregnant women at each routine prenatal visit are recommended.

Medication. For the initial episode of pyelonephritis, a first-generation cephalosporin is the drug of choice 1–2g every 6 hours. Ampicillin plus gentamicin is used for recurrences. Antibiotic suppression is continued throughout the remainder of the pregnancy after an episode of pyelonephritis. Nitrofurantoin 100 mg once or twice daily is a common suppression regimen.[8] Sulfa drugs need to be avoided in late pregnancy because of the increase risk of neonatal hyperbilirubinemia. Antipyretic agents are used as necessary for fever.

Hospitalization. Historically, all pregnant women with a diagnosis of pyelonephritis were admitted to the hospital for antibiotics and hydration. Intravenous antibiotic therapy continues for 24–48 hours after the woman becomes afebrile, and costovertebral angle tenderness subsides.[8] The complications, even though uncommon, are severe and can be life threatening. Recently, out patient protocols have been developed in an attempt to provide safe and effective outpatient care of these women.[47,48] The outpatient model includes intravenous (IV) hydration, 2g of IV ceftriaxone, observation for 2 hours and discharge. The clients return daily for intramuscular ceftriaxone until afebrile and then are placed on oral antibiotics.[47,48] Most providers are continuing to manage pregnant women with initial hospitalization. The efficacy of outpatient management needs continued evaluation.

Postpartum. About 2–4 percent of women develop a lower urinary tract infection postdelivery secondary to factors such as birth trauma, expected bladder hypotonia, residual urine, catheterization, anesthesia and vaginal examinations. Pyelonephritis can be a likely sequelae to these infections if not treated adequately. Antibiotic therapy for these infections continues for up to 10 days. Education of the new mother should include the importance of completing all medica-

tion to decrease incidence of recurrence. Since E. coli is the causative organism in most cases, sulfonamides, nitrofurantoin, ampicillin, or ephalosporins are used. Breastfeeding while taking sulfonamides is controversial, but the risk is low in healthy full-term infants.[49]

Women who experienced recurrent urinary tract infections or pyelonephritis during pregnancy need radiographic evaluation of the upper urinary tract 3 months postpartum to assess for structural abnormality.[8] Urine for culture and sensitivity should be obtained at the routine postpartum visit.

INTRA-AMNIOTIC INFECTION

Intra-amniotic infection (IAI) is any infection within the intrauterine structures. Although in the past, the terms *chorioamnionitis* and *amnionitis* were used interchangeably, each is a specific diagnosis dependent on the structures affected. The conditions are frequently not detected until after delivery.

The organisms most often isolated from the amniotic fluid of infected women are Group B streptococci, *Bacteroides* species, *Bacteroides bivius*, *Escherichia coli*, *Clostridium*, peptostreptococci, and *Fusobacterium*. *Mycoplasma hominis* and *Listeria monocytogenes* have also been isolated, but not necessarily from infected women. How these organisms may affect preterm labor and neonatal sepsis is not clear. Group B streptococci are currently the most common cause of sepsis and meningitis in neonates and young infants. Group A streptococci are not usually associated with neonatal sepsis.

Perinatal Group B Streptococcal Disease

Group B Streptococcus (GBS) is a leading cause of neonatal infection in the United States and a significant cause of maternal illness. GBS is a gram positive bacterium that colonizes in the vagina and when present during pregnancy attributes to maternal and/or neonatal infection.

Epidemiology

In most populations studied, from 10–30 percent of pregnant women were colonized with GBS in the vaginal or rectal areas.[50] Colonization rates can differ among ethnic groups, geographic areas, and by age; however, rates are similar between pregnant and nonpregnant women. The incidence of GBS is higher in African American women and women under 20 years of age.[50,51] The amniotic cavity protects the fetus from ascending pathogens; however, with rupture of the membranes and onset of labor, ascending infection from the lower genital tract can occur. Infants born to women who have positive GBS cultures prenatally have 29 times the risk of early onset disease than do infants born to women whose prenatal cultures were negative.[50]

The incidence of neonatal sepsis is only 1–2 percent; however, infection can be fatal or lead to permanent neurodevelopmental defects.[50,52] The origin of group B streptococci in the genital tract is unclear, but the gastrointestinal tract seems the likely source. Reinfection is common through either autoinfection or sexual intercourse.

Subjective Data

Women with colonies of group B streptococci in the genital tract are asymptomatic. With intra-amniotic infection, however, the client may report vague symptoms of fever and malaise, usually in the third trimester after membranes have ruptured.

Objective Data

Early diagnosis is difficult because symptoms do not occur until infection has progressed substantially and caused amniotis.

The earliest sign of infection is most likely fever. Uterine tenderness, foul smelling amniotic fluid, maternal leukocytosis and tachycardia are detected late in the infectious process.

Cultures can be done to isolate group B streptococci, but a minimum of 24 hours is needed for test results. Gram stains can provide immediate results but are not specific or reliable for group B streptococci.[50,52] Routine antenatal screening has not been effective in detecting women at risk for delivering an infected neonate. Maternal colonization is frequently transient and intermittent; therefore, a positive antenatal culture does not indicate that a culture will be positive at the time of labor.

Differential Medical Diagnoses

Pyelonephritis, bacterial vaginosis, gonorrhea.

Plan

Prevention. Research has focused on either inducing protective immunity in the neonate or eradicating colonization from the mother and/or neonate (chemoprophylaxis). Several vaccines to induce antibodies against GBS are being developed but may have limited effectiveness due to reduced transplacental transport of protective antibody before 32–34 weeks' gestation. Controversy has surrounded the screening, timing, and treatment of GBS to reduce neonatal GBS infection.

Psychosocial Interventions. All pregnant women need education especially in the third trimester on the potential for GBS infection and need to be aware of risk factors and screening recommendations. It is unclear whether a woman who has had a child with neonatal sepsis is truly at risk during a subsequent pregnancy, but emotionally she is clearly at risk. Any history of neonatal sepsis can cause apprehension. The provider must recognize this and be sensitive to the client's concerns and questions.

Screening. In May 1996, Centers for Disease Control and Prevention (CDC) in collaboration with the American College of Obstetricians and Gynecologists (ACOG) and the American Academy of Pediatrics (AAP) released recommendations on the prevention of perinatal Group B Streptococcal Disease. Until further data is available, both a screening based or a risk factor based approach is appropriate. The screening based approach recommends all pregnant women be screened at 35–37 weeks' gestation for anogenital GBS colonization. Obtain one or two swabs from the vaginal introitus and anorectum without using a speculum. Cervical cultures are not acceptable.[50] Appropriate nonnutritive moist swab transport systems (e.g., Amies') are commercially available.[50] Those women positive for GBS should be offered intrapartum penicillin. The other approach is to provide intrapartum chemoprophylaxis for women with risk factors without screening.

Medication. Antibiotic treatment of women who are colonized during prenatal screening is not effective in eliminating the organism or preventing neonatal disease. Antibiotic treatment prenatally is not recommended. Intravenous penicillin G is the drug of choice for intrapartum chemoprophylaxis in women with a documented positive culture for GBS. Ampicillin is an acceptable alternative as well as other agents such as Clindamycin when used if clinical amnionitis is present. Women who are treated based upon risk factors include those who 1) had a previous infant with invasive GBS disease, 2) had GBS bacteriuria during current pregnancy, 3) are less than 37 weeks' gestation, 4) have ruptured membranes 18 hours or more, or 5) have temperature equal to or greater than 38° C (100.4° F).[50] The presence of multiple gestation alone is not a criteria for intrapartum chemoprophylaxis but because of its frequent association with preterm birth may necessitate consideration for treatment.[51] If the prenatal screening results are unknown at the onset of labor, chemoprophylaxis should be given based upon intrapartum risk factors.[50,51]

Delivery. Critical to the implementation of the CDC guidelines is the notification of staff caring for the woman during the intrapartum period. A positive prenatal screening for Group B Streptococcus needs to be clearly documented on the chart. The woman needs to be counseled to the importance of knowing her GBS status and, if positive, needs to know to communicate that to staff in the intrapartum unit. Neonatal colonization usually occurs at the time of delivery, but cesarean birth does not reduce the vertical transmission or infection rates. Presence or suspicion of GBS is not an indicator for surgical delivery.[51]

Neonatal Follow-Up. Routine use of prophylactic antibiotic agents for infants born to mothers who received intrapartum prophylaxis is not recommended. For infants symptomatic of sepsis, several management approaches are being used.

Implications for Providers. Even with release of guidelines by national groups, controversy continues among professionals. Providers need to maintain current on the recommendations and accepted approaches within their practice sites. Clear documentation of any screening results and

RISKS ASSOCIATED WITH DELIVERING AN INFANT WITH PERINATAL GROUP B STREPTOCOCCAL DISEASE

Prenatal

< 20 years of age
African American ethnicity
Positive 35–37 week GBS culture
Previous delivery of GBS infected neonate (early onset)
Treatment of GBS bacteriuria in current pregnancy

Intrapartal

Membrane rupture > or = 18 hours
Fever > or = 38° C (100.4° F)
< 37 weeks' gestation

Adapted from Reference 50.

management plans are critical. Systems for communicating prenatal culture results to intrapartum physician and nursing staff must be established. Brochures have been developed by numerous public and private organizations to assist the provider counsel and educate women and their families.

Implications for Parents. Women and their families need to be aware of the strategies for the early detection, treatment and prevention of Group B Streptococcus transmission to the neonate. One volunteer organization, Group B Strep Association, has been formed to educate expectant parents about the implications of Group B Streptococcus on neonatal outcome.

BLEEDING

Bleeding any time during pregnancy is serious and potentially life threatening. It occurs in 10 to 20 percent of all pregnancies.[53] The amount of bleeding and the time it occurs determine the urgency and management plan.

SPONTANEOUS ABORTION

Spontaneous abortion is the termination of pregnancy before the point of fetal viability. Gestation should not be more than 20 weeks and conceptus should not weigh more than 500 g or be longer than 16.5 cm, crown to rump. *Miscarriage* is the lay term for spontaneous abortion.

Types of abortion are categorized according to signs and symptoms.

- A *threatened abortion* is possible pregnancy loss; however, pregnancy may continue without further problems. Slight bleeding usually occurs, and some uterine contractions are felt as abdominal cramping. Uterine size is compatible with dates, the cervical os is closed, and no products of conception are passed. Prognosis is unpredictable.
- An *inevitable abortion* is a pregnancy that cannot be salvaged. Moderate bleeding and moderate to severe uterine cramping occur, and the cervical os is dilated. Uterine size is compatible with dates. The products of conception are not passed. Prognosis is poor.
- In an *incomplete abortion,* some products of conception are passed. Moderate to severe uterine cramping and heavy bleeding occur. Uterine size is compatible with dates; the cervical os is dilated. Prognosis is poor.
- In a *complete abortion,* all products of conception are expelled. Bleeding may be minimal and uterine contractions have subsided. The uterus is normal prepregnancy size; the cervical os may be opened or closed.
- A *missed abortion* occurs when the embryo is not viable but is retained in utero for at least 6 weeks. Uterine contractions are absent. Bleeding may initially be absent, but spotting begins and later becomes heavier.
- *Habitual abortion* is the experience of three or more consecutive spontaneous abortions.

Epidemiology

A precise etiology of spontaneous abortion does not exist, but varied maternal and fetal factors are attributed to its incidence. Maternal age greatly increases the risk, i.e., a 40-year-old woman carries twice the risk of a 20-year-old.[8] Genetic abnormalities are the most common. Endocrinologic disorders, specifically elevated levels of luteinizing hormone, have also been associated with pregnancy loss.[54] Prior pregnancy loss is associated with increased risk for pregnancy loss, but consideration of the genetic and endocrinological factors makes this relationship unclear. Frequently, the embryonic sac is empty or a de-generated fetus is found; both conditions are referred to as *blighted ovum.* Another cause of spontaneous abortion is maternal infections. Both viral and bacterial infections can cause local infection of the conceptus, endometritis, or more generalized pelvic disease, all of which can lead to fetal death and abortion.

In addition, anatomic abnormalities of the reproductive tract are associated with abortion, usually in the second trimester. Some chronic diseases, such as diabetes, nutritional deficiencies, renal diseases, and lupus erythematosus, also affect a woman's ability to maintain her pregnancy. Moreover, lifestyle practices, such as smoking, substance abuse, and exposure to environmental hazards, are related to early pregnancy loss. Incidence reports reveal that about 20 percent of all pregnant women experience some cramping and bleeding in early pregnancy. About one half of those women continue through an uneventful pregnancy; the other half suffer pregnancy loss.

Subjective Data

Varying degrees of vaginal bleeding, low back pain, abdominal cramping, and passage of products of conception are reported. Usually the severity of cramping progresses, and a change is seen in the type of blood lost.

Many women in early pregnancy report "spotting," a brown-red vaginal discharge that stains underwear or toilet tissue. Vaginal bleeding that becomes bright red is usually significant. The amount of bleeding is ascertained by the saturation of sanitary napkins and the frequency with which the napkins must be changed. Saturation of one sanitary napkin every hour is significant.

Objective Data

Data are established using categorizations based on the client's signs and symptoms and diagnostic test results.

Uterine size is less than the expected gestational size.

Fetal heart tones are reassuring and dictate a conservative management plan; their absence beyond the tenth week of gestation may indicate a missed abortion.

Cervix may be dilated, soft or products of conception noted at the os; bleeding may be seen.

Real-time sonography will determine the presence of an embryonic sac and detect fetal cardiac motion, which is reassuring and dictates a "wait and see" management approach. If the β-hCG is greater than 1500 mIU/ml and if the pregnancy is intrauterine, the gestational sac should be visualized by transvaginal ultrasound.[8] Transabdominal ultrasound of the gestational sac may not be visualized until the B-hCG reaches 6000 mIU/ml. Absence of the embryonic sac in the uterus may indicate ectopic pregnancy and must be investigated further.

Serial β-subunit human chorionic gonadotropin (β-hCG) measurements scheduled at least 2 days apart correlate with appropriate rise in β-hCG. Blood is collected for each measurement and sent to the laboratory. β-hCG levels should double every 2 days in early pregnancy, peak at about 10 weeks, then gradually decrease during the remainder of pregnancy. Doubling of levels every 2 days indicates viability and favorable prognosis. Failure of the β-hCG level to double is suspicious of ectopic pregnancy or abortion. Although the client requires no specific instructions for this test, waiting the 2 days between specimens may be distressing to her.

Some providers use *progesterone* in addition to β-hCG levels to determine presence of a viable pregnancy.[8,55] Progesterone levels equal to or greater than 25ng/ml are suggestive of a viable intrauterine pregnancy.

Differential Medical Diagnoses

Malignancy, cervicitis, ectopic pregnancy, gestational trophoblastic disease (hydatidiform mole).

Plan

Psychosocial Interventions. Provide information for the client and her partner throughout all phases of threatened or eventual abortion. Reasons for blood tests and sonograms should be openly discussed. Explain to the client that precautions of bedrest and/or pelvic rest will continue until an asymptomatic period of at least 48 hours has elapsed.

The health care provider should be understanding of the many different responses to pregnancy loss. A response may be influenced by the value of the pregnancy to the client or couple, the desire for pregnancy, the length of gestation, history of other pregnancy losses, the couple's relationship, their social network and support, and religious beliefs (refer to Chapter 10, on Infertility).

Medication. In some cases, progesterone supplementation via vaginal suppositories has been used successfully for women with known luteal phase defect associated with spontaneous abortion defect.

Specific Interventions. Threatened abortion requires conservative "wait and see" management, unless symptoms threaten the life of the mother. Bedrest is not shown to affect outcome in threatened abortion but is commonly prescribed. The client at home on bedrest and/or pelvic rest should be instructed to maintain adequate hydration and report ominous signs or symptoms. The client should be evaluated weekly in the health office to determine complete blood count, serial β-hCG levels, any signs of infection, or a missed abortion.

- Bedrest requires that the woman be away from her job, have limited or no child care responsibilities at home, and rest in a horizontal position, except when bathing or using the toilet.
- Pelvic rest means no sexual intercourse; no douching or inserting anything into the vagina.
- Instructions for hydration are to drink a minimum of 32 ounces of noncaffeinated fluid every 24 hours.
- Clients are taught the signs and symptoms of infection and how uterine contractions and vaginal bleeding may progress.

Inevitable, incomplete, or missed abortion should be treated more aggressively as soon as a definitive diagnosis is made. To prevent infection and uterine hemorrhage, the uterus should be emptied of all products of conception. Whether instrumental evacuation is necessary in cases of complete abortion is controversial. If some products of conception remain in the uterus as evidenced by cramping and bleeding, enlarged and/or soft uterus, or fever, suction curettage is recommended. Removal of necrotic decidua decreases the incidence of postabortion bleeding and shortens the recovery period.

Missed abortion usually progresses to inevitable abortion, but a "wait and see" approach can be emotionally intolerable for some women. In such cases, suction curettage is recommended during the first trimester. In the second trimester, dilatation and evacuation may be performed or labor may be induced with an intravaginal prostaglandin E_2 (PGE$_2$) suppository. Some primary care providers use a laminaria to dilate the cervix overnight prior to the procedure, thereby facilitating a less stressful dilatation procedure. For some women, delaying the definitive diagnosis and treatment plan is necessary to help them accept the situation emotionally. The Rh factor should be assessed and immunoglobulin administered to Rh-negative, unsensitized women.

Follow-Up

Instruct the client about the danger signs of infection or incomplete evacuation of the uterus: fever, foul smelling lochia, excessive bleeding, back or abdominal pain.

Inform the client that she will need to use contraception for at least 4 to 6 months to allow for complete maternal healing and regeneration of endometrial lining. Advise her to have a gynecological exam within 2 to 3 weeks of the abortion.

If a woman has had repeated pregnancy losses, complete evaluation is recommended to determine possible causes; appropriate treatment may be instituted prior to future pregnancies (refer to Chapter 10, Infertility).

ECTOPIC PREGNANCY

Ectopic pregnancy is the implantation of a fertilized ovum outside the uterine cavity.[8,45] Most ectopic pregnancies occur in a fallopian tube, but may also occur in the cervix, on an ovary, or in the abdominal cavity. Following implantation, the embryo grows, but no decidua is present.[56] The structure of the implantation can sustain some growth; however, rupture is usually inevitable. Early signs of pregnancy, including uterine changes and amenorrhea, are present, secondary to hormonal influence. Ectopic pregnancy is a potentially life threatening condition and involves pregnancy loss.

Epidemiology

The etiology of extrauterine implantation originates with an interference in normal ovum transport. Women at risk are those who have used an intrauterine device or who have a history of infertility, pelvic inflammatory disease, tubal surgery (e.g., ligation or reconstruction), or ectopic pregnancy, the most common being history of tubal infection.[8,57]

Some risk, although low, is associated with abdominal or pelvic surgery, postacute appendicitis, intrauterine exposure to diethylstilbestrol (DES), or use of drugs that slow ovum transport (e.g., minipill).[56,57,58,59] Cesarean birth is not an associated risk factor.[60]

Incidence worldwide has increased but varies significantly among populations. In the United States, ectopic pregnancy occurs in approximately 1 in 50 pregnancies and is a leading cause of maternal mortality.[59,61] It is more prevalent in poor, less advantaged countries. Although maternal mortality has decreased in the United States, the actual number of ectopic pregnancies has increased. The increased incidence appears to be related to factors associated with infertility, such as chronic salpingitis, earlier detection by ultrasound, and sensitive β-hCG assays.[8,59]

Subjective Data

Classical and atypical presentations are used in diagnosis. The classical clinical presentation includes many of the early signs of pregnancy: 1 to 2 months of amenorrhea, morning sickness, breast tenderness. The most common presenting symptoms are abdominal pain and irregular vaginal bleeding.[8] Abdominal pain can be unilateral, and mild vaginal bleeding is possible. The client is motivated to seek emergency care when her pain becomes sharper and she experiences more generalized discomfort. She may report gastrointestinal disturbances and feelings of malaise and syncope. She may faint. Classically, pain is referred to the shoulder as the hemorrhage becomes extensive and irritates the diaphragm.

Atypical clinical presentations are not so clearly evident. Many clients report vague or subacute symptoms. They may report menstrual irregularity. Amenorrhea may not be obvious, as intermittent spotting or mild vaginal bleeding may mimic normal menses. Ectopic pregnancy should be considered in diagnosis when any woman of childbearing age reports mild or severe abdominal symptoms. Symptoms do not necessarily correlate with the severity of the condition; mild signs and symptoms may occur with massive hemorrhage.

Objective Data

Any sexually active woman with a missed menses is at risk for ectopic pregnancy. Use of current diagnostic methods has provided the early detection of ectopic pregnancy before symptoms occur or become severe. When symptoms do occur, they mimic other problems with similar complaints.

Physical examination may reveal symptoms of shock especially after hemorrhage. The woman in early gestation may appear in little discomfort. General signs of shock include cool, clammy skin and poor skin color and turgor. Late signs are hypotension and tachycardia. Abdominal examination may reveal some unilateral adnexal tenderness. A pelvic exam reveals a normal appearing cervix, but marked tenderness is noted. The vaginal vault may be bloody, usually brick red to brown in color. There may be vaginal tenderness. A tender adnexal mass may be palpated, and the uterus may be slightly enlarged and soft.

Levels of serial β-hCG are used to diagnose ectopic pregnancy. A small amount of functioning trophoblastic tissue, as is found in ectopic pregnancy, will produce a small amount of β-hCG without the amount of expected doubling increases associated with normal pregnancy. In a normal intrauterine pregnancy, hormone levels should double every 2–4 days with a predictable slope of increase. Low β-hCG levels are therefore suggestive of an ectopic pregnancy and should be followed by a repeated quantitative radioimmunoassay.

A sonogram is used to determine if the pregnancy is intrauterine, to assess the size of the uterus, and to detect presence of fetal viability.[56,59] If the β-hCG is greater than 1300 to 1400 mIU/ml at 35 days of gestation, and the pregnancy is intrauterine, a gestational sac should be visualized by transvaginal ultrasound.[8] Absence of an intrauterine gestational sac is diagnostic of ectopic pregnancy.

Culdocentesis may be done to detect intraperitoneal blood, which will be present following tubal pregnancy rupture. This procedure is carried out during a pelvic exam. The health care provider inserts a needle through the vaginal wall into the cul-de-sac and withdraws whatever fluid is present. Nonclotted blood indicates hemorrhage. The source of bleeding is then identified by means of laparoscopy or laparotomy, and measures are taken to control bleeding.

Differential Medical Diagnoses

Pelvic inflammatory disease, ovarian cyst, ovarian tumor, intrauterine pregnancy, recent spontaneous abortion, early hydatidiform degeneration, acute appendicitis, and other bowel related disorders.

Plan

Psychosocial Interventions. Inform the client about procedures and support her as early diagnosis and appropriate medical referral are pursued. Because laparoscopy is frequently necessary for a definitive diagnosis, prepare the woman for safe and timely transfer to a hospital. Information about the procedure and management plan should be clearly stated for the client and her partner, a family member, or friend.

Medication. Methotrexate is used in the nonsurgical management of ectopic pregnancy. The therapy is new for this condition and has been administered successfully via muscularly, local infiltration, or orally. It clears remaining trophoblastic tissue and may avoid the need for laparotomy.[8,62,63] The client eligible for methotrexate therapy must be hemodynamically stable and the mass must be unruptured, measuring fewer than 4 cm determined by ultrasound.[8] The severe side effects of bone marrow suppression, hepatotoxicity, stomatitis, pulmonary fibrosis, alopecia, and photosensitivity from methotrexate are uncommon in short-term therapy for ectopic pregnancy, but need to be administered with appropriate caution. Single dose methotrexate is 50 mg/m^2 of body surface area intramuscularly. For longer-term dosing, methotrexate, 1mg/k of body weight intramuscularly every other day, Leucovorin, 0.1 mg/kg intramuscularly every other day, is used to mitigate severe side effects.[8,59] Treatment continues until the β-hCG drops equal to or greater than 15 percent in 48 hours or 4 doses of methotrexate has been given.[8] Serum β-hCG should be monitored weekly until undetected; blood count, platelet count, and liver enzyme levels should also be monitored weekly.[8,56] Colicky pain secondary to the stomatitis can mimic ectopic rupture and must be differentiated by assessment for hypotension, tachycardia or falling hematocrit indicating hemorrhage. Clients should avoid gas producing foods such as beans or cabbage, which may also mimic ectopic rupture. Clients should also avoid sun exposure while taking the methotrexate because of the photosensitivity of the drug.

Evacuation of Conceptus. Immediately after ectopic pregnancy is diagnosed, the conceptus is evacuated. The success of conservative surgery is influenced by the condition of the client and the affected organ (e.g., fallopian tube, ovary), location of the conceptus, and the client's desire for future fertility. Two problems associated with surgery are uncontrolled bleeding and residual trophoblastic tissue. Because of the bleeding, a salpingectomy is necessary for many tubal ectopic pregnancies. A laparotomy should only be indicated in the case of uncontrolled hemorrhage or hemodynamic instability. Historically, treatment focused on prevention of death, but with the ability to perform linear salpingostomy, emphasis is now on facilitating rapid recovery, preserving fertility, and reducing costs.[8]

Follow-Up

Postoperatively, all Rh-negative unsensitized clients should be given Rh immunoglobulin. Discuss the normal body changes the client will experience. Instruct her concerning contraception, danger signals (e.g., signs of postsurgical infection or hemorrhage), and any further follow-up testing. The emotional needs of clients will vary. Pregnancy may not have been realized prior to diagnosis, and learning about the pregnancy and pregnancy loss in such a short period can be overwhelming. Pregnancy should be acknowledged and its meaning discussed. Explain to a client that having one ectopic pregnancy increases her chances for future ectopic pregnancies, however the risk is less with the use of methotrexate. Re-

view the signs and symptoms of repeated ectopic pregnancy with her. Advise her to practice contraception for at least 2 months to allow for adequate healing and tissue repair. In 20 percent of cases treated with methotrexate, residual tissue remains and causes hemorrhage and other complications.[8] Weekly blood tests for β-hCG levels should be monitored until β-hCG becomes undetectable. The initial follow-up visit should include discussion of the need for follow-up blood testing, emotional responses to the ectopic pregnancy, risk factors, and need for contraception.

Prevention of ectopic pregnancies through screening and client education is essential. Preventing tubal damage from, for example, sexually transmitted disease, can decrease the incidence of the disorder. Encouraging the use of condoms can decrease the incidence of many infections responsible for tubal scarring. Early detection and prompt treatment of gonorrhea and chlamydia, when they do occur, can decrease morbidity.

Selection of an appropriate contraceptive method is important. Because IUD use may be associated with infections and tubal pregnancy, women need to be informed of the risk and effect of an IUD on future pregnancies.

GESTATIONAL TROPHOBLASTIC DISEASE

Gestational trophoblastic disease is a group of neoplastic disorders that originate in the human placenta.[45,64] Gestational tissue is present but pregnancy is nonviable.

- *Hydatidiform mole.* The most common type of gestational trophoblastic disease, hydatidiform mole is a benign neoplasm of the chorion in which chorionic villi degenerate and become transparent vesicles containing clear, viscid fluid. Recently, two types of molar gestations have been distinguished: partial and complete. No fetus or amnion is found in the complete mole, but in the partial mole, a fetus or evidence of an amniotic sac is present.
- *Invasive mole* (chorioadenoma destruens). Invasive mole is a complete molar gestation that has invaded the myometrium, metastasized to other tissues, or both. Karyotyping reveals abnormal genetic material resulting from an empty egg or diploid sperm.

- *Choriocarcinoma.* This rare chorionic malignancy may follow any type of pregnancy, even years later. Half of choriocarcinomas occur following hydatidiform molar pregnancy.

Epidemiology

Etiology may be influenced by nutritional factors, such as protein deficiency. Such deficiencies would explain some of the race and geographical differences associated with gestational trophoblastic disease.

The incidence of molar pregnancy varies markedly around the world. Incidence in the Far East and Southeast Asia is 5 to 15 times greater than that in Western industrialized nations. The true incidence of partial mole is unknown, because many are diagnosed as spontaneous abortions and tissue karyotyping is not done. Moles do recur in subsequent pregnancies. Age is also a factor; older women have a greater incidence of molar pregnancy.

Subjective Data

Presenting symptoms are similar to those of spontaneous abortion. The client usually reports signs of early pregnancy (amenorrhea, breast tenderness, morning sickness) and presents with vaginal bleeding around the 12th week of gestation. Bleeding may begin as spotting, usually brownish rather than bright red. Some women experience severe nausea and vomiting and are treated for hyperemesis gravidarum. Fluid retention and swelling, similar to what is associated with pregnancy induced hypertension (PIH) later in a pregnancy, may occur with molar pregnancy in the second trimester. Uterine cramping may or may not be present.[64]

Objective Data

Physical examination may reveal what is sometimes a first sign of molar pregnancy: expulsion of grapelike vesicles with or without a history of vaginal bleeding. Vital signs are usually stable; no medical emergency exists. The abdomen is soft and nontender; in the vagina, bloody or clear vesicles may be present. The uterus is usually enlarged beyond the point of expected gestation and has a "doughy" consistency. Ovaries may be enlarged and tender secondary to theca lutein cysts, which develop from ovarian hyperstimulation of high human chorionic gonadotropin levels. No fetal heart tones or fetal activity is detected.

The sonogram shows the absence of the gestational sac and characteristic multiple echogenic regions within the uterus.[65]

Human chorionic gonadotropin levels are extremely high in molar pregnancies and continue to rise 100 days after the last menstrual period. No single value is diagnostic; therefore, serial values must be evaluated and compared with the normal pregnancy curve for β-hCG.

Differential Medical Diagnoses

Normal pregnancy, threatened abortion: error in dates, uterine myomas, polyhydramnios, multiple gestation.

Plan

Prompt identification of gestational trophoblastic disease and appropriate referral are essential to management.

Psychosocial Interventions. Explain the diagnostic procedures and follow-up blood work to the client. Explore the meaning of the client's pregnancy with her and her partner, a family member, or friend. Support them in their grieving. Accounting for religious beliefs and cultural practices is crucial in counseling women concerning the necessity of contraception. Reassurance about future pregnancies is appropriate, because prognosis is good even for women with invasive molar pregnancies.

Medication. If β-hCG levels either rise or plateau after evacuation, *chemotherapy* is indicated for potential metastatic disease. For women who wish to protect their fertility, single agent therapy is used, usually methotrexate administered orally.[45]

Other Interventions. Evacuation of the uterus is necessary as soon as the diagnosis is made. *Dilatation and curettage* (suction curettage) is the safest, most effective method of emptying the uterus. Labor induction with prostaglandins or oxytocin is not recommended because these agents are inefficient in emptying the uterus of all trophoblastic tissue. Hospital admission is necessary for adequate anesthesia and nursing surveillance.

A *chest x-ray* is ordered to establish a baseline if there is any question later of invasive disease.

Serial monitoring of β-hCG levels is done weekly until normal for 3 weeks and then monthly for 6 months after the evacuation procedure. Levels of β-hCG are used to detect residual trophoblastic tissue. If any tissue remains, β-hCG levels will not regress. A rising β-hCG level could indicate the presence of a new gestation and must be investigated prior to any extensive diagnostic imagining or therapeutic intervention.[8]

No further intervention is necessary if β-hCG levels decrease to normal, that is, become nondetectable. Pregnancy may be allowed after β-hCG levels remain normal for a minimum of 1 year. *Reliable contraception* must be used during this time because a positive pregnancy test cannot differentiate normal early pregnancy from beginning invasive disease. Reliable and safe contraceptives such as oral contraceptives, medroxyprogesterone acetate (Depo-provera), or Norplant are desirable.

PLACENTA PREVIA

In placenta previa, the placenta becomes implanted in the lower segment of the uterus and obstructs the presenting part prior to or during labor. When the cervix begins to dilate, the placenta is pulled away from the endometrial wall and bleeding can occur. Any significant bleeding that leads to hemorrhage can endanger the mother and, if allowed to persist, can interfere with uteroplacental sufficiency.

The three types of previa (total, incomplete, and marginal) are classified by the amount of cervix involved.

- In *total or complete previa,* the entire internal os is covered with placenta.
- In *incomplete (or partial) previa,* the internal os is only partially covered by the placenta.
- In *marginal or low lying previa,* the edge of the placenta is at the cervical os but does not obstruct any part of it.

The amount of cervical dilation can affect the classification system. Other systems are based on the amount of placental encroachment over the os at the point of full dilation.

Epidemiology

The etiology of placenta previa is unknown, but certain women are at greater risk than others. Parity is the most common risk factor; old fundal implantation sites are scarred and not suitable for implantation. Other uterine surgical scars, such as those from cesarean birth or myomectomy, increase the chance of placental malimplantation. Advanced maternal age, maternal smoking, and a history of induced or spontaneous abortion have also been reported to be risk factors for placenta previa.[66,67] Recent data show black and other minority women have a higher prevalence for previa than do white women.[67]

Incidence seems to vary with gestation, although the condition is reported in 1 of every 200 pregnancies.[67] Better diagnostic techniques have revealed gestational differences. For example, in the second trimester, placenta previa is a prevalent finding on sonogram, but as pregnancy progresses the incidence falls. In the third trimester, the lower uterine segment stretches and develops, making the placenta seem to migrate away from the internal os, and the previa resolves.

Subjective Data

The characteristic symptom of placenta previa is painless bleeding during the third trimester of pregnancy. Bleeding may occur as early as 20 weeks of gestation and without any precipitating event. Previa should be suspected in any bleeding that occurs after 24 weeks of gestation.[8] Blood is usually bright red. A woman may experience symptoms of shock, such as syncope. The first bleed, however, is usually not a significant amount.

Objective Data

Vital signs are stable; fetal heart tones are normal, and fetal activity is present. The uterus is nontender with a normal resting tone. Bright red blood is evident on sanitary napkins.

Diagnosis is best made by sonogram. No pelvic exam is done to avoid dislodging any clot that may have formed at the cervix. Historically, a sterile vaginal exam was done in a surgical suite to determine the diagnosis; if catastrophic bleeding occurred during the procedure, an emergency cesarean was performed. Now, however, with noninvasive accurate sonograms, such examination is rarely necessary or recommended.[8]

Differential Medical Diagnoses

Abruptio placentae, genital lacerations, excessive show, cervical lesions and/or severe cervicitis, nonvaginal bleeding (urinary or rectal).

Plan

The role of the primary care provider lies primarily in the early detection of placenta previa. Referral for appropriate intervention is necessary.

Medication. Not indicated.

Management. The medical plan depends on the extent of hemorrhage and length of gestation. If gestation is less than 36 weeks, an attempt is made to stabilize the mother, administer transfusions as needed, and maintain the pregnancy. Strict hospital bed rest is employed, and the mother and fetus are closely monitored. If bleeding stops and the hematocrit is greater than 30 percent, then gradual ambulation may be allowed. Some women may be allowed to return home with limited activity until further problems arise or labor begins.

Provide the client with clear instructions about pelvic rest and what to do if signs of impending labor or bleeding begins.

During the "wait and see" period, amniocentesis may be done weekly after 36 weeks to document fetal maturity. In addition, serial sonograms are done to determine placement of the placenta and to note any "migration." Later in the pregnancy, placental problems can lead to uteroplacental insufficiency and intrauterine growth retardation.

Sonography. Serial sonograms are also used to monitor fetal growth. If bleeding continues or recurs, then operative delivery may be forced.

Delivery. The amount of bleeding, general fetal condition, fetal presentation and gestation will affect delivery decisions. Once fetal maturity is accomplished, delivery is planned. The extent to which the os is covered by the placenta determines if vaginal delivery is considered. Cesarean delivery is usually recommended.[8]

Postpartum Follow-Up. It is the same as for other postpartum women. The amount of blood loss is associated with perinatal outcome, even though the number of bleeding episodes does not increase perinatal mortality or morbidity. A mother usually recovers readily from anemia and fluid loss. During the first month of life, the infant is at increased risk for death, compared with infants of the same gestational age and birth weight. The increased risk is probably related to transient episodes of fetal hypoxia.

ABRUPTIO PLACENTAE

Abruptio placentae is the partial or complete detachment of a normally implanted placenta at any time prior to delivery. Detachment occurs more frequently during the third trimester, but may occur anytime after 20 weeks of gestation. The proposed mechanism is that maternal arterioles become thrombosed and lead to degeneration of decidua and, subsequently, to rupture of one vessel. The resultant bleeding forms a retroplacental clot, which increases pressure behind the placenta and adds to the separation process.

The classification of abruptio placentae is based on the signs and symptoms of abruption in combination with selected laboratory findings.

- *Grade 1.* Slight vaginal bleeding may be evident. Maternal symptoms are consistent with amount of blood lost. Uterine tetany and tenderness, if present, are minor. The fetal heart rate is within normal limits, maternal blood pressure is unaffected and maternal fibrinogen level is normal.[8]
- *Grade 2.* Mild to moderate bleeding occurs. Uterine tenderness and tetany are present. Fetal heart tones are usually absent or show signs of distress. Maternal blood pressure is normal, but the pulse rate may be elevated. The fibrinogen level is usually reduced to 150 to 250 mg percent.[8]
- *Grade 3.* Uterine tetany and tenderness are present. Bleeding may be concealed or be moderate to severe in amount. Maternal hypotension

is usually present and fetal death common. Fibrinogen levels are often reduced to less than 150 mg percent and other clotting abnormalities are present.[8]

Epidemiology

The etiology of abruptio placentae is unknown. Maternal smoking, poor maternal nutrition, chorioamnionitis, and use of cocaine are risk factors for premature separation. Until recently, maternal age and multiparity have also been associated with increase incidence of abruption, but recent reports fail to show that relationship.[8] Conditions with underlying vascular involvement, particularly hypertension, can predispose a woman to abruption. Severe trauma, such as an automobile accident or injury secondary to domestic violence, has also been associated with abruption. The incidence of battering of women has grown and the incidence of battering during pregnancy is higher than other times.[68,69]

The true incidence is unknown because abruption occurs in varying degrees. Incidence ranges from 1 in 206 to 1 in 86 deliveries.[8] The disparity reflects variation in the criteria used for diagnosis.

Subjective Data

Symptoms of abruptio placentae can vary significantly depending on the extent and location of separation. The client may report labor pains with some continual cramping. With more severe abruption, severe, sudden, knifelike pain may be described. The client may experience no bleeding, a small amount of dark old blood, or profuse bleeding. Depending on the amount of blood lost from the systemic circulation, she may experience symptoms of shock, such as syncope.

Objective Data

Physical Examination. May reveal vaginal bleeding (dark old blood or bright red blood), uterine tenderness (local or generalized), increased uterine tone, occasional boardlike quality with little or no relaxation between contractions, lack of fetal heart tones, or signs of fetal distress (such as tachycardia, loss of beat-to-beat variability, or late decelerations). No vaginal or rec-

tal exam is done until placenta previa is eliminated as a diagnosis.

Sonogram. Frequently used to locate a retroplacental clot. A clot may not be seen on the sonogram in an early abruption, but if symptoms are severe, time is critical and diagnosis must be made on presumptive signs.

Differential Medical Diagnoses

Placenta previa, hematoma of rectus muscle, ovarian cysts, appendicitis, degeneration of fibroids.

Plan

Immediate identification of possibility or suspicion of abruptio placentae dictates prompt referral for appropriate stabilization and treatment.

Psychosocial Interventions. Allay the anxiety of the woman and her family. They need to be informed about impending diagnostic tests, possible hospitalization and surgery.

Management. Maintain respiratory and cardiovascular support (intravenous fluid, oxygen), as needed, until the client is transported to the hospital. Because of the potential for hemorrhage, development of a coagulopathy disorder is a risk. Hemorrhage may occur into the postpartum period.

Delivery. Delivery is necessary if severe symptoms are present and condition is life threatening for the mother or fetus. Whether the fetus is to be delivered by cesarean or vaginal birth will depend on the assessment of the mother and the fetus. If the mother's condition is stable, but the fetus is not viable, cesarean birth is not indicated. Cesarean delivery is indicated when there are signs of fetal distress, maternal hemorrhage, maternal coagulopathy, or poor progress of labor. Fetal well-being is assessed by electronic fetal monitoring. If both mother and fetus are stable, assessment for fetal maturity is done to assist in decisions of the timing of delivery.

Follow-Up

After delivery, care for women with abruptio placentae is the same as that for other postpartum women. It may be necessary to deal with pregnancy loss or in some cases, when the infant survives, maternal grieving may occur over loss of a "normal" pregnancy. Infants may need care in a newborn intensive care unit, which adds to family stress.

ANEMIAS

Anemia is the reduction of hemoglobin to below normal quantity.[70] In a normal pregnancy, concentrations of erythrocytes and hemoglobin fall because of a disproportional increase in the ratio of plasma volume to erythrocyte volume (physiological anemia of pregnancy). During pregnancy, plasma volume increases as much as 45 to 50 percent, but erythrocyte volume increases only 25 percent. Many women have borderline hemoglobin levels before pregnancy; therefore, they do not have the reserve necessary to support physiological changes. Hemoglobin concentration decreases after 8 weeks, drops to its lowest level at midpregnancy, and rises slightly or stabilizes near term. Hemoglobin and hematocrit values are expected to return to prepregnancy level by 6 weeks postdelivery unless there was severe blood loss during the intrapartal or postpartal period. Anemia is not a disease, but a symptom of an underlying condition.

IRON DEFICIENCY ANEMIA

In iron deficiency anemia, the hematocrit is less than 32 percent, or the hemoglobin concentration is less than 10.5 g/dL.[71] Many providers initiate treatment with a hematocrit of 34 percent.

Epidemiology

The cause of iron deficiency anemia is an inadequate iron supply usually secondary to poor dietary intake. Teenagers and women of low socioeconomic status are at greatest risk because of the likelihood of inadequate or improperly balanced diets.[71] Women with short intervals between pregnancies or who have histories of prolonged heavy menses are also at risk.

The incidence of iron deficiency anemia is highest among pregnant women. Approximately 30–50 percent of all women are anemic in pregnancy.[8,70,71]

Subjective Data

A woman may experience some fatigue or lassitude that may affect her ability to perform activities of daily living. In the second and third trimesters of pregnancy, she may notice shortness of breath on exertion.

Objective Data

All prenatal clients should be screened in the first trimester for anemia. Physical examination of a pregnant woman may suggest iron deficiency anemia; blood tests confirm it.

Physical examination may reveal pale conjunctiva and mucous membranes.[70] Grade II systolic heart murmur may also be detected. Fetal iron stores are protected at the expense of maternal stores.[71] Consequently, fetal effects are not noted unless the maternal hemoglobin level is below 7 g/dL.

Diagnostic tests show decreased serum iron levels; the number of reticulocytes is low. A complete blood count (CBC) with indices is done showing mature red cells as microcytic and hypochromic The mean corpuscular volume (MCV = $80–95u^3$) will be decreased; the mean corpuscular hemoglobin (MCH = 27–31 pg) will be decreased; the mean corpuscular hemoglobin concentration (MCHC = 32–36 percent) will be decreased; and the reticulocyte count (0.5–3.1 percent) will be either normal or low. Two very sensitive and reliable laboratory tests for diagnosis of iron deficiency are serum ferritin (concentration of less than 12 µg/L) and free erythrocyte protoporphyrin (FEP). In the FEP test look for a fivefold increase over the normal of 15 to 80 µg/dL.[71,72]

Differential Medical Diagnoses

Folate deficiency, thalassemia, sickle cell disease, aplastic anemia, HELLP Syndrome.

Plan

Psychosocial Interventions. Inform the client of her need to eat a well balanced diet, emphasizing foods that are high in iron. Explain how iron rich foods are important for her health during and after pregnancy.

Medication. Supplemental iron is administered. Whether it should be given to all pregnant women is controversial. The recommended daily dose of elemental iron for U.S. nonpregnant women is 60 mg. Most prenatal vitamins contain that amount of iron. Women with a hematocrit level of less than 32 percent should be treated for iron deficiency anemia.

The recommended dosage when deficiency is diagnosed is 120 to 180 mg of elemental iron per day in separated doses; this amount is equivalent to the iron contained in two or three 300-mg tablets of ferrous sulfate.[70] Total iron supplementation per day should include iron contained in prenatal vitamin and not exceed the 180 mg of elemental iron daily. For women who cannot tolerate oral iron therapy, parenteral administration may be necessary.

A side effect of iron supplementation is gastrointestinal disturbance. To enhance its absorption, iron should be taken 30 minutes prior to a meal, preferably with a source of vitamin C. Taking iron with milk, tea, or antacids should be avoided. This timing, however, may lead to gastrointestinal effects, disturbances that can be decreased by taking the iron after meals.[71] For pregnant women, taking iron following meals is less problematic because dietary iron absorption is much more efficient during pregnancy. Instruct the client to drink extra fluids (not tea) to offset problems with constipation. Some clients may not be able to tolerate the maximum daily dose. To maximize the woman's compliance, individualize administration and dosage. Spacing the doses throughout the day may also help absorption because only so much can be absorbed at one time.

Follow-Up

Schedule a repeat reticulocyte count in about 2 weeks. The count should rise significantly. All anemic women should be closely monitored for infection and signs of intrauterine growth retardation. Following delivery, these women should remain on iron therapy and be monitored for recovery. More than 2 years may be needed to replenish iron stores from dietary sources. Counseling women about this period is important if other pregnancies are planned.

FOLIC ACID DEFICIENCY

Folic acid is a B-complex vitamin essential for cell growth and division. It promotes the matura-

tion of red blood cells. Folic acid is stored in the liver for 4 to 6 weeks. Consequently, overt deficiency does not manifest until late in pregnancy or during the postpartum. Maternal folic acid deficiency in the first 8 weeks of gestation is associated with neural tube defects.[73,74,75]

Epidemiology

Folic acid deficiency is due to an inadequate iron supply usually secondary to poor dietary intake of folic acid. It is the most common cause of megaloblastic anemia.[71]

Teenagers and women of low socioeconomic status are at greatest risk for folic acid deficiency because of the likelihood of inadequate or improperly balanced dietary intake. Green vegetables, peanuts, and animal proteins, especially liver and red meats, are good sources of folic acid. Also at risk are women with hemoglobinopathies or those with a multiple pregnancy or pregnancies with a short interval between. Women taking hydantoin or ingesting ethanol are also at risk.

Folic acid deficiency in the United States is usually diet related. It is not unusual for folic acid deficiency to coexist with iron deficiency anemia. Folic acid deficiency is also associated with premature labor.[73,75]

Subjective Data

A client with folic acid deficiency may experience symptoms, including nausea, vomiting, and anorexia during pregnancy, and possibly experience symptoms of iron deficiency if it coexists.

Objective Data

Physical examination may reveal pale conjunctiva and mucous membranes, as well as a grade II systolic heart murmur. Signs of folic acid deficiency cannot be distinguished from those of iron deficiency anemia, as the two conditions are usually concurrent.

Diagnostic tests include determination of serum folate and RBC folate levels. Levels normally fall during pregnancy; however, a fasting folate level of less than 3 ng/mL in an anemic woman is a presumptive sign for diagnosis. Hypersegmented neutrophilic leukocytes and macrocytic red cells on peripheral smear are diagnostic, but definitive diagnosis is made by bone marrow examination. This should seldom be necessary.[71] The reticulocyte count will be depressed in the folic acid deficient client, but reticulocytosis usually occurs within 3 days after administration of a folic acid supplementation.

Differential Medical Diagnoses

Iron deficiency anemia, thalassemia, sickle cell anemia.

Plan

Prevention. For those women who have no history of neural tube defects (NTD), consumption of folate 0.4 mg/day is recommended.[73,74,75,76,77] Plans to fortify certain food sources such as breads and cereals are being considered and are available in some products.[77,78]

Psychosocial Interventions. Provide the client with information about foods that are high in folic acid. Explain to the client the importance of eating healthful foods every day to benefit herself and her fetus.

Medication. Prophylactic medication, a prenatal vitamin that contains 0.5 to 1.0 mg of folate, is given to most pregnant women. Prenatal vitamins that require a prescription usually contain 1 mg of folic acid. A full 1.0 mg per day is needed, if there is a deficiency. Women with significant hemoglobinopathies, on anticonvulsants such as Phenytoin, or have multiple gestation are advised to supplement with 1.0 mg daily of folic. Women who have had a previous infant affected by neural tube defect should be advised to supplement their diet with daily folate 4 mg/day 2–3 months prior to pregnancy. These women should continue folate 4mg/day during pregnancy.[74]

Follow-Up

The measures used for clients with folic acid deficiency are the same as those for women with iron deficiency anemia. The appropriate screening for iron deficiency should be performed and iron supplementation initiated when indicated.

THALASSEMIA

Thalassemia is an autosomal recessive genetic disorder that causes a reduction in or the absence of the alpha or beta globin chain in hemoglobin. Symptoms will depend upon the number and location of the missing proteins on the gene.[79] Either α- or β-thalassemia can occur.

Homozygous α*-thalassemia or* α*-thalassemia major* diagnosed women have short life expectancies and need expert obstetrical management. Women with α-thalassemia have signs and symptoms of hemolytic anemia, namely, hemosiderosis, a condition characterized by deposition in organs of the iron containing pigment hemosiderin, which is derived from hemoglobin degeneration. Symptoms may include chills, fever, hypotension, tachycardia, anxiety, nausea, vomiting, renal failure, and shock. Hydrops fetalis and stillbirth are associated with this condition.[79]

Heterozygous α*-thalassemia carrier.* Normal outcome is expected for mother and infant. Iron supplementation is given for documented iron deficiency anemia. If Asian, the partner should be screened for hemoglobinopathies due to the possibility of fetus being homozygous for α-thalassemia.

Heterozygous β*-thalassemia minor (*β*-thalassemia carrier).* Normal outcome is expected for mother and infant; is sometimes first identified in pregnancy. Women with the disorder are at risk for iron deficiency anemia and pregnancy induced hypertension. Folic acid and iron supplementation are necessary, only if indicated. Parenteral iron is contraindicated because of the possibility of exogenous hemosiderosis. This disorder is more common in the African American, Italian, and Asian populations.[76,79] Some forms can produce a child with major disease; therefore, partner should be screened for any hemoglobinopathies.

β*-Thalassemia major (Cooley's anemia),* *which is* homozygous β, is rare and is a life threatening condition; therefore, affected women usually do not reach childbearing age.

Management. Asymptomatic thalassemia carriers do not require any special testing but should receive serial ultrasounds to monitor fetal growth. Nonstress testing is also suggested to evaluate fetal well-being.[8] A good outcome is expected for both mother and infant. Administration of oral iron supplementation is controversial because hemosiderosis is possible.[9,79] Parenteral administration is contraindicated.[79] Further discussion is beyond the scope of this chapter; however, medical referral and genetic counseling is necessary.

SICKLE CELL ANEMIA

Sickle cell anemia is an autosomal recessive inherited disease that results from abnormal hemoglobin (hemoglobin SS) synthesis. Persons with sickle cell trait, on the other hand, are heterozygous (AS) for hemoglobin and may go undiagnosed because of the lack of symptoms. *Sickle cell trait (AS)*, however, may be identified with routine prenatal screening. *Hemoglobin C (Hemoglobin SC Disease)* is another variant in hemoglobin formation and in women who are heterozygous for both the S and C genes have hemoglobin SC disease. All women in high risk groups should be screened during the initial prenatal visit.

In sickle cell trait, anemia and crisis states do not usually occur except in extreme cases. There is no increased risk for the fetus.

Epidemiology

Sickle cell disease (sickle cell anemia) involves periods of hypoxia that lead to destruction of red blood cells, hemolytic anemia, and occlusion of blood vessels by abnormally shaped cells. Pregnancy can predispose to periods of hypoxia and trigger a crisis state. Infections, such as pyelonephritis, pneumonia, and osteomyelitis, occur more frequently among pregnant women with sickle cell disease. Other adverse effects that the disease has on pregnancy include an increased incidence of abortion, preterm labor, intrauterine growth retardation, and stillbirth.[80] Sickle cell disease is found almost exclusively in African Americans, but also among Greeks, Italians, Middle Easterners, and Asian Indians. Infants with sickle cell anemia will not show any signs of disease until the fetal hemoglobin has fallen to adult levels. In fact, some affected children do not demonstrate signs until adolescence.

Women with hemoglobin SC disease have less perinatal mortality than women with sickle cell anemia; there is an increased incidence of early spontaneous abortion and pregnancy induced hypertension.[8]

Sickle cell anemia is inherited as an autosomal recessive disorder. The disease occurs in 1 in 700 adult African Americans. The sickle cell trait is carried by 1 in 12 African Americans. Clinically significant hemoglobin SC disease occurs in 1 in 833 adult blacks in the United States.[8] The trait for hemoglobin SC occurs in 1 in 40 adult blacks.[8] One in every 625 black children born in the United States is homozygous for hemoglobin S.

Subjective Data

Women with sickle cell trait are usually asymptomatic

The client with sickle cell anemia reports multifocal pain, dyspnea, malaise, neurological symptoms, and gastrointestinal upset.

The crisis state is characterized by pain, dyspnea, and malaise. Pain can be multifocal, occurring in the extremities, chest, abdomen, or back. It frequently occurs in bones and joints. Neurological symptoms include headache, visual changes, and seizures. Liver and spleen involvement results in gastrointestinal symptoms, including nausea and vomiting or severe abdominal cramping.

Women with hemoglobin SC disease have only mild symptoms and frequently are undiagnosed until they experience more pronounced symptoms in pregnancy.

Objective Data

Physical examination of the mother in sickle cell crisis reveals symptoms in several systems.

- Skin is pale and possibly jaundiced.
- Visual acuity and peripheral vision may decrease.
- Signs of distress are apparent. The client experiences shortness of breath and possibly signs of pulmonary embolus or pneumonia.
- Abdomen may be distended with hepatomegaly and palpable spleen. Fundal height may be equal to or less than expected, depending on the client's general health prior to the episode.

- Kidneys are unable to concentrate urine and signs of kidney failure may be evident.
- Fetal heart tones, if present, may be elevated or lack variability.

With hemoglobin SC disease, a dramatic fall in hematocrit occurs in a crisis secondary to a marked sequestration of a large volume of RBCs in the spleen. During pregnancy these women may have a mild thrombocytopenia associated with increased splenic activity.[8]

A blood hemoglobin electrophoresis is done to determine the hemoglobin type. Electrophoresis confirms hemoglobin SS, AS or SC. During their initial prenatal visit, all African American women, women of Greek, Italian, Middle Eastern, or Asian Indian ancestry should be screened or have documentation of S and C hemoglobin.

Differential Medical Diagnoses

Malabsorption syndromes, alcoholic cirrhosis, hookworm infestation.

Plan

Psychosocial Interventions. Involve the client's family in every aspect of care. Provide information and clarification about the disease and its implication for pregnancy, delivery, and the fetus. The provider must be sensitive to the woman's possible fear of dying or fear of losing her infant. A crisis is painful and may be life threatening.

Education. Make the client with sickle cell anemia aware of the need to recognize symptoms of crisis or complication as soon as possible. Immediate attention can defer the effect on the fetus and frequently decrease the intensity of symptoms. Instruct the client to seek care at the first sign of a crisis. Teach the client the danger signs of pregnancy induced hypertension and signs and symptoms of infection. Early treatment of common infections, particularly vaginitis and cystitis, may decrease the incidence of more advanced infections, such as pyelonephritis and osteomyelitis.[80]

Genetic Referral. The partner of the woman with sickle cell anemia, sickle cell trait, or hemoglobin SC should be tested and, if both are affected and/or carriers, prenatal diagnosis of the fetus should be offered. Hemoglobin S can be identified through hemoglobin electrophoresis and DNA analysis of fetal blood.

Preconceptional Counseling. Ideally, those women affected by hemoglobinopathies are screened and are aware—prior to conception—of the risks of sickle cell anemia and hemoglobin SC disease to themselves and to a pregnancy. Determining both her own and the partner's status can assist the couple in making appropriate reproductive decisions for them.

Medication. There is no specific medication for sickle cell disease or the crisis state. Antibiotics are used for infection. Analgesics are used for pain during a crisis. Iron therapy should be initiated only if anemia is present. Some authorities are concerned about iron overload; therefore, iron supplementation is not given unless indicated by serum iron and ferritin levels.[8] Folate supplementation with good dietary habits and folic acid 1 mg/daily is recommended throughout the pregnancy.

Other Interventions. Prophylactic transfusions have been used throughout pregnancy with some success, but the practice is controversial.

Blood samples are taken throughout pregnancy to closely monitor cardiac, renal, and liver function. This procedure is especially critical during and after crises.

A *urine culture and sensitivity* should be performed at least once each trimester for women with sickle cell trait. Sickling can occur in the renal medulla, leading to reduced oxygen, necrosis of kidney tissue, and renal tubular dysfunction.[8] These factors predispose to an increased risk for bacteriuria, which, if undiagnosed, can progress to pyelonephritis.

An early sonogram is recommended to confirm dates; serial sonograms to assess fetal growth. Starting at 30 weeks, sonograms should be done weekly or biweekly to assess fetal well-being and amniotic fluid volume.

Sickle cell crisis requires hospitalization, enabling administration of transfusions, oxygen, intravenous therapy for hydration, and sedation and analgesia.

Delivery. Depends on the condition of both mother and fetus in relation to gestation and the risks and benefits that are presented. After 36 weeks, delivery should be initiated as soon as fetal lung maturity is documented. Vaginal delivery is preferred, if possible, and general anesthesia should be avoided because of the risk of hypoxia. During labor, fluid overload must be avoided and the woman should remain in the left lateral recumbent position as much that can be tolerated. Oxygen therapy may be necessary.

Follow-Up

After delivery, recommend genetic counseling to assist the client and her family to plan future pregnancies. The newborn is screened within the first few days of life. The woman is observed closely for postpartum hemorrhage.

Women with hemoglobin SC disease need the same program of prenatal care as outlined above for the woman with sickle cell anemia.[8]

PREGNANCY INDUCED HYPERTENSION

Pregnancy induced hypertension (PIH) is characterized by hypertension, proteinuria, edema, or all of these conditions, after 20 weeks of gestation. Previously, PIH was known as toxemia of pregnancy. Pregnancy induced hypertension is the same physiological condition as preeclampsia. *Eclampsia* refers to a convulsive state.

PIH is characterized by a blood pressure of 140/90 on two occasions at least 6 hours apart. Previously, a sustained rise of 30 mm Hg or more above baseline systolic blood pressure or a sustained increase of 15 mm Hg or more in baseline diastolic blood pressure was of diagnostic value. This criterion for diagnosis is no longer valid.[81] Proteinuria and edema in combination with hypertension have historically been referred to as the cardinal signs. PIH is a multiorgan disorder with various clinical signs. Proteinuria less than 300 mg in 24 hours and slight edema are present in mild PIH.

In severe PIH, the blood pressure is higher than 160/110 on two occasions at least 6 hours apart. Proteinuria is greater than 500 mg in 24-hour urine collection, and oliguria (less than 400 mL in 24 hours) is detected. Severe PIH is diag-nosed if pulmonary edema or thrombocytopenia with or without liver damage is present.

Endothelial Damage. The true cause of PIH continues to allude researchers. Much has been learned regarding the physiological changes. The latest theory focuses on the activation of the coagulation system and subsequent endothelial injury. Subsequent to an immunological disturbance triggered by abnormal placental implantation, substances are released that activate or injure endothelial cells. The effect of endothelial injury explains the multiorgan system involvement. Endothelial damage leads to subsequent platelet adherence, fibrin deposition, and the presence of schistocytes. The fluid shift from intravascular to intracellular spaces causes generalized edema. Hemoconcentration occurs because of the decreased blood volume in the intravascular space. Decreased blood flow to the liver leads to microembolization, ischemia, possible infarct, and tissue damage. Subcapsular hemorrhage may occur.

Thromboxane/Prostacyclin Imbalance. One explanation describes hypertension developing secondary to an imbalance in placental prostacyclin and thromboxane production. Prostacyclin is a potent vasodilator and inhibitor of platelet aggregation. A deficiency during pregnancy contributes to the occurrence of preeclampsia. Thromboxane, on the other hand, is a potent vasoconstrictor and stimulates platelet aggregation.

In normal pregnancy, thromboxane is increased: maternal plasma levels are higher late in pregnancy than in midpregnancy.[45,82] In normal pregnancy, prostacyclin and thromboxane levels are equal, but in a preeclamptic woman, the placenta produces seven times more thromboxane than prostacyclin. Vasoconstriction, platelet aggregation, and reduced uteroplacental blood flow result. This observation may explain some of the hematologic changes associated with PIH but does not identify the primary etiology of the disease.[83]

Vasospasm. The disease is characterized by generalized vasospasm and a constant degree of tension in the vascular system. As a result, blood pressure rises and blood flow to target organs is reduced, giving rise to the various signs and symptoms of pregnancy induced hypertension. In addition to the vascular system, the organs most affected are the brain, liver, kidneys, placenta, and lungs. Decreased blood flow to the brain leads to fluid shift, cerebral edema, and changes in sensorium. Cerebral edema also leads to central nervous system irritability, which can predispose to convulsions.

Kidneys. Decreased blood flow to the kidneys normally initiates production of renin and angiotensin I, which is converted to angiotensin II, the pressor agent that causes vasoconstriction and stimulates production of increased aldosterone. Aldosterone stimulates the reabsorption of sodium. In normal pregnancy, plasma renin and angiotensin II are elevated, but vasoconstriction does not occur because of the increased aldosterone. The higher levels of aldosterone indirectly increase blood volume and offset vasoconstriction. In PIH, the kidney becomes compromised.

Fetus. Decreased uteroplacental blood flow can decrease fetal oxygen and lead to fetal stress or distress. Prolonged vasoconstriction can contribute to intrauterine growth retardation and premature separation of the placenta (abruptio placenta).

Lungs. Fluid shift in the lungs leads to pulmonary edema.

Again, these changes help describe the events associated with PIH but are not unique occurrences to this disease and do not explain a primary etiology.[83]

Calcium. Recently, studies have reported an inverse relationship of maternal blood pressure and calcium intake. Women with preeclampsia have been hypocalcuric due to increased kidney reabsorption of calcium. Calcium supplementation has been shown to reduce both systolic and diastolic blood pressure. So far, there is no direct evidence that calcium supplementation affects long-term fetal outcome. Studies are presently in progress to determine the role of calcium supplementation in the prevention of PIH.[8,84] Also, the ability to predict PIH by determining levels of urinary excretion of calcium is being studied.[85]

Epidemiology

Although it is not known why pregnancy induced hypertension occurs, acceptable explanations are affected by several important observations.

- PIH occurs more frequently in primigravidas.
- PIH occurs more frequently with excessive placental tissue, as is seen in women with diabetes, gestational trophoblastic disease, and multiple gestation.
- PIH seems to have a genetic component. Some evidence has been found that the genetic composition of fetal tissue may predispose a woman to the development of eclampsia. An increased incidence of eclampsia among female relatives has been noted, but no conclusions have been drawn so far.
- Symptoms usually do not become evident until the third trimester, but there is evidence the process begins as early as the first trimester.
- Symptoms progress; early identification of symptoms and subsequent intervention can decrease the severity of disease and improve perinatal outcome.

Five to seven percent of all pregnant women experience pregnancy induced hypertension.[81,86] It is responsible for more than 25,000 deaths annually. Women at risk for developing PIH include those at extreme ends of the childbearing age range (teenagers and women older than 40), women with preexisting vascular or renal disease, obese women, and women with lupus erythematosus.

Subjective Data

The two most significant signs of PIH (proteinuria and hypertension) occur without the woman's awareness. By the time symptoms occur, PIH is severe. A woman may report headache, visual disturbances, facial, ankle, and finger edema, or severe heartburn with abdominal pain. Therefore, frequent prenatal visits for all pregnant women are recommended for blood pressure and proteinuria screening. All women should be informed of the danger signals and directed to seek evaluation immediately.

Objective Data

Neurological. Woman may exhibit a decreased attention span, disorientation, sleepiness, or decreased alertness. Brisk reflexes or clonus may herald an imminent convulsive state; however, many normal women have hyperactive reflexes.[81,87]

Assessment may thus be helpful in monitoring drug therapy, but it cannot be diagnostic for determining status of PIH.

Retinal Changes. May include edema and arteriolar spasm.

Lungs. Rales and rhonchi can be heard in affected lobes when pulmonary edema is present.

Liver. Hepatomegaly or upper right quadrant tenderness, or both, may be present.

Kidneys. Oliguria (less than 400 mL of urine in 24 hours) is associated with severe hypertension.

Fundal Height. Usually as expected by dates. A nonreactive nonstress test may indicate fetal compromise.

Blood Pressure. Must be carefully and consistently measured to be meaningful. Consistent measurements are those obtained in the same arm with the client in the same position, using appropriate size cuff, and taken at least 6 hours apart.[82,88]

Measurements are done to detect changes in blood pressure, urine, and fluid retention. The mean arterial pressure (MAP), or the average pressure in the arteries, is calculated from a blood pressure reading using the formula $MAP = D + 1/3 \, (S \, 2 \, D)$, where D is diastolic pressure, and S is systolic pressure.[82]

In normal pregnancy, cardiac output increases, but peripheral resistance decreases. Arterioles relax to compensate for increased blood volume. MAP should decrease, particularly in the second trimester. An elevated MAP is important to note but is not a valid predictor of impending PIH.[82]

- MAP should be 82 mm Hg or lower in the first and second trimesters and 89 mm Hg or lower in the third trimester.
- Weight is determined every visit; the client should gain no more than 4 pounds per month, or fewer than 2 pounds per week.
- A urine dipstick is done at every prenatal visit to screen for proteinuria; normal is negative or trace.
- The hematocrit is monitored to detect hemoconcentration; should not be greater than 42 percent.

Convulsive State. An emergency situation and can occur at any time, although the client has usually exhibited signs of severe PIH. Convulsive facial twitching and tonic–clonic contractions of the body occur. Gradually, movements subside, but the client may remain in a coma for an indefinite period. Following seizure, the client is hypoxic and acidotic and requires stabilization before delivery.

Differential Medical Diagnoses

Diseases that mimic severe PIH or HELLP syndrome (see subsequent discussion), including cholecystitis, viral hepatitis, idiopathic thrombocytopenia, hemolytic uremic syndrome, microangiopathic syndrome, fatty liver disease pregnancy and peptic ulcer. Other hypertensive disorders may occur and become evident during pregnancy. Other conditions with similar presenting symptoms such as appendicitis, kidney stones, pyelonephritis, and gastroenteritis are other possibilities.

Chronic (Essential) Hypertension. In this disorder, a blood pressure of 140/90 or higher develops before pregnancy, is recognized before 20 weeks of gestation, or continues indefinitely postpartum. Chronic hypertension is seen more frequently in multiparous older women who had hypertension in previous pregnancies. African American women are overrepresented in the incidence of maternal hypertension.[86] Fetal survival is related to clinical course, maternal renal function, and gestation at delivery. Clinical signs are different from those of pregnancy induced hypertension.

- Edema is usually absent.
- Proteinuria is absent.
- Hyperflexia does not occur.
- Weight gain is within normal limits.
- Physical signs associated with hypertension, such as retinal changes (arteriosclerosis and hemorrhages), occur.
- Fundal height may lag behind normal expectations, indicating possible intrauterine growth retardation.[86]

Chronic Hypertension with Superimposed PIH. Signs of pregnancy induced hypertension can occur in a woman who already has underlying hypertension. Proteinuria may or may not occur. Perinatal mortality increases significantly.

Late, Transient, Gestational Hypertension. Some women experience elevated blood pressure late in the third trimester, intrapartally, or within the first 24 hours postpartally. Other signs of preeclampsia or chronic hypertension are absent, and blood pressure usually returns to normal limits by 10 days postpartum. Whether the occurrence is a sign of underlying chronic hypertension is unclear.

HELLP Syndrome. HELLP is an acronym for hemolysis, elevated liver enzymes, and low platelets. Controversy surrounds the terminology, incidence, cause, diagnosis, and management of this syndrome. It is, however, considered a variant of severe preeclampsia and can develop prenatally, intrapartally, or postpartum.[89]

Symptoms and signs of HELLP syndrome include nausea, with or without vomiting, epigastric pain, upper quadrant tenderness, demonstrable edema, and hyperbilirubinemia. Blood tests reveal elevated serum glutamate-oxaloacetate transaminase (SGOT = 5–40 IU/L); elevated serum glutamate-pyruvate transaminase (SGPT = 5–35 IU/L); normal serum electrolytes; elevated blood urea nitrogen (BUN = 10–20 mg/dl), and creatinine (0.5–1.1 mg/dl); normal prothrombin time (PT = 11–12.5 seconds), partial prothrombin time (PPT = 60–70 seconds), and fibrinogen; a peripheral blood smear indicating burr cells, schistocytes, or both; and thrombocytopenia (platelet count below 100,000/mm^3). Proteinuria is 2+ or greater.[88]

Disseminated Intravascular Coagulopathy. Disseminated intravascular coagulopathy is associated with severe PIH and HELLP syndrome. Most authors, however, do not consider HELLP syndrome a variant of disseminated intravascular coagulopathy because coagulation parameters in HELLP (PT, PTT, and serum fibrinogen) are usually within normal limits. Opinions vary, but the true relationship between these two processes is unclear.

Plan

Prevention. Since the etiology of PIH/preeclampsia is unknown, efforts to prevent or reduce the incidence have been unsuccessful. The goal in management of PIH/preeclampsia is in the early detection and stabilization of the symptoms. There have been attempts to prevent the disease through dietary manipulation. In the past, high protein or low salt diets were used to correct abnormalities. Other dietary adjustments are being examined.

- *Calcium.* Calcium supplementation of 1500–2000 mg/d used in clinical trials in the hopes to reduce overall incidence; initiated prior to 20 weeks' gestation and continued throughout pregnancy. Results of clinical trials not available.
- *Magnesium.* Because of long successful history of using magnesium sulfate in treatment of PIH and preeclampsia, magnesium deficiency proposed as possible cause; studies have been conflicting; magnesium supplements are not recommended to prevent PIH/preeclampsia.[8]
- *Zinc.* Historically, zinc deficiency has been associated with PIH and preeclampsia, preterm delivery, and intrauterine growth retardation. At present, no adequate data support strong relationship between zinc deficiency and the prevention of PIH or preeclampsia.[8]

Psychosocial Interventions. The major role of the primary care provider in working with a client with a hypertensive disorder in pregnancy is providing education and support. Teaching about a healthy, balanced diet is important. The client may need to be taught to take her blood pressure or perform a dipstick urine test. All clients need to know the danger signals of PIH.

The provider must also be sensitive to the client's anxieties and concerns about the expected outcome and health of her unborn child. Women with PIH should be assisted and encouraged, within safety limits, to continue normal preparation for birth and the newborn.

Medication. Drugs are given to decrease seizure activity and reduce blood pressure.

ASPIRIN. Low dose aspirin therapy has been instituted if mild PIH is diagnosed because it is believed to decrease thromboxane production and platelet aggregation and may decrease the incidence of preeclampsia and fetal growth retardation.[81,90] No increased maternal or fetal risks have been demonstrated after administration of 60 to 80 mg of aspirin daily late in the third trimester in

TABLE 18–2. MONITORING NEEDED TO ADMINISTER MAGNESIUM SULFATE

Activity to Monitor	Sign of Toxicity
Deep tendon reflexes	Hypoactivity
Respirations	< 12 rpm
Urinary output	< 25 mL/h
Blood pressure	Significant drop (> 15 mm Hg)
Pulse	Tachycardia—sign of shock

Source: References 81, 87.

the woman at high risk for developing PIH. Women at high risk are those with chronic hypertension, a history of placental abruption, PIH in a previous pregnancy, or lupus erythematosus. More research is needed to define the length of therapy, the effective dose, and the appropriate client for this therapy. Aspirin therapy in normotensive women has not shown to be of benefit and is not recommended by the American College of Obstetricians and Gynecologists (ACOG).[81,90] The primary care provider should be in consultation with the obstetrician/obstetrical specialist if administering aspirin therapy.[81]

MAGNESIUM SULFATE. The drug of choice to control or prevent seizure activity (see Table 18–2).[81,87,91,92] It is usually given as a bolus and subsequently in continuous intravenous infusion. Because magnesium sulfate readily crosses the placenta, the newborn will be affected by the sedative properties of the drug. The newborn may exhibit hypotonia, suppressed respiratory effort at delivery, and poor sucking. These effects subside as the newborn excretes drug over the following 3 to 4 days.

ANTIHYPERTENSIVE THERAPY. Initiated to decrease blood pressure enough to protect maternal organs without causing hypotension and threatening fetal oxygen supply. Recently, *phenytoin* (*Dilantin*) has been suggested as an appropriate alternative for seizure control, had fewer side effects, and had better client acceptance. Cardiotoxicity is possible and, therefore, electrocardiographic monitoring during administration is recommended. Because of the known teratogenic effects during pregnancy, confining its use to the intrapartal period is necessary.[49,87]

HYDRALAZINE. The drug used most often, relaxes smooth muscle and causes vasodilation. Blood pressure drops quickly; therefore, the client must be closely watched every 2 to 5 minutes until stabilization occurs, which is within 1 hour. If not controlled or corrected, blood pressure can drop rapidly, lead to fetal hypoxia and subsequent distress.

Whether pregnant women with chronic hypertension should be treated with antihypertensive agents is controversial. Most specialists agree that therapy should be continued for women who are already on a treatment regimen including the possible use of diuretics. Therapy for women on reserpine or propranolol should, however, be changed because of their fetal side effects. For women not taking a drug, hydralazine (Apresoline) or methyldopa (Aldomet) is recommended. Treatment is generally initiated when the blood pressure is 150/110. Management is planned after accurate dates of pregnancy are determined.

Conservative Treatment. Intermittent bed rest, an adequate diet, and close monitoring are recommended for women with mild pregnancy induced hypertension. Bedrest assists the cardiovascular return of fluid from the extremities and increases blood flow to the heart and subsequently to the uterus, causing uterine relaxation. Bed rest, preferably in the left lateral position at least intermittently throughout the day, and limited physical activity induce diuresis and, usually, a drop in blood pressure. Sustained bedrest produces major side effects and should be avoided. Home care is successful when family support is adequate to afford the client appropriate rest. A client who is not hospitalized should visit the health office two to three times a week for evaluation. Antepartal self-monitoring needs to be taught to the client (see Table 18–3).

Antepartal monitoring of pregnant women with known chronic hypertension involves obtaining a baseline serum creatinine, uric acid, and creatinine clearance. In addition, a baseline sonogram is done to confirm dates; sonograms are repeated in the second and third trimesters, and fundal height is carefully determined at regular prenatal visits. Moreover, the client must be taught how to take her blood pressure twice a day.

Delivery. The only cure for PIH is delivery of the fetus. Primary goal of management is to allow

TABLE 18–3. ANTEPARTAL MONITORING OF PREGNANT WOMAN WITH MILD PREGNANCY INDUCED HYPERTENSION

Home	Office Visit
Check blood pressure once or twice a day	Check blood pressure
Check weight every day	Check weight
Perform urine dipstick twice daily	Perform urine dipstick (protein)
Observe symptoms: occipital headaches, blurred vision, irritability or emotional tension, scotoma, epigastric pain or any signs and symptoms of labor	Assess symptoms: occipital headaches, blurred vision, irritability or emotional tension, scotoma, epigastric pain or any signs and symptoms of labor
Record fetal movements daily	Obtain baseline serum creatinine, uric acid, creatinine clearance, total protein—repeat twice every week
	Obtain baseline liver enzymes, hematocrit, platelet count—twice a week
	Auscultate fetal heart tones, baseline fundal height, and weekly measurements
	Perform baseline nonstress test (NST) twice weekly
	Perform contraction stress test if NST is nonreactive
	Obtain baseline and serial sonograms
	Arrange for amniocentesis near term, starting at 33 weeks

Source: References 81, 82.

pregnancy to progress as far as possible without jeopardizing maternal or fetal well-being. Timing and mode of delivery depend on stability of the maternal–fetal unit, gestation, and the cervix. For the woman with eclampsia, delivery should occur as soon as possible after the woman and fetus are stabilized. If the cervix is favorable and other factors are controlled, labor is induced with intravenous oxytocin. Concurrently, magnesium sulfate therapy is administered to control or prevent seizures. Cesarean delivery is initiated if immediate delivery is indicated.

Some controversy exists as to use of epidural anesthesia. With proper blood pressure control, it can provide satisfactory anesthesia and permit the mother to be awake for delivery.

Hospitalization. Hospitalization is usually essential in the treatment of chronic hypertension with superimposed PIH. The intrauterine environment becomes increasingly hostile to the fetus, and each day is a delicate balance between the risks and benefits of intrauterine and extrauterine existence.

Severe PIH is treated aggressively, as hypertension poses an immediate threat to mother and fetus. Aggressive therapy includes maternal and fetal assessments, medications to prevent seizure activity and stabilize blood pressure, and preparation for delivery. Because of the

need for intensive and sometimes invasive monitoring techniques such as invasive hemodynamic monitoring, hospitalization is required with critical obstetrical care provided by appropriate medical and nursing staff.[93,94]

System Support. For the client with eclampsia, airway maintenance and oxygen are necessary. Hemodynamic monitoring is useful for appropriate fluid management.

Follow-Up

The prognosis for pregnancy depends on the severity of symptoms. With aggressive screening, identification, and treatment, maternal and fetal morbidity and mortality have decreased. Following delivery, most women recover quickly without any sequelae. The presence of contributing factors dictates the type of follow-up necessary. If underlying chronic hypertension or lupus erythematosus is suspected, then postpartal referral to an internist for assessment is needed.

Many women do not have problems with elevated blood pressure in subsequent pregnancies; however, all women should be informed of the possibility and the need for early prenatal care and evaluation.

Diabetes

Diabetes is a chronic disease characterized by a relative lack of insulin or absence of the hormone, which is necessary for glucose metabolism. In normal pregnancy profound metabolic alterations occur to support the growth and development of a fetus. Maternal basal metabolism increases as a response to fetal growth. The increase contributes to increased glucose utilization and the risk of maternal acidosis. Glucose rapidly moves from maternal circulation to the fetus by simple diffusion; insulin does not cross the placental membrane.

Insulin, however, is present as early as 12 weeks in the fetal pancreas; it is stimulated by glucose from the maternal circulation. The increase in glucose to the fetus results in accelerated growth of the fetus. Human placental lactogen (HPL) and growth hormone (somatotropin) increase in direct correlation with the growth of placental tissue; it rises throughout the last 20 weeks of pregnancy and causes an increase in insulin resistance. HPL stimulates the mobilization of free fatty acids for maternal use, which can lead to maternal ketoacidosis. The hormonal changes of pregnancy have conflicting but carefully balanced effects on carbohydrate metabolism. The increased estrogen acts as an insulin antagonist. Progesterone, on the other hand, augments insulin secretion while diminishing its peripheral effectiveness. In most cases, the maternal pancreas is able to increase insulin production to maintain normal glucose levels.[45,95,96,97]

The woman with undiagnosed diabetes is not able to cope with changes in metabolism resulting from insufficient insulin. The woman with suboptimal function who is not diabetic may not experience difficulty early in the pregnancy, but when pregnancy related hormones are produced by the enlarging placenta and reach certain levels, her pancreas will not be able to accommodate the increased insulin demand. The increased need for insulin and the tendency toward hyperglycemia emerge most often between 20 and 30 weeks of gestation.

In an attempt to predict client outcome and to establish treatment guidelines for diabetic clients, several classification systems are used.

TABLE 18–4. WHITE'S CLASSIFICATION OF DIABETES IN PREGNANT WOMEN

A	Chemical diabetes
B	Maturity onset (age > 20 years), duration < 10 years, no vascular change
C	Age 10–19 years, duration 10–19 years
D	< 10 years at onset; > 20 years' duration, benign retinopathy, calcified vessels of legs, hypertension
E	Overt diabetes at any age
F	Nephropathy
R, RF, H, T	Combined retinopathy, renal disease, arteriosclerotic heart disease, renal transplant

Adapted from Reference 96.

White's classification is based on age at onset of disease and degree of vascular involvement, but because of improved technology to monitor and treat mother and fetus the classification is infrequently used (see Table 18–4).[96] A simpler classification developed from the National Diabetes Data Group Classification of Diabetes Group has been used recently (see Table 18–5).

Diabetic Woman's Response During Pregnancy

A woman with diabetes may have several problems during pregnancy as a result of her diabetes, such as hypoglycemia, urinary tract infection, hypertension, hydramnios, and retinopathy.

Hypoglycemia. Hypoglycemia occurs primarily in the first trimester in insulin dependent, controlled diabetics. Because of its accelerated

TABLE 18–5. CLASSIFICATION OF DIABETES

A. Insulin-dependent type (type I)
B. Non-insulin-dependent type (type II)
   1. Nonobese
   2. Obese
C. Other types (secondary diabetes)
   1. Pancreatic disease
   2. Hormonally induced
   3. Chemically induced
   4. Insulin receptor abnormalities
   5. Certain genetic syndromes
   6. Others
D. Impaired glucose tolerance (subclinical diabetes)
E. Gestational diabetes (pregnancy induced glucose intolerance)

Source: References 8, 49, 96.

growth, the fetus uses glucose available in the maternal circulation, thereby decreasing the diabetic woman's need for insulin. Women accustomed to a consistent diet and insulin intake are not able to adjust to their reduced need for insulin. Consequently, they commonly develop hypoglycemia in the first trimester.

Urinary Tract Infection. Urinary tract infection is common in diabetics because more glucose is filtered due to their increased glomerular filtration rate. Glycosuria predisposes to bacterial infection.

Hypertension. Hypertension is related to the same factors that cause pregnancy induced hypertension. Diabetics have a predisposition to PIH.

Hydramnios. Ten to twenty percent of diabetics have hydramnios. The reason is poorly understood, but it is explained as caused by fetal glycosuria. The urine in amniotic fluid attracts water to balance the high osmolarity of the fluid.

Retinopathy. Diabetes is associated with retinal changes that may exacerbate during pregnancy and become more symptomatic.

Effects on Fetus and Neonate

The fetus who remains in an environment of maternal hyperglycemia may demonstrate macrosomia, teratogenesis, or death.

Macrosomia. The accelerated fetal growth that occurs when a mother is diabetic leads to a macrosomic or large-for-gestational-age infant.[45,49,98] Latina women with GDM are at higher risk for having a macrosomic infant.[99]

Teratogenesis. If significant maternal hyperglycemia continues, it can lead to maternal ketoacidosis and to movement of ketones across the placental membrane. These ketones have been associated with teratogenesis. Although rare, agenesis has been linked with ketosis between 5 and 6 weeks of gestation. Cardiac anomalies also occur. Ideally, preconception and early pregnancy glycemic control will prevent excess rates of congenital anomalies.[45,95,96] Unfortunately, even with improved care of women with diabetes, more infants are born today with birth defects caused by diabetes.[45] There is need for increased planning for pregnancy in diabetic women.[100]

Death. Among mothers who develop ketoacidosis, 50 percent of infants die. Early first trimester ketosis may cause early pregnancy loss. Hyperinsulinemia in the fetus may lead to delayed surfactant production in the lung and contribute to the incidence of respiratory distress syndrome.

Other Effects. Neonates of diabetic women have more problems with hypoglycemia, hypocalcemia, and hyperbilirubinemia in the first days of life.

Epidemiology

Diabetes is thought to have more than one cause. Insulin deficiency may be associated with damage to the pancreatic cells that make insulin, inactivation of insulin by antibodies, or increased insulin needs, as in pregnancy and obesity.

A genetic component, possibly an autosomal recessive trait, may exist but is not clearly understood. Diabetes is more prevalent in some families than others. Ethnicity may also be a factor. Latino women have a higher incidence of gestational diabetes mellitus.[99]

It is estimated that 2 to 3 percent of all pregnant women have diabetes mellitus; 90 percent of them have gestational diabetes. Annually, more than 90,000 women experience gestational diabetes in pregnancy.[96] Today, maternal mortality is negligible, but fetal mortality is 10 to 20 percent. Excluding death due to major congenital malformations, the perinatal mortality rate among newborns of diabetic women who receive optimal care approaches that observed during normal gestation.[45,96] In the early 1970s, 30 percent of all diabetic women died from complications related to diabetes in pregnancy; 65 percent of their infants died.

Subjective Data

Insulin Dependent Diabetes. A woman who is insulin dependent may experience more problems with nausea during early pregnancy. Insulin management is more difficult if she is nauseous and vomiting because eating patterns and insulin dosage are disrupted. If care is not taken, she may experience shock, coma, or both.

Gestational Diabetes. The client with gestational diabetes may be asymptomatic throughout the pregnancy.

Objective Data

Certain signs are common in women with diabetes in pregnancy.

- Insulin dependent women may have retinal changes that occurred during a previous pregnancy. Retinal changes are also seen in older women or women who have been diabetic since early childhood. Gestational diabetes does not generally cause retinal changes.
- Fundal height may be greater than, equal to, or less than expected by dates, depending on the uteroplacental unit. Beginning in the second trimester, fundal height will exceed expected height by dates. Evidence of excessive uterine fluid is a tympanic, tight abdomen.
- Excessive weight gain is common.
- Glycosuria is present.

Women with gestational diabetes may be asymptomatic throughout pregnancy or have only subtle signs. Therefore, earlier testing (prior to the 26–28 weeks' gestation) of symptomatic women will facilitate prompt intervention. Identification is a three-step process.

The first step is to identify the population at risk. The client's history may suggest gestational diabetes and warrant screening in the second trimester at 18–20 weeks' gestation. Some clinicians have suggested screening women at high risk of GDM at the initial prenatal visit, but this is controversial and has not been a reliable detection of GDM. High risk historical factors include the following:

- Family history of diabetes
- Poor obstetrical history, such as unexplained stillbirths or spontaneous abortions
- Previous unexplained birth of preterm or low birth weight infant
- Previous newborn weighing 4000 g or more
- Previous infant with major congenital anomaly

Risk factors in the current pregnancy: If any of these risk factors are present at any point in the pregnancy, the glucola screening should be considered.

- Maternal age more than 35 years
- Obesity (weight more than 200 pounds)
- Recurrent monilial vaginitis

- Glycosuria determined with urine dipstick on two consecutive occasions
- Hydramnios
- Excessive weight gain or fundal height greater than expected, or both

Finally, screen all prenatal clients. A reliable, specific, and cost effective screening for gestational diabetes is the 1-hour post-50-g glucola plasma screen.[96,101] Optimal time is between 26 and 28 weeks of gestation.

If the 1-hour plasma glucola is between 135–140 mg/dL, the client should undergo a 3-hour glucose tolerance test (GTT) to establish the diagnosis.[8,102] Experts in some countries are challenging all screening programs, but in the United States, universal screening has become standard practice with exception for some low risk populations such as teens. In clients with a 1-hour glucola screen above 185–190 mg/dl, the glucose tolerance test is unnecessary.[8,101] Some experts suggest that treatment should be initiated immediately without performing the GTT.[101] Other experts suggest performing a fasting blood glucose and if that level is 105 mg/dl or greater, treat the woman for GDM.[8] Two elevated values on the 3-hour GTT are diagnostic of gestational diabetes. There is recent consideration for lowering the criteria values for diagnosis but consensus does not exist at present.[102] If one value is elevated, repeat the screening at 32 to 34 weeks. (Refer to Table 16–7, page 458).

Elevated amniotic fluid insulin at 14–20 weeks' gestation may be predictive of gestational diabetes. Because amniocentesis is necessary to obtain the specimen of amniotic fluid, this is not recommended routinely.[103]

Differential Medical Diagnoses

Pancreatitis, malabsorption syndrome, hyperemesis gravidarum, hyperthyroidism.

Plan

Preconceptional Counseling. Because of the teratogenic effects of uncontrolled glucose in the first trimester of pregnancy, women with already existing diabetes need to be advised to obtain glucose control prior to pregnancy. Women on oral hypoglycemic agents should discontinue those agents and use insulin for glucose control prior to conception. Those on insulin may need to adjust doses in order to obtain closer glucose regulation than allowed in the nonpregnant condition.

Psychosocial Interventions. The primary care provider can play a major role in educating a client with diabetes and helping achieve healthy outcome.[104,105] Encourage the client to continue preparing for birth of the child. Do not discourage her from attending childbirth classes. Because of the frequent prenatal visits and additional testing, the client may require help in rearranging and adjusting work responsibilities. Much depends on the maturity and motivation of the client. Normal daily activity should be continued.

Educating the client about treatment is critical to the successful management of diabetes. With appropriate counseling and information, the client and her family will be able to deal with all changes in her body as well as in her lifestyle.

Medication. The main goal of treatment is control of blood glucose levels. Ideally, blood glucose should remain between 60–90 mg/dL fasting and 120 mg/dl 2-hours after meals; levels above 150 mg/dL have been associated with increased perinatal morbidity.[96] Glucose levels can be lowered through diet control and insulin administration if indicated.

Insulin requirements for the previously diagnosed diabetic woman frequently decline in the first trimester and then gradually increase during the remaining months of pregnancy.

For a woman who has gestational diabetes, insulin therapy is initiated if, on more than two episodes within a 2-week interval, glucose levels are above 120 mg/dL. Women who receive insulin should monitor their glucose levels at home daily; this includes a fasting level and at least one 2-hour postprandial level. Currently, insulin therapy is not recommended for all gestational diabetics, but it may be in some centers.

A mixture of intermediate and regular insulin is given in one to two subcutaneous doses daily. Beef and pork insulin have been replaced by semisynthetic human insulin preparations.[8] Because of less immunogenic properties of human insulin products compared to animal insulin, they are preferred during pregnancy.

Amounts are adjusted on the basis of daily glucose levels. Insulin dosages frequently are split between the morning and evening to provide around-the-clock coverage. Pregnant diabetics require a larger dose of insulin, and their needs increase throughout pregnancy. A decrease in insulin needs during the third trimester may signal placental dysfunction, not stabilization of the diabetic process. The use of the open-loop continuous subcutaneous insulin infusion pump therapy is gaining acceptance for pregnant women. Bolus amounts are necessary to cover meals and are determined by self-monitoring but, at all other times, the pump provides generally close to 1 unit of insulin per hour continuously.

Oral hypoglycemic agents have been associated with teratogenesis, and their use is contraindicated. Ideally, women with diabetes on oral hypoglycemic agents should be counseled about the teratogenic effects and be advised to switch to insulin for glucose control prior to pregnancy. The woman who was diabetic before pregnancy and taking an oral agent should immediately change to insulin on becoming pregnant.[49]

Diet. To accommodate pregnancy, 300 calories should be added to the diet of any woman each day. Diet counseling is initiated immediately after diagnosis of gestational diabetes. Ideally, a nutritionist should be available for instruction initially and consultation throughout pregnancy. The diet should contain 35 calories per kilogram of maternal weight (plus 300 calories for pregnancy), with 35 to 40 percent derived from complex carbohydrates. Additional fiber may help control glucose.

Some clients maintain adequate control of their diabetes with dietary changes alone. Differences occur in how to monitor glucose accurately in these clients. Some systems use weekly office visits and fasting blood sugar and 2-hour postprandial levels to monitor glucose. Other centers teach clients home glucose monitoring, which may be ordered two to four times a day, daily, or intermittently throughout the week. The provider must be sensitive to the women's ability to cope with frequent self-monitoring techniques required for glucose management. For some women, acceptance of the diagnosis and perception of the impact of GDM on herself and fetus will affect adherence to treatment regimes.[106]

Exercise. Exercise can be a healthy adjunct in controlling glucose levels if it is not prolonged, over strenuous, or contraindicated for other reasons.[96] It must be tailored to the individual's glucose-insulin balance with proper timing, intensity, and duration. The client should not exercise during states of fasting or hyperinsulinemia.

Monitoring Techniques. Several tests may be done throughout pregnancy to provide information about maternal and fetal health.

The *glycosylated hemoglobin A_{1C} (HbA$_{1C}$) test* measures glucose saturation of red blood cells, that is, the amount of glucose that will last the cell's lifetime. The test reflects serum glucose levels over the previous 4 to 6 weeks. Prolonged periods of hyperglycemia are evident in an elevated HbA$_{1C}$. The test is useful in evaluating past glucose control and client compliance. Any value less than 7.5 percent indicates good diabetic control; 7.6 to 8.9 percent, fair control; and 9 percent or higher, poor control. HbA$_{1C}$ does not correlate well with fetal well-being.

Routine urine screening is necessary because diabetic clients are predisposed to urinary tract infections.

An eye examination is recommended for established diabetics because of the proliferative retinopathy that occurs. Exacerbation occurs in about 15 percent of diabetics during pregnancy; laser coagulation may be required to control the process and prevent the possibility of blindness. Because GDM usually does affect the retina, history of GDM alone does not warrant retinal examination.

An early *sonogram* is recommended to confirm dates so that care may be planned and carried out at appropriate intervals. For established diabetics, *serial sonograms,* starting at 26 to 28 weeks in 4–6 week intervals, are helpful in monitoring fetal growth. All women with diabetes have several sonograms to assess fetal size, amniotic fluid volume, and status of the placenta. Exams can detect fetal macrosomia, the most common reason for shoulder dystocia at delivery.[8] Sonographic measurements of fetal abdominal circumference assist in detecting fetal macrosomia.[8]

Maternal assessment of *fetal activity* is also used to assess fetal well-being. The interval of maternal detection of cessation of fetal activity and

fetal death is shorter than in other complications of pregnancy. The woman should monitor fetal activity daily starting at 25 weeks' gestation. (See section on fetal movement counts Chapter 19.)

α-*Fetoprotein* (*AFP*) (triple screen) should be determined at 16 to 18 weeks of gestation to screen for spinal cord defects and Down syndrome. There is an increased incidence of neural tube defects in pregnant diabetics. Normal values of AFP for diabetic women are lower than for the nondiabetic population.[8]

Fetal echocardiography is done at 20–22 weeks' gestation in women with IDDM to detect presence of cardiac lesions, especially those of the great vessels and cardiac septum.

Serial nonstress testing (*NST*) should start at 32 weeks and continue until delivery. If the client has other vascular risks or is in poor glucose control, the NSTs should be started prior to 32 weeks' gestation and be done more frequently during the week. If the NST is nonreactive, the contraction stress test (CST) or biophysical profile (BPP) is done.[8] Although the contraction or oxytocin challenge test (CST) is a more sensitive means of detecting fetal problems, most centers rely on biweekly NSTs because the CST carries the risk of preterm labor. The BPP is not superior to the NST alone, but does provide further information and assurance in order to allow continuation of the pregnancy.[8] Doppler umbilical artery velocimetry studies are being used in some centers for antepartum fetal surveillance; more investigation is required for these studies to be used for reliable decision making regarding the pregnant woman with IDDM or GDM.[8]

The *glucose level in amniotic fluid* may be measured during amniocentesis. Normally, levels decrease as pregnancy progresses. An elevated amniotic fluid glucose level is associated with neonatal respiratory depression and low Apgar scores; this information may help in making decisions concerning delivery.

Delivery. Decisions concerning delivery can be difficult. Historically, the incidence of fetal death in the third trimester was decreased by arbitrary delivery at 36 to 37 weeks of gestation. Although infants survived, the incidence of respiratory distress syndrome and the complications of premature birth increased.

Newer technologies are used to document fetal maturity prior to delivery. The lecithin/ sphingomyelin (LS) ratio of the amniotic fluid of diabetic women is not a reliable determinant of fetal lung maturation; however, the presence of phosphatidylglycerol (PG) strongly correlates with maturity. Because PG is associated with false immature rate, other more dependable tests are being evaluated.[107] Samples are obtained by amniocentesis.

Increased chance of shoulder dystocia and cephalopelvic disproportion secondary to fetal macrosomia associated with traumatic birth and asphyxia in diabetic women. Vaginal delivery is attempted unless the fetus is estimated by sonogram to weigh more than 5000 g. In that case, a cesarean delivery may be initiated.[108,109]

Today, with more adequate assessment of fetal weight and well-being, clients may progress to term and deliver as normally as possible.

The key to intrapartum management of diabetic women is control of blood sugar within strict parameters. Clients are monitored with fingerstick blood samples every 1 to 2 hours and intravenous insulin is administered if necessary. An epidural is acceptable analgesia and anesthesia.

Follow-Up

After delivery, insulin needs drastically decrease. The established diabetic may not need to return to insulin therapy for a few days. She should, however, resume her usual prepregnant glucose monitoring routine. The gestational diabetic who has been taking insulin will not need to continue. Screen the gestational diabetic with a 100 gm 5-hour glucose tolerance test at the 6-week postpartum exam to assess for underlying diabetes. Encourage the diabetic women to breastfeed, as it helps use glucose.

The primary health care provider must discuss future childbearing plans and contraception with clients. The risks should be discussed candidly. The gestational diabetic can return to whatever contraceptive method she prefers. For the established diabetic, oral contraceptives may be contraindicated because of the increased risk of thromboembolic disease and vasculopathy. The low dose combination pill, minipill, or progestin implant may be used by well controlled diabet-

ics.[96] There is some evidence of deterioration in carbohydrate tolerance in depomedroxyprogesterone acetate (Depo-Provera) users as well as the progestin implant, Norplant. These are acceptable alternatives but are not suggested as first line choices.[8] Historically, intrauterine devices have been contraindicated for diabetics because of their association with infection, but this has recently been challenged.

Suggest sterilization if the woman has completed her family or the risks of future pregnancies warrant the procedure.

PRETERM LABOR AND BIRTH

A preterm birth is one that occurs prior to 37 completed weeks of gestation.[110] Premature/ preterm labor has its onset prior to 37 completed weeks of gestation.[45,110] The onset of labor, which is poorly understood no matter when it occurs, involves complex interaction among fetal, hormonal/endocrine, structural, and maternal changes. Low birthweight (LBW) infants weigh fewer than 2500 gm at birth, regardless of gestational age. Very low birthweight (VLBW) infants weigh fewer than 1500 gm at birth. In many discussions of preterm birth, low birthweight is used interchangeably. Infant weight has traditionally been used as the indicator for gestational age. Evaluation of programs, drug therapy, research, and policies have been developed using birth weight as the defining variable for prematurity. With the advent of sensitive pregnancy tests in correlation with accurate menstrual history and improved technology with sonography, gestational age can be accurately determined and differentiated from the premature infant. Low birthweight infants can be the result of prematurity, in some instances a result of a poor intrauterine environment, or a combination of those factors. There is no one explanation for the incidence of low birthweight or prematurity. Until preterm labor is better understood, prevention and treatment will be inadequate. Many of the factors are known, but how these factors interact in what order is yet unclear. For the sake of clarity, two categories of preterm birth have emerged: those that are spontaneous and those indicated. The spontaneous delivery includes delivery that spontaneously occurs after preterm labor, premature rupture of membranes, or premature dilation of the cervix. Indicated preterm births follow medical or obstetric disorder that places the fetus at risk such as diabetes, pregnancy induced hypertension, placenta previa, abruptio placenta, or intrauterine growth retardation. This section will focus on the spontaneous preterm birth.

Theories of Labor

Several theories to explain the onset and maintenance of labor have been proposed; however, none by itself adequately explains the process.

Uterine Stretch. The uterine stretch theory suggests that once the uterus reaches a certain size, it begins to contract to empty itself. The fact that premature labor occurs in most multiple gestations supports this theory; however, the theory does not explain why some women have excessively large newborns without premature labor or why women with small-for-gestational-age newborns have preterm birth.

Progesterone Withdrawal. Another theory is progesterone withdrawal. Historically, it was believed that progesterone decreased immediately prior to birth and triggered labor. Clinically, however, the decrease has not been demonstrated; administration of progesterone does not slow or stop labor.

Oxytocin Sensitivity. Oxytocin stimulation has also been proposed. More oxytocin receptors are present in the myometrium later in gestation; thus, the uterus becomes more sensitive to oxytocin as pregnancy progresses. Oxytocin causes increased uterine activity but not necessarily cervical changes. It plays a major role in the second stage of labor and postpartum but not in the initiation of labor.

Prostaglandins. The release of prostaglandins from the endometrium stimulates uterine activity, and prostaglandins have a significant role in the initiation of labor. (Oxytocin acts on the endometrium to release prostaglandins.) Use of prostaglandins any time during gestation induces labor.

Fetal Influence. Fetal-maternal communication is considered. The fetus may play a role in initiating labor. A stressor on the fetus will stimulate production of fetal cortisols. Cortisol production is communicated to the placenta or amniotic fluid, or both, thereby stimulating the production of prostaglandin precursors.

Preterm Labor Syndrome. This approach suggests that in response to an inflammatory insult, whether it be an infection or ischemia, the fetal membranes and decidua produce cytokines. These cytokines then stimulate the production of the precursors to prostaglandins, which stimulate the myometrial contractions and release the proteases that injure the membranes and underlying decidua. The result is cervical ripening, dilatation, and/or membrane rupture. An important concept is that the more advanced gestational age correlates with the responsiveness of the uterus to this insult, i.e., the women after 30–32 weeks' gestation will be more susceptible to this syndrome than the women at 22 weeks' gestation.

The risk to the fetus for preterm birth is associated with the immaturity of the organ systems. Conditions common in the premature infant are respiratory distress syndrome, intraventricular hemorrhage, bronchopulmonary dysplasia, patent ductus arteriosus, necrotizing enterocolitis, sepsis, apnea and retinopathy of prematurity. Some of the long-term effects are increased risk for neurodevelopmental handicaps such as mental retardation, cerebral palsy, seizure disorder, blindness, and deafness.

Epidemiology

The incidence of LBW and VLBW deliveries has changed little in the past 20 years, even though infant mortality has drastically decreased. Black infants have twice the risk as caucasian infants to be born at LBW. The reason for this remains unclear.

The causes of preterm labor are unknown, although several complications and conditions of pregnancy are associated with preterm birth (see Table 18–6).

Demographic risks for preterm labor include age under 17 years or greater than 34 years, African American ethnicity, and poor socioeconomic status.[111] These risk factors are probably not causative but do contribute to preterm labor

TABLE 18–6. PRINCIPAL RISK FACTORS FOR PRETERM LABOR AND BIRTH

Demographic Risks

Age: < 17 years or > 34 years
Low socioeconomic status
Unmarried
Race: African American
Low educational level

Medical Risks Predating Pregnancy

Parity: 0 or > 4
Nonimmune status for selected infections (e.g., rubella)
Genitourinary anomalies/surgery
Low birthweight, preterm birth
Multiple spontaneous abortions
Low weight for height
Selected diseases (e.g., hypertension)
Poor obstetric history
Maternal genetic factors

Medical Risks in Current Pregnancy

Multiple gestation
Hypotension
Hypertension/preeclampsia
First or second trimester bleeding
Spontaneous premature rupture of membranes
Anemia or hemoglobinopathy
Fetal anomalies
Hyperemesis gravidarum
Poor weight gain
Short interpregnancy interval: < 1 year
Selected infections
Placental problems
Oligohydramnios or polyhydramnios
Isoimmunization
Incompetent cervix

Behavioral and Environmental Risks

Smoking
Alcohol and other substance abuse
High altitude
Poor nutritional status
Exposure to diethylstilbestrol and other toxic compounds

Source: References 110, 111, 112, 115, 116, 117, 118, 121, 123.

because of their association with inadequate prenatal care, poor nutrition, or lifestyle.

Medical risks, such as hypertension and genetic disorders, which were present before a pregnancy occurred, are associated with indicated preterm birth. The most predictive risk factor for preterm delivery is history of previous preterm delivery.

Medical risks initiated by the current pregnancy constitute a considerable list. Renovascular disorders, such as abruptio placentae, are linked with preterm labor. Conditions that enlarge the uterus excessively, such as multiple gestation and macrosomia, are also associated with preterm labor. Any infection is a risk factor. Pyelonephritis during pregnancy has long been recognized as a risk factor (see Table 18–6).

Bacterial infection of the lower genital tract and amnion may lead to rupture of membranes and preterm labor. The most common causative organisms are ureaplasma, urealyticum, mycoplasma hominis, Bacteroides, and Gardnerella vaginalis.[112,113] It is unclear whether premature cervical dilatation and uterine activity lead to rupture of membranes or whether rupture of membranes from other factors leads to preterm labor. It has been proposed that infection promotes the release of prostaglandins, which stimulate uterine activity and cervical change. Data are not conclusive as to whether treating maternal infection will subsequently prevent preterm labor, but recent studies suggest that aggressive identification and treatment of bacterial vaginosis can reduce rates of premature delivery.[112,114,115]

Behavioral and environmental risks include smoking, alcohol consumption, and substance abuse. Such activities inject possible toxins into the maternal-fetal unit and possibly induce prostaglandin production. Many studies have linked occupational factors, especially prolonged periods of standing or walking, to the occurrence of preterm delivery and low birthweight infants.[116,117]

Premature birth occurs in 7 to 10 percent of all pregnancies and accounts for 50 to 70 percent of all perinatal deaths.[1,110]

Subjective Data

Some women fail to recognize the signs and symptoms of preterm labor perhaps because the symptoms of pelvic pressure, increase in vaginal discharge, backache, and menstrual-like cramps mimic symptoms that occur in normal pregnancy. Uterine contractions persistently occur with or without pain or discomfort. Clients may complain of low backache, a sense of lower abdominal pressure, or lower abdominal or thigh pain. Some women experience a change in vaginal discharge from creamy white to more mucoid, blood-tinged, or watery.

Objective Data

Cervical changes that indicate ripening (effacement, dilatation, or anterior position) and that occur prior to 35 weeks of gestation are signs of preterm labor. Cervical assessment has both objective and subjective qualities. Cervical dilatation of 3 cm or more is fairly straightforward but cervical consistency described as soft or firm is highly subjective and not reproducible among examiners.[8] Any uterine activity assessed by electronic monitor or by palpation should be timed and considered preterm labor until shown otherwise. Early engagement and zero station of presenting part may also be observed.

The diagnostic tests depend on the physical findings. A *transabdominal sonogram* may be ordered to confirm gestational dates and assist in decisions about timing delivery. Sonogram assessment will include placental location, estimation of fetal weight, and amniotic fluid volume to assess fetal well-being. Serial sonograms can help identify a growth-retarded infant who may not necessarily be preterm but, instead, small-for-gestational-age.

Transvaginal sonogram assessment of the length of the cervix has also been used to predict early labor since shortened cervical canal length is associated with preterm delivery.[118] A cervical length of 30 mm or more using transvaginal sonography is evidence that effacement has not occurred.[8] When the internal os has begun to open, the external os is closed, and the cervical canal is fewer than 18 mm, there is a funneling effect apparent on a transvaginal sonogram.[8] These observations are superior to digital examination in predicting which women will deliver prematurely.

Recently, testing for *fetal fibronectin* has shown to be helpful in predicting women with preterm contractions at high risk for preterm delivery.[119] The presence of fetal fibronectin, in the cervix or vagina is associated with chorioamionitis. The presence of the fetal fibronectin which normally is not detected in normal vaginal secretions after 22 weeks of gestation, indicates evidence of bacterial related membrane breakdown and associated preterm delivery.[119,120] A positive fetal fibronectin is associated with premature delivery within seven to fourteen days. Therefore, a positive fetal fibronectin may need a more im-

mediate aggressive treatment and monitoring while a negative fibronectin warrants a wait and see approach.[121,122]

Other assessments such as the presence of *meconium stained amniotic fluid or elevated amniotic fluid white blood count* have been linked to intrauterine infection and, thus, preterm delivery.[123,124] Implications of these two tests for the diagnosis or prognosis of preterm labor is unknown.

Sometimes, true preterm labor is diagnosed in *retrospect.* With the use of new tests, the goal is to improve the reliability and specificity of diagnosing preterm labor. Significant numbers of women experience painful regular contractions during pregnancy without having a preterm birth.

Criteria have been developed for defining preterm labor.

- Gestational age of 20 to 37 weeks
- Documented regular contractions on fetal monitor: at least four in 20 minutes or eight in 60 minutes
- At least one of following: rupture of membranes, documented cervical change, cervix at least 3 cm dilated or 80 percent effaced compared to initial cervical length (fewer than 30 mms), or fibronectin positive.[8,45]

Differential Medical Diagnoses

False labor/Braxton-Hicks contractions, urinary tract infection.

Plan

The primary care provider works with several team members in managing the care of a client in preterm labor. Because preterm labor is a multifaceted problem, it requires a multidisciplinary approach. All members of the team provide information and support to encourage the client to participate in her care. All work toward the term delivery of a normal infant.

Psychosocial Interventions. The best treatment for preterm labor is prevention. To meet that end, providing general health education about pregnancy, birth, and prenatal care is essential. Generally, to address the risk of having a low birth-weight infant, it is necessary to improve family planning services and provide accessible prenatal care for any woman regardless of her financial status. A client often needs assistance with lifestyle changes. Many of these risk factors, such as smoking, substance abuse, poor nutrition, and job related activities, are amenable to change. Educating and counseling women about these issues prior to and during pregnancy could have beneficial effects on the incidence of preterm labor.[125,126] In addition, helping the client to deal with stress, whether it is related to physical exertion from specific physical activities or occupational requirements or to emotional and financial factors, may lower the incidence of preterm labor.[116] Currently, however, the correlation between stress and preterm labor is unclear. All of these areas are difficult to research and only minimal attention has been given to them.

Identifying Infection. The incidence of preterm labor is linked with genital tract infection. Any client showing possible preterm labor should have cervical, vaginal, and urinary cultures done and be treated with appropriate antibiotics. The screening and antimicrobial treatment of *bacterial vaginitis* and bacteriuria have been reported to reduce the occurrence of preterm labor and birth.[114,127] Any client with suspicion of preterm labor should have a sterile speculum examination for pH, fern, pooled vaginal fluid to rule out premature rupture of membranes. Cultures should be collected from the outer one-third of vagina and perineum for group Beta Streptococcus, from the cervix for Chlamydia and N. gonorrhoea, and from the external cervical os and posterior vaginal fornix for fibronectin. Metronidazole is recommended for bacterial vaginitis because it is effective, does not eradicate the normal lactobacillus, and avoids issues related to penicillin allergies.[114] Prophylactic administration of antibiotic therapy is not recommended.[49]

Premature rupture of membranes (*PROM*) is the leaking of amniotic fluid prior to the onset of labor contractions, and with this discussion refers to PROM prior to 37 weeks of gestation. PROM associated with preterm labor is differentiated from PROM at term in that infection of the choriodecidual membranes has preceded the PROM as compared to chorioamniotitis, which occurs with rupture of the membranes at term. The most com-

mon presenting symptom is history of a sudden gushing fluid from the vagina followed by persistent, uncontrolled leakage. A sterile vaginal exam is done to collect fluid for testing. When applied to a dry slide, amniotic fluid will dry into a microscopic crystallization in a "fern" pattern. It can accurately confirm premature rupture of membranes in 85–98 percent of cases. The pH if amniotic fluid is present will be blue-green and range 6.5–7.75. A sonogram to determine amniotic fluid volume, fetal presentation, estimated fetal weight and gestational is done to prepare for delivery.

Diagnosing Preterm Labor. The diagnosis is frequently uncertain and, because the treatment incurs added risks, accurate diagnosis is critical but challenging because of lack of definitive tests. When cervical dilatation is 3 cm or more, the diagnosis of preterm labor is confirmed and the woman is a candidate for tocolysis. If the cervix is less than 3 cms, then the diagnosis is not confirmed; repeat the cervical exam in 30–60 minutes. There must be a cervical change of at least 1 cm, a dilation of 2 cms, or a positive fibronectin assay before preterm labor is confirmed in the woman with persistent contractions. When the cervix is fewer than 2 cms, monitor contraction frequency, assay fibronectin, and repeat cervical examine in 1–2 hours.[8]

Tocolytic Medication. Several types of drugs have been tried to interrupt preterm labor and prevent premature birth. At present, the role of any tocolysis is questionable. Studies are inconclusive and debatable; placebos have a high rate of effectiveness. Overtreatment is probably occurring in women in whom preterm labor has been misdiagnosed. There is evidence that tocolysis can delay delivery up to 48 hours and allow for the mother to be transferred to a setting where more risk appropriate care can be provided, if necessary. This delay also provides an opportunity to administer steroids.

Many drug therapies involve some type of home monitoring system once the client stabilizes. The question that arises is whether self-palpation (which she must be taught) is as effective in detecting uterine contractions as use of a uterine monitoring device. Most programs employing devices also include home visits or phone calls from nurses. It is difficult to determine which is more effective: the uterine monitor or nursing contact. More research is needed.

Magnesium sulfate competes with calcium in smooth muscle and reduces the force and frequency of uterine contraction. The client with premature contractions must be hospitalized and the magnesium sulfate administered parenterally, usually intravenously. The loading dose is usually 6 g magnesium sulfate in 10–20 percent solution over 15 minutes. Maintenance dose is 2 g/hr magnesium sulfate added to 1 liter dextrose with saline. The client must be closely monitored by specially trained personnel while receiving magnesium sulfate and be carefully weaned when therapy is discontinued.

Beta sympathomimetics, including ritodrine and terbutaline, are the most promising drugs currently available. They suppress the contractile response of the uterus.

- Ritodrine (Yutopar), the only FDA drug approved by the Food and Drug Administration for use in preterm labor, relaxes the uterus. Side effects are related to stimulation of the sympathetic nervous system: bronchial relaxation leads to pulmonary edema, hypotension can lead to fetal stress, glycogenolysis can lead to hyperglycemia, and cardiac stimulation leads to tachycardia. Ritodrine administration is initiated by intravenous therapy and requires hospitalization.[8,128]
- Terbutaline (Brethine), like ritodrine, is administered for uterine relaxation. Initially, it is given by subcutaneous injection 0.25 mg every 3 hours. Oral maintenance doses are continued unless uterine contractions return. Some evidence suggests that clients can learn to use a subcutaneous infusion pump and continue parenteral therapy at home; however, the advantage of the pump over oral dosing has not been substantiated.[49,128,129]

Antiprostaglandins, or prostaglandin synthetase inhibitors (e.g., indomethacin [Indocin]), have been tried for some clients resistant to beta-adrenergic drugs. The usual dose is a 50-mg loading dose orally or 50–100 mg dose rectally. Subsequently, 25–50 mg is administered orally every 4–6 hours, depending upon client response. Be-

cause prostaglandin is a strong stimulant of the uterine myometrium and indomethacin reduces the synthesis of prostaglandins, it has promise in the cessation of labor. They have limited use in short-term intervals because of their association with closure of the ductus arteriosus, neonatal pulmonary hypertension, and oligohydramnios.

Calcium channel blockers have been used to a limited extent to inhibit myometrial contractions. Oral nifedipine (Procardia) is being used with success for some women who do not respond to other therapies. It has become the drug of choice for some centers because of the low incidence of maternal side effects and ease of administration. Fetal side effects are not a concern. It cannot be given in combination with magnesium sulfate.

Oxytocin antagonists are being sought as an effective tocolytic. Atosiban (Antocin) is being studied in a number of trials across the United States. Atosiban displaces oxytocin and vasopressin from their receptor sites and, thus, reduces uterine contractility. There are minimal side effects, but effectiveness compared to other tocolytics is yet unknown.[128]

In general, tocolytic medications are not indicated when maternal conditions warrant early delivery for the benefit of the woman or the fetus. Tocolytics would be contraindicated in women with cardiac disease, significant hypertension related to chronic or pregnancy induced hypertension, or the occurrence of antenatal hemorrhage. From the fetal perspective, tocolysis is not indicated in gestation 37 weeks or greater, cervical dilatation greater than 3 cm, birth weight of 2500 gms or more, fetal distress, intrauterine growth retardation, or maternal infection. Tocolysis is also contradicted in the case of fetal demise or lethal anomaly.[8]

Risk Screening. Although not proven reliable or sensitive in predicting preterm labor, risk screening is used by most primary health care providers to try to identify at risk women and intervene to prevent preterm birth.[130,131] Risk screening should be done during the initial prenatal visit and again at 25 to 28 weeks of gestation. A uniform tool for risk screening is not currently available.[110,131] (See section on epidemiology for list of risk factors.) Cervical fetal fibronectin has limited value as a predictor of preterm delivery in a low risk population.[132] Further investigation of fibronectin and use of transvaginal measurement of the cervical canal as screening tools for identifying women at risk for developing preterm birth is being done.

Education. The major component of a program to prevent preterm labor is education of the client and staff. Comprehensive assessments and timely interventions throughout pregnancy by appropriate professionals are critical to improve the perinatal outcome.[133]

Client education includes instruction about a variety of preventive measures. Information is provided about the *signs and symptoms of labor.* All pregnant women should be instructed to notify the health care provider if leaking of fluid begins, vaginal spotting or bleeding develops, or uterine contractions occur every 10 minutes or more frequently. The client may need instruction to *time contractions* from the beginning of one contraction to the beginning of the next contraction.

A client may need to learn self-care strategies to *decrease uterine activity.* When uterine activity occurs, she should first lie down, preferably on her left side, drink fluids (at least 8 oz), palpate the uterus, and time contractions. The client must be instructed that if contractions do not subside in 30 to 60 minutes, she must be evaluated by a health care provider.

The client must also be informed about the specific *drug therapy* being administered, how to take it properly, when and the side effects.

The staff must be educated to be sensitive to a client's complaints and not to dismiss low backache, cramps, or descriptions of "the baby balling up" as normal discomforts of pregnancy. Emergency room caregivers and answering services should be apprised of the special needs of a preterm labor client.

Home Uterine Monitoring. Home uterine activity monitoring has been used in an effort to identify preterm labor for the purpose of diagnosing, monitoring, or adjusting tocolytic therapy.[134] Review of studies fails to demonstrate the effectiveness of uterine monitoring in the reduction of preterm birth.

Traditional Approach. The traditional plan of care comprises bed rest, hydration, and sedation.

- Bed rest assists the cardiovascular return of fluid from the extremities and increases blood flow to the heart and subsequently to the uterus, causing uterine relaxation. Bedrest remains one of the most widely prescribed medical interventions for preterm labor, even though it is costly, disruptive to families, and may either have no effect or negative effects on fetal outcomes.[135,136] Bedrest produces major side effects in every major organ system including cardiovascular deconditioning, diuresis with accompanying fluid, electrolyte, and weight loss, muscle atrophy, and psychological stress. Because of these physiological and psychological side effects of bedrest, the provider needs to anticipate and intervene to allay these effects. Assisting the woman and her family to arrange family activities and responsibilities to accommodate at least 3–4 periods of 20-minute rest periods in the recumbent position can relieve fatigue and pressure on the cervix. Home care including medical and nursing assessment, child care, homemaker services, supportive counseling, and instruction in stress relaxation are all interventions being utilized to assist preterm labor patients maintain bedrest.[137,138,139] Hospitalization to ensure bedrest is sometimes necessary.[135,136,140]
- Sedation reduces the client's anxiety and helps her to rest. If, however, delivery is imminent, sedation poses the risk of neonatal respiratory suppression.
- Hydration also increases blood flow to the uterus. Even though commonly prescribed, the effectiveness of hydration has not been well established and needs further investigation.[141]

Ultrasound. Transabdominal ultrasounds are used to assist in the diagnosis and monitoring of the woman with preterm labor. Sonography is done to assess placental location, determine amniotic fluid volume, estimate fetal weight and presentation, and assess fetal well-being. Information from sonography assists in making delivery decisions.[8] Transvaginal assessment of cervical length has also been used to identify women at risk for preterm birth. A cervical length of fewer than 30 mm at 24–28 weeks has been postulated to predict the occurrence of preterm birth. At present, this observation has not been tested in relation with any program of intervention.[8]

Cerclage. Cerclage late in pregnancy for excessive dilatation (CLIPED) historically has not been used but may be appropriate in some cases to delay delivery.[110,142] Clients must be free of infection and greater than 21 weeks of gestation.

Delivery. If labor is not halted, delivery management is based on fetal size and presentation. Delivery mode should be as atraumatic as possible; cesarean section is frequently performed with breech presentations. Cesarean sections should only be performed for the usual fetal and maternal indications.

Corticosteroid Administration. It is recommended to administer corticosteroids to the mother prior to delivery to stimulate surfactant production in the fetus and decrease the incidence of respiratory distress syndrome, intraventricular hemorrhage, and overall neonatal mortality. To be effective, corticosteriods must be given between 28 to 32 weeks of gestation, maternal infection must not be present, and membranes must be intact.[49] Administrating steroids in the case of rupture of membranes is controversial.[8] Women at risk for premature delivery are usually given dexamethasone, 6 mg every 6 hours for four doses, or betamethasone, 12 mg every 24 hours for two doses, both intramuscularly.[49,128,143] The major maternal side effect is potential pulmonary edema when given concurrently with tocolytics. Follow-up of children whose mothers have prenatal corticosteroids has not shown any untoward effects.[143] In addition to corticosteroids, most centers are using surfactant replacement in the newborn to prevent or decrease the problems of respiratory distress syndrome.[144] Exogenous replacement surfactant is even more effective when given to infants of mothers treated prenatally with corticosteroids.[45] Neither of these treatments replaces the natural lung maturity that occurs in utero.

Preterm labor is not stopped if severe uterine bleeding or maternal disease or infection is present. Premature rupture of membranes is associated with preterm labor and genital tract infection; therefore, once rupture is suspected, cervical cultures, including those for group beta streptococci, mycoplasma, gonorrhea, and chlamydia, should be obtained. Decision making with respect to delivery must balance the risk of prematurity with that of maternal/neonatal sepsis. Currently, the conservative approach of delaying delivery is more common, unless infection cannot be controlled with antibiotic therapy.

The client is hospitalized. Her temperature is monitored throughout the day, and the leukocyte count is evaluated every 2 to 3 days. An amniocentesis is considered to rule out subclinical infection. Tocolysis is contraindicated when chorioamnionitis is present.

SUBSTANCE ABUSE

Research has documented a causal relationship between a woman's health behaviors and the health of her unborn child. Ingestion of certain chemicals, legal and illegal, can be teratogenic. Indeed, the use of illegal chemicals (those that have no medically sanctioned use) is rising at an alarming rate in the United States. Cocaine, an amphetamine, is one example. Unfortunately, improper use of tobacco, alcohol, and caffeine is common and tolerated in our society. In addition, certain controlled substances, such as sedatives, amphetamines, and narcotics, are misused.

Pregnancy affects a woman's response to certain drugs. Consequently, an amount of drug taken during pregnancy may have different, more unpleasant effects than it would in the nonpregnant state. Drugs cross the placenta but may not be able to cross back. The fetus, which usually requires more time to detoxify and excrete drugs, becomes a reservoir.

The timing of drug ingestion may also determine the type and severity of damage. Because many women are polyusers, the problem is compounded. Mixed drug abuse may increase the incidence of adverse effects. It certainly complicates the primary care provider's ability to predict outcome and the counseling needs of clients. Research on drug abuse has been extensive, but inconsistent and, in many cases, inconclusive. To assess clients effectively and intervene appropriately so as to promote and maintain health, however, the provider must be knowledgeable about current, accurate information.

Epidemiology

Trying to explain or predict human behavior is a complex, usually unsuccessful endeavor. Because so many variables interact, research becomes difficult; however, research suggests that combination of biological, sociological, and psychological factors interact to determine the onset and severity of substance abuse. Addiction may have a genetic basis.

The *agent-host-environment theory* proposes that an individual is susceptible because of an inherited genetic trait, a milieu that participates in drug use, or both. It becomes repetitious, almost semireflexive behavior. A pleasurable drug reaction reinforces participation.

The *psychic pain theory* states that drug use is an attempt to relieve "psychic pain." Feelings of depression, loneliness, or anger may lead persons to self-medicate. Some describe the use of drugs as a way to control their lives, which otherwise seem out of control, or to combat feelings of powerlessness and helplessness.[145] Other researchers have proposed that women's *inability to develop adequate relationships as children* is linked to later substance abuse.[146] Substance abuse may be a harmful health behavior triggered in response to a major life stress or trauma. It has been reported that 70 percent of women report being raped or sexually abused prior to their substance abuse.[147,148]

In several recent studies of obstetrical populations, 10 to 15 percent of clients reported their drug use during pregnancy.[149] According to national estimates from the National Institute on Drug Abuse, 5.5 percent of all pregnant women use an illicit drug in pregnancy.[147] Black women are more likely to use drugs than are white or Hispanic women.[150] In reality, however, the incidence of drug use is higher, as many women deny use.[149] Routine prenatal toxicology has been proposed to increase the identification of women abusing drugs during pregnancy. The intent has been to anticipate the medical treatment for complications of pregnancy, such as preterm labor, and provide the appropriate education and referral.[149] There is much variance to the accuracy and usefulness of present urine and blood toxicology tests. Some states have enacted laws mandating prenatal drug screening and treatment, but there are legal/ethical pitfalls to this approach.[147] Coerced treatment has not shown to be effective in reducing perinatal substance abuse and has been challenged as to its legal justification.

Subjective Data

A client with substance abuse problems does not usually seek health care expressing her abuse as a chief complaint. Her complaints are usually vague, frequently cloaked by other problems for which she desires some relief. Often, she seeks prenatal care late or not at all. The client may arrive at the emergency room in labor or experiencing a complication of pregnancy that involves pain or bleeding.

Symptoms of withdrawal that may motivate a woman to seek care include nausea and vomiting, nervousness, tremors, and abdominal cramps. A woman abusing drugs often has a history of sexually transmitted disease. Because many of the same lifestyle factors for drug use are also the same risk factors for HIV, a history of positive HIV status is associated with substance use in women. Other clues that place a woman at risk for substance abuse include a history of a low birthweight infant, prostitution, poor self-care, parent or sexual partner who abuses drugs, or family violence.[147,151]

Objective Data

Effects of selected drugs in pregnancy and signs of recent drug use are listed in Tables 18–7 and 18–8, respectively. (See Chapter 23 for more details on drug use.)

Drug use is an important part of a client's history. The primary care provider must remember that the client may be involved in illegal activities, such as drug selling and prostitution, and may fear repercussions of seeking care. She often denies substance abuse. A caring, concerned manner is therefore critical to help the client feel "safe" and respond honestly. Indeed, many clients feel relieved because they want to discuss their problem. Pregnancy is the motivator for some who want to try treatment.[147] In settings where routine testing is done, the provider needs to inform the woman in a positive manner that routine testing will be done to assist in providing quality care and assuring for healthy outcome.

It is essential in discussions with clients about substance abuse to clarify the type of drug taken, the time during gestation when the fetus was exposed, and the amount of drug taken, it is

TABLE 18–7. INCIDENCE AND EFFECTS OF USE OF CERTAIN DRUGS IN PREGNANCY

Substance	Incidence	Possible Effect on Pregnancy
Nicotine	20–30% of women of childbearing age	Vasoconstriction: decreased uteroplacental blood flow, decreased birth weight, prematurity, abortion, abruptio placentae
Alcohol	96% of population at some time	Decreased folic acid and thiamine, inadequate weight gain, second-trimester abortion, fetal alcohol syndrome, alcohol-related birth defects
Caffeine	Average intake, 3 cups coffee daily	Fetal risks nebulous, caffeine present in newborn
Sedatives (barbiturates)	Widespread, not known	Teratogenic effects not known, newborn withdrawal, maternal seizures in labor
Amphetamines (cocaine)	1 in 10 newborns exposed to illegal drugs	Vasoconstriction: pregnancy-induced hypertension, abruptio placentae, abortion; maternal starvation: ketosis and dehydration, "snow-baby syndrome," neonatal cerebral hemorrhage, preterm birth, increased incidence of sudden infant death syndrome, neural tube defects, failure to thrive
Narcotics heroin morphine codeine meperidine opium	< 1% of pregnant women	Maternal and fetal withdrawal, abruptio placentae, abnormal presentation, preterm labor, premature rupture of membranes, intraamniotic infections, postpartum endometritis, urinary tract infection, septic thrombophlebitis, increased incidence of pregnancy-induced hypertension, intrauterine growth retardation, small-for-gestational-age infant, neonatal jaundice, congenital anomalies, including cardiac and genitourinary newborn infection
Marijuana (cannabis)	10% of all 18- to 25-year-olds	"Amotivational syndrome," no documented adverse effects on fetus, altered neonatal behavioral patterns

Source: References 150, 156.

necessary also to assess the client's concerns, level of knowledge, and fears. Such assessment depends on the adeptness of the provider. Questionnaires are available through drug and alcohol abuse centers to help the provider assess the type(s) and severity of an abuse problem.[147,150] Assessment tools to assess alcohol usage include the MAST (Michigan Alcoholism Screening Tool), the CAGE (Cut Down Annoyed Guilt Eye-opener), and the T-ACE (Tolerance Annoyed Cut Down Eyeopener). The DAST (Drug Abuse Screening Test) is available as a broad based screening instrument.[152] The Substance Abuse Subtle Screening Inventory (SASSI) is another

effective clinical tool, which has been positively compared to using urine toxicology.[153]

Ideally, the initial prenatal visit should provide an opportunity for all women to complete a confidential questionnaire that will provide a baseline for discussion. The provider should review the findings with the client in a private setting.[147]

The provider must not be judgmental toward clients who are abusing drugs. Many women use drugs to fill a need in their lives; they already suffer from low self-esteem and guilt feelings. Showing disapproval may increase their guilt, and the only way they may be able to deal with guilt

TABLE 18–8. SIGNS OF RECENT DRUG USE

Sedatives	Unsteady gait, odor of fresh or stale alcohol, nystagmus, slurred speech
Amphetamines	Anxiety, paranoia, tracks or needle marks, tattoos or self-scarring over arms (to disguise needle marks), nasal irritation, frequent purposeless movements, excessive fetal activity
Narcotics	Depressed mood, nodding, pinpoint pupils, tracks or needle marks, tattoos, skin abscesses/cellulitis, fingertip burns (diminished pain sensation)
Hallucinogens	Paranoia, anxiety, thought disorders, impaired judgment, fingertip burns

Source: References 150, 156.

is by using more drugs. The goal of therapy is to help the client deal with pregnancy by developing a trusting relationship with a person instead of the drug(s). Providing a full spectrum of medical, social, and emotional care is mandatory.

The interview should be done in a matter-of-fact manner. Questions should be phrased in a fashion that assumes drug use to decrease the client's defensiveness, for example, How many times do you drink beer in one week? In addition, the provider should ask about drinking and drug use prior to pregnancy. Evasive answers may indicate a problem. It is not necessary or wise for the primary care provider to seek a detailed account of drug usage at this initial interview. Referral and follow-up with substance abuse clinicians are ideal.

Differential Medical Diagnoses

Medical problems associated with substance abuse in pregnancy may include the following: sexually transmitted diseases including HIV infection and AIDS; uncertain date of last menstrual period; hepatitis; skin abscesses and cellulitis; anemia and malnutrition; tuberculosis; and urinary tract infections.

Plan

Substance abusers are not going to stop because of any one intervention or because someone tells them to stop. The success rates of treatment programs are dismal. Nevertheless, many woman can be helped, as can their children, and that is the focus of the primary care provider. Multifaceted programs are needed to more adequately promote the health of these women and their unborn children.

Psychosocial Interventions. The dangers of drug use in pregnancy need to be conveyed. Preconceptional counseling should include information about alcohol, smoking, caffeine, medications, and all other drugs, legal and illegal. The primary care provider should be supportive, yet provide clear directions to pregnant and prepregnant clients about avoiding smoking, drinking, and drugs. Substance abuse crosses all socioeconomic and cultural groups; screening is not limited to

low socioeconomic groups. Lack of insurance, lack of child care, lack of transportation, or homelessness are identified as barriers to substance abusing women seeking or staying in care. Removal of these barriers is important to any treatment intervention.[147]

Medication. See Chapter 23.

Legal Issues. Providers need to be aware of the laws and practices within their state and settings. Issues such as charting, confidentiality, and responsibilities for reporting vary by state.

Psychological Therapy. Once abuse has been identified, therapy should begin with the primary caregiver. Although the client may resist referral to a specialist and her personal freedom must be protected, adequate treatment is important. In addition to appropriate individual and/or group psychological therapy, a comprehensive program includes routine prenatal medical care, prenatal education, substance abuse education, parenting education, vocational training, housing if needed, and integration into self-help programs. Specialized programs for pregnant women are designed to deal with substance abuse as well as the high risk nature of pregnancy and birth. Case management and home visiting by caring, knowledgeable professionals have enhanced the effectiveness to perinatal substance abuse treatment.[146,147,154]

Preparation for delivery and the infant is a positive activity and should be encouraged. Special classes will help the client to prepare. Historically, these women do not receive gratification from infant care, but the programs preparing them for childbirth include strategies to boost self-esteem by helping the woman successfully parent her child.

A client should not be separated from her children, but instead should be involved in child care in a supportive, healthy environment. Children also need referral for close pediatric care.

Prenatal Care Issues. The types of drugs being used in pregnancy have variable effects on the women and her fetus.

Nicotine. Smoking cessation during pregnancy can reduce the risk of complications of pregnancy and incidence of low birthweight. One of the most effective strategies to assist people to quit smoking is having the medical professional advise cessation. Communities should have smoking cessation programs targeting pregnant women available at low or no charge from organizations such as the American Lung Association, the American Cancer Society, or the March of Dimes (refer to Chapter 23).

ALCOHOL. Heavy drinking is a risk to the fetus throughout the pregnancy, so reduction or elimination of alcohol at any time during gestation is beneficial to the fetus. Referral to appropriate counseling including self-help groups such as Alcoholics Anonymous can be helpful (refer to Chapter 23).

CAFFEINE. Reports suggest that moderate use of caffeine does not increase the risk of spontaneous abortion or growth retardation.[8] Women should be advised to curtail heavy consumption of caffeinated beverages and substitute with more nutritious fluids or water.

SEDATIVES (BARBITURATES AND BENZODIAZEPINES). When these drugs have been ingested in high doses prenatally and stopped abruptly, the withdrawal can be life threatening to mother and fetus. Cessation of these drugs should be done gradually under the supervision of the physician. The withdrawal symptoms are similar to opiate withdrawal.

AMPHETAMINES (COCAINE). Advise immediate cessation of subsequent drug; cocaine causes its effect quickly on the maternal system and fetus. Abruptio placenta is commonly associated with cocaine usage in pregnancy. Cocaine is associated with stillbirths, prematurity, impaired infant growth, central nervous system problems such as deficits, and microcephaly.[155]

NARCOTICS (HEROIN, MORPHINE, MEPERIDINE, OPIUM). Usually these women who are addicted to narcotics ingest periodic doses inconsistently. These peaks and nadirs of drug level create periods of fetal withdrawal and possible hypoxia. Methadone maintenance is given to stabilize the maternal addictive behavior and prevent periods of fetal binge and withdrawal. Methadone maintenance requires the women to be in a drug treatment program under the supervision of appropriate personnel. Hospitalization for initial

stabilization and orientation to the methadone is ideal but may not be available in many communities.[156] Some programs are available in outpatient settings. The initial dose is usually 10–20 mg, with additional doses of 5 mg every 4–6 hours depending on evidence of withdrawal symptoms.[156] The level of methadone should be approximately 20–40 mg/day and remain stable, particularly in the third trimester.[8] Enrolling pregnant women in a methadone maintenance program can reduce obstetrical complications, increase chance for participation in prenatal care, and enhance the opportunity to engage them into drug treatment program. Neonates of women using narcotics including methadone will demonstrate signs and symptoms of neonatal abstinence syndrome (NAS). NAS includes generalized disorders of the gastrointestinal tract, respiratory, and central nervous systems (see Table 18–9). Paregoric, phenobarbital, and diazepam are used to alleviate the withdrawal symptoms in the neonate.

MARIJUANA. Effects on pregnancy and fetus are not clear; advise to discontinue usage.

Delivery. Ideally, women who are abusing drugs in pregnancy are identified, and plans for con-

TABLE 18–9. NEONATAL ABSTINENCE SYNDROME

Gastrointestinal tract
  Excessive sucking
  Poor feeding
  Regurgitation/Projectile vomiting
  Loose stools/Watery stools
Respiratory system
  Frequent yawning
  Mottling
  Nasal stuffiness
  Sneezing
  Nasal flaring
  Respiratory rate > 60/min
Central nervous system
  Excessive high-pitched cry
  Hyperactive moro reflex
  Tremors
  Increased muscle tone
  Myoclonic jerks
  Generalized convulsions
  Shortened sleep periods after feeding

Source: Adapted from Weiner, Susan. (1992). Perinatal impact of substance abuse module 3. White Plains, New York: March of Dimes Birth Defects Foundation.

tinuation of care carry into the intrapartum period. Either urine or blood toxicology screening may be done upon admission. Frequency and type of maternal and fetal monitoring will be determined by the type and amount of prenatal drug(s) used.

Child Follow-Up. In general, infants born to mothers abusing drugs during pregnancy are at greater risk to experience lack of adequate parenting, possibly child neglect and abuse, as a result of attachment difficulties, mothers' disorganization and unpredictability. The incidence of long-term effects of developmental delays and learning disabilities of in utero exposure to drugs is controversial. Because of the many confounding factors associated with these women and their unstable, often impoverished lifestyle, establishing a causative link to the in utero exposure to drugs and subsequent behavior is impossible (refer to Table 18–9).

MULTIPLE GESTATION

Several complications of pregnancy are associated with multiple gestation. Spontaneous abortion, for example, is more than twice as common in multiple gestation. Visualization of twins on an early sonogram of a woman who later delivered a single newborn has occurred and is known as the vanishing twin syndrome. It is believed that one or more embryos can be reabsorbed without jeopardizing the remaining embryo. Fatty liver disease and pulmonary edema are also more frequent in multiple gestation.[157]

Overdistention can interfere with sustained functional labor contractions and affect dilatation and effacement; ineffective uterine activity results. It may also lead to uteroplacental insufficiency and fetal stress. Consequently, cesarean delivery is more common.[157] Varied factors related to gestational age, general maternal health, labor pattern, and the maternal-placental unit determine fetal compensation in labor. The incidence of postpartum hemorrhage from uterine atony is significantly increased secondary to overdistention of the uterus during pregnancy.

Development

Monozygotic (MZ) twins, also called identical twins, arise from a single fertilized ovum that divides during the early development phase into two embryos with identical genetic material.[45] The time of division determines fetal and placental morphology. Division occurring late, between 8 and 12 days' postfertilization, will result in incomplete separation and, thus, conjoined twins.[45]

Dizygotic (DZ) twins, also called fraternal twins, arise from multiple ova that are fertilized by multiple sperm. Multiple ovulation results from excessive gonadotropin stimulation. Fraternal twins are not true twins but siblings who share the same intrauterine environment. High order multiple gestations (more than three fetuses) can result from monozygotic, dizygotic, or mono- and dizygotic division.

With a multiple gestation, blood volume increases 500 mL more than a single gestation; the volume of amniotic fluid in twin gestation may reach 10 L.

Epidemiology

The incidence of multiple gestation worldwide has increased from 1 in every 80 pregnancies to 1 in 49.[158] The incidence of triplets is 1 in 1300 pregnancies, and that of quadruplets, 1 in 512,000 pregnancies. Incidence of multiple gestation varies among countries and races. Africa has the highest reported incidence, 1 in 22 pregnancies; Japan has the lowest incidence, 1 in 254 pregnancies. Within the United States, incidence varies among races: African Americans experience multiple gestation in 1 in 100 pregnancies; caucasian women, in 1 in 110 pregnancies. The risk of congenital anomalies in multiple gestation is 3 times greater than in a single gestation.

With identification of the vanishing twin syndrome, the incidence may be higher than previously thought. Early diagnosis by sonography has documented multiple gestations that resulted in single births.

A woman taking an ovulation induction drug or using an in vitro fertilization technique is at increased risk for multiple gestation.[158,159] Other factors increase the risk of multiple gestation: dizygotic twins are more likely to occur among female relatives, women of advanced maternal age, and multiparas.

Subjective Data

During early pregnancy, a woman with multiple gestation may experience more severe nausea and vomiting, which may last well into the second trimester. Hyperemesis gravidarum, probably related to increased human chorionic gonadotropin levels, may be the only diagnostic clue in the first trimester. The client may later experience excessive fetal movements. Neither sign, however, is reliable or helpful in early diagnosis.

Objective Data

The data used to diagnose the presence of a multiple gestation are collected by physical examination, maternal serum α-fetoprotein testing, and sonography.[45,158]

In the second trimester, examination may reveal signs suggestive of multiple gestation. The most common early sign is a fundal height greater than expected for dates. More than one heartbeat may be heard. Palpation of more than one fetus is not usually possible until the third trimester.

Maternal serum α-fetoprotein is measured between 15 and 18 weeks of gestation. If the α-fetoprotein level is elevated, multifetal gestation is suspected. Sonography is used for definitive diagnosis and to identify the number of fetuses.[45]

Differential Medical Diagnoses

Anemia, hyperemesis gravidarum, hyperthyroidism, gestational trophoblastic disease, gestational diabetes.

Plan

Clinical goals are to prevent premature birth and to detect fetal growth retardation early. The incidence of preterm delivery in multiple gestation is 20 to 50 percent. Fetal growth is usually satisfactory until 30 to 32 weeks of pregnancy. From 32 weeks onward, the total weight gain of fetuses is similar to the total weight gain of a single fetus. Head circumference is similar, but fetuses have a low weight.

Psychosocial Interventions. Support the client during diagnostic testing. Clarify the critical nature of such testing. Explain to her that a late diagnosis of multiple gestation is associated with a greater risk of poor perinatal outcome.

Maternal Assessment. Carefully evaluate the usual pregnancy changes with particular attention to signs and symptoms of pregnancy induced hypertension and preterm labor. In late pregnancy the incidence of PIH increases threefold; it also occurs earlier in pregnancy and is more severe.

The larger increase in maternal blood volume associated with multiple gestation increases the incidence of iron deficiency anemia.

Fetal Surveillance. Sonography and a nonstress test are among the tests that may be carried out.

Sonography is done early in the second trimester to assess fetal structures for anomalies, to determine placental placement, and to identify chorionicity and amnionicity.[45,158,160] Fetal anomalies occur more frequently in monozygotic twins.

After 28 weeks, sonograms are done every 2 to 3 weeks to assess fetal growth. Biparietal diameter alone is an inadequate predictor of growth; the percentage of weight difference among fetuses must be assessed. A 20 percent or less difference is acceptable.[160] Anything higher is suggestive of discordant growth.[45,158] Intrauterine growth retardation must be differentiated from discordant growth. Growth discordant twins have lower Apgar scores, longer hospitalization, and higher perinatal death rates.

Malpresentation, which is common, is detected by sonogram. The most likely presentation is vertex/vertex; however, interlocking fetal parts can affect delivery. Crowding provokes less desirable presentations, such as vertex/breech, breech/breech, vertex/transverse, or several other combinations. Cord prolapse and cord entanglement are usually associated with malpresentation. Also diagnosed by sonogram is twin transfusion syndrome. Twin transfusion syndrome is uncompensated, unidirectional blood flow from one fetus to another. The donor twin becomes hypovolemic with suboptimal growth; the recipient becomes hypervolemic and hydropic.

Nonstress tests start at 28 weeks and are done weekly. Each fetus should be monitored separately if possible.

Other tests that may be done are chorionic villus sampling and amniocentesis. These tests are carried out for the same reasons as for a single gestation pregnancy. Preterm labor, if present, is treated as usual. The lecithin/sphingomyelin ratio is used to make a decision about the timing of delivery, for example, in the case of a woman with twins and pregnancy induced hypertension. As no significant difference is found in the lecithin/sphingomyelin ratio among sacs of laboring women, only one sac needs to be tapped.

Selective Termination. Selective termination, the voluntary reduction of the number of embryos in a high order multiple gestation, is performed as early as possible in the first trimester, if desired.[45,158] The intent is to increase the chance for survival for the remaining embryos. Among the various methods used is injection of potassium chloride into the embryonic sac to allow natural reabsorption. The number of embryos to be terminated is controversial. Because the perinatal outcome is significantly less favorable for more than two fetuses, most recommend reduction to two embryos. Many ethicolegal questions arise. The client and her family must have a thorough knowledge and understanding of the procedure and its implications.

Comfort Measures. To address the intense discomfort associated with the exaggerated physiological changes of multiple gestation, various measures may be implemented. Nausea and vomiting may require intravenous hydration. Constipation, heartburn, sleeping disturbances, and low back pain interventions can be reviewed as usual. The overdistended uterus mechanically blocks the lower extremities, causing dependent edema and varicosities in the legs and labia. Maternity support hose may be recommended early in pregnancy. Maternity "sling" girdle has been helpful for some women to help support the gravid uterus and alleviate lower backstrain associated with multiple gestation. Exercises, particularly those to stretch and strengthen the lower back muscles, may be suggested.

Although excessive fetal movement is reported, it does not warrant intervention.

The health care provider can assist women in controlling and coping with changes with anticipatory guidance and education.[161]

Diet. In addition to foods that are rich in iron, recommend a supplement of 60 to 80 mg elemental iron per day. Encourage daily intake of prenatal vitamins with 1.0 mg folic acid. Monitor the woman's weight gain at each office visit. Normal weight women should gain 1.5 lb/wk after the 20 weeks of gestation.[162]

Bed Rest. Bed rest for women with a multiple gestation has been studied extensively with inconclusive results. Although bed rest has not prevented preterm birth, some evidence suggests that bed rest initiated at 26 to 32 weeks may increase birth weight and thereby improve perinatal outcome. Most providers limit a woman's activity based on her lifestyle and general health.

Preparation for Childbirth. Classes should be begun earlier than usual, as immobility can be a problem in the later weeks of gestation.[161]

Preterm Labor. Preterm labor is treated if signs occur. The use of tocolytic drugs to prevent preterm labor has not proven successful. Prophylactic cervical cerclage has also not been beneficial, unless the client is experiencing premature cervical dilatation.

Delivery. Decisions concerning delivery are based on gestational age, estimated fetal weights, presentations in relation to each other, and availability of adequate intrapartum monitoring. Cesarean birth is performed frequently because of malpresentations and because of concern for the ability of preterm and low birthweight fetuses to tolerate a difficult vaginal birth. An intrapartal sonogram is necessary to identify fetal presentations and establish a management plan for delivery.

Follow-Up

Because of the increased chance of uterine atony and early hemorrhage following a multiple birth, caution is exercised to identify and treat it as soon as possible.

Although breastfeeding decisions are based on the same reasoning as that used following the birth of a single infant, a woman with more than one newborn will probably need additional education and support. More patience and time are needed to establish adequate lactation and feasible routines. Lactation consultants, lay groups such as the LaLeche League, and informed nurses within the health care system are available for referral.

Attachment may take longer when more than one infant is involved. Neonatal illness and separation can also interfere in parent-child bonding. Other factors affecting attachment include the meaning of the pregnancy to the couple, maternal health, and the general living conditions. If one or more of the siblings is hospitalized, ill or dies, parents experience ambivalence in trying to grieve and at the same time celebrating the survival of one or more infants.

Most communities have lay groups of parents who have had multiple births, such as Mothers of Twins and Mothers of Multiples. These groups provide sympathetic counseling, practical suggestions on how to cope with more than one infant at a time, directions for obtaining equipment and supplies, and referral for financial assistance, which is frequently needed.

Nursing diagnoses

The following nursing diagnoses identified by the author are representative of those used in the health care plan of women with complications in pregnancy; however, these diagnoses by no means constitute an inclusive list.

- Acute pain related to
  —stretching of uterus
  —pressure on surrounding tissue from enlarging gestational sac or blood in peritoneum
  —uterine contractions and cervical dilatation
- Alteration in
  —nutrition related to lack of knowledge of healthy diet pattern
  —parenting related to negative experiences in pregnancy, highly stressful delivery, or both

- Altered nutrition, less than body requirements, related to fever, anorexia, or nausea of disease process
- Altered sexual patterns related to medically imposed restrictions, couple's fear of harming fetus, or both
- Altered maternal tissue perfusion related to hemodynamic changes
- Altered family processes related to hospitalization
- Altered health maintenance related to
  —lack of knowledge about drug therapy or instruction in self-care at home
  —lack of knowledge of medical management plan
  —denial of problem and delay or rejection of management plan
  —high risk lifestyle practices (shared needles, unprotected sexual intercourse)
- Anxiety (mild, moderate, severe) related to knowledge deficit about
  —the diagnosis, treatment, and meaning to pregnancy
  —preterm labor, its treatment, and the meaning to pregnancy
  —diabetes and its meaning to the pregnancy
- Body image disturbance related to
  —swelling and changes from disease process
  —physiological and anatomical changes of pregnancy
- Decreased appetite and inadequate fluid intake
- Decreased cardiac output related to hypovolemia
- Disturbance in self-esteem related to inability to conceive "normal" pregnancy
- Dysfunctional grieving related to anticipated loss of pregnancy and fetus
- Fear related to threat
  —to own well-being
  —of pregnancy loss or birth of defective child
- Fluid volume deficit related to
  —peritoneal or other abnormal blood loss
  —fluid shift out of the intravascular space

- Grieving related to actual pregnancy loss or threat to fetal safety
- Impaired health maintenance related to
  —inadequate support systems
  —lack of knowledge concerning necessary contraception and follow-up care postevacuation
- Impaired skin integrity related to skin eruptions from infection
- Ineffective coping related to the exaggerated discomforts of pregnancy
- Potential for
  —injury related to eclamptic seizures
  —inadequate parenting/attachment related to birth of more than one offspring
  —inadequate nutrition related to increased nutrient needs of more than one fetus

REFERENCES

1. Rosenberg, H., Ventura, S., Maurer, J., Heuser, R., & Freedman, M. (1996). *Births and deaths: United States, 1995* (Monthly Vital Statistics Report, 45, No. 3, Supplement 2, 1–40).
2. Atrash, H. K., Alexander, S., & Berg, C. J. (1995). Maternal mortality in developed countries: Not just a concern of the past. *Obstetrics & Gynecology, 86,* 700–705.
3. Singh, G. K., & Yu, S. M. (1996). Adverse pregnancy outcomes: Differences between U.S.- and foreign-born women in major U.S. racial and ethnic groups. *American Journal of Public Health, 86,* 837–843.
4. Edge, V., & Laros, R. K. (1993). Pregnancy outcome in nulliparous women aged 35 or older. *American Journal of Obstetrics and Gynecology, 168,* 1881–1885.
5. Fretts, R., Schmittdiel, J., McLean, F., Usher, R., & Goldman, M. B. (1995). Increased maternal age and the risk of fetal death. *The New England Journal of Medicine, 333,* 953–1002.
6. Guyer,B., Strobina, D. M., Ventura, S. J., & Singh, G. K. (1995). Annual summary of vital statistics. *Pediatrics, 96,* 1029–1038.
7. Heaman, M., Robinson, M., Thompson, L., & Helewa, M. (1994). Patient satisfaction with an antepartum home-care program. *JOGNN, 23,* 707–713.
8. Gabbe, S. G., Niebyl, J. R., & Simpson, J. L. (Eds.). (1994). *Obstetrics normal and problem pregnancies.* (3rd ed.). New York: Churchill Livingstone.
9. Prevention of hepatitis A through active or passive immunization: Recommendations of the advisory committee on immunization practices. (1996). *MMWR, 45* (No. RR–15), 1–30.
10. Freitag-Koontz, M. J. (1996). Prevention of hepatitis B and C transmission during pregnancy and the first year of life. *Journal of Perinatal and Neonatal Nursing, 10,* 40–55.
11. Hepatitis B vaccine. (1996). *MMWR, 45*(No. RR–12), 7–8.
12. Zuckerman, A. J. (1995). Occupational exposure to hepatitis B virus and human immunodeficiencey virus: A comparative risk analysis. *American Journal of Infection Control, 23,* 286–289.
13. Prevention of varicella: Recommendations of the Advisory Committee on Immunization Practices. (1996). *MMWR, 45*(No.RR–11), 1–25.
14. Grant, A. (1996). Varicella infection and toxoplasmosis in pregnancy. *Journal of Perinatal and Neonatal Nursing, 10,* 17–29.
15. Establishment of VARIVAX pregnancy registry. (1996). *MMWR, 45*(No. 11), 239.
16. Hedrick, J. (1996). The effects of human parvovirus B19 and cytomegalovirus during pregnancy. *Journal of Perinatal and Neonatal Nursing, 10,* 30–39.
17. Finch, C. (1995). Human parvovirus B19 in pregnancy. *JOGNN, 24,* 495–498.
18. Torok, T. (1990). Human parvovirus B19 infections in pregnancy. *The Pediatric Infectious Disease Journal, 9,* 772–775.
19. Hocke, C., Morlat, P., Chene, G., Dequae, L., Dabis, F., & The Groupe D'pidemiologie Clinique Du Sida En Aquitaine. (1995). *Obstetrics & Gynecology, 86,* 886–891.
20. HIV testing among women aged 18–44 years—United States, 1991–1993. (1996). *MMWR, 45*(No. 34), 733–737.
21. Dickover, R., Garratty, E., et. al. (1996). Identification of levels of maternal HIV-1 RNA associated with risk of perinatal transmission. *JAMA, 275,* 599–605.
22. Sperling, R. S., Shapiro, D. E., Coombs, R. W., et.al. (1996). Maternal viral load, zidovudine treatment, and the risk of transmission of human immunodeficiency virus type 1 from mother to infant. *The New England Journal of Medicine, 335,* 1621–1629.
23. Eyler, A. E. (1996). Current issues in the primary care of women with HIV. *The Female Patient, 21,* 14–28.

24. Chu, S. Y., Hanson, D. L., Jones, J. L., & The Adult/Adolescent HIV Spectrum of Disease Project Group. (1996). Pregnancy rates among women infected with human immunodeficiency virus. *Obstetrics, 87,* 195–198.

25. Zelewsky, M., & Birchfield, M. (1995). Women living with the human immunodeficiency virus. *JOGN, 24,* 165–172.

26. Brown, D., Rigby, F., & Elkins, T. (1996). HIV infection and physician responsibilities: A commentary on the ACOG Ethics Committee opinion #130. *Women's Health Issues, 6,* 106–108.

27. *Program advisory ZDV therapy for reducing perinatal HIV: Implementation in HRSA-funded programs.* (1996). Rockville, MD: U.S. Department of Health & Human Services.

28. Landers, D. V., & Sweet, R. L. (1996). Reducing mother-to-infant transmission of HIV—The door remains open. *The New England Journal of Medicine, 334,* 1664–1665.

29. Schwarz, R., & Moreno, J. (1996). HIV testing: The evolution of a policy. *Women's Health Issues, 6,* 109–111.

30. Study finds AZT reduces HIV transmission rate from mother to infant. (1994). *VOICE AWHONN, 2,* 1–2.

31. Kass, N. E., Faden, R. R., Gielen, A., & Campo, P. C. (1992). Pregnant women's knowledge of the human immunodeficiency virus: Implications for education and counseling. *Women's Health Issues, 2,* 17–25.

32. Bowd, A., & Loos, C. (1995). Gender differences in adoption of AIDS preventive behaviors: Implications for women's AIDS education programs. *Women's Health Issues, 5,* 21–26.

33. Lauver, D., Armstrong, K., Marks, S., & Schwartz, S. (1995). HIV risk status and preventive behaviors among 17,619 women. *JOGNN, 24,* 33–39.

34. Grumet, B. (1992). It's time for selected routine testing of newborns for human immunodeficiency virus. *Women's Health Issues, 2,* 12–16.

34. Wise, B. (1996). Pharmocologic update antiretroviral therapy in adults. *Journal of the American Academy of Nurse Practitioners, 8,* 329–342.

35. A new class of anti-HIV drugs debuts. (1996). *AJN, 96,* 59–63.

37. Collier, A., Coombs, R., et.al. (1996). Treatment of human immunodeficiency virus infection with saquinavir, zidovudine, and zalcitabine. *The New England Journal of Medicne, 334,* 1011–1017.

38. Baigis-Smith, J., Coombs, V.J., & Larson, E. (1994). HIV infection, exercise, and immune function. *IMAGE: Journal of Nursing Scholarship, 26,* 277–281.

39. Foley, M. E., Fahs, M. C., Eisenhandler, J., & Hyer, K. (1995). Satisfaction with home health-care services for clients with HIV: Preliminary findings. *Journal of the Association of Nurses in AIDS Care, 6,* 20–25.

40. Dimick, L. A., Levinson, R. M., Manteuffel, B. A., & Donnellan, M. (1996). Nurse practitioner's reactions to persons with HIV/AIDS: The role of patient contact and education. *Journal of the American Academy of Nurse Practitioners, 8,* 419–426.

41. Sherman, D. W. (1996). Nurses' willingness to care for AIDS patients and spirituality, social support, and death anxiety. *IMAGE: Journal of Nursing Scholarship, 28,* 205–213.

42. Landesman, S., Kalish, L., et. al. (1996). Obstetrical factors and the transmission of human immunodeficiency virus type 1 from mother to child. *The New England Journal of Medicine, 334,* 1617–1623.

43. Committee on Pediatric AIDS. (1995). Human milk, breastfeeding, and transmission of human immunodeficiency virus in the United Stattes. *Pediatrics, 96,* 977–979.

44. Bradley-Springer, L. A. (1994). Reproductive decision-making in the age of AIDS. *IMAGE: Journal of Nursing Scholarship, 26,* 241–246.

45. DeCharney, A. H., & Pernoll, M. L. (1994). *Obstetrics & gynecologic diagnosis & treatment* (4th ed.). Norwalk, CT: Appleton & Lange.

46. Hagay, Z., Levy, R., Miskin, A., Milman, D., Sharabi, H., & Insler, V. (1996). Uriscreen, a rapid enzymatic urine screening test: Useful predictor of significant bacteriuria in pregnancy. *Obstetrics & Gynecology, 87,* 410–413.

47. Brooks, A. M., & Garite, T. J. (1995). Clinical trial of the outpatient management of pyelonephritis in pregnancy. *Infectious Diseases in Obstetrics and Gynecology, 3,* 50–55.

48. Millar, L. K., Wing, D. A., Paul, R. H., & Grimes, D. A. (1995). Outpatient treatment of pyelonephritis in pregnancy: A randomized controlled trial. *Obstetrics & Gynecology, 86,* 560–564.

49. Rayburn, W. R., & Zuspan, F. P. (1992). *Drug therapy in obstetrics and gynecology* (3rd ed.). Baltimore: Mosby.

50. Prevention of perinatal Group B streptococcal disease: A public health perspective. (1996). *MMWR 45*(No.RR–7), 1–24.

51. ACOG Committee on Obstetric Practice. (1996). Prevention of early-onset Group B streptococcal disease in newborns. *Committee Opinion, 173,* 1–8.

52. Mahlmeister, L. (1996). Perinatal Group B streptococcal infections: The nurse's role in identification and prophylaxis. *Journal of Perinatal and Neonatal Nursing, 10,* 1–16.

53. Zinaman, M. J., Clegg, E., Brown, C. C., O'Connor, J., & Selevan, S. G. (1996). Estimates of human fertility and pregnancy loss. *Fertility & Sterility, 65,* 503–509.

54. Hasegawa, I., Tanaka, K., Sanada, H., Imai, T., & Fujimori, R. (1996). Studies on the dytogenetic and endocrinologic background of spontaneous abortion. *Fertility & Sterlitity, 65,* 52–54.

55. Lyon, D. (1995). Critical pathways in the management of first-trimester bleeding and pain. *The Female Patient, 20,* 19–27.

56. Maiolatesi, C., & Peddicord, K. (1996). Methotrexate for nonsurgical treatment of ectopic pregnancy: Nursing implications. *JOGNN, 25,* 205–208.

57. Brumsted, J. (1996, March). Managing ectopic pregnancy nonsurgically. *Contemporary OB/GYN,* 43–56.

58. Ankum, W. M., Mol, B. W. J., Van der Veen, F., & Bossuyt, P. M. M. (1996). Risk factors for ectopic pregnancy: A meta-analysis. *Fertility & Sterility, 65,* 1093–1099.

59. Powell, M. P., & Spellman, J. R. (1966). Medical management of the patient with an ectopic pregnancy. *Journal of Perinatal and Neonatal Nursing, 9,* 31–43.

60. Kendrick, J. S., Tierney, E. F., Lawson, H. W., Strauss, L. T., Klein, L., & Atrash, H. (1996). Previous cesarean delivery and the risk of ectopic pregnancy. *Obstetrics & Gynecology, 87,* 297–301.

61. Norwita, E. R. (1995). Persistent ectopic pregnancy. *The Female Patient, 20,* 66–74.

62. Rulin, M. C. (1995). Is aalpingostomy the surgical treatment of choice for unruptured tubal pregnancy? *Obstetrics & Gynecology, 86,* 1010–1013.

63. Gross, Z., Rodriquez, J. J., & Stalnaker, B. L. (1995). Ectopic pregnancy nonsurgical, outpatient evaluation and single-dose methotrexate treatment. *Journal of Reproductive Medicine, 40,* 371–374.

64. Soto-Wright, V., Bernstein, M., Goldstein, D. P., & Berkowitz, R. S. (1995). The changing clinical presentation of complete molar pregnancy. *Obstetrics & Gynecology, 86,* 775–779.

65. Teng, F., Magarelle, P. C., & Montz, F. J. (1995). Transvaginal probe ultrasonography diagnostic or outcome advantages in women with molar pregnancies. *Journal of Reproductive Medicine, 40,* 427–430.

66. Chelmow, D., Andrew, E., & Baker, E. (1996). Maternal cigarette smoking and placenta previa. *Obstetrics & Gynecology, 87,* 703–706.

67. Taylor, V. M., Peacock, S., Kramer, M. D., & Vaughan, T. L. (1995). Increased risk of placental previa among women of Asian origin. *Obstetrics & Gynecology, 86,* 805–808.

68. Huzel, P., & Remsburg-Bell, E. (1996). Fetal complications related to minor maternal trauma. *JOGNN, 25,* 121–124.

69. McFarlane, J., Parker, B., & Soeken, K. (1996). Abuse during pregnancy: Associations with maternal health and infant birth weight. *Nursing Research, 45,* 37–42.

70. Hoffman, J. (1993). Iron deficiency anemia: An update. *Journal of Perinatal and Neonatal Nursing, 6,* 13–20.

71. Mani, S., & Duffy, T. (1995). Anemia of pregnancy. *Clinics in Perinatology, 22,* 593–607.

72. Bushnell, F. K. L. (1992). A guide to primary care of iron-deficiency anemia. *Nurse Practitioner, 17,* 68–74.

73. Czeizel, A. (1995). Folic acid in the prevention of neural tube defects. *Journal of Pediatric Gastroenterology and Nutrition, 20,* 4–16.

74. Recommendations for the use of folic acid to reduce the number of cases of spina bifida and other neural tube defects. (1992). *MMWR, 41*(No. RR–14), 1–7.

75. Romanczuk, A., & Brown, J. (1994). Folic acid will reduce risk of neural tube defects. *MCN, 19,* 331–334.

76. Folic acid supplement recommended to avoid recurrent NTDs. (1993, February 8). *ACOG Newsletter.*

77. Romano, P., Waitzman, N., Scheffler, R., & Pi, R. D. (1995). Folic acid fortification of grain: An economic analysis. *American Journal of Public Health, 85,* 667–676.

78. Crane, N., Wilson, D., Cook, D. A., Lewis, C., Yetley, E., & Rader, J. (1995). Evaluating food fortification options: General principles revisited with folic acid. *American Journal of Public Health, 85,* 660–666.

79. Esposito, N. W. (1992). Thalassemia: Simple screening for hereditary anemias. *Nurse Practitioner, 17,* 50–61.

80. Smith, J., Espeland, M., Bellevue, R., Bonds, D., Brown, A., & Koshy, M. (1996). Pregnancy in sickle cell disease: Experience of the cooperative study of sickle cell disease. *Obstetrics & Gynecology, 87,* 199–205.

81. Hypertension in pregnancy. (1996). *ACOG Technical Bulletin 219,* 1–8.

82. Roberts, J. (1994). Current perspectives on preeclampsia. *Journal of Nurse-Midwifery, 39,* 70–90.

83. Queenan, J. T. (Ed.). (1994). *Management of high-risk pregnancy.* Boston: Blackwell Scientific Publications.

84. Bucher, H. C., Guyatt, G. H., Cook, R. J., Hatala, R., Cook, D. J., Lang, J., & Hunt, D. (1996). Effect of calcium supplementation on pregnancy-induced hypertension and preeclampsia. *JAMA, 275,* 1113–1117.

85. Suarez, V., Trelles, J., & Miyahira, J. (1996). Urinary calcium in asymptomataic primigravidas who later developed preeclampsia. *Obstetrics & Gynecology, 87,* 79–82.

86. Samadi, A. R., Mayberry, R. M., Zaidi, A. A., Pleasant, J. C., McGhee, N., Rich, R. J. (1996). Maternal hypertension and associated pregnancy complications among African-American and other women in the United States. *Obstetrics & Gynecology, 87,* 557–563.

87. Sisson, M., & Sauer, P. (1995). Pharmacologic therapy for pregnancy-induced hypertension. *Journal of Perinatal and Neonatal Nursing, 9,* 1–12.

88. Visser, W., & Wallenburg, H. C. S. (1995). Temporising management of severe pre-eclampsia with and without the HELLP syndrome. *British Journal of Obstetrics and Gynecology, 102,* 111–117.

89. Halligan, A., Shennan, A., Lambert, P. C., Swiet, M., & Taylor, D. J. (1996). Diurnal blood pressure difference in the assessment of preeclampsia. *Obstetrics & Gynecology, 87,* 205–208.

90. Morris, J., Fay, R., Ellwood, D., Cook, C., & Devonald, K. J. (1996). A randomized controlled trial of aspirin in patients with abnormal uterine artery blood flow. *Obstetrics & Gynecology, 87,* 74–78.

91. Roberts, J. (1995). Magnesium for preeclampsia and eclampsia. *The New England Journal of Medicine, 333,* 250–251.

92. The Eclampsia Trial Collaborative Group. (1995). Which anticonvulsant for women with eclampsia? Evidence from the collaborative eclampsia trial. *Lancet, 345,* 1455–1463.

93. AWHONN. (1994). Clinical Commentary: Invasive Hemodynamic Monitoring in High-Risk Intrapartum Nursing. Committee on Practice.

94. Harvey, M. (1992). Critical care for the maternity patient. *MCN, 17,* 296–309.

95. Chauhan, S., Perry, K., McLaughlin, B., Roberts, W., Sullivan, C., & Morrison, J. (1996). Diabetic ketoacidosis complicating pregnancy. *Journal of Perinatology, 16,* 173–175.

96. ACOG. (1994). Diabetes and Pregnancy Number 200. ACOG Technical Bulletin.

97. Rosenn, B., Miodovnik, M., Khoury, J., & Siddiqi, T. (1996). Counterregulatory hormonal responses to hypoglycemia during pregnancy. *Obstetrics & Gynecology, 87,* 568–574.

98. Marconi, A. M., Paolini, C., Buscaglia, M., Zerbe, G., Battaglia, F., & Pardi, G. (1996). The impact of gestational age and fetal growth on the maternal-fetal glucose concentration difference. *Obstetrics & Gynecology, 87,* 937–942.

99. Homko, C., Nyirjesy, P., Sivan, E., & Reece, E. A. (1995). The interrelationship between ethnicity and gestational diabetes in fetal macrosomia. *Diabetes Care, 18,* 1442–1445.

100. Rodgers, B., & Rodgers, D. (1996). Efficacy of preconception care of diabetic women in a community setting. *The Journal of Reproductive Medicine, 41,* 422–426.

101. Landy, H., Gomez-Marin, O., & O'Sullivan, M. J. (1996). Diagnosing gestational diabetes mellitus: Use of a glucose screen without administering the glucose tolerance test. *Obstetrics & Gynecology.*

102. Berkus, M., Langer, O., Piper, J., & Luther, M. (1995). Efficiency of lower threshold criteria for the diagnosis of gestational diabetes. *Obstetrics & Gynecology, 86,* 892–896.

103. Carpenter, M., Canick, J., Star, J., Carr, S., Burke, M. E., & Shahinian, K. (1996). Fetal hyperinsulinism at 14–20 weeks and subsequent gestational diabetes. *Obstetrics & Gynecology, 87,* 89–93.

104. York, R., Brown, L. P., Miovech, S., & Armstrong, C. L. (1995). Pregnant women with diabetes: Antepartum and postpartum morbidity. *The Diabetes Educator, 21,* 211–213.

105. York, R., Brown, L. P., Armstrong, C. P., & Jacobsen, B. S. (1996). Affect in diabetic women during pregancy and postpartum. *Nursing Research, 45,* 54–56.

106. Arstrong, C. (1996). Relationships between the perceived impact of gestational diabetes mellitus and treatment adherence. *JOGNN, 25,* 601–607.

107. Livingston, E., Herbert, W., Hage, M., Chapman, J. F., & Stubbs, T. M. (1995). Use of the Tdx-FLM Assay in evaluating fetal lung maturity in an insulin-dependent diabetic population. *Obstetrics & Gynecology, 86,* 26–29.

108. Coustan, D. R. (1996). Management of gestational diabetes mellitus: A self-fulfilling prophecy? *JAMA, 275,* 1199–1200.

109. Naylor, C. D., Sermer, M., Chen, E., & Sykora, K. (1996). Cesarean delivery in relation to birth weight and gestational glucose tolerance. *JAMA, 275,* 1165–1170.

110. Novy, M. J., McGregor, J. A., & Iams, J. D. (1995). New perspectives on the prevention of extreme prematurity. *Clinical Obstetrics and Gynecology, 38,* 790–808.

111. Miller, H. S., Lesser, K., & Reed, K. L. (1996). Adolescence and very low birth weight infants: A disproportionate association. *Obstetrics & Gynecology, 87,* 83–88.

112. Hillier, S., Nugent, R. P., Eschenbach, D. A., et. al. (1995). Association between bacterial vaginosis and preterm delivery of a low-birth-weight infant. *The New England Journal of Medicine, 333,* 1737–1742.

113. Goldenberg, R. L. (1996). Editorial: Intrauterine infection and why preterm prevention programs have failed. *American Journal of Public Health, 86,* 781–783.

114. Hauth, J. C., Goldenberg, R. L., Andrews, W. W., DuBard, M. B., & Copper, R. L. (1995). Reduced incidence of preterm delivery with metronidazole and erythromycin in women with bacterial vaginosis. *The New England Journal of Medicine, 333,* 1732–1736.

115. Kundsin, R. B., Leviton, A., Allred, E., & Poulin, S. A. (1996) Ureaplasma urealyticum infection of the placenta in pregnancies that ended prematurely. *Obstetrics & Gynecology, 87,* 122–127.

116. Ceron-Mereles, P., Harlow, S. D., & Sanchez-Carrillo, C. I. (1996). The risk of prematurity and small-for-gestational-age birth in Mexico City: The effects of working conditions and antenatal leave. *American Journal of Public Health, 86,* 825–831.

117. Henrikson, T. B., Hedegaard, M., Secher, N. J., & Wilcox, A. J. (1995). Standing at work and preterm delivery. *British Journal of Obstetrics and Gynecology, 102,* 198–206.

118. Iams, Jay, Goldenberg, R. L., Meis, P. J. et al. (1996). The length of the cervix and the risk of spontaneous premature delivery. *New England Journal of Medicine, 334,* 567–572.

119. Iams, J. D., Casal, D., McGregor, J. A., et.al. (1995). Fetal fibronectin improves the accuracy of diagnosis of preterm labor. *American Journal of Obstetrics and Gynecology, 173,* 141–145.

120. Morrison, J. C., Naef, R. W. III, Botte, J. J., Katz, M., Belluomini, J. M., & McLaughlin, B. N. (1996). Prediction of spontaneous preterm birth by fetal fibronectin and uterine activity. *Obstetrics & Gynecology, 87,* 649–655.

121. Goldenberg, R. L., Thom, E., Moawad, A. H., Johnson, F., Roberts, J., & Caritis, S. N. (1996). The preterm prediction study: Fetal fibronecting, bacterial vaginosis, and peripartum infection. *Obstetrics & Gynecology, 87,* 656–660.

122. Garite, T. J., & Lockwood, C. J. (1996). A new test for diagnosis and prediction of preterm delivery. *Contemporary OB/GYN, 41,* 77–93.

123. Yoon, B. H., Yang, S. H., Jun, J. K., Park, K. H., Kim, C. J., & Romero, R. (1996). Maternal blood C-reactive protein, white blood cell count, and temperature in preterm labor: A comparison with amniotic fluid white blood cell count. *Obstetrics & Gynecology, 87,* 231–237.

124. Mazor, M., Furman, B., Wiznitzer, A., Shoham-Vardi, I., Cohen, J., & Ghezzi, F. (1995). Maternal and perinatal outcome of patients with preterm labor and meconium-stained amniotic fluid. *Obstetrics & Gynecology, 86,* 830–833.

125. Eganhouse, D. J. (1994). A nursing model for a community hospital preterm birth prevention program. *JOGNN, 23,* 756–766.

126. Hueston, W. J., Knox, M. A., Eilers, G., Pauwels, J., & Lonsdorf, D. (1995). The effectiveness of preterm-birth prevention educational programs for high-risk women: A meta-analysis. *Obstetrics & Gynecology, 86,* 705–712.

127. Fiscella, K. (1996). Racial partners in preterm births. *Public Health Reports, 111,* 104–113.

128. Viamontes, C. (1996). Pharmocologic intervention in the management of preterm labor: An update. *Journal of perinatal and neonatal nursing, 9,* 13–30.

129. Romeo, C. C., & Jones, P. (1994). Home infusion therapies for obstetric patients. *JOGNN, 23,* 675–681.

130. ACOG Committee on Obstetric Practice. (1996). *Home uterine activity monitoring,* 172.

131. Edenfield, S. M., Thomas, S. D., Thompson, W. O., & Marcotte, J. J. (1995). Validity of the Creasy risk appraisal instrument for prediction of preterm labor. *Nursing Research, 44,* 76–81.

132. Hellemans, P., Gerris, J., & Verdonk, P. (1995). Fetal fibronectin detection for prediction of preterm birth in low risk women. *British Journal of Obstetrics and Gynecology, 102,* 207–212.

133. Jones, D. P., & Collins, B. A. (1996). The nursing management of women experiencing preterm labor: Clinical guidelines and why they are needed. *JOGNN, 25,* 569–592.

134. Lantz, M. E., & Porter, K. B. (1995). Home uterine activity monitoring update on the literature. *The Female Patient, 20,* 80–88.

135. Schroider, C. (1996). Women's experience of bed rest in high-risk pregnancy. *IMAGE: Journal of Nursing Scholarship, 28,* 253–258.

136. May, K. (1994). Impact of maternal activity restriction for preterm labor on the expectant father. *JOGNN, 23,* 246–251.

137. Grohar, J. (1994). Nursing protocols for antepartum home care. *JOGNN, 23,* 687–694.

138. Hart, M. (1996). Nursing implications of self-care in pregnancy. *MCN, 21,* 137–143.

139. Maloni, J. (1994). Home care of the high-risk pregnant woman requiring bed rest. *JOGNN, 23,* 696–706.

140. Stringer, M., Spatz, D., & Donahue, D. (1994). Maternal-fetal physical assessment in the home setting: Role of the advanced practice nurse. *JOGNN, 23,* 720–725.

141. Freda, M. C., & DeVore, N. (1996). Should intravenous hydration be the first line of defense with threatened preterm labor? A critical review of the literature. *Journal of Perinatology, 16,* 385–389.

142. Weinstein, L., Okin, C. R., & Fellens, T. E. (1996). The CLIPED procedure: An attempt to improve perinatal outcome in hopeless situations. *Journal of Perinatology, 16,* 27–30.

143. Corbett, J. V., & Omlin, K. (1995). Prenatal and postnatal use of corticosteroids. *MCN, 20,* 346.

144. Modanlou, H. D., Beharry, K., Padilla, G., & Iriye, B. (1996). Combined effects of antenatal corticosteroids and surfactant supplementation on the outcome of very low birth weight infants. *Journal of Perinatology, 16,* 422–428.

145. Kearney, M. H., Murphy, S., Irwin, K., & Rosenbaum, M. (1995). Salvaging self: A grounded theory of pregnancy on crack cocaine. *Nursing Research, 44,* 208–213.

146. Tiedje, L. B., & Starn, J. R. (1996). Intervention model for substance-using women. *IMAGE: Journal of Nursing Scholarship, 28,* 113–118.

147. Laken, M. P., & Hutchins, E. (1996). *Recruitment and retention of substance-using pregnant and parenting women.* Rockville, MD: U.S. Department of Health and Human Services.

148. Martin, S. L., English, K. T., Andersen, K. et. al. (1996). Violence and substance use among North Carolina pregnant women. *American Journal of Public Health, 86,* 991–998.

149. Miller, W. H., Cox, S. M., Harbison, V., & Campbell, B. (1994). Urine drug screens for drug abuse in pregnancy: Problems and pitfalls. *Women's Health Issues, 4,* 152–155.

150. Budd, K. (1995). Perinatal substance use: Promoting abstinence in acute care settngs. *AACN Clinical Issues, 6,* 70–78.

151. Koniak-Griffin, D., & Brecht, M. L. (1995). Linkages between sexual risk taking, substance use, and AIDS knowledge among pregnant adolescents and young mothers. *Nursing Research, 44,* 340–346.

152. Kinney, J. (1991). *Clinical manual of substance abuse.* St. Louis: Mosby Year Book.

153. Horrigan, T., Piazza, N. J., Weinstein, L. (1996). The Substance Abuse Subtle Screening Inventory is more cost effective and has better selectivity than urine toxicology for the detection of substance abuse in pregnancy. *Journal of Perinatology, 16,* 326–330.

154. Ludwig, M. A., Marecki, M., Wooldridge, P. J., & Sherman, L. M. (1996). Neonatal nurses' knowledge of and attitudes toward caring for cocaine-exposed infants and their mothers. *Journal of Perinatal and Neonatal Nursing, 9,* 81–95.

155. Billman, D. O., Nemeth, P. B., Heimler, R., & Sasidharan, P. (1996). Prenatal cocaine/polydrug exposure: Effect of race on outcome. *Journal of Perinatology, 16,* 366–369.

156. Weiner, S. M. (1992). *Perinatal impact of substance abuse module 3 nursing issues for the 21st Century.* White Plains, NY: March of Dimes Birth Defects Foundation.

157. Skupski, D. K. (1996). Maternal complications of twin gestation. *The Female Patient, 21,* 72–84.

158. Chervenak, F. A., Newman, R., Evans, M. I., Reece, E. A., & Devoe, L. D. (1993). Multiple Gestation, *The Female Patient, 18,* 14–33.

159. Corchia, C., Mastroiacovo, P., Lanni, R., Mannazzu, R., Curro, V., & Fabris, C. (1996). What proportion of multiple births are due to ovulation induction? A register-based study in Italy. *American Journal of Public Health, 86,* 851–854.

160. Chauban, S. P., Cowan, B., Brost, B., Washburne, J. F., Magann, E. F., & Morrison, J. C. (1996). Estimating birth weight in twins. *The Journal of Reproductive Medicine, 41,* 403–408.

161. Spillman, J. (1987, Mar.). The emotional aspect of multiple pregnancy—The midwife's in support of the family. *Midwives Chronicle & Nursing Notes,* 58–62.

162. Lantz, M. E., Chez, R., Rodriguez, A., & Porter, K. (1996). Maternal weight gain patterns and birth weight outcome in twin gestation. *Obstetrics & Gynecology, 87,* 551–556.

CHAPTER 19

ASSESSING FETAL WELL-BEING

Marion Herndon Fuqua

Highlights

*I*t is often a dilemma
for the client to make
the choices presented
by screening and as-
sessment tests.

- Nursing Diagnoses
- Pregnancy at Risk
- Sequencing Advanced Fetal Testing
- Fetal Movement Counts
- Fetal Heart Rate Assessment
- Nonstress Test and Contraction Stress Test
- Screening for Size/Dates Discrepancies
- Screening and Prevention of Rh Isoimmunization
- Maternal Serum Screening
- Ultrasonography
- Biophysical Profile Studies
- Doppler Flow Studies
- Amniocentesis and Chorionic Villus Sampling
- Percutaneous Umbilical Blood Sampling
- Development of Screening Technology

▶ INTRODUCTION

The assessment of fetal well-being is both a subjective and an objective task, the success of which depends on open communication between the health care provider and the client. Very simple noninvasive assessments, such as perception of fetal movement and fundal height measurement, have been used for years. Technological advances in assessing the fetus and improving the chances of fertility not only for older women but also for women with disease have required that the health care provider gain increasing knowledge and skill. Allowing advanced practice nurses to perform antepartum testing not only provides continuity of care by providing education and medical care to the mother and fetus but also provides access to care in outlying areas where care would not be available.

Technological advances in assessing the fetus may initiate a number of questions, often leaving the health care provider with further questions, and a client with new fears and anxieties about her pregnancy. Asking one question always leads to another, as Pandora's box is opened. As one author stated, "There is as yet an untested possibility that the reduction in mortality could be overshadowed by a higher incidence of long-term handicap because of a possible increase in the number of planned preterm deliveries of sick babies."[1] It will continue to be a struggle to decrease perinatal mortality without increasing the rate of inappropriate obstetric intervention.

Nursing Diagnoses for Fetal Assessment

Diagnosis, interpretation, and management or referral often are foremost in providing quality fetal assessment. Counseling, support, and education for mother and family are critical care elements that reduce anxiety about the unknown developing fetus and enable the health care provider to achieve continuity of care. The following list of nursing diagnoses, though by no means complete, does give insight into the time and attention needed for "supportive" care. Because the nursing diagnoses listed here apply to most of the tests described in this chapter, they are not repeated with the descriptions of the tests. Although only one or a few specific applications of the diagnosis may be given in this list, there are many other situations that are applicable.

Of utmost importance is to take into account racial-ethnic differences when counseling clients: a recent study revealed African American and Latina women to be less likely to use prenatal diagnosis as compared to white and Asian women, suggesting beliefs about testing, termination, and raising a disabled child may be unique to each racial-ethnic group; attitudes may be specific for the racial-ethnic group as opposed to socioeconomic status.[2] Cultural differences concerning pregnancy and disability do exist and need to be appreciated in order to provide information that enables the client to make an informed decision about fetal assessment. Variations in knowledge and access to prenatal diagnostic services influence a client's decisions as well and need to be assessed with each individual.[2,3]

GENERAL NURSING DIAGNOSES WITH FETAL TESTING[4]

- *High Risk for Injury.* An obvious risk of invasive assessment techniques, such as chorionic villus sampling and amniocentesis, is the potential for injury. Such potential also exists for client and fetus with substance abuse and with oligohydramnios (compressed cord). Each client identified as a substance abuser should be considered at risk for fetal insult, and depending on the clinical status, will dictate the surveillance needed to assess fetal well-being. A coordinated plan of care relies on a team approach, helping not only the client through a treatment program but also the fetus with a plan of care for assessment, depending on the status of the client. Refer to Chapter 18 as well on Substance Abuse.

- *Powerlessness.* Once advanced fetal assessments begin, particularly daily or biweekly, a client may feel as though her body cannot properly care for the fetus or provide an adequate environment. Powerlessness applies, for example, to an isoimmunized client who cannot control the hemolysis of fetal red blood cells or to the client who may be bleeding herself due to abruptio placentae or placenta previa. The client's control may be limited or lost because of the medical condition of the fetus or client.

- *Altered Comfort.* Comfort is disrupted by invasive tests or complete bed rest. Comfort is perceived differently by each individual and therefore should be explored with the client.

- *Anxiety.* Almost every woman with a normal pregnancy has some anxiety. Anxiety is heightened with complications and can be reinforced by additional fetal assessment. Some clients welcome the opportunity to follow their fetus more closely; others see testing as a reminder that their pregnancy is not normal. There may be uncertainty for the client about whether she will carry the fetus to term or whether delivery will be vaginal or cesarean.

- *Fear.* A woman with a history of fetal loss or complications is understandably fearful when faced with the possibility of fetal loss or fetal anomaly. Cultural and religious teachings or beliefs may increase fear if testing is not discussed thoroughly with the client.

- *Ineffective Individual Coping or Compromised, Disabled, or Ineffective Family Coping.* Coping skills may be increasingly stressed during pregnancy if testing or procedures are begun early in gestation or if roles within the family are disrupted (e.g., when a client is on strict bed rest or is hospitalized). If assessments are daily or weekly, continued support and encouragement are needed, as well as inquiries about how testing may be affecting the client, the father, and other family members. Ineffective coping may be encountered with fetal demise, termination of pregnancy, and fetal anomalies. Culture may influence coping mechanisms.

- *Noncompliance.* A knowledge deficit or cultural or religious beliefs may cause noncompliance in fetal testing. Noncompliance is also seen among substance abusers, particularly those who fear legal repercussions. Furthermore, noncompliance may occur if a client is unable or unwilling to give up her various roles, such as those of being a mother, wife, or businesswoman.

- *Spiritual Distress.* Spiritual distress is an obvious diagnosis for a client considering termination of pregnancy and may also be significant if blood products or fetal surgery is required. A client may interpret poor outcome or pregnancy problems as punishment for something she has done.

- *Grieving, Anticipatory and/or Dysfunctional.* Applicable for a client carrying a fetus with structural or chromosomal anomalies or in the event of fetal demise. Allow the client to grieve the loss of a "perfect infant." Be attuned to the client or family unable to grieve or voice feelings or for whom there are no support systems. If a client has experienced a prior pregnancy loss, assess whether she resolved her grief before the current pregnancy. Consider also when the fetus has a chromosomal or structural anomaly that is incompatible with life.

- *Social Isolation.* A client who is on strict bed rest or hospitalized may be socially isolated. Terminating a pregnancy without family or social support may also be difficult for a client. Fetal demise or an infant with an anomaly also causes isolation, as friends and family have difficulty responding to grieving parents.

- *Altered Parenting.* Parenting can be altered among substance abusers and women with problematic pregnancies. Testing and management may disrupt family roles and, consequently, future parenting. A client may associate the infant with the financial and psychological stresses of pregnancy and perceive the infant differently than she does her other children.

EMOTIONAL SUPPORT

- *Counsel the Client Before and After Each Test.* Prior to any test, ensure that the nature of the test, the information that it will provide, and the possibility of further intervention or testing are explained to the client. Counseling occurs before optional screening (e.g., α-fetoprotein) or testing to investigate a perceived risk to the client or fetus. It is often a dilemma for the client to make choices presented by some screening and assessment tests. Any risks to the client or fetus also are reviewed. To reinforce discussions and reduce anxiety, provide written information and answer questions thoroughly. Tell the client when test results are expected.

If maternal or fetal risk is the indication for assessment, for example, in cases of diabetes mellitus, the client needs to understand the particular risk, how it affects her pregnancy, and why various tests are important to assess fetal well-being. Depending on the clinical situation, several testing modalities are used. Often a client may become frustrated when one test cannot provide the necessary information, and it may be difficult for her to appreciate why different tests are required. If the health care provider explains the need for assessment, the benefits for both fetus and client, and encourages her to voice her opinions in the decision making process, the client will see herself as part of the solution, not the problem. Hence, the client is able to positively participate in the plan of care. If the client is upset over the need for tests or the results of tests, she may not "hear" what is being said. Therefore, include the support person or significant other in the counseling, and if possible, wait until the client is ready to hear available options. A support person can later help the client to recall the plan of care when her anxiety eases.

- *Acknowledge the Normalcy of Feelings of Guilt.* A client may feel guilty if she feels inconvenienced by testing but realizes its importance. Having to put the fetus first for 9 months can be stressful during a healthy pregnancy, much less a complicated one requiring invasive or time consuming procedures. With isoimmunization, for example, a client may feel guilty about her body "rejecting" or "harming" the fetus. Allow her to express those feelings. Reinforce the fact that she cannot control the actual isoimmunization process but can work with the health care team to provide the best care possible for her fetus and by doing so is helping her fetus.

- *Provide Support When an Infant Has a Chromosomal or Structural Anomaly.* The parents of a fetus with an abnormality may resent the invasive, lengthy procedures and wonder why they are necessary. The health care provider must be prepared to respond in such situations. The client must be informed of diagnoses and, where appropriate, referred to support groups for additional information. Support groups can be extremely helpful in assisting the client with the transition from being pregnant to caring for an infant with an abnormality. In addition, the client needs to grieve the loss of a "perfect child."

- *Provide Support If the Client Chooses Termination.* A client who chooses to terminate her pregnancy for any reason also needs support. This may be particularly true if termination is performed during the first or second trimester when the client has started "showing," heard the fetal heartbeat, felt movement, seen the fetus with ultrasound, and perhaps confided to friends and family that she is pregnant. The decision to terminate a pregnancy is likely to be a very difficult one.

- *Be Aware of Spiritual Distress.* Spiritual distress may be encountered when the client or fetus requires blood (as with isoimmunization) or blood products (Rhogam). Although it is difficult, the client and health care provider may need to consult with legal sources concerning client and fetus rights. Spiritual distress may also be encountered with termination of a pregnancy, spontaneous abortion, fetal demise, or neonatal death. Clients who have a fetus with a structural or chromosomal anomaly may feel this is due to punishment for something they have done "wrong," or as a reflection upon their value as an individual. This can have significant repercussions within the family unit. There may be situations in which the health care provider may not be able to attend to the needs of the client. Further psychological, spiritual, or financial intervention may be necessary. The health care provider can be a valuable mediator in such instances, especially by ensuring that appropriate follow-up for abnormal test results is made available to the client *before* she undergoes various tests.

INDICATIONS FOR FETAL ASSESSMENT

Routine Assessment

Routine fetal assessment begins at the first prenatal visit. Fundal height is measured or a bimanual examination is performed to assess uterine size. If applicable, the fetal heartbeat is auscultated and the client's perception of fetal movement is determined.

This routine standard of care continues for all pregnancies until delivery. Some women begin pregnancy with risk factors (e.g., diabetes) that warrant further fetal surveillance. Furthermore, complications of fetal or maternal origin may arise during pregnancy and require fetal testing. Surveillance or testing is done to monitor a fetus that may be at risk for poor outcome. Some tests, such as a α-fetoprotein, should be offered to all women as a screening method; a risk factor need not be present.

Advanced Assessment

In general, advanced assessment is indicated when there is the risk of uteroplacental insufficiency, but it also can be indicated because of fetal factors, such as decreased movement. Each clinical situation is individualized for client and fetus. While some risk factors can be identified at the initial prenatal visit, a significant percentage of problems arise in pregnancies without any risk factors.[5] Not all health care providers believe that each of the following conditions warrants testing. Moreover, protocols concerning the onset and frequency of indications that warrant particular tests vary among institutions. As technology progresses and the etiology of fetal compromise is further understood, the list may grow.

Fetal Conditions[5,6,7]
- Premature rupture of membranes
- Isoimmunization
- Decreased fetal movement
- Any irregularity of fetal heartrate heard with Doppler ultrasound
- History or presence of congenital anomalies
- Intrauterine growth retardation, presence or history of
- Abnormal amniotic fluid volume
- Premature rupture of membranes

Maternal Conditions[5-9]
- Advanced maternal age (for genetic screening)
- Unexplained vaginal bleeding
- Postdate pregnancy
- Multiple gestation
- Unexplained high α-fetoprotein
- Poor obstetric history, history of fetal loss
- Maternal substance abuse
- Nutritional and eating disorders
- Uterine structural anomalies

Significant Maternal Disease[6,7,10,11]
- Chronic hypertension
- Diabetes mellitus, insulin dependent or gestational
- Pregnancy induced hypertension
- Anemia
- Hemoglobinopathies
- Cardiac, renal, pulmonary, or connective tissue disease
- Hyperthyroidism
- Systemic lupus erythematosus

Advanced Assessment for Pregnancies at Risk

Disagreement exists about when advanced fetal assessment should begin, but the following guidelines generally can be used.

- *Have an Accurate Estimation of Gestational Age for the High Risk Pregnancy.* For example, a client with a previous ectopic should have an ultrasound done early in the first trimester to confirm an intrauterine pregnancy. Accurate dating is also important for clients with chronic diseases such as diabetes and hypertension, or a history of an IUGR infant.
- *Begin as Complications Arise.* For example, once intrauterine growth retardation or preeclampsia is diagnosed, fetal surveillance should begin.
- *Anticipate Events.* Begin 2 weeks before the time the problem arose during the previous pregnancy. Weeks and colleagues[12] suggest, however, that surveillance begin at 32 weeks with a history of demise, unless the fetal loss was before this in the previous pregnancy; then begin assessment 2 weeks prior to the diagnosis of the previous demise.[12]

- *Begin at 26 Weeks of Gestation in the Presence of Maternal Disease.* Testing should begin when a clinician would consider intervening on the behalf of the fetus, which is usually 26 weeks,[10] although Manning begins antenatal testing using the biophysical profile at 25 weeks.[13] Most fetuses have a placental reserve until 32–34 weeks' gestation, at which time surveillance can begin for various clinical indications, except when maternal disease is severe, and then begin testing at 26 weeks.[10]
- *Assess the Postdate Fetus (Gestational Age Greater than 40 Weeks).* If the only indication for assessment is postdates, then weekly surveillance is usually acceptable. The frequency of assessment ranges from daily to weekly depending on diagnosis severity (if applicable) and fetal and maternal status. Many centers begin testing at 41 weeks.[10]
- *Frequency of Testing.* This is based on the clinical condition of the mother and fetus. Some diseases dictate frequent testing as fetal compromise could be sudden, as in insulin dependent diabetes, and testing is usually twice weekly.[11] If the potential for compromise is rapid, such as with isoimmunization, testing may be daily or twice daily.[11]
- *Assess in the First Trimester If Fetal Therapy is Possible.* For example, the fetus who has alloimmune anemia requiring transfusion should be tested in the first trimester.[11] Once testing is initiated, various options are available if the fetus is compromised, although delivery may not be a feasible option, depending on gestational age of the fetus and the adequacy of the facility to care for a premature infant. With the advances in technology, intervention on behalf of the fetus does not necessarily indicate delivery.[11]

Surgical fetal therapy is being researched to correct potentially lethal anomalies, but is still investigational.[14] Currently there are several fetal conditions that can be successfully treated in utero through medical management of the mother. These include metabolic, endocrinologic, cardiovascular and hematologic disorders, as well as fetal infections, such as parvovirus and toxoplasmosis.[15] Treatment consists of medicating the mother for the specific condition; assessment to evaluate therapeutic fetal drug levels can be evaluated through percutaneous umbilical blood sampling.[15]

Stem cell transplantation is also under investigation. Stem cells are a unique group of bone marrow cells capable of self-renewal, multilineage proliferation, and differentiation.[16] These cells have been found in bone marrow, peripheral blood, fetal cord blood, and the fetal liver.[16] These cells could be infused into the fetus early in gestation intraperitoneally or via percutaneous umbilical blood sampling prior to target organ damage.[16] Genetic disorders for which this would be an option of treatment would be congenital bone marrow disorders, such as metachromatic leukodystrophy.[16]

SEQUENCING ADVANCED FETAL TESTING

Testing can begin for a variety of reasons at any gestational age. Some tests are more appropriate than others. The Appendix (at the end of this chapter) provides an algorithm of fetal testing that might be used once problems arise.[17] It is one of many available frameworks to be adjusted within institutional protocols. No single test can be regarded as the exclusive choice for assessing fetal well-being as each test reveals different parameters of fetal pathophysiology, often in a complimentary manner.[18]

FETAL ASSESSMENT

FETAL MOVEMENT

Maternal perception of fetal movement correlates with fetal well-being.[19] Fetal movement is usually perceived by the client at 16 to 20 weeks' gestation.[19] By the use of ultrasound, fetal movement has been noted as early as 6–8 weeks.[19,20] A normal fetus has coordinated movements by 16 to 20 weeks of gestation. Perceived fetal movement is most often related to trunk and limb motion and rollovers, or flips.[20] Generally, during the second half of pregnancy, fetal movement becomes more organized, and weaker movements are replaced by stronger movements, which increase in frequency and peak in the 32nd week.[19] Thereafter, fetal movement declines gradually by 40 weeks; however, at term the normal fetus has an average of 40 fetal movements a day.[19] After 36 weeks, only 15 percent of fetal movement is perceived by the client, and usually only those movements lasting beyond 20 seconds.[19] Maternal perception of movement may also diminish, as a result of decreasing amniotic fluid volume, improved fetal coordination, fetal sleep cycles, and increased fetal size, thereby decreasing uterine volume.[19]

Significance of Fetal Movement

Decreased fetal movement may be indicative of asphyxia and intrauterine growth retardation.[19] The compromised fetus decreases oxygen requirements by decreasing activity; documented cessation of activity is a possible indication of impending demise, and a decrease in activity is usually due to chronic, as opposed to acute, fetal distress.[20]

Even with a reassuring fetal heart rate, decreased fetal movement is a sensitive indicator of fetal distress. It should be a red flag to the clinician when the client reports decreased fetal movement, even in the presence of normal electronic fetal monitoring as a client's perception is often more reliable than electronic monitoring.[12] Clients with underlying "silent" problems but no obvious risk factors may be identified only through decreased fetal movement. Approximately 50 percent of stillbirths occur in the absence of any maternal or fetal risk factors.[20]

Factors That Decrease Fetal Movement

Maternal use of barbiturates, alcohol, methadone, narcotics, or cigarettes may decrease fetal movement; however, constant activity has been seen in fetuses of mothers addicted to narcotics.[21] The drug's effect depends on the amount used, concurrent use of other drugs, and the route by which the drug is taken (i.e., intravenous injection, inhalation, or oral).

Decreased movement, however, may be due to fetal sleep cycles or to inactivity during a particular time of day.[19] Fetuses do have circadian rhythms, and mothers note that fetal movement tends to be greatest during the evening.[19]

Fetal and placental factors associated with decreased fetal movement or abnormal patterns of fetal movement include anencephaly, ischemia, chromosome abnormalities, growth retardation and neuromuscular disease.[20] Some malformed fetuses, however, may have patterns of movement similar to those of normal fetuses.[20] A fetus with severe intrauterine growth retardation (characterized by fetal weight below the fifth percentile for the given gestational age) may have diminished activity. Mild growth retardation, on the other hand, does not appear to reduce the number of fetal movements.[20]

FETAL MOVEMENT COUNTS (FMCS)

Procedure. Instruct all clients to perform fetal movement counts (FMCs) after 28 weeks' gestation. To heighten client awareness of fetal movement, instruct her to do FMCs daily using a protocol such as the following. Several other counting methods have been devised.[7,20]

- Record the start time, then lie in the left lateral position, preferably after a meal or when the fetus is most active. A quiet location is best.
- Place a hand over the abdomen to palpate movement. You may also sit or stand if you are able to detect movement.
- Remain in this position until you have counted 10 fetal movements.
- Record the end time.

To ensure continuity, FMCs should be done at approximately the same time each day. If *10* movements are not obtained within *1 hour,* then further testing is indicated (e.g., a nonstress test).[20] Using this method, most clients feel 10 movements within 30 minutes; participation in FMCs is heightened when less than 1 hour is spent each day counting fetal movements.[20]

Fetal surveillance should be initiated within 12 hours of a client's perception of decreased activity; consider an NST.[20]

Advantages and Disadvantages. Performing FMCs is simple, inexpensive and does not require machinery. The client may proceed at her own convenience and in privacy. FMCs can promote maternal-fetal bonding.[20] Fetal compromise is often first realized when FMCs are initiated. Presence of adequate fetal movement offers some assurance of lack of fetal compromise.

There are also disadvantages to FMCs. A pregnant woman who is busy throughout the day and unable to lie quietly and focus on her fetus may feel less movement. An obese woman may feel less movement, although this has not been well documented. A client may become anxious if movement is difficult to palpate or perceive, particularly if the pregnancy is problematic or if there is a history of fetal demise.

Client Teaching and Counseling. Provide the client with detailed information concerning FMCs, including the significance of decreased fetal movement and the need to inform the health care provider promptly of any irregularity. Inquire about the client's FMCs at each visit to enhance the provider/client relationship and to stress the importance of FMCs.

FETAL HEARTRATE ASSESSMENT

Fetal heartrate should be auscultated by 12 weeks of gestation with Doppler ultrasound or at 17–19 weeks with DeLee fetoscope.[19] Auscultate the fetal heartrate (FHR) at each prenatal care visit for 1 full minute to note rate and rhythm. Take care not to mistake placental flow or maternal heart rate for FHR. Placental flow or souffle is a swishing sound different from the actual fetal heartbeat, which is a very distinct, clear beat. To ensure that the maternal heartrate is not confused with the FHR, palpate the client's pulse at the wrist while simultaneously auscultating the fetal heart through the abdomen with the Doppler or the fetoscope.

Procedure

Place a small amount of gel (with a water-soluble base) on the abdomen or directly on the Doppler. A fetoscope, which also can be used, does not require gel. Early in gestation (12 to 14 weeks), FHR is best auscultated just above the symphysis with the Doppler. As pregnancy progresses, the fetal heart is usually heard in the lower abdominal quadrants; however, toward the end of pregnancy if the fetus is not in the vertex position, the FHR is often auscultated near or above the umbilicus.[19] It is easiest to locate FHR with the client on her back, if she is able to tolerate that position. Most women can tolerate being supine for a few minutes. If the FHR is not found quickly, it may help

to locate the fetal back by performing Leopold's maneuvers.

Leopold's maneuvers are as follows:[19]

- Facing the client, gently outline the uterus with warm hands. Ascertain what part of the fetus is at the fundus: fetal breech feels nodular and large, and the fetal head feels hard, rounded, and generally more movable.
- Facing the client, gently but firmly palpate the sides of her abdomen using the palms of your hands. The fetal back will be a hard, resistant structure; the opposite palm should feel nodularity of the extremities, such as knees or elbows. If the fetus is not completely on its side, an additional moment of palpation may be needed to determine fetal orientation.
- Facing the client, grasp the lower portion of the maternal abdomen just above the symphysis pubis. If the presenting part is not engaged, it will be mobile. With careful palpation, noting cephalic prominence, it may be possible to determine whether the fetal head is extended or flexed.
- Facing the client's feet and using the tips of the first three fingers of each hand, gently but firmly palpate toward the axis of the pelvic inlet. If the fetal head presents, then the cephalic prominence will be noted first with one hand while the other hand will be able to descend more deeply into the pelvis.

In vertex presentation, the cephalic prominence will be on the same side as the arms and legs, thereby confirming flexion of the fetal head. Cephalic prominence on the same side as the back suggests extension of the fetal head, or face presentation. The ease with which the cephalic prominence is noted provides information regarding descent: if the cephalic prominence is palpable, then the vertex has not reached the level of the ischial spines.

These movements may be difficult to interpret if the placenta is anterior or if the client is obese.[19]

Interpretation of FHR

The FHR should be 120 to 160 beats per minute (bpm), with allowance for variations in normal accelerations.[19] A normal fetal heartrate at twenty weeks' gestation is 160.[22] As the fetus matures, so does the parasympathetic and sympathetic nervous systems, thereby decreasing the fetal heartrate.[22] *Bradycardia* is a baseline heartrate of 110 or below, *moderate bradycardia* as a baseline heartrate of 80–100 bpm, and *severe bradycardia* is a baseline heartrate of fewer than 80 bpm for more than 3 minutes.[19,22] *Mild tachycardia* is a baseline heartrate of 161 to 180 bpm, and *severe tachycardia* is a baseline heartrate of more than 180 bpm.[19] Decelerations or variables may be heard, but they are identified and validated only with external FHR monitoring.

If fetal heartrate or rhythm abnormalities are heard, then a nonstress test is warranted to ascertain the FHR baseline and any periodic patterns. Ultrasound is used to assess cardiac function and note any anomalies. If FHR is absent, a second Doppler or fetoscope (if applicable) may be helpful. Ultrasound is indicated to document fetal viability if the FHR is not heard by 12 weeks' gestation with Doppler, or 19 weeks with a DeLee fetoscope, or if it is absent after previously being documented.[19]

Factors That Influence Fetal Heartrate Detection

FHR may be heard earlier than 12 weeks with Doppler if the uterus is anteflexed, as opposed to being retroflexed, and if the client has little adipose tissue.[19] Adipose tissue may make it more difficult to hear the fetal heart early in gestation or later using a fetoscope.[19] The type and age of the Doppler used may also affect ability to hear the fetal heart early in gestation.

Advantages and Disadvantages

The procedure is noninvasive, and most clients enjoy hearing the fetal heart. Listening promotes bonding for mother, father, and siblings and may enable the mother to conceptualize her pregnancy early in gestation, prior to fetal movement. Often fetal movement can be heard with the Doppler and aids the client in recognizing fetal movement.

On the other hand, the client may be anxious if the fetal heart is not detected immediately or is not heard at all, or if the fetus moves and the FHR is temporarily lost.

Client Teaching and Counseling

Inform the client of the normal range of heartrate to decrease her anxiety; many women are unaware that FHR should be 120 to 160 bpm and worry that the fetal heart is beating too fast. Reassurance usually suffices.

NONSTRESS TEST AND CONTRACTION STRESS TEST

The nonstress and contraction stress tests both reflect the status of fetal cardiac physiology, as well as the fetal status of the central, peripheral, and autonomic nervous systems through heartrate monitoring.[7,10,21,23] The tests were developed to assess any indication of uteroplacental insufficiency, thereby predicting the fetus' ability to endure the stress of labor or the need for premature delivery if the fetus is distressed and could be better cared for outside the uterus.

NONSTRESS TEST

Mature reactivity is present in over 65 percent of fetuses tested using electronic fetal heartrate monitoring at 28 weeks.[21] The nonstress test (NST) can be performed reliably after 28 weeks of gestation when the aforementioned fetal systems, particularly the autonomic nervous system, usually reach acceptable maturity and can be assessed; the 26–27 week fetus is unlikely to have a reactive pattern. As technology expands, and the age of viability becomes earlier, ultrasound may become the primary method of assessment.[23] Because it is a noninvasive and simple procedure, the NST is appropriate for many clinical indications. In cases of serious fetal or maternal disease, additional tests may be performed.

Procedure. Ideally, the client has not been fasting and has not smoked recently as this may affect test results.[7] The procedure involves the use of a fetal heart monitor. Two belts are secured around the abdomen; one holds the tocodynameter over the fundus, which measures any uterine activity. The other belt holds a transducer over the fetal heart, which measures the fetal heartrate. Preferably, the client lies on her left side to avoid supine hypotension. Fetal heartrate, fetal movement, and uterine contractions (if they occur) are assessed over 20 minutes and recorded on a monitor strip. The client notes fetal movement by using a hand held "event marker" or by pushing a button on the monitor that marks the strip. Perceived fetal movement is thereby correlated with FHR. Fetal movement without an acceleration is atypical, and further workup is warranted.[10]

Interpretation. The NST may be interpreted as reactive or nonreactive. A *reactive NST* is characterized by two fetal heartrate accelerations that last 15 seconds and reach 15 beats above baseline FHR in 20 minutes (15-by-15 criteria).[7] If a reactive NST cannot be obtained after 20 minutes, then monitoring is continued another 20 minutes in order to take the fetal sleep-wake cycle into account.[7] According to one source, the NST can be continued for up to 120 minutes to reduce the potential for a false nonreactive test.[23]

In the second trimester, an acceleration of 10 beats may suffice as an adequate acceleration.[23] Research may continue in the area of defining varied criteria for assessing fetal well-being in the second trimester.

When the NST is reactive, or "negative," it can be repeated at weekly intervals; in most cases, fetal well-being can be relatively assured for 1 week.[23] Some clinical situations involving the client or the fetus may dictate more frequent testing, such as insulin dependent diabetes or other threats to the placenta.[11,23] The ideal interval for surveillance has not been established; weekly, biweekly, and daily testing are utilized, depending on the clinical situation; however, even with daily testing, fetal demise is encountered on rare occasions.[23] Frequency of testing is left to the discretion of the clinician, taking into account the clinical aspects of disease that affect maternal and fetal well-being.

A *nonreactive NST* is characterized by the absence of two fetal heartrate accelerations using the 15-by-15 criteria in a 20-minute time frame.[7] Other questionable patterns, such as lack of variability and presence of decelerations may be noted, however. Additional testing, such as a contraction stress test (CST) or biophysical profile, should be considered.[24]

Factors that influence reactivity include maternal sedatives, smoking, and hypoglycemia, fetal sleep cycles, and maternal or fetal disease and fetal anomalies.[23,25] Lengthening the NST may be reasonable in order to rule out *some* of these variables.

Periodic patterns that may be viewed during NSTs and CSTs and require evaluation include fetal bradycardia, tachycardia, decelerations, and lack of variability. The following definitions (variability, acceleration, deceleration, sinusoidal pattern), although helpful in understanding the fundamentals of interpreting FHR tracings, will neither replace diagnostic manuals nor diminish the expertise gained through experience in reading FHR tracings.

Variability. Short-term variability (*STV*), considered the most important indicator of fetal well-being, is the fluctuation of FHR from beat to beat, giving rise to a "saw-toothed" tracing. Variability reflects the pathway between the autonomic nervous system and the heart, and is an important index of cardiovascular function.[19] Short-term variability, however, can only be truly documented by using internal, not external, monitoring.

Long-term variability is the fluctuation of FHR over 1 minute. It is assessed by noting the difference between maximum and minimum FHR, excluding accelerations, decelerations, and patterns exhibited during contractions.[19]

Classification of Variability[19]

- *Absent.* FHR changes of 0–2 bpm.
- *Minimal.* FHR changes of 3–5 bpm.
- *Average.* FHR changes of 6–10 bpm.
- *Moderate.* FHR changes of 11–25 bpm.
- *Marked.* FHR changes of greater than 25 bpm.

Essentially, FHR changes of 6 to 25 bpm are reassuring; however, minimal or marked variability does not always imply fetal distress.[19] *Questionable tracings always require a second opinion concerning intervention or further diagnostic testing, such as CST or biophysical profile.*

Acceleration. Accelerations are increases in FHR over baseline, specifically a 15-bpm increase for 15 seconds; this usually assures the clinician of the absence of fetal acidosis.[25]

Deceleration. Decelerations are decreases of FHR below baseline; they can be early, late, or variable. *Early decelerations* usually occur as a vagal response to increased intracranial pressure with fetal head compression.[25] An early deceleration is uniform in shape with a contraction, beginning and ending with the contraction. It is shallow and symmetrical, and usually seen in the active phase of labor.[25]

Late decelerations are symmetrical decreases in the FHR beginning at or after the peak of the contraction; FHR does not recover until contraction ends.[19] Uteroplacental insufficiency should be questioned.[19] Hypoxia and possibly fetal myocardial depression have been postulated as well.[25] Markedly compromised fetuses frequently display subtle, shallow decelerations.[10]

Variable decelerations are usually due to cord compression. Variable decelerations have variable shape, depth, and duration and may occur at any time. Severe decelerations last more than 60 seconds with FHR fewer than 70 bpm.[19] There are varying opinions as to the clinical significance of variables noted during antepartum testing. Deep, prolonged variable decelerations not associated with fetal movement may suggest oligohydramnios or cord compromise; suspicious variable decelerations have been associated with growth retarded fetuses, those with decreased Wharton's jelly, as in the postdates fetus, and with diminished amniotic fluid.[10]

Sinusoidal Pattern. A sinusoidal pattern is characterized by a smooth, undulating FHR pattern, usually with an absence of variability.[25] Oscillations are 3 to 5 cycles per minute, with an amplitude of 5–15 bpm above and below the baseline.[25] Reactivity is absent, and the pattern lasts beyond 10 minutes.[25] The pattern may be seen with severe chronic, as opposed to acute, fetal anemia, and severe hypoxia and acidosis.[25] Sinusoidal patterns have also been noted with the use of alphaprodine and other medications, and in this circumstance do not indicate fetal compromise.[25]

Use of Vibroacoustic Stimulation. An artificial larynx, or acoustic stimulator, can be used to achieve a reactive tracing and reduce the length of the NST. No deleterious effects have been assessed, although research continues in this area.[26] If accelerations or fetal movement are not noted within 10 minutes during the NST, vibroacoustic stimulation is applied to the woman's abdomen over the fetal head for 1 to 3 seconds.[26] Acceptable accelerations usually result. One or two additional stimuli may be applied at 1- to 2-minute intervals if necessary. Induced accelerations appear to be valid in assuring fetal well-being.[7,25]

Advantages and Disadvantages. The advantages of the NST are that it is easily performed and noninvasive. Furthermore, hearing and seeing the FHR recorded on the tracing may promote maternal-fetal bonding.

A disadvantage of the NST is that it requires someone with expertise to read the results, particularly suspicious patterns. There is current investigation of computerized analysis of fetal heartrate, however.[23] This provides an objective reading of the "tracing" or "strip," as well as providing accurate measurements of the various numerical parameters of the fetal heartrate. Computerized systems would refine interpretation of fetal heartrate patterns (variability, accelerations, decelerations, and baseline rate).[23]

The NST can be a lengthy procedure, particularly if a protocol is not in place for the use of acoustic stimulation. Continuous FHR tracing may be difficult to obtain if the client is obese or if the fetus is fewer than 28 weeks' gestation. The NST is seldom reactive before 28 weeks,[24] and it cannot recognize impaired fetal growth or fetal anomalies.

Client Teaching and Counseling. Initially, to avoid client confusion and undue concern, explain the tracings of uterine activity and FHR. The client should also be told what the average FHR is and that variability is normal. Many women are alarmed when the FHR fluctuates (particularly with accelerations), or frightened if the FHR is temporarily "lost" as a result of a fetal or maternal position change. Explaining the different aspects of FHR monitoring can alleviate many fears. If vibroacoustic stimulation is used, have the client feel and hear the stimulus before applying it to the abdomen.

CONTRACTION STRESS TEST

Performed to note fetal response to uterine contractions, using the principle of induced stress to assess placental insufficiency. It is theorized that if the fetus is hypoxic or has uteroplacental insufficiency, late decelerations will occur with uterine contractions.[7,10,21] In many institutions, it is the test of choice. A CST may be indicated if a reactive NST cannot be obtained. If the CST is contraindicated, then a biophysical profile (BPP) or NST should be considered.[10]

Contraindications. Absolute contraindications are history of classical cesarean section, placenta previa or abruptio placenta, premature rupture of membranes, fundal presentation, and vasa previa.[10] Relative contraindications are premature labor, multiple gestation fewer than 36 weeks, and incompetent cervix.[7,10]

Procedure. The test procedure is much the same as that for the NST. The client is placed in a semi-Fowlers position to prevent supine hypotension. Attain an initial reading of blood pressure, pulse, and respirations. Blood pressure readings are taken every 10–15 minutes; maternal hypotension can decrease uteroplacental perfusion, and, therefore, lead to false-positive results.[10] The tocodynameter is applied to the fundus, and the transducer placed over the fetal heart. In obese clients, the transducer may have to be hand held to maintain a constant reading of the fetal heartrate.[10] A baseline tracing of the fetus is obtained for 15 to 20 minutes. Contractions are achieved by means of nipple stimulation, which causes the release of endogenous oxytocin, or through the use of intravenous oxytocin. Breast stimulation achieves adequate contractions 80 percent–100 percent of the time when utilized.[10] This eliminates the need for intravenous oxytocin, and also shortens testing time.[10] Spontaneous contractions are acceptable, provided criteria are met. Protocols vary among institutions.

To perform nipple stimulation, the client brushes one nipple with the palmar surface of the fingers, or rolls the nipple between the thumb and index finger through her clothing for 2-minute intervals, with 2-minute rests in between, alternating breasts.[10] If after 4 cycles adequate contractions have not occurred, one nipple can be stimulated continuously. If unsuccessful, bilateral continuous stimulation can be performed for 10 minutes.[10] Experienced nurses can titrate the amount of stimulation needed.[10] As a last resort, oxytocin infusion is begun. An intravenous line is started with a 21-gauge butterfly needle using half normal saline.[10] The oxytocin infusion is begun at 0.5–1.0 mU/min. The rate is doubled every 15–20 minutes until uterine response is noted; thereafter, smaller increments are used until criteria are met to evaluate tracing. Usually 4 to 8 mU is sufficient.[7] Once adequate contractions are achieved, the infusion is discontinued.[10] Regardless of the method used, the client is monitored until uterine activity returns to baseline; if late decelerations are noted, monitoring continues until the tracing is reactive and late decelerations are no longer present.[10]

Interpretation. Interpreting a CST requires three contractions, lasting at least 40 seconds each, within a 10-minute period.[10] Since contractions are recorded through external monitoring, the only criteria they must meet in regards to strength is that they are clearly recorded in order to interpret the tracing.[10] It is also important to note other aspects of the fetal heartrate strip, including reactivity.[7,10]

- *Positive CST.* Late decelerations in more than 50 percent of contractions, regardless of contraction frequency.[7,10] Delivery should be considered or further tests pursued, as the CST has a 30 percent false-positive rate.[10] If delivery is chosen, and reactivity is absent as well, abdominal delivery is considered as the fetus may not be able to tolerate the stress of labor.[10]
- *Equivocal CST with Hyperstimulation.* Late decelerations in the presence of hyperstimulation (more than 5 contractions in 10 minutes or contractions lasting longer than 90 seconds).[10] Retesting should be done in 24 hours, or other tests pursued, such as a BPP.
- *Equivocal Suspicious.* Late decelerations noted with less than 50 percent of contractions in absence of hyperstimulation.[10] A suspicious test can be extended by obtaining 10 additional contractions.[10] Extension may decrease a false-positive rate in the presence of a reassuring tracing.[10]

- *Negative or Normal CST.* No late or variable decelerations.[7,10] Subsequent testing is based on fetal and maternal conditions and the protocol of the institution.
- *Unsatisfactory CST.* Failure of adequate contractions to occur with either nipple stimulation or oxytocin infusion.[7] Consider a biophysical profile.

Advantages and Disadvantages of the Contraction Stress Test. The CST determines fetal ability to endure labor. If the fetus cannot tolerate the stress of contractions in a controlled testing environment, then it is unlikely the fetus could tolerate labor.[10] Therefore, this screening helps to avoid fetal distress. Some consider the CST more effective than the NST in evaluating the fetus.[10]

Nipple stimulation is less costly than oxytocin infusion and does not carry the possible complications associated with venipuncture, such as phlebitis and bruising. Hence, the client may prefer nipple stimulation if she is comfortable touching her breasts in a clinical situation. Providing the client with privacy may reduce feelings of self-consciousness.

Theoretically, the CST carries the potential to induce labor; therefore, it is contraindicated if contractions are to be avoided. In the event that contractions induce fetal distress, immediate intervention should be initiated. Another disadvantage is that the CST may take longer than the NST. Clients may become upset with the invasive procedure of oxytocin infusion, if needed.

Client Teaching and Counseling. Review those points included in the discussion of the NST. In addition, inform the client about the possible use of intravenous oxytocin. Clients should be aware that in most cases "manufactured" contractions do not prompt actual labor, but they may cause slight discomfort. Often contractions are painless.

SCREENING FOR SIZE/DATE DISCREPANCIES

The developing fetus has a genetically predetermined potential for growth but can be influenced by the mother's health, placental function, maternal substance use and abuse, nutrition, and perinatal infection.[27]

When gestational age does not correlate with the apparent size of the uterus or fetus, further evaluation is indicated. The discrepancy may be noted during a bimanual exam or fundal height measurement at a regular prenatal visit, or at delivery when the Dubowitz examination is performed to estimate gestational age of the newborn. If the infant appears smaller or larger than would be expected for the dates, it is very important to determine the actual gestational age of the infant to the best of one's ability. This can impact decisions for interventions if needed. Regardless of when the discrepancy is detected, its cause should be investigated.

PROCEDURES

It is helpful to have good estimates of gestational age by means of pelvic examination or ultrasound in the first or second trimester.[28] The last normal menstrual period is recorded and used as the basis for actual gestational age if the client is certain she remembers the first day of her last normal period and if her cycles are about 28 days long.

At each prenatal visit, fundal height is measured or uterine size is assessed to correlate size with gestational age. A measuring tape calibrated in centimeters is used; the distance between the top of the symphysis pubis and the top of the uterine fundus is measured. The general rule is to consider ultrasound if uterine size is 3 weeks above or below the calculated gestational age, or fundal height is 3 cm above or below the calculated gestational age.[27,28] Fundal height is most accurate when the bladder is empty.[19]

Gestational age can be determined and the fetus assessed for abnormalities using ultrasound. A discrepancy in size may simply be the result of incorrect menstrual dates. It is, however, important to rule out other etiologies. All clients who are at risk for IUGR should have an early ultrasound before 20 weeks, and serial ultrasounds done thereafter since fundal height measurement alone will miss one-third of IUGRs, and a single ultrasound in late pregnancy cannot detect IUGR.[27,29,30]

DIFFERENTIAL MEDICAL DIAGNOSES

Small-for-Gestational-Age (SGA). SGA is a clinically generic term that describes a fetus whose weight is less than 10th percentile without reference to etiology.[31] Most SGA babies are small but normal fetuses.[31] The fetus can be normal, but small; not normal and therefore small; or normal as seen clinically but whose growth potential has been retarded.[31]

Intrauterine Growth Retardation. Intrauterine growth retardation (IUGR) manifests as a fetal weight below the 10th percentile for age, but has clinical evidence of abnormal or dysfunctional growth.[19,30] Fifteen to 20 percent of IUGR fetuses are at risk for perinatal compromise and death.[30] Twenty-six percent of stillbirths can be related in some way to IUGR.[30] IUGR infants often have thermoregulatory difficulties and hypoglycemia not to mention that many IUGR babies are born prematurely, therefore having to cope with the sequellae of preterm birth as well.[27] The perinatal mortality and morbidity are significant.[30]

The etiology of IUGR can also be divided into three categories:[28]

Maternal—inadequate substrate is available as seen with smoking, cyanotic heart disease, antiphospholipid syndrome.

Placental—inadequate transfer of substrate due to placental insufficiency such as seen with essential hypertension.

Fetal—adequate substrate is present from the mother, and the placenta is functioning normally, but the fetus is unable to use the substrate, as seen with intrauterine infection or congenital anomalies.

Growth retardation can be asymmetric or symmetric:

Asymmetrical growth retardation occurs primarily during the middle of the second trimester or into the third trimester and results in decreased cell size. The fetus reacts to the insult by sparing certain cells by blood redistribution, particularly to the brain, heart, placenta and adrenal glands.[11,27] The diminished blood flow to kidney and lung results in decreased amniotic fluid and ultimately oligohydramnios.[30] The head is proportionally larger than the abdomen due to decreased abdominal circumference as liver glycogen stores are depleted.[27,28] Placental dysfunction is felt to be the main cause.[27] Fetal insult can result from abruption (abruption is also caused by maternal disease); placenta previa; placental, cord, or uterine abnormalities; multiple gesta-

tion.[31,32] Maternal diseases are also associated with asymmetrical IUGR: severe anemia, chronic hypertension, renal disease, vascular disease, malnutrition, and other chronic diseases.[31,32]

Symmetrical growth retardation occurs with fetal insult during the first trimester, when fetal growth is related to increase in cell number. There is inadequate growth of both the head and the body, all organs are proportionately reduced in size, and the absolute growth rate is decreased.[19,28] Sonography reveals symmetric growth lags in measurements of the biparietal diameter, femur length, and abdominal circumference.[27] Symmetric IUGR infants are less likely to be normal, and has several causes:[19,27,28,32]

- A first trimester infection, such as TORCH (toxoplasmosis, other infections, rubella, cytomegalovirus, herpesvirus)
- Congenital fetal anomalies
- Chronic maternal malnutrition
- First trimester radiation exposure
- Genetic disorders
- Maternal substance abuse

Large-for-Gestational-Age. A fetus may be large-for-gestational-age (LGA), or macrosomic, because of a pathological process, such as diabetes, or because of genetic reasons (e.g., parents of large stature).[32] An LGA fetus weighs more than 4500 g at birth or above the 90th percentile for age.[32]

Risk factors include genetic and congenital disorders, gestational or insulin dependent diabetes, obesity, multiparity, prolonged gestation, and previous delivery of infant weighing more than 4500g, and large maternal stature.[32] The incidence of stillbirth, birth trauma, and neonatal metabolic abnormalities is increased in LGA fetuses.[32]

The complications of an LGA fetus for the mother include increased risk of cesarean birth, postpartum hemorrhage, shoulder dystocia, perineal trauma, and operative vaginal delivery.[32] The fetus is at increased risk for stillbirth, anomalies, and shoulder dystocia.[32] The neonate is at increased risk for hypoglycemia, birth injury, hypocalcemia, polycythemia, jaundice, and feeding difficulties.[32] Long-term sequellae include an increased risk of obesity, type II diabetes, neurologic or behavioral problems, and childhood onset of cancer (leukemia, Wilms' tumor and osteosarcoma).[32]

Differential Diagnoses. Increased uterine size may indicate twins, inaccurate dating, polyhydramnios, uterine fibroids, or a fetal anomaly such as hydrocephaly. Decreased size may indicate fetal demise or oligohydramnios. Both polyhydramnios and oligohydramnios may signify serious fetal anomalies.[19,33]

INTERVENTIONS

Intrauterine Growth Retardation. Three variables are involved with treatment of IUGR: fetal environment, fetal assessment, and timing of delivery.[27,28] This is important as IUGR infants have a greater risk of stillbirth, hypoxia, neonatal complications, and cerebral palsy.[29]

Improving the fetal environment involves consideration of nutritional supplementation,[28] bed rest and stopping work (to increase uterine blood flow),[27,28] cessation of drug use (alcohol, street drugs, smoking),[27,28] and aggressive treatment of maternal disease (cardiac and renal conditions, hypertension, malabsorption syndrome).[27] Smoking is the most important risk factor for IUGR and cessation of smoking, even in late pregnancy, provides benefit.[29] Passive smoking has been found to decrease birthweight as well.[29]

Fetal assessment may require ultrasound or karyotyping. Ultrasound is indicated to assess fetal growth, and measurements may be repeated at 2-week intervals.[30,34] Several measurements can be used; biparietal diameter (BPD), abdominal circumference (AC), head circumference (HC), fetal ponderal index (relationship between weight and length), abdominal diameter-femur length ratio, and HC/AC ratio.[27,30] Abdominal circumference measurements are the single best predictor of IUGR; BPD alone is not sufficient to diagnose IUGR.[27,29]

Karyotyping and viral cultures from an amniotic fluid sample may be considered if a chromosomal anomaly is suspected.[27] Consider maternal serum TORCH titers, although their value is questionable.[27]

Other tests assessing fetal well-being are fetal movement counts, biophysical profile, Doppler flow studies, amniotic fluid volume assessment, CST, NST, or any combination of these tests.[27,28,30] Weekly fetal surveillance is indicated in IUGR, although biweekly assessment is considered with moderate IUGR.[28] Daily surveillance may be indicated, depending on the condition of the mother or fetus.[31]

In fetuses with severe IUGR, it has been noted that Doppler flow studies become abnormal first, prior to a reduction in fetal heartrate variability; fetal body and breathing movements were the last to be decreased.[27] Absence of fetal breathing and fetal movement over a period of time suggests severe compromise and impending fetal death.[30]

Aspirin therapy has been researched, but controversy exists on its effectiveness to decrease IUGR.[27,31] Delivery may be considered if no fetal growth occurs in a 2-week interval or if the fetus has a better chance of survival outside the uterus. Survival depends on the facilities available to care for the infant and gestational age.[27,29] Cesarean section is often utilized as the compromised fetus has difficulty tolerating the stress of labor.[27] Fetal lung maturity is often in question when considering interrupting a pregnancy; however, the stress of IUGR tends to accelerate fetal pulmonary maturity.[28]

Large-for-Gestational-Age Fetus. The mother is screened for gestational diabetes if the fetus is diagnosed as LGA, has no apparent anomaly, and parental stature is not a cause.[32]

Nutritional counseling for the mother includes information about appropriate weight gain and dietary needs of pregnancy. It is prudent to maintain caloric intake to no more than 2400 calories per day.[32] Ultrasound surveillance should be considered to provide a close follow-up of estimated fetal weight.

Delivery before the fetus reaches 4500 g may need to be considered to decrease the incidence of trauma. Establishing lung maturity first is essential. Cesarean birth may be considered if the estimated fetal weight is greater than 5000 g.[32] Each situation should be individualized, as ultrasound based estimates of fetal weight have an error range of plus or minus 10 percent to 15 percent.[32]

CLIENT TEACHING AND COUNSELING

Describe to the client the interventions that are to be carried out. Emphasize that these interventions will increase the chances of a healthy, term infant (if possible) to heighten her participation with the proposed plan of care. For a client whose fetal growth retardation is due to drug use, further discussion about drug use is necessary (see Chapter 18, Substance Abuse).

Many clients believe that a large infant is a sign of good health and that the mother has adequately cared for herself and her infant. The opposite, however, can be true for the mother of a small infant. When counseling clients, it may be difficult to overcome the negative connotations associated with a small infant. Educating the client concerning the underlying processes of abnormal growth patterns may encourage her participation in care.

After delivery, if the cause of the SGA or LGA infant is diagnosed, appropriate intervention or counseling should be initiated. For instance, a mother of an LGA baby should be screened for undiagnosed diabetes, even if previous screens were negative.[32] Both the mother of an LGA or IUGR baby should be encouraged to seek early prenatal care with subsequent pregnancies to establish accurate dating and to follow the growth of the fetus serially to assess any abnormal growth patterns. If maternal conditions exist that can be modified or controlled, such as eating disorders or maternal substance abuse, then the postpartum period is an excellent time for preconceptional counseling.[32] Open discussions concerning substance use may make the client aware of the need to prevent pregnancy and to seek counseling if she is dependent on a substance. Clients who use substances occasionally need to be aware of the potential teratogenic effect of one exposure.

SCREENING AND PREVENTION OF RH ISOIMMUNIZATION

Maternal sensitization, or isoimmunization, may occur with exposure to blood or blood products that contain an antigen not found in maternal blood cells. Exposure potentially prompts production of antibodies to that antigen.[19,35] Sensitization can occur following transfusion or exposure to fetal blood containing factors inherited from the father. The incidence of Rh isoimmunization has decreased because of the administration of Rh immune globulin (Rhogam) to unsensitized women. However, Rh isoimmunization does occur; it may increase due to sharing of needles among drug users,[36] or an Rh-negative woman may unknowingly abort an Rh-positive fetus.[19] Fetal sensitization can also occur according to the "grandmother" theory: an Rh-negative fetus is exposed to enough maternal Rh-positive red blood cells during delivery to cause fetal sensitization.[35]

Rh STATUS

Rh status refers to presence (Rh-positive) or absence (Rh-negative) of Rh antigen on the red blood cell. More than 400 antigens of the Rh factor have been identified.[19] They can all cause hemolytic disease; however, the D antigen causes 90 percent of cases of Rh isoimmunization.[35] Individuals lacking antigenic determinant D require two exposures to the Rh antigen to produce significant sensitization, unless the first exposure is massive.[35] Other antigens have various effects on fetuses as a result of diversified antibody responses and should be managed individually.[19] Because the vast majority of cases of isoimmunization are due to the D antigen, in the remainder of this section the D antigen is used as an example.

Initial Screening. For all clients, determine blood type, Rh status, and atypical antibody titer (indirect Coombs test) early in pregnancy.[5]

Interpretation of Results and Management. If the client is D-negative or has a positive antibody screen, determine the father's blood type and Rh and antigen status. If the father is D-negative and has no antigens to the corresponding antibodies that the mother has, then no further consideration is needed.[36] If, however, the father is Rh-positive and has a negative antigen screen, or if testing the father's blood is not possible, draw a maternal antibody titer at 28 weeks. If D antibody is absent, then give Rhogam.

Rhogam is given specifically to prevent isoimmunization to D antigen.[36] Rhogam is comprised of anti-D IGg antibodies and acts by binding with Rh-positive fetal cells if they are present in the maternal circulation. Through various means, it blocks maternal antigen processing.[35] Rhogam is of no value when isoimmunization has occurred. Rhogam is again given within 72 hours of delivery if the fetus is Rh-positive.[19] In addition, Rhogam is given to Rh negative clients who undergo bilateral tubal ligation after delivery, because in the future they may decide to have the ligation reversed. Breastfeeding is not a contraindication to administration of Rhogam.

If the client has a positive antibody screen and the father is positive for antigen, maternal antibody should be characterized and the titer determined.[35] Titers must be followed through gestation if it is determined that antibodies are IgG; IgG can cross the placenta and cause hemolytic disease in the fetus.[19,35] A rising or elevated titer (greater than or equal to 1:8 or 1:16, depending on the laboratory) indicates the need for further clinical assessment (see Management of an Isoimmunized Pregnancy later in this section).[35]

Of clinical importance is the need to notify the blood bank of the client's irregular antibody in the event a transfusion is needed at delivery.

Currently, the ability to determine fetal blood type through polymerase chain reaction is being studied, which would decrease the need of obtaining repeated maternal antibody titers and noninvasive fetal testing.[37] This is being studied using amniotic fluid obtained during amniocentesis for standard obstetric indications;[38] a realistic possibility for the future is to isolate fetal cells through a maternal blood sample.[39] Limited studies have confirmed the ability of PCR to determine fetal Rh status using fetal blood, amniocyte, and CVS samples, but more research is needed to have consistent accuracy to avoid mistyping an Rh-positive fetus as an Rh-negative fetus through these experimental techniques.[38]

Other Indications for Administration of Rhogam During Pregnancy. Rhogam should be given anytime there exists a potential for mixing Rh-positive fetal and Rh-negative maternal blood.[19,35] *If there is ever any doubt as to whether or not to give Rhogam, then it should be given.*[19,35]

- Chorionic villus sampling
- Therapeutic or spontaneous abortion
- Ectopic pregnancy
- Hydatidiform mole
- Amniocentesis
- Antepartum hemorrhage

- Fetal blood sampling
- External version
- Fetal death
- Fetal surgery
- Transfusion of D-positive blood to D-negative mother

Hemorrhage. If at any time during the pregnancy a large fetal-to-maternal hemorrhage is suspected, or copious bleeding occurs at delivery, as with manual removal of the placenta, the Kleihauer-Betke test is performed on a sample of maternal blood to measure fetal blood in the maternal system. If fetal blood is present in maternal blood, then 10 µg of Rhogam is given per milliliter of fetal blood in the maternal system. The standard dose is 300 µg, which is effective for 30 mL of fetal blood. If more than 30 mL of blood is present in the maternal system, then the volume of fetal red cells can be estimated by analysis of maternal blood; the dose of Rhogam is adjusted accordingly.[19,35]

PROCESS OF ISOIMMUNIZATION

If the client does not receive Rhogam and is exposed to D antigen on fetal cells, she will produce anti-D IgM antibodies. This initial response usually is not problematic (unless the exposure is massive), as IgM antibodies do not cross the placenta.[19,35] A second exposure to fetal cells with the D antigen will cause the development of IgG antibodies.[19,35] No amount of prophylaxis at this point will prevent a hemolytic response.[19,35]

Anti-D IgG antibodies cross the placenta readily, coat fetal cells if they have D antigen, and cause hemolysis.[19,35] If hemolysis is mild, the fetus may compensate by increasing its production of red blood cells. If hemolysis is severe, the fetus maximizes red blood cell production in the liver and spleen. The increased demands on the fetal liver result in enlargement, altered function, and decreased albumin production, which lead to leakage of fluid from the fetal vasculature. Ascites and effusions thereby develop. As hemolysis continues, anemia worsens; liver failure and circulatory compromise result. Ultimately cardiovascular collapse and fetal death occur. These events describe the process of fetal hemolytic disease, or hydrops fetalis.[19,35]

Management of an Isoimmunized Pregnancy.
Management begins with assessment of maternal blood type, presence or absence of Rh factor, and any atypical antibody titers at the first prenatal visit. Information from the client about a prior pregnancy, if applicable, or actual prenatal records from a previous pregnancy are helpful. Subsequent care employs methods of fetal monitoring.

Maternal antibody titers are assessed early in pregnancy. Each laboratory establishes its own thresholds for critical values.[38] Once this threshold is reached, ultrasound and amniocentesis should be considered to assess the possibility of severe hemolytic disease.[19,38] These titer values apply to anti-D sensitization only; other antibody responses may cause hydropic disease at titer of 1:8.[35] It is helpful for the laboratory to save each sample in the frozen state so that subsequent titers can be done in duplicate.[36]

Ultrasound should be used when the maternal titer rises and abnormalities, such as ascites, are noted. Ultrasound is helpful in monitoring the fetal condition through sonographic features such as cardiomegaly, ascites, pericardial effusions, hepatosplenomegaly, umbilical vein dilation, presence of subcutaneous edema, placental changes, and polyhydramnios.[36] The ultrasound may be done alone or with amniocentesis or percutaneous umbilic blood sampling(PUBS).[35]

Amniotic fluid assays and PUBS may begin early in the second trimester, depending on the extent of disease. Bilirubin, the byproduct of red blood cell destruction, can be measured spectrophotometrically in amniotic fluid or fetal blood. PUBS is used to monitor the fetal hematocrit, which truly determines the severity of fetal anemia, as compared to relying on amniotic fluid assays alone; amniotic fluid spectrophotometry is not accurate on fetuses fewer than 28 weeks.[19,35,38] Through monitoring of the bilirubin level and fetal hematocrit, the necessity and frequency of fetal transfusion can be assessed. The frequency of monitoring occurs at 1 to 3 week intervals, depending on the severity of disease.[35]

Nonstress tests are recommended as a hydrops affected fetus may exhibit sinusoidal or other ominous patterns during heartrate monitoring.[19] Diminished fetal activity, however, may precede changes detected by external monitoring.

Therefore, fetal movement counts between ultrasound exams are advised to monitor an affected fetus.[36]

Treatment of Isoimmunization. Transfusions may be administered using the intraperitoneal or intravascular route,[36] and are recommended if the fetal hematocrit is 2g/dL less than the mean for normal fetuses of the same gestational age.[19] Transfusion is at present the only method that will save a hydropic fetus if delivery is remote.[35] A combination of intraperitoneal and intravascular routes is advocated.[36] Other methods have been investigated to minimize fetal hemolysis, but none have been successful.[19,35]

Client Teaching and Counseling. For the unsensitized client, reinforce the need for Rhogam at 28 weeks and after delivery. Support and encourage the client be involved in her care, emphasizing the importance of prenatal care visits. A client considering home delivery needs to be aware of the importance of receiving Rhogam within 72 hours if the baby's blood type is unknown or if the infant is Rh-positive in order to prevent isoimmunization in the next pregnancy.

Some clients feel that if they miscarry early in gestation and all tissue is passed and bleeding stops, they do not need to be evaluated in the health care setting. Stress the importance of evaluation and, at the same time, the necessity of receiving Rhogam when miscarriage occurs.

In the event of isoimmunization, carefully discuss all procedures with the client to encourage her participation and fully explain the plan of care.

ABO INCOMPATIBILITY

ABO isoimmunization is not as severe because most antibodies to A and B antigens are IgM antibodies, which do not cross the placenta.[19] Usually, the mother is blood type O, with anti-A and anti-B in her serum, and the infant is blood type A, B, or AB.[19] Titers and amniocentesis are not required during pregnancy; however, treatment begins after delivery for the infant. Jaundice becomes clinically apparent as the infant's red blood cells are hemolyzed as a result of ABO incompatibility. The infant's bilirubin levels are monitored and phototherapy is used to treat jaundice. Occasionally, a transfusion is required for the infant.[19]

Client Teaching and Counseling. Most teaching centers on information concerning the infant's condition. The mother also needs reassurance. Emphasize to the client that her infant's condition is not her fault and that she should not feel guilty about the infant undergoing treatment. Providing her with written material that explains ABO incompatibility and treatment will help. The client needs to be prepared should the infant become frankly jaundiced. Tell her that the pediatrician may change the infant's feeding schedule or type of feeding to enhance the breakdown of bilirubin. Because the infant will be undergoing phototherapy a vast majority of the time, the mother will have less time to hold, feed, and bond with her infant. Assess this potential inability to bond and arrange to have the client provide as much care as possible. Also explain that the infant's eyes will be covered while undergoing phototherapy.

Discuss the possibility of transfusion. Discussion may assist the client in making decisions about problematic religious or cultural issues. Because transfusions can become a legal issue, every effort should be made to educate the client concerning the need for treatment. In this way, conflict may be avoided.

MATERNAL SERUM SCREENING

Maternal serum screening for fetal chromosomal anomalies should be offered to women of all ages at 15–16 weeks. Triple-marker screening consists of maternal serum alpha-fetoprotein (MSAFP), unconjugated estriol (uE3) and the b subunit of human chorionic gonadotropin (hCG) as a screen for Down syndrome and other fetal aneuploidies.[8,40,41] The triple screen may be able to detect up to 60 percent of trisomy-21 fetuses; low levels of serum chorionic gonadotropin have been associated with trisomy-18 and 13 fetuses.[9,19,40] Low levels of all three markers can be indicative of trisomy 18; low levels of MSAFP and uE3 and a high level of hCG can be indicative of trisomy 21.[8,42] The detection rate for other chromosome anomalies is unknown.[42]

α-Fetoprotein (AFP), a glycoprotein produced by the fetal liver, gastrointestinal tract, and embryonic yolk sac, increases in the amniotic fluid through urination, gastrointestinal secretions, and movement across fetal blood vessels.[19] AFP crosses the placenta and fetal membranes into the maternal bloodstream, resulting in a rise in maternal serum AFP (MSAFP).[19] The level can be measured by taking a sample of maternal blood between 16 and 18 weeks of gestation.[9]

Human chorionic gonadotropin (hCG) is secreted by synctiotrophoblasts and detectable in maternal serum 8 days after ovulation.[43] hCG is the most sensitive screening marker for the detection of Down syndrome; elevated levels are indicative of Down syndrome.[43]

Unconjugated estriol (uE3) is regulated by the placenta, fetal adrenal glands, and fetal liver.[43] The use of uE3 aids in the detection of trisomy 18, and lower levels are associated with Down syndrome.[43] Measurement of MSAFP was initially used to screen for open neural tube and ventral wall defects; since its introduction in 1983, other conditions have been associated with abnormal levels of MSAFP (see Etiology of an Abnormal Result).[8,9,43] Triple screening should be offered to all women. Clients with a personal or family history of neural tube defects or chromosomal anomalies should also be offered more appropriate methods for diagnosis of chromosomal or structural anomalies (e.g., chorionic villus sampling, amniocentesis, or ultrasonographic evaluation of fetus), depending on the client's risk factors, history, and age.[42,44]

INTERPRETATION

The levels of MSAFP, hCG and uE3 are reported as multiples of the median (MoM) and adjusted in the laboratory for maternal weight, presence of diabetes, gestational age, multiple gestation, and race.[8,43] In a singleton pregnancy, *elevated values of MSAFP* are greater than 2.0 to 2.5 MoM.[8] *Low values, however, are assessed with respect to maternal age* (maternal age dependent threshold); elevated values are not.[43] With respect to low values, normal ranges of MSAFP are established by each laboratory based on maternal age. Each laboratory generates its own medians based on the populations it serves.[8]

ETIOLOGY OF AN ABNORMAL RESULT

Elevated MSAFP levels are associated with underestimated gestational age; oligohydramnios; neural tube defects, genetic anomalies, multiple gestation; pilonidal cysts, open ventral wall defect; fetomaternal hemorrhage; renal, pulmonary, abdominal wall, esophageal, skin, and placental anomalies; liver necrosis, cystic hygroma, sacrococcygeal teratoma, osteogenesis imperfecta, and malignancy, cloacal exstrophy, low birthweight, decreased maternal weight.[19,43]

Low MSAFP levels are associated with chromosomal trisomies, gestational trophoblastic disease, fetal death, increased maternal weight, and overestimated gestational age.[19]

Although the triple screen was initially used to screen for trisomy 21, other chromosomal abnormalities have been associated with abnormal results.[41]

CLINICAL MANAGEMENT

Elevated markers, particularly MSAFP, require that the serum be retested if time permits.[3] If the second triple screen is also abnormal, ultrasound is performed alone or with amniocentesis.[3] Ultrasound can be used either to correct gestational age or to note a structural anomaly. Confirmation of gestational age is not advised if the risk is for trisomy 18 as these fetuses may already be growth retarded.[42]

If gestational age is incorrect or if another nonpathological cause of an abnormal value is noted (such as twins), the MoM is recalculated and usually found to be within normal limits. Underestimation of gestational age is the most common reason for an elevated MSAFP.[3] If a structural anomaly is noted, the fetus should be thoroughly assessed for other anomalies and amniocentesis offered to note genetic aberrations. If no anomaly is apparent and no other cause of an abnormal marker is found, amniocentesis is indicated.[3]

Amniocentesis is done to assess amniotic fluid AFP (AFAFP) and perform chromosomal analysis. A positive AFAFP is validated by measuring the amount of acetylcholinesterase (AChE) in the amniotic fluid sample.[3] AChE is present only if there is an open neural tube defect.[9] If the elevated AFAFP level is due to contamination with fetal blood, AChE will be absent. A low level of AChE or its absence suggests something other than open neural tube defect as the etiology of the elevated AFAFP.[3] As stated previously, a detailed ultrasonographic exam should follow the amniocentesis.[3]

Ninety to ninety-five percent of clients with abnormal MSAFP levels have a normal level of AFAFP. Even though the AFAFP is normal, the risk for IUGR, premature labor, neonatal death, preeclampsia, fetal demise, and abruption is greater; the causes are not well documented.[8,45] These clients should undergo high resolution ultrasounds and fetoplacental surveillance during the remainder of pregnancy.[3]

Amniocentesis is not a test to determine whether or not to consider termination. Rather, it should be seen as a diagnostic tool. Invasive genetic testing remains the gold standard for fetal diagnosis. Diagnosis of a fetal problem allows the health care provider to supply the client with options for the pregnancy. This may be a referral to a perinatologist for further care or planning of care for the infant at delivery and beyond; termination may be considered as well. By providing information to the health care provider as well as the client, pregnancy outcome and the plan of care can be optimized.[8] In the presence of an open neural tube defect, cesarean delivery appears to retain greater neurologic function and should be considered for clients carrying a fetus with a neural tube defect.[43]

ADVANTAGES AND DISADVANTAGES

Maternal serum screening can be done in the office or clinic. If subsequent testing due to abnormal values reveals a fetal problem, treatment (if possible) may be instituted; this also enables the client to be prepared and plan care for a child with a chromosomal or structural anomaly. This certainly is an advantage for the clinician when planning fetal surveillance, as well as the mode of delivery, and the care that will be needed by the neonate after delivery. Screening and diagnosis in the second trimester also allows the client the option of choosing termination.

For those who do not wish to have an invasive procedure, triple marker screening may be an option. Diagnosis and confirmation of abnormal results, however, would require amniocentesis.

There are disadvantages. Maternal serum testing screens for abnormalities; it is not diagnostic. Further intervention is required to assess the etiology. The high rate of false positive results may increase further if certain factors, for example, race and multiple gestation, are not taken into account, and clients may proceed with amniocentesis unnecessarily (see next section). Also, closed neural tube defects such as those associated with hydrocephaly cannot be detected by maternal serum testing.

Client Teaching and Counseling

Inform the client of possible test outcomes and clinical sequence of testing that would be advised in the event of abnormal test results prior to drawing MSAFP. Many clients can cope with having blood drawn, but the decision to do a chromosomal analysis may pose a cultural or religious dilemma for some. The sequence of events leading to diagnosis after an abnormal test result is often unanticipated. Some clients want to know if the fetus has an abnormality; others prefer not to know until the birth and may refuse further diagnostic testing. The health care provider may be caught in the middle as in the event of an abnormal MSAFP result, wherein the fetus will be assumed to be at risk.

ULTRASONOGRAPHY

Ultrasonography uses high frequency sound waves to produce an image. A transducer directs sound waves toward an object (e.g., the fetus). When the waves interface with solid structures, energy is reflected back to the transducer, which creates electrical voltage. That voltage produces an image on screen. Real-time ultrasound differs from conventional ultrasound. Real-time ultrasound uses a multiple-pulse system of sound waves to note movement, such as fetal breathing; conventional ultrasound uses only a single pulse.[34] Specialized training is needed to perform and interpret ultrasound. Abdominal ultrasound or a transvaginal probe may be used in assessment.

Ultrasound has no confirmed biologic adverse effects on the fetus.[34,36] This has led many to use ultrasound indiscriminantly. Clients often want an ultrasound just to know the sex of the baby. Currently, ultrasound should be used only to the medical benefit of a mother or fetus, although many health care providers use ultrasound routinely. Some feel it should be offered to all women in their second trimester to detect anomalies and to confirm gestational age.[8] With various changes in health care, however, the cost effectiveness of providing routine screening to all women remains an issue.[8] Some studies have found benefit to routine screening, while others found no difference in perinatal outcome.[8] *Routine ultrasound examination is not currently recommended by the American College of Obstetricians and Gynecologists.*[34]

Generally, ultrasonography should provide the information sought (e.g., possible source of bleeding), as well as various parameters depending on gestational age. The use of the term "level" is being phased out as it is more prudent to assess parameters that are appropriate for the gestational age. A distinction is made when a fetus is considered to be at risk for a structural anomaly, or if during a basic scan, there are questionable findings. In this case the client should be referred for a targeted ultrasound for specialized scanning.[46] The health care provider should not assume a lack of responsibility for being knowledgeable and competent when providing even a basic ultrasound, however, as most congenital anomalies occur in the absence of risk factors.[46] The following general criteria for ultrasound will no doubt change as ultrasound becomes more refined and is utilized more for prenatal diagnosis.

- *Basic Ultrasound.* Establishes gestational age, fetal presentation, documentation of fetal life, location of placenta, number of fetuses, measurement of multiple fetal body parts, and amniotic fluid volume; detects maternal pelvic masses and gross fetal anomalies.[34,46] To be performed by an appropriately trained operator.[34]
- *Targeted Ultrasound.* A targeted ultrasound establishes information obtained in the basic ultrasound and surveys or "scans" the fetal anatomy for malformations. To be performed by an operator with experience and expertise in this type of scanning.[34,44]

- *Limited Ultrasound.* Used when specific information is sought based on the clinical situation. Examples would be the following:[34]
  - Assessment of amniotic fluid volume
  - Fetal biophysical profile testing
  - Ultrasonography guided amniocentesis
  - External cephalic version
  - Confirmation of fetal life
  - Localization of placenta in event of antepartum bleeding
  - Confirmation of fetal presentation

INDICATIONS FOR ULTRASOUND

Gestational Age Determination. Ultrasound is used to establish gestational age in the first, second, or third trimester.

Scanning in the first trimester should obtain the following information.[34]

- Presence or absence in an intrauterine gestational sac
- Identification of embryo or fetus
- Fetal number
- Presence or absence of fetal cardiac activity
- Crown-rump length
- Evaluation of uterus and adnexal structures

Various parameters such as fetal heart activity and the presence of a gestational sac are noted earlier, using vaginal scanning as opposed to abdominal scanning.[34] Gestational age is most accurately assessed in the first trimester as there is minimal variation in fetal growth.[46] Gestational age is most accurately estimated by measuring crown-to-rump length (CRL) between 5 and 12 weeks,[30] gestational age can be calculated within 3–5 days 95 percent of the time.[30,34]

Scanning in the second trimester is often performed to determine gestational age when there is a discrepancy between uterine size and menstrual history. If a health care provider routinely performs only one ultrasound, an ultrasound done at 15–18 weeks not only provides an accurate measure of gestational age but allows surveillance of the fetal anatomy as well.[46] The most commonly used measurements are biparietal diameter (BPD), femur length(FL) or length of other long bones, and abdominal(AC) and head circumferences(HC).[30,34] Placental location is noted as well; however, the placenta "migrates"

during the pregnancy, and often what is seen as a marginal previa in the second trimester will be absent in the third trimester.[34] This is due to lengthening of the lower uterine segment later in pregnancy.[34]

Growth Assessment. Ultrasound is indicated when a discrepancy exists between estimated gestational age and uterine size. The ultrasound is done to rule out abnormalities or to correct errors in dating. It is used serially to diagnose intrauterine growth retardation in clients at risk for decreased uteroplacental perfusion, for example, those with hypertension or a history of fetuses with intrauterine growth retardation.[32] Serial ultrasounds may also be used for an obese client, because accurate assessment of uterine size by means of fundal height measurement is difficult in obese women.

Ratios of various measurements are often given to provide an index for growth. If not, they can be calculated and compared with standardized charts to determine appropriate growth for a particular gestational age.

Beyond the first trimester numerous variables are used to assess fetal growth, including BPD, FL, and AC. In the second and third trimesters, good estimates of gestational age are obtained from 12 to 20 weeks, using the BPD and FL. The BPD between 12–20 weeks is accurate for plus or minus 7 days.[30] FL can be measured accurately after 14 weeks.[30] In the third trimester, large variances of up to plus or minus three weeks occur, hereby decreasing the accuracy of third trimester dating.[34]

Detection of Fetal Anomalies. Fetal anomalies can be detected with ultrasound. Assessing fetal structures for anomalies is *fetal scanning.* Transabdominal scanning remains the standard, used at 18–22 weeks to assess the fetus for anomalies.[47] As technology advances, however, transvaginal sonography may become an equal option.[47] More than 80 percent of fetal anomalies develop before 12 weeks, and if detected, could allow early intervention.[47] It has been proposed to consider early screening for gross fetal anomalies and anatomic markers for genetic aberrations, then another scan at 18–22 weeks for complete assessment of all organs, particularly the fetal heart.[47] With a targeted assessment, craniospinal, cardiothoracic, urinary tract, and skeletal anomalies and gastrointestinal lesions should be detected.[47] The ultrasonographer should be experienced in performing these scans.[34] Fetal scans are indicated for women with a family history of disorder or anomaly of the abdominal wall or central nervous, renal, cardiac, or skeletal system.[34] Exposure to any teratogen that produces structural anomalies is also an indication for ultrasound.[34] Use and image interpretation will become more complex and diverse as technology advances.

Assessment of Amniotic Fluid Volume. Amniotic fluid volume can be assessed by ultrasound. Polyhydramnios has been associated with abnormal fetal position, operative delivery, and abruption.[48] Preterm delivery is also increased with polyhydramnios, which carries an increased perinatal mortality and morbidity rate.[48] A decrease in volume may indicate fetal compromise. Several studies have correlated decreased amniotic fluid volume with intrauterine growth retardation due to the adaptive response fetuses exhibit to hypoxemia; blood shunting to the vital organs (brain, adrenals, placenta, heart) and therefore away from the kidneys.[48,49] This shunting of blood away from the kidneys over a period of time results in oliguric oligohydramnios.[11] Oligohydramnios is also associated with intrapartum asphyxia and fetal death, correlating the presence of oligohydramnios with poor placental function.[48] In the absence of ruptured membranes and a functional genitourinary tract, the diagnosis of oligohydramnios indicates fetal compromise.[11]

Pregnancies complicated by extremes of amniotic fluid volume are also associated with fetal congenital anomalies; polyhydramnios has been associated with anomalies that obstruct fetal swallowing, such as diaphragmatic hernia; cardiac, intracranial, spinal and ventral wall defects have been reported as well.[33,48] Oligohydramnios has been associated with incidence of fetal urinary tract abnormalities; long-standing oligohydramnios restricts fetal movement, predisposing the developing fetus to orthopedic abnormalities due to compression, and interferes with normal fetal lung development resulting in pulmonary hypoplasia.[48] Oligohydramnios is considered to be an ominous sign, and a diagnostic workup should follow.

Polyhydramnios is defined as an amniotic fluid volume greater than the 95th percentile for a given gestational age; oligohydramnios is less than the 5th percentile for a given gestational age.[48] There is debate over the best method to measure amniotic fluid volume; the amniotic fluid index (AFI) appears to be less subjective. The AFI is the sum of the largest vertical pocket of fluid in each of the four quadrants of the uterus.[33] Generally, a total sum of 5 cm or less indicates severe oligohydramnios; 5.1 cm to 8.0 cm indicates moderate oligohydramnios, and 8.1 to 24 cm represents normal amniotic fluid volume.[33] Values greater than 24 cm, or more than 2000 ml indicate polyhydramnios.[33] These values are compared with established "normal" values for a given gestational age.[30,34] The "largest vertical pocket" was the original method, which assesses the vertical depth of the largest pocket visualized. If the largest pocket is less than 2cm, then oligohydramnios is present.[30]

Monitoring of a Post-Term Pregnancy. Surveillance should be considered for post-term pregnancy, defined as one that lasts beyond 42 weeks.[50] Perinatal mortality at 44 weeks is 4–6 times greater than for the fetus delivered at term.[50] Many providers initiate surveillance at 41 weeks.[50] The combination of monitoring amniotic fluid volume, the NST, biophysical profile and fetal movement counts is used to assess the post-term fetus.[50] Gestational age cannot be accurately determined at term.[50]

Detection of Placental Abnormalities. Ultrasound is used to grade the placenta.[51]

- *Grade 0.* The placenta is homogeneous, without calcifications, and with a smooth chorionic plate on the fetal side. A grade 0 is seen in the first and frequently in the second trimester; may be seen at term with maternal diabetes.
- *Grade I.* Echogenic densities are noted due to calcifications. The chorionic plate has an undulating appearance, which may remain unchanged until term.
- *Grade II.* More irregular surface with rounded areas; divisions of cotyledons are seen at chorionic surface but not extending to base plate or vascular complex of the myometrium.

- *Grade III.* Heterogeneous texture; lines of calcifications divide cotyledons, and maternal lakes are seen.

Some classify a pregnancy as high risk if a grade III placenta is present prior to 36 weeks because of the potential for fetal compromise; placental grading in relationship to gestational age may be indicative of IUGR, maternal diabetes, or placental vessel damage; however, the value of placental grading remains controversial.[11,31,34,51]

For women with a history of vaginal bleeding, ultrasound is needed to establish fetal viability and, if possible, to locate the origin of bleeding. Placenta previa or abruptio placentae may be diagnosed.

Documentation of Fetal Viability. When fetal heart tones are inaudible by Doppler at 12 weeks or with the DeLee fetoscope at 17 to 19 weeks, or if they are absent after previous documentation, ultrasound is indicated to verify cardiac activity.[19] A developing embryo can be seen as early as 34 days after the last normal menstrual period, and fetal cardiac activity has been documented 38 days after the last normal menstrual period.[30]

Detection of Ectopic Pregnancy. Ectopic pregnancy is always a possible diagnosis in the first trimester in a client with abdominal pain and a positive pregnancy test. Abdominal ultrasound may be attempted first, depending on the protocol of the institution. If abdominal assessment is unsatisfactory, a transvaginal probe is used.

Compilation of Biophysical Profile. The biophysical profile is compiled using ultrasound (see next section).

ADVANTAGES AND DISADVANTAGES

Abdominal ultrasound is not invasive, and may promote bonding, particularly before quickening. Abdominal ultrasound presents a problem for a client experiencing nausea and vomiting during pregnancy, because she must drink approximately 1 quart of water in the hour before examination. The transvaginal probe does not require a full bladder (as does abdominal ultrasound). Anxiety may be increased if clients are not given information during ultrasound concerning structures seen and the well-being of the fetus. Clients' fears are

lessened with positive feedback from the ultrasonographer, but due to the various levels of expertise, information may not be shared with the client until confirmed by a provider with clinical expertise in ultrasonography. Ultrasound must be performed and interpreted by a qualified individual. Depending on the test, expertise is required to collect correct data and interpret findings.

Loss of fetus or termination may be more difficult if the client has already viewed the fetus. If ultrasound has promoted bonding, a client may grieve more with demise or termination.

CLIENT TEACHING AND COUNSELING

Explain to the client what ultrasound is. Inform her that no cases of harm to a fetus have been documented. The client needs to be aware that a technician may perform the ultrasound, and, if so, that person can identify structures but cannot interpret findings. Depending on protocol, the radiologist, physician, or practitioner is responsible for discussing the results with the client.

For abdominal ultrasound, the client must drink approximately 1 quart of water 1 hour prior to procedure and, therefore, needs to be aware that there will be pressure on her bladder during ultrasound. If an ectopic pregnancy or any other diagnosis in which surgery may be indicated is to be ruled out, the bladder should be filled by catheter (usually by a technician), and the client should be informed of the need for catheterization.

For the client undergoing transvaginal ultrasound, explain that a probe will be inserted into the vagina. She can expect some pressure but should not be uncomfortable. Briefly describe the probe and reassure the client that the probe will not hurt the fetus or cause miscarriage. A full bladder is not necessary for transvaginal ultrasound.

Biophysical profile (BPP)

Real-time ultrasound allows assessment of various parameters of fetal well-being: fetal tone, breathing, motion, and amniotic fluid volume. These four parameters together with the NST constitute the biophysical profile; however, not all

TABLE 19–1. GUIDELINES FOR INTERPRETING THE BIOPHYSICAL PROFILE

8/8 (without NST), 10/10 (with NST), and 8/10 (with normal AFV)	Testing may be repeated.
8/10 with abnormal AFV	Consider delivery if gestation is greater than 36 weeks. If less than 36 weeks, serial testing is advised; consider delivery if the BPP is less than 6.
6/10 with normal AFV	If the gestation is longer than 34 weeks, consider delivery; if less than 34 weeks, repeat the BPP in 24 hours. Consider delivery if the BPP score is less than 6.
6/10 with abnormal AFV	Consider delivery if the gestation is longer than 26 weeks.
4/10 with normal AFV	Consider delivery if gestation is greater than 32 weeks. If less than 32 weeks, repeat the BPP on the same day; consider delivery if that score is less than 6.
4/10 with abnormal AFV	Consider delivery if longer than 26 weeks.
2/10	Extend the BPP to 60 minutes. Consider delivery if the score remains less than 6 and gestation is longer than 26 weeks.
0/10	Consider delivery if > 26 weeks.

Source: Reference 11.

facilities perform NST unless other parameters of the profile are abnormal. Manning advocates using the NST only when one of the four parameters of the BPP is abnormal.[13] BPP may best be used as a secondary method of testing fetal well-being, or perhaps used as an adjunct to NST. For some, the BPP is fundamental to fetal assessment, particularly in high risk pregnancies.[31]

PROCEDURE

Usually the profile is compiled in an outpatient testing center within a hospital. Skilled personnel are required to perform the NST, as well as to conduct and evaluate the ultrasound. Although the BPP is an advanced surveillance test, nurses with advanced training can perform the ultrasound, score the BPP, and in nonreassuring situations, initiate further assessment.[52]

SCORING

Each component of the BPP is scored as 2 (variable normal) or 0 (variable abnormal).[11] A total score of 10 is possible if the NST is used. Thirty minutes is allotted for testing, although fewer than 8 minutes is usually needed.[13] If the fetus is fewer than 32 weeks, BPP may need to be extended to 60 minutes.[53] In another scoring system under investigation, each component receives a score of 0, 1, or 2 and the placenta is graded; no advantage has been noted with this revised scor-

ing system.[11,13] The following criteria must be met to obtain a score of 2; anything less is zero.[11,13]

- *Gross Body Movements.* Three or more discrete body or limb movements.
- *Fetal Tone.* One or more full extension and flexion of a limb or trunk, or opening or closing of a hand.
- *Fetal Breathing.* One or more breathing movements of at least 30 seconds' duration.
- *Amniotic Fluid Volume (AFV).* One or more pockets of fluid measuring at least 2 cm in 2 perpendicular planes.
- *Nonstress Test.* Performed in the event one of the first four parameters are abnormal; graded as normal (2) or abnormal (0). A normal NST is characterized by two accelerations greater than 15 bpm over baseline, each lasting at least 15 seconds within a 20-minute period. An abnormal NST characterized by fewer than two episodes of accelerations or accelerations fewer than 15 bpm above baseline within 30 minutes.

INTERPRETATION

Results of the BPP should be considered in view of the clinical history and the facilities available to care for mother and fetus. The recommendations in Table 19–1 are to be used as guidelines within an existing protocol.[11]

Further testing, such as Doppler flow studies, may be required to validate clinical decisions.[7]

ADVANTAGES AND DISADVANTAGES

As with ultrasound, the BPP can enhance maternal bonding and help the client recognize fetal movement. The BPP has the sensitivity to predict poor fetal outcome in high risk pregnancies, as well as to permit assessment of amniotic fluid volume, placental characteristics, and the function of various fetal systems.

Research continues regarding questions of the effectiveness of the BPP as a screening test and the frequency with which it needs to be performed. Expertise is needed to perform and assess the BPP accurately. Computerized biophysical profiles are currently being utilized.[52] A modified version of the BPP, which assesses only the NST and AFV, has been found to be just as successful in terms of outcome and intervention rates when compared with a full BPP.[7,10]

CLIENT TEACHING AND COUNSELING

Provide information to the client about ultrasound (see preceding section), as the BPP is usually compiled through the use of abdominal ultrasound. If possible, point out the fetal anatomic structures and indicate the clinical parameters being assessed.

DOPPLER FLOW STUDIES

Doppler ultrasound velocimetry is used to obtain hemodynamic information.[54] By transmitting an ultrasound beam across a blood vessel, the velocity of blood flow can be measured.[55] Although previously used only to assess peripheral vasculature and cardiac function in children and adults,[42] Doppler ultrasound is now used to evaluate maternal and fetal blood flow. Umbilical arterial, aortic, cerebral, and uteroplacental circulation can be assessed.[18] There is also potential for using the cerebroplacental ratios as indicators of hypoxia and acidosis, as fetal circulation is redistributed in order to "shunt" blood to vital organs, such as the brain, in the presence of IUGR.[18,56] The brain sparing effect can vary based on gestational age, and has to be taken into consideration.[56] It has been postulated the brain sparing effect disappears prior to fetal demise.[56] If research continues to confirm

this theory, cerebral Doppler flow studies may be utilized to provide guidelines as relates to the critical time to interrupt pregnancy.[56] Its use is still under investigation, however, and should be used in conjunction with umbilical arterial Doppler indices.[18,55] The precise role of Doppler flow studies regarding screening, diagnosis, and management will continue to evolve.

Because diastolic flow normally increases in relation to systolic peak throughout pregnancy, monitoring a pregnancy at risk for compromise includes noting decreased diastolic flow.[54] Decreased diastolic flow indicates increased placental bed resistance and potential compromise for the fetus due to decreased placental perfusion. Decreased or absent diastolic flow indicates high resistance in the placenta and is often seen in pregnancies complicated by preeclampsia or intrauterine growth retardation.[54] These fetuses have higher rates of morbidity and mortality.[55] As placental insufficiency worsens, there is first a decrease in diastolic flow, then an absence, then reverse diastolic flow is seen.[56] Serial studies provide insight into worsening placental insufficiency; decreasing diastolic flow is associated with low birthweight and adverse perinatal outcome.[56] Absence of end-diastolic flow requires more frequent or further testing; the presence of reverse diastolic flow indicates serious fetal compromise, and requires further testing and/or intervention.[54,55]

If the potential for decreased placental perfusion exists, for example, in women with hypertension, Doppler can predict a poor outcome. Other maternal disease states in which Doppler detects the fetus at risk is fetal growth retardation, systemic lupus, antiphospholipid antibody syndrome and diabetes.[54] Some feel Doppler flow studies should be made available to all women who have high risk pregnancies.[1,57]

Controversy surrounds the ability of Doppler flow studies to detect fetal acidosis.[54] The NST and BPP appear to be able to more accurately assess asphyxia than the S/D ratio of umbilical arterial Doppler measurements, although others conclude Doppler flow studies may be a better indicator of acidemia than BPP.[18,56] Doppler assessment should be viewed with other clinical data in determining management of a compromised fetus; it should not be the sole parameter in determining fetal well-being, or the basis of clinical decisions.[56] It is not a sensitive screening tool to predict intrauterine growth retardation among unselected populations; rather, it identifies the fetus at risk for adverse perinatal outcome as it is a test of *placental* function as opposed to an assessment of the fetus.[54,56,57] Fetuses at risk for IUGR, however, may be examined every 2–4 weeks with Doppler ultrasound; if an abnormal flow is detected, surveillance of the fetus can increase to biweekly, or more frequently, if delivery is remote.[55]

Fetal Doppler echocardiography is also used. Fetal echocardiography should be recommended to clients who have a history of congenital heart disease, or maternal conditions that increase the risk of congenital cardiac anomalies such as diabetes, drug or teratogen exposure.[55]

INDICATIONS

Decreased placental perfusion caused by maternal disease or placental abnormalities is a potential indication for Doppler flow studies. Doppler has been used in pregnancies complicated by hypertension, diabetes mellitus, intrauterine growth retardation, and Rh isoimmunization.[54]

Arrhythmias detected with auscultation or electronic fetal monitoring can be identified using M-mode echocardiography.[55]

Fetuses diagnosed with cardiac anomalies can benefit from pulsed and color Doppler ultrasonography for accurate diagnosis and cardiac function.[55] Due to the differences in blood flow in the fetus versus the neonate, a congenital cardiac anomaly is not necessarily lethal in utero; care consists of accurate diagnosis of the abnormality, frequency of assessment, possible treatment prior to delivery, and how care will be provided to the neonate after delivery.[55]

PROCEDURE

Currently the umbilical arteries are the most widely used to assess fetal well-being with Doppler flow studies and seem to hold the greatest promise for clinical evaluation.[18,56] To evaluate the umbilical artery, the blood flow is assessed during systole and diastole with a Doppler probe, thereby creating a waveform that can be plotted and measured. The systolic/diastolic (S/D) ratio

is derived by dividing systolic peak by the end-diastolic component.[54]

A pulsed wave Doppler probe is used for flow studies. The client lies supine with the uterus slightly tilted, using a wedge or cushion. After transducer gel is placed on the abdomen, the fetus is located with Doppler probe. Flow within the umbilical artery is identified, and the difference between systolic and diastolic flow is displayed. Several readings are taken, and the S/D ratio calculated.[18,55]

The S/D ratio becomes irrelevant when diastolic flow is absent; therefore, other values are obtained.[58] The pulsatility index (PI), also known as the impedance index, is the S/D ratio divided by the mean velocity.[58] This requires computer assisted calculation of mean velocity, and is subject to experimental error.[58] It is the preferred index, however, for vessels of microcirculation or when diastolic flow is absent or reversed.[56] The resistance index (RI) is the S/D ratio divided by the systolic value.[19,58]

INTERPRETATION

The PI, RI, and S/D ratio all normally decrease during pregnancy due to decreased placental resistance.[56] Higher placental resistance is found in the presence of placental insufficiency, detected by a decrease in diastolic velocity.[56] The values for all three indices are calculated and compared with standardized charts for fetuses of the same gestational age.[55] Doppler indices are affected by gestational age, fetal breathing, fetal heartrate, and the location on the umbilical cord that is chosen to perform Doppler flow studies; Doppler indices are higher on the fetal end of the cord than the placental end, and this should be taken into consideration when interpreting values.[18,56]

As previously stated, absence of end-diastolic flow or presence of reverse diastolic flow is correlated with adverse perinatal outcome and has been associated with trisomy 13, 18, and 21, as well as congenital heart and kidney disease, and fetal infections.[18]

Reverse diastolic flow, which is caused by increased flow resistance in the placental bed, is an indication for hospitalization and evaluation for delivery. Reverse diastolic flow has been associated with fetal death.[54] Reverse flow may occur with an incompetent valve or abnormal ventricular function.[54] Other abnormalities seen are persistent diastolic notching, major left-to-right variance in indices varying with placental site, and deep transition of high impedance to low impedance.[58]

All abnormal results warrant further evaluation, such as fetal heartrate monitoring, biophysical profile, ultrasonography to monitor growth, or amniotic fluid indices.[54] Delivery should be considered when other tests indicate imminent fetal danger or when reverse diastolic flow is encountered.[54]

ADVANTAGES AND DISADVANTAGES

Doppler has the potential to detect fetal compromise in high risk pregnancies, it is noninvasive, it has no contraindications. In some instances of fetal compromise, changes in Doppler flow studies occur prior to detection of abnormalities with FHR monitoring.[54] Doppler flow studies may become abnormal 3 weeks before irregularities can be assessed using external fetal monitoring.[54] There are also several disadvantages. An experienced individual must perform the test; up to 1 hour is required for a premature fetus. To date, studies question the indications for Doppler use; therefore, it should be done as an adjunct with other studies.[54]

CLIENT TEACHING AND COUNSELING

Provide the same information given for ultrasound testing. The client needs to know why the test is being done, its implications, and how it complements other tests. Be sure to coordinate exams, counseling and planning sessions; if fetal echocardiography is used due to a cardiac abnormality, be sure to coordinate exams, counseling and planning sessions; if fetal echocardiography is used due to a cardiac abnormality, be sure to coordinate sessions with pediatric cardiologists and neonataologists to provide continuity for the client.[55]

AMNIOCENTESIS AND CHORIONIC VILLUS SAMPLING (CVS)

Both amniocentesis and CVS aid in the diagnosis of chromosomal abnormalities in a fetus. Generally, prenatal diagnosis is offered to clients who will be age 35 or older at delivery, because the risk of a chromosomal abnormality is equal to the risk of fetal loss associated with amniocentesis and chorionic villus sampling. Before these tests are done, fetal viability and normal growth must be established by ultrasound.

AMNIOCENTESIS

Amniotic fluid is withdrawn from the uterus, and the cells obtained are cultured to identify chromosomal and biochemical abnormalities; amniocentesis is performed at 15 to 18 weeks of gestation.[59] First trimester and early second trimester amniocentesis at 11–14 weeks has been investigated, although it appears that first trimester amniocentesis carries a higher fetal loss rate than CVS or traditional amniocentesis.[8,44,60] The volume of amniotic fluid is lower in earlier gestations, requiring the practitioner to carefully assess the amount of fluid withdrawn to avoid pulmonary complications and possible impaired development of extremities.[16,59] The general rule is to remove only 1 ml of fluid per week of gestation.[59]

Research continues as to the safety of *early* amniocentesis (prior to 15 weeks gestation). It is a desirable procedure due to the fact health care providers are already comfortable with it and the cost is lower compared to CVS.[60,61] Early amniocentesis is an alternative to CVS, but due to the restrictions involved with amniotic fluid volume and with membrane tenting due to a lack of fusion, it is unlikely amniocentesis will be performed at the gestational age of CVS.[61]

The majority of amniocenteses are performed to rule out chromosomal anomalies.[59] As with CVS, ultrasound must be performed prior to the procedure to confirm gestational age and fetal viability.

Amniocenteses is done with ultrasound guidance and surgical asepsis to avoid infection. After the abdomen is cleansed and the puncture site locally anesthetized, a 20- or 22-gauge, 3- to 6-inch needle is inserted. Amniotic fluid is aspirated and analyzed. After the procedure, fetal cardiac activity is verified, and the fetus is monitored for adverse effects.[19] The incidence of fetal-maternal hemorrhage is well documented; therefore, MSAFP should never be evaluated immediately after amniocentesis.[59] *Rhogam is administered to Rh-negative clients after the procedure.*[19]

Indications. A repeatedly elevated MSAFP or an initial low MSAFP, maternal age greater than 35 years, history of chromosomal anomaly in a child or close family member, parental balanced chromosomal rearrangement, dysmorphology noted on ultrasound, previous infant or fetus with an open neural tube defect, two or more unexplained spontaneous abortions, and a family history of detectable Mendelian disorders are indications for amniocenteses.[8,59]

Amniocentesis is not only used to obtain amniotic fluid for genetic studies but also for a variety of indications. Amniotic fluid can be analyzed for infection through the use of bacterial and viral studies, and biochemical analysis has made it possible to detect open neural tube defects and assess the status of fetal lung maturity[59] (see Assessing Fetal Lung Maturity in this section). Amniocentesis is also an avenue for fetal treatment, as used with amnioinfusion in the presence of severe oligohydramnios or release of fluid as seen with severe polyhydramnios.[33,59]

Although ultrasound has become more sophisticated at screening for anatomical landmarks associated with genetic anomalies, and the use of the triple screen has enhanced a noninvasive method for screening, amniocentesis remains the gold standard for fetal diagnosis of chromosomal abnormalities.[8]

Advantages and Disadvantages. Traditional amniocentesis is associated with a lower risk of complications than CVS, although the risk varies among institutions.[60] Early amniocentesis carries a higher fetal loss rate, and since it's fairly new, there is too little data to be reassured concerning values that have been set for AFAFP and AChE values.[60,61] There is an increased risk of membrane tenting, which may increase the number of needle insertions and may lessen the chance of the membranes resealing.[59] Since amniocentesis is a procedure many providers are already familiar with, however, the risks associated with early amniocentesis may decrease due to increased provider use. Early amniocentesis is also more readily available than CVS since providers are familiar with the procedure. If the client chooses to terminate the pregnancy, early amniocentesis has the same advantage of CVS to provide prenatal diagnosis in the first or early second trimester

when termination is safer to perform than during the late second trimester, as well as being less emotionally disturbing as fetal movement has not been perceived.[59]

Amniocentesis cannot detect a closed neural tube defect and is associated with some complications. If a fetal anomaly does exist and is not detected until the second trimester with amniocentesis, the client who chooses to terminate her pregnancy is at greater risk for complications than if she had terminated the pregnancy in the first trimester.[8,62]

Complications. Maternal risks include hemorrhage, uterine cramping, infection, injury to the abdominal wall, uterus, placenta, leakage of amniotic fluid, and blood group sensitization.[59] Fetal risks include pregnancy loss, needle injury, and infection.[59] Fetal injury does not occur often due to the use of ultrasound guidance; however, in the event the fetus rolls or brushes against the needle, experience with fetal tissue biopsy and fetal surgery has shown that fetal skin injuries generally heal without scarring.[59] Skilled practitioners quote a pregnancy loss associated with amniocentesis at 0.3 percent to 0.5 percent.[59]

Client Teaching and Counseling. Inform the client that she may experience uncomfortable pressure during the procedure, mild cramping up to 48 hours after the procedure, and slight bruising around the insertion site. Reassure the client that fetal heartbeat will be verified after the procedure. Instruct the client to telephone if she notes bleeding, leaking fluid, severe cramping, temperature higher than 100° F, chills, as well as lack of fetal movement if fetal movement has been noted by the client already. Advise the client to avoid strenuous activity or sexual intercourse for 48 hours after the procedure.[44]

Inform the client of the possible risks to herself and the fetus, the significance of abnormal values, and the possible consequences prior to the procedure. Be prepared to counsel the client concerning all possible options.

ASSESSING FETAL LUNG MATURITY

Amniocentesis is used in the third trimester to assess fetal lung maturity if delivery is a possibility prior to 37 weeks' gestation. The procedure is performed much in the same way as described for a second trimester amniocentesis. The fluid obtained can be analyzed through a variety of means to assess the risk of respiratory distress in the newborn. Several components are produced as the fetal lung matures, which are secreted in the tracheal fluid, and then released into amniotic fluid. This can then be assessed via amniocentesis. These components can be measured from fluid obtained from a vaginal pool, as in the case of ruptured membranes, but can give false readings on some tests.[19]

The following are methods to assess lung maturity: Lecithin-to-sphingomyelin Ratio (L/S ratio)—Prior to 34 weeks, lecithin and sphingomyelin are found in equal amounts in amniotic fluid. After 34 weeks, the level of lecithin begins to rise. If the L/S ratio is less than 2:1, there is a greater risk of respiratory distress than if the ratio were 2:1 or greater.[19] In the presence of a compromised fetus that could be better cared for outside the uterus, however, a L/S ratio of less than 2:1 may not weigh as significantly if the fetus is expected to deteriorate further if left in utero.[19]

Phosphatidyglycerol (PG)—PG enhances surface-active properties that aid in prevention of alveolar collapse. It is either reported as present or absent. The presence of PG provides assurance that respiratory distress is unlikely to develop but does not fully guarantee it.[19] PG can be evaluated from a vaginal pool specimen.[19]

Surfactant-Albumin Ratio—Has shown promise with its predictive value; a Tdx reading of 50 or more has predicted fetal lung maturity.[19]

Shake test—Performed with a 1:1 dilution of amniotic fluid and 95 percent ethanol. This is shaken for 20 seconds, and read at 15 minutes. A stable bubble over the entire surface is considered a positive reading for maturity.[63]

Tap test—Performed by mixing 1 ml of amniotic fluid with 1 drop of 6N hydrochloric acid and 1.5 ml of diethyl ether. The test tube is tapped three to four times, creating 200–300 bubbles. In the presence of maturity, the bubbles rise quickly to the surface and burst. If after 10 minutes there are five bubbles or fewer in the ether layer, then the test is positive for maturity.[63]

Each method has its own level of sensitivity, specificity, and predictive value.[63] Not all of the above methods are utilized in every institution;

the tap test was found to be a good alternative to other methods due to its accuracy, low cost and ability to be carried out "at the bedside," rather than requiring a laboratory facility for analysis.[63] The L/S ratio and presence of PG, however, is still the gold standard for many providers.

Corticosteroids were first used in 1972 for women who were anticipated to deliver prematurely to enhance fetal lung maturity; it was found that the incidence of early neonatal death, necrotizing enterocolitis, respiratory distress syndrome (RDS), and intraventricular hemorrhage (IVH) was decreased as well.[64] The use of corticosteroids, given to the mother to accelerate lung maturity in the fetus, is debated in perinatal centers, despite recommendations for use from a NIH Consensus Conference.[64] In summary, this conference recommended corticosteroid use for infants between 24 and 34 weeks' gestation who are at risk for preterm delivery, unless delivery is eminent.[64] In women with premature preterm rupture of membranes (PPROM) without indication of chorioamnionitis, corticosteroids are recommended if the fetus is between 24 and 32 weeks' gestation to decrease the incidence of IVH; data concerning decreased incidence for RDS was equivocal for women with PPROM.[64] The reader is referred to the source for exact protocols for administration.[64]

The use of surfactant, given to the infant through an endotracheal tube at delivery, is decreasing the incidence of neonatal mortality related to respiratory distress syndrome.[19] The use of corticosteroids antenatally complements surfactant therapy after delivery to reduce mortality in the infant.[64]

CHORIONIC VILLUS SAMPLING (CVS)

CVS is the isolation of cells derived from the same fertilized egg as the fetus; genetic analysis can then be performed on these cells.[62,65] CVS is performed between 10 and 12 weeks.[62] Sampling may occur transcervically or transabdominally; the techniques have equal loss rates.[62] With ultrasound for guidance, the villi are aspirated from the placenta and examined. A direct cell culture can be available in hours, but should be interpreted as a preliminary result as there has been a high rate of false mosaicism (the presence of one or more cell types).[44] Further cell culture is available in 5 to 14 days.[44] The methodologies and indications for transcervical and transabdominal CVS are slightly different.[44,60]

After the procedure, fetal cardiac activity is verified with ultrasound, and the fetus is monitored to note any adverse effects. In addition, Rhogam should be administered to unsensitized Rh-negative clients after the procedure.

MSAFP should be offered to all women at 15–16 weeks because CVS cannot detect open neural tube defects.[42,44] Amniocentesis is the preferred method of diagnosis if testing for open neural tube defects.[60]

Indications. Indications for CVS are maternal age greater than 35, previous child with a chromosome abnormality, balanced structural chromosome rearrangement in a parent, or family history of detectable Mendelian disorders.[8] If amniotic fluid is required for diagnosis, such as for neural tube defects, the client should be offered amniocentesis instead.[44,65] CVS is not utilized to diagnose fragile X syndrome.[62]

Contraindications. CVS is not recommended in the isoimmunized client as CVS may worsen sensitization.[60] Transcervical sampling is preferred with a posterior placenta, and retroverted uterus.[60] Transabdominal sampling is preferred with an anterior placenta and is the method of choice in clients who have active herpes lesions.[60]

Advantages and Disadvantages. Compared with amniocentesis, CVS permits quicker diagnosis (5 to 14 days for cell culture, depending on health care facility) and, thereby, earlier recognition of a fetal abnormality.[44] Earlier recognition is helpful if the client must make a decision concerning termination of the pregnancy. Termination during the first trimester presents fewer risks to the client and enhances her privacy, as pregnancy is not yet obvious to others.[65] Moreover, early diagnosis can be essential to recognize and treat various chromosomal anomalies.[8] Although there is a risk of pregnancy loss (see Complications), very few failures occur in actually retrieving villi and performing chromosomal analysis.[60]

One disadvantage of CVS is that currently it is only done in large facilities; not all facilities have the capability or staff with sufficient expertise. Another disadvantage is that CVS tests only for chromosomal anomalies and cannot detect anatomic aberrations, such as open neural tube defects. Also note the complications listed.

Complications. Pregnancy loss varies depending on the center and the expertise of the provider; CVS carries a slightly higher rate of procedure failure and fetal loss than amniocentesis, but the rate has not been found to be statistically significant.[60,62,65] The risk of fetal loss from CVS is approximately 0.5 to 1.0%.[65]

Fetal loss may also be coincidental. Women who are at increased risk for pregnancy loss secondary to their age or having a chromosomally abnormal fetus will have an increased rate of spontaneous abortion despite the risk of CVS or amniocentesis. Spontaneous fetal loss occurs with 0.5 percent of pregnancies.[65]

Clinical infection is reduced if transabdominal sampling is used for a client with cervicitis or vaginitis, although overall infection rates for CVS or amniocentesis has been less than 0.1 percent.[65]

Subsequent limb anomalies have been linked to CVS. Conflicting reports exist concerning the incidence and etiology of limb reduction, however. Theories suggest that vascular disruption may occur during the retrieval of chorionic villi, affecting formation of embryonic limbs or limbs that have already been formed.[65] Anomalies may also be related to gestational age at the time of CVS, catheter or needle size, and the clinician's experience in performing CVS.[60,62] Current data estimate the risk of limb reduction related to CVS at 0.03 percent–0.10 percent.[62] The risk of limb reduction has been higher when CVS is performed at less than 10 weeks' gestation.[60,62] It is recommended to perform CVS between 10–12 weeks after the last menstrual period and by experienced providers with a combined experience of 200–250 procedures.[8,60,65]

Client Teaching and Counseling. Advise the client to call if she experiences moderate vaginal bleeding, severe cramping, leaking fluid, temperature higher than 100° F, or chills. Cramping may continue for up to 48 hours after CVS. The client should avoid strenuous activity and sexual intercourse for 48 hours. Discuss each step of the procedure with the client to help decrease her anxiety.

The client should be aware of the potential risks to herself and the fetus. The consequences of an abnormal result should be discussed prior to the procedure. Be aware of all options available to the client; referrals to perinatologists and pediatricians are helpful for the client in becoming knowledgeable about her fetus. If the client chooses termination, counsel her appropriately and be knowledgeable about the location of centers for pregnancy termination.

PERCUTANEOUS UMBILICAL BLOOD SAMPLING (PUBS)

The terms PUBS and cordocentesis are used interchangeably in reference to the invasive sampling of fetal blood. PUBS was originally done using fetoscopy, and fetal loss was high (5 percent to 6 percent).[66] The use of ultrasound has decreased the risks of PUBS, however, and its use for a variety of indications has expanded in the last few years.[67] PUBS not only can be a method to assess fetal well-being but can provide fetal therapy as well.[66,67]

PROCEDURE

PUBS can be performed at approximately 16–18 weeks' gestation or later as clinical indications arise.[67] Ultrasound is used to assess fetal viability, position, biometry, location of the placenta, and presence of fetal anomalies.[68] The insertion site of the umbilical cord in the placenta is identified.[68] The maternal abdomen is cleansed and draped, just as for amniocentesis.[68] The operator and sonographer wear surgical cap, gown, and gloves if fetal transfusion is to be performed; only surgical gloves are necessary for blood sampling.[66] Under ultrasound guidance, a 20- to 25-gauge needle is inserted into the amniotic cavity and into the umbilical vein; the veins can be distinguished by their size, and the direction of blood flow using color Doppler.[68] Confirmation that the blood sample is of fetal origin is imperative.[67] A number of tests are available, including the Kleihauer-Betke test and comparison of mean corpuscular volume.[66,67]

Once the needle has been inserted into the umbilical vein, fetal blood is withdrawn into a syringe.[68] Samples can be evaluated for coagulation studies, blood group typing, complete blood count, karyotyping, and blood gas analysis.[68] Due to the risk of transplacental hemorrhage, Rh-negative clients are given Rhogam.[67] Intrahepatic fetal blood sampling and cardiocentesis have been researched as well, although the fetal loss rate is higher than for umbilical vein insertion.[68]

After the age of viability, a course of corticosteroids is advised prior to PUBS.[68] This is to enhance fetal lung maturity due to the risk of preterm labor, or for the need for immediate delivery in the event fetal distress occurs during or after PUBS.[68] For this reason, if the fetus is at the age of viability, PUBS should only be done in a hospital setting (as opposed to an outpatient setting) in order to deliver the fetus by cesarean section if needed.[68]

INDICATIONS[66,68]

- Cytogenetic diagnosis: for instance, when rapid karyotype is needed, or if one or more cell types is identified (mosaicism or pseudomosaicism) at amniocentesis or CVS
- Congenital infection: toxoplasmosis, rubella, cytomegalovirus, parvovirus, congenital syphilis
- Congenital immunodeficiency
- Coagulopathies
- Platelet disorders
- Hemoglobinopathies
- Severe IUGR: detect etiology, assess fetal hematologic and acid-base function
- Multiple gestation: twin to twin transfusion syndrome
- Fetal therapy: transfusions or pharmacologic agents when transplacental passage of the drug is poor
- Diagnosis and/or treatment: fetal anemia, nonimmune hydrops

COMPLICATIONS

Fetal loss varies, depending on indication, operator experience, technique, and gestational age at procedure.[68] Other complications can be hemorrhage, cord hematoma or thrombosis, which may obstruct blood flow and cause fetal distress, bradycardia, fetomaternal hemorrhage, chorio-amnionitis, premature rupture of membranes, and abruptio placentae.[67,68] It is debated whether or not there is an increased risk for preterm delivery.[67,68]

In general, fetal loss rates due to PUBS range from 1 to 4 percent and higher depending on the indication for PUBS.[66,67] With such a significant loss rate, only clients with clear indications should be offered this method of assessment.[67] Adequate imaging of the cord is not always possible, and another method of surveillance should be chosen, or PUBS should be postponed.[67] Aseptic technique, and limiting the number of puncture sites will reduce complications.[67] Transversing the placenta may worsen alloimmunization due to intermixing of fetal and maternal blood.[67]

ADVANTAGES AND DISADVANTAGES

Fetal karyotype can be obtained from a culture of fetal blood in 48 to 72 hours.[67] PUBS is used to assess the alloimmunized pregnancy at gestational ages fewer than 26 weeks, as the accuracy of spectrophotometric analysis of amniotic fluid has not been validated in assessing the status of fetal anemia.[67] The use of PUBS for fetal transfusion is lifesaving for the fetus with non-immune hydrops fetalis if the fetus is remote from term.[67]

The main disadvantage is fetal loss, as well as other complications noted.

CLIENT TEACHING AND COUNSELING

The client needs to be aware of the risks involved, as well as the need for immediate intervention in the event fetal distress is noted. Other options, if applicable, should be made available to the client. Counseling, and, therefore, fetal loss rates, need to be specific in regard to the indication for PUBS. Genetic studies versus transfusion for nonimmune hydrops are completely different indications and require specific counseling based on the status of the client and fetus.

POTENTIAL SCREENING METHODS FOR THE FUTURE

FETAL CELL ISOLATION FROM MATERNAL BLOOD

It is possible to assess fetal cells obtained from a maternal blood sample; screening for trisomy 21 is possible by this method.[44] Fetal cells may be present in maternal circulation as early as 6 weeks of gestation, and fetal nucleated red cells seem to hold the greatest promise for research.[39,69]

The development of PCR and fluorescence in situ hybridization (FISH) is under investigation to be able to provide this type of noninvasive screening to women.[69] PCR can detect one fetal cell in 10^{5th} to 10^{6th} maternal cells, and fetal DNA sequences have been detected in all three trimesters.[39] Fetal sex may be determined through use of polymerase chain reaction amplification (PCR) with Y-chromosome DNA primers.[66] FISH uses chromosome specific probes to detect fetal aneuploidies.[39,67] Currently, neither FISH nor PCR provides full cytogenetic diagnosis but may serve as screening tests for clinically significant aneuploidies.[69]

The greatest advantage is that information can be obtained in 2 to 3 days, and there are no risks to the fetus.[67] Enrichment of fetal cells will have to be refined as well in order to provide accuracy.[39] The National Institute of Health is currently sponsoring trials to evaluate efficiency of detecting fetal genetic abnormalities; the trials should be completed by 1998.[69] Research will continue in this area to refine a cost effective procedure, while providing a noninvasive test to assess the fetus.[44] Readers are referred to Carson and Buster, for a thorough but easy to read review of PCR and FISH.[70]

FETAL FIBRONECTIN AS AN INDICATOR OF PRETERM LABOR

Current research is attempting to identify markers that would predict preterm labor; fetal fibronectin is a protein produced by fetal membranes, and serves to bind the placenta and fetal membranes to the decidua.[71] It is found in cervicovaginal secretions until 16–20 weeks, then is no longer normally present until late in pregnancy.[71]

It has been postulated that if fibronectin is present in cervicovaginal secretions after 20 weeks, it may be the result of a destruction of the basement membranes, possibly due to bacterial colonization.[72,73] Fetal fibronectin has been found to be of value in predicting spontaneous preterm birth, particularly when combined with home uterine monitoring, but not in reducing spontaneous preterm birth.[71,73] Since research continues to identify interventions to prevent preterm birth, it may be ineffective to identify those at risk, with the possibility of intervening unnecessarily, and potentially causing more harm than good.[71] For the moment, the use of fetal fibronectin may be able to help researchers effectively target interventions that would be valuable in preventing preterm birth; if fibronectin is in fact related to bacterial colonization, research may focus on intervention specific to certain bacteria, or the inhibition of prostaglandin production after bacterial colonization.[73] One study suggests the endometrium may be colonized prior to conception.[72] The ramifications of this theory are far reaching. Research will continue in the realm of preterm birth to discover and understand the etiology, pharmacologic intervention, and ongoing surveillance needed to prevent preterm birth.

FETAL TISSUE BIOPSY

Fetal skin sampling is utilized to diagnose disorders that cannot be diagnosed by chorionic villus sampling or amniocentesis.[74] Initially, this procedure was done using fetoscopy, but is now done with ultrasound guidance.

The procedure is performed at 17–20 weeks. Gestational age, viability, fetal lie, placental location, and any abnormalities are assessed prior to the procedure with ultrasound.[74] The maternal abdomen is cleansed and locally anesthesitized. A trocar is introduced into the uterus, and a 2mm biopsy taken from the fetal thorax, back, buttocks, or scalp.[74] Ultrasound surveillance continues after the procedure to assess fetal status and note any bleeding.[74]

Fetal liver and muscle biopsy has been performed at 17–20 weeks, and 16–22 weeks, respectively, for diagnoses in which DNA analysis

is not able to assess for the detected mutation, such as carbamoyl-phosphate synthetase deficiency, glycogen-storage disease, and duchenne muscular dystrophy; there is not sufficient data for either procedure to cite complications.[66,74]

INDICATIONS

Utilized when histologic evaluation is required for diagnosis as is the case with several genodermatoses, which are severe and often fatal.[66,74] CVS and amniocentesis are not applicable to diagnose these disorders at this time, although may be diagnosable through DNA analyses in the future.[74]

COMPLICATIONS

The risks are much the same as for amniocentesis, with the addition of cosmetic or functional injuries.[66,74] In experienced centers, the fetal loss rate from fetoscopy and fetal skin sampling is less than 5 percent.[74]

PREIMPLANTATION GENETIC DIAGNOSIS

There have been 40 births (presumably more by the time of this printing) in which preimplantation genetic diagnosis has occurred utilizing FISH and PCR.[75] There are currently seven centers in the United States performing preimplantation diagnosis.[66] Diagnosis of Tay-Sachs disease and cystic fibrosis is possible by preimplantation diagnosis, for example.[76] Biopsy of the embryo occurs after in vitro fertilization as it reaches the eight cell stage.[76] One or two blastomeres are removed from the developing embryo and analyzed.[76] If analysis confirms that the blastomere is not affected with the disorder in question, then the developing embryo can be transferred to the uterus for implantation.[76] The entire process, after ovum harvesting for in vitro fertilization, takes approximately 48 hours.[76]

INDICATIONS[70]

- Avoidance of repeated pregnancy termination
- Necessity for early treatment
- Very high genetic risk
- Advanced maternal age
- Improving efficiency of infertility treatments

The benefit is to be able to detect disorders prior to implantation to avoid the need for pregnancy termination of affected fetuses. To date, there have not been any reports of physical anomalies of those infants born after preimplantation analysis.[70,76] Misdiagnosed embryos have been implanted, however.[75] As technology advances, genetic analysis prior to implantation may in fact become a method of "surveillance," just as CVS and amniocentesis are utilized. Several ethical issues are raised with this new technique and will need to be addressed as research continues.

REFERENCES

1. Alfirevic, Z., & Neilson, J. (1995). Doppler ultrasonography in high-risk pregnancies: Systematic review with meta-analysis. *American Journal of Obstetrics and Gynecology, 172,* 1379–1387.

2. Kuppermann, M., Gates, E., & Washington, E. (1996). Racial-ethnic differences in prenatal diagnostic test use and outcomes: Preferences, socioeconomics or patient knowledge? *Obstetrics and Gynecology, 87,* 675–682.

3. Covington, C., Gieleghem, P., Board, F., Madison, K., Nedd, D., & Miller, L. (1996). Family care related to alpha-fetoprotein screening. *JOGNN, 25,* 125–130.

4. Carpenito, L. (1993). *Nursing diagnosis: Application to clinical practice* (5th ed.). Philadelphia: J. B. Lippincott Company.

5. American Academy of Pediatrics and American College of Obstetricians and Gynecologists. (1992). *Guidelines for perinatal care* (3rd ed.). Elk Grove Village, New York: American Academy of Pediatrics.

6. Vintzileos, A. (1995). Antepartum fetal surveillance. *Clinical Obstetrics and Gynecology, 38,* 1–2.

7. Committee on Technical Bulletins of the American College of Obstetricians and Gynecologists. (1994). Antepartum fetal surveillance. *ACOG Technical Bulletin, 188,* 1–5.

8. Kuller, J., & Laifer, S. (1995). Contemporary approaches to prenatal diagnosis. *American Family Physician, 52,* 2277–2283.

9. Garber, A., Fox, M., & Tabsh, K. (1992). Genetic evaluation and teratology. In N. Hacker & G. Moore (Eds.), *Essentials of obstetrics and gynecology* (pp. 93–108). Philadelphia: W. B. Saunders.

10. Lagrew, D. (1995). The contraction stress test. *Clinical Obstetrics and Gynecology, 38,* 11–25.

11. Manning, F. (1996). Fetal biophysical profile scoring. In A. Fleischer, F. Manning, P. Jeanty, & R. Romero (Eds.), *Sonography in obstetrics and gynecology* (pp. 611–619). Stamford, CT: Appleton & Lange.

12. Weeks, J., Asrat, T., Morgan, M., Nageotte, M., Thomas, S., & Freeman, R. (1995). Antepartum surveillance for a history of stillbirth: When to begin? *American Journal of Obstetrics and Gynecology, 172,* 486–492.

13. Manning, F. (1995). Dynamic ultrasound-based fetal assessment: The fetal biophysical profile. *Clinical Obstetrics and Gynecology, 38,* 26–44.

14. Yankowitz, J. (1996). Surgical fetal surgery. In J. Kuller, N. Chescheir, & R. Cefalo (Eds.), *Prenatal diagnosis & reproductive genetics* (pp. 181–191). St. Louis: Mosby.

15. Hunter, S., & Yankowitz, J. (1996). Medical fetal therapy. In J. Kuller, N. Chescheir, & R. Cefalo (Eds.), *Prenatal diagnosis & reproductive genetics* (pp. 172–180). St. Louis: Mosby.

16. Wiley, J. (1996). Stem cell transplantation for the treatment of genetic disease. In J. Kuller, N. Chescheir, & R. Cefalo (Eds.), *Prenatal diagnosis & reproductive genetics* (pp. 243–269). St. Louis: Mosby.

17. Druzin, M. (1990). Fetal surveillance update. *Bulletin of the New York Academy of Medicine, 66,* 246–254.

18. Maulik, D. (1995). Doppler ultrasound velocimetry for fetal surveillance. *Clinical Obstetrics and Gynecology, 38,* 91–111.

19. Cunningham, G., Macdonald, P., Gant N., Leveno, K., & Gilstrap, L. (1993). *Williams Obstetrics,* (19th ed.) Norwalk: Appleton & Lange.

20. Rayburn, W. (1995). Fetal movement monitoring. *Clinical Obstetrics and Gynecology, 38,* 59–67.

21. Schifrin, B. (1995). Antenatal fetal assessment: Overview and implications for neurologic injury and routine testing. *Clinical Obstetrics and Gynecology, 38,* 132–141.

22. Williams, J., & Blanchard, J. (1996). *Electronic monitoring of the fetal heart.* London, England: Books for Midwives Press.

23. Paul, R., & Miller, D. (1995). Nonstress test. *Clinical Obstetrics and Gynecology, 38,* 3–10.

24. Farmakides, G., & Weiner, Z. (1995). Computerized analysis of the fetal heart rate. *Clinical Obstetrics and Gynecology, 38,* 112–120.

25. Committee on Technical Bulletins of the American College of Obstetricians and Gynecologists. (1995). Fetal heart rate patterns: Monitoring, interpretation and management. *ACOG Technical Bulletin, 207,* 1–9.

26. Smith, C. (1995). Vibroacoustic stimulation. *Clinical Obstetrics and Gynecology, 38,* 68–77.

27. Hansen, W. (1996). Intrauterine growth retardation. In J. Kuller, N. Chescheir, & R. Cefalo (Eds.), *Prenatal diagnosis & reproductive genetics* (pp. 124–133). St. Louis: Mosby.

28. Hamilton, L., & Hobel, C. (1992). Intrauterine growth retardation, intrauterine fetal demise, and post-term pregnancy. In N. Hacker and G. Moore (Eds.), *Essentials of Obstetrics and Gynecology* (pp. 281–288). Philadelphia: W. B. Saunders.

29. Holmes, R., & Soothill, P. (1996). Intrauterine growth retardation. *Current Opinion in Obstetrics and Gynecology, 8,* 148–154.

30. Manning, F. (1996). Intrauterine growth retardation: Diagnosis, prognostication, and management based on ultrasound methods. In A. Fleischer, F. Manning, P. Jeanty, & R. Romero (Eds.), *Sonography in obstetrics and gynecology* (pp. 517–540). Stamford, CT: Appleton & Lange.

31. Manning, F. (1995). Intrauterine growth retardation. In F. Manning (Ed.), *Fetal medicine: Principles and practice* (pp. 307–393). Norwalk, CT: Appleton & Lange.

32. Varner, M. (1994). Disproportionate fetal growth. In A. DeCherney & M. Pernoll (Eds.), *Current obstetric and gynecologic diagnosis and treatment* (pp. 344–356). Norwalk, CT: Appleton & Lange.

33. Queenan, J. (1996). Polyhydramnios. *Contemporary OB/GYN, 41,* 11–16.

34. Committee on Technical Bulletins of the American College of Obstetricians and Gynecologists (1993). Ultrasonography in pregnancy. *ACOG Technical Bulletins, 187,* 1–9.

35. Tabsh, K., & Theroux, N. (1992). Rhesus isoimmunization. In N. Hacker and G. Moore (Eds.), *Essentials of obstetrics and gynecology* (pp. 299–307). Philadelphia: W. B. Saunders.

36. Queenan, J. (1994). Diagnosis and treatment of Rh-erythroblastosis fetalis. *Contemporary OB/GYN, 39,* 48–62.

37. Van Den Veyver, I., Subramanian, S., Hudson, K., Werch, J., Moise, K., & Hughes, M. (1996). Prenatal diagnosis of the RhD fetal blood type on amniotic fluid by polymerase chain reaction. *Obstetrics and Gynecology, 87,* 419–422.

38. Yankowitz, J., & Weiner, C. (1996). Modern management of rhesus disease. *Current Opinion in Obstetrics and Gynecology, 8,* 139–141.

39. Ganshirt, D., Garritsen, H., & Holzgreve, W. (1995). Fetal cells in maternal blood. *Current Opinion in Obstetrics and Gynecology, 7,* 103–108.

40. Kellner, L., Weiner, Z., Weiss, R., Neuer, M., Martin, G., Mueenuddin, M., & Bombard, A., (1995). Triple marker (alpha fetoprotein, unconjugated estriol, human chorionic gonadotropin) versus alpha fetoprotein plus free beta subunit in second-trimester screening for fetal Down syndrome: A prospective comparison study. *American Journal of Obstetrics and Gynecology, 173,* 1306–1309.

41. Benn, P., Horne, D., Briganti, S., & Greenstein, R. (1995). Prenatal diagnosis of diverse chromosome abnormalities in a population of patients identified by triple-marker testing as screen positive for Down syndrome. *American Journal of Obstetrics and Gynecology, 173,* 496–501.

42. Coulson, C., Katz, V., & Kuller, J. (1996). Triple-marker screening for aneuploidy. In J. Kuller, N. Chescheir, & R. Cefalo (Eds.), *Prenatal diagnosis & reproductive genetics* (pp. 84–94). St. Louis: Mosby.

43. Committee on Educational Bulletins of the American College of Obstetricians and Gynecologists. (1996). Maternal serum screening. *ACOG Educational Bulletin, 228,* 1–9.

44. Wright, L. (1994). Prenatal diagnosis in the 1990s. *JOGNN, 23,* 506–515.

45. Wenstrom, K., Owen, J., Davis, R., & Brumfield, C. (1996). Prognostic significance of unexplained elevated amniotic fluid alpha-fetoprotein. *Obstetrics and Gynecology, 87,* 213–216.

46. Chescheir, N. (1996). Overview of obstetric sonography. In J. Kuller, N. Chescheir, & R. Cefalo (Eds.), *Prenatal diagnosis & reproductive genetics* (pp. 102–107). St. Louis: Mosby.

47. Rottem, S. (1995). Early detection of structural anomalies and markers of chromosomal aberrations by transvaginal ultrasonography. *Current Opinion in Obstetrics and Gynecology, 7,* 122–125.

48. Moore, T. (1995). Assessment of amniotic fluid volume in at risk pregnancies. *Clinical Obstetrics and Gynecology, 38,* 78–90.

49. Devoe, L., & Ware, D. (1994). Oligohydramnios: definition and diagnosis. *Contemporary OB/GYN, 40,* 31–40.

50. McMahon, M., Kuller, J., & Yankowitz, J. (1996). Assessment of the post-term pregnancy. *American Family Physician, 54,* 631–636.

51. DuBose, T. (1996). Extrafetal structures of pregnancy. In T. DuBose (Ed.), *Fetal Sonography,* (pp. 345–365). Philadelphia: W. B. Saunders Company.

52. Gegor, C., Paine, L., Costigan, K., & Johnson, T. (1994). Interpretation of biophysical scores by nurses and physicians. *JOGNN, 23,* 405–410.

53. DeVoe, C. (1995). Computerized fetal biophysical assessment.. *Clinical Obstetrics and Gynecology, 38,* 121–131.

54. Maulik, D. (1996). Doppler ultrasound in obstetrics. In G. Cunningham, P. Macdonald, N. Gant, K. Leveno, & L. Gilstrap (Eds.), *Williams Obstetrics* (Supp. 16), 1–14.

55. Reed, K. (1995). Using doppler ultrasound to detect fetal problems. *Contemporary OB/GYN, 40,* 15–28.

56. Mari, G., & Copel, J. (1996). Doppler ultrasound: Fetal physiology and clinical application. In A. Fleischer, F. Manning, P. Jeanty, & R. Romero. (Eds.), *Sonography in obstetrics and gynecology* (pp. 251–260). Stamford, CT: Appleton & Lange.

57. Divon, M. (1996). Umbilical artery Doppler velocemitry: Clinical utility in high-risk pregnancies. *American Journal of Obstetrics and Gynecology, 174,* 10–14.

58. Harman, C. (1996). Doppler ultrasound: Maternal applications. In A. Fleischer, F. Manning, P. Jeanty, & R. Romero (Eds.), *Sonography in obstetrics and gynecology* (pp. 225–245). Stamford, CT: Appleton & Lange.

59. Cabaniss, M. (1996). Amniocentesis. In J. Kuller, N. Chescheir, & R. Cefalo (Eds.), *Prenatal diagnosis & reproductive genetics* (pp. 136–144). St. Louis: Mosby.

60. Kuller, J. (1996). Chorionic villus sampling. In J. Kuller, N. Chescheir, & R. Cefalo (Eds.), *Prenatal diagnosis & reproductive genetics* (pp. 145–158). St. Louis: Mosby.

61. Smidt-Jensen, S., & Sundberg, K. (1995). Early amniocentesis. *Current Opinion in Obstetrics and Gynecology, 7,* 117–121.

62. American College of Obstetricians and Gynecologists. (1995). Chorionic villus sampling. *ACOG Committee Opinion, 160,* 1–3.

63. Crodriguez-Macias, K. (1995). A comparison for determining fetal pulmonary maturity. *International Journal of Obstetrics and Gynecology, 51,* 38–42.

64. NIH Consensus Development Panel on the Effect of Corticosteroids for Fetal Maturation on Perinatal Outcomes. (1995). Effect of corticosteroids for fetal maturation on perinatal outcomes. *JAMA, 273,* 413–417.

65. U.S. Department of Health and Human Services. (1995). Chorionic villus sampling and amniocentesis: Recommendations for prenatal counseling. *Morbidity and Mortality Weekly Report, 44,* 1–12.

66. Bahado-Singh, R., Morotti, R., Pirhonen, J., Copel, J., & Mahoney, J. (1995). Invasive techniques for prenatal diagnosis: Current concepts. *Journal of the Association for Academis Minority Physicians, 6,* 28–33.

67. Laifer, S., & Kuller, J. (1996). Percutaneous umbilical blood sampling. In J. Kuller, N. Chescheir, & R. Cefalo (Eds.), *Prenatal diagnosis & reproductive genetics* (pp. 151–158). St. Louis: Mosby.

68. Ghidini, A., Munoz, H., & Romero, R. (1996). Fetal blood sampling. In A. Fleischer, F. Manning, P. Jeanty, & R. Romero (Eds.), *Sonography in Obstetrics and Gynecology* (pp. 661–686). Stamford, CT: Appleton & Lange.

69. Norton, M., & Bianchi, D. (1996). Prenatal diagnosis using fetal cells in the maternal circulation. In J. Kuller, N. Chescheir, & R. Cefalo (Eds.), *Prenatal diagnosis & reproductive genetics* (pp. 228–234). St. Louis: Mosby.

70. Carson, S., & Buster, J. (1995). Diagnosis and treatment before implantation: The ultimate prenatal medicine. *Contemporary OB/GYN, 41,* 71–85.

71. Goldenberg, R., Mercer, B., Meis, P., Copper, R., Das, A., & McNellis, D. (1996). The preterm prediction study: Fetal fibronectin testing and spontaneous preterm birth. *Obstetrics and Gynecology, 87,* 643–648.

72. Goldenberg, R., Thom, E., Moawad, A., Johnson, F., Roberts, J., & Cartis, S. (1996). The preterm prediction study: Fetal fibronectin, bacterial vaginosis and peripartum infection. *Obstetrics and Gynecology, 87,* 656–660.

73. Morrison, M., Naef, M., Botti, J., Katz, M., Belluomini, J., & Mclaughlin, B. (1996). Prediction of spontaneous preterm birth by fetal fibronectin and uterine activity. *Obstetrics and Gynecology, 87,* 649–655.

74. Cadrin, C., & Golbus, M. (1996). Fetal tissue sampling. In J. Kuller, N. Chescheir, & R. Cefalo (Eds.), *Prenatal diagnosis & reproductive genetics* (pp. 159–171). St. Louis: Mosby.

75. Grifo, J., Tang, Y., Munne, S., & Krey, L. (1996). Update in preimplantation genetic diagnosis: Successes, advances, and problems. *Current Opinion in Obstetrics and Gynecology, 8,* 135–138.

76. Fries, M. (1996). Preimplantation embryo analysis. In J. Kuller, N. Chescheir, & R. Cefalo (Eds.), *Prenatal diagnosis & reproductive genetics* (pp. 236–242). St. Louis: Mosby.

APPENDIX: AN ALGORITHM OF FETAL TESTING THAT MIGHT BE USED WHEN A PROBLEM ARISES

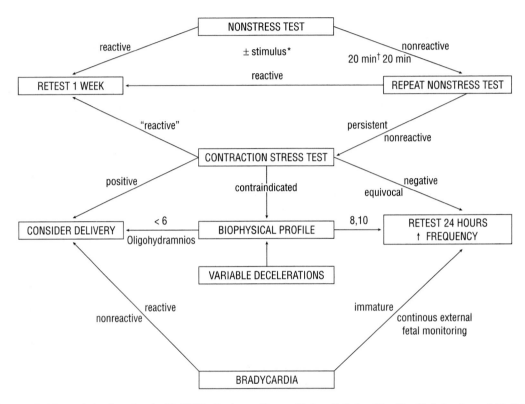

Reprinted with permission from Druzin, M. (1990). Fetal surveillance—Update. Bulletin of the New York Academy of Medicine, 66, *246–254.*

*Some institutional protocols may add vibroacoustic stimulation.

†If nonreactive after 20 minutes, may continue testing another 20 minutes.

CHAPTER 20

POSTPARTUM AND LACTATION

Kathleen M. Akridge

The support and experience previously provided by the extended family are not easily accessible for families of today.

Highlights

- The Puerperium
- Two-Week and Four- to Six-Week Assessments
- Postcesarean Section Assessments
- Normal Postpartum Assessments
    - Pelvic Musculature
    - Breasts
    - Contraception
- Postpartum Complications
    - Gestational Diabetes
    - Persistent Hypertension
    - Hemorrhage
    - Uterine Subinvolution
    - Mastitis
    - Metritis With Pelvic Cellulitis
    - Thyroiditis
    - Urinary Tract Infection
    - Acute Appendicitis
- Early Discharge
- Adjusting to Parenting
    - Barnard and Mercer Models
    - Factors Inhibiting Attachment
    - Family Relationships, Single Parent
    - Discipline and Parenting Skills
- Children With Malformations
- Postpartum Depression
- Perinatal Loss
- Breast- and Bottle-Feeding

► INTRODUCTION

Knowledge of the normal physiologic changes and complications of the postpartum period, parental roles, perinatal loss, and lactation is essential in managing the care of a client and her family postpartum. The health care provider must be familiar with assessment, diagnosis, management, and follow-up and know when referral is needed for further evaluation and management.

In the diagnosis and management of complications, it may be necessary to implement emergency measures until definitive care from a consulting medical professional arrives. The postpartum woman may be assessed in a hospital setting, alternative birthing site such as a birthing center, or the home.

The extended family of 40 or 50 years ago has been replaced by nuclear families and such nontraditional families as single-parent and blended (two partial families joined to become one) families. The support and experience previously provided by the extended family are not easily accessible for families of today. Early hospital discharge means that many of the nurturing and infant care skills previously taught by health professionals on the second postpartum day are now crammed into a short time frame just prior to hospital discharge, when the client's attention is often focused on what awaits her at home. To meet the health needs of today's new mother, many hospitals provide follow-up telephone calls or home visits.

Many women choosing to breastfeed may be deterred when faced with engorgement, tender nipples, and nonsupportive family and friends. Women who deliver twins may believe that breastfeeding is not possible. A unique opportunity exists to make this a successful experience for the breastfeeding family.

The postpartum experience is not always joyful. Many women or couples are left to deal with the loss of the fantasized infant as they struggle with the reality of a miscarriage, deformity, or perinatal death. Knowing how to help the woman and her family and suggest appropriate referral is imperative. There is a list of Support Groups at the end of this chapter.

Health care during the postpartum period focuses on evaluation of the physiological and psychological changes that normally occur. Any abnormal findings or dysfunctional behavior detected during the antepartum and postpartum periods should continue to be evaluated.

THE PUERPERIUM

Postpartum, also referred to as the *puerperium,* is the period from delivery of the placenta and membranes to the return of the woman's reproductive organs to their nonpregnant state. It generally lasts about 6 weeks and is divided into three segments. The immediate puerperium is the first 24 hours after delivery; the early puerperium extends from the second day postpartum to the end of the first postpartum week; and the remote puerperium continues to the end of the sixth week.

IMMEDIATE POSTPARTUM

- *Uterine Involution.* This process includes shedding of the decidua and endometrium. It is monitored by assessing the amount of lochia and uterine size and tone.

  - Immediately after delivery the uterus is approximately two-thirds to three-fourths of the way between the umbilicus and the symphysis pubis; after a few hours, the uterus rises to the level of the umbilicus and remains there or one fingerbreadth below for about 2 days before gradually descending into the pelvis. Any time the top of the fundus is above the umbilicus, bladder or uterine distention from blood or clots is possible.

- Lochia is the uterine discharge during the puerperium that escapes vaginally. Lochia rubra is the earliest lochia and is red because it contains blood and decidual tissue. It begins immediately after delivery and continues the first 2 to 3 days postpartum.

- *Vagina and Perineum.* These structures are quite stretched and edematous following a vaginal delivery. The vagina gapes at the introitus; it is also smoothwalled and generally lax. Hematoma should be suspected if the woman reports excruciating pain or is unable to void, or if a tense, fluctuant mass is noted. Inspect the episiotomy for hematoma. Vulvar and rectal hemorrhoids are often present and must be observed for evidence of thrombosis. After delivery, ice bags may be applied to the perineum and hemorrhoids for 30 to 60 minutes; ice bags are removed then to prevent a secondary effect, vasodilation.

- *Vital Signs.* Blood pressure, pulse, and respirations should be stabilized to within normal limits. Fever is indicative of infection, probably in the genitourinary tract.

- *Bladder.* The bladder is edematous, hypotonic, and congested immediately postpartum. Consequently bladder distention, incomplete emptying, inability to void, and excessive urine residual may develop unless the woman is encouraged to void periodically even when she does not feel the need.

- *Breasts.* Lactation naturally begins unless a lactation suppressant has been given. Colostrum is the first fluid the infant receives from the breast. Engorgement commonly occurs 48–72 hours after delivery. An ice bag applied to the breasts for 30–60 minutes and then discontinued for 1 hour before being reapplied may give the nonlactating woman some relief from engorgement. The use of cold cabbage leaves has gained in popularity as a reliable and safe way to treat engorgement. The cold cabbage leaves are applied to the breasts, leaving just the nipples exposed. The leaves are removed in about 20 minutes when they become wilted. A randomized study done by Nikodem, Danziger, et al. in Johannesburg found the use of cold cab-

bage leaves effective but not statistically significant in suppressing lactation.[1]

- *Abdominal Muscles.* The muscles are flabby, and all have some degree of diastasis recti. If the client elected to have tubal sterilization, part of the pre-operative counseling should include advising the client of a possible increase in pain or discomfort because of the abdominal surgery as well as from the postpartum afterpains. If cesarean section was performed, a dressing usually covers the incision, and it should be dry. Staples are generally used in the skin closure and are removed 5 to 7 days postoperatively. Obviously, women undergoing a cesarean birth will experience pain.

- *Postpartum Blues and Grief.* Descriptions are provided in the sections on Psychiatric Disturbances and Perinatal Loss.

EARLY PUERPERIUM

From the second postpartum day to the end of the first postpartum week additional changes evolve.

- *Uterus.* The uterus is approximately 12 weeks' size and is barely palpable just above the symphysis pubis.

- *Lochia Serosa.* The normal uterine discharge from the vagina that occurs during postpartum days 4 to 10 is lochia serosa. It contains primarily serous fluid, decidual tissue, leukocytes, and erythrocytes. Flow is decreasing. Encourage use of sanitary pads rather than tampons.

- *Vagina and Perineum.* The vagina remains smooth, and the perineum may be slightly uncomfortable. If an episiotomy was performed, the sutures will still be palpable. Attention should be given for signs of infection or hemorrhoids. Discourage douching as it may alter vaginal pH and wash out protective vaginal organisms. Bathing can soothe and cleanse the perineum. Oils and fragrances should not be used in bath water. If hemorrhoids are present, relief can be obtained with Tucks, Nupercaine ointment, dermaplast, increased fluid and fiber intake, stool softeners as needed, and warm or cool sitz baths. Urinary incontinence may indicate cystocele (see Chapter 13).

- *Breasts.* By this time, breasts contain milk for those women who are breastfeeding. Breast milk usually appears on postpartum days 3 to 5, and is a bluish white. A mother may need reassurance that the color is normal and her milk has not become "weak" (see Breastfeeding section).
- *Abdominal Muscles.* These muscles are lax, and a woman needs reassurance that it is normal. Walking and swimming may help tone muscles without exerting undue stress.
- *Diuresis and Profuse Perspiration.* These conditions are normal as long as the woman is afebrile.

LATE PUERPERIUM

From the end of the first postpartum week to the end of the sixth week maternal change continues.

- *Uterus.* The uterus returns to its nonpregnant size 4 to 6 weeks following birth.
- *Lochia Alba.* The last lochia, lochia alba, begins at about day 10 and continues until approximately day 35 postpartum. It is scant, composed primarily of leukocytes and decidual cells, and is creamy white.
- *Vagina and Perineum.* These structures begin to regain tone by 6 weeks postpartum. Rugae are normally present by that time. Atrophy, however, may still be evident in the lactating woman. Of concern are maintaining and strengthening vaginal tone, preventing pelvic relaxation, and promoting nonpainful resumption of intercourse.
- *Breasts.* The breasts begin to adapt to the nutritional needs of the baby, but engorgement and mastitis remain primary concerns. Assess the breastfeeding process and family support. The breasts of a nonlactating woman may contain milk for up to 3 months postpartum.
- *Renal System.* Urinary tract infection (UTI) may occur, and continuing assessment is of particular concern for clients with a history of UTI.
- *Abdominal Muscles.* Abdominal wall musculature becomes firmer by the end of the sixth postpartum week but may never regain its prepregnant appearance if the muscles remain weakened and stretched.

THE FOUR- TO SIX-WEEK POSTPARTUM ASSESSMENT

SUBJECTIVE DATA

Generally review the woman's systems. Specific determinations also need to be made:

- Number of weeks postpartum
- General adaptation to motherhood; assess client's rest and sleep habits, appetite, activity level, exercise program, and nutrition.
- Coping ability in caring for baby and making family adjustments or living as single parent.
- Problems with baby (feeding, health, first exam).
- Family adjustments caring for baby.
- Sexual activity (resumption, type of contraceptive used, dyspareunia and other concerns, including possible lack of desire, fear of discomfort or of becoming pregnant again).
- Family planning method desired; assess previous methods used, length of time used, satisfaction with methods, and reason for discontinuance.

Ask the client if she has called a health care provider or gone to an emergency room and whether she was admitted or readmitted. In addition, ask if she has had fever, chills, or flulike symptoms.

- *Breasts.* Assess for engorgement and breastfeeding concerns.
  - Determine when engorgement occurred, how long it lasted, if it has been treated and how and whether it continues to be a problem or has resolved.
  - If breastfeeding is discontinued, determine the length of breastfeeding and the reason for stopping.
  - If the client is currently breastfeeding, ask her about concerns, frequency, nipple soreness, breast care, and enjoyment of breastfeeding.
- *Lochia.* In the postpartum period, assess the duration of each lochia color in sequence, presence of odor, excessive bleeding, clots, and pain.
- *Return of Menses.* Several factors influence the return of menses, such as contraceptive method

and breastfeeding. Nonlactating women menstruate 6 to 8 weeks following delivery, and lactating women 2 to 18 months following delivery, depending on whether she is exclusively breastfeeding or if she is supplementing with formula. The first postpartum menstruation is heavier than normal menstruation and often anovulatory. Menses returns sooner in the multipara than the primipara.

OBJECTIVE DATA

Physical Examination

Generally assess the client.

- *General Appearance and Vital Signs.* Compare blood pressure with range before and during pregnancy. Compare weight with prepregnant weight and weight at delivery. Inquire as to rest/sleep and activity levels. Obtain 24-hour dietary recall to assess nutritional intake.
- *Neck.* Determine that the thyroid is nonpalpable. If thyromegaly or nodules are palpated, order thyroid function tests (TFTs) and refer client for medical evaluation (see Normal Postpartum Health Assessment).
- *Breasts.* Evaluation is influenced by whether the client is lactating.

  - Lactating breasts should be full, without erythema, masses, or lymphadenopathy. Milk should be easily expressed.
  - Nonlactating breasts are soft, without masses or lymphadenopathy. Bilateral galactorrhea may be present in nonlactating women for up to 3 months' postpartum; these women should return for evaluation of galactorrhea beyond 3 months' postpartum. Mechanical stimulation of nonlactating breasts may lead to persistence of milky discharge, but more serious causes should be ruled out.

- *Extremities.* Assess for varicosities and phlebitis.
- *Cardiovascular and Respiratory Systems.* Rate and rhythm should be regular without murmurs or extra heart sounds. Clear, equal breath sounds should be evident bilaterally. Blood volume returns to normal by approximately 1 week postpartum.

- *Abdomen and Musculoskeleton.* Assess for costovertebral angle tenderness (CVAT) and tenderness along paraspinous muscles. In addition, inspect for abdominal striae, diastasis, hernias, masses, tenderness, and lymph nodes. If she experienced a cesarean birth, assess healing. Abdominal musculature involution may require 6 to 8 weeks.
- *Genitalia and Reproductive Organs.* Several structures are involved.

  - External genitalia should be without edema or lesions and nontender.
  - Vagina should appear rugated, except in lactating women when rugae may be decreased secondary to hypoestrogenic state. Episiotomy site should be intact, well healed, and nontender.
  - Cervical internal os should be closed. If it is open, determine whether placental products have been retained. After childbirth, the cervix appears as a transverse slit. It appears stellate if severe lacerations were sustained during childbirth.
  - Uterine corpus at 4 to 6 weeks' postpartum is nonpregnant size. If uterine tenderness is detected, consider infection and prepare appropriate cultures (e.g., chlamydia, gonorrhea).
  - Involution of ovaries and fallopian tubes is complete by 6 to 7 weeks' postpartum.
  - Inspect rectum for hemorrhoids. Assess sphincter control, especially if third- or fourth-degree laceration was sustained during childbirth.
- *Psychological Factors.* Assess affect for mood of mother, and her interaction with infant or other indications of maternal-infant bonding. Inquire as to health of infant and whether infant has had a routine exam.

Diagnostic Tests

Various tests need to be performed.

- Compare antenatal and postnatal hemoglobin levels and hematocrits.
- Check immunity status for rubella and, if not immune (titer $\leq 1:10$), confirm that rubella vaccine was given prior to hospital discharge. Nursing mothers may be vaccinated.

- If client is Rh-negative, check Rh status of infant and, if clinically indicated, determine whether Rho(D) immune globulin was given to mother postpartum.
- Check when last Pap smear was done and results.
- If any sexually transmitted disease was detected during pregnancy, consider repeating tests.

PLAN

- *Psychosocial Intervention.* Counseling may be helpful about available social services, public health nursing, and child protective services (see Postpartum Depression Support Groups at the end of this chapter).
- *Family Planning.* Ask the client whether she was satisfied with previously used methods of contraception. Ask about her concerns regarding the method she wishes to use or is using now. Base your instructions about a method of contraception on the client's level of comprehension. Address safer sex as well as satisfaction with or changes in relationship with sexual partner.
- *Preventive Measures.* Encourage health maintenance/health promotion activities, such as breast self-examination, Kegel exercises, annual Pap examination, smoking cessation, weight reduction, and exercise. Reassure mothers of term and low-birthweight babies that it may take months for them to feel "normal" again.[2]

FOLLOW-UP

- *Pap Smear.* Perform if due or if previously abnormal. Performing a Pap smear prior to 8 weeks' postpartum increases the likelihood of an abnormal report.[3]
- *Colposcopy.* Perform or refer if clinically indicated.
- *Culture.* Culture for chlamydia or gonorrhea if indicated.
- *Urine Testing.* Monitor for urinary tract pathology by performing dipstick. Culture urine if bacteriuria occurred during pregnancy or if physical exam warrants.
- *Blood Tests.* Obtain hemoglobin level, hematocrit, or complete blood count if indicated.
- *Immunization.* Request rubella immunization if indicated.

- *Intravenous Pyelogram and Urology.* Consider referring client for intravenous pyelogram and urology consultation if she has a history of pyelonephritis or hematuria of unknown etiology during pregnancy.
- *Glucose Testing.* Request 75-g glucola (i.e., 2-hr oral glucose tolerance test) if the client was gestational diabetic. Protocols vary depending on the setting. A 3-hour test may be used. Since glucose tolerance testing in the immediate postpartum period is unreliable, however, there must be a wait of at least 6 weeks' postpartum for a reliable testing of carbohydrate intolerance.

NORMAL POSTPARTUM HEALTH ASSESSMENT

Essential aspects of normal postpartum health assessment are pelvic musculature and breast evaluations and contraception counseling. See Chapter 14 for information on breast self-examination. Evaluation of pelvic musculature and contraception counseling are discussed here.

PELVIC MUSCULATURE

Pelvic musculature is assessed following pregnancy to evaluate involution and resumption of nonpregnant function (see Chapter 13). The general function of pelvic musculature is to support pelvic organs and assist urinary continence.

Etiology of Relaxed Pelvic Musculature

Relaxed musculature may be related to childbearing, age, obesity, or lack of exercise.

- Closely spaced pregnancies or large fetuses can stretch and traumatize pelvic musculature and contribute to relaxation.
- Aging, because of decreased estrogen production, contributes to loss of elasticity.
- Obesity increases intraabdominal pressure and contributes to relaxation of vaginal muscles.
- Failure to perform Kegel exercises permits continued relaxation.

Subjective Data

A woman may report sensations of pelvic pressure, urinary incontinence, and lack of perineal support during defecation.[4] Specific information needs to be pursued.

- Involuntary loss of urine during an activity that increases intraabdominal pressure, e.g., coughing, sneezing
- Age of onset and circumstances of incontinence
- Increase in severity or number of pelvic symptoms, or both, such as loss of bladder control, incomplete emptying of bladder, a sensation of vaginal pressure, inability to defecate without use of counter pressure.
- Day and night voiding patterns
- Frequency and severity of wetting
- Amount of urine lost (drops, teaspoon, tablespoon, quarter of cup, layer of clothing soaked)
- History of and reasons for previous vaginal or urinary tract surgery
- History of lower back surgery (The pudendal nerve innervates pelvic floor muscles and could have been damaged in surgery.)
- Past history of stress urinary incontinence and method of treatment
- Fluid intake
- Medications including over-the-counter, currently being used
- Use of bladder irritants, such as caffeine, non-nutritive sweeteners

Stress urinary incontinence (SUI) and detrusor instability should be differentiated. SUI results from an incompetent urethra. Urine is lost immediately with an event that increases intraabdominal pressure.[4] With detrusor instability (involuntary contraction) the bladder itself is the cause of incontinence. A delay occurs between the precipitating event and urine loss; urine loss may also be sudden and without warning.[4]

Objective Data

Data are determined by preliminary diagnostic tests followed by measurement of pelvic muscle strength.

Preliminary Assessment. The first test requires that the client not urinate for 2 hours prior to the exam. She should stand with legs apart, hold a folded paper towel against her perineum, and cough vigorously. The amount of urine lost can be seen on the towel.[4]

The urine stop test assesses pelvic muscle strength. It has a negative correlation to the strength of pelvic muscles: the greater the time needed to stop urine flow, the weaker the musculature. The client sits on a standard commode with the knees about 16 inches apart to discourage use of gluteal or abdominal muscles. The examiner must be able to hear the onset of urination, and the client must be able to hear the "stop" command. Five seconds after onset of urination, the client is told to stop. Women with adequate muscle control should stop urination completely within 2 seconds.[4]

Digital Examination. Digital measurement of pelvic muscle strength scale assesses vaginal muscles. The examiner inserts index and middle fingers 6 to 8 cm into the introitus on an antero-posterior plane and ask the client to contract her vaginal muscles around the fingers for as long as possible and as forcefully as possible. The scoring criteria are pressure, duration of pressure, and alteration in plane of examiner's fingers.[4] Scores range from 1 to 4, with 4 denoting the greatest muscle strength (Table 20–1).

TABLE 20–1. PELVIC MUSCLE STRENGTH RATING SCALE

Characteristic	1	2	3	4
Pressure	None	Weak, feel pressure on fingers, but not all way around	Moderate, feel pressure all around	Strong, fingers compress override
Duration	None	< 1 s	> 1 < 3 s	> 3 s
Displacement in plane	None	Slight incline, base of fingers move up	Greater incline of fingers along total length	Fingers move up and are drawn in

From C. Sampselle and C. Brink (1990). Pelvic muscle relaxation. Journal of Nurse Midwifery, 35(3), 130. Copyright American College of Nurse Midwives. Reprinted with permission.

The next step is to assess for cystocele, ure-throcele, rectocele, and enterocele. Firmly exert pressure with fingers posterior to the vaginal wall and ask the client to bear down or cough. Observe the vaginal wall to detect an anterior bulge (cystocele or urethrocele). Continue pressing posteriorly with fingers while simultaneously separating them; ask the client to cough or bear down and observe the posterior wall for a bulge (rectocele or enterocele).

Women should be examined for pelvic organ prolapse in the lithotomy, sitting, and standing positions. Examining the client only in the lithotomy position will obscure some pelvic support defects. Each organ that descends within the vaginal canal should be graded according to the maximum degree of descent. Clinical grading is as follows:[5]

- Grade 0—no descent
- Grade 1—descent between ischial spines and hymen
- Grade 3—descent within hymen
- Grade 4—descent through hymen

Plan

Pelvic muscle exercise benefits women with cystocele, urethrocele, rectocele, or enterocele that bulges into the vaginal vault but not outside the introitus. It may be done in any position as long as knees are 16 to 18 inches apart. Instruct the client to contract vaginal muscles as tightly as possible for as long as possible; the goal is to hold each contraction for 5 to 10 seconds. Initially, the client should contract her pelvic muscles while slowly counting to 5, hold, and gradually release to the count of 5. The aim is 80 contractions per day (groups of 5 to 20 per session).[4]

Refer the client to a urologist or gynecologist if she has a "cele" that descends beyond the introitus (a third degree).

CONTRACEPTION COUNSELING

Assessment

Assess a woman's knowledge of and preference for available contraceptive methods (see Chapter 9). She should be instructed in her choice of a temporary or permanent method. Temporary methods include barrier, hormonal, and spermicidal devices and periodic abstinence. Permanent methods are female sterilization and male sterilization.

Reversible Contraceptive Methods

Combination Oral Contraception. If breastfeeding, a woman may begin low dose combination oral contraception ($\leq$ 35 mcg estrogen) 6 weeks' postpartum.[6] Starting a breastfeeding woman on combination pills before her 6-week exam increases the risk of lactation suppression.[7] If not breastfeeding, women may begin combination oral contraception 2 weeks' postpartum.[7] Starting the combination oral contraceptive pill before 2 weeks' postpartum increases the risk of thromboembolic disease.[7]

Progestin Only Contraceptives (POCs). Progestin only contraceptives such as the minipill, Norplant®, Progestasert IUD®, and Depo-Provera® are safe to use in breastfeeding women and may be administered at the time of discharge.[7] They do not interfere with milk production and may even increase milk production.

Diaphragm. The diaphragm should be fitted at the 6-week postpartum exam, as it can not be fitted properly before that time.[7] Episiotomies are also tender and attempting to fit a diaphragm before 6 weeks would only increase the client's discomfort. Fitting should also be deferred until that time because bleeding increases the risk of toxic shock syndrome.

Intrauterine Device (IUD). IUDs can be inserted immediately after the delivery of the placenta, within 48 hours postpartum, or at the 6-week postpartum exam. If immediate postdelivery insertion is done, Hatcher et al. recommend only the Paraguard® because it has been shown to be the safest and most effective IUD for postpartum women.[7] Expulsion rates are much higher in immediate postpartum insertion than at the 6-week exam.[7]

Spermicides. Because breastfeeding can cause a decrease in estrogen, spermicides may add comfort by relieving vaginal dryness during intercourse.

Lactation Amenorrhea Method (LAM). It should be stressed that breastfeeding is not an effective method of birth control but, if used solely to supply the infant with food, it is used to space pregnancies in many cultures. Breastfeeding can be used to delay subsequent pregnancies. It can be very effective if the infant is completely breastfed without any supplements.[7] Using fertility awareness methods, ovulation is much more difficult to assess for a woman who is breastfeeding. Basal body temperature can not be determined unless the woman has had 6 hours of uninterrupted sleep.[7]

Lactation Amenorrhea Method. An upward thermal shift in basal body temperature (BBT) occurs after ovulation; intercourse should be avoided until the third day after the temperature rise. Temperature is monophasic during the preovulatory period of lactation; sexual abstinence is indicated when using BBT until ovulatory cycles have resumed.[8]

Cervical mucus changes may be misleading during anovulatory postpartum, as dry mucus is similar to that of preovulatory days during an ovulatory cycle; profuse, thick mucus makes identification of mucous patterns for prediction of ovulation difficult.

- Take basal body temperature if cervical mucus appears or the cervix opens or becomes elevated.
- "Infertility" of breastfeeding can be reasonably assumed if cervical mucus remains tacky for 3 weeks and does not become clear and stretchy.[8] This is the strongest indicator of return to ovulation and fertility in women who are breastfeeding.
- With intermittent signs of cervical mucus discharge, begin BBT. When mucus lasts 3 or more days and its cessation is accompanied by continued low temperature, breastfeeding infertility can be assumed 2 days after mucus disappears.[8] To better assess mucus, coitus should be every other day so that the presence of ejaculate and sexual lubrication does not interfere with cervical mucus.

If weaning occurs slowly after 3 to 4 months, daily BBT should be continued and cervical mucus checked for onset of ovulation. Coitus is allowed throughout a 10-day weaning period. The couple should consider themselves fertile on the eleventh day until cervical and thermal signs show ovulation has occurred.[8] If weaning occurs naturally, the client should monitor for signs of ovulation after the ninth postpartum month.[8]

The importance of exclusive breastfeeding, as well as the importance of continuing breastfeeding to maintain postpartum infertility, should be taught to clients and their partners. Infants are not introduced to solid foods until approximately 6 months old and they may be slowly introduced to taking liquids by cup. Refer clients to breastfeeding support groups and local lactation consultants.

ASSESSMENT OF POSTOPERATIVE CESAREAN BIRTH AND STERILIZATION

Following cesarean birth, encourage ambulation to decrease risk of thrombosis and embolism. Assess for thrombophlebitis by checking the lower extremities for edema of the affected leg, positive Homan's sign, muscle pain in affected leg, tenderness, erythema, or induration along a vein in the affected leg. Give analgesics shortly before ambulation. Monitor intake and urinary output by measurement for 24–48 hours. Observe wound for infection. Encourage woman's contact with family and infant.

After female sterilization, clients should be aware that discomfort may be greater because of the surgical procedure, but mild analgesia, such as nonsteroidal anti-inflammatory drugs (NSAID), should provide relief. For women not obtaining relief with NSAID, medication like Tylenol #3®, Fioricet®, or Fioricet with codeine® can be used. Observe for infection, hematoma at incision site, including episiotomy (if performed). Encourage contact with infant prior to and after surgery.

TWO-THREE WEEK POSTPARTUM ASSESSMENT

Subjective Data

Several points of information may be gained from the mother or from hospital records at the 2–3 week postpartum asssessment. Generally review the woman's systems, with specific attention to the following:

- Type of birth (vaginal or cesarean); amount and color of vaginal bleeding, presence of foul odor or clots; length of labor and complications during labor, delivery, postpartum
- If cesarean birth, determine if staples removed. If episiotomy performed, assess for tears, lacerations
- Assess for amount and frequency of pain with urination; constipation; use of medications (prescription and over-the-counter) and reason for use; effectiveness of pain medication in obtaining pain relief; hemorrhoids; fever.
- Inquire regarding problems or concerns with baby (feeding, jaundice, colic, elimination patterns, assistance in caring for baby)
- Assess family adjustments: father's role, sibling behavior, extended family
- Support system during labor and delivery
- Weight and sex of baby
- Numbers of days in hospital, general well-being of both mother and baby
- Allergies
- Bladder and bowel function
- Diet/appetite, sleep patterns/fatigue

Review the mother's feelings about delivery. If mother experienced a cesarean birth, explore her understanding of the medical reasons.

Objective Data

Physical Examination

GENERAL APPEARANCE, VITAL SIGNS, WEIGHT. Does the woman appear rested, fatigued, depressed? Does she appear neat and well groomed or ill kempt? Compare blood pressure to range during pregnancy. Compare weight to prepregnant weight and weight at delivery.

NECK. Thyroid nonpalpable or palpable, but soft and without nodules. If thyromegaly or nodules palpated, evaluate for bruits, obtain thyroid function tests (TFT), and refer for medical evaluation. (See section Postpartum Thyroiditis for further information.)

CARDIOVASCULAR AND RESPIRATORY. Regular rate and rhythm without murmurs or extra sounds. Clear, equal breath sounds bilaterally.

BREASTS. 1) *Lactating:* Full, without erythema, masses, or lymphadenopathy. Milk easily expressed. 2) *Nonlactating:* Soft, without masses, lymphadenopathy. Bilateral galactorrhea may be present in nonlactating women for up to 3 months' postpartum.

ABDOMEN AND MUSCULOSKELETAL. Assess for costovertebral angle tenderness (CVAT) and tenderness along paraspinous muscles. Fundus is usually nonpalpable above the symphysis and is nontender to gentle palpation. If cesarean birth or sterilization performed, the incision is well healed without exudate, and nontender. Lower extremities are inspected for redness, warmth, and pain in calves. Assess for Homan's sign (pain elicited with dorsiflexion of foot).

GENITALIA/REPRODUCTIVE. Inspect perineum for swelling, hemorrhoids. If episiotomy noted, assess for edema, erythema, ecchymosis, approximation of edges. Bimanual is generally deferred until 6-week postpartum exam.

PSYCHOLOGICAL. Assess mother's feelings and understanding regarding labor and birth. Assess support system. Ask woman if sexual activity has been resumed. If sexual activity has been resumed, inquire as to any pain or discomfort. Inquire as to type of contraception being used or whether contraception is desired. If cesarean birth, review type of uterine incision with woman and the issue of vaginal birth after cesarean. Reassure regarding length of time to regain prepregnant weight may take one year.

Laboratory Tests. Determine rubella immunity and documentation of rubella vaccine given postpartum. For Rh-negative mothers, determine whether Rhogam® was given if infant Rh-positive.

Health Teaching. Review ways to ensure adequate rest (sleep when infant does, avoid late night television, limit visitations by family and friends). Encourage adequate fluid intake and frequent voiding to decrease uterine "afterpains." Change perineal pads frequently. Review perineal cleansing/sitz baths/warm water soaks. Assess whether prenatal vitamins are still being taken. If history of prenatal anemia or postpartum hemorrhage, inquire whether iron supplements are being taken and dosing used. Assess for adequate rest and nutritional needs to promote tissue healing.

SIX-WEEK POSTCESAREAN BIRTH ASSESSMENT

The 6-week postpartum evaluation of a woman who had a cesarean birth is the same as that of a woman who delivered vaginally, except that the abdominal incision is assessed following a cesarean birth as well as the perineum and vulva.

COMMON POSTPARTUM COMPLICATIONS

Table 20–2 summarizes the postpartum complications.

GESTATIONAL DIABETES

Gestational diabetes is carbohydrate intolerance that is induced by pregnancy (see Chapter 18).

Epidemiology

Among women with gestational diabetes, 40 percent may persist with diabetes in the postpartum; 60 percent of obese women with gestational diabetes develop diabetes later in life.[9]

Subjective Data

The client states she had diabetes during her pregnancy.

Objective Data

The 2 hour oral glucose tolerance test has traditionally been used to detect diabetes in nonpregnant women.[10] In women previously diagnosed with gestational diabetes, it is administered 6 weeks postpartum. The test measures the rate at which a concentrated amount of glucose is removed from the bloodstream (see Chapter 21). The healthy person almost immediately produces a surge of insulin that removes a large amount of the glucose, with insulin peaking in 30 to 60 minutes. Serum glucose levels return to normal within 3 hours.

If the test is performed, the procedure requires that for the 3 days preceding the test, the client consumes a diet containing at least 150 g of carbohydrate (300 g preferred) per day. After overnight fasting (12 hours), a sample of blood is taken. The client then drinks a preparation containing 75 g of glucose. She must drink all of the solution. A blood sample is then taken 2 hours later.

Counsel the client regarding the purpose of the test and the need for a high carbohydrate diet during the 3 days prior to the test. Remind the client that overnight fasting is required. In addition, advise her not to drink alcohol and caffeine the evening prior to the test and not to smoke during the 2-hour blood testing.

Differential Medical Diagnosis

Diabetes Mellitus
- *Normal Values.* Fasting, < 110 mg/dL, 2-hour plasma glucose, < 140 mg/dL.
- *Impaired Glucose Tolerance.* Fasting, ≥ 110 and < 126 mg/dL and 2-hour plasma glucose ≥ 140 and < 200 mg/dL after 75-g glucose load.[11]
- *Diabetic Values.* One of the following is needed for a positive diagnosis: unequivocal elevation of plasma glucose ≥ 200 mg/dL and classic symptoms of diabetes, including polydipsia, polyuria, polyphagia, and unexplained weight loss; fasting, ≥ 126 mg/dL on two occasions; 2-hour plasma glucose ≥ 200 mg/dL after 75-g oral glucose tolerance test.[11] Confirming the results by repeated testing on a subsequent day is recommended.

Plan

- *Postpartum Care.* In the gestational diabetic not requiring insulin (Class A), postpartum care is identical to that of the nondiabetic woman. Insulin requirements fall dramatically postpartum because of the decrease in placental hormones.[9] Insulin is no longer required postpartally in the woman with gestational diabetes requiring insulin (Class A_2). She should be advised to continue her self-monitoring of blood glucose to be sure she remains euglycemic. In the postpartum woman who had pregestational diabetes, insulin is given at approximately one-half of her prepregnancy dose.

TABLE 20–2. SUMMARY OF POSTPARTUM COMPLICATIONS

Complication	Signs Symptoms	Management
Postpartum Hemorrhage (early)	Soft, boggy uterus; Cool, clammy skin; Fever; Tachycardia; Vertigo; Tachypnea.	Maintain patient IV line and begin second line; Call physician; Type and cross for blood; Bimanual uterine massage if boggy uterus; Oxytocic agents; Elevate right hip; CBC and coagulation studies Meds: Oxytocin 10–40 units in 1000 ml of intravenous solution at 20–40 mU/min. until uterus firm, then continue for 24 hours postpartum or as directed by physician. Carboprost 250µg intramuscularly, repeated as necessary q15–90 minutes for maximum eight doses. Preferred over methergine. Methylergonovine maleate 0.2 mg intramuscularly.
Postpartum Hemorrhage (late)	Heavy lochia; Foul lochia; Fever; Opened cervical os; Pelvic or back pain; Uterine tenderness; Prolonged bleeding.	Bedrest; Physician consultation; Breastfeeding if possible. Meds: Methylergonovine maleate 0.2–0.4 mg po q16–8h for 2 days.
Subinvolution	Painless, heavy vaginal bleeding; Uterine size larger than expected; Uterine tenderness; Fever.	CBC; Endocervical cultures; Quantitative beta-HCG; Meds: Methergine 0.2mg q3–4h x 2 days; Augmentin 500 mg qid x 7–10 days; Tetracycline 500 mg qid x 10 days.
Mastitis	Flulike symptoms; Malaise; Fever and chills; Erythema and swelling of affected breast with possible pitting edema.	Milk culture; Bedrest; Continue breastfeeding; Ice packs/warm packs; Increased fluid intake; Meds: First choice—Dicloxacillin sodium 250–500 mg qid x 10 days Penicillin allergy: Cephoradine (Velosef) 500 mg q6h x 10 days
Metritis with pelvic cellulitis	Unilateral/bilateral abdominal pain; Foul lochia; Fever; Parametrial tenderness; Leukocytosis.	Endocervical cultures (GC & Chlamydia) & endometrial cultures (aerobic & anaerobic); Medical consultation; Hospitalization; Rest. Meds: (Intravenous)—Not in order of preference—Give until afebrile for 48 hours: Cefotetan 1–2 gms.q12h Cefoxitin 1–2 gms q6–8h Gentamicin 3–5 mg/Kg of body weight in 3 divided doses q8h. Obtain blood for peak gentamicin level 30 minutes to 1 hour after IV infusion. For trough levels, draw serum just prior to next dose. Clindamycin 150–160 mg q6h Oral: Erythromycin 500 mg qid x 10 days; Tetracycline 500 mg qid x 10 days; Augmentin 500 mg qid x 10 days; Cephalosporin 500 mg qid x 10 days.
Postpartum thyroiditis (thyrotoxicosis)	Weight loss; Increased fatigue; Palpitations; Heat intolerance; Sinus tachycardia.	Radioactive iodine uptake; Physician referral.
Postpartum thyroiditis (transient hypothyroidism)	Pronounced fatigue; Continued weight gain; Coarse hair; Dry skin; Delayed reflexes; Psychologic reactions mimicking depression.	Elevated TSH; Physician consultation Meds: Thyroxine therapy—begin with 0.1 mg/day.
Urinary tract infection	Spiking fever; Costovertebral angle tenderness; Dysuria; Urgency; Oliguria.	Urinalysis with culture and sensitivity; Meds: Macrobid 100 mg q12h x 3–5 days; Sulfamethoxazole/trimethoprim q12h x 3–5 days; Trimethoprim 100 mg q12h x 3–5 days.
Appendictis	RUQ or entire right abdominal tenderness; Positive Bryan's sign (pain elicited when enlarged uterus moved to right); Positive Alder's test (Pain elicited when clinician maintains constant pressure at area of maximal tenderness and woman rolls from supine to left position).	Endocervical and lochial cultures; CBC; UA; Medical referral; Hospitalization.

Source: References 13, 15, 16, 17, 18, 24, 25, 26, 27, 30.

- *Psychosocial Intervention.* Assess client's lifestyle and knowledge of diabetes and its management. If lifestyle changes are indicated, counsel the client about the specific change (e.g., diet or exercise). Provide clear, accurate information regarding nongestational diabetes and its usual signs and symptoms and management. Refer the client to support groups if indicated. Frank diabetes may develop as she ages.
- *Medication.* Medication is not usually needed after 1 to 2 days postpartum.
- *Follow-Up.* Refer client to a diabetologist if frank diabetes is revealed.

PERSISTENT HYPERTENSION

Persistent hypertension is blood pressure that remains significantly elevated in the postpartum period. It is usually indicative of chronic vascular disease. (See Chapter 21 for information about hypertension in nonpregnant women.)

Subjective Data

The client may report a family history of hypertension or a diagnosis of pregnancy-induced hypertension. She may have no specific symptoms.

Objective Data

Physical examination reveals a systolic blood pressure equal to or greater than 140, a diastolic blood pressure equal to or greater than 90, or both. No edema is evident. Reflexes are within normal limits. Other findings are normal.

Diagnostic tests include a urine dipstick for protein, baseline electrolyte, blood urea nitrogen (BUN), and creatinine levels, urinalysis for protein urea, and baseline albumin, calcium, and phosphorus levels. More extensive testing (e.g., electrocardiogram) if indicated by extent of findings.

Differential Medical Diagnoses

Essential hypertension, hyperaldosteronism, hyperthyroidism, pheochromocytoma, renovascular disease.

Plan

- *Psychosocial Intervention.* Determine stress levels and sources of stress and counsel client regarding ways to reduce stress. Referral for support and counseling may be appropriate.
- *Medication.* The safety of medications must be considered if the client is breastfeeding.
- *Lifestyle Changes.* Provide dietary counseling to help client reduce fat, sodium, and refined sugar intake. She should maintain adequate complex carbohydrate, protein, and polyunsaturated fats. Counsel regarding exercise for aerobic health. Lactating mothers require information about specific dietary modifications and exercise. Advise mothers to stop smoking; explain cardiovascular changes that occur with smoking. In addition, advise client not to consume alcohol.
- *Follow-Up.* Postpartum follow-up should occur 1 week after hospital discharge; if hypertension persists, consult with a physician or refer the client for management.

POSTPARTUM ECLAMPSIA

Definitions and Pathophysiology

Eclampsia usually complicates pregnancies after 20 weeks' gestation and usually closer to term. Eclampsia normally resolves with delivery. Postpartum eclampsia may occur within 10 days of delivery, but cases have been reported as late as 23 days' postpartum.[12,13] (See Chapter 18 for information about pregnancy induced hypertension.)

Subjective Data

Client may report severe and persistent occipital headaches, blurred vision, photophobia, scomata, epigastric or right upper quadrant pain.[12]

Objective Data

Physical Examination. Proteinuria, pedal edema, hypertension. Cunningham et al. consider diastolic blood pressure to be more reliable and state that any diastolic value of 90 mm Hg or more is abnormal.[14] Assess for brisk reflexes with clonus.

Diagnostic Tests. Urinalysis, serum uric acid, blood urea nitrogen (BUN), plasma glucose, liver function tests (to include SGOT, PT, PTT), electrolytes, serum creatinine, and fibrinogen. MRI of the brain with consultation.

Differential Medical Diagnoses

Cerebral venous thrombosis, intracerebral hemorrhage, hypertensive, encephalopathy, pheochromocytoma, tumors of the central nervous system, metabolic disorders, epilepsy.

Plan

Medical. Refer to physician for further management and hospitalization; consider neurological consultation. Medication used is identical to management of antepartum client and consists of anticonvulsant and antihypertensive therapy.

Psychosocial. Provide emotional support; address concerns of mother regarding her own safety as well as the care of her newborn.

POSTPARTUM HEMORRHAGE

Hemorrhage during the postpartum period is blood loss in excess of 500 mL in 24 hours. Blood is ideally, but not practically, measured by weighing pads and linens. The best method of estimation is use of laboratory data: There is a decrease in hemoglobin of 1 to 1.5 g/dL for every unit (450–500 mL) of blood loss.[15] If hematocrit, drawn on postpartum day 1 or 2, is 2 percent less than on admission, significant blood loss has occurred.[15] Factors contributing to hemorrhage are uterine atony, coagulopathy, birth canal trauma, and poor general health.

Early Postpartum Hemorrhage

Early hemorrhage refers to that which occurs during the first 24 hours postpartum. Several risk factors have been identified.

- Uterine overdistention (macrosomic infant, multiple fetuses, polyhydramnios)
- Midforceps delivery, forceps rotation
- Delivery through incompletely dilated cervix
- Intrauterine manipulation

- Use of drugs to induce or augment labor or of halogenated anesthetics
- History of previous postpartum hemorrhage
- Chorioamnionitis
- Retained placental tissue
- Coagulation defects
- Fibroids
- Placenta previa or abruptio placentae
- Interuterine rupture
- Uterine inversion

Subjective Data

The client may report vertigo, extreme fatigue, chills, or a history of anemia.

Objective Data

Physical examination reveals cool, clammy skin; fever; rapid, thready pulse; tachypnea; pallor of nail beds and mucous membranes. Bleeding may not be massive; however, a steady seepage may continue until significant hypovolemia has occurred. If uterine atony is the cause of blood loss, uterine assessment will show that the uterus feels boggy and that clots are easily expressed with massage.

The complete blood cell count (CBC) provides a reliable measurement of blood loss. Blood studies will show a decrease in the hemoglobin level of 1 to 1.5 g/dL for every unit (450–500 mL) of blood lost; the hematocrit will decrease by about 2 to 4 percent for same amount of blood loss.[15]

Coagulation studies are done to determine the nature and extent of coagulation disorders contributing to the abnormal bleeding. Consult with physician for management.

Differential Medical Diagnoses

Early postpartum hemorrhage secondary to uterine atony, early postpartum hemorrhage secondary to lacerations, hemorrhage secondary to blood coagulopathies.

Plan

Psychosocial Intervention. Provide emotional support. Inform the client in a calm tone of the procedures that are being instituted. Make instructions specific, for example, "I'm going to give you some oxygen through this mask. I want you to try to breathe normally so that the oxygen will help you." Encouraging the woman to breastfeed will help in the release of oxytocin and therefore help facilitate natural uterine contractions.

Other Interventions

- Maintain patent intravenous line and begin second intravenous line.
- Bimanual uterine massage.
- Elevate right hip (prevent vena cava syndrome).
- Oxygen therapy with face mask at 6–8 liters per minute; provide positive pressure ventilation if needed.
- Call physician and inform him/her of client's status and corrective measures already instituted.
- Assess client's response by monitoring vital signs.
- Insert Foley catheter to measure urinary output.
- Record intravenous fluids infused.
- Anticipate blood transfusion and request crossmatching of blood.

Medication

OXYTOCIN

- *Indication.* Uterine stimulation.
- *Administration.* Diluted in intravenous fluids per hospital or agency protocol; usually 10 to 40 units in 1000 mL of intravenous solution given at 20 to 40 mU/min.[15]
- *Side Effects.* Hypertension, uterine tetany, nausea, vomiting, bradycardia, tachycardia, premature ventricular contractions, water intoxication.
- *Contraindication.* Hypersensitivity to oxytocin.
- *Anticipated Outcomes on Evaluation.* Decreased uterine bleeding and increased uterine tone.
- *Client Teaching.* Inform the client that she will experience increased uterine contractions, which may be quite uncomfortable.

PROSTAGLANDINS

- *Indication.* Uterine contraction.
- *Administration.* Intramuscularly—Carboprost (Prostin 15/M; Hemabate) 250 µg, repeated as necessary every 15 to 90 minutes—up to maximum of eight doses.[15,16]

- *Side Effects.* Mild fever, diarrhea, abdominal cramping, vomiting.
- *Contraindications.* Hypersensitivity, respiratory disease.
- *Anticipated Outcome on Evaluation.* Decreased uterine bleeding.
- *Client Teaching.* Counsel the client regarding possible side effects, including abdominal cramps, low grade fever, and diarrhea.

Anesthesia/Analgesia. Choice of regional or general anesthesia depends upon client's stability, cause of hemorrhage, presence of underlying disease pathology, potential for further blood loss, need for additional surgery, and the expertise of the anesthesiologist.[16] Spinal or epidural anesthesia is imprudent unless client is hemodynamically stable.[16] If minimally invasive procedure will be needed to control the hemorrhage, and the woman is hemodynamically stable, a regional anesthetic with close monitoring of the woman may be appropriate.[16] A general anesthetic is less likely to interfere with hemodynamics than a regional block.[16]

METHYLERGONOVINE MALEATE (METHERGINE)

- *Indications.* Uterine and vascular smooth muscle constriction.
- *Administration.* Intramuscularly, orally, and, in an emergency, intravenously.

Intramuscular	0.2 mg, repeated in 2 to 4 hours[15]
Oral	0.2 to 0.4 mg every 6 to 8 hours, usually for 2 days
Intravenous	Hazardous; should be reserved for emergency control of postpartum hemorrhage. If methylergonovine maleate is given intravenously, 0.2 mg is infused over 60 seconds or longer.

- *Side Effects.* Headache, dizziness, nausea, vomiting, chest pain, palpitation, hypertension (especially when given intravenously).
- *Contraindications.* Hypertension, hypersensitivity to ergot alkaloids, respiratory disease, cardiac disease, peripheral vascular disease.
- *Anticipated Outcome on Evaluation.* Decreased uterine bleeding.

- *Client Teaching.* Inform the client about possible side effects and increased uterine cramping.

Follow-Up

Advise client to eat foods high in protein and iron to aid in tissue healing and build up body iron stores. Iron supplements will be needed for an additional 2 to 3 months postpartum.

Late Postpartum Hemorrhage

Late hemorrhage occurs after the first 24 hours and up to 1 month postpartum. Its usual onset is 6 to 10 days after delivery. Several risk factors have been identified:

- Retained placental tissue
- Uterine subinvolution
- Infection

Subjective Data

The client may report pelvic or back pain, uterine tenderness, or bleeding for more than 2 weeks.

Objective Data

Physical examination may reveal heavy lochia with a foul odor, fever, an open cervical os after the first week postpartum, and hematoma.

A complete blood count is ordered (see Early Postpartum Hemorrhage).

Differential Medical Diagnoses

Trauma, blood coagulopathy.

Plan

- *Psychosocial Intervention.* Provide emotional support by assisting to calm the client and her family—speaking calmly and giving information about procedures (see Early Postpartum Hemorrhage). She may need help obtaining child or infant care.
- *Medication.* Methylergonovine maleate was discussed under Early Postpartum Hemorrhage. Antibiotics should be added if endometritis is suspected (see Metritis with Pelvic Cellulitis).
- *Ultrasound.* Ultrasound examination is done to detect retained placental fragments.

Follow-Up

Consult with a physician to determine need for hospital admission or other management.

SUBINVOLUTION OF THE UTERUS

Subinvolution of the uterus is the arrest or prolongation of the normal involution process that occurs following pregnancy.[17] Complications of subinvolution include hemorrhage, pelvic peritonitis, salpingitis, and abscess formation.

Epidemiology

Several risk factors are identified in the etiology of subinvolution:

- Distended bladder
- Retained placental fragments
- Endometritis
- Cesarean birth
- Uterine myoma
- Multiparity

Subjective Data

The client may report painless, excessive vaginal bleeding; chills and fever; pelvic or back pain. Obtain sexual history from client—resumption of intercourse, use of sex toys, new partner, contraceptive used and type.

Objective Data

Physical examination of the genitalia and reproductive tract reveal whether the uterus is larger than expected for the period of puerperium and whether fundal height is normal—midway between the umbilicus and symphysis following the third stage of labor and at the level of the bony pelvis 2 weeks postpartum. The uterus should return to nonpregnant size at 4 to 6 weeks postpartum.[17] With subinvolution the uterus feels boggy and soft and may be tender. Uterine bleeding, excessive lochia, and leukorrhea are possible. Fever may also be present.

Diagnostic tests include serum blood tests, culture of cervical discharge, and ultrasound. Clients must be prepared for venipuncture.

- A complete blood count is performed to detect anemia and infection.

- An erythrocyte sedimentation rate (ESR) is a diagnostic evaluation for occult infective disease.
- Cervical discharge is cultured to identify a specific infective agent, such as chlamydia trachomatis or group B strep. Before a cervical specimen is obtained, the client should be informed about the use of the speculum, the testing to be done, and the reason for the test.
- Quantitative determination of the β subunit of human chorionic gonadotropin (hCG) assists the health care provider in detecting pregnancy, trophoblastic tumors, and tumors that ectopically secrete hCG. Explain the rationale for requesting the test to the client.
- Pelvic ultrasound is done to evaluate whether placental fragments were retained. Instruct the client to drink four glasses of water 1 hour prior to the ultrasound exam. While she is supine on examining table, the transducer is placed in contact with her skin and swept over the area being studied.

Differential Medical Diagnosis

Distended bladder, ovarian cyst, pelvic adhesions, malignant uterine tumors, cystitis, gestational trophoblastic disease, anemia, uterine leiomyoma, retained placental fragments.

Plan

Psychosocial Intervention. Inform the client about the diagnosis, suspected etiology, and plan of treatment. Explain that methylergonovine may cause painful uterine contractions. Advise her of the need to rest and avoid overexertion.

Medication. For information on methylergonovine maleate, see Early Postpartum Hemorrhage. If infection is suspected, treat presumptively with antibiotics.[17]

AMOXICILLIN CLAVULANATE POTASSIUM (AUGMENTIN)
- *Indication.* Broad spectrum antibiotic. Because augmentin contains a β-lactamase inhibitor, it is effective against bacteria that produce β-lactamase.
- *Administration.* One 500-mg tablet orally every 8 hours for 10 days.
- *Side Effects.* Nausea, vomiting, diarrhea, vaginitis, eosinophilia, leukopenia.

- *Contraindication.* History of penicillin allergy.
- *Anticipated Outcome on Evaluation.* Clinically decreased evidence of infection. Check culture and sensitivity report from earlier cultures to confirm effectiveness of chosen antibiotic.
- *Client Teaching.* Instruct the client to complete the 10-day medication regimen. Tell the client to telephone if side effects make compliance difficult or if no improvement in symptoms.

TETRACYCLINE
- *Indication.* Broad spectrum antiinfective.
- *Administration.* One 500-mg tablet orally every 6 hours for 10 days.
- *Side Effects.* Nausea, vomiting, diarrhea, increased BUN, rash, urticaria, photosensitivity, increased pigmentation, hepatotoxicity, pseudomembranous colitis.
- *Contraindications.* Hypersensitivity to tetracyclines, kidney dysfunction, pregnancy, lactation.
- *Anticipated Outcome on Evaluation.* Decreased clinical evidence of infection. Check culture and sensitivity report to confirm organism's responsiveness to tetracycline.
- *Client Teaching.* Explain to the client that effects of tetracycline decrease when antacids, dairy products, or kaolin/pectin are also consumed. Advise the client to avoid sun exposure (sunscreen does not seem to decrease photosensitivity), to contact the health care provider if significant diarrhea develops, and to complete the 10-day medication regimen.

DOXYCYCLINE
- *Indication.* Broad spectrum antibiotic/antiinfective.
- *Administration.* One 100-mg tablet orally every 12 hours for 10 days.
- *Side Effects.* Same as for tetracycline.
- *Contraindications.* Hypersensitivity to tetracyclines, pregnancy, lactation. Because elimination is primarily nonrenal, doxycycline, unlike tetracycline, may be used for clients with renal failure.
- *Anticipated Outcome on Evaluation.* Decreased clinical evidence of infection.
- *Client Teaching.* Emphasize the need to complete the 10-day medication regimen. Instruct the client to avoid sun exposure (sunscreen does not seem to decrease photosensitivity) and to take doxycycline with a full glass of

water. Do not lie down at least 1 hour after administration to avoid epigastric discomfort. In addition, let the client know that the drug may be taken with meals, as its absorption is not affected by food.

Hospitalization. Hospitalization may be necessary if infection is severe, if pelvic structures in addition to the uterus are involved, or if uterine bleeding is excessive.

Follow-Up

Reassess the uterus in 1 to 2 weeks. Report signs and symptoms of hemorrhage, pelvic peritonitis, salpingitis, or abscess to physician for further evaluation and management.

MASTITIS

Mastitis, an inflammation of the breast, may be caused by tight clothing, missed infant feedings, poor drainage of duct and alveolus, or an infecting organism (*Staphylococcus aureus, Escherichia coli, Streptococcus*).[17,18]

Infection may be transmitted from lactiferous ducts to a secreting lobule, from a nipple fissure to periductal lymphatics, or by hematogenic means. Five percent of lactating women develop mastitis.[19]

Subjective Data

A woman may report flulike symptoms, including malaise, fever, and chills. She may also describe a tender, painful area or lump in the breast.

Objective Data

Physical examination is usually sufficient to diagnose mastitis. Assess vital signs. Fever is often high; tachycardia is common. Examination of the breasts reveals increased warmth, redness, tenderness, and swelling. The affected lobule is often in the outer quadrant and wedge-shaped; the nipple is cracked or abraded; and the breast distended with milk. Suspect a breast abscess if there is no resolution of symptoms after several days of antibiotic therapy.[20] If an abscess has formed, pitting edema is possible

and fluctuation may be felt over the affected area. As an abscess usually requires both antibiotics and drainage for resolution,[20] the client should be referred to a physician for further management. The remainder of the exam is usually normal.

Diagnostic testing may include a culture and sensitivity, although it is seldom used. Diagnosis is generally made without culture. Culture and sensitivity identifies the causative infectious agent using an expressed sample of breast milk. Test results may not be available for 72 hours, however, antibiotic therapy needs to be started immediately.

Differential Medical Diagnoses

Clogged duct, simple breast engorgement, breast abscess, viral syndrome.

Plan

Psychosocial Intervention. Counsel the client regarding the etiology of mastitis. Unless she has been prescribed a sulfa drug (see the following), encourage her to continue breastfeeding emphasizing that her medication is safe to use during lactation. Inform the client of the signs and symptoms of worsening mastitis and the need to call the health care provider should they develop.

Medication. Sulfa drugs should not be prescribed if the nursing infant is less than 1 month old.[18]

DICLOXACILLIN SODIUM (DYNAPEN, DYCILL, PATHOCIL)
- *Indication.* Treatment of penicillinase-resistant organisms.
- *Administration.* 250 to 500 mg orally every 6 hours for 10 days.
- *Side Effects.* Nausea, vomiting, diarrhea, vaginitis.
- *Contraindication.* Hypersensitivity to penicillins.
- *Anticipated Outcome on Evaluation.* Resolution of mastitis.
- *Client Teaching.* Instruct the client to complete the 10-day medication regimen even if she feels better before medication is finished; if medication is not taken for all 10 days, the risk for relapse increases.[17,18,19] The medication is category B for pregnancy.

Cephalexin (Keflex) or Cephradine (Velosef)

- *Administration.* 500 mg every 6 hours for 10 days; inhibits cell wall synthesis.
- *Side Effects.* Nausea, anorexia, diarrhea, maculopapular and erythematous rashes, urticaria, anaphylaxis.
- *Contraindications.* Hypersensitivity to cephalosporins.
- *Anticipated Outcome.* Resolution of mastitis
- *Client Teaching/Counseling.* Finish all medication. If medication not taken for 10 days, there is an increase risk for relapse of infection.

Acetaminophen (Tylenol)

- *Indications.* Antipyretic and analgesic.
- *Administration.* 325–650 mg orally every 4 hours as needed, not to exceed 4 g per day.
- *Side Effects.* Few, if taken in therapeutic doses. Acetaminophen does not cause gastric bleeding or inhibit platelet aggregation. No relationship to Reye's syndrome has been found. Overdosage can cause hepatic necrosis.
- *Contraindication.* None is known.
- *Anticipated Outcome on Evaluation.* Decreased pain and fever.
- *Client Teaching.* Inform the client about the effects of overdosage; instruct her to take no more than 4 g per day. She should know the early symptoms of hepatic necrosis: nausea, vomiting, diarrhea, sweating, abdominal discomfort. Tell the client to telephone the health care provider if she experiences symptoms of overdosage.

Breast Care. Ice or warm packs may be applied to the breast, whichever is more comfortable. The client should continue to nurse her infant on both breasts, but begin on the unaffected breast and thus allow the affected breast to "let down." Review breastfeeding techniques with the client.

Complications of mastitis require special breast care measures.

- Candidal invasion, described as incredible pain like "hot cords," is a fungal infection of milk ducts. Nystatin cream (Mycostatin or Mycolog) should be massaged into the nipple and areola after each feeding. The infant must simultaneously be given oral nystatin or the mother will be reinfected.

Fluid Intake. The client should increase fluid intake.

Lifestyle Changes. Bed rest, with bathroom privileges, is necessary in the treatment of mastitis to prevent the client from becoming exhausted and thereby worsening the mastitis.[18]

Follow-Up

Referral to a breastfeeding support group or lactation consultant may be necessary (see Support Groups).

METRITIS WITH PELVIC CELLULITIS (ENDOMETRITIS)

This form of endometritis is inflammation of the decidua, myometrium, and parametrial tissues following childbirth.[17] Bacteria from an infected surgical incision and from a colonized cervix and vagina enter amniotic fluid during labor. Once in amniotic fluid, bacteria invade uterine tissue postpartum. Bacteria invade the remaining uterine decidua up to a few days postpartum.

Endometritis may have an early onset, generally following cesarean birth, or late onset, usually after vaginal delivery and tends to be mild.[17]

Epidemiology

Risk factors include cesarean birth, membranes ruptured for longer than 3 hours, prolonged labor, numerous cervical examinations, internal fetal monitoring, and cervical lacerations.[13,17]

Transmission occurs via several routes.

- Lymphatic transmission may be from an infected cervical laceration, uterine incision for cesarean birth, or uterine laceration.
- Direct invasion occurs when cervical laceration extends into connective tissue at the base of broad ligaments, providing direct access to infective organisms.
- Transmission may be secondary to pelvic thrombophlebitis. A thrombus may become purulent, resulting in necrosis of venous walls and pathogenic access to surrounding connective tissue.[17]

Metritis with pelvic cellulitis occurs among 3 to 6 percent of vaginal deliveries and 90 percent of operative deliveries done for cephalopelvic disproportion without perioperative prophylaxis.[13,17,21]

Subjective Data

A client may report unilateral or bilateral abdominal pain; foul smelling lochia; fever, which is minimal if confined to decidua, but more commonly 39° C (102.2° F) or higher; malaise; and anorexia.[17]

Objective Data

The client appears wan and lethargic. She also appears to have pain.

- Vital signs show a fever of about 38° C (100.4° F); tachycardia may or may not be present.
- Abdominal and musculoskeletal examinations reveal significant lower abdominal pain with tenderness and rebound. Paralytic ileus may cause distention and vomiting.[17]
- Genitalia and reproductive organs have parametrial tenderness on bimanual exam. The pelvic exam may be normal even with severe endometritis. Uterine subinvolution is possible. Discharge is increased, dark red/brown, and foul smelling. Cervical motion tenderness is also possible.

A complete blood count is ordered to detect infection or anemia. Leukocytosis (15,000 to 30,000 cells per microliter) may be noted on testing of the serum sample. The client should be counseled regarding the purpose of the test and the method used to obtain the serum sample.

Blood cultures are obtained to rule out bacteremia or septicemia. Explain the test procedure and purpose. Two specimens should be obtained, one for aerobic and one for anaerobic organisms.[13,17] Cleanse the rubber stoppers of the two specimen bottles with povidone-iodine and allow to air dry, then cleanse the stoppers with 70 percent alcohol. Using aseptic technique and universal precautions, obtain two venipuncture specimens after cleansing the puncture site with either povidone-iodine or 70 percent alcohol and allowing skin to dry for 1–2 minutes. The anaerobic bottle should be inoculated first, then the aerobic bottle, which is then vented with a special cotton plugged needle designed for that purpose. Mix both bottles gently, label, and send to the laboratory.[22]

Chest radiography is used to diagnose pulmonary diseases, to detect mediastinal abnormalities, and to assist in assessment of pulmonary status. Request upright anterior, posterior, and lateral views of chest. Inform the client about the test's purpose. She should be told that the radiology technician will ask her to remove her clothing to the waist, take a deep breath and exhale, and take a second deep breath and hold it while the x-ray is taken. Assure the client that the procedure takes only a few minutes, is painless, and may be safely performed during lactation.

Cervical cultures are done to identify *Neisseria gonorrhoeae, Chlamydia,* or other pathogens, such as group B streptococci and *Staphylococcus aureus.*

- A sterile speculum exam is conducted with the client in the lithotomy position. *No* lubricant is used on the speculum. Excess cervical mucus is gently removed with a large cotton tipped applicator. Next, a sterile swab, specific for the test desired, is inserted into the endocervical canal. The swab is not removed from the endocervical canal for several seconds to allow absorption of organisms. Swabs are placed into the appropriate culture container for transport to laboratory.
- Inform the client about the test, including its rationale. The health care provider obtaining the cultures should wear disposable gloves according to the facility's protocol and Centers for Disease Control guidelines.

A urine culture and sensitivity is done to diagnose urinary tract infection. Urine is collected in a sterile container. Ask the woman to thoroughly wash her hands with soap and water and dry her hands with a disposable towel. To prepare for urine collection, instruct the woman to remove the cap from the sterile container and place its outer surface down on a clean surface. Then she should cleanse the area around the urinary meatus from front to back with an antiseptic sponge. She should separate the labia with one hand before collecting the specimen. A small amount of urine is passed into the toilet bowl before the remaining urine is collected in a sterile container.

Differential Medical Diagnoses

Metritis with pelvic cellulitis, cystitis, pyelonephritis, mastitis, appendicitis, viral disease, septic pelvic thrombophlebitis, toxic shock syndrome, paralytic ileus.

Plan

Because of severe, life-threatening complications as noted previously, referral to physician for hospital admission is mandatory. Outpatient management for mild cases of late postpartum endometritis, after physician consultation, may be appropriate.[13] Close follow-up by telephone and returning to the office in 48 hours is mandatory.

Psychosocial Intervention. Inform the client of her diagnosis and treatment plan and inquire about her support systems.

Medication Interventions. Health care provider may choose one of the following as clinically indicated. Parenteral administration of antibiotics is mandatory in moderate to severe infections and should be continued until the client has been afebrile for 48 hours.[13] Oral antibiotics after parenteral treatment are not necessary and no longer recommended.[12,13,21] A recent study compared the use of once-daily and 8-hour dosing of gentamicin. No differences were found in development of complications, need for change in antibiotics, readmission, length of hospital stay, or length of time clients remained febrile once therapy was initiated.[23] A significant difference was found in the initial peak serum concentration, however, with 24 clients in the control group requiring dose adjustment for an initial peak serum concentration of less than $5.0 \mu g/ml$.[23]

ERYTHROMYCIN

- *Indication.* Infection.
- *Administration.* 500 mg orally every 6 hours for 10 days.
- *Side Effects.* Gastrointestinal disturbances, vaginitis. Cholestatic hepatitis is caused by erythromycin estolate but not by other forms of erythromycin. Symptoms of cholestatic hepatitis include nausea, vomiting, abdominal pain, jaundice, and elevated levels of serum bilirubin

and liver transaminases. Erythromycin can increase plasma levels and half-lives of theophylline, carbamazepine, and warfarin.
- *Contraindication.* Hypersensitivity to the drug.
- *Anticipated Outcome on Evaluation.* Resolution of infection.
- *Client Teaching.* Instruct the client to complete the medication regimen, even if she feels better sooner. Advise her to take the medication with a full glass of water; she should not take erythromycin with fruit juice.

AUGMENTIN. Augmentin is a broad spectrum antibiotic (previously discussed, p. 653) used to treat metritis with pelvic cellulitis.

CEPHALOSPORINS. The cephalosporins, including cephradine (Velosef), cephalexin (Keflex, Keftab, Ceporex), cefaclor (Ceclor), and cefadroxil (Duricef, Ultracef), are broad-spectrum antibiotics with β-lactamase activity.

- *Administration.* Cefaclor: 500 mg orally every 8 hours for 10 days, not to exceed 4 g per day. Cephradine and cephalexin: 500 mg orally every 6 hours for 10 days. Cefadroxil: initial loading dose of 1 g orally, then 1 to 2 g orally every day or every 12 hours for 10 days.
- *Side Effects.* Maculopapular rash, urticaria, and gastrointestinal upset. Discontinue medication if allergy symptoms appear (urticaria, rash, hypotension, difficulty breathing).
- *Contraindication.* Hypersensitivity to cephalosporins and pencillins.
- *Anticipated Outcome on Evaluation.* Resolution of symptoms and clinical improvement.
- *Client Teaching.* Stress the importance of completing the medication regimen. Instruct the client to report signs of allergy.

CEFOXITIN. 1–2 grams IV every 6–8 hours
- *Side Effects.* Maculopapular and erythematous rashes; uriticaria; pseudomembranous colitis; diarrhea; transient neutropenia; hemolytic anemia; hypoprothrombinemia; anaphylaxis; pain induration sterile abscesses at IV site; phlebitis; thrombophlebitis.

GENTAMICIN. Gentamicin is an aminoglycoside used in the treatment of endometritis. Onset of action is immediate after IV administration, but unknown if given intramuscularly. Peak serum levels occur in 30–90 minutes. Gentamicin efficacy in serious infections has been correlated with peak serum concentrations greater than 6µg/mL, and toxicity is increased when trough levels exceed 2µg/mL for prolonged periods. Aminoglycocide's bactericidal activity is concentration dependent, and bacterial growth is suppressed for long periods after administration. In addition, there is a phenomenon called "adaptive resistance," in which bactericidal activity of subsequent doses of an aminoglycoside is decreased by the initial dose. Clinical trials of single dose aminoglycoside therapy apply these principles of aminoglycoside action and have proven to be as effective as conventional multiple dose regimens with less nephrotoxicity.

- *Administration.* Gentamicin: 3–5 mg/Kg of body weight in three divided doses IV every 8 hours. For single dose therapy, 5 mg/Kg of body weight IV. Obtain blood for peak gentamicin level 30 minutes to 1 hour after IV infusion; for trough levels, draw blood just before the next dose. Do not collect blood in heparinized tube as the heparin is incompatible with the aminoglycoside. Monitor renal function (output, specific gravity, urinalysis, blood urea nitrogen [BUN], and creatinine levels, creatinine clearance). Evaluate the client's hearing during therapy.
- *Side Effects.* Neuromuscular blockade; ototoxicity (tinnitus, vertigo, hearing loss); nephrotoxicity (cells or casts in the urine; oligouria; proteinuria; decreased creatinine clearance; increased BUN, nonprotein nitrogen, and serum creatinine levels).
- *Interactions.* Cephalothin (increased nephrotoxicity); Dimenhydrinate (may mask symptoms of ototoxicity); General anesthetics, neuromuscular blockades (may increase neuromuscular blockade); Indomethacin (may increase serum peak and trough levels of gentamicin; monitor levels closely); I.V. loop diuretics (increased ototoxicity); other aminoglycosides, amphotericin B, anyclovor, cisplatin, methoxyflurane, vancomycin (increased ototoxicity and nephrotoxicity); Parenteral penicillins (gentamicin inactivation in vitro; do not mix together).

CLINDAMYCIN. Clindamycin is an anti-infective used in the treatment of postpartum endometritis.

- *Oral dosage.* 150–160 mg every 6 hours.
- *Parenteral.* IM or IV: 300–600 mg every 6–8 hours up to 4.8 grams per day in life threatening infections.
- *Side Effects.* Nausea, diarrhea, dysphagia, bloody or tarry stools, pain, anaphylaxis; sterile abscess with IM injection.

Conservative management with antibiotics usually produces a response in 48 hours. A poor response indicates abscess, retention of placental parts, or incorrect diagnosis.[13] Physician referral is mandatory.

Fluid Intake. Women with metritis with pelvic cellulitis should increase fluid intake.

Lifestyle Changes. Explain to the client and her partner the client's general need for rest, as well as her need for pelvic rest (including no sexual intercourse).

Follow-Up

Medical consultation is required. In addition, telephone the client daily and schedule a return appointment 48 to 72 hours after treatment begins. Complications of endometritis can be severe.

- With septic pelvic thrombophlebitis, pain typically develops after the second or third postpartum day. Fever spikes continue despite antimicrobial treatment. Diagnosis is established using computerized tomography or magnetic resonance imaging (MRI).[21] Refer the client for immediate medical treatment.
- Pelvic abscess is usually unilateral. Clinical presentation is 1 to 2 weeks postpartum and surgical drainage is most likely necessary, as rupture can cause peritonitis.[21] Referral to a physician is indicated.

POSTPARTUM THYROIDITIS

Postpartum thyroiditis is an autoimmune thyroid disease that results from transient rebound of the autoimmune process following delivery or abortion.[24] The thyroid is unable to regulate both the release of previously synthesized thyroid hormone as well as the synthesis of new thyroid hormone.[25] It is differentiated from other forms of thyrotoxicosis by the lack of thyroid pain, its transient symptoms with spontaneous remission, and elevated serum antibodies and thyroid hormones (hyperthyroid phase) with concomitant suppression of radioactive thyroid uptake.[24,25]

Epidemiology

The risk factors involved include a personal history of known or suspected thyroid disease (a genetic or family history is not a predictor); small, soft, diffuse goiter; any pituitary gland dysfunction; psychological distress that intensifies over time and requires intervention; and symptoms that persist despite the absence of external stressors or that persist after stressors abate.[24]

Postpartum women account for 10 percent of all individuals with thyroiditis.[26]

Subjective Data

A client may report symptoms of thyrotoxicosis during the first postpartum month and transient hypothyroidism with symptoms that peak after 3 to 5 months.

Thyrotoxicosis has a rapid onset in the latter half of the first postpartum month and persists for 2 to 4 months, usually resolving by the fourth postpartum month. The client reports weight loss, fatigue that occurs easily, heat intolerance, palpitations, hand tremors, nervousness, or other psychoneurotic reactions.[26,27]

In transient hypothyroidism, clinical signs peak between 3 and 5 months postpartum. The client shows progressive and pronounced fatigue, continued weight gain in the latter months of first postpartum year, coarse hair, dry skin, and psychological reactions that mimic depression. Any complaint of fatigue, palpitations, impaired memory, depression, or loss of attention span during the first year postpartum needs to be evaluated.[24,25,27]

Objective Data

Physical examination reveals signs unique to both phases of postpartum thyroiditis. In the thyrotoxicosis phase, the client exhibits sinus tachycardia, stare or lid lag, brisk reflexes, and a firm, nontender thyroid. Only 50 percent of women have thyroid enlargement.[27] The transient hypothyroidism phase involves delayed reflexes, psychomotor retardation, and psychological reactions that mimic depression.

The thyroid-stimulating hormone (TSH) test is done to diagnose primary hypothyroidism, differentiating primary from secondary hypothyroidism. In addition, an elevated level of serum thyroid-stimulating hormone is noted in the hypothyroid phase. The test procedure requires a blood sample. Inform the client of the venipuncture procedure and the rationale for the test, and explain test results to her.

The antithyroglobulin antibody test differentiates thyroid diseases such as Hashimoto's thyroiditis and thyroid carcinoma. A blood sample is also used in this test. Inform the client of the venipuncture procedure and the purpose of the antithyroglobulin antibody test.

Thyroid peroxidase antibodies (TPO) previously called antimicrosomal antibodies (MsAb) is a diagnostic evaluation for the presence of thyroid microsomal antibodies.[24] As a blood sample is required, advise the client about the venipuncture procedure. Tell the client that high antibodies to thyroid peroxidase indicate an increased risk for developing thyroid disease in the first year postpartum.[26,27] A TSH assay should be requested. Women with goiters and a high titer of thyroid peroxidase antibodies, but a normal TSH, should have the TSH remeasured in 3 months.[24]

The radioactive iodine uptake test (contraindicated for pregnant or lactating women) reveals increased uptake in hyperthyroidism of Graves' disease, but decreased uptake in hyperthyroidism of thyroiditis.[25] This diagnostic test evaluates the thyroid's ability to concentrate and retain iodine and is indicated in the diagnosis of thyroid disease.

The test procedure is done in conjunction with a thyroid scan and assessment of thyroid hormone levels. A fasting state is preferred. A liquid form or capsule of radioiodine is administered orally. The radioactivity of the thyroid gland is measured by scanning the gland 2, 6, and 24 hours later.

Provide the client with information about factors that interfere with, or lower, radioactive iodine uptake: iodized foods and iodine-containing medications (1 to 3 weeks' duration), vitamin preparations that contain minerals (1 to 3 weeks' duration), antithyroid medications (2 to 10 days' duration), thyroid medications (1 to 2 weeks' duration), antihistamines, corticosteroids, isoniazid, thiocyanate, perchlorate, sulfonamides, orinase, Butazolidin, adrenocorticotropin, aminosalicylic acid, coumadin anticoagulant.[28]

Medications and conditions that increase uptake include thyroid stimulating hormone, pregnancy, cirrhosis, barbiturates, lithium, phenothiazine, iodine-deficient diets, and renal failure.[28] Tell the client that the test is painless, but requires 24 hours to perform. Restrict iodine intake (e.g., iodized salt, seafood) for at least 1 week prior to the test.

Differential Medical Diagnosis

Graves' disease, postpartum depression, Sheehan's syndrome.

Plan

Psychosocial Intervention. Reassure the client regarding the validity of her symptoms. Explain to her the etiology and management of postpartum thyroiditis. Counsel the client regarding spontaneous resolution as well as possible recurrence of the condition with future births.

Medication. Levothyroxine (T4) is administered to treat hypothyroidism. Initial doses should be low, beginning with 0.1 mg/day, increasing gradually every 2 weeks until full replacement doses have been achieved.[24] Replacement doses have been achieved when repeat thyroid function tests are within normal limits.

- *Side Effects.* Rare when given in therapeutic doses. Excessive doses of levothyroxine may cause thyrotoxicosis; symptoms are anxiety, insomnia, tremors, tachycardia, angina, palpitations, hyperthermia, and sweating.
- *Contraindication.* None is known.
- *Anticipated Outcomes on Evaluation.* Reversal of signs and symptoms of hypothyroidism and a decline in serum TSH levels.
- *Client Teaching.* Instruct the client to take the medication on an empty stomach to enhance absorption; morning administration decreases sleeplessness. Medication should be kept in a light-resistant container. Advise the client to report excitability, irritability, or anxiety. Also advise her not to switch brands of levothyroxine unless approved by the health care provider.

Follow-Up

Referral to a physician is required. Regular checkups are scheduled for laboratory assessment of thyroid function. Physical and laboratory assessment should continue for 2 years postpartum. As the thyroid gland often recovers in 1 year, the health care provider can assess thyroid function and the need for continued thyroid replacement by halving the dose and repeating the TSH 6–8 weeks later.[24] If the TSH continues to be normal, one can assume normal thyroid functioning and the levothyroxine can be discontinued.[24]

URINARY TRACT INFECTION

Epidemiology

Risk factors for infection, caused by bacteria in the urinary tract (see Chapter 21), include trauma to the bladder or urethra, such as that resulting from catheterization; history of urinary tract infection; sickle cell trait; and diabetes mellitus. Infection is transmitted in vaginal secretions via sexual intercourse and perineal pads.

Subjective Data

A client may report dysuria, oliguria, urinary frequency or urgency, nausea and vomiting, chills, and abdominal pain or cramping.

Objective Data

Physical examination usually reveals that general appearance and vital signs are within normal limits. Fever, however, may be present and is indicative of upper urinary tract infection (pyelonephritis). The abdomen and musculoskeletal system exam is done to detect costovertebral angle tenderness and suprapubic tenderness.

A urinalysis determines the properties of urine and abnormal products. Pyuria (white blood cells in urine), hematuria (red blood cells in urine), and positive nitrite indicate a urinary tract infection and warrant a urine culture. The test procedure for urinalysis requires a routine urine sample obtained by voiding. Instruct the client about the purpose of the test and the method of collection.

A urine culture and sensitivity is done to diagnose bacterial infection and identify offending organisms (see Metritis With Pelvic Cellulitis for a description of the test procedure and client teaching).

Differential Medical Diagnoses

Urinary tract infection (lower or upper tracts); Chlamydia trachomatis.

Plan

Psychosocial Interventions. Provide the client with information and counsel her regarding the suspected diagnosis and pathophysiology of urinary tract infection.

Medication. One of the following drugs is administered. (*Amoxicillin* is no longer the first choice as many organisms causing urinary tract infections are resistant to ampicillin/amoxicillin.)

NITROFURANTOIN (MACROBID)
- *Administration.* One 100-mg tablet orally every 12 hours for 3–5 days.
- *Side Effects.* Gastrointestinal reactions (nausea, vomiting), headache, vertigo, drowsiness.
- *Contraindications.* Hypersensitivity to the drug, glucose-6-phosphate dehydrogenase (G6PD) deficiency, renal disease.
- *Anticipated Outcomes on Evaluation.* Resolution of client's symptoms and negative urine culture following treatment.
- *Client Teaching.* Advise the client to complete the 3–5 day medication regimen even if symptoms disappear before that time. Medication is taken with food or milk. The client should be told to return for a followup visit if indicated.

TRIMETHOPRIM-SULFAMETHOXAZOLE
(BACTRIM-DS, SEPTRA-DS, COTRIM-DS)
- *Administration.* One tablet orally every 12 hours for 3–5 days.
- *Side Effects.* Gastrointestinal reactions (nausea and vomiting), rash, blood dyscrasias (hemolytic anemia, leukopenia, thrombocytopenia).
- *Contraindications.* Hypersensitivity to trimethoprim or sulfonamides, G6PD deficiency, first

12 weeks or last trimester (28 to 42 weeks) of pregnancy, megaloblastic anemia.
- *Anticipated Outcomes on Evaluation.* Resolution of client's symptoms and negative urine culture following treatment.
- *Client Teaching.* Instruct the client to complete the 3–5-day medication regimen even if symptoms improve or disappear before that time. Medication should be taken with a full glass of water; water intake is increased to decrease crystallization in kidneys. Advise the client to avoid sunlight to prevent burns and to contact the care provider if side effects occur.

TRIMETHOPRIM
- *Administration.* One 100-mg to 200-mg tablet every 12 hours for 3 to 5 days.
- *Side Effects.* Exfoliative dermatitis, pruritus, rash, thrombocytopenia, leukopenia, nausea, vomiting, abdominal pain, increased AST (SGOT), ALT (SGPT), bilirubin, creatinine.
- *Contraindications.* Hypersensitivity, Creatinine clearance 15 ml/min, renal disease, hepatic disease, megaloblastic anemia.
- *Anticipated Outcomes.* Reduction in client's symptoms and negative urine culture following treatment.
- *Client Teaching.* Advise client to complete the course of treatment even though symptoms may disappear.

CEPHALOSPORINS
- Cephradine one 250–500 mg tablet every 6 hours for 3–5 days.
- Cephalexion one 250 mg tablet every 6 hours for 3–5 days.

For information on cephalosporins, see Endometritis.

Follow-Up

Review proper perineal hygiene with the client. In addition, reemphasize her need to increase fluid intake. (Additional follow-up is outlined in Chapter 21.)

ACUTE APPENDICITIS

The appendix may become inflamed as a result of obstruction of the appendiceal lumen by hardened stool, hypertrophy of lymph follicles in the wall of the appendix, or strictures.

Epidemiology

In a pregnancy and the puerperium, the appendix is atypically positioned, as it is in obese individuals. Chronic constipation is another risk factor. Adolescents and young adults, however, are at greatest risk; the incidence of acute appendicitis is rare among pregnant and postpartum women.

Subjective Data

The client may report loss of appetite, abdominal distention, and abdominal pain.

Objective Data

Physical examination may reveal the client to be distressed, obviously in pain. Her vital signs are likely to be within normal limits; temperature may be elevated.

Abdominal muscles do not show the classic signs of appendicitis (abdominal guarding and rigidity) in early puerperium, as the appendix does not return to its usual location until involution is completed (6–8 weeks).[29]

- Tenderness is common in the right upper quadrant or entire right abdomen when uterine size is 12 weeks or greater.
- Psoas, obturator, and Rovsing's signs are not predictive of appendicitis in pregnant or postpartum women.
- Bryan's sign is positive if moving the enlarged uterus to the right elicits pain,[29] and may be a more reliable indicator of appendiceal pathology.
- Alder's test requires the health care provider to maintain constant pressure at an area of maximum tenderness while the client rolls from the supine position onto her left side. Alder's test assists in differentiating pain of uterine etiology from that of extrauterine origin;[29] pain of uterine origin may be relieved by change in position, whereas pain of extrauterine origin will not be relieved regardless of position.

Examination of the genitalia and reproductive tract reveals that the lochia is not excessive and has no foul odor, the cervix is closed, and the uterus is nontender.

Diagnostic tests assess blood, urine, and endocervical tissue.

A complete blood count identifies anemia and specific infections. Leukocytosis is nonspecific and does not differentiate appendicitis from other inflammatory causes of abdominal pain. White blood cell (WBC) counts of 20,000 to 25,000/mm^3 and increased neutrophils are not uncommon in appendicitis during the first 10 to 14 days postpartum. A blood sample must be obtained, and the client counseled regarding the purpose of the test and the method used to obtain the sample.

The erythrocyte sedimentation rate (ESR) is used to monitor an inflammatory or malignant disease. The test also helps to detect and diagnose occult disease. A blood sample must be obtained, and the client counseled regarding the purpose of the test and method of collection.

Urinalysis determines the properties of urine, including abnormal products. Pyuria (white blood cells in urine), hematuria (red blood cells in urine), and positive nitrite are indicative of urinary tract infection and warrant urine culture. Sterile pyuria (> 5 WBCs per high-power field) and hematuria are seen in 15 to 30 percent of pregnant and puerperal women, in whom the appendix lies proximal to the ureter.[29] (See Urinary Tract Infection for details of the test procedure and nursing implications.)

The urine culture and sensitivity is discussed under Urinary Tract Infection.

Endocervical cultures are discussed under Endometritis.

Differential Medical Diagnoses

Appendicitis; endometritis; pyelonephritis; tuboovarian abscess.

Plan

Counsel the client and her family about the diagnosis and assist the family to arrange for child care. Immediate referral to a surgeon is mandatory, as complications include death and appendiceal perforation.

EARLY DISCHARGE

Early discharge follows a hospital stay of 48 hours or fewer. It subjects a woman and her infant to certain risk factors. For example, physical complications may occur: discomfort at an episiotomy or cesarean incision site, endometritis, mastitis. Physiologic changes may be affected: uterine involution, increased edema and hyperemia of the bladder with possible atony, and diuresis. The client will confront other changes, such as fatigue, meeting the needs of her infant, role conflict, and adjustment within parental and family relationships.[30]

Follow-up care in the home or by telephone should be pursued to assess the health needs (physical, psychosocial, and educational) of the mother, the family, and the infant in the early puerperium and to implement nursing plans to meet assessed needs. Criteria for prospective payment and a shorter hospital stay will need to be complied with as insurance policies may differ with both hospital stay and home visits.[31,32] Referral to support groups may be helpful (see Support Groups at the end of this chapter).

A study conducted by the National Center for Health Statistics looked at risk factors for poor health and discharge timing on 9953 women in 48 states who had a live birth. These women were cared for either by midwives or physicians. Clients of midwives who were discharged early were more likely to have either private insurance or none at all. Clients of midwives who remained in the hospital for an extra night were more likely to have not attended childbirth classes, or were multiparous with birth intervals fewer than 24 months. These criteria differed from that of physicians' use of hospitalization stays for clients. Clients of physicians who were discharged early tended to have Medicaid, and had birth intervals greater than 24 months. Clients of physicians who remained in the hospital for an extra night tended to have attended childbirth classes and had more than a high school education.[33] With the push for short hospital stays by insurance companies,[31] more must be done to assist the new mother in the care of her newborn.

If discharge is anticipated within 24 hours of delivery, the American Academy of Pediatrics Committee on Fetus and Newborn and the American College of Obstetricians and Gynecologists' Committee on Obstetrics have established the following guidelines:[34]

- Mother had an uncomplicated vaginal delivery following a normal antepartum course and was observed after delivery for a sufficient time to ensure that her condition is stable. Pertinent laboratory data, including a postpartum hemoglobin and hematocrit, was obtained and, if appropriate, RhIg administered.
- Family or other support system should be available to the mother for the first few days following discharge.
- The mother should be aware of possible complications and how to notify the practitioner.
- Procedures for readmission of obstetric patients should be consistent with hospital policy, as well as local and state regulations.

For early infant discharge, the following criteria should be met:[34]

- Antepartum, intrapartum, and postpartum course for both mother and infant should be uncomplicated.
- Maternal readiness to assume independent care of her newborn should be assessed with return demonstration on feeding techniques, skin and cord care, measurement of temperature with a thermometer, ability to assess infant well-being and recognize common neonatal illness. Family members who will care for the infant should attend prenatal childbirth or infant care classes in which problems within the first few days after birth are discussed.
- The infant was born at term, is of appropriate weight, and has a normal examination.
- The infant should be able to maintain normal body temperature and suck and swallow normally.
- Mother and family should be aware of a physician directed source of continuing medical care for both mother and infant and arrangements should be made for an examination of the baby 48 hours after discharge.

- Laboratory data should be reviewed, to include the following: maternal testing for syphilis and hepatitis B surface antigen, cord or infant blood type and direct Coombs test (if the mother is Rho[D] negative, or is type O, or if screening had not been performed for maternal antibodies), infant hemoglobin or hematocrit and blood glucose as clinically indicated, and screening tests as required by law.
- Initial hepatitis B vaccine administered.

Within 48 hours after discharge, the following assessments of the infant should be done:

- Evaluation of condition by history and physical examination, to include assessment for adequate nutrition and hydration, normal stool pattern, jaundice, quality of mother-infant interaction, and infant behavior.
- Review of laboratory data prior to discharge.
- Screening tests for PKU, hypothyroidism, and other metabolic disorders as indicated by state law and clinical judgment.
- Health maintenance planning, to include emergency services, preventive care and immunizations, periodic evaluations, and necessary screening.

These recommendations have been further validated by a study conducted by Soskolne, Schumacher, Fyock, et al. Based on their findings, the authors recommended that all infants born either preterm, low birthweight, or with possible physiological abnormalities not be discharged prior to 72 hours.[35]

HOME VISITS

Home visits are made within the first week of discharge, and should be available to any childbearing family. The family should live within a reasonable radius of the health agency. If they do not, referral to a closer agency is indicated.

FOLLOW-UP TELEPHONE CALLS

Telephone calls are made within the first week after hospital discharge to all families who elect not to have home visits.

MATERNAL ASSESSMENT

Physical inspection, psychological evaluation, and assessment of feeding technique are parts of the maternal exam and can be assessed during home visits.

Physical Examination. Focus on answering the following questions:

GENERAL APPEARANCE AND VITAL SIGNS
- Does the client appear rested or exhausted?
- Are her blood pressure and pulse within her normal limits, based on her baseline vital signs as an inpatient (assuming no pregnancy induced hypertension)?
- Does the client complain of chills or fever? If so, determine her temperature.
- In a client with a history of pregnancy induced hypertension, how does current blood pressure compare with in-hospital blood pressure?

BREAST HEALTH AND CARE
- Is the client lactating?
- Are the breasts soft, or hard and painful (engorged)?
- Is the client wearing a supportive bra?
- If the client is breastfeeding, how often is the infant nursing?
- Is the client experiencing pain or nipple tenderness when she breastfeeds?
- Does the client feel comfortable with breastfeeding or insecure or worried?

ABDOMEN AND MUSCULOSKELETAL SYSTEM
- Does the client have discomfort or difficulty urinating?
- Is she constipated or does she have hemorrhoids?
- If the client had cesarean birth, how does the incision appear? Are staples present? What is the color of the skin and skin integrity? Is the incision draining? If so, what color is the drainage?
- Is there any back or neck pain or pain in the lower extremities?
- Is there swelling in the lower extremities?

GENITALIA AND REPRODUCTIVE ORGANS
- What is the fundal height?
- Is there uterine tenderness?
- How much lochia is evident and what color is it? Has there been any change in these qualities?
- If an episiotomy was done, is the incision erythematous? draining? intact?

Psychological Evaluation. Assess the client's ability to cope: What is her financial status? Did she recently relocate? Are her family and significant other supportive? What is her housing situation? Is she homeless, or living in overcrowded conditions?

Provide anticipatory guidance for a client concerning her neonate's behavior. Assess her and her family's knowledge of neonatal and infant development and infant cues. Assess their adjustment to the infant.

Feeding Technique. Assess feeding technique—breast or bottle—during follow-up visits or phone calls. Who is the primary provider of care for the infant? Does another person in the client's family influence infant feeding, for example, the type of milk given, the frequency of feedings, the introduction of solids?

Breastfeeding technique may be assessed by asking specific questions. How often does the infant nurse? How is the infant held when breastfed? Do her breasts feel soft after feeding? Ask the client to describe the infant's suck: Is it strong and vigorous, or does the infant frequently stop sucking and cry? How many wet diapers does the infant have in a day? Infants that are getting enough breast milk have 6 to 8 wet diapers a day. Are supplemental feedings given? If so, ask the client the reason for supplementation.

Consider observing the mother and infant during a feeding session to assess the effectiveness of breastfeeding technique. Bottle feeding technique may also be assessed by questioning. How often is the infant fed and by whom? What type of milk is given—commercially prepared formula or table milk? How is the infant held during feeding? Is the bottle propped? Is the nipple properly positioned? Are solids given? If so, why and how is infant fed the solid food?

Environment. Do people smoke in the home? Recent studies have confirmed the effect of tobacco smoke to respiratory ailments in children exposed to passive smoke as well as the increased risk of SIDS.[36,37] The risk of SIDS appears to be proportional to the number of cigarettes from all adults the infant is exposed to.[37]

Infant Care. Assess the client's or caregiver's knowledge of infant cues, infant sleep and wake states, and child developmental stages (see Neonatal Assessment, which follows). Inquire as to infant's position (prone, supine, side lying). In

healthy infants, the American Academy of Pediatrics recommends infants no longer be placed in the prone position for sleep.[38] Instead, healthy infants should be placed in the supine or side lying position.[38,39] Placing healthy infants in the supine or side lying position is associated with a lower risk of SIDS. Infants in whom the prone position is still recommended are premature infants with respiratory distress, infants with symptoms of gastroesophageal reflux or with certain upper airway anomalies, infants with Pierre Robin Syndrome.[38]

Health Teaching. Provide the client with information about exercise and rest, nutritional needs, postpartum sexuality and fertility, health care, and the nurturing needs of the infant. (Refer to Adjustment with the Infant's Father for specific information.)

NEONATAL ASSESSMENT

Physical inspection, home safety assessment, and identification of engagement and disengagement cues are parts of the neonatal evaluation, which should be assessed during a home visit.

Physical Examination. The physical examination is directed to answering several questions.

GENERAL APPEARANCE AND VITAL SIGNS

- Has the infant gained weight since hospital discharge? Although 5–10 percent of birth weight may be lost by both bottlefed and breastfed infants, the newborn should return to or exceed birth weight by the first week of life.[18] Weigh the infant if a portable scale is available.
- Does the infant appear healthy?
- When awake, does the infant appear alert, wan, irritable?
- What color is the infant's sclera? If yellow, was bilirubin tested prior to discharge?
- When is the infant's follow-up appointment?
- Is the infant's skin clean, without lesions, bruises, or unexplained markings?

Cardiovascular and respiratory assessments include the infant's apical pulse and respiratory rate. If either is elevated, inquire regarding infant's sucking strength, frequency of feedings, and type of cry (absent, weak, vigorous). If assessment indicates possible infection, refer the client and infant for follow-up.

Abdominal assessment determines the amount and frequency of the infant's voidings and the amount and consistency of stool. Assess the abdomen for softness and tenderness.

In a male infant the circumcision site, if present, is assessed for type of discharge and evidence of healing. If circumcision was not done, instruction should be given regarding proper care: Wash external penile skin only, as foreskin of infants and young children cannot be retracted.

Genitalia of a female infant may show a small amount of vaginal blood, which is the result of maternal estrogen in utero.

Home Safety. A hazard-free environment is important. Anticipatory guidance is useful for potential safety problems at different developmental stages of the infant and child. Suggest client not leave infant unattended on bed, table, swing. If client's nails are long, suggest she trim them to keep from scratching or otherwise injuring infant. Suggest to the client, for example, that she tie knots in plastic bags before throwing them away, use child-safety gates, and select toys with no sharp edges or separable, hazardous parts. Keep loose objects from edge of table, sink, or store where a small child can reach up to grab and cause injury.

Child Development. The health care provider should observe nonverbal and verbal cues used by the infant to initiate or stop interaction with the caregiver. An infant's demonstration of disengagement behaviors warrants cessation of caretaking activity and then reassessment of the infant. Evaluate the infant's sleep states (deep or light sleep) and awake states (drowsy, quiet alert, active alert, crying). An infant is most conducive to learning and taking in environmental stimuli when in an active alert state. Point out the infant's engagement and disengagement cues to the mother or care provider.

ENGAGEMENT CUES
- Verbal cues are feeding sounds (sucking) and crying.
- Nonverbal cues are rooting; alerting signs; facial brightening; smooth cyclic movements of the extremities; mutual gaze; feeding posture; brow raising; and facing gaze (infant looks at parent's or caregiver's face).[40]

DISENGAGEMENT CUES
- Verbal cues are spitting; vomiting; hiccoughs; whimpering; crying during caregiving activity; and fussing.
- Nonverbal cues are lip compression; clenching eyes; gaze aversion; yawning; tongue show; increased foot movement; and hand-to-ear movement.[40]

ADJUSTING TO PARENTING

Parenting is a skill that is often learned, to varying degrees of success, by trial and error. Attachment is a process whereby affection develops between infant and parent or caregiver. The process of attachment has been defined as an emotional or affectional commitment to an individual, facilitated by positive interaction between the two and mutually satisfying experiences.[41] Maternal attachment begins during pregnancy as the result of fetal movement and maternal fantasies about an infant.[42,43,44]

A mother's attitudes about pregnancy may influence her feelings about the infant. Maternal grief over the loss of a fantasized perfect child may result in delayed bonding or attachment if, for example, the infant is born prematurely or with obvious birth defects. The infant's behavior can also affect maternal bonding. The infant's crying, avoidance of eye contact, refusal of breast, or withdrawal of a hand when touched is negative reinforcement for a mother.

Nursing Child Assessment Satellite Training tools have been developed to enable the health care provider to identify families that need intervention.[40]

BARNARD MODEL FOR ATTACHMENT AND PARENTING

Adaptation is a result of caregiver-environment-infant interaction. Kathryn Barnard noted that the infant has the tasks to produce clear clues and to respond to the caregiver. If the infant is unable (due to immaturity, illness, or other physical/neurological problems), the adaptive process is interrupted. The mother/caregiver, in turn, cannot respond to the infant's needs, resulting in feelings of maternal inadequacy. Tasks for the mother/caregiver include being able to respond to the infant's cues, to allay distress, and to provide a growth-stimulating environment. Failure interferes with the infant's ability to adapt. The infant, in turn, becomes frustrated, and learns inappropriate interaction behaviors.[40] The environment is also influential. For example, the family is impacted by the actual birth of the child, or social deprivation, or an alternate family style, such as single parenting.

Stress or interference may cause parental insensitivity to an infant's cues, failure of the infant to give reliable cues, and failure of the infant to respond to the parent.

MERCER MODEL FOR ATTACHMENT AND PARENTING

Mercer's definition of attachment—a process affected by positive feedback through mutually enjoyable experiences—stresses "process" (progressive nature, occurring over time), "positive feedback" (social, verbal, nonverbal, real or perceived responses of one partner to another), and "mutually satisfying experience" (environment can have positive or negative impact on the mother-infant interaction).[41]

Four stages of attachment are identified:

- *Anticipatory.* Mother seeks out role model.
- *Formal.* This stage begins with the birth of the child and continues for 6 to 8 weeks; the mother's behaviors are affected primarily by the expectations of others.
- *Informal.* Mother begins to develop her own unique role behavior.
- *Personal.* Mother feels comfortable with role and others accept her role performance.[45,46]

INHIBITORS OF ATTACHMENT

Maternal Factors. Among high risk and low risk women and partners, parental competence is a major predictor of parent-infant attachment.[47] Facilitating parental competence thereby increases parent-infant attachment.[47,48] Parental competence may be defined as the real or perceived ability to care for the physical and psychosocial needs of the infant.

Several factors inhibit attachment and decrease competence.

- Medication, such as narcotics, sedatives, and some forms of anesthesia
- Physical problems from pregnancy, such as long labor, difficult delivery, or chronic illness
- Lack of experience in caring for newborns/older infants
- Learned maternal behaviors that have a negative influence
- A negative self-concept
- Lack of a positive support system
- Grieving a significant loss
- Anticipatory grieving over an imagined loss of infant, resulting from, for example, complicated pregnancy or postnatal problems
- Psychological unpreparedness due to premature birth
- Escape mechanisms, such as alcoholism and drugs[43]

Infant Factors. Several factors may inhibit attachment.

- Neonatal complications in full-term infants
- Infant abnormalities
- Immaturity resulting from premature birth
- Multiple births
- Feeding difficulties[43]

Paternal Factors. A father may exhibit behaviors that inhibit his attachment with the infant.

- Difficulty adjusting to new dependent
- Failure to relate to newborn
- Escape mechanisms, such as alcohol and drugs
- Separation from mother and child because of business or military responsibilities[41]

Hospital Factors. Hospital procedure may inhibit attachment.

- Separation of infant and mother immediately after birth, at night, and for long periods during day
- Policies that discourage or inhibit unwrapping and exploring the infant, limiting mother's caretaking
- Restrictive visiting policies
- Hospital/intensive care environment
- Staff behavior not supportive of mother's caretaking attempts and abilities[43]

PARENTS OF INFANTS WITH MALFORMATIONS

Stages of Adjustment. A wide range of change occurs during adjustment.

- Shock, irrational behavior
- Denial
- Grief/anger/anxiety
- Equilibrium; lessening of anxiety and intense emotional reactions
- Reorganization[49]

Long-Range Impact. Caring for a child with malformation affects all aspects of the parents' lives.

- Financial cost for surgery, medical care for chronic problems, or early stimulation, for example, physical therapy sessions
- Guilt over time spent with affected infant compared with that spent with other child(ren)
- Social support from family and friends having adverse effect on family relationship

Therapeutic Approach. The health care provider should realize that the infant is a complete distortion of the parents' fantasized infant and that a therapeutic approach is necessary to address their feelings.

- Parents must mourn the loss of the fantasized child before they can fully attach to the living "defective" infant.
- Guilt accompanies their mourning.
- Resentment and anger are often directed at health care personnel. Allow parents to express their feelings and take the time necessary to experience the full extent of their grief.
- The demands of the "imperfect" newborn retard mother's attempt to mourn the fantasized child.
- Mourning is asynchronous; that is, progress through the stages of mourning varies for each parent.[49]
- Parents should not be given conflicting information concerning their infant.
- The health care provider may be a role model for parents by responding to the infant with smiles; the infant's positive features should be pointed out to parents.
- Social services may provide financial assistance, and a support group social, interpersonal, or medical support.

- Arrange for home care visit to ensure after discharge care is being implemented.[50]

FAMILY RELATIONSHIPS

The Secundigravida. The concerns of a woman experiencing her second pregnancy are primarily for her other child and the expectation of caring for two children.

- Concern for first child may cause grieving over the dyadic relationship with the first child and her anticipation of the first child's pain.
- Managing the care of two children may cause a mother to feel overwhelmed. She may have increased expectations of the first child and may doubt her own ability to love two children equally.
- Assist the parents in developing confidence in parenting skills through parenting classes that include information about infant and child behavior, home visits, and telephone calls.
- The second pregnancy may not be as exciting or as desired as the first. The mother may not be totally engrossed in mothering her second baby as she was with the first. She may feel sad or guilty.
- Maternal self-perception changes[51,52] and she sees herself as experienced. She recognizes her needs as separate from those of her role as mother.

Readjustment with the Infant's Father. A negative effect of childbirth may be the breakup of the marriage or relationship. The mother may lack support in child care and household tasks. Spouse abuse or child abuse may increase. In assessing the couple, focus on their sharing of tasks, sexual relationship, leisure activity, and financial management.

- Sharing of family tasks and responsibilities often occurs following agreement before childbirth on the division of tasks. Equal sharing of child and infant care may be agreed on, or the parents may prefer that the father be primary caregiver for the older child or children. Other parents may prefer that the father assume more household tasks and the mother have the responsibility for infant and children.

- Assess the parenting roles of the mother and father. Assess their self-expectations and their expectations of each other. Parenting behavior can be adaptive (constructive) or maladaptive (nonconstructive, harmful). A recent study looked at fathers' parenting attitudes during the first year of their child's life. Findings revealed a lack of knowledge of behavior of 3-month old infants and a strong belief in corporal punishment.[53] The health care provider may need to identify normal infant and child behaviors and developmental tasks to the parent or caregiver. Alternative forms of discipline for an older child (e.g., "time out") may need to be discussed. Refer parent or caregiver to parenting classes through, for example, churches or March of Dimes.
- The sexual relationship may be safely resumed 2 weeks postpartum.[54] Physiological responses in the puerperium may cause a decrease in the intensity of the sexual experience. The decrease is due to thin vaginal walls in the hypoestrogenic state, especially during lactation; delayed congestion of the labia majora and minora until the plateau phase, and decreased strength of orgasmic contractions. Sexual activity is decreased because of fatigue, weakness, vaginal discharge or spotting, perineal pain, tight or lax vaginal muscles, breast discomfort, and decreased vaginal lubrication. Client teaching may include suggestions to enhance sexual comfort and "safer sex" behaviors and precautions.
  - Saliva (after postpartum exam) or water-soluble gel (Astroglide®, Replens®, K-Y jelly®) may be used for lubrication.
  - Lubricated condoms may provide comfort.
  - The female-superior or side-to-side positions may help control the depth of thrusting.
  - Gentle rotation of two fingers around the vagina may aid vaginal relaxation.
  - Other displays of affection (holding, cuddling) are pleasurable if intercourse is not desired.
  - The woman may assist partner to orgasm with masturbation or fellatio. Her partner may help her also achieve orgasm without intercourse.
  - The client should perform Kegel exercises to regain vaginal tone.

- A nutritious diet will promote healing and a sense of well-being.
- Leisure time for the couple should include time alone. They may enlist the help of family and friends to watch the infant and children. Encourage communication between the couple ("I love you," "You are special to me," "Thanks for your help"). Simple gestures of affection (romantic card or flowers for him or her) provoke loving feelings.
- Management of finances may require referral to a community food bank, social services, or the Women, Infants, and Children Program (WIC).

Single Parent/Working Mother. Address the parent's child-rearing difficulties, financial insecurity, role conflict, or social isolation.

- Encourage the parent to verbalize feelings on how absence of one parent may affect parent-infant relationship or child development.
- Identify for the working mother the positive aspects of separation (daily break from infant and child care while at work).
- Stress the importance of quality rather than quantity of time spent with the infant and children.
- Assist the parent in developing confidence in parenting skills through parenting classes that include information about infant behavior, home visits, and telephone calls.
- Encourage inexpensive activities that are relaxing and enjoyable for parent and infant.
- Financial insecurity may benefit from referral to community food bank, social or legal services, or WIC. In addition, referral for housing or job training may be necessary.

A parent experiencing role conflict and uncertainty concerning responsibilities may benefit from assistance in establishing priorities and assigning appropriate tasks to older children. Referral to appropriate resources may also be necessary to develop essential skills in caretaking and home management.

Social isolation and loneliness may be eased by client's involvement in parental and social groups (apartment complex, church, extended family) and support groups (see list of Support Groups at the end of this chapter).

Lesbian Families. Such families may include legal guardian relationships, working collectives, roommates, ex-lovers now considered family members, and couples with or without children.[55]

The health care provider should be knowledgeable regarding lesbian issues and health care concerns, comfortable providing health care to the gay population, and supportive of the lesbian family.[56]

Lesbian concerns range from unique to common:

- Fear of custody battles require referral for legal advice on custody, because a nonbiological lesbian parent may not have a legal right to parent a child if the biological parent, her partner, dies.[55,57]
- Fear of HIV infection is possible. An alternative insemination/unscreened donor may have been used for conception. One partner may use intravenous drugs or may have intercourse with men. The mother may receive fluid (vaginal fluid, menstrual blood) from an HIV-infected partner. One means of exchanging fluid is sharing a dildo without using a condom.[58] If HIV infection is a concern, counsel women regarding safer sex (see Chapter 11).
- Battering—physical, emotional, or verbal—is possible. (See page 671 for assessment tool for abuse.) Refer the woman for counseling, to a shelter, or to a support group. The woman may decide not to provide information on abuse if she is lesbian, as her sexual preference may then be included as part of her medical record and thus be subject to review by future insurers, physicians, and nurses.
- Alcoholism affects lesbian relationships and families as it does heterosexual relationships and families.
- Support may be lost from family and friends and her job.[55,58]

A role model should be available to assist with maternal tasks.

- Determine the coparent's involvement in infant care and with partner.
- Encourage the partner's role in parenting.
- Encourage the partner's presence during health care visits.
- Referral to appropriate support groups may be helpful.

Families with Human Immunodeficiency Virus Infection. HIV-infected families are those families in which one or more persons are infected with the virus. Persons may be asymptomatic carriers or exhibit AIDS, having been diagnosed with opportunistic infections and malignancies. The epidemiology of AIDS is described in Chapter 11.

The health care provider must maintain a nonjudgmental attitude and should not assume heterosexuality. Do not record the client's sexual preference in her records without her permission. Offer nonheterosexual educational materials and, if necessary, educate yourself about lesbian lifestyles. Review availability of HIV testing if the client expresses concern. Identify what the family sees as its needs; many HIV-infected families are living in unsanitary, crowded, and physically hazardous environments and may not be enrolled in basic public assistance programs. Establish a trusting relationship; be aware of family member attempts to manipulate.

Teach clients about infection control, such as hand washing, avoiding exchange of body fluids or sharing of razors and toothbrushes, wrapping soiled peripads in sturdy plastic containers, and cleaning soiled surfaces with a dilute bleach solution of 1 part bleach to 10 parts water. Review safer sex practices with clients.

Advise clients to contact the health care provider should they note signs of infection: fever, foul smell of lochia, excessive amount of bleeding, return of bright red bleeding. Clients should also contact the health care provider if there are signs of worsening HIV infection: fatigue, anorexia, weight loss, sore throat, cough, dermatologic disorders, or unusual vaginal discharge. The infant's health care provider should be contacted if the infant exhibits fever, poor feeding, oral thrush, diarrhea, cough, or flulike symptoms.

Instruct the client on how to avoid other infection, for example, not ingesting raw meat or eggs to avoid *Salmonella* infection, not emptying cat litter to avoid the risk of toxoplasmosis, not sharing needles, and discontinuing substance abuse, including tobacco and alcohol.[59,60]

Families with Domestic Violence. More than 2.5 million women experience some form of violence each year.[61] Physical abuse during pregnancy ranges from 8–17 percent.[61] Child abuse often coexists or increases with spouse abuse.[62] Family violence is a major factor contributing to poverty and homelessness of women.[63]

Make an assessment for evidence of domestic violence, using Abuse Assessment Screen:[64]

- Have you ever been emotionally or physically abused by your partner or someone important to you?
- Within the last year, have you been hit, slapped, kicked, or otherwise physically hurt by someone?
- Since you've been pregnant, were you hit, slapped, kicked, or otherwise physically hurt by someone? If yes, by whom? Total number of times.
- Were you ever forced to have sexual activities? If yes, by whom? Total number of times.
- Are you afraid of your partner or anyone you listed above?

It is also imperative to screen for child abuse. Parents who were abused as children are six times more likely to abuse their children.[65] Kemper[65] states the following screening questions are asked at her clinic: As a child,

1. How often did your parents ridicule you in front of friends or family?
   Frequently   Often   Occasionally
   Rarely   Never
2. How often were you hit with an object such as a hairbrush, board, stick, wire, or cord?
   Frequently   Often   Occasionally
   Rarely   Never
3. How often were you thrown against walls or down stairs?
   Frequently   Often   Occasionally
   Rarely   Never
4. Did your parents ever hurt you when they were out of control?
   Yes   No
5. Do you feel you were physically abused?
   Yes   No
6. Do you feel you were neglected?
   Yes   No
7. Do you feel you were hurt in a sexual way?
   Yes   No
8. Would you like more information about free parenting programs, parent hotlines, or respite care?
   Yes   No

Once abuse has been identified, assess the potential for danger for the client. An increase in the severity or frequency of abuse, attempts at choking the woman by her partner, threats or attempts on her part to commit suicide, attempts or threats on his part to commit suicide are some indicators that the client is in danger and consideration for her safety must be undertaken. She should be encouraged to think of a safety plan that may include the following:

- Hiding money
- Hiding extra set of house or car keys
- Set up a code with family/friends
- Ask neighbor to call police if violence begins
- Remove weapons
- Have available social security numbers (his, client's, childrens'), rent and utility receipts, birth certificates (client's and childrens'), driver's license, bank account numbers, insurance policies and numbers, marriage license, valuable jewelry, important phone numbers.[66]

Offer information on available shelters, legal and criminal assistance.

When child abuse screenings are positive, it is important to follow up with open ended questions or statements. Ask the parent how the family might best address the issue. Acknowledge the individual's courage in facing and identifying problems, as well as the family's strengths. Follow-up with the family is essential.

Child or spouse abuse should be considered when a child or adult presents with an injury or symptom that is not consistent with the clinical evidence, illogical or changing explanations for an injury are given by the parent, or when there is concomitant abuse of the child's mother.[67] Individuals should be interviewed separately to provide privacy and convey a sense of respect for the person as an individual.

Empowering strategies to use for the survivor of abuse include acknowledging the abuse, listening, avoiding blame, exploring options, and making referrals.[68]

Homeless Families. More than two thirds of homeless families are headed by single women.[46] Approximately one third of homeless people are women.[69] Their education most likely does not exceed high school.

Health issues for homeless families are staggering.

- Social isolation
- Lack of access to health care
- Physical violence on the streets and in shelters
- Spouse abuse, child abuse, or both
- Substance abuse
- Chronic health problems
- Obesity
- Inadequate diet: insufficient iron, folic acid, calcium; excessive intake of saturated fats[70,71,72]
- Parasites
- Infectious diseases
- Exposure to the elements

Arrange for nursery services so that the client may attend classes in parenting skills and learn about infant behavioral cues. Identify and prevent family violence with counseling or referral. Identify and teach basic foot care: keep feet clean and dry; use proper technique for cutting toe nails; use appropriate footwear; wear clean dry socks.[63] Evaluation and care are provided at times and locations convenient to the population to be served. Assist in providing nutritional information to volunteers at "soup kitchens." Refer families to community resources for lodging and job training. WIC, substance abuse programs, and domestic violence programs may also be suggested.

Discipline and Parenting Skills in Families. Parenting involves caring for your children physically and emotionally in a loving manner so that they are able to become responsible, caring adults. Parenting is not an innate behavior but a learned art. For some, parenting is learned from one's own parents. One may then decide which parenting behaviors to keep and which ones to avoid. At best, this may stimulate a new parent to learn alternative parenting styles by attending parenting classes. At worst, a new parent stays with the parenting style he/she was exposed to and may have unrealistic behavior expectations of his/her child. Developing a sense of self-esteem and self-worth in the child is enhanced by discipline, provided that the discipline is supportive and develops problem solving skills.[73] Yet many parents attempt to accomplish this task with little knowledge of normal developmental stages of infants and children leading to unrealistic expectations.

Brazelton defines discipline as "teaching," not punishment.[74] Brazelton states that children sense a need for discipline, and toward the end of the second year, will make this need known by obvious testing. He further states that self-discipline, which is the goal of discipline, comes in three stages: trying out limits, teasing to elicit a response from others as to what is and is not allowed, and internalizing these previously unknown boundaries.[74]

Problem solving is one way to discipline by allowing parents and child to work together to reach a decision.[75] Spanking and hitting are not constructive forms of discipline, are demeaning to children, and may inhibit the development of a guilty conscience.[75] Brazelton gives the following guidelines for discipline:[74]

- Respect a child's stage of development
- Fit the discipline to the child's stage of development
- Discipline must fit the child
- When your child is with other children, try not to hover
- Model behaviors for the child
- After the discipline is over, help her explain what it's all about
- Use a time-out, but for a brief period only
- Ask the child's advice about what might help next time
- Physical punishment has very real disadvantages
- Watch out for mixed messages (e.g., telling a child "Don't do that" when you really aren't sure or don't mean it)
- Stop and reevaluate whenever discipline doesn't work
- Pick up the child to love her afterward
- Remember to reinforce the child when he isn't teasing you by commenting on how well he is controlling himself

Brazelton lists behaviors exhibited by children when parents are too strict. The following behaviors should warrant closer observation of the child and family and may require intervention:

- A child who is too good or too quiet, or who doesn't dare express negative feelings
- A child who is too sensitive to even mild criticism

- A child who doesn't test you in age appropriate ways
- A child without a sense of humor and joy in life
- A child who is irritable or anxious most of the time
- A child who shows symptoms of pressure in other areas—feeding, sleeping, or toileting—and who may regress to an earlier kind of behavior, acting like a baby or a much smaller child.[74]

PLAN

The plan to assist families in their adjustment to parenting should offer many alternatives to address the multitude of needs.

- *Practical Guidance.* This can include the simple suggestion to lay out clothes at night for the next day to decrease tension in the morning while dressing the infant and older child (children) for day care or school.
- *Child Development and Behavior.* Teaching a client about child development enables her to better understand older children and the new infant; counseling should address infant's cues and states.
- *Referral.* Individual counseling may be necessary for a client who feels excessively guilty or angry about her first child's reactions to the infant. After counseling the client regarding daily nutritional needs of adults, infants, and children, referral for specific dietary needs may be helpful. Refer the client for legal assistance and domestic violence counseling and assistance if appropriate (see Parenting/Family Support Groups at end of chapter).

PSYCHIATRIC DISTURBANCES

Psychiatric disturbances occur during the puerperium. The disturbances are classified on the basis of their severity:

- *Maternity Blues or "Baby Blues."* Transient, emotional disturbances commonly occurring around the second or fourth postpartum day, lasting from a few hours to 2 weeks.

- *Postpartum Depression.** Characterized by lowered mood, irritability, fatigue, feelings of worthlessness, sleeping and eating changes, and subtle changes of personality.
- *Postpartum Psychosis.** Severely impaired ability to perform daily living tasks.[76]

Epidemiology

Etiology and Risk Factors. Schaper, Rooney, et al. administered the Edinburgh Postnatal Depression Scale (Table 20–3) to 1139 women in an attempt to determine the extent of postpartum depression as well as to identify risk factors. Factors that were statistically significant were marital status (separated, divorced, widowed), marital instability, lack of medical insurance, and a history of depression.[77] This confirms some of the risk factors identified by Boyer (see Table 20–4).

MATERNITY BLUES. Maternity blues are the mildest form of depression and are usually self-limiting. They begin on the second or third postpartum day and last up to 14 days.

Psychological factors are rapid hormonal changes (decreased estrogen, human placental lactogen, progesterone, human chorionic gonadotropin, plasma renin, aldosterone);[76,78] lack of sleep and less effective sleep; and increased energy expenditure. Psychological factors include the conflict caused by cultural expectations to bear children and pursue personal goals and the economic cost of childbearing and childrearing.

POSTPARTUM DEPRESSION. Postpartum depression has a slow, insidious onset over several weeks postpartum. It usually begins within 2 or 3 weeks postpartum and may last up to a year. There is no definite etiology.

Physiological Factors. Although the etiology of postpartum depression includes hormonal, neurotransmitter, genetic, and psychological factors,[79] the exact etiology remains unclear.[78,80] Risk factors for development of postpartum depression include the presence of anxiety or depression during pregnancy, family history of depression, increased marital conflict and/or dissatisfaction,

---

*Conditions are prolonged beyond usual period expected for "blues."

TABLE 20–3. EDINBURGH POSTNATAL DEPRESSION SCALE (EPDS)

Name:

Address:

Baby's age:

As you have recently had a baby, we would like to know how you are feeling. Please **<u>underline</u>** the answer which comes closest to how you have felt **in the past 7 days,** not just how you feel today. In the past 7 days:

*1. I have been able to laugh and see the funny side of things.
    As much as I always could
    Not quite so much now
    Definitely not so much now
    Not at all

2. I have looked forward with enjoyment to things.
    As much as I ever did
    Rather less than I used to
    Definitely less than I used to
    Hardly at all

*3. I have blamed myself unnecessarily when things went wrong.
    Yes, most of the time
    Yes, some of the time
    Not very often
    No, never

4. I have been anxious or worried for no good reason.
    No, not at all
    Hardly ever
    Yes, sometimes
    Yes, very often

*5. I have felt scared or panicky for no very good reason.
    Yes, quite a lot
    Yes, sometimes
    No, not much
    No, not at all

*6. Things have been getting on top of me.
    Yes, most of the time I haven't been able to cope at all
    Yes, sometimes I haven't been coping as well as usual
    No, most of the time I have coped quite well
    No, I have been coping as well as ever

*7. I have been so unhappy that I have had difficulty sleeping.
    Yes, most of the time
    Yes, some of the time
    Not very often
    No, not at all

*8. I have felt sad or miserable.
    Yes, most of the time
    Yes, quite often
    Not very often
    No, not at all

*9. I have been so unhappy that I have been crying.
    Yes, most of the time
    Yes, quite often
    Only occasionally
    No, never

*10. The thought of harming myself has occurred to me.
    Yes, quite often
    Sometimes
    Hardly ever
    Never

Response categories are scored 0, 1, 2, and 3 according to increased severity of the symptom. Items marked with an asterisk are reverse scored (i.e., 3, 2, 1 and 0). The total score is calculated by adding together the scores for each of the ten items. Users may reproduce the scale without further permission providing they respect copyright (which remains with the *British Journal of Psychiatry*) by quoting the names of the authors, the title and the source of the paper in all reproduced copies.

From J. L. Cox, J. M. Holden, R. Sagovsky (1987), Detection of Postnatal Depression: development of the 10-item Edinburgh Postnatal Depression Scale. British Journal of Psychiatry, 150, *786. Copyright 1987 by the British Journal of Psychiatry. Reprinted by permission.*

low levels of social and partner support.[80,81,82] Studies indicate that postpartum adolescents have significantly lower rates of depression if the adolescent receives support from her mother and the infant's father.[82,83] They, as did adult mothers with depression, reported more negative feeding interactions with their infants and reported less confidence in their mothering skills than adolescents without depressive symptoms.[83]

POSTPARTUM PSYCHOSIS. Postpartum psychosis has its onset within a few weeks or, at most, 3 months postpartum; the affected woman is 16 to 20 times more likely to require hospital admission in the 3 months postpartum than in an equivalent period preconceptionally. Primiparas are at greatest risk. The symptomatology may resemble that of maternity blues.[79]

Physiological factors are theorized; there is no definite etiology. Theories involve hormonal, neurotransmitter, and genetic factors. Psychological factors reflect no definite etiology; the primary risk factor seems to be a history of manic-depressive psychosis or unipolar disorder with psychotic features.[80,81]

Incidence. Incidence varies among the three classifications. Maternity blues affect 50 to 70 per-

TABLE 20–4. RISK FACTORS FOR POSTPARTUM DEPRESSION

1. Woman feels increased anxiety/worry during this pregnancy.
2. Woman has history of perimenstrual mood swings.
3. Woman has history of depression following previous pregnancy.
4. Woman does not feel in control of life.
5. Woman perceives self as nervous person or a worrier.
6. Woman believes she has lack of family or friends she can call for support.
7. Woman expresses feelings of depression or sadness with this pregnancy.
8. Woman regrets she is pregnant and feels child unwanted.
9. Woman had unhappy childhood.
10. Woman has financial/housing/personal problems.
11. Woman has history of emotional problems.
12. Woman was previously treated for mental illness.
13. Woman feels anger at life situation or at family or acquaintances.
14. Woman blames self when things go wrong.
15. Woman feels unloved by infant's father.

Note: Preliminary research done by D. Boyer suggests that women with three to six risk factors are at risk for postpartum depression, and women with more than six risk factors are at high risk.

From D. Boyer (1990). Prediction of postpartum depression. In 1990, NAACOG's Clinical Issues in Perinatal and Women's Health Nursing, 1 (3), 364. Copyright 1990 by NAACOG. Adapted by permission.

cent of postpartum women. Postpartum depression affects 10 to 15 percent of women during the first 3 months postpartum; 25 percent of these women are likely to develop chronic, severe depression.[80,84] Postpartum psychosis affects 1 to 2 per 1000 new mothers.[80]

Subjective Data

Current Symptoms. Symptoms may be similar among the three classifications; however, distinct differences are reported by clients. It is important to identify the major problems causing the client to seek help: severe mood swings, hyperactivity, irritability, depression, obsessional thoughts, insomnia, lack of appetite, difficulty with concentration, hallucinations, delusion, inability to care for herself or child, suicidal or homicidal thoughts.

MATERNITY BLUES. Women with maternity blues report weeping, often alternating with periods of elation; irritability; anxiety; headaches; confusion; forgetfulness; depersonalization; disturbances in sleep pattern; and fatigue.[78,81]

POSTPARTUM DEPRESSION. Women with postpartum depression report symptoms similar to those of maternity blues but without periods of elation. In addition, these symptoms are more intense and last longer. The client considers herself a failure as a mother; she looks for reasons for the perceived failure and associates it with real or imagined character weaknesses and questions self-worth. She experiences excessive fatigue and excessive weight gain or weight loss. Thinking and speaking may be slow. Suicide is a serious hazard and the method is often well planned.[78,80]

POSTPARTUM PSYCHOSIS. Women with postpartum psychosis report variable symptoms. Three expressions, or phases, of psychosis are possible: manic phase, delirious state, and psychotic depression.

- Manic phase, with symptoms similar to those of the manic phase of bipolar disorder is characterized by racing thoughts, hyperactivity, and mood swings.
- Delirious state symptoms include confusion, dissociative episodes with confusion, dissociative episodes with hostility, and anxiety.
- Psychotic depression symptoms include suicidal tendencies, desire to harm the infant or others, psychomotor retardation, and prominent delusions that are often related to the infant.[76,80]

History of Present Illness. Ask the client to describe the onset of symptoms. What symptoms were present during pregnancy or after the infant's birth? When were symptoms more severe or less severe, and how long did they last? Have symptoms caused her to make unexpected changes in lifestyle?

Past Psychiatric Condition. Ask the client if she has a history of depression, bipolar disorder or other psychiatric illness. Were any of the illnesses related to childbearing? Did she receive any psychotropic medication? Did the medication help?

Medical-Surgical-Obstetrical History. Was the pregnancy planned or unplanned? Were there complications with this pregnancy? Have the client describe her labor and delivery. Does she have a history of medical illness (thyroid disease, other endocrinological problems)? Did the newborn have any serious health problem?

Family History. Does any family member have psychiatric problems (depression, bipolar disorder, schizophrenia, alcoholism or other substance abuse, anorexia nervosa, bulimia)? What type of help was received? Was medication received and what was the response? What was the client's childhood like? Ask her to describe her relationship with parents and her perceptions of their effectiveness as role models. Is there a history of physical or sexual abuse?

Social History. With whom does the client live? Is there someone with whom she can share the responsibility of caring for the child and house? Are there financial problems? Is she planning to work full- or part-time outside the home or full-time in the home? Is her partner emotionally supportive?

Objective Data

Physical Examination. Excessive weight loss or gain is possible. Affect may be flat; speech and thinking processes may be slow; the woman may be weepy, agitated, or irritable. She may exhibit confusion, hostility, or anxiety. The remainder of the physical examination is most likely within normal limits.

Edinburgh Postnatal Depression Scale. The Edinburgh Postnatal Depression Scale (EDPS) is employed in determining objective data (see Table 20–4). The scale has a higher sensitivity (95 percent) than the Beck Depression Inventory (68 percent)[85] and is used to detect major postpartum depression and changes in the severity of depression. It can also be used to monitor the effectiveness of treatment. The scale has been administered 6 weeks postpartum, but recent study showed significant positive correlation between EPDS scores at 5 days and 6 weeks.[86]

Ask the client to complete the scale alone, without other family members present. She should underline those responses that come closest to how she felt during the previous 7 days; she should answer all 10 items. A score of 12/13 indicates the likelihood of depression, but not its severity. Have the client verbalize her feelings by responding to open ended questions.

Differential Medical Diagnoses

Maternity blues, postpartum depression, postpartum psychosis.

Plan

Psychosocial Intervention. During the antepartum period, provide the client with information related to maternal changes that could occur after birth: mood swings and lifestyle changes. Suggestions should include coping strategies related to the birth:

- Get plenty of rest.
- Allow family and friends, if available, to help with household tasks and the care for older children.
- Eat a well-balanced diet that is low in salt and sugar and high in complex carbohydrates, protein, and green leafy vegetables.
- Drink plenty of fluids, especially water, and limit caffeine intake.
- Continue prenatal vitamins.
- Perform light exercise daily.
- Ensure some personal time and adult relationships.
- Avail oneself of support groups and other community resources (see Breastfeeding/ Information Support Groups at the end of this chapter).

Medication Interventions. It is imperative that postpartum women be screened and treated for postpartum depression so they can function in their role as mother, providing the love so necessary in an infant's and child's life. Beck analyzed 19 studies on postpartum depression published between 1983–1993. Beck found that postpartum depression has a significant effect on mother-infant interaction.[87]

Antidepressants are most useful in women with pronounced vegetative signs of depression: fatigue, poor concentration, hopeless and helpless feelings, irritability, suicidal thoughts, no appetite. Medication should be continued for 9–12 months after remission of symptoms.[80,81] Conditions requiring prompt psychiatric referral include suicidal and/or homicidal ideation, evidence or concern of psychotic symptoms, severe impairment of functional capabilities, avoidance of infant or overconcern of infant's health, failure to respond to therapeutic trial of antidepressants, and comorbid substance abuse.[81] Lithium, an antimanic, or carbamazepine, an anticonvulsant, are used to manage manic episodes. Antipsychotic drugs may be prescribed for women with postpartum psychoses who are experiencing hallucinations or other distortions of reality.

TRICYCLIC ANTIDEPRESSANTS. Tricyclic antidepressant administration is begun after physician consultation and referral. More sedating tricyclic antidepressants, such as doxepine (Sinequan), trazodone (Desyril), and imipramine (Tofranil) are useful for women with insomnia, agitation, and anxiety attacks.[76]

Doxepin and Trazodone are Category C drugs, and the American Academy of Pediatrics states that the effect on a nursing infant are unknown but may be of concern.[88] Imipramine is a Category D drug during pregnancy, and the American Academy of Pediatrics classifies it as an agent whose effect on the nursing infant is unknown but may be of concern.[88] Less sedating tricyclic antidepressants, such as desipramine (Norpramine) and protriptyline (Vivactyl) are more useful for clients with severe fatigue, difficulty waking up in the morning, or concern they may not hear their infant cry if they are too sedated.[76] Desipramine is a Category C drug, and the American Academy of Pediatrics lists it as an agent whose effect on the nursing infant is unknown but may be of concern.[88] While Protriptyline is also listed as a Category C drug, no data are available regarding the safety of use during lactation.[88]

- *Administration.* Initially, 25 mg per day, increasing by 25 mg in divided doses every other day as tolerated until a therapeutic range is reached. Blood levels must be drawn to determine the therapeutic range. The dosage range for doxepin, imipramine, and desipramine is 150 to 200 mg per day.[76]
- *Side Effects.* Oversedation, dry mouth, constipation.
- *Contraindications.* Hypersensitivity to tricyclic antidepressants, urinary retention, narrow-angle glaucoma. Concomitant use of a tricyclic antidepressant and a monoamine oxidase (MAO) inhibitor can lead to severe hypertension from excessive adrenergic stimulation of the heart and blood vessels. Tricyclics potentiate activity of direct-acting sympathomimetic and anticholinergic drugs and decrease response to indirect-acting sympathomimetic drugs.
- *Anticipated Outcome on Evaluation.* Remission of symptoms of depression.
- *Client Teaching.* Include information on relieving side effects. If the client feels oversedated, the dosage can be increased more slowly and the majority of dose taken at night. Dry mouth can be moistened by chewing gum or sucking lemon drops. Constipation can be relieved by drinking more fluids and eating more fiber. Psyllium laxatives, such as Metamucil, are also helpful. Advise clients that there is a 2- to 3-week lag time before depression clinically improves.

SEROTONIN REUPTAKE INHIBITORS. Selective serotonin reuptake inhibitors are also indicated to treat depression. They have fewer and less noticeable side effects and a wider margin of safety. Fluoxetine (Prozac) is administered initially, 20 mg in the morning with dosage increased according to response; it may be given in divided doses in the morning and at noon. The dosage should not exceed 80 mg per day.

Sertraline (Zoloft) administration begins at 50 mg orally daily. As the therapeutic response may take 2–4 weeks, dosage adjustments can be made after that time frame. The dosage range is 50 to 200 mg daily.

Paroxetine (Paxil) administration begins at 20 mg orally daily. Dosage may be increased in 10-mg increments up to a maximum of 50 mg daily.

All three medications are listed as Category B drugs in pregnancy, but the American Academy of Pediatrics classifies them as agents whose effects on the nursing infant are unknown but may be of concern.[88]

- *Side Effects.* Nervousness, anxiety, insomnia, headache, somnolence, tremor, nausea, vomiting, dry mouth, arrhythmias, dyspepsia, weight loss, rash pruritus, urticaria. Selective serotonin uptake inhibitors may prolong the half-life of diazepam. Use with tryptophan can cause agitation, gastrointestinal distress, and restlessness. Avoid use with tricyclic antidepressants because of the increased adverse effects on the central nervous system. Interaction with warfarin or other highly protein-bound drugs can increase serum level. Advise the client of the 2–4 week lag before clinical improvement of depression.
- *Contraindications.* Hypersensitivity to any of the selective serotonin re-uptake inhibitors. In addition, the drug should not be used within 14 days of cessation of MAO inhibitors. Cimetidine may increase the plasma concentration of paroxetine.

- *Anticipated Outcome on Evaluation.* Remission of symptoms of depression.
- *Client Teaching.* Include information about side effects.

TETRACYCLIC. (Remeron) Is an antidepressant recently released. It is an antagonist of 5-Ht2 and 5-Ht3 receptors, as well as H1 receptors.

It is a Category C drug for pregnancy, and it is unknown if mirtazapine is excreted in breast milk.

- *Administration.* 15 mg at bedtime, adjustments to dosing should not be made before 1–2 weeks of therapy. Usual dosage range is 15–45 mg daily.
- *Side Effects.* Somnalence, increased appetite and weight gain, dry mouth, constipation, dizziness. It can cause agranulocytosis, and can cause an additive effect if taken with alcohol and CNS depressants. It should be used with caution in clients with kidney and liver impairment or a history of seizures, or if antihypertensives are used.
- *Contraindications.* Concomitant use of MAO inhibitors, alcohol, diazepam or other CNS depressants.
- *Anticipated Outcome on Evaluation.* Abatement of depression.
- *Client Teaching.* Include information concerning side effects and contraindications.

LITHIUM. Lithium is indicated if antidepressant treatment precipitates a manic episode, with symptoms of racing thoughts, hyperactivity, pressured speech, increased energy, and impulsive behavior.[76] Discontinue use of antidepressant if manic episodes occur, and begin lithium. Long-term use of lithium can induce goiter and has been associated with degenerative renal changes. Therefore, baseline thyroid function tests (T_3, T_4, thyroid stimulating hormone) and renal function tests (BUN, creatinine) should be obtained as a baseline. Thyroid stimulating hormone and renal function tests should then be done every 6 months. Lithium is a Category D drug for use during pregnancy, and the American Academy of Pediatrics considers lithium to be contraindicated during breastfeeding because of the potential for lithium induced toxicity in the breastfeeding infant.[88]

- *Administration.* Therapeutic range: 0.5 to 1.0 mEq/L; higher levels can produce toxicity (nausea, vomiting, diarrhea, shakiness) and extremely high levels can produce death. Subther-

apeutic levels do not provide an adequate clinical response.[76] Serum values should be drawn weekly, then every 2 to 3 months. Lithium is the drug of choice for clients with postpartum psychosis with manic features.

- *Side Effects.* Nausea, vomiting, diarrhea, thirst, polyuria, lethargy, slurred speech, muscle weakness, fine hand tremor. When administered above the therapeutic range, lithium may cause headache, persistent gastrointestinal upset, confusion, hyperirritability, drowsiness, dizziness, tremors, ataxia, dry mouth, hypotension, rash, and pruritus.
- *Contraindications.* Hepatic disease, renal disease, pregnancy, lactation, severe cardiac disease.
- *Anticipated Outcome on Evaluation.* The abatement of manic symptoms.
- *Client Teaching.* Include information related to side effects.

CARBAMAZEPINE. Carbamezepine (Tegretol) can be used by clients who cannot tolerate or who do not respond well to lithium. Because carbamazepine has been associated with the development of potentially fatal blood cell abnormalities (leukopenia, thrombocytopenia, agranulocytosis, aplastic anemia), a baseline complete blood cell count should be obtained followed by complete blood counts every four weeks.

Carbamazepine is a Category C drug, and although it is excreted into breast milk, the amount is low and accumulation does not seem to occur. The American Academy of Pediatrics considers its use to be compatible with breastfeeding.[88]

- *Indications.* Seizure disorders, trigeminal and glossopharyngeal neuralgias, bipolar disorder.
- *Administration.* Initially 200 mg orally per day, gradually increasing by 200 mg per day in divided doses. Optimal dosage is 600 to 1800 mg per day. The serum therapeutic level is 4 to 12 µg/mL.[76]
- *Side Effects.* Sedation, ataxia, nausea, and vomiting. Carbamazepine accelerates the metabolism of oral contraceptives and coumadin-type anticoagulants.
- *Contraindications.* Hypersensitivity to carbamazepine or tricyclic antidepressants, bone marrow depression, and concomitant use of MAO inhibitors.
- *Anticipated Outcome on Evaluation.* Abatement of manic behaviors.

- *Client Teaching.* Include information concerning side effects and contraindications.

ANTIPSYCHOTIC DRUGS. Antipsychotic drugs such as trifluoperazine (Stelazine), haloperidol (Haldol), and thioridazine (Mellaril) are also prescribed. See the current *Physicians' Desk Reference* (PDR) or a pharmacotherapeutic resource for detailed information. Psychiatric referral is mandatory.

Follow-Up

Postpartum depression poses serious sequelae for mother, infant, and family during the first postnatal year. Depressed mothers may not pick up on their infants' cues, thus failing to meet their infants' needs.[87]

Use of appropriate medication to alter mother's mood and enhance her sensitivity to her infant's cues will help strengthen the bond between the mother-infant dyad. Home visits, telephone calls, and psychiatric referral may be part of follow-up care.

Consider telephone calls 3 days after hospital discharge and a home visit 7 days after discharge to assess the client's adaptation to motherhood and family responsibilities. If she is adapting well, repeat contact after another 7 to 10 days. On the other hand, if she is experiencing difficulty, refer her to appropriate agencies or support groups (see Breastfeeding Information/Support Groups at the end of this chapter).

- Cognitive and supportive therapies help identify and correct distorted perceptions of reality and encourage the partner or other family member(s) to assist with household and child care tasks.
- Concurrent marital therapy, in conjoint sessions, is especially helpful if the partner exhibits narcissistic behavior or is a substance abuser.[76]
- Support groups (group therapy) complement individual therapy. They help decrease the sense of isolation.
- Hospitalization should include admission of both mother and infant.[84]

PERINATAL LOSS

Perinatal loss involves perinatal mortality, both stillbirth and neonatal death.[89] A perinatal loss may also involve a perceived loss, including loss of expectation or giving one's infant up for adoption.

Stillbirth or neonatal death (death within the first 30 days of life) is obviously a loss for the mother and the family. Less obvious may be the loss felt by a woman who miscarries or elects to terminate a pregnancy. All of these losses are irrevocable.

Loss of expectation is also a real loss for some women and their families. It may be experienced in the birth of a viable infant who is premature or has congenital anomalies or deformities. Loss of expectation may also be experienced when the birthing act causes losses that precipitate maternity blues even though the infant is healthy. For example, postpartum fatigue may make daily tasks difficult to perform and contribute to postpartum blues or depression.

The woman or couple who gives up an infant for adoption experience loss, especially if they bonded with the infant before birth. Giving up the infant does not eliminate these bonds.[90]

Epidemiology

In 1990 the United States ranked 17th among other nations in infant mortality, with a rate of 10.4 per 1000 live births.[91] Despite a decline in infant mortality to 7.9 per 1000 live births, the United States slipped to 18th place among world nations in 1995.[92] Low birthweight infants are 5–10 times more likely to die during their first year of life than infants of normal weight.[93] The infant mortality rate for African Americans (16.8 per 1000 live births) remains at twice that of white infants (6.9 per 1000 live births).[93]

Out of 3.3 million babies born alive in the United States, 30,000 die during the first 28 days of life from genetic disease and congenital malformations; they constitute 10 percent of total neonatal deaths.[94,95] Approximately 33 percent of stillbirths have a congenital defect.[95] Miscarriages occur in approximately 43 percent of pregnancies; approximately 50 percent are caused by chromosomal anomalies.[96]

Subjective Data

A client may report sadness, loss of appetite, inability to sleep, increased irritability or hostility toward others, preoccupation with the lost infant, inability to return to normal activities, and somatic distress.[97] The client may also have feelings of guilt and preoccupation with her negligence or minor omissions.[90,97]

Objective Data

Data are determined concerning the client and her family's grieving by means of observation and counseling. The primary health care provider can then help them cope with their loss. If the health care provider is to assist the family through its grieving process, he/she must realize mothers and fathers grieve differently.[98] Mothers express more grief and grieve longer than do fathers.[98] This difference in grieving may also lead to sexual problems. The father may desire sexual activity because he perceives coitus as a way to share and comfort as well as be comforted.[98] The mother may perceive this desire as callousness.

Phases of Mourning. Progression through the five stages of mourning varies among individuals and regression may occur. Perinatal grieving involves acute grief, which is most intense during the 4- to 6-week period following loss and less intense in the subsequent 4 weeks. The normal grief reaction may last from 6 months to 2 years or may never resolve. The anniversary of the loss may reactivate grief reactions.[98]

- The shock and numbness stage (denial) is expressed as impaired normal functioning. The individual has difficulty making decisions and may be aloof.
- Searching and yearning (anger) constitute the second stage of mourning. Anger and bitterness can be transferred to other people, especially health care professionals. Restlessness and guilt feelings may also be experienced.
- Bargaining, which is usually a brief phase, attempts to delay loss.
- Disorganization (depression) is the phase when the reality of the loss occurs. Depression may occur as the full impact of loss is felt. Guilt feelings remain.
- Resolution may be seen as the individual begins to function better at home and at work. Self-confidence increases. The individual is able to place the loss in perspective with life.[99,100]

Parental Tasks. Following perinatal loss, parents must work through the loss and make it real. The parents must allow the normal grief reaction to progress. During this time, parents should meet their own needs as well as those of their other children and communicate their feelings to the children.

Multiple Gestation. Parents who experienced a multiple gestation may have an additional or more acute sense of loss from conflicting emotions. Parents need to grieve their deceased infant(s) before relating to the survivor(s). Parents may experience grief from loss of prestige as parents of twins. In addition, they may have a sense of inadequacy, as the death of one child may be perceived as the inability to raise more than one child.

Plan

Psychosocial Interventions. Measures are directed toward helping parents work through loss and make it real. Their coping abilities are assessed and, if indicated, the parents are referred to support groups for counseling.

- Telephone parents (especially important on what had been due date or on the anniversary of death) to reevaluate coping and readjustment. Call during the evening to involve the partner. Provide parents with the phone number of the hospital's maternity floor.
- Advise parents to join support groups (see Parental/Family Support Groups and Perinatal Loss Support Groups at the end of this chapter).
- Provide anticipatory guidance, counseling parents about the normalcy of grief, its stages, and the varying duration. Warn parents of an emotional roller coaster of "good" days and "bad" days—days when a sight, smell, or sound may bring back a flood of memories and tears. Most difficult time is 2 to 4 months after death (acute grief).
- Prepare parents to deal with reactions of others, especially well meaning but insensitive comments.
- Advise couple that it is not uncommon for sexual intimacy to be compromised by avoidance, depression, or disinterest for up to 2 years after the death of a child.[98]
- Facilitate communication and expression of grief with such open ended statements as "Some fathers have said . . . Tell me how you feel."
- Ask the father how he's doing—avoid expressing concern for just the mother.

- Recommend postponing pregnancy until both parents have worked through their grief.
- Provide suggestions for dealing with grief.

  - Communicate with partner, family, and friends; talk about the infant or child who died.
  - Eat a well-balanced diet and drink adequate fluids; avoid caffeine and alcoholic beverages.
  - Exercise daily.
  - Avoid tobacco as it depletes the body of vitamins, increases stomach acidity, decreases circulation, and can cause palpitations.
  - Rest daily; rest at night even if unable to sleep.
  - Clarify values; don't be persuaded to act or think as you think you should behave. Ignore "shoulds" (e.g., "I should be strong and not cry").
  - Ease marital stress. Realize that no two people grieve the same way. Take the time to share thoughts and feelings each day and listen to what your partner is saying. Express affection for each other and other family members throughout the day.
  - Recognize and respect the need for solitary time.
  - Keep mementos of the baby. Some hospitals provide a picture, lock of hair, or ID bracelet.
  - Read books, poems, and articles that comfort; avoid "scare" literature and technical medical bulletins.
  - Keep a diary or journal of thoughts, memories, and mementos.
  - Write poems or letters to the infant.
  - Avoid making big decisions or changes for 24 months, and do not let others make decisions for you; put away baby clothes and articles when you are ready.
  - Accept help from others; request help from clergy if desired.[95,101]

Medication. Medication is not indicated.

Follow-Up

Follow-up involves continuing observation for resolution of grief. Grief is completed when an individual is able to turn outward and think of others and to formulate plans for the future. Give couple a list of resources they can turn to when they are ready. (See Resources at end of this chapter.) If grief remains unresolved, refer parents to a skilled professional counselor. Unresolved grief may be observed in several behaviors:

- Persistent yearning for recovery of lost objects
- Overidentification with the deceased
- Inability to cry or rage despite desire to do so
- Misdirected anger or ambivalence toward infant
- Lack of support group/person
- Presence of secondary gain, e.g., increased attention to mother

BREASTFEEDING

In 1984, 25 percent of American women breastfed for 6 months; in 1987, the number of women breastfeeding infants at 6 months dropped to 21 percent and to 19.7 percent in 1992.[18] In Third World countries and in acute poverty-stricken areas in the United States, an infant who is bottle fed has a greater morbidity and mortality risk within the first year than an infant who is breastfed.[102,103] Despite the increased safety of commercial infant formulas, breastfeeding has distinct advantages for both mother and infant, and almost no contraindications. Human milk is physiologically compatible with the human infant's digestive tract, and provides the exact balance of nutrients, electrolytes, and immunological factors necessary for optimal growth and development. Even the act of suckling employs the use of different muscles and feeding mechanism than bottle feeding.[18,104] Breastfeeding is more convenient for the mother, nothing to heat or spoil, no extra bottles to transport. An emotional bond develops between mother and nursing infant that does not occur when an infant is bottle fed.[18,57]

A mother who is breastfeeding for the first time may not have the support of family and friends, and needs encouragement, support, and accurate information to become self-assured about breastfeeding. Teaching should ideally begin during the pregnancy. The health care provider should help the first-time breastfeeding mother and her infant to successfully breastfeed.

TYPES OF BREASTFEEDING

Unrestricted Breastfeeding

The infant is put to breast immediately after delivery and then on demand. Breast milk is the major source of nourishment for the first year of life or longer.

The advantages of this type of breastfeeding are that less illness occurs during first year of life,[18] infant has mouth-nipple contact and body contact, and the breast is associated with comfort as well as food. The disadvantage is that breastfeeding requires the mother's dedication.

Token Breastfeeding

Restrictions are placed on the duration of breastfeeding and the length of each time at the breast; feedings are scheduled. The mother may pump her breasts and store the milk for others to give (e.g., daycare providers). Weaning occurs by the third month or earlier.

The advantage is that other family members can participate in feeding the infant. The disadvantages are that the milk supply may decrease, the infant is more susceptible to illnesses, and the infant learns bottle-sucking techniques, which may lead to nipple confusion.

BREAST ANATOMY

Breast tissue comprises glands, supporting connective tissue, and fatty tissue. The primary structures are skin, subcutaneous tissue, and the corpus mammae.

The skin includes the nipple, areola, and general skin. Each nipple contains 15 to 25 milk ducts; each of the tubuloalveolar glands opens separately onto the nipple. The nipple also contains smooth muscle fibers, sensory nerve endings, and sebaceous and apocrine glands. Nipple erection is caused by tactile, sensory, or autonomic sympathetic stimuli. Montgomery's tubercles contain the ductular openings of sebaceous and lactiferous glands. They secrete a substance that protects and lubricates the nipple and areola during pregnancy and lactation.

Subcutaneous tissue lies just below the dermis.

The corpus mammae is divided into the parenchyma and stroma. Parenchyma includes the ductular-lobular-alveolar structures. The lactiferous ductal system connects the alveoli to the nipple. Fifteen to twenty tubuloalveolar glands are embedded in fat.[18] They open into lactiferous ducts, which open into lactiferous sinuses, which, in turn, open onto the nipple. The stroma comprises connective tissue, fat, blood vessels, nerves, and lymphatics.

PHYSIOLOGY OF LACTATION

Lactation is hormonally controlled. The physiological changes that occur are directed toward mammogenesis, lactogenesis (milk secretion), and galactopoiesis (milk maintenance). Most milk is synthesized in the acini and smaller milk ducts during suckling.[18]

Mammogenesis

Mammogenesis is the development of the mammary glands to their functional state.

Estrogen stimulates parenchymal proliferation and ductal growth. Luteal and placental hormones increase ductular and lobular formation; placental lactogen, prolactin, and chorionic gonadotropin accelerate mammary growth.[18] Prolactin (from the anterior pituitary gland) stimulates glandular production of colostrum; human placental lactogen stimulates secretion of colostrum by the second trimester;[18] and progesterone stimulates lobular growth.

Lactogenesis

Milk production by the mammary glands proceeds in two stages.

Stage I of lactogenesis begins 12 weeks before parturition and is preceded by significant increases in lactose, total proteins, and immunoglobulins and decreases in sodium and chloride.[18] Stage II clinically begins on days 2 and 3 postpartum with copious milk secretion; mature milk is established in approximately 10 days.[18]

Galactopoiesis

Prolactin stimulates and sustains lactation (milk secretion); oxytocin stimulates milk ejection. An intact hypothalamic-pituitary axis regulates prolactin and oxytocin levels and is essential for the maintenance of milk secretion. Ejection reflex is dependent on receptors in the canalicular system of the breast. Dilation or stretching of the canalicules causes a reflex release of oxytocin. Tactile receptors for both oxytocin and reflex prolactin release are located in the nipple.[18]

Prolactin secretion is controlled by prolactin inhibitory factor (PIF) produced by the hypothalamus.[105] Suppression of PIF allows the anterior pituitary gland to secrete uninhibited amounts of prolactin. Catecholamine levels in the hypothalamus control PIF. Drugs and events that decrease catecholamines also decrease PIF, thereby causing an increase in prolactin.[18] Among nonnursing mothers, prolactin levels drop to normal in 2 to 3 weeks, independent of lactation suppression therapy.

Release of oxytocin into the circulation is stimulated by sucking. Two minutes of sucking may be required for a full oxytocin response.[106] Release of oxytocin peaks 6 to 10 minutes after sucking begins.[106] The hormone causes the ejection of milk (milk ejection reflex) from alveoli and smaller milk ducts into larger lactiferous sinuses and ducts. It also stimulates myometrial contraction and uterine involution.

Composition of Human Milk

Milk varies with the stage of lactation, time of day, sampling time during a given feeding, maternal nutrition, and the individual. Initially, colostrum is produced. A transitional phase in production leads to secretion of mature milk.

Colostrum. A yellowish, thick fluid produced during the first postpartum week. It contains higher concentrations of sodium, potassium, and chloride than mature milk. Protein, fat-soluble vitamins, and minerals are also in larger concentration than in transitional or mature milk. This high-protein, low fat milk meets the needs and reserves of the newborn.[18] The mean energy value is 67 kcal/100 mL of mature milk. Colostrum facilitates the establishment of bifidus flora in the digestive tract and the passage of meconium. It contains abundant antibodies.

Transitional Milk. Secreted beginning 7 to 10 days postpartum and continuing until 2 weeks postpartum. The concentration of immunoglobulins decreases, although lactose, fat, and total caloric content increase. Water-soluble vitamins increase and fat-soluble vitamins decrease to approach the level found in mature milk.[18]

Mature Milk. The only necessary source of nutrition for an infant's first 4 to 6 months of life and should be the primary source for the first year.[18,107,108]

- Water is the major constituent. A lactating woman requires an increased water intake. If water intake is decreased, sensible and insensible water loss are decreased before water for lactation is decreased.
- Lipids, the second most plentiful constituent, and the most variable, provides the major portion of kilocalories. It is almost completely digestible.
- Proteins constitute 0.9 percent of human milk content.[18]
- The predominant carbohydrate is lactose. Synthesized by the mammary gland, it is specific for newborn growth and enhances calcium absorption. Lactose appears to be critical for the prevention of rickets, as human milk is relatively low in calcium.
- Minerals essential to the newborn are potassium and iron.
  - Potassium levels are higher than sodium in breast milk (similar to intracellular fluids). Sodium levels in cow's milk are 3.6 times greater than those in human milk.[18]
  - The concentration of exogenous elemental iron in human milk is 100 µg/1100 mL.[18] Normal infants need 8 to 10 mg per day in the first year of life. Prepared formulas provide 10 to 12 mg per day; infants breastfed for the first 6 months are not at increased risk for iron-deficiency anemia or depletion of iron stores.[18,109] Although its concentration in human milk is low, iron is absorbed more readily than iron from other sources. Thus, infants are not at risk for iron deficiency anemia or depletion of iron stores if they are breastfed totally during the first 6 months of life.
  - An adequate supply of vitamins A, E, and C is present in breast milk. The amount of vitamin A in mature human milk is 280 IU and in cow's milk, 180 IU; an infant consuming 200 mL of breast milk every day obtains an adequate amount of vitamin A.

- Serum levels of vitamin E in breastfed babies rise quickly at birth and are maintained by approximately 4 weeks postpartum with only breast milk intake.[18]
- Vitamin C and other water-soluble vitamins in human milk reflect maternal dietary intake.[18] Human milk is an excellent source of these water-soluble vitamins.[18]

Resistance Factors and Immunological Significance

Breastfeeding significantly decreases infant morbidity and mortality by protecting against enteropathogens that may contaminate other food or formula. The protective factors contained in breast milk are both cellular and humoral.[18]

Cellular factors include macrophages, polymorphonuclear leukocytes, and lymphocytes. These cells are phagocytes and they stimulate antibody formation. The humoral factors are immunoglobulins.

- Immunoglobulin A (IgA) is the most important immunoglobulin in terms of biological activity, and it is the most concentrated. IgA also has antitoxin activity against *Escherichia coli* and *Vibrio cholerae* and thereby prevents diarrhea.[18,102]
- Bifidus factor is responsible for the growth of *Bifidobacterium bifidum,* the predominant bacteria in the gut of breastfed infants. The flora of bifid bacteria inhibits pathogenic *Staphylococcus aureus, Shigella,* and *Protozoa* and encourages growth of *Lactobacillus bifidus,* which crowds out other bacteria. Lysozyme and lactoferrin act directly to inhibit pathogen growth. The resistance factor protects against *Staphylococcus* infection.[18,102,108]
- Breast milk contains antibodies against poliovirus, coxsackievirus, echovirus, influenza virus, and rhinovirus and, thus, helps to prevent viral infections.[18,102]
- Breast milk protects against the development of allergies. An infant begins to produce antibodies to cow's milk (which is the basis of formula) within 18 days of ingestion. Syndromes associated with cow's milk allergy include gastric enteropathy, atopic dermatitis, rhinitis, chronic pulmonary disease, eosinophilia, and failure to thrive.[18,102]

CONTRAINDICATIONS TO BREASTFEEDING

Breast Cancer. Controversy regarding the role of prolactin in the progression of mammary cancer may be a reason to contraindicate breastfeeding for pregnant women.[18] Breastfeeding may offer a small protective effect against the development of breast cancer.[18,110]

Hepatitis B Virus. Breastfeeding permitted in protected infants—rapid schedule of immunization (0, 1, and 2 months) of infant would be indicated.[103] Milk donors should be screened for this virus or milk should be pasteurized.[103]

Cytomegalovirus. Breast milk also contains appropriate antibodies that protect the infant against cytomegalovirus. There does exist a risk for the infant who is exposed to virus but not a daily dose of antibodies, and risk for severe infection is especially great in premature infant of nonimmune mother.[18,104]

Human Immunodeficiency Virus. For women in the United States who test positive for HIV, breastfeeding is contraindicated.[18,103,111] Breastfeeding, however, remains the feeding method of choice in countries where the death rate in the first year of life is 50 percent, compared with the 18 percent risk of dying from AIDS when born to an infected mother.[18]

Augmentation or Reduction Mammoplasty. If milk ducts were cut during mammoplasty, breastfeeding may not be possible.[18] Incisions around the areola usually indicate that some milk ducts were cut and possible nerve damage occurred.[110]

Active Tuberculosis. Breastfeeding is permitted if the mother's skin test is positive, and if at the same time there is no radiologic indication of disease and the client has started antituberculin medication. If the mother has a positive tuberculin skin test and positive chest film, she may breastfeed if she is taking antituberculous medication and the sputum culture is negative.[18,103] The American Academy of Pediatrics considers INH, rifampin, ethambutal, and streptomycin compatible with breastfeeding.[88] If the sputum culture is positive, breastfeeding may be possible after the mother has taken medication for at least 1 week. Limited isolation from the mother with active disease may be required. The breastfeeding infant may be treated prophylactically by the pediatrician.

ELEMENTS OF BREASTFEEDING

Compression of Lactiferous Sinuses. Externally, the infant's mouth should cover the lactiferous sinuses, whereas internally, the correct movement of the infant's tongue provides areolar compression between the infant's tongue and palate. The lactiferous sinuses lie underneath the areola; compression of the lactiferous sinuses removes milk from the breast. Sucking may need to continue for 2 minutes for the full response to oxytocin release.

Number of Feedings per Day. A minimum of eight feedings are necessary in 24 hours, with each feeding providing a minimum of 5 to 10 minutes of swallowing at each breast. The milk ejection reflex takes 2 to 3 minutes before it is effective;[18] limiting nursing to 2 to 3 minutes does not permit the infant to obtain milk. Suck efficiency is critical to breastfeeding success.

Systematic Assessment of Infant at Breast.[106] Assessment of a breastfeeding session requires direct observation. Observe positioning and alignment, areolar grasp, and sucking.

POSITIONING AND ALIGNMENT. The infant should be relaxed, in a responsive state, and displaying early hunger cues—rooting and hand-to-mouth activity. Crying is a late hunger cue.

The infant's body should be flexed with the head and trunk aligned so that the head is straight on the breast, not turned laterally or hyperextended (head and body are at breast level). The infant should be brought to the breast, not the breast to the infant. Proper alignment decreases traction on the mother's nipples; the areola and nipple are more easily kept in the infant's mouth; swallowing is facilitated.

The mother's hand should cup her breast, with her fingers supporting the lower portion of the breast and her thumb resting on the upper portion. The infant should be permitted to grasp at least one-half inch of areolar tissue. This position is the "C-hold," and permits the mother to support her breast without distorting the nipple.

The traditional "scissors" or "cigarette" hold in which the breast is held between the mother's middle and index fingers has two disadvantages: 1) the mother's fingers cannot spread apart as far as in the C-hold and may interfere with the infant's latching on, and 2) breast tissue can be restricted by the scissors hold to such a degree that ducts become plugged.[107]

AREOLAR GRASP. The infant must have a correct mouth opening, correct lip flanging, and correct tongue placement. To elicit the grasp gently, tickle the infant's lips with the nipple to stimulate the mouth to open. When the mouth is opened wide, quickly pull the infant close to the breast and center the nipple in infant's mouth. Move the infant's head and trunk as a unit to avoid hyperflexion, hyperextension, or lateral turning of the head. Avoid holding the back of the infant's head to maneuver it onto the breast, because it does not allow the mother to feel rapid arm motion and erodes her confidence if the infant latches on. Placing a hand on the mother's arm and moving it quickly toward her breast allows the mother to feel the quick arm movement.

BREASTFEEDING PROBLEMS. May be determined during systematic assessment of the infant at the breast.

- Problems with grasping the areola may be caused by "prissily pursued" lips. The infant appears to be drinking through a straw. Only the nipple is grasped, and the mother often experiences nipple pain. The infant receives little milk because the lactiferous sinuses are not compressed. Break the suction by inserting a finger into the corner of infant's mouth and stimulate the mouth to open wide. Alternate sucking of the nipple and the areola through pursed lips will traumatize the nipple and the suck will become inefficient.[106] Friction may abrade the mother's areolar tissue and result in ineffective sucking.
- Another grasping problem is negative pressure in an infant's intraoral cavity, which results in retention of the nipple and areolar tissue in the infant's mouth. This counteracts the naturally retractile nature of nipple tissue, helps to refill the lactiferous sinuses with milk from the lactiferous ducts, and conveys milk to the oropharynx. Negative pressure is achieved when an infant forms an effective seal with the border of his or her mouth.

- Sore nipples cause discomfort, and breastfeeding should not hurt. If the mother has sore, cracked nipples, the cause must be found: Review positioning and latch-on of the infant. A variety of measures may be tried to relieve sore nipples.

  - Rule out problems such as monilia. The mother may complain of severe nipple itching or a severe pain when infant nurses. The infant may or may not show signs of thrush. The mother and infant should be treated simultaneously, the mother with Nystatin cream or Mycolog cream rubbed into the nipple after each feeding and the infant with oral Nystatin.[18]
  - Some milk may be expressed before feeding to stimulate the milk ejection reflex, thus allowing for softening of the areola before the infant latches on.
  - Some milk may be expressed onto the nipples after feedings and allowed to air dry.
  - The flaps of the nursing bra may be left open after feedings.
  - Nursing pads with plastic liners should be avoided. Nipple shields also compound the problem by increasing nipple irritation and confusing the baby so that the baby sucks improperly and further irritates the nipple.[18,104]

SUCKING. Correct sucking requires that the infant's tongue cover the mandibular-alveolar ridge on the lower gum line and curve beneath the areolar tissue.

Evaluate tongue placement by gently pulling infant's lower lip downward. Incorrect tongue placement is indicated by clicking or smacking sounds and drawing in of cheek pads with each suck, or by the loss of large amounts of milk over the infant's chin.[106,107] A short tongue or one with a short lingual frenulum may not extend over the lower alveolar ridge.

Evaluate areolar compression by carefully noting the type of sucking and swallowing. A sustained slower mandibular motion indicates nutritive sucking; rapid mandibular motion indicates nonnutritive sucking. Audible swallowing is the most reliable indicator of milk intake. Documentation of an infant's breastfeeding should state: "Breastfed with audible swallowing at each breast."[106]

Breastfeeding Positions. Whichever position (four are listed below) the mother uses to nurse her infant, she should be comfortable. Pillows should be used to help support her arm and help her hold the baby close to her breast, relaxed and without muscle strain.

- *Cradle Hold.* The mother sits up, the infant faces her, and the infant's head or arm rests on the mother's forearm or in the crook of her arm. The cradle hold is a good choice for a mother whose infant has low muscle tone, for example, an infant with Down syndrome.
- *Football Hold.* The mother sits up, the infant's head faces her breast, and the body is tucked under her arm at her side. The baby's bottom should be resting on a pillow near the mother's elbow to provide additional support for the mother and avoid muscle strain. The football hold is a good choice for a mother who recently had abdominal surgery, as the position does not put pressure on the incision.
- *Side-Lying Position.* Both the mother and infant lie on their sides, facing each other, with the infant's feet pulled in close to his or her body. Pillows under the mother's head, behind her back, and under the knee or her upper leg may provide comfort. This position is more restful for mothers and has been found to significantly reduce fatigue among new breastfeeding mothers.[112]
- *Slide-Over Position.* This position is especially useful with infants who refuse one breast. The mother can begin nursing the infant on the preferred side, then slide the infant over to the less preferred side once the milk ejection reflex has occurred. The infant's body position is not changed; he or she merely "slides over."

Breast Preparation. To prepare breasts for feeding, first assess them by palpating the tissue and inspecting the nipples and areolae; then teach the mother proper care of the breasts.

Palpate to detect inelastic breast tissue. Skin that is taut and firm and difficult to pick up is more prone to engorgement. Tissue can be improved by prepartum massage (see Chapter 7) and measures to prevent engorgement.[18]

Assess the nipples and areolae by gently compressing each areola between the thumb and forefinger. The normal nipple everts with gentle pressure; the inverted or tied nipple inverts more with gentle pressure.[18] Inverted nipples may be treated with a nipple shell worn during last trimester (see the list at the end of this chapter). Exercises to evert the nipple are rarely successful and can lead to premature labor.[18]

Stress the importance of avoiding soap and other drying agents on the nipples. Teach the mother to wash breasts with water only.[18,107] Routine use of ointments and creams is discouraged, as some have irritants, such as lanolin;[18,19,107] Vitamin E or hormone creams or ointments are unsafe on the nipples unless prescribed for a specific problem, and they then should be used only in minute amounts.[18,107] Sebaceous glands and tubercles of Montgomery are easily plugged by repeated application of oily substances.

Extrinsic Factors Contributing to Breastfeeding Problems. Separation at any time, delayed feedings, and introduction of bottle feedings interfere with breastfeeding.

Separation of mother and infant interferes with milk ejection reflex; the infant is not able to nurse on demand, causing a delay that contributes to milk stasis and engorgement. If in the mother's absence, the infant learns to suck on a bottle, then sucking at the breast becomes incorrect, causing pain and trauma.

Delaying first feedings to a healthy infant—an infant is most receptive to nursing in the first 90 minutes after birth—can erode the mother's self-confidence when a sleepy infant is later brought to her to feed. Delay can also decrease the milk ejection reflex.

Limiting the frequency and duration of feedings contributes to breastfeeding problems. The milk ejection reflex occurs 2 to 3 minutes after sucking is initiated.[18] Limiting nursing interferes with the reflex and the infant's milk supply. The limited feedings contribute to milk stasis and engorgement and sore nipples.

Introducing bottles to an infant interferes with the milk ejection reflex by suggesting to the mother that her milk is insufficient. Bottles cause the infant to become confused as sucking at the breast differs from sucking on a commercial nipple or pacifier. An infant may reject the breast or, on the other hand, suckle frequently and for prolonged periods to be satisfied.

Breastfeeding Infants in Multiple Births. The advantages of breastfeeding infants in a multiple birth are similar to those of breastfeeding a single child: breastfeeding provides a perfect food that is easily digested and provides immunities; the milk is easily accessible; financial savings are substantial; and a special relationship is promoted between mother and infants. A disadvantage may be that the mother finds breastfeeding multiple infants exhausting. The mother may find a support group helpful (see Support Groups and Resources, A).

The amount of milk produced is influenced by the size of the infants and the number of breastfeeding sessions. The mother should begin breastfeeding at the earliest possible time. An electric piston-type pump (Medela or Ameda/Egnel) may be needed if infants are unable to suckle.[113] Optimal milk production with minimum pumping will most likely involve five pumping sessions per day, at least 10 to 15 minutes per breast. A minimum total of 100 minutes pumping over 24 hours is recommended;[113] short, frequent sessions to express milk are more effective and stimulate more milk production than longer sessions with longer intervals.[113] It is not necessary for the mother to waken at night and pump.[113]

If only one infant can feed and the other is hospitalized the mother has two options: 1) Nurse twin A while simultaneously pumping for twin B. Breast milk obtained can be taken to twin B. This schedule is rigorous and may be exhausting for the mother. 2) Begin pumping for twin B a few days prior to the infant's discharge.

Feedings may be simultaneous or individual. Simultaneous feedings are advantageous because both feedings are completed in one session. Simultaneous feedings save time and may take advantage of simultaneous letdowns. A disadvantage is that the mother loses individual time with each infant.

Individual feedings are advantageous because modified scheduling may be employed. For example, the hungrier infant sets the pace, and the second infant is awakened for feedings. A disadvantage of this type of feeding is that it is time consuming.

Simultaneous Feedings. Proper positioning is particularly important for breastfeeding two infants so that the mother does not bear the weight of the infants. Pillows should support the infants' weight.

- The double football hold is used for simultaneous feedings. The head and neck of each infant are supported by the mother's hands, with each infant's body tucked under one of the mother's arms and their feet toward her back. The infants' abdomens face up or are rotated in toward the mother's chest or side. An advantage of the double football hold is that the mother can assist with head control; the more difficult to manage infant should be placed on the side easiest for the mother to manage.[113] The mother should not bend over to nurse but, instead, bring the infants close to her.
- In the combination cradle/football position, twin A is held like football and approaches the breast at 12 and 6 o'clock. Twin B is cradled across the mother's chest with her or his abdomen tucked in tightly toward the mother's abdomen and approaches the breast at 9 and 3 o'clock.[113] Two advantages of this position are that it is the most inconspicuous for nursing outside the home, and it is easily mastered if one or both infants have difficulty latching onto the breast.
- In the parallel hold both infants are angled in the same direction. Twin A is cradled, held with legs behind twin B; the legs simultaneously support twin B's head. The advantage of the parallel hold is that the weight of one twin keeps the second infant attached to the breast. In addition, the mother's arms can rest comfortably on pillows.[113]
- In the crisscross hold both infants are in cradle position, with the legs of one crossing over those of the other. The infants are in the crook of the mother's arms and are rotated toward her abdomen. The mother supports the infants by holding their buttocks. A disadvantage is that this position is difficult for infants to maintain; it requires head control.[113]
- "V" position is similar to crisscross. The mother is lying nearly flat on her back with pillows under her head. The infants' heads are at their mother's breasts, forming a "V," with their knees touching her upper abdomen.[107] This position allows the mother to rest more comfort-

ably; it can be used for night feedings. The disadvantage is that it requires infants to have more head control and assistance in grasping the nipple.[113]

DRUG TRANSMISSION IN BREAST MILK

Transmission of a drug in breast milk from mother to infant depends on several factors:

- Absorption of drug by mother's body: half-life or peak serum time, absorption rate, route of administration
- Lipid solubility and plasma protein binding properties of drug
- Movement of drug from maternal plasma to milk; cell diffusion or active transport
- Amount of drug ingested by infant
- Concentration of drug in milk
- Size and relative metabolic maturity of infant
- pH of substrate[18,114]

The effect of the drug can be minimized in several ways:

- Do not use a long-acting form of the drug. Infants have difficulty with excretion and detoxification usually occurs in liver; however, the infant liver is immature.
- Schedule the doses so that the least amount of the drug enters the milk: Have the mother take medication immediately after breastfeeding.
- Choose drug that passes least into milk.
- Advise the mother to take medication as directed and to watch the infant for unusual signs and symptoms or a change in feeding pattern or activity. She should contact her health care provider if she has any concerns or questions.

Contraindications. Certain drugs are contraindicated while breastfeeding:

- Alcoholic beverages (interfere with ejection reflex)
- Chronic aspirin use may cause metabolic acidosis in infant and affect platelet function (aspirin or acetaminophen in single dose is not significantly transferred)
- Cocaine
- Chloramphenicol (potential for bone marrow toxicity)

- Cimetidine (unknown effect in nursing infant)
- Cyclosporine
- Doxorubicin
- Gold salts (rash, kidney and liver inflammation)
- Iodine (preferentially concentrated in milk with concentrations 20 to 30 times those of maternal serum)
- Lithium (infant hypotonia, lethargy)
- Methotrexate
- Minor tranquilizers (barbiturates, benzodiazepines)
- Narcotics (methadone for maintenance therapy reported safe)
- Phencyclidine (PCP)
- Thiouracil (not, however, propylthiouracil)
- Tobacco (smoking more than 20 cigarettes per day decreases milk supply; passive, inhaled smoke increases risks for allergies, sudden infant death syndrome, pneumonia, and bronchitis)[107,114,115,116,117]

Drugs requiring temporary interruption are radiopharmaceuticals including indium-111 and gallium-67.[115]

The effects of metoclopramide on nursing infants are unknown. No adverse effects have been reported; however, there is the potential for central nervous system effects.[115]

Drugs that have caused significant effects in some nursing infants and should be used with caution include clemastine, phenobarbital, primidone, and sulfasalazine.[115]

A mother who uses recreational drugs should not breastfeed.

Amphetamines (crack, speed, ups, uppers) are excreted in breast milk; levels in milk exceed those in maternal serum. Abstinence from amphetamines is recommended until more information is available.

Cocaine (snow, coke, crack, champagne, tool, pearl flake, blow, gold dust, dama blanca) appears to be excreted in breast milk.[118] Cocaine intoxication has been reported in 2-week-old infants. Mothers should not apply cocaine to sore nipples.[118] Seizures, apnea, and cyanosis were reported in an 11-day-old infant whose mother applied cocaine to sore nipples.[118]

Heroin ("H," junk, smack, China white, black tar) crosses into breast milk to cause addiction in breastfed infants.[118]

Hallucinogens have not been reported in breast milk. Hallucinogens include LSD (acid, lysergic diethylamide), mescaline (peyote), psilocybin (found in certain mushrooms) and Ts and blues (combination of pentazocine and tripelennamine).[118]

Marijuana (dope, weed, herb, grass, pot, hashish, hash) has unknown long-term effects on infants; the concentration transferred into breast milk is eight times that in maternal blood.[118]

Compatible Drugs. Certain drugs are usually compatible with breastfeeding:

- Amoxicillin
- Azithromycin
- Cefoxitin
- Cisplatin
- Diltiazem
- Erythromycin
- Hormones (oral contraceptives, including those with estrogen which may decrease milk production)
- Ibuprofen
- Labetalol
- Methimazole
- Mexilitine
- Minoxidil
- Piroxicam
- Procainamide
- Propranolol
- Suprafen
- Terbutaline
- Ticarcillin
- Tolmetin
- Verapamil.[18,107,114,115]

BREAST PUMPS

Mothers of preterm infants or of newborns hospitalized for other reasons and mothers who work may use breast pumps. An infant's suckling, however, remains the most efficient pump. Infants suck at approximately 55 to 220 mm Hg.[119] Pumps that match suckling stimulate the milk ejection reflex and promote milk production most effectively. The vacuum produced by a pump should not exceed the vacuum created by an infant.

Infants nurse in a burst-pause pattern. Suckling has three phases: suction, release, and relaxation. The actions are carried out approximately

60 times per minute.[119] Infants apply suction for less than 1 second each time.[120]

A correctly fitting flange surrounds the areola and allows the nipple to move back and forth during pumping. The flange should engulf and firmly support the breast and allow maximum nipple stretch, yet be small enough to provide gentle nipple friction.

There are different types of pumps. An electric pump obtains more milk and is easier to use than a hand-operated pump or manual expression.[121] The double pump expresses milk most quickly and can be rented for about one dollar per day. An intermittent draw pump is less likely to cause trauma and provides better stimulation of the milk ejection reflex.[121]

Manual expression of milk might be necessary in the event a part of the mechanical pump is lost or the pump is left at home. To manually express (pump) milk, the mother first washes her hands. She positions her thumb and first two fingers about 1 to 1½ in. behind her nipple, forming a "C" with her hand. She should then push straight into the chest wall and roll her thumb and fingers forward. The movement is repeated rhythmically; the thumb and fingers are rotated to milk other sinuses. She should express each breast until milk flow decreases, then gently massage the breasts to stimulate milk ejection.[107]

Not recommended for pumping breasts is the bicycle horn pump. It cannot be sterilized, milk can be easily contaminated, and it has no collection mechanism for milk. It is difficult to clean, can damage breast tissue, and it expresses milk ineffectively.

Using a Pump. Practicing with pump before actual need for milk will facilitate successful use. A woman should become knowledgeable about the pump several weeks before milk is actually needed; she should practice putting the pump together and using it. Hands should be washed before beginning breast pumping, and manufacturer's instructions followed for cleaning the pump.

The mother moistens the breast with water (to form a seal), centers the nipple in the proper size nipple adapter, and begins pumping at the lowest setting. To stimulate the milk ejection reflex she should interrupt milk expression several times to gently massage the breast. She should switch breasts when milk flow begins to decrease.

Storing Milk. If milk is to be used within 48 to 72 hours refrigeration is sufficient for storage. Milk should be frozen if storage will be longer than 24 hours. Do not freeze in glass containers but in rigid polyprophylene plastic containers to maintain stability of cells and immunoglobulins.[102] Frozen milk can be stored for 1 month in the freezer compartment of a refrigerator or 6 months in a deep freeze. Methods of thawing milk can adversely affect anti-infective factors. Frozen milk should be thawed in the refrigerator and used within 24 hours. Thawing milk in warm water can cause contamination, and subjecting milk to microwave temperatures of 72° to 98° C can result in a marked decrease in anti-infective factors.[102]

RETURNING TO WORK AND BREASTFEEDING

Pumping/Expressing Milk. Advise the client to begin freezing milk for later use approximately 14 days before returning to work. She should pump at least three times per day, after breastfeeding the infant. A formula is used to estimate the amount of milk needed per feeding:

$$\frac{\text{infant weight} \times 2.5}{\text{number of feedings}} = \text{ounces per feeding}$$

For example, for a 10-pound infant,

$$\frac{10 \times 2.5}{8} = \frac{25}{8} = \begin{array}{l}\text{approximately 3 oz of milk}\\ \text{milk needed per feeding}\end{array}$$

A Nuk-type nipple should be used when bottle feeding, as it most closely resembles breast.

Baby's Refusal of Bottle. Refusing to drink from a bottle occurs most often among infants approximately 3 months old. Using a bottle along with breastfeeding in the first month of life increases the likelihood of nipple confusion; poor suckling at breast results and establishment of a milk supply that meets the infant's needs is delayed.[121] Someone other than mother should use a second feeding skill with the infant, for example, offering milk in a cup or spoon rather than the bottle.[121]

Preparing for Absence. Some guidelines might help the client adapt to the challenges of breastfeeding and spending time away from the infant.

- Suggest to the client that she pack an extra bra and wear a two-piece outfit to facilitate pumping and to camouflage leakage of milk.
- Advise the client to ensure that the infant's caregiver is comfortable with the mother's desire to breastfeed and knows how to handle breast milk.
- Suggest to the client that she pack several diaper bags to obviate the need to return home for forgotten articles.
- Refer the client to a breastfeeding support group (see Breastfeeding Information/Support Groups at the end of this chapter).

BOTTLE FEEDING

Although breast milk is the perfect food for infants, not all mothers choose or are able to breastfeed their infants. Formula feedings should be given to an infant for the first year of life. If the infant is allergic to cow's milk, soy-based formulas may be used.

An amendment was passed in 1980 by Congress to the Food, Drug and Cosmetic Act specifying new regulations for commercially prepared infant formula. This act, the Infant Formula Act of 1980, gave the Food and Drug Administration (FDA) the authority to establish quality-control procedures for infant formula, to establish recall procedures, to establish and revise nutrient levels, and to regulate labeling. Manufacturers were also required to analyze each batch of formula to ensure all nutrients were present in the correct amounts, to ensure that the formula was stable over the period of recommended shelf life, and to make all records available to the FDA. The year 1986 saw the requirement for standard labeling of nutrition information and directions for preparation become mandatory.[116]

Calories are provided to the infant in the form of carbohydrates, protein, and fat. By the end of the second week in life, full-term infants require 100–110 Kcal/kg/day of fluids to maintain cellular growth and function. Preterm infants weighing fewer than 2500 grams may require 110–150 Kcal/kg/day to achieve satisfactory growth. Fluid requirements are higher than in full-term infants because of greater fluid loss. Because of the immature digestive system, premature infants will require different formula than full-term infants.[122]

TEACHING BOTTLE FEEDING

- Point the nipple directly into the mouth and on top of the tongue, rather than toward the palate. The nipple should be full of milk at all times to avoid ingestion of air. The nipple hole should be large enough so that milk flows in drips when inverted; if it is too large, the infant can drink too fast and regurgitate or overeat.
- Stroke, cuddle, and talk to the infant during feedings.
- Never prop bottles or feed infant in totally recumbent (flat) position which can result in positional otitis media.
- Avoid warming bottles in a microwave oven, as milk can become too hot and burn the infant. Formula should be at room temperature.
- Avoid reusing milk from a previous feeding.

NURSING DIAGNOSES

The following nursing diagnoses identified by the author are representative of those used in the health care plan of women during postpartum and lactation; however, they by no means constitute a complete list.

- Alteration in parenting related to: conflict of roles; fatigue; poor nutrition; work overload; lack of support of significant others; unrealistic expectations for self, partner, child
- Disturbance in self-concept, maternal role performance, related to: discrepancy between perceived and actual role behaviors; fatigue; inability to achieve self-ideal mothering roles
- Altered family processes: poverty; economic crisis; loss of home
- Ineffective family coping, disabling: rejection; abandonment; abuse
- Altered nutrition, more than body requirements: knowledge deficit regarding components of daily nutritional requirements; lack of storage/cooking facilities

- Compromised family coping related to: lack of support or positive reinforcement for primary caregiver; psychological illness of family member; conflict of roles (mother, career, and wife); fatigue/poor nutrition/work overload; minimal reserves (financial, housing, child care)
- Impaired parenting related to lack of effective role-model
- Impaired home maintenance related to: morbidity of parent (depression); knowledge deficit of management problems and solutions
- Impaired social interaction with infant related to: fatigue, illness; role conflicts; work overload; negative infant behaviors; minimal support of significant others; unwanted pregnancy
- Disturbance in self-concept, maternal role performance, related to: discrepancy between perceived and actual role behaviors; fatigue; inability to achieve self-ideal mothering roles.

SUPPORT GROUPS AND RESOURCES

Breastfeeding Information/Support Groups

Ameda/Egnell
765 Industrial Drive
Cary, IL 60013
(800) 323–8750

Breast pumps and breastfeeding accessories

Gentle Expressions
Graham-Field
400 Rabro Drive East
Hauppauge, NY 11788
In New York: (800) 632–8390
Outside New York: (800) 645–8176

International Childbirth Educators' Assn.
P. O. Box 20852
Milwaukee, WI 53220
(414) 476–0130

International Lactation Consultant Organization
P. O. Box 4031
University of Virginia Station
Charlottesville, VA 22903

La Leche League International
9616 Minneapolis Ave. Box 1209
Franklin Park, IL 60131–8209
(708) 455–7730

Medela, Inc.
P. O. Box 660
McHenry, IL 60051–0660
(800) 435–8316

Breast pumps, breast pump rentals (including double pumping system), breastfeeding products.

Women, Infants, and Children (WIC) and Food Stamp Programs (administered by local health departments).

Cesarean Birth Support Groups

Cesarean Prevention Movement
P. O. Box 152
Syracuse, NY 13210
(315) 424–1942

Cesarean Support Education and Concern
22 Forest Road
Framington, MA 01701
(508) 877–8266

Parenting/Family Support Groups

Al-Anon Family Group Headquarters
P. O. Box 862, Midtown Station
New York, NY 10018
(212) 302–7240
(800) 356–9996

Alcoholics Anonymous
475 Riverside Drive
New York, NY 10163
(212) 870–3400

(Resource material and referral service)

Alcoholics Anonymous (Gay AA groups)
P. O. Box 90
Washington, DC 20044–0090

Association of Birth Defect Children
Orlando Executive Park
5400 Diplomat Cir., Ste. 270
Orlando, FL 32810
(407) 629–1466

Association of Maternal and Child Health Programs
1350 Connecticut Ave. NW, Ste. 803
Washington, DC 20036
(202) 775–0436

Council of Families with Visual Impairment
26616 Rouge River Dr.
Dearborn Heights, MI 48127
(800) 424–8666

Custody Action for Lesbian Mothers
P. O. Box 281
Narbeth, PA 19702

Center for Sickle Cell Disease
2121 Georgia Ave., SW
Washington, DC 20059

Fragile X Foundation
1441 York St., Ste. 215
Denver, CO 80206
(800) 688–8765

Fragile X Program
Duke University
P. O. Box 3364
Durham, NC 27710
(919) 684–5513

Klinefelter Syndrome & Associates
P. O. Box 119
Roseville, CA 95661–6119

(Enclose stamped, self-addressed envelope)

Lesbian Mothers' National Defense Fund
P. O. Box 21567
Seattle, WA 98111
(206) 325–2643

Little People of America, Inc.
7238 Piedmont Dr.
Dallas, TX 75227–9324
(800) 24–DWARF

National Association of Developmental Disabilities Council
1234 Massachusetts Ave. NW, Ste. 103
Washington, DC 20005
(202) 347–1234

National Association of Lesbian/Gay Alcoholism Professionals (NALGAP)
1147 South Alvarado Street
Los Angeles, CA 90006

Recovery center with services available to gay, lesbian, and bisexual alcoholics and addicts.

National Association for Sickle Cell Disease
3345 Wilshire Blvd., Ste. 1106
Los Angeles, CA 90010–1880
(800) 421–8453

National Center for Lesbian Rights
1663 Mission Street, 5th floor
San Francisco, CA 94103
(415) 621–0674

Nonprofit, public interest law firm dedicated to preserving and increasing the legal rights of lesbians and gay men.

National Center on Child Abuse and Neglect Department of Health & Human Services
U.S. Children's Bureau/NCCAN
P. O. Box 1182
Washington, DC 20013–1182
(703) 385–7565
(800) 394–3366

Information on programs in individual states, publications, and training materials

National Coalition against Domestic Violence
(202) 638–6388
(303) 839–1852

National Domestic Violence Hotline
(800) 333–7233

Makes referrals to lesbian or lesbian-friendly support and shelter services

National Gay and Lesbian Task Force (NGLTF)
1734 14th Street NW
Washington, DC 20009–4309
(202) 332–6483

National Information Center for Children and Youth with Disabilities
Box 1492
Washington, DC 20013
(703) 893–6061
(800) 999–5599

National Organization for Rare Disorders (NORD)
P. O. Box 8923
New Fairfield, CT 06812–1783
(203) 746–6518
(800) 999–NORD

National Organization for Victim Assistance (NOVA)
(202) 232–6682
(800) TRY–NOVA

Neurofibromatosis, Inc.
8855 Annapolis Rd., Ste. 110
Lanham, MD 20706–2924
(301) 577–8984
(800) 942–6825

Parents Anonymous
520 S. Lafayette Park Pl., Ste. 316
Los Angeles, CA 90057
(213) 388–6685

Parents of Down Syndrome Children
C/O The Arc
11600 Nebel Street
Rockville, MD 20852
(301) 984–5792

Parent Care
9041 Colgate Street
Indianapolis, IN 46268–1210
(317) 872–9913

For parents of premature and high risk infants

Parents Helping Parents
535 Race Street, Ste. 140
San Jose, CA 95126
(408) 288–5010

(Provides help with families of children with special needs, physical, mental, emotional, or learning disabilities; preemies; long-term, chronic, or terminal illness

Spina Bifida Association
4590 MacArthur Boulevard, Suite 250
Washington, DC 20007
(202) 944–3285
(800) 621–3141

Support Organization for Trisomy 18/13
2982 S. Union St.
Rochester, NY 14624
(716) 594–4621

Your Twins/NOMOT (National Organization of Mothers of Twins Clubs, Inc)
P. O. Box 23188
Albuquerque, NM 87192–1188
(505) 275–0955

Postpartum Depression Support Groups

Depression after Delivery (D.A.D.)
P. O. Box 1282
Morrisville, PA 19067
(212) 295–3394
(800) 944–4773

Postpartum Support International
927 North Kellogg Ave.
Santa Barbara, CA 93111
(206) 881–6580 or (805) 967–7636

Perinatal Loss Support Groups

SIDS Alliance
10500 Little Patuxent Pkwy, Ste. 420
Columbia, MD 21044
(410) 964–8000
(800) 221–SIDS

The Compassionate Friends
P. O. Box 3696
Oak Brook, IL 60522–3696
(708) 990–0010

International Council for Infant Survival
8178 Nadine River Cir.
Fountain Valley, CA 92708
(800) 247–4370

(Offers consolation and information to members of families who have lost a child to sudden infant death syndrome and who may blame themselves for the death)

Resolve through Sharing
La Crosse Lutheran Hospital
1910 South Avenue
La Crosse, WI 54601
(608) 785–0530 ext. 3693

SHARE
St. John's Hospital
800 East Carpenter
Springfield, IL 62769
(217) 544–6464

REFERENCES

1. Nikodem, V., Danziger, D., Gebka, N., & Gulmezoglu, A. (1993, June). Do cabbage leaves prevent breast engorgement? A randomized, controlled study. *Birth, 20*(2), 61–64.

2. Gennaro, S., & Krouse, A. (1996). Patterns of postpartum health in mothers of low birth weight infants. *Health Care for Women International, 17,* 35–45.

3. Rarick, T., & Tchabo, J. (1994, May). Timing of the postpartum Papanicolaou smear. *Obstetrics and Gynecology, 83*(5, Part 1), 761–764.

4. Sampselle, C., & Brink, C. (1990, May/June). Pelvic muscle relaxation: Assessment and management. *Journal of Nurse Midwifery, 35*(3), 127–132.

5. ACOG. 1995. Oct. Pelvic organ prolapse. *ACOG Technical Bulletin* (No. 214), Washington, DC: ACOG.

6. Erwin, P. (1994, January/February). To use or not use combined hormonal oral contraceptives during lactation. *Family Planning Perspectives, 26*(1), 26–30, 33.

7. Hatcher, R. A., Stewart, F., Trussell, J., Koval, D., Guest, F., Stewart, D. K., & Cates, W. (1994). Postpartum contraception and lactation. In *Contraceptive Technology* (16th ed.), pp. 433–452. New York: Irvington.

8. Davis, M. S. (1992). Natural Family Planning. In NAACOG's Clinical Issues in Perinatal and Women's Health Nursing. (3)2:280–292.

9. Reece, E., Homko, C., & Hagay, Z. (1995, July). When the pregnancy is complicated by diabetes. *Contemporary Obstetrics and Gynecology, 40*(7), 43–44, 46, 48, 50, 52, 57–58, 60–61.

10. American Diabetes Association (1996, January). Office guide to diagnosis and classification of diabetes mellitus and other categories of intolerance. *Diabetes Care,* 19 (Suppl. 1) S-29.

11. American Diabetes Association. (1997, July). Report of the expert committee on the diagnosis and classification of diabetes mellitus. *Diabetes Care, 20*(7), 1183–1197.

12. Lubarsky, S., Barton, J., Friedman, S., Nasreddine, S., Ramadan, M., & Sibai, B. (1994, April). Late postpartum eclampsia revisited. *Obstetrics and Gynecology, 83*(4), 502–505.

13. Drulinger, L. (1994, February). Postpartum emergencies. *Emergency Medicine Clinics of North America, 12*(1), 219–237.

14. Cunningham, F. G., MacDonald, P., & Gant, N. (1997). Hypertensive disorders in pregnancy. In *Williams Obstetrics,* (20th ed.) pp. 693–744. Stamford, CT: Appleton & Lange.

15. Akins, S. (1994, March/April). Postpartum hemorrhage: A 90s approach to an age-old problem. *Journal of Nurse Midwifery, 39*(Suppl. 2), 123S–134S.

16. Leonard, R., Robert, K. and O'Grady, J. (1995, April). Postpartum hemorrhage: Working with the anesthesiologist. *Contemporary OB & GYN 40*(4):46–48, 51, 55, 58.

17. Cunningham, F. G., MacDonald, P., & Gant, N. (1997). Infection and disorders of the puerperium. In *Williams Obstetrics,* (20th ed.), pp. 693–744. Stamford, CT: Appleton & Lange.

18. Lawrence, R. (1994). *Breastfeeding: A guide for the medical profession* (4th ed.). St. Louis: C. V. Mosby.

19. NAACOG. (1991, November). Facilitating breastfeeding. *OGN nursing practice resource.* Washington, DC: Author.

20. Scott-Connor, C., & Schorr, S. (1995, October). The diagnosis and management of breast problems during pregnancy and lactation. *The American Journal of Surgery, 170,* 401–405.

21. Calhoun, B., & Brost, B. (1995, June). Emergency management of sudden puerperal fever. *Obstetrics and Gynecology Clinics of North America, 22*(2), 357–367.

22. Fischbach, F. (1996). Microbiologic studies. In *A manual of laboratory and diagnostic tests* (5th ed., pp. 441–511). Philadelphia: Lippincott-Raven.

23. Del Priore, G., Jackson-Stone, M., Shim, E., Garfinkel, J., Eichmann, M., & Frederiksen, M. (1996, June). A comparison of one-daily and 8-hour Gentamicin dosing in the treatment of postpartum endometritis. *Obstetrics and Gynecology, 87*(6), 994–1000.

24. Gerstein, H. (1994). Screening for postpartum thyroid dysfunction. *Comprehensive Therapy, 20*(6), 331–335.

25. Bishnoi, A., & Sachmechi, I. (1996, January). Thyroid disease in pregnancy. *American Family Physician, 53*(1), 215–220.

26. Cunningham, F. G., MacDonald, P., & Gant, N. (1997). Endocrine disorders. In *Williams obstetrics* (20th ed., pp. 1223–1238). Stamford, CT: Appleton & Lange.

27. Solomon, B., Fein, H., & Smallridge, R. (1993, February). Usefulness of antimicrosomal antibody titers in the diagnosis and treatment of postpartum thyroiditis. *Journal of Family Practice, 36*(2), 177–182.

28. Fischbach, F. (1996). Nuclear medicine studies. In *A manual of laboratory and diagnostic tests* (5th ed., pp. 617–682). Philadelphia, PA: Zippincott.

29. Brennan, D. F. (1989, January). Postpartum abdominal pain. *Annals of Emergency Medicine, 18*(1), 83–89.

30. Stover, A., & Marnefon, J. (1995, October). Post-partum care. *American Family Physician, 52*(5), 1465–1472.

31. Solomon, G. (1996, April 25). Length of hospital stay for mothers and newborns. Letter to the editor. *N Engl J. Med, 334*(17), 1134.

32. Parisi, V., Meyer, B., & Maffetone, M. (1996, April 25). Length of hospital stay for mothers and newborns. Letter to the editor. *N Engl J Med, 334*(17), 1135.

33. Margolis, L., & Kotelchuk, M. (1996, January/February). Midwives, physicians, and the timing of maternal postpartum discharge. *Journal of Nurse Midwifery, 41*(1), 29–35.

34. American Academy of Pediatrics, American College of Obstetricians and Gynecologists. (1992). *Guidelines for prenatal care* (pp. 107–111). Elk Grove Village, IL: American Academy of Pediatrics.

35. Soskolne, E., Schumacher, R., Fyock, C., Young, M., & Schork, A. (1996, April). The effect of early discharge and other factors on readmission rates of newborns. *Archives of Pediatric and Adolescent Medicine, 150,* 373–379.

36. Bakoula, C., Kafritsa, Y., Kavadias, G., Lazopoulou, D., Theodoridou, M., Maravelias, K., and Matsaniotis, N. (1995, July 25). Objective passive smoking indicators and respiratory morbidity in young children. *Lancet, 346*(8970): 280–281.

37. Klonoff-Cohen, H., Edelstein, S., Lefkowitz, E., Srinivasan, I., Kaegi, D., Chang, J., & Wiley, K. (1995, March 8). The effect of passive smoking and tobacco exposure through breast milk on sudden infant death syndrome. *JAMA, 273*(10): 795–798.

38. Long, C., and Barron, D. (1992, September, October). SIDS and infant positioning: implications for critical care. *Pediatric Nursing, 18*(5): 524–528.

39. Dwyer, T., Ponsonby, A., Blizzard, L., Neuman, N., & Cochrane, J. (1995, March 08). The contribution of changes in the prevalence of prone sleeping position to the decline in sudden infant death syndrome in Tasmania, *JAMA, 273*(10): 783–789.

40. Barnard, K. (1978). *Learning resource manual.* Seattle, WA: University of Washington, Nursing Child Assessment Satellite Training.

41. Mercer, R. T. (1983). Parent-infant attachment. In L. Sonstegard, K., Kowalski, & B. Jennings (Eds.). *Women's health: Vol. II. Childbearing* (pp. 17–42). New York: Grune & Stratton.

42. Cranley, M. S. (1981). Roots of attachment: The relationship of parents with their unborn. In *Birth defects: Original article series, 17*(6), 59–82. March of Dimes Birth Defects Foundation.

43. Cropley, C. (1986). Assessment of mothering behaviors. In S. H. Johnson (Ed.), *Nursing assessment and strategies for the family at risk* 2nd ed., pp. 15–40. Philadelphia: Lippincott.

44. Davis, M., & Akridge, K. (1987, November/December). The effect of promoting intrauterine attachment in primiparas on postpartum attachment. *JOGNN, 16*(6), 430–437.

45. Mercer, R. T. (1985, July/August). Process of maternal role attainment over the first year. *Nursing Research, 34*(4), 198–204.

46. Mercer, R. (1990). *Parents at risk.* New York: Springer Publishing Company.

47. Mercer, R. T. & Ferketich, S. (1990, March). Predictors of parental attachment during early parenthood. *Journal of Advanced Nursing, 15*(3), 268–280.

48. Muller, M. (1996, February). Prenatal and postnatal attachment: a modest correlation. *Journal of Obstetric, Gynecologic, and Neonatal Nursing, 25*(2): 161–166.

49. Klaus, M., & Kennell, J. (1983). Adjusting to malformation. In *Bonding: The Beginnings of parent-infant attachment* (pp. 140–161). St. Louis: C. V. Mosby.

50. Sokol, M. (1995, January). Creating a community of caring for families with special needs. *Journal of Obstetric, Gynecologic, and Neonatal Nursing, 24*(1), 64–70.

51. Merilo, K. (1988, May–June). Is it better the second time around? *MCN, 13*(3), 200–204.

52. Sammons, L. N. (1990). Psychological aspects of second pregnancy. In S. Flagler (Ed.), *Psychological aspects of pregnancy: Vol. 1(3), NAACOG's clinical issues in perinatal and women's health care* (pp. 317–324). Philadelphia: Lippincott.

53. Tiller, C. (1995, July/August). Thather's parenting attitudes during a child's first year. *Journal of Obstetric, Gynecologic, and Neonatal Nursing, 24*(6), 508–514.

54. Cunningham, F. G., MacDonald, P., & Gant, N. (1997). The puerperium. In *Williams obstetrics* (20th ed.), pp. 533–546). Stamford, CT: Appleton & Lange.

55. Zeidenstein, L. (1990, January/February). Gynecological and childbearing needs of lesbians. *Journal of Nurse Midwifery, 35*(1), 10–18.

56. Harvey, S. M., Carr, C., & Bernheine, S. (1989, May/June). Lesbian mothers: Health care experiences. *Journal of Nurse Midwifery, 34*(3), 115–119.

57. Boston Women's Health Book Collective. (1992). *The new our bodies, ourselves: A book by and for women.* New York: Touchstone.

58. Loring, M., & Smith, R. (1994, May/June). Health care barriers and intervention for battered women. *Public Health Reports, 109*(3), 328–338.

59. Bastin, N., Tamayo, O. W., Tinkle, M., Amaya, M. S., Treejo, L. R., & Herera, C. (1992, March/April). HIV disease in pregnancy: Part 3. Postpartum care of the HIV-positive woman and her newborn. *Journal of Obstetric, Gynecologic, and Neonatal Nursing, 21*(2), 105–111.

60. Enfantis, J. (1990). In-patient maternity care for the HIV-positive woman and her newborn. In B. P. Sinclair, & A. M. McCormick (Eds.), *AIDS in women: Vol 1(1). NAACOG's clinical issues in perinatal and women's health care* (pp. 47–52). Philadelphia: Lippincott.

61. The Jacobs Institute of Women's Health Care. (1995). Violence against women. In J. Horton (Ed.), *The women's health data book* (3rd ed., pp. 121–127). Washington, DC: Author.

62. Quillian, J. (1996, April). Screening for spousal or partner abuse in a community health setting. *Journal of the American Academy of Nurse Practitioners, 8*(4), 155–160.

63. Norton, D. & Ridenour, N. (1995, March). Homeless women and children: The challenge of health promotion. *Nurse Practitioner Forum, 6*(1), 29–33.

64. Quillian, J. (1995, July). Domestic violence. *Journal of the American Academy of Nurse Practitioners, 7*(7), 351–356.

65. Kemper, K. (1995). Psychosocial screening. In Parker, S. & Zackerman, B. (Eds.). *Behavioral and Developmental Pediatrics* (pp. 30–34). Boston: Little, Brown and Company.

66. McFarlane, J., & Parker, B. (1994). Abuse during pregnancy: A protocol for prevention and intervention. In K. Damus & M. Freda (Eds.), *Abuse during pregnancy* (pp. 14–40). White Plains, NY: March of Dimes Foundation.

67. Newberger, E. (1995). Physical abuse. In Parker, S. & Zuckerman, B. (Eds.). *Behavioral and Developmental Pediatrics* (pp. 232–238). Boston: Little, Brown and Company.

68. Yan, M. (1995). Wife abuse: Strategies for a therapeutic response. *Scholarly Inquiry for Nursing Practice: An International Journal, 9*(2), 147–158.

69. Robert Wood Johnson Foundation. (1991). *Challenges in health care: A chartbook perspective 1991* (pp. 80–81). Princeton, NJ: Author.

70. Bachrach, L. L. (1987). Homeless women: A context for health care. *The Milbank Quarterly, 65*(3), 371–396.

71. Drake, M. A. (1992, May–June). The nutritional status and dietary adequacy of single homeless women and their children in shelters. *Public Health Reports, 107*(3), 312–319.

72. Wiecha, J. L., Dwyer, J. T., & Dunn-Strohecker, M. (1991, July–August). Nutrition and health services needs among the homeless. *Public Health Reports, 106*(4), 364–374.

73. Campbell, J. (1992). Parenting classes: Focus on discipline. *Journal of Community Health Nursing, 9*(4), 197–207.

74. Brazelton, T. B. (1992). Discipline. In *Touchpoints* (pp. 252–260). New York: Addison-Wesley.

75. Sieving, R., & Zirbel-Donisch, S. (1990, November/December). Development and enhancement of self-esteem in children. *Journal of Pediatric Health Care, 4*(6), 290–296.

76. Casiano, M. E. (1990). Outpatient management of postpartum psychiatric disorders. In D. M. Semprevivo (Ed.), *Postpartum depression: Vol. 1(3), NAACOG's clinical issues in perinatal and women's health* (pp. 395–401). Philadelphia: Lippincott.

77. Schaper, A., Rooney, B., Kay, N., & Silva, P. (1994, August). Use of the Edinburgh postnatal depression scale to identify postpartum depression in a clinical setting. *Journal of Reproductive Medicine, 39*(8), 620–624.

78. Leopold, K. & Zoschnick. (1997, August). Postpartum depression. *The Female Patient, 22:* 40–44, 47–49.

79. Boyer, D. (1990). Prediction of postpartum depression. In D. M. Semprevivo (Ed.), *Postpartum depression: Vol. 1(3), NAACOG's clinical issues in perinatal and women's health nursing* (pp. 359–368). Philadelphia: Lippincott.

80. Alley, S., O'Donnell, J., & Bope, E. (1995, October). Postpartum depression. *The Female Patient, 20:* 17–18, 20, 59–60.

81. Stowe, Z., and Nemeroff, C. (1995, August). Women at risk for postpartum-onset major depression. American Journal of Obstetrics and Gynecology, 173-(2): 639–645.

82. Barnet, B., Joffe, A., Duggan, A., Wilson, M., & Repke, J. (1996, January). Depressive symptoms,

stress, and social support in pregnant and post-partum adolescents. *Archive of Pediatric and Adolescent Medicine, 150:* 64–69.

83. Panzarine, S., Slater, E., & Sharps, P. (1995, August). Coping, social support, and depressive symptoms in adolescent mothers. *Journal of Adolescent Health Care, 17*(2): 113–119.

84. Kumar, R. (1990). An overview of postpartum psychiatric disorders. In D. M. Semprevivo (Ed.), *Postpartum depression: Vol. 1(3). NAACOG's clinical issues in perinatal and women's health nursing* (pp. 351–358). Philadelphia: Lippincott.

85. Harris, B., Huckle, P., Thomas, R., Johns, S., & Fung, H. (1989). The use of rating scales to identify post-natal depression. *British Journal of Psychiatry, 154,* 813–817.

86. Hannah, P., Adams, D., Lee, A., Glover, V., & Sandler, M. (1992, June). Links between early post-partum mood and post-natal depression. *British Journal of Psychiatry, 160,* 777–780.

87. Beck, C. (1995, September/October). The effects of postpartum depression on maternal-infant interaction: A meta-analysis. *Nursing Research, 44*(5): 298–304.

88. Briggs, G., Freeman, R., & Yaffe, S. (1994). *Drugs in Pregnancy and Lactation* (4th ed.). Baltimore, MD: Williams & Wilkins.

89. Cunningham, F. G., MacDonald, N. G., & Gant, N. (1989). Obstetrics in broad perspective. In *Williams Obstetrics* (18th ed., pp. 1–6). East Norwalk, CT: Appleton & Lange.

90. Rubin, R. (1984). *Maternal identity and the maternal experience.* New York: Springer Publishing Company.

91. U.S. Bureau of the Census. (1995). *Statistical abstract of the United States* (115th ed., no. 1363). Washington, DC: Author.

92. Horton, J. (Ed.). (1995). Reproductive health. In *The women's health data book* (2nd ed., pp. 1–30). Washington, DC: The Jacob's Institute of Women's Health.

93. U.S. Bureau of the Census. (1995). *Statistical abstract of the United States* (115th ed., No. 120). Washington, DC: Author.

94. Lynch, M. (1989, March/April). Congenital defects: Parental issues and nursing supports. *Journal of Perinatal and Neonatal Nursing, 2*(4), 53–59.

95. Limbo, R., & Wheeler, S. R. (1986). *When a baby dies: A handbook for healing and helping.* LaCrosse: Gunderson Clinic, Ltd.

96. Cunningham, F. G., MacDonald, P., & Gant, N. (1997). Abortion: In *Williams obstetrics* (20th

ed., pp. 579–606). East Norwalk, CT: Appleton & Lange.

97. Kennell, J., Slyter, H., & Klaus, M. (1970, August 13). The mourning responses of parents to the death of a newborn infant. *NEJM, 283*(7), 344–349.

98. Wallerstedt, C. & Higgins, P. (1996, June). Facilitating perinatal grieving between the mother and father. *JOGNN, 25*(5): 389–394.

99. Limbo, R., & Wheeler, S. R. (1986). Coping with unexpected outcomes. In *NAACOG update series: Vol. 5 (Lesson 3).* Princeton, NJ: Continuing Professional Education Center.

100. Szgalsky, J. (1989, October). Perinatal death, the family, and the role of the health professional. *Neonatal Network, 8*(2), 15–19.

101. Staudacher, C. (1987). Surviving the loss of a child. In *Beyond grief: A guide for recovering from the death of a loved one* (pp. 99–126). Oakland, CA: New Harbinger.

102. Orlando, S. (1995, September). The immunologic significance of breast milk. *Journal of Obstetric, Gynecologic, and Neonatal Nursing, 24*(7), 678–683.

103. Goldfarb, J. (1993, March). Breastfeeding: AIDS and other infectious diseases. *Clinics in Perinatology, 20*(1), 225–243.

104. Newman, J. (1990, February). Breastfeeding problems associated with the early introduction of bottles and pacifiers. *Journal of Human Lactation, 6*(2), 59–63.

105. Blackburn, S., & Loper, N. (1992). The postpartum and lactation physiology. In *Maternal, fetal and neonatal physiology: A clinical perspective* (pp. 136–155). Philadelphia: W. B. Saunders.

106. Shrago, L. (1990, May/June). The infant's contribution to breastfeeding. *JOGNN, 19*(3), 209–215.

107. Mohrbacher, N., & Stock, J. (1991, August). *The breastfeeding answer book.* Franklin Park, IL: La Leche League International.

108. Dewey, K., Heinig, J., & Nommsen-Rivers, L. (1995, May). Differences in morbidity between breast-fed and formula-fed infants. *Journal of Pediatrics, 126*(5, Part 1), 696–702.

109. Schulz-Lell, G., Buss, R., Oldigs, H. D., Dörner, K., & Schaub, J. (1987, July). Iron balances in infant nutrition. *ACTA Paediatrica Scandinavica, 76*(4), 585–591.

110. Speroff, L., Glass, R. H., & Kase, N. G. (1994). The breast. In *Clinical gynecologic endocrinology and infertility* (5th ed., pp. 547–582). Baltimore: Williams & Wilkins.

111. American College of Obstetricians and Gynecologists. (1992, June). *Human immunodeficiency*

virus infections (Technical Bulletin, No. 169). Washington, DC: Author.

112. Milligan, R., Flenniken, P., & Pugh, L. (1996, May). Positioning intervention to minimize fatigue in breastfeeding women. *Applied Nursing Research, 9*(2), 67–70.

113. Sollid, D., Evans, B., McClowry, S., & Garrett, A. (1989, July). Breastfeeding multiples. *Journal of Perinatal and Neonatal Nursing, 3*(1), 46–65.

114. Anderson, P. (1993, January). Medication use while breastfeeding a neonate. *Neonatal Pharmacology Quarterly, 2*(2), 3–14.

115. Toll, L. (1990, June). A review of the new AAP guidelines of drugs and human milk. *Journal of Human Lactation, 6*(2), 73–74.

116. Bronner, Y. L., & Paige, D. M. (1992, March/April). Current concepts in infant nutrition. *Journal of Nurse-Midwifery, 37*(Suppl. 2): 43S–58S.

117. Hill, P., & Aldag, J. (1996). Smoking and breast-feeding status. *Research in Nursing and Health, 19,* 125–132.

118. Hansen, B., & Moore, L. (1989, December). Recreational drug use by the breastfeeding woman. *Journal of Human Lactation, 5*(4), 178–180.

119. Zinamon, M. J. (1987, October). Breast pumps: Ensuring mothers' success. *Contemporary OB/GYN, 30*(Special Issue), 55–57, 60–62.

120. Walker, M. (1987, July–August). How to evaluate breast pumps. *MCN, 12*(4): 270–276.

121. Auerbach, K. (1990, January/February). Assisting the employed breast-feeding mother. *Journal of Nurse Midwifery, 35*(1), 26–34.

122. Darby, M., & Loughead, J. (1996, March/April). Neonatal nutritional requirements and formula composition: A review. *Journal of Obstetric, Gynecologic, and Neonatal Nursing, 25*(3), 209–217.

PRIMARY CARE CONDITIONS AFFECTING WOMEN'S HEALTH

IV

CHAPTER 21

COMMON MEDICAL PROBLEMS: CARDIOVASCULAR THROUGH HEMATOLOGICAL DISORDERS

Elaine Ferrary • Judy Parker-Falzoi

*C*oronary artery disease was once considered a male affliction, although women are now recognized to be at equal, and in some circumstances, greater risk. Men and women however, may differ in onset, distribution, and presentation of this disease.

Highlights

- Cardiovascular Disorders
- Dermatoses
- Ear, Nose, and Throat Disorders
- Endocrine Disorders
- Gastrointestinal Disorders
- Hematological Disorders

► INTRODUCTION

A number of disorders or medical problems are seen in practice that are clinically significant to women or are normal in any general population. It is, of course, beyond the scope of this text to touch on all medical concerns. But an effort has been made in this edition to expand and discuss subjects of interest to primary care providers. For convenience, coverage of these common concerns—listed alphabetically by medical area—has been divided into Chapters 21 and 22. In Chapter 21 cardiovascular disorders; dermatoses; ear, nose, and throat disorders; endocrine disorders; gastrointestinal disorders; and hemato-

logical disorders are covered. In Chapter 22 musculoskeletal injuries, neurological disorders, ophthalmologic disorders, pulmonary disorders, and urinary tract disorders are discussed. Chapter references provide guidance in finding more in-depth information, and the index should be consulted for the location of specific problems.

The provider's level of comfort and competence in managing medical problems depends on experience, medical resources, location of practice, access to diagnostic testing, practice protocols, and scope of practice.

CARDIOVASCULAR DISORDERS

The four cardiovascular disorders considered here are coronary artery disease, hyperlipidemia, hypertension, and mitral valve prolapse.

CORONARY ARTERY DISEASE

Coronary artery disease (CAD) is caused by altered blood flow in the coronary arteries and, consequently, reduced oxygenation of the myocardium. Myocardial ischemia occurs when oxygen demand exceeds oxygen supply. The supply-demand balance may be disturbed by coronary atherosclerosis, vasospasm, thrombus formation, or cardiomyopathy.

Epidemiology

Coronary artery disease was once considered a male affliction, although women are now recognized to be at equal and, in some circumstances, greater risk.[1,2,3,4] Men and women, however, may differ in the onset, distribution, and presentation of this disease.

The incidence of coronary artery disease is distributed throughout the population. It is the leading cause of death in women older than 50. More than 500,000 Americans die each year of heart attacks. Almost half are women.[2] CAD is the most common cause of heart attacks. It is more prevalent among minorities, particularly African Americans.

Modifiable Risk Factors. Factors that may influence the development of CAD include cigarette smoking, obesity, physical inactivity, hypertension, and hyperlipidemia.

Cigarette smoking is largely responsible for cardiovascular events in premenopausal women.[1,2,5] It increases the risk of CAD two to three times that of a nonsmoker, but the risk is reversible within a year of cessation of smoking. Smoking low-tar and low-nicotine cigarettes does not reduce the risk of cardiovascular events. With the substantial increase in the number of women smoking, the incidence of CAD is rising. Moreover, women who smoke *and* use oral contraceptives are more likely to have a heart attack.[2,4,5] In addition, the use of estrogens by smokers may exacerbate the chance of thrombus formation.

Obesity also presents a formidable risk. Clients who are more than 30 percent overweight are more likely to develop heart disease even if it is their only risk factor.[1,2,4,6]

Physical inactivity—a sedentary lifestyle—contributes to CAD by unfavorably altering serum lipid ratios.

Hypertension and hyperlipidemia and their specific contributions to risk are discussed later under Cardiac Disease.

Nonmodifiable Risk Factors. Nonmodifiable risk factors for CAD are family history, age, gender, and diabetes.

A strong family history of CAD is significant. Early sudden cardiac death of a first-degree relative warrants a more aggressive approach in controlling modifiable risk factors, even if the client is asymptomatic.[1,2,3]

Age and gender differences are difficult to distinguish because research studies on women and cardiovascular disease are inadequate. Current research shows that the average age of onset of CAD among men is between 40 and 44 years. Women tend not to develop heart problems until after menopause, most likely because of the cardioprotective effects of estrogen. After menopause the risk of CAD increases steadily. If menopause is iatrogenic (the uterus and ovaries are surgically removed), the risk of a heart attack rises more sharply than if menopause occurs naturally. Exogenous estrogen replacement after menopause may reduce the risk of cardiovascular events by as much as 50 percent.[2,4] (Also refer to Chapter 15, Estrogen Replacement Therapy.)

Morbidity and mortality associated with myocardial infarction are higher among women, because of the failure to identify CAD earlier in women. Anginal symptoms more likely are attributed to noncardiac causes.[4]

Diabetes mellitus not only increases the risk of CAD, but is a major predictor of mortality following a myocardial infarction.

Subjective Data

Women are likely to report chest pain (angina) as their first symptom. Men typically present with a myocardial infarction or sudden cardiac death. A thorough history includes the onset, character, location, radiation, frequency, duration, precipitating factors, relieving factors, and associated symptoms. If the client reports a clear relationship between her symptoms and physical exertion, a cardiac origin is highly suspected.

Intensity of pain does not always correlate with severity of disease. Angina may be described as a minor ache or crushing chest pain. Clients may relate only associated symptoms such as dyspnea and diaphoresis with exertion. Treatment of silent ischemia is based more on objective than on subjective findings.

Objective Data

Physical Examination. May reveal nothing abnormal; however, signs of CAD may include the following:

- *General Appearance.* Obese, anxious, dyspneic.
- *Vital Signs.* High or low blood pressure, tachycardia or bradycardia, fever.
- *Skin.* Cyanosis, diaphoresis.
- *Eyes.* Arcus senilis, xanthomas, hypertensive retinopathy.
- *Neck.* Jugular venous distention, carotid bruits.
- *Chest.* Rales, rhonchi, wheezes, or diminished breath sounds.
- *Heart.* Murmurs, gallops, rubs, clicks, irregular rhythms, displaced point of maximal impulse (PMI), heaves, and thrills.
- *Vascular System.* Absent or diminished peripheral pulses, edema, mottling.
- *Abdomen.* Hepatomegaly, bruits.

Diagnostic Tests. Laboratory testing includes a *CBC* and *kidney and liver function tests* to determine underlying disease and identify risk factors.

The chest x-ray assists in differential diagnosis and in evaluating the progress of disease. It may reveal increased pulmonary markings or cardiomegaly.

Electrocardiography (ECG) permits myocardial ischemic changes to be seen in ST segment elevation or, more commonly, depression. Dysrhythmias, such as atrial fibrillation or atrial flutter, may be detected. This noninvasive test is essential to detection of myocardial ischemia; however, a normal ECG does not rule out diagnosis of infarction or ischemia. The procedure lacks specificity and sensitivity in women, particularly younger women, those with atypical chest pain and breast attenuation.[1,2,4]

Exercise tolerance testing (ETT), a stress test, identifies the location of ischemic vessels by recording the changes that occur during exercise on an ECG. When evidence of ischemia is presented early in testing, the likelihood of multivessel involvement is increased. Approximately 40 percent of women have a false-positive reading.[4,6]

Nuclear perfusion studies have low false-positive rates in women when corrected for breast attenuation.[2] Pharmacologic studies are recommended when exercise testing does not yield conclusive information or the client is deconditioned or disabled, prohibiting her from sustaining a level of exertion necessary to complete the testing. A day is usually required to complete the test.

Cardiac catheterization, is the most definitive test to determine the location and extent of CAD. In experienced laboratories it is performed with low mortality (0.2 percent) or severe vascular complications (0.7 percent).[6] A catheter is threaded through to the coronary vessels retrograde usually from the femoral arteries.

The client should anticipate an overnight stay and that a standard preoperative workup is done. Specific preoperative and postoperative teaching should be done by the cardiologist or designated staff member.

Echocardiography is the most sensitive, noninvasive diagnostic test used to measure cardiac size and function. It determines abnormalities in the motion of the myocardium, abnormalities in structure and ventricular function, and hypertrophy. The procedure is noninvasive. In the future, exercise echocardiograms may be more sensitive in detecting CAD than stationary echocardiograms or electrocardiograms.[2,4,6]

Differential Medical Diagnoses

Thoracic outlet syndrome, mitral valve prolapse, anemia, substance abuse, costochondritis, gastroesophageal reflux disorder, panic disorder.

Plan

As interventions are employed, continued surveillance of symptoms, medications, and risk factors is required.

Psychosocial Interventions. Provide anticipatory guidance about diagnostic testing and the nature of the disease. Assist clients in gaining a sense of control over the disease through risk reduction. Clients need to know the risks and benefits of all treatment options to make informed decisions about their lives and health.

Medication. Coupled with a reduction in modifiable risk factors, medication is a viable option for up to two thirds of clients with CAD. In weighing medical against surgical intervention, the key factors are the extent and location of damage.[1,2,3,4,6]

- *Nitrates.* Nitrates may be used independently or with other medications. Nitrates are used as an antianginal agent because of their vasodilating effect.
  - *Administration.* Sublingual, topical, transdermal, and oral (long-acting or chewable tablet) forms are available. The sublingual form acts within 15 seconds and has a 15- to 30-minute duration of action. Ointments and transdermal patches may last 12 hours or longer.
  - *Side Effects.* Headaches are common. They may be relieved by changing the dosage, route of administration, or if taken with acetaminophen. Other reactions to nitrates are hypotension, dizziness, and palpitations.
  - *Contraindications.* Do not administer to clients with severe hypotension.
  - *Anticipated Outcome on Evaluation.* Anginal episodes decrease or are eliminated.
  - *Client Teaching.* Include information about all possible side effects and indications for intermittent use of nitrates as needed.

- *Aspirin.* Aspirin lowers the risk of myocardial infarctions in persons at increased risk for atherosclerosis and thrombogenesis, including persons who have had a myocardial infarction, unstable angina, or postcoronary artery bypass grafting.[1,2,6] Aspirin inhibits platelet aggregation and prevents formation of arterial thrombi on atherosclerotic plaques. It is recommended for men at risk for CAD or for men older than 40 with known cardiac disease; aspirin appears to have the same therapeutic benefits for women. It is considered prudent therapy for women with known cardiac disease.[1,2]
  - *Administration.* One enteric coated 325-mg aspirin is taken daily.
  - *Side Effects.* Gastrointestinal upset and bleeding.
  - *Contraindications.* Do not administer to clients with ulcerative disease and coagulopathies.
  - *Anticipated Outcomes on Evaluation.* Progression of atherosclerotic disease slows,

and the likelihood of thrombolic events decreases.

- *Client Teaching.* Include information about the side effects of aspirin. Medication needs to be used consistently to be an effective preventive measure.

- **β-*Adrenergic Receptor Antagonists.*** Beta blockers may be indicated for hypertension and ischemic heart disease. These drugs attenuate increased blood pressure and heart rate during activity, thereby decreasing the workload of the heart. They have been shown to decrease mortality postmyocardial infarction.[2,3]

  - *Administration.* The new β_1 selective agents block myocardial receptors with little effect on bronchial or smooth vascular muscle—a benefit to those with asthma or claudication.[1]
  - *Side Effects.* Depression, impotence, peripheral vascular ischemia, and palpitations are known to occur. The beta blocker may decrease the effectiveness of other medications such as oral hyperglycemic agents.
  - *Contraindications.* Do not administer to clients with heart failure, sick sinus syndrome with atrioventricular block, bradycardia (fewer than 50 beats per minute), and asthma.
  - *Anticipated Outcomes on Evaluation.* Symptoms of angina, as well as blood pressure, decrease.
  - *Client Teaching.* Plan to continue indefinitely. Review, and encourage client to report any side effects at all visits.

- *Calcium Channel Blockers.* Calcium channel blockers decrease vascular resistance, thereby increasing blood flow. They are also used for hypertension. Some calcium channel blockers are used for rate control in specific cardiac arrhythmias. Eighty percent of the dose is orally absorbed, but because of extensive hepatic metabolism, a much smaller dose reaches the systemic circulation.

  - *Side Effects.* Side effects are specific to the agent and include hypotension, dizziness, constipation, headache, and peripheral edema.
  - *Contraindications.* Use with caution if clients have hypotension, heart failure, and slow or altered cardiac conduction.
  - *Anticipated Outcomes on Evaluation.* Episodes of angina and blood pressure decrease.

- *Client Teaching.* Make clear to the client that calcium channel blockers are more expensive than other antihypertensive medications, but are usually effective with qd or bid dosing and are associated with fewer side effects.

Surgical and Other Interventions. In percutaneous transluminal coronary angioplasty (PTCA), a balloon is introduced into an artery and inflated at the site of an atherosclerotic plaque. In dilating the vessel, the balloon flattens the plaque against the arterial wall, reducing its thickness. About one third of arteries restenose. Complications include acute restenosis or vessel dissection, with the possibility of open heart surgery or death.[3,4,6]

Coronary artery bypass grafting (CABG) is performed for select groups of clients with multivessel disease, left main coronary artery disease, or ventricular aneurysm. Generally, anginal symptoms markedly improve and improvement persists at least 10 years. Surgical risks may be increased or decreased, depending on the extent of disease and the presence of other underlying medical problems at the time of surgery.[4,6]

Lifestyle/Dietary Changes. Such changes can dramatically reduce morbidity and mortality. Primary prevention focuses on modifying risk factors: hypertension, hyperlipidemia, cigarette smoking, obesity, and physical inactivity.[1,2,3,4,7] Advise the client to follow a low-cholesterol and low-fat diet (see Hyperlipidemia).

Physical activity is tailored to the individual client, considering her overall physical condition and cardiac history. Advise the client to avoid exertional activities during extreme weather conditions or after a heavy meal. The client should always carry nitroglycerin and alert the health care provider to any change in symptoms. Advise the client about cardiac rehabilitation programs, especially if she is having difficulty returning to an acceptable level of physical activity.

Cigarette smoking is a significant risk factor and should be discontinued.[5] Involve the client in a smoking cessation program.

HYPERLIPIDEMIA

Hyperlipidemia is an increased plasma lipid concentration of cholesterol, triglycerides, or both. Water-insoluble lipids are carried in the bloodstream by lipoproteins, which are complex molecules made up partly of cholesterol and tri-glycerides. Lipoproteins transport both dietary and endogenous lipids from sites of absorption or synthesis to sites of storage or metabolism.

High levels of low-density lipoprotein are injurious to the vascular intima and lead to the deposition of cholesterol. This and other thrombotic events combine to form atherosclerotic plaques within the vessel, narrowing the lumen and eventually reducing blood flow to many tissues.[8]

Classification of Lipoproteins

Four principal classes of lipoproteins have been determined.[8]

- Chylomicrons are the major transporters of dietary triglycerides.
- Very low density lipoproteins (VLDLs) are responsible for the transport of endogenous triglycerides.
- Low density lipoproteins (LDLs) are the major transporter of cholesterol.
- High density lipoproteins (HDLs) collect cholesterol from the tissues to return it to the liver, thereby acquiring the pseudonym "good cholesterol."

Epidemiology

Genetic factors and lifestyle are major forces in the development of hyperlipidemia.

Risk factors are a high-fat diet, genetic predisposition, sedentary lifestyle, cigarette smoking, and underlying diseases (diabetes mellitus, hypothyroidism, chronic renal disease, liver or gastrointestinal disorders). These may all contribute to an alteration in lipid values.

Levels of LDLs and HDLs are predictors of risk (see Table 21–1). Although LDL level is a powerful predictor of CAD in men, HDL level appears to be a better predictor of risk for CAD in women. Even with a higher average total cholesterol and higher LDL levels, women have fewer cardiovascular events than men, possibly due to their higher HDL levels.[2,8,9] A ratio of 4 or less is considered acceptable; a ratio of 6 or above warrants an aggressive approach.[8,9] Research is almost exclusively based on men; until further studies of women are completed, it is considered clinically prudent to apply to women the same

recommendations used in the care of men. Hyperlipidemia can occur in pregnant women. Treatment is usually not indicated. Follow-up at 6 months postpartum or at cessation of breastfeeding is recommended.

Hyperlipidemia occurs in 25 percent of the U.S. adult population.[8,9]

Subjective Data

The client reports a first-degree relative with known hyperlipidemia, a family history of premature CAD, or a medical condition associated with hyperlipidemia. An extensive diet, exercise, and health belief history is key in assessing the client's current status and future teaching needs.

Objective Data

Although the physical examination may be entirely normal (see Coronary Artery Disease), physical findings that are consistent with hyperlipidemia are obesity, xanthomas, lipemia retinalis, corneal arcus, and hepatosplenomegaly.

Hyperlipidemia Screening. Diagnostic laboratory testing includes screening asymptomatic clients for hyperlipidemia every 5 years (see Table 21–1). It is done more often if there are additional risk factors.

The test procedure, a fasting serum lipid profile study, involves venipuncture, which is more accurate than a fingerstick. The blood sample is drawn after a minimum of 8 hours of fasting. Values that classify clients as moderate to high risk

TABLE 21–1. CLASSIFICATION OF LIPIDS

	Level (mg/dL)		
	Desirable	Borderline	High Risk
Total cholesterol	< 200	200–239	> 240
High density lipoprotein cholesterol	> 40	35–55	< 35
Low density lipoprotein cholesterol	< 130	130–159	> 160
Triglycerides	< 250	250–500	> 500

Source: References 8, 9.

are based on at least two separate studies by venipuncture, drawn 2 months apart. If the difference is less than 30 mg/dL, the two values are averaged. If the difference is more than 30 mg/dL, another sample is obtained and the three values are averaged.[8]

Inform the client that she may drink water when fasting. Fasting is most important in the assessment of hypertriglyceridemia. A random (nonfasting) total cholesterol can be done as a screening measure in low-risk individuals.

The client should understand that every 1 percent decrease in a high serum cholesterol reduces her risk for coronary artery disease by 2 percent. Significantly elevated triglycerides should be treated to prevent pancreatitis.

Differential Medical Diagnoses

Diabetes mellitus; liver disease (obstructive, hepatocellular, or hepatic storage disorder); hypothyroidism; renal disease (nephrosis and renal failure); hormonal imbalance (estrogens, progestins, and androgens); hyperuricemia; acute intermittent porphyria; alcoholism.

Plan

A majority of clients with hyperlipidemia are managed by their primary care provider. Treatment must be individualized with respect to age, risk factors, clinical status, and the presence or extent of CAD (see Table 21–2).

Psychosocial Interventions. Support and encourage clients who are changing their diet and level of physical activity to reduce lipid blood levels. Clients should have realistic expectations and be given objective evidence of their efforts. If medications are indicated, reinforce the information that nonpharmacological interventions are also essential to lowering lipids. Some individuals may have a genetic predisposition to elevated serum cholesterol and, consequently, have less response to nonpharmacologic interventions. Avoid attributing high levels to noncompliance without adequate evaluation.

Medication. Consider discontinuing medications that may adversely influence lipid levels. Medication chosen to lower lipid levels is specific to the client and the desired effect on lipid profile. Adherence to any drug regimen necessitates that the client be informed of the benefits of the drug, its potential side effects, cost, and convenience. A motivational feedback mechanism is provided by repeated serum cholesterol evaluation, which reflects the progress made.

- *Antioxidants.* Vitamin E and other antioxidants inhibit either oxidation of LDL cholesterol or its uptake into the endothelium of coronary arteries. Reliable research data in this area are lacking. No policy recommendations have been made.[8]
- *Psyllium.* Psyllium hydrophilic mucilloid is the active ingredient in many bulk-forming laxatives (e.g., Metamucil). It binds with cholesterol

TABLE 21–2. RECOMMENDED INTERVENTIONS FOR GROUPS AT RISK FOR CORONARY ARTERY DISEASE

Client Group	Recommendations
1. All adults > 20 years of age	Measure TC[a] every 5 years
2. TC < 200 mg/dL	Desirable range General dietary and risk reduction counseling Repeat in 5 years
3. TC 200–239 mg/dL	Borderline high risk; confirm with fractionated lipid profile
4. If no CAD and fewer than two risk factors	Phase 1 diet Reevaluate in 1 year; goal is to lower LDLs < 160
5. If definite CAD or two risk factors and LDLs > 160	Lower LDLs < 130 by diet
6. If definite CAD or two risk factors and LDLs > 190	Give medication; goal is to lower LDLs < 160 if no CAD or fewer than two risk factors; otherwise lower < 130
7. TC > 240 mg/dL	High risk; same as for groups 3–6

[a]TC, total cholesterol; CAD, coronary artery disease; LDL, low density lipoprotein.
Source: References 8, 12, 19.

for removal via the gut. Psyllium hydrophilic mucilloid is an option for clients with mild to moderately elevated lipid levels and for whom a bulk laxative is indicated. Dosage varies with the individual: Begin with the smallest recommended dose and increase as needed. Drink sufficient fluids to avoid constipation and gas pains.

- *Bile Acid Sequestrants (Cholestyramine and Colestipol).* These agents reduce cholesterol by binding bile acids in the gut.[8,9,10]

  - *Administration.* A powder, which is mixed with a liquid, or chewable bars are taken in two to four divided doses. Usual dosage for cholestyramine is 12–24 g p.o.; for colestipol is 15–30 g.
  - *Side Effects.* Gastrointestinal complaints are common. Bile acid sequestrants may interact with fat-soluble vitamins. Triglycerides tend to increase.
  - *Contraindications.* Do not administer to pregnant women.
  - *Anticipated Outcome on Evaluation.* Both LDL and total cholesterol levels decrease.
  - *Client Teaching.* Usually lower cost than other anticholesterol agents. Require much cooperation on the client's part. Also advise the client that the preparations have a gritty quality and should be taken several hours apart from other medications.

- *Nicotinic Acid (Niacin).* Nicotinic acid reduces cholesterol by inhibiting its synthesis in the liver.[8,9,10]

  - *Administration.* Usual drug dosage is 2–3 g t.i.d. in three divided doses. Start with the smallest dose and gradually increase as tolerated until the desired effect is achieved.
  - *Side Effects.* Pruritus, gastrointestinal distress, and severe flushing are known side effects.
  - *Contraindication.* Do not administer to clients with liver abnormalities.
  - *Anticipated Outcome on Evaluation.* All lipoprotein levels are normal.
  - *Client Teaching.* Advise the client that nicotinic acid is the least expensive of the medications. Flushing, a side effect, may be controlled by not drinking alcohol or warm fluids

and taking one 325-mg aspirin tablet 30 minutes before the nicotinic acid, if there is no contraindication to the use of aspirin.

- *Gemfibrozil (Lopid).* Gemfibrozil is a fibric acid derivative that is indicated primarily to lower plasma triglycerides. It also lowers cholesterol, but to a lesser extent, and may raise high density lipoprotein.[8,9,10]

  - *Administration.* Give 600 mg orally twice daily, 30 minutes prior to a meal.
  - *Side Effect.* Gastrointestinal distress is known to occur.
  - *Contraindications.* Do not administer to clients with impaired renal or hepatic function or to pregnant or breastfeeding women.
  - *Anticipated Outcome on Evaluation.* Total cholesterol decreases, with a greater effect on triglycerides.
  - *Client Teaching.* Counsel the client to be alert for drug interactions.

- *Probucol (Lorelco).* Probucol lowers serum cholesterol levels by reducing low density lipoprotein concentrations.[8]

  - *Administration.* A 500-mg tablet is taken twice daily with meals.
  - *Side Effects.* Probucol is generally well tolerated. Side effects are infrequent; however, diarrhea may occur. Ventricular arrhythmias may be a serious side effect.
  - *Contraindications.* Do not administer to pregnant or breastfeeding clients. Safe use has not been established.
  - *Anticipated Outcomes on Evaluation.* All cholesterol levels, including that of HDL, decrease.
  - *Client Teaching.* Inform the client that a favorable decline in cholesterol levels should be seen in about 2 months. It is generally thought that if probucol is not effective after 4 months, it should be discontinued. Probucol accumulates slowly in adipose tissue and may persist 6 months or longer after the last dose. Advise clients to discontinue use at least 6 months prior to conception.

- *Hydroxymethylglutaryl Coenzyme A (HMG-CoA) Reductase Inhibitors.* These agents reduce cholesterol by inhibiting the enzyme that catalyzes the rate-limiting step in cholesterol synthesis. Slowing down the rate of cholesterol synthesis decreases the release of cholesterol into the bloodstream.[8,9,10]

- *Administration.* These medications are taken once a day with the evening meal or twice daily with meals. Lovastin is usually given as 20–80 mg p.o. in one or two doses; Simvastatin as 40–80 mg p.o. in one or two doses; Pravastatin as 40 mg p.o. in one to two doses. Atorvastatin 10–40 mg p.o. in one dose.
- *Side Effects.* Myalgias and elevated liver enzymes are known side effects; however, the inhibitors are generally well tolerated.
- *Contraindication.* Consult with a physical/ hepatologist when clients have known liver disease. Avoid concommitant use with potentially hepatotoxic drugs, e.g., INH.
- *Anticipated Outcome on Evaluation.* Cholesterol levels decrease.

Surgical Intervention. None known.

Lifestyle Changes. Physical activity might include 30 minutes of aerobic exercise daily to increase HDL levels and facilitate weight loss.

Cigarette smoking increases LDL levels. Encourage your client to discontinue smoking.

Dietary Interventions. Refer to the American Heart Association's progressive dietary plan for hyperlipidemia. Clients may benefit from consultation with a dietitian, especially if the diet becomes more complex with additional restrictions imposed because of other illnesses.[8,10] Dietary measures are safe and cost effective and may eliminate the need for drugs to lower cholesterol.

Phase I of American Heart Association diet calls for considerable restriction of fats and carbohydrates. All family members should be involved. Meet with them collectively or at least with the primary meal provider. Emphasize the foods that can be eaten rather than those that cannot.

- *Fat* intake is reduced to 30 percent or less of the diet. A high-fat diet without cholesterol raises serum cholesterol levels by increasing bile reabsorption from the gut, which, in turn, limits the amount of cholesterol that can be excreted. Decrease saturated fats to 10 percent of caloric intake.
- *Cholesterol* is limited to no more than 300 mg per day.
- *Complex carbohydrates* include water-soluble fiber and are increased in small amounts as tolerated.
- *Weight* is maintained at ideal body weight.
- A *food diary* is recorded to target problem areas and provide feedback for the client and provider.
- A specific *food plan* is described during dietary counseling. For example, recommend mozzarella cheese made with skim milk or any dairy product with less than 1 percent fat. Recommend chicken or fish instead of beef. Offer suggestions on how to cook meat (broil, boil) to reduce fat content.

Phase II of the American Heart Association diet further restricts fat intake to 20 to 25 percent of total calories. Saturated fats are reduced to 6 to 8 percent of total fat intake and cholesterol to 150 to 200 mg per day.

Follow-Up

Ascertain whether the expectation of a 10 to 20 percent decrease in total cholesterol was reached after approximately 6 weeks of dietary modification. Before considering any change in the treatment plan, individuals who have no additional risk factors should continue dietary interventions for at least 6 months. Most medications reduce total cholesterol an average of 20 to 25 percent, and triglycerides 40 to 50 percent, within 6 weeks. Much remains to be learned concerning the management of hyperlipidemia as it relates to age and risk of CAD.

HYPERTENSION

Hypertension (HTN) is a systolic blood pressure (SBP) of 140 mm Hg or greater, a diastolic blood pressure (DBP) of 90 mm Hg or greater, or both on three separate occasions two weeks apart (see Table 21–3).

Epidemiology

Essential hypertension is idiopathic and most common. It affects approximately 50 million

TABLE 21–3. CLASSIFICATION OF BLOOD PRESSURE FOR ADULTS AGED 18 YEARS AND OLDER

Category	Systolic, mm Hg	Diastolic, mm Hg
Normal	< 130	< 85
High normal	130–139	85–89
Hypertension		
Stage 1 (mild)	140–159	90–99
Stage 2 (moderate)	160–179	100–109
Stage 3 (severe)	180–209	110–119
Stage 4 (very severe)	> 210	> 120

Source: The fifth report of the Joint National Committee on Detection, Evaluation, and Treatment of High Blood Pressure (JNCV). (1993). Archives of Internal Medicine, 153.

Americans. Risk factors are a genetic predisposition, age older than 40, minority status, alcoholism, less educated, and/or lower socioeconomic group.[11,12] Although nicotine transiently increases blood pressure, prolonged use is not associated with an increased prevalence of hypertension. Hypertension is the leading risk factor for coronary heart disease, congestive heart failure, stroke, retinopathy, and renal disease.

Women have less hypertension before menopause, possibly due to higher levels of estrogen or lower levels of androgen or because of lower blood volume.[12]

Reversible risk factors include medication, alcohol abuse, excessive dietary sodium, and obesity.

Secondary hypertension, which is uncommon, may be caused by polycystic kidneys, renovascular disease, aortic coarctation, Cushing's syndrome, and pheochromocytoma.

Subjective Data

A client with hypertension is most often asymptomatic but may complain of chest pain, headache, visual or neurological changes. She may report a family or personal medical history of hypertension, diabetes, kidney disease, hypothyroidism, cardiovascular disease, or stroke. Be alert for deviations from usual blood pressure readings or a history of elevated blood pressure. Note results and side effects of previous treatments. Identify risk factors including recent weight gain or loss, changes in exercise or diet, increased sodium, alcohol intake, smoking or recreational drug use. Obtain a complete psychosocial history including socioeconomic status, emotional stress, coping mechanisms, and cultural habits. List all prescription and nonprescription medications that may contribute to hypertension.[11,12,13,14]

Objective Data

Physical Examination. May include the following:

- *General.* Obesity (note pattern), pallor, sweating.
- *Fundoscopic.* Arteriovenous compression or nicking, hemorrhages, exudates, or papilledema.
- *Neck.* Thyroid abnormalities, carotid bruits, jugular/venous distention.
- *Lungs.* Wheezes, rales, or rhonchi.
- *Heart.* Murmurs, rubs, gallops, displaced PMI, regular rate and rhythm.
- *Abdomen.* Bruits, masses, hepato-splenomegaly, or enlarged kidneys.
- *Vascular.* Absent or diminished pulses.
- *Extremities.* Edema, cyanosis, clubbing.

Blood pressure findings that are abnormal are episodic elevations, discrepancies between blood pressures in contralateral arms, and decreased pressures in the lower extremities. Specific measures may be taken to ensure accurate blood pressure readings.

- Seat the client with her arm supported and positioned at the level of her heart.
- Cigarettes should not be smoked or caffeine ingested within 30 minutes of the measurement.
- Have the client rest for about 5 minutes before measuring blood pressure.
- Use appropriate cuff size. The rubber bladder should be two-thirds the size of the arm.
- Check readings in both arms. Note any discrepancies.

Diagnostic Tests. Laboratory tests include a CBC, chemistries to evaluate kidney and liver function, lipid profiles, and urinalysis. These are done to provide baseline values for the selection and surveillance of medications, and monitor for sequelae from hypertension.

The electrocardiogram (ECG) is used to detect left ventricular hypertrophy (LVH), the result of cardiac adaptation to increased pressure and increased afterload imposed by an elevated blood pressure.[11,12,13,14] Left ventricular hypertrophy is a significant independent risk factor of cardiac dysrhythmias, congestive heart failure, and sudden death.

Differential Medical Diagnoses

Pheochromocytoma, thyroid disease, renal disease, Cushing's syndrome, primary aldosteronism, alcoholism, iatrogenic.

Plan

The goal of intervention is to prevent the morbidity and mortality associated with high blood pressure. The severity of hypertension, evidence of target organ damage and other risk factors for cardiovascular and cerebrovascular disease guides intervention.

Psychosocial Interventions. Involve the client in decisions concerning treatment. Acknowledge hypertension as a chronic disease that can be controlled but not cured. Contract with the client for follow-up at predetermined intervals.

Medication. Medication for moderate or severe hypertension decreases potential cardiovascular mortality and morbidity. Clients with mild hypertension benefit from medication in that it arrests the progression to a more severe condition and reduces the risk of cerebrovascular accidents. In individuals with a blood pressure persistently higher than 94 mm Hg, the benefits of drug therapy outweigh the risks[11,12,13,14,15] (see Table 21–4).

Single-dose therapies are usually a first choice to improve compliance and reduce side effects and expense. When choosing a drug, consider concomitant medical problems, e.g., beta blockers can mask hypoglycemic problems in diabetes and worsen asthma; some calcium channel blockers can exacerbate migraines (nifedipine), even though some are used for migraine prophylaxis. Also consider race: African Americans are more likely to respond favorably when diuretics are used with calcium channel blockers.[16,17,18,19,20]

- *Diuretics.* Diuretics reduce blood pressure by decreasing volume and thereby decreasing preload. They are classified by mechanism and site of action.

  Thiazides and sulfonamides are relatively contraindicated in persons with sulfa allergies. These agents may raise lithium blood levels and serum cholesterol. Concomitant administration of nonsteroidal anti-inflammatory drugs may antagonize thiazide or sulfonamide effectiveness or cause electrolyte disturbances and sexual dysfunction.

  Potassium-sparing agents are used with caution with clients who are renal compromised or are using angiotensin converting enzyme inhibitors (ACEI). These agents can also potentiate the effectiveness of ACEI and calcium channel blockers.

  Loop diuretics cause electrolyte disturbances. Potassium supplementation is often required.
- *Angiotensin-Converting Enzyme Inhibitors.* Angiotensin-converting enzyme (ACE) inhibitors are indicated to suppress the renin-angiotensin-aldosterone system. Structure, absorption, and duration of action differ slightly among these drugs. They are particularly effective for congestive heart failure.

  Administer ACE inhibitors once or twice daily. Although they are generally well tolerated, adverse effects may include cough (persistent and nonproductive), angioedema, hypotension, rash (most common with captopril), and hyperkalemia. Monitor renal function. Avoid potassium containing salt substitutes.[16,17]
- *Beta Blockers.* Beta blockers and calcium channel blockers (see Coronary Artery Disease) are also used for hypertension (see Table 21–5). Beta blockers have been shown to decrease morbidity and mortality and remain initial drugs of choice after diuretics.[1]

TABLE 21–4. ANTIHYPERTENSION AGENTS*

Type of Drug	Usual Dosage Range, Total mg/	Doses per Day	Mechanisms	Comments
Initial Therapy∧				
Diuretics				For thiazide and loop diuretics, lower doses and dietary counseling should be used to avoid metabolic changes
Thiazides and related agents			Decreased plasma volume and decreased extracellular fluid volume; decreased cardiac output initially, followed by decreased total peripheral resistance with normalization of cardiac output; long-term effects include slight decrease in extracellular fluid volume	More effective antihypertensive than loop diuretics except in patients with serum creatinine ≥ 221 μmol/L (2.5 mg/OL)
Bendroflumethoazide	2.5–5	1		Hydrochlorothiazide or chlorthalidone is generally preferred; used in most clinical trials
Benzthiazide	12.5–50	1		
Chlorothiazide	125–500	2		
Chlorthalidone	12.5–50	1		
Cyclothiazide	1.0–2	1		
Hydrochlorothiazide	12.5–50	1		
Hydroflumethiazide	12.5–50	1		
Indapamide	2.5–5	1		
Methyclothiazide	2.5–5	1		
Metolazone	0.5–5	1		
Polythiazide	1.0–4	1		
Quinethazone	25.0–100	1		
Trichlormethiazide	1.0–4	1		
Loop diuretics			See thiazides	Higher doses of loop diuretics may be needed for patients with renal impairment or congestive heart failure
Bumetanide	0.5–5	2		Ethacrynic acid is only alternative to patients with allergy to thiazide and sulfur-containing diuretics
Ethacrynic acid	25.0–100	2		
Furosemide	20.0–320	2		
Potassium sparing			Increased potassium resorption Aldosterone antagonist	Weak diuretics
Amiloride	5–10	1 or 2		Used mainly in combination with other diuretics to avoid or reverse hypokalemia from other diuretics
Spironolactone	25–100	2 or 3		Avoid when serum creatinine ≥ 221 μmol/L (2.5 mg/dL)
Triamterene	50–150	1 or 2		May cause hyperkalemia, and this may be exaggerated when combined with ACE inhibitors or potassium supplements
Adrenergic inhibitors			Decreased cardiac output and increased total peripheral resistance; decreased plasma renin activity; atanolol, betaxolol, bisoprolol and metoprolol are cardioselective	Selective agents will also Inhibit Beta-receptors in higher doses, e.g., all may aggravate asthma
Beta-Blockers				
Alenolol	25–100+	1		
Betaxolol	5–40	1		
Bisoprolol	5–20	1		
Metoprolol	50–200	1 or 2		
Metoprolol (extended release)	50–200	1		
Nadolol	20–240+	1		
Propranolol	40–240	2		
Propranolol (long acting)	50–240	1		
Timolol	20–240	2		

TABLE 21–4. ANTIHYPERTENSION AGENTS (CONTINUED)

Type of Drug	Usual Dosage Range, Total mg/	Doses per Day	Mechanisms	Comments
Adrenergic inhibitors (cont.)				
Beta-Blockers with ISA				
Acebutolol	200–1200+	2	Acebutolol cardioselective	No clear advantage for agents with
Carteolol	2.5–10+	1		ISA except in those with
Penbutolol	20–80+	1		bradycardia who must receive a
Pindolol	10–80+	2		Beta-blocker; they produce fewer
				or no metabolic side effects
Alpha-beta Blocker			Same as Beta-blockers, plus	Possibly more effective in blacks
Labetalol	200–1200	2	Alpha$_1$-blockade	than other Beta-blockers
				May cause postural effects,
				titration should be based on
				standing blood pressure
Alpha$_1$-Receptor blockers				
Doxazosin	1.0–16	1	Block postsynaptic	All may cause postural effects;
Prazosin	1.0–20	2 or 3	Alpha$_1$-receptors and	titration should be based on
Terazosin	1.0–20	1	cause vasodilation	standing blood pressure
ACE Inhibitors			Block formation of angiotensin II,	Diuretic doses should be reduced
Benazepril	10.0–40+	1 or 2	promoting vasodilation and	or discontinued before starting
Captopril	12.5–150+	2	decreased aldosterone; also	ACE inhibitors whenever
Cilazapril	2.5–5.0	1 or 2	increased bradykinin and	possible to prevent excessive
Enalapril	2.5–40+	1 or 2	vasodilatory prostaglandins	hypotension
Fosinopril	10.0–40	1 or 2		Reduce dose of those drugs
Lisinopril	5.0–40+	1 or 2		marked with a + in patients
Perindopril	1.0–16+	1 or 2		with serum creatinine ≥ 221
Quinapril	5.0–80+	1 or 2		μmol/L (2.5 mg/OL
Ramipril	1.25–20+	1 or 2		May cause hyperkalemia in
Spirapril	12.5–50	1 or 2		patients with renal impairment
				or in those receiving
				potassium-sparing agents
				Can cause acute renal failure in
				patients with severe bilateral
				renal artery stenosis or severe
				stenosis in artery to solitary
				kidney
Calcium antagonists			Block inward movement of	These agents also block slow
Diltiazem	90–360	3	calcium ion across cell	channels in heart and may
Diltiazem (sustained release)	120–360	2	membrane and cause	reduce sinus rate and produce
Diltiazem (extended release)	180–360	1	smooth-muscle relaxation	heart block
Verapamil	80–480	2		
Verapamil (long acting)	120–480	1 or 2		
Dihydropyridines	2.5–10	1		Dihydropyridines are more potent
Amlodipine	5–20	1		peripheral vasodilators than
Felodipine	2.5–10	2		diltiazem and verapamil and
Isradipine	60–120	3		may cause more dizziness,
Nicardipine	30–120	3		headache, flushing, peripheral
Nifedipine	30–90	1		edema, and tachycardia
Nifedipine (GITS)				

(Continued)

TABLE 21–4. ANTIHYPERTENSION AGENTS (CONTINUED)

Type of Drug	Usual Dosage Range, Total mg/	Doses per Day	Mechanisms	Comments
Supplemental Therapy				
Centrally acting alpha agonists				
Clonidine	0.1–1.2	2	Stimulate central alpha-receptors	Clonidine patch is replaced
Clonidine (patch)∞	0.1–0.3	1 wkly	that inhibit efferent	once/wk
Guanabenz	4–64	2	sympathetic activity	None of these agents should be
Guanfacine	1–3	1		withdrawn abruptly; avoid in
Methyldopa	250–2000	2		patients who do not adhere to
				treatment
Periperal-acting adrenergic antogonists				
Guanadrel	10–75	2	Inhibits catecholamine release	May cause serious orthostatic
Guanethidine	10–100	1	from neuronal storage sites	and exercise-induced
				hypotension
Rauwolfia alkaloids				
Rauwolfia serpentina	50–200	1	Depletion of tissue stores of	
Reserpine	.05–.25	1	catecholamines	
Direct vasodilators				
Hydralazine	50–300	2–4	Direct smooth-muscle	Hydralazine is subject
Minoxidil	2.5–80	1 or 2	vasodilation (primarily	phenotypically determined
			arteriolar)	metabolism (acertylation)
				For both agents, should treat
				concomitantly with diuretic
				and Beta-blocker due to fluid
				retention and reflex
				tachycardia

*In all patients, lifestyle modifications should also be advised. ACE indicates angiotensin-converting enzyme; ISA intrinsic sympathomimatic activity and GITS, gastrointestinal therapeutic system.

∧The lower dose indicated is the preferred initial dose, and the higher dose is the maximum daily dose. Most agents require 2 to 4 weeks for complete efficacy, and more frequent dosage adjustments are not advised except for severe hypertension. The dosage range may differ slightly from the recommended dosage in the *Physicians' Desk Reference* or package insert.

+Indicates drugs that are excreted by the kidney and require dosage reduction in the presence of renal impairment (serum creatinine $\geq$ 221 μmol/L $\geq$ 2.5 mg/OL⎟).

∞Weekly patch is 1, 2, 3, equivalent to 0.1 to 0.3 mg/d/.

A 0.1-mg dose may be given every other day to achieve this dosage.

The fifth report of the Joint National Committee on Detecting, Evaluation, and Treatment of High Blood Pressure. (JNCV). 1993. Archives of Internal Medicine, 153, 154–183.

Figure 21–1 summarizes the management of care, balancing lifestyle changes and medications.

Lifestyle/Dietary Changes. Dietary modification may be an essential lifestyle change. Weight should be kept within 15 percent of desirable weight. Encourage a low fat, low salt diet, high in fiber. Avoid caffeine and encourage smoking cessation.[5] Advise the client to limit alcohol intake.

Physical activity may include a 30-minute aerobic exercise program at least three times a week. The program should be initiated gradually. An overall increase in physical activity is encouraged; the benefits are numerous.

- High-density lipoprotein levels increase.
- Arterial blood pressure decreases.
- Glucose intolerance improves.
- Stress decreases.

Advise the client to stop smoking. Cessation reduces the risk of coronary artery disease. The most successful strategies are those that involve both pharmacological and behavioral methods.[5]

TABLE 21–5. ANTIHYPERTENSIVE DRUG THERAPY: INDIVIDUALIZATION BASED ON SPECIAL CONSIDERATIONS (GUIDELINES FOR SELECTING INITIAL THERAPY)*

Clinical Situation	Preferred	Requires Special Monitoring	Relatively or Absolutely Contraindicated
Cardiovascular			
Angina pectoris	Beta-Blockers, calcium antagonists		Direct vasodilators
Bradycardia/heart block, sick sinus syndrome	. . .		Beta-blockers, labetalol, verapamil, diltiazem
Cardiac failure	Diuretics, ACE inhibitors		Beta-Blockers, calcium antagonists, labetalol
Hypertrophic cardiomyopathy with severe diastolic dysfunction	Beta-Blockers, dilitiazem, verapamil		Diuretics, ACE inhibitors, Alpha₁-blockers, hydralazine, minoxidil
Hyperdynamic circulation	Beta-Blockers		Direct vasodilators
Peripheral vascular occlusive disease	. . .	Beta-Blockers	
After myocardial infarction	Non-ISA Beta-blockers		Direct vasodilators
Renal			
Bilateral renal arterial disease or severe stenosis in artery to solitary kidney	. . .		ACE inhibitors
Renal insufficiency			
Early (serum creatinine. 130–122 μmol/L (1.5–2.5 mg/ol)	. . .		Potassium-sparing agents, potassium supplements
Advanced (serum creatinine, ≥ 221 μmol/L (≥ 2.5 mg/ol/L)	Loop diuretics	ACE inhibitors	Potassium-sparing agents, potassium supplements
Other			
Asthma/COPD	. . .		Beta-Blockers, labetalol
Cyclosporine-associated hypertension	Nifedipine, labetalol	Verapamil,† nicardipine,† diltiazem†	
Depression	. . .	Alpha₂-Agonists	Reserpine
Diabetes mellitus			
Type I (insulin dependent)	. . .	Beta-Blockers	
Type II	. . .	Beta-Blockers, diuretics	
Dyslipidemia	. . .	Diuretics, Beta-blockers	
Liver disease	. . .	Labetalol	Methyldopa
Vascular headache	Beta-Blockers		
Pregnancy			
Preeclampsia	Methyldopa, hydralazine		Diuretics, ACE inhibitors
Chronic hypertension	Methyldopa		ACE inhibitors

*ACE indicates angiotensin-converting enzyme; ISA, intrinisic sympathomimetic activity; and COPD, chronic obstructive pulmonary disease.
†Can increase serum levels of cyclosporine.
The fifth report of the Joint National Committee on Detection, Evaluation and Treatment of High Blood Pressure, (JNCV). 1993. Archives of Internal Medicine, 153, *154–183.*

Biofeedback and relaxation have been demonstrated to have modest results in reducing blood pressure in selected groups and may be the most useful treatment for mild hypertension.

Follow-Up

Arrange for periodic evaluation for target organ damage and continue to reinforce lifestyle modification, education, client that HTN is the leading cause of heart disease and stroke.[11] Intervals between office visits vary and depend on the degree and lability of hypertension. Adjust medication after 3 to 4 weeks if the client's response is inadequate.

Address reasons for unresponsiveness to therapies (see Table 21–6). For clients who are following nonpharmacological therapeutic recommendations in addition to medications, a trial of step-down therapy and drug withdrawal

Lifestyle Modifications:
   Weight Reductions
   Moderation of Alcohol Intake
   Regular Physical Activity
   Reduction of Sodium Intake
   Smoking Cessation
   Avoid Caffeine

If Inadequate Response
   Continue Lifestyle Modifications
   Initial Pharmacologic Selection:
   Diuretics of β-blockers are preferred because reduction in morbidity and mortality has been demonstrated; ACE inhibitors, calcium anagonists, α-receptor Blockers, and α-β-blockers have not been tested therefore not shown to reduce morbidity and mortality

If Inadequate Response

Increase Drug Dose	or	Substitute Another Drug	or	Add 2nd Agent From Different Class

If Inadequate Response
   Add 2nd or 3rd agent and/or diuretic if not already prescribed

Figure 21–1. Managing lifestyle changes and pharmacotherapy with hypertensive clients. *(Source: The Fifth Report of the Joint National Committee on Detection, Evaluation, and Treatment of High Blood Pressure (JNCV) 1993.)*

may be considered after blood pressure has been at goal level for 1 year.

MITRAL VALVE PROLAPSE

Mitral valve prolapse (MVP) is a relatively benign and common disorder. Its distinguishing pathology is ventriculovalvular disproportion. The chordae tendinae, which suspend the mitral valve, are too large for the left ventricular cavity. Valve leaflets are also enlarged and thickened. The primary causative factor seems to be characteristic dysgenesis of collagenous valvular tissue.[21,22]

Epidemiology

Mitral valve prolapse is a genetic disorder of autosomal dominance; offspring have a 50 percent chance of being affected if one parent has the disorder.[21] MVP occurs in several connective tissue diseases, other cardiovascular processes, and miscellaneous muscular and thyroid abnormalities.[22]

Studies show that MVP is the most common valvular abnormality in the United States, with

TABLE 21–6. POSSIBLE CAUSES OF HYPERTENSION TREATMENT FAILURE

1. Nonadherence
   A. Side effects
   B. Cost
   C. Frequency of dosage
2. Drug related
   A. Inappropriate choice or combination
      Blacks and older clients tend to do better with diuretics and calcium channel blockers.
   B. Rapid inactivation
   C. Drug interactions
      Sympathomimetics
      Antidepressants
      Adrenal steroids
      Nonsteroidal anti-inflammatory drugs
      Nasal decongestants
      Oral contraceptives
3. Associated conditions
      Increasing obesity
      Excessive alcohol intake
      Renal insufficiency
      Renovascular hypertension
      Malignant/accelerated hypertension
4. Volume overload
      Inadequate diuretic therapy
      Excess sodium intake
      Fluid retention from reduction of blood pressure
      Progressive renal failure
      Congestive heart failure

Source: Adapted from the Joint National Committee on Detection, Evaluation and Treatment of High Blood Pressure (JNCV). (1993). Archives of Internal Medicine, 153, 154–183.

about 5 percent of the general population affected.[21,22] Mitral valve prolapse is encountered at all ages and appears to be equally common in women and men.[22] Prevalence varies from 2 to 40 percent, depending on the method of diagnosis (auscultation or echocardiography).[21,22] The prevalence of "clinically significant" MVP is estimated to be 2 to 4 percent.

Complications are mitral regurgitation, infective endocarditis, thromboembolism, and cardiac arrhythmias. They may occur, but usually are not serious and can either be prevented or treated. Sudden death is rare. The role of MVP in thromboembolic disease is less clear. It is often considered a factor in unexplained cerebral ischemic events; however, the incidence of transient ischemic attacks is quite low, at 0.02 percent. With no complications, activities and exercise are not limited.

Mitral regurgitation is caused most often by MVP, although only a very small percentage of clients with MVP progress to mitral regurgitation. Moreover, a small number within that group become hemodynamically impaired.[21,22]

Anxiety is not a causative factor in the development of MVP but it can be a manifestation. Heart, hormone, and chemical disturbances may account for the symptomatology of panic disorder; however, they are not yet understood.

Subjective Data

A client with mitral valve prolapse is usually asymptomatic; however, she may report chest pain and/or palpitations. The exact etiology of pain is unknown. The chest pain is atypical for angina and usually nonexertional. It may result from mechanical stress on the papillary muscle, from coronary artery spasm or embolism, left ventricular dysfunction, rate-related supply/demand imbalance, independent coronary artery disease, or extracardiac conditions. Heart palpitations are also common. Other symptoms include complaints of fast heart rate, skipped beats, lightheadedness, fatigue, weakness, dyspnea, anxiety, and postural phenomena.

Objective Data

Mitral valve prolapse is identified by means of physical examination, electrocardiogram, and echocardiogram. Laboratory tests are done to rule out other suspected medical problems.

Physical Examination. Usually normal unless MVP is associated with other conditions. Cardiac symptoms include an isolated, high-pitched, mid- to late systolic click. The client may have a late systolic murmur (late or pansystolic murmurs indicate mitral regurgitation). Chest auscultation is best done with the diaphragm over the cardiac apex. Examine the client in the supine and left lateral recumbent positions. The click is heard earlier and occupies much of systole when sitting or standing. Postural auscultation is the key to diagnosis. If the client is squatting, the click may be closer to S2. Murmur often disappears during pregnancy because of expanding blood volume and the subsequent increase in left ventricular cavity size.

Diagnostic Tests. See Coronary Artery Disease and Hypertension sections for tests done to rule out medical problems that may be associated with MVP.

Electrocardiogram abnormalities are present in up to 50 percent of clients, but do not usually account for subjective complaints.[21,22]

The echocardiogram confirms the diagnosis and extent of disease. It is recommended to determine whether mitral valve leaflets have hypertrophied, which increases the risk of infective endocarditis and progression to mitral regurgitation. Obtaining an echocardiogram to confirm MVP is not universally accepted.[21,22]

Differential Medical Diagnoses

Marfan's syndrome, rheumatic fever, trauma, hypertrophic cardiomyopathy, atrial septal defect, anorexia nervosa, pectus excavatum, connective tissue disorders, anxiety or depressive disorders.

Plan

Psychosocial Interventions. Educate the client about her common, benign condition. The valve functions properly, and usually no treatment is needed. Mitral valve prolapse does not appear to alter the course of pregnancy. Periodic auscultatory examinations are necessary to note any changes.

Medication. Although not usually required, medications may be prescribed.

β-*Adrenergic or calcium channel blockers* are usually effective in controlling symptoms (palpitations).[21,22] Their use is described under Coronary Artery Disease.

Anxiolytic drugs are recommended **only** if there is an underlying anxiety disorder.

Anticoagulants and antiplatelet medications are a possible therapeutic intervention for those at high risk for thromboembolic disease. Their effectiveness in terms of primary prevention remains unknown.

Antimicrobial prophylaxis is recommended for clients with mitral valve prolapse **and** mitral regurgitation or those who have MVP associated with thickening and redundancy of the valve leaflets. Prophylaxis is **not** recommended for prolapse without valvular regurgitation[21,22,23]

TABLE 21–7. RECOMMENDED PROPHYLAXIS FOR DENTAL, ORAL, OR UPPER RESPIRATORY TRACT PROCEDURES IN PATIENTS WHO HAVE MITRAL VALVE REGURGITATION[a]

Drug	Dosing Regimen
Amoxicillin[b]	3.0 g orally 1 hour before procedure; then half the dose 6 hours after initial dose
In Amoxicillin/Penicillin-Allergic Patients	
Erythromycin[c]	Erythromycin ethylsuccinate (E.E.S.) 800 mg or erythromycin stearate (Erythromycin Stearate Filmtab) 1.0 g orally 2 hours before procedure; then half the dose 6 hours after initial dose
or	
Clindamycin (Cleocin)	300 mg orally 1 hour before procedure; then half the dose 6 hours after initial dose

[a]Prolapse alone does not warrant medication.
[b]The antibiotics amoxicillin, ampicillin, and penicillin V are equally effective in vitro against beta hemolytic streptococci (the most common cause of endocarditis following dental procedures); however, amoxicillin is now recommended because it is better absorbed from the gastrointestinal tract and provides higher and more sustained serum levels.
[c]These forms of erythromycin are recommended because of more rapid and reliable absorption.
Source: References 21, 22, 23.

(see Table 21–7). Prophylaxis may prevent risk of endocarditis in clients with valvular disease who must undergo procedures that may cause transient bacteremia, although bacterial endocarditis may occur despite preventive measures. Guidelines for administration have been established and are considered standard practice; however, controlled clinical trials are inadequate. Bacteremia should be considered if a client experiences unexplained malaise or fever following a surgical or dental procedure. Poor dental hygiene or periodontal infections may produce bacteremia in the absence of dental procedures.

Surgical Interventions. Valve repair or replacement is indicated for symptomatic and hemodynamically significant mitral regurgitation. The procedure depends on the extent and etiology of disease.

Follow-Up

Recommend follow-up in 2 to 5 years for asymptomatic clients without murmurs.

DERMATOSES

Skin problems account for many primary care visits. Rashes or lesions may appear on exposed areas of the body or on the face and may cause the client embarrassment and concern. She is likely to seek attention promptly and may expect rapid resolution. The provider needs to be a "derm detective," taking a thorough history and using observational skills. Knowing the correct term to describe the lesion and looking at the pattern of distribution often lead to the correct diagnosis (see Table 21–8).

SCALING MACULES, PATCHES, AND PLAQUES

Superficial Fungal Infections

Superficial mycotic infections of the skin are identified according to the area of the body affected. There are two main classes of organisms, Tinea and Candida. The lesions are varied in appearance, but almost all caused by Tinea have a scaly appearance. These scales may be scraped and examined for hyphae under a microscope using KOH.

Epidemiology. Tinea and candidal dermatophyte infections are common in adults and children and in hot, humid climates. Diabetics, the obese, and women who exercise to the point of profuse sweating may be especially prone to recurrent candidal infections. Exposure to infected pets, especially cats, may precede ringworm.[1,2,3]

Subjective/Objective Data and Associated Findings, and Differential Diagnoses for Specific Disorders. See Table 21–9.

DIAGNOSTIC TESTS. Tinea versicolor, Tinea corporis (ringworm), and Tinea pedis are usually diagnosed on the basis of history and characteristic appearance/distribution. Scales on the lesion may be scraped onto a slide, covered with KOH, and examined under the microscope for hyphae if diagnosis in doubt. Tinea capitis (scalp ringworm) and Tinea unguium (nail fungus) are diagnosed by fungus culture before treatment is begun.

Plan

PSYCHOSOCIAL. Fungal infections may cause body image disturbance and concern regarding contagion. Nail infections may require months of treatment before resolution. Reassurance about self-limited nature of most common dermatoses is helpful to the client. Be open to these issues.

TABLE 21–8. DERMATOLOGIC TERMINOLOGY

Lesion: general term for a single small area of affected skin
Rash: collective term for many lesions that may occur singly, in clusters, or are confluent

Primary Lesions

Macule: small flat area of color change no larger than 2 cm; usually smooth but may have fine scale
Patch: macule larger than 2 cm, usually arising from enlarging macules
Papule: small palpable mass less than 1.5 cm, usually elevated; may be skin colored or pigmented
Plaque: flattopped palpable lesion larger than 1.5 cm; a papule that has enlarged in length and width
Nodule: papule that has enlarged in three dimensions, length, width, and depth and is larger than 1.5 cm
Wheal: pale pink slightly elevated fluid filled papule
Vesicle: fluid filled papule; small blister
Bulla: vesicle larger than 1 cm; may represent coalescence of vesicles
Pustule: vesicle containing polymorphonuclear leukocytes; therefore, appears white; does not by itself signify infection
Purpura: microvascular disruption characterized by hemorrhage into the skin producing ecchymoses (> 3 mm) or petechiae (< 3 mm)

Secondary Lesions

Scale: loose fragments of keratin; appears on a rapidly proliferating epithelium
Crust: dried exudate that develops when the epithelium has been disrupted and plasma exudes to the surface
Erosion and Ulcer: represent epithelial and dermal disruption, respectively; may have a soft base or crust
Excoriation: scratch marks
Lichenification: thickening of skin from chronic rubbing

Using these terms along with a description of the distribution, color, and associated findings make an algorithmic approach to diagnosis possible.
Subjective Data. Key questions to ask for all common dermatoses:
What did the rash look like when it first appeared?
Has the rash spread?
What past or current treatment? Results?
Previous occurrence?
Pruritic? Painful?
Any other household members with similar rash?
Recent history of new medication or cosmetic?
Any other symptom or medical problem?

Source: Reference 1.

Tinea Versicolor

MEDICATION. Oral Ketoconazole 400 mg

- *Administration.* One dose of oral ketoconazole followed by application of selenium sulfide shampoo head to toes at bedtime. In A.M. shower, working up lather, then rinse. Encourage client to work up sweat the day following ketoconazole ingestion. Ketoconazole is delivered in sweat to the skin. Treatment may be repeated in 1 week for a maximum of three treatments.[2]
- *Adverse Effects.* Ketoconazole may cause disulfram reaction with alcohol ingestion. Other adverse effects include headache, nausea, vomiting, elevation of liver enzymes, pruritis.
- *Contraindications.* Ketoconazole can be hepatoxic. Assess for history of liver disease. Draw baseline liver enzymes.
- *Interactions.* Decreased absorption with antacids and H2 blockers. May alter levels of dilantin and increase effects of hypoglycemic agents and coumadin.

Follow-up. Advise client to call to schedule appointment if no response after 3 weeks of treatment. Advise client it may take months for pigment to return to previous shade.

Tinea Corporis (Body Ringworm)

MEDICATION. Topical antifungal such as Miconazole 2 percent, available over-the-counter.

- *Administration.* Advise client to apply 2–3 times per day and continue application 3–5 days after lesions disappear.
- *Adverse Effects.* Pruritic rash, irritation.
- *Contraindication.* Known sensitivity to miconazole.

DIET/LIFESTYLE. Advise client that household pet may be source of infection. Follow-up with veterinarian is suggested.

Follow-Up. Advise her to schedule appointment if no response to therapy after 1 week treatment.

Tinea Capitis (Scalp Ringworm)

Note: Organism should be identified by fungal culture before therapy is begun. Topical antifungals will not eradicate infection but twice weekly shampooing with Selenium 2.5 percent will decrease shedding of spores.

TABLE 21–9. SCALING MACULES, PATCHES, AND PLAQUES

Diagnosis	Subjective Data	Objective Data Distribution	Differential DX
Tinea versicolor	Mildly pruritic	Pale macules that do not tan Fine scale when scraped (KOH +) Young adults *Mainly on trunk*	Vitiligo (no pigmentation)
Tinea corporis (ringworm)	Mildly pruritic May have cat	Annular lesion with scaly border and central clearing or scaly patches with distinct border *Exposed areas*	Psoriasis (on knees, elbows) Secondary Syphilis (on palms, soles) Pityriasis rosea (more lesions)
Tinea capitis (scalp ringworm)	Usually asymptomatic May have asymptomatic carrier in family	Scaly plaque of alopecia or broken hairs Kerion formation may occur (inflamed, boggy nodule) Cervical adenopathy Diagnosis on basis of fungal culture *Scalp*	Seborrheic dermatitis (oily scales) Impetigo (more inflamed, honey colored crust)
Tinea pedis (athlete's foot)	May have intense itching and burning	Scaling and fissuring of toe webs or scaling, thickening and cracking of skin of heel and sole KOH positive *Feet, toes*	Contact dermatitis (appears on dorsum of foot) Dyshidrosis (KOH neg., vesicles)
Tinea unguium	Usually asymptomatic Often history of Tinea pedis	Thickened, yellow crumbly nails Keratin and debris under nail Diagnosis by fungal culture *Finger and toenails*	Psoriasis (pitting of nails) Candidiasis (no debris)
Pityriasis rosea	Occasional pruritis History of larger lesion preceding eruption	Fawn colored, oval scaly macules or papules in Christmas tree pattern on back Spring and fall Young adults female more than male *Trunk distribution*	Secondary Syphilis (nonpruritic on palms and soles, RPR+) T. corporis (fewer lesions)
Eczema and Nummular Eczema	Pruritic History of atopy (asthma, allergy)	In flare, weepy, inflamed, lichenified skin Often Dennie's lines (infraorbital fold) and nasal crease May have secondary impetigination *Distribution Eczema—face, sides of neck, flexural aspects of knees, elbows, wrists* *Nummular: Backs of hands, fingers, extensor aspects of forearms, legs*	Contact Dermatitis (differentiated by history and distribution) Psoriasis (silvery scales)
Seborrheic dermatitis	Pruritis in hairy areas Chronic	Yellow, grayish greasy scales in irregular patches Dandruff on scalp *Seborrheic areas of body: scalp, eyebrows, nasolabial folds, presternal and pubic regions*	Psoriasis (red plaques with silvery scales) Tinea capitis (positive fungal culture)
Psoriasis	May or may not be pruritic Family history First eruption 12–20 yrs old	Begins as pink macules covered by fine silver scale Enlarges to coalesce to well demarcated plaques that are raised from the surrounding skin Pinpoint bleeding with removal of large scale (Auspitz's sign) Pitting of nails *Characteristic distribution: knees, elbows (extensor surface) scalp, lumbosacral area, and often gluteal folds*	Seborrheic dermatitis (see previous) Nummular eczema (see previous)

TABLE 21–9. SCALING MACULES, PATCHES, AND PLAQUES (CONTINUED)

Diagnosis	Subjective Data	Objective Data Distribution	Differential DX
Discoid lupus	Asymptomatic Onset in 40s	Red, scaly, round or oval plaques 5–20mm diameter with well-defined border Scales are tacklike May result in alopecia and scarring with hypo- or hyperpigmentation *Characteristic butterfly pattern on face, also on scalp, hairline, ears*	Seborrheic dermatitis (scales greasy)

Source: References 1, 3, 6, 9.

MEDICATION. Oral griseofulvin is the medication of choice.

- *Administration.* Griseofulvin microsize 500 mg or 330 mg ultramicrosize po daily for 1 month. Should be taken with meal having highest fat content to minimize GI distress.
- *Adverse Effects.* Headache (usually resolves within a week), nausea, vomiting, rash, photosensitivity, granulocytopenia, hepatotoxicity. Draw baseline complete blood count (CBC) with differential and liver enzymes before initiation of therapy. Can potentiate the effects of alcohol.
- *Contraindications.* Known hypersensitivity, liver failure, porphyria. Use caution if allergic to penicillin (griseofulvin produced by Penicillium).
- *Expected Outcome.* It may require 3 months to eradicate infection.

DIET/LIFESTYLE. Griseofulvin has slightly metallic taste. Encourage client to maintain adequate nutrition as sense of taste may be altered. Stress importance of adherence to daily dose to prevent relapse. Advise client to avoid overexposure to sunlight. Alcohol should be avoided during treatment. Stress importance of personal hygiene and scalp care, not sharing combs, brushes, hats, towels.

Follow-Up. Evaluate after 1 month for response to therapy. Repeat CBC with differential and liver enzymes. Refer to physician or dermatologist if abnormal test results or if condition not improved or worse.

Tinea Pedis (Athlete's Foot)

MEDICATION. Topical antifungal such as miconazole 2 percent (available over-the-counter).

- *Administration.* Apply two to three times per day after feet are washed and dried completely. Continue to use for 7–10 days after lesions disappear. If macerated tissue between toes, advise client to apply aluminum subacetate (Domeboro) soaks for 20 minutes two to three times a day to help dry lesions before applying miconazole.
- *Adverse Effects.* Contraindications, see Tinea Corporis.
- *Expected Outcome.* May take several weeks to eradicate infection. Advise client infection may recur. Some become chronically affected and may need systemic therapy such as griseofulvin (see previous discussion) 500 mg po daily for one month, itraconazole (see following) 200 mg daily for 1 month. May require up to 3 months systemic therapy.

DIET/LIFESTYLE. Educate client regarding conditions that lead to infection, e.g., trapped moisture between toes, going barefoot in community showers and bathing places. Advise client to wear cotton socks, change several times a day if profuse sweating of feet, dry between toes thoroughly.

Follow-Up. Evaluate response to therapy in 1 week. Refer to physician if no improvement or if secondary infection.

Tinea Unguium

Note: Must establish diagnosis by fungal culture before beginning treatment.

MEDICATION. Initial treatment of choice is griseofulvin, 1.0–1.5 g/d (see previous discussion), but toenail infections may require 12 months of treatment.

Itraconazole (Sporonax) has recently been approved for treatment of fungal nail infections. Advise client medication is expensive but may resolve infection in shorter time than griseofulvin.

- *Administration.* Itraconazole 200 mg once daily after meal with highest fat content.

- *Adverse Effects.* Nausea, vomiting, headache, rash, elevated liver enzymes.
- *Interactions.* Coadministration with terfenadine, astemizole, cisapride may cause serious cardiac arrhythmias and even death. Coadministration with midazolam or triazolam may potentiate sedative effects. May enhance anticoagulant effect of coumadin; may enhance hypoglycemic effect of oral hypoglycemic agents.
- *Contraindications.* Hepatic disease, pregnancy or women at risk for pregnancy, nursing mothers.
- *Expected Outcome.* Mean time to complete cure 10 months but may clear after 3–4 months. Often recurrent.

DIET/LIFESTYLE. Advise client to file nails daily. In clients who acquired infection from artificial nails, advise them infection may recur if artificial nails worn again.

Follow-Up. Evaluate client after 1 month. Repeat liver enzyme tests. Refer to physician or dermatologist if not responding to therapy in expected time frame or if condition worsens.[2,3,6]

PITYRIASIS ROSEA

The cause of pityriasis is unknown. Because it is generally a disease of children and young adults, does not recur and often follows an upper respiratory infection, a viral etiology is possible. It could also be a postviral immunological reaction.[1]

Epidemiology

Most common in young adults and 50 percent more common in females. Usually occurs in fall or spring. Concurrent infections in households occur but are not common (less than 2 percent in married couples).[6]

Subjective/Objective Data, Associated Findings and Differential Diagnoses

See Table 21–9.

Diagnostic Tests. Pityriasis resembles the rash of secondary syphillis but is usually differentiated by distribution, lack of palm, sole involvement. An RPR titer should be drawn if diagnosis is in doubt or if client is at risk for syphillis.

Plan

Psychosocial Interventions. Reassure the client that this is a self-limited problem and is not thought to be contagious. Lesions may remain hyperpigmented in Asian, Latino, and African American clients; may persist for several weeks.

Medication. Topical steroid creams, low to midpotency (e.g., 1 percent hydrocortisone, triamcinolone 0.1 percent), depending on degree of inflammation, applied two to three times daily in thin film (see Table 21–10).

Colloidal oatmeal baths (Aveeno) may provide relief from pruritis. Packets may be purchased without prescription for nominal cost. Advise client to mix with tepid water and soak two to three times per day for 10–15 minutes.

- *Adverse Effects.* See Table 21–10.
- *Contraindication.* Sensitivity to steroid cream. Use cautiously if possibility of fungal or bacterial skin lesion, if impaired circulation (may increase risk of skin ulceration).
- *Expected Outcome.* Advise client rash may take 6 weeks to clear.

Follow-Up

Advise client to call or schedule visit if rash worsens or if persists more than 6 weeks.

ATOPIC DERMATOSES: ECZEMA AND NUMMULAR ECZEMA

Atopic dermatitis is a chronic disease with exacerbations and remissions throughout the lifetime of the client. It is usually diagnosed in infancy. Its most prominent feature is uncontrolled scratching that seems to arise spontaneously. This is known as the itch-scratch cycle, the more the skin is rubbed or scratched, the more highly pruritic it becomes. Nighttime scratching to the point of excoriation of the skin can occur.

Nummular eczema appears most commonly as coinshaped lesions on the extensor surfaces of forearms and legs. Eczema in adults affects mainly the flexural aspects of elbows, wrists and knees. The epidemiology and treatment is the same for both. See Eczema and Nummular Eczema.

TABLE 21–10. TOPICAL CORTICOSTEROIDS

Generic Name (Brand Name)	Potency Class	Indications and Comments
*Hydrocortisone 0.5 & 1.0% cream and lotion	Low	Seborrhea, mild eczema, mild contact dermatitis Available over-the-counter
*Desonide 0.05% (Tridesilon)	Low	As for hydrocortisone, but more efficacious, especially for lesions on face By prescription Expensive.
Triamcinolone acetonide 0.1% ointment, cream, lotion (Kenalog, Aristocort)	Medium	Eczema and nummular eczema, Pityriasis rosea, psoriasis, contact/allergic dermatitis, dyshydrosis Use lotion on scalp
*Mometasone furoate 0.1% cream and lotion (Elocon)	Medium	Same as Triamcinolone
Fluocinolone acetonide 0.025% cream and ointment (Lidex)	Medium	Same as Triamcinolone
Betamethasone dipropionate 0.05% cream and lotion (Diprosone, Maxivate)	High	Psoriasis, discoid lupus Eczema, severe contact/allergic dermatitis
Amcinonide 0.1% ointment, cream, lotion (Cyclocort)	High	Same as Betamethasone
Fluocinonide 0.05% gel, ointment, cream and lotion (Lidex)	High	Same as Betamethasone
Clobetasol propionate 0.05% cream, ointment (Temovate)	Ultra	Limit use to two continuous weeks Cannot occlude
Halobetasol propionate 0.05% cream, ointment (Ultravate)	Ultra	Slightly more effective in psoriasis than Clobetasol Same as Clobetasol

*Not fluorinated
NOTE: Vehicle choice depends on distribution, extent, area of body, and cosmetic consideration.

Ointment:	Use where additional moisturizing desired		Lotion:	Use for hairy areas or where large areas involved
	Use if client reports stinging with cream			May be drying to the skin
	Can be occlusive, for given strength more efficacious than creams			Short exposure time, may rub off before absorbed
	Can cause maceration, acne		Gel:	Use when drying effect desired, good for scalp
	May not be suitable for cosmetic reasons			
Cream:	Usually best vehicle choice			
	Mild emollient			
	Can be comedogenic			

Size of dispenser usually small (15 grams) and large (60 grams). For an adult of average size, it takes 20–30 grams to cover body once. One arm is covered by about 3 grams in one application. One palm requires about 0.5 grams in one application.

Adverse effects. Topical steroids may cause local irritation, overgrowth of bacteria or fungus, acneiform eruption, hypopigmentation, striae, miliaria. Advise client to use sparingly and never on mucous membranes or in genital area. Can be systemically absorbed if not used carefully. Midpotency to high potency steroids on face can cause hypopigmentation, rosacealike rash. Striae formation in the genital-groin area can occur with fluorinated topical steroids; therefore, only hydrocortisone should be used in these areas.
Source: References 1, 6.

Epidemiology

It is estimated that 20 percent of the population carries a genetic trait for atopy, which is inherited in an autosomal dominant pattern. Its expression in the form of eczema is about 25 percent of the individuals who inherit this atopic diathesis. Most clients with eczema note flares in times of stress and fatigue.

Serum IgE levels are often elevated in individuals with severe disease. They may also have asthma and/or hay fever. Nummular eczema is more common in young adult women and elderly men.[1]

Subjective/Objective Data and Differential Diagnoses

See Table 21–9. See Eczema and Nummular Eczema.

Plan

Psychosocial Interventions. Stress management and helping the client get restful, restorative sleep are key. An exercise and fitness program and courses in meditation, yoga, or biofeedback may be necessary. Since this is more often than not a lifetime problem with unexplained recurrences, the client may experience a feeling of helplessness. She may also have body image concerns. Use of make-up may have to be limited. It is important to be sensitive to these issues and to provide support.

Medications. Steroid creams and/or ointments are the cornerstone of treatment. See Table 21–10 for list. Potency of steroid is determined by severity of presentation. Start with midpotency if possible but may initially require high potency topical steroid for 2–3 weeks twice a day, then taper to every other day, then to weekends only. As soon as inflammation subsides, have client switch to emollients, such as Eucerin or Aquaphor. Tapering steroid use is important to minimize rebound flares. See Pityriasis roseae and Table 21–10 for discussion of topical steroids.

Severe or extensive outbreak may require oral prednisone taper. Start with 40 mg, then taper down by 10 mg amounts every 2 to 3 days over a period of 10–14 days.

- *Administration.* Take indicated dose in A.M.
- *Adverse Effects.* Insomnia, headache, nervousness, hypertension, acne, delayed healing, thrush, fluid retention, weight gain, hyperglycemia, hypokalemia, muscle weakness.
- *Contraindications.* Presence of systemic fungal infection, known hypersensitivity to prednisone. Use with caution if GI ulceration, renal disease, hypertension, diabetes, osteoporosis, congestive heart failure, tuberculosis, glaucoma, cirrhosis of the liver, hypothyroidism, and psychotic tendencies as it may exacerbate these conditions.

- *Client Teaching.* Advise client to take in A.M. to avoid sleep disturbance, not to discontinue abruptly. Advise client on adverse effects, reassure that these are temporary and resolve after completing taper.

Acute weeping lesions may be treated with aluminum subacetate solution (Domeboro soaks) or colloidal oatmeal (Aveeno) in tepid baths or as wet dressings for 10–15 minutes two to three times a day. Skin is rinsed, patted dry, and topical steroid is applied after bathing or soaking.

If yellow, honey colored crusts or pustules appear, secondary impetigination may have occurred. Antistaphylococcal medications such as dicloxacillin 250 mg QID or erythromycin 250 mg QID (if allergic to penicillin) may be prescribed for 7 days.

Adverse effects of both antibiotics include nausea, vomiting, diarrhea. Contraindicated in those clients with known hypersensitivity.

Systemic antihistamines, such as Hydroxyzine 25 mg may help to control pruritis especially at night. It may be taken every 6 hours.

Adverse effects include drowsiness, dry mouth, blurred vision, constipation, and urinary retention.

- *Contraindications.* Known hypersensitivity. Use with caution in pregnancy and in clients with glaucoma or urinary retention.
- *Client Teaching.* May potentiate effects of barbiturates, alcohol, tranquilizers, or other central nervous system depressants.

LIFESTYLE MODIFICATIONS. See prior discussion of psychosocial interventions. It may be helpful for the client to keep a symptom diary including cosmetic use, foods eaten, stressful events when she first notes flare-up to increase insight and sense of control. Modifications in skin care such as use of moisturizers or emollients such as Eucerin or Aquaphor several times a day, avoidance of prolonged hot water baths and of wool clothing next to skin are helpful. She should keep her fingernails trimmed and filed. Lowering of the thermostat in winter prevents overheating and perspiring, especially at night. Prompt showering after workouts helps eliminate irritative properties of perspiration.

Follow-Up

During flare-ups, evaluate client every week for response to therapy. Telephone contact is also helpful to provide support. Have client call at first signs of flare.[1,6]

SEBORRHEIC DERMATITIS

Seborrheic dermatitis is a more localized form of chronic atopic dermatitis that is usually confined to the scalp. It may spread to the forehead and eyebrows. On the body it may appear in the groin, axillae, and the presternal region. The hallmark of seborrhea is greasy yellow or grayish scales overlying irregular reddish patches of skin. Blepharitis is a complication of seborrheic dermatitis. (See discussion in Common Ophthalmologic Problems.)

Epidemiology

Genetic predisposition that begins in puberty and persists. More common in men. Flares occur in cold weather months, when the air is dry. Clients with Parkinson's disease or HIV infection may be more at risk.[6]

Subjective Data/Objective Data/ Differential Diagnoses

See Table 21–9, Seborrheic dermatitis.

Plan

Psychosocial Interventions. Due to scalp and face involvement, may be source of great distress to client. It is highly visible and often gives appearance of poor hygiene. Client will need reassurance and prompt resolution. Like eczema, condition may be exacerbated by emotional stress, food allergies, and fatigue.

Medication. Daily use of tar or selenium shampoo with twice weekly use of ketoconazole 2 percent (Nizoral) shampoo if moderately severe. Advise that shampoos may cause pruritis. Topical application of low potency steroid lotion or cream in small amounts may be used on areas of marked inflammation after shampooing (see Table 21–10). Advise client to avoid fluorinated steroids on face.

Treatment of the scalp may improve affected areas of the face. On intertriginous areas, shampoos may be used but avoid greasy ointments. Advise client to avoid using ketoconazole shampoo on genital area.

Lid margins may be cleaned with baby shampoo (Johnson & Johnson) applied undiluted with a cotton swab at night.

Diet/Lifestyle. Advise client that hygiene and environment play a role in exacerbations. Sweat retention tends to make it worse as well as lapses in daily shampoo routine. Stress reduction, adequate rest, nutrition, and hydration promote healthy skin and scalp.

Follow-Up

Have client telephone or schedule visit to discuss response to therapy after 1 to 2 weeks, depending on severity of presentation.

PSORIASIS

Psoriasis, like eczema, is a lifelong, chronic disease (with acute flares) whose course is unpredictable. It is characterized by red plaques that are covered with silvery or white scales. Its cause is unknown but about 30 percent of clients have a family history. Immunologic factors may also play a role. Clients with psoriasis have an increased incidence of HLA antigens.[1]

Epidemiology

Onset is often in young adulthood, but may also appear initially in children or older adults. It is not uncommon and 1–2 percent of the U.S. population may be affected. Clients with AIDS may experience an abrupt onset of psoriasis. Ten to fifteen percent of clients with psoriasis may also have psoriatic arthritis with polyarticular involvement.[1,6]

Subjective/Objective Data, Associated Findings/Differential Diagnoses

See Table 21–9, Psoriasis.

Plan

Psychosocial Interventions. Because psoriasis typically affects exposed areas of the body, it can have a huge impact psychologically. Early onset appears to have the greatest negative effect on the quality of life, impacting both social and occupational sectors. Some may fear stigmatization by others due to fear of AIDS.[9]

Medication. Mid- to high potency topical steroids are most often used (see Table 21–10).

- *Administration.* Use twice daily for 2–3 weeks. Greater penetration may be achieved by removal of the superficial scale by soaking or by use of a keratolytic agent such as salicylic acid. (See discussion of salicylic acid use in section on warts.) Switch to lower potency steroid combined with nightly application of tar gel product such as Estar or Psorigel. Warn client that tar is messy to apply and will stain clothes and sheets.

  Because topical corticosteroids do not produce long-term remission and may make psoriasis more difficult to treat in the long run, some recommend using occlusion alone to treat isolated patches. Sheets of Duoderm may be placed over the lesion and left on for a minimum of 5 days. This treatment should be repeated over several weeks. Improvement may be noted in 3 to 4 weeks.

  Oral steroids are seldom used by the primary practitioner due to frequent rebound flares and worsening of the condition. Scalp lesions may be treated with tar shampoos (Neutrogena T/Gel) used daily or 2 percent ketoconazole (Ni zoral) shampoo by prescription used twice weekly.

  If psoriasis affects more than 30 percent of the body, refer to a dermatologist for light therapy with UVB three times a week for PUVA (psoralen plus UVA). PUVA may increase the risk of cataract formation and skin cancer. Other therapies used by dermatologists include methotrexate, cyclosporine, and synthetic retinoids. Refer to pharmacology text for further information on these agents.[1,6]

  Oral antihistamines at bedtime such as hydroxyzine (Atarax) 25 mg may be helpful if pruritis is severe or interferes with rest.

- *Expected Outcome.* Advise client psoriasis is a chronic condition with periods of flare and remission.

Diet/Lifestyle. Some clients may find exposure to sunlight is beneficial but warn them about harmful effects of prolonged exposure such as skin cancer and premature aging of the skin. Sunscreen should always be worn. Advise client to try to avoid trauma to affected areas and to resist rubbing and scratching in order to avoid secondary infection. Arthritis associated with psoriasis often improves with successful skin treatment.

Follow-Up

Follow weekly during flares. If client referred to dermatologist, request treatment plan to ensure continuity of care.

DISCOID LUPUS

The cause of discoid lupus is not known but it is theorized that exposure to sunlight leads to DNA damage in epithelial cells. The changed DNA may trigger an autoimmune response. Lupus occurs along a continuum moving from discoid lupus which is confined to the skin to systemic lupus.[1] (See section on Autoimmune Disease.)

Epidemiology

Discoid lupus first appears in young adults with equal frequency in men and women. A familial pattern has been observed. It is a lifelong disease with exacerbations occurring after sun exposure. Ten percent of those with systemic lupus (SLE) also have the discoid lesions. In time, some with solely cutaneous involvement may develop SLE, but this is uncommon.[1]

Subjective/Objective Data/Associated Signs/Differential Diagnosis

See Table 21–9, Scaling macules, patches and plaque Discoid lupus.

Plan

Clients should be referred to the dermatologist for biopsy. An ANA titer may also be ordered to define the extent of disease.

Psychosocial Interventions. Discoid lupus can cause scarring, patchy alopecia, and loss of pigment (especially in darker complexioned individuals). The cosmetic results can be devastating. Aggressive and early treatment may help avoid scarring and permanent alopecia. Be supportive and alert to the need for psychological counseling.

Medications. High potency topical steroids are initial treatment (see Table 21–10). Applied to skin and covered with occlusive dressing, such as Duoderm. Dermatologist may inject triamcinolone 2.5–10 mg/ml once a month into lesions before advancing to systemic medications such as antimalarials.

- *Expected Outcome.* Discoid lesions usually respond to triamcinolone injection.
- *Client Teaching.* Client should be aware of medications that can increase sensitivity to sunlight including doxycycline, thiazides and piroxicam.
- *Lifestyle.* The client should avoid outdoor activities during times of the day when sunlight is strongest. Advise use of sunscreen with high SPF always. Protective clothing should be worn.

Follow-Up

Request visit notes and treatment plan from dermatologist. Some clients may be managed by primary care provider after initial referral.

VESICULAR DERMATOSES: CONTACT DERMATITIS

Contact dermatoses can be classified into two main types: irritant and allergic. Eighty percent are due to exposure to common universal irritants, such as soap, solvents, and detergents. The most common contact allergens include poison ivy, poison oak, nickel, latex, hair dye, topical medications, perfumes, cosmetics, and adhesive tape. Allergy to an antibiotic may cause dermatitis. The presentation of contact dermatoses may be acute as in poison ivy or subacute if repeated exposure has occurred and sensitization has developed over time.

Epidemiology

The elderly may be more prone to contact dermatitis due to thinning of the skin and loss of protective moisture. Certain occupations, especially those requiring contact with irritants and allergens cited previously, are at increased risk.[1,4,6]

Subjective/Objective Data, Associated Features, Differential Diagnosis

See Table 21–11, Contact or allergic dermatitis.

Plan

The first step in treatment is to remove the offending agent. Client may have to be referred to dermatologist for patch testing if diagnosis of agent unclear.

Psychosocial Interventions. This is usually a self-limited problem, which is resolved in 2 to 3 weeks once the offending agent is removed. Practitioner should be aware, however, that removal of the offender may cause distress, by necessitating a change in lifestyle, occupation, or grooming.

Medications. If lesions are weeping, apply wet dressings (Burow's soaks) 30–60 minutes several times a day. After soaking a topical steroid in a drying vehicle, such as Lidex gel 0.5 percent may be applied. If highly inflammatory and pruritic, mid- to high potency topical steroid cream may help. See Table 21–10. Taper down to mid- to low potency after 2 weeks. If acute severe reaction with extensive skin involvement, oral prednisone taper may be needed. Start with 40–60 mg and taper down by 10 mg every 3 days. See section on eczema for discussion of oral prednisone.

Oral antihistamines such as hydroxyzine (Atarax) 25 mg may be needed to control pruritis.

- *Expected Outcome.* Usually resolves in 2–3 weeks.
- *Lifestyle.* As noted, may require client to change or modify work, grooming, or hobby, depending on offending agent. Prevention is key.

Follow-Up

Evaluate client after 1 week of treatment for response. Refer to dermatologist if not responding to treatment or if patch testing indicated.

VESICULAR DERMATOSES: SCABIES

Scabies is an intensely pruritic dermatitis caused by infestation with the mite Sarcoptes scabei. The female mite burrows under the skin and deposits eggs, which hatch and mature over a 3-week

TABLE 21–11. VESICULAR DERMATOSES

Diagnosis	Subjective Data	Objective Data Distribution	Differential DX
Contact or allergic dermatitis	Pruritic Burning History of trigger	Weeping, encrusted vesicles and bullae in acute stage May have linear streaking pattern *Distribution asymmetric and pattern may be diagnostic* *Look for site of contact*	Impetigo (positive culture) Scabies (location, no weeping)
Scabies	Pruritis especially at night History of contagion, overcrowded living	Excoriations and vesiculopapular lesions and burrows *Distribution is diagnostic; webs of fingers, toes; heels of palms, buttocks, breasts, elbows, axillae* *Rarely on face* *Early in course lesions isolated*	Eczema (distribution, scaling, history)
Herpes Simplex labialis	Burning, tingling often precedes eruption Recurrent Triggered by stress, sunlight	Small grouped vesicles on erythematous base Blisters fragile and may present as erosion *Distribution: vermillion border of lip, rarely in mouth*	Aphthous ulcers (ulcers only on oral mucosa or gingiva)
Herpes Zoster	Very painful Usually not recurrent	Grouped, tense vesicles in linear pattern *Distribution: typically only face or trunk spreading over 1–2 dermatomes*	Poison ivy, oak (vesicles confluent not grouped)
Dyshidrosis	Very pruritic Recurrent Triggered by stress Common in young adults	Tapioca vesicles 1–2 mm that may coalesce to form blisters that dry and become scaly or fissured *Distribution is characteristic: palms, fingers, soles of feet*	Tinea pedis (between toes) Secondary syphilis (+RPR, not vesicular) HSV if immunocompromised

Source: References 1, 6.

incubation period, causing intense pruritis. It can be passed on by person to person contact or through bedding and clothes. It spreads on the skin by fingernail contamination.

Epidemiology

All ages affected and all socioeconomic groups. Less common in African Americans.[1]

Subjective/Objective Data/ Differential Diagnoses

See Table 21–11, Vesicular Dermatoses: Scabies.

Diagnostic Tests. Usually diagnosed on basis of history and appearance of burrows in characteristic locations, webs of fingers, genitalia. Burrows can be opened with scalpel blade at the end or dark point, and mite can be placed on slide and examined under oil immersion for confirmation.

Plan

Psychosocial Interventions. May cause embarrassment to client due to concern over hygiene. Client education important concerning mode of transmission, occurrence in all socioeconomic groups.

Advise her that partner may be infected (common site is penile shaft and glans) and should be treated.

Medication. Permethrin Cream (Elimite) 5 percent. Applied neck to toes, with special care to include webs of fingers and toes, axillary, gluteal folds, under breasts. Advise client not to wash hands after application, should be left on overnight 8–12 hours then rinsed. Single application is usually effective.

- *Adverse Effects.* Usually mild stinging, pruritis.
- *Contraindications.* Known sensitivity to permethrin or chrysanthemums.

- *Expected Outcome.* Single application usually effective if applied thoroughly and as directed. Pruritis may persist especially if atopic history, but client is no longer contagious after 24 hours of treatment completion. Topical low- to mid-potency steroid cream may be used after treatment if inflammation and pruritis persist. Oral antihistamines such as 25 mg hydroxyzine (Atarax) taken at bedtime may relieve pruritis (see Table 21–10).

Lifestyle Modification. Instruct client to wash all bedding, clothes and towels in hot soapy water and dry on hottest dryer setting. Nonwashable items may be placed in airtight plastic bag for 2 weeks or sent to dry cleaner. Advise client of possibility of reinfection if partner is not treated. Advise her she may spread infestation to others up to 24 hours after completion of treatment. No special attention is needed for furniture or inanimate objects.

Follow-Up

Advise client to call to schedule visit if treatment is not effective.

VESICULAR DERMATOSES: HERPES SIMPLEX

Herpes simplex (cold sore or herpes labialis) is a recurrent infection caused by the virus Herpesvirus hominis. It appears as tightly clustered vesicles on the vermillion border of the lips, but may appear on other areas of the face. The blisters are fragile, and most common presentation is a secondary erosion that forms a crust. Following the initial infection, the virus remains dormant in the dorsal root ganglia and reactivates during times of stress, trauma, head colds, fever, and exposure to sunlight. The first episode may be asymptomatic.

Epidemiology

Herpes simplex infection is transmitted by exposure to a clinically infected person, an asymptomatic virus shedder, or reactivation of a latent infection. Appearance of the vesicle occurs 3–5 days after exposure and lasts 5–10 days. Contagion is possible during the first few days of vesi-cle appearance. Vesicles usually appear in the same site with recurrent infections. Lesions may not clear in immunocompromised individuals.[1]

Subjective/Objective Data/ Differential Diagnoses

See Table 21–11, Vesicular Dermatoses: Herpes Simplex.

Diagnostic Tests. Usually diagnosed on basis of prior history but can be confirmed by opening vesicle dome with small needle, swabbing fluid exudate with sterile swab, and sending for viral culture.

Plan

Psychosocial Interventions. Client may be concerned about appearance and about contagion. Discuss importance of frequent handwashing to prevent autoinoculation and refraining from oral sex. Advise her that lesion usually resolves in a week. Be sensitive to issues of possible sexual transmission and address them accordingly. Client education very important to clear up misconceptions between Type I and Type II Herpes. See discussion of HSV in chapter on Vaginitis and Sexually Transmitted Disease.

Medication. Acyclovir 200 mg 5 times a day or 400 mg three times a day is usually reserved for initial gingivostomatitis to shorten duration of symptoms and viral shedding. Its benefits are more modest for recurrent episodes and treatment must be initiated at earliest sign of lesion. Can be taken prophylactically before menses or prolonged exposure to sunlight.

In immunocompromised individuals, 5 percent acyclovir ointment may be used as topical treatment if oral acyclovir has been shown to be ineffective, but it is not approved for use in noncompromised individuals because of concerns of mutagenicity of the drug and promotion of resistant strains.

Warm compresses may be applied to lesions for comfort and removal of exudate. Advise client to discard after use to prevent spread of virus. Topical over-the-counter preparations such as Blistex may be beneficial to keep lesion moist and prevent painful cracking and fissuring.

Lifestyle. Advise client to apply sunscreen before exposure to sunlight. May also apply warm, moist cloths, but advise client these may contain virus and should not be handled by other household members. Careful and frequent handwashing is the key to prevent spreading to vulnerable contacts such as the elderly and infants.

Follow-Up

Advise client to call to schedule visit if not cleared in 7–10 days.

VESICULAR DERMATOSES: HERPES ZOSTER

Shingles or Herpes Zoster is a painful vesicular eruption along a dermatome, It is caused by reactivation of the varicella-zoster virus whose first appearance causes chicken pox.

Epidemiology

In younger adults, thoracic dermatomes are most often affected. In older adults, the area of distribution of the trigeminal nerve is frequently involved. If more than two dermatomes are affected, individual may be immunocompromised.

Postherpetic neuralgia is an excruciatingly painful complication, especially if the trigeminal nerve is involved. The infection may also spread to the eye and cause a dendritic pattern conjunctivitis. Disseminated zoster in immunocompromised individuals may be life threatening.[1,6]

Subjective/Objective Data/ Differential Diagnoses

See Table 21–11, Vesicular Dermatoses: Herpes Zoster.

Diagnostic Tests. History and appearance are usually diagnostic, but a viral culture will confirm diagnosis. (See previous discussion on Herpes Simplex for method of culture.) Confirmation by culture is especially important if vesicles cross several dermatomes. If this is the case and the culture is positive for Herpes Zoster, client should be evaluated for immunocompromise.

Plan

Refer immediately to ophthalmologist if eye appears to be involved. Refer to physician if appears to be disseminated, involves more than two dermatomes, or appears on face or scalp.

Psychosocial Interventions. Facial appearance may cause body image disturbance. Reassure client that infection usually resolves in 2 to 3 weeks and does not recur (unless immunocompromised).

Medication. Oral Acyclovir 800 mg five times a day for 7 days if started within the first 72 hours may accelerate clearing and reduce pain. (See discussion of acyclovir in chapter on Vaginitis and Sexually Transmitted Disease.)

No method of treatment has been effective in reducing incidence of postherpetic neuralgia. Clients 60 years old and older and immunocompromised clients are at greatest risk for this painful condition.

Colloidal oatmeal soaks (Aveeno) or calamine lotion may be soothing to the skin.

Follow-Up

Evaluate client in 1 week for response. Refer to physician immediately if condition does not improve.

DYSHIDROSIS (DYSHIDROTIC ECZEMA)

Dyshidrosis or pompholyx is a very common eczematous dermatitis of the hands and feet. It has the characteristic appearance of tapioca grains on the sides of the fingers. It is intensely pruritic.

Epidemiology

First appearance is usually in young adulthood and in times of stress. Its course and recurrence is unpredictable, but episodes tend to decrease in late adulthood. Often associated with atopy and nickel allergy.[1]

Subjective/Objective Data/ Differential Diagnoses

See Table 21–11, Vesicular Dermatoses: Dyshidrosis.

Diagnostic Tests. Diagnosis is usually made on the basis of history and characteristic appearance. Because of its appearance on palms and soles, an RPR to rule out secondary syphillis is suggested. May coexist with Tinea pedis (athlete's foot) so KOH prep may be indicated.

Plan

Psychosocial Interventions. Clients who internalize stress to a great degree or who are obsessive-compulsive may need referral for psychological counseling. Fissuring and chapping of the skin may be disfiguring. Advise client prevention of flares is key. See lifestyle measures following.

Medication. Mid- to high potency steroid cream or ointment may be helpful to decrease[1] pruritis and to treat peeling and fissuring, which occur after vesicular stage. If weepy and eczematous, advise application of cool, moist compresses or Burow's soaks (Domeboro) twice a day for 15 minutes to dry, debride, and reduce swelling before application of topical steroid (see Table 21–10). Oral steroids are generally not used because of chronicity of condition.

Advise client that dyshidrosis may not respond well to topical steroids, except for relief of pruritis and inflammation. Acute flares usually resolve within 2–3 weeks.

Lifestyle. Avoiding irritants is the key to preventing flares. Advise client to wear cotton gloves inside latex or plastic gloves when hands are immersed in water. Always use hand cream after washing hands, especially those creams containing emollients, such as Eucerin and Aquaphor.

Follow-Up

Evaluate client after 7–10 days of therapy for response.

PUSTULAR AND NODULAR DERMATOSES

Acne Vulgaris

Acne is a common skin condition under the influence of hormonal and genetic factors. It usually starts with stimulation of the sebaceous glands by androgen; therefore, its appearance coincides with puberty. Sebaceous glands increase in size,

and output of sebum rises to a point where plugging of the follicle occurs.

Bacteria, mainly *Propionibacterium* acnes, causes breakdown of the sebum, disruption of the follicle wall into the dermis, and subsequent inflammation.[5]

Epidemiology. First appears in mid- to late adolescence and usually wanes in severity in 20s but can persist in women into their 40s. Begins with oily skin and plugged follicles known as whiteheads (closed comedones) and blackheads (open comedones) over the nose and forehead. The sebum inside the plugged duct may cause irritation to adjacent skin and produce inflammatory lesions, nodules, and pustules. Severe cystic acne is more common in males and is rarely found in women. Women often find acne worsens just before menses and may improve (or become worse) with pregnancy. Its course during a lifetime is unpredictable but appearance of cysts and family history of scarring are bad prognosticators.[1,5,6]

Subjective/Objective Data/Differential Diagnoses. See Table 21–12, Pustular and Nodular Dermatoses, Acne Vulgaris.

DIAGNOSTIC TESTS. Diagnosis is made on basis of history and appearance. Pustular lesions resistant to treatment may have to have exudate sent for culture and sensitivity.

Plan

PSYCHOSOCIAL INTERVENTIONS. Acne is an overwhelming concern to adolescents and young adults. In a 1994 survey by the AMA, 89 percent of girls worried about their complexion and half believed it was the first thing people noted about them.[5] Depending on its severity, it can lead to depression and social isolation. The practitioner must be alert to these concerns and anticipate any need for psychological counseling. Be supportive of appropriate coping mechanisms.[5]

MEDICATIONS. Treatment is directed to predominant type of lesion. The aim is to prevent scarring. Be sure to ask the client about efficacy of past and present treatments. Advise her to avoid astringents unless skin is very oily and use only on oily spots.

TABLE 21–12. PUSTULAR AND NODULAR DERMATOSES

Diagnosis	Subjective Data	Objective Data Distribution	Differential DX
Acne Vulgaris	Usually onset at puberty. May have mild pain, itching May have history of topical or oral steroid use	Inflammatory, open and closed comedones, papules and pustules nodules, and cysts with scarring but hallmark is comedone *Distribution: face, neck, upper back, chest, shoulders*	Folliculitis (hairy areas, rare on face)
Rosacea	Middle-aged onset History of flushing, burning, esp. with hot food and drink	Inflammatory papules, flushing, telangiectases Comedones absent Often associated with seborrhea and blepharitis *Distribution: only on face*	Acne vulgaris (comedones prominent)
Impetigo	Pruritis	Pustules (may have macules and vesicles also) Honey colored crust When crust removed leaves denuded area *Distribution: often on face*	Contact Dermatitis (trigger, linear pattern)
Folliculitis	Itching and burning History of hot tub use, diabetes, excessive sweating	Pustules at base of hair follicle May have erythema of surrounding skin *Distribution: hairy areas of body*	Acne (see above) Impetigo (see above) Pseudofolliculitis (pustules at side not in follicle, caused by ingrown hair)
Furuncles and Carbuncles	Painful Common in diabetics, obese with oily skin, staph carriers	Abscess of hair follicle with enlarging, conical shape May coalesce to form carbuncle Becomes flocculent with purulent discharge *Distribution: most common sites are hairy areas exposed to irritation, friction, moisture as face, neck, axillae, buttocks, groin, upper back*	Inflamed epidermal cyst (history of cyst, cheesy exudate) Acne (not in follicle)
Warts	No symptoms unless on sole of foot (painful)	Flesh colored papule or nodule 1–10mm that may form mosaic Surface is rough, verrucated (sawtoothed), or flat May be pedunculated or have cauliflowerlike appearance Plantar warts resemble corns or calluses *Distribution: anywhere on body but commonly on hands, face, neck, upper trunk, soles of feet, genital area*	Squamous cell cancer (biopsy always if in doubt)

Source: References 1, 6, 8, 10.

Choice of vehicle for topical agents depends on appearance of skin. Creams and lotions moisturize, but creams are heavier and may be more appropriate for very dry or irritated skin. Gels and solutions are alcohol based and tend to dry the skin. Client preference should also be taken into consideration.

For the comedonal stage, over-the-counter products that contain salicylic acid (Stridex), resorcinol, and/or sulfur (Sulforcin), benzoyl peroxide (Fostex, Clearasil Maximum Strength) are fairly effective if used on a regular basis. Alpha-hydroxy acids loosen follicular plugging.

- *Administration.* Dab directly on individual lesions twice daily after washing and drying skin.
- *Adverse Effects.* May sting or burn.

The most effective agent is topical tretinoin (Retin-A) because it unplugs comedones and prevents new ones from forming. It is considered appropriate for almost all acne.

- *Administration.* Start with lowest concentration 0.025 percent gel or cream applied once daily at bedtime after washing and drying skin to remove dirt and make-up. Choice of vehicle depends on whether client's skin is dry (cream preferred) or oily (gel is drying). May be used every other day if used in combination with antibiotic (see following).

- *Adverse Effects.* Include burning, peeling, and redness.
- *Contraindications.* Include known sensitivity to Vitamin A/retinoic acid.
- *Client Teaching.* Warn client to avoid contact with eyes and mucous membranes. Apply sparingly, total amount used should be equivalent to size of one or two peas. Do not dot on lesions but lightly spread on skin. Advise her it may initially cause exacerbation of inflammatory lesions 7–10 days after starting but resolves over several weeks. Avoid prolonged exposure to sunlight and always wear sunscreen SPF 15 or higher. Concentration can be increased if needed to 0.05 percent or 0.1 percent gel or cream.

If client is able to tolerate, benzoyl peroxide can be used in the morning and tretinoin at night. Benzoyl peroxide (concentrations 2.5 percent gel and liquid, 5 percent and 10 percent gel, liquid and cream) is effective against *Propionibacterium* acnes and inflammation, and tretinoin speeds cell turnover and prevents new comedones.

- *Administration.* Advise her to start with application of medications on alternate nights until she has adjusted to irritating effects of each, then proceed to use of benzoyl peroxide in morning and tretinoin at night.
- *Adverse Effects.* Local stinging and burning.
- *Contraindications.* Known sensitivity to either agent.
- *Client Teaching.* Avoid eyes, mouth, angles of nose, mucous membranes. Wash hands after using each.

This can be a very effective treatment and can result in dramatic clearing after 6–8 weeks.[5]

Topical antibiotics such as clindamycin (Cleocin T) available 10 mg/ml as gel, lotion, or cream and erythromycin (A/T/S, Erycette) 2 percent gel, ointment, or solution may be used in combination with tretinoin.

- *Administration.* Antibiotic is applied twice a day and tretinoin at night. When used simultaneously, apply antibiotic first, allow to dry, then apply tretinoin.

- *Adverse Effects.* Local irritation, stinging, burning.
- *Contraindication.* Known sensitivity to ingredients.
- *Client Teaching.* See aforementioned. If rash appears, discontinue at once and call provider.

In more difficult cases, a benzoyl peroxide-erythromycin gel combination (Erythromycin/BP gel) can be used in the morning with tretinoin at night. Initially, start using each on alternating nights until adjustment to irritating effects. Contraindication is known sensitivity to any ingredients.

- *Expected Outcome.* Advise client it may take at least 4 weeks to achieve desirable results.

If papules and pustules predominate and there is scarring, consider adding an oral antibiotic, such as erythromycin 250 mg QID, tetracycline 500 mg po BID, or minocycline 100 mg BID. Minocycline is the least photosensitizing of the tetracyclines, is somewhat more effective than tetracycline, and can be taken with food.

- *Adverse Effects.* Include lightheadedness, change in skin pigmentation if taken over long periods of time, development of vaginal yeast infection.
- *Contraindications.* Is known sensitivity to tetracyclines and pregnancy (teratogenic).[5]

Topical antibiotic preparations may be used such as erythromycin gel or clindamycin (Cleocin T) but be aware that *Propionibacterium* acnes can develop resistance to both these preparations. Use erythromycin gel in combination with benzoyl peroxide as discussed previously.[5]

NOTE: If client is taking oral contraceptives, switch to lower androgenic pill, such as Devulen 1/35.

DIET/LIFESTYLE. There is no evidence that chocolate or fatty foods make acne worse. Nor does vigorous scrubbing or sun tanning make it better. Gentle cleansers, such as Dove, Basis, or Neutrogena are recommended. Advise client never to pick or squeeze pimples; it can lead to scarring. Review current cosmetic products. Changing to oil free make-up can lessen comedone formation. Reassure client best results come from adherence to agreed upon treatment plan and patience, may take 4–6 weeks to see improvement.

Follow-Up. Refer clients with severe or cystic acne to dermatologist. After 1 week of treatment plan, evaluate client, then again at 1 month.

ROSACEA

Rosacea is a chronic skin condition that develops in middle age. It may progress through four stages:

Stage I: Prerosacea—transient flushing and erythema of the face and neck
Stage II: Vascular rosacea—persistent erythema and telangiactasia
Stage III: Inflammatory rosacea—multiple inflammatory papules and pustules
Stage IV: Glandular hyperplastic rosacea— (usually in men) lymphedema and hypertrophy of connective tissue[10]

Epidemiology

It is estimated 10 percent of the population may be affected, women three times more often than men. Genetic pattern common especially in those of Celtic or northern European origin. Its cause is unknown, and its course is unpredictable. Vasomotor lability in response to heat may play a role.[10]

Subjective Data/Objective Data/ Differential Diagnoses

See Table 21–12, Pustular and Nodular Dermatoses: Rosacea.

Diagnostic Tests. Diagnosis is usually made on the basis of history and appearance. If lupus or cutaneous sarcoidosis is suspected, diagnosis is made by biopsy and client should be referred to dermatologist.

Plan

Psychosocial Interventions. Rosacea is a chronic disease, and treatment is continuous. Reassure client that early intervention and prevention of flares help. Body image concerns and embarrassment should be addressed. A glandular, hyper-

plastic stage (usually seen in men) may cause rhinophyma in which nose appears enlarged and bright red or violaceous. Client may be suspected of being a heavy drinker because of flushed appearance of skin.

Medications. Topical clindamycin and errthromycin may be beneficial (see discussion of both these agents in section on acne). Metronidazole gel 0.75 percent has been shown in some studies to be comparable in efficacy to oral tetracycline.[10]

- ▪ *Administration.* Applied twice daily.
- ▪ *Adverse Effects.* Transient redness, burning, irritation.
- ▪ *Contraindications.* Allergy to metronidazole or its component ingredients. Use cautiously if history of blood dyscrasias; may potentiate oral anticoagulants.
- ▪ *Client Teaching.* Avoid contact with eyes.
- ▪ *Oral Antibiotic.* Tetracycline 500 mg BID or if gastric upset, Minocycline 50–100 mg BID
- ▪ *Administration.* Twice a day for 6–8 weeks. Advise client not to take with food. May taper dose down to maintenance dose of Tetracycline 250–500 mg or Minocycline 50 mg every other day.
- ▪ *Adverse Effects.* Photosensitivity, light-headedness, dizziness, diarrhea, anorexia.
- ▪ *Contraindications.* Pregnancy, known sensitivity.

Diet/Lifestyle. Discuss triggers of flushing and erythema such as excessive cold, wind, heat, alcohol, and spicy foods. Some studies have shown that prolonged exposure to computer screens may aggravate rosacea.[10]

Follow-Up

Evaluate client in 1 week for tolerance of therapy, then again at 1 month. Refer to dermatologist if condition worsens or rhinophyma (enlarged red nose).[10]

IMPETIGO

Impetigo is a contagious infection of the skin that is caused by Staphylococcus aureus coagulase positive and/or group A beta hemolytic Streptococcus. Most cases of impetigo today are due to Staphylococcus. The lesions may be vesicles, pustules, and/or bullae, but the diagnostic feature is honey colored crust.

Epidemiology

Most common in childhood, especially on the face around the nares, but in adults can occur on any exposed surface. It can spread to others. Secondary impetigination can occur with eczema or other vesiculobullous dermatoses and is treated as impetigo.

Subjective Data/Objective Data/ Differential Diagnoses

See Table 21–12, Pustular and Nodular Dermatoses: Impetigo.

Diagnostic Tests. Diagnosis is usually based on history and appearance. Treatment is empiric with broad spectrum antibiotic covering staph and strep, but culture and sensitivity of exudate may be helpful if resistant organisms in community are a concern.

Plan

Psychosocial Interventions. Reassure client impetigo responds very quickly to oral antibiotics.

Medication. Dicloxacillin 250 mg po QID for 7 days or if allergic to penicillin, erythromycin 250 mg QID for 7 days. (See previous discussion of Dicloxacillin under Mastitis, chapter on Postpartum and Lactation. Erythromycin discussed earlier under Eczema.)

In areas where erythromycin resistant staphylococcus, Ciprofloxacin 250 mg po BID for 7 days is a reasonable but expensive alternative.

Adverse effects include GI upset, headache, dizziness, nightmares.

Contraindicated in known sensitivity, nursing mothers.

If impetigo is localized to small area, mupirocin 2 percent ointment (Bactroban) may be used topically three times a day.

- *Adverse Effects.* May cause local stinging. If no response in 3 days, switch to oral antibiotics and culture.
- *Expected Outcome.* Rapid resolution of infection.

Lifestyle. Warm, moist compresses may be used to soften and remove crusts. Advise client to separate washcloths and towels from other household members.

Follow-Up

Advise client to call or to schedule visit if not resolved in 5–7 days.

FOLLICULITIS

Folliculitis is an infection or inflammation of the hair follicle caused by *Staphylococcus aureus* (or if arises after use of hot tub, *Pseudomonas aeruginosa folliculitis*), by a fungal dermatophyte, by oils (industrial or cosmetic), or perspiration. The causative agent can be differentiated on the basis of history, location of the pustules, bacterial culture, KOH preparation and fungal culture, and lack of response to antibacterial therapy.

Epidemiology

Bacterial folliculitis is more prevalent in diabetics. Common sites are the groin and exposed areas of the arms and legs. Folliculitis may appear during the first week of oral steroid therapy (steroid acne) or may flare when dose is tapered. Hot tub folliculitis appears in 1 to 4 days after use of a contaminated tub. The rash is tender and pruritic.

Fungal folliculitis is characterized by the clustering of the follicular pustules, commonly on the hands, arms, legs, and scalp. In women, infection often occurs when the dermatophyte from Tinea pedis is spread to the legs when shaving. The follicles cluster on the lower legs. Fungal folliculitis can also arise from misdiagnosed Tinea corporis that is treated with steroids. Pustular follicles then arise on the face and dorsum of the hand.

Pseudofolliculitis is caused by ingrowing hairs. Pustules and papules are located beside the follicle but not in the follicle.[6]

Subjective Data/Objective Data/ Differential Diagnoses

See previous discussion and Table 21–12, Pustular and Nodular Dermatoses: Folliculitis.

Diagnostic Tests. Bacterial culture and sensitivity, fungal culture and/or KOH prep are ordered as appropriate. Often empiric treatment is started based on history and appearance while waiting for culture result.

Plan

Psychosocial Interventions. Because pustules appear on exposed areas, client may have body image concerns.

Medication. If bacterial in origin dicloxacillin 250 mg QID for 14 days (see discussion under Impetigo). Small areas may be treated with muciprocin 2 percent ointment (see discussion under Impetigo).

Fungal folliculitis usually responds only to oral antifungals such as griseofulvin (see Tinea Pedis). Confirm by fungal culture before starting therapy.

Folliculitis on the back, which has been diagnosed as acne and does not respond to acne treatment, may be due to *Pityrosporum orbiculare,* which is treated with topical 2.5 percent selenium sulfide (Selsun) applied for 15 minutes daily for 3 weeks.

Medication is not indicated for irritant folliculitis, except for use of drying soaks such as Burow's or benzoyl peroxide.

Aluminum subacetate (Burow's) soaks or compresses twice a day for 15 minutes provides soothing relief to skin, especially if exudative.

Lifestyle. Control of blood sugars is helpful in diabetics. Advise women who acquire infection as a result of shaving legs to use depilatory until resolved or use disposable shavers. Treat water in hot tubs with appropriate chemicals. If irritant folliculitis is caused by occupational exposure to oil, suggest client wear protective clothing and gloves. She may need to switch to oil free make-up.

If excessive perspiration is the cause, suggest client shower promptly after exercise, avoid tight, occlusive clothing, lose weight if indicated.

Follow-Up

Evaluate client in 7 days for response to therapy. Culture if not responding and consider referral to dermatologist if immunocompromised.

FURUNCLES AND CARBUNCLES

A furuncle (abscess or boil) is an infection of the hair follicle. It is more extensive and deep seated than folliculitis and involves the adjacent tissue. Furuncles develop acutely with sudden onset of pain and tenderness. If the furuncles enlarge and coalesce, they may form a carbuncle.

Epidemiology

Furuncles are caused by *Staphylococcus aureus.* Heat and moisture favor their development, especially where trauma has occurred. Immunocompromised individuals are at higher risk for development. At risk for recurrent infections are chronic nose and throat carriers of Staph.

Subjective Data/Objective Data/ Differential Diagnoses

See Table 21–12, Furuncles and Carbuncles.

Diagnostic Tests. Bacterial culture of exudate after incision and drainage is recommended. Treatment is started immediately and is modified if needed based on sensitivity.

Plan

Psychosocial Interventions. Furuncles often develop in the axillae and the anogenital area causing pain and embarrassment. Be alert also to hygiene and body image concerns.

Medications. Dicloxacillin 250–500 mg four times a day for 10–14 days. If sensitive to penicillin, erythromycin 250 mg four times a day or ciprofloxacin 250 mg twice a day. (See previous discussions of these agents in sections on Folliculitis, Impetigo.)

If client is chronic carrier, application of 2 percent muciprocin (Bactroban) ointment to nares, anogenital area, axillae may help eliminate carrier state.[1,6]

Local Measures. Warm soaks applied for 20–30 minutes three times a day may help immobilize lesions and prevent spread. Advise client not to manipulate furuncles to minimize risk of much deeper and even systemic infection. Floculant lesions may have to be incised, drained, and packed.

Lifestyle. Because furuncles may develop in moist, warm areas, advise client to wear loose clothing, fabrics that allow perspiration to evaporate, avoid use of petroleum, oil based cosmetics, lotions.

Follow-Up

Evaluate client in 1 week for response to therapy. If furuncle incised and drained, schedule client for daily evaluation to change packing, irrigate. Refer to physician if infection recurs. Client or intimate contacts may be staph carriers.

WARTS (HUMAN PAPILLOMAVIRUS)

Warts are benign tumors of the skin caused by the Human Papillomavirus. There are more than 63 types of HPV and some have premalignant potential. Cutaneous warts fall into three broad classifications:

Common warts
Plantar warts of the foot
Flat warts

They can occur on any part of the body including the hands, face, feet. Mucosal warts arise on mucous membranes such as the conjunctiva, oral mucosa, larynx, and the anogenital area.[8] (See discussion of genital warts in chapter on sexually transmitted disease.)

Epidemiology

Warts often arise in childhood and regress spontaneously, usually in 1 to 2 years. In adults, they are less likely to regress. They are caused by a virus and have an incubation period of 2–18 months. Warts are contagious by fomites, by autoinoculation from one area to another, and from person to person. Warm, moist environments subjected to trauma or friction favor the growth. A single very small papule may grow to 5–10 mm, and new warts may cluster around to form a mosaic of 3 cm. It is estimated that more than 24 million U.S. citizens have common cutaneous warts, a level of epidemic proportions.

Subjective/Objective Data/ Differential Diagnoses

See Table 21–12, Pustular and Nodular Dermatoses: Warts.

Diagnostic Tests. Usually diagnosed on basis of appearance. Biopsy indicated if located on sun damaged skin; if large, chronic wart in elderly; if color, border change; if long standing wart of finger (high potential for squamous cell cancer).

Plan

Psychosocial Interventions. Concern about appearance leads many women to seek treatment. Depending on location, warts may also interfere with work, hobbies, or activities of daily living. Reassure client that, even though common cutaneous warts are benign, you appreciate her concern regarding possible malignancy or skin cancer. Give client realistic expectations of successful treatment. It may take several visits to eradicate lesions. Give client option of no treatment by pointing out possibility of spontaneous regression, possibility of skin damage, scarring from treatment.

Treatment. Any suspicion of squamous cell carcinoma must be biopsied. Any mucosal wart should be excised immediately and sent to the pathologist.

There are three mainstays of treatment for cutaneous warts: salicylic acid, cantharidin, and liquid nitrogen cryotherapy.

Salicylic acid is available over-the-counter under various trade names (Compound W, Wart-Off, Freezone).

- *Administration.* Apply to the entire area after bathing and soaking the wart for several minutes. Pat dry and use applicator to cover the wart. Adjacent skin should be avoided, may use petrolatum to protect. Use every night and rinse off in morning. For warts on soles of feet (plantar warts), may cover with occlusive dressing or salicylic plaster. Apply daily. Remove dead skin by filing off with pumice stone. Frequency of treatment is dependent on tenderness and results.
- *Adverse Effects.* Warn client about local irritation. Contraindicated if allergic to aspirin.
- *Client Teaching.* May require repeated treatments, less effective than cathardin but less painful.

Cantharidin (Cantharone) is not available at all pharmacies. It is a blistering agent that must be formulated from its ingredients by the pharmacist and is for office use only.

- *Administration.* Solution is applied to wart with a wooden applicator and left on for 24 hours under an occlusive dressing. It is applied in the office. Solution is removed with mild soap and water the next day. It is reapplied weekly depending on results.
- *Adverse Effects.* Moderate to severe pain may develop 12 to 24 hours after treatment.[8]
- *Contraindications.* Known sensitivity to agent. Use with caution if client is diabetic, or has impaired circulation.

See Chapter 11 (Vaginitis and Sexually Transmitted Diseases) for discussion of liquid nitrogen cryotherapy.

Lifestyle. Advise client that warts are contagious and may be spread to other areas of the body or to other close contacts after a break in the skin or maceration. A single wart may contain millions of infectious virions.[8] Treatment of plantar's warts may require client to stay off feet or use crutches. Assess effect on occupation and activities of daily living.

Follow-Up

Evaluate response to therapy after 1 week. Advise client to call if significant pain develops after office treatment. Refer insulin dependent diabetics, those who do not respond to treatment to dermatologist.

ANOGENITAL PRURITIS

Anogenital pruritis is a diagnosis of exclusion after all other causes of pruritis have been ruled, such as viral or bacterial infection, infestation, sensitivity to soaps or chemicals, psoriasis, or atrophic vaginitis. Poor hygiene may be at fault.

Epidemiology

Pruritis vulvae is not uncommon in women. It does not involve the anal area in most cases.

Subjective Data

Intense pruritis, especially at night. Client may report scant white discharge.

Objective Data

Absence of physical findings is the rule. May see excoriations, erythema, and/or fissuring.

Differential Diagnoses

Candidiasis, pediculosis, contact or allergic dermatitis, psoriasis, seborrhea, atrophic vaginitis, human papilloma virus.

Plan

Psychosocial Interventions. Condition may be extremely embarrassing to client and may lead to social isolation in extreme cases.

Medication. Pramoxine cream or lotion or hydrocortisone-pramoxine 1 percent cream, lotion or ointment applied three to four times a day for up to 4 weeks. Wash hands after use and avoid contact with eyes.

- *Adverse Effects.* May burn or sting.
- *Contraindications.* Known sensitivity.
- *Client Teaching.* Scrupulous hygiene.

Diet/Lifestyle. If constipation present, may be exacerbating pruritis. Follow high fiber diet, drink plenty of fluids. Advise cleaning skin after every bowel movement with moistened soft cloth. Sitz baths may also relieve discomfort.

Follow-Up

Re-evaluate after 7–10 days for response to therapy.

CELLULITIS

Cellulitis is an infection of the skin and subcutaneous tissue without purulent formation.

Epidemiology

Cellulitis may follow superficial injury to the skin, folliculitis, stasis ulcer. Often the initial insult may be inapparent. It is caused primarily by gram positive cocci, such as staphylococcus or streptococcus.

Subjective Data

Client complains of pain and tenderness.

Objective Data

Diffuse border of warm, red skin.

Diagnostic Tests. Diagnosed on basis of appearance. Bacterial culture from injection and aspiration of saline rarely yield valuable results and may further spread cellulitis.

Differential Diagnoses

Severe contact dermatitis may resemble cellulitis but is pruritic and not as painful.

Plan

Psychosocial Interventions. Reassure client that with prompt treatment and adherence to treatment plan, cellulitis resolves promptly.

Medications. See prior discussion of Impetigo.

Diet/Lifestyle. Advise client to apply warm soaks at least three times a day, elevate extremity. If legs or feet affected, limit ambulation as much as possible.

Follow-Up

Mark area affected and evaluate within 1 to 2 days by telephone contact or office visit. Close follow-up needed for frail and/or elderly client, client with hand or anogenital involvement.

DERMATOLOGICAL CONDITIONS NEEDING REFERRAL

ERYSIPELAS

Erysipelas is a form of cellulitis that appears on the cheek, first near the nasolabial fold. Over a period of a few days, it spreads rapidly to form a smooth, erythematous hot area. It is caused by beta-hemolytic streptococcus. The client may appear toxic on presentation with chills, fever, and pain. If erysipelas is not treated immediately, it can spread systemically and be fatal.

Epidemiology

Can occur at any age. Older clients and those who are immunocompromised are at greatest risk. Occurs after break in skin or trauma.[6]

Subjective Data

Client may report first appeared as small papule near nose and spread rapidly. May complain of chills, fever, and malaise.

Objective Data

Edematous, sharply marginated hot red area, which may have vesicles or bullae on surface. May pit to finger pressure.

Diagnostic Tests. White count and erythrocyte sedimentation rate are elevated. Blood culture may be positive for strep.

Differential Diagnoses

Urticaria following insect bite (resolves over next 24 hours). Cellulitis has less definite margin.

Plan

Refer to physician immediately. Client is put on bed rest with head of bed elevated. May require hospitalization and intravenous penicillin or erythromycin therapy.

ERYTHEMA NODOSUM

The lesions of erythema nodosum are large 4–10 cm red, painful slope shouldered or flattopped plaques that appear on the anterior lower legs and less commonly on the thigh. The most common causes of this inflammatory vascular reaction include reactions to medications such as sulfa, penicillin, progestins; infections such as streptococcus, deep mycoses, tuberculosis, hepatitis B, and syphilis; autoimmune disease and malignancies such as sarcoidosis, leukemia, and inflammatory bowel disease.

Epidemiology

More common in women. May appear in pregnancy.

Subjective Data

Client may report fever, malaise and joint pain before appearance of nodules.

Objective Data

Usually bilateral distribution on anterior lower leg or around ankle. Warm to touch, 4–10 cm in size, tender.

Differential Diagnoses

Cellulitis does not appear as multiple lesions. Erythema multiforme has a more general distribution.

Plan

Psychosocial Interventions. Erythema nodosum may be the presenting sign of a chronic, serious disease. Psychosocial support for such a diagnosis should be anticipated.

Treatment is based on underlying cause. Consult with the physician regarding further workup. Comfort measures include nonsteroidal anti-inflammatory agents and, in some cases, bed rest.

PALPABLE PURPURA

Purpura arises from the escape of the red blood cells into the skin due to an immune complex mechanism or trauma. It has two forms, petechiae (3 mm or less) and ecchymoses (larger than 3 mm). Purpura do not blanch with pressure. Nonpalpable purpura are caused by platelet abnormalities, actinic purpuras, and use of steroids. The most common cause of nontraumatic palpable purpura is a cutaneous vasculitis secondary to infection, connective tissue disease, or medication sensitivity. Noninflammatory etiologies include subacute bacterial endocarditis, amyloidosis, and embolic disease. Some palpable purpura are idiopathic. Serious causes and any underlying blood dyscrasia must be ruled out.[7]

Epidemiology

Depends on underlying cause.

Subjective Data

A careful history will often lead to diagnosis. Key items are recent onset of pharmacotherapy, fever, history of collagen vascular disease, malignancy, sexually transmitted disease, travel history and insecticide exposure.

Objective Data

Careful examination of the skin, heart, lungs, abdomen, joints, and genitalia. Laboratory tests may include CBC, ESR, blood cultures, ANA, rheumatoid factor, BUN, creatinine, and urinalysis. Range of tests depends on likely etiology and client's presentation. Skin biopsy may be needed if cause is not self-limited such as drug reaction or infection.

Differential Diagnoses

Cutaneous vasculitis, bacteremia, Rocky Mountain spotted fever, subacute bacterial endocarditis, amyloidosis, trauma, cholesterol emboli, disseminated intravascular coagulation, pseudopurpura such as Kaposi's sarcoma, Sweet's syndrome (fever, rash on upper body 5–10 days after upper respiratory infection; may be marker of leukemia).[7]

Plan

Consultation with physician to outline diagnostic tests and possible further referral.

SKIN CANCER

Skin cancer is the most common type of cancer in the United States. Its incidence has increased dramatically in the last 10 years, over 65 percent for nonmelanoma cancers.

The three most common types are basal cell cancer, squamous cell cancer, and malignant melanoma. Basal and squamous cell cancers are more common; however, malignant melanoma accounts for almost all the deaths. Women, because of their sun bathing, are particularly at risk.

The United States Public Health Service's Healthy People 2000 program recommends annual skin examinations for adults over 50 years old with risk factors for skin cancer.[11]

BASAL CELL SKIN CANCER

Basal cell cancer (BCC) arises from epidermal keratinocytes. It grows by direct extension and destruction of surrounding tissue. Metastasis is uncommon.[11]

Epidemiology

Risk factors are similar for all types of skin cancer:

- Fair skin that burns easily and tans poorly (see Table 21–13)
- Substantial time spent outdoors, particularly occupational, for example, farmers and sailors
- History of childhood sunburns
- Family history of skin cancer
- X-ray, radiation burn sites, UV light therapy, chronic venous stasis ulcers
- Arsenic ingestion (rare)
- Immunosuppression

Fair skin and sun exposure are the key risk factors. More than 90 percent of basal cell cancer occurs on sun exposed areas of the head and neck but are rare on the back of the hand. The cancer may occur at sites of previous trauma, such as in thermal burns and scars. Basal cell cancer has many clinical forms, which vary in appearance and malignant potential.

It is estimated that one in seven Americans will develop basal cell cancer. It is the most common type of skin cancer in the United States. Basal cell cancer is common among caucasians and rare among African Americans. It may occur at any age. The incidence markedly increases after age 40 but basal cell carcinomas are becoming increasingly common in 20–30 year olds.[6,11,12]

TABLE 21–13. SKIN CANCER PREVENTION GUIDELINES

1. *Avoid sun exposure*
   - Skin types I–IV are especially susceptible.
   - Protect infants and children. Children cannot protect themselves and significant increased risk may be associated with exposure in first decade.
   - Use caution with sun-sensitizing medications: tetracycline, tricyclics, antihistamines, antipsychotics, hypoglycemics, diuretics, antineoplastics, retin A.
2. *Avoid tanning salons. Artificial sunlight is no safer than sunlight.*
3. *When you must be in the sun, protect yourself*
   - Avoid peak times for ultraviolet B: 10 A.M. to 2 P.M.
   - Wear protective clothing: hats, especially broad brimmed; light-colored clothing.
   - Beware of reflective surfaces: snow and cement.
   - **Use sunscreen or sun block whenever going outdoors:** Choose strong enough sun protective factor (SPF). See guidelines below. Apply adequate amounts of sunscreen; manufacturer's directions are more than most people use. Apply lotion 30–60 minutes before expected sun exposure, as it takes time for *para*-aminobenzoic acid (PABA) to bind in the stratum corneum. Reapply at least every 40–80 minutes and more frequently if swimming or perspiring.
4. *Types of sunscreens/sunblocks*
   - Chemical sunscreens
     - PABA and PABA esters: they are the first choice because they effectively block ultraviolet B (UVG), which is associated with skin cancers.
     - Non-PABA sunscreens include benzophenones and cinnamates, which weakly block UVB; use if allergic to PABA.
   - Physical sunblocks: zinc oxide and titanium dioxide; opaque and often cosmetically unacceptable.
5. *Skin type and choice of sun protection factor (SPF)*

Skin Type	Skin Color and Sunburn History	SPF
I	Very fair: always burns, never tans	≥15
II	Fair: burns easily, tans minimally	≥15 or more
III	Light brown: burns moderately, tans gradually and uniformly	10–15
IV	Moderate brown: burns minimally, always tans well	6–15
V	Dark brown: rarely burns, tans profusely	6–15
VI	Deeply pigmented: never burns	Low

Source: References 11, 13, 18.

TABLE 21–14. DIFFERENTIAL DIAGNOSES OF DYSPLASTIC NEVI

Sign	Common Mole	Dysplastic Nevi
Shape	Round or oval	Irregular
Margins	Sharp, well circumscribed	Hazy, indistinct
Color	Light brown to black, uniform pigmentation	Variegated tan, dark brown on pink background
Topography	Flat or smooth dome shape	"Fried egg" shape, papular center with macular periphery or pebble contour
Size	Usually < 6 mm	Usually > 6mm, up to 12 mm
Number	Usually 12–25	One or many, often > 100
Location	Usually face and upper extremities	Mostly on covered areas: buttocks, scalp, and female breasts
Age of onset	Few appear after early adulthood	Continue to appear after age 35

Source: Reference 19.

Subjective Data

Basal cell cancer is primarily asymptomatic; its course is unpredictable. The lesion may remain small with almost no perceptible growth for years or it may grow rapidly. Symptoms such as enlargement, change in color, pain, itching, and bleeding should be investigated. If a client is uncertain about how long a crust lesion has been present, have her return for follow-up in 2 weeks. If the suspicious lesion remains unchanged, refer her for biopsy.[11]

Objective Data

Because the early stages of skin cancer are primarily asymptomatic, screening is crucial. A complete physical exam reveals more than six times the pathology revealed by exams limited to normally exposed sites.

Physical examination should employ a magnifying lens and good lighting to observe suspicious lesions. It is helpful to wet the lesion with oil or an alcohol swab and stretch the lesion between two fingers to check for color patterns. Look for signs of dysplastic nevus syndrome (see Table 21–14). In addition to good visualizations, careful palpation for lymphadenopathy is necessary.

Basal cell cancer usually begins as a small shiny papule that enlarges over months and develops telangiectasias and a pearly border. After time, it develops a central ulcer that recurrently crusts and bleeds. Less common forms of basal cell cancer appear as flat plaques. Keep in mind that the lesion may take many forms. A basal cell carcinoma of the eyelid may have the appearance of a sty that recurs on the lower lid.[11]

Diagnostic tests may be performed by a dermatologist following referral. A suspicious lesion is evaluated and skin biopsy may be necessary.

Differential Medical Diagnoses

See Table 21–15.

Plan

Psychosocial Interventions. Help the client to understand the importance of compliance with referrals and treatment regimens. Reassure her that prompt referral and treatment results in a high rate of cure, about 90–95 percent.

TABLE 21–15. DIFFERENTIAL DIAGNOSIS OF SKIN CANCER

Benign skin lesions	Nevi, seborrheic keratosis, cysts, skin tags, dermatofibromas, keloids
Dermatoses	Seborrhea, eczema, psoriasis, human papilloma virus, fungi
Lesions with premalignant potential	Actinic keratosis, leukoplakia, dysplastic nevus syndrome
Skin cancers	Basal cell cancer, squamous cell cancer (Bowen's, Paget's), malignant melanoma, mycosis fungoides (rare T-cell lymphoma that originates in skin)
Cutaneous metastasis	3–5% of those with metastatic disease develop secondary skin cancers

Source: References 12, 13, 14, 16, 17.

The following organizations provide materials for client and health care education on skin cancer:

National Cancer Institute
Cancer Information Service
31 Center Drive (MSC 2580)
Bldg. 31, Room 10A07
Bethesda, MD 20892–2580
Phone: (800)4–CANCER (422–6237)

Skin Cancer Foundation
245 Fifth Avenue, Suite 2402
New York, NY 10016
Phone: (212) 725–5176

Medication. None is administered.

Surgical Interventions. Surgical excision may be recommended following skin biopsy.

Lifestyle Changes. There is no safe tan. Sun exposure accelerates photoaging.[13] Convincing young women to avoid sun tanning is *very* difficult because of cultural norms and feelings of invulnerability. In prevention education, an emphasis on photoaging may be more effective. All people wrinkle; the question is how much and how soon. Have the woman look at how smooth and soft the skin of her upper inner arm is and compare it with that on the back of her hand. This demonstrates photoaging. Encourage all women to follow the skin cancer prevention guidelines in Table 21–13.[11,13]

Also encourage the client to stop smoking.

Follow-Up

Referral to a dermatologist is necessary after identification of a suspicious lesion.

SQUAMOUS CELL CANCER

Squamous cell cancer (SCC) arises in the epithelium. Like basal cell cancer, squamous cell cancer is most common on areas exposed to the sun; however, distribution is somewhat different. SCC is commonly found on the scalp, the back of the hand, the ear and the lower lip. It often arises from a precursor lesion called *actinic keratosis.* Actinic keratosis, a premalignant skin condition

of the elderly, may appear as flat tan or brown spots with adherent scales and mild surrounding erythema. These often feel rough. Induration, inflammation, and oozing suggest degeneration into malignancy. Squamous cell cancer arising from actinic keratoses is not aggressive but can eventually metastasize.

Squamous cell cancers that arise at thermal burn sites or sites of chronic inflammation have a higher metastatic potential than squamous cell cancers evolving from actinic keratoses.[14]

Epidemiology

The etiology of squamous cell cancer differs somewhat depending on the type; however, all of these cancers usually appear on sun exposed areas of fair-skinned persons. These types (simplified here) and their locations include Bowen's disease, on the trunk and extremities; erythroplasia of Queyrat, on the glans penis; Paget's disease, on the areola, nipple, and vulva; and extramammary Paget's disease, on the anogenital region, axilla, external ear canal, and eyelids.

Paget's disease of the areola manifests as a sharply demarcated area of erythema and scaling, often with oozing and crusting. It is associated with breast cancer, but easily confused with eczema. By contrast, eczema is bilateral and resolves with treatment; Paget's lesions are mostly unilateral and progressive.

Squamous cell cancer is common in the oral cavity of women who smoke and drink, often on the posterior lateral borders of the tongue. Leukoplakia, a white opaque patch found on the lips, oral mucosa, and vulva, is a precursor lesion that may degenerate into squamous cell cancer.

Hairy leukoplakia is different from leukoplakia; it is unique to AIDS and associated with the Epstein-Barr virus and human papillomavirus. White and hairy papillary projections are found primarily on the lateral border of the tongue.

Incidence reports show that squamous cell cancer is the second most common skin cancer among the general population. It is the most common among African Americans, especially those with a history of a scarring process, such as a burn or leg ulcer.[14]

Subjective Data

Squamous cell cancer is primarily asymptomatic, but a client may report itching, irritation, bleeding, or a change in skin appearance.

Objective Data

See Objective Data under Basal Cell Cancer.

Physical examination reveals a variable appearance among clients, but the lesions usually begins as a reddish papule or plaque with a scaly or crusted surface. It may mimic dermatitis. Later, the lesion may appear nodular or warty. Eventually, it ulcerates and invades underlying tissue.

Lesions on the lower lip may start with a thickened, dry, scaly surface on the vermillion border. Later it may progress to a nodule. Lesions of the lower lip, especially those on the inside mucous membrane, are very aggressive and demand prompt referral for treatment.[14]

Diagnostic evaluation and management are carried out by a dermatologist.

Differential Medical Diagnoses

See Table 21–15.

Plan

Psychosocial Interventions. Emphasize the importance of skin cancer prevention (see Table 21–13). Some actinic keratoses may regress if the client avoids sun exposure. Stress the importance of the treatment regimen outlined by the specialist. Refer her to the resources listed for basal cell cancer.

Medication. Methotrexate or 5-fluorouracil (Efudex) may be injected by the dermatologist after biopsy for certain selected types of lesions. Failure to respond necessitates excision of the lesion.[14]

Surgical Interventions. Excision, cryosurgery, or electrodesiccation and curettage may be performed depending on the extent of the lesion.

Lifestyle Changes. See those recommended for clients with basal cell cancer.

Follow-Up

Continue to monitor the client for new lesions every 3 months and teach her how to perform monthly self-examinations of the skin.

MALIGNANT MELANOMA

Malignant melanoma (MM) arises from melanocytes. It is associated primarily with sun exposure. Because most malignant melanomas arise from pigmented moles, any change in a mole is always of concern. Removal of benign moles does not decrease the risk for malignant melanoma. It may develop anywhere there are melanocytes or pigmented skin, such as mucous membranes, eyes, and the central nervous system. Malignant melanoma may arise de novo, that is, from sites where no mole is visible.

Malignant melanoma is deadly. Early identification and prompt surgical excision offer the only change for cure. The radial growth phase is a "window of opportunity" during the first several months to years of a malignant melanoma. A mole removed while it is less than 0.76 mm deep is associated with a 95 percent cure rate. Excision of vertical growths greater than 4 mm results in only 50 percent survival at 5 years.[15,16]

Dysplastic nevus syndrome (DNS) is a familial syndrome found in 2 to 5 percent of the population. Individuals with dysplastic nevus syndrome have at least 6 percent lifetime risk for malignant melanoma. Clients exhibit large asymmetric and irregularly pigmented nevi. If they have two close family members with malignant melanoma, their lifetime risk for developing malignant melanoma is over 50 percent and may approach 100 percent.

Epidemiology

An epidemic of skin cancers has occurred since the 1920s when tans became "fashionable." More than 500,000 new skin cancers are diagnosed each year in the United States. Malignant melanoma accounts for only 3 percent of these cancers, yet it is responsible for three-quarters of the deaths from skin cancer.[11]

The most important risk factor for melanoma is skin color. It is rare in African Americans. In nonblacks major risk factors include number of moles, tendency to freckle, tendency to burn in sunlight, past history of sunburns (especially in childhood), family history of atypical nevi, family history of malignant melanoma. Immune dysfunction may also be a risk factor. Research indicates that immunocompromise may allow transformation of dysplastic nevi into malignant melanoma.[16]

In a recent survey, nonmelanoma skin cancers increased by 65 percent, while the number of cases of melanoma grew by 21 percent in the same 9-year period. The lifetime risk of developing invasive malignant melanoma is one in 87 in 1996 and is expected to be one in 75 by the year 2000.[17] It is now the leading cause of cancer deaths in women younger than 35.

Subjective Data

Four major symptoms are enlargement, color change, pain (sometimes "itch"), and bleeding. Most clients present with only one symptom, and any symptom warrants referral for evaluation. Refer to a dermatologist all women with a family history of dysplastic nevus syndrome, especially if they also have a family history of melanoma.

Objective Data

A physical examination will help identify suspicious changes. The ABCDs (asymmetry, border, color, diameter, surface/sensation) can assist practitioners, as well as clients, in performing skin exams (see Table 21–16).

Physical examination focuses on sun exposed areas (back, head, and neck) where most malignant melanomas occur. Acrolentiginous melanoma is a rare, but rapidly fatal lesion, occurring most often among African Americans on their palmar, plantar, or nail bed surfaces. Each of the several types of melanoma has its own particular idiosyncrasies and growth patterns. Be suspicious of variegated color, irregular borders and surfaces, and an increase in size (see Table 21–16).

Small dysplastic nevi may be difficult to differentiate from common moles on physical exam. If the client has a family history of dysplastic nevus syndrome and any questionable lesion, refer her to a dermatologist.

Diagnostic tests are conducted by a dermatologist. Refer any suspicious lesion for evaluation and probable biopsy.

Differential Medical Diagnoses

See Table 21–14.

Plan

Psychosocial Interventions. Educate the client about moles and reassure her that not all moles are harmful. In general, people are born without moles. Small, flat, tan "common" moles develop in childhood and increase in size and number after puberty. They may become smooth domes. By early adulthood, individuals average 12 to 25 moles. In individuals who live long lives, the moles recede and disappear before death.

Medication. Refer to dermatologist.

Surgical Intervention. Surgical excision may be performed.

Lifestyle Changes. Encourage the client to follow skin cancer prevention guidelines (see Table 21–13). She should also perform monthly self-exams of the skin and stop smoking.

Follow-Up

Refer a client with any suspicious lesion to a dermatologist. If dysplastic nevus syndrome is suspected, refer the client. With numerous dysplastic nevi, baseline photographs and perhaps serial photodocumentation are needed.

TABLE 21–16. ABCDs OF SKIN CANCER

A	Asymmetry	One half shaped unlike the other
B	Border	Irregular, notched, or scalloped
C	Color	Haphazard shades of brown, red, blue, gray
D	Diameter	Greater than 6 mm (size of the tip of a pencil eraser)
S	Surface or sensation	Surface distortion may be subtle or obvious, assess by focusing light at side of lesion; sensation refers to itch, burn, or pain

Immunocompromised clients may be seen every 3 to 4 months by the dermatologist. Family members of clients with dysplastic nevus syndrome must be screened; often an early operable melanoma is found in a distant relative. All women should be taught the ABCDs of melanoma (see Table 21–16). A complete skin exam should be conducted at the time of the client's annual physical. Encourage women to examine their skin monthly at home.

Ear, nose, and throat disorders

These disorders are frequently encountered in primary care, the most common being the common cold, otitis media, acute sinusitis, and pharyngitis.

THE COMMON COLD

The common cold is a mild, self-limited condition caused by a viral infection of the upper respiratory mucosa. The nasal mucosa is prominently involved.

Epidemiology

Studies of the common cold demonstrate that age and environmental contacts are the two major factors influencing the extent of illness.[1,2] Numerous groups and hundreds of viral strains cause "cold" symptoms. Rhinoviruses are the most common group. Others include coronaviruses, respiratory syncytial virus, adenovirus, echovirus, coxsackievirus, and parainfluenza virus.[1,2,3]

Transmission is primarily via direct contact with infected secretions, usually hand-to-hand and subsequent hand-to-face contact. It is evident that good handwashing is crucial in breaking the chain of transmission. Less often, transmission occurs via respiratory droplets from coughs or sneezes. Crowds and poor ventilation promote transmission. The incubation period is usually 48 to 72 hours.[1,2,3]

Incidence of the common cold among average adults is 2 to 4 colds per year; the average child has 6 to 12 colds per year; parents of small children have about 6 colds per year.[1,2] People seek primary care most often for viral upper respiratory conditions. The vast majority of these illnesses are benign and self-limited; however, they have a major social and financial impact. They are responsible for more absences from work and school than any other type of illness.[1,2,3]

Subjective Data

The client's chief complaints are malaise, rhinorrhea, and a "scratchy" throat. Nasal secretions are usually clear and copious at onset, changing to mucoid appearance later in the illness. Mucopurulent secretions *do not* necessarily indicate a secondary bacterial infection. Fever is rare in adults. Symptoms peak in 2 to 4 days, then gradually resolve. The total course of the illness is usually 5 to 10 days. When nasal symptoms last longer than 10 to 14 days, the client needs to be evaluated for sinusitis or allergies.[1,2,3]

Objective Data

Physical examination reveals a benign general appearance. Fever is either low grade or absent. Nasal mucosa is often edematous with clear discharge.

The pharynx appears to have mild erythema. Lymphoid hyperplasia of the posterior pharynx is more common than tonsillar enlargement. Lymph nodes are usually nonpalpable, but small anterior cervical nodes may be palpable. Lungs are clear.

Differential Medical Diagnoses

Bacterial infections (*Mycoplasma pneumoniae, Chlamydia psittaci,* group A beta hemolytic streptococcus); viral syndromes (Epstein-Barr or mononucleosis, cytomegalovirus); allergic rhinitis (seasonal, associated itching and copious clear nasal discharge).[2,3] Colds resolve in a few days; other syndromes are more severe and/or long lasting.

Plan

A large part of intervention is helping the client care for herself.

Psychosocial Interventions. Educate the client on the expected course of her illness and the need for

TABLE 21–17. OVERVIEW OF ORAL MEDICATION TYPES USED FOR THE COMMON COLD[a]

Class	Indications	Side Effects	Contraindications
Decongestants	Shrink swollen nasal mucosa	Neurologic agitation, increased blood pressure	Avoid with hypertension.
Antihistamines	Dry up mucous membrane secretions	Drowsiness (no effect on blood pressure)	Avoid with asthma and history of asthma "flair" with use of antihistamines. Avoid giving with sedating medications or alcohol.
Antipyretics/analgesic	Relieve discomfort or fever	Gastrointestinal irritation with nonsteroidal anti-inflammatory drugs	Aspirin is associated with Reye's syndrome; use acetaminophen, especially in clients under age 18.

[a]Numerous drugs are included in each class. See specific pharmacotherapeutics texts for details.
Source: References 1, 2, 3.

self-care. Empower her to pursue self-care when appropriate. Provide information about viral and bacterial infections.[1,2,3]

Medication. See Table 21–17.

Lifestyle Changes. Lifestyle changes may help prevent the spread of colds. Advise clients to practice good handwashing and to avoid hand-to-face contact. Increasing fluid intake helps keep secretions loose and moving. Physical activity may be carried out as tolerated.

Strongly encourage cessation of smoking, as it increases the risk for secondary bacterial infections affecting ears, sinuses, and the lungs.

Follow-Up

Teach clients to look for pain (in ear, face, or chest), fever (fever higher than 102° F or fever that recurs after initial few days), and distressing cough that is associated with dyspnea, fever, or localized chest pain, or that is persistent and progressive.[1,2]

OTITIS MEDIA

Otitis media (OM) is an acute infection of the middle ear. The majority of infections are caused by eustachian tube dysfunction, which in adults is caused primarily by edema from viral upper respiratory infections and allergies. Barotrauma (flying/scuba diving) and cancer can also impair eustachian tube function. Chronic negative pressure in the middle ear leads to serious effusion and overgrowth of respiratory tract bacteria, with subsequent purulent discharge and inflammation.[2,4]

Epidemiology

Studies indicate that otitis media is a bacterial disease of the respiratory tract mucosa. The three primary pathogens are *Streptococcus pneumoniae, Hemophilus influenzae,* and *Moraxella catarrhalis* (previously *Branhamella catarrhalis*). Resistant strains of *M. catarrhalis* and *H. influenzae* can produce β-lactamase, which inactivates penicillin and amoxicillin.[2,3,4]

Otitis media is most often a secondary bacterial infection following a viral upper respiratory tract infection or problems with allergies.

Incidence reports show otitis media most common among children; however, at least 4.4 percent of the adult population has one episode per year.[2]

Subjective Data

Usually the client reports a history of viral respiratory infections, allergies, or barotrauma. She describes unilateral or bilateral ear pain associated with decreased hearing. Systemic symptoms are uncommon in adults. New onset of recurrent otitis media with no preceding history of upper respiratory infections or allergies may be indicative of cancer, especially in women who smoke and drink alcohol.

Objective Data

Data are gathered primarily from physical examination of the ears.

Physical examination reveals a general benign appearance. Vital signs are usually normal, fever rare. The external canal of the ear should appear normal, with no tragus or mastoid tenderness. Otoscopy is used to evaluate five parameters of tympanic membrane appearance:

Otoscopic Exam

- *Color.* Erythema is consistent with acute infection.
- *Contour.* The membrane may be bulging in acute suppurative otitis media, and retracted in serous otitis.
- *Translucence.* The membrane may be thick and opaque in chronic otitis.
- *Structural Changes.* An irregular light reflex or blisters indicate infection.
- *Mobility.* A light reflex should move with insufflation; immobility is consistent with infection.[5]
- *Mastoid.* Should not be tender.
- *Nasal Cavity.* Turbinate may be erythematous, gray, and boggy. A clear discharge may be present.
- *Oropharynx.* May be benign or changes are consistent with allergic rhinitis or pharyngitis.
- *Neck.* Nodes may be present.

If the canal is obscured by copious purulent drainage and the possibility of rupture exists, do not instill anything into the ear or attempt to clean it out.

Diagnostic tests are not usually indicated. An audiogram may be helpful in assessing hearing, and tympanometry may help assess mobility.

Differential Medical Diagnosis

Several conditions of a serious nature should be considered.

External otitis is also called "swimmer's ear." The canal is usually swollen with exudate and tender with external manipulation of the ear. *Treatment with otic drops, usually Cortisporin otic suspension, is required.*

Serous otitis media is characterized by a retracted tympanic membrane, possibly an air-fluid level, and often decreased hearing. There is no erythema, and the condition is common with allergies and upper respiratory infections.

Mastoiditis is a life threatening condition caused by the spread of infection from the middle ear to the air cells of the mastoid process. Any

tenderness over the mastoid should lead to suspicion of mastoiditis. Refer the client immediately for hospitalization.

Meningitis usually causes the client to appear toxic; severe neck pain occurs with flexion.

Malignant otitis externa is associated with a 50 percent fatality rate and is seen in diabetics and in those immunocompromised with external otitis. Refer the client to a physician immediately.[2,4,5,6]

Plan

Medication. Use of antibiotics and other medication is debatable. In European countries, such as The Netherlands, antibiotics are not prescribed because improvement is seen in 10 days regardless of treatment. In this country, however, it is felt that the risk of suppurative complications is too great, supporting aggressive treatment with antibiotics.[4,6]

In general, the first choice is amoxicillin (Polymox) 250 or 500 mg orally three times daily for 10 days; the second choice is trimethoprim-sulfamethoxazole double-strength tablets (Bactrim DS) twice daily for 10 days. Third-choice antibiotics include cefaclor (Ceclor), amoxicillin/clavulanate potassium (Augmentin), Azithromycin (Zithromax), and Clarithromycin (Biaxin) can also be used. For analgesia, acetaminophen and NSAIDs usually suffice. Decongestants have never been proven to shorten the course of otitis media and are used only symptomatically for nasal congestion. Refer to a pharmacotherapeutics text for details.

Tympanostomy (myringotomy) is not usually required for adults. Refer the client to an ear, nose, and throat specialist if she does not improve after two or three 10-day treatment regimens.

Lifestyle Changes. Advise the client to avoid vigorous nose blowing and to increase fluid intake. Encourage the client to stop smoking, as smoking increases the risk of otitis media.

For fluid behind the ear, teach the client to carry out gentle autoinsufflation: She manipulates the posterior pharynx (swallowing, chewing gum, yawning) to speed drainage of fluid from the middle ear.

Follow-Up

Ask the client to return to the clinic if acute symptoms, such as pain, are not improved in 48 hours or if she is not asymptomatic in 10 days.[2,4]

ACUTE SINUSITIS

Acute sinusitis is infection of one of the four sinuses: maxillary, frontal, ethmoid, and sphenoid. The mucosal lining becomes swollen and occludes air exchange and mucous drainage, resulting in inflammation, bacterial replication, and purulent discharge.[7,8]

Epidemiology

Studies reveal that numerous conditions can predispose an individual to acute sinusitis. The most common risk factors are viral upper respiratory infections, allergic rhinitis, and dental extraction and abscesses. Barotrauma (flying or diving), foreign bodies, tumors, and polyps are less common but they can block the ostia (or openings) to the sinuses.[2,7,8]

The primary organisms causing acute sinusitis are *Streptococcus pneumoniae, Haemophilus influenzae, Moraxella catarrhalis,* group A streptococci, and staphylococci.[2,7,8] Organisms involved in chronic infections include those already listed as well as mixed anaerobes, which are often difficult to treat.

Incidence reports show acute sinusitis as a common condition; it complicates about 0.5 percent of all upper respiratory infections.

Subjective Data

Taking a detailed history is imperative, as a physical exam is of limited use in making the diagnosis. The classic history is a preceding upper respiratory infection lasting 5 days or longer, with subsequent development of copious yellow-green nasal discharge and intense, localized facial pain, worse on forward bending. Discomfort is often intense and constant. Depending on which sinus is infected, the pain may be referred to the teeth or palate (maxillary), the eyebrow area (frontal), or behind the eyes or at the top of the head (ethmoid and sphenoid). Note whether symptoms are unilateral or bilateral. Some infections present with only a history of purulent nasal discharge and fatigue, with no associated face pain.

Infection can be acute (1 day to 3 weeks), subacute (3 weeks to 3 months), or chronic (more than 3 months). The time frame is important to ascertain, and then treat the infection aggressively, as chronic infection is more difficult to treat and at times can require surgical intervention.[9,10]

Objective Data

Physical Examination. Reveals a benign general appearance. Vital signs are usually normal; fever is rare. If fever is high, consider referral. (Caution: Clients are in pain and may be taking analgesics that mask fever; ask if they have taken any acetaminophen, aspirin, or NSAIDs in the previous 4 hours.)

Abnormal eye movements, facial edema, and erythema around the eyes suggest spreading cellulitis; immediate referral is necessary.[2,7,8]

A purulent nasal discharge and edematous turbinates may be noted, as may a purulent postnasal drip.

Sinuses are difficult to assess; percussion for tenderness and transillumination are often unreliable.[2,7,8]

Diagnostic Tests. Since plain films of the sinus offer only low specificity and sensitivity, more clinicians are using computed tomography (CT) scans (without contrast) when such tests are indicated. CT scans offer good visualization of the ostiomeatal complex, the openings of the anterior ethmoid maxillary, and frontal sinuses.[2,8,9] Nasal endoscopy allows direct visualization of the anatomic and pathologic features of the nose.[9]

Differential Medical Diagnosis

Viral upper respiratory infections, allergic rhinitis, rebound medicamentosa from topical decongestants, dental extractions and abscesses, nasal polyps and tumors.[2,7,8]

Plan

Psychosocial Interventions. Encourage the client to comply with the antibiotic regimen. Educate her about the warning signs and symptoms of complications: facial swelling, visual problems, high fever, increased pain.[8,9]

Medication. Antibiotics, decongestants, and analgesics may be helpful.

The *antibiotic* of first choice is amoxicillin, 500 mg orally three times daily for 21 days. An alternative is trimethoprim-sulfamethoxazole double strength (Bactrim DS) twice daily for 21 days.[7,8,11]

Decongestants may help to shrink tissue and drain infection. Monitor hypertensive clients closely.

Analgesics include NSAIDs, which help to ease the pain and edema.

Antihistamines are usually avoided, as they may dry mucous membranes and impair ciliary movement to clear sinuses.

Surgical Interventions. Surgical management may be recommended by an ear, nose, and throat specialist if the client's symptoms do not improve.

Lifestyle Changes. Use of a room humidifier, hot showers, and nasal saline nose drops may keep mucous membranes moist and draining. Application of warm packs to the affected area may provide comfort. Increasing fluid intake also helps to keep secretions loose. Advise physical activity as tolerated, and discourage smoking.

Follow-Up

Consider the potentially lethal complications of acute sinusitis, including periorbital cellulitis and abscess leading to meningitis, osteomyelitis, or cavernous sinus thrombosis. Refer clients to a physician if they appear toxic, have a high fever, or exhibit redness or swelling around the eyes, difficulty moving the eyes, or double vision.

Symptoms should improve greatly 48 hours after starting antibiotics. If not, refer the client to a physician. All symptoms should resolve before completion of medications. If not, or if they recur, refer the client to a physician. Rule out tumors and polyps if acute episodes recur or if symptoms persist with treatment.[2,7,8,11] Assess for and treat allergic rhinitis after acute symptoms resolve.

PHARYNGITIS

Pharyngitis, an inflammatory condition of the pharynx, has numerous causes. Three causes discussed here in depth are group A beta hemolytic streptococci (GABHS), infectious mononucleosis, and *Neisseria gonorrhoeae* (see Table 21–18).

Epidemiology

Identification of GABHS necessitates immediate treatment, because these organisms can cause rheumatic fever if untreated and if associated with local suppurative complications such as tonsillar abscess.[12,13] Infectious mononucleosis is acute infection with the Epstein-Barr virus. Although pharyngitis caused by mononucleosis cannot be treated, it should be identified so that the client can be monitored for potentially lethal complications, such as airway compromise and splenic rupture. Pharyngitis caused by *N. gonorrhoeae* may be confused with pharyngitis caused by GABHS or mononucleosis, but it must be identified so that sexual partners can be treated.[2,12,13]

Transmission of GABHS (scarlet fever) occurs primarily among children of school age or people living under crowded living conditions, such as college dormitories and military barracks. Mononucleosis is primarily a disease of the young passed through mucous membrane secretions. Gonorrheal pharyngitis is most commonly seen among homosexual males, but should be considered in any sexually active adult with a sore throat who fails to respond to treatment.[2,12,13]

Incidence reports show that GABHS are responsible for about one third of the sore throats seen in primary care. GABHS commonly occur among children between 3 and 15 years of age; however, these organisms cause 5 to 20 percent of sore throats among persons older than 15.[12,13] Ninety percent of the population has had mononucleosis by age 40. Most adults are not aware that they had it in childhood. The infection tends to be more severe if contracted as an adult.[12,13]

Gonorrhea is responsible for about 1 percent of pharyngitis infections among adults treated in primary care.

TABLE 21–18. DIFFERENTIAL DIAGNOSIS OF PHARYNGITIS

Bacterial Diseases	Viral Diseases	Other Diseases

GABHS[a]
Large tonsils beefy red ± exudate
Fever (>101 °F)
Nodes anterior and very tender
Rash, scarlatina sandpaperlike
Often headache
Often vomit once
No cough
	Mononucleosis
	Large tonsils, palatine petechiae ±exudate
	Fever may or may not occur
	Nodes posterior or generalized
	Rash, faint, maculopapular
	Headache may or may not occur
	Persistent anorexia/fatigue
	Rare cough
	30% splenomegaly
	10% hepatomegaly
		Mycoplasma
		Rarely diagnosed in absence of
		  bronchitis/pneumonia
		Candida
		"Thrush," rule out AIDS, cancer, and
		  diabetes
		Allergies
		Consider if "cold lasts >3 weeks," worse
		  in morning and nighttime, postnasal
		  drip

Gonorrhea 1% of sore throats in adults ±exudate History of oral sex	**Common cold** URI caused by rhinovirus, etc. usually nasal symptoms may be hoarse	**Spirochetes** Syphilis Acute necrotizing ulcerative gingivitis Ulcers on gums "Trench mouth"
Diphtheria Pseudomembrane Unimmunized population	**Herpes simplex** Ulcers on gums, hard palate tissue and lips	**Dehydration**
Haemophilus influenzae Rare in adults Epiglottis in children	**Coxsackievirus** Ulcers on soft palate and tonsillar pillars	**Irritant gases** **Trauma**

Group D and C streptococci
Rarely cause suppurative complications,
  therefore not treated
	Cytomegalovirus
	Mononucleosis-like syndrome may be
	  asymptomatic or quite ill, will shed
	  virus, dangerous to pregnant women
	  with no immunity
		Foreign body
		Neoplasm

Tuberculosis	**Measles, mumps, rubella, varicella**	

[a]GABHS, group A beta hemolytic streptococci; URI, upper respiratory infection.
Source: References 1, 2, 12, 13.

Subjective Data

Histories reported by women vary, depending on the etiology of pharyngitis. Pharyngitis caused by GABHS is associated with a classic history of sudden onset of malaise, fever (usually higher than 101° F), tender anterior cervical nodes, headache, and a severe sore (not "scratchy") throat. Nasal symptoms are infrequent and cough is rare. Often a woman has been exposed to small children. If an abscess is present, the client may experience excruciating unilateral pain and may report drooling or spitting saliva, rather than swallowing it. Ask the client about a history of abscesses, as recurrence is common.

Infectious mononucleosis in adults usually presents with a history of gradual onset of fatigue that becomes severe (sleeping 12 to 14 hours per day). Appetite decreases. Sore throat begins, and the client complains of "aches" around the neck caused by prominent neck adenopathy. Fever is variable; temperature may be normal to greater than 103° F. Side tenderness and jaundice may be caused by hepatosplenomegaly. Symptoms are most prominent in the first 2 weeks, and gradual full recovery usually occurs in 6 weeks.[2]

Gonorrheal pharyngitis may be mild or severe. The diagnosis is suspected if a client reports a new sexual partner and oral sex. The diagnosis is primarily suspected if persistent sore throat is not cured by usual management.[11]

Objective Data

Because physical examination cannot differentiate between viral and bacterial causes of pharyngitis, specific laboratory tests are required for diagnosis.

Physical Examination. Findings depend on the etiology (see Table 21–19). The client may be flushed, appear sick and have fever. A fine, red, sandpaper-like rash is consistent with GABHS (scarlet fever). A maculopapular rash is consistent with mononucleosis and hemorrhagic

TABLE 21–19. DIFFERENTIAL DIAGNOSIS OF INFECTIOUS PHARYNGITIS: EXUDATIVE VERSUS NONEXUDATIVE

Exudative	Nonexudative
Group A beta hemolytic streptococci	Rhinovirus
Mononucleosis	Coronavirus
Adenovirus	Respiratory syncytial virus
Neisseria gonorrhoeae	Influenza virus
Mixed anaerobic bacteria	Parainfluenza virus
Herpes simplex virus	

Source: References 1, 2, 12, 13.

pustules with gonorrhea. Jaundice can occur in mononucleosis.[2]

Nasal congestion and a hoarse voice are primarily of viral origin and are rare in pharyngitis caused by GABHS, mononucleosis, or gonorrhea. "Hot potato" voice and drooling are red flags and may indicate an abscess. In pharyngitis caused by GABHS, tonsils are often large and beefy red with a thick white exudate. Suspect an abscess or peritonsillar cellulitis if the soft palate shows unilateral bulging, the uvula is deviated or edematous, or if the client will not open her mouth because of pain.[3,12,13] Never force a client's mouth open; if epiglottis is present it may cause spasm and occlusion of the airway.

Neck adenopathy is nonspecific. As a rule, however, large, very tender anterior nodes are consistent with pharyngitis caused by GABHS or gonorrhea; posterior cervical nodes and generalized adenopathy are more consistent with pharyngitis caused by mononucleosis.

The lungs should be clear. Abdominal examination may reveal side tenderness, indicating hepatosplenomegaly from mononucleosis or the mononucleosis-like cytomegalovirus.

Genitalia are examined only if gonorrhea is suspected.

Diagnostic Tests. Specific for bacterial and viral infections. For pharyngitis caused by GABHS, in-office rapid strep tests or cultures are helpful. The white blood cell count may be slightly elevated in streptococcal pharyngitis, but may be greater than 15,000 if an abscess exists.

For infectious mononucleosis, the mononucleus spot test (or heterophile antibody test) often does not turn positive for 5 to 12 days or longer after onset of illness. The CBC is usually normal or shows a slightly decreased white blood cell count with a predominance of lymphocytes and monocytes. The diagnosis may be made with a blood smear showing 20 percent atypical lymphocytes. If the client exhibits the classic clinical picture of mononucleosis but the monospot remains negative, consider ordering a battery of tests to rule out cytomegalovirus, toxoplasmosis, and histoplasmosis.

For gonorrheal pharyngitis, order a throat culture; use calcium alginate swabs, plate on Thayer Martin medium, and incubate.

Differential Medical Diagnoses

See Tables 21–18 and 21–19.

Plan

Psychosocial Interventions. Explain to the client her condition or the differential diagnoses being considered if tests were inconclusive. Inform her about the course of treatment to expect and the red flag symptoms that should prompt her to call the health care provider.

Medication. Refer to a current pharmacotherapeutics text for details.

For pharyngitis caused by GABHS, penicillin V (Betapen-VK) 250 to 500 mg orally four times daily for 10 days (administer erythromycin if the client is allergic to penicillin V).

NOTE: Although amoxicillin is effective against GABHS, do not give it when the strep test is negative and mononucleosis cannot be ruled out as cause of exudative pharyngitis. Clients with mononucleosis develop a total body maculopapular rash if given amoxicillin.[12,13]

For pharyngitis caused by infectious mononucleosis, analgesics such as ibuprofen may be given. Steroids may be used if tonsillar enlargement threatens the airway.[12,13]

For gonorrheal pharyngitis, if uncomplicated, inject ceftriaxone sodium (Rocephin) 125 to 250 mg (by weight) intramuscularly (see Chapter 11 for recommendations). Also administer oral doxycycline (Vibramycin) or tetracycline (Achromycin) to treat the possibility of concurrent chlamydial infection.

Surgical Interventions. Surgery may be needed if abscess is present. Refer the client for needle aspiration and possible incision and drainage.

Lifestyle Changes. If pharyngitis caused mononucleosis is diagnosed, encourage the client to listen to her body and to rest when she feels tired. She should avoid vigorous activity for about 6 weeks and protect her sides because of the risk of rupturing the spleen.[2] Otherwise, activity is as tolerated. Warn the client to avoid hepatotoxins, such as alcohol. The client may use warm saline gargles and lozenges if she feels they help.

If gonorrheal pharyngitis is diagnosed, education about safer sex practices should be discussed and all sex partners should be tested and treated.

If pharyngitis caused by GABHS is diagnosed, decreased activity and alcohol avoidance are recommended. In general, encourage clients to increase fluids and nutrition. Discourage smoking.

Follow-Up

Follow-up is specific to the condition.

Pharyngitis caused by GABHS should improve greatly in 48 hours; otherwise have the client return to rule out abscess or other infection.

Clients with pharyngitis caused by mononucleosis are sickest on about days 4 to 8 of illness and should be followed on the basis of the clinical picture. Observe for airway obstruction, hepatitis, and splenic enlargement.

Clients with gonorrheal pharyngitis are at risk for numerous complications, such as disseminated gonococcal infection with bacteremia and purulent arthritis.[63] Ensure that all sexual contacts are treated.

ENDOCRINE DISORDERS

The four most commonly occurring endocrine disorders discussed in this chapter are hypothyroidism, hyperthyroidism, thyroid nodules, and diabetes.

HYPOTHYROIDISM

Hypothyroidism is a clinical syndrome associated with subnormal levels of circulating thyroid hormones. A client may be asymptomatic; the condition may be mild to severe. Myxedema is the advanced form of hypothyroidism characterized by proteinaceous infiltration of the skin and subcutaneous tissues with multiple organ system involvement.[1,2,3,4]

Epidemiology

The cause differs among the four types of hypothyroidism: primary, secondary, goitrous, and transient.

Primary hypothyroidism is characterized by atrophy or destruction of thyroid tissue due to an autoimmune response. Primary hypothyroidism accounts for more than 90 percent of hypothyroid disease. Primary hypothyroidism may also be iatrogenic (following radioiodine therapy or thyroidectomy for hyperthyroidism), idiopathic, or the result of a congenital disorder (cretinism).[1,3,4]

Secondary hypothyroidism results from insufficient stimulation of an intrinsically normal gland. It may occur in primary disorders of the pituitary or hypothalamus, which result in deficiencies of thyroid-stimulating hormone (TSH) or thyrotropin-releasing hormone (TRH).

Goitrous hypothyroidism is due to defective thyroid hormone synthesis and is characterized by development of a goiter. Goitrous disorders include Hashimoto's thyroiditis; iodine deficiency; acquired hypothyroidism, caused by the use of goitrgens (propylthiouracil, methimazole, lithium, or iodine); peripheral resistance to thyroid hormone; and infiltrative disorders (amyloidosis, sarcoidosis, lymphoma, or malignancy). Transient hypothyroidism can occur as the result of pregnancy or significant illness. It usually resolves within 6 months of onset, and close monitoring is all that is required.[2,5]

Routine screening of asymptomatic adults is not recommended. It may be clinically prudent, however, to screen those at increased risk, namely, elderly women, newborns, those with a strong family history of thyroid disorders, postpartum women 4 to 8 weeks after delivery, and clients with autoimmune disease.[1,2]

The onset of hypothyroidism is most common in women between 30 and 60 years of age. It develops in both men and women. It is a common disorder of the elderly. The prevalence of thyroid disease in clients more than 60 years of age is about 4 percent, eight times higher than in the general population.[2,5]

Subjective Data

Hypothyroidism is easily misdiagnosed because its presentation is nonspecific and it involves multiple organ systems. Less than one-third of the elderly manifest typical symptoms: cold intolerance; weight gain; dry skin; weakness; fatigue; hoarseness; inattention or difficulty concentrating; dizziness; constipation; athralgias; muscle cramps; menstrual irregularities, particularly menorrhagia; galactorrhea and depression.

Objective Data

Physical Presentation. Depends on the progression of disease from a subclinical one to a medical emergency, such as that which often precedes myxedems coma.

Physical Examination
- *General Appearance.* Flat affect; low pitched, slow speech.
- *Vital Signs.* Bradycardia, hypertension.
- *Skin.* Thin, brittle nails with transverse grooves; dry, scaly cool skin with a diffuse wavy pallor.
- *Head.* Coarse, dry, brittle hair with alopecia; facial edema; enlarged tongue; thinning or absence of the lateral eyebrows.
- *Neck.* Normal, enlarged, small, or absent thyroid; thyroid nodules; tracheal deviation.
- *Chest.* Exertional dyspnea, pleural effusions.
- *Heart.* Cardiomegaly, arrhythmias.
- *Abdomen.* Gastrointestinal hypomotility, ascites.
- *Neurologic Exam.* Cerebellar dysfunction, delayed deep tendon reflexes, parathesias, peripheral neuropathies.
- *Endocrine System.* Galactorrhea.

Diagnostic Laboratory Tests. Reveal levels of circulating thyroid hormones. The active thyroid hormones are tetraiodothyronine (thyroxine or T4) and triiodothyronine (T3). Both T3 and T4 circulate in the serum, bound to three proteins: thyroxine-binding globulin (TBG), thyroxine-binding prealbumin (TBPA), and albumin. The small fractions of T3 and T4 that circulate free (not bound to protein) are the active forms. Alterations in TBG (e.g., with pregnancy, estrogen replacement, or the use of oral contraceptives) may change total circulating T3 and T4 levels but do not affect free unbound forms.

Primary hypothyroidism is confirmed by a high level of thyroid-stimulating hormone (TSH) and a low level of free T4. A serum TSH is the most sensitive test; it is elevated in more than 95 percent of clients with hypothyroidism.[1,2,4,5,6]

Secondary hypothyroidism is differentiated from primary hypothyroidism by the thyrotropin-releasing hormone (TRH) test of pituitary-thyroid regulation. If secondary hypothyroidism is suspected, the client should be referred to an endocrinologist.

Differential Medical Diagnoses

Cardiac disorders, renal disorders, neuromuscular disorders, and depression are common diagnostic considerations.

Plan

Psychosocial Interventions. It may be necessary to address acute anxiety reactions, which are often among the manifestations of this multisystem disorder. Reassure the client that her symptoms will gradually abate with treatment. Depressed clients may benefit from short-term counseling.

Medication. Levothyroxine (Levoxine, Synthroid), a synthetic T4 hormonal replacement, is the medication of choice.

- *Administration.* Begin with levothyroxine 25 to 50 mcg daily and increase by 25 mcg every 6 weeks according to TSH levels. Dosages need to be adjusted with caution in the elderly and in clients with cardiac disease.[1,3,4]
- *Side Effects.* Palpitations and dysrhythmias are known to occur, particularly in clients with cardiac disease.
- *Contraindications.* Contraindications are outweighed by the risk of not treating the hypothyroidism. Use caution, however, in clients with cardiac disease and the elderly.
- *Evaluation of Drug Action.* To ensure equilibrium, measure serum TSH values no sooner than every 6 weeks after initiating therapy and again 3 to 4 months after a maintenance dose is reached. Annual TSH values are done to monitor therapy, as needs may change with time.
- *Client Teaching.* Review with the client signs and symptoms of hypothyroidism and hyper-

thyroidism, which may indicate the need for medication change.

The decision to treat subclinical hypothyroidism must be evaluated on an individual basis. If the client is symptomatic, a trial of levothyroxine may be indicated. If the client has coexisting medical problems, a referral to an endocrinologist is indicated.[1,4]

Lifestyle Changes. The daily medication regimen and chronic condition may cause the client to alter her self-perception. Encourage positive, affirming activities. Diet and exercise are not restricted.

Follow-Up

Once the maintenance dose has been established, annual visits are all that may be required to check the TSH level and reinforce client teaching.

HYPERTHYROIDISM (THYROTOXICOSIS)

Thyrotoxicosis is a hypermetabolic state that results from an excess of circulating thyroid hormone. Excessive thyroid hormone does not always result from thyroid gland hyperactivity; thus thyrotoxicosis, not hyperthyroidism, is the preferred term.

The most common condition is Graves' disease, an autoimmune disorder. Thyroid-stimulating immunoglobulin (TSIs) binds to thyroid cell receptors and stimulates overproduction of thyroid hormones T4 and T3. The cause of TSI production is unknown. Graves' disease is characterized by diffuse thyroid enlargement (goiter), hyperthyroidism, ophthalmopathy, and occasionally pretibial myxedema.[1,7,8]

Other causes of thyrotoxicosis include toxic multinodular goiter, toxic adenoma, subacute thyroiditis, autoimmune thyroiditis, and excessive exogenous thyroid hormone.[1]

Epidemiology

Graves' disease, which accounts for up to 90 percent of all cases of thyrotoxicosis, appears to be familial in origin. Family history also shows an increased incidence of other autoimmune disorders. Toxic multinodular goiter is usually seen after age 50 in individuals with preexisting non-

toxic goiter. Silent thyroiditis occurs fairly frequently in postpartal women.

Graves' disease occurs predominantly among women 20 to 40 years old. Up to 2 percent of women are affected. Either sex at any age may be affected.[1,2,4,7,8]

Subjective Data

Clients may report tremulousness; palpitations; heat intolerance; increased perspiration; eye irritation, excessive lacrimation, photophobia, and diplopia; dyspnea; unexplained weight loss, despite increased appetite; frequent bowel movements; fatigue; weakness, especially of the proximal muscles; and decreased menstrual flow or amenorrhea.

Objective Data

Symptoms are related to excessive sympathomimetic activity and increased catabolic activity. The elderly do not usually present with classic symptoms. Cardiac symptoms, including atrial fibrillation, are more common among the elderly, whereas goiter and eye symptoms may be absent.

Physical Examination
- *General Appearance.* Rapid, rambling, anxious speech.
- *Vital Signs.* Tachycardia, systolic hypertension, widened pulse pressure.
- *Skin.* Warm, smooth, moist skin and onycholysis.
- *Eyes.* Exophthalmus, proptosis, upper lid retraction, periorbital swelling.
- *Neck.* Enlarged, soft thyroid gland, nodules, thyroid bruits.
- *Chest.* Tachypnea.
- *Heart.* Atrial fibrillation, hyperdynamic apical impulse, systolic flows murmur.
- *Vascular System.* Bounding peripheral pulses.
- *Abdomen.* Hyperactive bowel sounds.
- *Musculoskeletal System.* Myopathy, especially in the proximal lower extremities.
- *Central Nervous* System. Fine tremor, hyperreflexia.

Diagnostic Laboratory Tests. Show an elevated serum free T4 and a low TSH. If results are normal yet suspicion remains high, refer the client to an endocrinologist for further evaluation. Additional studies might include a serum T3 or thyrotropin-releasing hormone test. Dopamine hydrochloride and corticosteroids can suppress TSH levels.[1,2,4]

Differential Medical Diagnoses

Amphetamine or cocaine abuse, anxiety states/panic disorder, chronic obstructive pulmonary disease, pheochromocytoma, myeloproliferative disease, diabetes.

Plan

Treatment must be individualized with consideration to the etiology and severity of disease, client's age, concomitant disease, and risks and benefits of therapeutic modalities.

Psychosocial Interventions. Reassure the client that her condition is not a malignant process and can be treated quite effectively.

Medication. Antithyroid drugs, beta blockers, and radioactive iodine are used.

Antithyroid Drugs. Antithyroid drugs are not without significant side effects; in rare cases potentially fatal reactions can occur. The client should be referred to an endocrinologist for treatment. Methmazole (Tapazole) 5–20 mg/day initially; 5–20 mg/day maintenance; thought to be the more potent than PTU; may be given in one daily dose. Propylthiouracil (PTU) 300–600 mg/day initially; 50–200 mg/day maintenance; must be given in three equally divided doses because of its shorter half-life; PTU is the drug of choice in pregnancy as it is more highly protein bound and crosses the placenta less readily. The medication may be reduced by half when the client's symptoms have resolved, the goiter has decreased, and the T4 has normalized. It is not useful to check labs more often than every 4–8 weeks. Drug therapy is maintained for 1 year. Approximately 50–60 percent of clients will experience a relapse.[1,4,8,9]

- *Side Effects.* The most frequent side effects are rash, malaise, fever, urticaria, arthralgia, gastrointestinal disturbances, and loss of taste. Transient leukopenia occurs in approximately 12 percent of adults.

- *Contraindication.* Do not administer antithyroid drugs to clients with cardiac disease.
- *Anticipated Outcome on Evaluation.* Level of circulating thyroid hormone decreases as evidenced by a return to normal TSH level.
- *Client Teaching.* Inform the client that although the duration of therapy is controversial, it is rarely longer than 2 years.

Beta Blockers. Beta blockers are indicated to alleviate symptoms of thyrotoxicosis: tachycardia, palpitations, hypertension, tremor, heat intolerance, and anxiety. Beta blockers are used as an adjunct to radioactive iodine until its therapeutic effect is achieved. Propranolol (Inderal) is the most commonly used beta blocker. The goal is to titrate the dose to maintain a heartrate between 70–90 and decrease other symptoms. The usual dose is 160 mg/day in either divided doses or long acting preparation. See section on hypertension for further discussion of beta blockers.

Radioactive Iodine. Radioactive iodine is the treatment of choice for clients over age 40. The client is referred to an endocrinologist for administration.[1,4,8,9]

- *Administration.* The tracer dose of radioactive iodine in tablet form is administered and followed by irradiation.
- *Side Effects.* Within the first year, hypothyroidism occurs in 10 percent of those treated. The likelihood of hypothyroidism developing increases by 5 percent each subsequent year over the next 20 years.
- *Contraindication.* Radioactive iodine is never administered to pregnant women.
- *Anticipated Outcome on Evaluation.* If an adequate dose of RAI is given, it will be 100 percent effective. Approximately 20 percent of clients require a second dose. Complete resolution of symptoms occurs within 6 months of treatment.
- *Client Teaching.* Inform the client that RAI is inexpensive and effective. Many clients then exhibit hypothyroidism and require T4 replacement. Periodic testing for hypothyroidism (TSH level) should be done indefinitely. The amount of radiation received is comparable to the amount necessary to perform a barium

enema. Clients should not become pregnant for 6 months after treatment.

- *Surgical Interventions.* Surgical intervention is limited and controversial. It may be an option for pregnant women or for those who do not respond to antithyroid medications.[4]

Follow-Up

The treatment will dictate the follow-up. Educate the client about the symptoms of hyper- and hypothyroidism.

THYROID NODULES

A thyroid nodule is a mass that presents as a single palpable nodule or as a part of a multinodular gland. The diagnostic challenge is to distinguish a benign nodule from a malignancy.

Epidemiology

Studies often reveal a history of radiation exposure. The period of latency ranges from 5 to 35 years, with an average of 20 years. A family history of thyroid malignancies or endocrine tumors is common. About 20 to 30 percent of persons exposed to ionizing radiation develop palpable thyroid abnormalities; 50 percent have nodules. Of those nodules, 30 to 50 percent are malignant. Single nodules are more likely to be malignant than is a multinodular gland.[1,4]

Incidence reports reveal that about 4 percent of the adult population has thyroid nodules; the incidence increases to 5 percent among individuals older than 60 years. Nodules are four times more common in women than men; however, malignant nodules are more common in men. At least 95 percent of all palpable nodules are benign.[1,4]

Thyroid cancer is rare, and deaths from thyroid cancer are even rarer.

Subjective Data

A client may report a medical history of thyroid disorders, endocrine tumors, and/or head or neck irradiation. Although most women are asymptomatic, a client may have hoarseness, vocal cord paralysis, and dysphagia.

Objective Data

Physical Examination. May be unremarkable or reveal symptoms of hypo- or hyperthyroidism. Nodules range from barely palpable to visible; their physical characteristics do not secure a diagnosis of benign or malignant. Although nodules may be tender, most are nontender. Thyroid malignancy is suggested by a solitary firm nodule with associated nontender cervical lymphadenopathy.

Diagnostic Methods. These include thyroid function tests, biopsy, and imaging. Laboratory tests usually show normal thyroid function.[1,4]

A fine-needle aspiration biopsy is the most reliable diagnostic method. If the aspirate shows malignancy, the probability is that it is 95 percent correct. If suspicious, a 45 percent chance of malignancy is probable. Biopsy determines which nodules will be surgically excised; biopsy is the only definitive evaluation and surgery the definitive treatment.

The test procedure requires an experienced cytologist. It is safe, inexpensive, and accurate. A fine-needle aspiration biopsy followed by a thyroid scan for suspicious lesions seems to be the most cost effective approach.

Ultrasonography determines consistency but does not define benign versus malignant disease. It is used as a guide for fine-needle aspiration.

Radionuclide imaging classifies nodules as "hot" or "cold." A malignant lesion incorporates less iodine than normal thyroid tissue; therefore, it should appear "cold." This technique is not sensitive; although a "hot" nodule reduces the likelihood of malignancy, it does not exclude the possibility.[1,4]

Thyroid suppression is controversial and logistically difficult to interpret because of clinical limitations in sizing nodules.

Differential Medical Diagnoses

Hemorrhagic cysts, Hashimoto's thyroiditis.

Plan

Psychosocial Interventions. Inform the client that although it is rare for a nodule to be malignant, the risk is real.

Surgical Interventions. Surgical management of thyroid cancer is controversial. It is generally agreed that the nodule be removed and suppressive therapy utilized. The amount of thyroid to be removed (one lobe or total thyroidectomy) and the method of follow-up may vary.

Follow-Up

Refer all clients with thyroid nodules to an endocrinologist who will manage treatment.

DIABETES MELLITUS

Diabetes mellitus is a chronic disorder that is characterized by hyperglycemia; associated with major abnormalities in carbohydrate, fat, and protein metabolism; accompanied by a marked propensity to develop relatively specific forms of renal, ocular, neurologic, and premature cardiovascular diseases.

Diabetes is diagnosed by clinical signs and symptoms of polyuria, polydipsia, polyphagia, weight loss, and/or blurred vision with persistent hyperglycemia; fasting plasma glucose levels exceed 110 and/or random plasma glucose levels exceed 126 on at least three separate occasions.[1,2,10,11,12]

The causes of diabetes are unknown, although current thought includes genetic predisposition, unknown precipitating events, and progressive autoimmune destruction of pancreatic beta cells.

Epidemiology

Diabetes can be classified into two types: type I or insulin-dependent diabetes and type II or noninsulin-dependent diabetes. Other types of diabetes can be associated with other specific conditions or syndromes (pancreatic, endocrine, medications) and are beyond the scope of this book.

Type I (Insulin-Dependent) Diabetes

Type I diabetes accounts for 3 percent of all new cases of diabetes diagnosed each year in the United States. Its annual incidence rate in the under 20 age group is 15 per 100,000. Type I can develop at any age, although generally most cases are diagnosed when the client is under 30.[1,2,10]

Clients with type I are insulinopenic. Insulin therapy is essential to prevent rapid and severe dehydration, catabolism, ketoacidosis, and death. They are usually lean and often have experienced significant weight loss, polyuria, and polydipsia before presentation.

Type II (Noninsulin-Dependent) Diabetes

Type II diabetes is characterized by fasting hyperglycemia and insulin resistance. It is usually diagnosed after age 40 but can occur at any age. It affects an estimated 85–90 percent of the 6 million Americans diagnosed with diabetes. Because type II diabetes is a slowly progressive disease, the number of individuals with undiagnosed DM is thought to be nearly the same as the number diagnosed.[1,2,10,11]

The likelihood of developing type II is approximately equal by sex but is greater in African Americans, Hispanics, and Native Americans. Obesity (more than 20 percent over ideal body weight), a family history of diabetes, age 40 or over, hypertension, hypercholesterolemia, gestational diabetes or having one or more infants weighing more than 9 pounds at birth are major risk factors.[1,2,10,13]

Type II diabetes is characterized by insulin resistance and is present in the majority of all clients with fasting blood sugars (FBS) greater than 110. Sites of insulin resistance include hepatic and peripheral tissues. Postbinding abnormalities are primarily responsible for insulin resistance. Impaired binding may be secondary to associated obesity and hyperinsulinemia but may also contribute to impaired tissue insulin sensitivity. Diet recall may reveal high fats, sweets, and starches. There is evidence that weight reduction, exercise, and diet change are beneficial in primary and secondary prevention of NIDDM.[1,2,10,12,13,14]

The American Diabetes Association recommends screening adults with one or more risk factors every 3 years.

Impaired Glucose Tolerance

Impaired glucose tolerance is characterized by a fasting plasma glucose level of > 110 mg/dl and < 126 mg/dl on two separate occasions.

These clients may develop type II diabetes and should be monitored closely.

Subjective Data

The client may report a history of weight loss, polydipsia, polyuria, polyphagia, blurred vision, endocrine disorders, alcoholism, pancreatitis, gestational diabetes, medications (e.g., steroids, thiazide, diuretic), frequent urinary tract infections, yeast vaginitis, poor healing wounds, or a family history of diabetes.

Objective Data

- *General.* Recent weight gains or losses.
- *Eyes.* Fundoscopic-diabetic retinopathy.
- *Mouth/Throat.* Candidiasis.
- *Gastrointestinal.* Diminished bowel sounds. Right upper quadrant tenderness (pancreatitis).
- *Genito-Urinary.* Vulvo-vaginal candidiasis.
- *Neurological.* Decreased sensation peripherally, gait disturbances, carpal tunnel syndrome.
- *Extremities.* Decreased pulses, poor healing wounds, temperature or color changes.
- *Diagnostic.* Fasting blood sugar > 110 mg/dl on two separate occasions or random BS over 200. Glycosolated Hemoglobin greater than 8. Oral glucose tolerance testing is useful to confirm the diagnosis of gestational diabetes and evaluate clients with complications suggestive of diabetes (background retinopathy, neuropathy).
- *Other Lab.* Elevated amylase (pancreatitis) or cholesterol (especially triglycerides).

Differential Medical Diagnoses

Medication induced diabetes (steroids, thiazide, diuretics), hypothyroidism, hyperthyroidism, human immunodeficiency virus (HIV), substance abuse.

Plan

The goals are to achieve normal metabolic control, reduce the potential for development of complications, promote a reasonable body weight, and encourage healthy eating habits. The Diabetes Control and Complications Trial (DCCT)[11] showed an overall reduction in potential compli-

cation when these goals are achieved. Before treating, assess the client's self-care attitudes, abilities, and priorities.

Treatment modalities include dietary modifications, increased physical activity, pharmacologic intervention, and intensive and continued client education.[13,15]

Psychosocial Interventions. The diagnosis of diabetes is a lifelong, life altering one. Explore the client's perception of her self-image, her health beliefs, and her perception of diabetes. Consider a referral to a diabetes support group.

Dietary Interventions. The client should be encouraged to follow a low fat, no added salt diet and to avoid sweets. Consider a referral to a nutritionist and the local chapter of the American Diabetes Association or the local diabetes educators in your community.

Physical Activity. Encourage the client to develop a regular exercise plan based on her current fitness level. Establish fitness goals and follow-up at regular visits.[15]

Pharmacologic Intervention. The Type I diabetic is essentially insulinopenic and requires exogenous insulin. The type II or NIDDM diabetic will require pharmacologic intervention when diet modification and increased physical activity fails to control glucose levels alone. The physiologic abnormalities of NIDDM progress gradually over time and then lose efficacy. Five years of success on a given treatment is what may reasonably be expected.[10]

Oral Agent Therapy

- *Sulfonylureas.* All sulfonylureas act by increasing the secretion of insulin in response to fasting blood glucose levels. They reduce the fasting hyperglycemia but have little effect on postprandial glucose.[1,16] In choosing a sulfonylurea (or any agent), expense, ease of dosing, and comorbid conditions, must be considered. See Table 21–20.
- *Acarbose (Precose).* Acarbose, taken at the beginning of a meal, interferes with hydrolysis of dietary disaccharides and complex carbohydrates, delaying absorption of glucose and other

TABLE 21–20. INSULIN ORAL AGENT THERAPY

First Generation Sulfonylureas		
Agent	Dose Range (mg)	Doses/Day
tolbutamide (Orinase)	500–3000	bid or tid
tolazamide (Tolinase)	100–1000	qd or bid
acetohexamide (Dymelor)	250–1500	qd
chlorpropamide (Diabinese)	100–500	qd
Second Generation Sulfonylureas		
glipizide (Glucotrol)		
glipizide XL (Glucotrol (XL)	2.5–40	qd or bid
glyburide (Micronase,	5–20	qd
Diabeta)	1.25–20	qd or bid
micronized glyburide		
(Glynase PresTab)	0.75–12	qd
gliperamide		
Other Agents		
acarbose (Precose)	25–50	tid with meals
metformin (Glucaphage)	1000–2550	bid or tid

Source: References 2, 7, 8, 9, 10, 11, 13.

monosaccharides. It can be helpful in lowering postprandial plasma glucose concentrations.

- *Administration.* Acarbose is taken at the beginning of a meal. The recommended starting dose is 25 mg t.i.d. and increasing at 4- to 8-week intervals, depending on postprandial blood glucose concentrations and tolerance, up to 50 mg t.i.d. for clients weighing fewer than 60 kg, or 100 mg t.i.d. for heavier clients.[16]
- *Adverse Effects.* Unabsorbed carbohydrates undergo fermentation in the colon, leading to gastrointestinal distress, which may diminish with time. Acarbose may decrease intestinal absorption of iron and cause anemia.
- *Interactions.* Acarbose may increase the risk of hypoglycemia when taken with other hypoglycemic agents. Oral treatment of hypoglycemia must be with glucose because sucrose may not be adequately hydrolyzed and absorbed. Acarbose may decrease the bioavailability of metformin, and their gastrointestinal adverse effects may be additive; concurrent use should probably be avoided.[16]

- *Metformin (Glucaphage).* A biguanide hypoglycemic agent for treatment of clients with NIDDM not adequately controlled by diet alone. Metformin is absorbed from the gastrointestinal tract over approximately 6 hours and excreted by the kidneys without being metabolized. It decreases glucose production in the liver and increases glucose uptake but does not cause clinical hypoglycemia. It has no effect on pancreatic insulin secretion and requires the presence of insulin to be effective. It is used to overcome insulin resistance. In a study by DeFronzo et al., the substitution of metformin for glyburide resulted in little benefit.[17,18,19]

  - *Administration.* Metformin is available in 500 mg and 850 mg tablets. The starting dose is 500 mg b.i.d. with the morning and evening meal. The usual dosage is 850 mg b.i.d., and the maximum is 850 mg t.i.d.
  - *Adverse Effects.* Metformin can cause a metallic taste, diarrhea, nausea, vomiting, and anorexia. Most of these symptoms diminish or disappear with a decreased dose or discontinuance of the drug.
  - *Lactic Acidosis.* All biguanides inhibit lactate metabolism, and increased concentrations of the drug associated with renal impairment can cause lactice acidosis. Even a temporary reduction in renal function, such as occurs after angiography, can cause lactic acidosis. The drug should be discontinued 2 days before such procedures and restarted only after renal function returns to normal. Increased alcohol intake, conditions associated with hypoxemia (heart failure, shock, hepatic failure) or surgery are indication for stopping metformin.[17,18,19]

Combination Therapy

The combination of *metformin and glyburide* was found superior to treatment with either drug alone.[18] This has been shown to lower plasma glucose and glycosylated hemoglobin values in clients with NIDDM who had poor responses to maximal doses of a sulfonylurea. It is recommended to start with either a sulfonylurea or metformin, increase as indicated and add the second agent

TABLE 21–21. REGULAR INSULIN THERAPY

	Onset of Action	Peak	Duration
Short Acting regular and semilente	30–45 minutes	2–3H	5–6H
Intermediate Acting NPH and lente	2–3H	6–9H	12–14H
Long Acting ultralente	slow	none	18–24H

Note: H=hour
Source: Reference 2.

when the maximum dosage has been reached. Due to the progressive nature of diabetes in some clients, oral agents will fail and insulin should be started. For most, this will mean a permanent commitment to insulin.

The combination of a *sulfonylurea and insulin* has been used as a transitional step between management by oral agents and aggressive insulin therapy.[1,10,20] The combination recommended by the American Diabetes Association is half the dose of the oral agent in the morning and 0.2 units/kg at bedtime. See Tables 21–20 and 21–21.

Insulin Therapy

Insulin-Dependent Diabetes (type I). In these clients, the production of insulin by the beta cell is lost and the client becomes dependent on the use of exogenous insulin. Understanding the actions of the various insulins is crucial to designing an insulin program that will mimic the body's own insulin release.

Intensive insulin therapy in three or more injections a day, with home glucose monitoring, will provide ideal control. The basal dose of insulin is given as either a long-acting or intermediate-acting insulin. A bolus dose is given premeal to mimic the endogenous release of insulin at mealtimes. Before adjusting doses, confirm diet and exercise patterns, recent illnesses or stressors, any hypoglycemia or hyperglycemia events, or other medication changes.

Non-Insulin-Dependent Diabetes. These clients may require exogenous insulin to supplement de-

creased endogenous production or decreased insulin response. The American Diabetes Association recommendations for starting dose in NIDDM is 0.5 per kilogram of an intermediate-acting insulin in a single or two doses. It is best to match the peak action of insulin to the rise in glucose that occurs in the early morning hours between 3 and 8 A.M. Therefore the P.M. dose would be administered at bedtime.

Follow-Up

Follow-up should be individualized based on the client's current needs. Regular screening for microvascular and macrovascular complications.[21,22,23] Regular review of the client's home glucose monitoring diary and technique as well as reinforcement of dietary and exercise recommendations. If diabetes is difficult to control, consider other medications as the cause—thiazide diuretics and beta blockers can cause hyperglycemia. Beta blockers can also mask the signs and symptoms of hypoglycemia.

GASTROINTESTINAL DISORDERS

This section covers the following disorders: gastroesophageal reflux disease, peptic ulcer disease, gallbladder disease, irritable bowel syndrome, anal fissures, and hepatitis.

GASTROESOPHAGEAL REFLUX DISEASE

Gastroesophageal reflux disease (GERD) is a clinical syndrome characterized by heartburn, a burning sensation resulting from the backward flow of gastric contents into the esophagus. The most common form is idiopathic lower esophageal sphincter incompetence. It is primarily a motility disorder. Contributing factors include gastric hyperacidity, impaired esophageal clearance, increased volume of gastric contents, and altered mucosal resistance.[1,2,3]

Etiology reveals that hiatal hernias predispose to GERD, but are not pathognomonic.

Pregnancy and obesity may exacerbate symptoms. Cigarette smoking, chocolate, fatty foods, caffeine, alcohol, and some medications (tetracycline, doxycycline, quinidine, slow-release potassium supplements, iron, calcium channel blockers, and nonsteroidal anti-inflammatory drugs) also aggravate GERD. Delayed gastric or esophageal emptying and prolonged exposure to gastric acid increase the frequency and severity of symptoms, complications, and recurrence of gastroesophageal reflux.[1,2,3]

Epidemiology

GERD is common at all ages, but more prevalent among persons 60 to 70 years old. Incidence is reported to be as high as 30 to 40 percent in the general population and accounts for almost half of all noncardiac chest pain.[1,2,3,4] GERD is reported in 46 percent of all asthmatics. The higher incidence of GERD among asthmatics may be related to medications.

Early diagnosis and appropriate treatment can prevent secondary complications, such as esophageal strictures, ulcers, Barrett's esophagus, bleeding, pulmonary disease, and hoarseness.

Subjective Data

The client describes a burning sensation or pain underneath the sternum followed by a bitter taste. It may be related to certain foods. Intensity varies, but the sensation usually increases after eating, with forward bending, when supine, or with vigorous exercise. Less common symptoms that may be reported are odynophagia, dysphagia, and pulmonary manifestations, such as nocturnal coughing, wheezing, and hoarseness.

Objective Data

Physical examination is usually benign.

Endoscopy. The most definitive approach to diagnosis. It allows direct visualization and biopsy. Endoscopy is usually performed under conscious sedation.

Advise the client of the risks and benefits of the procedure. It is associated with increased risks for clients who have cardiopulmonary disease, are elderly, or otherwise debilitated.

Upper Gastrointestinal X-ray. Determines the extent of damage to esophageal mucosa. It detects ulcers, strictures, hiatal hernias, and masses. Double-contrast studies are more sensitive and specific than single-contrast studies. They have a sensitivity of 80 to 90 percent, which decreases with ulcers less than 5 mm in diameter. Barium is used as contrast in x-rays of the upper gastrointestinal tract.

A 24-Hour pH Monitor (a portable unit). Useful in determining the total acid exposure and identifying episodes of nocturnal reflux. The pH probe is manually placed in the esophagus; reflux is defined by a distal esophageal pH less than 4.

The Bernstein Test. Used to demonstrate the relationship of symptoms to pain. Symptoms are simulated: hydrochloric acid and normal saline are alternately infused into the esophagus, while the patient's response is recorded. The test is potentially uncomfortable for clients.

Esophageal Manometry. Indicated for clients who are not responding to conventional medical therapy or for whom surgery is being considered. Lower esophageal pressure is measured, and esophageal peristalsis and the competence of the lower esophageal sphincter are assessed. Normal lower esophageal sphincter pressure ranges between 10 and 25 mm Hg. A pressure of 6 mm Hg or less or inappropriate sphincter relaxation is also highly diagnostic.

Differential Medical Diagnoses

Peptic ulcer disease, esophageal strictures, Barrett's esophagus, angina, pancreatic disease, esophageal candidiasis, Zollinger-Ellison syndrome, respiratory disease.[1,2,5,6]

Plan

In determining the management of symptoms, consider their severity, the cost of procedures, the risk-benefit of diagnostic testing, the age and health status of the client, and the cost of medications.

Psychosocial Interventions. Involve the client as an active partner in management. She should know that the condition is chronic but manageable.

Medication. Medications are not corrective but protect the mucosa from chronic insult. They suppress and neutralize acid and are cytoprotective.

Antacids neutralize gastric acid.

Alginic acid (Gaviscon) forms a foamy coating over gastric contents, protecting the esophageal mucosa during regurgitation.

H2 receptor agonists block parietal cell actions and thereby decrease gastric acid formation. Few side effects are noted; however, close observation for drug interactions is important.

The dopamine antagonist/protokinetic agent metoclopramide hydrochloride (Reglan) increases esophageal sphincter pressure and enhances gastric emptying. It is associated with central nervous system, and other side effects. It may be given in conjunction with an H2 blocker.

Cisapride (Propulsid) is a prokinetic drug that has the ability to correct the pathologic motility abnormality and has a low side effect profile.

The *"acid proton pump" inhibitor omeprazole* (Prilosec) inactivates the hydrogen-potassium ATPase enzyme that drives the proton pump of the parietal cell. It is indicated for intractable reflux esophagitis, Zollinger-Ellison syndrome, and hyperhistaminic states.

Cholinergic drugs (e.g., bethanecol hydrochloride) increase lower esophageal sphincter pressure.

Anticholinergic agents reduce acid secretion but are rarely used because of their adverse effects.

Sucralfate (Carafate tablets) binds bile salts and pepsin, aids mucosal regeneration, and enhances prostaglandin synthesis, making it cytoprotective.

Misoprostol (Cytotec), a synthetic prostaglandin analog, reduces mucosal injury related to use of nonsteroidal anti-inflammatory drugs. Diarrhea may preclude prolonged use.

Surgical Interventions. Surgery may be indicated for clients who have evidence of reflux and failed a 6-month trial of medical management.[1,2,3] Surgery is reserved for those who have not responded to simple therapeutic maneuvers or medications, or have advanced disease or complications, such as esophageal stricture, severe bleeding, and pulmonary aspiration. A hi-

atal hernia is not an indication for surgery. Surgery is effective in 90 percent of cases; the Nissen fundoplication procedure restores sphincter competence.

Lifestyle/Dietary Changes. Lifestyle and dietary changes may be effective initial and adjunctive therapies.[1,2,3] Controlled studies, however, show their benefits are limited.

The diet should not include offending foods (spicy foods, high-fat foods, citrus juices, chocolate, peppermint, onions, and caffeine). Ideal body weight should be maintained and alcohol eliminated. Advise the client to take the following measures:

- Avoid recumbent positions within 3 hours of a meal.
- Elevate the head of the bed on 4- to 6-in. blocks or on a bed wedge.
- Avoid bending forward.
- Discontinue cigarette smoking and use of all nicotine products.
- Avoid constricting clothing.

Follow-Up. Follow-up to determine response to therapy, to reinforce nonpharmacologic measures, and to assess for respiratory symptoms.

PEPTIC ULCER DISEASE

Peptic ulcers are small sores, or lesions, in the lower end of the esophagus or the lining of the stomach, duodenum, or jejunum. The two main types of peptic ulcer disease (PUD) are duodenal and gastric.

Pepsin, the chief enzyme of gastric juices, combines with hydrochloric acid to digest food in the stomach. Normally the lining of the stomach resists corrosion, but for unclear reasons, resistance can break down and an ulcer develops. Because most clients with these ulcers demonstrate normal acid production, research is directed toward mucosal defense mechanisms.[1,5,6,8,9]

Epidemiology

Peptic ulcer disease affects approximately 4 million Americans a year. It occurs more frequently in men.[8,9]

Risk factors include cigarette smoking, medical or family history, and medication. Nonsteroidal anti-inflammatory drugs (NSAIDs)/aspirin or steroids in high doses or used long term can contribute to the development of PUD, particularly among women older than 65 years. The risk is the same for plain or buffered aspirin but less if it is enteric coated, because with the coating the tablet dissolves in the small intestine.

Medical conditions predisposing individuals to PUD are hyperparathyroidism (secondary to increased calcium, which increases gastric secretion), cirrhosis, renal failure and chronic steroid use. The evidence that increased stress causes or activates ulcer formation is not conclusive.

In clients older than 50, it is necessary to rule out gastric cancer as an etiology, especially if symptoms have a recent onset or are persistent despite treatment.[8,9]

Transmission may involve *Helicobacter pylori* (*Campylobacter pyloris*), although its role in the pathogenesis of ulcers is unclear. Investigators believe that gastroduodenal mucosa infected with the organism is more likely to undergo ulceration.[5,6] It is agreed that it is the causative organism in type B antral gastritis.[6,7]

Subjective Data

Less than half of clients with PUD present typically. Clinical features in the elderly are often vague or may be absent until a complication occurs.

Gnawing, burning, epigastric or upper abdominal pain radiating to the back may awaken clients in the night or early morning. Typically, symptoms of a peptic ulcer are brought on by an empty stomach and may be relieved by eating.

On the other hand, gastric ulcers are usually aggravated by eating. Pain begins almost immediately after eating. It is not uncommon for months or years to pass without pain. Associated symptoms include dyspepsia, heartburn, and nausea or may be more severe with vomiting and weight loss. Bowel habits generally remain unaltered.[8,9]

Objective Data

Diagnostic tests and other procedures are the sources of objective data. Physical examination rarely helps in diagnosis. Epigastric tenderness is neither specific nor sensitive. Rectal exam may be hemocult positive. The sensitivity is 10–70 percent.[10]

Diagnostic laboratory tests are used to evaluate a client for complications, such as bleeding, or indications of malabsorption. Blood is drawn for CBC and chemistries.

The upper gastrointestinal series and endoscopy are explained under Gastroesophageal Reflux Disease.

H. pylori is diagnosed by endoscopic biopsy, serum IGG or by breath test.

Differential Medical Diagnoses

Esophageal stricture, Barrett's esophagus, angina, respiratory disease, gallbladder disease, gastroesophageal reflux disease.

Plan

Psychosocial Interventions. Provide information and support concerning diet and possibly long-term medications. The role of stress is controversial.

Medication. See Gastroesophageal Reflux. If H. pylori is diagnosed, a 2-week course of clarithromycin (Biaxin) and omeprazole (Prilosec) 20 mg qd should relieve symptoms. Less expensive courses are often for longer periods of time and require tid and qid dosing.[1,6,9]

Ulcer recurrence may be prevented with chronic H2 blockers at half the initial therapeutic dose among persons at high risk for recurrence (asthmatics, cigarette smokers, and diabetics) or clients at high risk for complications (renal transplant recipients and clients with systemic disease)[5,6,7] (see Table 21–22).

Dietary Interventions. Have the client eliminate from her diet any offending foods and alcohol. Frequent, small bland meals with milk were encouraged for years; however, there is no evidence this will promote healing. Milk may exacerbate symptoms as it stimulates acid secretion.

TABLE 21–22. MANAGEMENT OF PEPTIC ULCER DISEASE

Symptoms consistent with peptic ulcer disease

+

Absence of complications[a]

+

Age < 50 years

↓

Avoid exacerbating agents, e.g., aspirin, alcohol, smoking

Treat empirically with
   H2 blocker ⟶ Symptoms persist/worsen

↓ ↓

Therapeutic response at 2-week follow-up	Endoscopy/x-ray
Continued for total of 6–8 weeks	If biopsy needed, refer to GI specialist

[a]History of GI/peptic ulcer disease, bleeding, weight loss, persistent pain, vomiting.
Source: References, 1, 5, 6.

Follow-Up

Follow-up differs for gastric and duodenal ulcers. Gastric ulcers take longer to heal and require a full 8 weeks of treatment. Duodenal ulcers may heal more quickly but recur in about 80 percent of clients within 1 year and are more likely to be a chronic condition. Refer clients with ulcers that are unresponsive (persistent symptoms) to a GI specialist.

GALLBLADDER DISEASE

The two gallbladder diseases discussed in this chapter are cholecystitis and cholelithiasis.

Cholecystitis is acute inflammation of the gallbladder, usually caused by a gallstone blocking the outlet of the gallbladder or cystic duct. Edema, infection, and ulceration result. If this process continues, necrosis, perforation, and peritonitis may result.

Cholelithiasis is the presence or formation of gallstones. Generally, gallstones form whenever cholesterol is oversaturated. Gallstones are classified by composition.[1,8,9,11]

Cholesterol stones constitute 80 percent of all gallstones in the United States and contain, in addition to cholesterol, bile acids, calcium salts, proteins, and phospholipids.

Pigment stones are black or brown. Black pigment is more common in the United States, brown among native Asians.

Epidemiology

The incidence of gallstones in the United States is approximately 10 percent. Eighty percent of stones are thought to be the cholesterol type.[1,9]

Risk factors are multiparity, use of estrogens (including oral contraceptives), obesity, rapid weight loss, high-fat diet. Crohn's disease (involving the ileum or ileal resection), regional enteritis, cirrhosis, diabetes, a family history of gallbladder disease, total parenteral nutrition, and solid organ transplant. There is a 50 percent chance of recurrence with a previous history of gallbladder disease.[1,9]

Gallbladder disease occurs primarily among overweight women 40 to 65 years of age. The incidence among women is almost three times that among men and increases with age.[1,8]

Subjective Data

Initially, a client reports diffuse, intermittent right upper quadrant pain, an ache or pressure that occurs at night or early in the morning. It progresses to a continuous, more severe pain and may radiate to the epigastrium or right shoulder. Onset of pain may be sudden and last from 20 minutes to 5 or 6 hours; it may continue as a dull ache for 24 hours or longer. Intervals between episodes vary considerably, from weeks to years. Pain may be accompanied by nausea, vomiting, constipation, or fever.[1,8,11]

Objective Data

Physical examination during the acute phase of disease maybe helpful along with diagnostic tests.

Physical Examination. Not helpful in the nonacute phase. During the acute symptom phase, specific changes may be observed:

- *General.* Restless, fever, jaundice.
- *Eyes.* Icteric.
- *Chest.* Clear to auscultation, splinting with respiration.
- *Abdomen.* RUQ tenderness; Murphy's sign; a palpable globular mass may be found behind the lower border of the liver.

Diagnostic Laboratory Tests. May reveal elevations of serum transaminases, alkaline phosphatase (due to obstructed biliary tract), or serum lipase or amylase (gallstone pancreatitis). An increase in white blood cells with a left shift denotes cholecystitis or cholangitis.

Ultrasonography is used to diagnose gallstones. It is a quick and inexpensive way to evaluate the liver, pancreas, and other abdominal organs. It is now the diagnostic test of choice.

Endoscopic retrograde cholangiopancreatography (ERCP) aids in the diagnosis of common duct calculi, biliary dilatation, cystic duct obstruction and cancer.

An *oral cholecystogram* is a diagnostic evaluation for cholelithiasis. The client takes iopanic or tyropanoic acid tablets the night before the exam. The dye concentrates in the gallbladder and permits its visualization the following day. The method is well tolerated. It is 90 to 95 percent accurate in detecting stones.

Differential Medical Diagnosis

Angina, peptic ulcer disease, esophageal spasm, appendicitis, intestinal obstruction, gastroesophageal disease, pancreatitis, myocardial ischemia, pyelonephritis.

Plan

Psychosocial Interventions. Discuss with the client that surveillance of recurrence alone may be suitable management for infrequent symptoms and little disability.

Medication. Medication is limited to comfort measures. A client who has asymptomatic gallstones can be monitored and will not necessarily require intervention. Use of oral bile salts is limited to clients with small radiolucent stones (indicating cholesterol composition) and a functioning gallbladder and to clients with mild or infrequent symptoms. Oral salts are also given to clients who refuse surgery or who are poor surgical candidates. The medication is taken daily for 6 months to 2 years. Treatment requires follow-up visits and ultrasound examination. Medication is expensive.[1,8,11]

Bile salts alter the ratio of bile acids to cholesterol and lecithin as well as reduce HMG-COA reductase activity, thereby reducing hepatic cholesterol synthesis.

Surgical Interventions. The laparoscopic approach to cholecystectomy is the treatment method of choice. It reduces postoperative pain as well as hospitalization and at-home recovery time.

Lithotripsy, extracorporeal shock-wave therapy of gallstones, is gaining popularity but its use is limited. Its distinct advantage is that it is noninvasive. More research is needed to determine the rate of recurrence, adverse sequelae, and cost effectiveness.

Follow-Up

Refer clients with acute cholecystitis to a collaborating physician, gastrointestinal specialist, or surgeon for evaluation and treatment. Acute cholecystitis can be a life threatening emergency. Major complications are perforation of the gallbladder with resultant peritonitis and internal biliary fistula. Fever, severe pain, and elevated white blood cell counts are indications for prompt surgical referral. The size, number, and location of gallstones influence the decision to treat aggressively versus conservatively. A more aggressive approach will likely be based on greater pain and disability from biliary attacks.

IRRITABLE BOWEL SYNDROME

The etiology of irritable bowel syndrome (IBS) is probably multifactorial. Contraction of colonic smooth muscle is controlled by cyclic alterations of smooth muscle membrane potential. In IBS, the normally orderly movement of colonic contents is altered. The entire gut, particularly the colon, is affected.[1,8,12,13]

Epidemiology

Etiology reveals a threefold increase in psychiatric illnesses (anxiety, hysteria, and depression) among persons with irritable bowel syndrome. When psychiatric illness is a cofactor, clients are more often middle-aged.[1,11]

Irritable bowel syndrome occurs most often among women between the ages of 20 and 50 years, but it may develop at any age. It is one of the most common reasons for referral to gastrointestinal specialists. About 30 percent of the general population may have symptoms, but only 14 percent seek medical attention.

Subjective Data

A careful history is the key to diagnosis. Acute stressful events, such as acute illness, job demands or loss of job, financial pressures, and illness or death of a close friend or relative, seem to precipitate attacks. Poor dietary habits may also be influential. About 50 percent of clients report nausea, heartburn, and dyspeptic symptoms. Colic abdominal pain varies in intensity. It may be precipitated by eating, but is typically relieved by a bowel movement. A client may experience diarrhea, constipation, or both. In addition, she may report abdominal distention, increased amounts of rectal mucus, and a feeling of incomplete evacuation. The condition does *not,* however, awaken clients from sleep, does *not* usually result in any appreciable weight loss (if any, it is less than 10 percent of body weight) and does *not* cause rectal bleeding.[12,13]

Objective Data

Diagnosis is often made only after other gastrointestinal disorders have been excluded. Consequently, expensive and unnecessary testing may occur. A detailed history guides the workup.

Physical Examination. May reveal diffuse abdominal tenderness. A rectal exam is essential. Hemorrhoids and anal fissures are evaluated.

Diagnostic Laboratory Tests. CBC, chemistries, urinalysis, and examination of stools for ova and parasites (particularly Giardia). Stools for culture, white blood cells, red blood cells. An erythrocyte sedimentation rate is done to rule out inflammatory bowel disease. A lactose tolerance/hydrogen breath test may be done.

Flexible sigmoidoscopy is used to rule out polyps, malignancy, and inflammatory bowel disease. The procedure is usually well tolerated. In the absence of organic lesions, irritable bowel syndrome is strongly suspect.

A colonoscopy is indicated for clients older than 40 years or with a strong family history of colon cancer. The test rules out polyps and malignancy. The client is given a cathartic 24 hours

prior to procedure to evaluate bowel debris. Usually the procedure is performed utilizing conscious sedation.

Differential Medical Diagnoses

Laxative abuse, lactose intolerance, Crohn's disease, ulcerative colitis, colon cancer, parasitic infestation, sorbitol intolerance, thyroid disorders, diabetes, eating disorders.

Plan

Psychosocial Interventions. Although symptoms can be stress related, overemphasizing the role of stress can induce confusion and guilt in the client. She should know that irritable bowel syndrome is a chronic condition that can be managed. Reassure her that her condition is not cancer and will not progress to inflammatory bowel disease. Symptoms are controllable, although it may take time and a trial-and-error approach to find the right therapeutic management for an individual. A plan should focus on diet and lifestyle. Discuss stress reduction techniques.

Medication. Medications that may be used address a variety of symptoms.[1,8,12,13]

Psyllium is a bulk laxative that improves regularity and is the main pharmacotherapeutic intervention.

Calcium channel blockers decrease smooth muscle response to neurohumoral stimulation.

Nitrates stimulate production of cyclic guanosine monophosphate within the cell, inhibiting smooth muscle contractions.

Anxiolytics are nonspecific in their action and reserved for underlying anxiety disorders.

Lopraumide HCl, 4 mg initially followed by 2 mg after each unformed stool will control diarrhea.

Antispasmodic agents such as dicyclomine hydrochloride (Bentyl) are used for abdominal pain and cramping.

A tricyclic antidepressant or *selective serotonin reuptake inhibitor* is used when depression, with or without anxiety, is present.

Lifestyle/Dietary Changes. These changes include modifications in diet, exercise, and elimination.

A low-residue diet is recommended for diarrhea and a high-fiber diet for constipation. Advise the client to avoid gas-producing foods (e.g., cabbage and beans) and to eat at regular hours; to chew food thoroughly; and to increase intake of fluids, especially fruit juices and water.

Daily exercise is helpful. Also advise the client to avoid straining at bowel movements; the urge to defecate should be promptly followed by elimination.

Follow-Up

A diagnosis of irritable bowel syndrome does not require frequent x-rays or colonscopic examinations. The frequency of follow-up visits depends on the severity of the client's symptoms. Systems are reviewed, the effectiveness of intervention assessed, and a physical examination done. Encourage the client to return should her symptoms exacerbate or change. Irritable bowel syndrome is a chronic illness that requires support and reinforcement of the prescribed therapeutic regimen.

ANAL FISSURES

An anal fissure is a linear ulcer on the margin of the anus.

Epidemiology

Anal fissures are a secondary irritation from diarrhea or straining related to constipation, laxative overuse, or trauma. Their exact incidence is unknown.

Subjective Data

A client may report bleeding and pain with and often after defecation. Pain may be severe and last 30 minutes or more following bowel movement. Pruritis ani may occur.[1]

Objective Data

Internal hemorrhoids may be found. Lateral traction on buttocks should expose the fissure. If not, inspection with an anoscope should aid in visualization. In the acute stage, tissues are erythematous and inflamed. Chronic fissures may erode the anoderm and expose the base of the internal sphincter.

Differential Medical Diagnoses

Primary lesion of syphilis, tuberculosis ulcerations, herpes, malignant epithelioma, abscesses, anorectal fistulas, cancer, Crohn's disease.

Plan

Psychosocial Interventions. Address the client's acute fear of cancer that may be aroused by her pain or bleeding. Reassure her that symptoms will resolve and can be prevented.

Medication. Stool softeners and lubricating anesthetic ointments (short-term) are used for severe pain. Avoid laxatives and suppositories.

Surgical Interventions. An internal sphincterotomy is usually performed to decrease the pressure of chronic fissures in the anal canal. A short 2- to 3-day hospital stay is required, the wound heals quickly, and the procedure is curative in 90 to 95 percent of cases.

Lifestyle/Dietary Changes. Advise the client to follow a high-fiber diet and increase fluids. Sitz baths are of no proven value.

Follow-Up

Most symptoms resolve within 2 to 4 weeks. If, however, no improvement occurs, refer the client to a surgeon.

HEPATITIS

Hepatitis is an inflammation of the liver caused by any one of several viruses or other factors. Five different viruses—hepatitis A, B, C, D, and E are responsible for most liver infections. Some lead to chronic hepatitis, a disease that can lead to cirrhosis, hepatic cancer, and death. Hepatitis A is the most common form. It does not produce long-term complications, and recovery is usually complete in 1 to 2 months. Hepatitis A is spread through a fecal-oral route and is most contagious in the late incubation period before symptoms develop. Infected individuals do not remain carriers.

Hepatitis B is spread through blood and body fluids. It can develop into chronic hepatitis in approximately 6–10 percent of those infected, which can lead to cirrhosis or hepatocellular carcinoma.[8,9] Symptoms are similar to hepatitis A, although fever is less likely.

Hepatitis C is spread through contaminated needles, blood transfusions (especially prior to 1992) and possibly sexual contact. Fifty to 80 percent or greater of those with acute infection progress to chronic disease, with 20–30 percent advancing to cirrhosis.[8,9] Liver cancer is also possible. Symptoms are similar to hepatitis B. No vaccine has been developed.[1,8]

Hepatitis D occurs in conjunction with hepatitis B. Transmission is from contaminated needles; sexual contact is less likely. There is no vaccine for hepatitis D, although vaccination against hepatitis B is protective.[8,9,14]

Hepatitis E is a virus spread similarly to hepatitis A. No cases have been reported in the United States. A vaccine has not been developed.[8,9,14]

Epidemiology

It is estimated that 200,000–300,000 persons become infected with HBV each year in the United States, with the greatest number of cases in the 20–39 age group. Approximately 1.0–1.25 million people have chronic, asymptomatic HBV infection. Fifty to 67 percent of acute HBV infections are asymptomatic. Routine screening for hepatitis B virus (HBV) infection in the general population is not recommended.[1,8,9] Certain high risk groups may be screened to assess eligibility for vaccination. High risk groups include IV drug users, heterosexual contact with HBV-infected individuals, heterosexual contact with at risk individuals (IV drug users), multiple sexual partners, and male homosexual activity.

The number of cases of hepatitis A each year is unknown. Approximately half of all reported hepatitis cases in the United States are attributable to hepatitis A, with the greatest number of cases in the 20–39 age group.[1]

Four million Americans are estimated to have hepatitis C.

Subjective Data

The client may complain of fatigue, lack of appetite, nausea and vomiting, muscle and joint aches, low grade fever, rash and jaundice.

Objective Data

Exam may be normal in acute phase

- *General.* Client may be ill appearing and/or jaundiced.
- *Eyes.* Icteric in acutely ill.
- *Oropharynx.* Pharyngitis may be present in hepatitis A.
- *Lungs.* Rhonchi and/or wheezing.
- *Heart.* Sinus tachycardia associated with fever.
- *Abdomen.* Striae, decreased bowel sounds, diffuse or right upper quadrant tenderness, hepatomegaly, and possibly splenomegaly.
- *Extremities.* Joint tenderness and possibly joint swelling.

Diagnostic Tests. Most laboratories offer acute and convalescent hepatitis panels that include hepatitis A and B. Polymerase chain reaction (PCR) to detect hepatitis C remains an investigational tool at present and is not generally available.[8] Anyone who received a blood transfusion before 1992 needs to be tested for hepatitis C, according to August 1997 Public Health Service advisory committee.

The screening test for HBV infection is the identification of HbsAg. The immunoassays have a sensitivity and specificity of greater than 98 percent.

Chemistry panels to assess electrolyte and liver function, complete blood count to assess for anemia, platelet counts and coagulation screen to assess clotting abilities and liver function.

Differential Diagnoses

Drug induced hepatitis, gallbladder disease, other viral syndromes, and metastatic cancer.

Plan

Treatment is supportive. Encourage small frequent meals earlier in the day. Nausea progresses throughout the day. Clients unable to tolerate PO fluids will require IV fluids and antiemetics. No specific drug therapy is available for uncomplicated hepatitis. Avoid exposure to hepatotoxic drugs.

Psychosocial. Counseling concerning high risk behaviors and the possibility of transmission. Encourage client to have sexual partner(s) tested if indicated. If possible, the client should avoid sex as long as HBsAg is in the serum.

Medication

VACCINES. The hepatitis B vaccine has a 85–95 percent protective efficacy when administered in three intramuscular doses.[1,8,9] Injection into the deltoid muscle is recommended as injection into the buttocks has been associated with a suboptimal response. Soreness at the injection site is the most common side effect. RecombivaxHB and Engerix-B are the vaccines licensed for use in the United States. They may be used interchangeably at any point in the vaccination schedule. Both are given in a three-dose series, with the second and third doses administered 1 and 6 months after the first dose. The recommended dose is 1 mL. Pregnancy and lactation are not contraindications.[1] Preexposure prophylaxis is recommended in health care workers, male homosexuals, dialysis clients, neonates, and children.[1,8,9]

The hepatitis A vaccine has been proven efficacious in children; clinical trial in adults have not been performed. The vaccine produces seroconversion rates of 90–100 percent after one dose and 99–100 percent after two doses in healthy adult volunteers. Immune globulin with the first dose may be necessary for high risk individuals.[1,8,9]

HBIG is used in postexposure situations (e.g., sexual contacts, needle sticks). The adult dose is 0.06 ml per kg intramuscularly.[1,4] Ideally, it is given within 2 days of exposure and again 1 month later. It is not useful after 1 week postexposure.

Follow-Up

Follow-up to provide continued support, check for resolution of acute symptoms, and to follow liver enzymes and coagulation panels one to two times a week. As symptoms resolve, the interval between visits may be lengthened. Recheck liver function studies, hepatitis convalescent panels, and coagulation studies 6 months after resolution of acute symptoms. Refer clients with evidence of chronic disease to a hematologist. Chronic carriers and their families need to be counseled to avoid transmission risks, anxiety and/or depression related to the diagnosis.

HEMATOLOGICAL DISORDERS

The last section of this chapter covers most of the common and a few of the rarer disorders of the blood. It begins with an overview of anemia and then differentiates among iron deficiency anemia, thalassemia, anemia of chronic diseases, and finally less common anemias: glucose-6-phosphate dehydrogenase deficiency; sickle cell anemia, and sickle trait; anemia caused by vitamin B_{12} deficiency; and folate deficiency.

OVERVIEW OF ANEMIA

Anemia is a *sign* of an *underlying* problem; it is not a diagnosis. Identifying anemia is the beginning of a workup, much as identifying a fever is the start of a diagnostic workup. Correcting the anemia may be of little importance compared with finding its cause.[1,2]

In general, anemia is defined either as a reduction in red blood cell (RBC) volume measured by hematocrit (Hct) or a decrease in the percent concentration of hemoglobin (Hgb) in the peripheral blood. The World Health Organization defines anemia in women as a hemoglobin less than 12 g/dL and in pregnant women as a hemoglobin less than 11 g/dL.[1,3] Clinical practice sites and laboratories may vary in their parameters.[1,2]

Laboratory values may be affected by age, sex, altitude, smoking, and hydration state. Beware of "spurious anemia" caused by hemodilution during pregnancy and congestive heart failure. Look at the individual's clinical picture.[2,3] All blood cell types (RBCs, white blood cells [WBCs], and platelets) are derived from the pluripotent stem cells in the marrow. Pancytopenia, or a decrease in all cell types—WBCs (leukopenia), RBCs (anemia), and platelets (thrombocytopenia)—requires referral to a hematologist.[2]

TABLE 21–23. DIFFERENTIAL DIAGNOSES OF ANEMIA BY ERYTHROCYTE MORPHOLOGY

Microcytic Anemia (MCV[a] < 80)	Macrocytic Anemia (MCV > 100)	Normocytic Anemia (MCV 80–100)
Iron deficiency	B$_{12}$ deficiency	Anemia of chronic disease[b]
Thalassemias	Folate deficiency	Endocrinopathy
Anemia of chronic disease[a]	Liver disease	Hemolysis
Sideroblastic	Alcoholism	Myeloma
Aluminum toxicity	Myelodysplastic syndromes	Renal disease
	Marked reticulocytosis	Sideroblastic[a] anemia
	Spurious anemia	Bleeding
		Aplastic anemia

[a]Mean corpuscular volume.
[b]Some overlap can occur depending on stage of disease.
Source: References 1, 2, 3.

Three mechanisms cause anemia: blood loss; decreased red cell production, usually as a result of insufficient building supplies such as iron, vitamin B$_{12}$, and folate; and increased red cell destruction (hemolysis). To determine the mechanism, ask the following three questions.[2,3]

What Is the Mean Corpuscular Volume? Mean corpuscular volume (MCV) is one of three RBC indices and indicates blood cell size. Normal MCV is approximately 80 to 100 fL. According to the MCV, anemias are categorized as microcytic, normocytic, or macrocytic (see Table 21–23).

What Is the Reticulocyte Count? Reticulocytes are immature RBCs that retain nuclear particles for 24 hours after leaving the marrow. Normally, reticulocytes constitute about 1 to 1.5 percent of circulating RBCs.[2,3] Increased reticulocyte count (> 3 percent) may be an indication of rapid bleeding or hemolysis as the body attempts to replenish lost RBCs. Reticulocyte counts less than 1 percent may indicate nutritional deficiencies or marrow dysfunction.[2,3]

What Is the Clinical Picture? Based on the client's demographic characteristics and problem list, certain types of anemia would be suspected (see Table 21–24).

Among the many types of anemia (most of them rare), three account for approximately 90 percent of the anemias in the United States. They are iron-deficiency anemia (IDA), thalassemia, and the anemia of chronic diseases (ACD).[1,2]

IRON-DEFICIENCY ANEMIA

Iron-deficiency anemia can be caused by inadequate dietary intake of iron or by loss of iron through bleeding. Because the body aggressively recycles iron, adults with reasonable nutrition do

TABLE 21–24. DIFFERENTIAL DIAGNOSIS SUGGESTED BY CLINICAL PICTURE

Female	Iron deficiency
Race	
Blacks	G6PD,[a] thalassemia, hemoglobinopathies
Mediterranean origin	G6PD, thalassemia
Southeast Asians	Hemoglobinopathies (e.g., HgB E)
Infections	G6PD, immune hemolysis
Thyroid disease	IDA, pernicious anemia
Alcoholism	Bleeding, folate deficiency, IDA, sideroblastic anemia, hemolysis, hypersplenism
Renal failure	Decreased production, hemolysis, bleeding
Connective tissue disorders	Anemia of chronic diseases, IDA, hemolysis
Cancer	Anemia of chronic diseases, hemolysis
Lead exposure	Sideroblastic anemias, IDA
Drugs	
Sulfa	G6PD
Dilantin	Megaloblastic anemia (folate), pure red cell aplasia
Antitubercular drugs	Sideroblastic anemia
Gold	Aplastic anemia

[a]G6PD, glucose-6-phosphate dehydrogenase deficiency; IDA, iron-deficiency anemia.
Source: References 2, 3.

not experience deficits. Nutritional inadequacies occur primarily in infants, children, and pregnant women. In a woman who is not pregnant, blood loss is assumed to be the cause of iron-deficiency anemia.[1,2,3] In premenopausal women, menstruation is the primary cause of blood loss. In postmenopausal women and in men, IDA is presumed to result from occult gastrointestinal blood loss (rule out colon cancer) until proven otherwise.[1,2,3]

Epidemiology

Studies reveal that IDA among pregnant women is caused by nutritional deficits, and among nonpregnant women, primarily by blood loss. Risk factors for bleeding include frequent heavy menses, miscarriages, abortions, deliveries, and surgeries. On average, women lose about 50 mL of blood per month as a result of menses; women with heavy menses may lose five times this amount. Oral contraceptive use decreases menstrual blood flow 30 to 60 percent and thus protects against IDA. Progestin-containing contraceptive methods may also decrease blood loss.[2] Risk factors for occult bleeding include GI disorders (Crohn's diverticulosis) and a family history of colon cancer or hemolytic anemias.[2,3]

Incidence reports show that IDA is the most common nutritional disorder in the world. It is seen primarily in children; however, it is estimated to occur in 20 percent of adult women, 50 percent of pregnant women, and 3 percent of adult men.[1]

Subjective Data

Subjective data vary for premenopausal and postmenopausal women. Premenopausal women report heavy or frequent menses. Acute loss of large volumes of blood may cause the sudden onset of shortness of breath, faintness, thirst, weakness, and rapid pulse. More commonly, however, blood loss is slow and subtle, especially in postmenopausal women. In that manner, the body is able to adjust to the gradual decrease in RBCs; no symptoms develop until the hemoglobin is 6 to 8 g/dL. In severe chronic cases, symptoms may include fatigue, dysphagia, sore tongue or mouth, and pica.

History-taking should focus on sources of blood loss or hemolysis. Ask about blood dona-

tions, recent surgeries, epigastric burning or pain, melena (rectal bleeding), family history of colon cancer, medications, diet, smoking, alcohol use, NSASD use, previous anemia, and splenectomy.[2,3]

Objective Data

Physical Examination. May reveal nothing abnormal. Occasionally, however, signs of anemia may be detected.

- *General Appearance.* Fatigue, tachypnea.
- *Vital Signs.* Increased pulse and respirations; may be orthostatic, with decreased blood pressure on standing.
- *Skin.* Pallor, tenting, pale palpebral conjunctiva, nails with spooning, separation, and ridges.
- *Mouth.* Angular stomatitis (sores at corners of mouth), cheilosis (red, sore lips), glossitis (beefy red tongue consistent with vitamin B_{12} deficiency).
- *Chest.* Rapid respiratory rate, rales.
- *Heart.* Flow murmurs, tachycardia.
- *Abdomen.* Splenomegaly (hemolysis), hepatomegaly (liver disease, alcoholism), masses (colon cancer), epigastric tenderness (gastritis).
- *Pelvic Exam.* Rule out mass.
- *Rectal Exam.* Rule out mass, guaiac stool.
- *Central Nervous System.* Altered mental status (rule out lead poisoning and vitamin B_{12} dementia), paresthesia (pernicious anemia).[2,3]

Diagnostic Tests. Performed in stages; avoid the expensive shotgun approach to ordering tests.

Initial laboratory tests include a baseline complete blood cell count (CBC) with indices (MCV, mean corpuscular hemoglobin [MCH], mean corpuscular hemoglobin concentration [MCHC]) and reticulocyte count. A fecal test for occult blood is done on the basis of the clinical picture.[1,2,3]

Initial findings are evaluated. If data reveal microcytic (MCV < 80), hypochromic anemia with a low reticulocyte count, the diagnosis is most likely IDA. Confirm the diagnosis prior to treatment by ordering an iron panel, which usually comprises a serum iron, total iron binding capacity (TIBC), and percent saturation. Also order a serum ferritin test. (*Note:* Iron-deficiency anemia usually occurs gradually. Consequently, laboratory values change slowly over time. The continuum of change begins with decreased serum ferritin and progresses to decreased serum iron, increased TIBC with decreased percent saturation, and finally to decreased MCV and hemoglobin [indices usually are normal until hemoglobin is 10 g/dL].)[2,3]

Consult the physician if laboratory data are not consistent with the clinical picture or the hematocrit is less than 25 percent/dL. Also plan consultation if the client has a positive stool guaiac, history of bleeding, family history or a family history of colon cancer.

Follow-up tests are crucial to ensure that the diagnosis is correct and that anemia is resolving with treatment. At 1 week, the reticulocyte count should increase 5 to 10 percent; at 1 month, the hemoglobin should increase 2 points; at 2 to 3 months, all normal levels should be reached. Iron is continued another 3 months or more.[1,2,3]

Differential Medical Diagnoses

See Tables 21–23 and 21–24.

Plan

Psychosocial Interventions. Reassure the client with iron-deficiency anemia secondary to menses or pregnancy that her condition is common. Advise her that it takes at least 6 months to completely refill iron stores. Stress the importance of follow-up laboratory tests to confirm the diagnosis. Encourage compliance with oral iron and dietary measures. If the client is postmenopausal, explain the need for further testing to locate the source of blood loss.[1,2,3]

Medication. Ferrous sulfate is given once iron-deficiency anemia has been documented, confirmed by laboratory tests, and the underlying cause has been diagnosed and treated.

- *Administration.* A 325-mg tablet is taken three times a day, with 500 mg vitamin C (to aid absorption), for a minimum of 6 months.[1,2,3] Also see Chapter 5, Menstruation and Related Problems and Concerns.
- *Side Effects.* The most frequent are gastrointestinal: nausea, constipation, and black stools. The difficulty tolerating iron may be minimized

if the client consumes the dose with food, starting slowly with one tablet per day, increases her fluid intake, and increases her dietary fiber. Increase the dose as tolerated.

- *Contraindications.* Do not administer iron if a deficiency has not been documented by laboratory tests. Iron overload can be fatal and hard to reverse. Mistakenly treating other types of anemia, such as sideroblastic anemia and anemia of chronic diseases, with iron can lead to overload and death.[2,3]
- *Client Teaching.* After diagnosis, explain to the client that follow-up and treatment will continue for about 6 months. Stress the importance of obtaining follow-up laboratory tests at 1 and 3 months and continuing medications as ordered. Advise the client to keep iron out of the reach of children.

Dietary Interventions. The diet should include foods high in iron: lean meats, egg yolk, shellfish, leafy greens, raisins, and dried apricots and peaches. Advise the client to avoid taking iron with tea, antacids, or dairy products.

The iron supplement contained in multivitamins (18 mg iron) will not correct iron-deficiency anemia but will help prevent recurrences of the problem in menstruating women. The average American diet contains 10 to 15 mg of iron per day; only about 1 to 2 mg per day is absorbed. Dietary measures alone are usually insufficient to correct the iron losses from heavy menstruation. Generic one-a-day multivitamins with iron are a reasonable approach to avoiding IDA in otherwise healthy women, but will not correct an anemia.[1,2]

Follow-Up

All clients should be retested to confirm the IDA diagnosis and to determine if the anemia is improving. (As stated earlier, after 1 month with adequate treatment the hemoglobin should increase 2 points; at 2 to 3 months the ultimate goal of the hemoglobin within normal range should be reached. Iron supplementation is continued for 3 months thereafter.) If the client is compliant, yet no improvement occurs, reconsider the diagnosis.

THALASSEMIA

Thalassemia encompasses a group of hereditary anemias in which synthesis of one or both chains of the hemoglobin molecule (α and β) is defective. A low hemoglobin level and a microcytic, hypochromic anemia result. Individuals who are heterozygous for α- or β-thalassemia have *thalassemia minor;* those who are homozygous have *thalassemia major.* β-Thalassemia major (Cooley's anemia) is a fatal condition. The most severe form of α-thalassemia major results in hydrops fetalis syndrome.

Epidemiology

In the United States, β-thalassemia minor occurs primarily among African-Americans and persons of Mediterranean descent. α-Thalassemia occurs primarily among Southeast Asians. Its transmission is genetic. β-Thalassemia minor is a silent "carrier" state in which the individual fails to produce a β hemoglobin chain. The body compensates by selectively producing hemoglobin A_2, which does not require a β chain.[2,3] α-Thalassemia minor is a more benign state and more difficult to diagnose, as hemoglobin A_2 does not increase and other confirmatory tests are not readily available for adults.[2,3] β-Thalassemia affects fewer than 1000 Americans.[1]

Subjective Data

Thalassemia minor is an asymptomatic condition, diagnosed inadvertently primarily by abnormal laboratory findings.

Objective Data

Physical examination reveals nothing abnormal.

A routine CBC will indicate a combined extremely low MCV (usually less than 65 fL) and only a slightly decreased hemoglobin (usually between 10 and 12 g/dL).[2,3]

Hemoglobin electrophoresis can confirm a diagnosis of β-thalassemia because of the increased level of hemoglobin A_2; the test cannot confirm α-thalassemia. The clinical picture and other laboratory results must be evaluated.

The test for α-thalassemia is not easily available. If, however, a client has a clinical picture consistent with β-thalassemia trait (very low MCV and mild anemia) yet hemoglobin electrophoresis does not show an increase in hemoglobin A_2, suspect the α-thalassemia trait. Refer the client for genetic counseling.

Differential Medical Diagnoses

See Table 21–23.

Plan

Psychosocial Interventions. Make the appropriate genetic counseling referral and support the client as she makes decisions regarding childbearing. Reassure her that she is not "sick" and does not need lifelong treatment for anemia.

Medication. None is required. Caution the client that blindly and constantly supplementing her diet with iron tablets is dangerous and a needless expense.[2,3]

ANEMIA OF CHRONIC DISEASES

Anemia of chronic diseases (ACD) is a common but poorly understood condition. It is seen in clients with cancer or chronic inflammatory disorders, such as lupus and rheumatoid arthritis. Despite adequate iron supplies, the body cannot use its stored iron. Red blood cells may be normocytic or microcytic; no uniform hematologic picture can be outlined.[2,3]

Epidemiology

The cause of anemia of chronic diseases is unknown, although it is associated with chronic inflammatory conditions.

Subjective Data

The condition is usually asymptomatic. When anemia becomes severe, symptoms relative to the coexisting chronic disease may exacerbate. In addition, symptoms of anemia, such as fatigue and shortness of breath, may be present.

Objective Data

For information on the physical examination, see Iron Deficiency Anemia.

No specific diagnostic tests are conclusive; the anemia is primarily a diagnosis of exclusion. A CBC may reveal normocytic or microcytic anemia; however, no consistent pattern is found in other tests. The serum ferritin is usually adequate. For diagnosis, refer to a physician.

Differential Medical Diagnoses

See Table 21–23.

Plan

Psychosocial Interventions. Support the client in dealing with chronic illness.

Medication. None is required. Caution the client to avoid taking iron unless prescribed: excess intake may cause iron overload.[2,3] Ask the client if she is taking a nonsteroidal anti-inflammatory drug. Gastrointestinal bleeding and subsequent iron deficiency may confuse the clinical picture.

Follow-Up

Consultation with a physician is necessary for all clients with ACD. If anemia is severe, refer the client to a hematologist.

LESS COMMON ANEMIAS

These rarer but still prevalent anemias are usually caused by dietary deficiencies and/or genetic inheritance.

Glucose-6-Phosphate Dehydrogenase Deficiency

Glucose-6-Phosphate Dehydrogenase Deficiency (G6PD deficiency), which is inherited, causes a hemolytic anemia. The enzyme protects RBCs against breakdown by free oxygen. Until an acute hemolytic episode is triggered, the client remains asymptomatic. Hemolysis can be precipitated by viral or bacterial infections or by certain oxidizing drugs.

Glucose-6-phosphate dehydrogenase deficiency is usually discovered accidentally; for example, a pregnant woman who is followed with serial hematocrits may be diagnosed when a marked anemia develops after treatment with an antibiotic, such as sulfa. If hemolysis is severe,

she is referred to a hematologist. The woman is instructed to avoid aspirin, sulfa, nitrofurantoin, primaquine, phenacetin, and some vitamin K derivatives.[2,3]

Glucose-6-phosphate dehydrogenase deficiency is seen primarily in African Americans and persons of Mediterranean descent.[2,3]

Sickle Cell Anemia

Sickle cell anemia is an inherited disease seen primarily in clients of African descent. People with *sickle cell trait* have erythrocytes containing 20 to 40 percent hemoglobin S, with the remaining hemoglobin appearing as normal adult.

Epidemiology. Sickle cell anemia and sickle cell trait are caused by various genetic defects in hemoglobin chains. Sickle cell disease (Hgb SS) occurs in 1 in every 375 African Americans, 1 in 3000 Native Americans, 1 in 20,000 Hispanic Americans, and 1 in 60,000 whites.[1] Occasionally, sickle cell trait occurs in persons of Mediterranean, Arabian, or East Indian descent.[1,2,3]

Subjective Data. Most often persons with sickle cell trait are asymptomatic; occasionally, however, episodes of hematuria, increased bacteriuria, and pyelonephritis during pregnancy are associated with this trait. Clients with sickle cell anemia will report frequent painful crises.

Objective Data. Examination is usually benign in sickle cell trait and between sickle cell disease crises. See Tables 21–23 and 21–24 for differential diagnoses.

Plan. Management consists primarily of documenting the condition, encouraging genetic counseling, and reassuring the client that sickle cell trait is benign.[2,3] Clients in acute crisis should be referred for emergency management.

Vitamin B$_{12}$ Deficiency

Anemia caused by vitamin B$_{12}$ deficiency is megaloblastic, most often caused by pernicious anemia and occasionally by gastrointestinal disorders that result in gastrectomy. Lack of dietary vitamin B$_{12}$ is rarely a problem, as body stores last 3 to 5 years. Vitamin B$_{12}$ absorption, however, may be affected. It requires the intrinsic factor produced by the stomach lining and an intact ileum, where absorption actually occurs. Pernicious anemia is an autoimmune disorder that usually becomes symptomatic around age 60 when the stomach is unable to produce intrinsic factor; as a result, the small intestine is unable to absorb vitamin B_{12}. The "classic triad" of vitamin B_{12} deficiency includes weakness, sore tongue, and paresthesias (particularly loss of vibratory sense). The Schilling test is used for diagnosis. Treatment involves monthly vitamin B_{12} injections.[2,3]

Folate Deficiency

Folate deficiency, related primarily to inadequate nutrition, may cause a megaloblastic anemia. Folate does not accumulate in the body; therefore, the anemia is more common than that caused by vitamin B_{12} deficiency. Folate deficiency most commonly occurs during pregnancy and among alcoholics. Lab work reveals a megaloblastic anemia (MCV > 100) and a decreased folate level. Diagnosis is confirmed by an appropriate clinical response to administration of folic acid, usually 1 mg per day. Management should also address the underlying condition, such as alcoholism. Sources of folic acid (leafy vegetables, fruits, nuts, and liver) should be increased in the diet. Certain drugs, for example, dilantin and trimethoprim, inhibit folate absorption.[2,3] It is interesting to note that the macrocytic anemias caused by vitamin B_{12} and folate deficiency can cause false-positive Pap smears. Abnormal Pap smears should be repeated after adequate treatment with vitamin B_{12} or folic acid.[2,3]

REFERENCES

Cardiovascular Disorders

1. Smith, M. A., & Johnson, D. G. (1991). Evaluation and management of coronary artery disease: Guidelines for the primary care nurse practitioner. *Nurse Practitioner Forum, 2*(1), 19–26.
2. Villablanca, A. (1996). Coronary heart disease in women: Gender differences and effect of menopause. *Postgraduate Medicine, 100*(3), 191–202.
3. McGovern, P., et al. (1996). Recent trends in acute coronary heart disease. *New England Journal of Medicine, 334*(14), 884–890.
4. Hennekens, C., et al. (1996). Coronary disease: The leading killer. *Patient Care,* 116–141.
5. Agency for Health Care Policy and Research Smoking Cessation Clinical Practice Guideline. (1996). *Journal of American Medical Association, 275*(16), 1270–1280.
6. Wexler, A., et al. (1991). Difference in use of procedures between women and men hospitalized for CAD. *New England Journal of Medicine, 325*(4), 221–230.
7. James, T., & Eaton, C. (1995). Exercise prescription. *American Family Physician, 52,* 543–550.
8. Second report of the expert panel on detection, evaluation, and treatment of high blood cholesterol in adults (Adult Treatment Panel II). (1993). *NIH Publication* No. 93–3096.
9. Woodhead, G. (1996). The management of cholesterol in coronary heart disease risk reduction. *Nurse Practitioner, 21*(9), 45–53.
10. Prisant, L. (1996). Hypercholesterolemia: A rational use of cholesterol—Lowering diets and drugs. *Consultant,* 1123–1138.
11. The fifth report of the Joint National Committee on detection evaluation, and treatment of high blood pressure (JNCV). (1993). *Archives of Internal Medicine, 153,* 154–183.
12. Kaplan, N. (1995). The treatment of hypertension in women. *Archives of Internal Medicine, 155,* 563–567.
13. Moser, M. (1996). Management of hypertension, Part I. *American Family Physician, 53*(7), 2295–2302.
14. Moser, M. (1996). Management of hypertension, Part II. *American Family Physician, 53*(7), 2553–2560.
15. Levy, D., et al. (1996). The progression from hypertension to congestive heart failure. *JAMA, 275*(20), 1557–1562.
16. Weir, M., et al. (1995). Differing mechanisms of actions of angiotensin-converting enzyme inhibition in Black and White hypertensive patients. *Hypertension, 26*(1), 124–130.
17. Gullickson, C. (1993). Client-centered drug choice: An alternative approach in managing hypertension. *Nurse Practitioner, 19*(2), 35–41.
18. Blake, G. (1994). Primary hypertension: The role of individualized therapy. *American Family Physician, 50*(1), 138–146.
19. Newton, J., et al. (1993). Treatment of mild hypertension study. *JAMA, 270*(6), 713–724.
20. Davis, B., et al. (1996). Rational and design for the anti-hypertensive and lipid lowering treatment to prevent heart attack trial (ALL HAT). *American Journal of Hypertension 9*(4), 342–360.

21. Sorrentino, M. (1993). Mitral valve prolapse. *Post Graduate Medicine, 93*(6), 63–80.

22. Noble, J., (1996). Textbook of Primary Care Medicine. St. Louis: Mosby Year Book Inc.

23. Auten, G., et al. (1996). Endocarditis: Current guidelines on prophylaxis, diagnosis, and treatment. *Consultant*, 973–993.

Dermatoses

1. Lynch, P. (1987). *Dermatology for the house officer* (2nd ed.). Baltimore: Williams & Wilkins.

2. Segal, R., et al. (1993). Once weekly treatment with oral ketoconazole for superficial fungal infection. *Journal of American Academy of Dermatology, 28*(1), 126–127.

3. Bergus, G., & Johnson, J. (1993). Superficial tinea infections. *American Family Physician, 48*(2), 259–268.

4. Eaglstein, W., McKay, M., & Pariser, D. (1994). The problems that plague aging skin. *Patient Care, 28*(9), 89–119.

5. Berson, D., Draelos, Z., & Webster, G. (1995). Saving face: A treatment update for acne. *Patient Care, 29*(19), 20–44.

6. Goldstein, S., & Odom, R. (1996). Skin and appendages. In L. Tierney, S. McPhee, & M. Papadakis (Eds.), *Current medical diagnosis and treatment* (35th ed.). Stamford, CT: Appleton & Lange.

7. Stevens, G., & Adelman, H. (1995). Palpable purpura: An algorithmic approach. *American Family Physician, 52*(5), 1355–1362.

8. Miller, D., & Brodell, R. (1996). Human papillomavirus infection: Treatment options for warts. *American Family Physician, 53*(1), 135–143.

9. Gupta, M., & Gupta, A. (1995). Age and gender differences in the impact of psoriasis on quality of life. *International Journal of Dermatology, 34*(10), 700–703.

10. Faria, D., & Krull, E. (1996). Recognizing and managing rosacea. *Hospital Medicine, 32*(2), 35–40.

11. Daniel, C., Dolan, N., & Wheeland, R. (1996). Don't overlook skin surveillance. *Patient Care, 30*(11), 90–107.

12. Hacker, S., Browder, J., & Ramos-Caro, F. (1993). Basal cell carcinoma. *Postgraduate Medicine, 93*(8), 101–111.

13. Browder, J., & Beers, B. (1993). Photoaging. *Postgraduate Medicine, 93*(8), 74–92.

14. Hacker, S., & Flowers, T. (1993). Squamous cell carcinoma of the skin. *Postgraduate Medicine, 93*(8), 115–126.

15. Edwards, L., Glass, F., Levine, N., & Sober, A. (1996). Melanoma: A strategy for detection and treatment. *Patient Care, 30*(11), 126–153.

16. Roth, M., & Grant-Kels, J. (1996). Pigmented skin lesions: How to distinguish the benign from malignant melanoma. *Consultant, 36*(7), 1516–1524.

17. Rigel, D. (1996). Malignant Melanoma: Perspectives on incidence and its effects on awareness, diagnosis, and treatment. *CA—A Cancer Journal for Clinicians, 46*(4), 195–198.

18. Marks, R. (1996). Prevention and control of melanoma: The public health approach. *CA—A Cancer Journal for Clinicians, 46*(4), 199–216.

19. Runkle, G., Zaloznik, A. (1994.) Malignant Melanoma. *American Family Physician 49*(1), 91–98.

Ear, Nose, and Throat Disorders

1. *Report of the U.S. Preventive Services Task Force: Guide to clinical preventive services.* (1996). Alexandria: Internal Medical Publishing, Inc.

2. Noble, J. (Ed.). (1996). *Textbook of primary care medicine.* St. Louis: Mosby Year Book, Inc.

3. Mays, M., & Lether, S. (1996). Primary care for women: Management of common respiratory problems. *Journal of Midwifery, 41*(2), 139–154.

4. Papeas, D., et al. (1996). Acute otitis media: Update on how and when to give antibiotics. *Consultant*, 721–728.

5. Wautzman, A. (1996). Otoscopic examination: What to look for in the external ear. *Consultant*, 933–942.

6. Ostrowsky, V. (1996). Pathologic conditions of the external ear and auditory canal. *Post Graduate Medicine, 100*(3), 223–237.

7. Guarderas, J. (1996). Rhinitis and sinusitis: Office management. *Mayo Clinic Proceedings, 71*, 882–888.

8. Schwartz, R. (1994). The diagnosis and management of sinusitis. *Nurse Practitioner, 19*(12), 58–64.

9. Lockey, R. (1996). Management of chronic sinusitis. *Hospital Practice, 31*(3), 141–151.

10. Chester, A. (1996). Chronic sinusitis. *American Family Physician, 53*(3), 977–987.

11. Douville, L. (1995). Pharmacologic highlights: Management of acute sinusitis. *Journal of the American Family Academy of Nurse Practitioners, 7*(8), 407–411.

12. Ruoff, G. (1996). Recurrent Streptococcal Pharyngitis. *Post Graduate Medicine, 99*(2), 211–222.

13. Gwaltney, J., et al. (1996). Rational Management of Sore Throat. *Patient Care*, 76–93.

Endocrine Disorders

1. Rakel, R. (Ed.). (1996). *Textbook of primary care medicine.* Philadelphia: W. B. Saunders Co.
2. Report of the U.S. Preventative Services Task Force (1996). Guide to Clinical Preventative Services. Alexandria Internal Medical Publishing.
3. Heitman, B., & Irizussy, A. (1995). Hypothyroidism: Common complaints, perplexing diagnosis. *Nurse Practitioner, 20*(3), 54–60.
4. American Association of Clinical Endocrinologists. (1995). *AACE clinical practice guidelines for the evaluation and treatment of hyperthyroidism and hypothyroidism.*
5. Brody, M. (1995). Thyroid screening. *Postgraduate Medicine, 98*(2), 54–66.
6. Pittman, J. (1996). Evaluation of patients with mildly abnormal thyroid function tests. *American Family Physician, 54,* 961–966.
7. Behnia, M., & Gharib, H. (1996). Primary care diagnosis of thyroid disease. *Hospital Practice,* 121–134.
8. Hewnessey, J. (1996). Diagnosis and management of thyrotoxicosis. *American Family Physician, 54*(4), 1315–1324.
9. Wartofsky, L. (1996). Treatment options for hyperthyroidism. *Hospital Practice,* 69–82.
10. Noble, J. (1996). Textbook of Primary Care Medicine. St. Louis: Mosby Year Book Inc.
11. Cefalu, W. (1996). Treatment of type II diabetes. *Postgraduate Medicine, 99*(3), 109–122.
12. American Diabetes Association (1997, July). Report of the expert committee on the diagnosis and classification of diabetes mellitus. *Diabetes Care, 20*(7), 1183–1197.
13. Fahey, P., et al. (1996). The athlete with type I diabetes: Managing insulin diet and exercise. *American Family Physician, 53*(5), 1611–1618.
14. Karl, D., et al. (1996). Diabetes mellitus: Lessons from the DCCT and how to implement them. *Consultant,* 1670–1681.
15. Hirsch, I. (1996). Surveillance for complications of diabetes. *Postgraduate Medicine, 99*(3), 147–162.
16. Abramowicz, M. (1996). Acarbose for diabetes mellitus. *The Medical Letter, 38*(967), 9–11.
17. Abramowicz, M. (1995). Metformin for noninsulin dependent diabetes mellitus. *The Medical Letter, 37*(948), 41–42.
18. Defronzo, R., et al. (1995). Efficiency of metformin in patients with non-insulin-dependent diabetes mellitus. *New England Journal of Medicine, 333,* 541–549.
19. Cefalu, W., et al. (1996). What's new about the new oral diabetes drugs. *Patient Care,* 40–66.
20. Johnson, J., et al. (1996). Efficiency of insulin and sulfonylurea combination therapy in type II diabetes. *Archives Internal Medical, 156,* 259–264.
21. Brown, D. (1996). Diabetic retinopathy: How and when to screen. *Consultant,* 1412–1422.
22. Will, J., et al. (1996). The contributions of diabetes to early deaths from ischemic heart disease: U.S. gender and racial comparisons. *American Journal of Public Health, 86*(4), 576–579.
23. Ziemer, D. (1996). Diabetes in urban African Americans, the management of type II diabetes in a municipal hospital setting. *The American Journal of Medicine, 101,* 25–33.

Gastrointestinal Disorders

1. Shaw, B. (1996). Primary care for women: Management and treatment of gastrointestinal disorders. *Journal of Nurse, Midwifery, 41*(2), 155–172.
2. Barr, L. (1996). Gastroesophageal reflux: Recognizing a typical prevention. *Post Graduate Medicine, 99*(4), 231–237.
3. Kahrilas, P. (1996). Gastroesophageal reflux disease. *JAMA, 276*(12), 983–988.
4. Regueico, M., et al. (1996). Current guidelines for GERD. *Contemporary Internal Medicine, 8*(3), 61–69.
5. Khulusi, P., et al. (1995). Prospective screening of dyspeptic patients by helico bacter pylori serology. *The Lancet, 346,* 1315–1318.
6. Fay, M., & Jaffe, P. (1996). Diagnostic and treatment guidelines for helico bacter pylori. *The Nurse Practitioner, 21*(7), 28–35.
7. Robinson, M. (1995). Prokinetic therapy for gastroesophageal reflux disease. *American Family Physician, 52*(3), 957–962.
8. Noble, J. (Ed.). (1996). *Textbook of primary care medicine.* St. Louis: Mosby Yearbook Inc.
9. Rakel, R. (Ed.). (1996). Conn's Cure and Therapy. Philadelphia: W. B. Saunders Co.
10. *Report of the U.S. Preventative Services Task Force: Guide to Clinical Preventative Services.* (1996). Alexandria: Internal Medical Publishing, Inc.

11. Kowdley, K. (1996). Update on therapy for hepatobiliary disease. *The Nurse Practitioner, 21*(7), 78–88.
12. Cerda, J., et al. (1996). Effective, compassionate management of IBS. *Patient Care,* 131–146.
13. Thompson, W. (1994). Irritable bowel syndrome: Diagnostic and therapeutic dilemma. *Contemporary Internal Medicine, 6*(4), 45–56.
14. Bryan, J. (1995). Viral hepatitis: Update on hepatitis D and E. *Consultant, 18* 46–1850.

Hematological Disorders

1. *Report of the U.S. Preventive Services Task Force: Guide to clinical preventative services.* (1996). Alexandria: Internal Medical Publishing.
2. Rakel, R. (Ed.). (1996). Conn's Current Therapy. Philadelphia: W. B. Saunders Co.
3. Noble, J. (Ed). (1996). *Textbook of primary care medicine.* St. Louis: Mosby Yearbook Inc.

CHAPTER 22

COMMON MEDICAL PROBLEMS: MUSCULOSKELETAL INJURIES THROUGH URINARY TRACT DISORDERS

Judy Parker-Falzoi • Elaine Ferrary

*7*0–90% of the population will experience low back pain during their lifetime. It is second only to the common cold in lost days of work and is the leading cause of disability in those under 45 years of age.

Highlights

- Musculoskeletal Injuries
- Neurological Disorders
- Ophthalmologic Disorders
- Pulmonary Disorders
- Urinary Tract Disorders

► INTRODUCTION

This chapter continues the coverage of usual medical problems found in the general primary care practice. Chapter references provide guidance for finding more in-depth information.

Musculoskeletal Conditions

Whether physically active or sedentary, clients often visit a primary care setting complaining of aches in muscles, back, arms, wrists, legs. This section discusses the following: ankle sprain and knee sprain, acute low back pain, carpal tunnel syndrome, bursitis, fibromyalgia, gout, osteoarthritis, rheumatoid arthritis, and systemic lupus erythematosus.

MUSCULOSKELETAL INJURIES: ANKLE SPRAIN AND KNEE SPRAIN

Ankle sprain and knee sprain are the two most common sports related injuries. The lateral ligaments of the ankle are most often involved in a sprain. Knee sprain typically involves the medial or lateral collateral ligament or the meniscus.

Epidemiology

Five percent of all sports related injuries involve the ankle.[1] Once an ankle injury has occurred, the ankle is twice as likely to be injured again.[2] Activities that involve running and jumping such as basketball, volleyball, and dance place the female athlete at risk for ankle sprain. Knee injuries occur in sports where the leg is planted and the body pivots, such as basketball, skiing, tennis, ice skating, and dance.

Subjective Data

Ask the client to describe in detail the circumstances of the injury. Most ankle sprains occur when the foot is plantar-flexed and inverted. Eversion injuries are usually more severe and may involve fracture of the ankle mortise joint. The client may have continued her activities and noted pain and swelling only after several hours. Any report of a popping noise at time of trauma is significant for extensive ligament tear and disruption in both knee and ankle injuries. Ask about treatment following trauma (ice, elevation, medication) and any history of previous injuries.

Objective Data: Ankle Sprain

Physical Examination. Observe for deformity, ecchymosis, and swelling. Observe gait if client is able to bear weight.

- *Range of Motion.* Move the joint through its range of motion if possible (the client may have to be distracted). In assessing the ankle, cradle it in your hand and palpate the medial and lateral malleoli and the fifth metatarsal. Flex and extend the ankle. Assess resistance to anterior and varus stress.

Grade I sprain:	Mild pain and tenderness; little or no swelling
Grade II sprain:	Slight to moderate instability; moderate pain and tenderness; moderate swelling and ecchymosis
Grade III sprain:	Significant instability; marked pain and tenderness; marked swelling and ecchymosis

Grade III sprains must be referred to orthopedist.

Diagnostic Tests. Films are indicated if the client has point tenderness of the medial or lateral malleolus and if she is unable to bear weight right after the injury. X-ray the foot if there is tenderness at the base of the fifth metatarsal.

Differential Medical Diagnoses

Ankle fracture (x-ray confirms), fracture of the fifth metatarsal (x-ray confirms), gout (not associated with trauma).

Plan

Psychosocial Interventions. If client is a competitive athlete or dancer, injury may cause great anxiety and possibly loss of income. Reassure her that with rest and careful rehabilitation, recovery is usually complete.

Medication. Nonsteroidal anti-inflammatory drugs such as Ibuprofen 600 mg orally three times a day for 7–10 days (see Table 22–1). If NSAIDs contraindicated, acetaminophen may be used for pain control. If sprain is severe, short-term use of narcotic analgesics may be indicated. Consult physician.

Lifestyle. Rest, ice, compression and elevation (RICE) are ordered for the first 48–72 hours postinjury to reduce swelling and pain. If the sprain is grade II, nonweight bearing is advised for 72 hours. Begin gentle range of motion exercises after 48 hours. Start strengthening exercises as soon as pain and swelling subside. Begin with calf and peroneal muscle stretches. Pool exercises may help if pain and stiffness prevent full stretches. Cross training by cycling and stationary cross country ski machines increases all over muscle tone and endurance. Encourage client to recondition slowly and not overdo. Advise her that pain of re-injury may be masked by analgesics.

Wrapping with elastic bandage is not considered effective support when client is returning to previous level of activity. If used in combination with high-top shoes efficacy is increased. Taping is often used but may lose support capability during exercise. Lace-up supports and semirigid stirrup supports have been shown to prevent re-injury.[2]

Follow-Up

Evaluate after 72 hours. Clients with grade I injuries may be able to start rehabilitation at this point. Grade II sprains should be examined for compartment syndrome, manifested by increased swelling, pain, and restriction of movement. Reassess grade II sprains at 7 days post injury for possible return to weight bearing and rehabilitation or if indicated, referral to Orthopedics/Physical Therapy.

Objective Data: Knee Sprain

Physical Examination

- *Range of Motion.* Ask the client to flex and extend the knee. Typically, she will not be able to extend fully. If the patella was dislocated at the time of trauma (common in women), it will relocate on extension.
- *Palpation.* Client will complain of intense pain when the patella is pushed laterally. Palpate the knee for tenderness and effusion. (See discussion of technique in section on bursitis.) Large effusions appear just above the patella and are obvious. Small effusions can be detected by applying pressure to the lateral patella and observing for a bulge medially. Assess for instability during varus and valgus stress, with the ankle held under the elbow of the examiner and with the client supine. Joint laxity indicates injury to the medial collateral ligament.

The most reliable and accurate test for instability of the cruciate ligament is Lachman's test. The client is supine and flexes the knee 15–20 degrees. The examiner places one hand on the proximal tibia and one hand on the distal femur. She or he shifts the tibial plateau anteriorly while holding the femur stationary. A soft end point to the maneuver or anterior translation indicates a tear of the anterior cruciate ligament.

Diagnostic Tests. X-ray the knee only if there was direct trauma to the patella and if a fracture or avulsion injury is suspected. For soft tissue injuries with high suspicion of cruciate ligament tear, MRI is indicated.

Differential Medical Diagnoses

Knee fracture (x-ray confirms). Bursitis (palpable swelling and warmth on the patella, may not have history of trauma), meniscal tear (swelling and pain along joint line, locking or popping with varus/valgus stress) cruciate ligament tear (laxity with full extension on Drawer sign test and Lachman's maneuver).

TABLE 22–1. CLASSIFICATION OF NONSTEROIDAL ANTI-INFLAMMATORY DRUGS

Classification	Dosage	Advantages	Disadvantages
I. Salicylate Preparations Aspirin (enteric coated tablets) 325/500/650mg	1 G QID Extended 1.6 G BID	Inexpensive Effective in OTC, readily available	High incidence GI distress Increased bleeding time Tinnitus Bronchospasm More frequent doses needed
Nonacetalated Salsalate (Disalcid) 500/750 mg	3–4 G/day in 2–3 doses	Fewer GI effects Less effect on kidney function Does not increase bleeding time Less effect on beta blockers, diuretics, ACE-I	Tinnitus Vertigo Moderately expensive
Diflunisal (Dolobid) 250/500 mg	500 mg BID	Twice a day dosing Less effect on kidney function, beta blockers, diuretics, ACE-I	GI distress May potentiate warfarin Headache Tinnitus Moderately expensive
II. Acetic Acid Naproxen (Naprosyn) 250/375/500 mg	250–500 mg BID	Available OTC in 125 mg tablet Effective first line drug Also effective vs migraines	GI distress Fluid retention May increase LFTs Moderately expensive
Sulindac (Clinoril) 150/200 mg	150–200 mg BID	Least effect on kidney function Does not affect platelet aggregation	GI distress Potentiates warfarin May cause hepatitis Very expensive
Diclofenac (Voltaren) 25/50/75 mg	150–200 mg qd in 2 or 3 doses	Useful in ankylosing spondylitis	GI effects Headache Dizziness May cause hepatitis Very expensive
Indomethacin (Indocin) 25/50/75 mg	25–50 mg TID	Useful in gout Very inexpensive	GI effects Headache Agranulocytosis and anemia Increases warfarin and lithium levels

III. Propionic Acid
Ibuprofen
(Motrin, Advil)
400/600/800 mg
	1.2–3.2 G in 3–4
	doses
		Effective first line drug
		Fairly inexpensive
		Lowest incidence of GI and hepatic
		   effects
		Available OTC in 200 mg dose
			GI effects
			Fluid retention
			May induce meningitis in clients
			   with SLE

Ketoprofen (Orudis) 25/50/75 mg	50–75 mg TID-QID	Available OTC in 12.5 mg dose	Expensive Increased risk of GI bleed Tinnitus Dizziness
Oxaprozam (Daypro) 600 mg	1200 mg	Once a day dosing	Very expensive GI effects
IV. Pyranocarboxylic Acid Etodolac (Lodine) 200/300 mg	300–400 mg TID	Does not lower prostaglandins therefore fewer GI effects	Expensive

TABLE 22–1. CLASSIFICATION OF NONSTEROIDAL ANTI-INFLAMMATORY DRUGS (CONTINUED)

Classification	Dosage	Advantages	Disadvantages
V. Enolic Acid Piroxicam (Feldene) 10/20 mg	20 mg once a day	Once a day dosing	Avoid in elderly Increased incidence of GI effects Potentiates warfarin
VI. Nonacid Nabumetone (Relafen) 500 mg	1–2 G once a day	Decreased incidence of GI effects	Expensive

Key: RA = rheumatoid arthritis; OTC = over-the-counter (available without prescription); LFTs = liver function tests; CNS = central nervous system; SLE = systemic lupus erythematosus.

Note: All nonsteroidal anti-inflammatory drugs have analgesic, antipyretic properties. All may cause rash, inhibit platelet aggregation, lower the effectiveness of antihypertensive agents, cause gastric irritation, kidney damage, bone marrow suppression, anorexia, and nausea. As a general rule, they should not be prescribed to those individuals taking anticoagulants.

Source: References 27, 28, 29.

Plan

Refer client with patellar fracture and cruciate and collateral ligament tears to orthopedist immediately.

Psychosocial Interventions. See section under Ankle Sprain.

Medication. See Ankle Sprain.

Lifestyle. RICE for first 72 hours. Knee immobilizer more effective than elastic bandage. Continue immobilizer or wrap until ligament tenderness and swelling have resolved (may take 2–6 weeks). Weight bearing as tolerated. Isometric quadriceps exercises with tensing of the quadriceps muscle 10 times every hour. Gradual rehabilitation lasting about twice as long as the period of immobilization. Advise client to start with straight leg raising 10 repetitions three times a day; may add handweight held on the quadriceps as tolerated (avoid ankle weights). Taping 6 inches above and below the joint line or use of short padded knee brace may be indicated when client resumes previous activity to prevent re-injury.[3]

Follow-Up

Evaluate in 72 hours for decrease in swelling and pain. If range of motion has decreased and pain has increased refer to physician for possible referral to orthopedics. Meniscal tears that do not respond may require arthroscopy.

ACUTE LOW BACK PAIN

Acute low back pain is a very common, usually benign and self-limited disorder. It may arise as a result of myofascial strain, degenerative change, or injury to the spine with or without nerve impingement. It may also accompany a serious underlying systemic disorder.

Epidemiology

Seventy to 90 percent of the population will experience low back pain during their lifetime. Fifty percent of those of working age will report back problems each year. It is second only to the common cold in lost days of work and is the leading cause of disability in those under 45 years of age.

The estimate of the social and medical costs of back pain in the United States ranges from $20–$50 billion.[4,5]

Subjective Data

The health history is key to rule out more serious underlying disorders. Important information includes age, provocative event, onset, character and radiation of pain, previous history of cancer or other serious medical condition, unexplained weight loss, pain that is worse at rest, response to self-care or previous therapy, history of intravenous drug use, history of urinary disorder. Only 2 percent of acute low back pain is due to nonmechanical causes, such as systemic disease or infection.

Typically the client reports onset after physical activity such as heavy lifting. It is made worse by twisting or bending. The pain may be localized to the lumbarsacral spine or may extend down the posterior thigh to the knee. Disc herniation with sciatic impingement causes unilateral radiation below the knee with numbness or weakness. Cauda equina compression, a surgical emergency, causes saddle anesthesia, bilateral leg weakness, and loss of bladder and/or bowel control. The client is referred immediately to a neurosurgeon.

Other elements to elicit in the health history include occupational history, present work status, any pending litigation or compensation issues, previous rehabilitation for back problems, substance abuse, and depression.

Objective Data

Physical Examination

- *General Appearance.* Observe posture, gait; ask client to walk on toes, on heels, balance on one foot.
- *Spine.* Inspect for deformity. Observe range of motion for limitation. Palpate for tenderness.
- *Lower Extremities.* Observe for quadriceps wasting. If there are lower extremity symptoms or signs, test deep tendon reflexes and great toe dorsiflexion strength.

  Palpate the spine for tenderness.

  The straight leg raising test is positive if the nerve root is irritated. It has low specificity but high sensitivity for herniation at the L4-5 and L5-S1 level. The client is supine, and the examiner raises the leg. It is positive if radicular pain is elicited before the leg reaches 60 degrees or fewer.
- *Abdomen.* Examine for tenderness and auscultate for abdominal bruit.

Diagnostic Tests. Radiologic studies are not routinely ordered unless pathological fracture, infection, tumor or traumatic injury is suspected. In the latter case, imaging may be important if litigation is a possibility. Anteroposterior and lateral lumbar films are the selected views.

MRI in clients with nerve root impingement signs is usually ordered only if results would change the course of therapy or if surgery is being considered.

Radionuclide bone scan is ordered only if high suspicion for osteomyelitis or metastasis.

Complete blood count may be indicated if infection is suspected.[4,6]

Differential Medical Diagnoses

Myofascial strain, herniated disk, compression fracture, fibromyalgia, osteoarthritis, spondylolisthesis, ankylosing spondylitis (rare in women), osteomyelitis, iatrogenic (from excessive bed rest or inactivity), pyelonephritis, bleeding aortic aneurysm, cancer of the pancreas, PID, tumor of the pelvis, multiple myeloma, various psychosocial factors such as mood disorder, drug seeking behavior, interpersonal or occupational stress.

Plan

Psychosocial Interventions. Reassure the client that acute low back pain is in most cases a self-limited problem. In 90 percent of the cases, it resolves within 6 weeks, no matter what interventions are used. The drug seeking client, the client with depression, should be referred appropriately.

Medication. NSAIDs or analgesics such as acetaminophen are used to manage pain. See previous discussion of these medications.

MUSCLE RELAXANTS. If muscle spasms are present, muscle relaxants may be used for 2–3 days.

CYCLOBENZAPRINE (FLEXERIL) 10 MG
- *Administration.* One tablet orally four times a day.
- *Contraindications.* Hyperthyroidism, congestive heart failure, cardiac disease, use of monoamine oxidase inhibitors.
- *Adverse Effects.* Drowsiness, dizziness, tachycardia, hypotension, dyspepsia.

METHOCARBAMOL (ROBAXIN) 750 MG
- *Administration.* Two tablets orally four times a day.
- *Contraindication.* Known hypersensitivity.
- *Adverse Effects.* Drowsiness, dizziness, bradycardia, hypotension, gastrointestinal upset.

NOTE: Warn client not to use these medications with alcohol.

BENZODIAZEPINES. Sciatic pain from nerve root impingement may not respond to above drugs, and a brief course of a benzodiazepine such as diazepam and bed rest with hips and knees slightly flexed may offer the only relief. These are controlled substances and can only be prescribed by the physician. Refer to a pharmacology text for further information.

Nonpharmacological Interventions. A recent study in Finland showed that individuals who continued ordinary activities as tolerated had a more rapid recovery than those who were put on strict bed rest or were treated with back mobilizing exercises.[7]

Local application of ice for 15–30 minutes four times a day may be beneficial. Heat is not indicated early in the course of treatment because it may exacerbate the pain.

Bed rest with bathroom privileges for more than 3 days may lead to more disability from deconditioning. Exercises are not indicated during the acute phase of pain and muscle spasm, but passive flexion and extension of the spine may provide relief. It is recommended to do these for 5 minutes every hour as tolerated.

Diet/Lifestyle. The working client should return to work within 4 to 7 days. If her job involves heavy lifting, a review of proper body mechanics is indicated. Referral to a physical therapist may be necessary for a program of exercises and work conditioning. The obese client will benefit from weight loss. Strengthening of the abdominal muscles is indicated for all clients with chronic low back pain. Swimming pool exercises such as walking with water resistance against the trunk are helpful when weightbearing exercises are not well tolerated due to lower extremity weakness.

Follow-Up

Re-evaluate the client after 2 weeks for response to therapy and return to normal activities. Refer to a physician those who complain of no improvement or a worsening of symptoms. A study in North Carolina showed that primary care providers provide the least expensive, most cost effective treatment for acute low back pain.[8]

CARPAL TUNNEL SYNDROME

Carpal tunnel syndrome is the most common entrapment neuropathy and is caused by compression of the medial nerve at the wrist. It is considered to be a work related repetitive use disorder; however, no well controlled research studies have been able to document this.[9]

Epidemiology

Carpal tunnel syndrome (CPS) is most prevalent in middle-aged women. The incidence has been calculated at 125 per 100,000 population in a study of the period 1976–1980. The highest reported incidence was reported in meatpackers. Occupational and recreational activities that entail repetitive wrist movements, vibrations, use of force as in grasping and pinching, and awkward wrist position place the individual at highest risk.[9,10]

Diabetes, rheumatoid arthritis, collagen vascular disorders, pregnancy, menopause, and hypothyroidism are medical conditions associated with CPS.

Subjective Data

The client complains of numbness, tingling, and pain in the hand that may radiate to the wrist and distal arm. The diagnostic hallmark is numbness and pain that wakes her up at night. Pain also occurs with activities that involve flexion or extension of the wrist. Fine motor coordination may be affected, causing her to drop things. The numbness and tingling is relieved by shaking the wrist in the manner of shaking down a mercury thermometer. When asked to pinpoint the areas of the hand most affected, she will identify the thumb, index, and middle fingers. She may not have pain.

Objective Data

Physical Examination. Examine base of thumb for thenar atrophy.

Tinel's and Phalen's tests are sensitive and specific in the diagnosis.

Phalen's sign is positive when flexing the wrist 90 degrees for 30–60 seconds causes numbness and tingling in thumb and first two or three fingers.

Tinel's sign is positive when tingling symptoms are reproduced by tapping with fingers or reflex hammer over the carpal tunnel.

Assess grip and pinch strength and sensitivity to touch. Assess for associated medical conditions such as rheumatoid arthritis, hypothyroidism, and diabetes.

Diagnostic Tests. Electromyography and nerve conduction studies will confirm the diagnosis. In most primary care settings, this is not ordered unless other complicating factors such as cervical disc disease or possible work compensation is at issue. Diabetics may also require more extensive studies and referral to a neurologist if there is a question of peripheral neuropathy.

Differential Medical Diagnoses

Cervical radiculopathy (pain above the shoulder, numbness and tingling occurs with cough, sneeze). Ulnar neuropathy (pain in ulnar nerve distribution). Thoracic outlet syndrome (weakness of hand muscles, sensory loss over ulnar region of hand and forearm). Peripheral neuropathy of diabetes (history, numbness not position dependent).

Plan

Psychosocial Interventions. The diagnosis of CPS may have serious implications for the client's occupational or recreational activities. It is important to be sensitive to these issues and provide reassurance and support. Early intervention and ergonomics are key.

Medication. Nonsteroidal anti-inflammatory drugs may help in early disease and during acute flares. See Table 22–1. Steroid injections of the wrist by an experienced practitioner thoroughly familiar with the carpal tunnel may relieve pain and numbness for weeks to years. Usual dose is triamcinolone 20–40 mg. See discussion of steroid injections under Bursitis.

Vitamin B_6 (pyridoxine) has no therapeutic effect in documented clinical trials. In large doses, it can be neurotoxic. Those who do report decrease in symptoms may have underlying peripheral neuropathy.

Diet/Lifestyle. Ergonomic interventions such as positioning keyboards to minimize wrist flexion, wearing wrist support during provocative activities will usually help. Wrist splinted in neutral position with palmar support worn at night is useful in early disease.

Follow-Up

Re-evaluate client in 10–14 days. If no improvement is noted or if client has long standing history, refer to orthopedic surgeon. Age of 50 years, duration of disease more than 10 months, and unrelenting numbness and tingling are poor prognosticators for success of conservative management. The client with probable co-existing morbidity as indicated by positive rheumatoid factor or antinuclear antibody is referred to a rheumatologist.

BURSITIS

Bursitis is an inflammation of the bursa, the fibrous sac that lies between some tendons and bones and acts as a cushion. The bursa is lined with a membrane that secretes synovial fluid. The most common causes of bursitis include trauma (acute and repetitive injury), infection, and arthritic conditions. The shoulder, the elbow, the hip, the knee, and the ankle are affected sites.

Epidemiology

Shoulder and knee pain are two of the most frequently cited reasons for primary care visits, with bursitis accounting for 0.4 percent of all visits.[11] Clients of all ages and levels of activity are affected; the daily jogger, the dance student, the golfer or softball player, the client with osteo- or rheumatoid arthritis, the child care provider who spends a lot of time on her knees. Runners are especially at risk, as are women with heavy, adipose legs.

Subjective Data

The client notes an abrupt onset of swelling and localized point tenderness over the affected bursa. There is usually an aching pain and pain on range of motion, but inflammation of the olecranon bursal sac (resembling a goose egg at the tip of the elbow) may cause no pain. The client typically has a history of repeated minor trauma or overuse.

Be sure to ask her about any recent unexplained fever, history of rheumatoid arthritis, systemic lupus erythematosus, or gout, past medical history, surgical history, occupational and recreational activities.

Objective Data

Physical Examination. Inspect the affected site for swelling, erythema. Observe the client moving the adjacent joint through active range of motion for limitations.

SHOULDER PAIN. Two tests are particularly useful for evaluating shoulder pain, the crossover test and the Apley scratch test.

- *Crossover Test.* Client reaches across the chest to touch the opposite shoulder (indicates acromioclavicular pathology).
- *Apley Test.* Client reaches behind neck to touch opposite superior scapula (abduction and external rotation). Client places arm and hand behind back and touches opposite inferior scapula (adduction and internal rotation).[12]

KNEE. To evaluate the knee, ballotte the patella. This is done by milking the fluid into the space between the patella and the femur. Start about 15 cm above the superior margin of the knee and slide index finger and thumb along the sides of the femur. While maintaining pressure on the kneecap, tap the patella. An effusion is present if the fingers on either side of the patella feel the tap. In bursitis no effusion is present, and the fluid cannot be milked into the space beneath the patella.

HIP. The evaluation of the hip for trochanteric or ischial bursitis includes full active and passive range of motion of the hip and palpation of the greater trochanter and ischial tuberosity for point tenderness.

ALL AFFECTED JOINTS. Observe for erythema. Palpate the site for crepitus, tenderness, warmth. Note degree of range of motion if possible for comparison on follow-up. Test extremity for strength and pain at extremes of range of motion. If bursitis is chronic, supporting muscles may have atrophied from underuse and weakness.

Diagnostic Tests

ARTHROCENTESIS. If infection is suspected, aspirate fluid must be sent for analysis: cell count, appearance, culture, microscopy (presence of crystals), gram stain.

COMPLETE BLOOD COUNT. To rule out infection.

OTHER TESTS. May include an erythrocyte sedimentation rate, antinuclear antibody, rheumatoid factor, and/or uric acid based on differential diagnosis.

RADIOGRAPHS. Usually not necessary unless there was acute trauma that preceded the pain, obvious deformity, instability, or conservative treatment for 2–3 weeks has failed.

MRI. Indicated only when surgery is considered.

BONE SCAN. In the case of lower extremity pain if the diagnosis is in doubt and the management would be changed, a bone scan may be indicated to rule out stress fracture, avascular necrosis, osteomyelitis.

Differential Medical Diagnoses

Osteoarthritis, rheumatoid arthritis, gout (see discussions of these conditions for defining features).

Upper extremity pain: fracture, shoulder dislocation, rotator cuff tear, adhesive capsulitis; referred pain from neck injury, Pancoast tumor of the lung, pneumonia or pleural effusion.

Lower extremity pain: sciatica, lumbar disc disease, avascular necrosis of the femoral head, pelvic stress fracture, pelvic tumor, meniscal tear, ligamentous injury or tear, Achilles tendinitis, Reiter's syndrome.

Plan

Psychosocial Interventions. If occupational or recreational factors have contributed to development of bursitis, the client may have concerns about future disability. Advise her that with rest, medication and following suggested rehabilitation, bursitis can be managed and controlled without permanent damage.

Medication. NSAIDs are the first line medications for control of pain and reduction of inflammation. The usual course of treatment is for 4–6 weeks if the symptoms have been present for fewer than 3 weeks and there is no significant loss of motion in the joint (see Table 22–1).

INFECTIOUS BURSITIS

ANTIBIOTICS. In the case of infectious bursitis, consult with a physician. If outpatient treatment, start patient immediately on antibiotic that covers staphylococcus, such as dicloxacillin 500 mg QID or cephalexin 500 mg QID, pending culture result. Continue antibiotics for 14 days. Consult pharmacology text for further information on these medications.

CHRONIC BURSITIS

STEROID INJECTION. In chronic bursitis or when conservative management fails, injection of a corticosteroid such as betamethasone 6 mg or triamcinolone 20–40 mg mixed with 3 cc of lidocaine into the bursa at the point of maximal tenderness provides rapid pain relief. Only those practitioners experienced in the procedure should attempt this.

- *Adverse Effects.* Complications include infection, tendon rupture, fat atrophy, skin pigment change, hyperglycemia. Client must be informed of possible adverse effects before the procedure.

Follow-Up

Injection can be repeated in 30 days for a maximum of three in a year.[11]

Nonpharmacological Treatment. The acronym PRICEMM is helpful to guide the treatment of bursitis (protection, relative rest, ice, compression, elevation, medication, and modalities).[11]

- *Protection.* For heel and knee bursitis, foam padding or bracing of the site can protect from friction injury. Retrocalcaneal bursitis often results from poorly fitting shoes or worn heel counters. Ice skaters and distance runners are groups at risk.

  Bursitis of the hip, especially ischiogluteal bursitis (Weaver's Bottom), is aggravated by prolonged sitting and is distinguished by pain in the gluteal region. Client may benefit from sitting on a foam pad or "doughnut" cushion.

  Clients with bursitis of the shoulder may use a sling to support the weight of the arm, but this must be removed three or four times a day to prevent adhesive capsulitis.

- *Relative Rest.* Encourage the client to engage in alternative exercise activities such as swimming, cycling, or ski machines.

  In the case of shoulder bursitis, the client should perform pendulum circles with the affected arm three times a day. Later, advance to more frequent light resistance range of motion exercises using a towel or elastic bands. Do these for 10 minutes twice a day.

  For bursitis of the knee, strengthening the quadriceps and the hamstring muscles is important.

- *Ice.* Massage ice on affected site for 10 minutes twice a day or more, especially before aggravating activities.

- *Compression and Elevation.* Ace bandage is applied and extremity is elevated.

- *Modalities* may include ultrasound and/or high voltage electrical stimulation under the direction of a physical therapist. Also if muscle weakness or loss of range of motion, refer for physical therapy.[11]

Diet/Lifestyle. If the client is obese, weight loss and exercise are encouraged to prevent future exacerbations or progression to chronic bursitis. Dedicated athletes should cross train in activities that do not stress the affected site, may benefit from referral to sports medicine clinician. Clients whose occupation aggravates the bursa, such as workers who must raise the arm over the head repetitively, should start on a program to strengthen surrounding muscle groups.

Follow-Up

Re-evaluate in 7 days or in 3–4 weeks if steroid injection. Continue therapy for 14 more days if response noted. If no improvement noted, consult with physician for further workup, need for steroid injections, or referral.

FIBROMYALGIA

Fibromyalgia (also called fibrositis) is a common, often underdiagnosed, pain syndrome characterized by generalized migratory pain and fatigue. It is considered a soft tissue rheumatic disease.

It is defined by tender points on the axial skeleton in all four body quadrants. There are several other syndromes often associated with fibromyalgia, including migraine headaches, irritable bowel syndrome, and affective disorders. It has been theorized that the neurotransmitter serotonin may be involved.[13,14]

Epidemiology

Fibromyalgia is more common in women than in men. The prevalence increases with age, especially in those 45–55 years old. It is estimated that 3 percent to 6 percent of the population including children meet the 1990 American College of Rheumatology's diagnostic criteria (see following).[13]

Subjective Data

The client's history supplies important clues to the diagnosis. The usual presenting complaints are widespread "joint" pain and overwhelming fatigue. The client may have visited several other providers and/or the emergency room to find an explanation for her condition. She may have been prescribed nonsteroidal anti-inflammatory drugs, which did not provide lasting pain relief.

It is important to review all systems because a constellation of other disorders has been associated with fibromyalgia. Their presence is not required for diagnosis but strongly suggests it.

Neurological: higher incidence of migraine and tension headaches; fleeting parasthesias; difficulty concentrating; short-term memory difficulty; sensitivity to loud noise.

Cardiopulmonary: noncardiac chest pain, palpitations, mitral valve prolapse. Higher incidence of multiple chemical and environmental sensitivities, rhinitis, nasal congestion.

Gastrointestinal: irritable bowel syndrome, heartburn, esophageal dysmotility.

Genitourinary: dysmenorrhea, urinary frequency, urgency, interstitial cystitis.

Psychologic: higher incidence of depression and somatization.

Objective Data

Physical Examination

CRITERIA FOR DIAGNOSIS. History of pain for at least 3 months in all four quadrants of the axial skeleton.

Pain in 11 of 18 paired tender points elicited by 4kg (about 8 pounds) of firm digital palpation pressure:

> Occiput
> Cervical spine C5-C7
> Trapezius muscle
> Supraspinatus muscle
> Second rib at costochondral junction
> Lateral epicondyle
> Upper outer gluteal muscle
> Greater trochanter
> Knees at medial fat pad

Examine all joints identified as painful for swelling, warmth, synovitis, instability, and deformity.

Diagnostic Tests. There is no specific laboratory or diagnostic test to establish the diagnosis. Diagnosis is based on history, presence of trigger points, and absence of inflammation. A few screening tests are helpful including complete blood count, erythrocyte sedimentation rate, blood chemistry panel, and thyroid panel. Imaging studies are usually not necessary or helpful.

Differential Medical Diagnoses

Rheumatoid arthritis, systemic lupus erythematosus (joint inflammation, elevated sedimentation rate); hypothyroidism (high TSH); polymyalgia rheumatica (shoulder and girdle pain and weakness, anemia, high sedimentation rate, age greater than 50); polymyositis (weakness).

Plan

Psychosocial Interventions. The client may feel overwhelming relief that a diagnosis has been made. Reassure her that although fibromyalgia is a chronic disease for which there is no cure, it is not progressive. She can make an enormous difference in the quality of her life by adopting healthy lifestyle measures. Encourage her to take an active role in devising the plan of care.

Medication

AMITRYPTILINE. 10 mg orally 1–2 hours before bedtime. Dosage may be increased by 10 mg qhs per week to a maximum of 70 to 80 mg qhs.

- *Mechanism of Action.* Amitryptiline is a tricyclic antidepressant that affects serotonin activity and is thought to potentiate endogenous opioids (endorphins). These two mechanisms may account for amitryptiline's analgesic effect in chronic pain syndromes.[14]
- *Adverse Effects.* Include vivid dreams or nightmares for the first few nights, hungover feeling in the morning. Other adverse effects include dry mouth, constipation, nausea.

    Contraindicated in those who are hypersensitive to tricyclic antidepressants. Also in recovery phase of myocardial infarction (may induce arrhythmias).
- *Expected Outcome.* Client will note improved and more restful sleep. Advise her it may take several weeks and some titration of the medication to achieve maximal effect.
- *Client Teaching.* Advise client to keep sleep diary and note dosage at which sound sleep with minimal hangover is achieved. Advise her of additive effects of alcohol, antihistamines, sedatives, and tranquilizers.

CYCLOBENZAPRINE (FLEXERIL). 10 mg taken at bedtime may be prescribed if client unable to tolerate amitriptyline. Titrate to maximum dose of 40 mg. Contraindications, adverse effects, client teaching similar to amitriptyline.

NONSTEROIDAL ANTI-INFLAMMATORY. Medications may be tried but advise client they may be ineffective.

ANTIDEPRESSANTS. Such as the selective serotonin reuptake inhibitors may be helpful in certain clients. See discussion of these in the chapter on Psychosocial Health Concerns.

NARCOTIC ANALGESIC. Should be avoided.

Lifestyle/Diet. The cornerstone of treatment is promotion of adequate rest and appropriate exercise. Advise client to avoid caffeine and alcohol before bedtime. Encourage her to start a daily program of low impact aerobic and stretching exercises. Examples include water exercises, stationary cycling, cross country skiing machines. Massage therapy may also be effective. Advise client results do not occur overnight, may take several weeks or months before significant difference is appreciated.

Follow-Up

Regularly scheduled visits during flares are recommended, at 1- to 2-week intervals. During each visit, focus on self-help strategies such as time management to ensure adequate sleep and daily exercise routine. Encourage client to keep diary of activities and symptom occurrence.

GOUT

Gout is first and foremost a disease a disease of abnormal uric acid metabolism. It is characterized by increased production or reduced excretion of uric acid from the blood stream. The excess uric acid is converted to sodium urate crystals that precipitate and become deposited in joints or other tissue.

There are four stages of gout: asymptomatic hyperuricemia, acute gouty arthritis, symptom free periods between attacks, and chronic tophaceous gouty arthritis.[15]

Epidemiology

Gout is more common in men than in women. In women, the onset is after menopause. There is primary gout, which is due to an inborn error of metabolism, and secondary gout, which may have a genetic predisposition. It is an acquired hyperuricemia from diuretic use, myeloproliferative disorders, chronic renal disease, hypothyroidism, alcoholism, and psoriasis. Transplant recipients may have decreased renal function and take medication that decreases uric acid excretion (especially cyclosporine). They are at high risk of developing gout.

Subjective Data

In the first stage of gout, the client will be asymptomatic. Hyperuricemia is detected during routine blood and urine screening.

In the acute attack, the client will complain of sudden onset of severe monarticular pain with swelling and erythema. She may report a low grade fever and malaise. The joints most commonly affected are the first metatarsophalangeal joint, the ankle, the elbow, and the knee. The attack may have followed an episode of excessive alcohol intake, high purine diet, initiation of diuretic therapy for hypertension, renal dysfunction, surgery, or infection. Typically the initial attack is followed by a period of remission of months to years.

If the client reports a history of gout, she may present with polyarticular symptoms that may be indistinguishable from rheumatoid arthritis.

Be sure to include thorough sexual history, illicit drug use, surgical history (especially joint replacement), and risk of immunocompromise.

Objective Data

Physical Examination

- *General appearance.* Typically, the initial attack is monoarticular and affects the great toe (podagra).
- *Inspection.* The affected joint will be quite swollen and perhaps dusky red.
- *Palpation.* Joint is warm or even hot to touch and exquisitely tender. The client may not be able to tolerate anything touching the site, such as sheets, socks or other articles of clothing.

    Tophi, nodular deposits of monosodium urate monohydrate crystals, may be found on the helix of the ear, the ulnar aspect of the forearm, Achilles tendon, and olecranon bursa.
- *Range of motion.* It may not be possible to move the joint through its range of motion due to pain.

Diagnostic Tests

ARTHROCENTESIS. Diagnosis is confirmed by aspiration of the joint and microscopic inspection for crystals. If a reliable history of recurrent gouty attacks is given, it may not be necessary to tap the joint.

SERUM URIC ACID LEVEL, CBC, ESR. May be drawn, but these tests do not confirm diagnosis. Serum uric acid is almost always elevated > 6.0 mg/dl in women.

X-RAYS. Generally not indicated for the acute attack but in later disease may show punched out areas in the bone due to radiolucent urate tophi.

Differential Medical Diagnoses

Cellulitis (client able to move joint through range of motion, pain is superficial), septic joint (differentiated by arthrocentesis), pseudogout (crystals in aspirate are calcium pyrophosphate, uric acid level is normal), rheumatoid arthritis (differentiated by aspirate).[16]

Plan

Psychosocial Interventions. If the client has a high alcohol intake, advise her that alcohol may precipitate gouty attacks and should be used with caution. If she is unable to control her intake, refer for substance abuse counseling. The transplant recipient who develops gout as a result of her medication may be coping with anger and despair.

Medication. Pharmacological intervention is based on stage of illness.

Asymptomatic Hyperuricemia. Asymptomatic hyperuricemia requires no medication. See following for diet and lifestyle management. If client is taking diuretic, it may contribute to hyperuricemia.

Acute Gout. The acute attack is treated with an *NSAID,* often indomethacin 25–50 mg TID continued until the attack resolves (5–10 days). In clients unable to take NSAIDs (e.g., transplant recipients) intraarticular injection of triamcinolone 10–40 mg (depending on the size of the joint) is effective and provides relief in 6–12 hours. Joint aspiration is required, however, to rule out the septic joint.

COLCHICINE. May also be used in the acute attack, but it has fallen out of favor due to the high incidence (80 percent) of significant and often serious gastrointestinal symptoms, such as nausea, vomiting, diarrhea, and abdominal cramping. It is most effective if taken early in the attack (first few hours).

- *Administration.* 0.5–0.6 mg po every hour until pain is relieved or until nausea or diarrhea. Not to exceed 8 mg total dose. See following for discussion of colchicine.

Chronic Gout. Repeated attacks are treated with *colchicine* 0.6 mg BID. Specific indications are mild hyperuricemia and frequent attacks.[15]

- Exact mechanism of action of colchicine is unknown but may involve leukocyte migration and reduction of lactic acid produced by leukocytes, resulting in decreased deposition of uric acid.

- *Adverse Effects.* Vomiting, diarrhea, abdominal pain, nephrotoxicity, myopathy, confusion, peripheral neuritis, bone marrow depression.
- *Contraindications.* Serious renal, hepatic, and cardiac disease. Also those with blood dyscrasias or inflammatory bowel disease.
- *Expected Outcome.* Suppression of acute attacks.
- *Client Teaching.* Advise client to report any adverse effects, e.g., dysphagia (sore throat), rash, unusual bleeding, weakness, numbness.

URIC ACID LOWERING AGENT. Uric acid lowering agent such as *allopurinol* may be indicated if serum uric acid levels remain high (8.5–9.0 mg/dl) after diet modification and alcohol avoidance. Monitor CBC, serum uric acid levels, hepatic and renal function at onset of treatment and periodically thereafter.

- *Dosage* is 100–300 mg orally per day.
- *Mechanism of Action.* Allopurinol is a xanthine oxidase inhibitor that reduces uric acid production.
- *Adverse Effects.* Headache, sleepiness, rash, Stevens-Johnson syndrome, nausea, vomiting, diarrhea, metallic taste, agranulocytosis, anemia, bone marrow depression, elevated liver enzymes.
- *Contraindications.* Known hypersensitivity, hemochromatosis. Use with caution in pregnancy, breast-feeding, renal impairment, bone marrow depression.
- *Client Teaching.* Advise client to discontinue medication immediately at first sign of rash (occurs most often in those taking diuretics or those with renal impairment). Advise client to drink 10–12 glasses of water per day to maintain urine output.

TRIAMCINOLONE. If client is unable to take NSAIDs, steroid injection of triamcinolone 10–40 mg, depending on the size of the joint, may provide relief. Before injection, joint aspiration for gram stain and microscopic examination for crystals should be done to rule out sepsis (see further discussion under bursitis).

PREDNISONE. Oral prednisone 40–60 mg/day, tapered over a week, if several joints are affected (see previous discussion under asthma for information on steroid taper).

Diet/Lifestyle. The obese client should be advised on weight loss. Stress the importance of avoiding liquid fad diets or fasts. Hyperuricemia is associated with obesity and hyperlipidemia. Dietary sources of purines do not cause gouty attacks, but a low cholesterol diet is important in maintaining health. A high liquid intake is important to aid urate excretion and minimize formation of urate stones in the kidney. Bed rest is important in the acute attack. Cold compresses and elevation of the extremity may increase comfort.

Follow-Up

Evaluate the client in 7–10 days. After the initial attack if a second attack occurs within 6 months, refer to a rheumatologist.

OSTEOARTHRITIS

Osteoarthritis, or degenerative joint disease, usually becomes symptomatic at age 40–50 years old. The onset is insidious, the changes in joints slowly progressive. It begins with joint space narrowing followed by osteophyte formation. Virtually all individuals over the age of 70 are affected.

Epidemiology

The 1984 National Health and Nutrition Examination Survey (NHANES) showed that 12.1 percent of the population aged 25 years to 74 years have arthritis. It is the most common cause of limitation of activities, surpassing heart disease, cancer, and diabetes. The client with arthritis will visit her primary care provider an average of four times a year for this problem. Both men and women are affected equally, with onset earlier in men. The knee is the most common joint affected in women, especially obese women.[17,18]

Subjective Data

Important areas to cover in the symptom history include onset, nature and duration of the pain. Be sure to include issues of lifestyle, obesity, and/or occupational factors that may contribute to the condition.

The client complains of increased pain with use. Although she may find pain is more severe in the knee or the hip, the hands and feet are the most common sites of early arthritic changes. She may also note morning stiffness. This usually lasts fewer than 30 minutes. Going up or down stairs, bending, or kneeling may have become increasingly difficult. A family history of arthritis or a previous injury to the affected joint may exist. Ask her about former or current activities, such as jogging, weight or fitness training, or dancing.

Objective Data

Physical Examination. The physical exam focuses on the affected joint(s).

GAIT. Observe the client's gait for antalgia.

Inspect for erythema, deformity, muscle atrophy, or swelling.

Palpate the joint for warmth, swelling, tenderness. *Inflammation* manifested by warmth, swelling, or effusion requires further evaluation to rule out infection, inflammatory processes such as rheumatoid arthritis or gout, or autoimmune disease (see following Differential Medical Diagnoses).

RANGE OF MOTION. Move the joint through its active and passive range of motion, noting limitation, crepitus, and client's expression of pain.

Diagnostic Tests. The most important question to answer before ordering a specific test or an x-ray is whether the outcome of the test will alter the plan of care or the prognosis of the client. If the pain is recent in onset (i.e., within last few weeks) and the joint does not appear inflamed or unstable, no further diagnostic tests are indicated.

RADIOGRAPHIC EVALUATION. Indicated if the pain has persisted despite conservative management, if trauma preceded the pain, or the joint appears unstable.

LABORATORY TESTS. Erythrocyte sedimentation rate (ESR), antinuclear antibody titer (ANA), serum uric acid, and/or rheumatoid factor should be drawn if a high suspicion of rheumatoid arthritis, gout, or systemic lupus erythematosus is raised. These tests should not be used to screen because of their low specificity.

Arthrocentesis. Fluid aspirate must be tested to rule out infection if the joint is warm, an effusion is present, and the client reports a history of fever, recent unprotected sex, or sexually transmitted disease.

Differential Medical Diagnoses

See Table 22–2.

Diagnosis is usually based on physical exam, lack of systemic or constitutional symptoms such as malaise or fever, and minimal joint inflammation.

TABLE 22–2. COMPARISON OF OSTEOARTHRITIS AND RHEUMATOID ARTHRITIS

	Osteoarthritis	Rheumatoid Arthritis
Onset	Age 50–55 years old (men often earlier)	Age 20–60 yrs old
M/F ratio	Men = Women	Women two to three times more than men
Constitutional symptoms	Absent	Present
Joints affected	Hips, knees, spine, DIP, PIP, MTP	Wrists, MCP, PIP, MTP
Pattern	Asymmetrical, often monoarticular in weightbearing joints	Symmetrical, often polyarticular
Other signs	Crepitus Heberden's nodes on dorsum of DIP Osteophyte formation and joint space narrowing on x-ray	Swelling, warmth, tenderness Deformities such as swan's neck and boutonniere of fingers Rheumatoid nodules on bony prominence especially elbows
Laboratory tests	None indicated	Elevated sedimentation rate +Rheumatoid factor

Key: DIP = Distal interphalangeal joint; PIP = Proximal interphalangeal joint; MTP = Metatarsophalangeal joint; MCP = Metacarpophalangeal joint.
Source: References 17, 18, 22.

Rheumatoid arthritis presents with the warm spongy joint enlargement of synovitis as opposed to the bony hard and cool enlargement in osteoarthritis.

Systemic lupus erythematosus usually features discoid skin lesions or malar rash and complaints of extreme fatigue, anorexia, and weight loss.

Gout has an acute onset usually with monarticular involvement, especially the first metatarsophalangeal joint.

Other bone diseases. Always be alert to the possibility that pain, especially back pain, may be due to other bone diseases such as osteoporosis, metastatic neoplasia, or multiple myeloma. Suspicion is raised by history and lack of response to conservative therapy.

Plan

Psychosocial Interventions. A diagnosis of arthritis for a woman in her 30s or 40s is distressing in view of the chronicity and progressive character of the disease process. Reassure her that with pharmacological management of her pain and with promotion of overall fitness and control of body weight, arthritis need not significantly alter her lifestyle.

Medication. Analgesics such as acetaminophen and nonsteroidal anti-inflammatory drugs are the cornerstones of pain management.

ACETAMINOPHEN. 325 mg–650 mg p.o. every 4 hours not to exceed 4 grams per day for 1 month or 2.6 grams daily for long-term use.

- *Adverse Effects.* Usually mild but may include nausea, abdominal pain, mental changes, difficulty in urination, rash.

  Contraindicated with known allergy to medication, active liver or kidney disease.
- *Client Teaching.* Advise that many OTC medications contain acetaminophen. Include the amounts in calculation of daily dose. Warn of risk of liver damage if history of heavy or binge drinking, liver disease.

  NOTE: Acetaminophen does not have anti-inflammatory properties. Several studies have shown, however, that it may be as effective as an NSAID in relieving pain of osteoarthritis.[19]

NONSTEROIDAL ANTI-INFLAMMATORY DRUGS. See Table 22–1 for dosage and comments.

- *Adverse Effects.* Predominantly GI distress, GI bleeding, peptic ulcer formation. Also headache, peripheral edema, tinnitus, prolonged bleeding time, bronchospasm.
- *Contraindications.* Known sensitivity or allergy to NSAID or aspirin. Active GI, liver disease or kidney disease, diabetes with renal insufficiency, asthmatics who experience bronchospasm with aspirin or NSAID.
- *Client Teaching.* Advise client she may take acetaminophen 325–650 mg p.o. in intervals between NSAID dosages (if 8–24 hours) to manage acute flare-ups. Always advise to take with food, to stop medication if GI distress. If client on antihypertensive agent, NSAID may lower its effectiveness. May potentiate anticoagulants, hypoglycemic effects of insulin and oral hypoglycemics.

  NOTE: The lowest effective dose of NSAID should be prescribed to minimize GI toxicity. Also select an agent that has a low incidence of adverse GI effects. In individuals at high risk for development of ulcers and for whom NSAIDs are the agent of choice, misoprostol (a prostaglandin E analogue) 0.1 mg–0.2 mg four times a day reduces the frequency of gastropathy by stimulating mucus and bicarbonate secretion, enhancing mucosal blood flow, and inhibiting acid se-cretion. Misoprostol is contraindicated in pregnancy.[18]

  Intra-articular injection of steroids is usually not indicated unless there is an associated synovitis caused by accumulation of intra-articular debris, evidence of tendinitis, or trochanteric bursitis. Steroid injection is difficult and should be attempted only by the skilled practitioner after consultation with physician and appropriate radiologic studies.

Diet/Lifestyle. The Framingham Knee Osteoarthritis study found that weight loss significantly decreased the risk of symptomatic knee osteoarthritis in women.[20] Osteoarthritis develops in the weight-bearing joints, and decreasing the stress on these joints can delay disease progression. Therefore, if the client is obese, advise her a sensible weight loss program will be of great benefit.

Recent studies have also shown that walking 1 mile four to seven times per week significantly decreased lower body disability, especially in

African Americans.[21] Specific exercises that strengthen supporting muscles such as the quadriceps are beneficial. Clients can be shown how to do these exercises while sitting down. Non-weightbearing exercises such as swimming and stretching promote and maintain flexibility. Canes and walkers can reduce joint load and improve mobility in those with advanced disease. Client teaching on proper body mechanics in the use of assistive devices is required. Referral to a physical or occupational therapist may be indicated, especially if limitations in activities of daily living are noted. This service is often covered by insurance.

Alternating heat for 15 minutes followed by ice for 15 minutes may relieve pain and muscle spasm. Advise client with co-existing diabetes or peripheral vascular disease not to exceed exposure times. Various over-the-counter heat generating creams such as capsaicin cream (Zostrix) are also available. Advise client it may be helpful to use cream, apply ice, or take medication before aggravating activity such as shopping or housework.

Follow-Up

Follow-up at 1 to 2 weeks for evaluation of therapy and any adverse effects of medications. If high risk for GI bleed, obtain baseline CBC. Monitor renal function, liver function and CBCs at 3-month intervals if on daily medication. Refer to orthopedic surgeon if pain is intolerable with medication or if significant loss of movement and disability.

RHEUMATOID ARTHRITIS

Rheumatoid arthritis (RA) is a chronic inflammatory disease of the joints affecting the synovial membrane and tendon sheath. There is no known cause. Although RA has systemic manifestations, the hallmark of the disease is synovitis of the peripheral joints in a symmetric distribution. This usually results in cartilage destruction, erosion of the bone, and joint deformities. The course is unpredictable. Some individuals have mild disease with little joint damage, while others experience crippling disease and nerve compression syndromes.

Epidemiology

In a survey of British patients, where 24 percent complained of joint pain, 1 percent had rheumatoid arthritis.[17] Women are more commonly affected than are men. The disease usually develops between the ages of 35 years old to 50 years old. There is often a positive family history.

Subjective Data

The client commonly reports a prodrome of extreme fatigue, anorexia, weight loss, weakness, and mild musculoskeletal pain. She may have a history of low grade fever. Inflammatory changes of swelling and erythema in several joints such as the hands, wrists, and knees appear in a symmetric pattern. These changes may emerge gradually over a period of weeks or months. In a small percentage of patients, the onset is acute and is usually accompanied by fever, lymphadenopathy, and splenomegaly.[22] The defining features of rheumatoid arthritis are morning stiffness lasting more than 1 hour and symmetric peripheral joint swelling and pain.

Objective Data

Physical Examination. Inspection of the affected sites reveals swelling and often erythema. Palpation elicits tenderness, and the joint is warm to touch. Range of motion may be limited due to accumulation of synovial fluid and pain. If disease is in later stages, soft tissue contractures can result in deformities. Examples of these are radial deviation of the wrist with ulnar deviation of the fingers, swan neck and boutonniere deformities of the digits involving the PIP and DIP joints. Deformities can also develop in the feet.

Extraarticular manifestations of disease process include rheumatoid nodules on extensor surfaces, especially the elbow and lower arm, the Achilles tendon and the occiput; muscle atrophy; rheumatoid vasculitis; pleuropulmonary inflammation; scleritis; osteoporosis.

Diagnostic Tests. Results of diagnostic tests may be misleading, and no test is specific for diagnosis. The American Rheumatism Society's revised criteria for diagnosis include morning stiffness, arthritis of three or more joints, arthritis of hand joints, symmetric pattern, rheumatoid nodules, presence of rheumatoid factor, and radiographic changes. Four of the seven criteria must be present for diagnosis.[22]

Two-thirds of clients test positive for rheumatoid factor but 5 percent of the normal population may test positive also.[22] Other disease entities with similar presentation may generate rheumatoid factor, such as systemic lupus erythematosus, sarcoidosis, mononucleosis, hepatitis B. High titers are predictive of more severe disease. Therefore, rheumatoid factor is not useful as a screening test but can confirm diagnosis and identify those at high risk for more severe systemic disease course.

COMPLETE BLOOD COUNT. May reveal a normochromic normocytic anemia. Erythrocyte sedimentation rate is increased in active disease.

RADIOGRAPHIC EVALUATION. Generally not helpful in early disease, but as disease progresses may reveal osteopenia and bony erosions. They may be of value in consideration of drug therapy or surgery.

Differential Medical Diagnoses

Osteoarthritis has minimal joint inflammation, lacks constitutional symptoms, and affects weightbearing joints (see Table 22–2).

Systemic lupus erythematosus has a similar presentation and age of onset and may be differentiated by malar rash or characteristic discoid lesions, positive antinuclear antibody and antibody to double stranded DNA.

Gout is monarticular, more common in men.

Plan

Psychosocial Interventions. Diagnosis of a chronic disease with an unpredictable course is a major life stressor in addition to the pain and fatigue that accompany it. Reassure the client that the goals of therapy include pain management, preservation of function, and control of destructive processes. Be alert for signs of depression that may necessitate referral for counseling. Encourage the client to join a support group. Reassure her that even though you may refer her to a rheumatologist and/or physical therapist, you

will continue to provide primary care and case management.

Medication. First line drugs for early disease are the *nonsteroidal anti-inflammatory agents.* (See Table 22–1 and discussion in the section on osteoarthritis.)

If first line therapy fails, referral to a physician or to a specialist in connective tissue disease is indicated. Disease modifying medications such as gold compounds, antimalarial such as hydroxychloroquine, methotrexate, and sulfasalazine may be prescribed. Consult pharmacology text for further discussion of these medications.[26]

Nonpharmacological Interventions. Include referral to a licensed physical therapist for pain management, physical conditioning, and preservation of function. The therapist can provide a home therapy routine as well as adaptive devices to assist with activities of daily living.[23]

Lifestyle/Diet. Although diet claims for relief and even cure of arthritis abound, there is no scientific basis for these claims. Advise that a sensible diet, which includes a wide variety of foods, and a program of physical conditioning and overall health maintenance assures the best outcome. Encourage adequate rest periods to decrease joint inflammation.

Follow-Up

Once the initial diagnosis is made, follow-up is based on disease progression. All clients should be reevaluated in 1 to 2 weeks for response to therapy. Most clients have a disease pattern of periodic exacerbations with periods of remission. About 15 percent have remission after an initial flare without major deformity developing. Predictors of future disability include age, female sex, radiologic pathology, increased titers of rheumatoid factor.[22]

SYSTEMIC LUPUS ERYTHEMATOSUS

Systemic lupus erythematosus (SLE) is a disorder of unknown etiology that can affect almost any organ system. It is characterized by damage to cells and tissue caused by immune complexes and pathogenic autoantibodies.

Epidemiology

SLE is generally a disease of women in their childbearing years; 90 percent of all cases fall into this category. It is more common in African Americans. The prevalence in the United States is 15 to 50 per 100,000 in urban areas. There appears to be a genetic predisposition.[24]

Subjective Data

The client may present with only a malar or discoid rash or she may complain of generalized joint pain and malaise. Most experience arthralgias, myalgias, and intermittent arthritis as the earliest manifestation. Multiple system involvement may also be indicated by chest pain and nonspecific gastrointestinal complaints (anorexia, weight loss, nausea). Be sure to ask about medication use. Several drugs cause a syndrome resembling lupus, especially procainamide and hydralazine. Other drugs that have been implicated more rarely include isoniazid, chlorpromazine, d-penicillamine, methyldopa, and oral contraceptives. Discontinuation of the offending drug usually resolves clinical symptoms in a few weeks.[24,25]

Objective Data

Vital Signs. Temperature may be slightly elevated.

Physical Examination. If suspicion of SLE is high, a thorough head to toe physical exam is indicated, including weight.

- *Skin.* The rash of SLE is more often malar in a butterfly shape than discoid (as in discoid lupus). It is flat or slightly raised, erythematous, appearing over the cheeks and the bridge of the nose but can extend to the chin, ears, or any sun exposed area. Client may also have aphthous ulcers in the buccal mucosa and vasculitic skin lesions such as purpura, infarcts (splinter hemorrhages) of skin, digits, or nails and leg ulcers. Twenty percent of those with SLE have discoid lupus lesions. (See discussion of discoid lupus in dermatology section.) The client may have patchy alopecia.[24]
- *Eyes.* The eye and retina should be examined for episcleritis, conjunctivitis, swelling of the optic disc, and vascular abnormalities.
- *Heart.* Cardiac involvement is indicated by the presence of a pericardial friction rub, gallop rhythm, or new onset of murmur.
- *Lungs.* Pulmonary manifestations include adventitious lung sounds, pleural rub, and increased respiratory rate.
- *Abdomen.* Palpate the abdomen for tenderness and note any guarding. Clients with SLE are at risk for peritonitis and pancreatitis.
- *Musculoskeletal Exam.* Musculoskeletal manifestations include joint swelling, especially the proximal intraphalangeal (PIP), metacarpophalangeal (MCP) joints of the hands, the wrists, and knees. The client may have only hand and feet puffiness and tenosynovitis.
- *Neurological Exam.* Perform a thorough neurological examination, concentrating on cognitive function, cranial nerves for palsy, and cerebellar dysfunction.

Diagnostic Tests

Urine pregnancy test for all women of childbearing age.

Routine urinalysis to detect proteinurea, hematuria.

Antibody to double stranded DNA (most specific test to detect SLE).

Antinuclear antibody (ANA, most sensitive test to detect SLE). Antinuclear antibody titer may remain positive for years.

Chest x-ray if indicated to detect effusion.

ECG, echocardiogram if indicated to detect pericarditis, endocarditis, valvular abnormality.[25]

Flat plate of the abdomen if ascites, liver enlargement.

Complete blood count to detect anemia.

Serum chemistries to assess renal and hepatic function.

Differential Medical Diagnoses

Rheumatoid arthritis; skin disorders such as urticaria, erythema multiform, rosacea; scleroderma; multiple sclerosis. Always consider drug induced lupus from procainamide, hydralazine, and less frequently isoniazid, chlorpromazide, d-penicillamine, methyldopa, oral contraceptives.

If client is diagnosed with SLE, she is referred to a physician for further management.

She may be followed by a rheumatologist, nephrologist, cardiologist, pulmonologist, or neurologist based upon the stage and manifestation of disease.

Plan

Psychosocial Interventions. SLE is a chronic disease with no known cure. Its course is unpredictable with emissions and flares. The overall survival is about 70 percent over 10 years.[24]

The client will need a high degree of support and empathy from the provider. She may go through denial, anger, despair. If pregnant, she will need information and counseling on how the pregnancy may affect the course of her disease. She may have to consider terminating the pregnancy. Assure her that even though she is seen by various specialists, you are available for support and education.

Medication. Drug therapy based on systemic manifestations of disease.

ANTI-INFLAMMATORY AGENTS. Most clients with mild SLE are treated with nonsteroidal anti-inflammatory drugs and topical corticosteroids for joint pain and skin rashes.

SYSTEMIC STEROIDS. Those with complications of disease such as thrombocytopenic purpura, hemolytic anemia, myocarditis, pericarditis, and nephritis are treated with glucocorticoids. During acute exacerbations, doses may be given every 8–12 hours. When disease is controlled, one morning dose of prednisone or other short-acting glucocorticoid is given and tapered down to the lowest dose that suppresses acute flare.[24,25]

AZOTHIOPRINE. Cytotoxic agents such as azothioprine in cases of lupus nephritis may prevent renal failure, but their use is controversial and may cause serious side effects.

NOTE: See previous discussion of oral steroids and pharmacologic text for further information on above medications.

Experimental Therapy. Newer experimental treatment modalities include plasmapheresis, total lymph node irradiation, intravenous gamma globulin, and cyclosporine.[24]

Diet/Lifestyle. The practitioner can be a very important resource for the client in promoting healthy diet and lifestyle to retard disease progression. Infection and renal disease are the major causes of death in those with SLE. Adequate rest and nutrition, a positive outlook, protection of joints, regular exercise as tolerated, use of sunscreen on skin are key to maintaining optimum health in the presence of illness.

Follow-Up

The practitioner should continue to follow the client for routine health care including an annual well woman exam, mammogram, and treatment of episodic illness.

NEUROLOGICAL DISORDERS

The term *neurological disorders* casts a broader net than one might first suppose, since within its boundaries can be found everything from the common headache to seizures and Parkinsonism. This section encompasses information on headache; fever; dizziness and vertigo; Bell's palsy; two alterations in consciousness—syncope and seizures—and Parkinsonism and essential tremor.

HEADACHE

Headache is one of the most common complaints leading to office and emergency room visits. It accounts for many lost work days and disruptions in family relationships.

In 1988, the Headache Classification Committee of the International Headache Society adopted 13 categories to help clarify the confusing differential diagnosis of headache.[1] This section focuses on the two most common types: tension and migraine.[2] Most experts agree that tension and migraine headaches are on a continuum, with some overlap and shared characteristics and etiologies.

Prior to discussing the common and more benign headaches, it is best to understand less common headache variants and potentially more dangerous headaches requiring referral and further diagnostic testing. Less than 5 percent of headaches fall into a category that has been labeled traction or inflammation.[2]

TABLE 22–3. RED FLAG SYMPTOMS
FOR DANGEROUS HEADACHES

No recognizable benign pattern for headaches

Client description: "Worst headache ever"

Onset of headache with exertion (cough, strain, Valsalva maneuver)

Vomiting without nausea

Personality changes (decreased alertness or cognition)

Any abnormality on physical exam
  Neck not supple, pain with flexion
  Fever
  Focal neurological signs

Seizure(s)

Sudden change in headache pattern especially in those over age 50

Progression of symptoms

Traction and inflammation headaches are precipitated by organic conditions, for example, brain tumors, bleeding, meningitis, and temporal arteritis. Often, no characteristic history indicates the cause, but red flag signs may be present[3] (see Table 22–3).

UNCOMMON HEADACHE VARIANTS

Several uncommon headache variants must be considered in diagnosis: cluster headaches, complex migraines, and headaches caused by pseudotumor cerebri, temporal (giant cell) arteritis, and subarachnoid hemorrhage.

Keep in mind that systemic illnesses can affect headaches and that anxiety about the cause of the headache may magnify or distort the clinical features. Look at the total picture including the possibility of referred pain from sinus infections or dental infections.

Cluster Headaches

Cluster headaches are an uncommon variant type of migraine. Reports show that 90 percent occur among men. Attacks usually begin between ages 20 and 40 and occur in "clusters," usually nightly in 6-week cycles. The pain often begins 1 to 2 hours after falling asleep and wakes the client up. Excruciating pain lasts about 1 hour and is described as "boring" around one eye. Tearing and nasal congestion often occur on the affected side. In contrast to migraine, those affected are restless, often getting out of bed and pacing. Cluster headaches are frequently triggered by alcohol or histamine. Refer the client to a neurologist.[3]

Complex Migraine Headaches

Complex migraines are associated with focal neurological signs, which may continue after the prodrome and into or past the headache phase. They may be confused with stroke. Always refer the client to a neurologist.

An unusual variation in young people is the basilar migraine. The client may complain of vertigo, double vision, numbness and may have an ataxic gait, visual field changes, and changes in level of consciousness.[4]

Pseudotumor Cerebri

Headaches may be caused by pseudotumor cerebri (benign intracranial hypertension). The intracranial hypertension, often of unknown etiology, is most often seen among children or obese young women. It has been associated with use of tetracycline, vitamin A, corticosteroids and oral contraceptives as well as pulmonary disease and endocrine disturbances. A client is in no apparent distress. She may report "mild headache"; papilledema is noted on the physical exam. Partial or complete visual loss may occur if not treated. Refer the client to a neurologist immediately.

Temporal Arteritis

Headaches may also result from temporal (giant cell) arteritis. The arteritis is of unknown etiology and occurs primarily after age 50. Clients may have associated fever, malaise, and muscle aches, especially in the shoulders and hips. Clients usually, although not always, have a headache. Visual symptoms such as diplopia occur among 50 percent. Temporal arteritis is also associated with proximal muscle weakness (polymyalgia rheumatica). Tenderness over the temporal artery and rarely the occipital artery may be elicited. The erythrocyte sedimentation rate is dramatically elevated, often greater than 100 mm per hour. Refer the client to a neurologist immediately. Treatment with steroids is initiated to prevent blindness.

Subarachnoid Hemorrhage

Subarachnoid hemorrhage may be reported as a sudden onset of the "worst headache of my life."

This may be followed by nausea, vomiting, and a decreasing level of consciousness. The hemorrhage is usually secondary to trauma, a ruptured aneurysm or congenital arteriovenous malformation. Subarachnoid hemorrhage is most common between ages 25 and 50. The individual may collapse and lose consciousness. Neck stiffness and neurological signs almost always occur. Refer the client to a neurologist immediately or an emergency room for an emergent CT scan.

TENSION HEADACHES

The pathophysiology of tension headaches is poorly understood. Although once referred to as muscle contraction headaches, current research indicates that muscle contraction is not always present with this type of headache. Stress or tension is almost always involved, but the exact pathophysiology is unknown. Tension headaches can be episodic or chronic daily headaches.

Epidemiology

Studies reveal that tension headaches are the most prevalent of all headache types. They are more common in women than in men and decrease in frequency with age.[3] Episodic tension headaches are the classic stress-related headaches. Chronic daily headaches, on the other hand, are often associated with depression that requires treatment.

Subjective Data

A headache history, taken with interest and concern, is the key to the diagnosis. Patterns should be established (see Table 22–4). Rule out a history of trauma, neurological signs, and concurrent disorders.

Have the client keep a headache diary. She should record the day and time of the headache and surrounding events, such as diet, physical activity, and menstrual cycle. She should note aggravating and relieving factors. Have her record the time and dose of any medication taken, both prescribed and over-the-counter.

When taking a history, it is important to have a client identify different types of headaches, as

TABLE 22–4. HEADACHE SYMPTOM PATTERNS IN HISTORY

Symptom	Migraine Headache	Tension Headache	Traction and Inflammation
Onset	10% have aura; may awake with headache	Gradual; often begin during times of stress	Varied (tumors may have periods of pain remission, but pain returns with increased severity)
Duration	Usually 8–12 hours; range 3 hours to rarely 3 days	Usually 8–12 hours; may last days, weeks, months	Varied, but tumor symptoms progressive
Frequency	Usually one or two per month or fewer with pain free periods; rarely one per week	Wide range (daily to rarely)	Varied
Pain location	Approximately 60% unilateral; may switch side or become bilateral	Approximately 90% bilateral; frontal area, "hat band" area, or back of neck	Often unilateral
Pain quality	Throbbing; moderate to severe	Constant; nagging to severe	Varied
Associated symptoms	Nausea, vomiting photophobia, phonophobia	Varied from mild intolerance to light and noise to nausea and anorexia	Varied (vomiting without nausea, personality change, focal neurological signs)
Triggers	Stress; menses; alcohol; food; "letdown" after stress	Stress	None known (mass lesion headache worse after cough or Valsalva maneuver)
Relieving factors	Rest in dark room; sleep	Relaxation exercise; Tylenol/NSAID[a]	Varied

[a]Nonsteroidal anti-inflammatory drug.

she may easily have more than one. Ask her to describe specific symptoms (see Table 22–4).

Objective Data

Data are based on a complete physical examination and, in some instances, diagnostic tests. Physical examination includes examination of the nervous system and eyes, nose, and throat (see Table 22–5).

Usually no diagnostic tests are indicated for tension headaches. For any patient older than 40 with a new type of headache, order a CBC and erythrocyte sedimentation rate to rule out temporal arteritis.

TABLE 22–5. PHYSICAL EXAM FOR HEADACHE

General appearance: Note affect, photophobia.

Vital signs: Blood pressure and temperature must be charted.
  Blood pressure—Hypertension (HTN) rarely causes headaches; pain with diastolic > 120–140. HTN may aggravate migraine.
  Temperature—Fever, rule out meningitis, arteritis, sinusitis, abscess.

Mental Status: Usually assessed within framework of interview.

Cranial Nerves[a]	Head, Eyes, Ears, and Throat
(If normal, efficient charting states "cranial nerves II–XII intact.")	
I. Olfactory: usually not done	
II. Optic: visual acuity, visual fields by confrontation	Disc flat (rule out papilledema)
III,IV,VI. Oculomotor, trochlear, abducens PERRLA,[b] EOMs, note ptosis of upper lids	
V. Trigeminal Motor—palpate masseter, open and close jaw Sensory—touch forehead, cheek, jaw	Palpate "click" from temporomandibular joint Palpate temporal area (rule out arteritis)
VII. Facial Observe facial symmetry Raise eyebrows, frown Close eyes, resist opening Smile, puff out cheeks	Check tenderness over sinuses (rule out sinusitis)
VIII. Acoustic: hearing watch tick	Look at tympanic membrane
IX,X. Glossopharyngeal, vagus Symmetrical movement soft palate	Check teeth
XI. Spinal accessory Atrophy, shrug upward against hands Turn head against your hands	Check nodes Check neck stiffness Bruits Tender neck muscles
XII. Hypoglossal Tongue movement, fasciculations	

Screening motor and cerebellar function
  Walk: note gait, heel/toe walk
  Hop on one foot, Romberg
  Deep knee bend, check arms pronator drift
  Finger to nose

Screening sensory
  Pain and vibration (tuning fork), hands and feet
  Stereognosis

Reflexes
  Check deep tendon reflexes, Babinski, and other systems if indicated by history

[a]For efficiency, examine cranial nerves and head, eyes, ears, nose, and throat system simultaneously.
[b]PERRLA, pupils equal, round, reactive to light and accommodation; EOM, extraocular movement.

TABLE 22–6. DIFFERENTIAL DIAGNOSES OF HEADACHES

Tension Headache	Vasomotor	Traction and Inflammation Headache
Episodic/chronic	Migraine	Mass lesions (tumors, hematomas, edema)
Temporomandibular joint (TMJ) syndrome	With aura	Head, eye, ear, nose, and throat diseases, such as
Chronic myositis	Without aura	sinusitis, tooth abscess
Cervical osteoarthritis	Complicated	Temporal arteritis
	Perimenstrual headache	Cranial neuralgias
	Cluster	Occlusive vascular disease
	Hypertension	Pseudotumor cerebri
	Fever (toxic vascular)	

Differential Medical Diagnoses

See Table 22–6.

Plan

Psychosocial Interventions. It is crucial to reassure the client that tension-type headaches are usually not associated with any severely negative consequences. A thorough physical exam can greatly decrease the woman's anxiety level. Once reassured, she can better focus on lifestyle changes and stress management techniques that might help to decrease the frequency of headaches.

Medication. Nonsteroidal anti-inflammatory drugs (NSAIDs) are very helpful for tension headaches as well as migraine and perimenstrual headaches. Ibuprofen (Advil, Motrin) is the first choice; naproxen sodium (Naprosyn) is helpful for perimenopausal headaches. Refer to the previous discussion of NSAIDs in section on Musculoskeletal Disorders.

- *Side Effects.* Gastrointestinal distress and bleeding may occur.
- *Contraindications.* Do not administer to those clients with a history of peptic ulcer disease, bleeding disorders, pregnancy, kidney problems, or allergic reactions to NSAIDs.
- *Anticipated Outcome on Evaluation.* Headache is relieved.
- *Client Teaching.* Advise the client that NSAIDs are most effective when taken at onset of pain. Encourage her to break the pain cycle and give adequate amounts of medication. Nar-

cotics should not be given for this diagnosis, as clients may become physically dependent and experience withdrawal and rebound headaches.

NOTE: Chronic daily headaches are often drug-rebound headaches caused by overuse of analgesics, especially narcotics, acetaminophen, and ibuprofen. Anyone taking these medications more than four times a week is at risk.

Lifestyle/Dietary Changes. The client may require support in evaluating current life situation and stressors. Help her to prioritize activities and to let go of unnecessary tasks and difficulties. Teach general stress management principles and coping mechanisms. Refer the client for counseling if indicated.

Dietary changes are not applicable unless over- or undereating is a source of tension or stress.

Exercise or other physical activity is an effective stress reducer. Encourage and support lifestyle changes that incorporate 30 minutes of aerobic exercise 3 to 5 days a week.

Follow-Up

Plan a follow-up visit 2 weeks after the initial visit to support and reassess the client. If headaches have not significantly improved or if the client has experienced any new symptoms, such as those listed in Table 22–4, refer her to a neurologist. Keep in mind that most depressed clients will present for care with a physical complaint and that headache is one of the most common complaints.[5]

MIGRAINE HEADACHES

Migraine headaches are recurrent episodic accompanied by nausea and/or vomiting and photophobia. According to the IHS classification at least two of the following features must also be present: unilateral location, pulsating quality, moderate to severe intensity, and aggravated by physical activity.[1]

The pathogenesis of migraine is thought to be composed of three phases. The first phase begins in the brainstem. The second phase involves vasomotor activation (constriction and dilatation) of arteries both inside and outside the brain. The third phase starts with activation of the brain's head and face pain processing center and the subsequent release of neuropeptides. Pain can be generated during any one of these phases. Most studies of the etiology of migraine pain now focus on disturbances in serotonergic mechanisms as the primary cause.[4,6]

In migraines with an aura, previously called "classic migraines," focal neurological symptoms usually precede the headache and may last up to about 20 minutes. Auras are often visual; they may include visual field deficits, a scintillating scotoma (a luminous patch with irregular outline in the visual field), or a fortification spectrum (a dark patch with zig-zag outline). Other neurological auras, such as aphasia and hemiplegia, occur occasionally. When the aura fades, the headache usually begins.

Migraines without an aura, previously called "common migraines," have the features of classic migraines, such as throbbing pain, nausea, vomiting, photophobia, and phonophobia, but no aura.[7]

Perimenstrual headaches occur either 2 to 3 days before onset of menses or during the first days of flow. They are frequently severe, usually without aura, and accompanied by nausea and vomiting. It is hypothesized that they are related to fluctuations in estrogen and serotonin levels. Many women consider them as part of premenstrual syndrome (PMS) and may fail to report them.[3]

Epidemiology

The overall incidence of migraine is about 10 percent of the population. There is usually a strong positive family history. It is more common in women than in men by a ratio of 3:1. Onset is often in childhood, usually at the time of puberty, generally decreases in frequency after menopause. Pregnancy may relieve or intensify migraine.[3,4] The use of oral contraceptives may be a risk factor for more frequent, more intense migraines; on the other hand, oral contraceptives may make migraines better. Women with neurological symptoms accompanying the headache (other than visual aura) should not take oral contraceptives. Those on hormone replacement with estrogen who report new onset of migraine or an increase in incidence may need an adjustment in dosage or a change from conjugated to pure estrogen.[3]

Subjective Data

Obtaining a complete history is essential (see Table 22–4). The history is used to differentiate between migraines and tension headaches because their treatments differ. The criteria for migraine without an aura include a recurring idiopathic headache with at least two of the following: nausea (with or without vomiting), unilateral pain, throbbing, photophobia or phonophobia, association with menstrual cycle, positive family history.

Objective Data

A physical examination is done (see Table 22–5). For recurrent migraines, no diagnostic workup is necessary. For an initial diagnosis, a CBC and chemistries may be helpful. Anemia, electrolyte imbalance, and increased calcium can aggravate migraines.

Differential Medical Diagnoses

See Table 22–6.

Plan

Psychosocial Interventions. Psychosocial intervention is critical, especially for a client who has migraines with an aura, as these can be very frightening. Reassure the client that she is not having a stroke and involve her as an active participant in measures to prevent and abort attacks.

Medication. See Table 22–7.

Lifestyle/Dietary Changes. Focus primarily on what triggers the migraine. Often there is a "let-down" trigger; for example, the headache starts Saturday morning following a stressful week. Counsel the client to readjust her lifestyle and help her with stress management.

Diet may be a factor in the occurrence of migraines. The most common triggers are chocolate, alcohol, and aged cheeses (see Table 22–8). Ask the client to keep a diary of foods eaten and to avoid foods associated with the onset of migraine. Encourage her to eat at regularly scheduled intervals; a drop in blood sugar level may trigger a headache.

Advise the client that physical activity, including aerobic exercise for 30 minutes three to five times a week, helps to reduce stress.

Follow-Up

Teach the client the warning signs of headaches with serious underlying causes (see Table 22–3). If such a warning sign occurs, refer her to a neurologist immediately. Otherwise, arrange to see the client about every 4 to 6 weeks until the migraines improve. If no improvement is seen in 8 weeks or the migraines worsen, refer her to a neurologist.

FEVER

Body temperature is regulated between 97–99 degrees Fahrenheit (36–37.2 degrees Centigrade). When heat production exceeds heat dissipation, for example during vigorous exercise, the core body temperature may rise above this range until regulatory mechanisms such as sweating, hyperventilation, and vasodilatation promote heat loss and return the body temperature to normal. A sustained elevation of body temperature is called fever and represents a regulated rise to a new set point.[11] Fever of unknown origin (FUO) is a temperature greater than 101° F (38.2° C) that occurs on several occasions during a 3-week period in a person whose diagnosis is not apparent after 1 week or more of study.[12] It should be noted that in the vast majority of occurrences the diagnosis is either readily apparent after a history and physical exam or becomes evident within a few days.

TABLE 22–7. OVERVIEW OF MEDICATIONS FOR MIGRAINES[a]

Abortive Measures: Appropriate for clients experiencing occasional headaches, not more than one a month.

NSAIDs[b]: Very effective, especially if taken early because they block the sterile inflammation of migraines. Any NSAID may be tried. Naproxen sodium (Naproxyn, 550 mg p.o. b.i.d.) helpful for women suffering with perimenstrual vascular headaches.

Antiemetics: Oral or per rectum. Prochlorperazine (Compazine) suppositories are an example. Help nausea and aid client in "sleeping off" the headache.

Ergots: Potent vasoconstrictors. May be given intramuscularly, orally, sublingually, by inhalation, or rectally. Most helpful if client has "aura" and can take immediately. Example: Ergotamine tartrate SL (Ergostat) 2 mg at onset and 1 mg every 30 minutes until headache is relieved or to a maximum of 6 mg per day, 12 mg per week.

A widely recognized, effective treatment for acute migraine is dihydroergotamine mesylate (D.H.E. 45 injection) given 1 mg IM. Give antiemetic first or concurrently.

Caution. Be familiar with doses of medications used. Overuse can lead to "ergotism" (prolonged vasoconstriction that can cause tissue ischemia and gangrene). Beta blockers increase the risk for ergotism; simultaneous use is contraindicated.

Serotonin agonist: Sumatriptan (Imitrex) 6mg subcutaneously or 100 mg orally. May repeat dose in 1 hour if headache not relieved or if it recurs. Maximum dose is 12 mg s.q. or 300 mg p.o. in 24 hours.

Caution. Not to be used within 24 hours of an ergot preparation. First dose should be given under observation by health care provider due to adverse effects of general feelings of heaviness and sensation of chest tightness and pressure. Should not be given to those with coronary artery disease or at high risk of unrecognized cardiovascular disease, e.g., postmenopausal women, women with hypertension, obesity, diabetes, strong family history, or smokers.

Preventive Measures: Indicated for three or more attacks per month or one prolonged attack per month. Give adequate trial of 3–6 months of therapy.

Beta blockers: Numerous types (propranolol, long-acting preparation increases compliance). Effective in 50 percent of cases.

Caution. Contraindicated with such conditions as asthma and congestive heart failure.

Tricyclics: Numerous types (amitriptyline [Elavil] often used, starting with a 25-mg dose at bedtime, increasing as necessary).

NSAIDs: Ibuprofen, naproxen sodium, aspirin. Observe for gastrointestinal side effects.

Calcium channel blockers: Numerous types (verapamil [Calan, Isoptin] p.o. 240–360 mg per day). Usually ordered by neurologist.

Methylsergide (Sansert): **Last choice.** Ordered only by a neurologist. Can cause fibrosis of heart valves and peritoneum if given longer than 6 months.

[a]Please consult a current pharmacotherapeutics text for details.
[b]Nonsteroidal anti-inflammatory drugs.
Source: References 7, 8, 9, 10.

TABLE 22–8. DIETARY FACTORS AND MIGRAINE HEADACHES

Direct Vasoactive Substances	Indirect Triggers
Tyramine	Caffeine withdrawal
Aged cheeses	Nicotine
Pickled foods	Hypoglycemia
Fresh baked bread	Ice cream
Marinated foods	Medications
Red wines	Griseofulvin
Nitrates (cured meats)	Trimethoprim
Aspartame	Indomethacin
Avocados	Nifedipine
Bananas	Ergotamines
Nuts	Nitroglycerin preparations
Chocolate	Hormones
Monosodium glutamate (MSG)	H-2 receptor antagonists, e.g., cimetidine, ranitidine
Alcohol	Monoamine oxidase inhibitors

Epidemiology

The febrile response in children is greater than in adults; in the elderly it may be absent even in bacterial illnesses.

The setting in which the fever occurs is also important. Acute fever in a traveler to southeast Asia or Africa may be due to malaria or an insect borne virus. A college student with fever is likely to have a viral infection or mononucleosis. An elderly person recently hospitalized may have urinary tract infection (UTI), pneumonia, phlebitis, or wound infection. Someone with an immune disorder may have an infection caused by an opportunistic agent.[11]

Subjective Data

A symptom history may suggest the cause of fever, especially upper respiratory congestion, myalgias, gastrointestinal upset, ear pain, cough, painful or frequent urination, or rash.

In the absence of these symptoms, inquire about recent use of major tranquilizers such as haloperidol and fluphenazine or antibiotic use. Neuroleptic malignant syndrome is a rare but potentially life threatening reaction to these drugs. Serum sickness may follow antibiotic treatment and is usually accompanied by rash and arthralgias. Also inquire about illicit drug use, possible occupational exposures to infected animals or chemicals.

Elderly patients may report no other symptom than fever but suspect tuberculosis (TB), occult neoplasm, or urinary tract infection.

Objective Data

Physical Examination. A thorough head to toe exam of all organ systems is necessary if the etiology of the fever is not elicited by the history. If the fever is high (greater than or equal to 102° F or 39° C) with few systemic complaints, look for a bacterial infection of the chest, throat, or abdomen. If there is a low grade fever (less than or equal to 101.5° F or 38.6° C) associated with systemic complaints and few focal findings, think virus.

Do not neglect the dental exam. Abscessed devitalized teeth may cause fever without pain.

Fever after an upper respiratory infection suggests sinusitis. Shaking chills suggest pyelonephritis or pneumonia.

Diagnostic Tests. Laboratory studies are indicated by the results of the history and physical. These may include *complete blood count with differential, urinalysis; monospot* (detects mononucleosis); *erythrocyte sedimentation rate* (elevated in inflammatory condition such as rheumatoid arthritis, inflammatory bowel disease); *liver function tests* (elevated in hepatitis); *antistreptolysin; titers* (elevated in recent streptococcal infection); *Lyme titer;* and *cultures* of blood, stool, urine, and throat.

Radiographic Studies. A chest x-ray or flat plate of the abdomen may also be useful.

If endocarditis is suspected, order an *ECG* (electrocardiogram) and possibly an *echocardiogram* if valvular involvement is likely.

Tuberculosis skin test with controls should be placed when appropriate and especially if no obvious etiology is found.

Human immunodeficiency virus (HIV) test is indicated if high risk behaviors elicited by history.

Differential Medical Diagnoses

See Table 22–9.

TABLE 22–9. DIFFERENTIAL DIAGNOSIS OF FEVER

Etiology	Symptoms and Associated Factors	Physical Findings
Upper Respiratory Infection:		
Viral	Mild fever Temp 101.5° F (38.6° C) Sore throat, rhinitis, ear fullness Systemic symptoms	Cough, oropharynx injected (no exudate)
Bacterial	High fever—Temp 102° F (39° C) More common in children Pronounced localized symptoms	Tonsillar exudate Bulging tympanic membrane
Other Viral Syndromes (influenza gastroenteritis)	Mild fever Muscle aches, nausea, vomiting, diarrhea	Minimal physical findings
Drug Reaction	Often high fever Occasionally rash Use of OTC or prescription drug	Fever abates when drug stopped

Urinary Tract Infection	Often high fever and chills, backache, urinary frequency and
	  urgency
	Often hematuria
		Costovertebral angle and suprapubic
		  tenderness

Chronic Hepatitis	Intravenous drug use Low grade fever Fatigue, anorexia	Right upper quadrant tenderness Hepatomegaly Jaundice
Tuberculosis	Low grade fever Weight loss Night sweats May have been incarcerated	Chest findings, + skin test for purified protein derivative (PPD)
Infectious Mononucleosis	Young adult Low grade fever Fatigue	Pharyngitis Adenopathy Splenomegaly

Chronic Fatigue Syndrome	Debilitating fatigue lasting more than 6 months
	Mild recurrent or persistent low grade fever for 6 months
	Sore throat, muscle weakness, myalgia, migratory arthralgia
	  without swelling or redness
	Neuropsychologic complaints
		Nonexudative pharyngitis
		Posterior or anterior cervical adenopathy
		  2 cm or more
		Low grade fever on 2 separate occasions

Note: For a diagnosis of chronic fatigue syndrome, the 1988 CDC guidelines require that all other clinical conditions that produce these symptoms must be excluded.[28]
Other occult infections, inflammatory conditions, and causes of low grade fever of unknown origin in adults include the following: sinusitis, dental abscess, diverticulitis, subacute bacterial endocarditis, osteomyelitis, inflammatory bowel disease, lymphoma, carcinoma, connective tissue disorder, pulmonary emboli, and hepatobiliary disease.
Source: References 11, 12, 14, 26.

Plan

Psychosocial Interventions. Reassure the client that you will continue to follow her closely and inform her of all test results. Answer all questions as fully and candidly as possible and provide an office telephone number.

Medication. Antipyretics such as acetaminophen or ibuprofen may be taken for comfort and are best given on a regular schedule every 6 hours as opposed to as needed. The etiology of the fever will guide the prescription of other medications.

Lifestyle/Diet Changes. Tepid water baths and plenty of fluids (at least 8 ounces of water or juice every hour while awake) will promote comfort and prevent dehydration. Ask client to keep temperature diary by checking body temperature at least three times a day before taking antipyretic medications.

Follow-Up

Telephone follow-up within 2 to 3 days. Schedule appointment in 1 week to review findings and assess response to any medications prescribed. If no obvious cause is found after completion of initial diagnostic testing, consult with physician.

DIZZINESS/VERTIGO

Dizziness is a sensation of disequilibrium or altered orientation in relation to one's surroundings. Dizziness as lightheadedness must be distinguished from vertigo. Dizziness may be a sensation of generalized weakness (presyncopal lightheadedness) or an inability to maintain balance (disequilibrium). Vertigo is a hallucination of movement. With objective vertigo, the client has the sensation of the room spinning; with subjective vertigo, she has the feeling of her own body spinning when the eyes are closed.[13,14]

Epidemiology

Dizziness as a chief complaint accounts for over 7.8 million office visits per year. Up to one-third are diagnosed as vestibular in origin, one-fifth are attributed to hyperventilation, and the remainder to neurologic, psychiatric, and cardiovascular etiologies. It is a frequent complaint of the elderly and may be a predictor of risk for falling, morbidity, and/or functional decline.[15]

The key to differentiating self-limiting versus more serious causes of dizziness is to obtain a thorough history and perform a careful examination.

Subjective Data

The client may have difficulty clarifying what she means by "feeling dizzy." Important questions include the following: Are you spinning? Is the room spinning? Is the dizziness most noticeable when you first stand, sit up, or turn your head? Did the dizziness start suddenly or has it gone on for awhile? How long does the feeling last? What makes the dizziness decrease? What kind of medicines are you taking and for how long?

Significant associated symptoms will assist in the correct diagnosis, especially nausea, tinnitus, ear fullness, one-sided weakness, double vision, facial numbness, numbness or tingling of the extremities. It is also important to ask if the dizziness has been followed by loss of consciousness or seizure activity. If pregnancy is a possibility, a sexual history and evaluation of contraceptive measures are needed.

Objective Data

Physical Examination
- *Vital signs.* Postural blood pressure readings.
- *Head and neck.* Auscultate for carotid bruit. Examine ear canal and tympanic membrane. Test hearing acuity with 512 Hz tuning fork.
- *Full neurological exam,* including evaluation of the cranial nerves (sensory and motor), assessment of cerebellar function, and sensory/motor function. Observe gait for spasticity, ataxia, antalgia, and foot drop.
- *Specific provocative tests and maneuvers* may also aid in correct diagnosis. Having the client *hyperventilate* for a minute or two may reproduce symptoms if no focal abnormalities are found on exam. The *Dix-Hallpike maneuver* is done on clients with positional vertigo (those whose vertigo disappears at rest). It involves rapid change from the sitting position to lying down with the head turned to one side and the neck extended over the end of the exam table 30–45 degrees. A diagnosis of paroxysmal positional vertigo can be established with any of the following findings:
  - *Subjective vertigo.*
  - *Nystagmus* preceded by a latent period of several seconds after completion of the Dix-Hallpike maneuver. Care should be used in doing this maneuver and should not be performed on frail patients or those with atherosclerotic disease.[15]

Diagnostic Tests

ECG. If a cardiovascular cause of dizziness is suspected, a 12 lead electrocardiogram (ECG) is appropriate to rule out arrhythmias and conduction disorders.

HEAD CT. If focal neurological deficits are found during the physical exam, computed tomography (CT) of the head and/or audiogram may be ordered to rule out hemorrhage or tumor.

Pregnancy test, beta human chorionic gonadotropin (HCG), is ordered as needed for women of reproductive age.

Differential Medical Diagnoses of Dizziness/Lightheadedness and Vertigo

See Table 22–10. Consult with physician if cardiac etiology or if focal neurological findings.

Psychosocial Interventions. If a benign or self-limiting etiology is found, client reassurance is most important. The elderly may need family support with medication use. Emphasize importance of making the home environment safer to

TABLE 22–10. DIFFERENTIAL DIAGNOSES OF DIZZINESS/LIGHTHEADEDNESS AND VERTIGO

Condition	Symptoms	Provocative Factors	Physical Findings
Positional vertigo	Recurrent Not associated with tinnitus or hearing loss Short duration episodes	Positional change (head-turning)	Nystagmus and vertigo a few seconds after provocative position change
Otitis media	Persistent vertigo Earache	Upper Respiratory Infection	Dull or red tympanic membrane
Meniere's syndrome	Sudden onset of vertigo Not precipitated by sudden movement Recurrent Tinnitus Nausea/vomiting Duration: hours to days	Menses Emotional stress	Nystagmus Hearing deficit
Labyrinthitis	Sudden onset of vertigo Lasts hours to days Nausea/vomiting May have hearing loss	May be precipitated by viral infection	Physical exam normal
Acoustic neuroma	Gradual onset Persistent vertigo Chronic unilateral hearing deficit Tinnitus Facial numbness on affected side	None	Hearing loss Palsy or spasm of facial nerve
Brainstem dysfunction (vertebrobasilar insufficiency or tumor)	Elderly with acute onset of vertigo Normal hearing Paresthesia Blurred vision Diplopia Slurred speech	None	Vertical or lateral nystagmus
Dizziness/Lightheadedness Psychogenic	Recurrent Persistent Multiple complaints Not associated with posture	Emotional stress	Normal PE
Hyperventilation syndrome	Recurrent circumoral or digital paresthesia	Emotional stress and anxiety	Symptoms reproduced by hyperventilation
Reactive hypoglycemia	Recurrent. Onset 2–4 hrs. after meals Trembling	Carbohydrate ingestion	Sweating Tachycardia
Orthostatic hypotension	Recurrent giddiness on standing	Erect posture Anti-HTN medications	Drop in blood pressure on standing
Drugs	Persistent lightheadedness without true vertigo	Medication	
Sick sinus syndrome	Recurrent dizziness Syncope palpitations	None	Irregular pulse Bradycardia

Source: Adapted from R. Seller. Differential Diagnosis of Common Complaints (1993). (2d ed). Philadelphia: W. B. Saunders Company.

prevent falls. If referral to a cardiologist, neurologist or ear, nose, throat (ENT) surgeon is indicated, reassure the client that you will be available for her other health needs and as a resource.

Medication. Positional vertigo: Meclizine HCL 25 mg, one p.o. every 6 hours as needed for dizziness.

- *Adverse Effects.* Drowsiness, dry mouth, blurred vision, nausea, constipation, diarrhea.
- *Contraindications.* Known hypersensitivity. Use with caution in elderly due to sensitivity to antihistamine effects; may increase dizziness, cause sedation or hyperexcitability. Use with caution in glaucoma, asthma.
- *Client Teaching.* May potentiate effects of alcohol or other central nervous system (CNS) depressants.

If otitis media is diagnosed, appropriate antibiotics are given (see discussion of otitis media in Respiratory Infections).

Meniere's disease is treated with diuretics, such as hydrochlorothiazide 50–100 mg daily (see previous discussion of diuretics under hypertension) and a low salt diet.

Lifestyle Changes. If vertigo is acute, bedrest and a low salt diet are helpful. Advise the client to use care in movement. Driving may have to be curtailed until the symptoms resolve. Provocative head maneuvers such as the Dix-Hallpike (five repetitions performed twice a day) may habituate the vestibular response of positional vertigo.

Follow-Up

Refer those with labyrinthine, cardiovascular, psychiatric, and neurologic disorders to a physician. Telephone follow-up to assess alleviation of acute symptoms may be warranted. Anyone who is not referred should be seen within 7–10 days.

BELL'S PALSY

Bell's palsy is an idiopathic facial paralysis of the seventh cranial nerve. Its pathogenesis is unknown. There is no evidence to support the theory that it is related to reactivation of the herpes simplex virus.

Epidemiology

The incidence of Bell's palsy is about 1 in 60 or 70 persons over a lifetime. It can occur at any age and is common worldwide. The median age is 40 years old. The incidence appears to increase in pregnancy, especially the third trimester. Ten percent of patients have a recurrence. Hypertension and diabetes are more prevalent among those with Bell's palsy.[16]

Subjective Data

The client may report a sudden onset of pain behind the ear that precedes the paralysis by a day or two. Taste sensation may be diminished or absent. She may also find that her sense of hearing is heightened. She may complain of tearing and inability to close the eye on the affected side. Eating may be difficult.

Objective Data

Physical Examination. The affected side of the face is expressionless with smoothing of forehead wrinkles and flattening of the nasolabial fold. The corner of the mouth sags on the affected side, and the mouth is drawn to the unaffected side. The ipsilateral eyebrow may be raised or lowered. The client will be unable to wink, but on attempt, the eye will rotate upward. There may be a pooling of tears in the lower eyelid. Either side of the face can be affected and the extent of paralysis can range from mild to complete.

A complete neurological exam to determine if other neurological deficits are present is necessary. The ear and surrounding area should also be evaluated.

Differential Medical Diagnoses

Herpes zoster may also produce a facial palsy, but a vesicular eruption is present. Acoustic neuromas can produce palsy, but hearing loss accompanies this disorder. Bilateral palsy, facial weakness that progresses slowly over several weeks and/or persists more than 6 months, focal neurological signs discovered during the physical exam suggest other more serious diagnoses, such as stroke or infarct, tumor, or multiple sclerosis.

Plan

Psychosocial Interventions. Client reassurance of good recovery in several weeks to months is important. Eighty percent have full recovery in a few months.[16] Incomplete paralysis in the first week is the most favorable prognostic sign. Body image may suffer as client waits for resolution.

Medication. Use of steroid taper starting with 60 (4–5 days) mg p.o. daily individual doses over the first 4–5 days and then tapered over the next 7–10 days may be beneficial, but studies supporting this are inconclusive. The placebo effect of giving medication may provide patient support, and steroids may relieve pain if it is present.

Lifestyle/Comfort Measures. Liquid tears may protect the eye from excessive drying, and an eye patch should be worn at night.

Follow-Up

Telephone follow-up is suggested within 2 weeks. The client should return for office evaluation in 6–8 weeks. Consult with physician if residual paralysis.

ALTERATIONS IN CONSCIOUSNESS: SYNCOPE

Syncope is sudden loss of consciousness and postural tone that resolves rapidly and spontaneously. It arises from an interruption in the flow of blood to the brain. If cerebral tissue is deprived of glucose or oxygen for more than 5 seconds, syncope can occur. If the event lasts more than 15 seconds, tonic movements can occur that may resemble seizure activity.[14] The challenge to the provider is to determine if syncope is due to underlying cardiovascular disease or another serious cause.

Epidemiology

Syncope is a relatively common complaint and may account for 3 percent of emergency room visits and up to 6 percent of hospital admissions. Most studies show that in at least 40 percent of individuals with syncope, no cause will be identified.[17] Up to half of all adults will experience a syncopal episode during their lives. In the elderly, the incidence is increased because of decreased blood flow to the brain, a result of the aging process.[18,19]

Subjective Data

A complete history including a detailed account of the syncopal episode, premonitory symptoms, and postsyncopal recover period is crucial to identifying a potential cause. Other factors to note are associated symptoms such as angina, palpitations, nausea, visual changes, numbness in the face or extremities.

Ask if the event was preceded by exertion, heat exhaustion, dehydration or emotional stress. Tachyarrhythmias usually have an abrupt onset with no warning and lead to a fall, which may result in injury. Neurogenic syncope or seizure may be preceded by an aura and followed by confusion, drowsiness, and incontinence. Often the event is not witnessed and details may not be provided.

Ask the client about her medications purchased over-the-counter.

Past medical history may elicit key factors such as history of myocardial infarction or seizure disorder.

Objective Data

Physical Examination. Thorough cardiac and neurologic exams are key.

CARDIOVASCULAR. Blood pressure readings in both arms sitting, supine, and standing must be obtained. The client's blood pressure is measured in both arms 5 minutes after she has stood up from a supine position. A fall of 30 mmHg in the systolic blood pressure is significant for orthostatic hypotension. Important parts of the exams to differentiate cardiac from noncardiac causes include heartrate and rhythm to detect arrhythmia, presence of bruit or murmur, character of peripheral pulses, presence of edema or adventitious lung sounds indicating congestive heart failure.

NEUROLOGICAL. Includes evaluation of gait, presence of nystagmus, assessment of cranial nerves, cerebellar function, mental and/or emotional status.

Diagnostic Tests

12 LEAD ECG. The single most important diagnostic test to differentiate cardiac from noncardiac

causes of syncope is the 12 lead ECG. If the office ECG is normal and a cardiac cause is strongly suspected, ambulatory ECG (Holter monitoring), may be necessary.

ECHOCARDIOGRAM. If a murmur is auscultated and the syncopal event occurred with exertion, an echocardiogram may detect left ventricular outflow tract abnormality.

Carotid dopplers are indicated if a carotid bruit is detected.

Routine blood tests are usually not helpful unless anemia, hypoglycemia, or electrolyte abnormality is strongly suspected.

Head CTs are not helpful in diagnosis unless focal neurological findings are present; likewise electroencephalograms (EEG) are generally not diagnostic.

Differential Medical Diagnoses

Cardiac causes of syncope can be due to obstruction, ischemia, or arrhythmia. Clients with obstructive causes often report syncope with exertion. This occurs when cardiac output is fixed by aortic stenosis or hypertrophic obstructive cardiomyopathy. The latter is the most common cause of sudden death in young athletes.[18] Pulmonary hypertension can also cause exertional syncope.

Bradyarrhythmias from complete heart block or other high grade atrioventricular block can present with syncope unrelated to posture. Sick sinus syndrome (characterized by sinus bradycardia and sinus pause that is preceded by supraventricular tachycardia) is suspected in the client who complains of palpitations just prior to the syncope.

Tachyarrhythmias, especially self-terminating ventricular tachycardia, are common in clients with coronary artery disease and reduced left ventricular function. It can be life threatening if the rhythm converts to ventricular fibrillation. Torsades de Pointes, an arrhythmia associated with prolongation of the QT interval, is a cause of syncope. It may result from certain medications such as antiarrhythmic agents, antidepressants; the interactions of common drugs such as terfenadine with erythromycin; from metabolic abnormalities (hypokalemia, hypomagnesemia, hypocalcemia); and drug use (cocaine, sympathometrics).

Wolf-Parkinson-White syndrome, a supraventricular tachycardia, can be diagnosed by 12 lead ECG.

Ischemic events such as acute angina and infarct can present as syncope. The client may have not have had any preceding chest pain.

Consider cardiac origin of syncope in any client with organic heart disease, especially the elderly and in those with no premonitory symptoms who collapse abruptly.

Cerebrovascular disease causing temporary interruption of blood flow to the vertebral or basilar arteries is detected by neurological exam. Focal findings may include vertigo, cranial nerve abnormalities, and bilateral sensory motor abnormalities.

Noncardiac causes include vasovagal syncope, which is the most common type in healthy young women. It is often preceded by pain, fear, emotional stress. It may be accompanied by tonic clonic movements or muscle twitches and may be mistaken for seizures. Rapid recovery and lack of confusion or drowsiness differentiate it from seizure activity.

Situational syncope is also mediated by autonomic reflex mechanisms. Examples include cough, micturition, and defecation syncope.

Drug related syncope can be caused by diuretics, antihypertensives, antiarrhythmics, cocaine or alcohol.

Clients with frequent syncopal episodes of unknown origin may have underlying psychiatric problems.[14,17,18]

Plan

Consult with physician for further diagnostic workup and referral of any client with cardiac or neurological causes of syncope.

Psychosocial Interventions. Reassurance is offered to the client with noncardiac, nonneurologic syncope. If an underlying psychiatric disorder is suspected, suggest referral for counseling.

Medication. The client who is referred to cardiology or neurology may be placed on a variety of medications, depending on the underlying etiology of the syncope. The practitioner should become familiar with these agents and provide medication teaching if needed. Be especially alert for interactions with other medications the client may be prescribed or take as over-the-counter remedies.

If the cause of the syncope is a result of medications the client was taking at the time of the event, adjustment in dosage or stopping the medication may be necessary.

Lifestyle Changes. If substance abuse is present, advise the client of the consequences of continued abuse and refer to appropriate drug treatment program. Recommend stress reduction measures. In the elderly or frail client who is at risk for recurrence, fall precautions are needed. Some clients may have to stop driving.

Follow-Up

Telephone or office follow-up in 7–10 days is recommended for those not scheduled for further workup. Alert them that recurrent syncope requires further diagnostic testing.

ALTERATIONS IN CONSCIOUSNESS: SEIZURES

A seizure is a paroxysmal, transient change in neurologic function caused by a disturbance in the electrical activity of the brain. Chronic, recurrent seizures are diagnosed as epilepsy. Seizures are classified as simple, complex partial, absence, and generalized tonic-clonic seizures. The seizure may entail a brief lapse of attention or a period of several minutes of loss of consciousness with abnormal movements.[20,21]

Epidemiology

Epilepsy is usually diagnosed between 5 and 20 years of age but can start later in life as a result of trauma or disease. Epilepsy affects about 0.5 percent to 2 percent of the population of the United States.[20]

Subjective Data

First ask the client whether she has ever been diagnosed with a seizure disorder and if she is still taking anticonvulsant medication. If the answer is no, then a detailed account of events or sensations that preceded and followed the seizure is key. A febrile illness, headache, mental confusion suggest an acute infection. Headache with vomiting and a neurological deficit point to a tumor or an intracranial bleed. Recent heavy use of alcohol or barbiturates with sudden withdrawal can trigger seizures. It is also important to ask about prior history of head trauma, kidney disease, or cardiovascular disease. Assess risk factors for human immunodeficiency virus (HIV). In the elderly patient, Alzheimer's disease may be a cause.

Some clients may have a prodrome or premonition of an impending seizure but memory of this may be lost in the postictal state.

Prodromal symptoms include headache, mood change, fatigue, and myoclonic jerking. These precede the seizure by several hours and are not considered part of the aura that immediately precedes the seizure.

If the seizure was witnessed, ask for a description. Partial seizures affect only part of the brain. Simple partial seizures may be characterized by focal motor symptoms such as convulsive jerking or altered sensation such as parasthesias or tingling that spread to other parts of the extremity or body. Consciousness is not impaired. Complex partial seizures are characterized by impairment of consciousness along with the symptoms and signs of simple seizures.

Generalized seizures involve the whole brain. Absence seizures have an abrupt onset of unresponsiveness to external stimuli that may be very brief. Typically, they begin in childhood. Myoclonic seizures are distinguished by single or multiple myoclonic jerks. Tonic-clonic seizures (grand mal) are characterized by sudden loss of consciousness, rigidity (tonic phase) lasting about a minute followed by clonic jerking of the muscles lasting 2 to 3 minutes. Immediately after the seizure, the client may recover consciousness, fall asleep, or have another seizure. The postictal state is characterized by stupor or confusion. Often the client is incontinent during the seizure or may have suffered injury from a fall or from tongue biting.[20,22]

Objective Data

Physical Examination. A complete neurological and cardiovascular exam may reveal no abnormalities especially in younger women.

Note body temperature. Assess for nuchal rigidity.

Examine the skin for signs of alcohol or drug abuse (jaundice, needle marks). Subcutaneous nodules and cafe au lait spots may indicate the presence of neurofibromatosis.

Perform a complete cardiovascular examination to distinguish seizure from syncope. (See previous section on syncope.)

A thorough neurological examination may reveal focal neurological deficits that point to a space occupying lesion, such as tumor or abscess, chronic subdural hematoma, or to arteriovenous malformation. Assess mental status, especially in the elderly, for signs of Alzheimer's disease.

Diagnostic Tests. Diagnostic tests are selected on the basis of prior history and physical exam. Blood chemistries that measure liver and kidney function, blood glucose, and anticonvulsant medication levels may be indicated as well as a complete blood count. In high risk populations, an HIV test may be appropriate. If cardiovascular cause suspected, an ECG is needed to complete the workup.

Any woman with a new onset seizure needs an EEG and a CT scan with and without contrast or magnetic resonance image (MRI).

Differential Medical Diagnoses

- *Syncope.* See previous section on syncope.
- *Transient Ischemic Attacks.* These last longer than seizures and are accompanied by weakness or numbness, not by abnormal motor activity.
  - *Migraine headache* can present with aura preceding the headache that can make it difficult to distinguish from partial seizures. There are also migraine equivalents, which may be characterized by hemiparesis, numbness, and/or aphasia without headache. Usually the symptoms and signs develop more slowly (over several minutes) and the time factor helps distinguish from seizure activity.
- *Panic Attacks.* These may be harder to distinguish from absence or simple seizures but psychiatric history may provide clues.
- *Orthostatic Syncope.* Usually occurs after a change in posture, lasts a few seconds, and is

followed by prompt recovery as opposed to postictal confusion.

- *Pseudoseizures.* May be hysterical conversion reaction or malingering. They are usually neither preceded by a tonic phase nor followed by postictal behavior. The EEG is usually normal.
- *Generalized Tonic-clonic Seizures.* May occur 48 hours after *withdrawal* from *alcohol* in the client with a history of chronic or high intake. Treatment with anticonvulsants is generally not required unless status epilepticus occurs. As long as the client abstains from alcohol, seizure should not recur.

Plan

Referral. Refer to a physician any client who is suspected to have had a seizure. MRI, CT scan, and/or EEG may be ordered before referral to a neurologist. If the underlying cause is infection, admission to the hospital may be indicated. If the underlying etiology is cardiovascular, refer to a cardiologist for further workup. The client with an alcohol withdrawal seizure should be referred for detoxification and rehabilitation.

Medication. Anticonvulsant medication is selected by the neurologist, based on the type of seizure. Once stabilized on a dose, she usually returns to the care of the primary care provider.

The practitioner should be familiar with the more commonly prescribed anticonvulsant medications discussed subsequently. For more complete information, consult a pharmacology reference.

The drugs of choice for simple and complex partial and tonic-clonic seizures are phenytoin and carbemazeine.

PHENYTOIN. 300–400 mg p.o. per day as single dose or divided tid.

- *Administration.* It takes 5–10 days to reach a state drug level. Client may be admitted to the hospital for loading until a steady state is achieved and seizures are controlled. Optimum serum drug level is 10–20 µg/ml.
- *Adverse Effects.* Gingival hyperplasia, hirsutism, skin rash, ataxia, slurred speech, nystagmus, hypotension, nausea, vomiting, hepatic toxicity, and blood dyscrasias.

Toxicity signs include drowsiness, nausea, vomiting, nystagmus, slurred speech, ataxia, and tremors. Overdose can be lethal due to respiratory and circulatory collapse.

- *Contraindications.* Known hypersensitivity, sinus bradycardia, and heart block. Use with caution in hepatic, renal dysfunction, and in the elderly.

    Phenytoin has potentially serious interactions with many other medications. Consult a pharmacology reference for further information.

- *Client Teaching.* Emphasize adherence to prescribed doses of medication, signs of toxicity, interactions with other medications and over-the-counter drugs. Advise client not to drink alcohol while taking medication; it will decrease effectiveness and may increase adverse CNS effects. Advise client on oral contraceptives that phenytoin may decrease contraceptive effects, and discuss alternative methods. Medication should be taken with food to minimize GI effects. Encourage client to wear Medic Alert tag.

CARBAMAZEPINE. 600–1200 mg p.o. in divided doses (usually twice a day).

- *Administration.* Steady state levels achieved in 3–4 days. Therapeutic range is 4–12 µg/ml in serum.
- *Adverse Effects.* Diplopia, nystagmus, dysarthria, ataxia, drowsiness, nausea, blood dyscrasias, hepatotoxicity.

    Signs of toxicity include impaired breathing, respiratory depression, tachycardia, shock, arrhythmias, impaired consciousness, psychomotor disturbances, nausea, vomiting, oliguria, or anuria.

- *Contraindications.* Known hypersensitivity to carbamazepine and to tricyclic antidepressants; past or present history of bone marrow depression; use of monoamine oxidase inhibitors within the last 14 days (can cause hypertensive crisis). Use with caution if hepatic, cardiac, or renal dysfunction; increased intraocular pressure; elderly (may cause agitation, confusion, activate latent psychosis).

    Consult pharmacology reference for interactions with other medications.

- *Client Teaching.* See discussion of phenytoin.

VALPROIC ACID. For absence seizures, myoclonic seizures, and certain tonic-clonic seizures.

- *Administration.* Usual dose is 750–1250 mg in three doses. It takes 2–4 days to reach the steady state. Therapeutic range is 50–100 µg/ml.
- *Adverse Effects.* Weight gain, hair loss, tremor, drowsiness, nausea, vomiting, diarrhea, hepatic toxicity, thrombocytopenia.

    Toxicity is indicated by somnolence and coma.

- *Contraindications.* Known hypersensitivity and hepatic dysfunction. Use with caution in clients on anticoagulants.
- *Interactions.* Valproic acid may potentiate the effects of monoamine oxidase inhibitors, antidepressants, and anticoagulants. May cause absence seizures if used with clonazepam.
- *Client Teaching.* Teach client importance of taking as prescribed. Advise client of adverse effects. Take with food to minimize GI effects. Swallow—do not chew—to avoid mucosal irritation and unpleasant taste. Encourage client to wear Medic Alert tag.

    Newer anticonvulsants such as felbamate, gamapentin, and lamotrigine have been approved for adjunctive therapy for partial and secondarily generalized seizures. Felbamate is now under review because of reports of aplastic anemia. Consult a pharmacology text for further information.[21]

Diet/Lifestyle. The client with well controlled seizure disorder is capable of leading a normal life, including work, school, and driving (depending on state laws). She should be counseled regarding the importance of healthy eating and rest patterns to maintain optimal health. Confront possible alcohol and illicit drug use openly and advise client of risks. Preconception counseling and consultation with the neurologist before pregnancy is advisable.

Follow-Up

For the person with an isolated seizure and no further workup scheduled, telephone follow-up in 7 days is suggested. Follow-up office visit in 3 months is warranted as well as immediate follow-up should the seizure recur. Telephone follow-up is advised after client is seen by neurologist or other specialist to become familiar with treatment plan. Request written plan from consultant.

PARKINSONISM AND ESSENTIAL TREMOR

Tremor is a purposeless, rhythmic movement resulting from the involuntary alternating contraction and relaxation of opposing groups of skeletal muscles. Essential or familial tremor is usually inherited and has no other associated features. Parkinsonism is a movement disorder characterized by tremor, rigidity, and bradykinesia. It is slowly progressive and caused by an imbalance of the neurotransmitters dopamine and acetylcholine.

Epidemiology

Essential tremor and Parkinsonism are common disorders. Familial essential tremor is often inherited in an autosomal dominant pattern. It can appear at any age. Parkinsonism affects 1 in 100 adults over 50 years of age. It can be found in equal numbers of males and females and occurs in all ethnic groups.[23]

Subjective Data

Important questions to ask the client: What parts of the body are involved? Does the tremor occur with movement (intentional tremor) or at rest? Does the tremor only affect one side of the body or is it symmetrical? Does any other member of the family have a similar disorder? Does emotional stress make the tremor worse and does alcohol make it less noticeable? Are there any other associated complaint such as hoarseness, dysphagia, drooling, depression, nightmares, slowed movement, problems cutting food, turning in bed, and buttoning clothing? Do you use caffeine, stimulant drugs, drink alcohol, take theophylline, anticonvulsants?

Objective Data

Physical Examination. A complete neurological exam is performed, including assessment for cognitive impairment.

Begin with observation of the client's gait, posture, and facial expression. The client with Parkinson's disease takes small, shuffling steps, with little swinging of the arms. The posture is stooped. She may have difficulty stopping and turning around. The facial expression may be fixed with little blinking. Examine the skin for signs of seborrhea of the scalp and face (common in Parkinson's disease).

Examine the mouth and lips for tremor and drooling.

Assess the extremities for strength and deep tendon reflexes. There is usually no weakness and no alteration of deep tendon reflexes.

Observe the tremor. The benign essential tremor will involve one or both hands and/or the head. It persists at rest but worsens with use of the affected hand. No other abnormalities are noted during the exam (see Table 22–11).

The tremor of Parkinson's disease often becomes less apparent with activity. In early disease, it is confined to one limb or one side of the body. Emotional stress may exacerbate it.

Assess for rigidity. The client with Parkinsonism exhibits increased resistance to passive movement. She may have difficulty arising from a sitting position.

Assessment of cognitive function may be incorporated into the rest of the exam. If deficits are found, more in depth testing may be needed such as the Folstein Mini-Mental Status Examination (see Table 22–12).

Diagnostic Tests. Selected on basis of examination findings but may include rapid plasma reagent (RPR), vitamin B-12 and folate levels, complete blood count (CBC), blood chemistries for electrolyte levels and liver function, thyroid stimulating hormone (TSH).

Differential Medical Diagnoses

Huntington's disease involves rigidity and bradykinesia but is distinguished by choreic movements, which are irregular and jerky, as opposed to tremor, which is rhythmic. It is an inherited disease.

Depression may present with expressionless face and slowed movement. It can be difficult to distinguish from early Parkinson's disease and may coexist at the time of diagnosis.

Plan

Consult with the physician if Parkinsonism is suspected. Initial management may be at the primary care level.

TABLE 22–11. CHARACTERISTICS OF TREMOR AND PARKINSONISM

	Essential Tremor	Parkinsonism	Other
Body part affected	Hands, head	Pill-rolling tremor of thumb, finger	Intentional tremor of multiple sclerosis, brain lesion may involve legs
Aggravating Factors	Emotional stress, use of limb	Conspicuous at rest and stress	
Ameliorating Factors	Alcohol use	Lessens with use of limb and disappears with sleep	Alcohol withdrawal worsens intentional tremor
Associated Features	None	Bradykinesia, stooped posture, mask-like face, small handwriting, cognitive impairment	

Source: Reference 20.

Psychosocial Interventions. Reassure the client with essential tremor that though the tremor may become progressively worse with age, no other functional abnormalities are associated with this disorder. Provide emotional support to the client and her family affected with Parkinsonism. This is a progressive, debilitating illness. Not only does it affect motor function; 15–30 percent of clients develop dementia.[23] Anticipatory guidance is key to the plan. Refer family to support and information groups, such as the Parkinson's Disease Foundation, the National Parkinson's Foundation, the American Parkinson's Disease Association, Inc.

Medication. Essential tremor is treated with *propranolol* starting dose 60 mg p.o. titrating up for effect to maximum dose of 240 mg. See previous discussion of beta blockers in section on hypertension.

TABLE 22–12. FOLSTEIN MINI-MENTAL STATE EXAMINATION

Maximum Score	Client Score	Questions
5		"What is the (year) (season) (date) (day) (month)?"
5		"Where are we?" Name of (state) (county) (city or town) (place, such as hospital or clinic) (specific location, such as floor or room).
3		The examiner names three unrelated objects clearly and slowly, then asks the client to name all three of them. The client's response is used for scoring. The examiner repeats them until client learns all of them if possible.
5		"Begin with 100 and count backwards by subtracting 7." Stop at 65 (5 responses).
3		If the client learned the three objects above, ask her to recall them now.
2		The examiner shows the client two simple objects, such as a wrist watch and pencil, and asks her to name them.
1		"Repeat the phrase, 'No ifs, and, or buts.'"
3		The examiner gives the client a piece of blank paper and asks her to follow the three-step command: "Take the paper in your right hand, fold it in half, and put it on the floor."
1		On a blank piece of paper, the examiner prints the command "Close your eyes," in letters large enough for the client to see clearly, then asks her to read it and follow the command.
1		"Make up and write a sentence about anything." This sentence must contain a noun and a verb.
1		The examiner gives the client a blank piece of paper and asks her to draw a symbol (two interlocking pentagons). All 10 angles must be present and 2 must intersect.
Total Possible = 30	Client's Total =	(If total score is 23 or below, further evaluation may be indicated)

Folstein, et al. Mini-Mental State. Journal of Psychiatric Research. Vol. 12; pp. 189–198. 1995.

Pharmacologic intervention for Parkinsonism is based on restoring dopaminergic function through the use of levodopa (which is metabolized to dopamine) combined with carbodopa (a dopa-decarboxylase inhibitor), which inhibits levodopa metabolism outside the brain.[23]

PARKINSONISM MEDICATION

CARBODOPA-LEVODOPA (SINEMET OR SINEMET CR)

- *Administration.* Available in several dosage combinations and as an immediate release and a controlled release form. Consult with physician regarding preferred form. Dosage will depend on stage of disease and diurnal progression of symptoms. See pharmacology text or reference 23 for further discussion on adjusting dosage.
- *Adverse Effects.* Worsening of Parkinsonism symptoms, dyskinesias, cardiac rhythm irregularities, orthostatic hypotension, spasm or closing of eyelids, severe nausea and vomiting. In clients with dementia, may cause hallucinations and psychosis.
- *Contraindications.* Known hypersensitivity, asthma, emphysema, severe cardiovascular disease, narrow-angle glaucoma, malignant melanoma, history of myocardial infarction.
- *Expected Outcome.* Improvement in ability to perform activities of daily living.
- *Client Teaching.* Adverse effects, signs of toxicity (muscle twitching and blepharospasm are early signs).

Selegiline, a monoamine oxidase-B inhibitor, is under investigation as a neuroprotective agent that may delay the progression of disability and the need for levodopa. Refer to pharmacology text for further discussion and current research on this medication.

Other medications may be added based on associated symptoms and progression of disease. These are best initiated in consultation with neurologist.

Lifestyle/Diet. Clients with essential tremor should be advised to avoid self-medication with alcohol. If tremor is not well controlled with medication, client may have problems with handwriting and other manual skills. Be sensitive to impact on social and professional life.

Help with activities of daily living in the form of assistive devices may help client with Parkinsonism maintain independence. These measures may include rails and banisters in the home, eating utensils with large handles, nonskid mats for table and bath, communication devices to enhance speech. Client may need special texturized diet if swallowing difficulties are present.

Occupational and physical therapy referrals may be appropriate.

Follow-Up

The client diagnosed with essential tremor should be seen in 2 weeks for response to medication and possible adjustment of dosage.

Client with Parkinsonism should be seen within 2–3 days of initiation of carbodopa-levodopa to assess response and to observe for toxicity. If referred to neurology, request copy of plan. Continue to provide primary care services.

DEMENTIA/ALZHEIMER'S DISEASE

Dementia is a progressive organic mental disorder with characteristic behaviors and cognitive decline. The hallmark is short-term memory loss, but associated features may include impaired judgment, impaired abstract thinking, language or motor function disturbance, and/or personality change. It must be distinguished from delirium or acute confusional state, which are usually reversible when the underlying cause is corrected. A major irreversible cause of primary dementia in the elderly is Alzheimer's disease. Other causes of dementia are listed in Table 22–13.

Epidemiology

Dementia affects one in ten American adults over the age of 65. It is probably the most feared problem of aging. Alzheimer's accounts for 60 percent to 70 percent of irreversible dementia. It is age related, has an insidious onset, and may follow a familial pattern. Recent studies indicate that women who take estrogen long after menopause (a decade or more) may be less likely to develop Alzheimer's disease.[24]

Multi-infarct dementia accounts for 15–20 percent of dementias, is more common in men, and is associated with hypertension and transient ischemic attacks (TIAs). According to recent studies, about 11 percent of dementias are reversible or partially reversible. The clients more likely to have a reversible dementia are those with recent acute onset, rapid deterioration, atypical presentation, multiple drug use or polypharmacy, history of depression, and onset younger than 60–70 years old.[25,26]

Subjective Data

The first symptom noted is forgetfulness or loss of short-term memory. This must be distinguished from the benign senescent forgetfulness that sometimes accompanies aging and from depression. Progression of symptoms differentiates benign senescent forgetfulness from the short-term memory loss of Alzheimer's. The family may begin to note increasing difficulty with daily activities such as balancing the checkbook, dressing appropriately, cooking. The client may have some loss of expressive and comprehensive language including word finding difficulty. She may have undergone a personality change, becoming more irritable and impatient; she may be paranoid in her thinking at times. At this point, the family may bring the client in for evaluation. The client herself may have no specific complaint but may become agitated when asked simple questions that she is unable to answer. It is important to review prescription and nonprescription medications taken and alcohol intake.

Objective Data

Physical Examination
- *General Appearance.* Begin with careful observation of the client paying special attention to gait, affect and facial expression, initiation or fluency of speech. Physical appearance may resemble Parkinsonism with stooped gait, mask-like face, and slowed movement.
- A *complete cardiovascular exam* focuses on blood pressure and the presence of carotid bruits.
- The *neurological exam* focuses on motor, sensory, hearing, vision, cranial nerves, tremor, reflexes, and cerebellar function.

  The client in the early stages of Alzheimer's may have an essentially normal exam up to this point.

Diagnostic Tests. A Folstein or other Standard Mini-Mental Test (see Table 22–12) to assess cognitive function will aid in the diagnosis, but be aware that educational and cultural differences may make scoring difficult.

Standard lab tests to order include CBC, B12 and folate, thyroid function, biochemical profile. Consider an RPR or HIV test if high risk for syphilis or acquired immunodeficiency syndrome (AIDS) dementia.

Order CT or MRI if tumor, subdural hematoma, stroke, hydrocephalus, or multi-infarct dementia is suspected. There is no imaging modality available to definitively diagnose Alzheimer's disease.

Differential Medical Diagnoses

The client with normal pressure *hydrocephalus* may have gait disturbance (broad-based stance) and incontinence.

Creutzfeldt-Jacob disease is a rare, rapidly progressive fatal neurological disease characterized by behavior change, myoclonus, and rigidity.

TABLE 22–13. CAUSES OF DEMENTIA

Probably Irreversible Causes (in order of decreasing prevalence)
Alzheimer's disease
Multi-infarct dementia
Alcohol
Parkinson's disease
Huntington's disease
Mixed (Alzheimer's and multiinfarct)
Trauma
Anoxia

Potentially Reversible Causes
Depression
Normal-pressure hydrocephalus
Drugs
Neoplasm
Metabolic
Infections
Subdural hematoma

Source: Adapted from Clarofiglo, A., Treatable vs. Untreatable Dementia, Clinical Geriatrics. *Vol. 4 #1; p. 47; Jan. 1996.*

Parkinson's disease may manifest with early symptoms of dementia when neuromuscular features are not prominent.

Huntington's disease is diagnosed on basis of family history and the accompanying movement disorder. Onset is 20–50 years of age.

Korsakoff's syndrome due to chronic alcohol use involves memory loss and some impairment of cognitive function. It is associated with thiamine deficiency and has a sudden onset.

Tumor, multi-infarct, subdural hematoma are differentiated on the basis of the imaging modality used.

Plan

Psychosocial Interventions. This may be the most important area for the practitioner. See Table 22–14. The diagnosis must be made clear. It should also be emphasized that maintaining optimal health status for the client will improve the quality of life for both family and client. A Medic-Alert bracelet should be worn. Refer client and family to the Alzheimer's Association, 70

East Lake St., Suite 600, Chicago, IL 60601, telephone 800–621–0379.

Medication

DONEPEZIL HCL (ARICEPT)

- *Mechanism of Action.* Cholinesterase inhibitor that has shown some benefit in enhancing cognitive function in those with mild to moderate Alzheimer's.
- *Administration.* Starting dose is 5 mg once a day in the evening. May increase to 10 mg each evening after 4–6 weeks of therapy.
- *Adverse Effects.* Nausea, vomiting, diarrhea, muscle cramps, fatigue, anorexia, insomnia.
- *Contraindications.* Known sensitivity to donepezil or piperidine derivative. Cautious use if other serious medical conditions such as sick sinus syndrome, ulcers, asthma, urinary or intestinal obstruction.

TACRINE (THA)

- *Mechanism of Action.* A centrally acting anticholinesterase inhibitor may improve cognition in early Alzheimer's.
- *Administration.* Starting dose 10 mg QID (taken between meals if tolerated). Increase in 40 mg/d increments no sooner than every 6 weeks to maximum dose 160 mg/d.
- *Adverse Effects.* May cause hepatic failure (dose related), vomiting, diarrhea, agitation, confusion, dizziness, insomnia, somnolence, hallucinations, purpura.
- *Contraindications.* Hepatic disease, inability to adhere to weekly monitoring of liver function. Cautious use if other serious medical.conditions such as sick sinus syndrome, ulcers, asthma, urinary or intestinal obstruction.
- *Expected Outcome.* May improve cognitive function in early disease.
- *Client/Family Teaching.* Prepare client and family that they may see no improvement. Only about one-third of clients respond. Very expensive. Must have liver function test levels drawn every week for first 18 weeks of therapy, then every 3 months. Must have weekly levels when dose increased. Advise family to monitor urine output (may cause outflow obstruction). Advise family abrupt discontinuation can cause acute degeneration of cognitive function.

TABLE 22–14. WORKING WITH FAMILIES OF CLIENTS WITH DEMENTIA

1. Discuss diagnosis and prognosis
2. Refer family members to the Alzheimer's Association and to support groups for the families of clients with dementing illnesses.
3. Recommend reading material to provide the family with information about dementing illnesses and coping strategies (titles may be obtained from Alzheimer's Association).
4. Refer the family to attorneys, financial planners, and other professionals to help maintain client's personal affairs.
5. Discuss difficult decisions including tube feeding and institutionalization with family members at an early stage.
6. Watch for caregiver stress or elder abuse.
7. Emphasize three principles: (a) the need to provide structure for the client, (b) the need to limit goals and expectations for the client, and (c) the necessity of establishing and maintaining a "no-fail" environment for the client.

"No-Fail" environment means providing a low-demand environment in which the client is less likely to become frustrated by her own limitations or cognitive deficits. Examples of "no-fail" measures are offering finger-food when she is no longer able to use utensils, asking questions she is likely to be able to answer, maintaining a schedule of activities of daily living that maximizes her best time of day.

Source: Stewart, J., Management of Behavior Problems in the Dementia Patient. American Family Physician. Vol. 52 #8; pp. 2311–2317. 1995.

Antidepressants, such as secondary amine *tricyclic antidepressants* (nortriptyline and desipramine) or one of the selective *serotonin reuptake inhibitors,* may improve quality of life significantly in early disease. See chapter on Psychosocial Health Concerns for further information on these medications.

Diet/Lifestyle. See Table 22–14. A healthy and varied diet, adequate rest, maintenance of regular elimination, and skin hygiene are vitally important areas for the client, especially when she is unable to provide these for herself. Advise family to avoid using antihistamines for sleep problems. These medications have a high potential to cause confusion. Instead suggest limiting chocolate, colas, tea, and coffee that contain caffeine. Providing a safe environment is key as well as including client in family or community activities as much as possible.

Follow-Up

Once the diagnosis is made, a follow-up visit in 2 weeks is suggested to ascertain how the client and her family are adjusting to the diagnosis. Consult with physician if signs of psychosis appear or if increasing agitation and behavioral disturbances. Regularly scheduled visits every 3 months or more often based on the client's status.[27]

OPHTHALMOLOGICAL DISORDERS

CONJUNCTIVITIS

The most common eye problem encountered in primary care is a red eye. The redness is caused by injection of the conjunctival, episcleral or ciliary blood vessels. In evaluating the client, it is important to remember that common problems are common; that is, that conjunctivitis caused by a virus, bacteria, or allergen is usually the diagnosis. It is imperative, however, to rule out other more serious disorders. As always, a good history and physical exam are keys to diagnosis.

Epidemiology

Several species of bacteria normally colonize the conjunctival sac, most commonly *Staphylococcus* *albus* and *aureus, Corynebacterium,* and *Streptococcus.* Acute bacterial conjunctivitis may be caused by an overgrowth of *Staphylococcus aureus.* It may also be caused by *pneumococcal infection,* especially in colder weather, and by *Haemophilus* in warmer regions of the United States. In younger individuals, Haemophilus is more often the causative organism than Staphylococcus aureus. Other bacteria implicated in acute conjunctivitis include *Neisseria gonorrhoeae, Neisseria meningitidis, Escherichia coli,* and *Proteus* species. Chronic bacterial conjunctivitis is usually caused by *Staphylococcus aureus* or *epidermidis* or by *Streptococcus pyogenes.* It is often associated with blepharitis.

Sexually active young adults are at risk for inclusion conjunctivitis caused by *Chlamydia* contamination of the eye after sexual contact and at risk for the hyperacute conjunctivitis caused by *Neisseria gonorrhoeae.* Alcoholics and other individuals with nutritional deficiencies are at risk for all types of infectious conjunctivitis.

Viruses are the causative organism in most cases of infectious conjunctivitis. Most commonly implicated are the adenoviruses. A more serious form of viral keratoconjunctivitis is caused by the Herpes simplex virus that may spread to the eye after contact with genital lesions. Herpes zoster may also spread to the eye.

Seasonal or vernal conjunctivitis is less common in women than in men, occurs in the spring, and may have associated photophobia. Allergic conjunctivitis is associated with a history of asthma or atopy.[1,2,3]

Subjective Data

Important questions to ask:

Do you wear contact lenses? Contact lens wearers are at higher risk for infectious conjunctivitis, especially bacterial. Often they continue to wear the lens and are at risk for infection by anaerobes and for corneal ulceration.

When did the redness first appear? Which eye? The onset of viral and acute bacterial conjunctivitis as well as inclusion conjunctivitis is abrupt, often affecting one eye and after several days spreading to the other eye by autoinoculation. Irritant conjunctivitis follows contact with a trigger such as a chemical.

Is there any change or loss of vision? Blurred vision may occur with inclusion conjunctivitis. Epidemic keratoconjunctivitis caused by several *adenovirus* types may be associated with formation of a pseudomembrane that reduces vision. *Herpes* infection of the eye may also cause decreased visual acuity especially if not treated promptly.

Any discharge? Copious, thick exudate is the hallmark of gonococcal conjunctivitis. Mucopurulent to mucoid discharge accompanies other forms of infectious conjunctivitis. Allergic conjunctivitis causes tearing.

Any pain? Foreign body sensation? Pruritis? Gonococcal conjunctivitis is accompanied by discomfort, swelling of the eyelid, and tenderness. Chronic bacterial conjunctivitis and *Herpes* virus keratoconjunctivitis may cause a foreign body sensation. If treatment of *Chlamydial* conjunctivitis is delayed, iritis may develop resulting in photophobia. Allergic conjunctivitis is characterized by often intense pruritis.

Previous eye injury, head trauma, infection, or surgery? Viral conjunctivitis often follows an upper respiratory infection. Previous eye surgery may put client at risk for bacterial conjunctivitis. Eye injury puts client at risk for subsequent iritis and corneal abrasion (which must be differentiated from the red eye of conjunctivitis).

Any contact with infected genital secretions? Always retain high suspicion of sexually transmitted etiology of conjunctivitis in sexually active client. *Gonococcal, Chlamydial,* and *Herpes* virus conjunctivitis require prompt diagnosis and referral to an ophthalmologist to prevent serious consequences including loss of vision.

Any chronic disease? Medications taken routinely? Immunocompromised individuals are at higher risk for infectious conjunctivitis. Clients with psoriasis or seborrhea are more prone to chronic conjunctivitis. Conditions associated with increased risk of iritis include *Herpes zoster, Herpes simplex* infections, *Lyme disease, tuberculosis, syphilis,* and *autoimmune disease* such as inflammatory bowel disease and sarcoidosis.

Any association with occupation or hobby? Welders who do not wear protective eyeglasses are at risk for a punctate keratitis (arc welder's eye), which presents with redness and photophobia. Irritant or allergic conjunctivitis may follow accidental exposure to chemical used in a hobby or craft.

Any family member with similar problem? Viral conjunctivitis is highly contagious.

Objective Data

Physical Examination. Appearance of the eye and lids. Conjunctival (bulbar and palpebral) injection is the hallmark of conjunctivitis. Lids may be very swollen in gonococcal conjunctivitis, erythematous in chronic bacterial conjunctivitis with crusting at the base of the eyelash (see Table 22–15).

Chlamydial inclusion conjunctivitis produces follicles on the palpebral conjunctiva, especially on the lower lid. Marked swelling of the conjunctiva occurs in allergic conjunctivitis. Examine for exudate. The exudate of gonococcal conjunctivitis is thick, copious and accumulates in the lashes. Acute bacterial conjunctivitis is characterized by thinner mucopurulent discharge. The exudate of viral and allergic conjunctivitis is watery.

Compare pupils for equality of size, important in differentiating conjunctivitis from iritis and glaucoma. Conjunctivitis causes no inequality. In iritis, pupil is small and unequal.

Examine for swelling of preauricular nodes present in viral conjunctivitis, including Herpes keratoconjunctivitis.

Evert eyelid to examine for foreign body that may have triggered injection of the conjunctiva.

Evaluate extraocular movements, test pupillary reaction, visual fields.

Direct ophthalmoscopy of fundus and disc. Flashlight examination of anterior chamber.

Diagnostic Tests

VISUAL ACUITY. It is imperative to assess visual acuity. If this is not done, a serious mistake in diagnosis may occur, placing the practitioner at risk for negligence. If the client has forgotten or lost her corrective lenses, a pinhole disk may be used to optimize acuity.

Client with chemical conjunctivitis caused by acid or alkali needs pH measurement of conjunctival secretion after initial irrigation with large amounts (one to two liters) of normal saline or water. If pH is less than or greater than 6.8–7.0, continue to irrigate to prevent permanent damage and refer immediately to the ophthalmologist.

FLUORESCEIN STAINING. Fluorescein staining of conjunctiva and examination by slit lamp or Wood's Lamp for epithelial staining defect if corneal injury suspected. Fluorescein staining assists in the diagnosis of Herpes keratoconjunctivitis, which has a characteristic dendritic appearance.

If gonococcal or Chlamydial infection suspected, confirmation by stained smear and culture is needed. Prompt diagnosis and treatment prevent blindness.

Acute bacterial conjunctivitis and chronic conjunctivitis are usually diagnosed by examination and history; however, if there is doubt about the causative organism a culture and sensitivity should be obtained.

Differential Medical Diagnosis

Iritis presents with intense photophobia, redness localized around the cornea, and smaller unequal pupil of the affected eye (see Table 22–16).

Acute angle closure glaucoma causes diminished vision, hazy or steamy cornea, dilated unequal pupil in the affected eye, with redness around the cornea.

Scleritis, an inflammatory condition of the deeper vessels of the sclera, is characterized by pain, no exudate, and a localized redness, often most intense in the superior globe of the eye.

Corneal abrasion and foreign body are diagnosed by history, foreign body sensation, and epithelial staining defect on staining and slit lamp or Wood's Lamp examination.

Plan

The client with acute angle closure glaucoma, foreign body that has penetrated the cornea or is not removed by irrigation, iritis, scleritis, or keratoconjunctivitis caused by Herpes virus or arc welding is referred immediately to an ophthalmologist.

Psychosocial Interventions. Reassure client eye tissue heals very quickly; with adherence to treatment regimen, good outcome is expected. Client may be sensitive about appearance, especially if exudate present. She should avoid mascara and eyeliner until conjunctivitis resolved. She may need a work excuse if she works in health care setting, food service, or child care. If conjunctivitis is due to sexually transmitted disease, advise client that partner(s) need treatment.

Medication

VIRAL CONJUNCTIVITIS

NORMAL SALINE EYE DROPS

- *Administration.* Two drops each eye every 2 to 3 hours for as long as needed.
- *Side Effects.* May experience transient stinging of eyes.
- *Contraindication.* None.

TABLE 22–15. OBJECTIVE FINDINGS IN CONJUNCTIVITIS

	Viral	Bacterial	Chlamydia	Allergic
Exudate	Serous	Copious mucopurulent or mucoid NOTE: Gonococcal conjunctivitis drainage is copious and purulent	Thin, serous	Watery profuse
Unilateral vs Bilateral	Bilateral NOTE: HSV unilateral	Unilateral	Often unilateral	Bilateral
Associated Features	Enlarged preauricular nodes Pharyngitis Abrupt onset Palpebral conjunctiva injected HSV: Dendritic pattern if fluorescein stained	Blepharitis Hordeolum Eyelids stuck together	Urethritis Prominent follicles upper and lower lids Nontender preauricular node May have mild keratitis	Asthma Atopy Itchy eyes Swollen eyelids Chemosis (edema) of cornea and conjunctiva

Key: HSV: Herpes Simplex Virus
Source: References 1, 2, 4.

TABLE 22–16. DIFFERENTIAL DIAGNOSES OF RED EYE

	Conjunctivitis	Corneal Abrasion	Iritis	Acute Glaucoma
Signs and Symptoms				
Pain	Mild	Moderate to severe	Moderate to severe	Severe (often with nausea and vomiting)
Foreign Body Sensation	Mild	Moderate to severe	None	None
Vision	Normal	Blurred	Blurred with photophobia	Greatly reduced
Pupil Size	Normal	Normal	Small in affected eye	Dilated
Incidence	Common	Common	Infrequent	Rare
Other Information	May follow upper respiratory infection	Hx important for foreign body, abrasion, contact lens wear, use of arcwelding equipment		Anterior chamber shallow

Source: Stokes, H. Conjunctivitis in Dornbrand, L., Hoole, A., and Pickard, C. Manual of Clinical Problems in Adult Ambulatory Care 2d ed. Boston; Little Brown and Company. 1992. p. 27.

- *Expected Outcome.* Advise the client it may take 7–10 days before conjunctiva clear.

NOTE: Ophthalmologists recommend that antibiotic eye drops not be used for the treatment of viral conjunctivitis due to the potential for allergic response. Agents such as sodium sulfacetamide and erythromycin have low potential; gentamicin, neomycin, and tobramycin have high potential. If it is difficult to distinguish whether conjunctivitis is due to virus or bacteria or if client at risk for bacterial superinfection, treat with low potential agent and evaluate after 3–5 days for response.

ALLERGIC CONJUNCTIVITIS

NAPHAZOLINE HYDROCHLORIDE. Ophthalmic solution 0.1 percent.

- *Administration.* Instill 1–2 drops each eye every 3–4 hours for relief of itching and redness.
- *Adverse Effects.* Transient stinging, pupillary dilation, hyperemia, increased or decreased intraocular pressure.
- *Contraindications.* Sensitivity to ingredients, history of glaucoma.
- *Expected Outcome.* May be recurrent problem, but medication should relieve symptoms.
- *Client Teaching.* Advise client to report blurred vision, eye pain, lid swelling and discontinue use if occurs. Use of cool compresses as needed for added comfort. May add oral antihistamine such as Benadryl if severe itching.

CHEMICAL CONJUNCTIVITIS. Cool compresses for 15–20 minutes several times a day and use of top-

ical vasoconstrictor solution such as naphazoline hydrochloride solution (see prior information).

NOTE: If chemical trigger is acid or alkali, immediately irrigate eye with normal saline or water, measure pH. When neutral pH achieved, examine fluorescein-stained eye with slit lamp and/or refer to physician.

ACUTE BACTERIAL CONJUNCTIVITIS

SODIUM SULFACETAMIDE. (Sulamyd—10 percent) solution.

- *Administration.* Two drops in the eye every 3 hours while awake for 5–7 days.
- *Adverse Effects.* Blurred vision, transient burning and stinging. Hypersensitivity, intense itching and/or burning.
- *Contraindication.* Known sensitivity to sulfonamides.
- *Expected Outcome.* Symptoms usually resolve in a couple of days.
- *Client Teaching.* Advise client not to let dropper touch eye, remove exudate with warm, clean cloth before instilling drops. Teach signs/symptoms of sensitivity and advise client to discontinue use immediately and call practitioner if sensitivity develops. Wait 10 minutes before using another eye preparation.

HYPERACUTE BACTERIAL CONJUNCTIVITIS. Hyperacute bacterial conjunctivitis due to Neisseria gonorrhoeae must be referred to ophthalmologist for topical and systemic antibiotic therapy to prevent corneal damage and systemic spread.

NOTE: If client allergic to sulfonamides, erythromycin ophthalmic ointment may be used four times a day for the same duration of time. See following for adverse effects and client teaching.

Chronic Bacterial Conjunctivitis

erythromycin ophthalmic ointment

- *Administration.* Apply to lower lid inner canthus to outer canthus four times a day for at least 2 weeks.
- *Adverse Effects.* Blurred vision, transient burning and stinging.
- *Contraindication.* Known sensitivity to erythromycin.
- *Expected Outcome.* Reduces bacterial count but may recur.
- *Client Teaching.* Advise client to clean eyelashes with neutral soap such as baby shampoo (see Blepharitis for details) before applying ointment. Advise client scrupulous hygiene may help prevent recurrence.

Inclusion Conjunctivitis (Chlamydial Conjunctivitis). Requires referral to ophthalmologist for systemic therapy and confirmation of diagnosis. If there is any doubt about the diagnosis, refer. Sexually active women may have no associated symptoms, such as vaginal discharge. Diagnosis is based on suspicion, prominent follicles on lower palpebral conjunctival sac, and confirmation by Giemsa-stained conjunctival scraping. Treatment is with Doxycycline 100 mg twice a day for 3–5 weeks.

Lifestyle. Clients with infectious conjunctivitis should avoid spread by not sharing towels, washcloths, make-up. Advise client to discard any eye make-up used at time of onset of symptoms.

Frequent handwashing is emphasized, and always after touching eyes. May not return to work until exudate resolved if employed in health care, child care, or food service.

Clients with allergic conjunctivitis should try to determine trigger(s) and avoid as much as possible.

If conjunctivitis is associated with sexually transmitted disease, advise client on other risks of unprotected sex such as pelvic inflammatory disease, sterility, HIV infection.

CORNEAL ABRASION

Corneal abrasion is caused by disruption of the epithelial covering of the cornea. It may follow trauma, any superficial contact such as with dust, debris or prolonged exposure to ultraviolet light such as sunlight, sunlamp, or welder's arc.

Epidemiology

Contact lens wearers are at higher risk for abrasion (and ulceration) not only because insertion of the lens may result in abrasion but because the cornea over time may become less sensitive to insult and treatment may be delayed. Clients in occupations involving prolonged exposure to dirt, dust, debris, sunlight, and wind are also at higher risk for corneal abrasion.

Subjective Data

Client reports history of trauma, severe pain, foreign body sensation, and photophobia.

Objective Data

Physical Examination. Diffuse or localized redness. May have profuse tearing. Client may be unable to open eye for examination if pain severe. Oblique illumination of the cornea by penlight may reveal irregular area on corneal surface. Always evert eyelid to examine for foreign body.

Diagnostic Tests

Visual Acuity. Is recorded. (Practitioner may have to instill one to two drops topical ophthalmic anesthetic such as procainamide before starting examination.)

Fluorescein Staining. Fluorescein strip is dampened with sterile normal saline and lightly touched to the conjunctival surface of lower lid. After stain is blinked into surface of eye, cornea is examined with slit lamp or Wood's lamp. Epithelial staining defect appears as deep green with cobalt blue filter.

Differential Medical Diagnoses

Herpes simplex keratitis. Suspect if previous history of herpes keratitis, coexisting fever blister or herpes genitalis, vague or absent history of trauma, dendritic corneal stain pattern.

Ultraviolet keratitis. History of exposure to sunlight, snow, sunlamp, or welder's arc without adequate eye protection. Symptoms occur 6–12 hours after exposure. Client complains of intense pain and photophobia and may be unable to open eyes. Staining reveals diffuse punctate pattern of both corneas.

Plan

Refer immediately any client with herpes keratoconjunctivitis or ultraviolet keratitis to physician and/or ophthalmologist. Consult with physician if corneal abrasion. Deep or extensive abrasions, corneal ulceration, contact lens wearers should always be referred for follow-up with ophthalmologist.

Psychosocial Interventions. Reassure client that cornea heals very rapidly but emphasize strict adherence to treatment plan to prevent complications such as ulceration and infection.

Medication

ERYTHROMYCIN OPHTHALMIC OINTMENT. Is used to prevent injection.

- *Administration.* Apply to lower lid and with firm pressure place sterile dry dressing over eye to prevent lid movement. Tape is placed from cheek to forehead to secure bandage.
- *Adverse Effects.* Transient stinging of eye.
- *Contraindication.* Sensitivity to erythromycin (rare).
- *Expected Outcome.* Superficial abrasion usually heals within 24–48 hours without complication.
- *Client Teaching.* Advise patient not to drive. She should rest at home, not remove bandage, and keep unaffected eye closed as much as possible. She should be seen the next day by the practitioner (if skilled in using slit lamp) or referred to an ophthalmologist (always if contact lens wearer).

Lifestyle Changes. If the client is a contact lens wearer and has recurrent episodes of conjunctivitis, irritation, or abrasion, advise her to return to ophthalmologist or optometrist who originally prescribed lenses for further evaluation.

Follow-Up

Client is always examined the next day using slit lamp or Wood's lamp after fluorescein staining. If staining defect remains or if client continues to complain of foreign body sensation or pain, consult with physician immediately. Request copy of visit note and treatment plan if referred to ophthalmologist in order to assure continuity of care.

DISORDERS OF THE EYELID: HORDEOLUM AND CHALAZION

A hordeolum is an abscess of the meibomian gland (internal hordeolum) or the gland at the base of the lash (external hordeolum or sty). It can occur on the upper or the lower lid. It is caused by Staphylococcus. If the abscess is internal it can press on the conjunctiva and cause a cellulitis of the lid.

A chalazion is a granulomatous inflammation of the meibomian gland that is caused by an internal hordeolum.

Epidemiology

Both conditions are common in children and adults. Clients with compromised immunity such as diabetics may be more prone to develop hordeolum.

Subjective Data

The client with hordeolum may complain of pain in proportion to the degree of swelling. If a chalazion is large, it may press on the eyeball and cause pain, conjunctival injection or even blurring of vision.

Objective Data

Hordeolum causes a red, tender swelling of the lid, usually arising from the skin surface. If the hordeolum is internal (less common), it is larger and can press on the conjunctiva. If the entire lid becomes swollen, it can progress to a cellulitis. Chalazion is a small nontender nodule that can be palpated within the upper or lower eyelid. If the lid is everted, a corresponding area of redness is seen. A chalazion may become infected, and the presentation would be similar to a hordeolum with painful swelling.

Physical Examination. Inspection of the eyelid and everting the lid usually confirm the diagnosis. If the hordeolum is internal, the cornea should be examined for abrasion (see previous section on corneal abrasion).

Diagnostic Test. None is indicated.

Differential Medical Diagnoses

Chalazion and hordeolum are often confused. Chalazion tend to be smaller and chronic; they are usually not painful unless they are quite large. Hordeolum presents with pain and localized redness.

Blepharitis (see following) involves the whole eyelid and is usually accompanied by scaling, itching, and burning.

Plan

Psychosocial Interventions. Both hordeolum and chalazion can be disfiguring and cause body image concerns. Reassure the client that if conservative measures do not resolve the conditions, prompt referral to the ophthalmologist will follow.

Medication and Treatment

HORDEOLUM
- Bacitracin or erythromycin ophthalmic ointment instilled into the conjunctival sac every 3 hours. (See above discussion of erythromycin ointment in section on conjunctivitis.)

SODIUM SULFACETIMIDE SOLUTION (SULAMYD-10)
- If drops preferred and client not allergic to sulfa, may be prescribed, two drops in affected eye every 3 hours while awake. (See previous discussion in section on conjunctivitis.)
- Warm compresses applied for 15 minutes to the affected eye three or four times a day are also helpful to reduce swelling. If the acute stage is not resolved within 48 hours, refer to an ophthalmologist for incision and drainage.

CHALAZION
- Erythromycin ophthalmic ointment. If the chalazion is large or if it appears to be infected,

inflamed, or affects vision, treat with erythromycin ophthalmic ointment and refer to an ophthalmologist.
- Small chalazion may be treated with warm compresses as above.

Lifestyle. Ophthalmic ointment may cause blurred vision and impair driving and close work. Advise client not to rub, scratch or touch eye, wash hands before and after applying medication or compresses.

Follow-Up

If hordeola recur client may have a chronic Staphylococcal infection of the eyelid. In addition, recurrent eyelid lesions may be basal cell carcinoma. Refer to the ophthalmologist.

BLEPHARITIS

Blepharitis is an inflammation of the lid margins that is usually chronic. There may be acute exacerbations and infectious flare-ups.

There are two types of blepharitis, anterior and posterior. Anterior blepharitis involves the eyelid skin, lashes, and glands. It may be chronic with swelling of the lids along the lash line and scaling of the skin. It is often associated with seborrhea and dandruff. There can be acute flare-ups of anterior blepharitis caused by staphylococci.

Posterior blepharitis is an inflammatory condition of the eyelids caused by dysfunction of the meibomian glands.

Epidemiology

Blepharitis is the most common disorder of the eyelids. The client often has associated seborrhea, dandruff, and/or acne rosacea.

Subjective Data

The client usually complains of burning, itching, and irritation. She may also have noted mucous discharge if the meibomian glands are inflamed.

Objective Data

Physical Examination. In anterior blepharitis, the client's eyes are red-rimmed and the conjunctiva may be injected. Scales may be seen clinging to the eyebrows and eyelids. If there is an acute flare, there may be a loss of lashes. The redness and crusting will be more pronounced.

In posterior blepharitis, telangiectasias can be seen on the lid margins. The openings of the meibomian glands may be plugged, inflamed, and exudative. Associated tears may be greasy. There may be mild entropion of the lid margin.

Diagnostic Test. Usually not indicated. Physical exam confirms the diagnosis.

Differential Medical Diagnoses

See previous section on hordeolum and chalazion page 830.

Plan

Psychosocial Interventions. Reassure the client that even though this is a chronic condition, flare-ups can be minimized with meticulous hygiene and self-care. Body image concerns should be explored because of the scaling and redness of the lids.

Medication and Treatment

ANTERIOR BLEPHARITIS

- If the client has frequent exacerbations, nightly application of erythromycin or bacitracin ophthalmic ointment applied with a cotton swab to the lid margin may be indicated. (See previous discussion of these medications in section on conjunctivitis.)
- Tar or selenium shampoo daily controls scaling of the scalp.
- Acute flare of anterior blepharitis is treated with sodium sulfacetamide (Sulamyd-10) drops every 2 to 3 hours while awake or erythromycin ointment applied four times a day. (See previous discussion of these medications in section on conjunctivitis.)
- The cornerstone of treatment is scrupulous hygiene of the scalp, eyebrows, and lid margins. Scales should be removed from the lashes and eyebrows with a damp cotton applicator dipped in baby shampoo twice a day. Advise the client to pull the lower lid down so that lash margins are thoroughly scrubbed. Follow with warm water cloth to rinse. If scales adhere to lashes, advise client to apply warm compresses for several minutes before swabbing with baby shampoo to loosen scales.

POSTERIOR BLEPHARITIS

- Inflammatory flares may require systemic therapy with erythromycin 250 mg four times a day or tetracycline 250 mg twice a day. (See previous discussion of these medications under common dermatological conditions.)
- Consult with physician regarding use of topical steroid drops.
- Mild posterior blepharitis may only require daily expression of meibomian glands by gentle pressure to lids followed by cleansing regimen as described previously.
- Client with associated entropion may require referral to ophthalmologist for surgery if lashes rub on cornea.[4]

Lifestyle Modifications. Advise the client to use hypoallergenic cosmetics and not to share eye make-up. She should avoid rubbing the eyes and wash hands often especially after touching eye area.

Follow-Up

During acute flares evaluate for response to therapy in 1 week. Encourage client to call if inflammation starts in order to initiate therapy promptly.

UVEITIS

Uveitis is an inflammation of the uveal tract of the eye, which includes the iris, ciliary body, and choroid. Uveitis is most often confined to the anterior structures of the iris and ciliary body. Posterior uveitis is rare and usually does not present with a painful red eye but with complaint of decreased vision and spots in the visual field.[5]

Epidemiology

In the client without accompanying systemic illness, the most common cause of acute anterior uveitis is trauma. Systemic disorders associated with anterior uveitis include the HLA-B27 complexes (sarcoidosis, psoriasis, inflammatory bowel disease, ankylosing spondylitis, Reiter's syndrome). Herpes simplex and herpes zoster may also cause anterior uveitis. Posterior uveitis may be caused by sarcoidosis (usually bilateral involvement), tuberculosis, syphilis, toxoplasmosis, leprosy. In many cases of anterior uveitis, no underlying cause is determined.[4,5]

Subjective Data

In anterior uveitis, the client complains of eye pain, redness, photophobia, and blurred vision. She may deny history of trauma or coexisting illness. In *posterior uveitis,* the client presents with complaint of gradual diminution of vision, spots appearing in the visual field, and no inflammation or pain.

Objective Data

Physical Examination. In *acute anterior uveitis,* the affected pupil is small and may be irregular. The conjunctiva is injected around the limbus. Profuse tearing may be present. In *posterior uveitis,* the eye appears normal or quiet.

Diagnostic Tests

Visual Acuity. Always record visual acuity. If client has forgotten or lost corrective lenses, a pinhole disk may be used to optimize acuity. Acuity in the affected eye is diminished from baseline.

Slit Lamp Examination. Slit lamp examination of the anterior chamber reveals inflammatory cells and flare.
NOTE: Practitioner who is not skilled in the use of a slit lamp should not attempt to examine the client without confirmation of findings made by physician.

Plan

Refer immediately to ophthalmologist. Treatment involves use of topical mydriatic and cycloplegic agents that dilate the pupil and paralyze the ocular muscles of accommodation and use of topical corticosteroids to suppress inflammation.

GLAUCOMA

Glaucoma is a condition of abnormally elevated pressure within the eye caused by an obstruction of outflow of the aqueous humor. Acute (angle closure) glaucoma occurs when the obstruction arises from the iris and blocks the exit of aqueous humor from the anterior chamber. It is acute in onset occurring with pupillary dilatation and is an ophthalmology emergency. The client must be referred immediately to prevent vision loss and damage to the optic nerve. Open angle glaucoma develops slowly from an obstruction within the

canal of Schlemm. Over time it too can cause optical nerve damage and blindness if not detected and treated appropriately.

Epidemiology

Glaucoma is the second most common cause of irreversible blindness in the United States. Acute angle closure glaucoma occurs less often than open angle glaucoma. Far-sighted women in their 50s are most likely to be affected as are Asians who may have a narrow anterior chamber angle.[4,6]

Open angle glaucoma is more common among African Americans with earlier onset, and more severe damage at time of diagnosis. The risk of glaucoma increases with age and has an hereditary pattern. Risk factors for damage to the optic nerve due to open angle glaucoma include the following: elevated intraocular pressure; enlargement of the optic cup; vascular abnormalities, e.g., hypertension, diabetes, migraine; myopia; and use of steroids.[4]

Subjective Data

Acute angle closure glaucoma presents with sudden onset of extreme pain and blurred vision. Client may associate onset with sitting in darkened theater, time of stress, or having pupil dilated during ophthalmoscopic examination. She may experience nausea and abdominal pain.

Open angle glaucoma has an insidious onset and there are no symptoms in the early stages. Later the client may note constriction of the visual field with central vision preserved. She may note haloes around lights if the intraocular pressure is markedly elevated.

Objective Data

Physical Examination. *Acute angle closure glaucoma* causes a red eye, steamy appearing cornea, and a moderately dilated pupil that is nonreactive to light. The globe feels hard when lightly touched. The client with *open angle glaucoma* has a normal appearing eye. The nurse practitioner in primary practice may not be skilled in tonometric measurement to assess intraocular pressure but she/he can perform the most useful method of screening, ophthalmoscopic examination of the optic disk. The average cup to disk ratio is 0.3 and is equal bilaterally. Examine disk for narrow rim and hemorrhage. An enlarged cup or an asymmetric cup-to-disk ratio is grounds for referral to an ophthalmologist for visual field and tonometric analysis.[6]

Assessment of visual fields by confrontation may be done but may not be reliable. Constriction of vision is gradual and subtle. Thorough examination is done with specialized equipment usually not found in primary practice and requires 10–20 minutes per eye.

Diagnostic Tests

VISUAL ACUITY. Central vision is usually preserved, but every good eye exam begins with acuity.

VISUAL FIELDS BY CONFRONTATION. Detects tunnel vision through use of special instrument used by trained personnel in optometrist or ophthalmologist's office.

TONOMETRY. Hand held tonometers are available and safe to use if the practitioner is trained and skilled in their use. The most accurate measurement is done by applanation tonometry as opposed to Schiotz tonometry, which may underestimate pressure. Normal intraocular pressure is 10–21 mm Hg. Diagnosis is not made on a single reading. It is important to note that client may have optic nerve damage with pressure below 22 mm Hg.[6]

Differential Medical Diagnoses

See Table 22–16.

- *Acute Angle Closure Glaucoma.* Client complains of intense pain and photophobia, pupils are unequal, cornea has steamy appearance.
- *Optic Neuritis.* Sudden loss of vision, pain especially with eye movement, usually central vision lost. Associated with underlying disorder as multiple sclerosis, sarcoidosis, systemic lupus erythematosus.

Plan

The client with acute angle closure glaucoma is referred immediately to a physician. It is an ocular emergency and is usually treated by laser iridotomy to reduce pressure. Subsequent treatment is the same as open angle glaucoma.

If open angle glaucoma is suspected, the client is referred for outpatient ophthalmologic evaluation as soon as possible.

Psychosocial Interventions. A diagnosis that carries with it the risk of blindness is very frightening. Reassure the client that with early diagnosis, treatment, and careful follow-up, glaucoma can be managed. A high level of compliance is necessary and the medications can be very expensive. Assessment of the client's support system and social situation is important to promote a favorable outcome.

Medication. Treatment for open angle glaucoma usually begins with a *topical beta adrenergic blocker* such as timolol or betaxolol. The mechanism of action is to reduce production of aqueous humor.

TOPICAL BETA ADRENERGIC BLOCKER
- *Administration.* One drop to the conjunctival sac twice a day. Advise client to press on the lacrimal sac after instillation to decrease systemic absorption.
- *Side Effects.* Bronchospasm, exacerbation of congestive heart failure, cardiac condition disturbance, depression, confusion, hypotension.
- *Contraindications.* Known hypersensitivity, severe bradycardia, overt cardiac failure, second and third degree heart block, asthma, severe chronic obstructive pulmonary disease.
- *Expected Outcome.* Ophthalmologist will monitor response to therapy and adjust dosage until maintenance drug regimen is determined. The practitioner should assess adherence and barriers to the treatment plan. He/she should examine the optic disc during periodic screenings between eye doctor visits for any changes.
- *Client Teaching.* Inform the client that glaucoma can be managed but not cured. Therefore, adherence to dosage and administration of eye drops is crucial. Inform client to report any adverse effects promptly.

MIOTICS PILOCARPINE. This is the most widely used agent. It lowers intraocular pressure through contraction of the sphincter muscle of the iris, resulting in pupil constriction.

- *Administration.* One or two drops in the eye four times per day.

- *Side Effects.* Blurred vision, increased bronchial secretions, nausea, vomiting, diarrhea.
- *Contraindications.* Known hypersensitivity, overt congestive heart failure.
- *Expected Outcome.* See aforementioned.
- *Client Teaching.* See prior information. Warn patient about blurred vision and driving or operating equipment.
- *Surgical Interventions.* Argon laser trabeculectomy may be performed on those for whom optimal pressure has not been achieved with topical medications or who are unable to tolerate these agents. It is done on an outpatient basis under topical anesthesia. Glaucoma filtration surgery is reserved for those clients who have failed all other methods. It involves establishing an alternative exit for aqueous humor. It can be done on an outpatient basis.[6]

Follow-Up

Request notification from ophthalmologist of any change in treatment regimen and timing of follow-up visits. Assess client adherence to plan of care.

CATARACTS

A cataract is an opacity of the lens of the eye. Because lens fibers are produced throughout a lifetime and none is lost, the density of the lens increases with age. A cataract may or may not be associated with visual impairment. The specific changes in vision that result are loss of contrast sensitivity and glare.

Epidemiology

Incidence of cataract increases with age after the age of 50. It is estimated from several studies that the prevalence is close to 50 percent in individuals over 75 years old. Risk factors associated with development include exposure to ultraviolet-B radiation, diabetes, smoking, heavy alcohol use, history of trauma, retinal detachment, prolonged systemic steroid therapy, and certain systemic illnesses such as diabetes, myotonic dystrophy, and atopic dermatitis.

Subjective Data

The client may complain of impaired vision, "like a fog over my eyes." The location of the opacity often determines whether near vision or far vision is affected. The client with a central opacity complains of glare because pupillary constriction causes light to enter the area most opacified. She may report that she sees better in low light than in well lighted rooms. She may have stopped driving at night due to the glare from oncoming headlights. Color vision may be impaired. There is no complaint of pain or redness.

Objective Data

Physical Examination. Conjunctiva are clear.

- *Funduscopic Examination.* As the cataract becomes denser, the retina becomes harder to visualize.

Diagnostic Tests
- *Visual Acuity.* May or may not be affected depending on location of opacity.

Differential Medical Diagnoses

Glaucoma, retinal vascular occlusive disorders, macular degeneration.

Plan

Refer client to an ophthalmologist for further evaluation. Other retinal disorders may be present.

Psychosocial Interventions. Reassure the client that early detection and regular follow-up with an ophthalmologist improves outcome. Advise client surgery may not be indicated immediately.

Medication. None.

Nonsurgical Measures. Changing eyeglass prescription as needed, especially when myopia is induced by the cataract. Bifocals, magnifying lenses, and appropriate lighting may be helpful until surgery is performed.

Surgery. The decision to perform surgery is based on clinical judgment and visual acuity, usually when acuity is reduced to 20/50 or less (based on state driving laws requiring better vision to drive). The latest technique involves ultrasonic fragmentation of the lens nucleus with implantation of an intraocular lens. Postoperative complications include risk of infection, glaucoma, retinal detachment, hemorrhage, posterior capsular opacification. In 95 percent of cases acuity is improved.[7]

Lifestyle. Before surgery client may have curtailed some activities such as night driving, hobbies, reading. She may experience the loss of independence or income.

Follow-Up

Usually followed by ophthalmologist for 6–8 weeks after surgery. The practitioner should continue to monitor vision and perform functional assessments at each visit after release from the surgeon. Be alert for posterior capsular pacification, which can develop several months to several years after removal of the lens. Signs and symptoms same as for cataracts.

PULMONARY DISORDERS

This section on disorders associated with the lung covers asthma and influenza as well as the lower respiratory tract infections, pneumonia and acute bronchitis.

ASTHMA

Asthma is a chronic inflammatory disorder of the airways. Chronic inflammation is responsible for increased airway hyperresponsiveness to a variety of stimuli, for recurrent symptoms, airway narrowing, and respiratory symptoms. Inflammation is responsible for acute bronchoconstriction, swelling of the airway wall, chronic mucus plug formation, and airway wall remodeling.[1,2,3] Asthma can begin in response to sensitizing agents and the development of atopy later in life. Atopy is considered to be the strongest risk factor for the development of asthma.[1,4,5]

It is important to understand that any client with asthma, regardless of severity, may develop an acute severe asthma exacerbation. The clients most at risk are those with a history of multiple hospital admissions, past intubation, multiple pysch/social problems, a recent decrease in corticosteroids, and noncompliance with lifestyle modifications and medications.

Effective management of asthma relies on four integral components: measurement of lung function to assess and monitor the client's asthma; pharmacologic therapy; environmental measures to control allergens and irritants; and client education.[1,2,5]

An acute asthma exacerbation has an early and late phase response. The early /bronchoconstrictive phase is characterized by the rapid development of reversible airway obstruction in response to a stimulus, usually within minutes but may occur up to 2 hours later.

The late phase response can occur 6 to 12 hours later. It is an inflammatory response less likely to respond to bronchodilators.

Epidemiology

Asthma morbidity and mortality are on the rise. From 1980 to 1987, the prevalence rate of asthma in the United States increased 29 percent, and death rates for asthma as the first listed diagnosis increased 31 percent. In 1988, asthma related health care costs exceeded $4 billion in the United States.[1,2,5] Asthma is associated with predisposing and causal factors and can vary in severity (see Table 22–17).

Subjective Data

The client may report a history of any of the following: chest tightness, shortness of breath, dyspnea on exertion, or a nonproductive cough. The symptoms may occur with exercise, exposure to animals with fur, smoke, pollen, changes in temperature, strong emotional expression, aerosol chemicals, and dust mites. Many clients will have a history of childhood asthma, a history of seasonal allergies, and/or a family history of asthma.

Objective Data

Physical Examination. The physical examination between exacerbations may be normal.

Evaluate the client for signs of atopy: eczema, allergic conjunctivitis, rhinitis, coughing, sneezing.

TABLE 22–17. AGENTS CAUSING ASTHMA IN SELECTED OCCUPATIONS

Occupation or Occupational Field	Agent
laboratory animal workers, veterinarian	dander and urine proteins
food processing	shellfish, egg proteins, pancreatic enzymes, papain, amylase
dairy farmers	storage mites
poultry farmers	poultry mites, droppings and feathers
granary workers	storage mites, aspergillus, indoor ragweed, and grass pollen
research workers	locusts
fish food manufacturing	midges
detergent manufacturing	*Bacillus subtilis* enzymes
silk workers	silk-worm moths and larvas
bakers	flour, amylase
food processing	coffee bean dust, meat tenderizer (papain), tea
farmers	soy bean dust
shipping workers	grain dust (molds, insects, grain)
laxative manufacturing	ispaghula, psyllium
sawmill workers, carpenters	wood dust (western red cedar, oak, mahogany, zebrawood, redwood, Lebanon cedar, African maple, eastern white cedar)
electric soldering	colophony (pine resin)
cotton textile workers	cotton dust
nurses	psyllium, latex
	Inorganic Chemicals:
refinery workers	platinum salts, vandium
plating	nickel salts
diamond polishing	cobalt salts
manufacturing	aluminum fluoride
beauty shop	persulfate
welding	stainless steel fumes, chromium salts
	Organic Chemicals:
manufacturing	antibiotics, piperazine, methyldopa, salbutamol, cimetidine
hospital workers	disinfectants (sulfathiazole, chloramine, formaldehyde, glutaraldehyde)
anesthesiology	enflurane
poultry workers	aprolium
fur dyeing	paraphenylene diamine
rubber processing	formaldehyde, ethylene diamine, phthalic anhydride
plastics industry	toluene diisocyanate, hexamethyl diisocyanate, dephenylmethyl isocyanate, phthalic anhydride, triethylene tetramines, trimellitic anhydride, hexamethyl tetramine
automobile painting	dimethyl ethanolamine diisocyanates
foundry worker	reaction product of furan binder

Source: International Census Report on Diagnoses and Treatment of Asthma. (1992). (NIH Publication No. 92–3091).

During an exacerbation, the client may exhibit signs of acute respiratory distress such as wheezing, coughing, tachycardia, and anxiety.

Diagnostic Tests. In clients with mild to moderate asthma, all laboratory tests may be normal. Well controlled asthma blood gases will be normal.

During an exacerbation, mild to moderate hypoxia and hypocapnia with a respiratory alkalosis may be present. During a severe exacerbation, respiratory acidosis may be present.

Measurement of lung function for diagnosing asthma is analogous to measurement in other chronic disease. For most, peak expiratory flow

(PEF) correlates well with FEV1.[1,2,3] Regular home monitoring can help clients detect early signs of deterioration.

Differential Medical Diagnoses

Cardiac disorders, allergic rhinitis/sinusitis, sarcoidosis, chronic obstructive pulmonary disease, airway obstruction, cystic fibrosis pulmonary embolism, gastroesophageal disorders, cough associated with angiotensin converting enzymes inhibitors, obesity.

Plan

Treatment must be individualized with consideration to medication, risk reduction and severity of disease.

Psychosocial Intervention. Clients with asthma frequently have poor recognition of their symptoms and poor perception of severity, especially if their asthma is severe and long standing.[2] Clients frequently are concerned with lost time from work and decreased productivity. The client may also need to consider a job change away from triggering agents.

Medication. Medication choice focuses on airway inflammation associated with both acute and chronic asthma. The trend is to focus on preventive use of avoidance strategies and anti-inflammatory drugs to treat the underlying disease process rather than only the acute consequences. See Tables 22–18, 22–19, 22–20, and 22–21. Clients with asthma are at risk for flus and pneumonia; consider influenza and pneumovax vaccines.

Client Education. Stress avoidance of known triggers, proper use of metered dose inhalers, and use of peak flow monitors, and smoking cessation.

Follow-Up

Follow-up of acute exacerbations should be individualized based on severity and client comfort and reliability.

Asymptomatic clients should be followed on as an needed basis with emphasis placed on continued client education.

TABLE 22–18. TOLERANCE OF NONSTEROIDAL ANTI-INFLAMMATORY DRUGS IN ASPIRIN-INDUCED ASTHMA

Precipitate Asthma Exacerbations	Well Tolerated (Cause no bronchoconstriction)
Salicylates	Sodium salicylate
Aspirin	Choline salicylate
Diflunisal	Choline magnesium
Salesate (salicylsalicylic acid)	Salicylamide
Polycyclic acids	Dextropropoxyphene
Acetic acids	Azapropazone
Incomethacin	Benzydamine
Suliudac	Chloroquine
Tolmetin	Paracetamol*
Arylaliphatic acids	
Naproxen	
Diclofanac	
Fenoprofen	
Ibuprofen	
Ketoprofen	
Tiaprofenic acid,	
Fluribrofen	
Enolic acids	
Piroxicam	
Fenamates	
Mefanamic acid	
Flufenamic acid	
Cyclofenamic acid	
Pyrazolones	
Aminopyrine	
Noramaidopyrine	
Sulfinpyrazone	
Phenylbutazone	

*When beginning therapy, give half a tablet of paracetamol and observe patient 2 to 3 hours for symptoms that occur in no more than 5 percent of patients.
Source: References 1, 3, 18.

INFLUENZA

Influenza, an acute, usually self-limiting, upper respiratory infection, may be caused by influenza A, B, or C virus. Strains of the A virus are the most common and most virulent. B virus infection has some increased association with Reye's syndrome. C virus infection is a mild illness, usually not significant or identified clinically.

Epidemiology

Etiology of the influenza virus reveals the unique ability to vary antigenically from year to year, hence the terms antigenic drift (minor variations) and antigenic shift (major variations). Prior

TABLE 22–19. DIAGNOSE AND CLASSIFY SEVERITY OF ASTHMA

	Clinical Features Before Treatment	Medication Required to Maintain Control
Step 4 **Severe** **Persistent**	Continuous symptoms Frequent exacerbations Frequent nighttime asthma symptoms Physical activities limited by asthma symptoms PEF or FEV • ≤60% predicted; • variability>30%	Multiple daily long-term preventive medications: high doses inhaled corticosteroid, long-acting bronchodilator, and oral corticosteroid long term
Step 3 **Moderate** **Persistent**	Symptoms daily Exacerbations affect activity and sleep Nighttime asthma symptoms >1 time a week daily use of inhaled short-acting B-agonist PEF or FEV • >60% – <80% predicted; • variability >30%	Daily long-term preventive medications; inhaled corticosteroid and long-acting bronchodilator (especially for nighttime symptoms)
Step 2 **Mild** **Persistent**	Symptoms ≥1 time a week but <1 time per day Exacerbations may affect activity and sleep Nighttime asthma symptoms >2 times a month PEF or FEV • ≥80% predicted; • variability 20–30%	One daily long-term preventive medication; possibly add a long-acting bronchodilator to anti-inflammatory medication (especially for nighttime symptoms)
Step 1 **Intermittent**	Intermittent symptoms <1 time a week Brief exacerbations (from a few hours to a few days) Nighttime asthma symptoms ≤2 times a month Asymptomatic and normal lung function between exacerbations PEF or FEV • ≥80% predicted; • variability <20%	• Intermittent quick-relief medication taken as needed only; inhaled short-acting B-agonist • Intensity of treatment depends on severity of exacerbation; oral corticosteroids may be required

Source: Asthma Management and Prevention: Global Institute for Asthma. 1995, December. (NIH Publication No. 90-3659A).

exposure provides limited immunity. Epidemics occur every 2 to 3 years; about every 10 years, the strains vary dramatically and produce a "pandemic."[3,6]

Transmission is primarily through aerosolized particles from a cough or sneeze, although the virus can be spread by clothing or hand contact. The incubation period is about 18 to 72 hours. Infectious viral shedding occurs for 10 days but is most prominent in the first 48 hours of illness.

In an epidemic year, 20 to 30 percent of the population may contract influenza. Deaths are usually due to pneumonia (influenza pneumonia is the sixth leading cause of death in the United States) or to cardiovascular decompensation related to the influenza.[3,6]

Groups at risk for influenza complications include persons over 65, persons with chronic cardiac or pulmonary disorders, persons with chronic metabolic disorders (e.g., diabetes mellitus), renal dysfunction, immunosuppression, and nursing home residents.[3,5,6,7]

Subjective Data

History reveals the four hallmarks of influenza: headache, myalgias, especially in the legs and back; fever, often to 102° F to 104° F for 3 to 4 days or longer; and nonproductive cough, which usually is not prominent at the beginning of illness but increases over time. Watery eyes and dry throat may be present, but nasal symptoms are usually absent.

TABLE 22–20. TREATMENTS IN THE STEPWISE APPROACH TO LONG-TERM MANAGEMENT OF ASTHMA

	Long-Term Preventive	Quick-Relief
Step 4 **Severe** **Persistent**	Daily medications: • **Inhaled corticosteroid,** 800–2000 mcg or more, and • Long-acting bronchodilator; either long-acting inhaled B-agonist, sustained-release theophylline, and/or long-acting B-agonist tablets or syrup, and • Corticosteroid tablets or syrup long-term.	• Short-acting bronchodilator: **inhaled B-agonist** as needed for symptoms
Step 3 **Moderate** **Persistent**	Daily medications: • **Inhaled corticosteroid,** 800–2000 mcg and • Long-acting bronchodilator, especially for nighttime symptoms; either long-acting inhaled B-agonist, sustained release theophylline, or long-acting B-agonist tablets or syrup.	• Short-acting bronchodilator: **inhaled B-agonist** as needed for symptoms, not to exceed 3–4 times in 1 day
Step 2 **Mild** **Persistent**	Daily medications: • Either **inhaled corticosteroid,** 200–500 mcg, **cromoglycate, nedocromil,** or sustained-release theophylline • If needed, increase inhaled corticosteroids, if inhaled corticosteroids currently equal 500 mcg, increase the corticosteroids up to 800 mcg, or add long-acting bronchodilator (especially for nighttime symptoms); either long-acting inhaled B-agonist, sustained-release theophylline, or long-acting B-agonist tablets or syrup.	• Short-acting bronchodilator: **inhaled B-agonist** as needed for symptoms, not to exceed 3–4 times in 1 day
Step 1 **Intermittent**	None needed	• Short-acting bronchodilator: **inhaled B-agonist** as needed for symptoms, but less than once a week • Intensity of treatment will depend on severity of attack • Inhaled B-agonist or cromoglycate before exercise or exposure to allergen

Source: Asthma Management and Prevention: Global Institute for Asthma. 1995, December. (NIH Publication No. 96-3659A).

Objective Data

Physical Examination. The client may be flushed and sweating. She appears ill. High fever is common, usually greater than 102° F, but rarely 106° F or higher. Heart and respiratory rates are increased.

The eyes, ears, nose, and throat usually appear normal. The lungs are clear. If crackles or rhonchi are heard, obtain a chest x-ray to rule out influenza pneumonia.

Monitor the heart to assess cardiovascular status. Influenza may precipitate cardiovascular failure in cardiac clients.

Diagnostic Tests. Usually not required unless the fever lasts longer than 4 days, in which case a white blood cell count should be ordered. If the WBC is greater than 12,000, suspect pneumonia and order a chest x-ray.

Differential Medical Diagnoses

Parainfluenza virus, respiratory syncytial virus, adenovirus, other viral syndromes. In the absence of an epidemic, it is difficult to identify influenza from many other viral syndromes. Note that influenza is always associated with cough.

Plan

Psychosocial Interventions. Inform the client about the expected course of disease, and teach the warning signs of influenza pneumonia and cardiac complications. Reassure her that taking acetaminophen is permitted. Aspirin, however, should be avoided because of its association with Reye's syndrome. Comfort will be increased and myalgia decreased if fever is controlled.

Medication. Medication is administered for prophylaxis and treatment.

TABLE 22–21. LONG-TERM PREVENTIVE MEDICATIONS FOR ASTHMA

Name and also Known As	Generic Name	Mechanism of Action	Side Effects (risk for serious side effects)	Long-Term Effect	Quick-Relief Effect
Corticosteroids adrenocorticoids flucocorticoids	**Inhaled:** beclomethasone budesonide flunisolide fluticasone triamcinolone **Tablets or syrups:** Prednisolone prednisone methylprednisolone	**Anti-inflammatory agent:** Prevents and suppresses activation and migration of inflammatory cells; reduces airway swelling, mucus production, and microvascular leakage; increases responsiveness of smooth muscle beta receptors	**Inhaled** corticosteroids (+) have few known adverse effects. Use of spacers and mouth washing after inhalation help prevent oral candidiasis. Doses above 1 mg a day may be associated with skin thinning, easy bruising, and adrenal suppression. **Tablet or syrup** corticosteroids (+++) used long term may lead to osteoporosis, arterial hypertension, diabetes, cataracts, hypothalamic-pituitary-adrenal axis suppression, obesity, skin thinning, or muscle weakness.	**Inhaled:** Yes+++ **Tablets or syrups:** Yes++	**Inhaled:** No **Tablets or syrups:** ++ yes (over hours)
Sodium cromoglycate cromolyn cromolyn sodium cromones		**Anti-inflammatory agent:** inhibits activation of, and mediator release from, inflammatory cells.	(–) Minimal side effects. Cough may occur upon inhalation.	+ Yes	– None
Nedocromil cromones nedocramil sodium		**Anti-inflammatory agent:** inhibits activation of, and mediator release from, inflammatory cells.	(–) None known	+ Yes	– None
Long-action, beta-agonists long-acting beta-adrenergics sympathomimetics	**Inhaled:** salmeterol formoterol **Sustained-release tablets:** terbutaline salbutamol	**Bronchodilator:** Opens airways by relaxing airway smooth muscle, enhancing mucociliary clearance, and decreasing vascular permeability.	**Inhaled** beta-agonists have fewer, and less significant, side effects than tablets. **Tablet** beta-agonists (+) may cause cardiovascular stimulation, anxiety, pyrosis, skeletal muscle tremor, headache, or hypokalemia.	**Inhaled:** Yes ++ **Tablets:** Yes+/–	Not to be used to treat attacks
Sustained-release theophylline amiophyline methylxanthine xanthine		**Bronchodilator** with uncertain anti-inflammatory effect; Inhibits early and late reactions to allergen.	(++) Nausea and vomiting are most common. Serious effects occurring at higher serum concentrations, include seizures, tachycardia, and arrhythmias. Theophylline monitoring is often required; see text.	+ Yes	++ Yes

Ketotifen	**Antiallergic agent**	May cause sedation and weight gain.	+ Yes children	– None
Short-acting beta-agonists adrenegics beta-stimulants sympathomimetics albuteral bitolteral fenoherol isoetharine metaproterenol pibuteroll salbutamol terbutaline	**Bronchodilator:** Open airways by relaxing airway smooth muscle, enhancing mucociliary clearance, and decreasing vascular permeability.	**Inhaled** beta-agonists have fewer, and less significant, side effects than tablets or syrups. **Tablet or syrup** beta-agonists (+) may cause cardiovascular stimulation, skeletal muscle tremor, headache, and irritability.	**Inhaled:** +/– some **Tablets or syrups:** +/– some	**Inhaled:** +++ Yes **Tablets or syrups:** ++ Yes
	Bronchodilator: Reduces vagal tone to airways. Slower onset of action than beta-agonists.	(–) Minimal mouth dryness or bad taste in the mouth.	–	++
	Bronchodilator	(++) Nausea, vomiting. At higher serum concentrations: seizures, tachycardia, and arrhythmias; theophylline monitoring may be required—see text.	+/–	+
	Bronchodilator that also treats anaphylaxis and angioedema.	(++) Similar, but more significant effects than beta-agonist. In addition; convulsions, chills, fever, and hallucinations.	Not recommended for long-term treatment.	In general, not recommended for treating asthma attacks if beta-agonists are available.

Source: Asthma Management and Prevention: Global Institute for Asthma. 1995, December. (NIH Publication No. 96—3659A).

AMANTADINE. Amantadine (Symmetrel) is the only drug approved for both prophylaxis and treatment in influenza A; it is not effective against influenza B.

- *Administration.* For prophylaxis, administer for 2 weeks with a late vaccine in the midst of an outbreak. For treatment amantadine must be given within 24 to 28 hours of the onset of symptoms.

  The usual adult dose for those 65 years or younger is 200 mg bid for 10 to 14 days.
- *Side Effects.* Side effects are infrequent and cease when medication is stopped. The client may experience central nervous system symptoms, including nervousness, dizziness, and insomnia.
- *Contraindications.* Do not administer to any client with renal compromise or clients older than 65 years.
- *Expected Outcomes.* When used for treatment, amantadine should decrease the severity and duration of illness.
- *Client Teaching.* When amantadine is given for prophylaxis, inform the client that it is 70 to 90 percent effective in preventing influenza A and it is only protective for the duration of therapy. It does not replace the vaccine as it fails to work against influenza B.

INFLUENZA TRIVALENT VACCINE. The high risk groups for whom annual administration of vaccine is currently recommended are persons with congenital or acquired heart disease, chronic lung disease, chronic renal disease, chronic severe anemia, and immunocompromising illness (diabetes, cancer). Others for whom the vaccine is indicated are persons over 60, those living in chronic care/nursing homes, family members of high risk groups and health care workers.

- *Administration.* Influenza trivalent vaccine (two strains of A and one of B) is administered annually beginning in September. Vaccinations begin protection in 2 weeks; protection peaks in 1 to 2 months and gradually declines over time. Vaccines may be given anytime after an outbreak begins but should be supplemented with 2 weeks of amantadine treatment until the vaccine can induce a response.

- *Side Effects.* Side effects are rare with modern inactivated vaccines. Less than 5 percent of recipients develop a febrile reaction; some local soreness may be noted.
- *Contraindications.* Those with an egg allergy or febrile illness.
- *Expected Outcome.* The vaccine will be 80 percent effective in preventing disease. If the disease is contracted, the course of illness will be less severe.
- *Contraindications.* There are no contraindications to administering the vaccine in combination with other childhood and adult vaccines provided they are given at separate sites.
- *Client Teaching.* Encourage the client to obtain the vaccine annually in September rather than waiting for symptoms to appear. Stress that influenza is contagious.

Lifestyle Changes. Encourage the client to increase intake of fluids to prevent dehydration, to get adequate bed rest, to avoid contact with others; discourage smoking.

Follow-Up

Influenza pneumonia occurs approximately 1 week after the onset of influenza symptoms. It is characterized by severe dyspnea, cyanosis, and often scanty blood-tinged sputum. The lungs may sound clear, evaluation by chest x-ray and pulse oximetry will assist in determining severity of illness. Pneumonia, which can occur at any age, accounts for one-half of the deaths associated with influenza. If you suspect pneumonia, refer the client for possible hospital admission.

Preventing influenza is crucial. Only 20 percent of the high risk population is vaccinated against this deadly disease, and amantadine is underused in epidemics. To facilitate implementation of a vaccination program in an office setting, one staff member should be designated to head the effort each fall. During that season, charts of high risk clients should be flagged and posters placed in waiting and exam rooms. Consider becoming involved in a communitywide education effort.

LOWER RESPIRATORY TRACT INFECTIONS: PNEUMONIA AND ACUTE BRONCHITIS

Pneumonia is defined as an acute infection of the alveolar spaces or interstitial tissues (or both) of the lung. There are four classifications of pneumonia: typical, or classic bacterial, pneumonia; atypical pneumonia; aspiration pneumonia; and hematogenous pneumonia. This section focuses on the two types seen most often in primary care, typical and atypical.

Acute bronchitis has been defined as an acute, usually transient, inflammation of the tracheobronchial tree.[8] It most often occurs in response to a viral infection, to a noxious stimulus, or to the use of certain medications, such as angiotensin-converting enzyme inhibitors. Secondary bacterial bronchitis can be a complication of a viral respiratory infection. Invaders include the usual respiratory pathogens, such as Streptococcus pneumonia, Hemophilus influenza, Chlamydia pneumonia, and Mycoplasma pneumonia (see Table 22–22).

Epidemiology

Studies show more than 4 million cases of pneumonia are diagnosed annually; of these approximately 800,000 require hospitalization.[3,8,9] It is the most common cause of infectious death in the United States. The very young, the very old, and the immunocompromised are most at risk. Acute bronchitis is more common; a large percentage of cases are caused by viral pathogens or atypical pathogens.

Subjective Data

The symptoms reported by clients with pneumonia and acute bronchitis are compared in Table 22–23.

Pneumococcal pneumonia has a classic history of a sudden onset of rigor and fever of 101° to 106° F. Clients report a rusty colored or purulent sputum, chest pain, and shortness of breath.

Mycoplasma pneumonia, on the other hand, has a less dramatic clinical picture and history. The cough is paroxysmal and may be nonproductive. Fatigue and shortness of breath are common.

TABLE 22–22. PNEUMONIA PATHOGENS OBSERVED IN PRIMARY CARE

Classic	Atypical
Common	
Streptococcus pneumoniae (also called pneumococcal)	Mycoplasma pneumoniae
	Viral
Uncommon	
Haemophilus influenzae	Legionella pneumophila
Staphylococcus aureus	Chlamydia psittaci
Klebsiella pneumoniae	Francisella tularensis

Source: References 10, 11, 19, 20, 21.

Questions to ask include the following: How long has the cough lasted? Was the cough preceded by a URI? Have you missed work or school? Do you have an underlying respiratory disorder? Did the cough begin abruptly? Did the cough begin after the initiation of a new medication?

Objective Data

Physical Examination. Positive findings on exam can be found in Table 22–23.

Diagnostic Tests

Labwork. Is ordered only if pneumonia is suspected. The serum white blood count is often higher than 12,000 in pneumonia and normal in bronchitis. Cold agglutinins are found in 75 percent of cases of Mycoplasma pneumonia (titer of 1:64 or greater). Arterial blood gases can be useful in determining severity of illness.

Chest X-ray. Is indicated if pneumonia is suspected and will guide treatment and follow-up. Lobar or segmental consolidation is strongly suggestive of Pneumococcal pneumonia. The chest x-ray may be false negative if the client is dehydrated.

Gram Stain. A gram stain of sputum may be helpful if an adequate sample is obtained. Good smears have fewer than 10 squamous epithelial cells and more than 25 neutrophils per high power field. These results can guide empirical therapy if one organism predominates. Gram-positive diplococci suggests Streptoccus pneumonia; Gram-negative coccobacilli suggests Haemophilus influenzae; absence of a predominant bacterium with neutrophils suggests Mycoplasma pneumoniae.

TABLE 22–23. HISTORY AND EXAMINATION TO DIFFERENTIATE PNEUMONIA AND ACUTE BRONCHITIS

Symptoms/Signs	Bronchitis	Pneumonia
History		
Onset	Gradual, over 5–10 days, usually preceded by URI*	Acute onset, ± preceding URI
Fever	Mild or absent	Usually 101–106 °F
Chills	Mild, recurring, or intermittent	True "rigor," teethrattling chill
Chest pain	Vague "tightness" or chest congestion	Intense, pleuritic, localized
Sputum	Scant to copious	"Rusty" colored in pneumococcal or mucopurulent
Dyspnea	Rare	Common
Examination		
General appearance	Not toxic, no apparent distress	Often toxic, weak, may use accessory muscles
Vital signs	Often normal	Often tachycardia, tachypnea, fever
HEENT*	Heart	Normal or findings consistent with URI
Lungs		Crackles, won't clear with cough; signs of consolidation (E to A changes, dull to percussion) ± rub
Heart	At normal baseline	Tachycardia

*URI, Upper respiratory infection; HEENT, head, eyes, ears, nose and throat.
Source: References 7, 8, 9, 11, 20, 21.

A sputum culture, if carefully obtained, will confirm the diagnosis and is critical for immunocompromised clients.

Differential Medical Diagnoses

Asthma, exposure to noxious substances, allergic rhinitis, gastroesophageal reflux disorder, medication induced, aspiration, other infectious causes, pulmonary edema and foreign body.

Plan

Psychosocial Interventions. Reassure the client and teach her the warning signs of potential complications. In addition, advise her to notify the health care provider immediately if symptoms of complications develop (see Table 22–24).

Medication. Antibiotics and metered-dose inhalers (MDIs) are used in treatment. Pneumonococcal vaccine is used in prevention.

Antibiotics. See Table 22–25. There is great debate in the literature concerning the use of antibiotics in bronchitis. Most literature is advocating a watch and wait approach. If the client develops symptoms of complications or shows no improvement in 3 days, the use of antibiotics should be considered. When considering the use of extended spectrum antibiotics such as clarithromycin or azithromycin, consider the cost as well as efficacy.

- *Metered-Dose Inhalers.* MDIs can be useful in treating the cough associated with acute bronchitis. (See Table 22–21.)
- *Pneumococcal Polysaccharide Vaccine.* It is recommended for healthy adults over 65; anyone with heart, lung, liver, or renal disease; diabetics; alcoholics; immunocompromised adults (including clients with HIV and splenectomized clients); and children older than 2 years who have risk factors such as sickle cell disease, HIV, and nephrotic syndrome.

TABLE 22–24. CRITERIA FOR OUTPATIENT MANAGEMENT OF PNEUMONIA*

1. Able to take fluids and oral medications
2. Not toxic, no respiratory distress, only single lobe involvement
3. No underlying chronic disease, such as chronic obstructive pulmonary disease or diabetes
4. Pneumonia not related to aspiration (alcoholism or sedation, for example)
5. Adequate support system at home to provide care, observation, and immediate transportation to hospital if condition worsens.

*Client must meet the following criteria.
Source: References 10, 11, 19, 20, 21.

TABLE 22–25. ANTIBIOTICS FOR LOWER RESPIRATORY INFECTIONS*

Pneumococcal pneumonia	Penicillin V (betapen) 250–500 mg p.o.q.i.d. × 14 days
Mycoplasma pneumonia	Erythromycin 250–500 mg p.o.q.i.d. × 14 days
Pneumonia, etiology unknown	Erythromycin 250 mg p.o.q.i.d. × 14 days
Bronchitis	Usually of viral origin; no antibiotics indicated. If mycoplasma bronchitis or secondary bacterial bronchitis is suspected, erythromycin 250 mg p.o. q.i.d. × 10 days is treatment of choice. Smokers are highly likely to develop a secondary bacterial bronchitis. Trimethoprim-sulfameth oxazole or amoxicillin may be administered to treat mixed organisms or *Haemophilus influenzae.*

*For details see a current pharmacotherapeutics text.
Source: References 8, 10, 11, 19, 20, 21.

Recent recommendations are to revaccinate after 6 years individuals at highest risk and to revaccinate without waiting those individuals who are highest risk who have received the 14-valent vaccine.[5] Refer to a current pharmacotherapeutics text.

- *Administration.* The vaccine is given in a single intramuscular dose.
- *Side Effects.* Side effects are minor and local. Fifty percent of clients experience pain or redness at the site of injection; one percent have a fever or rash.
- *Contraindication.* Do not administer to any client who has had a known reaction to the vaccine or an egg allergy.
- *Expected Outcome.* Overall, the vaccine has a protective effect in 64 percent of recipients.[5]
- *Client Teaching.* Encourage the client to receive the vaccine if she is in a high risk category. Emphasize that more than 500,000 cases of pneumonia occur every year with a 5 percent mortality rate. Discuss the side effects with the client.

Lifestyle Changes. Advise the client to humidify the environment if possible, to increase the intake of fluids, to get proper nutrition, and to rest. Cough suppressants are used only if the cough is excessive and disrupts rest. Discourage smoking.

Follow-Up

Any client with pneumonia should be reevaluated every 24 hours. Most clients with pneumonia should be afebrile in 72 hours. Refer for hospitalization any client who does not rapidly improve. Possible complications of pneumonia include pleural effusion, emphysema (suspect a lung abscess if fever persists), disseminated intravascular coagulation, and nephritis.[9,10,11,12]

Clients with bronchitis should gradually improve and the cough resolve over the course of several weeks. Any client with a cough lasting more than 6 weeks requires a chest x-ray to rule out other conditions such as lung cancer, lymphoma, tuberculosis, and pulmonary edema. If the x-ray is negative, consider asthma.

CHRONIC OBSTRUCTIVE PULMONARY DISEASE

Chronic obstructive pulmonary disease (COPD) refers to several pulmonary disorders with airway obstruction as the common denominator. The two most common disorders, emphysema and chronic bronchitis, will be addressed here. Chronic bronchitis is characterized by cough and hypersecretion (phlegm production) for at least 3 months of the year for 2 consecutive years with airway obstruction documented by spirometry. Emphysema is characterized by abnormal permanent enlargement of the airspaces distal to the terminal bronchiole, destruction of their walls, and without obvious fibrosis. Most clients with COPD demonstrate features of coexistent chronic bronchitis (pink puffer) and emphysema (blue bloater). Pure forms of chronic bronchitis and emphysema are rare.[3,13]

Cigarette smoking is the single most important risk factor for the development of COPD. Clients with COPD may exhibit signs of bronchial hyperresponsiveness with episodes of wheezing in addition to their baseline airway obstruction.[3,5,14]

Epidemiology

COPD is the fourth leading cause of death in the United States; more than half of patients with COPD die within 10 years of diagnosis. Cigarette smoking is the most common cause of COPD. Cigar and pipe smoking also increase risk but to a lesser extent. Host susceptability is a key factor since approximately 15 percent of smokers develop COPD. Males are affected more often than females, but this is changing as more females continue to smoke. Chronic exposure to coal, cement, grain dusts, or acid fumes, could result in chronic bronchitis.[3,5,13,14]

Subjective Data

The client will give a history of smoking or chronic occupational exposure. She will usually be over 50 but may be significantly younger relative to the age of onset and number of cigarettes per day.

Chronic bronchitis is characterized by cough, phlegm production (white/gray, worse in the morning), and dyspnea. Clients with emphysema will complain of dyspnea and little productive cough.

Objective Data

Physical Examination
- *General.* Normal body weight with chronic bronchitis. Weight loss with emphysema.
- *Skin.* Cyanosis with advanced disease.
- *Neck.* Jugular venous distention.
- *Lungs.* Tachypnea, accessory muscle use, pursed lip breathing, wheezing, rhonchi that shift with cough, decreased breath sounds.
- *Heart.* Positive S-3 or S-4 with advanced disease.
- *Abdomen.* Accessory muscle use. Enlarged liver with advanced disease.
- *Extremities.* Lower extremity edema with advanced disease.

Diagnostic Tests. Pulmonary function tests (PFTs) to assess for obstruction. Arterial blood gases to assess oxygenation. An oxygenation saturation of less than 88 percent and a PaO_2 of less than 55 is indicative of severe hypoxemia requiring supplemental oxygen.[3,5,14,15,16] A complete blood count (CBC) may demonstrate polycythemia. A chest x-ray may demonstrate overdistended lungs.

Differential Medical Diagnoses

Asthma, congestive heart failure, sarcoidosis, interstitial lung disease, cystic fibrosis, sleep apnea, and cardiac disease.

Plan

Encourage smoking cessation. Studies show a significant improvement in lung function and slowing of the rate of decline in FEV1.[3,5,13]

Psychosocial Interventions. Involve the client in decisions concerning treatment. Acknowledge COPD is a chronic debilitating disease that can be treated and quality of life can be improved. Discuss the possibility of progression of the disease. Discuss with the client and her significant others advanced directive wishes.

Depression, fear and chronic fatigue are common occurrences in clients with COPD and are frequently related to the client's emotional state not pulmonary dysfunction.[5,13,15,16] Inability to carry out activities of daily living can lead to low self-esteem. Assess the client's emotional state at frequent intervals.

Medication

BRONCHODILATORS. Beta-agonists (e.g., albuterol) are effective in hyperreactive clients. They have a rapid onset of action. Caution must be used in clients with cardiac disease.[1,2,3,4,17,18]

ANTICHOLINERGICS (IPRATROPIUM). In stable COPD, ipratropium is a more potent bronchodilator. Ipratropium and albuterol have an additive effect when combined.[13]

METHYLXANTHINES. Theophylline has a narrow therapeutic range and can have potentially life threatening interactions with other drugs. Long acting preparations can have a positive effect on nocturnal symptoms. Caution must be used in clients with cardiac and/or hepatic disorders.[1,2,3,4,17,18]

CORTICOSTEROIDS. The efficacy of corticosteroids in COPD has not been established. Inhaled corticosteroids are beneficial in clients with underlying hyperreactive/inflammatory processes. See Table 22–21.

OTHER MEDICATIONS. Encourage the client to receive the *influenza vaccination* annually. The client should receive *amantadine* for any high risk exposures (see Influenza section).

The client should receive a *Pneumovax* injection at the time of diagnosis and every 6 years after. These injections will decrease the risk of further lung damage and possible progression of COPD.[5,6,7]

Oxygen. Home oxygen therapy has been documented to increase the life span and improve quality of life in hypoxemic clients.[3,15,16] Oxygen is indicated when the PaO_2 reaches 55 or below and/or the O_2 saturation reaches 88 percent or below. The dosage of oxygen should be the liters per minute needed to attain a PaO_2 between 65 and 80 mm Hg.[15] The usual dose is 2 liters per minute.

Lifestyle/Dietary Changes. Encourage the client to increase her hydration to two to four liters in 24 hours to thin secretions and facilitate expectoration. The client with COPD has increased nutritional needs at a time when her disease may make her feel anorexic secondary to increased work of breathing, diaphragm pressure. Encourage the client to eat small, frequent, high calorie meals. A nutrition consult may be helpful. Encourage frequent regular exercise. The American Lung Association and local hospitals frequently offer support groups.

Follow-Up

Regular follow-up to assess for progression of disease, nutritional status, psychosocial status, medication usage, and polycythemia. Annual pulmonary function tests and arterial blood gases to assess the client's current status, or they may be required to document the continued need for oxygen therapy.

URINARY TRACT DISORDERS

This section discusses three common disturbances: urinary tract infection, interstitial cystitis, and urinary incontinence.

URINARY TRACT INFECTION

Urinary tract infection (UTI) denotes the presence of microorganisms anywhere from the kidney (acute pyelonephritis), to the bladder (cystitis), to the distal urethra (urethritis). Urine is sterile, with the possible exception that the normal urethra may be colonized by diphtheroids,

lactobacillus, and alpha hemolytic streptococci. Ascent of pathogenic bacteria typically begins with the rectal flora moving upward to the vaginal introitus, distal urethra, bladder, and finally, occasionally, the kidney. The population of bacteria established in the bladder may double every 40 minutes.[1]

With repeated infections, it is important to differentiate between reinfection and relapse. Reinfection usually occurs more than 2 weeks after adequate antibiotic treatment. Relapse refers to recurrence of the same organism, usually from an incompletely treated focus in the kidneys.[1,2,3]

Epidemiology

Etiology. In a bladder infection, a combination of specific host and pathogen factors are involved. In healthy women, a few serotypes of *Escherichia coli* are responsible for more than 85 percent of bladder infections, yet these serotypes constitute only 1 percent of rectal flora. A specific interrelationship between bacterial adhesion and epithelial cell receptors in women may predispose them to infection.[2]

Periurethral cells in infection-prone women more readily bind *E. coli* cells than do periurethral cells in women who are not prone to infection. In women with recurrent UTIs, periurethral tissue is laden with pathogenic bacteria. Any additional factor, such as the motion of sexual intercourse, may cause these women to develop infection. Surface mucin that coats the bladder helps prevent bacterial attachment. That lining may decrease with age and falling estrogen levels, however.[2] Risk factors for infection vary depending on the location of infection (see Table 22–26).

Sexual activity places women at risk for all types of UTIs. The risk for cystitis is highest with vaginal intercourse. Any manipulation of the urethra, however, such as oral sex and masturbation, has some associated risk. Voiding prior to intercourse has not been shown to decrease risk of infection; however, voiding after intercourse decreases infection rates.[2] Diaphragm and spermicide use greatly increases risk. Recent studies suggest that diaphragm spermicides may predispose women to UTIs by altering vaginal flora.[2]

TABLE 22–26. RISK FACTORS FOR URINARY TRACT INFECTIONS

Cystitis	Acute Pyelonephritis	Urethritis
Childhood UTI[a]	Childhood UTI	New sex partner
Sexual activity ("honeymoon cystitis")	Prior history of pyelonephritis	Male partner with recent dysuria (rule out
Diaphragm use	Three UTIs in past year	sexually transmitted diseases)
Spermicide use	Known structural abnormality or stone	
	Urban indigent	
	Immunocompromised status	
	Pregnancy	

[a]Urinary tract infection.
Source: Reference UTD2.

Transmission. Most often women serve as their own reservoir for pathogenic bacteria. Bacterial growth in the urinary tract of women is primarily related to urethral manipulation, most often as a result of intercourse. Residual urine, blockage of urine flow, or decreased voiding due to dehydration can also promote bacterial growth. Common pathogenic organisms in the urinary tract of women are listed in Table 22–27.

Urethritis may be caused by sexually transmitted diseases; primarily gonorrhea, chlamydia, and herpes. Urethritis and dysuria in males are usually secondary to sexually transmitted diseases; therefore, male partners with suspected urinary tract infections should be carefully assessed and treated for sexually transmitted diseases as appropriate. Some men develop dysuria in the presence of *Ureaplasma urealyticum,* which is not currently considered a cause of sexually transmitted disease.

Incidence. Approximately 40 percent of women will experience a lower urinary tract infection.[3] Among women with a UTI, 10 to 20 percent with an acute uncomplicated infection will have a re-

currence.[3,5] UTIs may occur at any time in the life span, but are more common with increasing age. The high prevalence rate with increased age is associated with falling estrogen levels, bladder emptying problems, an increase in chronic systemic problems, concurrent diseases, bowel incontinence, overuse of catheters, and poor nutrition.[4]

Subjective Data

After data are collected, the primary care provider must discern whether symptoms are vaginal or urinary (see Table 22–28) and whether the upper urinary tract is involved (see Table 22–29). It is important to review a woman's history of UTIs or urinary problems and any recent medications; antibiotics will yield negative urine findings, and medications such as pyridium can make urine orange or green. Be sure to ask about over-the-counter medications such as those containing phenylpropanolamine or pseudoephedrine, which may impair bladder emptying.[5]

An accurate sexual history is crucial. Women do not always volunteer important infor-

TABLE 22–27. COMMON PATHOGENIC ORGANISMS IN WOMEN

Gram-Negative Pathogens	Gram-Positive Pathogens
Escherichia coli (responsible for >85% of UTIs)[a]	*Staphylococcus saprophyticus* (previously thought not to be a
Proteus mirabilis (a urea-splitting organism, associated with stone formation)	pathogen; now second most common cause of UTI in women)
Klebsiella species	*Staphylococcus aureus*
	Group A beta hemolytic streptococci
	Enterococci

[a]Urinary tract infections.

TABLE 22–28. HISTORICAL CLUES TO DYSURIA

Cystitis	Vaginitis	Urethritis
Abrupt onset	Gradual onset	Gradual onset
Internal dysuria	External dysuria	Internal dysuria
Change in voiding: frequency, urgency, small volumes, possibly nocturia and/or incontinence	No change in voiding pattern	May have some change in voiding pattern, no nocturia
Symptoms aggravated by voiding	Symptoms more continuous	Symptoms primarily associated with voiding
May have grossly bloody or odorous urine	No change in urine appearance	No change in urine appearance
No vaginal discharge	Vaginal discharge odor, itch, or irritation	May or may not have vaginal discharge or bleeding
10% complain of suprapubic tenderness	No abdominal symptoms	Abdominal pain if associated with pelvic inflammatory disease

mation such as having vaginal discharge or a new sex partner and, consequently, need to be questioned carefully. Women can usually discern whether dysuria is internal or an external burning as the urine passes over the labia. Vaginal infections, such as *Trichomonas, Candida,* bacterial vaginosis, and herpes simplex, may cause external dysuria.

Most often, urethritis in women is caused by *Chlamydia trachomatis,* the most prevalent bacterial sexually transmitted disease in the United States. Infrequent infections of the urethra may include *Neiserria gonorrhoeae, Trichomonas,* herpes simplex, and *Candida.*

Dysuria occurring gradually over 5 to 7 days is more characteristic of urethritis and

TABLE 22–29. DIFFERENTIATION OF UPPER AND LOWER URINARY TRACT INFECTIONS BY MEANS OF HISTORY AND PHYSICAL EXAMINATION

Lower UTI[a] (Cystitis)	Upper UTI (Acute Pyelonephritis)
Usually sudden onset	Often gradual onset over >5 days
Dysuria and voiding symptoms	± Voiding symptoms
No systemic symptoms	Fever, chills, nausea, vomiting
No costovertebral angle tenderness	Often costovertebral angle tenderness
Serum WBC count normal	Serum WBC count often elevated
No WBC casts	May have WBC casts

[a]UTI, urinary tract infection; WBC, white blood cell.

acute pyelonephritis than cystitis, which usually has an abrupt onset. Urethritis symptoms, such as dysuria, with no recognized pathogens and no pyuria may be secondary to trauma or postmenopausal estrogen deficiency.[1]

Accurate discrimination between upper and lower UTIs by means of a history or physical exam is difficult. Of women diagnosed with lower UTI (cystitis), 30 percent actually have occult pyelonephritis.[5] Because pyelonephritis can cause permanent renal damage or death, if untreated, it is crucial to try to make the correct diagnosis using a history (see Table 22–29). Differences may distinguish lower UTI (cystitis) from upper UTI (acute pyelonephritis). The typical presentation of acute pyelonephritis is abrupt onset of fever and flank pain; it may also be associated with generalized symptoms, such as nausea, vomiting, and chills. Pain may be perceived as low back or abdominal. Women with acute pyelonephritis may have no symptoms of dysuria or other common bladder symptoms.

History must confirm the presence or absence of any systemic symptoms: fever, chills, nausea, vomiting, diarrhea, headache, or malaise. Be sure to ask about any previous history of pyelonephritis or kidney stones. Cystitis is rarely associated with fever or systemic symptoms; therefore, the presence of fever or systemic symptoms is strongly suspicious of pyelonephritis. Risk factors for upper UTIs also need to be assessed (see Table 22–26).

Objective Data

Physical Examination. The client is generally assessed; occasionally a pelvic exam is necessary.

- *General Appearance.* A client with acute pyelonephritis may appear toxic.
- *Vital Signs.* Blood pressure and temperature are elevated.
- *Costovertebral Angle Tenderness.* Determine whether it is present.
- *Abdomen.* Check for suprapubic tenderness; a more extensive exam is done if the abdomen is very tender or if the bladder is palpable from distention.
- *Pelvic Exam.* A pelvic exam may or may not be indicated based on the history and results of lab tests. When it is done, examine Skene's and periurethral glands. A pelvic exam may be necessary if the client has a history of external dysuria or gradual-onset dysuria especially with vaginal discharge or other vaginal symptoms; new or multiple sex partners; or internal dysuria (but the urinalysis appears benign with no pyuria).

Diagnostic Tests. Methods of testing include urine dipstick urinalysis, urine culture and sensitivity, vaginal wet mounts, and various cultures. The leukocyte esterase dipstick has a sensitivity of 75–90 percent in detecting pyuria associated with infection. A positive dipstick correlates with five white blood cells (WBC) per high powered field (HPF).[1,3,5]

Urinalysis is the cornerstone of diagnosis. It is important to teach women how to collect a urine specimen* and to examine urine within 1 hour of collection, because bacteria multiply (see Table 22–30).

---

*Studies reported in the *Journal of Pediatrics, American Journal of Medicine,* and *New England Journal of Medicine* have shown that the procedure to obtain a clean catch urine specimen does not reduce bacterial contamination of urine cultures. A study of 100 women was reported in 1993 by the University of Virginia Health Sciences Center. It confirmed that to obtain a good urine sample for culture, it is not necessary to first clean the urinary meatus or to hold the labia apart while voiding.

A *urine culture and sensitivity test* is beneficial in determining the type of bacteria and its sensitivity to antibiotics. It was previously believed that a true infection was represented by a colony count of 10^5 microorganisms. Current research, however, shows that by using a colony count of 10^5, health care providers miss the diagnosis of acute bacterial cystitis in about half the women presenting with clinical symptoms. A colony count of 10^2 (100 colonies) in a symptomatic female is considered sufficient to cause a true, treatment-worthy infection.[1,5]

Traditionally urine cultures were done prior to and following treatment of any urinary tract infection. As a result of cost-benefit analysis, a more rational approach is recommended, based on the individual's clinical profile.[1,5]

With uncomplicated cystitis, urine pretreatment cultures are not recommended unless the diagnosis is in question. The purpose of posttreatment cultures is to rule out relapses or untreated foci of infection.

Pretreatment urine cultures are recommended in specific circumstances.

- All complicated urinary tract infections, including suspected pyelonephritis, history of structural abnormalities, and history of frequent urinary problems/infections
- Uncertain diagnosis
- Symptoms present longer than 7 days
- History of UTI within preceding 3 weeks (possible relapse)
- History of recent catheterization or urologic surgery
- Pregnancy or suspected pregnancy
- Diabetes or other immunocompromising disorders

Posttreatment cultures are recommended in the following circumstances.

- Failure to improve with treatment
- Diagnosis of acute pyelonephritis
- Presence of complications

Vaginal wet (KOH and saline) mounts are used to rule out *Trichomonas, Candida,* and *bacterial vaginosis* (see Chapter 11).

STD cultures are done to rule out *gonorrhea* and *chlamydia.*

TABLE 22–30. URINALYSIS FINDINGS ALTERED BY URINARY TRACT INFECTIONS[a]

Color/appearance	Often dark, turbid with foul smell; may be grossly bloody (hemorrhagic cystitis)
Dipstick	
Specific gravity	If too dilute, may be false-negative reading (i.e., low count of WBCs RBCs, bacteria).
pH	If very high pH, may be associated with urea stone-forming *Klebsiella;* low pH retards bacterial growth
Nitrites	Confirms presence of bacteria that convert nitrates to nitrites (does not always mean infection if asymptomatic; see asymptomatic bacteriuria section)
Protein	May have 1+ or 2+ protein with lower UTI; however, 3+ or 4+ urine deserves special attention and follow up to rule out kidney damage. Vaginal secretions may contaminate urine and give false positive for some protein; deserves follow-up
Leukocyte esterases	Quick way to determine pyuria, not as accurate as microscopic.
Microscopic Exam	Usually performed on spun urine; in women, normal urinary sediment may contain one or two RBCs and up to 4 WBCs per high-power field
RBCs	40–60% of women with cystitis have some microscopic hematuria; most common cause of hematuria is infection; also seen with stones, glomerulonephritis, neoplasm, tuberculosis
WBCs	May come from any part of urinary tract; "clumping" may be seen in infection; presence of 5–10 WBCs per high-power field is suspicious for UTI, although false positives are common in women
Bacteria	Usually visible in true infection
Casts	RBC and/or WBC casts indicate kidney involvement
Epithelial cells and mucous	Large amounts of either suspicious for vaginal contamination

[a]WBC, white blood cell; RBC, red blood cell; UTI, urinary tract infection.

Differential Medical Diagnoses

Primary differential diagnoses are urethritis, cystitis, and pyelonephritis (see Tables 22–28 and 22–29). Differential diagnoses also include asymptomatic bacteriuria, interstitial cystitis, and renal calculi.

Asymptomatic Bacteriuria. Asymptomatic bacteriuria is defined as bacteria in the urine with no symptoms of urinary tract infection. Whether to treat is debatable. Current recommendations are to treat pregnant women as if the condition were a urinary tract infection. Elderly women, who have a high incidence of bacteriuria, have not been harmed by asymptomatic bacteriuria nor do they benefit from treatment. In fact, treatment is expensive and may cause drug toxicity.[6]

Interstitial Cystitis. Interstitial cystitis is a syndrome of painful bladder without infection, characterized by urinary frequency, urgency, nocturia, and bladder pressure sensations that are often relieved by voiding. The urologist diagnoses interstitial cystitis by excluding other causes of painful bladder (cancer, tuberculosis, cystitis, herpes). Diagnosis is supported when cystoscopy reveals mucosal bleeding after distention of the bladder. Etiology is uncertain. (See page 853 in this chapter on Interstitial Cystitis.)

Renal Calculi. Renal calculi, called kidney stones, may cause intermittent flank pain or pain that radiates around to the abdomen. They are associated with hematuria. Clients may develop superimposed urinary tract infections. Most calculi are composed of calcium oxalate and phosphate and can be visualized on x-ray of the kidney, ureter, and bladder. Uric acid stones, on the other hand, do not show up on x-rays and are associated with urea-splitting bacteria, such as *proteus mirabilis.* UTIs with *Proteus* must be evaluated to rule out calculi.[7]

Plan

Psychosocial Interventions. Discuss pain/discomfort management with the client and explain the mechanisms of urinary tract infections. Reassure her that a UTI is not a sexually transmitted disease, although intercourse may be mechanically related to the condition. Inform the woman so that she can identify her own precipitating factors and use appropriate preventive measures.

TABLE 22–31. TREATMENT OPTIONS FOR UNCOMPLICATED AND RECURRENT CYSTITIS

Uncomplicated Cystititis: Rare or Infrequent Episodes of Cystitis	

First-Line Medications

1. Single-dose therapy — No longer recommended due to low rates of cure.
2. Three-day treatment
   - Advantages — New area of study that combines decreased cost and decreased side effects.
   - Disadvantages — Twice the side effect rates as single dose; more research on effectiveness needed.
   - Medications of choice — TMP/SMX double-strength tablets b.i.d. × 3 days or nitrofurantoin (Macrodantin) 50–100 mg q.i.d. × 3 days.
   - Client teaching — Call to return to clinic quickly if not improved or symptoms reappear.
3. Traditional 7- to 10-day treatment
   - Advantages — Only a 5% failure rate; most research done with this approach.
   - Disadvantage — Twice the side effect rate of single dose, increased cost, decreased compliance.
   - Medication of choice — TMP/SMX DS b.i.d. × 7 days or nitrofurantoin 50 mg q.i.d. × 7 days.
   - Client teaching — Encourage finishing medication as ordered; if side effects occur, stop medications and telephone primary health care provider.

Second-Line Medications

Several new, expensive medications are now available for urinary tract infections. They should be reserved for clients with allergies or with resistant organisms, e.g., ciprofloxacin (Cipro) 250 or 500 mg b.i.d. × 7 days or norfloxacin (Noroxin) 400 mg b.i.d. × 7 days.

Recurrent Cystititis: Arbitrarily Defined as Three or More Episodes of Cystitis Per Year	

1. Postcoital prophylaxis
   - Indications — Highly effective for the 85% of women who have onset of symptoms 24 to 48 hours after intercourse; intercourse does not occur as frequently as daily.
   - Medications — Oral antibiotic is taken just prior to or just after intercourse.
   - Options — 50 mg nitrofuraniton, 250 mg cephalosporin, half single-strength TMX/SMX.
2. Intermittent self-start therapy
   - Indications — Client must be motivated and reliable about following directions. Home dipslide cultures are prepared by client at onset of symptoms and the client self-starts traditional first-line antibiotics as prescribed; dip slides are inexpensive and save cost of two office visits; client must demonstrate a clear knowledge of the procedures and the signs of relapse and pyelonephritis.
   - Medications — 3-day course of traditional antibiotics. TMP/SMX double strength b.i.d. × 3 days or nitrofurantoin 50–100 mg q.i.d. × 3 days p.o.
3. Low-dose continuous prophylaxis
   - Indications — Method of choice with high or daily sexual frequency; absence of any infection must be documented by urine culture prior to start.
   - Medications — Cephalexin (Keflex) 250 mg, trimethoprim 100 mg, TMP/SMX 1/2 tablet single strength. Given daily at bedtime or three times weekly; nitrofurantoin avoided, as long-term exposure may cause hypersensitivity reactions in the lung and kidney maybe an option during pregnancy; breakthrough infections treated with the full traditional 7-day therapy as indicated.

[a]See a current pharmacotherapeutics text for details.
[b]TMP/SMX, trimethoprim—sulfamethoxazole (Bactrim).
Source: References 1, 2, 3, 5.

Medication. Table 22–31 lists the management options for cystitis and Table 22–32 describes outpatient management of acute pyelonephritis.

Surgical Interventions. Women with recurrent cystitis rarely have anatomic abnormalities that require surgical intervention. Referral to a urolo-gist, however, is suggested for women with recurrent problems who have a history of childhood infections, more than one episode of acute pyelonephritis, possible nephrolithiasis, relapsing infections, infections caused by *Proteus mirabilis,* or painless hematuria. Prolapse of the bladder, uterus, or rectum in older women may

TABLE 22–32. ACUTE PYELONEPHRITIS: OUTPATIENT MANAGEMENT[a]

Criteria for Outpatient Management[b]
1. Diagnosis is secure (consult with physician)
2. No underlying, complicating disease, such as diabetes
3. Not pregnant
4. No history of recent urinary tract instrumentation
5. Not toxic, must be able to tolerate oral therapy and fluids
6. Follow-up must be easily accessible in 24 hours
7. Culture and sensitivity must be sent the day treatment is initiated

Medications
1. Must be broad spectrum (ampicillin and first-generation cephalosporins should not be used) trimethoprim— sulfamethoxazole (Bactrim) double strength b.i.d. or ciprofloxacin hydrochloride (Cipro) 500 mg b.i.d. for 14 days
2. Addition of a stat dose of intramuscular gentamicin (dose based on weight) or ceftriaxone 1 GM, IM used by some clinicians
3. Client should improve substantially in the first 24 hours; consult/refer if not improved.

[a]Consult a pharmacotherapeutics text for details.
[b]Woman must meet these criteria to attempt outpatient management.

cause bladder outlet obstruction and impaired emptying resulting in urine stasis and increasing the risk of infection. These women may benefit from referral for urodynamic studies.[5]

Lifestyle Changes. Teach the client healthy voiding practices: void at first urge, void after intercourse. Encourage the client to make these practices routine. Advise her to maintain adequate hydration and to avoid use of contraceptive methods associated with increased UTI risk, such as a diaphragm.

Older women may benefit from use of estrogen cream therapy, 2 grams intravaginally twice a week. A recent trial also demonstrated a reduced risk of urinary tract infection in women who drank cranberry juice daily.[4]

Follow-Up

Women should feel much improved within 24 to 48 hours of starting medication; if not, they should be instructed to telephone or return to the clinic. Teach clients the warning signs and symptoms of pyelonephritis and instruct them to telephone immediately if any of the symptoms develop.

For management of urethritis and vaginitis, see Chapter 11. For pregnant women, aggressive screening for urinary tract infection and treatment is recommended. UTIs and asymptomatic bac-

teriuria in pregnancy are associated with increased fetal and maternal morbidity.

INTERSTITIAL CYSTITIS

Interstitial cystitis is a chronic, painful bladder disorder whose course is unpredictable. It is characterized by urinary frequency, urgency, nocturia, and suprapubic pain in the absence of urinary pathogens. The etiology is unknown, but most accepted theories involve an initial insult to the bladder wall by toxin, allergen or immunologic agent that causes an inflammatory response.

Interstitial cystitis is frequently misdiagnosed as psychogenic in origin or goes undiagnosed for years. It can profoundly affect the client's ability to work, maintain a home, family, and satisfying sexual relationship. There is no uniformly effective treatment; however, an individualized management plan that actively involves the client helps prevent permanent disability.[8,9,10]

Epidemiology

Interstitial cystitis affects one in 350 individuals, 90 percent of whom are women.[9] Median age at diagnosis in one large study was 42 years old; however, nearly 30 percent were younger than 30 years old at onset of symptoms. A few studies point to a genetic link and a higher than expected prevalence in Jewish women.[11]

Other factors associated with significant risk of development include hysterectomy, irritable bowel syndrome, hypersensitivity to medications, history of migraine, chronic fatigue syndrome, and fibromyalgia.[11,12]

Theories of Etiology. Currently accepted theories of the origins of interstitial cystitis include infection by bacteria or virus, lymphatic obstruction, inflammation and autoimmunity, and reflex sympathetic dystrophy.

Scanning electron microscopy has shown microbes embedded in the bladder mucosa. The most common organism was found to be Gardnerella vaginalis. Appropriate antibiotic therapy has failed to consistently relieve symptoms.

Defects in the glycosaminoglycans layer of the bladder, which constitutes a protective mucosal barrier, has been noted in many studies. Whether this is cause or effect is unknown.

Reflex sympathetic dystrophy with the bladder as the target organ is another consideration. It is hypothesized that the pain is ischemic and arises from excessive sympathetic vasomotor activity. This constant stimulation leads to changes in the lining of the bladder.

Most researchers agree that the cause is multifactorial. The most consistent findings on biopsy of the bladder are a high number of mast cells in the detrusor muscle and a disruption in the protective glycosaminoglycans layer. Current treatment modalities are based on these theoretical causes.[8]

Subjective Data

The client may have consulted several health care providers in the past several months or years without getting relief from her symptoms. She will report urgency, frequency, and acute suprapubic pain. She may have to void every hour while awake and several times at night. She may complain of painful intercourse. Because of these disruptions in her life, she may be sleep deprived, anxious, depressed, and suffer from social isolation. She may describe periods of flare in symptoms right before her menses, at menopause, with certain foods, and/or at times of stress.

Be sure to ask about coexisting conditions such as migraine headaches, irritable bowel syndrome, fibromyalgia, chronic fatigue syndrome, allergies and hypersensitivities to foods and medications. Review gynecologic history for previous urinary tract infections, pelvic inflammatory disease, vaginal infections, bladder instrumentation, hysterectomy, laporoscopic procedures. Ask her about both traditional and nontraditional treatments she has tried and the outcomes.

Objective Data

Physical Examination. The physical exam focuses on the abdomen and pelvis.

- *General Appearance.* The client may seem anxious. Her gait may be slow and measured to avoid jarring pain.
- *Vital Signs.* Afebrile.
  - Palpate the back for costovertebral angle and lower back tenderness.

- Percuss the abdomen for bladder distension and palpate for suprapubic tenderness and masses.
- *Pelvic Exam.* Because interstitial cystitis is a diagnosis of exclusion, a complete pelvic exam is indicated to rule out infection, pelvic inflammatory disease, uterine and adnexal masses. Be sure to examine the urethra, Bartholin's and Skene's glands.

Diagnostic Tests. Urinalysis to detect infection, hematuria. Urinanalysis will be normal with interstitial cystitis.

Pregnancy test, wet prep, gonorrhea, and/or chlamydia cultures as indicated by exam.

Differential Medical Diagnoses

- *Cystitis.* Presence of white blood cells and bacteria in urine sediment.
- *Renal Calculi.* Presence of hematuria, colicky flank pain.
- *Pelvic or vaginal infection* indicated by exam, wet prep, cultures.
- *Pelvic masses* such as fibroid tumor, ovarian cyst detected by examination, history.
- *Genital herpes* indicated by history and presence of lesions.
- *Tubercular cystitis* and bladder detected on cystoscopy (see following).

Diagnosis/Management. The client is referred to the urologist for cystoscopy under general anesthesia. Diagnosis is made on the basis of presence of fissures, hemorrhage, and/or ulcers in the bladder wall and biopsy showing inflammatory process (presence of mast cells).

Psychosocial Interventions. Reassurance and support of the client are the first steps in alleviating some of her discomfort. She may feel overwhelming relief that her pain is considered real and not "all in her head." Actively involve her in the plan of care. Ask her to keep a diary of voiding patterns, symptoms, and flares with pain scales and associated conditions such as onset of menses, periods of high stress. When the diagnosis is confirmed by a urologist, refer her to the Interstitial Cystitis Association, a nonprofit organization that provides information and support and funds research.

The Interstitial Cystitis Association
P.O. Box 1553
New York, NY 10159–1553

Medication. There is no definitive medical treatment for interstitial cystitis. Occasionally, the dilatation of the bladder during diagnostic cystoscopy results in relief of symptoms.

DIMETHYLSULFOXIDE (**DMSO** SOLUTION). One of the experimental modalities of treatment uses dimethylsulfoxide (DMSO solution) a solvent thought to have anti-inflammatory properties. A urologist instills 30–50 cc into the bladder at weekly intervals. Results have not been consistent in relieving symptoms, and the client often relapses when installations are stopped.[13]

AMITRIPTYLINE. 10 mg to 75 mg po at night is used for its analgesic and anticholinergic properties.[14] See previous discussion of amitriptyline in section on fibromyalgia.

NIFEDIPINE (PROCARDIA OR ADALAT). A *calcium channel blocker* such as nifedipine (*Procardia or Adalat*) 30 mg sustained release one tablet by mouth each day or night may be used. A calcium channel blocker. It is thought to act by relaxing detrusor muscle and vascular smooth muscles.[15] See previous discussion of calcium channel blockers in section on hypertension.

HYDROXYZINE (ATARAX). 25–50 mg po at night may be prescribed for its anticholinergic property of inhibiting mast cell production.[16] See previous discussion of hydroxyzine in section on common dermatoses.

Lifestyle Changes. Because no medication appears to show consistent relief of symptoms, an individualized approach to the client involving a self-care regimen is recommended.

The most effective plans include the following:

- *Dietary Modifications.* Avoidance of high acid foods and fluids that contain high fat and low carbohydrates. See Table 22–33. Addition of high fiber foods to diet. Eating several small meals per day instead of large meals.
- *Nutritional Supplements.* Vitamins A, B₆, and C may have protective effects on the bladder.

TABLE 22–33. DIETARY MODIFICATIONS FOR INTERSTITIAL CYSTITIS

Foods to Avoid	
Chocolate	Alcoholic beverages
Soy sauce	Hot, spicy foods
Fruits, especially citrus or foods with citric acid	Coffee, tea, all caffeine
	Carbonated soft drinks
Artificial sweeteners	Avocado
Brewer's yeast	Cheese (especially aged)
Chicken liver	Corned beef
Fava and lima beans	Mayonnaise
Pickled herring	Onions (small amount for flavoring acceptable)
Rye bread and rye products	
Yogurt	Vitamins with aspartate, yeast, synthetic Vitamin D
Sour cream	
High animal protein meals	Fermented foods
Vinegar and vinegar products	Tap water
Sprouts of any kind	Foods with molds
Foods with chemical additives	Fried foods
Hydrogenated fats including margarine or shortening	Smoked foods

Foods to Add	
Rice	Pasta
Potatoes	Vegetables
Chicken	Watermelon
Meat	Grapefruit

Note: There are no controlled studies suggesting that dietary changes can relieve symptoms; however, many clients identify acid foods or fluids with exacerbation of symptoms.
Source: Adapted from Reference 12.

Vitamin E is a natural vasodilator. Magnesium may have antianxiety properties.

- *Stress Reduction.* Stress is the most significant factor for flare of symptoms. Adequate rest, exercise, participation in support group, and relaxation techniques such as yoga and deep-breathing are recommended.
- *Bladder Retraining.* Used when pain is absent or at lower level. Method is to increase time between voids in intervals, for instance 10–15 minutes longer each time.

Set goal with client for target time between voids based on voiding pattern before treatment began. Teach her how to do Kegel's exercises. (See discussion in section that follows on urinary incontinence.)[12]

Follow-Up

Continue to follow for primary health care. As with other pain syndromes, it is better to schedule client for regular visits to assess response to therapy. A suggested interval may be every 2 weeks at the beginning of the treatment plan and then monthly. Maintain close communication with urologist.

URINARY INCONTINENCE

Urinary incontinence (UI) is the involuntary loss of urine that is demonstrable and that is sufficient to be a social or hygienic problem.[17,18] It is a common and costly problem in younger and older women. It has significant psychosocial and economic impact on the individual, her caregivers, and society. It is estimated that less than half the individuals with UI consult health care providers about the problem. This may be due to its acceptance as a natural condition of aging, the availability of absorbent products (minipads and Depends), and lack of information on treatment options and benefits.[17]

Appropriate management can result in significant improvement. Development of an effective treatment plan depends on accurate identification of the subtype of urinary incontinence.

Subtypes of Urinary Incontinence. Control of bladder function is maintained by voluntary and involuntary mechanisms. The detrusor muscles of bladder and internal urethral sphincter are under autonomic nervous system control, which may be modulated by cerebral cortex connections. The external urethral sphincter and pelvic floor muscles are under voluntary control.

Other factors that contribute to urinary continence include adequate estrogen, which may help maintain bladder sphincter tone; adequate bladder capacity, elasticity, and smooth muscle tone; maintenance of an acute posterior urethravesicular angle to support the bladder neck and urethra.

Subtypes of urinary incontinence are based on compromise of aforementioned mechanisms.

Urge incontinence is the involuntary loss of urine associated with a strong desire to void. It is caused by *detrusor instability* due to involuntary detrusor contractions. These involuntary contractions may be caused by a neurological disorder

such as stroke or multiple sclerosis, or occur as part of the aging process.

Stress urinary incontinence (SUI) is involuntary loss of urine during coughing, sneezing, laughing, or other physical activities that increase intraabdominal pressure. The most common cause of SUI in women is urethral hypermobility or significant displacement of the urethra and bladder when intraabdominal pressure is increased. Other causes include intrinsic urethral sphincter weakness, which may be congenital or acquired after trauma or radiation therapy, multiple incontinence surgical procedures, spinal cord lesion, or hypoestrogenism.

In older women UI is most often a combination of urge and stress incontinence. It is important to identify which component is most bothersome in order to target treatment.

Overflow incontinence is the result of overdistention of the bladder. It usually presents with frequent or constant dribbling or urge/stress incontinence symptoms. It is caused by underactive or a contractile detrusor or by bladder outlet obstruction. Medications (diuretics, anticholinergics, psychotropics, alpha-adrenergic blockers), neurologic conditions such as diabetic neuropathy, spinal cord injury, or radical pelvic surgery causing prolapse of pelvic organs may impair or alter the innervation of the detrusor muscle. Overflow incontinence secondary to outlet obstruction is rare in women.

Other types of incontinence include functional incontinence caused by factors outside the urinary tract such as chronic physical or cognitive impairment and unconscious or reflex incontinence common in paraplegics.[17]

Epidemiology

Urinary incontinence affects about 13 million Americans, predominantly women and the elderly. It is estimated that 17–46 percent of noninstitutionalized women over 60 years old are incontinent. Between 25–30 percent report incontinence frequently either daily or weekly. Of the homebound elderly, 53 percent are incontinent. UI is a major cause of institutionalization. The estimated health care costs of UI are $10 billion in the community and $5.2 billion in nursing homes.[17]

Risk factors for development of UI in women include increasing age, increased parity, immobility, impaired cognition, obesity, medications (diuretics, anticholinergic agents, psychotropics, narcotic analgesics, alpha-adrenergic blockers), hysterectomy, smoking, alcohol use, fecal impaction, estrogen depletion, pelvic muscle weakness, and childhood nocturnal enuresis. Of these factors that are modifiable, obesity and hysterectomy may have the most impact on prevention of daily incontinence.[17,20]

Subjective Data

Information should include a focused medical, neurologic, and genitourinary history that includes the above cited risk factors and a review of medication use, both prescribed and over-the-counter.

Ask detailed questions about the associated symptoms and factors of her incontinent episodes including the following:

- Duration and characteristics (stress, urge, dribbling)
  - What symptoms are most bothersome to the client
  - Frequency, timing, and amount of continent and incontinent voids, e.g., dribbles in underpants vs soaking through clothing
  - Triggers of incontinence (cough, exercise, surgery, trauma, new medication)
  - Other lower urinary tract symptoms such as nocturia, dysuria, hesitancy, weak and/or thin stream, hematuria, suprapubic pain
  - Fluid intake, especially coffee or other caffeine containing foods and fluids
  - Alterations in bowel, sexual function
  - Previous treatment and outcome
  - Amount of absorbent pads, briefs (Depends) used
  - Expectations of treatment
  - Psychosocial evaluation of mental status, mobility, living environment

Objective Data

Physical Examination

- Vital signs for hypertension, elevated temperature.
- Gait for mobility.

- Neuromuscular assessment to detect abnormalities that suggest multiple sclerosis, stroke, spinal cord lesion, and to assess cognition, strength, and manual dexterity.
- Cardiovascular status for presence of edema that may contribute to nocturia.
- Lungs for crackles or wheezes that may indicate congestive heart failure, chronic obstructive pulmonary disease, asthma that may contribute to cough.
- Abdominal examination to assess for organomegaly, masses, diastesis recti, bladder distension, or other factors that may affect intraabdominal pressure.
- Rectal examination to assess sphincter tone, presence of fecal impaction, rectal mass.
- Pelvic examination to assess perineal skin, genital atrophy, pelvic organ prolapse (cystocele, rectocele, uterine prolapse), pelvic mass. Palpate anterior vaginal wall for discharge from urethra or tenderness, which suggests diverticulum, carcinoma, or inflammation of the urethra.

Diagnostic Tests

Urinalysis to detect hematuria (infection, cancer, stone), glucosuria (polyuria), pyuria, and bacteria.

COUGH STRESS TEST. Test is done when bladder is full but before urge to void is strong. Done in lithotomy position. Examiner observes for urine loss from urethra while client coughs vigorously. If instant loss, SUI likely. If leakage delayed or persists after cough, detrusor instability may be cause of UI. If no leakage and symptoms suggest SUI, perform test in upright posture.

POSTVOID RESIDUAL (PVR). Can be done by catheterization or pelvic ultrasound. Observation of urine stream can be noted for hesitancy, straining, slow or interrupted stream. Measure postvoid residual within a few minutes after voiding. It is generally accepted that PVRs fewer than 50 cc are normal. If repetitive PVRs range from 100–200cc, then inadequate emptying. One measure of PVR may not be sufficient.

If transient, reversible, or modifiable causes of UI have been detected, client may need no further evaluation and may be treated with trial of medications and behavioral modalities described subsequently.

Plan

Those who should be referred to a urogynecologic specialist include the following:

- Those whose UI persists after initial therapeutic trial
- Uncertain diagnosis (lack of correlation between symptoms and findings)
- Consideration of surgical referral especially if failure of previous surgery
- Hematuria without infection
- Comorbid conditions such as incontinence with recurrent symptoms of urinary tract infection, persistent difficulty emptying bladder, history of radical pelvic surgery, symp-tomatic pelvic prolapse, abnormal PVR, neurological condition.[17]

Psychosocial Interventions. Because urinary incontinence is so common and underreported, it is suggested that questions about bladder function be a routine part of the annual gynecologic exam for women of all ages. Not only can this lead to prompt treatment of reversible causes of UI but also can relieve client hesitancy in bringing the subject up.

Client education about causes and initial therapy are important in order to reassure her that certain modalities may relieve or resolve her incontinence. Be realistic. In some clients, incontinence may never be cured but may only be manageable. Advise client that corrective surgery or bladder tuck may not cure incontinence. Be sure to refer her to support groups such as

Help for Incontinent People (HIP), Inc.
P. O. Box 544
Union, SC 29379

Medication
Stress Urinary Incontinence

ESTROGEN. Postmenopausal women in whom stress incontinence is related to intrinsic sphincter atrophy may benefit from estrogen replacement as the initial therapy. (See hormone replacement therapy in chapter on Climacteric, Menopause, and the Process of Aging.) The estrogen may be administered orally, transdermally, or transvaginally. Some reports suggest topical estrogen may bring faster relief by local effect. Remember women with intact uteri should be given a progestin.

- *Expected Outcome.* Advise her that beneficial effects may not occur earlier than 6–12 weeks after initiation of treatment.

ENTEX. (Phenylpropanolamine) Sympathomimetic drug with alpha-adrenergic against activity that helps increase bladder outlet resistence. 25–100 mg sustained release orally twice daily.

- *Adverse Effects.* Nausea, dry mouth, insomnia, rash, pruritis, restlessness. NOTE: Phenylpropanolamine did not cause significant increases in blood pressure during evaluation period of studies in which it was used to treat incontinence.[17]
- *Contraindications.* Known hypersensitivity to ingredient. Caution in hypertension, hyperthyroidism, cardiac arrhythmia, angina.
- *Expected Outcome.* Advise client complete cure is rare but may note some subjective improvement.

  NOTE: Estrogen may be added as an adjunctive agent if single agent fails for postmenopausal women.

IMIPRAMINE. Alternative is imipramine (Tofranil). An anticholinergic and alpha-adrenergic agonist. May be of benefit. No large scale studies to support its use.

- *Administration.* 75 mg p.o. daily if first line medications fail or are contraindicated. Nighttime dose may be used to avoid daytime drowsiness.
- *Adverse Effects.* Nausea, drowsiness or insomnia, weakness, fatigue, postural hypotension.
- *Contraindications.* Known hypersensitivity to tricyclic antidepressants, recovery phase of myocardial infarction. Caution in cardiovascular disease.

URGE INCONTINENCE WITH DETRUSOR INSTABILITY

ANTICHOLINERGIC AGENTS. First line medications are anticholinergic agents that work by blocking bladder contractions and relaxing sphincter muscle.

OXYBUTYNIN. (Ditropan) 2.5–5.0 p.o. three times a day.

- *Adverse Effects.* Dry skin, dry mouth, blurred vision, change in mental status, nausea, constipation.
- *Contraindications.* Known hypersensitivity, narrow angle glaucoma (not wide angle), gastrointestinal or urinary obstruction, myasthenia gravis.
- *Expected Outcome.* Advise improvement usually modest.

PROPANTHELINE. Second line anticholinergic is Propantheline (Pro-Banthine) 7.5–30 mg p.o. three to five times a day.

- *Adverse Effects.* Urinary retention, blurred vision, dry mouth, nausea, constipation, tachycardia, drowsiness, confusion.
- *Contraindications.* Known hypersensitivity, narrow angle glaucoma, urinary or gastrointestinal obstruction, myasthenia gravis.
- *Expected Outcome.* Advise degree of improvement may be modest.

Both the aforementioned medications should be used only in conjunction with voiding schedule or behavioral interventions as discussed subsequently. Client must be carefully monitored for urinary retention.

TRICYCLIC ANTIDEPRESSANTS. Tricyclic antidepressants such as Imipra-mine (see prior discussion) as smooth muscle relaxant may also be effective.

OVERFLOW INCONTINENCE DUE TO DETRUSOR HYPOMOBILITY (WHEN OBSTRUCTION IS RULED OUT). Is usually the result of neurological disorders such as diabetic neuropathy. Anticholinergics and tricyclic antidepressants should be avoided. Pharmacologic intervention is usually ineffective except for Bethanecol.

BETHANECOL. (Urecholine) 10–25 mg three to four times a day.[19]

- *Mode of Action.* Cholinergic agonist that stimulates muscarinic receptors of parasympathetic nervous system. Increases tone of detrusor muscle resulting in contraction, decreased bladder capacity, and subsequent urination.
- *Adverse Effects.* Abdominal pain, diarrhea, bradycardia, hypotension, bronchoconstriction.
- *Contraindications.* Known hypersensitivity, coronary artery disease, peptic ulcer, parkinsonism, asthma.
- *Expected Outcome.* Advise client may be ineffective. Check postvoid residual urine volumes before and after treatment to assess efficacy.

Behavioral Interventions
- *Habit training* is targeting scheduled voids to match client's voiding habits as observed by caregiver. It can achieve good results with those who are homebound and have a caregiver.

- *Bladder training* is recommended for management of urge incontinence and mixed stress and urge incontinence. Client is advised to resist urge to void or postpone voiding and urinate on a fixed schedule. Initial goal is usually set for 2–3 hours between voids while awake. Adjustment of fluid intake may be needed. Goal is to increase intervals over a period of several months.
- *Pelvic muscle exercises* are especially useful for stress urinary incontinence and urge incontinence. The first step is to make the client more aware of muscle function. The examiner teaches the woman how to do the exercises by inserting the gloved finger into vagina and instructs client to tighten muscles around finger. Client is advised to sustain contraction for at least 2–4 seconds followed by an equal period of relaxation. She is instructed to perform these exercises with five repetitions every half-hour during the day, or alternatively, for 10 minutes twice a day. The key is consistency. Advise her to contract these muscles before and during situations when leaking occurs (e.g., cough, sneeze, laughter, exercise).

A recent study in one small group of 23 women indicated that long-term outcomes of pelvic floor muscle exercises compared with surgery are equal.[21]

Other behavioral modalities that may be of benefit include *biofeedback, vaginal weight training* and *pelvic floor electrical stimulation.* These may be used in conjunction with pelvic muscle exercises. Consult physician or urogynecologist for referral.

Diet/Lifestyle. Client education regarding factors that may impact incontinence include the following:

- Avoiding excessive alcohol and caffeine.
- Use of fiber and stool softeners to avoid constipation.
- Medications that may have adverse effects on incontinence including diuretics, psychotropic agents, narcotic analgesics, over-the-counter products for appetite control and colds, calcium channel blockers.
- Control of blood sugar to prevent polyuria.
- If prescribed diuretics are part of treatment for co-existing medical conditions, edema dosages

may be minimized by use of non-pharmaco-logic interventions such as use of support stockings, leg elevation, and sodium restriction.

- Barriers to reaching toilet and environmental alterations such as bedside commode.

Follow-Up

Telephone follow-up in 1 week to assess adherence and barriers to treatment plan. Office visit in 2 weeks. Try initial treatment for 4–6 weeks. If no improvement, refer to physician or urogynecologist for further urodynamic studies.

REFERENCES

Musculoskeletal Conditions

 1. Baker, C., & Todd, J. (1995). Intervening in acute ankle sprain and chronic instability. *The Journal of Musculoskeletal Medicine, 12* (7), 51–68.
 2. Rifat, S., & McKeag, D. (1996). Practical methods of preventing ankle injuries. *American Family Physician, 53*(8), 2491–2498.
 3. Birrer, R., & Poole, B. (1995). Athletic taping, part 3: The knee. *The Journal of Musculoskeletal Medicine, 12*(7), 43–45.
 4. U.S. Department of Health and Human Services, Public Health Service, Agency for Health Care Policy and Research. (1994). *Clinical practice guideline No. 14: Acute low back pain problem in adults* (Publication No. 95–0642). Rockville, MD: Author.
 5. Wheeler, A. (95). Diagnosis and management of low back pain and sciatica. *American Family Physician, 53*(2), 1333–1341.
 6. Gillette, R. (1996). A practical approach to the patient with back pain. *American Family Physician, 53*(2), 670–676.
 7. Malmivaara, A., et al. (1995). The treatment of low back pain—Bed rest, exercises, or ordinary activity? *New England Journal of Medicine, 332*(6), 351–355.
 8. Carey, T., et al. (1995). The outcomes and costs of care for acute low back pain seen by primary care practitioners, chiropractors, and orthopedic surgeons. *The New England Journal of Medicine, 333*(14), 913–917.
 9. Dawson, D. (1993). Entrapment neuropathies of the upper extremities. *New England Journal of Medicine, 329*(27), 2013–2018.
10. Katz, R. (1994). Carpal tunnel syndrome: A practical review. *American Family Physician, 49*(6), 1371–1379.
11. Butcher, J., Salzman, K., & Lilligard, W. (1996). Lower extremity bursitis. *American Family Physician, 53*(7), 2317–2324.
12. Glockner, S. (1995). Shoulder pain: A diagnostic dilemma. *American Family Physician, 51*(7), 1677–1687.
13. Clauw, D. (1995). Fibromyalgia: More than just a musculoskeletal disease. *American Family Physician, 52*(3), 843–851.
14. Godfrey, R. (1996). A guide to the understanding and use of tricyclic antidepressants in the overall management of fibromyalgia and other chronic pain syndromes. *Archives of Internal Medicine, 156*(10), 1047–1052.
15. Calin, A. (1995). Managing hyperuricemia and gout: Challenges and pitfalls. *Journal of Musculoskeletal Medicine, 12*(2), 42–46.
16. Hench, P., Meislin, H., Weiss, J., & Zink, B. (1993). Hot joint: Narrowing the differential. *Patient Care, 27*(9), 100–123.
17. Litman, K. (1996). A rational approach to the diagnosis of arthritis. *American Family Physician, 53*(4), 1295–1310.
18. Hooker, R. (1996). Osteoarthritis of the hip and knee. *Clinician Review, 6*(1), 54–68.
19. Jobanputra, D., & Nuki, G. (1994). Nonsteroidal anti-inflammatory drugs in the treatment of osteoarthritis. *Current Opinion in Rheumatology, 6,* 433–439.
20. Felson, D., Zhang, Y., Anthony, J., Naimark, A., & Anderson, J. (1992). Weight loss reduces the risk for symptomatic knee osteoarthritis in women. The Framingham Study. *Annals of Internal Medicine, 116*(7), 535–539.
21. Clark, D. (1996). The effect of walking on lower body disability among older blacks and whites. *American Journal of Public Health, 86*(1), 57–61.
22. Lipsky, P. (1994). Rheumatoid arthritis. In K. Esselbacher et al. (Eds.), *Harrison's principles of internal medicine* (13th ed.). New York: McGraw-Hill, Inc.
23. Newcomer, K., & Jurisson, M. (1994). Rheumatoid arthritis: The role of physical therapy. *The Journal of Musculoskeletal Medicine, 11*(1), 14–26.
24. Hahn, B. (1994). Systemic lupus erythematosus. In K. Esselbacher et al. (Eds.), *Harrison's principles of internal medicine* (13th ed.). New York: McGraw-Hill, Inc.
25. Spiera, H., & Rothschild, J. (1995). When systemic lupus erythematosus involves the heart. *The Journal of Musculoskeletal Medicine, 12*(1), 54–69.
26. Abramowicz, M. (1994). Drugs for rheumatoid arthritis. *The Medical Letter, 36*(935), 101–106.

27. Heigh, R. (1994). Use of NSAIDs. *Postgraduate Medicine, 96*(6), 63–67.

28. Furst, D. (1994). Are there differences among non-steroidal antiinflammatory drugs? *Arthritis & Rheumatism, 37*(1), 1–9.

29. Langman, M., et al. (1994). Risks of bleeding peptic ulcer associated with individual non-steroidal anti-inflammatory drugs. *Lancet, 343,* 1075–1078.

Neurological Disorders

1. Olsen, J. (1988). Classification and diagnostic criteria for headache disorders, cranial neuralgias and facial pain. *Cephalgia, 8* (Suppl.7), 9–96.

2. Pearce, J. (1994). Headache. *Journal of Neurology, Neurosurgery and Psychiatry, 57,* 134–143.

3. Barrett, E. (1996). Primary care for women. Assessment and management of headache. *Journal of Nurse-Midwifery, 41*(2), 117–124.

4. Patterson, L. (1995). Headache. In D. Lemcke, J. Pattison, L. Marshall, & D. Cowley. (Eds.), *Primary care of women* (1st ed.). Norwalk, CT: Appleton & Lange.

5. Ryan, C. (1996). Evaluation of patients with chronic headache. *American Family Physician, 54*(3), 1051–1057.

6. Raskin, N. (1994). Headache In Esselbacher et al. (Eds.), *Harrison's principles of internal medicine* (13th ed.). New York: McGraw-Hill, Inc.

7. Welch, K. (1995). Helping patients fend off migraine. *Emergency Medicine, 27*(1), 45–64.

8. Abramowicz, M. (1995). Drugs for migraine. *The Medical Letter, 37* (943), 17–20.

9. Baumel, B. (1994). Migraine: A pharmacological review with newer options and delivery modalities. *Neurology, 44* (Suppl. 3), S13–S18.

10. Cady, R., Rubino, J., Crummett, D., & Littlejohn, T. (1994). Oral sumatriptan treatment for recurrent headache. *Archives of Family Medicine, 3* (9), 766–772.

11. Gelfand, J., Dinarello, C., & Wolff, S. (1994). Fever, including fever of unknown origin. In K. Esselbacher et al. (Eds.), *Harrison's principles of internal medicine* (13th ed.), New York: McGraw-Hill, Inc.

12. Seller, R. (1993). Fever. In R. Seller "Differential diagnosis of common complaints" (2nd ed). Philadelphia: W. B. Saunders.

13. Burke, M. (1995). Dizziness in the elderly: Etiology and treatment. *The Nurse Practitioner, 20*(12), 28–35.

14. Seller, R. (1993). Dizziness, lightheadedness, and vertigo. In R. Seller (Ed.), *Differential diagnosis of common complaints* (2nd ed.). Philadelphia: W. Saunders Company.

15. Browder, J. (1992). Dizziness. In L. Dornbrand, A. Hoole, & G. Pickard (Eds.), *Manual of clinical problems in adult ambulatory care* (2nd ed). Boston: Little, Brown and Company.

16. Victor, M., & Martin, J. (1994). Disorders of the cranial nerves. In K. Esselbacher et al. (Eds.), *Harrison's principles of internal medicine* (13th ed.). New York: McGraw-Hill, Inc.

17. Chen, L., & Goldschlager, N. (1995). Syncope: A directed search for cardiac and noncardiac causes. *Consultant, 35*(5), 655–666.

18. Kwiatkowski, T., & Alagappan, K. (1996). Syncope: An overview for the primary care physician. *Primary Care Update Ob/Gyns, 3*(3), 101–107.

19. Hart, G. (1995). Evaluation of syncope. *American Family Physician, 51*(8), 1941–1948.

20. Dichter, M. (1994). The epilepsies and convulsive disorders. In K. Esselbacher et al. (Eds.), *Harison's principles of internal medicine* (13th ed.). New York: McGraw-Hill, Inc.

21. Wilder, B. (1995). The treatment of epilepsy: An overview of clinical practices. *Neurology, 45*(Suppl.2), S7–S11.

22. Aminoff, M. (1996). Epilepsy. In L. Tierney, S. McPhee, & M. Papadakis (Eds.), *Current medical diagnosis & treatment* (35th ed.). Stamford, CT: Appleton & Lange.

23. Stacy, M., & Brownlee, H. (1996). Treatment options for early Parkinson's disease. *American Family Physician, 53*(4), 1281–1287.

24. Tang, M., Jacobs, D., Stern, Y., Marder, K. Schofield, P., Gurland, Andrews, H., & Mayeux, R. (1996). Effect of estrogen during menopause on risk and age at onset of Alzheimer's disease. *Lancet, 348,* 429–432.

25. Clarfield, A. (1996). Treatable vs untreatable dementia. *Clinical Geriatrics, 4*(1), 44–53.

26. Resnick, N. (1996). Geriatric medicine and the elderly patient. In L. Tierney, S. McPhee, & M. Papadakis (Eds.), *Current medical diagnosis & treatment* (35th ed.). Stamford, CT: Appleton & Lange.

27. Stewart, J. (1995). Management of behavior problems in the demented patient. *American Family Physician, 52*(8), 2311–2317.

28. Griffith, C. (1996). Chronic fatigue syndrome: New insights into an enigmatic illness. *Physician Assistant, 20*(2), 38–54.

Ophthalmological Disorders

1. Schachat, A. (1995). The red eye. In L. Barker, J. Burton, & P. Zieve (Eds.), *Principles of*

ambulatory medicine (4th ed.). Baltimore: Williams & Wilkins.

2. Small, R. (1995). Ophthamology in primary care: Office work-up for the red eye. *Consultant, 35*(3), 321–327.

3. Donnenfeld, E., Kaufman, H., & Schwab, I. (1993). Conjunctivitis: Update on diagnosis and treatment. *Patient Care, 27*(1), 22–46.

4. Riordan-Eva, P., & Vaughan, D. (1996). Eye. In L. Tierney, S. McPhee, & M. Papadakis (Eds.), *Current medical diagnosis and treatment* (35th ed.). Stamford, CT: Appleton & Lange.

5. Nishimoto, J. (1996). Iritis. *Postgraduate Medicine, 99*(2), 255–262.

6. Rosenberg, L. (1995). Glaucoma: Early detection and therapy for prevention of vision loss. *American Family Physician, 52*(8), 2289–2298.

7. U.S. Department of Health and Human Services, Public Health Service, Agency for Health Care Policy and Research. (1993). *Clinical practice guideline No. 4: Cataract in adults: Management of functional impairment* (Publication No. 93–0542). Rockville, MD: Author.

Pulmonary Disorders

1. *Global initiative for asthma, Global strategy for asthma management and prevention NHLBI/Who Workshop report.* (1995, January). (NIH Publication No. 95, 36–59). Bethesda, MD: National Heart, Lung and Blood Institute.

2. *International Concensus report on diagnosis and treatment of asthma.* (1992). (NIH Publication No. 92–3091).

3. Noble, J. (Ed.). (1996). *Textbook of primary care medicine.* St. Louis: Mosby Yearbook Inc.

4. Milve, S. (1995). Acute asthma exacerbations: Strategy for early assessment and aggressive management. *Consultant,* 1787–1796.

5. Report of the U.S. Preventative Services Task Force. (1996). *Guide to clinical preventative services.* Alexandria, VA: Internal Medical Publishing, Inc.

6. Reece, S. (1995). Preventing influenza and its complications: A Public Health Initiative for the Year 2000. *The Nurse Practitioner, 20,* 32–44.

7. Osguthospe, N., et al. (1995). An immunizing update for primary health care providers. *The Nurse Practitioner, 20,* 52–66.

8. Davis, A. (1996). Acute bronchitis in adults and children. *Patient Care,* 102–127.

9. File, T. (1996). Community-acquired pneumonia: What's needed for accurate diagnosis. *Post Graduate Medicine, 99*(1), 95–107.

10. Cunha, B. (1996). Community-Acquired Pneumonia. *Post Graduate Medicine, 99*(1), 109–122.

11. Cunha, B. (1996). Community-acquired pneumonia: New bugs, new drugs. *Patient Care,* 142–162.

12. Fine, M., et al. (1996). Prognosis and outcome of patients with community-acquired pneumonia. *JAMA, 275*(2), 134–141.

13. Friedman, M. (1995). Changing practices in COPD: A new pharmacologic treatment algorithm. *Chest, 107*(5), 194–197.

14. Ziment, I. (1995). The B-agonist controversy: Impact in COPD. *Chest, 107*(5), 198–205.

15. Pfister, S. (1995). Home oxygen therapy: Indications, administrations, recertifications, and patient education. *Nurse Practitioner, 20*(7), 44–55.

16. Fitzgerald, D., et al. (1996). Office evaluations of pulmonary function: Beyond the numbers. *American Family Physician, 54*(2), 525–534.

17. Inteciano, B. (1993). Metered-dose inhalers. *Archives Internal Medicine, 153,* 81–85.

18. Craig, T. (1996). Drugs to be used with caution in patients with asthma. *American Family Physician, 54,* 947–953.

19. Cunha, B. (1996). Atypical pneumonia. *Post Graduate Medicine, 99*(1), 123–132.

20. Wisinger, D. (1993). Bacterial pneumonia. *Post Graduate Medicine, 93*(7), 43–52.

Urinary Tract Disorders

1. Thompson, C. (1995). Urinary tract infections. In D. Lemcke, J. Pattison, L. Marshall, & D. Cowley (Eds.), *Primary care of women* (1st ed.). Norwalk, CT: Appleton & Lange.

2. Lerner, S. (1995). Recurrent urinary tract infections in otherwise healthy adult women. *Nurse Practitioner, 20* (10), 48–56.

3. Williams, D. (1996). Urinary tract infection. *Postgraduate Medicine, 99*(4), 189–204.

4. Nygaard, I., & Johnson, J. (1996). Urinary tract infections in elderly women. *American Family Physician, 53*(1), 175–182.

5. Staam, W., & Hooten, T. (1993). Management of urinary tract infections in adults. *New England Journal of Medicine, 329* (18), 1328–1334.

6. Medillo, K. (1995). Asymptomatic bacteruria in older adults: When is it necessary to screen and treat? *Nurse Practitioner, 20* (8), 50–66.

7. Eisenstein, B. (1994). Diseases caused by Gram-negative enteric bacilli. In K. Esselbacher, et al. (Eds.), *Harrison's principles of internal medicine* (13th ed.). New York: McGraw-Hill, Inc.

8. Ratliff, T., Klutke, C., & McDougall, E. (1994). The etiology of interstitial cystitis.

Urologic Clinics of North America, 21(1), 21–30.

 9. Barger, M., and Woolner, B. (1995). Primary care for women. Assessment and management of genitourinary tract disorders. *Journal of Nurse-Midwifery, 40*(2), 231–245.

10. Ratner, V., Slade, D., & Greene, G. (1994). Interstitial cystitis. A patient's perspective. *Urologic Clinics of North America, 21*(1), 1–5.

11. Koziol, J. (1994). Epidemiology of interstitial cystitis. *Urologic Clinics of North America, 21*(1), 7–20.

12. Whitmore, K. (1994). Self-care regimens for patients with interstitial cystitis. *Urologic Clinics of North America, 21*(1), 121–130.

13. Childs, S. (1994). Dimethyl sulfoxide (DMS02) in the treatment of interstitial cystitis. *Urologic Clinics of North America, 21*(1), 85–88.

14. Hanno, P. (1994). Amitryptilline in the treatment of interstitial cystitis. *Urologic Clinics of North America, 21*(1), 89–91.

15. Fleichman, J. (1994). Calcium channel blockers in the treatment of interstitial cystitis. *Urologic Clinics of North America, 21*(1), 107–111.

16. Theoharides, T. (1994). Hydroxyzine in the treatment of interstitial cystitis. *Urologic Clinics of North America, 21*(1), 113–119.

17. U.S. Department of Health and Human Services, Public Health Service, Agency for Health Care Policy and Research. (1996). *Clinical practice guidelines No. 2, 1996 update: Urinary incontinence in adults: Acute and chronic management.* (Publication No. 96–0682). Rockville, MD.

18. Haab, F., Zimmern, P., & Leach, G. (1996). Female stress urinary incontinence due to intrinsic sphincteric deficiency: Recognition and management. *The Journal of Urology, 156*(1), 3–17.

19. Mold, J. (1996). Pharmocology of Urinary Incontinence. *American Family Physician, 54*(2), 673–686.

20. Brown, J., Seeley, D., Fong, J., Beach, D., Ensrud, K., & Grady, D. (1996). Urinary incontinence in older women: Who is at risk? *Obstetrics and Gynecology, 87*(5), 715–721.

21. Bo, K., and Talseth, T. (1996). Long-term effect of pelvic floor muscle exercise 5 years after cessation of organized training. *Obstetrics and Gynecology, 87*(2), 261–265.

CHAPTER 23

PSYCHOSOCIAL HEALTH CONCERNS

Angela Carter Martin

*F*or a woman to achieve changes for herself and her family, she must acknowledge her self-worth. The health care provider can play a vital supporting role.

Highlights

- Stress
- Abuse of Women
    - Sexual Harassment
    - Violence
    - Sexual Abuse
- Substance Abuse
    - Smoking Cessation
- Mental Health Problems
    - Depression
    - Anxiety
    - Post-Traumatic Stress Disorder
    - Anorexia Nervosa
    - Bulimia
    - Binge-Eating disorder
- Homelessness

▶ INTRODUCTION

In the last 20 years, women have striven to legitimately and fully participate in the social, political, and economic systems in our country. Technological advances, improved living conditions, and decreased mortality related to pregnancy and childbirth have contributed to a life expectancy for a woman to 78.9 years.[1] Despite these advances, women continue to experience excessive stress and mental health problems that are associated with alienation, powerlessness, and poverty.[2]

To thoroughly address women's health, the primary care provider must consider the potential psychosocial problems that women face. Women experience higher rates of selected mood and anxiety disorders than do men.[3] Other specific problems are sexual harassment, physical and verbal abuse, and sexual assault; unwanted pregnancy; substance abuse; and eating disorders. Identifying women at risk for these health problems and managing their care are important roles for primary care providers.

Prevention of these complex psychosocial problems requires that women, and society as a whole, acknowledge their existence. Community education, referrals, support systems, and counseling offer women the opportunity to learn new skills and behaviors that can reduce the incidence of psychosocial problems and their associated mortality and morbidity. With resources available in the community, primary care providers can support women in their efforts to prevent or reduce the numbers of complex psychosocial problems they face. For a woman to achieve changes for herself and her family, she must believe in her self-worth. The primary care provider can play a vital supporting role.

STRESS

Stress is a unique and individual expression in response to any number of events. It occurs when the adaptive or coping mechanism is overwhelmed by events. An event is not always negative; it may be positive, such as marriage or a promotion.

Stress is the result of an intertwining of forces: stressors, perceptions of those stressors, emotional and physiological responses to those perceptions, and efforts to cope.[4] The degree to which a certain stressor causes stress is determined by the perception of that stressor.[4] Stressors may include interpersonal problems, time demands, and internal conflicts.[4]

Risk factors are poor support systems, ineffective coping skills and psychopathological conditions. No precise data are available about the incidence of stress; however, all individuals experience it to some degree.

Subjective Data

A woman may react to stress by becoming anxious or depressed, developing physical symptoms, or using substances. Women who are victims of violence or abuse often display signs of excessive stress early in the abuse or in reaction to acts of violence. See Abuse of Women, Sexual Abuse or Rape, Anxiety, Depression, and Substance Abuse sections.

Objective Data

See Abuse of Women, Sexual Abuse or Rape, Anxiety, Depression, and Substance Abuse sections.

Differential Medical Diagnoses

Coronary heart disease, chronic pain, headaches, hypertension, asthma, rheumatoid arthritis, irritable bowel syndrome, ulcers, eczema, anxiety, depression, muscular tension, insomnia, fatigue.

Plan

Psychosocial Intervention. Discuss with the client ways to avoid a stressful situation. If a stressful situation is unavoidable, discuss ways to minimize stress by altering the stressor.[4] If a stressor is unavoidable, the client needs to develop coping skills to deal with it. Coping is through a healthy lifestyle (sleep, balanced nutrition, exercise, relaxation).[4] Help the client to identify self-induced stress caused by unrealistic expectations and to correct the stress producing thoughts.[4] Encourage the client to develop a relaxation program; it might include progressive muscle relaxation, meditation, and breathing exercises. Time management and assertiveness training may also be helpful.

Follow-Up

If physical causes for the client's symptoms do not exist, refer the client to a mental health specialist for a complete psychological evaluation.

Abuse of Women

SEXUAL HARASSMENT

Sexual harassment encompasses unwelcome sexual advances, requests for sexual favors, and other oral or physical conduct or written communications of an intimidating, hostile, or offensive nature or action taken in retaliation for reporting such behavior, regardless of where such conduct might occur.[5,6] Sexual harassment is a common experience, affecting 42 percent of women in occupational settings and 73 percent of women during medical training.[6] Sexual harassment occurs most often among women working in a male dominated profession but may occur in any work environment. Sexual harassment occurs in all age groups, with 50 percent of younger women, ages 11 to 16 years, reporting such abuse.[7] Few women file complaints against the perpetrator. It is thought that women frequently fail to report sexual harassment because they prefer to have the abuse stopped rather than to see the perpetrator punished.[6]

Subjective Data

A woman may express an inability to concentrate, reduction in confidence, decreased motivation that affects her job, tension, nervousness, anger, fear, or helplessness. These feelings may or may not carry over into her home. Physical complaints may include nausea, loss of appetite, headaches, chest pain, and chronic fatigue, which may lead to use or abuse of alcohol, prescriptive drugs, or nonprescriptive drugs to reduce stress related symptoms.

The history includes several specific points of information.

- *Chief complaint,* with brief description in chronological order of present problem, document dates when harassment began and what action, if any, the client has taken to stop the harassment
- *Medical history* noting childhood illnesses; injuries (be observant for injuries that are not consistent with explanation); hospitalizations and surgeries; previous major illnesses; allergies; habits (start with less offensive), including caffeine, tobacco, alcohol, and illicit drugs; and medications, prescriptive and nonprescriptive
- *Family medical history* noting substance abuse and any mental health problems
- *Social history* noting family relationships (married/separated/divorced/single); support system; occupational history (time at present job, recent loss of job or job change); and economic status
- *Subjective psychological functioning,* with cognitive abilities (orientation to present, memory, history of psychiatric illness) and cultural implications, evaluate for anxiety and depressive symptoms
- *Lifestyle history* noting nutrition and rest and exercise patterns

Objective Data

A thorough physical examination and wide range of diagnostic tests complete the diagnostic process.

Physical Examination
- *General Appearance.* The client may appear disheveled or be well groomed, may be over- or

underweight, and may appear anxious or nervous.

- *Eyes.* Circles may be visible under eyes. Eyes may be red and puffy from lack of sleep or crying.
- *Neck.* Neck muscles may be tense and tender from stress or tension.
- *Skin.* Observe for bruising, lacerations, burns, dryness, or cold and clamminess.
- *Nails and Hair.* The nails and hair may be dull and brittle.
- *Chest.* Note any increase in respiratory rate.
- *Vascular System.* Note any increase in blood pressure and heartrate.
- *Abdomen.* Bowel sounds may be hypoactive or hyperactive. Abdomen may be tender on palpation.
- *Musculoskeletal System.* Examination may reveal bruising, redness, edema, joint pain or swelling, poor posture, tense muscles, or limited range of motion.
- *Nervous System.* Poor coordination, unsteady gait, abnormal cranial nerve evaluation, sluggish speech, flight of ideas, inability to concentrate, and poor memory are possible findings.
- *Genitalia.* If indicated. See Sexual Abuse.

Diagnostic Tests (depending on the clinical presentation)

- Electrocardiogram
- Electroencephalogram, if indicated
- Complete blood count to rule out anemia and infection
- Thyroid panel to rule out thyroid disease
- Other lab tests as necessary for health promotion/maintenance and/or to evaluate symptoms

Nursing Implications

Throughout the physical examination, validate all normal findings and reassure the client. Before laboratory tests, explain the test, review what the process involves and why the test is being done. Explain any abnormal findings completely.

Differential Medical Diagnoses

Depression, chronic fatigue syndrome, gastroenteritis, dyspepsia/ulcers, migraine or cluster headaches, panic/anxiety attacks, stress.

Plan

Psychosocial Intervention. Listen carefully to the client's description of the harassment. Provide information about the emotional, physical, economic, and family effects of harassment. Validate the connection between physical and emotional symptoms and the harassment. Explore the impact of harassment on marital and family life.[8] Validate the client's experience and help her resist devaluing herself. Discuss options and their ramifications. Encourage assertiveness training and stress management, and review existing coping skills. Help refine coping skills as needed. Often feelings of empowerment will alleviate symptoms of depression and anxiety.

Follow-Up

Refer the client to a psychotherapist or other mental health professional for individual or group counseling. Referral for legal counsel may also be appropriate.

VIOLENCE

Abuse occurs in many forms, from forceful physical abuse to less obviously damaging verbal abuse. Intent to hurt the victim ranges from slapping, beating, pushing, biting, and threatening to attack with a weapon. Psychological aggression and abuse not only refer to verbal abuse, such as insults, constant negative feedback, screaming, and swearing, but may include depriving a woman of sleep and food. This violence often involves a combination of abusive acts.[9] Most violent acts committed against women involve intimates.[10] Women report less than half of all incidents of violence committed by intimates to authorities.[11]

Epidemiology

Etiology. Violence and abuse are often the result of inefficient coping and stress reducing skills. Frequently, the abuser's behavior is the result of learning; the abuser may have witnessed abuse or been abused.[9,12]

The battering cycle, or cycle of violence, is characterized by tension building incidents.[12,13] Tension builds with acts of intimidation and initial, though lesser, physical abuse (shoving, pushing, name calling). As it escalates, the woman first tries to placate her partner. When this does not work, she withdraws to prevent a confrontation. During this time, the woman's repressed anger can contribute to her sense of guilt and low self-esteem. He may become more aggressive as she withdraws.

Explosion occurs following mounting tension with physical and verbal attack and subsequent injury. The woman often feels she was at fault and the outburst was justified. The explosive phase usually lasts 24 hours or fewer, which allows the abuser to release tension.

During the honeymoon that follows the explosion, the abuser repents and promises never to abuse again.[13] The abused woman wants to believe that the abuse will stop and stays in the relationship.

In the repetitive cycle, abuse does not stop with one incident, but increases in frequency and severity. Learned helplessness, low self-esteem, feelings of guilt, lack of resources, and anticipatory fear eventually immobilize a woman to the point where she feels there is no way to escape.[9,13] The abused woman usually has a small social network with whom she can confide but probably will not because of her shame and guilt. She is usually dependent on her abuser, both emotionally and financially, and makes excuses for the abuser's behavior.[13] The abused woman is caught between maintaining the relationship, economic survival, and the well-being of her partner and children on the one side, and her own physical and emotional well-being on the other.[14]

Risk Factors. History of abuse as a child, poor self-esteem, substance abuse or dependence, limited resources, and absence of support persons are risk factors.[15]

Incidence. Violence against women is a major health problem. An assailant attacks a woman somewhere in the United States every 15 seconds. Between 2 and 4 million women are physically battered each year.[16] Minority women are particularly at risk for such abuse.[17,18] In a study of prevalence of violence against women in a primary care setting, over 25 percent of women respondents had experienced physical and emotional partner abuse in the previous year, and the abuse was disclosed to primary care physicians only 28 percent of the time.[19] Approximately 30 percent of women who use emergency rooms do so because of spousal or partner abuse.[20] One-half of all homicides of women are committed by a current or former boyfriend.[21]

Subjective Data

Few women who seek medical care will state the cause of their injuries. Health care providers seeing nonacutely ill women in an office setting will not be confronted with any specific sign or symptom suggestive of battering.[9,17]

Vague symptoms may present during the tension building phase secondary to increased stress. Symptoms may include backaches, headaches, fatigue, anxiety, stress, insomnia, anorexia, indigestion, hypertension, allergic skin reactions, palpitations, hyperventilation, chest pain, choking sensation, claustrophobic feelings, and pelvic pain.[21,22]

In relating her history, a client may be hesitant, embarrassed, or evasive. She can look depressed, abuse alcohol and medications, and have a history of suicide attempts.[21,22,23] Gathering a complete social history, including substance use and abuse, family situation, and support systems is important. If the client reports abuse, documentation of all details is important. Explore any history of prior episodes of abuse with the client.

Indicators of possible battering include change in appointment pattern (increased or frequently missed appointments), complaints of problems at home or with partner (partner jealous, possessive), making excuses for partner's behavior, and ambivalent statements about battering or signs of fear when discussing it.[24,25] Provide the client with privacy while interviewing. If the abuser is with her, try to speak to her alone without raising the abuser's suspicion.

Objective Data

Do a complete physical exam and carefully document the findings. Assure the client that the assault was not her fault. Explicitly document the extent and types of abuse and note if the client's explanation is not consistent with her injuries.

Encourage the client to respond to questions; however, if she becomes upset, explain concern and describe the cycle of violence, emphasizing its repetitive and escalating nature.

In the physical examination, a body map documenting the current injuries, healing injuries, and scars will be helpful in describing the client's presentation in the future. Take photographs if written consent given. Try to photograph the client's face or attach some type of identifying information, e.g., driver's license when taking photographs.

- *General Appearance.* The client may appear well groomed or chaotic with torn clothes. She may be nervous and emotional or calm and collected. There may be injuries that require immediate attention or no visible signs of injury.
- *Head, Face, and Throat.* These are the most typical locations of injury.[9]
- *Skin.* Note any lacerations, burns, and bruises of the skin, both old and new. Be sure to examine all areas covered by clothing. If the patient has not changed clothes, inspect clothes for evidence of violence.
- *Chest.* Chest exam may reveal difficulty breathing because of pain from fractured ribs.
- *Vascular System.* Look for elevated blood pressure and heartrate.
- *Abdomen.* Abdominal pain may be evident with palpation. In pregnant women, the breast and abdomen are targets of assault.[26,27]
- *Genitalia.* See the section on Sexual Abuse.
- *Musculoskeletal System.* Look for fractures of the extremities, ribs, and skull; pain with palpation, redness, swelling, and bruising.

All primary care providers should be knowledgeable about specific legal guidelines in their state. Notify police when the law requires it or if a client requests legal assistance.[28,29]

Differential Medical Diagnoses

Trauma not related to abuse, suicide attempt, self-mutilation.

Plan

Because of their potential for early contact with victims, primary care providers are in an excel-

lent position to intervene in the cycle of domestic and/or family violence.

Psychosocial Intervention. Ideally, intervention should begin during the tension building phase or immediately after an abusive incident.

Identification of the Problem

Many primary care providers fail to recognize the signs and symptoms of abuse. Explore all suspicions of abuse, even at the risk that the abuse does not exist.[22,24]

- Support the client in acknowledging a problem
- Affirm that abusive behavior is unacceptable
- Assist the woman to gain access to available community resources, such as housing, counseling, legal services (The provider does not, however, initiate contact).[21,29]
- Help the client to identify options, as she may believe she has none
- Assist the client to develop an escape plan if she plans to stay in the abusive situation. (This includes placing clothes, money, and copies of necessary documents in an easily accessible, secret, and secure place.)[30]

Follow-Up

Counseling is essential; also, encourage clients to consider asking for professional help. Often, however, the client is not ready to seek assistance. Providers respect the client's decision. Abused women will often leave and return several times to an abusive relationship before deciding that the relationship should be ended.[28] Pursue treatment of all injuries and order x-rays as needed.

SEXUAL ABUSE OR RAPE

Sexual abuse or rape is forced sexual intercourse perpetrated against the will of a victim.[31,32] Force may be employed by physical violence, coercion, or threat of harm. Acquaintance rape usually occurs in a dating situation and is perpetrated by someone the woman knows and trusts.[28,31] Sexual assault involves actions other than rape: sodomy, forced anal intercourse; oral copulation, forced copulation of mouth of one person with sexual organ or anus of another; rape with a foreign object, forced penetration of genital or anal openings with a foreign object; and sexual battery, unwanted touching of an intimate part for sexual arousal.

Burgess and Fawcett have published a comprehensive sexual assault assessment tool that addresses the many complicated social, medical and psychological effects of sexual assault on a woman.[33] Primary care providers may find this tool helpful for documentation.

Epidemiology

Etiology. Rape challenges a woman's ability to maintain her defenses and arouses feelings of guilt, anxiety, and inadequacy.[31,32] The overwhelming experience heightens her sense of helplessness and intensifies her conflict about dependence and independence. The survivor's response is determined by her stage in life, her defensive structures, and her coping ability.

Rape trauma syndrome comprises the sequential reactions of the survivor in dealing with her experience. The syndrome, described as a two- or three-stage process, helps explain how rape victims respond to the traumatic experience of rape.

The immediate response, or acute phase, occurs immediately after the assault or the disclosure of assault.[31,32] The survivor's lifestyle is completely disrupted and reactions are tearfulness and agitation or a relaxed calm.[29] This stage can last as long as 3 to 6 months, with typical symptoms being anxiety, fears and phobias, suspiciousness, major depressive symptoms, feelings of inferiority, inability to think clearly, and difficulty functioning at home, work, or school.[31,32] In addition, feelings of guilt, shame, embarrassment, and self-blame are common. Psychophysiological disturbances affect eating, sleeping, gastrointestinal function, and sexual intimacy.[34] Ensuring safety and regaining control over her life are the survivor's main emotional needs during this time.[31,32] Medical attention is important as 66 percent of women will show trauma of a mild to moderate degree, and 4.5 percent will have serious physical injuries.[35]

The middle phase, or readjustment stage, is a period of transition when the survivor rationalizes that she could have prevented the assault and develops unrealistic plans to avoid another.[31,32]

The final stage, or reorganization phase, may last 2 years or longer and is difficult and painful.[31] During this stage, the survivor begins to deal with the reality of her victimization and may make changes in lifestyle, relationship, and work.[31]

Along with a two or three stage model of recovery, other authors discuss recovery within the broader content of post-traumatic stress disorder (PTSD) as described in the *Diagnostic and Statistical Manual of Mental Disorders.*[36] See Post-traumatic Stress Disorder for a complete discussion. Another mental health disorder that may occur as an outcome of rape is acute stress disorder, differentiated from post-traumatic stress disorder by the time symptoms are exhibited. The symptoms last for at least 2 days but do not persist longer than 4 weeks after the traumatic event.[37]

Risk Factors. Any woman is at risk; however, dating situations, unfamiliar partners, alcohol and drug use, and miscommunication create additional risk.

Incidence. Rape is one of the most frequently committed and underreported violent crimes in the United States. Taking unreported rapes into consideration, one of every three women will be raped during her lifetime.[12] A rape of a woman is reported every 6 minutes.[38] About 12.1 million U.S. women (one of every eight adult women) have been forcible rape victims during their lives.[39] A woman may be raped at any age, but the highest risk occurs between the ages of 15 and 24.[15] Unmarried, separated or divorced women and nonwhite women are the most frequent victims of rape and attempted rape.[11]

Subjective Data

A client may report various physical and psychological problems. Explore a history of sexual abuse in any woman who presents with multiple physical complaints, even if associated with functional limitations.[40]

Careful recording of the details of the assault, along with the client's gynecological, sexual, and social histories, is essential. If the assault occurred within the last 72 hours, refer the client to a designated sexual assault center with trained sexual assault examiners for the completion of the assessment.[41] Primary care providers who work in rural areas may not have access to such expertise. Providers in such settings should be knowledgeable in the assessment of sexual assault. The following information is for educational purposes of nonexpert examiners and for the assessment of victims who report the assault later. Detailed forms are available for the documentation of such an assessment.[33]

Symptoms may include headaches, sleep disturbance, loss of appetite with weight loss or gain, nausea, vomiting, constipation, diarrhea, sexual dysfunction, menstrual irregularities, abnormal vaginal discharge, and urinary dysfunction. The client may report difficulty in relationships with others and in functioning at home, work, or school.

The history of assault will include date, time, location, description, use of a weapon, and type of weapon; the part of the body penetrated, the object used to penetrate (body part or foreign object); occurrence of ejaculation; and involvement of alcohol or other drugs. Record any information about the assailant. Question the client about her activities after the assault: Did she shower, change clothes, urinate, or defecate?

The past medical history includes dates of immunizations, especially tetanus and hepatitis. Prior HIV titer or status if known.

The obstetric and gynecologic history includes the date of the client's previous menstrual period, pregnancies, abortions, and miscarriages; contraceptive methods used; and history of sexually transmitted infections.

The sexual history includes information about the client's sexual activity: Was she sexually active within 1 week before or after assault? Has she been the victim of past sexual assaults (give dates)? Does she have any HIV high risk sexual contact.

The social history includes information about whether the survivor lives alone, has a support system, wants someone notified, needs social service assistance, or wants police notified if they are not aware of assault.

Objective Data

Document findings from the physical examination and any forensic tests conducted.

Complete a thorough physical examination and sexually transmitted disease (STD) testing after treating major injuries, no matter how much time has elapsed since the assault. If the woman has not showered or changed clothes since the assault, have her disrobe while standing on a sheet to collect any evidence. Then, give her a gown. Place any clothes that may contain evidence in a labeled paper bag.

Physical Examination

- *General Appearance.* The survivor may be calm and relaxed or tearful and emotional. Notice torn and stained clothes; injuries may be visible.
- *Head, Face, and Throat.* There may be lacerations, abrasions, and bruising. Dried secretions may be present on the face, mouth, or ears. The client may complain of headaches.
- *Chest.* There may be bruising, lacerations, and abrasions and tenderness on palpation. Note any increased respiration, difficulty breathing, or hyperventilation.
- *Abdomen.* Bruising, lacerations, abrasions, and tenderness may be evident, indicating potential internal injuries.
- *Musculoskeletal System.* Look for potential fractures by examining skin for lacerations, abrasions, bruising, and the back and extremities for tenderness.
- *Gastrointestinal.* Symptoms may include anorexia, nausea, vomiting, and abdominal or rectal pain.
- *Genitalia and Reproductive Tract.* The perineum, rectal area, and vagina may have bruises, lacerations, and abrasions. Bartholin's and Skene's glands and the urethral meatus may be tender. Uterine size, shape, and consistency may be abnormal. Note any tenderness with cervical motion and uterine and adnexal palpation. Watch for tears or pain on rectovaginal examination as suggestive of internal pelvic trauma.
- *Psychiatric.* The client may report symptoms of anxiety, depression, suicidal ideation, mood swings, phobias, sexual difficulties, uncontrollable memories or flashbacks, substance abuse, detachment from others or dissociative symptoms.

Use a body map to document all injuries, including their size, location, and coloration.

Photographs of abrasions, with some form of identification appearing on the photographs, may be helpful if the victim plans legal action. Obtain written consent.

Diagnostic Tests. Complete within 24 to 72 hours of the assault. Forensic specimen collection is best when done by an experienced practitioner.[41] All laboratory findings are documented in the medical record. Use a Wood's light to check the perineum and thighs for blood or semen.

Obtain gonorrhea and chlamydia cultures from the endocervix, vaginal vault, rectum, and oropharynx, as indicated by history or evidence of penetration.

Collect urine for microscopic examination and pregnancy test. Obtain cervical and rectal swabs for evidence of herpes simplex virus. Determine HIV status at this time.

Wet mount specimens can show trichomonas, clue cells, and motile sperm for up to 72 hours. Include the pH of vaginal discharge and presence of positive whiff test.

Collect a vaginal smear to detect sperm and p30 prostate specific antigen; considered more reliable than phosphatase determination.

Bloodwork includes blood type/Rh, hepatitis antigen, rapid plasma reagin (RPR), and HIV antibody titer serum.

Collect fingernail scrapings from each hand and save in separately labeled bag.

Collect hair samples by combing both head and pubic hair; specimens placed in labeled bags.

Blood and dried fluids found on the survivor's body and clothing collected and labeled for DNA fingerprinting. Saliva is collected for blood group antigen testing.

Nursing Implications

In caring for a victim of sexual abuse or rape, it is important to understand that evaluation and treatment of the survivor require a multidisciplinary approach. If possible, a rape counselor who is present during the entire evaluation process can be helpful to provide client support.

If a woman calls and reports rape, instruct her to avoid showering or changing her clothes. Encourage her to go to the emergency room nearest her or to the health care provider's office.

Before taking a complete history, explain the process and that the information will help in her medical management as well as for forensic use. Determination of rape occurs in a court of law; therefore, the wording in the history should reflect only the client's report of the incident.[41] It is important to record, sign, and date all information. Ask the client to sign a consent form and release of information form. Reassure the woman that answers to questions, especially those covering her sexual history, will ensure proper medical treatment. Throughout her visit, explain each procedure and why it is being done, and restore her sense of control. Give her options and seek consent with each procedure. Reinforce that rape was not her fault. Provide information about available social services, including a crisis hotline. Assist her to decide whether to report the crime, and encourage her to seek follow-up care.

Differential Medical Diagnoses

Trauma not related to sexual assault.

Plan

Psychosocial Intervention. Refer the client for counseling. Women who do not deal realistically with rape and resolutions of issues may develop severe, long-term sequelae, such as depression, substance abuse, anxiety disorder, and suicide.[40] If the woman desires legal action, assist the woman in contacting the proper authorities.

Medication. Offer medication for sexually transmitted diseases or possible pregnancy.

Treatment for STDs (antibiotic prophylaxis) should be offered because of the 5 percent risk that infection was transmitted.[35,41] Six to twelve percent of victims contract chlamydia and/or gonorrhea; 3 percent contract syphilis, according to the Centers for Disease Control.[35] Other infections are commonly contracted, like trichomonas, bacterial vaginosis, and herpes (see Chapter 11 for treatment guidelines. Note: New CDC Guidelines are due late Fall 1997). Review the risks and benefits of both treatment and observation. If the client refuses prophylactic antibiotics, then do follow-up cultures at the 6-week visit. If the client consents to prophylactic antibiotics, then treat her according to current Centers for Disease Control

(CDC) guidelines for chlamydia, gonorrhea, syphilis, and trichomoniasis.

Offer postcoital contraceptive (PCC) medication to the client unless pregnancy exists or suspected. The risk of pregnancy with one act of intercourse varies from 0 percent to 26 percent, depending on the cycle day of exposure relative to ovulation. PCC medication reduces the risk of pregnancy by 75 percent.[41] Postcoital contraception is a safe, effective tool in avoiding unintended pregnancy. It is offered at the time of assault, regardless of the cycle phase.[35]

The most common regimen is taking two Ovral tablets (ethinyl estradiol 50 g and 0.5 mg norgestrel progestin) within 72 hours of coitus and two more 12 hours after the first dose (see Chapter 9, Emergency Contraception for a review of this treatment). Perform a pregnancy test before any administration of medication. A history of thrombosis or perhaps of hypertension would be potential contraindications. Review with the client the side effects, including nausea and vomiting; and danger signs, including abdominal pain, chest pain, headache, blurred vision, and leg pain. Other alternatives suggested are Lo-Ovral, Levelen, Nordette, Triphasil yellow pills, or Tri-Levlen yellow pills given in appropriate doses (4 pills each time).[42] Offer hepatitis B and tetanus vaccination if indicated.

Follow-Up

A telephone call or return office visit within 24 to 48 hours of initial treatment allows for ongoing evaluation of problems and concerns. Schedule an appointment for 1 week after initial treatment to evaluate physical and emotional status. If the client has no complaints, defer the physical exam. Review all laboratory findings with the client. Inquire about counseling. If the client does not participate in counseling, encourage her to begin and provide a referral. Schedule the last visit at 4–6 weeks. At that time, complete a repeat physical exam, collect specimens for repeat cultures for STDs, rapid plasma reagin, and HIV antibody. Repeat HIV testing in 3 month intervals up to 1 year following exposure. Perform a pregnancy test as needed.

Golding found that a sexual assault history with physical symptoms often correlate with im-

paired functioning, and personal and social costs to the woman.[40] In following women with a history of assault, the researcher points to the importance of primary care provider's role in helping affected women recover from the assault. If the trauma remains unresolved and/or the abuse is chronic, referral to community services and mental health care is necessary.

SUBSTANCE ABUSE

ALCOHOL, COCAINE, SEDATIVES-HYPNOTICS, CANNABIS, OPIATES AND TOBACCO

The DSM-IV makes a distinction between substance abuse and substance dependence. Primary care providers will regularly see clients with both conditions. Substance abuse will be the primary focus of this section. Information on treating substance dependence is available from any psychiatric textbook or substance treatment manual. A maladaptive pattern of psychoactive substance use is indicated by at least one of the following: the client continues to use a psychoactive or potentially addicting substance despite her awareness of persistent or recurrent social, occupational, psychological, or physical problems that are caused or exacerbated by its use; the client continues to use the substance in situations where use is physically hazardous; some symptoms of disturbance occur within a 12-month period; the client does not fulfill criteria for psychoactive substance dependence.[37] Substance abuse is multidimensional with interacting factors that predispose the client to addictive use. Gender, age, race, physiology, and genetics all contribute to development of addictive disease.[28,37]

Epidemiology

Etiology. Substance abuse and the risk factors for addiction are in many instances predictable. Clients who have a family history of addiction are at risk for addiction to drugs and compulsive behaviors.[28,37]

Female physiology may be influential. Women develop adverse health consequences from the use and abuse of alcohol and other drugs over shorter time periods and with lower consumption than men. Studies have documented that women have a physiological response to alcohol that is significantly different from men. Women enter substance abuse treatment at generally the same ages as men, but with shorter histories of substance use and more severe consequences.[43-45] One recent study indicates that alcoholic women showed deterioration of muscles, including the heart muscle, equal to that of men even though the women's lifetime dose of alcohol was 60 percent that of men.[46]

Psychological factors are influential. Psychopathology and psychological conflicts place women at risk for substance abuse. Traditional patterns of women's socialization include the belief that the needs of spouse, children, and others come first and that the expression of such feelings as anger and competition is unfeminine. Women may attempt to deal with their negative feelings through pharmacological suppression or drinking.[43]

Risk Factors. Specific risk factors exist.

- An addictive parent
- Divorce or separation
- Living alone with children
- Lesbian lifestyle
- Reliance on pharmacological agents or alcohol to relax, sleep, feel more comfortable in social settings, or control unpleasant feelings
- Adolescent smoking

Incidence. Approximately 17 million Americans (6.8 percent) have symptoms of alcoholism.[47] Historically, men have higher rates of alcoholism and other substance abuse; the incidence of substance abuse is gender related. Women, however, represent a growing percentage of drinkers. Among younger women in the general population, the proportion of drinkers is beginning to approximate that of men. In addition, rates of substance abuse in women may be underreported. By the year 2000, assuming a constant rate of alcoholism, there will be half again as many elderly alcoholics.[48] Though older women drink less and have fewer drinking problems than older men, their use of prescribed psychoactive drugs is thought to cause more problems.[49,50,51]

In 1993, approximately 11.7 million Americans reported that they currently used illegal drugs.[1] Women used virtually the same types of illegal drugs as did men, but they used them less frequently than men did (4.1 percent versus 7.4 percent in 1993).[1] Adolescent drug use is up 105 percent since 1992. The annual results of the National Household Survey on Drug Abuse show the percentage of adolescents between the age of 12 and 17 who admitted to using illegal drugs in the month preceding the survey increased from 5.3 percent in 1992 to 10.9 percent in 1995.[52] Use of all types of drugs is reported to have increased, but heroin use is estimated to have doubled since the mid-1980s. Purer products and a decline in the price are thought to be a factor.[53] Women are more likely than men to become addicted to prescription drugs and use them with alcohol, as they outnumber men in their reported abuse of over-the-counter medications in combination with alcohol.[54] Tobacco addiction causes a number of preventable deaths in the United States. While the prevalence of smoking has declined to nearly 23–25 percent of the U.S. population and the health risks associated with smoking are widely known, millions of Americans continue to smoke.[1] Between 1965 and 1985, the percentage of women who were defined as heavy smokers increased from 13 percent to 23 percent.[1]

Subjective Data

Careful observation and listening may reveal symptoms of abuse of a specific substance. Histories are also essential. Symptoms of abuse are often specific to a particular substance.

Alcohol abusers often report gastritis, vomiting, and diarrhea. They may lose or gain weight. In addition, a client may report nervousness, anxiety, depression, sleep disturbances, pelvic pain, abnormal vaginal discharge, infertility, or sexual dysfunction.

Cocaine abuse may lead to sinusitis and upper respiratory infection, allergic rhinitis, nasal congestion, and epistaxis. Weight loss may be experienced. Abstinence from cocaine may produce anxiety, fatigue, depression, irritability, and sleep disturbances.

Abuse of sedatives-hypnotics (benzodiazepines) may cause headaches, nausea, paranoia, and sleep disturbances. Withdrawal may cause insomnia and irritability. When used with alcohol, sedatives-hypnotics increase central nervous system depressant effects.

Cannabis (marijuana) abuse may provoke fatigue, decreased motivation, panic attacks, anxiety, and paranoia.[55]

Abuse of opiates produces an initial sense of euphoria, followed by a sense of tranquility and then sleepiness. Tolerance and dependence develop requiring higher doses to maintain the desired level of euphoria. Opiates do not directly cause serious organ damage.[55]

Use of tobacco causes many effects on the body. Chronic cough, wheezing, dyspnea, sore throat, and bad breath are rarely mentioned as complaints by clients. Clients do become concerned, however, about chronic obstructive pulmonary disease, asthma, cardiovascular disease, lung cancer and other potentially fatal illnesses, all of which have been associated with tobacco use. Tobacco products also contain nicotine, which is known to cause addiction and withdrawal.[55]

Histories are the best indicators of early substance abuse. Screening for substance abuse focuses on adverse consequences (e.g., family or marital problems, seizures or withdrawal symptoms) rather than on physical or laboratory findings.[56] An alcohol history may use a screening questionnaire such as the CAGE, questionnaire which looks at patterns and consequences, or the Short Michigan Alcoholism Screening Test (SMAST) which deals with consequences. Diagnosis should not rest solely on the questionnaire; rather, the questionnaire is used to determine the index of suspicion for abuse.[56,57] Clients will often describe starting out experimenting with a substance, like tobacco, to go on to using more and more to achieve the same effects.

The health care provider should always approach the client in a nonbiased manner. When questioning about abuse *always* begin with questions about less sensitive substances: How many cups of coffee do you drink per day? How much tobacco do you use per day? How many drinks per day? Then ask about tolerance (How many drinks does it take for you to feel high?) and the occurrence of blackouts. Inability to remember what happened when drinking is a probable sign of alcoholism.[37,55]

The drug history includes information about prescription medication, over-the-counter medication, and illicit drugs (substance abuse may progress from alcohol, to cannabis, to cocaine, etc.). Inquire if one drug is taken in conjunction with another or with alcohol. Previous treatment for substance abuse should be noted. Has the client tried to quit smoking in the past? If so, how did she quit and how long did she maintain nonuse of the substance.

The social history includes information about marital or family problems, job or promotion loss due to poor performance or absenteeism, financial difficulties and multiple arrests for disorderly conduct or driving under influence of a drug. Inquire about behavior changes, such as termination of old friendships and loss of interest in favorite pastimes.[58]

Past medical histories include questions about accidental injuries and illnesses related to abuse. For example, individuals who abuse cocaine have frequent urinary tract infections, sinusitis, nosebleeds, and burns if the drug is smoked; alcohol abuse may cause gastroenteritis, ulcers, hepatitis, and pneumonia; and cannabis frequently causes urinary tract infections.[55] Smoking causes increased rates of upper respiratory and lung infections. A history of pneumonia or chronic bronchitis may be elicited.[55]

The reproductive system and sexual history includes questions about pregnancies, abortions, sexually transmitted infections, pelvic inflammatory disease, abnormal Pap smears, menstrual irregularities, sexual dysfunction, and STD and HIV risk factors. Substance use and abuse decrease inhibitions. Consequently, a woman is more likely to engage in sexual intercourse, which may increase the risk of sexual abuse. Substance abuse may lead to frequent partners if sex is exchanged for substance; intravenous drug use increases the risk of hepatitis B and HIV infection.[55]

Family medical history includes information about mental illness, dysfunctional family, and substance abuse. Exposure to second-hand smoke should be noted.

Objective Data

Although histories and observation are important investigative tools, diagnosis is rarely made without laboratory tests and physical examination.

Alcohol. Alcoholism may be diagnosed with the use of physical examination and a variety of diagnostic tests: blood, liver, electrolyte, thyroid, glucose, and stool.

Physical Examination[55,56]

- *Skin.* Hair loss, cigarette burns, seborrheic dermatitis, palmar erythema, infections, thrombosed and spider veins (particularly on the chest) may be evident.
- *Head and Eyes.* Poor dentition is likely, with possible lesions on the posterior lateral tongue (increased risk for oropharyngeal cancer with alcohol and tobacco abuse) and alcohol odor to the breath. The face may be red and puffy; signs and symptoms of sinusitis present; the nose enlarged with prominent veins; the eyes puffy with erythematous conjunctiva, yellow sclera or dilated pupils; the voice hoarse with or without cough; and the parotid gland enlarged.
- *Chest.* The client may complain of a chronic cough. Auscultation of rates "E" to "A" changes indicate possible pneumonia. Point tenderness may be caused by ribs fractured during falls. Symptoms of chronic bronchitis, asthma, tuberculosis, noncardiogenic pulmonary edema may be noted.
- *Vascular System.* Examination may reveal cardiac arrhythmia, tachycardia, and hypertension. Symptoms may be suggestive of mitral value disease.
- *Abdomen.* The liver is palpable and tender in hepatitis. The spleen may be enlarged. Ascites may be present. Abdominal pain suggests gastritis, ulcers, duodenitis, esophagitis, ileitis, irritable bowel syndrome, or pancreatitis.
- *Musculoskeletal System.* Bruises or fractures indicate trauma. An abnormal gait and decreased muscle strength are related to myopathy. Gout causes red, tender, and edematous joints.
- *Genitalia and Reproductive Tract.* Menstrual irregularities, unplanned pregnancy, abnormal vaginal discharge, and pelvic pain with adnexal and cervical motion tenderness are possible findings.
- *Nervous System.* Examination may reveal abnormal cranial nerve findings, ataxia, positive Romberg, peripheral neuropathy, cerebral degeneration, myopathy, optic neuropathy, and presence of tremors or seizures.

Diagnostic Tests

- *Blood Tests.* Blood alcohol level may be elevated, positive toxicology screen for multiple substances; hemoglobin and hematocrit decreased (anemia); mean corpuscular volume increased (common finding in alcohol abuse); prothrombin time prolonged; platelets decreased (clotting disorder); elevated uric acid.
- *Liver Function Tests.* Serum g-glutamyltransferase (SGGT) (most sensitive), alanine aminotransferase (ALT), aspartate aminotransferase (AST), lactate dehydrogenase (LDH), amylase, alkaline phosphatase, total bilirubin, cholesterol, and triglycerides all increased (indicative of alcoholic liver disease).
- *Electrolytes.* Serum magnesium, calcium, phosphorus, and potassium usually decreased.
- *Thyroid Function.* Abnormal (especially in stimulant users).
- *Glucose.* May be increased or decreased; further evaluation by HgbA1C or GTT may be indicated.
- *Stool.* Occult blood present.

Sedatives-Hypnotics. Sedative-hypnotic abuse may be detected by symptoms similar to a state intoxication followed by drowsiness. Withdrawal from sedatives (benzodiazepines)-hypnotics can be fatal. Detoxification from sedatives-hypnotics should always be in an inpatient setting.[55] Many times there are no obvious physical findings, except in an overdose. Clients who overdose are seen in the emergency room.

Cannabis. Cannabis abuse may be detected by means of physical examination, with close attention to the eyes, and an electrocardiogram.

Physical Examination

- *General Appearance.* Dreamlike state.
- *Skin.* Burns on fingers or around mouth if cannabis is smoked.
- *Eyes.* Conjunctival injection often the only objective sign.
- *Vascular System.* Tachycardia and hypertension (especially if multiple drugs are used). A diagnostic electrocardiogram may show nonspecific ST-T wave changes related to rate.

Opiates. Opiates can be taken orally (oxycodone, hydromorphone), injected intravenously (IV) (heroin, morphine, or merperidine), or smoked (heroin). Unlike alcohol, opiates do not produce serious organ pathology.[55] Clients may have constipation, respiratory depression and anorexia from the substances used to cut the heroin.[59] The use of IV injection via shared needles places the client at risk for hepatitis B, human immunodeficiency virus (HIV) infection, endocarditis, local injection site infections, and other problems associated with contaminated IV injection.[55]

Cocaine. Cocaine can be smoked, snorted, or injected IV.[59] Cocaine abuse may be detected by examining the nose, chest, and cardiovascular system and by carrying out various diagnostic tests.

Physical Examination
- *Nose.* Nasal bleeding, erythematous nostrils, nasal septal atrophy with perforation.
- *Chest.* Increased respiratory rate, abnormal breath sounds.
- *Vascular System.* Increased heartrate, palpitations, cardiac arrhythmias, hypertension (possibly), elevated body temperature.
- *Extremities.* Track marks.
- *Neurological.* Jitterness, symptoms of depression.

Tobacco. Tobacco is consumed in a variety of products. It can be snuffed, chewed, and smoked. Tobacco can be easily detected by smell. Tobacco and cigarette stains can be seen on the teeth and fingers. Use can cause sore throat, cough, dyspnea and frequent respiratory infections.[59] Cough may be the only indication of cancer. Bloody sputum is a serious complaint.

Physical Examination
- *HEENT.* Irritation of the nasal passages, postnasal exudate on the posterior pharynx, tenderness of the sinuses, bad breath, stained teeth.
- *Chest.* Increased respiratory rate, dyspnea, orthopnea, inspiratory and expiratory wheezes, rhonchi and increased A-P diameter of the chest, angina.
- *Vascular System.* Evidence of peripheral vascular disease may be observed; claudication may occur. Clubbing of the finger may have occurred.

Diagnostic Tests
- Hepatitis panel
- Rapid plasma reagin (RPR)

- HIV infection
- Urine toxicology (for cocaine, cannabis, sedatives)
- See Chapter 21 for respiratory disease tests.

Nursing Implications

The primary health care provider's role is to help the client recognize and accept the negative relationship between her substance abuse and the consequences of abuse.[55] If substance use causes problems (physical, mental, legal, or financial), then use is abuse. The client needs to be told that a problem exists and given evidence to support this conclusion. Subsequently, the client should be directed to the proper resources. Primary care providers should also be familiar with symptoms of withdrawal for each of the substances abused. Treatment should be individualized, multifaceted, and continue indefinitely for maximum success.[55] If, on the other hand, substance use is detected, the woman should be educated about the potential problem of abuse to prevent it.

Differential Medical Diagnoses

Excessive stress, depression, anxiety, hyperthyroidism, viral or bacterial gastroenteritis, upper respiratory infection, chronic sinusitis, lower respiratory tract illness, emphysema not caused by smoking.

Plan

Psychosocial Interventions. Involve others close to the client in the treatment plan and inform them about the disease process. Use a positive approach and emphasize that the disease is treatable. Physician/psychiatric consultation is recommended for evaluation for dual-diagnosis disorders.

Dealing with denial is critical. Review all physical, emotional, financial, spiritual, and psychological effects of the substance abused to date. The first priority is to stop substance use, not to determine the cause of abuse. Total abstinence is the ideal; however, ability to abstain does not mean elimination of the problem. The inability of a woman to use a substance in moderation indicates that a problem may exist.

Contracts with self may be useful if the client is motivated to change her behavior. A contract should have realistic goals within a definite time. One way to help a woman realize that she has a problem is to have her contract to use a limited amount of substance (within reason) for a set time (3 months) in her usual pattern. If she finds she is using more than she contracted to use, then a potential problem exists. Four *A* activities are advised by the National Cancer Institute to help people stop smoking:

*A*sk all women if they smoke; ask routinely.

*A*dvise smokers to stop and give reasons.

*A*ssist the woman in stopping. Give self-help suggestions, a quit date, a plan, suggest nicotine gum/patch.

*A*rrange follow-up to review progress.[59]

See addendum at chapter's end for additional information on smoking cessation.

Medication. Disulfiram is recommended for alcohol abuse; the use of sedatives is not desirable. Disulfiram 500 mg, administered orally daily (after abstention for 12 hours) and reduced to 250 mg after 1 week, may be a deterrent. Disulfiram blocks metabolism of alcohol with acetaldehyde buildup, resulting in headaches, flushing, and nausea. Extreme side effects include hypertension, shock, and coma. The client must be taught about the medication and its potential danger. Side effects, without concomitant alcohol use, include impotence, liver damage, drowsiness, and fetal anomalies if taken by pregnant women. Contraindications are pregnancy, cardiac disease, and psychoses.[55]

To avoid withdrawal symptoms, nicotine is available in a gum or transdermal patch for those trying to stop smoking. Use of these products is controversial in pregnancy.[59] Many of these products are now available without a prescription. Other agents that are used include Clondine, a centrally acting adrenergic blocking agent; Lobeline, nicotine imposter; and antidepressants, especially if smokers also exhibit symptoms of depression.[55] See addendum at chapter's end for additional smoking cessation information.

Since detoxification from the other substances requires hospitalization, specific drugs and therapies are not discussed in this chapter. The primary care provider who is required to manage in-client detoxification should consult psychiatric and pharmacotherapeutics references.

Follow-Up

Refer the client for psychiatric consultation or other mental health services. Along with mental health resources, a client often needs help accessing financial aid, job training, and insurance benefits.[59] Women in all socioeconomic groups may face legal problems with child custody, drug theft, and driving infractions; therefore, they may need information about the legal system. Encourage the client to become involved in Alcoholics Anonymous or a similar group, especially those who have little family or friend support to help with behavior changes.[59] Significant others should become involved in a support group that deals with enabling behaviors. Biofeedback and relaxation training may also be helpful.

At first, the client should be followed closely. A minimum of one weekly visit is recommended, with additional phone contact if necessary.

Follow-Up for Tobacco Addiction. Continuous monitoring of the client who is trying to quit is essential. Clients should be told the symptoms of nicotine withdrawal, prescribed a nicotine withdrawal agent if no contraindications, and scheduled for a visit at 2 weeks. Women may find it more difficult to quit than men because of a lack of social support, more reliance on cigarettes to cope with stress, anxiety, and fear of weight gain.[56] Relapses in women occur in situations involving negative mood states such as excessive stress, conflicts, especially with others, and loss.[56] Repeat visits, as necessary should be made up to 1 year to reinforce and support the client's efforts. Structured programs for smokers have been shown to be the most effective.[55] Weight gain averages about 5 pounds. Support clients with ways to avoid high calorie foods and encourage them to increase exercise as needed.[59]

MENTAL HEALTH PROBLEMS

DEPRESSION

The *DSM-IV* (*Diagnostic and Statistical Manual of Mental Disorders,* 4th ed.) classification of depression is descriptive, considering clinical features of the depressive disorder.[37] Depression, classified as a mood disorder, includes major depression and dysthymic disorder.

Major depression occurs as a single episode or recurrent condition independent of life events. The client either has a depressed mood or loses interest or pleasure in all or almost all her usual activities and experiences four of the following conditions: significant weight loss or gain or changes in appetite; sleep disturbances; psychomotor agitation or retardation; fatigue or loss of energy; feelings of worthlessness or inappropriate guilt; diminished ability to concentrate; recurrent thoughts of death. Symptoms must have been present during the same 2-week period and represent a change from previous functioning.[37]

Dysthymia is a chronic, less acute mood disorder. The client must experience depressed mood for more than 2 years without being symptom free for more than 2 months and have two of the following conditions: poor appetite or overeating; sleep disturbance; low self-esteem; fatigue; poor concentration or difficulty making decisions; feelings of hopelessness.[37] Dysthymia is frequently a consequence of a preexisting, chronic nonmood disorder, such as anorexia nervosa, psychoactive substance dependence, or anxiety disorder.[15]

Everyone may experience some depressive symptoms following some traumatic or notable life event. Mild depressive episodes are usually related to some type of loss and are often accompanied by anger and guilt. The symptoms are usually self-limited and no treatment is necessary.

Epidemiology

Etiology. Current theories of depression focus on different factors, but the cause of depression is believed to be multifactorial.

Psychological models include psychosocial stresses and developmental problems (personality defects, childhood events).[15,28] Sense of loss, failure to live up to one's ego ideal, and a sense of hopelessness and helplessness are all important concepts in the etiology of depression.[28] Often, loss or perceived loss precedes the onset of depression. Loss may involve a person, expectation, or job. Common ideals are to be loved, to be good and kind, to be recognized for achievements, and to attain goals.[28] With disappointments and failures comes the feel-

ing of not living up to one's ego ideals. Guilt felt because of failure can lead to anger and self-hatred with feelings of hopelessness and helplessness. These feelings are related to one's negative self-concept, negative interpretation of one's experiences, and negative view of the future.

Biological models include genetic and biochemical factors. Depression appears to have some familial pattern or predisposition; however, the exact familial role is not known.[28] The biochemical model postulates a decrease in available biogenic amines at the postsynaptic membrane.[28] Many studies have used this model with inconsistent results.

Risk Factors. Risk factors include a family history of depression, poor self-concept or self-esteem, female gender, chronic nonmood disorders, substance abuse, loss or death, and stressful life event. Suicidal risk factors include previous attempted suicide, depression, dysfunctional family, battering, alcoholism, and chronic illness.

Incidence. Women continue to have higher rates of depression than do men despite improvement in their economic status and opportunities for self-development.[60] Reports reveal that 21 percent of women and 13 percent of men will have a major depressive episode in their lifetime; 13 percent of females and 8 percent of males suffer from depression in the United States over a given 12-month period.[3] Reproductive events, such as menarche, menopause, childbirth, and infertility, are associated with 30 percent of women's depressions.[55]

Subjective Data

Women frequently report somatic symptoms rather than depression, and several conditions are typically revealed in history taking, including chronic illness and substance abuse.

Symptoms that the depressed woman frequently reports include headaches, constipation, sleep disturbance, loss of energy, change in appetite with weight loss or increase, decreased libido, and chronic pain. These symptoms are somatic complaints, and a woman will more often present with them than complaints of depression. Unidentifiable somatic complaints frequently indicate depression and fatigue, but often women with these symptoms are labeled hypochondriacal or neurotic.[61] When asked about her feelings, a woman may admit to sadness; crying spells; feelings of guilt, worthlessness, or hopelessness; loss of interest in daily events; or withdrawal from work and recreation. She may complain of difficulty concentrating and thinking or an inability to make decisions.

History incorporates five areas: medical, family medical, gynecologic obstetric, social, and psychological.

Medical history is taken with the realization that any illness may cause depression, but chronic illness is the most likely cause. Questions regarding hospitalizations and injuries may provide important clues, especially if injuries are related to events such as violence or numerous accidents. Substance use should be included in the history, as it is often related to depression. In addition, include prescription and over-the-counter medications that are being taken, because some are associated with symptoms of depression. Stimulants can cause depression during withdrawal; certain antihypertensive agents, oral contraceptives, and corticosteroids may also cause depression.

Family medical history includes questions about the family's history of depression, mental illness, suicide, and substance abuse.

Gynecologic obstetric history includes the date of the previous menstrual period and cycle length to determine the possibility of premenstrual syndrome (PMS); PMS is associated with depression.

Social history includes marital status, family satisfaction, past or present violence or abusive home or work problems, job changes, economic status, and support systems. Recent losses and major stressors should be assessed.[56]

Psychological history includes information about previous psychiatric illness, suicide attempts, and cognitive abilities (memory and thought process). Always ask about suicidal ideation, what means would be used, if a plan has been established, and when the plan is to be carried out.[15]

Objective Data

A physical examination is done, as are several diagnostic tests, including those ruling out substance abuse.

Physical Examination. Begins with evaluation of the client's general appearance. She may be over-

or underweight, be unkempt, have poor affect, or move sluggishly.

- *Skin, Nails, and Hair.* Hair may be dirty and uncombed, and nails brittle and dry. Scars may be visible on the wrist or other parts of body.
- *Eyes.* The eyes may appear dull with fixed gaze, poor eye contact, circles under eyes from lack of sleep, and pale conjunctiva and mucosa.
- *Mouth.* Oral hygiene may be poor.
- *Neck.* Thyroid may be palpable or with nodules.
- *Nervous System.* See Substance Abuse and Violence sections. Mental status may require qualitative scales to determine degree of depression.

Diagnostic Tests. Are varied. Hematocrit and hemoglobin tests rule out anemia. The thyroid panel rules out thyroid disease. See Substance Abuse section for specific tests.

Nursing Implications

The health care provider must give full attention to the client in the privacy of an office. If the client does not feel comfortable, she will probably not be honest about her problem. A nurse practitioner may provide care for a mildly depressed woman usually in collaboration with a physician, but referral should be made to a qualified mental health professional for a seriously depressed woman. It is critical to know when to refer. *Always refer a client if suicidal ideation is expressed.*

Differential Medical Diagnoses

Chronic illness, hypothyroidism, depressive side effects from medication, premenstrual syndrome, substance abuse.

Plan

Psychosocial Intervention. The type of intervention depends on the type of depression. Individuals with major depression may benefit from antidepressant medication, education, supportive counseling, psychotherapy, and family therapy.[55,62,63] Individuals with dysthymia are often given antidepressant medication for symptom relief but are not as responsive as clients with major depression.[55,63] The client with dysthymia should also receive psychotherapy or supportive counseling.[28] The client with reactive depression usually requires no antidepressant medication but responds well to education, supportive counseling, and family therapy. When precipitated by an illness, depression often resolves as the illness improves.

Client education should include information about depression and the relationship of its symptoms to medical illness, stressors, and situational crisis. It should be stressed that depression is a medical illness, not a character defect or weakness. Treatments are effective, and there are many treatment options. An effective treatment can be found for nearly every client. Recovery is the rule, not the exception. The goal is complete symptom remission. Recurrence is a risk; therefore, the client should be encouraged to return with any recurrent signs and symptoms.[62,64] Teaching stress reduction, coping styles, and assertiveness may be beneficial.[65] Help the client identify and express her feelings of anger, hostility, sadness, and anxiety.

Supportive counseling focuses on encouraging the client to develop a social network and increase her activity. Participation in support groups may be beneficial for the client and her family. When appropriate, always involve persons who are important in the client's life.

Family counseling may be beneficial because episodes of depression have been associated with family dysfunction.[28] Psychotherapy's goal is to correct specific aspects of depression, including thoughts, behavior, and affect.[28,62] Its purpose is not to change the client's personality.

Treatment of Depression. Consists of three phases (see Table 23–1).[64] Acute treatment (6 to 12 weeks) aims at remission of symptoms. When medication is used, it should be individualized to the client to optimize treatment benefits and lower risk. Considerations in choosing a medication include short- and long-term side effects, past experience with medications, possible drug interactions, presence of other conditions, and age. Acute treatment should be monitored every 1 to 2 weeks. Evaluation at 6 weeks determines if the client is responding. If the desired response occurs, continue treatment for 6 weeks. If the client experiences some improvement, but not the desired response, consider adjusting the dosage.

If there is no response, the treatment may need to be changed. Continue to monitor every 1 to 2 weeks. Consult if the desired response does not occur.

Continuation treatment (4 to 9 months) aims at preventing relapse. Medication should be continued at full dosage.

Maintenance treatment aims at preventing recurrences in clients with prior episodes. Clients who have has three or more major depressive episodes should continue medication for at least 1–2 years. Current recommendations for clients who have had three or more episodes in 5 years is life long drug therapy.[63]

The objective throughout each treatment phase is attainment of a sustained asymptomatic state. The essential features of the plan should include education; regular monitoring of side effects and depressive symptoms; and adjustment or changes in the plan if response is not timely or complete.[62]

Medication. Medication includes antidepressant drugs, which work to elevate mood. Three major types are tricyclic antidepressants (TCAs), monoamine oxidase inhibitors (MAOIs), heterocyclic antidepressants and selective serotonin reuptake inhibitors (SSRIs). Most antidepressants may take several weeks before clinical improvement. Consequently, tell the client not to expect sudden improvement. Stress compliance. Instruct the client to avoid alcohol and other mood altering substances.[63] Tables 23–1, 23–2, and 23–3 provide overviews of the side effect profiles, pharmacology and treatment regimes of antidepressant medications.[63,64]

Caution clients to notify the provider if they have thoughts of suicide. Consultation with a physician is indicated.

Follow-Up

Initially, follow-up should be weekly, with telephone backup. The health care provider may counsel the reactive depressed client without referral for therapy. The client with major depression or dysthymia, however, should be referred for family counseling and psychotherapy. If a client exhibits a personality disorder or suicidal tendencies or the cause of depression is unidenti-

TABLE 23–1. SIDE EFFECT PROFILES OF ANTIDEPRESSANT MEDICATIONS

Drug	Anticho-linergic[b]	Drowsiness	Insomnia/ Agitation	Orthostatic Hypotension	Cardiac Arrhythmia	Gastro-intestinal Distress	Weight Gain (>6 kg)
Amitriptyline	4+	4+	0	4+	3+	0	4+
Desipramine	1+	1+	1+	2+	2+	0	1+
Doxepin	3+	4+	0	2+	2+	0	3+
Imipramine	3+	3+	1+	4+	3+	1+	3+
Nortriptyline	1+	1+	0	2+	2+	0	1+
Protriptyline	2+	1+	1+	2+	2+	0	0
Trimipramine	1+	4+	0	2+	2+	0	3+
Amoxapine	2+	2+	2+	2+	3+	0	1+
Maprotiline	2+	4+	0	0	1+	0	2+
Trazodone	0	4+	0	1+	1+	1+	1+
Nefazodone hydrochloride	1+	2+	0	2	—	1+	0
Bupropion	0	0	2+	0	1+	1+	0
Fluoxetine	0	0	2+	0	0	3+	0
Paroxetine	0	0	2+	0	0	3+	0
Sertraline	0	0	2+	0	0	3+	0
Monoamine oxidase inhibitors (MAOIs)	1	1+	2+	2+	0	1+	2+

Column groups: Central Nervous System (Anticholinergic, Drowsiness, Insomnia/Agitation); Cardiovascular (Orthostatic Hypotension, Cardiac Arrhythmia, Gastrointestinal Distress); Other (Weight Gain).

[a]0 = absent or rare, 1+,2+ = inbetween, 3+,4+ = relatively common.
[b]Dry mouth, blurred vision, urinary hesitancy, constipation.
From U.S. Department of Health and Human Services, Public Health Service, Agency for Health Care Policy and Research. (1993). *Clinical practice guideline No. 5. Depression in primary care: Detection, diagnosis, and treatment (Publication No. 93–09553). Rockville, MD: AMPCR; Drug Insert from Bristol-Myers Squibb Company. Revised October, 1995, Princeton, NJ. Serzone (Nefazodine hydrochloride) Tablets.*

fiable, a referral to a mental health professional should also be made.[55,62,64] After medication is determined, collaboration with a physician and follow-up may be indicated.

The suicidal client should always be referred. If a client contacts the provider and states she is suicidal, find out her location, keep her on the line, and telephone emergency medical services if another line is available. If she has not yet attempted suicide, try to persuade her to postpone suicide for a set period; if she has attempted suicide, try to find out what method was used.

ANXIETY

Anxiety may be defined as a normal emotional experience (part of normal stress reduction), a pathological cognitive/physiological symptom, or an abstract theoretical construct.[15,28,37] *DSM-IV* classifies anxiety disorders as panic disorder, agoraphobia, social phobia, simple phobia, obsessive-compulsive disorder, post-traumatic stress disorder, and generalized anxiety disorder. The disorders may overlap. With striking regularity, concomitant medical illness occurs in psychiatric clients.[62] Indeed, medical illness may cause psychiatric symptoms or exacerbate underlying psychiatric symptomatology.[61,64]

Types of Anxiety Disorders

Four types of anxiety are described below.

Panic disorders are short-lived, recurrent, unpredictable episodes of intense anxiety

TABLE 23–2. PHARMACOLOGY OF ANTIDEPRESSANT MEDICATIONS

Drug	Therapeutic Dosage Range (mg/d)	Average (Range) Elimination Half-Life[a]	Potentially Fatal Drug Interactions
Tricyclic Antidepressants			
Amitriptyline (Elavil, Endep)	75–300	24 (16–46)	Antiarrhythmics, MAOIs
Clomipramine (Anafranil)	75–300	24 (20–40)	Antiarrhythmics, MAOIs
Desipramine (Norpramin, Pertofrane)	75–300	18 (12–50)	Antiarrhythmics, MAOIs
Doxepin (Adapin, Sinequan)	75–300	17 (10–47)	Antiarrhythmics, MAOIs
Imipramine (Janimine, Tofranil)	75–300	22 (12–34)	Antiarrhythmics, MAOIs
Nortriptyline (Aventyl, Pamelor)	40–200	26 (18–88)	Antiarrhythmics, MAOIs
Protriptyline (Vivactil)	20–60	76 (54–124)	Antiarrhythmics, MAOIs
Trimipramine (Surmontil)	75–300	12 (8–30)	Antiarrhythmics, MAOIs
Heterocyclic Antidepressants			
Amoxapine (Asendin)	100–600	10 (8–14)	MAOIs
Bupropion (Wellbutrin)	225–450	14 (8–24)	MAOIs (possibly)
Maprotiline (Ludiomil)	100–225	43 (27–58)	MAOIs
Trazodone (Desyrel)	150–600	8 (4–14)	—
Selective Serotonin Re-uptake Inhibitors (SSRIs)			
Fluoxetine (Prozac)	10–40	168 (72–360)[b]	MAOIs
Paroxetine (Paxil)	20–50	24 (3–65)	MAOIs[c]
Sertraline (Zoloft)	50–150	24 (10–30)	MAOIs[c]
Nefazodone hydrochloride (Serzone)	300–500	11–24	MAOIs
Monoamine Oxidase Inhibitors (MAOIs)[d]			
Isocarboxazid (Marplan)	30–50	Unknown	For all three MAOIs: Vasoconstrictors,[e] decongestants,[e] meperidine, and possibly other narcotics
Phenelzine (Nardil)	45–90	2 (1.5–4.0)	
Tranylcypromine (Parnate)	20–60	2 (1.5–3.0)	

[a]Half-life is affected by age, sex, race, concurrent medications, and length of drug exposure.
[b]Includes both fluoxetine and norfluoxetine.
[c]By extrapolation from fluoxetine data.
[d]MAO inhibition lasts longer (7 days) than drug half-life.
[e]Including pseudoephedrine, phenylephrine, phenylpropanolamine, epinephrine, norepinephrine, and other drugs.
From U.S. Department of Health and Human Services, Public Health Service, Agency for Health Care Policy and Research. (1993). *Clinical practice guideline No. 5: Depression in primary care: Detection, diagnosis, and treatment (Publication No. 93–09553). Rockville, MD: AMPCR; Drug Insert from Bristol-Myers Squibb Company. Revised October, 1995, Princeton, NJ. Serzone (Nefazodone hydrochloride) Tablets.*

accompanied by physiological symptomatology. Episodes of apprehension, fear, and a sense of doom may be precipitated by a stimulus or may arise spontaneously.[37]

Generalized anxiety is the most common anxiety disorder.[66] It is defined as unrealistic or excessive anxiety and worry about two or more life circumstances occurring for 2 months or longer.[37] This disorder does not develop into panic attacks or phobias, is not due to physiological effects of a substance or a general medical condition.[37]

Phobic disorders use the mechanism of displacement. Clients transfer their feelings of anxiety from the true object to one that can be avoided.[37] Agoraphobia or a specific phobia can develop.

Obsessive-compulsive disorder involves an irrational idea or impulse that persistently intrudes into awareness.[36] The client recognizes its absurdity, but anxiety is relieved only with ritualistic performance, impulse, or entertainment of an idea.[15,28]

Post-traumatic stress disorder is discussed later in this section.

TABLE 23–3. IDEAL PHARMACOLOGICAL TREATMENT OF DEPRESSION

Acute phase: 6–8 weeks at full therapeutic doses; aim is remission of symptoms

Continuation phase: 4–9 months at full dose for all patients; aim is to prevent relapse

Maintenance phase: 1–2 years at full dose for patients with three or more prior depressive episodes, or lifelong if more than two episodes in 5 years; aim is to prevent recurrence of future depressive episodes

Source: Reproduced with permission from E. Herbindal and D. Gourley. (1996). Textbook of Therapeutics: Drug and Disease Management. Baltimore: Williams & Wilkins.

Epidemiology

Risk factors. Physical and mental illness, life situations or crises, and family history of anxiety disorders are risk factors for anxiety.

Incidence. Incidence varies among the four types of anxiety. Clinically significant anxiety disorders are seen in about 5–10 percent of persons presenting for ambulatory care.[56]

Panic disorder. Ratio is 2:1 for prevalence among women; onset younger than 25; affects 1.5 to 3.5 percent of population.[37] First-degree relatives of people with panic disorders have a 17 percent risk of being affected.[56]

Generalized anxiety. Questionable slight predominance among women; one year prevalence rate was approximately 3 percent with a lifetime prevalence rate of 5 percent in a community sample.[3]

Phobic disorder. Depends on type of phobia (animal phobias and agoraphobia are more common among women).[37]

Obsessive-compulsive disorder. Occurs equally in women and men; was once thought to be rare, but recent community studies identified a lifetime prevalence of 2.5 percent in the United States; highest rates among young, divorced, separated, and unemployed.[3,37] About 10 percent of the population in general have specific phobias.[3]

Subjective Data

The client may report dyspnea, shortness of breath or smothering sensation, palpitations, tachycardia, chest pain, flushing, sweating or cold clammy hands, abdominal discomfort, diarrhea, nausea, dry mouth, difficult swallowing, urinary frequency, headache, muscle tension, aches, soreness, trembling, twitching, or shakiness.[37]

Psychological complaints may include restlessness, fatigue, sleep disturbances, irritability or edginess, exaggerated startle response, difficulty concentrating, fear of being in places or situations from which escape might be difficult.

Anxiety produces symptoms that involve multiple organ systems and causes confusion and frequent medical consultation and testing. Moreover, certain medical conditions and medications produce symptoms of anxiety disorders.[37,55] In taking a history, explore the client's chief complaint, including precipitating factors, duration of symptoms, and use and effectiveness of self-treatment.

Past medical history includes chronic disease, illness, hospitalizations, and surgeries.

Medication use includes present and past prescription medications and over-the-counter medicines. Medications such as bronchodilators, caffeine, thyroid preparations and sedatives-hypnotics can cause anxiety states.

Habits include caffeine intake and use of tobacco, alcohol, and illicit substances.

Family medical history includes chronic diseases, substance abuse, and mental illness.

Gynecologic/obstetric history includes date of last (previous) menstrual period, cycle, and premenstrual symptoms.

Social history includes support systems, lifestyle, abusive home life, and job.

Psychiatric history includes previous depressive episode, peptic ulcer disease, migraine headaches, ulcerative colitis, or irritable bowel syndrome.

Objective Data

An extensive physical examination is done and a variety of diagnostic tests are performed.

Physical Examination

- *General Appearance.* The client may appear restless, trembling, or emotional.
- *Eyes.* Circles under the eyes indicate a lack of sleep. Nystagmus may be elicited with different maneuvers.
- *Ears.* Rule out otitis externa or media.

- *Mouth.* Rule out large tonsils, lesions, and polyps in throat causing difficult swallowing.
- *Neck.* Enlarged, tender, or nodular thyroid indicates thyroid disorder.
- *Skin.* Skin may be cold, clammy, sweaty, flushed, or pale.
- *Chest.* Respiratory rate may be increased. The client may hyperventilate. Wheezing may indicate asthma.
- *Vascular System.* Blood pressure and heart-rate may be increased. A murmur, gallop, or click may indicate mitral valve prolapse or arrhythmias. Rule out heart disease with chest pain.
- *Abdomen.* The client may experience pain with palpation. Bowel sounds may be absent or hyperactive.
- *Musculoskeletal System.* Gait may be unsteady. Joints may be red and edematous and a source of pain. Muscle strength may be abnormal. Signs of trauma may be evident.
- *Nervous System.* Examination may reveal hyperreflexia, positional vertigo, and abnormal cranial nerve findings.

Diagnostic Tests
- Electrocardiogram
- Electroencephalogram
- Urinalysis to rule out urinary tract infection and diabetes
- Thyroid panel as indicated
- Complete blood count to rule out anemia and infection
- Electrolytes as indicated
- Glucose tolerance test to rule out diabetes and hypoglycemia
- Upper and lower GI series if indicated

Nursing Implications

Showing genuine concern and empathy increases the chance that the client will perceive the health care provider as sympathetic to her problem. Use open ended questions when interviewing to allow the client to disclose information she may not otherwise have revealed. Permit the client to ventilate her concerns and, at the same time, to prioritize them. Reassuring her may also be helpful.[28]

Differential Medical Diagnoses

Hyperthyroidism, hypoglycemia, cancer, organic brain syndrome, depression, substance abuse, hypertension, side effects of prescription or over-the-counter medication, physical or sexual abuse.

Plan

Psychosocial Intervention. During an acute anxiety episode, stay with the client, decrease environmental stimuli, and, above all, remain calm. Counseling that focuses on the present, using reflection and clarification, is most effective.[28] Deal with issues of fears, self-concept, self-esteem, problem solving, and coping mechanisms. Acknowledge and express acceptance of anxiety. Relaxation techniques and imagery may help decrease anxiety. Assist the client to identify sources of anxiety, to develop plans to deal with them, and to modify her lifestyle. Generally, it is important to emphasis healthy lifestyle behaviors; avoiding stress when possible, decreased caffeine, no alcohol or illicit drugs, proper exercise and sleep. Social support is known to be helpful in reducing anxiety symptoms. Knowing that she has a condition that is treatable provides immense relief, as many people think they are going crazy.[59]

Medication. Medication categories include benzodiazepines, tricyclic antidepressants, monoamine oxidase (MAO) inhibitors and beta-adrenergic blocking agents. If the client's symptoms are not related to a specific syndrome other than anxiety, the client is usually treated with psychotropic medications (see Table 23–4). If a primary care provider selects one of the benzodiazepines (BZDs), it should be considered only for clients with disabling or severe symptoms and for clients who are unlikely to abuse it.[55,64] Duration of therapy should be short and dosage tailored to the individual. Progress must be monitored.[55] Addiction and withdrawal are possible. Beta-adrenergic blockers (propranolol) can be used to reduce peripheral somatic symptoms, but they are considered less effective than other anti-anxiety agents.[55,63,67] Antidepressants may also be used, especially if the anxiety is related to depression (see Depression).

TABLE 23–4. DOSING OF ANTIANXIETY MEDICATIONS[a]

Antianxiety Agent	Initial Dose[b]	Titration[b]	Maximum Dose[c]
BZDs:			
Alprazolam	0.25 mg tid	0.25–0.5 mg/d q 2–4 d	1 mg qid
Chlordiazepoxide	5 mg tid	5–10 mg/d q 2–4 d[d]	100 mg qhs
Clonazepam	0.5 mg bid	0.5–1.0 mg/d q 2–4 d[d]	3 mg bid
Clorazepate	7.5 mg bid	3.75–7.5 mg/d q 2–4 d[d]	60 mg qhs
Diazepam	5 mg bid	2–5 mg/d q 2–4 d[d]	40 mg qhs
Lorazepam	1 mg tid	0.5–1.0 mg/d q 2–4 d	5 mg bid
Oxazepam	10 mb tid	10–15 mg/d q 2–4 d	30 mg tid
Buspirone	5 mg tid	5 mg/d q 2–3 d	20 mg tid
Beta-blockers:			
Atenolol	25 mg qam	25 mg/d q 3–4 d	100 mg qam
Propranolol	10 mg tid	20–40 mg/d q 2–3 d	120 mg tid
TCAs:			
Clomipramine	25 mg qhs	25 mg/d q 2–4 d	250 mg qhs
Imipramine[e]	25–50 mg qhs	25 mg/d q 2–4 d	300 mg qhs
Nortriptyline	25 mg qhs	25 mg/d q 2–4 d	150 mg qhs
MAOIs:			
Phenelzine	15 mg qam	15 mg/d q 3–4 d[f]	45 mg bid
Tranylcypromine	10 mg qam		30 mg bid
SSRIs:			
Fluoxetine	20 mg qam	20 mg/d q 2–4 wk	80 mg qam
Fluvoxamine	50 mg qhs	50 mg/d q wk	150 mg bid
Paroxetine	20 mg qam	10 mg/d q wk	50 mg qam
Sertraline	50 mg qam	50 mg/d q wk	200 mg qam

[a]These are intended as general guidelines only. Elderly patients usually require approximately one-half the doses required for younger adults.
[b]SRI- and TCA-treated PD patients require lower initial doses and slower titrations (see text).
[c]BZD-treated PD patients may require higher doses (see text).
[d]After initial response, titrate q 1–2 weeks because of long half-life.
[e]Similar dosing strategies for amitriptyline, desipramine, and doxepin.
[f]Until 60 mg/d, then increase further only if there is no improvement after 8–12 weeks.
Source: (Reproduced with permission, from E. Herfindel and D. Gourley. (1996). Textbook of Therapeutics: Drug and Disease Management. *Baltimore: Williams & Wilkins.*

Common side effects of BZDs are dizziness, drowsiness, fatigue, confusion, disorientation, and, above all, psychological addiction. Contraindications are pregnancy, known hypersensitivity to BZDs, and use with alcohol and other central nervous system depressants. Weekly follow-up visits are encouraged. Discontinue medication as soon as possible. Provide information about side effects and contraindications and when to contact provider. Emphasize the need to use an effective contraceptive and avoid alcohol and other central nervous system depressants. Caution clients not to drive or use potentially dangerous equipment because of the sedative effects of anxiolytic agents.

Common side effects of beta blockers are masking of hypoglycemic symptoms in diabetics, bradycardia, and hypotension.[63] They are contraindicated in clients who have congestive heart failure, greater than first-degree A-V block, and asthma.[63,67] Tricyclic antidepressants can cause sedation, orthostatic hypotension, and anticholinergic effects. A small number of clients may experience a worsening of their anxiety symptoms while taking TCAs.[63]

Another medication used as an anxiolytic, but unrelated to benzodiazepines or barbiturates, is busperone (Buspar). Buspar requires several weeks to achieve its full effect. The dosage is increased daily (by 5mg/day) to a maximum of 20 mg po every 8 hours. Dizziness, headaches, GI upset, nervousness are selected side effects. It is contraindicated if the women is receiving MAOI. Advantages of Buspar are that it causes less sedation, and no withdrawal symptoms or tolerance are reported.[56,67] Currently, it is the treatment of choice for generalized anxiety disorder (GAD).

A word of caution is needed regarding MAO inhibitors. These drugs can cause serious interactions with other drugs and certain foods. A specialist should prescribe MAOIs and follow women during the treatment, ideally. MAOIs are the treatment of choice for social phobia, but SSRIs may be effective. Thus SSRIs should be considered first; they have fewer side effects. SSRIs may also be helpful for panic disorder.[63]

Other Treatment. Psychotherapy is often helpful in the treatment of anxiety disorders. Interpersonal dynamic and cognitive-behavior therapies are used in conjunction with medication. Clients with dual diagnoses or personality disorders should be referred to a mental health specialist for consultation.

Follow-Up

Follow-up is weekly; however, during an acute episode, daily clinic visits may be necessary. Referral depends on the health care provider's expertise, the severity of the client's symptoms and functional impairment, her response to intervention, and her receptiveness and motivation.[55] Consultation with a physician, referral, or both are indicated when medication is used or if signs of underlying physical or emotional problems are present. Immediately refer a client with any suicidal ideation.

POST-TRAUMATIC STRESS DISORDER

Symptoms of post-traumatic stress disorder (PTSD) develop following a psychologically distressing event that is outside the range of usual human experience.[37] The affected client reexperiences the traumatic event, avoids stimuli associated with the event, and exhibits a numbed general responsiveness and increased arousal.[37] The trauma that is experienced may be a serious threat to life or physical integrity, a serious threat or harm to someone close to the client, sudden destruction of one's home or community, or recently seeing someone injured or killed.[37]

Subjective Data

According to *DSM-IV,* a client must meet the following diagnostic criteria for PTSD: a person must have experienced a traumatic event in which both of the following were true: 1) the person experienced, observed, or was involved with an event(s) where harm or death were threatened and 2) intense fear, helplessness or horror were the primary affects. Symptoms may include any of the following: 1) persistent distressing memories of the event, 2) recurrent upsetting dreams, 3) reliving the experience as if it were happening now, 4) psychological distress following cues that remind the client of the event, 5) persistent avoidance of specific things that remind the client of the event, and 6) symptoms of increased arousal, e.g., insomnia, exaggerated startle response.

Objective Data and Differential Medical Diagnoses

See Anxiety, Depression, and Substance Abuse sections.

Plan

Psychosocial Intervention. Focus on counseling that emphasizes the here and now and strengthens existing defenses.[15,28] Helping clients to clarify the problem allows them to begin viewing it within its proper context and facilitates decision making.[28] Instructing clients about stress reduction techniques and encouraging them to develop relaxation and exercise programs may help them to reduce stress by providing other outlets for their feelings.

Medication. Medication may include limited use of sedatives for acute anxiety symptoms. (See Anxiety section.)

Follow-Up

Group and individual psychotherapy are usually needed for PTSD. Refer the client to a psychiatrist or mental health counselor for psychotherapy and medication. As with anxiety, referral for other manifestations of stress depends on the health care provider's expertise, the severity of symptoms and functional impairment, the client's response to intervention, and her receptiveness and motivation.[55]

EATING DISORDERS

Eating disorders are complex psychological problems that have genetic, neurochemical, developmental, sociocultural, behavioral, and familial components. For additional information about the developmental aspects of an eating disorder, see Chapter 4. Disorders discussed in this chapter are anorexia nervosa, bulimia and binge-eating disorder.

The largest percentage of clients with eating disorders are female.[37] The contemporary American body is seen as lean, strong, feminine and graceful. The focus on this ideal has led many women to strive for unrealistic goals for their body shape. As a result, 50 percent of American women are on a diet at any given time, with Americans spending over $5 billion annually on dieting products.[28]

A client's symptoms of an eating disorder can vary throughout the disease course. For example, a client may exhibit behaviors seen in different types of eating disorders, or her behavior may change over time from that which is more typical of anorexia to that which is typical of bulimia.

Several characteristics, however, are frequently reported by women with an eating disorder. For example, one or both parents or a sibling is preoccupied with weight and food. Or a crisis, such as loss, may precipitate an eating disorder; loss may be real (death) or psychological (breakup of a relationship or a move from familiar surroundings).

Another characteristic is family chaos, such as alcoholism, drug addiction, violence, sexual abuse, compulsive gambling, affective disorder, and depression. The client's behavior is a symptom of the family's ineffective coping style, not the cause of it. She has learned that unpleasant emotions, such as anger, disappointment, sorrow, and loss, are to be avoided. Consequently, she becomes accomplished at denial and may be unable to recognize the normal range and expression of human emotions.

In addition, a client's independence or autonomy from her family may have been stifled, allowing little control over her life. Control of her body is control of something. Finally, the common denominators of any eating disorder are low self-esteem and a distorted body image.[68]

Eating disorders include a wide spectrum of gross disturbances in eating behaviors. Generally, however, anorexics control weight by restricting food intake and by excessive exercise; bulimics alternate strict dieting with episodes of binging and purging; binge eaters also alternate strict dieting with binges but do not purge. It is important to differentiate binge-eating disorder from obesity: although the two have similar long-term health risks, *obesity* is a term based on weight that does not address psychological issues.

Dr. Kim Yeager described the "Female Athlete Triad" as disordered eating, amenorrhea, and premature osteoporosis seen in young women who are athletes.[69] These women are at increased risk for development of amenorrhea, with decreased estrogen levels that can lead to premature osteoporosis.

Unfortunately, predictors of outcome and prognosis for clients with anorexia and bulimia vary considerably because of diverse methodology, inconsistent utilization of diagnostic criteria, and lack of specifically defined criteria for recovery, relapse, and recurrence.

DSM-IV also includes the category Eating Disorders Not Otherwise Specified. Binge-eating disorder is one example of such a disorder. It is characterized by normal or excess weight in a person who has binge eating episodes, but does not engage in purging behaviors.[37] One consistent finding of studies is that the prevalence of eating disorders is increasing.[28]

ANOREXIA NERVOSA

Essential features of anorexia nervosa according to *DSM-IV* criteria are refusal to maintain body weight above minimal normal weight for age and height; intense fear of gaining weight or becoming fat, even though underweight; distorted body image ("feel fat" when obviously underweight or even emaciated); and amenorrhea (absence of at least three consecutive menstrual cycles when otherwise expected to occur or menstruation that occurs only following hormone administration).[37]

The *DSM-IV* specifies two types of anorexia nervosa: the restricting type in which clients do not regularly engage in binge eating or purging behavior and the binge eating/purging type in which clients do engage in binge-eating or purging behavior.

The client is preoccupied with food, weight, and diet (e.g., she counts the calories in one Lifesaver candy when keeping a food diary) and weighs herself more than once a day. She exhibits compulsive behaviors and low self-esteem. The client hoards food, has bizarre eating behavior, and limits selections to a few low calorie foods. She may overexercise to the point of exhaustion or injury.

Epidemiology

Risk Factors. Among the risk factors are female gender (20:1 female:male ratio); age range of 15 to 50; career choice that stresses thinness, competition, perfection, or self-discipline (modeling, theater, ballet, competitive athletics); parent or sibling with eating disorder, affective disorder, or substance abuse problem; psychiatric illness or depression; or being achievement oriented, compliant, "model" child, or perfectionist. A tremendous toll is taken on the families and clients affected by this illness. Mortality from anorexia nervosa is estimated to be between 6–10 percent.[28] Some studies suggest an increased incidence of eating disorders among young women with insulin-dependent diabetes; this association remains controversial.[70]

Incidence. Approximately 0.3–1 percent of the female population will develop anorexia nervosa usually between the ages of 13 and 20. Onset is usually early to late adolescence. Anorexia nervosa usually occurs among white females of middle-upper socioeconomic status.

Subjective Data

The client may report feeling bloated, fatigue, constipation, diarrhea, decreased libido, cold intolerance, insomnia, sore tongue, frequent upper respiratory infections, muscle weakness and cramps, dizziness, social isolation, nausea, fainting spells. She may deny hunger or exhaustion. Amenorrhea or infertility is associated with anorexia and bulimia.[28,71] An October 1990 study from Canada found that 7 percent of women aged 21–39 at an infertility clinic were currently suffering from anorexia or bulimia, a rate two to four times that in the general population; this study also demonstrated that women had failed to discuss their eating disorder with their gynecologists.[71] Attention should be paid to the client who presents with amenorrhea. An evaluation should begin when clients report missing 3–6 menstrual cycles.

Subtle clues may be detected by a health care provider who is attuned to the client. For example, the client may be oversensitive when weighed or have excessive concerns about being overweight, even if she appears normal or under normal weight. She may request advice about fad diets and weight loss programs, may claim she "does not have enough time to eat," may dress in oversized clothes or layers of clothing to hide weight or health (yet she denies a problem), and may be compulsive about exercise. A wide discrepancy may exist in caloric intake and expenditure, leading to caloric deficit and subsequent weight loss.

Thorough medical and psychosocial histories are of utmost importance. Various screening tools are available and most often used in psychotherapy: Eating Attitudes Test (EAT), Diagnostic Survey for Eating Disorders (DSED), Eating Disorder Inventory (EDI), and Bulimia Test (BULIT). A pertinent history that is applicable to any eating disorder addresses five topics.

Attitude. Weight attitudes and problems may be detected by asking several questions. Do you like yourself at current weight? What would you like to weigh? What was your weight in the past month? The past 6 months? What are your highest and lowest weights? Have you always been over/underweight? Are other family members over/underweight?

Diet History. Ask the client to complete a 24-hour dietary intake record of the previous day including breakfast, lunch, dinner, snacks; caffeine (sodas, tea, coffee); alcohol, recreational drugs, and tobacco; and medications (prescription and over-the-counter). Ask the client the following: What constitutes a binge? A reasonable meal? Note her reluctance or resistance to respond during the diet history. Assign the client the task of keeping a food/mood diary for several days: time of day eating occurred, food or beverage consumed, amount eaten, calories, food group supplied, how quickly meal was eaten, degree of hunger, feelings and circumstances that prompted eating, where eating took place, names of persons who ate with client, activities while eating (e.g., sitting, standing, walking, lying down).

Exercise. Describe frequency (per day or week) and type of exercise. Differentiate compulsive exercise and athletic exercise. The athlete participates in purposeful training with an athletic goal and has high exercise tolerance, good muscle development, body fat within normal limits, and, most importantly, an accurate body image. The pressure to excel, especially among elite athletes, has brought attention to the "female athlete triad": disordered eating, amenorrhea, and osteoporosis. This is especially common among athletes competing in appearance or endurance sports. Parents, coaches, athletic trainers, team physicians, and athletic association administrators must also recognize their roles in the development of this pattern and consider the lifelong consequences for the athlete.[59,69] If the client is a competitive athlete, she must learn at what point exercise loses its beneficial quality and becomes harmful. Reasons for excessive exercise should be evaluated: Is it the demand of a coach or sport or is it compulsive behavior to manage anxiety or purge the effects of eating? Also, can the athlete with an eating disorder stop dieting, binging, or purging when the season is over? Does the athlete realize that the behavior may compromise, rather than enhance, performance?

Menstrual History. At what age did menarche occur and at what age did regular menses begin? Is the client currently menstruating? Has the client experienced a recent change in menstrual pattern (in 20 percent of anorexics, this may be the first sign before low body weight)? What contraceptive method does she use? How many pregnancies? Abortions?

Social History. Does the client live alone? Does she cook or eat alone? Have friends and family complained of a change in her behavior? Ask the client to describe the number and character of her relationships. How many hours per week does she devote to school, work, or both?

Psychological History. Has she undergone a recent crisis? Has she ever had psychological counseling? Is she now undergoing counseling? Does she have symptoms of depression or anxiety? History of substance abuse?

Binging/Purging History. Does she vomit frequently or use laxatives, diuretics, or appetite suppressants? Does she use syrup of ipecac? Ipecac is an inexpensive, over-the-counter drug that can be lethal. Repeated use results in chronic absorption causing myopathy, which is reversible on discontinuation of the drug. Potentially fatal cardiomyopathy, however, may also be a consequence of chronic use.[72]

Objective Data

Data are determined by means of specific calculations to measure body fat and mass, physical examination, and several diagnostic tests to identify anemia and rule out imbalances in body chemistry and other metabolic reasons for weight loss.

Measurements

Measure frame size and compare height and weight with standardized height/weight tables (see Chapter 5 for discussion of ideal body weight). Measure percentage of body fat using skin fold calipers.[55] Plot body mass index [weight (kg)/height cm^2]; indexes greater than 27.2 and 26.9 indicate obesity in men and women, respectively.[55] A BMI below 22 should raise a suspicion; a BMI of 15 means starvation.

Calculate ideal body weight. For women, this is 100 pounds plus 5 pounds for every inch over 5 ft; for men, 110 pounds plus 5 pounds for every inch over 5 ft (see Chapter 5).

Physical Examination

- *General Appearance.* The client appears pale and emaciated, and manifests delayed sexual maturation.
- *Skin.* The client may have lanugo (fine, downy hair that covers extremities and face), brittle nails, dry skin, hair loss or thinning, and carotenemia evidenced by yellowing palms and soles.

- *Throat.* Buccal mucosa may be erythematous.
- *Breasts.* Breasts may be atrophied or poorly developed.
- *Vascular System.* Arrhythmias (secondary to electrolyte abnormalities) and peripheral edema may be detected.
- *Abdomen.* The abdomen may appear scaphoid. Bowel sounds may be hypoactive.
- *Genitalia and Reproductive Tract.* The client may have primary or secondary amenorrhea, irregular menses (may not be identified if she takes oral contraceptives), and decreased fertility.[59,73] Preterm birth and stillbirth are associated with anorexia and pregnancy.
- *Rectal Area.* Hemorrhoids (secondary to constipation) may be present.
- *Musculoskeletal System.* The client may exhibit overuse injuries (stress fractures, joint or tendon problems). A client with severe anorexia is at risk for osteoporosis.
- *Nervous System.* Determine if the client is suicidal.
- *Endocrine System.* Thyroid abnormalities may be detected.

Diagnostic Tests

- *Urinalysis.* A urinalysis is done to evaluate carbohydrate metabolism and specific gravity. Elevated ketones and protein indicate low carbohydrate metabolism (due to poor intake). Specific gravity is increased if the client is dehydrated and decreased if she is drinking excessive water (common before being weighed). A urine pregnancy test is done if amenorrhea is a symptom and the client is sexually active.
- *Blood Chemistry.* A complete blood count is done to determine anemia and neutropenia. Electrolytes are evaluated. Individuals who vomit and use laxatives and/or diuretics usually will have significant and sometimes life threatening electrolyte imbalances. Decreased potassium may cause arrhythmia, then death. In addition, decreased calcium, magnesium, chloride, sodium, albumin, and globulin and increased BUN are typical with anorexia nervosa.
- *Liver Function Tests.* To help rule out other causes of weight loss, some values may be affected by malnutrition.
- *Endocrine Tests.* Levels of follicle-stimulating hormone and luteinizing hormone may be decreased. Prolactin, thyroid-stimulating hormone, and thyroxine levels may be normal. Thyroid function tests may be borderline low.[70]
- *Electrocardiogram.* An electrocardiogram is indicated to determine the presence of arrhythmias, especially if the health care provider suspects poor follow-up or severe disease.

Differential Medical Diagnoses

Weight loss: rule out anorexia nervosa, hyperthyroidism, malabsorption syndrome, mesenteric artery syndrome, Addison's disease, Alzheimer's disease, Crohn's disease, depression, ischemic heart disease, carcinoma, other chronic diseases.[55]

Amenorrhea, primary: rule out pituitary adenoma, ovarian failure, genital tract obstruction. (See Chapter 8.) Amenorrhea, secondary: rule out pregnancy, pituitary failure, weight loss or decreased body fat due to body building or sports. (See Chapter 8.)

Plan

Psychosocial Interventions. It is vital that a trusting relationship be established between the primary health care provider and the client; this process takes time. Support the client, and remain nonjudgmental if she reveals bizarre food habits. Help the client to find appropriate alternative coping behaviors and reestablish a healthy attitude regarding food and weight. In addition, act as role model by accepting your body size and weight and by maintaining healthy eating and exercise habits.

Since the woman with anorexia nervosa is at risk for serious health consequences, consultation with a mental health professional and a primary care physician is advised. Coordination of care between providers is critical. Other resources are essential, for example, individual and/or group therapy (group therapy reduces secrecy and allows sharing of concerns), assertiveness training, self-esteem and body image groups, family therapy.

Medication. Tricyclic antidepressants may be prescribed if major depression is present, and monitored by a psychiatrist. A small volume is prescribed to avoid lethal dose if the client is suicidal. (See Depression section.)

Diet. Diet modification includes psychological measures, as well as careful nutritional planning, preferably by a nutritionist. Goals are to help the client understand basic nutritional education, her own nutritional requirements and the relationship between dieting and disordered eating patterns. A computer nutritional analysis is helpful in comparing the client's intake with healthy percentages of fat, carbohydrates, and protein. Estimate her basal metabolic rate.[74] This method provides reality based information to help dispel the client's nutritional myths.

Contract negotiation between client and health care provider focuses on an acceptable weight range and plan for exercise, food intake, and follow-up. Self-contract enhances the client's control in that she is responsible both for changing her behavior and identifying the reward to reinforce health promoting behavior. The ultimate responsibility for recovery lies with the client. If, however, the provider feels the client is endangering herself (low weight, excessive purging, refusing to eat, suicidal gestures), the provider must recommend inpatient therapy, which requires breaking confidentiality.

The American Diabetes Association's guidelines are used in nutritional planning. The client chooses foods in all food groups. Urge her to use servings, *not* calories, as a basis for planning: no fewer than 2 or 3 servings of meat or other protein, 6 to 11 of grains, 2 to 4 of fruits, 3 to 5 of vegetables, and 2 to 3 of milk. Smaller, more frequent meals may be more acceptable to a client who "feels full" quickly. Incorporate previously "forbidden" foods, that is, carbohydrates, into plan. Increase calories enough to elicit a 1- to 2-pound per week increase in weight.

Exercise. Exercise should be modified. Encourage the client to decrease the amount and intensity; for example, change from high-impact aerobics to strengthening/stretching, low-impact aerobics, or walking several times a week. If the client refuses to decrease exercise, she must substantially increase her food intake.

Follow-Up

Monitor the client's well-being. Assess weight weekly; the client should wear similar clothes each time. If the client weighs herself several times daily, encourage her to limit weighing to once a day or less.

Hospitalization criteria are made clear to client at her initial visit. This places the responsibility for control on the client.

MEDICAL INDICATIONS FOR HOSPITALIZATION. Severe emaciation (weight less than 85 percent of ideal body weight), laboratory tests showing decreased sodium and potassium, abnormal electrocardiogram, minimal or no food intake, persistent weight loss, and need to facilitate differential diagnosis. Medical complications include the following: weight loss greater than 30 percent of body weight over 3 months, heartrate less than 40 beats/min., temperature less than 36° C, systolic BP less than 70 mm Hg, serum potassium less than 2.5 Meq/L despite oral K+ supplementation, severe dehydration, systemic illness.[28]

PSYCHIATRIC INDICATIONS FOR HOSPITALIZATION. Moderate to severe depression (suicide risk); inability to function at home, work, or school; inability of family or current living arrangement to provide adequate psychological environment for improvement to occur; and lack of improvement in outpatient treatment.[28]

The prognosis for recovery from anorexia nervosa is poor, thus requiring long-term treatment and follow-up. Some clients may fully recover after one incidence, others may recover and relapse many times, still others continue to have symptoms over a number of years with gradual physical deterioration. The long-term mortality is estimated to be over 10 percent.[37]

BULIMIA

Specific criteria characterize bulimia.[37] Most characteristic, perhaps, are the recurrent episodes of binge eating. A binge is described as the rapid consumption of a large amount of food in a discrete period. To be diagnosed with bulimia, a client must have had, on average, a minimum of two binge-eating episodes per week for at least 3 months. During binges, clients often consume high calorie, sweet, salty, or starchy food (junk food) that is easily and rapidly eaten. The binge is terminated by abdominal discomfort, sleep, social interruption, or induced vomiting. The client feels a lack of control over eating behavior during binges. Moreover, the client is often self-critical and depressed following a binge.

In addition, self-induced vomiting, use of laxatives or diuretics, strict dieting or fasting, or vigorous exercise is used to prevent weight gain. The client is persistently overconcerned with body shape and weight. Frequent weight fluctuations (10 pounds per month) due to alternating binges and fasts are common; most bulimics are within the normal weight range. Bulimics also exhibit poor impulse control (promiscuity, shoplifting, self-mutilation) and may be multiple substance abusers (most frequently sedatives, amphetamines, cocaine, or alcohol).

Epidemiology

Bulimia occurs most often among females aged 13 to 50. Males are also diagnosed but to a lesser degree.

Risk Factors. Obesity during adolescence (may have started restrictive diet, now out of control), substance abuse, depression, and family history of alcoholism or affective disorder are risk factors.

Incidence. The condition is estimated to occur among 1 to 3 percent of adolescent and young women; the rate in males is estimated to be approximately one-tenth of that in females.[37]

Onset occurs in adolescence and early adulthood or during developmental transitions (college, marriage, breakup of relationship). Mortality is rare. It is usually related to unintended aspiration of vomitus or electrolyte abnormalities that cause cardiac arrhythmias or sudden death.

Subjective Data

The client usually acknowledges and is disturbed by her abnormal eating behavior. Negative thoughts, routine stress, diet hunger can lead to binges.[56] She usually feels shame and self-loathing afterwards. She may report abdominal distention, cramping, and constipation secondary to chronic laxative abuse. She may seek advice or prescriptions for laxatives, diuretics, or diets. The client may also describe muscle weakness and fatigue, depression, chronic pharyngitis, difficulty swallowing, esophageal irritations, frequent dental problems, shortness of breath, palpitations, and chest pain. She may spontaneously regurgitate food, may skip heartbeats, and may be able to consume large amounts of food that are inconsistent with her weight.

She may be secretive and plan binges. Family or roommates report that the client is frequently in the bathroom after meals with the shower or water running. She may steal money to buy food or steal food or laxatives. Binges may cost significant amounts of money; consequently, the woman is always without funds.

Weight fluctuations occur as a result of binges, which vary from 1000 to 5000 calories. Bingeing and purging may be carried out from a few times per month to 20 times per day. Injuries result from excessive exercise (3 to 5 hours per day); the client may be an aerobics instructor at more than one fitness center. She may be a high achiever, but passive and nonassertive.

Objective Data

A complete physical examination is done as are several diagnostic tests.

Physical Examination

- *General Appearance.* The client appears to be of normal weight for her height, although she may be slightly overweight.
- *Skin.* There may be scars on the dorsum of the hand from induced vomiting.
- *Head.* Examination may reveal bilateral parotid gland enlargement and "chipmunk" appearance.
- *Eyes.* Conjunctival hemorrhages may result from forceful vomiting.
- *Throat.* The dental enamel on inner aspects of the teeth may be eroded.
- *Chest.* Aspiration pneumonia from vomitus is most likely to occur with concomitant alcohol or drug ingestion.
- *Breasts.* Striae may be the result of weight fluctuations.
- *Vascular System.* Examination may reveal arrhythmias and peripheral edema secondary to laxative withdrawal (related to electrolyte disturbances). Sudden death may result from the cumulative ingestion of syrup of ipecac.

- *Abdomen.* There may be esophageal tears or rupture. Abdominal striae and poor musculature are due to rapid weight changes.
- *Genitalia and Reproductive Tract.* Pregnancy is a risk if the client vomits after taking oral contraceptives. In pregnancy, severe electrolyte imbalance can be lethal to the fetus.[56] Other associated reproductive complications are low birthweight, low APGAR scores, stillbirth, cleft palate, and abnormal presentation during labor.
- *Rectum.* Tearing and fissures may be caused by frequent enemas or hemorrhoids.
- *Musculoskeletal System.* Overuse injuries may be evident.
- *Nervous System.* Convulsions may be due to electrolyte imbalances.
- *Endocrine System.* Menstrual irregularities may be experienced. Conceiving may be difficult. The client who is an insulin-dependent diabetic is at risk for hyper- or hypoglycemia and ketoacidosis.

Diagnostic Tests
- Urinalysis
- Complete blood count (anemia, neutropenia)
- Electrolytes (decreased chloride, increased phosphorus, decreased total protein)
- Liver function tests (especially with alcohol or substance abuse)
- Electrocardiogram (indicated especially with ipecac use)
- Amylase test (differing reports use it as an indication of bulimia)
- Chest x-ray (may be indicated to rule out aspiration pneumonia)

Differential Medical Diagnoses

Digitalis or pilocarpine toxicity, gastrointestinal carcinoma, malignant hypertension, pyloric obstruction, mesenteric artery syndrome, metabolic alkalosis, migraine, pinealoma, postconcussive syndrome, posterior fossa tumor.[55]

Plan

Psychosocial Intervention. Psychotherapy is required for treatment. Mental health professionals often use cognitive-behavior therapy to modify eating and weight control behaviors and promote changes in attitudes that contribute to the disor-

dered eating. For interventions appropriate for the primary care provider, see the Anorexia section.

Medication. See Depression section.

Diet. Dietary intervention includes identifying "triggers." In addition, the client should be instructed in several steps toward recovery: to keep binge foods out of sight (or not purchase them); to be with other people at times known to be vulnerable (weekends, evenings) or to change her environment; to learn to nurture self in ways other than eating (taking bubble baths, reading, pursuing hobbies, telephoning a friend).[74] The client should plan three to four regularly scheduled meals per day and eat them regardless of binges and purges. Nonemaciated bulimics should be encouraged to maintain weight or to gain gradually by consuming no fewer than 1800 to 2400 calories per day.

Lifestyle Changes. See Anorexia.

Follow-Up

Follow-up is weekly or every 2 weeks to assess the client's weight. More crucial than weight evaluation, however, is monitoring the frequency of binge/purge behavior, exercise, and abuse of laxatives, appetite suppressants, and diuretics.

Hospitalization criteria are described under Anorexia. Hospitalization is not usual for bulimia unless bingeing and purging are almost totally interfering with the woman's life. Suicidal ideation requires hospitalization. Severity of the eating disorder, financial resources, and ability to manage the client in an outpatient setting will influence the decision to hospitalize a client with bulimia. Morbidity and mortality rates associated with this disorder are not known.

BINGE-EATING DISORDER

Binge-eating disorder was added to the fourth edition of the *Diagnostic and Statistical Manual of Mental Disorders.* It is characterized by clients who eat large quantities of food and calories, but do not attempt to prevent weight gain by purging, fasting, or excessive exercise. Previous description of this problem included compulsive overeating and pathological overeaters. The binge eating occurs, on average, at a minimum of 2 days a week for 6 months. Food is used to cope with stress, emotional conflicts, daily problems, boredom, depression, anxiety, loneliness, and anger.[37,75,76]

Not all clients diagnosed with binge-eating disorder are overweight. Researchers identified the incidence of binge-eating disorder to be approximately 1.2 percent with the typical subject being of normal weight, any race, and any age.[77] Another research study found women who were diagnosed with binge-eating disorder to have higher rates of other types of psychopathology such as anxiety or mood disorders.[78]

Epidemiology

Binge eating disorder is thought to begin during early childhood when eating patterns are developed. The condition continues through life. A parent may comfort an infant by feeding; a family may use eating as an escape from feelings or as an activity when bored. The client as a consequence responds to external cues (sight or smell of food) rather than internal cues (hunger or satiation following eating). Weight gain may be unremarkable until metabolic needs decrease as a young adult.

Studies drawn from weight-control programs have shown the overall prevalence to be 15 percent to 30 percent (with a mean of 30 percent), with females 1.5 times more likely to meet diagnostic criteria for this disorder than males.[37]

Subjective Data

From the client's history, it becomes evident that she reports a lack of control over her eating; she eats little in public, yet high weight is maintained due to private binges. One study found that obese subjects who failed to lose weight underreported their actual calorie intake and overestimated their physical activity.[79] The client binges on any available food, most likely at night or on weekends. She has a long history of unsuccessful diets and restricts social activities because she is embarrassed about her weight (inability to fit in normal size seats). The client may attribute social and career failures to weight (false belief that she would be a better person if thin) and may fear medical complications such as diabetes, hypertension, and heart disease.

Objective Data

A physical examination and several diagnostic tests are done.

Physical Examination

- *General Appearance.* The client appears healthy, but has excessive body fat on the extremities as well as the trunk.
- *Vital Signs.* Tachycardia and hypertension (use appropriately sized blood pressure cuff) are possible.
- *Skin.* Skin breakdown is observed at intertriginous areas (beneath abdomen, vulva, groin, breasts, axillae); wound healing is poor. If obesity is accompanied by androgen excess, acne and hirsutism of the face, lower abdomen, thighs, and chest may be observed.
- *Chest.* Respirations are increased. There is dyspnea on exertion.
- *Breasts.* Hair surrounds the areolae in women with androgen excess.
- *Vascular System.* Varicosities and thrombophlebitis may be present.
- *Abdomen.* Abdomen is protuberant.
- *Genitalia and Reproductive Tract.* There may be a history of pregnancy or delivery complications, newborn complications, or male hair pattern in females (if androgen excess).
- *Musculoskeletal System.* Examination may reveal osteoarthritis (especially of the hips and knees), sciatica, and lower extremity injuries.
- *Nervous System.* Depression may be revealed.
- *Endocrine System.* Hyperglycemia and amenorrhea are possible findings.

Diagnostic Tests

- Complete blood count
- Glucose and lipid profiles (cholesterol, high density and low density lipoproteins, fasting triglycerides)
- Electrolyte analysis (especially if using fad diets)
- Urinalysis
- Electrocardiogram
- Endocrine studies when indicated (follicle-stimulating hormone, thyroid-stimulating hormone, prolactin, luteinizing hormone, free testosterone, dehydroepiandrosterone sulfate)

Differential Medical Diagnoses

Obesity with amenorrhea—rule out polycystic ovary syndrome/anovulation; obesity due to compulsive eating disorder; complications of obesity, such as hypertension, gallbladder disease, hyperlipidemia, and non-insulin-dependent diabetes.

Plan

Psychosocial Interventions. See Anorexia section. Suggest to the client that she join a support group, such as Overeaters Anonymous.

Medication. Since many clients will also have an Axis I diagnosis, antidepressants may be indicated (see Depression). The role of SSRIs is increasing in management of overeating.[35] These drugs are effective in reducing appetite, as well as being safe. Medical therapy should not be used, however, without appropriate education, and lifestyle and nutritional changes.[80] Regain of weight is a consistent problem after drug therapy is stopped and long-term therapy should be considered for women who have a history of repeated losses and gains.

Diet. Dietary interventions are numerous (also see Anorexia). No fewer than 1200 calories should be consumed per day; otherwise, essential nutrients are restricted and metabolism decreased, possibly prompting a binge.

Suggest to the client that she replace problem behaviors with alternative behaviors.[81] Provide accurate information regarding weight loss programs, including the risks involved with fad diets or "powdered formula" diets. The following questions are helpful in evaluation of weight loss programs.[82]

- Is this a diet the client could live with indefinitely?
- What is the recommended rate of weight loss?
- Does the program take individual differences into account to determine caloric needs?
- To what extent does the plan educate the client about nutrition, behavior modification, and the importance of exercise?
- Does the program put the client in contact with professionals such as physicians, registered dietitians, and psychotherapists?
- What percentage of clients reach goal weight and maintain their losses?

- Does the program offer a maintenance plan once weight is lost?
- What is the nature of the advertisements and endorsements?
- How much does the program cost?

Exercise. Exercise needs to be incorporated into lifestyle. Inform the client about the health benefits of regular exercise. Exercise increases basal metabolic rate, which increases calorie use and promotes weight loss. Exercising at least four times per week for 20 to 30 minutes is recommended.

Devise a mutually acceptable plan for aerobic exercise; calculate the target heartrate.[55] Weight loss cannot occur and be maintained if the client is unwilling to continue exercise and reasonable caloric restriction.

Explain to the client that weight may not change drastically; rather, she should use as a guide how she feels physically and how her clothes fit. Encourage the client to wear flattering clothing to boost self-esteem.

Follow-Up

Follow-up visits are scheduled for every 2 weeks or monthly to evaluate weight and blood pressure and review exercise, dietary goals, and compliance problems. Self-monitoring, setting goals, social support, and the length of treatment are associated with successful loss of weight, whereas physical activity, continuing in a program, and self-monitoring are important to successfully keeping the weight off.[35]

HOMELESSNESS

Approximately 2 million men, women and children are homeless at some time each year.[83] The number of women and children living without a permanent place of dwelling is the fastest growing population among the homeless. Exactly how many women are homeless is not known. Women often remain out of sight to protect themselves against the possibility of violence.

Reasons for homelessness are complex; poverty, violence, substance abuse and mental illness are often cited as major causes.[84] The

Stewart B. McKinley Homeless Act (Public Law 100-77) defined the homeless person as one who does not have a fixed, regular, and adequate nighttime dwelling. This dwelling may be 1) a supervised or publicly operated shelter designed for temporary living quarters, 2) an institution serving as temporary residence for those requiring institutionalization, or 3) any public or private place not intended for regular sleeping quarters.[85]

Rarely does the literature on homeless persons distinguish health problems of women from those of men. Women who are homeless are at risk for the same health problems as women who are not homeless. Due to their poverty, sense of powerlessness and inability to access health care, however, women are particularly at risk for conditions and diseases that might be preventable if detected earlier. Pregnant women are particularly vulnerable to complications during pregnancy, labor, and the postpartum periods.[86] It is important for primary care providers to note that the use of screening tests is correlated more with access to preventative health care than to income or minority status.[87] Homeless women are likely to experience malnutrition and related problems such as anemia. Other common health problems are infections, communicable diseases, skin complaints, poorly managed diabetes and hypertension. Exposure to the elements, especially hypothermia, is also common.[88]

Along with physical problems, women who are homeless experience stress, anxiety, and depression. They are also at risk for abuse and trauma, both physical and psychological.[89] Use of drugs and alcohol are common.[90] These psychological problems are complicated by a lack of resources. Homeless women often do not have health insurance and are unable to pay for many of the traditional treatments for mental health problems.

Primary care providers must work with community agencies to devise practice models that improve accessibility to care and follow-up. Systems of care that improve access to care are located in many urban areas throughout our country. Funding, especially for health care services, continues to be a problem. Any system of care

should focus on early identification of the at-risk population, provision of services that are required to reduce morbidity and mortality from acute and chronic diseases, and follow-up. Practices located near homeless shelters and streets where homeless women and their families are likely to be found will increase access to preventative health care services. Primary providers must also examine their attitudes and beliefs regarding homeless women and look for ways to create therapeutic client-provider relationships and implement health care services.

REFERENCES

1. Horton, J. (Ed.). (1995). *The women's health data book: A profile of women's health in the United States.* Washington, DC: The Jacobs Institute of Women's Health.

2. Dennerstein, L. (1995). Mental health, work and gender. *International Journal of Health Services, 25,* 3, 503–509.

3. Kessler, R., McBonagle, K., Zhao, S., Nelson, C., Hughes, M., Esheleman, S., Wiltchen, H., & Kendler, K. (1994). Lifetime and 12-month prevalence of DSM-III-R psychiatric disorders in the United States: Results from the National Cormorbidity Survey. *Arch General Psychiatry, 51,* 8–19.

4. Manderono, M., & Brown, M. (1992). A practical, step by step approach to stress management for women. *Nurse Practitioner, 17,* 18–28.

5. U.S. Federal Aviation Administration. (1994). *Stopping sexual harassment in the workplace.* Washington, DC: Office of Civil Rights.

6. Charney, D., & Russell, R. (1994). An overview of sexual harassment. *American Journal Psychiatry, 151,* 10–17.

7. Roscoe, B., Strouse, J., & Goodwin, M. (1994). Sexual harassment: Early adolescents' self-reports of experiences and acceptance. *Adolescence, 29,* (115), 515–523.

8. Shrier, D. (1990). Sexual harassment and discrimination. *New Jersey Medicine, 87,* 105–107.

9. Council on Scientific Affairs, American Medical Association. (1992). Council reports violence against women. *Journal of the American Medical Association, 267,* 3184–3189.

10. Straus, M., & Gelles, R. (1990). *Physical violence in the American family.* New Brunswick, NJ: Transaction Publishers.

11. Bachman, R. (1994). *Violence against women.* (NCJ Publication No. 145325) Bureau of Justice

Statistics, U.S. Department of Justice. Washington, DC: U.S. Government Printing Office.

12. Straus, M., & Smith, C. (1993, Spring). Family patterns and primary prevention of family violence. *Trends Health Care Law Ethics, 8*(2), 17–25.

13. Walker, L. E. (1984). *The battered woman syndrome.* New York: Springer.

14. Moss, V., & Taylor, W. (1991). Domestic violence. *AORN Journal, 53*(5), 1158–1164.

15. Keltner, N., Schwecke, L., & Bostrom, C. (1995). *Psychiatric nursing.* St. Louis: Mosby.

16. U.S. Department of Health and Human Services. (1992). *Healthy people 2000: National health promotion and disease prevention objectives.* Boston: Jones & Bartlett.

17. Quillian, J. (1996). Screening for spousal or partner abuse in a community health setting. *Journal of the American Academy of Nurse Practitioners, 8*(4), 155–160.

18. Grisso, J., Schwarz, D., Miles, C., & Holmes, J. (1996). Injuries among inner-city minority women: A population-based longitudinal study. *Am J Public Health, 86* (1), 67–70.

19. Mazza, D., Dennerstein, L., & Ryan, V. (1996). Physical, sexual, and emotional violence against women: A general practice-based prevalence study. *Med J Aust, 164* (1), 14–17.

20. Centers for Disease Control and Prevention. (1993). Emergency department response to domestic violence. *Morbidity and Mortality Weekly Report, 42*(32), 617–620.

21. American Medical Association. (1992). American Medical Association diagnostic and treatment guidelines on domestic violence. *Archives of Family Medicine, 1,* 39–47.

22. Candib, L. (1990). Naming the contraindications: Family medicine's failure to face violence against women. *Family Community Health, 13,* 47–57.

23. Bergman, B., & Brismar, B. (1991). Suicide attempts by battered wives. *Acta Psychiatrica Scandinavica, 83*(5), 380–384.

24. DeLahunta, E. (1995). Hidden trauma: The mostly missed diagnosis of domestic violence. *Am J Emergency Med, 13*(1), 74–76.

25. Freund, K. M., & Blackhall, L. J. (1990). Detection of domestic violence in a primary care setting. *Clinical Research, 38,* 738A.

26. Campbell, J., & Humphreys, J. (1993). *Nursing care of survivors of family violence.* St. Louis: Mosby.

27. McFarlane, J., Parker, B., & Soeken, K. (1996). Abuse during pregnancy: Associations with maternal health and infant birth weight. *Nursing Research, 45*(1), 37–42.

28. Stuart, G., & Sundeen, S. (1995). *Principles and practice of psychiatric nursing.* St. Louis: Mosby.

29. Jezierski, M. (1992). Guidelines for intervention by ED nurses in cases of domestic abuse. *Journal of Emergency Nursing, 18*(1), 28A–30A.

30. Burg, M. (1996). Laminated cards for helping battered women. *MCN, 21,* 159–160.

31. Dunn, S. F., & Guilchrist, V. J. (1993). Sexual assault. *Primary Care, 20*(2), 359–372.

32. Burgess, A., & Holmstrom, L. (1979). *Rape, crisis and recovery.* New York: Prentice Hall.

33. Burgess, A., & Fawcett, J. (1996). The comprehensive sexual assault assessment tool. *Nurse Practitioner, 21*(4), 66–86.

34. Robinson, J., (1990). Rape: A crime with health consequences. *The Female Patient, 15,* 25–32.

35. Carlson, K., & Eisenstat, S. A. (1995). *Primary care of women.* St. Louis: Mosby.

36. Van der Kolk, B.A. (1994). The body keeps score: Memory and the evolving psychobiology of post-traumatic stress. *Harvard Review of Psychiatry, 1,* 253.

37. American Psychiatric Association. (1994). *Diagnostic and statistical manual of mental disorders* (4th ed.). Washington, DC: Author.

38. Vachss, A. (1993). *Sex crimes.* New York: Random House.

39. National Victim Centers. (1993). Rape in America: A Report to the Nation. Arlington, VA.

40. Golding, J. (1996). Sexual assault history and limitations in physical functioning in two general population samples. *Research in Nursing and Health, 19,* 33–44.

41. Beebe, D. (1991). Emergency management of the adult female rape victim. *American Family Physician, 43,* 2041–2046.

42. Hatcher, R., Trussell, J., Stewart, F., & Stewart, G. et al. (1994). *Contraceptive technology.* New York: Irvington Publishers, Inc.

43. Blume, S. B. (1994). Women and addictive disorders. In N. S. Miller (Ed.). *Principles of addiction medicine* (Sec. 16, Ch. 1, pp. 1–16). Chevy Chase, MD: American Society of Addiction Medicine, Inc.

44. Nespor, K. (1990). Treatment needs of alcohol-dependent women. [Special issue: Between life and death: Aging]. *International Journal of Psychosomatics, 37*(1–4), 50–52.

45. Reed, B. G. (1987). Developing women-sensitive drug dependency treatment services: Why so

difficult? *Journal of Psychoactive Drugs, 19*(2), 151–164.

46. Urbano-Marquez, A., Estruch, R., Fernandez-Sola, J., Nicholas, J., Pare, J. C., & Rubin, E. (1995). The greater risk of alcoholic cardiomyopathy and myopathy in women compared with men. *Journal of American Medical Association, 274,* 149–154.

47. Bucholz, K. (1992). Alcohol abuse and dependence from a psychiatric epidemiological perspective. *Alcohol Health Res World, 16*(3), 197.

48. Council on Scientific Affairs, American Medical Association. (1996). Alcoholism in the elderly. *JAMA, 275*(10), 797–801.

49. Gomberg, E. S. 1995). Older women and alcohol: Use and abuse. *Recent Dev Alcohol, 12,* 61–79.

50. Hill, S. Y. (1995). Mental health and physical health consequences of alcohol use in women. *Recent Dev Alcohol, 12,* 181–197.

51. Brennan, P., Moos, R., & Kim, J. (1993). Gender differences in the individual characteristics and life contexts of late-middle-aged and older problem drinkers. *Addiction, 88,* 781–790.

52. Virginian-Pilot. (1996, August 21). Teen drug use up 105% since 1992. No. 275, D1.

53. The fear of heroin is shooting up. (1996, August 26). *Newsweek,* 56.

54. Kinney, J. (1991). *Clinical manual of substance abuse.* St. Louis: Mosby-Yearbook.

55. Goroll, A., May, L., & Mulley, A. (1995). *Primary care medicine.* Philadelphia: J. B. Lippincott.

56. Lemcke, D., Pattison, J., Marshall, L., & Cowley, D. (1995). *Primary care of women.* Norwalk, CT: Appleton & Lange.

57. Ewing, J. (1984). Detecting alcoholism: The CAGE questionnaire. *JAMA, 252,* 1905–1907.

58. Bell, K. (1992). Identifying the substance abuser in clinical practice. *Orthopaedic Nursing, 11,* 29–36.

59. Seltzer, V., & Pearse, W. (1995). *Women's primary health care.* New York: McGraw-Hill.

60. Leon, A., Kerman, G., & Wickramaratane, P. (1993). Continuing female predominance in depressive illness. *Am J Public Health, 83,* 754–757.

61. Betrus, P., Elmore, S., & Hamilton, P. (1995). Women and somatization: Unrecognized depression. *Health Care for Women International, 16,* 287–297.

62. Perry, M., & Anderson, G. (1992). Assessment and treatment strategies for depressive disorders commonly encountered in primary care settings. *Nurse Practitioner, 17,* 25–36.

63. Herfinkel, E., & Gourley, D. (1996). *Textbook of therapeutics: Drug and disease management,* 6th ed. Baltimore: Williams & Wilkins.

64. U.S. Department of Health and Human Services, Public Health Service, Agency for Health Care Policy and Research. (1993). *Clinical practice guideline No. 5: Depression in primary care: Detection, diagnosis, and treatment* (Publication No. 93–09553). Rockville, MD: *AMCPR.*

65. Hassell, J. (1996). Improved management of depression through nursing model application and critical thinking. *Journal of the American Academy of Nurse Practitioners, 8*(4), 161–166.

66. Wittchen, H., Zhao, S., Kessler, R., & Eaton, W. (1994). DSM III-R generalized anxiety disorder in the National Comorbidity Survey. *Arch Gen Psychiatry, 51*(5), 355–364.

67. Levine, G. N. (1996). *Commonly prescribed drugs* (2nd ed.). Stanford, CT: Appleton & Lange.

68. Dolan, B., & Gitzinger, I. (1994). *Why women? Gender issues and eating disorders.* New Jersey: The Athlone Press.

69. Yeager, K. K., Agostini, R., Nattiv, A., & Drinkwater, B. (1993). Female athlete triad: Disordered eating, amenorrhea, osteoporosis. *Medicine and Science in Sports and Exercise, 25*(7), 775–777.

70. Rodin, G. M., & Daneman, D. (1992). Eating disorders and insulin dependent diabetes mellitus: A problematic association. *Diabetes Care, 15*(10), 1402–1412.

71. Stewart, D. E., Robinson, G. E., Goldbloom, D. S., & Wright, C. (1990). Infertility and eating disorders. *American Journal of Obstetrics and Gynecology, 163*(4), 1196–1199.

72. Dresser, L. P., Massey, E. W., Johnson, E. E., & Bossen, E. (1993). Ipecac myopathy and cardiomyopathy. *Journal of Neurology, Neurosurgery, and Psychiatry, 56*(5), 560–562.

73. Speroff, L., Glass, R., & Kase, N. (1994). *Clinical gynecology, endocrinology and infertility* (4th ed.). Baltimore: Williams & Wilkins.

74. Kinoy, B. (1994). *Eating disorders: New directions in treatment and recovery.* New York: Columbia University Press.

75. Giannini, A., Newman, M., & Gold, M. (1990). Anorexia and bulimia. *American Family Physician, 41*(4), 1169–1176.

76. Fairburn, C. (1995). *Overcoming binge eating.* New York: The Guilford Press.

77. Brewerton, T., Dansky, B., O'Neil, P., & Kirkpatrick, D. (1993, May). *Prevalence of binge eating disorder in U.S. women.* Paper presented at the American Psychiatric Association's Annual Meeting, San Francisco.

78. Specker, S., de Zwaan, M., Raymond, N., & Mitchell, J. (1994). Psychopathology in sub-

groups of obese women with and without binge eating disorder. *Compr Psychiatry, 35*(3), 185–190.

79. Litchtman, S., Pisarska, K., Berman, E., Pestone, M., et al. (1992). Discrepancy between self reported and actual caloric intake and exercise in obese subjects. *The New England Journal of Medicine, 327*(27), 1893–1898.

80. Marcus, M. D., et al. (1990). A double-blind, placebo-controlled trial of fluoxetine plus behavior modification in the treatment of obese-eaters and non-binge-eaters. *American Journal of Psychiatry, 147,* 876–881.

81. Brownell, K., & Fairburn, C. (Eds.). (1995). *Eating disorders and obesity: A comprehensive handbook.* New York: Guilford Press.

82. Special report: Choosing a weight-loss program. (1990). *Tufts University Diet and Nutrition Letter, 8*(6), 36.

83. Aday, L. A. (1994). Health status of vulnerable populations. *Annual Rev Public Health, 15,* 487–509.

84. Anderson, D. G. (1996). Homeless women's perceptions about their families of origin. *Western Journal of Nursing Research, 181*(1), 29–42.

85. Institute of Medicine. (1988). *Homelessness, health, and human needs.* Washington, DC: National Academy Press.

86. Killion, C. K. (1995). Special health care needs of homeless pregnant women. *Adv Nurs Sci, 18*(2), 44–56.

87. Lane, D., Polednak, A., & Burg, M. A. (1992). Does breast cancer screening differ between users of county-funded health canters and women in the entire community? *American Journal of Public Health, 82,* 199–203.

88. Drapkin, A. (1990). Medical problems of the homeless. In C. L. Canton. (Ed.), *Homeless in America.* New York: Oxford University Press.

89. North, C. S., Smith, E. M., & Spitznagel, E. L. (1994). Violence and the homeless: An epidemiologic study of victimizations and aggression. *Journal of Traumatic Stress, 7*(1), 95–110.

90. Wiecha, J. L., Dwyer, J. T., & Dunn-Strobecker, M. (1990). Nutrition and health services needs among the homeless. *Public Health Report, 106*(4), 364–374.

91. Brideau, D. J. Jr. (1997). Using nicotine replacement therapies. *Patient Care, 31,* 31–44.

92. Hurt, R. D., Sacks, D. P., Glover, B. D. et al. (1997). A comparison of sustained release bupropion and placebo for smoking cessation. *The New England Journal of Medicine, 337,* 1195–1202.

93. Briggs, G. G., Samson, J. H., Ambrose, P. J., et al. (1993). Excretion of buproprion in breast milk. *Ann Pharmacother, 27,* 431–433.

BIBLIOGRAPHY

Alexander-Mott, D., & Lumsden, B. (Eds.). (1994). *Understanding eating disorders: Anorexia nervosa, bulimia nervosa, & obesity.* Washington, DC: Taylor & Francis.

Ehhrenfeld, P. (Ed.). (1991, Spring). Calling on coaches: Athletes need help. *American Anorexia/Bulimia Association, Inc. Newsletter.*

Fallon, P., Katzman, M., & Wooley, S. (Eds.). (1994). *Feminist perspectives on eating disorders.* New York: Guilford Press.

Glasser, I. (1994). *Homelessness in global perspective.* New York: G. K. Hall & Co.

Herron, D. G. (1991). Strategies for promoting a healthy dietary intake. *Nursing Clinics of North America, 26*(4), 875–884.

Johnson, M. (1992). Tailoring the preparticipation exam to female athletes. *The Physician and Sportsmedicine, 20*(7), 61–72.

National Institutes of Health & National Institute of Mental Health. (1995). *Depression: What every woman should know* (Publication No. 95-3871). Washington, DC: U.S. Government.

Silverstein, B. (1995). *The cost of competence: Why inequality causes depression, eating disorders, and illness in women.* New York: Oxford University Press.

Seltser, B., & Miller, D. (1993). *Homeless families: The struggle for dignity.* Urbana & Chicago: University of Illinois Press.

Szmukler, G., Dare, C., & Treasure, J. (Eds.). (1995). *Handbook of eating disorders: Theory, treatment, and research.* New York: Wiley.

Thompson, J. K. (Ed.). (1996). *Body image, eating disorders, and obesity: An integrative guide for assessment and treatment.* Washington, DC: American Psychological Association.

Walsh, B.(1993). Binge eating in bulimia nervosa. In C. Fairburn, & G. Wilson (Eds.), *Binge eating: Nature, assessment and treatment.* New York: Guilford Press.

Welch, S., & Fairburn, C. (1994). Sexual abuse and bulimia nervosa: Three integrated case-control comparisons. *American Journal of Psychiatry, 151,* 402–407.

Werne, J. (Ed.). (1996). *Treating eating disorders.* San Francisco: Jossey-Bass Publishers.

Zerbe, K. (1993). *The body betrayed: Women, eating disorders, and treatment.* Washington, DC: American Psychiatric Press.

ADDENDUM TO SMOKING CESSATION

Additional information on this subject has been added prior to press date.

Smoking cessation success may be enhanced by using behavioral therapy alone or in conjunction with nicotine replacement products or even a non-nicotine antidepressant. First, assess the woman's readiness to quit, then help her plan a specific quit program. The provider must prepare her for withdrawal symptoms that may sabotage her earnest attempts. Assure her it takes most people several attempts. A partial list of withdrawal symptoms includes irritability, restlessness, hunger, drowsiness, difficulty concentrating, sleep disturbances, and strong cravings for nicotine.[91] Direct nicotine absorption into the circulation in concentrations sufficient to alleviate symptoms can occur through buccal (gum), nasal mucosa (spray), or skin (patch). Available nicotine replacement systems include nicotine inhalation system (Nicotrol inhaler), nicotine nasal spray (Nicotrol NS), nicotine polacriliex (Nicorette gum), and nicotine transdermal system (Nicoderm, Nicotrol, Prostep, Habitrol, etc).[91] In the heaviest smokers, the nicotine nasal spray seems to be most effective.[91]

The FDA has not approved nicotine replacement therapy for pregnant women, however, continued heavy smoking during pregnancy may have higher associated risks than the short-term use of nicotine replacement, providing replacement is followed by complete nicotine abstinence. Lower nicotine levels in replacement therapy may mean less uterine vasoconstriction.[91]

A non-nicotine alternative antidepressant to aid in smoking cessation has recently become available. Bupropion hydrochloride (Zyban) was shown in a recent study to be effective for smoking cessation while having minimal side effects along with reduced weight gain. Bupropion is not recommended for pregnant or lactating women (FDA Category B in pregnancy). Risks and benefits of use with the individual smoker must be weighed.[92,93]

Readers are urged to read references 91–93 carefully for more detailed information and resources on helping smokers with this difficult addiction. This is an area in which providers can have a real impact.

CHAPTER 24

HEALTH CARE CONCERNS FOR WOMEN WITH PHYSICAL DISABILITY AND CHRONIC ILLNESS

Kathleen J. Sawin

*B*eing disabled does not contradict responsible, effective parenting, yet judgmental attitudes continue.

Highlights

- Discrimination
- Culture and Disability
- Negative Attitudes Among Health Care Workers
- Women Who Are Lesbians
- Health Promotion
- Access Issues/Barriers
- Sexuality
    Communication and Education
    Body Image
    Service Animals
    Spasticity
    Spinal Cord Injury
    Joint Inflexibility and Pain
    Multiple Sclerosis
    Diabetes Mellitus
    Epilepsy
    Urinary and Bowel Appliances
    Pelvic Radiotherapy
    Cystic Fibrosis
    Cognitive Impairment
    Menarche
    Personal Attendant
    Sexual Activity
    Abuse
- Issues of Aging/Menopause
- Eliciting a History; Physical Examination
- Management of Contraception
- Pregnancy; Parenting
- Future Research
- Resources

► INTRODUCTION

The unmet needs of women with physical disabilities include accessibility to gynecologic care, sexuality and birth control counseling, and accessibility to professionals with a knowledge of how disability impacts primary care.

DISCRIMINATION

The discrimination that women with disabilities and chronic illness face is twofold: first, they are women, and second, they are individuals with disabilities. Narrow negative social attitudes set unnecessary barriers to the optimal growth and development of these women and the health care they obtain. An example is the stereotypic image of American women as having two major functions—caretaker and object of beauty. The ideal woman is physically "perfect,"[1,2,3] but women with disabilities are seen as dependent and nonproductive and judged incompetent to perform women's work.[4]

The Americans with Disabilities Act (ADA) became law in 1990. Discrimination in employment against qualified persons with disabilities is against the law, enforced by the U.S. Equal Employment Opportunity Commission and related agencies. As of July 26, 1994, this law applied to all employers with 15 or more employees.

IMPACT OF DISABILITY

Specific disabilities (spinal cord injury, cerebral palsy, multiple sclerosis, or disabling arthritis) prevent women, it is thought, from meeting society's major functions. Attractive women who use wheelchairs are seen as less than whole. For example, a comment overheard in a family planning clinic concerned a very attractive 19-year-old woman who had recently sustained a spinal cord injury and now used a wheelchair for mobility: "She used to be so pretty." In fact, the accident left no scar but changed only her mode of mobility.

ECONOMICS

Women experience greater effects from disability than do men in that they earn less, work less, and are studied less.[2,5–9] When rehabilitation services are provided, women are more likely to be rehabilitated for homemaking and much less likely to be rehabilitated for competitive employment.[10] High divorce rates are associated with disability; the highest rates are when the woman is the disabled spouse.[11] Nearly half live alone.[12] Economic status may even have an impact on a women's adaptation to disability. In addition, women with disability face extraordinary barriers in accessing health insurance.[13]

CULTURE AND DISABILITY/ILLNESS

CULTURE AND DISABILITY

Culture shapes women's experience with disabilities. Little is written about the experience of disability for women in diverse cultures. The more the disability experience is divergent from the societal norm of the referent culture group, however, the more issues women will face. For women who are immigrants, the experience is more difficult as the woman must deal with her marginality, social isolation, and alienation in a foreign culture.[14,15] The devaluation of self is not only rooted in the chronic illness experience but also from the definition of self that is constructed in dealing with the migration experience.

For African American women with disabilities, there may be issues of role conflict, employment and sexuality.[16] African American women may experience greater difficulty with multiple role conflict. They tend to have more roles, more children, greater environmental stress and may be more likely to be single parents. The kinship network of the African American woman, however, is a positive protective factor. If the disability causes collapse of that network, health care providers need to aggressively assist the woman to repair or renew her support network. Employment is a challenge for African American women. Women of color with disabilities have lower employment income levels than all other men and women. They earn \$.22 for every dollar earned by a white nondisabled man.[16] The evidence indicates that many African American women are traditional in their sexual practices. If the woman is hesitant to participate in oral sex behaviors, masturbation, or experiment with alternative methods of sexual intimacy, she may be at risk for sexual dissatisfaction. Health professionals need to assess the woman for the discrepancy between her ideal and real experiences. Assistance that helps decrease the discrepancy will optimize the woman's adjustment. Further, emphasis needs to be placed on conditions that unequally affect African American women, such as sickle cell. Lupus strikes most during the childbearing age, and African American women are over represented.[17]

Activists and scholars writing about the civil rights movement of individuals with disabilities reject the traditional view of disability as physically defective and needing to be fixed. Instead these activists are asserting that individuals with disabilities are a legitimate cultural minority. This philosophy is based on the belief that most of the problems faced by individuals with disabilities are not caused by the body "but by a society that refuses to accommodate our differences." This culture proposes that medical needs are only a small part of the disability experience, with the larger, more pressing problems being social and political.[4]

NEGATIVE ATTITUDES AMONG HEALTH CARE PROVIDERS

Health care providers have negative attitudes toward women with disabilities,[13,18,19] expect less of them,[20] and overestimate the negative impact of disability on family life.[4,21] Often, health care providers speak without sensitivity. They are frequently unaware of how many adults with disabilities live independently in the community, use adaptive equipment, modify homes, and use attendant care.[22] Moreover, professionals are more aware of predominately male disabilities and underestimate the frequency of disabilities among women.[2,9,13]

Health care providers have strong influence on knowledge, beliefs, and expectations of women with physical disabilities and chronic illness as they strive to maintain reproductive health.[13] Inservice training sessions for primary care providers and women's centers are needed to address access and attitudinal barriers.[21,23]

ASEXUAL MISPERCEPTION

Women with disabilities, especially those growing up with a disability, are seen by health care providers as asexual.[24-30] To the contrary, these women have numerous needs. Thirty-two women with disabilities reported, unanimously, their need for health care providers to see them as sexual beings.[20] Denying the sexuality of a woman limits the services that are provided for her.[2,9,13,29]

LOWERED EXPECTATIONS

Health care providers are among those who often send the message that a woman's body is unacceptable.[24,25,30] Expectations are that women with disabilities are less likely to marry or have children; they may be seen as more dependent, weak, and less able to care for themselves or a child.[3,30,31] In fact, a significant factor in whether young women with disabilities have active social lives was their parent's expectations.[30] Unfortunately, although these parents had educational goals for their daughters, only a small, percentage expected their daughters to be socially active.[30]

- School nurses given the same vignette about young adolescents with and without disabilities starting their menstrual period for the first time at school held different expectations for knowledge, self-care, and independence based only on the adolescents' use of a wheelchair for mobility.[32]
- Characteristically, clinic and hospital personnel talk to the person who is accompanying the individual with a disability, not to the individual herself. In addition, they frequently "talk down" or use language patterns appropriate for a child.[9,20]

SURMISED RETARDATION

Often women are treated as if physical disability means mental retardation, especially if their speech is impaired. Frequently, inebriation is assumed in addition to low IQ. Talking more loudly or more simply is a frequent reaction to speech disability.

PERCEIVED PARENTHOOD CONFLICT

Conflict is perceived between carrying out the responsibilities of parenthood and complying with a medical regimen. Mothers report that health care providers seem unable to recognize the profound interrelationship between their mothering responsibilities and chronic illness or disability. Many women hold the opinion that it is a contradiction to be both an effective mother and a "good patient."[33]

WOMEN WHO ARE LESBIANS

If women with disabilities/chronic illnesses experience double discrimination, women in the lesbian community are even more disadvantaged. Although literature exploring issues for lesbians with disabilities is very limited, a few recent authors help us understand these women's experiences.[34-37] Themes identified include 1) a sense of voicelessness in social and political arena, 2) difficulties in dealing with health care professionals, 3) discrimination in the workplace, 4) anger at public ignorance and injustice, and 5) physical abuse. One women with a stroke who had two prior experiences with physical attacks and "gay bashing" indicated "I feel even more vulnerable in a wheelchair."[36] Further, the family, a source of support for many individuals, may not be a positive factor for some women as they report the overwhelming feelings of powerlessness being both disabled and lesbian within the traditional family. Women report discriminatory practices in the workplace, which frequently seem insurmountable. Thus, economic dependence complicates the situation. This economic issue may be a factor in some of the anger voiced by women who had worked hard to escape poverty only to have a chronic illness/disability "pulling me back."[36] Women report both negative and positive experiences when relating to health care providers, although the overwhelming reaction is one of "not being listened to" and "not feeling safe or respected."[38] Both of these lead to "health care hop-

ping" and lack of continuity of care. Women report how powerful the acceptance is when they can introduce their girlfriend to their health care provider and "its ok."[35,36] Many lesbians with disabilities experience negative repercussions, however, when they "come out" with health care providers.[35]

Lesbians with disabilities indicate that their "safe haven" is the lesbian community. They report total acceptance and caring here that they do not find in the disability or conventional communities.[37] They indicate a pervasive able-bodyism in the feminist movement that excludes women with disabilities. According to these authors, feminists are reluctant to encompass women with disabilities because they perceive them as dependent, passive, and needy. They are seeking to portray a more powerful, competent, appealing female image.

Some lesbians with disabilities report a spiritual experience from the community support and others report religion itself used as a coping mechanism. The women interviewed by Marshall indicated that their partners figured most prominently in how they dealt with their disabilities.[36] Lesbians with disabilities are diverse, and their needs will need to be individually heard. The health care provider can "give all women a voice," listen and convey acceptance to women's diversity, and affirm women moving on to action from anger. The provider can do none of this, however, if lesbians with disabilities remain "invisible." Unapproachable health care providers add to the unaddressed health care needs of this population. For example more than 50 percent of lesbians have not had a Pap smear in the last 12 months.[35] The interventions addressed for all lesbians (see Chapter 7) are core to establishing a message of effective communication, approachability, and effectiveness when working with women with disability. To do this, providers need to increase their sensitivity. As one women indicated,

> The pious compassion shown to disabled people cannot be demonstrated to lesbians and gays. Conversely, the violent hostility shown gays and lesbians is hidden due to our disability. In a word, we are different. However, we are proud of our nonstereotypical multi-identities, and this power will force

our communities to expand their own horizons of the "acceptable." All disabled people are viewed as asexual, but we challenge that oppression twice. Our social challenge is that our sameness and our difference are included. We are in the struggle and we are OUT about it."[38]

Health Care Providers need to create an environment where women feel safe to voice their concerns and have their unique health care needs met.[39] REGARD, a self-advocacy organization for disabled lesbians and gays, works to establish knowledgeable providers. In addition, disabled lesbians have been totally excluded from the small numbers of studies that have explored lives of women with disabilities. In order to achieve optimal health, lesbians need to be included—in our expectations and our research.[38]

INEFFECTIVE TERMINOLOGY

Language is a powerful communicator of negative attitudes. Communication needs to be inclusive; Limiting, stereotypic terms must be avoided. See Table 24-1.

HEALTH PROMOTION

A Health People 2000 priority goal is to reduce health disparities among Americans. "The health promotion and disease prevention needs of people with disabilities are not nullified because they were born with an impairing condition or have experienced a disability or injury that has long-term consequences. In fact, the need for health promotion is accentuated."[40] Identifying interventions to support health promoting behaviors in persons with disabilities is the top priority of researchers in rehabilitation nursing.[41] There is a growing emphasis both from clinicians/researchers[41–43] and National Institutes of Health[44] to generate knowledge about an area ignored until recently—health promotion or wellness needs of women with disabilities/chronic illnesses. The Center for the Study of Women with Disabilities has been created at Baylor University, NIH has held a consensus conference on the Health of Women with Disabilities, and organizations such as the Spina Bifida Association and the American

Epilepsy Society have created an organizational committee or task force to address the unique needs of this population.

Nosek et al.[2] interviewed 31 women about wellness issues. The concepts of coherence, self-regulation, competence, resilience, empowerment, and health awareness have been cited in existing models of wellness. These women's experience indicated that resilience was the relevant concept in their lives. Their lines of defense emerged as an important part of this resilience as their boundaries were continually threatened by insensitive behaviors of medical professionals and overwhelming overprotectiveness by family. Women who were identified as high in wellness tended to be assertive, resourceful and pro-active in their search for knowledge and answers to the barriers they experienced.

Health promotion in women with disabilities embraces all activities traditionally encompassed in health promotion programs but also may include complementary therapies and programs aimed at specific disabilities such as Stay Well! The Polio Network's Manual for a Health Promotion Program.[45]

NUTRITION

Evidence[46,47] supports that 0.4 mg (400 micrograms) per day of folic acid, will significantly reduce the number of cases of neural tube defects (NTDs). Because NTDs occur in the early days of pregnancy before women are even aware of even being pregnant, the USPHS recommends that ALL women of childbearing age in the United states who are capable of becoming pregnant should take a multivitamin containing 0.4 of folic acid a day to reduce the risk of having a pregnancy affected with spina bifida or NDT. Women who have had a prior pregnancy affected by NTDs are considered high risk, should be placed on higher daily doses of folic acid (4mg), and need to plan with their health care provider for any anticipated pregnancies. Providers need to be aware that high doses of folic acid may mask vitamin B_{12} deficiency.[47] Obesity may put women at two to four times higher risk for NTD despite folic acid supplementation.[48] Thus, preconceptual counseling for weight reduction has even more impact if the client seeks conception.[49]

TABLE 24–1. LANGUAGE GUIDELINES FOR USE WHEN INTERACTING WITH WOMEN WHO HAVE A DISABILITY

1. Where possible, emphasize an individual, not a disability. Say "people or persons with disabilities" or "person who is blind" rather than "disabled persons" or "blind person." (Many individuals prefer to use the words *physically challenged* to describe this population.)

2. Avoid using emotional descriptors such as unfortunate, pitiful, and so on. Do not refer to or focus on a disability unless crucial for the purpose of communication. Emphasize abilities, such as "walks with crutches (braces)" rather than "is crippled"; "is partially sighted" rather than "partially blind."

3. Talk directly to the person with a disability. If using an interpreter, speak facing the person with hearing impairment.

4. Avoid labeling persons into groups, as in "the disabled," "the deaf," "retardate," and "the arthritic"; instead, say "people who are deaf," "person with arthritis," and "persons with disabilities."

5. Do not sensationalize a disability by saying "afflicted with," "victim of," and so on. Instead, say "person who has multiple sclerosis" or "person who has polio."

6. Avoid portraying persons with disabilities who succeed as superhuman. This implies that persons who are disabled have no talents, or unusual gifts.

7. Avoid use of "confined to wheelchair." Instead, consider "wheelchair user." Indeed many individuals are liberated by a wheelchair rather than limited by the chair.

8. Wheelchairs are extensions of a person's personal space. Ask permission before leaning on or moving equipment, such as a wheelchair.

9. After an initial greeting, sit down so that a person using a wheelchair won't have to crane his/her neck to make eye contact.

10. Shake whatever a person offers in greeting—a hand, prosthesis, or elbow.

11. When speaking with a person with a hearing loss, try to keep your face out of the shadows and your hands away from your mouth as you speak.

12. If you are speaking to someone and a sign language interpreter is present, remember to look at and talk to the person, not the interpreter.

13. If someone's ability to read, write, or handle documents is limited, be prepared to provide assistance in completing paperwork.

14. When someone with a disability enters your clinic, don't assume she needs your help. Greet the person and tell her you're available for assistance.

15. Always speak directly to a person with a disability. Don't assume a companion is a conversational go-between.

16. When you offer to assist someone who is visually impaired, allow the person to take your arm so you can guide, rather than propel her.

17. Act naturally. Do not be afraid to use expressions such as "Would you like to see that?" or "Let me run over there." On the other hand, don't ask personal questions you wouldn't ask someone without a disability.

18. Service animals are working when they are with their owners. Don't touch the animal without the owner's permission.

19. When speaking with a person with speech difficulty, talk normally. Don't pretend to understand when you don't. If necessary, ask the person to repeat. She has experienced this before and knows problems can arise.

Specific Language Guidelines

Disability (disabled, physically disabled). General term used for a (semi)permanent condition that interferes with a person's ability to do something independently—walk, see, hear, learn, lift. It may refer to a physical, mental, or sensory condition. Preferred usage is as a descriptive noun or adjective, as in persons who are disabled, people with disabilities, or disabled persons. Terms such as the disabled, crippled, deformed, and invalid are inappropriate.

Handicap. Often used as a synonym for disability. Usage, however, has become less acceptable (one origin is from "cap in hand," as in begging). Except when citing laws or regulations, *handicap* should not be used to describe a disability. This word can be used to describe the society or environment that limits accessibility.

Mute or Person Who Cannot Speak. Preferred terms to describe persons who cannot speak. Terms such as *deaf-mute* and *deaf* and *dumb* are inappropriate. They imply that persons without speech are always *deaf.*

Nondisabled. In a media portrayal of persons with and without disabilities, *nondisabled* is the appropriate term for persons without disabilities. Able-bodied should not be used, as it implies that persons with disabilities are less able. *Normal* is appropriate only in reference to statistical norms.

Seizure. Describes an involuntary muscular contraction symptomatic of the brain disorder epilepsy. Rather than saying "epileptic," say a "person with epilepsy" or "person with a seizure condition." The term *convulsion* should be reserved for seizures involving contractions of the entire body. The term *fit* is used by the medical profession in England, but it has strong negative connotations.

Spastic. Describes a muscle with sudden, abnormal involuntary spasms. It is not appropriate for describing a person with cerebral palsy. *Muscles* are spastic; people are not.

Speech Impaired. Describes persons with limited or difficult speech patterns.

Cesarean Birth. Should be used to describe a surgical birth. Avoid "section," it depersonalizes. Grapefruits get sectioned; women give birth.

Source: Adapted from Guidelines for reporting and writing about people with disabilities. *(1987). Media Project, Research and Training Center on Independent Living (348 Haworth Hall, University of Kansas, Lawrence, KS 66045); Sawin, K. J. (1986).* Physical disability in contemporary women's health. *Menlo Park, CA: Addison-Wesley; and* Disability etiquette. *Virginia Commonwealth University: Office of EEO/Affirmative Action Services.*

Efforts need to be made to broadly disseminate this information to the general public and to those using contraception services.[50] One such model is the "train the trainer" model used in select public health departments. One professional in each agency participates in training and is then responsible to document educating others in the home agency. This work, underwritten by the March of Dimes at the local level, may be an effective model using agencies, organizations, and schools.

PHYSICAL ACTIVITY SPORTS

Individuals with disabilities have demonstrated physiological responses to exercise similar to women without disabilities. In addition, exercise has been shown to yield positive overall fitness and psychological outcomes. Although most of the studies have been done on men, the data suggest normal wheelchair propulsion is not sufficient to maintain physical condition and training programs yield positive changes in physical conditioning.[51] Research is needed that explores the responses of women with disability to a variety of recreational and sports programs and the interaction of women's health status with these programs. The opportunities for physical activity or women with disabilities need to be expanded.[52]

ACCESS ISSUES/BARRIERS

The characteristics of medical systems sometimes constitute barriers to women with physical disabilities. Several women report dissatisfaction with services they receive from their provider, such as a different provider each time, procedures in some offices that prohibit staff from offering assistance to women in mounting an exam table, staff unwilling to offer assist with dressing, and appointments denied because the women use wheel chairs.[13]

Health care clinics that have architectural barriers limit the independence of women with mobility limitations. Access to buildings via appropriately constructed ramps and to elevators is critical to quality care, as is easy access to bathrooms, examination rooms, and scales. Most medical facilities have numerous architectural

barriers such as nonelevating exam tables and lack of platform scales to weigh persons who use a wheelchair. Even if the facility is architecturally accessible, furniture placement can make the examination room functionally unaccessible. Women experience difficulty obtaining reliable information regarding contraception and often get conflicting recommendations. A truly accessible environment regards women with disabilities as experts on the functioning of their own bodies and is sensitive to histories of traumatic interactions with medical environments. These settings actively develop policies that will increase access to reproductive health services for women with disabilities.[13,20]

In addition very little attention has been given to determining if access issues for women are different than for men. For mothers, daycare access, school, public playgrounds, and affordable housing are all fundamental access issues that are usually not on the list for "assessing accessibility" for most organizations.[51]

SPECIAL PROBLEMS

Sight and Hearing Impairment. Deaf or blind clients are limited in their ability to communicate with providers if interpreters are not available. If a woman provides an interpreter, she loses the option of having private interaction with the provider. If sign language is used in relating issues of sexuality and sexual intercourse, it should be remembered that sign communication is easily interpreted "across the room"; therefore, attention must be given to interview area.[52]

General Considerations

Specific educational resources are listed prior to the References, at the end of this chapter.

Providers may feel that once a woman experiences a disability, she should return to the homemaker role, even when the disability is not severe. Women who report that their sense of self-esteem is tied to work are least likely to report a specific disability.[53]

Severe Disability. Women institutionalized with severe multiple disabilities, including cognitive impairment, may have such clinical problems as vaginal discharge, menstrual cycle dysfunction, and oligomenorrhea. Sensitive onsite management is essential.[54] The severity of physical impairment, however, is not a good predictor of the impact of a disability on a woman.[50,51,53]

Providers need to assess the assumptions they hold. They may be surprised to learn that the severity of physical impairment is not a good predictor of impact of the disability on women.[20,25,55] In fact, fatigue and pain have been found to be predictors of health outcomes even after the impact of functional ability has been taken into consideration.

SEXUALITY

COMMUNICATION AND EDUCATION

Communicating and obtaining information about sexuality are among a woman's greatest concerns. The subject of sexuality and disabled women has been studied little, perhaps because of the erroneous assumption that among clients with a disability, sexuality adjustment is less an issue for women than for men.[11] Women report that professionals rarely initiate discussion of sexuality issues.[20,29,56]

The health care provider needs to take responsibility for initiating discussions of sexuality, but also important is offering "assistance rather than avoiding or overemphasizing the issue."[11] Assumptions should not be made at either extreme: none of these women has sexuality issues, or all of them do. Instead, assess each individual.

Some authors propose that the primary barriers to full expression of sexuality are the negative attitudes of others, especially family members and medical and rehabilitation professionals. The attitude that the disability has somehow "neutered" the woman interferes with her belief in her right to sexual feelings and expression.[2,3,27,29,30,51,54]

From their in-depth qualitative interviews, researchers[2] identified tasks important to developing a wellness perspective of sexuality among women with physical disabilities (see Table 24–2). These characteristics of being a "well woman," however, are not all of the story. The study found that examination of wellness cannot focus only on the individual and cannot be

TABLE 24–2. WELLNESS PERSPECTIVE OF SEXUALITY AMONG WOMEN WITH PHYSICAL DISABILITIES

Having a Positive Sexual Self-Concept
  She appreciates her own value
  She asserts her right to make a choice
  She feels ownership of her body
  She is able to restrict the limitations resulting from her disability to physical functioning only and does not impose those limitations to her sexual self
  She is accepting, not ashamed, of her body

Having Sexual Information
  She has general information about sexuality and is able to apply to herself
  She actively seeks information about how her disability affects her sexuality

Having Positive, Productive Relationships
  She feels generally satisfied with her relationships
  She is able to communicate effectively with others
  She feels stability in her relationships
  She is able to control the amount and nature of contact with others

Managing Barriers
  She is able to recognize psychological, physical and sexual abuse and its exploitation, and take action to reduce or eliminate it, or neutralize its impact.
  She has learned to reduce her vulnerability
  She understands her disability related environmental needs and seeks information on how to meet these needs
  She recognizes her right to live in a barrier free environment and takes action to achieve it
  She confronts societal barriers by using good communication skills to educate her partner, friends, and family

Maintaining Optimal Health and Physical Sexual Functioning
  She participates in health maintenance activities and engages in health promoting behaviors
  She feels congruity between her values/desires and her sexual behaviors
  She manages her environment to optimize privacy for intimate activities
  She is satisfied with the frequency and quality of sexual activity
  She is able to communicate freely with her partner about limitations and devices, and about what pleases her sexually

Source: Adapted from Nosek, M. A., Howland, C. A., Young, M. E., Georgiou, D., Rintala, D. H., Foley, C. C., Bennett, J. L., & Smith, Q. (1994). Wellness models and sexuality among women with disabilities. Journal of Applied Rehabilitation Counseling (25), 50–57.

framed in a deficiency model if solutions are to be found. It is important to study the context. These researchers concluded that the roots of problems are to be found in the macro system that insists on a normative group against which all others are to be compared and found deficient. The way a social problem is defined determines policy, strategies for change, and criteria for evaluation.

In the quantitative portion of this study, 475 women with disabilities were compared with a population of 425 women without disabilities. There was no difference between groups in sexual desire. Further, there was no impact of the severity of disability on sexual activity. Women with disabilities did report lower amounts of sexual activity, sexual response, and sexual satisfaction. Women with disabilities since childhood had more sexual thoughts and higher desire. No differences were found in sexual frequency, arousal, or satisfaction. The psychological factors predicted the greatest amount of sexual variance, 35 percent of variance in sexual satisfaction and 40 percent of the variance in sexual activity.[2] Other researchers agree, reporting decreased function without changes in interest or importance of sexual activity.[55]

In a study of adolescents with disabilities, Meeropol found few of the adolescents or their parents ever talked to a nurse or physician for sexuality information, and one quarter of the adolescents and 40 percent of their parents wished that a health care professional had offered this information.[56]

As long as women with disabilities are viewed as deviant from the social norm based only on disability, they will continue to be invisible.[2] The Syndey Manifesto, a statement of the World Assembly of Disabled Peoples International held in Sydney in 1994, summarizes the rights of women with disabilities. This Manifesto asserts that each time issues for women are considered, the woman with disabilities needs to be included.

Questions on How Sexuality Is Affected. The specific effects of a disability on sexual activity need to be communicated to a woman. For example, in some conditions spasticity might be experienced with orgasm.[57] The PLISSIT Model. This model, used to order levels of intervention for clients with sexual issues, is helpful for health care providers (see Chapter 6). PLISSIT is derived from "Permission giving, provision of Limited Information and Specific Suggestions, Intensive Therapy." All providers need to be skilled in permission giving, reinforcing the ability for a woman with a disability to be a sexual person and to be involved in sexual activ-

ities. The professional needs to understand and convey to women with disabilities that any manifestation of sexuality that is acceptable and satisfying to the individual or individuals involved is normal.

BODY IMAGE

Concerns about body image exist for some women with disabilities. The reactions of others may suggest to a woman that her body is unacceptable.[30]

Perceived Lack of Control. Issues such as physical dependency, bladder incontinence, spasticity, or other involuntary movements, which are not seen as adult conditions, may make the woman with a disability seem like an infant. The lack of control can lead to a mind-body split. "It was like my body belonged to the doctors, it wasn't mine any more." "Once I put my feet up in the stirrups, I had no control—my body belonged to them [examiners]."[20]

APPLIANCES. The need to use appliances or equipment may interfere with a woman's sense of self as sexually desirable.

SOURCE OF TROUBLE. The body may have a history of "causing" trouble. If a child grew up with a disability, her body may have caused parents trouble and could have become the "enemy."

SERVICE ANIMALS

The use of service animals is growing in popularity. These animals, most often dogs or monkeys, assist their owners in a wide variety of tasks from alerting a woman with hearing impairment that someone is at the door to retrieving objects for a woman with mobility impairment. In addition, women report they feel less vulnerable if their service animal is a large dog that barks loudly at strangers.

SPASTICITY

Spasticity can be elicited by a variety of tactile stimulations. Each woman needs to determine the ability of a variety of sexual activities to produce this response. Slow building stimulation may produce less spasticity than more intense stimulation. Women with spasticity might experience spasticity with orgasm.[53] The knee-chest position during sexual activities may facilitate decrease in spasticity.

SPINAL CORD INJURY

Because a women's fertility is not affected in a spinal cord injury, many providers and researchers have assumed no sexuality problems exist. Spinal cord injury precipitates specific physiological changes that reflect the level of cord injury and the completeness of the lesion. Some authors categorize lesions as above thoracic 10, between thoracic 10 and 12, and distal to thoracic 12.[57] Women with complete lesions experience neither traditional orgasm, nor clitoral or vaginal sensation;[53,58-61] however, women with spinal cord injury do report satisfying pleasurable orgasm-like sensations from stimulation of the breasts, ears, or other sensitive areas.[59] Even women with complete lesions report psychological and even physical sensations of orgasm or "intense pleasure" during sex.[60,62,63] These orgasm experiences are not related to type or level of SCI.[63] In addition, menstrual discomfort may remain, even if altered.[60] Vaginal lubrication may occur via reflex for women with lesions at T9–T11 or above [61,62,64] and has also been reported in relation to masturbation unrelated to level of lesion.[63] In addition, some women report cervical and vaginal pressure.[65] Arousal was present in women regardless of level of lesion and not correlated with type of stimulation (vaginal, cervical, or hypersensitive area). Clearly, the mechanism of sexual response in women with spinal cord injuries does not totally follow the traditional physiological model. Further research is needed to understand the physical and cognitive processes women experience.[66,67,68]

Change in Patterns. Adjustment in the first years after injury are most difficult. Some women report issues revolving around physical problems (bladder control, dry vagina), but issues regarding social interaction (attitudes of others) are numerous.[11] Changes in the reproductive system are listed:

- Temporary cessation of menses is normal for 60–90 percent of women for several months following injury. Cessation of menses may persist for up to 2 years, with the average duration being 6 months. For 89 percent of women, menses returns by 1 year.[61,64,65]

- Patterns of sexual activity for women with a disability may be decreased. Many women report the lack of a partner. It is important, however, to remember that the problem is universal. Participants in a Sexual Attitude Reassessment (SAR) workshop reported they were not as active as they wished (women without disability 56 percent, women disabled 57 percent).[55]

- Alternative areas of sexual stimulation and strategies for sexual expression need to be identified, including alternative positions, such as side lying, knee-chest positions, and chair sitting, for paraplegics and quadriplegics[57] and the stuffing technique (of flaccid penis) for women whose partner is paraplegic. If graphic depiction of positions for sexual intercourse would be helpful, the health care provider needs to communicate the appropriate resources.[57]

- The normal sexual responses that may occur are opening of the labia, contraction of the outer third of the vagina, expansion of the inner two-thirds of the vagina, and uterine contraction.

  - Resumption of ovulation is unpredictable. It may occur before menstruation[65]
  - Women at or approaching climacteric may become menopausal[61]
  - Many women (69 percent in a large SCI follow up study) are satisfied with postinjury sexual experience although many were not satisfied with information provided in rehabilitation SCI[66]

Autonomic Dysreflexia. A potentially fatal complication for women with spinal cord injury, autonomic dysreflexia, occurs if the lesion is complete and above T-6 and can lead to a stroke.[27]

Autonomic dysreflexia is a physiological reflex response to stimulation. Stimulation may be caused by conditions such as skin breakdown, bladder hyperdistention often due to kinked tubing, bowel distention, severe constipation, pelvic examination, labor, or intercourse positions.

Patterns of response vary among individuals; however, among all who have a complete lesion, the pathway within the cord that transmits sensations to higher levels is blocked. So, too, is the mechanism that relays messages downward from the brain. Consequently, blood pressure is not suppressed, and blood pressure rises with sustained reflex. As long as the sensation continues, the blood pressure continues to rise. Normal blood pressure for women with spinal injury is often lower than normal, for example, 90/60. Blood pressure in early dysreflexia might be 140/83. At this level, a woman could have significant symptoms of dysreflexia.

Dysreflexia is often overlooked by health care providers who do not know about the altered blood pressure norm. Headache, sweating, goose flesh above the level of lesion, flushed face, and nasal stuffiness are other signs of this potentially lethal complication.

Sources of stimulation can be additive. For example, if a client is slightly constipated or sitting or lying on an object, or her urine drainage system is slightly kinked, an additional stimulation such as a pelvic exam, sexual intercourse, or labor contraction could trigger dysreflexia. If dysreflexia occurs, the total situation must be assessed for hidden problems.

- If dysreflexia occurs during a procedure, *have the client sit up immediately.* Blood pressure increases when a person is lying down. A semi-sitting position is helpful to prevent dysreflexia during pelvic exams. Labor in that position might be helpful if it is comfortable.
- Monitor blood pressure during labor contractions.
- Assist the client in establishing effective bowel and bladder routines, which can prevent or reduce accidents and decrease the chance of additive dysreflexia episodes.
- Take extreme care to protect skin when transferring the client to an examining table.
- May need medication for acute episodes or on a long-term basis. Unresponsive dysreflexia is a medical emergency.

A woman with a spinal cord injury who is educated about the symptoms of autonomic dysreflexia needs to be listened to. She may have a card with treatment outlined or a hotline for contacting a rehabilitation consultant. Discuss the pattern of autonomic dysreflexia with all women with spinal cord injury before high risk situations (pelvic examination, labor, catheter change, etc.) occur.[13]

Ask the client about the frequency of the symptoms, triggering factors, and usual treatment. Were there any episodes in which she did not respond? Does she take medications routinely?

Latex Allergy. Since 1991, the Centers for Disease Control and Prevention (CDC) has been receiving an increasing number of reports of latex related allergy. Individuals (especially children) with spina bifida or myelomeningocele (a congenital spinal cord injury) have the highest incidence of latex allergy, varying from 12 percent to 40 percent of the population.[69–71] This condition also occurs in some women with multiple congenital malformations, especially multiple urinary anomalies, and in some health care providers with increased latex exposure. Reaction varies from mild wheal and flare episodes to anaphylatic reactions.[72–74] The latter are most frequently related to surgery. In addition, 3–17 percent of health care workers develop latex allergy.[75]

Most children/adolescents who have developed this allergy have reacted to balloons and gloves; however, condoms, dental dams, and urinary catheters have also created allergic response. Women with spina bifida are considered high risk and should be tested for latex allergy (RAST—radioallergosorbent testing).[76,77] Health care providers need to be alert to the possibility of latex sensitivities in their clients. Avoidance of latex materials (condoms, diaphragms, latex gloves) may be recommended for all individuals with spina bifida. Many settings that provide services to at-risk patients have converted to a nonlatex environment.[71] Staff in hospitals, clinics, dentists' offices, and especially ORs need to be well versed in precautions.[70,72] The Spina Bifida Association of America has a comprehensive list of nonlatex options, which is updated every 6 months[77] and a short well done video useful to both families and professionals (see Resource list). Individuals with a confirmed allergy should wear a medic alert bracelet and carry an epinephrine autoinjector kit.[80]

JOINT INFLEXIBILITY AND PAIN

Arthrogryposis congenita, sickle cell anemia with joint involvement, arthritis, severe scoliosis, amputation, and dwarfism may result in joint inflexibility and pain. With respect to sexual activity, careful assessment of physical parameters, such as range of motion, is helpful. Discussion about alternative positioning may follow. The importance of extended foreplay, possible gentle warming up and stretching, warm showers, and use of vibration, massage, or masturbation to achieve orgasm may also be considered. Prolonged rest should be avoided in order to decrease likelihood of joint stiffness. Sexual activity may augment an overall sense of comfort, as orgasm releases endorphins. The client may profit from some helpful suggestions.

- Choose the time of day for sexual activity relative to pain history.
- Consider a warm shower or compress in foreplay if effective in pain relief.
- Consider medicine for pain relief before intercourse if pain is limiting.
- Consider referral to a physical therapist for comprehensive muscle assessment in complex cases.

Assess social support. Data indicate that after controlling for physical limitations and social integration, social support was found to influence the outcome in women with arthritis.[78–81]

Encourage a positive, proactive attitude. Self-assessed health status is a powerful predictor of function.[82]

MULTIPLE SCLEROSIS

MS is the most common neurologic disease among young adults. Women are affected twice as often as men. Female sex hormones, estrogen and progesterone, may be involved. Clinical symptoms often appear during changes in hormonal balance during the menstrual cycle, after pregnancy, and during the climacteric.[83]

The symptoms of multiple sclerosis may vary greatly and may include spasticity, dry vagina, fatigue, muscle weakness, pain, bladder and bowel incontinence, and difficulty achieving orgasm.[84–87] No change, however, occurs in fertility or menstruation. Balance and fatigue may necessitate energy sparing sexual activities and positions for intercourse. A water-soluble lubricant may be used if the vagina is dry. Vibrators have been found to be helpful to those who tried them, as a way to increase stimulation and achieve orgasm.[84]

Data indicate that about half of women who have multiple sclerosis report changes in their sexual life.[85] The duration of MS, degree of disability, number of exacerbations in the last year, disability score, and presence of bowel problems or fatigue have little impact on the presence of sexual dysfunction, although the amount of sexual activity may decrease. Corticosteriods are most often used to reduce sexual malfunction but improved function in one study in only 24 of 60 subjects.[84]

Mattson reports that most women were interested in lovemaking, although interest did vary with disease activity. Eighty-eight percent of women in his study were satisfied and 95 percent of their partners were satisfied with sexual activity. Few women indicated dysfunction caused marital problems.[84] Some clients have irregular ovulation. This may lead to an abnormal secretion of hormones within the pituitary-gonadal axis, which in turn results in irregular menses and possible infertility.[83] Corticosteroids started for other symptoms have resulted in improved sexuality for many women.[84,86,87]

Life stressors, in addition to the disease, have a significant impact on women's sense of mastery. Thus, it might be helpful to have a shift from the emphasis of managing the physical condition to managing the uncertainty and assisting people with MS to achieve a better sense of mastery.[88] Professional help is rarely sought for dysfunction. Sensitive professionals need to address this subject openly with women and their partners.

DIABETES MELLITUS

The effect of diabetes on the sexuality of women is unclear, although sexual changes have been identified among men who have diabetes. Therefore, because genitosexual innervation appears to be analogous in males and females,[89] the potential for dysfunction among women also exists; however, data indicate that diabetic women do not differ in sexual function from their healthy controls.[89]

Spontaneous remission of sexual dysfunction reported on 6-year follow-up was related to improvement in the overall marital and social situations. Acceptance of illness (as judged by interviewer) and psychological distress were strong predictors of sexual function. From these data, it appears that sexual function is related to psychological adjustment to chronic illness.[90]

EPILEPSY

Women with epilepsy have normal fertility.[91] Several concerns exist for these women, however, including the effect of their hormones and menstrual cycle on seizures, contraception, fertility and sexuality issues.[92] Some experts now estimate up to 50 percent of women experience variations in seizure frequency with hormonal changes.[93] Many of the antiepilepsy drugs (AEDs) taken to control seizures have teratogenic potential, especially if the young woman is on more than one medication.[94] Infant malformations occur more in women using polytherapy rather than monotherapy. Safe sex becomes critical as the best outcomes of pregnancy are when the pregnancy is planned. Most women with epilepsy need to begin planning with their gynecologist and neurologist 6–12 months prior to conception. If a trial of decreasing or eliminating an AED is undertaken, it must be done with a slow taper and enough time off medication to evaluate effectiveness.[91,95] After the pregnancy, it is too late to change medications or try to reduce the number as the risk of prolonged convulsions is also a risk for the fetus.

Callanan and Stalland[92] recommend that women chart their seizures in relation to their menstrual cycle and/or ovulation to see if a pattern emerges. Some women would benefit from supplemental hormonal therapy. Puberty, a time of severe hormonal changes, should be monitored closely. The adolescent developmental tasks and emotional status further complicate the health care providers ability to identify patterns or cycles. All women, including adolescents, capable of becoming pregnant should be taking folic acid. Select AEDs have been shown to lower folic acid levels, which increases the risk for neural tube conditions. Genetic counseling may be helpful to determine patterns of birth defects in the family.[91]

A healthy development of sexuality has been affected for some women with epilepsy. These women report problems with self-image and self-confidence with occasional social isolation.

Women report these issues relate to the frequency of their seizures.[92] Some sexuality issues may be related to AEDs. A major initiative focusing on women has been underway in the organizations serving individuals with epilepsy. Focus groups of women with epilepsy identify the same issues of concerns as other women with disabilities: to be taken seriously and considered equal partners in health care, to have options in treatment and lifestyle, and to have a more informed public and health care provider.[96]

URINARY AND BOWEL APPLIANCES

Apparatus may discourage sexual activity. Steps, however, can be taken to ease discomforts.

- Foley catheters can be taped out of the way or removed, but may need to be reinserted soon after sexual activity; individuals using intermittent catheterizations should catheterize before sexual activity to prevent urine leakage.
- Stomal appliances can be ignored, changed, covered, or removed before sexual activity, based on what has been ordered and individual preference.
- Clients should be told that masturbation and coitus may stimulate bladder or bowel incontinence.
- Discussing how to tell potential partners about bladder and bowel issues may be critical. Role playing may be helpful.

PELVIC RADIOTHERAPY

Radiation may cause vaginal constriction resulting in dyspareunia.

CYSTIC FIBROSIS

Young women with cystic fibrosis are living into their third decade and beyond. Their pattern is parallel to other women with disabilities, however. Single women with cystic fibrosis start dating at a later age, have dated less often, felt less attractive, had less sexual desire and had more sexual issues than a comparison group of women without cystic fibrosis.[97] These authors conclude the tendency to overprotect these women may interfere with their sense of autonomy and self-worth. In addition, women who had a defiant attitude toward their chronic illness did better. This attitude is an example of "healthy denial" defined by this author not as denial of the illness but denial of the illness to impact normal function despite challenges. Women who were married differed from their single peers; they had later onset of illness, better physical health, and better sexual health.

WOMEN WITH COGNITIVE IMPAIRMENT

It is difficult for women with cognitive impairment to achieve sexual options available to other women with disabilities. Issues of sexual education, effective birth control, sexual expression, and pregnancy are complex. Even when parents verbalize the opinion that young adults with cognitive impairment should have sexual options, it is difficult for the same parents to prepare their own children to make sexual decisions,[98] consider teaching their teen the appropriate use of masturbation,[99] or teach abuse prevention skills.

CHANGES IN MENARCHE

It appears that some variations in menarche occur among women with select disabilities. For example, individuals with Down syndrome and spinal bifida experience menarche 11 months earlier than a comparison group of nondisabled subjects; however, others with genetic disabilities may have delayed menarche.[54,100] Individuals with blindness experience menarche earlier than normal. Head injury is also associated with precocious puberty.[101] Most women with spinal cord injury report the same or more discomfort with their menses after injury.[60] For some women with mobility impairments, lack of manual dexterity and difficulty transferring can impair independence and may lead a woman to seek a means to reduce or eliminate the menstrual cycle. Nosek[9] indicates the practice is wide spread in well meaning parents of women with cognitive impairment. Her point is that no research exists on the long-term effects of these drugs for women with decreased mobility. Depo-Provera, for example, may have serious cardiovascular side effects such as thrombophlebitis and pulmonary embolisms. Women and their families must carefully weigh the risks and benefits of interventions to manage menstrual hygiene with potential long-term effects.

PERSONAL CARE ATTENDANT

Many women with mobility or sensory limitations employ a personal care attendant. She may address some unique sexuality issues; for example, she may place the cervical cap or diaphragm and carry out the bowel or bladder program before sexual activity. Spouses and significant others often function as personal care attendants, but it can be difficult to be both care provider and lover. Each couple needs to address this issue. If both the woman and her partner are disabled, the attendant may assist in positioning the couple. The political issues surrounding reimbursement, regulation, and licensing of personal care attendants may dramatically affect the quality of life for women with disabilities.[102]

PLANNING SEXUAL ACTIVITIES

Women report a need to avoid spontaneity and instead plan for sexual activity. This need, however, can be seen as a benefit: because many disabled persons must communicate with their partners about sexual possibilities and restrictions, this opens up avenues for communication in other areas of the relationship. Unfortunately, many people who are totally physically independent may never experience such communication.[25]

ABUSE

Women with physical and cognitive disabilities may be at higher risk for abuse.[4,19,103,104]

There is combined cultural devaluation of women, devaluation based on age, and devaluation of disability. The woman with disability often has experienced overprotection and has internalized social expectations. Combine this with a lack of knowledge, overcompliance, an unrealistic view that everyone is a friend, limited social opportunity, constant negative feedback (women with disability are ugly, worthless, etc.), low self-esteem, and limited or no assertiveness or refusal skills, and it is understandable this population has a high incidence of abuse.[30,105] Women may not report abuse because of fear of not being believed due to their devalued status.[103] If a disabled teenager or adult feels undesirable, she may become vulnerable to exploitation, particularly in sexual relations.[19] In a national survey of over 800 women, Nosek[2] found women with disabilities 1½ times more likely to have been abused than their nondisabled peers; 50 percent of women with disability and 34 percent of women without disability reported abuse. These researchers proposed that women who get little information regarding sexuality are vulnerable to exploitation. Children who undergo frequent physical examinations or therapy can come to feel that their body causes pain, or is connected with unpleasant experiences. This feeling may yield a child or teen who feels disconnected from her body, at risk for abuse.[30] In a qualitative study of 31 women with disabilities, the disability itself did not seem to be related to the abuse experience.[104] These researchers concluded that it is the asexual, dependent, passive stereotype of women with physical disability that may be the root of the vulnerability to sexual abuse rather than the disability itself.

It is important that the health care provider acknowledge the sexuality of women with disabilities, teach healthy sexuality in the context of family, reinforce a positive sense of self, learn to recognize signs of abuse, listen to the patient, and act on reports of abuse. Assessment of abuse and treatment interventions for women with disabilities will be the same as their peers without disabilities. Prevention, however, is the major key.[105]

Educational programs need to be developed to address skill building in coping with potential or real abuse and orientation to sexuality rights and responsibilities.[105]

In addition, health care providers need to include sexual assertiveness skills in sex education or family life education curricula. The optimal time for this education is in childhood or adolescence. The vast majority of shelters for women who have been abused are unaccessible.[104] Professionals need to seek out opportunities to act as a consultant to schools and community groups that serve this population (YWCA, Independent Living Center, local school districts, and schools).

ISSUES OF AGING/MENOPAUSE

People with disabilities are now living into "old age." Postpolio syndrome is a reality for many women in their 50s. We do know that the major causes of death to persons with spinal cord injuries are respiratory infections, urinary tract infections and external causes such as suicide. There is little data, however, explaining why most other people with lifelong disabilities die. Individuals with disabilities and chronic illness are asking questions such as the following: What are the implications of aging to 60 if you have had osteoarthritis since 20? What is menopause like for women with disabilities,[9] or what are the implications on joint health of walking for many years with altered gait or of the early transition to wheelchair as primary source of mobility?

We know that the use of long-term steroids in women with lupus may compound osteopenia and that calcium supplementation with vitamin D needs to be included unless creatinine clearance or calcium excretion is impaired.[106] Further, women with physical disabilities are less likely to ambulate, participate in physical exercise, and are more likely to have a history of phlebitis. They enter menopause with fewer years of weight bearing and little or no participation in aerobic activity.[107] Thus, they are at risk for obesity, cardiovascular deconditioning, and cardiovascular illnesses. There are simple noninvasive assays to measure bone health. These data need to be collected both to describe this problem for the population and to treat individual women.

Menopause can also bring decreased skin turgor and strength, loss of elasticity and decreased blood supply. This can put a woman with disability at increased risk for skin breakdown.[106] It is also clear that menopause may occur earlier in women with Down syndrome.[108]

Women who would benefit from estrogen replacement have often been eliminated from consideration due to concerns over thrombotic events. The transdermal estrogen therapy, however, may be a safe option for many, especially if the thrombosis history is old.[109] Management in collaboration with gynecologist, geriatrician, and physiatrist consultants may optimize care for elderly women with disabilities.

Children or young women who survived polio may experience postpolio syndrome characterized by increased joint weakness and joint stiffness when they reach midlife (40–60 years of age). We need further research to know how the aging trajectory differs for people with disabilities since childhood or young adult. In addition, we know little about the impact of lifelong disability or chronic illness on menopause or about sexuality issues in those aging with disability.[110]

PHARMACOLOGICAL AGENTS

A number of drugs may have a negative impact on sexual function. A full assessment of both prescription and over- the-counter drugs is critical when addressing issues of sexuality with women who have a disability.[27]

HISTORY

INSPECTION OF SELF

Examiners should look at their own attitudes and expectations before eliciting a history from women with disabilities, to determine potential problems. Do not vary the history protocol to omit potential issues. If you usually ask about first sexual experiences, birth control, episodes of unwanted intercourse, or satisfaction with intimate relationships, also ask women with disabilities. In doing so, it is important to watch your "handicapism" terms and use inclusive and sensitive language (see Table 24–1).

SEXUAL EDUCATION HISTORY

The woman's knowledge of sexuality is pertinent. What was her family life while in school? Does she understand what implications her disability has for sexuality, contraception, birth control, and routine health needs? Ask if sexual information given either in adolescence or during rehabilitation was sufficient. From discussions with the client, determine knowledge deficits. In addition, identify unmet sexual and health needs. Include review of condition specific issues such as dysreflexia for women with spinal cord injury, latex allergy for women with spina bifida, or spasticity

issues for women with cerebral palsy. Ask all women about any allergy type reactions to latex products (balloons, rubber products, condoms, for example).

PROBLEMS PRESENTED

Ask the client what problems the disability has presented and how she has overcome these barriers.

PHYSICAL EXAMINATION

PHYSICAL ACCESSIBILITY OF CLINIC

Physical Layout. In assessing the physical layout of a clinic, determine wheelchair accessibility, for example, ramp dimensions, bathrooms, and doorways. Using a wheelchair may be helpful in assessing the environment. Lack of accessibility promotes the dependence of clients.[9,13,19,111,112]

The Americans With Disabilities Act, enacted in 1990, mandates that all new buildings meet minimal accessibility standards. Section 504 of the Persons With Disabilities Act of 1978 applies to all facilities receiving any federal funds. The regulations do not require that a facility have special programs or services. The regulations do, however, require that the same services offered to women without disabilities must be offered to women with disabilities.[113] For example, if women without disabilities are weighed, accurate mechanisms are needed to weigh women with disabilities. Wheelchair accessible scales can be used to weigh ambulating women as well. If the clinic offers Pap smears and pelvic examinations, it needs to offer women with disabilities the same services and to make necessary accommodations.

Accessible Supportive Examination Table. A table at wheelchair height facilitates transfer of women with motor disabilities. One such table[19] adjusts to wheelchair height to facilitate transfer to the table; it provides arm rests to support women with cerebral palsy and spasticity who may fear falling off the table when severe or unexpected spasms occur. The absence of leg support, however, may be a major drawback for women with leg weakness or paralysis. Examination tables that have leg support but are not at wheelchair height may be preferred in some settings. Each setting needs to assess its target population for services and provide the most accessible examination table.

Client's Equipment. The health care provider must realize that the wheelchair, crutches, and/or other equipment are part of the client's personal space. Ask permission from the client before sitting or leaning on the equipment or moving it, particularly when the client is in it or on the examination table, where she may want her equipment close by. The use of service animals needs the same sensitivity. Do not approach, speak to, or pet these animals without their owner's permission. Such activities only detract the animals from their jobs—caring for the person with a disability.

Special Equipment. Equipment such as nonlatex gloves, plastic catheters, and nonlatex pads needs to be available.

PSYCHOLOGICAL ACCESSIBILITY

It has been suggested that the client may find it more difficult to gain psychological accessibility to the health care provider than physical accessibility to the clinic. Providers must limit stereotypes, actively pursue optimal communication procedures, value mutual problem solving and goal setting, and use every opportunity to reaffirm normalcy. In a clinical setting, guidelines are needed to enhance accessibility, beginning with the first telephone contact. Proposed guidelines have been delineated by the Task Force on Concerns of Physically Disabled Women.[111] When the first appointment is made, clients should be asked the following:

- Do you have a physical disability? If so, ask the client to specify if it is difficult getting around, hearing, or seeing, and so on.
- What accommodations will be necessary for your visit to the clinic? Arrangements may need to be made that will allow for a longer visit.

Altered Pelvic Examination

Mutual Problem Solving. A health care provider must be aware that a client with disabilities may need an altered pelvic examination.[111,112] Discussion with the client should attempt to solve problems she might have had during previous pelvic

exams. Ask what positions caused problems and what worked best for her. Additional personnel may be needed to assist in supporting the client (e.g., holding legs) during the exam. The client should collaborate in deciding the need. She may prefer to bring a family member or friend with her to the exam.

- *Altered Range of Motion.* A side-lying position or speculum exam with "handle up" may be necessary because of alterations in range of motion.
- *Spasticity.* Women with cerebral palsy report spasms, especially adductor spasms, which may be controlled if the woman takes the knee-chest position, with an assistant "hugging" her,[112] or the side-lying position, with the bottom leg flexed and upper leg on the examiner's shoulder (similar to left lateral delivery position).[114] Keeping the woman's extremities close to the body decreases movement that may stimulate additional spasms.
- *Amputation and Decreased Range of Motion.* The client may be examined in a semisitting position. She may choose to hold the stump herself and place the other leg on the examiner's shoulder or she may choose to have assistance with holding her stump so she can hold a mirror and participate in the examination.
- *Specific Examination.* Examination of the genitalia must include inspection of the vaginal walls for atrophic changes, determination of intravaginal tone, and assessment of hair distribution in the genital region to help rule out possible endocrinopathies.[27] Some examiners find a "handle up" technique helpful for women with limited range of motion. This handle-up technique may also make viewing a midposition or anteverted cervix easier.

In patients who have a history of autonomic dysreflexia, spasticity, or pain on insertion of the speculum, xylocaine gel applied generously to the perineal area can make the exam more effective and comfortable if the gel will not interfere with any specimens needed. All movements in the examination should be gradual to allow patient accommodation.

Some authors suggest select use of the Q-Tip Pap smear for the rare woman with disabilities who is unable to tolerate a speculum examination.

This technique is much less accurate, however, and every effort should be made to assist the client and her family to understand the implications of its use.[115]

Reaffirming Normalcy. During the pelvic examination, reaffirm the client's identified normalcy and healthy status. This makes a strong positive impact on her perception of self.

BREAST SELF-EXAMINATION

In some rehabilitation and primary care settings, breast self-examination is not discussed with women with disabilities, even when they present for gynecologic examinations. Women with intact manual dexterity and sensation, however, can be taught breast self-examination. Moreover, some women with impaired sensation can perform a modified examination, or an attendant or partner can perform it. If neither of these plans is acceptable, more frequent examination by a health care provider should be considered.[112]

CONTRACEPTION

LACK OF INFORMATION

Information on contraception is often not offered to women with disabilities.[29,56,116] It is important, however, for health care providers to examine the options with clients. The choice may be a balance of risk factors,[116] for example, the risk of pregnancy versus the risk of the contraceptive method. If oral contraception or an intrauterine device (IUD) is considered and the method carries risk, consultation with or referral to a gynecologic specialist needs to be initiated.

Discussion of alternatives needs to take place with the woman who is allergic or whose partner is allergic to latex. Contraceptive options may be significantly restricted for women with mobility impairment or with a latex allergy. Joint management with a physician colleague is indicated.

ADOLESCENTS

To prove that they are normal, adolescents with chronic illness or disability often increase their sexual behavior. Consequently, they are at in-creased risk of pregnancy, sexually transmitted diseases, and abuse. Primary care of all adolescent women with chronic illness and disability must include assessment of the potential for sexual activity or actual sexual activity and the need for contraception.

TIMING OF DISABILITY

It is not clear what impact the timing of disability onset has on a woman's satisfaction with contraception and sexuality information. Women whose onset of disability is after menarche are identified by some as having special needs for contraception and sexuality.[55] Other data suggest that women who grow up with their disability do not have adequate sexuality and contraception counseling.[20,112] The need for sexuality and contraception counseling must be assessed regardless of the time of onset.

BARRIER METHODS

Barrier methods are often an optimal choice. If a client has manual limitations and, consequently, difficulty manipulating a barrier device, it is important to determine the availability of a partner or personal care attendant and their roles. A client may need to explore ways to ask her partner to assist with a barrier method. Many women have not considered asking a personal care attendant to assist with placement of a contraceptive device before sexual activity.

- *Condoms.* Condoms, which also provide protection against AIDS and other sexually transmitted diseases, are an option. Water-soluble lubricants can ease vaginal dryness. Caution should be taken to identify women who have, or whose partners have, latex allergies. A nonlatex condom (Avante) is now available. Testing is still underway to determine effectiveness against STDs and HIV, and FDA approval is pending for these purposes. Another nonlatex condom (Tactylon) is currently under development and being tested with release expected in the near future.
- *Cervical Cap.* For some women, a cervical cap is attractive, as it can be inserted in the morning by a personal care attendant and removed 24 hours later, eliminating the need for assistance during lovemaking.[112]

- *Diaphragm.* An increase in urinary infections is associated with the arch diaphragm. It may present particular problems and not be appropriate for women with urinary stasis. Caution should be taken to identify women who have, or whose partners have, latex allergies.

IMPLANTED AND INJECTED HORMONAL CONTRACEPTIVES

Norplant may be an option for some women if memory or manual dexterity is an issue. The presence of erratic bleeding, however, may be problematic for these women.[117] Depo-Provera, although only recently approved for contraceptive use by the Food and Drug Administration, is widely used in other countries. This contraceptive has been prescribed for women, including adolescents, with cognitive impairment; 5105 woman-months of experience were reported without pregnancy or side effects.[118]

Parents of youth with cognitive impairment reported high satisfaction with this method.[118] The Committee on Drugs of the American Association of Pharmacists (AAP) has found no evidence that Depo-Provera is harmful.[119] For teens with moderate or severe retardation, the benefits probably outweigh the risks.

An additional benefit of injected hormones is derived by women with severe mobility restrictions. If these women are dependent on others for menstrual hygiene care, the possible lack or decreased frequency of menstrual periods may increase their functional status.[117] Depo-Provera can be associated with decreased circulating estradiol and thus may cause vaginal dryness. More serious is the hypothetical concern about the effect of decreased estradiol on bone mass.[110]

Women with disability who are active in the political arena warn that we do not have enough data on either of these methods to be clear about their long-term impact for women with disabilities and recommend cautious use until more data are available.[9]

SEXUALLY TRANSMITTED DISEASES

Little is written about how women with disabilities/chronic illness experience STDs. If sensation is impaired, however, women may have special issues with STDs. For example, if women with disabilities have HSV, they may have limited ability to promptly respond to a prodome if it is tingling or itching in the affected area. Inability to identify developing "painful" lesions may have severe consequences to these women. These women will need to learn to identify and monitor more subtle cues. Many of these women may be in the habit of frequent visual skin inspection but may need to include genital area in this visual check.[117]

SPECIFIC CONDITIONS AND CONTRACEPTIVE NEEDS

Although research is limited, the data that are available for the most frequent disabilities and chronic illnesses are reported here and may be presented in discussions with clients. Because women with disabilities are considered high risk medically, joint management with a physician colleague or referral for a form of contraception other than a barrier method is recommended.

Spinal Cord Injury

The fertility of women with spinal cord injury is unaffected. Their decreased mobility and the increased incidence of deep vein thrombosis place them at high risk with respect to hormonal contraceptives, especially those containing estrogen. Birth control pills and Norplant are absolutely contraindicated if the woman is receiving antihypertensive medication or if she is known to have circulatory problems.[24]

Many women have healthy pregnancies and vaginal births. Some complications (urinary tract infections, immobility, skin breakdown) do occur, but in studies that have been conducted, the incidence is low.[6,10]

Intrauterine devices pose a risk because of the woman's decreased sensation and ability to determine warning signs of infection. Some women, however, indicate that dysreflexia is triggered by the "pain" that the patient is unable to perceive. The women may thus be able to "identify" infection with the occurrence of dysreflexia. In addition, they propose that checking the IUD string placement could be carried out by their partners. In a large follow-up study of women with spinal cord injury, the IUD was actually the preferred method.[66]

Most women with paraplegia can usually manage barrier methods with no or minimal assistance in positioning legs for effective insertion. Women with higher spinal cord lesions require assistance from a partner or an attendant.

Multiple Sclerosis

The menstrual and fertility patterns of women with multiple sclerosis rarely change.[24] Oral contraceptive use has no effect on the risk of developing multiple sclerosis. Smoking, however, may be a risk factor.[83,118,120]

The risk of pregnancy is not totally clear. Data are conflicting. Some studies show no effect on multiple sclerosis; others indicate exacerbation of the condition during pregnancy and postpartum.[119] A series of recent studies indicate pregnancy does not influence long-term prognosis.[120,121,122] In fact, Verdu, in a study of 200 women with multiple sclerosis, found women who had one pregnancy after onset of multiple sclerosis were dependent on a wheelchair after 18.6 years versus 12.5 for other women without pregnancy.[123] Cook et al. found the pregnancy year may be a higher risk, but it did not have a negative impact on the long-term rate of problems. There was an exacerbation of multiple sclerosis symptoms, however, in 20–40 percent of patients in the first 3 months postpartum.[120]

At present, there is significant evidence that hormonal therapy alters the course of multiple sclerosis.[118] Such therapy is contraindicated only for women with paralysis or restricted mobility. Of concern is one study that reported 54 percent of subjects used no contraception because of fear of side effects.[111]

Cystic Fibrosis

Women with cystic fibrosis now live until their 30s, and with increasing technology, the age of survival may increase even further in the next few years. Pregnancy can be a significant risk for both mother and infant.

Data on hormonal contraception are conflicting. The method may cause bronchial mucus to become scant, and it may support the development of endocervical polyps.[124] Pulmonary function and respiratory symptoms were not affected in a small study of 10 young women 15 to 24 years old. Nevertheless, hormonal contraception should be used only with extreme caution and very close monitoring of pulmonary status. There is no contraindication to the use of barrier methods among women with cystic fibrosis.[124]

Rheumatoid Arthritis

Rheumatoid arthritis is known to improve during pregnancy. Some evidence is reported that the onset of arthritis may be delayed by hormonal contraceptives.[119,124] Hormonal therapy, however, has not been shown to affect active disease.

Barrier methods may be difficult for some women to use if they experience weakness and decreased manual dexterity.[124] An intrauterine device may worsen existing anemia.

Cerebral Palsy

The effect of cerebral palsy on contraception varies greatly. If the client is paralyzed or has decreased mobility, hormonal contraception is risky. Independent use of barrier methods, especially the diaphragm or cervical cap, may be troublesome for women with spasticity; however, these methods are viable with partner participation.

Epilepsy

Estrogen levels are related to seizure threshold in women with epilepsy. Seizures vary during the menstrual cycle: incidence is highest during the estradiol spike before ovulation and the rapid drop in progesterone immediately before and during menstruation.

The relationship between oral hormonal therapy and seizures is less evident; however, no strong evidence has been found against the use of hormonal contraception.[124] Most reports of interaction between hormonal agents and seizure medication indicate accelerated breakdown of estrogens and recommend the use of 50 mg estrogen.[5,86,90,119,124] Breakthrough bleeding is a common sign that the anti-epileptic drug is lowering the effect of the BCP and a signal that a higher dose pill needs to be considered.[90]

An intrauterine device should not be used. Two reports indicate grand mal seizures with insertion.[124] In addition, infection potentially caused by an IUD may decrease medication control.

Inflammatory Bowel Disease

Data are limited on the relationship between inflammatory bowel disease and use of contraception. It is known, however, that the majority of women with inflammatory bowel disease worsen with pregnancy.[118] It is, therefore, important that the disease be stable for a year before pregnancy is even considered.

Barrier methods are recommended for contraception. A review of the literature indicates that the use of oral hormonal contraceptives is advised only with reservations; that is, low dose estrogen or progestin-only oral contraceptives may be taken with close monitoring of the disease by the consulting physician. With active disease or in the presence of malabsorption, hormonal therapy may be ineffective or dangerous.[118]

Down Syndrome

Fertility is unaffected. For many women with Down syndrome, the choice of contraception is affected by mobility, chronic illness, and cognitive factors. In the use of contraception, informed consent is a critical aspect.

- Oral hormonal contraception requires that a woman's memory skills be adequate for the regimen.
- Implants may be attractive to some.
- Women who have multiple disabilities (motor and cognitive) may not be able to manage a diaphragm.
- Adolescents and young women need comprehensive ongoing sex education and accessible adults to assist with problem solving and skill development.

Women with Sickle Cell Disease

Contraception for women with sickle cell disease is important for two reasons: 1) women with this condition can get pregnant and 2) their pregnancies are high risk and need careful planning. All barrier methods, most low dose pills, Norplant and Depo-Provera are options to consider for women with this condition. An IUD is contraindicated because of its association with infections and the complications of infections in women with sickle cell condition.[125]

Women with this condition need to consider genetic counseling before pregnancy is attempted. The transmission risk may be as high as 100 percent or as low as 0 percent. All children of women with sickle cell disease will have the sickle cell trait.[125]

Women with Lupus

Oral contraceptives increase risk of hypertension, thrombosis, and disease exacerbation. Barrier method in combination with spermicide is safest. Permanent sterilization may be an option chosen by some women.

Pregnancy

CONFRONTING NEGATIVE ATTITUDES AND BARRIERS

Disability is not a contraindication to responsible, effective parenting, yet judgmental attitudes continue.[20,112,114,125–127] Moreover, few agencies exist to assist the increasing number of pregnant women and mothers with disabilities. The majority (81 percent) of registered nurses, nurse practitioners, and occupational and physical therapists indicate their experience, education, and training have not prepared them adequately for this high risk population.[114]

Education of Health Care Providers

Programs must be developed to address health care providers' lack of information about the needs of mothers with disabilities. Information that is modified to answer questions about the unique situation of women with disabilities is needed. What are the emotional and physical changes of pregnancy? What are the special demands of labor and delivery? What are the adaptive parenting skills and equipment necessary for responsible parenting?

Consumer Guidance

Little information is provided to parents by professionals. One study found that women with rheumatoid arthritis depended on lay resources rather than on health professionals for guidance in nutrition; use of alcohol, tobacco, and nonprescription drugs; sexuality; consequences of a pregnancy on their disability or disease; and infant care techniques, equipment, and devices.[114] Health care providers who are involved in coordinating care and have no disability related experience must consult with others. For example, consideration should be given to speaking with a colleague in rehabilitation or an experienced, active consumer with disabilities.

Case Management

During pregnancy, case management may be indicated for a woman with disabilities. The case manager is responsible for assuring that the client's unique health care needs are being met, especially if numerous agencies are involved.

Partner Preparation

It is important for the health care provider to assess whether a woman's partner needs preparation. The partner may require information from the provider about the woman's special needs in order to give realistic support and avoid unnecessary restrictions. A typical concern of any couple experiencing pregnancy—hesitancy to have sexual relations for fear of hurting the baby—may be expanded for couples in which the woman has a disability; they may be afraid of hurting the woman.[114]

Although it is especially important for health care providers to interact with partners, data indicate that women with disabilities feel their partners are unwanted by health care providers during labor and delivery.[126,127] A prenatal care provider or case manager may need to initiate educational sessions to discuss attitudinal barriers. These activities should be organized well before delivery. If the partner also has a disability, special considerations may be needed to facilitate his involvement.

ACCESSIBILITY TO LABOR AND DELIVERY FACILITIES

Several questions should be asked about the structure of health care facilities and their accessibility to women with mobility and sensory impairment. Are labor and delivery rooms and bathrooms large enough to transfer women from a wheelchair? Are large showers available without a raised lip, which would prevent a woman from rolling her wheelchair into the shower? Are select rooms large enough to accommodate wheelchairs, consumer owned specially padded commode chairs, leg braces, crutches, and other equipment?

Specific Adaptive Needs of Client

Determine what the client needs with respect to her condition. Is a pressure relief mattress or raised toilet seat needed? Does she want to bring equipment from home? Plan a tour of the hospital during the fifth or sixth month of pregnancy so that the need for special equipment can be identified, and the equipment ordered.

Accessibility to Equipment

Having necessary equipment within reach is critical to the well-being and comfort of the client.[114]

Education for All Staff

Housekeeping personnel may need to know that a wheelchair positioned in a particular way next to a bed allows a woman to be independent. To move the chair makes the woman essentially a prisoner, as it removes her independence. Nursing staff may need to review prevention of skin shearing, management of dysreflexia, and implications of contraction monitoring.

PRENATAL AND PERINATAL PERIODS

The effects of a disability on the course of pregnancy are summarized in Table 24–3. Generally, in perinatal management, a health care provider needs to determine if a woman with a disability has access to a role model who has the same disability as she or if the client needs case management services.[128]

TABLE 24–3. EFFECT OF DISABILITY ON COURSE OF PREGNANCY AND LABOR/DELIVERY/POSTPARTUM

Disability/Condition	Pregnancy	Labor/Delivery/Postpartum
Spinal Cord Injury	May increase risk for skin problems. Women with SCI have the same problems as nondisabled women (UTIs, constipation, incontinence).[132,133,135] Data is scarce. Recent evidence indicates frequency of these problems is increased in women with SCI.[132,135] Some women do report having to change their regular urinary management during pregnancy.[136] Anemia, cardiac irregularity and toxemia may occur.[66] Management of anemia with iron may increase constipation. Consider this possibility proactively and take action to prevent it.[61] Assess women's ability to catherize and perform self-care as pregnancy progresses. May need temporary assistance.[132] It is not clear if patients with asymptomatic bacteriuria are at high enough risk of pyelonephritis to warrant antibiotic suppression or whether suppressive therapy would be more effective than frequent cultures. To decrease the risk of bacteriuria, SCI women should minimize residual volume and avoid continuous bladder catherization.[133] Nausea/vomiting can be especially uncomfortable with limited mobility.[66] Women who are wheelchair users may already experience orthostatic edema which may be accentuated increasing not only edema but also risk of skin problems. Frequency of weight shifts/position changes may need to increase. Need close monitoring of skin daily.[132] Autonomic dysreflexia increased.[61,62,132] Eighty-five percent of clients with SCI at T=6 or above will experience autonomic dysreflexia at some time.[132] Medication may be needed to control. Weekly exam after 28 weeks and antepartum anesthesia consultation for epidural block to prevent dysreflexia.[132,135] Psychosocial issues common in pregnancy similar to psychosocial issues generally experienced in pregnancy. Report feelings of powerlessness.[114]	No premature deliveries, infant outcomes were near normal weight,[66,133] no major complications.[66,133,134] Vaginal delivery the norm. Cesarean birth reserved for obstetrical indications. Lochial flow and sanitary pads put skin at risk. Frequent perinatal care necessary.[129] Silk sutures should be considered for women having episiotomies. Reabsorbable sutures should not be used for episiotomy since denervated regions do not absorb catgut suture.[134] Bladder/bowel, skin circulatory problems improve in postpartum.[132] If environment not accessible may need extra assistance in transferring.[132] Labor/birth in semi-sitting position.[61,126] Women with high lesions may need help in positioning. Autonomic dysreflexia increased in second stage labor.[61] Early identification and treatment essential for maternal/fetal health. Can lead to subarachnoid hemorrhage.[133] Aggressive labor management is critical. Epidural anesthesia often effective.[61,135] If does not respond to regional, potent short acting hypotensive appropriate.[133] Blood pressure monitoring frequently is not continuously. Critical to avoid known causes. Often misinterpreted as pre-eclampsia. Unlike toxemia, the BP increases with contractions and falls between contractions.[61,133,134] Treatment is different. Mothers with dysreflexia have no response to magnesium sulfate.[61] Can be triggered by catheterization, enema, insertion of uterine catheter if fetal monitor used, contractions or insertion of IV lines.[133] May also occur if woman sits on episiotomy or during breast feeding. Need to assess carefully for rebound hypotension in postpartum period.[132] Assess labor/delivery bed/table for skin risks. Pad delivery tables. Stirrups not recommended if woman has spasticity.[134] Respiratory rate less than 12 or greater than 16 indicates abnormal bleeding patterns and needs further evaluation. Pulse oximetry in labor and administration of supplemental oxygen may be necessary. Women with high lesions or above may be at risk for respiratory insufficiency.[132] At risk for unattended labor[132] although 66 percent are aware of onset of labor.[66] Report being victims of inadequate environmental design that hindered mobility.[127] Increased powerlessness if partner blocked from participation in labor and delivery.[114] Breastfeeding is possible. Women with high lesions and above may need special assistance with positioning and feeding. Breastfeeding feeding is possible. Women with SCI above T–6 may experience decreased milk production 6 weeks after delivery.[66,134,141] Early mobilization is recommended to prevent DVT.[61]

(Continued)

TABLE 24–3. EFFECT OF DISABILITY ON COURSE OF PREGNANCY AND LABOR/DELIVERY/POSTPARTUM (CONTINUED)

Disability/Condition	Pregnancy	Labor/Delivery/Postpartum
Rheumatoid Arthritis	Seventy-five percent will experience remission of disease. ADL easier to perform due to decreased joint stiffness, swelling, increase in grip strength.[118] May have overwhelming fatigue. Need to continue supervised exercise routine. For those with hand/shoulder involvement, dressing may become difficult.[79, 80]	Joint contracture may limit positioning. Pain needs to be carefully assessed. Ninety-five percent will experience flare up to symptoms[79, 80]
Multiple Sclerosis	Pregnancy and postpregnancy stress may increase symptoms but do not influence long-term prognosis.[120,121,122]	Risk for exacerbation of symptoms may be greater in the postpartum. Twenty to 40 percent of patients may have exacerbations in first 3 months postpartum.[120] Women who have been on long-term corticosteroids at the time of delivery may have relative adrenal insufficiency and should be given supplemental corticosteroid for 24 hours.[120] No contradiction to Breastfeeding unless drugs are toxic to the baby. Limb weakness or gait disturbances may necessitate assistance with childcare.[120]
Impaired Vision	Changing body may dramatically affect ability to function (center of gravity changes may alter her relation to object). Use tactile models. Assist to palpate abdomen. Lack of material in braille or on audiotape necessitates increased individual teaching. Birth rehearsal in labor room helps orient self to room, bed, bathroom.	Needs lots of labeling of people/equipment. Introduce self and identify function. Get women's input on amount of light needed in labor/delivery areas. Important to describe baby and his/her specific reactions/behaviors/facial expressions. Will assist mom to attach.[114] May use tactile calibrated bottle.[114]
Impaired Hearing	Talk to woman even if interpreter used eye to eye contact; get attention before proceeding.	Visual interaction critical. Assess light needed. Assess if needs to be in room where nurses station can be seen.[113]
Systemic Lupus	Lupus the great imitator so diagnosis difficult. Placenta impairment can be a direct result of disease inflammatory process or the thrombotic effects of lupus. Exacerbations of SLE first trimester or first 6 weeks postpartum. Drug therapy is individualistic and somewhat controversial.[143] Most women can achieve successful pregnancy. Fetal (fetal loss, preterm birth) and maternal (lupus flares, worsening renal function) morbidity remain major problems. Needs frequent monitoring, frequent assessment and control of maternal lupus activity. May need to adjust medication to avoid fetal tetratogenicity. Assess for interuterine problems.[144] Corticosteroid treatment is continued for many women without negative effect on the fetus. Needs close collaboration among specialists (internist, rheumatologist, obstetrician and neonatologist).[145] Careful management and close monitoring have substantially improved fetal outcomes. A series of studies suggest adding doppler flow assessment of placental perfusion after the fourteenth week of pregnancy and treatment with heparin for women with antiphosphlipid syndrome and previous history of thrombotic event. Pregnancy loss was significantly reduced.[146]	There is increased risk of spontaneous abortion and premature birth in women with SLE. Premature births occur most often with the lupus flares.[142,147] Intrapartum major goal to prevent infections—meticulous hand washing, limiting the number of vaginal exams and paying strict attention to sterile technique for any invasive procedure. Potential renal involvement requires frequent BP monitoring (screen at least hourly—more if any abnormal findings), hourly urinary protein, abnormal DTRs and clonus, and women's affect to assess for superimposed preeclampsia.[145] At risk for postpartum exacerbation. Intensive nursing care for 24–48 hours. Infant care complicated by fatigue.[145] Newborns need to be assessed for neonatal lupus and congenital cardiac problems.[147] Cesarean birth is needed only for obstetrical issues. Mothers who are being treated by immunosuppressive drugs should not breastfeed.[146] If breastfeed follow infant growth closely.[142]
Sickle Cell	While a women with this condition can have a healthy baby there are risks, thus preconceptual and prenatal care are critical.[148] Women may have to discontinue some medications and consider treatment options. Emotional support as well as aggressive treatment of acute events optimizes outcomes.[149,150]	Women with this condition have a higher rate of preterm deliveries, preeclampsia, pain crisis and pulmonary complications and SGA babies.[151] Neonates have more jaundice, anemia, and respiratory distress.[150,153] Newborn screening should be standard in all settings.[154] Emotional support as well as aggressive treatment of acute events optimize outcomes.[150]

Epilepsy

Although many women with epilepsy have been pressured to terminate a pregnancy because of the provider's or family's assumption that they could not have a healthy baby, over 90 percent of women with epilepsy will have normal healthy infants.

In over half of women studied, seizure frequency does not change during pregnancy. When the frequency did change, roughly half of the women had increases in frequency and half had decreases. If seizures increased, they occurred most often in the end of the first trimester and the beginning of the second. Women taking valproate (depakote, depakene) or carbamazepine (Tegretol) during the first trimester have a 0.5 to 2 percent risk of having a child with neural tube disease. The drugs most likely to cause severe congenital problems, Trimethadione (Tridione) and paramethadione (paradione), are rarely prescribed today.[92]

It is recommended that women with epilepsy see their neurologist monthly during pregnancy.[155]

Blood levels of AEDs need to be monitored more frequently in pregnancy and in the postpartum period due to frequent reduction in medication blood levels even when doses are constant or elevated.

Women with seizures have a 2–3% percent higher rate of birth defects with cleft lip, cleft palate, heart defects and spina bifida. All AEDs appear to increase the risk. There is an increased risk of seizures in the immediate postlabor and delivery phase. There is a slight chance of increased infant bleeding in the neonatal period. Some suggest the mother take supplement vitamin K1 during the last week of pregnancy and the infant be given a vitamin K shot after birth.[92,155]

Mothers taking AEDs can breastfeed. It may be helpful to have the father give a nighttime bottle as fatigue is related to increased seizure activity. Growth of the infant needs to be closely monitored and a 2 week checkup is critical.[92]

Diabetes
(see chapter 21 on medical problems)

Self-Assessment

The client should be able to identify the stressors and fears, both general and specific, that are related to her disability.

Staff Assessment

A woman's muscle strength, activities of daily living, and child care skills must be assessed. Determinations may be made by direct observation, reports of activities, and a child care activity assessment tool.[129–130] Or, referral may be made to a physical or occupational therapist, depending on resources and the severity of the woman's limitations. Assessment needs to be made early in pregnancy in order to design adaptive equipment. For example, one woman with minimal distal muscle strength who wished to breastfeed was able to place the child at the breast and initiate nursing but did not have the strength to hold the child throughout nursing. Believing that she could not breastfeed, she switched to formula. If she had been assessed early in pregnancy, her strength deficiency might have been identified and referral made to a rehabilitation engineer to design or modify a fabric infant carrier that would support the child during nursing. Most women with a disability are able to nurse their newborns. Indeed, the convenience of breastfeeding can be an advantage for women with mobility limitations.[131]

Dependency Increase

If a woman's dependency increases during pregnancy, there is a need to assess her specific level of function. Similarly, assess the body image issues generated by pregnancy.

Normal Emotional Changes

Reassure the client of the normalcy of emotional fluctuations during pregnancy.

Cesarean Birth

If cesarean birth is a possibility, discuss the options available, including father participation.[112,129]

Breastfeeding

This normal and healthy method in infant feeding is preferred by an increasing number of women with disability and chronic illness despite being discouraged by many health care providers. Breastfeeding is generally not contraindicated for women with spinal cord injury, multiple sclerosis, arthritis or epilepsy[66,92,95,120,134] but is contraindicated for women with sickle cell disease.[125] Women with lupus with taking immunosuppressive medications should not breastfeed.[146] Women with lupus not on these medications need to have close monitoring of their child's growth while breastfeeding.[142] Some women may need adaptive equipment or counseling about specific strategies to make breastfeeding successful.[137]

PARENTING

Health care providers unfamiliar with the adaptive skills of women with disabilities often question the ability of these women to care for their babies.[138,139] In fact, there are over 8 million families with children in which one or both parents has a disability. Many social institutions, however, such as family court, social services, and health care providers continue to have discriminary attitudes. Availability of a role model with a disability similar to the woman's can be very helpful to both the health care provider and the client. The roles of the parents and other caregivers must be assessed. Moreover, for the provider without expertise in infant care issues, consultation with a pediatric nurse practitioner, pediatrician, occupational therapist, rehabilitation consultant, or rehabilitation engineer may be helpful. In addition, an independent living center or a program that focuses on promoting positive parenting for women with disabilities, such as Through the Looking Glass, may be consulted.[129,130]

ADAPTATION OF THE FAMILY

Videotaped Evidence

A videotape study of parents with disabilities was conducted and several findings were reported.[129]

- Infants adapt extremely early to their mothers who have physical disabilities.
- Mothers develop the ability to read their infants' states and teach them to assist with necessary movement.
- Children differentiate between care providers. For example, an active toddler lies still during a long diapering by the blind father but resists and struggles from the outset with the sighted mother.

Equipment as Part of the Environment

It is common for children to consider a parent's equipment, such as wheelchairs and reachers, as ordinary parts of their environment without negative connotations. A toddler was overheard talking with her mom during a basketball tournament in which there was a wheelchair division. While observing a game played by nondisabled college students, she said, "Mom, what are they doing?" "Playing basketball, Honey." "But Mom, where are their wheelchairs?" Frequently, support services in both the health and social service arena are uninformed about resources that would make parenting and caretaking more effective for women with disabilities. Consultation with agencies that are knowledgeable in this area is critical to success.

Animals

If a woman with a disability uses a guide dog or other animal to assist with impaired mobility, close assessment must be made of its impact on child care.

Equipment Adaptation for Child Care

A woman with impaired mobility can alter equipment or procedures to assist with child care.[114]

- Women with mobility impairment may face special adaptation needs as parents.[114] Women who previously used a manual wheelchair may choose to use an electric wheelchair to free hands for child care.
- Furniture may need to be altered so that the woman can wheel up to the crib, changing table, or reclined stroller and be able to change the baby without moving her/him. Furniture

may also be altered to create firm raised edges for infant safety and to assist the woman with decreased hand or arm strength.

- Velcro can be sewn on the clothes of both mother and baby for necessary alterations. For example, breastfeeding may be made easier if the mother's bra and blouse have Velcro fasteners. Also, Velcro fasteners on the infant's clothes assist the mother in dressing her baby.[125]
- Bottle holders and bottle devices, such as a tactile calibrated bottle, may be helpful, as may adapting a breastfeeding position in the wheelchair.[114]

Impaired Vision and Hearing

A woman with impaired vision or hearing can also adapt procedures for child care.[114] The provider may need to facilitate the mother's interaction with her infant. The Brazelton tool is used to teach a mother about the states of the infant.[140] For a woman with impaired vision, the focus is on her hearing and touching and how they increase interaction with the infant. On the other hand, for women with hearing impairment, a visual role model, tactile stimulation, and musical toys are used. If both parents have sensory impairment, referral to an infant stimulation program should be considered.

Monitoring devices in a room or on a child can be helpful. Audiovisual resources may be useful.

Women with Epilepsy

Infant care is often more of a concern of the family and friends than of the woman with epilepsy. The health professional needs to evaluate the real risks with the woman based on the type of seizure she experiences. Women with seizures at night may not need to adjust their daytime activities dramatically. Developing a reality based concrete safety plan is recommended.[96] Women can change the baby on a mat on the floor, use plastic bottles and containers, have two adults when giving an infant or child a bath, always feed the child in an infant seat, highchair or appropriate chair, use a playpen for a safe play area, keep extra clothes on each level of the house to avoid stair climbing, use disposable diapers, move the child by stroller instead of being hand carried, and use microwave rather than conventional stove.[156]

FUTURE RESEARCH NEEDED

Several major official and voluntary organizations now have initiatives to explore the experiences of women with disabilities. This work, however, is early in its development. The research agenda developed by the National Center for Medical Rehabilitation Research, which called for "urgent and immediate need for development of an appropriate model of rehabilitation that addresses woman's unique role physically and also addresses the needs within the structure of her own environment," is still a timely call to action.[157] The current work raises as many questions as it answers. Researchers call for major initiatives in the significant area affecting the lives of people with disabilities. They identify the major focus areas as childhood, sexuality, contraception, sexually transmitted diseases, fertility, marriage, pregnancy, labor and delivery, parenting, decision to become a parent, parenting abilities, and influences of parent with disability on children.[158,159] The near future, it is hoped, will bring answers to many of the questions currently being raised.

SUMMARY

Women with disabilities are women first. Their similarities with other women are more common than their differences. One woman writes the following:

> We want to know that you value us as people and not just as examples of cultural diversity. We want you to know that life with a disability can be just fine. Sure, there are attitudinal and environmental barriers that make life difficult for us sometimes, but those obstacles are out there, not inside of us. Just imagine for a moment a woman in a wheelchair carrying a tiny baby. This woman is not being discharged from a maternity hospital where every woman must ride in a wheelchair. She is at the grocery store with her baby in an infant carrier and a cart full of groceries. Imagine her getting her self, her baby, her wheel-

chair, and her groceries into the car alone and driving away. Imagine her independent, sexual, competent, mature, busy, happy, and, like all new parents, exhausted! To you she may be an amazement, but to me, I just feel like myself.[126]

If approached with

- a willingness to listen and hear the issues and concerns of these women;
- a willingness to see the woman as a true participant/partner in planning and one who may have more medical information about her disability than the provider does;
- an awareness of one's own comfort level with uncertainty and individuals with disability, and
- a nonjudgmental approach

the sensitive clinician can create a quality experience for the individual and build a new reality for women with disabilities and chronic illnesses.

RESOURCES FOR WOMEN, THEIR FAMILIES, AND PROFESSIONALS

RESOURCE LIST

General

Materials from the Center for the Research on Women with Disabilities, Department of Physical Medicine and Rehabilitation, Baylor College of Medicine, 6910 Fannin, Suite 310-South, Houston, Tx 77030. (Fact Sheet, Research Summary, and Bibliography.)

Haseltine, F. P., Cole, S. S., & Gray, D. B. (1993). *Reproductive issues for persons with physical disabilities.* Baltimore: Paul H. Brooks Publishing Co.

Krotoski, D. M., Nosek, M. A., & Turk, M. A. (Eds.). *Women with physical disabilities.* Baltimore: Paul H. Brooks Publishing Co.

Lollar, D. J. (Ed.). (1994). *Preventing secondary conditions associated with spina bifida or cerebral palsy.* Washington, DC: Spina Bifida Association of America (1–800–621–3141).

Resources for Rehabilitation. (1994). *A woman's guide to coping with disability.* Lexington, MA: Resources for Rehabilitation. [Excellent detailed resource list per disability].

Recognizing Accomplishment

Driedger, D., & Gray, S. (1992). *Imprinting our image: An international anthology by women with disabilities.* Charlottetown, Prince Edward Island: Gynergy Books.

National Clearinghouse on Women and Girls With Disabilities. (1990). *Bridging the gap: A national directory of services for women and girls with disabilities.* New York: Education Equity Concepts, Inc.

Shapiro, J. P. (1993). *No pity: People with disabilities forging a new civil rights movement.* New York: Times Books, Random House.

Physical Accessibility of Health Care Setting

Duffy, Y. (1981). *All things are possible.* Ann Arbor, MI: Garvin & Associates.

Ferreyra, S., & Hughes, K. (1982). *Table manners: Guide to the pelvic examination for disabled women and health care providers.* [477 Fifteenth Street, Oakland, CA 94612. *Sex education for disabled people* ($3.50). Written by two differently abled women. Advocates a cooperative approach.]

Haseltine, F. P., Cole, S., & Gray, D. B. (1993). *Reproductive issues for persons with physical disabilities.* Baltimore: Paul H. Brooks Publishing Co.

Task Force on Concerns of Physically Disabled Women. (1978). *Within reach: Providing family planning services to physically disabled women.* New York: Human Sciences Press.

Task Force on Concerns of Physically Disabled Sexuality. (1978). *Toward intimacy: Family planning and sexuality concerns of physically disabled women.* New York: Human Sciences Press.

Parenting and Infant Care

Campion, M. J. (1990). *The baby challenge: A handbook on pregnancy for women with a physical disability.* New York: Tavistock/Routledge.

Cheatham, D., King, E., & Bartz, A. (1995). *Childbirth education for women with disabilities and their partners: A training manual for professionals.* Columbus, Oh: Nisonger Center Publications.

Cochrane, G. M., & Wilshere, E. R. (Eds.), (1988). *Parents with disabilities.* Oxford, England: Nuffield Orthopaedic Center.

Conine, T. A., Carty, E., & Safarik, P. (1988). *Aids and adaptations for disabled parents: An illustrated manual for service providers and parents with physical or sensory disabilities* (2nd ed.). Vancouver: School of Rehabilitation Medicine, University of British Columbia.

Mathews, J. (1992). *A mother's touch: The Tiffany Callo story.* New York: Henry Holt & Company.

National Newsletter for disabled parents and concerned professionals. *Through the Looking Glass,* 801 Peralta Avenue, Berkeley, CA 94707.

Rogers, J., & Matsumura, M. (1991). *Mothers to be: A guide to pregnancy and birth for women with disabilities.* New York: Demos Publication.

Ware, N. A., & Schwab, L. O. (1971). The blind mother providing care for an infant. *New Outlook Blind, 65,* 169–173.

Abuse

Berkowitz, C. D. (1990). Sexual abuse in the physically and developmentally disabled. *Nurse Practitioner Forum, 1*(2), 98–101.

Cole, S. (1986). Facing the challenges of sexual abuse in persons with disabilities. *Sexuality and Disability, 7,* 71–87.

Blackburn, M. (1995). Sexuality, disability and abuse: Advice for life . . . not just for kids. *Child care, health and development, 21*(5), 351–361.

Schor, D. P. (1987). Sex and sexual abuse in developmentally disabled adolescents. *Seminars in Adolescent Medicine, 3*(1), 1–7.

White, R., Benedict, M.I., Wulff, L., & Kelley, M. (1986). Physical disabilities as risk factors for child maltreatment: A selected review. *American Journal of Orthopsychiatry, 57*(1), 93–101.

Woodhead, H. C., & Murph, J. R. (1985). Influence of chronic illness and disability on adolescent sexual development. *Seminars in Adolescent Medicine, 1*(3), 171–176.

Sex Education

Baugh, R. J. (1984). Sexuality education for the visually and hearing impaired child in the regular classroom. *Journal of School Health, 54*(10), 407–409.

Dickman, I. R. (Ed.). (1975). *Sex education and family life for visually handicapped children and youth: A resource guide.* New York: Siecus.

George Washington University. (1979). *Who cares? A handbook on sex education and counseling services for disabled people.* Washington, DC: Author.

Krajicek, M. J. (1982). Developmental disability and human sexuality. *Nursing Clinics of North America, 17*(3), 377–386.

Kroll, K., & Klein, E. L. (1992). *Enabling romance: A guide to love, sex, and relationships for the disabled (and the people who care about them).* New York: Harmony Books.

"Managing Menstruation for Children with Spina Bifida" and "Family Planning for Teenagers with Spina Bifida." (1994). Appendix in L. Furman, & J. C. Mortimer. (1994). Menarche and menstrual function in patients with myelomeningocele. *Developmental Medicine and Child Neurology, 36,* 910–917.

McDermott, S., Kelly, M., & Spearman, J. (1994, Winter). Evaluation of a family planning program for individuals with mental retardation. *Sexuality and Disability, 12*(4), 307–327.

Muccigrosso, L. (1991) Sexual abuse prevention strategies and programs for persons with developmental disabilities. *Sex Disabil, 9,* 261–272

Rabin, B. J. (1980). *The sensuous wheeler: Sexual adjustment for the spinal cord injured.* San Francisco: Multi Media Resource Center.

Sandowski, C. (1989). *Sexual concerns when illness or disability strikes.* Springfield, IL: Charles C Thomas.

Smith, K., Wheeler, B., Pilecki, P., & Parker, T. (1995). The role of the pediatric nurse practitioner in educating teens with mental retardation about sex. *Journal of Pediatric Health Care, 9*(2), 59–66.

Sloan, S. (1995). *Sexuality and persons with spina bifida.* Washington, DC: Spina Bifida Association of America.

Spica, M. M. (1992). Educating the client on the effects of COPD on sexuality: The role of the nurse. *Sexuality and Disability, 10,* 91–101.

Whitaker, V., & LaVerne, A. (1993). A breast self-examination program for adolescent special education students. *Family & Community Health, 16*(2), 30–40.

1993. Whole issues of the journal *Sexuality and Disability* dedicated to sexual counseling for people with disabilities (includes a SIECUS annotated bibliography).

For Teens and Their Families

Kaufman, M. (1995). *Easy for you to say. Questions and answers for teens living with chronic illness or disability.* Toronto, Canada: Key Porter Books, Ltd.

A frank and explicit question and answer book addressing issues that teens with disabilities or chronic illness and their families face. Includes sections on overprotectiveness, sexuality, coping with medical personnel, work, school, and peers.

Kriegsman, K. H., Zaslow, E. L., & D'Zmura-Rechsteiner, M. A. (1992). *Taking charge: Teenagers talk about life and physical disability.* Bethesda, MD: Woodbine House.

Available from the American Spina Bifida Association. Much acclaimed primer for older school-age and teenage patients.

Ochs, V. (1995). *Protecting your child in an unpredictable world.* New York: Penguin Books.

Basic Bookshelf—United Cerebral Palsy Association, The Materials Mailing Center, P.O. Box 10485, Lancaster, PA 17605–0485. A wide variety of books for children, teens and young adults with disabilities and their parents (Sets for: New Parents, Adult Issues).

Spina Bifida Association of Kentucky's Transition to Independence Project, 982 Eastern Parkway, Box 18, Louisville, KY 40217–1566, 502–637–7363.

Hardin, P. (1995). *Building skills: A guide for parents and professionals working with young people who have spina bifida.*

Denniston, S., & Enlow, C. (1995). *Making choices: A journal workbook for teens and young adults with spina bifida that provides opportunities for making choices about their lives.*

Hardin, P. (1995). *Becoming the me I want to be: A guide for youth with spina bifida and their parents.*

Newsletters (available without charge and of interest to providers and families)

Children's and Youth's Health Issues. Published by the Institute for Health and Disability. University of Minnesota, 420 Delaware St, SE, Box 721, Minneapolis, Minnesota 55455. Web address: www.peds.umn.edu/centers/ihd/

The WOW Connection. The newsletter of Winners On Wheels, 2842 Business Park Avenue, Fresno, CA 93727. WOW is a nonprofit organization for children and youth who use wheelchairs. This is a social and recreational program to develop youngsters self-esteem and independence. Web address: www.wowusa.com.

College Information

Albrecht, A. (1996, September). School daze: What I wish I had known before I started college. *Exceptional Parent,* 64–67.

Back to School. (1996, May/June). *Sports 'N Spokes,* 11–17.

An article listing financial assistance available to students with disabilities at colleges or universities across the country. Also describes characteristics of a school that may be of interest to young women with disabilities (Disabled Student Services, Wheelchair Sports, Attendant Care).

How to choose a college: Guide for the student with a disability. One free copy is available from HEATH Resource Center, One Dupont Circul, Suite 800,

Washington, DC 20036. 1–800–544–3284. (HEATH is a newsletter addressing postsecondary education for persons with disabilities.)

Popular Press Artzicles

Klein, B. S. (1992, November/December). We are who you are: Feminism and disability. *Ms, 3,* 70–74

King, Y. (1993). The other body: Reflections on difference, disability and identity politics. *Ms, 3*(5), 72–75.

Mairs, N. (1996). Young and disabled: What it's like to seek friendship and love, work and happiness if you are young and disabled. *Glamour, 94*(1996, Mar), 196–199.

Perry-Sheridan, N. (1995, October). I was told not to have children. *Parents, 70,* 121–2+.

Rousso, H., Omalley, S. G., & Severance, M. (1988, July/August). Disabled, female and proud. Stories of ten women with disabilities. *The Exceptional Parent,* 44–47.

Equipment/Latex Free Products

Examination table custom designed for women with special needs. Contact Dr. Sandra Welner, Department of Obstetrics and Gynecology. Suite 5W33 Washington Hospital Center. Washington, DC 20010.

Avanti brand polyurethane condom (Schmid Laboratories). Has had limited testing that supports the prevention of pregnancies and STDs. A 1995 *Consumer Reports* article questioned just how much protection is offered. To date, the FDA has not allowed the manufacturer to make any effectiveness claims.

Reality Female Condom is made of polyurethane. Laboratory testing showed that Reality was an effective barrier to HIV and also to a virus particle that is smaller than the hepatitis B virus, the smallest virus known to cause an STD (1–800–643–0844, The Female Health Company).

Fisher, D. (1996). *Latex allergy: A resource book.* Maternal Child Nursing Department, Medical College of Virginia/Virginia Commonwealth University School of Nursing, Richmond, Virginia.

Latex allergy: A video. Available from the Spina Bifida Association of America, 4590 MacArthur Blvd NW, Suite 250. Washington, DC 20007–4226 (12 minute video suitable for professional and lay audiences). For an extensive list of products updated every 6 months contact Spina Bifida Association of America. Web address: www.infohiway.com/spinabifida/

Organizations

Coalition Sexuality and Disability	212–242–3900
National Information Center for Children and Youth with Disabilities	1–800–999–5599
National Center for Youth with Disabilities	1–800–333–6293
SIECUS Sex Information and Education Council of the U.S.	212–819–9770
Through the looking Glass	510–525–8138
National Women's Health Network	202–347–1140
National Organization on Disability (DOD)	1–800–248–2253
Antiepileptic Drug and Pregnancy Register	1–800–233–2334

There are national groups for most chronic illness or disability conditions. Contact your local library OR 1–800–555–1212 for current addresses or toll free number.

REFERENCES

1. Deegan, M. J. (1981). Multiple minority groups: A case study of physically disabled women. *Journal of Sociology and Social Welfare, 8,* 274–297.
2. Nosek, M. A., Howland, C. A., Young, M. E., Georgiou, D., Rintala, D. H., Foley, C. C., Bennett, J. L., & Smith, Q. (1994). Wellness models and sexuality among women with physical disabilities. *Journal of Applied Rehabilitation Counseling, 25* (1), 50–58.
3. Blackwell-Stratton, M. Breslin, M. L., Mayerson, A. B., & Bailey, S. (1988). Smashing icons: Disabled women and the disability women's movements. In M. Eine, & A. Asch (Eds.), Women with disabilities: *Essays in psychology, culture, and politics* (pp. 306–332). Philadelphia: Temple University Press.
4. Gill, C. J. (1996). Becoming visible: Personal health experiences of women with disabilities. In D. M. Krotoski, M. A. Nosek, & M. A. Turk (Eds.), *Women with physical disabilities.* Baltimore, Paul H. Brookes, Publishing Co.
5. Altman, B. M. (1996). Causes, risks and consequences of disability among women. In D. M. Krotoski, M. A. Nosek, & M. A. Turk (Eds.), *Women with physical disabilities.* Baltimore, Paul H. Brookes, Publishing Co.
6. Dangoor, N. & Florian, V. (1994). Women with chronic physical disabilities: Correlates of their

long-term psychosocial adaptation. *Int. J. Rehabil. Res, 17,* 159–168.

7. Vash, C. L. (1982). Employment issues for women with disabilities. *Rehabilitation Literature,* 43, 198–207.

8. Perlman, L., & Arneson, D. (1982). *Women and rehabilitation of disabled persons.* A report of the sixth annual Mary E. Switzer Memorial Seminar. Washington, DC: National Rehabilitation Association.

9. Nosek, M. (1992). Primary care issues for women with severe physical disabilities. *Journal of Women's Health, 1* (4), 245–248.

10. U.S. General Accounting Office. (1993). *Vocational rehabilitation: Evidence for federal program's effectiveness is mixed.* (GAO Pub. No: PEMD–93–19).

11. Drew, J. (1990). *Implications for nursing practice: A five-year review of recent spinal injury research.* Paper presented at 16th Annual Conference, Association of Rehabilitation Nursing, Phoenix, AZ.

12. McNewil, J. M. (1993). Current Population Reports, Americans with disabilities 1991–1992. Washington, DC: U.S. Bureau of the Census.

13. Nosek, M. A., Young,, M. E., Rintala, D. H., Howland, C. A., Foley, C. C., & Bennett, J. (1995). Barriers to reproductive health maintenance among women with physical disabilities. *Journal of Women's Health, 4,* 505–518.

14. Anderson W., Westbrook, M. T., & Adamson, B. J. (1989). Gender differences in allied health student's knowledge of disabled women and men. *Women & Health, 15* (4), 93–110.

15. Anderson, J. M. (1991). Immigrant women speak of chronic illness: The social construction of the devalued self. *Journal of Advanced Nursing, 16* (6), 710–717.

16. Alston, R. J., & McCowan, C. J. (1994). African American women with disabilities: Rehabilitation issues and concerns. *Journal of Rehabilitation 60,* 36–40.

17. Brown, C. N. (1996). *Pregnancy and women with lupus: Answering questions and dispelling myths.* Unpublished Paper. Virginia Commonwealth University.

18. Zwerner, J. (1982). Yes we have troubles but nobody's listening: Sexual issues of women with spinal cord injury. *Sexuality and Disability, 5* (3), 158–171.

19. Welner, S. L. (1993). Gynecologic care of the disabled woman. *Contemporary OB/GYN, 38* (1), 55–67.

20. Sawin, K. J. (1982). *Disabled women's perception on a health care visit for a physical examination.* Paper presented at 8th Annual conference, Association of Rehabilitation Nursing, Denver, CO.

21. Saxton, M. (1996). Teaching providers to become our allies. In D. M. Krotoski, M. A. Nosek, & M. A. Turk (Eds.), *Women with physical disabilities.* Baltimore, Paul H. Brookes, Publishing Co.

22. Kirshbaum, M. (1988). Parents with physical disabilities and their babies. *Zero to Three, 8* (5), 7–11.

23. Sawin, K., & Conti, A. (1994). *Curriculum to increase sensitivity towards needs of women with disabilities for primary care and women's health care providers.* Unpublished document, Virginia Commonwealth University School of Nursing.

24. The Boston Women's Health Book Collective. (1992). *The new our bodies, ourselves.* New York: Simon & Schuster.

25. Bogle, J. E., & Shaul, S. L. (1981). Body image and the woman with a disability. In D. G. Bullard, & S. E. Knight (Eds.), *Sexuality and Physical Disability.* St. Louis: C. V. Mosby.

26. DeHaan, C. B., & Wallander, J. L. (1988). Self concept, sexual knowledge and attitudes, and parental support in the sexual adjustment of women with early- and late-onset physical disability. *Archives of Sexual Behavior, 17,* 145–161.

27. Zasler, N. D. (1991). Sexuality in neurologic disability: An overview. *Sexuality and Disability, 9,* 11–27.

28. Drench, M. E. (1992). Impact of altered sexuality and sexual function in spinal cord injury: A review. *Sexuality and Disability, 10,* 3–14.

29. Nosek, M. A., Rintala, D., Young, M. E., Howland, C. A., Foley, C. C., Rossi, D., & Chanpong, G. (1996). Sexual functioning among women with physical disabilities. *Archives of Physical Medicine and Rehabilitation, 77,* 107–115.

30. Nelson, M. R. (1995). Sexuality in childhood disability. *Physical Medicine and Rehabilitation: State of the Art Reviews, 9* (2), 451–462.

31. Duffy, Y. (1981). *All things are possible.* Ann Arbor, MI: A. J. Garvin & Associates.

32. Tsy, A. M., & Opie, N. D. (1986). Menarche in the severely disabled adolescent: School nurses' attitudes, perceptions and perceived teaching responsibilities. *Journal of School Health, 56* (10), 443–447.

33. Thorne, S. E. (1990). Mothers with chronic illness: A predicament of social construction.

Health Care Women International, 11 (2), 209–221.

34. O'Toole, C. J., & Bregante, J. L. (1993). Disabled lesbians: Multicultural realities. in M. Nagler (Ed.), *Perspectives on disability.* Palo Alto, CA: Health Markets Research.

35. Stevens, P. (1994). Lesbians' health-related experiences of care and noncare. *Western Journal of Nursing Research, 16* (6) 639–659.

36. Marshall, A. (1995). *Disability within the lesbian community.* Unpublished manuscript. Virginia Commonwealth University.

37. O'Toole, C. J. (1996). Disabled lesbians: Challenging monocultural constructs. *Sexuality and Disability, 14* (3), 221–235.

38. Hevey, D., cited in O'Toole, C. J., & Bregante, J. L. (1993). *Disabled lesbians: Multicultural realities, perspectives on disability* (261–272). Palo Alto, CA: Health Markets Research.

39. Eliason, M. J. (1996). Lesbian and gay family issues. *Journal of Family Nursing, 2* (1), 10–29.

40. USDHHS, PHS. (1992). *Healthy people 2000: National health promotion and disease prevention objectives.* Boston: Jones and Bartlett.

41. Gordon , D. L., Sawin, K. J., & Basta, S. M. (1996). Developing research priorities for rehabilitation nursing. *Rehabilitation Nursing Research, 5* (2), 60–66.

42. Stuifbergen, A. K. (1996). Health promotion services and research: Opportunities for rehabilitation nursing. *Rehabilitation Nursing Research, 5* (2), 34, 42.

43. Murphy, K. P., Molnar, G., & Lankasky, K. (1995). Medical and functional status of adults with cerebral palsy. *Dev Med Child Neurol, 37* (12), 1075–1084.

44. Krotoski, D., Nosek, M. A., & Turk, M. A. (1996). *Women with physical disabilities.* Baltimore: Paul H. Brookes Publishing Co.

45. Roller, S. (1996). Health promotion for people with chronic neuromuscular disabilities. In D. M. Krotoski, M. A. Nosek, & M. A. Turk (Eds.), *Women with physical disabilities.* Baltimore, Paul H. Brookes, Publishing Co.

46. Recommendations for the use of folic acid to reduce the number of cases of spina bifida and other neural tube defects. (1992). *Morbidity and Mortality Weekly Report, 11* (41), 1–7.

47. Use of folic acid for prevention of spina bifida and other neural tube deficits 1983–1991. (1991). *MMWR, 40* (30), 513–516.

48. Shaw, G. M., Velie, E. M., & Schaffer, D. (1996). Risk of neural tube defect-affected pregnancies among obese women. *Journal of the American Medical Association, 275* (14), 1093–1096.

49. Murphy, F. A. (1996). Commentary. *APNSCAN: Literature Review for the Advanced Practice Nurse, 12,* 3.

50. Stengel, P. J. (1996). A train the trainer project on preconceptional counseling the role of folate in the prevention of neural tube defects. Thesis. Virginia Commonwealth University.

51. DePauw, K. P. (1996). Adapted physical activity and sport. In D. M. Krotoski, M. A. Nosek, & M. A. Turk (Eds.), *Women with physical disabilities.* Baltimore, Paul H. Brookes, Publishing Co.

52. Henderson, K. A., & Bedini, L. A. (1995). I have a soul that dances like Tina Turner, but my body can't: Physical activity and women with mobility impairments. *Res. Q. Exerc. Sport. 66,* 151–161.

53. Mudrick, N. R. (1933). Predictors of disability among midlife men and women: Differences by severity of impairment. *Community Health, 13* (2), 70–84.

54. Furman, L. M. (1989). Institutionalized disabled adolescents: Gynecologic care. *Clinical Pediatrics, 28,* 163–170.

55. Harrison, C. A., Glass, R. G., & Soni, B. (1995). Factors associated with sexual functioning in women following spinal cord injury. *Internal Medical Society of Paraplegia, 33,* 687–692.

56. Meeropol, E. (1991). One of the gang: Sexual development of adolescents with physical disabilities. *Journal of Pediatric Nursing, 6 (4),* 243–249.

57. Berhard, E. J. (1989). The sexuality of spinal cord injured women: Physiology and pathophysiology. A review. *Paraplegia, 27* (2), 99–112.

58. Cole, T. M. (1975). Sexuality and the spinal cord injured. In R. Green (Ed.), *Human sexuality: A health practitioner's text* (2nd ed., pp. 146–169). Baltimore: Williams & Wilkins.

59. Page, R. C., Cheng, H., Pate, T. C., Mathus, B., Pryor, D., & Ko, J. (1987). The perception of spinal cord injured persons toward sex. *Sexuality and Disability Journal, 8* (2), 112–132.

60. Kettl, P., Zarefoss, S., Jacoby, K., German, C., Hulse, C., Rowley, F., Corey, R. Sredy, M., Bixler, E., & Tyson, K. (1991). *Female sexuality after spinal cord injury. Sexuality and Disability, 9,* 287–295.

61. Yarkony, G. M., & Chen, D. (1995). Sexuality in patients with spinal cord injury. *Physical Medicine and Rehabilitation: State of the Art Reviews, 9* (2), 325–344.

62. Sipski, M. L., Alexander, C. J., Rosen, R. C. (1995). Physiological parameters associated with

psychogenic sexual arousal in women with complete spinal cord injuries. *Archives of Physical Medicine and Rehabilitation, 76,* 811–818.

63. Donohue, J., & Gebhard, P. (1995). The Kinsey Institute/Indiana University report on sexuality in spinal cord injury. *Sexuality and Disability, 13* (1), 7–85.

64. Boone, T. (1995). The physiology of sexual function in normal individuals. *Physical Medicine and rehabilitation: State of the Art Reviews, 9* (2), 313–323.

65. Whipple, B., Richard, E. Tepper, M., & Komisaruk, R. (1996). Sexual response in women with complete spinal cord injury. In D. M. Krotoski, M. A. Nosek, & M. A. Turk (Eds.), *Women with physical disabilities.* Baltimore: Paul H. Brookes, Publishing Co.

66. Charlifue, S. W., Gerhart, K. A., Menter, R. R., Whiteneck, G. G., & Manley, M. (1992). Sexual issues of women with spinal cord injury. *Paralegia, 30,* 192–199.

67. Sipski, M. L., Alexander, C. J., & Rosen, R. C. (1995). Orgasm in women with spinal cord injuries: A laboratory-bases assessment. *Archives of Physical Medicine and Rehabilitation, 76,* 1097–1102.

68. Sipski, M., & Alexander, C. J. (1993). Sexual activities, response and satisfaction in women pre- and post-spinal cord injury. *Archives of Physical Medicine and Rehabilitation, 74,* 1025–1029.

69. Pearson, M. L., Cole, J. S., & Jarvis, W. R. (1994). How common is latex allergy? A survey of children with myelodysplasia. *Developmental Medicine and Child Neurology, 36,* 64–69.

70. Banta, J. V., Bonanni, C., & Prebluda, J. (1993). Latex anaphylaxis during spinal surgery in children with myelomeningocele. *Developmental Medicine and Child Neurology, 35* (6), 543–548.

71. Gleeson, R. M. (1995). Use of non-latex gloves for children with latex allergies. *Journal of Pediatric Nursing, 10* (1), 65–66.

72. Barton, E. C. (1993). Latex allergy: Recognition and management of a modern problem. *Nurse Practitioner, 18* (11), 54–85.

73. Sussman, G. L., & Beezhold, D. H. (1995). Allergy to latex rubber. *Annals of Internal Medicine, 122* (1), 43–46.

74. Tosi, L., Slater, J. E., Shaer, C., & Mostello, L. A. (1993). Latex allergy in spina bifida patients: Prevalence and surgical implications. Journal of Pediatric *Orthopedics, 13* (6), 709–712.

75. Taylor, J. S., & Praditsuwan, P. (1996). Latex allergy. Review of 44 cases including outcome and frequent association with allergic hand eczema. *Archives of Dermatology, 132,* 265–271.

76. Fisher, D., & Sawin, K. (1997). Latex allergy: A curriculum for nursing. Department of Maternal Child Nursing. Virginia Commonwealth University.

77. Shaer, C., & Meeropol, E. (1995). Latex (natural rubber) allergy in spina bifida patients. *Spina Bifida Insights.* Included in the Latex Packet along with a list of latex containing products. Packet available from the Spina Bifida Association of America 1–800–621–3141.

78. Goodenow, C., Reisine, S. T., & Grady, K. E. (1990). Quality of social support and associated social and psychological functioning in women with rheumatoid arthritis. *Health Psychology, 9,* 226–284.

79. Dale, G. D. (1996). Intimacy and rheumatic disease. *Rehabilitation Nursing, 231,* 38–40.

80. Crotty, M., McFarlane, A., Brooks, P. M., Hopper, J. L., Bieri, D., & Taylor, S. L. (1994). The psychosocial and clinical status of younger women with early rheumatoid arthritis: A longitudinal study with frequent measures. *British Journal of Rheumatology, 33,* 754–760.

81. Brown, S., & Williams, A. (1995). Women's experience of rheumatoid arthritis. *Journal of Advanced Nursing, 21,* 695–701.

82. Reisine, S. T., Grady, K. E., Goodenow, C., & Fifield, J. (1989). Work disability and women with RA: The importance of disability, social, work and family factors. *Arthritis and Rheumatism, 32* (5), 538–543.

83. Swain, S. E., (1996). Multiple sclerosis, Primary health care implications. *Nurse Practitioner, 21,* 40–54.

84. Mattson, D., Petrie, M., Srivastave, D., & McDermott, M. (1995). Multiple sclerosis, Sexual dysfunction and its response to medications. *Archives of Neurology, 52,* 862–868.

85. Stenager, E., Stenager, E. N., Jensen, K., & Boldsen, J. (1990). Multiple sclerosis: Sexual dysfunctions. *Journal of Sex Education and Therapy, 16,* 262–269.

86. Hatzichristou, D. G. (1996). Preface to the special issue: Management of voiding, bowel and sexual dysfunction in multiple sclerosis: Towards a holistic approach. *Sexuality and Disability, 14* (1), 3–7.

87. Lundberg, P. O., & Hulter, B. (1996). Female sexual dysfunction in multiple sclerosis: A review. *Sexuality and Disability, 14* (1), 65–72.

88. Crigger, N. J. (1996). Testing an uncertainty model for women with multiple sclerosis. *Advanced Nursing Science, 18* (34), 37–47.

89. Kolodny, R. C. (1980). *Sexual problems in diabetes and selected endocrine disorders.* Paper presented at 1st Annual conference on sexuality and Physical Disabilities: Medical Aspects and Clinical Care, Ann Arbor, MI.

90. Jensen, S. B. (1986). The natural history of sexual dysfunction in diabetic women. A 6-year follow-up study. *Acta Medica Scandinavia, 219* (1), 73–78.

91. Hauser, W., & Hesdorffer, D. C. (1991). *Facts about epilepsy.* Landover, MD: Demos Publications.

92. Callanan, M., & Stalland, N. (1996). Issues for women with epilepsy. In N. Santilli (Ed.), *Managing Seizures Disorders.* Landover, MD: Lippincott-Ravin Publishers.

93. Shafer, P. O. (March 1996). Women's issues: Momentum growing in search for answers. *Epilepsy USA,* 6.

94. Dodson, W. E. (1996). Issues in the comprehensive management of epilepsy in children and young adults. In N. Santilli (Ed.), *Managing Seizures Disorders.* Landover, MD: Lippincott-Ravin Publishers.

95. Santilli, N. (1996). Selection and discontinuation of antiepileptic drugs. In N. Santilli (Ed.), *Managing Seizures Disorders.* Landover, MD: Lippincott-Ravin Publishers.

96. Shafer, P. O., Austin, D. R., Callanan, M., & Clerico, C. M. (1996). Safety and activities of daily living for people with epilepsy. In N. Santilli (Ed.), *Managing Seizures Disorders.* Landover, MD: Lippincott-Ravin Publishers.

97. Coffman, C. B., Levine, S. B., Althof, S. E., & Stern, R. (1994). Sexual adaptation among single young adults with cystic fibrosis. *Chest, 86* (3), 412–418.

98. Shepperdson, B. (1995). The control of sexuality in young people with Down's syndrome. *Child Care, Health and Development, 21* (5), 333–349.

99. Blackburn, M. (1995). Sexuality, disability and abuse: Advice for life . . . not just for kids. *Child Care, Health and Development, 21,* (5), 351–361.

100. Evans, A. L. (1988). Sexual maturation in girls with severe mental handicap. *Child Care, Health and Development, 14,* 59–69.

101 Sockalosky, J. J., & Kriel, R. L. (1987). Precocious puberty after traumatic brain injury. *Journal of Pediatrics, 100,* 373.

102. Nosek, M. A. (1993). Personal assistance: Its on the long-term health of a rehabilitation hospital population. *Archives of Physical Medicine and Rehabilitation, 74* (3) 127–133.

103. Cole, S. S. (1993). Facing the challenges of sexual abuse in persons with disabilities. In M. Nagler (Ed.), *Perspectives in disability* (2nd ed., pp. 273–282). Palo Alto, CA: Health Markets Research.

104. Nosek, M. A. (1995). Sexual abuse of women with physical disabilities. Physical Medicine and Rehabilitation: State of the Art Reviews, 9 (2), 487–501.

105. Elvik, S. L., Berkowitz, C. D., Nichols, E. L., & Inkelis, S. H. (1990). Sexual abuse in the developmentally disabled: Dilemmas of diagnosis. *Child Abuse Neglect, 14* (4), 497–502.

106. Julkunen, H. A., Kaaja, R., & Friman, C. (1993). Contraceptive practice in women with systemic lupus erythematosus. *British Journal of Rheumatology, 32,* 227–230.

107. Welner, S. (1996). Contraception, sexually transmitted diseases and menopause. In D. M. Krotoski, M. A. Nosek, & M. A. Turk (Eds.), *Women with disabilities.* Baltimore: Paul H. Brooks, Publishing Co.

108. Carr, J., & Hollins, S. (1995). Menopause in women with learning disabilities. *J. Intellect. Disabil. Res, 39,* 137–139.

109. Stampfer, M. J., Colditz, G. A., Willett, W. C. et al. (1991). Postmenopausal estrogen therapy and cardiovascular disease. *New England Journal of Medicine, 325,* 756–762.

110. Pitzele, S. K. (1996). Chronic illness, disability and sexuality in people older than fifty. *Sexuality and Disability, 139* (4), 309–311.

111. Task Force on Concerns of Physically Disabled Women. (1978). *Within reach: Providing family planning services to physically disabled women.* New York: Human Sciences Press.

112. Sawin, K. J. (1986). Physical disability. In J. Griffith-Kinney (Ed.), *Contemporary women's health.* Reading, MA: Addison-Wesley.

113. Enforcement of nondiscrimination on the basis of handicap in federally assisted programs (1990, December 19), *Federal Register, 55* (244), 52136.

114. Carty, E. M., Tali, C. A., & Hall, L. H. (1990). Comprehensive health promotion for the pregnant woman who has disabilities. *Journal of Nurse-Midwifery, 35* (3), 133–190.

115. Ware, L., Muram, D., & Gale, C. L. (1992). Q-Tip Pap smear: Should it be done routinely in

patients who have developmental disabilities? *Sexuality and Disability, 10,* 189–192.

116. Pope, A. M., & Tarlov, A. R. (1991). *Disability in America: Summary and recommendations: Toward a national agenda for prevention.* Washington, DC: National Academy Press.

117. Welner, S. L. (1993). Management approaches to sexually transmitted diseases in women with disabilities. In F. P. Haseltine, S. S. Cole, & D. B. Gray (Eds.), *Reproductive issues for persons with physical disability.* Baltimore: Paul H. Brooks Publishing, Co.

118. Neinstein, L. S, & Katz, B. (1986). Contraceptive use in the chronically ill adolescent female: Part II. *Journal of Adolescent Health Care, 7,* 350–360.

119. Hatcher, R. A., Trussel, J., Stewart, F. Stewart, G. K., Kowal, D., Guest, F., & Cates, W. (1994). *Contraceptive technology* (16th rev. ed.). New York: Irvington.

120. Cook, S. D., Troiano, R., Bansil, S., & Dowling, P. C. (1994). *Multiple sclerosis and pregnancy. Advanced Neurology, 64,* 83–95.

121. Villard-Makintosh, L., & Vessey, M. P. (1993). Oral contraceptives of reproductive factors in multiple sclerosis incidence. *Contraception, 47* (2), 161–168.

122. Stenager, E. Stenager, E. N. & Jenson, K. (1994). Effect of pregnancy on the prognosis for multiple sclerosis. A 5-year follow up investigation. *Acta Neurol Scand, 90* (5), 305–308.

123. Verdru, P., Pol, T., D'Hooghe, M., & Carton, H. (1994). Pregnancy and multiple sclerosis: The influence on long term disability. *Clinical Neurology and Neurosurgery, 96,* 38–41.

124. Neinstein, L. S., & Katz, B. (1986). Contraceptive use in the chronically ill adolescent female: Part I. *Journal of Adolescent Health Care, 7,* 123–133.

125. Earles, A., Lessing, S., & Vichinsky, E. (Eds.). (1994). A parents' handbook for sickle cell disease, Part II. Sacramento, CA: State of California Department of Health Services, Genetic Disease Branch.

126. Craig, D. I. (1990). The adaptation to pregnancy of spinal cord injured women. *Rehabilitation Nursing, 15* (1), 6–9.

127. Wasser, A. M., Killoran, M. M., & Bansen, S. S. (1993). Pregnancy and disability. *AWOHNNS Clinical Issues in Perinatal and Women's Health, 4* (2), 328–337.

128. Corbin, J. M. (1987). Women's perceptions and management of pregnancy complicated by chronic illness. *Health Care Women International, 8* (5–6), 317–337.

129. Kirshbaum, M. (1988). Parents with physical disabilities and their babies. *Zero to Three, 8* (5), 7–11.

130. Connie, T. A. (1988). *Aids and adaptations for disabled parents: An illustrated manual for service providers and parents with physical or sensory disabilities* (2nd ed.). Vancouver: School of Rehabilitation Medicine, University of British Columbia.

131. Asreal, W. (1987). The rehabilitation team's role during the childbearing years for disabled women. *Sexuality and Disability, 8,* 47–62.

132. Sauer, P. M., Harvey, C. J. (1993). Spinal cord injury and pregnancy. *Journal Perinatal Neonatal Nursing, 7* (1), 22–24.

133. Cross, L. L., Meythaler, J. D., Tuel, S. M., & Cross, A. L. (1992). Pregnancy, labor and delivery post spinal cord injury. *Paraplegia, 30,* 890–902.

134. Cross, L. L., Meythaler, J. D., Tuel, S. M., & Cross, A. L. (1991). Pregnancy following SCI . *Western J. Med., 154* (5), 607–611.

135. Crosby, E., St-Jean, B., Reid, D., & Elliot, R. (1992). Obstetrical anesthesia and analgesia in chronic spinal cord-injured women. *Canadian Journal of Anaesthia, 39,* 487–494.

136. Jackson, A. B. (1996). Pregnancy and delivery. *Sexuality and Disability, 14* (3), 211–219.

137. Thomson, V. M. (1995). Breastfeeding and mothering one-handed. *Journal of Human Lactation, 11* (3), 211–215.

138. Reinelt, C., & Fried, M. (1993). "I am this child's mother": A feminist perspective on mothering with a disability. In Nagler, M. (ed.) Perspectives on Disability, Palo Alto, CA: Health Markets Research.

139. Kirshbaum, M. (1996). Mothers with physical disabilities. In D. M. Krotoski, M. A. Nosek, & M. A. Turk (Eds.), *Women with physical disabilities.* Baltimore: Paul H. Brooks Publishing Co.

140. Brazelton, T. B. (1973). Neonatal behavioral assessment scale. Philadelphia: J. B. Lippincott.

141. Westgren, N. Hultling, C., Levi, R., & Westgren, M. (1993). Pregnancy and delivery in women with a traumatic spinal cord injury in Sweden, 1890–1991. *Obstetrics & Gynecology, 81,* 926–930.

142. Sala, D. J. (1993). Effects of systemic lupus erythematosus on pregnancy and the neonate. *Journal of Perinatal Nursing, 7* (3), 39–48.

143. MacMullen, N. J. & Dulski, L. A. (1996). Systemic lupus erythematosus what are the perinatal implications? *Mother Baby Jorunal, 1* (5) 7–10, 20–22.

144. Tincani, A., Faden, D., Tarantini, M., Lojacono, A., Tanzi, P., Gastaldi, A., DiMario, C. Spatola, L., Cattaneo, R., & Balestrieri, G. (1992). Systemic lupus erythematosus and pregnancy: A prospective study. *Clinical Exp Rheumatol, 10* (5), 429–431.

145. Derkesen, R. H. (1991). Systemic lupus erythematosus and pregnancy. *Rheumatology International, 11* (3), 121–125.

146. Buchanan, N., et al. (1992). A study of 100 high risk lupus pregnancies. American Journal of Reproductive Immunology, 28, 192–194.

147. Zurier, R., et al. (1987). *Systematic lupus erythematosus.* New York: Wiley.

148. Smith, J. A., Espeland, M., Bellevue R., Bonds, D., Brown, A. K., Koshy, M. (1996, Feb.). Pregnancy in sickle cell disease: Experience of the Cooperative Study of Sickle Cell Disease. *Obstet Gynecol 87* (2), 199–204.

149. Helman, N. S. (1990). Sickle cell disease and pregnancy. *NAACOGS Clin Issue Perinat Women's Health Nurs, 1* (2), 194–201.

150. Koshy, M. (1995). Sickle cell disease and pregnancy. *Blood Rev 9* (3), 157–164.

151. Seoud, M. A., Cantwell, C., Nobles, G., & Levy, D. L. (1994, May). Outcome of pregnancies complicated by sickle cell and sickle-C hemoglobinopathies. *Am J Perinatol 11* (3), 187–191.

152. Larrabee, K., & Cowan, M. (1995). Clinical nursing management of sickle cell disease and trait during pregnancy. *J. Perinat Neonatal Nurs, 9* (2), 29–41.

153. Brown, A. K., Sleeper, L. A., Pegelow, C. H., Miller, S. T., Gill, F. M., & Waclawiw, M. A. (1994). The influence of infant and maternal sickle cell disease on birth outcome and neonatal course. *Arch Pediatr Adolesc Med, 148* (11, 1156–1162.

154. Sickle Cell Disease Guideline Panel. (1993, April). Sickle cell disease: Screening, diagnosis, management and counseling in newborns and infants. *Clinical Practice Guideline No. 6* (AHCPR Pub No. 93–0562). Rockville, MD: Agency for Health Care Policy and Research, Public Health Service, U.S. Department of Health and Human Services.

155. Yarby, M. S., & Lannon, S. L. (1992). Epilepsy, pregnancy and parenting. Morris Plains, NJ: Park Davis.

156. Stalland, N., & Shafer, P. O. (1996). When the parent has epilepsy. In N. Santilli (Ed.), *Managing seizures disorders.* Landover, MD: Lippincott-Ravin Publishers.

157. Gordon, D. (1996). Foreward to D. M. Krotoski, M. A. Nosek, & M. A. Turk (Eds.), *Women with physical disabilities.* Baltimore: Paul H. Brooks, Publishing Co.

158. Graves, W. H. (1993). Future directions in research and training in reproduction issues or persons with physical disabilities. In F. P. Haseltine, S. S. Cole, & D. B. Gray (Eds.), *Reproductive issues for persons with physical disability.* Baltimore: Paul H. Brooks, Publishing Co.

159. Gray, D., & Schimmel, A. B. (1993). Future directions for research on reproductive issues for people with physical disabilities. In F. P. Haseltine, S. S. Cole, & D. B. Gray (Eds.), *Reproductive issues for persons with physical disability.* Baltimore: Paul H. Brooks, Publishing Co.

EMERGENCY CHILDBIRTH

Mary Beth Bryant McGurin • Brenda T. Brickhouse

INTRODUCTION

When a woman presents complaining of labor, the health care provider must quickly perform an assessment appropriate to the specific needs of the client; that is, the provider must determine whether delivery of the infant is imminent or if there is time for further assistance to be obtained. The nature of the assessment and interventions depends on the resources available. Arrangements should be made for car or ambulance transportation to the nearest facility equipped for maternal and newborn care.[1,2]

ASSESSMENT OF LABOR STATUS

MOTHER'S HISTORY AND SUBJECTIVE ASSESSMENT OF CURRENT STATUS

Ask the client her due date, gravida, and para. If she has had previous pregnancies, were they vaginal or Cesarean births? Has she been receiving regular prenatal care, and has she had any complications during this pregnancy? Ask if she has medical problems or if special tests were done for her or the fetus during pregnancy. Some complications that can impact delivery are not viewed as

such by women, especially if they do not feel ill (i.e., hypertension, urinary tract infection, twins, fetal abnormalities). Ask the client the time of the onset of contractions and the status of the fetal membranes. If her membranes have ruptured did she note the color? Was the amniotic fluid clear or meconium stained? Brownish-green amniotic fluid indicates the fetus has been stressed and passed meconium; the infant may need airway clearance and resuscitation immediately after birth. How long have her membranes been ruptured? Membranes ruptured longer than 24 hours place mother and infant at risk for infection and sepsis. Ascertain the presence or absence of vaginal bleeding, fetal activity, history of allergies, and use of any medications or drugs. Has she had an ultrasound during her pregnancy; if so, was she told she had a placenta previa? If she has a placental previa, vaginal examination is contraindicated and immediate transport by ambulance is indicated. Ask the client if she feels the urge to bear down or have a bowel movement during contractions; this would indicate that the fetal presenting part is in the vaginal vault (putting pressure on the wall of the rectum) and birth is imminent.

ANXIETY LEVEL

Determine the client's ability to cooperate during examination and delivery by her response to questions and directions, degree of physical relaxation (resting between contractions) versus tension and fear (thrashing, uncontrolled bearing down), and tone of verbalizations (calm versus frantic).

The authors wish to acknowledge the contribution of Mary Beth Bryant McGurin who prepared this Appendix for the 1st edition.

PHYSICAL ASSESSMENT

Examination of the client should include her vital signs, notation of fetal position and presentation, fetal heart rate and the duration, and quality of uterine contractions. If there are no contraindications to pelvic examination, the degree of cervical dilatation, effacement, status of the membranes, and type and station of the presenting part should be determined.

1. *Is the infant's head visible?* Inspect the vulva: bulging of the perineum, anal sphincter, or both, with separation of labia, revealing protruding membranes or crowning of the fetal head, indicates that birth is imminent.
2. *Is amniotic fluid or blood present?* Leaking amniotic fluid, bloody show (blood-tinged mucus), or both indicate only that labor is in progress, not necessarily that birth is imminent. As discussed earlier, note the color of the amniotic fluid if the sac appears to have ruptured. Frank vaginal bleeding (blood flowing like a menstrual period) or dried blood on the legs indicates a possible abnormality of the placenta. *Do not* insert the fingers, a speculum, or any other object into the vagina (see Abnormal Bleeding later in this appendix).
3. *Are uterine contractions effectively dilating the cervix?* Palpate the abdomen. Uterine contractions that begin every 2 minutes, last 60 to 90 seconds, and are hard (indentation is not elicited by fingertips pressing on abdomen during peak of contraction) indicate that active labor is in progress. If the client is bearing down and pushing with contractions, the fetal head is probably already out of the uterus (i.e., the cervix is fully dilated) and into the vaginal vault. Delivery is probably imminent. If sterile gloves are available and there is no frank vaginal bleeding, gently insert the index and middle fingers of one hand into the vagina until the fetal presenting part or cervix is palpable. Instruct the client to breathe slowly during the exam and to relax her buttocks; tell her what you

are checking for. A gravid cervix is very soft, often indiscernible from the vaginal wall, but easily distinguishable from the fetal presenting part, which is firmer. If the cervix can be felt between your fingers and the fetal presenting part, then you may have time to attempt transportation by ambulance to the closest facility offering maternity services. If only the fetal head is palpable deep in the vagina close to the perineum, the cervix is completely dilated, and delivery is imminent.

4. Is *the fetus tolerating the intrauterine environment?* Fetal well-being is assessed to ascertain measures that need to be taken before birth, to decrease stress to the fetus, and after delivery, to facilitate the transition to extrauterine life. If not already known, ask when the infant is due to be born and if there are any known or suspected problems with the infant. The gestational age of the fetus and any physical challenges will determine how much stress the infant can tolerate. (*Note:* Estimation of the gestational age of the fetus by measurement of fundal height is not accurate during the late stages of labor.) Between contractions, perform Leopold's maneuvers to determine which side of the abdomen to listen to for fetal heart sounds; that is, the side where you can feel a smooth, firm fetal back. Listen with the bell side of the stethoscope in the lower abdomen on that side. Count heartbeats for 15 to 30 seconds and multiply to obtain the beats per minute. If the fetal heartrate is less than 100 bpm or if amniotic fluid is meconium stained (green or brown), the fetus is or has been stressed; be prepared to resuscitate the infant immediately after birth. If birth does not seem imminent, turn the client onto her side (preferably left) to allow better blood flow to her uterus and the fetus. Auscultate the fetal heartbeat every 5 to 10 minutes. Also ask the client if the fetus has been moving in the last few hours, another measure of fetal well-being. A stressed, compromised fetus will not be as active as usual.

PROVISION OF EMOTIONAL SUPPORT AND RELAXATION COACHING

Enhance the client's ability to cooperate during the examination and delivery by teaching her how to gain some measure of control with her breathing. Encourage her to open her mouth and pant or blow slowly during contractions. She is probably frightened and uncomfortable. Acknowledge that everything possible will be done to help her. Ask her to keep her eyes open and to watch for directions. Maintain eye contact, speak calmly, and give simple directions. Have any available support person stay by her upper body to hold her hands and assist with instructions. Give frequent feedback and reassurance that they are both doing a good job. Ideally transport of the laboring woman should be done by emergency service providers. However, if you are transporting the woman and delivery of the fetus begins, stop the vehicle; this facilitates balance and concentration for you and mother.

PREPARATION FOR DELIVERY

ASSEMBLY OF AVAILABLE SUPPLIES

Where delivery is taking place will determine the type and amount of assistance and equipment available. If a readymade delivery kit is available, open it and place it to one side within easy reach. If no kit is readily available, have someone get the following items for you if possible: eight or more towels, sheets, or blankets (warm two of them); bulb syringe; sterile scissors; three cord clamps, kelly clamps, or shoestrings; two pair of sterile gloves; bowl or sealable plastic bag; sanitary pads; 3-cc syringe with needle; alcohol wipes; 1000 mL 5% dextrose in half-normal saline or in lactated Ringer's; intravenous catheters; intravenous tubing; other intravenous start supplies; two vials oxytocin (Pitocin, 10 units each) or 0.2 mg (1 cc) of methylergonovine maleate (Methergine); hot water bottle (filled) or heat pack. *Note:* If no supplies are available, use whatever cloth is available to protect your hands from contact with body fluids.

POSITIONING OF MOTHER AND DRAPING

Wash hands. Position the client lying on her back on a firm surface, with her knees bent and spread apart and her upper body elevated if possible. (This position provides maximum control in an emergency situation.) Observe the perineum while maintaining intermittent eye contact with the client and her support person.

INTRAVENOUS INFUSION

Start an intravenous infusion at a keep-vein-open rate; draw up both vials of oxytocin to be added to the intravenous fluid immediately following delivery of placenta.

DELIVERY OF THE INFANT

DELIVERY OF PRESENTING PART AND CLEARANCE OF AIRWAY

To avoid explosive delivery of the head (causing perineal tears), have the client pant or blow during contractions and give gentle, short pushes only between contractions. Place the hand most comfortable for you on the presenting part, usually the crown of the head, as it protrudes from the vagina during each contraction. Most practitioners use their nondominant hand, leaving their dominant hand to handle equipment or supplies. Maintain gentle, even pressure on the head, with the length of the fingers allowing the head to slide out of the vagina slowly. (It may take several contractions to complete delivery of the head.) If the amniotic sac is intact over the infant's face, remove it with your fingers. As soon as the head is born, place the fingertips of one of your hands on the back of the baby's head and then slide them down the curve of the baby's back at the level of the top of the shoulder and sweep them in both directions feeling for the umbilical cord. If found, pull the cord gently over the head. If the loop is too tight, have the mother pant or blow while you clamp the cord in two places; cut between the two clamps. Wipe the baby's face and head and wipe off fluid from the nose and mouth with a soft absorbent cloth. Gently suction the baby's mouth and nose with a soft rubber bulb syringe. With the next contraction, the head will align with the infant's body and externally rotate.

DELIVERY OF BODY

Shift slightly toward the back of the infant's head. Place your hands on each side of the head so that your fingers point toward the face, with the little fingers closest to the perineum. With contraction, or gentle pushes from the mother, exert downward and outward pressure on the side of the head with your top hand until the infant's anterior shoulder has slipped out from under the mother's symphysis pubis bone and can be seen. Then apply upward and outward pressure on the sides of the head with your bottom hand, and with both hands lift the infant's head toward the ceiling. As the infant is being born, slide your bottom hand down close to the perineum so that the shoulder, arm, elbow, and hand are held close to the infant's body, controlled, and born into the palm of your hand. The thumb on your bottom hand will be on the infant's back, your fingers will be across the infant's chest, and the infant's head will be resting on your wrist. Slide your top hand down the infant's back, slip your index finger between the infant's legs as the buttocks clear the perineum, and grasp the infant by the ankles. *Note the time of delivery.*

IMMEDIATE INFANT CARE

Move the infant in a smooth arc into a football hold by allowing the head and shoulders to pivot in your hand while swinging the legs and torso around; the infant's back is supported by your lower arm, and the lower half of the infant's body is tucked between your upper arm and side. Keep the infant's head in a downward position and turned to the side. Stay close enough to the mother so that there is no tension on the umbilical cord.

Suction the infant's mouth and nose gently with a bulb syringe (or wipe out with a cloth) and dry the infant. If you did not do so earlier, clamp the umbilical cord in two places about 6 in. from the infant's body and cut between the clamps. If clamps are not available, tie with shoestrings. (Not with thread!) If the infant does not breathe spontaneously and start to cry, dry the skin vigorously, rub the back, and flick the foot with your finger. Initiate infant CPR (rescue breathing and chest compressions) if necessary. When the infant does cry, place her or him on the mother's chest, skin to skin, and cover with warm blankets so that the infant's scalp is covered but the face can be seen. Use a hot water bottle or heat pack covered with a towel, if necessary and available, to keep the infant warm. Observe the infant for cyanosis or lethargy; stimulate as above if needed. Assign APGAR scores at 1 and 5 minutes. (Refer fo Appendix B.)

DELIVERY OF PLACENTA

Observe the vaginal opening for lengthening of the cord or increased bleeding, which indicate placental separation. Do *not* pull on the cord; instead, wait for uterine contractions to push out the placenta with attached membranes, and place it in a bowl or plastic bag. Transport to the hospital with the infant. Note any tears in the perineum.

IMMEDIATE POSTDELIVERY CARE OF MOTHER

CONTROL OF BLEEDING

Locate the grapefruit-sized uterine fundus under the umbilicus and massage it with one hand to keep it firm while supporting the uterus with the other hand just above the symphysis pubis. If oxytocin is available and an IV is running, introduce 20 units of oxytocin into the bag, and allow the IV to run open for about 5 minutes or until the uterus remains firm. If no IV is running, give 10 units (1 cc) oxytocin or 0.2 mg (1 cc) methylergonovine maleate IM into the buttocks or thigh. Even if medications are not available, vaginal bleeding should be minimal if the infant is put to breast, and the uterus is kept well contracted with massage every 10 to 15 minutes. Place a sanitary pad or folded cloth firmly against the perineum. Record blood pressure, pulse, and respirations every 15 minutes; the urinary bladder should be checked for distention and emptied if needed. If the uterus is soft or is above the umbilicus, it has lost its muscle tone and is full of clots. The fundus needs to be massaged (with support from the opposite hand just above the pubic bone to prevent eversion of the uterus into the vagina) until clots are expelled and the fundus is firm. If the uterus is displaced to one side of the midline, the urinary bladder is distended and needs to be emptied.

PHYSICAL AND EMOTIONAL RECOVERY

If the mother experiences severe shaking chills, reassure her that this reaction is normal after the hard work and anxiety of delivery. Slow, deep breathing may help alleviate the "shakes" and increase relaxation. Cover her with available blankets. Reinforce what a wonderful job she did during her labor and delivery. Encourage her to interact with her infant and support person. Assist the mother to breastfeed if she is planning to nurse. Notify the receiving health care facility of the impending arrival and condition of the mother and infant.

ABNORMAL CONDITIONS

BREECH PRESENTATION

When initially assessing the client's vaginal opening, note that instead of the top of the infant's head, the buttocks may present first (breech presentation), often accompanied by meconium. This delivery should only occur in a hospital. Only attempt a breech delivery if there are no other alternatives. Immediately activate Emergency Medical Services (EMS). Prepare the client and supplies as usual; allow the infant's legs, buttocks, and trunk to deliver spontaneously. When the baby is born up to the umbilicus, the remainder of the baby needs to be delivered in 3 to 5 minutes to prevent anoxia. In this event, gently pull down a loop of cord to prevent tension on the cord. If the arms do not deliver spontaneously,

reach up for the hands, one at a time, and sweep them down over the face. The body will turn to one side and the shoulders will deliver, the top shoulder followed by the bottom shoulder. The head is ready to deliver when the back is up (toward the ceiling). Put two fingers in the vagina below the head and press downward to make enough room for the baby to breathe. Have the mother push until the face starts to deliver. Then she should pant and the back of the head can be delivered slowly. Support the body in the palm of your gloved hand and on your lower arm, and try to bring the infant's arms out with the other gloved hand. Transport to the nearest hospital's obstetric unit with the mother's buttocks elevated; be prepared to resuscitate the infant if the head does deliver en route. Alert the receiving facility of impending arrival.

OTHER ABNORMAL PRESENTATION SITUATIONS

If the infant's arm protrudes from the vagina, transport the mother immediately to the nearest hospital's obstetric unit. This woman will not deliver spontaneously.

If a loop of umbilical cord protrudes from the vagina, cover it with moistened cloth (preferably with normal saline). Have the client assume the knee–chest position on the stretcher or car seat. (This is difficult to do, and the client and her support person will need much reassurance!) Insert your gloved hand into the vagina, and attempt to hold the presenting part off the prolapsed cord until you reach the delivery room, where staff are prepared to perform a Cesarean delivery.

If the mother is carrying more than one fetus, deliver subsequent infants just as the first. Remember that twin babies are likely to be smaller and in need of warmth and possible resuscitation.

ABNORMAL BLEEDING

If before or during delivery you observe blood flow rather than blood-tinged mucus, suspect a placental abnormality. Transport the client to the nearest hospital's obstetric unit while maintaining her in shock position (head down, hips elevated, covered with blankets). Record blood pressure, pulse, respirations, and fetal heart rate every 10 minutes. Monitor contractions and deliver the infant as indicated, being prepared to resuscitate the infant as needed and to treat the mother for shock if pulse rises and blood pressure drops. If the mother bleeds after delivery despite breastfeeding or nipple stimulation and your best efforts to keep her fundus firm, look for perineal lacerations, and apply a peripad or folded cloth snugly to the vulva. Bring all blood-soaked pads or material to the hospital. Always call the receiving facility to alert them of the arrival time and condition of the client and infant.

REFERENCES

1. Bidwell, D. (1990). Congratulations—It's a baby! *Emergency Medical Services, 19*(10), 21–24.
2. Varney, H. (1997). *Varney's Midwifery* (3rd ed.). Sudbury, MA: Jones and Bartlett Publishers.

IMMEDIATE ASSESSMENT OF THE NEWBORN

Martha Edwards Hart

INTRODUCTION

Newborn assessment is an ongoing process incorporating the basic principles of health care and promotion.

- *Purposes*
  a. To provide baseline information.
  b. To identify problems with transition from intra- to extrauterine life.
  c. To document individual variation and reactivity.
- *Principles*
  a. Follow a systematic approach, progressing from noninvasive to invasive, clean to dirty, and head to toe.
  b. Anticipate, on the basis of history.
  c. Do no harm.
  d. Attend to instinctive feelings that something may be wrong.
- *General Guidelines*
  a. Maintain universal precautions and neutral thermal environment.
  b. Focus on ABCs of cardiopulmonary resuscitation.
  c. Assess symmetry.
  d. If an external abnormality is visible, closely assess internal organs.
  e. Measure lesions, graph vital statistics, and document and interpret findings.

REVIEW OF HISTORY FOR RISK FACTORS (SEE CHAPTER 12))

- *Maternal.* Age; past medical history; social, developmental, and occupational history.
- *Obstetric.* Parity; last menstrual period (LMP); previous menstrual period (PMP); history of prematurity; medical complications and outcome of previous or current pregnancy.
- *Perinatal.* Intrapartum events; gestational age; condition at birth.

APGAR SCORES

EVALUATION OF INITIAL NEONATAL TRANSITION PERIOD

The acronym *APGAR*[1,2] facilitates assessment of five components of neonates' responses: appearance, pulse, grimace, activity, and respiration.

INTERPRETATION

- The APGAR is scored at 1 and 5 minutes of life.
- Five signs are evaluated and scored 0, 1, or 2.
- *10–10, Best Possible Condition.* As most healthy newborns are acrocyanotic, expect a score of 8 or 9.

APGAR SIGNS

Signs	0	1	2
Appearance (color)	Blue/pale	Body pink Extremities blue	Completely pink
Pulse (heart rate)	Absent	< 100	> 100
Grimace (reflex irritability)	No response	Grimace	Cough, sneeze, cry
Activity (muscle tone)	Limp	Some flexion	Flexed, active motion
Respiration (breathing efforts)	Absent	Weak, irregular gasping	Strong cry

- When the 5-minute score is 6 or less, some states require a 10-minute score. It is useful to obtain additional scores every 5 minutes until 20 minutes has passed or until two successive scores of 7 or higher are obtained.
- *0–2, Severe Asphyxia.* Infant is at high risk; requires resuscitation and further evaluation.
- *3–4, Moderate Asphyxia.* Infant is at moderate risk; probable resuscitation and further evaluation.
- *5–7, Mild Asphyxia.* Infant is at risk; possible intermittent resuscitation, and with or without further evaluation.
- *8–10, No Asphyxia.* Infant is at minimal risk; routine elective procedures.

Physical examination

Abnormal findings are noted in parentheses.

GENERAL SURVEY

- *State.*[3] Deep or light sleep; drowsy; quiet or active alert; crying.
- *Reactivity.* State changes, interactive capacity, self-consolability.
- *Color.* Pink, acrocyanosis; mottling (plethora, pallor, jaundice, cyanosis).
- *Posture.* Flexed (asymmetry, restricted movement).
- *Skin.* Smooth, elastic, warm, moist; vernix; lanugo; desquamation; Mongolian spots; milia; nevi; edema or petechiae over presenting part (pustules, lacerations, ecchymosis, rashes, café-au-lait spots, hemangiomas, meconium staining, pitting edema, poor turgor, scaling, sweating).
- *Respirations at Rest.* Rate = 30–60; symmetric; diaphragmatic or abdominal (flaring; grunt-

ing; intercostal, supraclavicular, or substernal retractions).

HEENT, MOUTH, AND NECK

- *Head.* Occipitofrontal circumference: 32.5–37 cm. Round; symmetric; molding; overriding or slightly open sutures; caput succedaneum = scalp edema, may cross suture line; cephal hematoma = subperiosteal hemorrhage, does not cross suture line (irregularities; craniotabes; depressions; asymmetry; fracture; fixed widely spaced/closed sutures). Fontanelles soft, flat, may bulge with crying; anterior = diamond; posterior = triangle (sunken; bulging at rest; enlarged; absent anterior; third fontanelle).
- *Face.* Symmetric; intact (asymmetry with movement, micrognathia; clefts).
- *Eyes.* Symmetric; lids easily open; positive blink; pupils round, equal, and reactive to light; positive red reflex; blue-gray or brown iris; no discharge; cornea and lens clear and intact; sclera bluish white; minor hemorrhages; pale pink conjunctiva; subconjunctival hemorrhage; chemical conjunctivitis; nystagmus; strabismus (asymmetry; short palpebral fissures; hypertelorism; fused edematous, drooping, or inflamed lids; setting sun sign; unequal, constricted, or poorly reactive pupils; pinkish or clefted iris; blue or jaundiced sclera; corneal opacities or ulcerations; purulent discharge; persistent uncoordinated movements).
- *Ears.* Well formed; symmetric; upper pinna at or above outer canthus of eye; curved pinna, firm cartilage; patent canals; positive response to noise (asymmetric; low-set; rotated; very large or small; malformed; preauricular, auricular skin tags, sinuses).
- *Nose.* Midline; intact; no discharge; bilateral nasal patency; obligatory nose breather (flat-

tened nasal bridge; flaring; clefts; chloanal atresia).

- *Mouth and Throat.* Pink, moist mucosa; sucking blisters; positive suck, root, and gag reflexes; transient circumoral cyanosis; midline mobile tongue; well-formed palate and gums; Epstein's pearls; inclusion cysts; teeth; scant saliva (clefts; thrush; tongue protrusion; long frenulum; macroglossia; high arched palate; excessive mucus).
- *Neck.* Short, straight, full range of motion; intact clavicles (webbing; masses; edema, venous distention; limited range of motion; torticollis; crepitation; fractures; opisthotonus).

CHEST

- *Thorax.* Symmetric; cylindrical; circumference at nipple line = 30–33 cm (bulging, depressed sternum; retractions; tachypnea; apnea).
- *Nipples.* Present; symmetric placement; supernumerary; enlarged; milky secretion (asymmetry; purulent drainage).
- *Breath Sounds.* Auscultate for vesicular or clear bilaterally (expiratory grunting; rales/crackles; rhonchi/wheezes; decreased, unequal).
- *Heart Sounds.* Rate = 120–160; auscultate for two clear, distinct sounds: S_2 slightly sharper, higher pitched than S_1; regular rhythm; point of maximal impulse (PMI) = lower left sternal border (displaced, distant, muffled, extra sounds; bradycardia/tachycardia; irregular rhythm; hyperactive precordium).

ABDOMEN

- *Contour.* Protuberant; symmetric; cylindrical shape; diastasis recti; prominent superficial veins (asymmetry; distention; flat; scaphoid; masses; visible peristalsis).
- *Bowel Sounds Present in All Four Quadrants.* Intermittent tinkling (hyperactive or absent).
- *Liver.* Palpate 1–2 cm below right costal margin; sharp edge (enlarged; round edge).
- *Kidneys.* Palpate oval structure in posterior flanks 1–2 cm above umbilicus; often difficult to palpate (enlarged; absent).
- *Umbilical Cord and Umbilicus.* Two arteries; one vein; gelatinous, bluish-white; skin clear and dry; umbilical hernia (two vessels; thin cord; foul odor; discharge; meconium stained).
- *Femoral Pulses and Lymph Nodes.* Palpate strong, regular pulses bilaterally (absent, irregular, weak, bounding, absent pulses; enlarged nodes).
- *Rectum and Anus.* Patent; positive anal wink (imperforate anus; fistulas; decreased tone); document passage and character of stools; meconium = dark green, tarry, thick viscous; mucus plug (foul odor; diarrhea; mucus; blood).

GENITOURINARY TRACT

- *Urination.* Confirm; clear; yellow; full stream (bladder distention; abnormal stream; blood-tinged).
- *External Genitalia.* Confirm appropriate for given gender (ambiguous; fecal urethral discharge).
  - *Male:* Observe urinary stream; meatus at tip of penis, glans covered by prepuce (epispadias = dorsal; hypospadias = ventral surface; phimosis); scrotum—pink to brown; symmetric; pendulous; rugation; testes descended or descending bilaterally; edema or bruising if breech (hydrocele = positive transillumination; hernia = negative transillumination; undescended or absent testes).
  - *Female:* Observe presence and position of urethra; introitus posterior to clitoris; labia majora meet midline; labia minora prominent; edema; hymenal tags; pseudomenstruation; mucoid, milky discharge (absent vagina or meatus).

BACK

- *Back and Spine.* Midline; straight; intact; easily flexed; symmetric; lanugo; pilonidal dimple (asymmetry; abnormal curvature; masses; pilonidal cyst, sinus, dimple, hair tufts; spina bifida).
- *Buttocks.* Symmetry; Mongolian spots (asymmetric gluteal folds).

EXTREMITIES

- *General.* Appearance, symmetry, size, length, and range of motion.

- *Fingers and Toes.* All present.
- *Hands and Feet.* Palmar and plantar creases; fisted hands (Simian crease; dysplastic nails; tightly fisted hands, obligatory palmar thumb; metatarsus varus; club feet; rocker-bottom feet; absent digits, abnormal spacing).
- *Arms.* Occasional tremors; easily adduct from trunk; full range of motion at elbow (fracture; palsy; paralysis).
- *Legs.* Mild medial rotation; transient in utero positioning = breech, "frogs legs"; symmetry of medial thigh skinfolds (asymetric size/ appearance; limited range of motion).
- *Hips.* Tests[2] to evaluate:
  - *Ortolani's Maneuver—Abduct, Up and Out.* Flex knees and hips, placing fingers bilaterally on greater trochanters, thumbs gripping medial aspect of femurs; adduct and abduct (positive jerking motion as femur passes over acetabulum).
  - *Barlow's Test—Up and Back, "Piston."* Flex hip and knee 90 degrees; gently attempt to slip femur head onto posterior tip of acetabulum by lateral pressure of thumb and by rocking knee medially with knuckle of index finger (palpable or audible hip click; movement is not normally felt).
- *Peripheral Pulses.* Present; symmetric; strong (absent; varied strength).

NERVOUS SYSTEM

- *Character of Cry.* Strong, lusty (weak, high-pitched, constant or none).
- *Reflexes.* Assess symmetry and strength of responses.
  - *Asymmetric Tonic Neck ("Fencing").* With the infant supine, turn head to one side. The infant may extend arm and leg on side head is turned toward with flexion of opposite arm and leg.
  - *Moro or Startle.* Abrupt position change or noise elicits extension and abduction of arms and extension of fingers with subsequent flexion or drawing in; infant may habituate or diminish response with repeated attempts.
  - *Rooting.* Stroke side of cheek, lips, or mouth with finger or nipple and head turns toward the stimulus, mouth opens, and sucking begins.
- *Sucking.* Finger or nipple in mouth elicits sucking movements.
- *Swallow.* Assess coordination of suck or swallow with first oral feeding.
- *Extrusion.* Solid object placed on tongue causes tongue to push outward to remove it.
- *Palmar and Plantar Grasp.* Finger placed in palm and base of toes elicits grasp of finger and brief downward curling of toes.
- *Babinski.* Stroke up lateral aspect of feet and toes fan up and out.
- *Pull to Sit or Traction.* With the infant supine, grasp the arms and pull to sitting position; the head lags, then is brought up and held briefly; note position and tone.
- *Glabellar or Blink.* Tap forehead at bridge of nose with finger to elicit bilateral blink.
- *Galant or Trunk Incurvation.* With infant in ventral suspension over examiner's hand, gently stroke, with finger of other hand, paravertebral portion of spine to elicit curvature toward stimulus.
- *Placing or Stepping.* Holding infant upright on flat surface elicits "stepping" movements with alternating flexion and extension of feet (may also elicit this response by stroking dorsum of foot while holding infant upright).

ESTIMATION OF GESTATIONAL AGE

Use Dubowitz or Ballard clinical assessments of physical characteristics and neuromuscular maturity[4,5] to classify neonates by gestational age and to determine potential mortality and morbidity risks.

REFERENCES

1. Apgar, V. (1996). The newborn (APGAR) scoring system: Reflections and advice. *Pediatric Clinics of North America, 13,* 645.
2. NAACOG. (1991). *OGN Nursing Practice Resource: Physical assessment of the neonate.* Washington, DC: Author.

3. Brazelton, T. B. (1973). *Neonatal behavioral assessment scale.* Philadelphia: J. B. Lippincott/ Spastics International Medical Publishers.
4. Dubowitz, L. M. S., Dubowitz, V., & Goldberg, C. (1970). Clinical assessment of gestational age in the newborn infant. *Journal of Pediatrics, 77,* 1.
5. Ballard, J. L., Khoury, J. C., Wedig, K., Wang, L., Eilers-Walsman, B. L., Lipp, R. (1991). New Ballard score, expanded to include extremely premature infants. *Journal of Pediatrics, 3,* 417.

BIBLIOGRAPHY

Coody, D., et al. (1996). Perinatal Conditions. In *Pediatric Primary Care: A Handbook for Nurse Practitioners.* Philadelphia: W. B. Saunders.

Reimann, D. & Coughlin, M. (1996). Newborn Adaptation to Extrauterine Life. In *Perinatal Nursing.* AWHONN Philadelphia: Lippincott.

Witt, P. (1993). Physical Assessment of the Newborn. In *Core Curriculum for Neonatal Intensive Care Nursing.* AWHONN Philadelphia: W. B. Saunders.

SELECTED LABORATORY VALUES

Ellis Quinn Youngkin

Chem 6 (1)a

Sodium	135–145 mEq/L (mmol/L)
Potassium	3.6–5.1 mEq/L (mmol/L)
Chloride	101–111 mEq/L (mmol/L)
Carbon dioxide	21–31 mEq/L (mmol/L)
Glucose (fasting)	65–110 mg/dL
Blood urea nitrogen	6–22 mg/dL

Chem 12 (1)

Creatinine (2)	0.6–0.9 mg/dL (in females)
Urate	2.3–6.9 mg/dL
Calcium	8.9–10.5 mg/dL
Phosphate	2.5–4.6 mg/dL
Anion gap (2)	8–14 mEq/L (mmol/L)
Osmolality	280–295 mmol/kg
Iron (2)	80–150 µg/dL
Cholesterol	≤ 200 mg/dL
Alkaline Phosphatase (2)	30–120 U/L
AST (SGOT) (2)[b]	8–40 U/L
ALT (SGPT) (2)	9–24 U/L (in females)
Protein (total)	6–8 g/dL

Lipid Profile (3)

Cholesterol	150–200 mg/dL
Triglycerides	40–150 mg/dL
Phospholipids	150–380 mg/dL
LDL-CHO (1)	< 130 mg/dL
HDL-CHO (1)	> 35 mg/dL
Cholesterol/HDL ratio (1)	≤ 4.4

Thyroid Profile (1)

TSH	0.32–5.00 µIU/mL
T_3 uptake	30–42%
T_4 total	4.5–12 µg/dL
FTI (calc)	5–12 µg/dL
Free T_4	1–3 ng/dL
Free T_3	0.2–0.6 ng/dL

Other Values

Prolactin (6)	< 20 ng/dL
FSH (5)	FSH (mIU/mL)
Follicular	4–13
Luteal	2–13
Midcycle	5–22
Postmenopausal	20–138
LH (5)	(mIU/mL)
Follicular	1–18
Luteal	0.4–20
Midcycle peak	24–105
Postmenopausal	15–62
Progesterone (2)	< 150 ng/dL (follicular)
	approx. 300 ng/dL (luteal)
	2000 mg/dL (midluteal)
Estrogen (2)	24–68 pg/mL (days 1–10 of menstrual cycle)
	50–186 pg/mL (days 11–20 of menstrual cycle)
	73–149 pg/mL (days 21–30 of menstrual cycle)
Testosterone (2)	30–95 ng/dL (females)
Free testosterone (4)	100–200 pg/dL
DHEA-S (4)	80–350 µg/dL (decreases with age)
Androstenedione	< 250 ng/dL
17-Hydroxyprogesterone (4)	15–70 ng/dL (follicular phase)
	35–290 ng/dL (luteal phase)
Cortisol (4)	
8:00 AM	5–25 µg/dL
4:00 PM	3–12 µg/dL
10:00 PM	< 50% of AM value

After ACTH stimulation test: plasma cortisol should increase 2–3 times over baseline at 30 and 60 minutes (4)

Dexamethasone suppression test	5+ µg/dL cortisone = test failure
Albumin (3)	3.5–5.0 g/dL

Anemia Workup (3)

Complete blood count		Reticulocyte count	0.5–2%
Red blood cells	$4.2–5.4 \times 10^6/mm^3$	Iron	60–190 µg/dL
Hemoglobin	12–16 g/dL	Total iron binding capacity	250–420 µg/dL
Hematocrit	37–47%	Transferrin	200–400 µg/dL
MCV	$80–95 \ \mu m^3$	Transferrin saturation	30–40%
MCH	27–31 pg	Ferritin	10–150 ng/mL (in females)
MCHC	32–36 g/dL	Hemoglobin electrophoresis	
White blood cells	$5000–10,000/mm^3$	Hgb A_1	95–98%
Differential		Hgb A_2	2–3%
Neutrophils	55–70%	Hgb F	0.8–2%
Lymphocytes	20–40%	Hgb S	0%
Monocytes	2–8%	Hgb C	0%
Eosinophils	1–4%	Platelet count	$150,000–400,000/mm^3$
Basophils	0.5–1%		

[a](1) Medical College of Virginia, Virginia Commonwealth University Hospitals Laboratory, September 1992. (2) *Clinical laboratory tests,* Springhouse Corp., 1991. (3) Pagana, K. D., & Pagana, T. J. (1997). *Mosby's diagnostic and laboratory test reference* (3rd ed.). St. Louis: Mosby. (4) Speroff, L., Glass, R., & Kase, N. (1994). *Clinical gynecologic endocrinology and infertility* (5th ed.). Baltimore: Williams & Wilkins (pp. 669, 969, 975, 989). (5) Nicoll, D., McPhee, S., Chou, T., & Detmer, W. (1997). *Pocket guide to diagnostic tests* (2nd ed.). Stamford, CT: Appleton & Lange.

[b]AST(SGOT), aspartate aminotransferase (serum glutamic-oxaloacetic transaminase); ALT(SGPT), alanine aminotransferase (serum glutamic–pyruvic transaminase); LDL-CHO, low-density lipoprotein cholesterol; HDL-CHO, high-density lipoprotein cholesterol; TSH, thyroid-stimulating hormone; T_3, triiodothyronine; T_4, thyroxine; FTI (calc), free thyroxine index (calculated); FSH, follicle-stimulating hormone; LH, luteinizing hormone; DHEA-SO_4, dehydroepiandrosterone sulfate; MCV, mean corpusacular volume; MCH, mean corpuscular hemoglobin; MCHC, mean corpuscular hemoglobin concentration; Hgb, hemoglobin.

INDEX

Page numbers followed by *t* and *f* indicate tables and figures respectively.

Continued on next page

Contents at a Glance

Continued from previous page

BONUS CONTENT ON THE WEB
Visit www.samspublishing.com/register to register your book and gain access to exclusive bonus content:

Adobe®
Photoshop® Elements 4
and Premiere® Elements 2

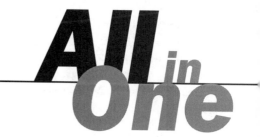

Chuck Engels

With contributing authors
Jennifer Fulton
Scott M. Fulton III
Steve Grisetti

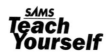
SAMS
Teach
Yourself

Sams Publishing, 800 East 96th Street, Indianapolis, Indiana 46240 USA

Adobe® Photoshop® Elements 4 and Premiere® Elements 2 All In One

International Standard Book Number: 0-672-32876-3

Library of Congress Catalog Card Number: 2005935743

Printed in the United States of America

First Printing: February 2006

09   08   07   06   4   3   2   1

Trademarks

Warning and Disclaimer

Bulk Sales

Sams Publishing offers excellent discounts on this book when ordered in quantity for bulk purchases or special sales. For more information, please contact

U.S. Corporate and Government Sales
1-800-382-3419
corpsales@pearsontechgroup.com

For sales outside of the United States, please contact

International Sales
international@pearsoned.com

Senior Acquisitions Editor
Linda Bump Harrison

Development Editors
Jon Steever
Alice Martina Smith

Managing Editor
Charlotte Clapp

Project Editor
Seth Kerney

Copy Editors
Benjamin Berg
Megan Wade

Indexer
Ken Johnson

Technical Editors
Greg Perry
Doug Nelson

Publishing Coordinator
Vanessa Evans

Multimedia Developer
Dan Scherf

Book Designer
Gary Adair

Page Layout
Nonie Ratcliff

About the Author

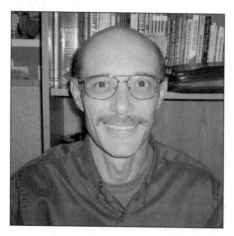

Chuck Engels graduated from Trans American School of Broadcasting in Wausau, Wisconsin. He worked in the radio industry for five years and studied theater and film at the University of Minnesota. Chuck has spent the past 18 years in the transportation industry, in management, and in software development. He currently lives near Atlanta, Georgia, with his wife and three children. He is a senior programmer and analyst in the software development department for an Atlanta-based freight transportation company. Chuck co-authored *Adobe Premiere Elements 2 in a Snap* with Steve Grisetti. Chuck is also involved in the media department for a 10,000-member church, and is an active member and regular contributor to the Adobe Premiere Elements User Forum. Chuck also hosts two websites where users can share their videos, tips, and tricks; learn more about video editing; and compete in video contests (http://www.chuckengels.com/PremierVideo and http://www.videoinasnap.com).

About the Contributing Authors

Steve Grisetti earned a master's degree in writing for television and film from Ohio University. He has taught college-level courses in television and video production and adult education classes on Photoshop and principles of design. Steve spent nearly 10 years in the Los Angeles–based entertainment industry, working on the sets and in the production offices of several large television and film companies. He is currently employed as a graphic designer in the marketing and communications department of a Milwaukee-based investment firm. Steve co-authored *Adobe Premiere Elements 2 in a Snap* with Chuck Engels. He also serves as host on Adobe's official Premiere Elements Support Forum (http://www.adobeforums.com/cgi-bin/webx?14@@.3bb574e6).

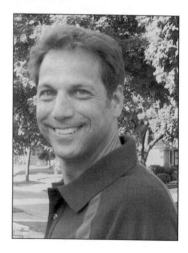

Jennifer Fulton, iVillage's former "Computer Coach," is an experienced computer consultant and trainer with more than 20 years of experience. Jennifer is also the best-selling author of more than 100 computer books written for both the education and retail markets, including *How to Use Dreamweaver and Fireworks, Adobe Photoshop Elements 3 in a Snap, Digital Photography with Photoshop Album in a Snap, Paint Shop Pro 8 in a Snap, Sams Teach Yourself Adobe Photoshop Elements 2 in 24 Hours, Sams Teach Yourself Windows Me in 10 Minutes, How to Use Microsoft Publisher 2000, How to Use Microsoft Office XP, Easy Microsoft Outlook 2000, Sams Teach Yourself Excel 2000 in 10 Minutes, Microsoft Office 2000 Cheat Sheet,* and *The Complete Idiot's Guide to Upgrading and Repairing PCs.* This book draws heavily on her most recent book, *Adobe Photoshop Elements 4 in a Snap.*

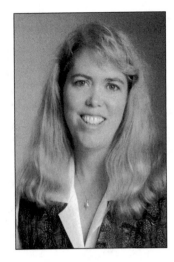

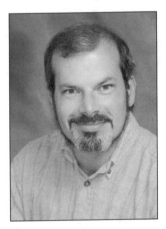

Scott M. Fulton III is a 22-year veteran technology author, currently featured online at InformIT.com and *Tom's Hardware Guide*. In the 1980s, as "D. F. Scott," he launched one of the world's first online technology news sources for *Computer Shopper* magazine, long before the Internet gave birth to the World Wide Web. In the 1990s, Scott published a dozen books and hundreds of articles, many on the topic of high-level programming. In 1994, just after they married, Scott and Jennifer formed Ingenus, a technology editorial partnership in the Midwest. But their greatest success to date is their daughter, Katerina, who at age eight is in the process of forming an art school, a radio station, and a presidential campaign exploratory committee. Scott is the co-author of *Adobe Photoshop Elements 4 in a Snap.*

v

Dedication

This book is dedicated to my God and Savior; my wife, Criss;
and my children, Heather, Britt, and Josh. Without your love,
support, and sacrifice, none of this would have been possible.
I humbly thank you all.
—Chuck Engels

Acknowledgments

In any major undertaking, there are many people who knowingly or unknowingly play big roles. The following people have played their parts well and to them I am truly thankful: Linda Harrison, for her help and support through this entire process. Alice Martina Smith, Seth Kerney, Ben Berg, Megan Wade, and Greg Perry, for giving such great advice and timely help to make this book the best. To Steve Grisetti, Jennifer Fulton, and Scott Fulton, thanks for the great material you created on these fantastic products. Without your contributions, this book would never have happened. The Media Department at Trinity Chapel, especially Tres, Rich, Hector, and Pastor Randy; you have inspired me more than you will ever know. A special thanks to Glenn Henderson, Ian Peters, and Bishop Jim Bolin, three great spiritual leaders. To everyone who prayed for me; your prayers were answered, and I thank you. To all of my fellow Premiere Elements forum members I thank you for letting me be a part of your world.
—Chuck Engels

We Want to Hear from You!

As the reader of this book, *you* are our most important critic and commentator. We value your opinion and want to know what we're doing right, what we could do better, what areas you'd like to see us publish in, and any other words of wisdom you're willing to pass our way.

You can email or write me directly to let me know what you did or didn't like about this book—as well as what we can do to make our books stronger.

Please note that I cannot help you with technical problems related to the topic of this book, and that due to the high volume of mail I receive, I might not be able to reply to every message.

When you write, please be sure to include this book's title and author as well as your name and phone or email address. I will carefully review your comments and share them with the author and editors who worked on the book.

Email: graphics@samspublishing.com

Mail: Mark Taber
           Associate Publisher
           Sams Publishing
           800 East 96th Street
           Indianapolis, IN 46240 USA

Reader Services

For more information about this book or another Sams Publishing title, visit our website at www.samspublishing.com. Type the ISBN (excluding hyphens) or the title of a book in the Search field to find the page you're looking for.

✔ Start Here

In my humble opinion, there has never been a better one-two punch in consumer graphic and video editing software. The Adobe Photoshop Elements 4.0/Adobe Premiere Elements 2.0 bundle outdoes them all.

Photoshop Elements, the offspring of the well-known professional graphics software Photoshop, is packed full of the same features as its professional counterpart. The same goes for Premiere Elements, the offspring of Premiere Pro. These two applications have retained much of the functionality, features, look, and feel of their Pro versions at a fraction of the cost. Premiere Elements even has much of the functionality and many of the features of Adobe's other pro digital video editing software, such as Encore DVD.

These two applications together give you the ability to create graphics, enhance and print photos, create slideshows, create DVD movies, and so much more. They are separate programs that have been integrated to give you a smooth workflow with time-saving steps. You can move images and video between the two with a few mouse clicks. You can take a still image captured from a video in Premiere Elements, send it to Photoshop Elements for enhancement, and send it back to Premiere Elements easily.

If you have used photo- or video-editing software before, or if this is your first attempt, you will enjoy the ease of use, professional features, and especially the finished product. In this chapter, we will take you through some of the things you need to know about Photoshop Elements 4.0 and Premiere Elements 2.0 before you get started. If you have used earlier versions of either application, you can jump right into a task if you like. Also, if you are familiar with photo- and video-editing software, you will probably do just fine. To learn what's new and get a quick overview of these two highly functional programs, read this chapter to discover Photoshop Elements 4.0 and Premiere Elements 2.0. As you continue through the many tasks in this book, notice that it is split up into three parts, just like this chapter: Part I, "Working with Photoshop Elements," Part II, "Working with Premiere Elements," and finally Part III, "Putting It All Together: Working with Photoshop Elements and Premiere Elements."

Working with Photoshop Elements

You might not have discovered it yet, but Photoshop Elements is actually two programs designed to work seamlessly together: the Editor and the Organizer. You use the *Editor* to make changes to digital images, such as brightening and sharpening them. You use the *Organizer* to catalog your images so that you can quickly locate and edit, print, or email them when needed.

▶ KEY TERMS

Editor—The portion of Photoshop Elements you use to make changes to images.

Organizer—The portion of Photoshop Elements you use to categorize your collection of graphic images.

Given the recent advancements in the field of digital photography, you might be surprised at how easy it is to take a bad picture. Even when your digital camera is taking pictures in Automatic mode, it might not properly compensate for less-than-favorable lighting conditions, unexpected movement of your subject matter, or poor composition. Luckily, in the digital world of photography, you can correct most mistakes with the help of a *graphics editor* such as the Photoshop Elements Editor.

▶ KEY TERM

Graphics editor—An application that allows you to edit your digital images.

Perhaps you don't use a digital camera; the quality of film photography is often far superior to that of digital images. Unfortunately, when you scan a photo print into a digital file, you often lose the qualities that made the original print superior in the first place—its sharpness, depth of tone, and color. Again, with the aid of graphic editors such as the Photoshop Elements Editor, you can restore the beauty your prints might have lost in translation. In this book, you'll learn everything you need to know about working with digital images, including how to use the Organizer and the Editor to categorize and manipulate them.

The Nature of Digital Photography

If you use a digital camera, you are more likely to print your photos at home rather than have a photo shop print them. Your computer essentially becomes the film lab, making you responsible for the touch-ups and corrections you'd otherwise trust to a lab technician. Don't let this new responsibility overwhelm you. As you'll learn in this book, the *Editor* provides many simple-to-use tools for fixing just about any problem in a digital image. When working with digital images, keep these things in mind:

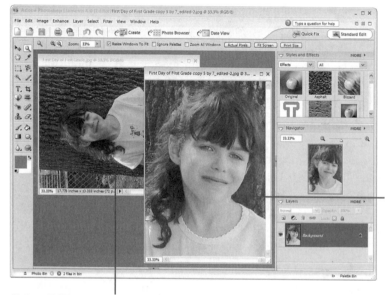

After Brightening and Cropping, the Image Is Ready for Printing

Before Editing, This Image Is Dark and Rotated Incorrectly

With the Editor, you become your own photo lab technician.

- **Film can record more detail than digital media**—To compensate, always take photos at your digital camera's highest *resolution*. Yes, this means you won't be able to store as many photos on the camera's memory card, but the photos you do save will be worth printing.

▶ KEY TERM

Resolution—In digital images, the number of pixels per inch/centimeter. The higher an image's resolution, the more detail it can contain.

▶ TIP

If you're given a choice of formats to use with your digital camera, choose RAW. If your camera doesn't use RAW, choose the TIFF format over JPEG because RAW and TIFF save more photographic detail than JPEG does.

- **Digital photos accumulate quickly**—Early on, you should develop a plan for managing your images, such as importing photos from your camera directly into the Organizer, a process that copies the images to the hard disk, renames them (if desired), and even fixes any red eye (again, if you choose that option). You should then back up these new, original images onto a CD-R, DVD-R, or other high-volume, permanent storage medium. If you select the **Move Files** option when you copy the new images to optical disc, the images are removed from the hard disk (saving space), but you can still review, print, and edit the images from the CD or DVD using the Organizer.

  Next, in the Organizer, you should review the *thumbnail* of each new image, selecting the best ones to keep and deleting the rest of the image files from the hard disk (if they are still there) and the *catalog*. As you review the images, you can tag those you do keep with special markers that identify their content. These *tags* will help you later locate these images in the catalog. You'll find that the Organizer is uniquely designed to help you with all the stages in this process.

- **Before making changes to your images, save copies of them, but do not edit your original images**—Before beginning to edit images, save them in PSD (Photoshop) format. This format allows you to use all of Photoshop Elements's tools to make your images picture perfect. When you're done editing, resave your images in a universal format such as TIFF or JPEG so they're easier to share and print than your edited PSD versions. Using the Organizer, back up the PSD and TIFF/JPEG versions of your edited images onto a CD-R, a DVD-R, or other storage medium.

- **Printing quality photos requires a printer designed and tested not only for color, but also for use with photo paper**—A printer specifically designed for printing photos is a good addition to your computer family if you want to print good-looking photos for albums, scrapbooks, and picture frames at home. As an alternative to buying your own color photo printer, consider a do-it-yourself printing kiosk that lets you insert a CD-R or PhotoCD and print photos on high-quality photo paper. Find a kiosk in your neighborhood (many discount department stores and drug stores have one) and study the instructions so you can save your photos in a compatible format on a compatible medium. For occasional photo printing needs, online services such as Adobe Photoshop Services enable you to upload your photos over the Internet, have them printed on quality stock, and have them delivered to you for a reasonable fee.

▶ **NOTE**

For optimum results, use only the photo paper that's compatible with your particular printer. Another consideration when printing photos at home is longevity. Archival inks and papers, though expensive, produce the best results.

- **If you intend to use the Editor to repair images scanned from old prints, invest in a quality scanner with high resolution**—Some premium scanner models include special features such as a film reader for scanning film strips and slides.

Using Photoshop Elements to Organize Photos

After beginning your foray into digital photography, it won't take long before you'll realize that your collection of images is getting almost too big to manage. This is where the Photoshop Elements Organizer comes in: Its purpose is to provide the tools you need to catalog images so you can locate them quickly, regardless of where they are stored—on the hard disk, a CD-R, a DVD, or a digital camera's memory card. Basically, you import images into the Organizer's catalog and then tag them with special markers that indicate what those images contain (for example, **Fourth of July**, **Oklahoma City**, or **Granddad and Nana**) or their purpose (for example, **Family Reunion Invitation**). Next, you'll use these markers to locate specific images for editing, printing, or using in *creations*. If you choose to edit an image, the Editor portion of Photoshop Elements appears, displaying its unique set of tools designed for making changes to images. To learn how to start the Editor and the Organizer, see **Using the Welcome Window**, later in this chapter.

▶ **KEY TERM**

Creations—Greeting cards, calendars, web galleries, slideshows, and other things you can make with the images in the catalog.

Using Photoshop Elements to Edit Photos

As you learned earlier, the portion of Photoshop Elements that enables you to edit and create graphic images is called the Editor. Although you can use the Editor to create buttons, banners, and other graphical gadgets for your web pages, its main purpose is to edit images. You can use the Editor's tools to retouch photographs, add text and other objects, and apply special effects. You'll learn how to start the Editor in **Using the Welcome Window**, later in this chapter. Right now I want to show you how a graphics editor such as the Editor can make your images look better.

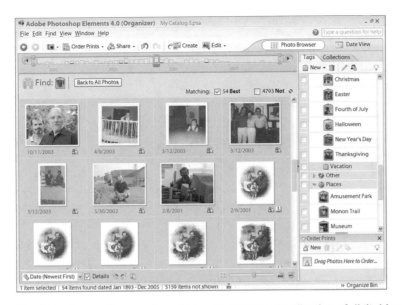

The Organizer enables you to quickly categorize your collection of digital images.

How to Use Layers

While editing or building an image, the Editor enables you to place data on multiple *layers*. The key purpose of layering is to give you a way to isolate individual parts of an image. For example, you might place your subject on a separate layer so you can lighten, recolor, resize, or position just it and not the entire photograph. In addition, data on upper layers obscures data on the layers below them, so you could copy a person onto a lower layer to place him behind other people or objects in a photograph. After using layers to manipulate elements of an image individually, you merge them together to create a flattened, single-layer image ready for printing or sharing.

▶ **KEY TERM**

Layer—A component of an image that contains its own data that can be manipulated separately from other data in an image.

▶ **NOTES**

After editing a PSD image, merge all the layers into a single background layer by selecting **Layer**, **Flatten Image**. If the results look good, save the image immediately in a shareable format such as JPEG or non-layered TIFF. (Retain the layer data in the PSD file by not saving over it.)

If you're still working in the PSD file, you can merge selected layers to reduce file size and make a complex image easier to work with. Of course, merge layers only when you're done with them. You can merge selected layers by selecting **Layer**, **Merge Layers**.

Merge only visible layers by selecting **Layer**, **Merge Visible**. Merge the current layer with the layers below it by selecting **Layer**, **Merge Down**, or merge the current layer with layers linked to it by selecting **Layers**, **Merge Linked**. For the **Merge Down** and **Merge Linked** commands to work, the bottommost layer must be a raster layer. If it's a shape or text layer, simplify the layer first (which converts it to raster data) by selecting **Layer**, **Simplify Layer**.

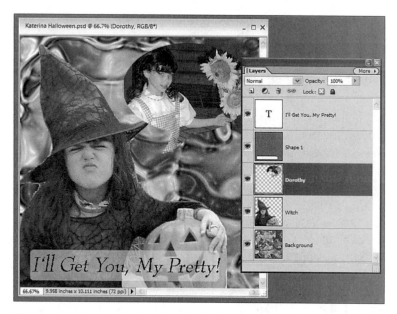

You can build a complex image by isolating each element on its own layer.

▶ NOTE

When you select a region of an image to restrict editing to that region, you're also restricting your edits to that region on the currently selected layer—unless you specify otherwise when making the selection.

Layers are listed in the **Layers** palette. A digital photograph starts out with a single layer called the *background layer*. The background layer is locked and cannot be moved within the layer stack; if you try to erase pixels on a background layer, they are not made transparent, but instead are changed to the current background color. Also, the background layer's opacity (transparency) and blend mode (how its pixels blend with layers below) cannot be changed. If you want to make changes to the background layer, you must first convert it to a regular image layer by selecting the layer and choosing **Layer**, **New**, **Layer from Background**. The name of the current layer is highlighted in the **Layers** palette; with a few exceptions, any changes you make apply only to the current layer. To select a layer for editing, click its name in the **Layers** palette. To select only the opaque pixels on a layer, press **Ctrl** and click the layer's thumbnail on the **Layers** palette.

▶ **KEY TERM**

Background layer—The lowest layer in an image; it cannot be moved in the layer stack until it is converted to a regular layer.

When needed, you can add layers to an image, including image layers (which contain a portion of an image), fill layers (filled with color, gradient, or pattern), and vector layers (which are created automatically when you add text or shapes to an image). You can also add an adjustment layer to test an adjustment (such as a brightness change) without making that adjustment permanent and control the amount of an adjustment or to apply the same adjustment to several layers at once.

The **Layers** palette shows you which layers are on top of others and which are beneath, with upper layers obscuring the layers beneath them. Move layers up or down the layer stack by dragging them on the **Layers** palette; to hide a layer temporarily, click its **Visible** icon. You can control how much a layer blocks the data in the layers below it by moving its **Opacity** slider at the top of the **Layers** palette. A layer that's 100% opaque is like new paint on a wall—it completely blocks the wall color beneath. Set the opacity to 50%, and the layer covers lower layers only partially—like a sheer veil. You can also control which areas of an image layer are seen by applying a *clipping mask*, which you'll learn how to do in 🔲 **Mask an Image Layer**. In a similar manner, a mask on a fill layer, which blocks the fill from covering portions of the layers below. On an adjustment layer, a mask can act as a blanket, protecting selected parts of a layer from changes such as a color adjustment.

▶ **NOTES**

To add a new layer, click the **New Layer** icon at the top of the **Layers** palette. The layer is added above the current layer in the **Layers** palette. To rename a layer, double-click its name on the **Layers** palette, type a new name, and press **Enter**. To delete the currently selected layer, click the **Delete Layer** button on the **Layers** palette.

To duplicate a layer and its contents, select the layer and choose **Layer**, **Duplicate Layer**; type a name for the layer and click **OK**. You can also use this command to copy a layer and place it in another image. You can quickly duplicate a layer by dragging it onto the **Create New Layer** button on the **Layers** palette. To copy a layer into another image quickly, drag the layer from the **Layers** palette and drop it in the other image window.

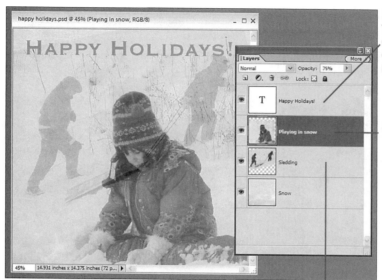

Because the Text Is Fully Opaque, It Obscures the Layers Below

The Partially Opaque Pixels of the Playing in Snow Layer Only Partially Obscure the Sledding Layer Below

Upper layers can obscure lower layers, depending on their opacity.

The Transparent Pixels in the Sledding Layer Allow the Snow Layer to Show Through Where Needed

If a layer is locked so you can't make changes to it, the **Lock** icon displays to the right of the layer name. When the layer is locked, you cannot change its blend mode, opacity, or layer style. You also can't remove a locked layer from an image. Although the background layer is always locked, you can lock any layer by selecting the layer and then clicking the **Lock All** button at the top of the **Layers** palette. Click the icon again to unlock the layer. You can lock just the transparency of a layer if you want by clicking the **Lock Transparent Pixels** button at the top of the **Layers** palette. When a layer has locked transparency, you cannot edit the opacity of a pixel on that layer, but you can change the pixel's color, brightness, or saturation. The **Lock** icon appears on the layer, but you can tell that the layer is only partially locked by moving the mouse pointer over the **Lock** icon and reading the message that appears.

When you select a layer in the **Layers** palette, any layers linked to the active layer display the **Link** icon. When layers are linked, they work together as a group. You can move, copy, rotate, resize, skew, or distort the linked layers as if they were one. To link layers, select them by pressing **Ctrl** and clicking each layer; then click the **Link Layers** button at the top of the **Layers** palette. A link icon appears on the selected layers. Click the **Link Layers** button again to unlink the layers if you want to resize, rotate, skew, distort, copy, or move a single layer rather than the linked group.

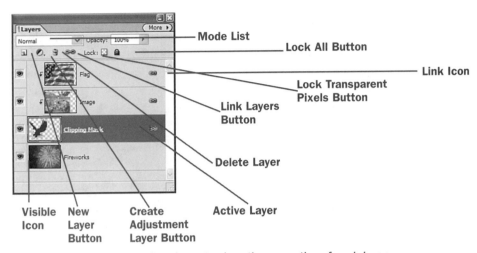

Mode List — Normal

Lock All Button

Link Icon

Lock Transparent Pixels Button

Link Layers Button

Delete Layer

Visible Icon | New Layer Button | Create Adjustment Layer Button | Active Layer

The Layers palette uses various icons to show the properties of each layer.

Another way you can change how an upper layer's data affects the layers below it is through that layer's blend mode. By default, the blend mode for each new layer is set to Normal, which means that layer's pixels block data but do not blend with the data on layers below it. You can change a layer's blend mode by activating that layer in the Layers palette and selecting the blend mode you want to use from the Mode list at the top of the Layers palette. Refer to the Sams Publishing website (www.samspublishing.com) for this book for a description of each blend mode and how it causes the pixels on the layer to blend with pixels on the layers below it.

About Selecting a Portion of a Photo

The Editor enables you to select a portion of a layer or layers to isolate that part of an image for editing. For example, if you select a portion of a layer and then begin painting, the paint affects only the selected area on that layer and none of the pixels outside it. Here, the selection acts as a kind of painter's tape, preventing the paint from spilling outside its borders and affecting the pixels you don't want to change. This same protection applies to any adjustment you might apply; for example, if you adjust the brightness after making a selection, only the pixels within the selected area are affected. You might also select an area when you want to delete, copy, rotate, resize, or move its pixels to another image or layer.

▶ **NOTE**

The Editor provides several tools for selecting the area you want to affect: the **Marquee** tools (which help you select a regularly shaped region such as a rectangle or circle), the **Selection Brush** tools (which enable you to paint or scribble over an area to select it), the **Lasso** tools (which enable you to select any region you can draw freehand or by tracing the edge of an object), and the **Magic Wand** (which selects pixels of a similar color with a single click). You'll learn how to use each of these tools later in this book.

The Editor gives you a variety of tools you can use to select the area you want to affect. You can combine tools, if you like, to select a complex area. Buttons on the **Options** bar (for all the selection tools but the **Selection Brush** tools) allow you to add, subtract, or intersect an existing selection. The selected area is marked with a *selection-marquee* so you can easily see the area you selected and distinguish it from the rest of the image (the unselected area).

▶ KEY TERM

Selection marquee—Moving dashes that mark the boundary of a selection.

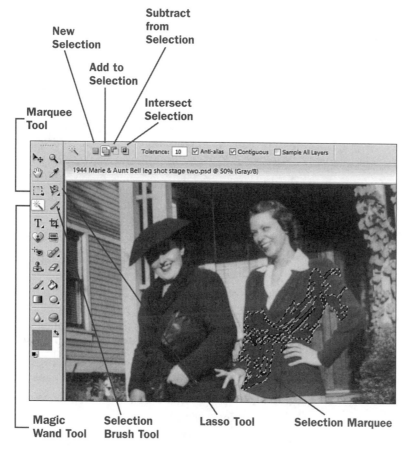

With a selection tool, you define where changes are to take place.

After you make a selection, the selection remains until you remove it. You can't make changes to the area outside a selection, so you'll need to remove the selection to affect other areas. To remove a selection, press **Esc** or choose **Select, Deselect**. To reselect the previous selection, choose **Select, Reselect**. To hide the marquee temporarily (but keep the selection in place), choose **View, Selection**.

You can modify a selection in many ways. You can move the selection marquee if needed to position the selected area precisely. Just click any of the selection tools, click inside the marquee, and drag the marquee into position. You can feather its edge to soften it, expand or contract it by a certain amount, smooth a selection's curved edges, or select just the area at the edges of a selection to create a border. To select everything *but* the current selection, invert the selection by choosing **Select, Inverse**.

Filters, Effects, and Layer Styles

Professional photographers often attach a filter to the front of the camera lens to bend the light coming into the camera and create visual effects. In the Photoshop Elements Editor, a *filter* can also be used to create a visual effect far beyond the capability of a mere lens attachment. For example, you can use a filter to change your image as though it were rendered by a watercolor brush, sketched with a charcoal pencil on coarse-bond art paper, or burned into a plate of steel with a blowtorch. You can also use filters for less artistic reasons, such as blurring the background around a subject, sharpening a photo, or removing scratches and small blemishes. You choose a filter from the **Filter** menu and configure its options using the dialog box that appears. You can also select a filter from the **Styles and Effects** palette by selecting **Filter** from the first drop-down list and then double-clicking the filter you want to apply. You'll learn how to apply various filters in upcoming tasks.

▶ KEY TERM

Filter—A series of computer instructions that modifies the pixels in an image.

▶ NOTE

Filters typically work only on RGB color images, although most work on grayscale images as well. See **19** Change Color Mode for help in changing color modes. In addition, you can't apply a filter to text unless you convert that text to raster data first. If you want to apply the filter to only a portion of an image, select that area first and then apply the filter.

Effects are time-savers—typically, an effect is a collection of several filters and other image adjustments applied automatically in a particular sequence to create a special effect. Effects can be applied to an entire layer, to a selection, to text, or to a flattened image with no layers. You can't make adjustments to an effect as you can with a filter; effects are a take-it-or-leave-it kind of thing. To apply an effect, select **Effects** from the first drop-down list on the **Styles and Effects** palette. Then double-click the effect thumbnail to apply that effect.

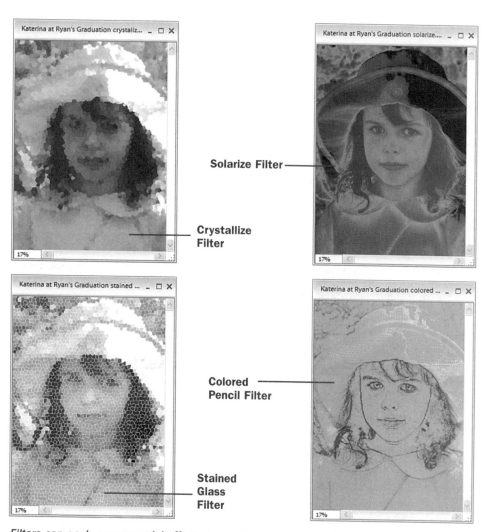

Solarize Filter

Crystallize
Filter

Colored
Pencil Filter

Stained
Glass
Filter

Filters can apply many special effects to your images.

Most effects are applied to a copy of the current layer, but some effects are applied to the entire image, after first merging the layers. You can narrow the list of effects by selecting an effects group from the second drop-down list. If an effect's name includes the notation (**selection**), the Editor will flatten all layers first, insert a new layer above the flattened layer, and apply the effect on that new layer within the selection. If an effect's name includes the notation (**type**), that effect can be applied only to a text layer. If an effect's name includes the notation (**layer**), that effect will be applied to a new layer above the current one.

▶ KEY TERM

Effect—A combination of filters and other image manipulations applied together auto-matically.

A *layer style* is often applied to the edges of objects or text on a shape or text layer. These "edge styles" are listed in the first grouping in the **Layer Style** list box on the **Styles and Effects** palette. For example, you can add a bevel layer style to apply a chiseled look to your text. You can also apply a layer style to the object itself, filling that object with a special texture or pattern. For example, using the **Orange Glass** layer style, you can make an object or some text look as if it were made from orange glass. These filler styles are listed in a second group-ing in the **Layer Style** list on the **Styles and Effects** palette.

▶ KEY TERM

Layer style—A design that's applied to layer data, meaning either all the objects on a layer, such as text or drawn objects, or to the layer as a whole. As new data is added to the layer, the style is applied to that data as well.

To apply a layer style, simply select an appropriate layer (a text layer, for exam-ple, for an edge style) and click the layer style you want to apply from those listed in the **Styles and Effects** palette. If you apply a layer style to a regular layer instead of to a shape or text layer, the layer style may replace all the data on that layer, depending on what that data is. If the layer is filled with an image, for example, the filler styles typically replace the image and fill the layer. If the layer contains pixels you've painted or drawn with the **Brush** or **Pencil** tool, or if it contains objects you've simplified to bitmap data, the filler styles fill only the interior of those drawings and not the entire layer. If you later change the bitmap data (for example, paint with a brush on the layer), the layer style is applied to the new data as well. Layer styles are cumulative, so the order in which they are applied to a layer is often important because that order can produce different results. With filters, effects, and layer styles, it's typically best to apply the filter, effect, or style you're thinking about and then use the **Undo** button to remove it if it doesn't work out as you thought. To remove a layer style after it is applied, select **Layer, Layer Style, Clear Layer Style**.

▶ TIPS

You can adjust the scale of a layer style after applying it if you don't like the result. For example, if you apply the **Puzzle** layer style (it's grouped with the other **Image Effects** layer styles) and want the puzzle pieces to look smaller, select **Layer, Layer Style, Scale Effects**. Then select a percentage (less than 100% makes the pattern smaller; more than 100% makes it bigger).

When a layer style is added to a layer, a small, cursive *f* appears next to the layer's name on the **Layers** palette. Click this **f** to display the **Style Settings** dialog box, which enables you to make small changes to the layer style. Right-click the **f** and select **Clear Layer Style** to remove the layer style altogether.

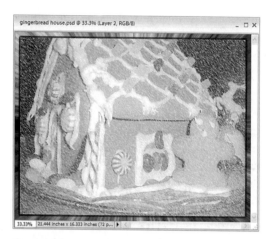

The Blizzard effect adds a chilly air to this scene, whereas the Angled Spectrum layer style applied to the border adds whimsy.

When to Use the Photoshop File Format

Your digital camera stores its photos in one of the universal image formats: perhaps JPEG, TIFF, or a version of RAW format customized by your specific camera manufacturer. Your digital scanner probably uses one of these formats as well. RAW format is uncompressed and can be considered a "digital negative" of your image, provided you have a program that can read the format. (Photoshop Elements can read most RAW formats, but you should check first before recording images you might want to edit later in RAW format.) But none of these formats is appropriate for saving work in progress—images with multiple layers, such as text, shape, and image layers.

True, TIFF format is capable of storing layer data. But a layered TIFF file might not be readable by some programs and will probably be considerably larger than Photoshop Element's default format—Photoshop (PSD) format. When you save an image in Photoshop format, all the image data is saved, such as layers, masks, saved selections, areas of transparency, and hidden data. When you complete your work on an image, you can merge all the layers and data into a single layer and then save the single-layer image in a smaller, universal format such as JPEG or non-layered TIFF. If you want the file to be usable on another computer and want the layers preserved, you can choose not to merge the layers and save them in a layered TIFF file that should be readable by most graphics editors. Even so, a lot of graphics editors these days can read PSD files easily, so converting your file to a layered TIFF might not be necessary.

Using the Welcome Window

Every time you start Photoshop Elements, you're greeted by the **Welcome** window. You can use its controls to start either the Editor or the Organizer, so you can quickly locate an image for editing, review a tutorial on an unfamiliar feature, watch the product overview, or start a new image or creation. To dismiss the **Welcome** window, click its **Close** button; to redisplay the **Welcome** window at any time, select **Window, Welcome** from the menu bar.

The buttons at the top of the **Welcome** window provide quick access to the most common tasks you'll want to perform at the start of a work session, such as importing images into the Organizer catalog, editing an image using **Quick Fix** or **Standard Edit** mode, beginning a new image, or starting a creation. You'll learn the specific steps for performing each of these actions in upcoming tasks.

To view the product overview, click the **Product Overview** button. To start a tutorial, click the **Tutorials** button at the top of the window. To open your web browser and display Adobe's home page, click the **Adobe** button at the bottom of the window.

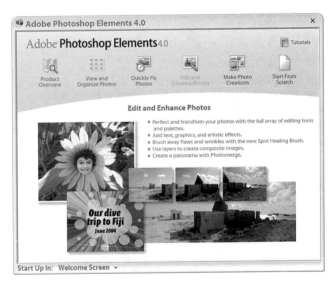

*The **Welcome** window provides a quick way to start your image editing session.*

Changing Preferences

Like most other programs, Photoshop Elements enables you to tweak its default settings to suit your needs. To change preferences in the Editor or the Organizer, select **Edit**, **Preferences** and then select the type of preferences you want to change from the submenu that appears. For example, in the Editor, select **Edit**, **Preferences**, **Saving Files** to change the way in which images are saved; in the Organizer, select **Edit**, **Preferences**, **Scanner** to change the default file type and resolution for images scanned into the Organizer catalog. The **Preferences** dialog box is then displayed with the appropriate page open.

▶ TIP

If you want to reset the currently displayed set of preferences back to default settings, in the Organizer, click **Restore Default Settings**. In the Editor, you can't reset to the defaults, but you can reset it to the way the dialog box looked before you opened it by clicking **Reset**.

After making changes to a set of preferences, save those changes by clicking **OK**. To change from one set of preferences to another in the Editor **Preferences** dialog box, select the set of options you want to view from the drop-down list at the top of the dialog box or click the **Next** button to view the next set of preferences in the list. Return to a previous set of preferences by clicking **Prev** instead. To change to a different preference set in the Organizer **Preferences** dialog box, select that set from the list on the left.

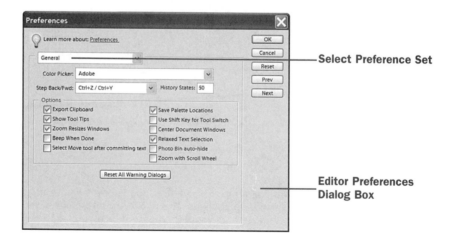

Select Preference Set

Editor Preferences
Dialog Box

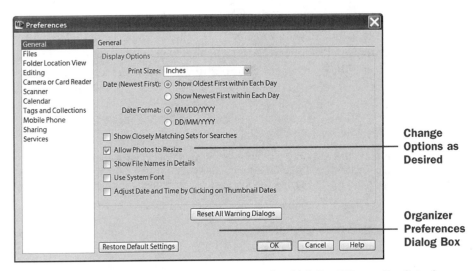

Use the **Preferences** dialog box to change the way in which the Editor or the Organizer perform basic tasks.

How to Undo Mistakes

Like a lot of programs, both the Editor and the Organizer remember the changes
you make to an image or the catalog and enable you to undo those changes as
needed. When you click the **Undo** button on the **Shortcuts** bar or select **Edit**,
Undo XXX from the menu (where *XXX* is the name of the action you want to
undo), Photoshop Elements undoes the most recent change. To undo the next
most previous change, click **Undo** or select **Edit**, **Undo** again. Whatever can be
undone can also be redone. Just click **Edit**, **Redo** or click **Redo** to undo the most
recent undo operation and return the image to the state it was in before you
clicked **Undo**.

▶ **TIP**

If you save an image while you're working on it, you can still undo changes you've made.
After you close the image, you can't undo the changes. This is true in the Organizer as
well: Changes to the catalog can be undone until you either close the catalog and open
a different one or simply exit the Organizer.

If you want to undo multiple changes in the Editor, use the **Undo History** palette.
Select **Window**, **Undo History** to display the palette. Changes are listed in the
order in which they occurred, with the most recent change appearing at the bottom. Drag the slider up from the bottom to undo changes, or simply select any
change from the list. All the changes made up to that point are undone in one
step (changes that have been undone appear faded to indicate that they no
longer apply to the current image). You can still redo the changes by dragging

the slider back down or clicking a change that's lower in the list than the last retained change. To clear the history list of all changes for the current image, click the **More** button and select **Clear Undo History** from the **More** menu.

▶ **NOTES**

To change the limit for the number of changes to an image the Editor can undo, select **Edit, Preferences, General.** Then adjust the **History States** value (the maximum value is 100) and click **OK.**

If you have several images open, the Editor remembers separate change histories for each image. When you display the **Undo History** palette, it lists only changes for the current image. Again, after an image is closed or you exit the Editor, you won't be able to undo your changes.

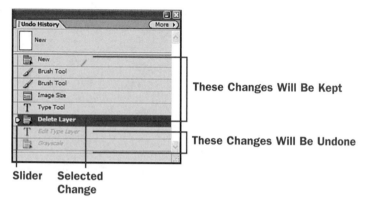

These Changes Will Be Kept

These Changes Will Be Undone

Slider   Selected
          Change

*The **Undo History** palette enables you to undo multiple changes in one step.*

Working with Premiere Elements

It really is pretty amazing when you think about how far video technology has come in such a short time. Just a little more than 20 years ago, broadcast professionals were editing analog video using what was essentially a mechanical controller between two VCRs. (And, before that, editors were literally cutting and splicing tape—a primitive age best forgotten.) The innovation of computer-based, nonlinear digital editing has not only changed the way video is assembled; it has changed our entire concept of the editing process.

Nonlinear editing takes a process that was once stressful, time-consuming, and expensive, and turns it into something that is intuitive, simple, and above all, easily revisable. There's more freedom to be creative, to try new things, to experiment, and to play.

Before Premiere Elements, most video-editing software aimed at consumers was designed with an easy-to-use interface as its priority. Adobe, however, took a different tack. Using as its base its top-of-the-line prosumer video-editing software, Premiere Pro, Adobe stripped back a few higher-end and professional features (features you will probably never miss), made many of the features more user-friendly, and produced an application that combines both a relatively simple, intuitive interface with the power and customizable features of a professional editing package. A product that's easy to learn—and yet capable of going as deep as the user dares to dig.

But dig a little deeper and you'll find even more. And more. In fact, every time you think you've discovered everything this program can do, you round a corner and find even more features, more things to customize, and more tricks, tweaks, and new applications. Premiere Elements can take you as far as you dare to go with your videos.

And that's the good news.

The bad news, though, is now that you are armed with Premiere Elements 2.0 and this book, you're never again going to have an excuse for creating a less-than-dazzling video. No more shoot-and-play home movies. No more boring family vacation videos.

Such is the responsibility that comes with a master's knowledge.

What Is Nonlinear Editing?

Throughout most of the past half century, video editing was done using a linear system. In other words, if you had a scene at the beginning of a videotape and you wanted to cut from it to a scene at the end of a videotape, you had to locate and dub the first scene onto a master tape, then *physically wind the tape* to the other end, locate the next scene, and then dub it onto the master. It took a lot of time and effort and, as whenever such logistics are challenging, it stifled, at least to some small degree, the creative process.

Nonlinear editing, which professionals began to incorporate into their workflow in the late 1980s, is about having an easier and more efficient way to access, juggle, and trim video clips. With nonlinear editing, rather than your video clips being stored in a linear format (such as on a videotape), scenes or clips are stored in an easily accessible catalog or bin where they can be quickly grabbed in any order, thrown together, cut, trimmed, rearranged, and reassembled. Your project can then be easily previewed, test-driven, undone, redone, revised, tweaked, and massaged until it is precisely the movie you want to make—and all with little more effort than editing text in a word processor.

▶ KEY TERM

Nonlinear editing—A computer-based video-editing system in which collected media can be easily assembled, trimmed, and re-ordered indefinitely.

This innovation gives you total creative freedom to experiment, to dream, to pull together in seconds what used to take minutes or hours—and then to throw it all away and try it again without even working up a sweat. That's total creative freedom, unhindered by any logistics.

And there's another advantage to nonlinear editing: The process is *nondestructive*. Simply put, this means that no matter what or how much you cut, trim, or manipulate your video project, the original clips remain unaltered. You can safely experiment with dozens of clips and effects assemblages, knowing that nothing you do will affect the original footage. The original clips remain fresh and unchanged, ready to be reused or reassembled into the next draft. Nothing is risked; nothing that's done can't be undone. It's like sketching with a pencil attached to the world's most efficient eraser!

▶ NOTE

In addition to the nondestructive nature of the nonlinear editing process, Premiere Elements offers the option to Undo (**Ctrl+Z**) all the way back to the most recent opening of your project. You can also jump back to certain points in your work by locating these points in the **History** panel.

A Few Key Premiere Elements Terms You Ought to Know

Before you begin to explore this program, several key features and terms—some unique to or uniquely used by Premiere Elements 2.0—crop up regularly. You'll definitely want to be clear on their definitions before you move forward:

- **Timeline**—This is where it all happens. The *Timeline* is the set of video and audio tracks where your clips assemble to become your video project. It's where you paint your masterpiece of sounds and images in time. Premiere Elements offers one of the most versatile timelines available at this level of software, with the potential for a virtually unlimited number of video and audio tracks.

  The vertical hairline that moves along the **Timeline** and indicates what part of the project is currently being viewed in the **Monitor** panel is called the current time indicator, or *CTI* for short.

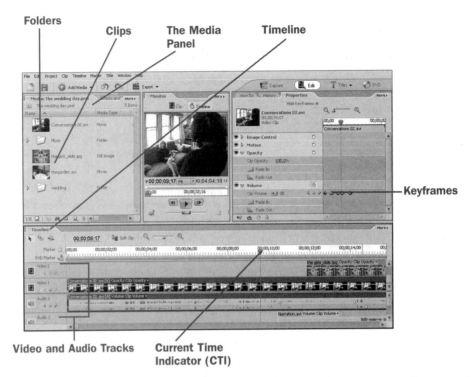

*Get familiar with the Premiere Elements **Edit** workspace and some common terms used there.*

▶ KEY TERMS

Timeline—The linear panel in which audio and video clips are assembled to create a video project.

CTI—The current time indicator is the vertical hairline that indicates your frame position on the **Timeline** (also known as the *playhead*).

- Clip—Although this word usually refers to a segment of video footage, Premiere Elements also uses the word to describe audio, photos, graphics, and other media you use in your video project. The reason for using *clips* as a universal term for your media is that, as far as your **Timeline** is concerned, all media is handled the same way. All clips—all media added to the Timeline—can be trimmed, sliced, effected, and transitioned into and out of.

▶ KEY TERM

Clip—Any graphic, still, audio, or video segment placed on the **Timeline** in a video project.

- **Folders**—*Folders* are one of the most useful and underused features of the **Media** panel (the panel to which all your clips are added when you import them into your project and from which you drag clips to the **Timeline**) and a feature Adobe has been incorporating into virtually all its products. What do you do when you've captured dozens of clips for your project and you're going crazy sifting through them all every time you want to locate one for a scene you're building? Add a folder to the **Media** panel. In fact, add several folders. Even add folders within folders. Name them. Drag your clips into them. When every set of clips is neatly categorized, you're just a few clicks away from any clip you want.

▶ KEY TERM

Folders—A sorting system used in the **Media** panel (similar to Windows Explorer's folder system) in which clips can be stored in collections and subcollections for easy access and categorization.

- **Scrubbing**—This term is used to describe the process of moving the **CTI** back and forth across the **Timeline** to locate a scene or to test a cut, transition, or effect. Premiere Elements offers a variety of ways to do this at a variety of speeds, including keyboard shortcuts and mouse controls. *Scrubbing* is something you'll be doing countless times as you build your project, and you'll very quickly be operating the controls without even thinking about it. But the important thing for now is that when someone mentions scrubbing, you know what he is talking about.

▶ KEY TERM

Scrubbing—Manually moving the **CTI** back and forth along the **Timeline** to locate a specific clip or frame or to test a transition. Watch the video in the **Monitor** panel as you scrub on the **Timeline**.

- **Video tracks**—Think of your *video tracks* as a stack of clips. Most of the time, you'll only see the clip on the top of the stack. But if you resize the top clip or make portions of it transparent, the clip below shows. Resize or reshape many layers or add transparency to them and you can see down through several layers of video clips at the same time. You can add a virtually unlimited number of video and/or audio tracks to your Premiere Elements project. When you start seeing how useful tracks can be, you'll wonder how you ever edited without them. (See **91** **Add, Delete, and Size Tracks**.)

- **Keyframing**—An important tool in Premiere Elements that, once mastered, will give you an amazing amount of control over virtually every other feature and effect in the program. The principle of keyframes is basically this: You indicate the frames on your **Timeline** in which you want an effect to occur or a position or effect to change; Premiere Elements automatically creates the movement, effect, or animation transitioning between these frames. *Keyframing* shows up in many of this book's tasks. After you develop an understanding of how the process works, you'll find a universe of ways to customize your effects, animation, and transitions with them. (See **119 Pan and Zoom a Photo a la Ken Burns**.)

▶ KEY TERM

Keyframing—The method used by Premiere Elements (as well as Premiere Pro and After Effects) for creating motion paths and transitioning effects. Points representing precise settings for effects or positions are placed on the **Timeline**, and the program automatically creates a movement or transition between those points.

- Rendering—In common video-editing use, this term refers to the process of converting nonvideo clips (such as photos) or clips that have had **Transitions** or effects applied to them into frames of video. But there's another definition of this term that comes up regularly. As you add nonvideo media (such as photos and graphics) to your **Timeline**, you'll notice a red line appearing on the **Timeline** above the clips. The red line indicates that this segment of your timeline has not yet been hard rendered. So how does this affect your life? Well, when you first play back a still or clip that's been effected or keyframed (or a transition that has been added between two not-yet-rendered clips), you might be a little disappointed with the preview. That's because Premiere Elements is desperately trying to create these changed frames on the fly—and depending on how intensely you've affected the clips and how powerful your computer is, the result can look rather ragged and choppy. *Rendering* this segment creates a temporary file to which the program can refer that displays a much clearer preview of what your final output will look like. This type of hard rendering is easy. Just press the **Enter** key and watch as the red line turns green. Of course, if you change the effect or transition, you'll need to re-render the segment. Rendering usually takes only a few seconds. When it's done, you can see exactly what this portion of your video will look like when you're finished.

▶ KEY TERM

Rendering—The process in which Premiere Elements creates video frames from stills or transitioned or effected video clips.

Starting Premiere Elements 2.0

When you first launch Premiere Elements, you will find yourself at the *splash screen*. As you can see, this screen offers three main options: **New Project**, **Open**

Project, and **Capture Video**. On the right side of the screen, at the very top, are two other icons, **Tutorials** and **Setup**.

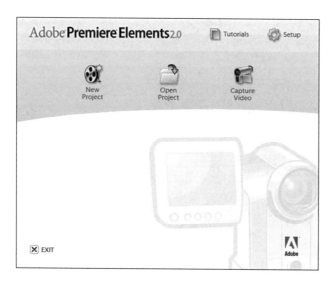

This is the splash screen; it is your starting point whenever you open Premiere Elements.

Use the **New Project** option to start a brand new project. You are asked to name your project before going to the Premiere Elements workspace. Use the **Open Project** option to open an existing project. When you click this icon on the splash screen, the **Browse** dialog box opens so you can select the project you want to open. The **Capture Video** option takes you right to the **Capture** window, ready to capture (import) video. See **77 Capture Digital Video Using FireWire** and **78 Capture Digital Video Using USB** for further instructions.

▶ NOTES

Premiere Elements project files end in **.prel**. When looking for existing project files, look for files with the **.prel** extension.

Premiere Elements Version 1 users beware: If you open a version 1 project and save it in version 2, you will not be able to open that project in version 1 again. To preserve the version 1 file, open it and choose **File**, **Save As** to save the file as a version 2 file, leaving the version 1 file unaltered.

When you click the **Tutorials** icon, you are taken into the Premiere Elements workspace and the **Tutorial** project opens. This is a short project, complete with Help, that introduces you to many of the concepts involved in creating a movie. The **Setup** window allows you to set the format for your projects: NTSC or PAL, Standard or Widescreen. (Get to this screen by clicking the **Setup** icon in the upper-right corner of the splash screen.) This is where you select a default format for your first and future projects. By selecting the **New Preset** button, you can change some of the settings and create your own customized preset format, making that the default for your projects. Click **New Project** to begin.

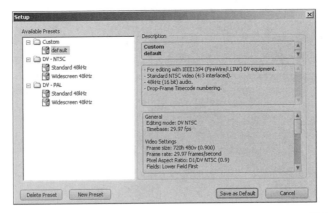

*This is the splash screen's **Setup** window; you can select NTSC (the television system primarily used in North America and Japan) or PAL (the television system used in most of Europe) settings for your projects.*

Understanding the DV-AVI Workflow

When working with Premiere Elements, as with any video-editing software, it's important to understand the difference between digital and analog video. In simple terms, it's the difference between an old-fashioned clock and a digital watch or between a record album and a CD.

In the old days (actually more like 10 years ago), consumer camcorders recorded video the way tape recorders record sound: Impulses of light and sound were translated into electronic pulses that were recorded magnetically onto a moving tape. Naturally, the quality of those pulses was limited by the camera's optics, the quality of the recording head, and the quality of tape. But the biggest liability was that every time a copy was made of the video, it was merely an analog attempt to reproduce an analog signal. With each copy, the quality of the recording diminished. Every generation of the video was a continually degraded approximation of the generation before.

Digital video was a major step forward for video quality. Rather than simply capturing electronic impulses of light and sound, digital video takes approximately 25 or 30 snapshots of more than 450,000 *pixels* of light and thousands of samplings of sound every second and records them not as electronic pulses but as binary code—exactly the same binary code your computer uses. The quality of this data is limited only by the camera's light and sound sensors. More importantly, when a copy is made, rather than simply approximating the original recording, the data itself is transferred from one source to another—meaning that each copy of the digital data is *identical* to the original recording!

▶ KEY TERMS

Digital video—Also called DV, it is video that records sound and motion as computer data, or chains of 1s and 0s.

Pixel—The basic building block of digital images. Although they seem to be painted with continuous color, digital images—on television, on your computer, or in your digital camera—are actually composed of tiny rectangles (pixels) of various settings of red, green, and blue. In most cases, pixels are so small that they blend into a smooth flow of color. However, when an image is stretched beyond its intended resolution, or *overrezzed*, the pixels become visible, and the image appears jagged or *pixelated*.

When transferred into your computer using an IEEE-1394 connection (commonly called *FireWire*) or *USB Video Class 1.0*, the video data stream from your digital camcorder remains virtually unchanged. The computer merely packages the digital video (DV) data into *DV-AVI* clips. You can edit those clips, cut them, and reassemble them. When you output the data back to your camcorder, it comes out in the same type of binary code stream as it went in. In other words, when working from a digital video camcorder and using a DV-AVI workflow, your camcorder and computer speak the same binary language.

▶ KEY TERMS

FireWire—Initially a brand name for Apple's high-speed data connection, it has become universal shorthand for any OHCI-compliant IEEE-1394 connection. It is also the current standard for transferring digital video data from a camcorder to a computer and back again.

USB Video Class 1.0—A relatively new high-speed standard for transferring digital video from specially equipped camcorders to a computer over a USB 2.0 connection.

The two forms of digital video available on consumer camcorders are miniDV and Digital8. The differences are minor. They both use exactly the same method for coding and transferring the digital video information, and they both create identical DV-AVI data streams when connected to a computer. The only difference is in the media themselves. MiniDV uses a small cassette specifically designed to work in miniDV camcorders. Digital8 uses slightly cheaper 8mm videocassettes (Hi-8 tapes are recommended). Additionally, many Digital8 camcorders can also play 8mm and Hi-8 analog tapes, an advantage when it comes to transferring video from these tapes into a computer.

DV-AVI is the *lingua franca* of PC-based video editing. All video-editing applications speak it fluently, and it is the highly recommended format for transferring files between your camcorder and the editing program on your computer and back again.

Premiere Elements, like virtually all PC-based nonlinear editors, uses a *DV-AVI* workflow. That means that no matter what you put into it—photos, graphics, or other video file formats—Premiere Elements assimilates it as some form of DV-AVI (ultimately delivering the final product as a DV-AVI). This is one of the reasons Premiere Elements can sometimes find it challenging to work with *MPEGs*, QuickTime, Windows Media, and other video files.

▶ KEY TERMS

DV-AVI—A PC-based video file format, designated by the file extension **.avi**, but distinguished from other kinds of AVI files by its use of the near-lossless DV codec, or file compression system. Because of its perfect balance of size and quality, it is the preferred video format for PC-based video editors, as well as being the universal language that all PC-based video-editing software speaks.

MPEG—A video file format developed by the Motion Picture Experts Group, MPEG uses a temporal compression system, a system of compressing the file by reusing repeated elements from frame to frame, that produces very small files—although they are sometimes technically challenging to edit. Although Premiere Elements 2.0 can work with MPEGs, you should consider them to be chiefly a *delivery* format (the files you burn to your DVDs) and not the preferred format for editing.

A number of products are available that convert analog video into digital files for your computer. Although Premiere Elements 2.0 is capable of handling a wide variety of video file types, it's always to your advantage to use a product that produces DV-AVI files. We recommend a few modestly priced pieces in **80 Capture Analog Video**.

For more information on transferring your camcorder's video into your computer, see **77 Capture Digital Video Using FireWire**. And for information on capturing video from DVD and MicroMV camcorders, as well as from unusual sources such as digital still cameras and picture phones, see **84 Add Media with the Adobe Media Downloader**.

A Word About System Requirements

Although Premiere Elements will work on most computers sold in the past five years or so, it is definitely to your advantage to have a more powerful system. DV-AVI video files devour huge chunks of hard drive space (at a rate of about a gigabyte of space for every five minutes of video), and the process of capturing, manipulating, effecting, rendering, and outputting those files, particularly on longer projects, can be very processor- (and hard drive space) intensive.

Intel P4 processors running at more than 1GHz, but less than 2.4GHz, will power the program, but to a limited degree. AMD processors require the SSE2 instruction set as noted in the following paragraph. You might have to shut down background processes in your operating system to capture and output, and rendering larger files can take a frustratingly long time if you're using one of these slower processors. (See **83 About Troubleshooting Capture Problems.**)

Intel P4 or above processors running at more than 2.4GHz should run the program effectively, with 3+GHz Hyper Threading Pentium 4, D, or M (including dual core) and Athlon XP 3000s, Athlon 64, and AMD Opteron and higher having more than adequate power to run all of the program's features. (Note that Premiere Elements works only with Athlons that use the SSE2 instruction set. A BIOS update might be required on some older machines, and pre-XP Athlon chips might not be able to run the program at all.)

Likewise, although 256MB of RAM is the minimum required by Adobe to run the program, at least 512MB is highly recommended and 1–2GB of RAM is ideal.

A large hard drive is also very important, not just because video files are huge but because Premiere Elements requires large amounts of free, contiguous hard drive space to write temp files and to use as *scratch disk* space. Maxing out a hard drive is something most people don't consider, but, especially with larger projects, it happens more often than you'd expect. At least 60GB of *free* space is recommended for a typical project, although high-demand projects might require more.

▶ **KEY TERM**

Scratch disk—An area of your hard drive in which Premiere Elements writes temporary files while rendering and encoding your project. Often the amount of scratch disk space needed to render and encode a project exceeds the size of the output file.

Although a second hard drive, one dedicated to your captured video and video temp files, is ideal (and is standard equipment for most professional editors), most desktop computers sold in the past year or two are more than capable of handling the video files and operating system on a single hard drive. However, if you experience data flow problems (such as dropped frames or interrupted capture or output), know that the installation of a second, video-dedicated hard drive often remedies the problem. (See **83 About Troubleshooting Capture Problems.**)

Finally, a nice, large monitor is definitely to your advantage when you're editing video. There's a lot going on onscreen, and you can greatly benefit from as much real estate as possible to allow for viewing all your timelines and having ready access to your tools and folders. Although a 17-inch monitor set to 1024×768 resolution will give you enough room to see everything, a 19-inch monitor with resolution settings at 1280×960 or higher allows you much more room to work.

For the truly ambitious, Premiere Elements supports dual monitors so you can place your **Monitor** panel on one screen and your controls and tools on the other. Whatever you choose, you'll find that you'll appreciate every pixel of screen space you can afford.

Putting It All Together

You will come to truly enjoy the ease of using Photoshop Elements and Premiere Elements side by side. In most cases, you will want to have both programs open at the same time, especially while working in Premiere Elements.

Of course, you can move files between the two programs in the usual way—that is, you can save a file in one program and then use **File**, **Open** or **File**, **Add Media** to get the file into the other program. With Photoshop Elements and Premiere Elements, however, there's an even simpler way. From the Premiere Elements main menu, select **File**, **New**, **Photoshop File**. This command opens a new blank image in the Photoshop Elements Editor.

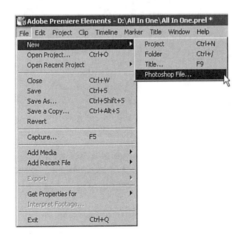

Open a new Photoshop file from Premiere Elements.

From the Photoshop Elements Organizer, select any images in the organizer you want to add to a current open project in Premiere Elements. Then, from the Photoshop Elements Organizer's main menu, select **File**, **Send to Premiere Elements**. All the selected images are added to the **Media** panel in your Premiere Elements project. You can send a single image, a group of Photoshop Elements images, a collection, or the entire contents of the Organizer.

PART I

Working with Photoshop Elements

IN THIS PART:

2

Importing Items into the Organizer Catalog

IN THIS CHAPTER:

By now you have probably accumulated quite a collection of digital images and are more than ready to start organizing them using the Photoshop Elements's Organizer. With the Organizer, you can quickly categorize your images and easily locate them later. At the heart of the Organizer is its catalog—in the catalog, you can organize all your images, regardless of their location, into whatever categories you choose. For example, if you want to organize all the photos of your son into a single grouping, you can do so even if those photos are stored in various locations on the hard disk and on several CDs or DVDs. To keep the Organizer running smoothly, you must keep its catalog in order, so in this chapter you'll learn not only how to add images to the catalog, but also to remove them when needed, to update the catalog when an image's location has changed, and to back up the catalog periodically (a process that backs up the catalog information *and* the media files it references). Finally, you'll learn how to back up the images themselves onto CD-ROM or DVD—something you might do to easily share images or take them to a kiosk (such as a Kodak Picture Maker) for printing.

❶ Import Media from a Folder, CD-ROM, or DVD

→ SEE ALSO

❷ Import Images from a Digital Camera

❸ Import and Separate Multiple Scanned Images

You might have recently received some photos by email and saved those photos to the hard disk, or you might have gotten a CD or DVD of photos from a friend or a photo processing lab. Because Organizer can categorize your images, you don't have to organize them on the hard disk into particular folders. For example, you could have simply saved all the email images with your other photos in the **My Pictures** folder, or you could have created a special folder just for those photos. When importing images from a CD or DVD, you can choose to keep the photos *offline*, and not copy them to the hard disk. If you choose to do this, low-resolution thumbnails of the images are created and displayed in the catalog; if you attempt to edit an offline image, you'll be prompted to insert the CD or DVD on which it's stored.

▶ KEY TERM

Offline—Images in the Organizer catalog that are stored on a CD-ROM or DVD, and not copied to the hard disk.

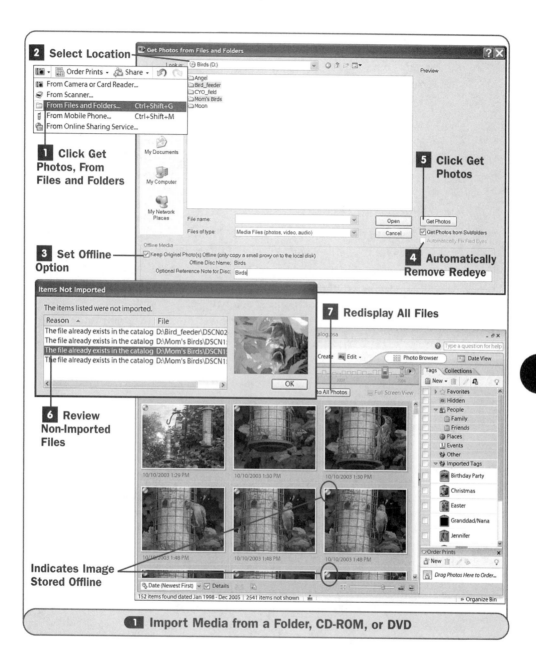

■1 Import Media from a Folder, CD-ROM, or DVD

▶ **TIP**

If you open a non-cataloged image in the Editor and make changes to it, you can add the image to the catalog when you save your changes. Just enable the **Include in the Organizer** option in the **Save As** dialog box.

1 Click Get Photos, From Files and Folders

In the Organizer, click the **Get Photos** button on the **Shortcuts** bar and then select **From Files and Folders** from the list that appears. You can also choose **File, Get Photos, From Files and Folders** from the menu bar.

If you've already inserted the CD or DVD, you can import the images by selecting **Organize and Edit pictures using Adobe Photoshop Elements** from the **What do you want to do?** list in the dialog box that Windows automatically displays.

2 Select Location

From the **Look in** drop-down list in the **Get Photos from Files and Folders** dialog box, select the drive that contains of the images you want to import. For example, if the files are located on the main drive, select **Local Disk (C)**. Select the folder that contains the images to import. Select multiple folders by pressing **Ctrl** and clicking each one. If you want to import the contents of any subfolders of selected folders, enable the **Get Photos from Subfolders** check box. If you're importing from a CD or DVD, and it doesn't contain any folders, skip this part.

3 Set Offline Option

If you're importing images from a CD or DVD and you want to keep the images offline (that is, you want to keep only low-resolution images in the catalog and leave the larger original images on the CD or DVD), enable the **Keep Original Photo(s) Offline** check box and type a name for the disc in the **Optional Reference Note for Disc** text box. If you do not enable the **Keep Original Photo(s) Offline** check box, the Organizer copies the files from the CD or DVD to the hard disk.

4 Automatically Remove Redeye

If the files you're importing are already on the hard disk, or if they're being copied there from a CD or DVD, you can have the Editor automatically remove red eye from the eyes of any people in the photos, before importing them into the catalog. Select the **Automatically Fix Red Eyes** option.

▶ **TIP**

The **Automatically Fix Red Eyes** option is perfectly safe; Photoshop Elements has an excellent red-eye fixer, and it saves its result in a new version of the image file in a version set. If you don't like the results for some reason, you can always delete the extra version of the image and go back to the original version.

5 Click Get Photos

Click **Get Photos** to begin the importing process. The **Getting Photos** dialog box appears, displaying each photo as it's added to the catalog. You can click **Stop** if you want to interrupt the importing process for some reason; only photos already imported at that point will appear in the catalog.

6 Review Non-Imported Files

After the import process is complete, the **Items Not Imported** dialog box might appear; it lists any files that were not imported because they were in an unsupported format or already in the catalog. Review the list and click **OK**.

7 Redisplay All Files

The Organizer might display a reminder telling you that the only images being displayed right now are those you have just imported; click **OK** to dismiss this warning box.

If you kept the images offline, a small CD icon appears in the upper-left corner of each small thumbnail. To redisplay all files in the catalog, click the **Back to All Photos** button on the **Find** bar.

▶ **NOTE**

Before importing images into the catalog, you can use the Editor to rename, resize, retouch, and reformat them at the same time. For example, you could copy images from your camera onto the hard disk and then rename them. See **17** **Rename, Resize, Reformat, and Retouch a Group of Images**. After processing the images and saving the results to the hard disk, import the images into the catalog by completing the steps in this task.

If the imported images contain metadata keywords (tags), the **Import Attached Tags** dialog box appears. You can add new tags to the **Organize Bin** to match the attached photo tags, or associate the attached tags with existing tags in the **Organize Bin**.

---

2   **Import Images from a Digital Camera**

→ SEE ALSO

1 Import Media from a Folder, CD-ROM, or DVD
3 Import and Separate Multiple Scanned Images

2 (margin tab)

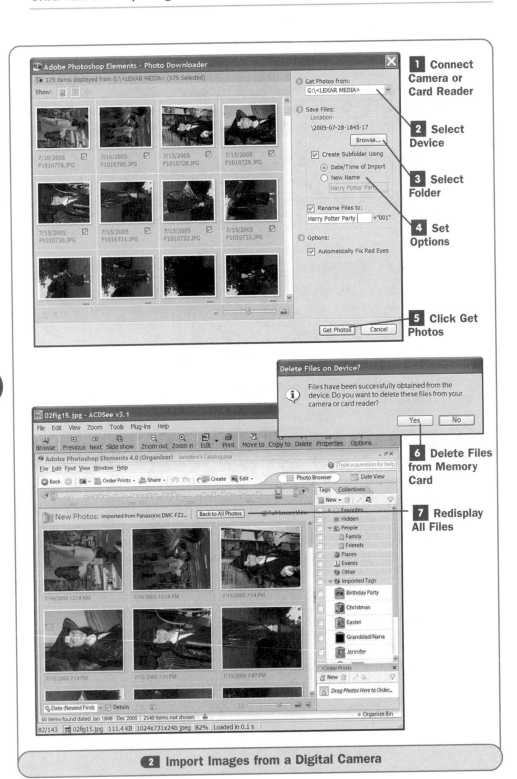

1 Connect Camera or Card Reader

2 Select Device

3 Select Folder

4 Set Options

5 Click Get Photos

6 Delete Files from Memory Card

7 Redisplay All Files

2 Import Images from a Digital Camera

You can import images directly from a digital camera and add them to the Organizer catalog. The method you use to do that, however, varies as much as digital cameras vary from one another. For a great many cameras, when you connect them to your computer using a USB, SCSI, or FireWire cable, Windows automatically detects the camera, reads its memory card, and displays the contents in a new drive window (a virtual drive) within **My Computer**. For example, your computer might have only one hard disk—drive C—but when you connect your digital camera, Windows presents you with a window that displays all the files on drive D, which is really the memory card inside your camera. At the same time, Photoshop Elements detects the virtual drive and launches its **Photo Downloader** to help you import the images into the catalog.

This same process occurs if you use a memory card reader. When you take the memory card out of the camera, insert it into the reader, Windows treats the contents of the memory card as a virtual (pretend) drive D or other drive letter. Once again, Photoshop Elements detects the virtual drive and launches the **Photo Downloader**.

1 Connect Camera or Card Reader

Connect the camera or the card reader to the computer, if it's not already connected. Adobe's **Photo Downloader** should automatically start and display the **Adobe Photo Downloader** dialog box. If Windows pops up a box asking if you want to use Adobe Photoshop Elements to organize and edit your files, click **Yes**, and the Downloader will start.

If the **Photo Downloader** does not start automatically, you can start it manually. In the Organizer, click the **Get Photos** button on the **Shortcuts** bar and select **From Camera or Card Reader** from the list that appears. You can also choose **File, Get Photos From Camera or Card Reader** from the menu bar. The **Get Photos from Camera or Card Reader** dialog box (which looks similar to the **Adobe Photo Downloader** dialog box shown here) appears.

▶ NOTE

If you can't get the Downloader to appear, use the driver that came with the camera to read its memory card. After copying the images to the hard disk using the camera's software, follow the steps in **1** Import Media from a Folder, CD-ROM, or DVD to import those images into the catalog.

2 Select Device

The card reader or camera should already be listed in the **Get Photos from** drop-down list. If not, open the list and select your camera or card reader (or its virtual drive letter) from the devices listed. After the memory card has been read, its images appear on the left side of the dialog box.

▶ **TIP**

You can change the camera preferences, such as the default folder in which images are stored, using the **Preferences** dialog box. Select **Edit, Preferences** from the Organizer main menu and then click **Camera or Card Reader.**

3 Select Folder

Your digital images will be copied to the **My Documents\My Pictures\ Adobe\Digital Camera Photos** folder. To change to a different folder, click the **Browse** button, select the folder into which you want to copy the new image files, and click **OK**.

4 Set Options

You can place the images you are importing into a subfolder of the folder you selected in step 3: First, enable the **Create Subfolder Using** check box. Then select either the **Date/Time of Import** option (if you want the subfolder to use the current date and time as its name) or **New Name** (if you want to name the subfolder yourself). If you chose the **New Name** option, type a name for the subfolder in the text box provided.

Because digital camera image files are typically given nondescript names such as **DSC00035.jpg**, you might want to tell the Organizer to rename the files as it imports them into the catalog. Just enable the **Rename Files to** check box and type a descriptive name in the text box. Organizer automatically adds a three-digit number to this description to create the filename. For example, if you type **Aunt Jane's Bday 2007** as the filename (notice the space I added at the end to separate the name from the number Organizer adds), files will be named **Aunt Jane's Bday 2007 001, Aunt Jane's Bday 2007 002**, and so on.

To automatically fix red eyes in any of your subjects, before importing the photos, select the **Automatically Fix Red Eyes** option.

▶ **TIP**

If you choose the **Automatically Fix Red Eyes** option, Photoshop Elements removes red-eye from each image and saves the result in an image file in a version set with the original image. If you don't like the results for some reason, you can always delete the extra version of the image and go back to the original version.

5 Click Get Photos

Click the **Get Photos** button to begin the importing process. The files are copied to the hard disk; if Organizer is not already started, it is started for you automatically. The **Getting Photos** dialog box appears, displaying each photo as it's added to the catalog. Click **Stop** if you want to interrupt the importing process for some reason; only photos already imported at that point will appear in the catalog.

▶ **NOTE**

If the imported images contain metadata keywords (tags), the **Import Attached Tags** dialog box appears. You can add new tags to the **Organize Bin** to match the attached photo tags, or associate the attached tags with existing tags in the **Organize Bin**.

6 **Delete Files from Memory Card**

After the files are imported into the Organizer, You might see a dialog box listing images that were not imported; typically, this is because the images are already in the catalog. If so, make a note of the images that were not imported and click **OK** to continue. Next, you'll see a dialog box asking whether you want to remove the images from the camera's memory card. Click **Yes** or **No** as desired.

7 **Redisplay All Files**

The Organizer might display a reminder telling you that the only images being displayed right now are those you have just imported; click **OK** to dismiss this warning box. To redisplay all files in the catalog, click the **Back to All Photos** button on the **Find** bar.

3

---

3 **Import and Separate Multiple Scanned Images**

→ **SEE ALSO**

55 Restore Quality to a Scanned Photograph

Although you can scan a photograph directly into the Organizer, using the **Get Photos, From Scanner** command, you might not want to. For example, if you think you'll need to edit the scan to remove spots and other imperfections or to improve the scan's color and contrast, why not import the scan directly into the Editor? After making changes, you can add the image to the Organizer when you save your edits.

Another reason why you might want to scan directly into the Editor is to exploit its capability to deal with multiple-image scans. If you've got multiple photographs to scan, you can lay them all on the scanner bed and perform a single scan. The Editor can then break up these images for you, creating the separate image files you need.

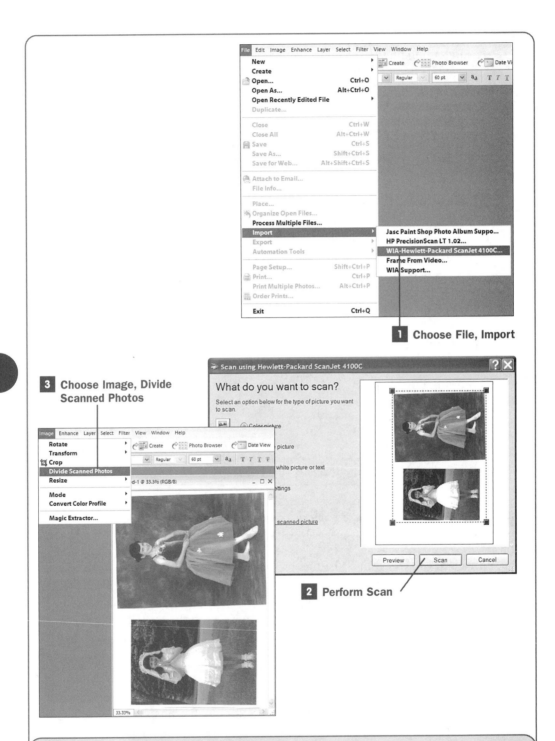

1 Choose File, Import

3 Choose Image, Divide Scanned Photos

2 Perform Scan

3 Import and Separate Multiple Scanned Images

4 **Click Save**

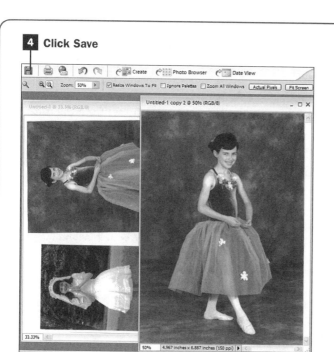

5 Save Image in Catalog

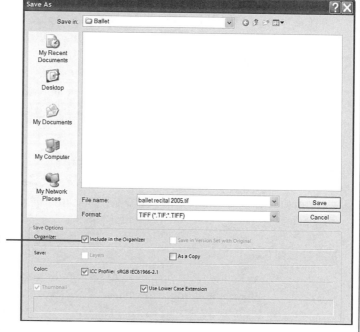

1 Choose File, Import

Lay the photograph(s) you want to scan on the scanner bed, leaving a small amount of space between them. This space enables the Editor to separate the images later on.

Choose **File, Import** from the menu bar and select your scanner from the list that appears. The program for your scanner automatically appears. My scanner happens to appear twice in the list—because it is *WIA* compliant, I'll choose that option.

▶ KEY TERM

WIA and TWAIN— Technologies that allow graphical software programs to communicate directly with digital cameras and scanners. TWAIN was replaced by WIA in Windows Me and Windows XP.

▶ TIP

If your scanner is not listed, select **WIA Support** from the menu. This option enables you to access the WIA support built into Windows, which might be able to clear up the problem by scanning for WIA- and TWAIN-compliant devices.

3

2 Perform Scan

The dialog box that appears displays the options available to your particular scanner. Shown here are the generic Windows scanning options. Adjust the options as desired (in this dialog box you'd click **Adjust the quality of the scanned picture**) and click **Scan** to scan the image(s) into the Editor.

I would choose as a minimum 70–100 PPI resolution for onscreen images, and 200–300 PPI for images you intend to print. Choosing higher resolutions for a scan can help you fix problems caused by scanning, such as moiré patterns.

3 Choose Image, Divide Scanned Photos

The image(s) appear in the Editor in a single, unsaved file. If you scanned multiple images, choose **Image, Divide Scanned Photos** from the menu. The Editor creates separate image files for you.

4 Click Save

None of the image file(s) are saved at this point. If you scanned multiple images, close the original scan window (the one with the multiple scanned images). Click **No** because you do not want to save this file.

Click each of the other image window(s), make changes as desired, and then click the **Save** button on the **Shortcuts** bar to save the image. The **Save As** dialog box appears.

▶ **TIP**

Scanned photographs often suffer from low brightness, poor contrast, low saturation, lack of sharpness, and may even contain moiré patterns. See **55** Restore Quality to a Scanned Photograph for help in improving your photographs after you scan them.

5 Save Image in Catalog

Select the folder in which you want to save the image from the **Save in** list, and type a name for the image in the **File name** box. Select an image type from the **Format** list. Select other options as desired, but be sure to enable the **Include in the Organizer** option so that the image is placed in the Organizer catalog. Click **Save** to save the image.

4 Locate Moved Files

As you are probably well aware by now, the Organizer catalog is not a collection of media files, but rather a listing of those files and their various locations on your hard disks, CDs, and DVDs. The Organizer is designed to keep track of any changes you initiate within its program (such as renaming, deleting, or editing images), but it is unaware of any file maintenance activities you perform on its media files outside of the program. If, for example, you use **My Computer** to move a file from one folder into another, the Organizer assumes that the file has simply disappeared. Similar problems arise if you rename or delete a file outside of the Organizer. Follow the steps in this task to remedy the problem, and reconnect the image thumbnail to its actual file on the hard disk.

To properly rename a file so that the Organizer keeps track of the modification, make the change within the Organizer using the **File, Rename** command. Move a file using the **File, Move** command. To delete a file from the Organizer catalog and from the hard disk (if you so choose), select it and press **Delete**.

▶ **TIP**

To tell Organizer to check for missing files periodically and to automatically reconnect them, choose **Edit, Preferences, Files** from the Organizer menu. Enable the **Automatically Search for and Reconnect Missing Files** option and click **OK**.

4

1 Select Moved Item

You may not know that a file's not connected to the catalog until you try to use it. Sometimes, a missing file icon will appear at the bottom of the image in the photo well. However you've identified a an image in the Organizer as being disconnected from its actual file, click the item in the Organizer to select it.

2 Choose File, Reconnect, Missing File

Choose **File, Reconnect, Missing File** from the menu bar. If you've moved a lot of files, you don't have to select any files in the catalog, but just choose **File, Reconnect, All Missing Files** instead. Typically, Organizer searches the hard disk so fast that it finds the missing file(s) right away, but if needed, click the **Browse** button in the searching box to display the **Reconnect Missing Files** dialog box.

3 Locate Actual File

In the **Reconnect Missing Files** dialog box, the original location and thumbnail of the missing image appear on the left. On the right side of the dialog box, the matching image and its new location appear. If Organizer didn't find the file (for example, you not only moved it, you also renamed it), from the drop-down list on the **Browse** tab, navigate to the folder in which the file is now located and select the file itself. You can select multiple files from the list on the left and choose the folder they are in on the right to reconnect a group of files.

4 Click Reconnect

Click the **Reconnect** button to update the file's location in the catalog. If you can't relocate the missing file and you no longer want the disconnected item in the catalog, click **Delete from Catalog** instead of **Reconnect**.

5 Click Close

You can reconnect files in other folders while the **Reconnect Missing Files** dialog box is open; just repeat steps 3 and 4. When you're through reconnecting files, click **Close**.

6 View the Result

After the file's new location is updated in the catalog, its thumbnail appears as normal in the photo well and the missing file icon is removed.

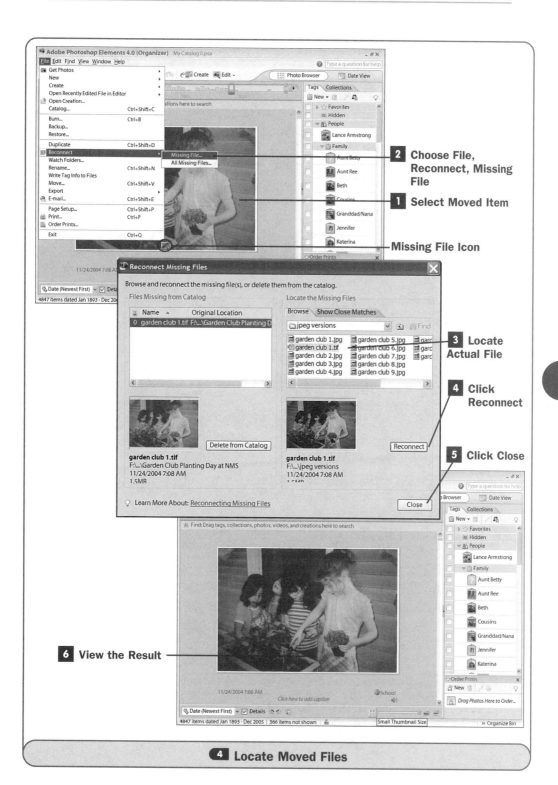

2 **Choose File, Reconnect, Missing File**

1 **Select Moved Item**

Missing File Icon

3 **Locate Actual File**

4 **Click Reconnect**

5 **Click Close**

6 **View the Result**

5 | Back Up the Organizer Catalog

After you've imported lots of images into the Organizer catalog and have used its features to organize your images, you won't want to risk losing your hard work. True, the catalog does not contain the images themselves (only a listing of their locations and names), so if something were to happen to the catalog, you wouldn't lose any photographs. What you would lose, however, are the *properties* of each image, such as the various tags and collections to which an image is associated, plus any audio captions or text notes you've appended to the images. You would also lose your creations and organizational information, such as an item's location, file size, file type, and thumbnail. If something happened to the catalog (but your media files were still okay), you could always reimport all your media files and then retag, annotate, and caption them, but that would be a lot of work. Therefore, periodically, you should back up *both* the Organizer catalog *and* your media files onto CD, DVD, or another drive in case something happens to your media files or the catalog. Lucky for you, the Organizer provides an easy method for you to do both in one simple process.

5

▶ **KEY TERM**

Properties—Information associated with each media file, such as its creation date, modification date, tags, collections, audio or text captions, or notes.

1 **Choose File, Backup**

In the Organizer, choose **File, Backup** from the menu bar. The first page of the **Burn/Backup** wizard appears.

2 **Choose Backup the Catalog**

In Step 1 of the **Burn/Backup** wizard, select the **Backup the Catalog** option and click **Next** to continue. The **Missing Files Check Before Backup** dialog box might appear; if it does, use it to reconnect any moved files before continuing with the backup or simply click **Continue**. See **4** **Locate Moved Files**.

▶ **NOTES**

If something occurs to the catalog later on (such as a power surge that damages the file), you'll be prompted to recover the file—a process that fixes the damage. Simply choose **File, Catalog** from the menu, click the **Recover** button, and then click **OK**.

If the catalog file is so badly damaged that it can't be repaired using this method, create an empty catalog first by choosing **File, Catalog** and clicking **New**. Then choose **File, Restore** from the menu, locate the incremental backup file (if any, because it must be restored first), and click **Restore**. After the incremental backup file's restored, you'll be prompted to select the full backup file so that its data can be restored as well.

3 Select Backup Type

In Step 2 of the **Burn/Backup** wizard, select the type of backup you want to perform: To back up the entire catalog and all your media files, select **Full Backup**. To make an incremental backup that contains any new media files added to the catalog since the last backup, select **Incremental Backup**. Click **Next**.

4 Choose Backup Drive

In Step 3 of the **Burn/Backup** wizard, select the drive to which you want to copy the catalog and media files from the **Select Destination Drive** list. If you select a CD or DVD drive, you'll be prompted to insert the disc. Do so and click **OK** to return to the **Burn/Backup** wizard.

5 Set Options

If you are backing up the data onto a CD or DVD, type a **Name** for the disc. You can also adjust the write speed by selecting a different speed from the **Write Speed** list. You might do this if you have been having trouble with your CD-R drive and want to compensate for that by having the computer write the data more slowly.

If you are backing up to another hard drive and not a CD-ROM or DVD, you must select a folder into which you want the data copied. If you are performing an incremental backup, the folder you select must be different from the one you originally selected when you did the full backup. Click the **Browse** button next to the **Backup Path** text box, select a folder, and click **OK**.

If you're performing an incremental backup, you must tell the Organizer where the original backup file is located. Click the **Browse** button next to the **Previous Backup File** text box, select the file that contains the original backup, and click **OK**. If you backed up previously onto and a CD or DVD, you'll be prompted to insert that disc so that the Organizer can determine the backup set to which you want to add. You'll remove the disc later so that you can insert a new disc on which to copy the incremental backup.

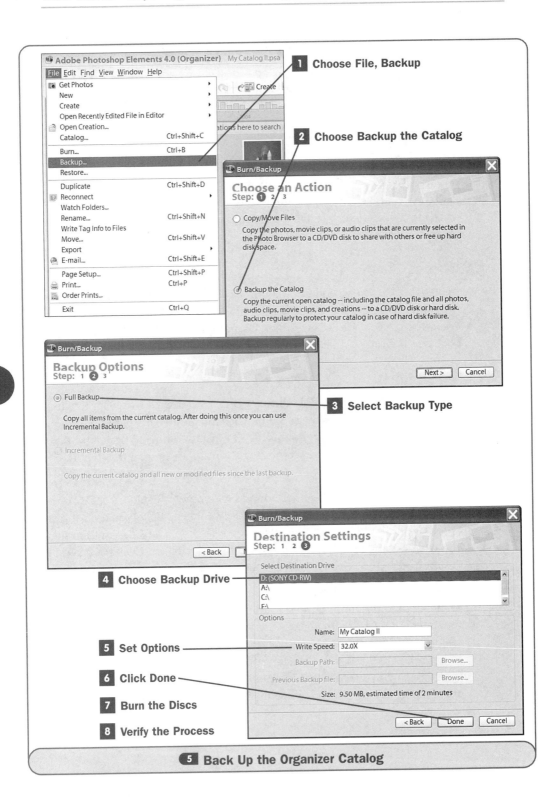

1 Choose File, Backup

2 Choose Backup the Catalog

3 Select Backup Type

4 Choose Backup Drive

5 Set Options

6 Click Done

7 Burn the Discs

8 Verify the Process

5 Back Up the Organizer Catalog

6 Click Done

Click **Done** to begin the backup process. If you are backing up the data onto a CD or DVD, you'll see a dialog box telling you how many discs you'll need to complete the backup. Click **Yes** to continue, and then follow the onscreen instructions.

If you are performing an incremental backup, the original backup disc is probably still in the drive (if you backed up to CD or DVD). If so, you'll be prompted at the proper time to remove the first disc and insert an additional disc on which to store the incremental backup. When the backup is complete, be sure to label any removable discs with the date and time of the backup.

7 Burn the Discs

The Organizer takes a moment to calculate how many discs you'll need and displays that information in the next dialog box. Click **Burn** to initiate the copy/move process. After a disc is completed, you'll see a reminder to label the disc properly.

8 Verify the Process

A message appears asking whether you want to verify the new disc. This process takes a while, but it also guarantees that the discs were created properly and can be read (which is time well spent if you later have to recover items from the discs). Click **Verify** to continue. At the end of the verification process, you'll be told whether everything is okay. If the verification detects any errors, repeat these steps to create a new series of discs. Otherwise, click **Don't Verify** to continue. window.

Click **OK** to continue. If an additional disc is needed to copy or move the files, you'll be prompted to insert additional discs until the procedure is complete.

5

3

Organizing Items in the Catalog

IN THIS CHAPTER:

After importing images into a catalog, you can begin to work with them in the Organizer. In this chapter, you'll learn how to review images one at a time in an automated slide show, group different versions of the same image, and categorize images. You group similar media files together by adding the same tag or collection marker. For example, you might add a **John** tag to several audio files, movie files, and images that feature your son, John. Similarly, you might add a **Calendar** collection marker to the images you're gathering for a calendar you want to make. Finally, you'll learn how to annotate your images with a written caption or note.

▶ NOTE

The tasks in this chapter assume that you are using the Organizer in **Photo Browser** view. If you're currently displaying items in **Date View** (on a calendar), you can change to **Photo Browser** view by clicking the **Photo Browser** button at the right end of the **Shortcuts** bar.

---

6   Review Images

✔ BEFORE YOU BEGIN	→ SEE ALSO
10 Add a Text Caption or Note	**71** Print Images Using an Online Service
	162 Create a Slide Show in Photoshop Elements

You can automatically review each image in a group with a full-screen *photo review*. The ideal time to perform a photo review is just after importing a set of images into the catalog because you can stop the review when needed to edit, rotate, or delete an image; mark an image for printing; or add a tag or collection marker. You can also skip to a particular image when desired. In addition, you can split the screen and compare two images when needed. In this task, you'll learn the ins and outs of conducting your own private photo review.

▶ KEY TERM

Photo review—A controllable slide show in which each image is displayed onscreen, one at a time, in whatever order and at whatever speed you want.

▣ Select Photos to Review

Photo review includes in its review only the images currently being displayed in the Organizer. So, if you've just imported some images you want to review, you can skip this step, because the newly imported images are the only ones currently showing. Otherwise, to limit the display, you can use the **Find** bar to show just the photos to review. You can also select the images to review by pressing **Ctrl** as you click each one, or by pressing **Shift** as you click the first and last photo in a group.

▶ TIP

Even if they are shown, audio and creation files are excluded from the photo review. Video files, however, are played during the review in their entirety.

2 Click Full Screen View

Click on the **Options** bar at the bottom of the photo well. The **Full Screen View Options** dialog box appears.

3 Set Options

To play music while you're reviewing your photos, select a music file from the **Background Music** list or click **Browse** to locate the file. Select the number of seconds you want each image to appear onscreen from the **Page Duration** list. To fade in and out between images, select **Fade Between Photos**.

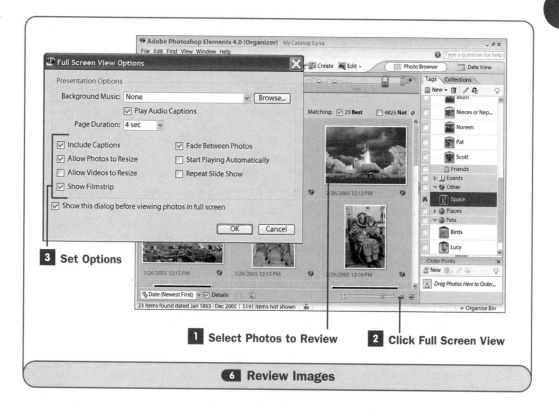

3 Set Options

1 Select Photos to Review

2 Click Full Screen View

6 Review Images

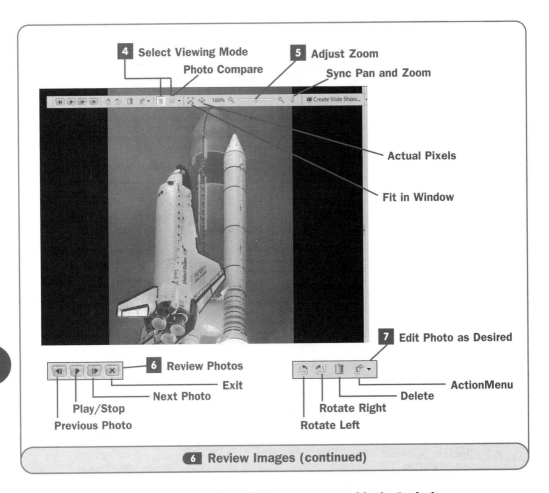

To display text captions you've added to images, enable the **Include Captions** option. To play audio captions you attached to any of these images, select **Play Audio Captions**. To allow photos to resize to fill the window, enable the **Allow Photos to Resize** option. To allow video files to resize to fill the window, enable the **Allow Videos to Resize** option. This option, however, can make low-resolution videos very grainy and hard to see.

To start the slide show automatically, select **Start Playing Automatically**. If you want the slide show to automatically repeat itself over and over until you stop it manually, enable the **Repeat Slide Show** option. To show the filmstrip (so you can view images in any order by selecting the one to view) select **Show Filmstrip**. Click **OK**.

4 Select Viewing Mode

If the slide show has started, you won't be able to set any options until you click **Stop**. Normally, each image is displayed one at a time during the show, but to display images side by side, click the **Photo Compare** button on the **Photo Review** toolbar (which you can display by moving the mouse at any time) and select either **Side by Side** or **Above and Below**.

5 Adjust Zoom

Adjust the zoom as desired: click the **Actual Pixels** button to display the photo in its original size (for a high-resolution photo, you'll have to scroll to see it all); click **Fit in Window** to shrink the photo so that all of it is displayed. You can also drag the **Zoom** slider to the left or right to adjust the zoom level. Click the **Sync Pan and Zoom** button to synchronize scrolling and zooming when displaying two images at a time.

6 Review Photos

Click **Play** to begin the slide show. Click **Stop** to pause the slide show temporarily to perform some action such as tagging an image, and then click **Play** to resume. If you do nothing but watch, each image is displayed and then you're returned to the photo well (unless you selected the **Repeat Slide Show** option in step 3, in which case the slide show will continue to repeat until you exit the photo review or stop it by clicking **Stop** on the review toolbar). If the filmstrip is displayed on the right, you can skip to an image at any time by clicking its thumbnail. You can also use the **Next Photo** and **Previous Photo** buttons to skip photos. The slide show will simply resume from that point.

If you're displaying two images at a time, you must switch from image to image manually. Click a pane to make that pane active (the active pane appears with a blue border), and then press ← or → on your keyboard, click **Next Photo** or **Previous Photo,** or click a thumbnail on the filmstrip to display that image in the active pane.

7 Edit Photo as Desired

If you're using **Photo Review** mode, click **Stop** to pause the slide show so that you can edit the displayed image. If you're using **Photo Compare** mode, click the pane that contains the image you want to edit.

Click the **Rotate Left** or **Rotate Right** button in the **Photo Review** toolbar to rotate the image sideways. Click **Delete** to remove the image from the catalog (and from the hard disk, if you want). Click the arrow on the **Action Menu** button to display a list of actions you can take, such as adding a tag

6

or collection marker to the current image, or marking an image for printing later on. Click the **Create Slide Show** button on the right side of the toolbar to create a slide show using these images.

When you're through, click the **Exit** button to stop the review and return to the main Organizer window. If you used the **Action Menu** to mark photos for printing, a dialog box appears. Click **Print** to print those photos locally; click **Order Prints** to send the images to an online service for printing.

---

7   Create a Tag

→ **SEE ALSO**

8 Create a Collection

To identify the content of images so that you can locate them when needed, you assign tags to those images. To make your various tags markers easier to use, you'll want to keep them organized by category. The **Tags** tab of the **Organize Bin** has several pre-existing tag categories for you to use: **Favorites**, **Hidden**, **People**, **Events**, **Other**, and **Places**. There are some subcategories in the **People** category as well: **Family** and **Friends**. To this list you can add as many categories and subcategories as you want. Although you can use the category and subcategory tags the Organizer provides to mark your images, you'll probably want to create at least a few tags that are more specific than just **Family** or **Events**.

When you create a new tag for your images, you assign it a unique name, add a descriptive note if desired, and select the category in which you want the tag to appear. New tags appear in the **Organize Bin** under the category you choose, at first with a generic icon that has no picture. The first time you assign the new icon to a photo, that photo is automatically applied as the icon for that tag. When you assign a group of photos to a new tag collectively, its icon is borrowed from the newest photo in that group. This task shows you how to create new tag categories and tag markers.

1   Click Tags Tab

To create a new tag category or subcategory, in the Organizer, click the **Tags** tab on the **Organize Bin**.

2   Click New Button

To create a new category or subcategory for tags, click the **New** button at the top of the **Organize Bin** and then select **New Category** or **New Sub-Category**. The **Create Category** or **Create Sub-Category** dialog box appears.

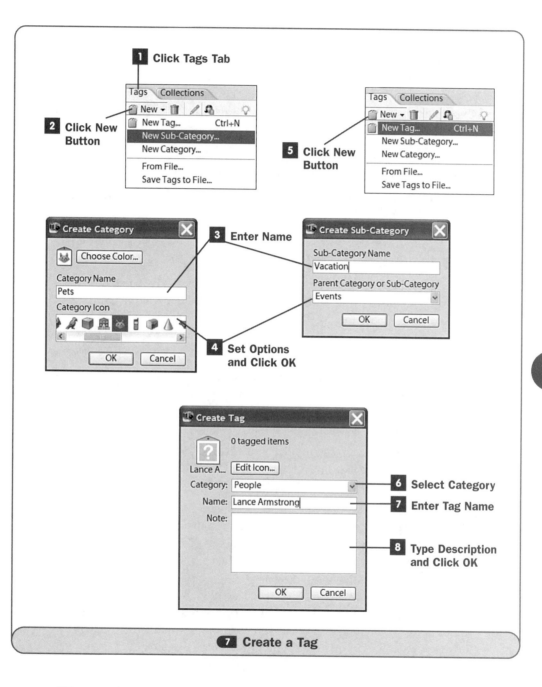

1 Click Tags Tab

2 Click New Button

5 Click New Button

3 Enter Name

4 Set Options and Click OK

6 Select Category

7 Enter Tag Name

8 Type Description and Click OK

7 Create a Tag

3 Enter Name

Type a name for the new tag category or subcategory in the text box provided.

4 Set Options and Click OK

When creating a tag category, select the icon you want to represent the category from those shown in the **Category Icon** list. You can also change the color that appears at the top of the tags in this category by clicking the **Choose Color** button, selecting a color from the **Color Picker** that opens, and clicking **OK** to return to the **Create Category** dialog box.

If you're creating a tag subcategory, select the category to which you want to assign it from the **Parent Category or Sub-Category** list.

Click **OK**. The new category/subcategory marker appears on the **Organize Bin**.

5 Click New Button

After creating any needed tag categories or subcategories, you can add new tags to the **Organize Bin**. Click the **New** button at the top of the **Organize Bin** and choose **New Tag**. The **Create Tag** dialog box appears.

6 Select Category

Open the **Category** drop-down list and select the tag category or subcategory to which you want to assign this new marker.

7 Enter Tag Name

Type a name for the new tag marker in the **Name** text box. The name can include spaces if you like, but you are limited to 63 characters.

8 Type Description and Click OK

Click in the **Note** box and type a description of the tag if desired. This note appears only when you select a tag and click the **Edit** button (the pencil icon) at the top of the **Organize Bin**, so it's of limited use. Click **OK** to create the new tag marker. The marker appears on the **Organize Bin** underneath the category or group you selected in step 6. The marker is now ready to be assigned to any item you want—although you've probably noticed that its icon is blank at the moment. When you assign a new marker to a photo for the first time, the marker will grab that photo for its icon. See **9 Attach a Marker to an Item**.

To remove a marker you no longer want, select it and click the **Delete** button (the trash icon) on the **Organize Bin**. The marker is automatically removed from any items to which it may have been assigned. To replace one marker with another, select both in the **Organize Bin**, right-click, and choose **Merge**

Tags. Select the marker to keep and click **OK**. Items with the other marker are automatically tagged with the marker you kept, and the other marker is removed from the **Organize Bin**.

You can enlarge the size of the icon that appears next to a tag by choosing **Edit**, **Preferences**, **Tags and Collections**, and choosing the last option from the **Tag Display** frame. Notice that you can also forgo the photo icon altogether and display a small folder icon instead.

▶ TIP

You can drag existing tags on top of a category or subcategory on the **Organize Bin** to move that marker to that category/subcategory. To change any of the attributes associated with a category or subcategory, select it and click the **Edit** button (the pencil icon) at the top of the **Organize Bin**. To remove a category or subcategory and the tags within it, click the **Delete** button (the trash icon) instead.

---

8 Create a Collection

✔ BEFORE YOU BEGIN	→ SEE ALSO
7 Create a Tag	**9** Attach a Marker to an Item

Collection markers appear on the Organize Bin. You can organize collection markers into groups if you like, but by their very nature (gathering together a special group of images for a specific purpose such as an upcoming family reunion), collections are unique and you'll probably find that you don't need to group them much, although you'll learn how to do so in this task.

Creating a collection marker is similar to creating a tag (see **7** Create a Tag). It's after you create a collection marker and apply it that you'll discover the key differences between the two: Photos in a collection are organized *in sequence*, by number, unlike a set of photos that share the same tag (which are shown in the catalog using the chosen sort order). The sequence is important when you want to organize a group of photos, perhaps for a slideshow or other creation where sequence is critical. The Organizer provides no collection groups initially, although you can easily create the ones you need, and place into them any existing collections group.

1 Click Collections Tab

To create a new collection group (or subgroup, which is even more rare), click the **Collections** tab.

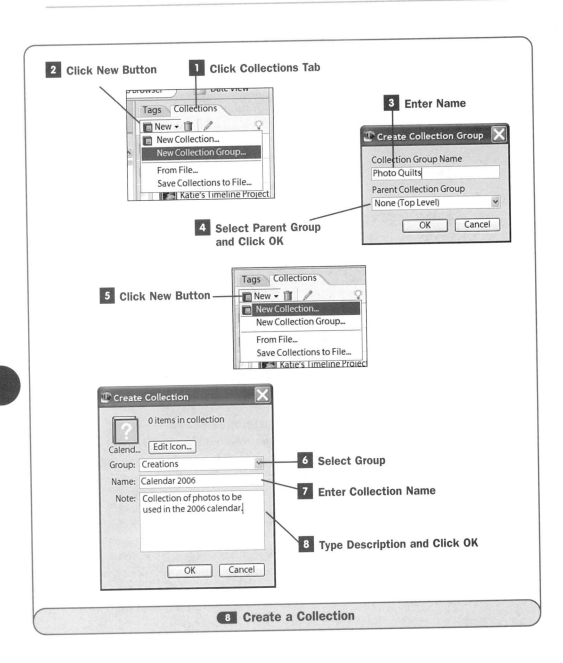

2 Click New Button **1** Click Collections Tab

3 Enter Name

4 Select Parent Group and Click OK

5 Click New Button

6 Select Group

7 Enter Collection Name

8 Type Description and Click OK

8 Create a Collection

2 **Click New Button**

To create a collection group or subgroup, click the **New** button on the **Organize Bin** and select **New Collection Group**. The **Create Collection Group** dialog box appears.

3 Enter Name

Type a name for the new collection group in the text box provided.

4 Select Parent Group and Click OK

To create a collection subgroup, select an existing group from the **Parent Collection Group** list. To create a collection group, leave this option set to **None**. Click **OK**. The new collection group/subgroup appears on the **Organize Bin**.

5 Click New Button

After creating any needed collection groups or subgroups, you can add new collection markers to the **Organize Bin**. Click the **New** button at the top of the **Organize Bin** and choose **New Collection**. The **Create Collection** dialog box appears.

6 Select Group

Open the **Group** drop-down list and select the collection group or subgroup to which you want to assign this new collection marker. If you don't want to group the new collection with other collections, choose **None (Top Level)** from this list.

7 Enter Collection Name

Type a name for the new collection marker in the **Name** text box. The name can include spaces if you like, but you are limited to 63 characters.

8 Type Description and Click OK

Click in the **Note** box and type a description of the collection if desired. This note appears only when you select a collection marker and click the **Edit** button (the pencil icon) at the top of the **Organize Bin**, so it's of limited use. Click **OK** to create the new collection marker. The marker appears on the **Organize Bin** underneath the group you selected in step 6 (if any). The marker is now ready to be assigned to any item you want—although you've probably noticed that its icon is blank at the moment. When you assign a new marker to a photo for the first time, the marker will grab that photo for its icon. See **9 Attach a Marker to an Item**.

8

▶ **NOTES**

To remove a collection marker you no longer want, select it and click the **Delete** button (the trash icon) on the **Organize Bin**. The marker is automatically removed from any items to which it may have been assigned. To replace one marker with another, select both in the **Organize Bin**, right-click, and choose **Merge Collections**. Select the marker to keep and click **OK**. Items with the other marker are automatically tagged with the marker you kept, and the other marker is removed from the **Organize Bin**.

You can drag existing collection markers on top of a group or subgroup on the **Organize Bin** to move that marker to that group/subgroup. To change any of the attributes associated with a group or subgroup, select it and click the **Edit** button (the pencil icon) at the top of the **Organize Bin**. To remove a group or subgroup and the collection markers within it, click the **Delete** button (the trash icon) instead.

9   **Attach a Marker to an Item**

✔ **BEFORE YOU BEGIN**

8 Create a Collection

8

To organize your media files into logical groups such as vacation photos, photos of the family dog, audio files of your daughter, movies of friends, and so on, assign tag and collection markers to them. After a marker has been associated with your media files, you can search for items with a particular marker and display just those files onscreen. For example, if you have a tag called **Hattie**, you could use it to instantly display photos of your pet Scottie dog.

▶ **TIP**

You can create new tags using the names of the folders in which images reside. Just display images by **Folder Location** by choosing that option from the **Photo Browser Arrangement** list at the left end of the **Options** bar, and click the **Instant Tag** button (located just after the folder name at the top of a folder group). A tag is created using the name of the folder, and all the images in that folder are automatically marked with the new tag.

1   **Select Items**

In the Organizer, select the item(s) you want to mark. To select multiple items, press **Shift** and click the first and last item in a contiguous group, or press **Ctrl** and click each item you want. If items are sorted by folder or import batch, you can click the gray bar above a group to select all items in that group.

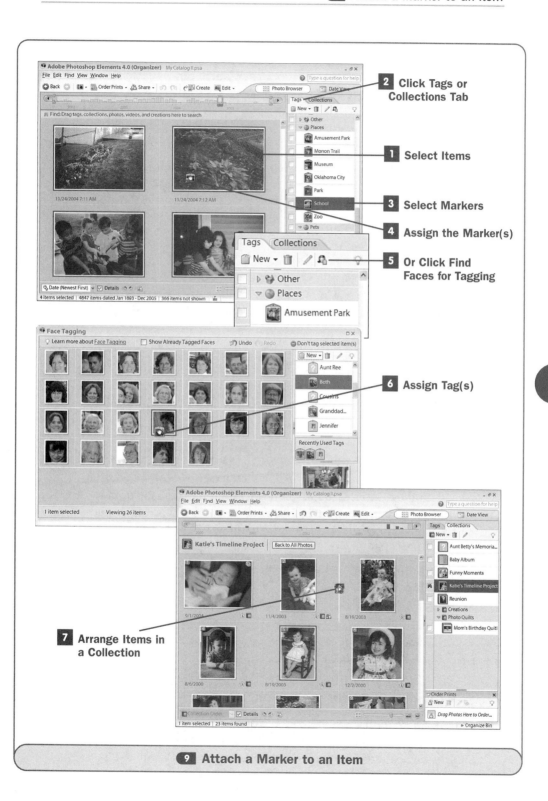

2 Click Tags or
Collections Tab

1 Select Items

3 Select Markers

4 Assign the Marker(s)

5 Or Click Find
Faces for Tagging

6 Assign Tag(s)

9

7 Arrange Items in
a Collection

9 Attach a Marker to an Item

2 Click Tags or Collections Tab

To assign a tag, click the **Tags** tab on the **Organize Bin**. To assign a collection marker, click the **Collections** tab instead.

3 Select Markers

In the **Organize Bin**, press **Ctrl** and click each marker you want to assign to the selected items. (You can assign multiple tags or multiple collection markers in one step, but not both.)

4 Assign the Marker(s)

Drag the selected marker(s) onto any one of the selected items and drop the markers on the item. If you're assigning a new marker to an image for the first time, that image is used as the marker's photo icon. If you selected multiple images, the first image in the group is the one used. The markers you assigned appear as icons underneath the selected items.

5 Or Click Find Faces for Tagging

To use the faces in the selected photos you selected to help you assign tags (not collection markers), skip steps 2–4 and instead, after selecting images, click the **Find Faces for Tagging** button at the top of the **Organize Bin**.

6 Assign Tag(s)

Organizer searches the selected image(s) for faces and displays them in small thumbnails in the **Face Tagging** dialog box (if a face is turned partially away from the camera, it might not be picked up). Drag a tag from the list on the right and drop it on a thumbnail to assign the tag to that image. To view the image from which a face thumbnail was pulled, click the thumbnail. The thumbnail is removed from the **Face Tagging** dialog box, unless you've selected the **Show Already Tagged** Faces option. Continue until you've tagged all your images, then click **Done**.

▶ **NOTE**

You can review a group of photos and assign tags or collection markers to them during the review. See **6 Review Images.**

7 Arrange Items in a Collection

After assigning a collection marker to a group of items (images, sound files, and/or video files), you can display that group in **Collections Order** view by clicking the box in front of the collection name on the **Organize Bin**.

Rearrange the items in a collection in any order you want by simply dragging them in the photo well. As you rearrange the items, the number assigned to each item (which appears in the upper-left corner of the item and denotes its position within the collection) changes.

10 Add a Text Caption or Note

With a text caption, you can provide a title for your "works of art" (your photographs). An image's caption appears in the photo well when you display the image using **Single Photo** view, and below each image in a photo review (see **6** **Review Images**). In addition, captions can be printed on a contact sheet and made to appear in various creations, such as a slide show, photo book, video CD, calendar, or HTML Photo Gallery. For longer descriptions or stories about an image, you can enter a note. Notes do not appear in the photo well, but only within the **Properties** pane.

▶ TIP

When searching for a particular image, you can search for text contained in its filename, caption, or note.

10

1 Select Image(s)

In the Organizer, click the image to which you want to add a caption. If you want to add the same caption to multiple images, select them now.

2 Click Show or Hide Properties Button

If it's not already displayed, click the **Show or Hide Properties** button on the **Options** bar to display the **Properties** pane. You can also choose **Window, Properties** from the menu.

3 Type Caption and/or Note

If you selected one image, click the **General** button at the top of the **Properties** pane. Then type your **Caption**, such as **Alyce on Big Bear Mountain, July 2005** or **We watched the rain under the protection of a large maple tree.** Your caption can include up to 2000 characters, including spaces, but you'll want to keep it short so it displays fully onscreen and in creations. Longer descriptions can be typed in the **Notes** section if you like.

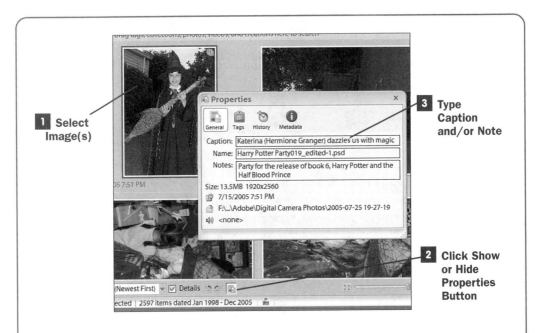

1 Select Image(s)

3 Type Caption and/or Note

2 Click Show or Hide Properties Button

10

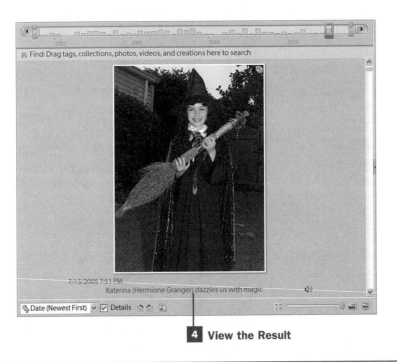

4 View the Result

10 Add a Text Caption or Note

If you selected multiple images, click the **Change Caption** button. Type your **Caption**, select **Replace Existing Captions** (otherwise, if an image already has a caption, it won't be replaced), then click **OK**.

Close the **Properties** pane by clicking its **X** button or by clicking the **Show or Hide Properties** button on the **Options** bar.

▶ TIPS

You can also enter text captions by double-clicking an image to display it in **Single Photo** view. Click where it says **Click here to add caption**, type a caption, and press **Enter**.

You can delete a text caption from either the **Caption** text box in the **Properties** pane, or from **Single Photo** view. Click the caption and then use the mouse to highlight the entire caption. Press **Delete** to remove the caption.

4 View the Result

Notes can only be seen in the **Properties** pane, and they are not used in creations. To view an image's caption, change to **Single Photo** view by double-clicking the image in the photo well or by clicking the **Single Photo View** button on the **Options** bar.

11

11 Make a Creation

→ SEE ALSO

9 Attach a Marker to an Item

Organizing images is just one of the things Organizer helps you excel at; another is being creative. Using the images in the catalog, you can make a variety of creations, including slide shows, VCD (a collection of slide shows playable on your TV), calendars, photo books, greeting cards, and an HTML photo gallery (a browsable gallery of images). You can share creations you make in a variety of ways, such as emailing them to friends, burning slide shows or VCDs onto a CD, printing album pages, calendars, and cards at home, or uploading calendars and photo books to Adobe Printing Services for professional services.

You make creations using the **Creations Wizard**; the wizard steps you through the process of arranging your photos, selecting a template, choosing options, and saving, emailing, printing, or uploading the result. In this task, you'll learn the basic steps in making a calendar. Although each creation type has its own set of options, the process is similar for each type.

2 Click the Create Button

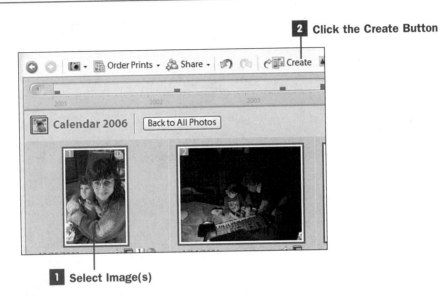

1 Select Image(s)

3 Select Creation Type

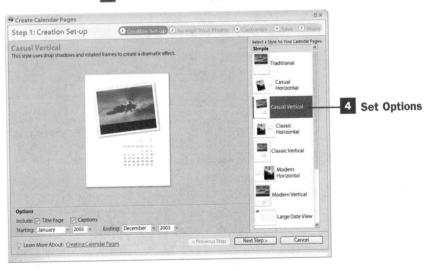

4 Set Options

11 Make a Creation

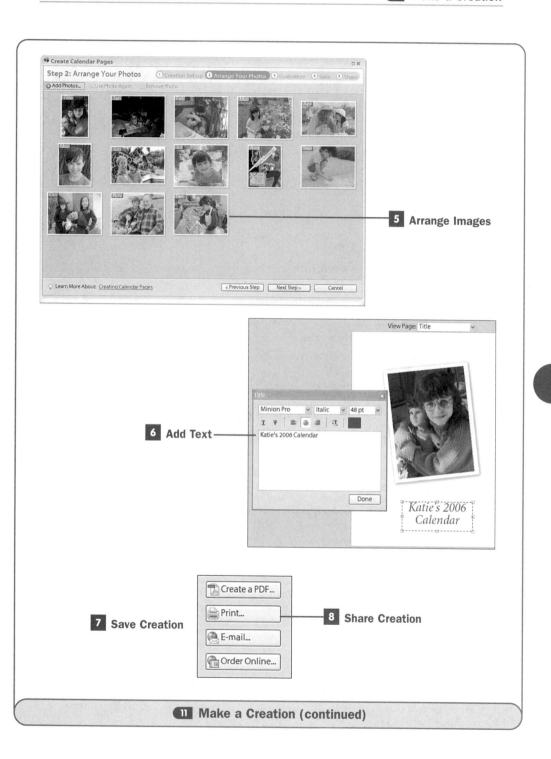

5 Arrange Images

6 Add Text

7 Save Creation

8 Share Creation

11 Make a Creation (continued)

▶ **TIP**

To help you arrange multiple photos for a creation, create a collection first, and use the collection to arrange them in the order you want. See 🔟 **Attach a Marker to an Item.**

1 **Select Image(s)**

In the Organizer, select the image(s) you want to use in the creation.

2 **Click the Create Button**

Click the **Create** button on the **Shortcuts** bar.

3 **Select Creation Type**

On the first page of the **Creations Wizard**, select the type of creation you want to make from those listed on the left. As you make a selection, a description of that choice appears on the right. Small icons appear above this description, indicating your choices (such as printing, burning to CD, ordering online, and so on) for this particular creation. Hover the mouse over an icon to see the choice it represents. Click **OK**.

11

▶ **NOTES**

VCDs, slide shows, and HTML photo galleries are not created using the **Creations Wizard**. If you choose **Slide Show** and click **OK** in step 3, a dialog box of options appears. Select the options you want for the slide show, and click **OK** to display the **Slide Show Editor**, which allows you to customize the transitions between each image, add music, text, and graphics.

If you choose **VCD with Menu** in step 3, the slide show(s) you selected appear; arrange the slide shows in the order in which you want them to appear on the VCD, select the VCD format, and click **Burn**.

If you choose **HTML Photo Gallery** in step 3, a dialog box appears in which you can choose the type of web page banner (heading) you want, adjust the size of the image thumbnails on the page(s), adjust the quality of the larger photos that appear when a thumbnail is clicked, and choose custom colors and fonts. Make your selections, choose a site folder in which to save the web pages that will be generated, and click **Save**.

4 **Set Options**

In Step 1 of the **Creations Wizard**, select a template from the list on the right. Set other options as desired. For example, in the calendar shown here, you can add a title page (you'll need an extra photo), image captions, and adjust the length of the calendar. Click **Next Step**.

5 Arrange Images

In Step 2 of the **Creations Wizard**, images appear in the order in which they were selected. Drag and drop images to rearrange them as desired. Click **Next Step**.

6 Add Text

In Step 3 of the **Creations Wizard**, you add text to the creation. Just double-click where indicated and type your text, set formatting by choosing the font, style, and size of the text, and click **Done**. Some creations have multiple pages; click the → to flip through pages and add text as needed. You can also resize and move images on each page if you like. Click **Next Step**.

7 Save Creation

In Step 4 of the **Creations Wizard**, type a name for the creation in the box provided or select **Use Title for Name** to use the name from the **Title Page** as the creation's name. To display all the images you used in the creation in the photo well after the creation is saved, select **Show these photos in my Photo Browser when finished**. Click **Next Step**.

8 Share Creation

In Step 5 of the **Creations Wizard**, select how you want to share the creation. For example, to resave the creation in PDF format and attach it to an email message, click **Email**. Some creations are designed specifically to be printed professionally, although you can still print them at home if you want. To order a professionally printed copy of such a creation, click **Order Online**. (See **71** **Print Images Using an Online Service** for more information on using an online service.) Options that are not applicable for this creation are grayed out. If you don't want to share the creation, click **Done**.

The creation appears with a special icon in its upper-right corner to help identify it as a creation. To redisplay all your creations, search by media type. See **12** **About Finding Items in the Catalog**. You can also mark creations with tag or collection markers to help you locate them again. To edit a creation, double-click its thumbnail in the photo well. To display the items used in a collection in the photo well, right-click its thumbnail and choose **Show Creation Items in Photo Browser**.

11

12   About Finding Items in the Catalog

Just because your catalog may have countless rows of thumbnails does not mean that it is less manageable, or that your media files are more difficult to find than when you had only a few dozen thumbnails to contend with. After each image file has been imported, the catalog automatically begins tracking that the item's filename, location, file date, and file type, and (in the case of images) the *Exchangeable Image File (EXIF)* data (also called *metadata*) that your camera/scanner stored in the file when the image was shot or scanned. This data typically includes the resolution, color gamut (color range), image size, compression, shutter speed, and f-stop of the image. An EXIF-aware application such as Photoshop Elements can use this data to adjust the image so that it appears, when displayed or printed, as closely to the way the image looked when shot as possible. In addition, through the **File Info** dialog box in the Editor, and the **Properties** pane in the Organizer, Photoshop Elements can amend the EXIF metadata to include tags, collection markers, title, description, and copyright information. Also, as you edit an image, its edit history is stored in the image's metadata. So, without doing any work other than importing a media file, you can locate an item immediately if you know any of its file data.

12

▶ KEY TERM

EXIF (Exchangeable Image File)—Data attached to a photo file that contains the key settings the camera used when the photo was shot.

▶ NOTE

EXIF data such as image resolution will not be saved in a scanned image if you use Microsoft Office Document Imaging to perform the scan. It's best to use the software that came with the scanner. In addition, some scanners might not be capable of recording EXIF data—see the scanner documentation.

The true organizational magic begins, however, when you associate any number of markers to the items in the catalog. The markers enable you to keep track of what's important about a particular item—for instance, whether it's a holiday, party, or other special event, or whether the shot was taken indoors or outdoors. You can add notes and captions to your catalog items, making it even easier to locate a particular media file when needed. In upcoming tasks, you'll learn how to search for items in the catalog using the tags and collection markers you've assigned. You'll also learn how to search for items based on their file date, filename, caption, note, media type (such as creation, movie, audio file, and so on), and history (not just when an item was imported or edited, but also when it was sent via email, shared online, or printed).

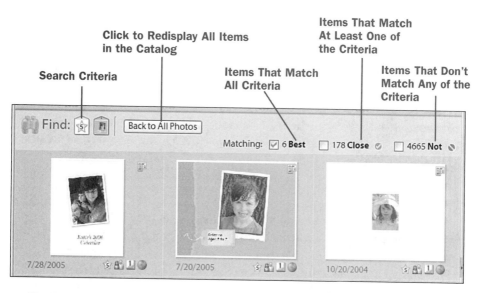

Search Criteria

Click to Redisplay All Items
in the Catalog

Items That Match
All Criteria

Items That Match
At Least One of
the Criteria

Items That Don't
Match Any of the
Criteria

The Find bar shows you the criteria for the currently displayed items.

When you perform a search of the catalog, the search criteria are displayed on the **Find** bar. For example, if you're searching for items with certain collection or tag markers, those markers appear in the **Find** bar. If you're looking for the photos you used in a particular slideshow, the **Find** bar reads **Used in** along with the name of that slideshow. If you're looking for only those items to which you've attached audio captions, the **Find** bar reads **Items with Audio Captions**. Underneath the **Find** bar, in the photo well, are the items that match your search. This means that, when you see something in the **Find** bar, all items in the catalog are not currently being shown; to display all items, click the **Back to All Photos** button on the **Find** bar. There is one exception here you should note: If you use the **Timeline** to limit the items displayed in the photo well, nothing appears on the **Find** bar to notify you that all items are not currently being shown. To clear the **Timeline** limitations and redisplay all items, choose **Find, Clear Date Range**.

▶ NOTES

You can review the results of a previous search by clicking the **Back** button on the **Shortcuts** bar. You can return to the current search by clicking the **Forward** button.

If you always want to display both matching and closely matching items when you conduct a new search, choose **Edit, Preferences** and select the **General** tab. Select the **Show Closely Matching Sets for Searches** option and click **OK**.

When there's an active search in progress, the **Find** bar displays the number of matches and non-matches. After you perform a search, the matching items are displayed in the photo well and a check mark appears next to the *XX* **Best** box on the **Find** bar (where *XX* represents the number of exact matches to all your criteria). To display exact matches and items that match at least one of the criteria, enable both the *XX* **Best** and *XX* **Close** boxes. To show only those items that do not match any of the criteria, disable the *XX* **Best** and *XX* **Close** boxes, and enable the *XX* **Not** box instead. If you enable the *XX* **Not** box and the *XX* **Best** box, *all the items in the catalog* will appear, but the non-matches will show a red **Not** icon (a circle with a slash) similar to the one on the **Find** bar. Matches won't have this icon.

Normally, you cannot mix and match different types of search criteria. For example, if you're searching for items that contain one or more tags, and you begin a search for items you emailed to someone, the Organizer clears the current search by tags and processes your search by email as a new search. However, using an item's metadata (its file date, shutter speed, aperture, tags, collection markers, edit history, and so on), you can create a unique search that combines the elements of these other, separate searches. For example, you can look for an item created on July 12th, marked with a **Party** tag, and shot with a large f-stop of F4 or lower (which may indicate minimal available light, such as an indoor shot).

There are so many ways to search for items in the catalog that we could not cover them all in the upcoming tasks. Because these search methods are really simple, I'll cover them briefly here. To locate items of a similar type (all creations or all videos), choose **Find**, **By Media Type**, then choose the type from the list that appears. For example, choose **Find**, **By Media Type**, **Videos**. To find images with similar content, select some sample images that show the content you want to find, and then choose **Find**, **Items by Visual Similarity with Selected Photo(s)**. Or just drag the similar images to the **Find** bar and drop them to create a search. With this type of search, it's best to select several items with similar content, because that makes it easier for Organizer to find more of the same. To find items with a date or time set to **Unknown**, select **Find**, **Items with Unknown Date or Time**. You might do this to locate and change items with unknown dates/times to something more specific.

To display images that have been edited and saved together with their originals in a version set, choose **Find**, **All Version Sets**. This command, however, does not display items you've grouped together manually in stacks. To display items that have not yet been tagged so that you can mark them, choose **Find**, **Untagged Items**. Items with collection markers and no tags will appear, along with items that have no markers at all. To find items that do not have a collection marker (but may or may not have a tag), choose **Find**, **Items Not in any Collection** instead.

4

Creating, Opening, and Saving Images

IN THIS CHAPTER:

The Editor comes with many tools for creating and manipulating graphics. With its help, you can restore old photographs, insert your missing brother into a family photo, or create a web page background. Before you can perform any of this graphics wizardry however, you must first open the image you want to work on or tell the Editor you want to start from scratch on a new image. In the tasks presented in this chapter, you will learn not only how to start something new, but also how to locate and open image files already saved to the hard disk. In addition, you'll learn how to save new or edited images in a variety of graphic formats and to perform simple image tasks such as resizing, renaming, and applying automatic image corrections.

▶ **NOTE**

Although you don't have to use the Editor to make changes to an image, if you use another program, you should initiate the edit from within the Organizer: First, select your preferred editor on the **Editing** page of the **Preferences** dialog box. Then select an image in the catalog and choose **Edit, Edit with XX**. If you don't initiate edits from within the Organizer, it won't know you've made changes to an image, and its thumbnail will not show correctly in the catalog. To manually update a thumbnail you've edited outside the Organizer without its knowledge, choose **Edit, Update Thumbnail**.

---

13   **Create a New Image**

→ **SEE ALSO**

35 About Color Management
157 Create a Graphic with Transparent Areas in Photoshop Elements
159 More Images Between Premiere Element and Photoshop Elements

---

As with other programs, if you want to use Photoshop Elements to create new art, such as a decorative Windows wallpaper or a Web page button, you must start with a new, empty image file. You might also create a new image file when you want to combine portions of several photographs into a photo collage, scrapbook page, or panorama. After creating a new image file, you should save it in Photoshop format as described in **14** **Save an Image**.

When you create a new image file, you set several initial parameters, such as the image's width and height. You are not stuck with your initial choices; you can change your selections later on as you work. For example, it's easy to resize a photograph to make it bigger or smaller as needed. In addition to width and height, you determine how finely detailed the image will be (its resolution). Finally, you'll select the background color and the image *color mode*. As you make your selections, the resulting file size (taking into account only a single, basic background layer) is displayed at the bottom of the dialog box. If necessary, reduce the image size, resolution, or color mode to make the file size more manageable for your system.

1 Click New Button

2 Enter Name

3 Select Preset

5 Adjust Resolution

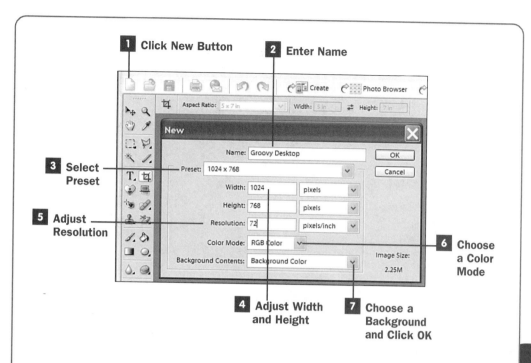

6 Choose a Color Mode

4 Adjust Width and Height

7 Choose a Background and Click OK

13

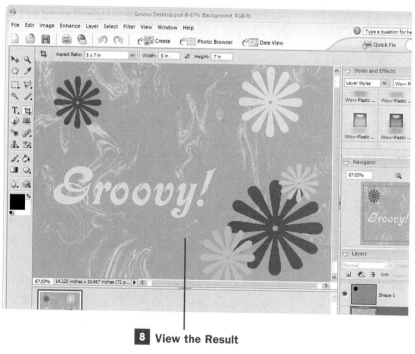

8 View the Result

13 Create a New Image

► **KEY TERM**

Color mode—Determines the number of colors an image can contain.

► **NOTE**

Before beginning any editing within the Editor for the first time, you should calibrate your monitor so that the colors you see onscreen will match what you get when you print a completed image. See 🔲 **About Color Management**.

1 Click New Button

In the Editor, change to **Standard Edit** mode and click the **New** button on the **Shortcuts** bar, or choose **File, New, Blank File** from the menu. The **New** dialog box appears.

2 Enter Name

Type a name for the new image in the **Name** box. The name you type will serve as the file's temporary name until you actually save the file. Because this is only a temporary name, you can skip this step if you like, and enter the permanent name for the file when you save it later on.

3 Select Preset

Open the **Preset** drop-down list and select one of the many common image types, such as a 5-by-7-inch photo or an 800-by-600-pixel Web background. You can modify the **Width, Height**, and **Resolution** settings that appear by following steps 4 and 5; otherwise, skip to step 6.

► **TIP**

To create a new image that uses the same dimensions as a currently open image, select the image's name from the bottom of the **Preset** list.

4 Adjust Width and Height

If your chosen preset doesn't match the image size you want exactly, select new **Width** and/or **Height** values.

5 Adjust Resolution

Depending on how detailed you want the image to appear, adjust the **Resolution** value. If the image will only be viewed onscreen or on the Web, an image resolution of 72 pixels per inch is sufficient; for images you intend to print, consider at least 300 PPI.

6 Choose a Color Mode

Open the **Color Mode** drop-down list and select the color mode you want to work with: **RGB Color** (for color images), **Grayscale** (for images in black, white, and grays), or **Bitmap** (for images in black and white only).

7 Choose a Background and Click OK

Open the **Background Contents** drop-down list and select the color you want to fill the bottom layer of your image—the background layer. You can choose **White**, **Background Color** (which makes the background the same color as the current background color as shown on the **Toolbox**), or **Transparent**. (The **Transparent** option is not available in **Bitmap** color mode.) After selecting a background, click **OK** to create the blank canvas for the new image onscreen.

8 View the Result

An image window opens with the dimensions and colors you choose. Use the Editor's tools to fill the image with color or data copied from another image. Apply filters, effects, or layer styles. After you've worked a little in your image, you'll want to save it so you don't lose your work. The best format for works in progress is Photoshop (*.psd), as explained in **14** Save an Image. After you work on the image, save the result in PNG, JPEG, or non-layered TIFF format, leaving your PSD image with its layers (if any) intact so that you can return at a later time and make different adjustments if you want.

Here, I created a quick image for use as a Windows background. I filled it with a purple background color, painted it with green and yellow droplets, and applied the **Glass**, **Wave**, and **Liquify** filters. Then I added some flowers using the **Custom Shape** tool, and some text.

14

14 Save an Image

→ **SEE ALSO**

17 Rename, Resize, Reformat, and Retouch a Group of Images
19 Change Color Mode

After copying files from a digital camera onto your computer or scanning images using a scanner, your first step should be to perform some type of backup. Typically, this involves burning copies of the image files onto a CD-R. See **2** Import Images from a Digital Camera for how to bring images into the catalog from your camera, and **5** Back Up the Organizer Catalog for help on making the backup copies of the catalog and its images.

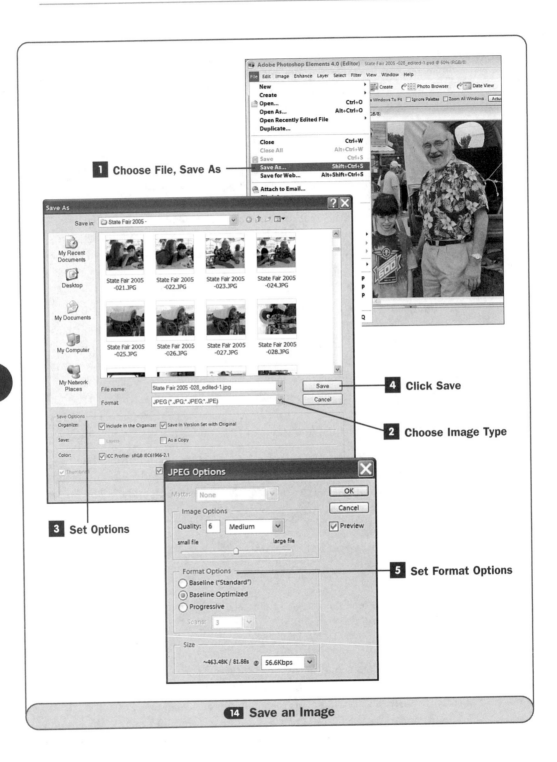

1 Choose File, Save As

4 Click Save

2 Choose Image Type

3 Set Options

5 Set Format Options

14 Save an Image

After importing an image into the catalog, backing it up, and beginning work on any touchups, you will most likely want to open the image in the Editor and save it in the Photoshop image format (PSD) by following the basic steps in this task. Using Photoshop PSD format ensures that you have access to all of the Editor's features, such as layers, transparency, vector objects, and masking, while also preserving the integrity of your original image's data. As you work on an image, you might want to save the image at various stages to which you can return later on, but not save these intermediate images in the Organizer, in a version set with the original image. To do this, select the **As a Copy** option from the **Save As** dialog box, as explained here in step 3. To make sure that this intermediate copy is not stored in the Organizer under its own thumbnail, be sure to deselect the **Include in the Organizer** option as well. When you are done working on an image, resave the Photoshop PSD file in a smaller, shareable format such as TIFF, JPEG, GIF, or PNG, again using the steps shown here. For this final, flattened copy of your image, be sure to select the **Save in Version Set with Original** and **Include in the Organizer** options in step 3, which will place the final version with the original under a single thumbnail in the catalog, where you can easily find them.

▶ TIPS

Photoshop Elements fully supports EXIF and PIM (Epson's Print Image Managing System, which its printers use to match printed output to how to an image looks onscreen), which means that you will not lose important digital camera data when you save your original file in Photoshop format.

If you have several photos that are similar to one another—such as several shots taken at around the same time—you can have the Editor make the same corrections to all of them simultaneously, and automatically save the results in whatever format you choose. See **17** Rename, Resize, Reformat, and Retouch a Group of Images for details.

1 Choose File, Save As

To save changes and replace the current file, click the **Save** button on the **Shortcuts** bar, or choose **File, Save** from the menu. To save changes in a different file so you keep your original file intact (for example, to save your working PSD image in a flattened, sharable format such as JPEG as shown here), choose **File, Save As** instead. The **Save As** dialog box appears.

▶ NOTE

When you send an image from the catalog to the Editor for changes, you can click the **Save** button if you like, since it will automatically bring up the **Save As** dialog box, with options set so that you do not overwrite your original file with your edits.

2 Choose Image Type

From the **Format** drop-down list, choose the image type you want to use. If you're just beginning edits on an image, save the working file by choosing **Photoshop (*.PSD; *.PDD)**. If you're saving the final version of an image, select a type that matches your purpose, such as a web-compatible format (GIF, JPEG, or PNG), an email-friendly compressed format (JPEG or PNG), or high quality printer-friendly format (TIFF).

3 Set Options

Change to the folder in which you want to save the image. If this is the first time saving a new image file, type a filename in the **File name** text box. Normally, you do not have to edit the filename of an existing file when you save it because the options you select change the filename for you, as described below. Set options as desired:

- **As a Copy**—Select this option to save a copy of the image so that you don't overwrite the existing file. *The current image is kept open so that you can continue working,* but the image as it looks right now is saved in a new file with *copy* added to the original filename. Use this option to save copies of your working image at various stages in the editing process. Doing so allows you to go back to an earlier version if some of your edits don't work out.

- **Include in the Organizer**—Select this option to add the image to the Organizer catalog (if it isn't there already). By default, this option is already checked, but you can disable it if you like.

- **Layers**—Select this option when the format you've chosen supports layers (Photoshop PSD or TIFF format) *and* you want to make certain that the full content and identity of all layers are saved in your file. (This option is disabled if the format you select does not support layers.) With the **Layers** option disabled, the Editor merges all content in the file into a single layer before saving.

▶ NOTES

Typically, you'll enable the **Layers** option when saving a working Photoshop PSD image file; although you can enable this option when saving in TIFF, you probably won't want to since it makes the file larger than a regular TIFF and may also make it incompatible with some graphics programs. Layering is especially important when you're creating an image made up of parts of other images.

If you turn off the **Layers** option when saving a layered image, the **As a Copy** option is turned on for you. This prevents you from saving a merged (flattened) version of your image over top of the copy that contains the separate layers. So when you disable the **Layers** option, your layered, working image is kept open, and a merged, flattened copy is saved to the disk with a different filename.

14

- **Save in Version Set with Original**— Select this option to group the edited version of an image with its original version in the Organizer catalog, in a single version set. When this is done, both items share the same thumbnail in the catalog. In addition, when you chose this option, **edited-1** (or another number, if you've edited this image several times) is added to the original filename, creating a separate file so that you do not overwrite your original or other edited copies in the version set.

- **ICC Profile**— Select this option to include the ICC color profile being used by your system, along with the other image data, in the image file. Knowing the name of this profile will help your printer or other computers render the image as you are seeing it now, rather than making color adjustments you don't want. See **35** **About Color Management**.

- **Thumbnail**—Select this option to save an image preview for applications that do not produce such previews for themselves. Admittedly, the number of applications that *can't* generate an image preview for themselves has grown quite few in recent years, but for these few, you might want to generate the preview for them. Normally, this option is on, but if you've changed your file-saving preferences so that image previews are not automatically created when you save, you'll be able to optionally save or not save a preview for particular images. Not saving a preview makes the image file smaller; however, having a preview enables you to view an image's content in the **Open** dialog box before you actually open the file. This option, by the way, has *nothing* to do with the Organizer's thumbnails, which it creates automatically when an image is added to the catalog.

▶ NOTES

To change your preferences for saving files (such as whether image previews are created), choose **Edit**, **Preferences**, **Saving Files** from the menu.

Not all image formats support the inclusion of thumbnails. For those formats, the **Thumbnail** option is not available.

- **Use Lower Case Extension**— Select this option to use lowercase letters in the filename extension—something that might be important if you intend to use the image on the Web or on a Linux computer, or if you're burning the image to a CD so that it can be read on a computer with a different operating system (such as a Mac). By default, this option is enabled, and it's typically best to leave it like that.

14

4 Click Save

Click the **Save** button. If you see a note reminding you that you're saving this image as part of a version set, click **OK** to continue.

5 Set Format Options

If you selected a particular file format from the **Format** list in step 2 (such as TIFF, JPEG, GIF, or PNG), an **Options** dialog box appears, allowing you to set options relating to that file format. Select an option, then click **OK**.

15 | Zoom In and Out

Whether you're making changes to a photograph or some artwork you've created yourself, you must be able to view the image clearly to make precise changes. Typically, this means zooming in on some area that doesn't look right so that you can discern the problem, and later zooming back out again to see whether the change you made looks right when the image is viewed at its regular size. To zoom in on an image and back out again, use the **Zoom** tool. If you don't want to switch tools, you can also zoom in and out using the **Navigator** palette.

1 Click with the Zoom Tool

Open an image in the Editor and then click the **Zoom** tool in the **Toolbox**. Press **Alt** while clicking with the **Zoom** tool to zoom out. Click the **Zoom In** or **Zoom Out** button on the **Options** bar to determine the direction of the zoom, then click the point you want to zoom in on (or away from) within the image window. Drag an area with the **Zoom In** tool to zoom in on that area.

▶ TIPS

To resize the image window as you zoom, enable the **Resize Windows to Fit** option on the **Options** bar. To allow the image window to expand below free-floating palettes, enable the **Ignore Palettes** option. To zoom all open image windows by the same amount, enable the **Zoom All Windows** option. (This option works only if you zoom using the **Zoom In** or **Zoom Out** buttons, and not the **Zoom** slider.)

To zoom in and out without actually selecting the **Zoom** tool first, press and hold **Ctrl+spacebar** and click the image to zoom in. Press and hold **Alt+spacebar** and click the image to zoom out.

Zoom Out

Zoom In

2 Or Choose a
Zoom Amount

3 Or Zoom to a
Set Size

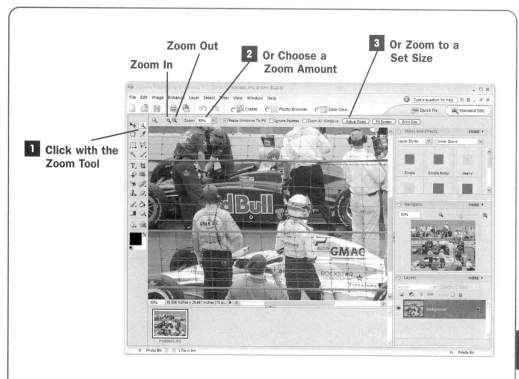

1 Click with the
Zoom Tool

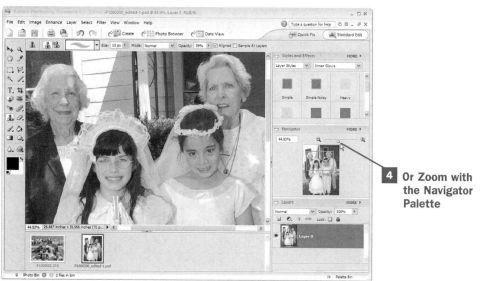

4 Or Zoom with
the Navigator
Palette

15

15 Zoom In and Out

2 Or Choose a Zoom Amount

You can also zoom by dragging the **Zoom** slider on the **Options** bar, or typing a percentage in the box and pressing **Enter**.

3 Or Zoom to a Set Size

To view the image at 100% (based on roughly 72 PPI, or optimum screen resolution), click the **Actual Pixels** button on the **Options** bar. To zoom the image as large as possible to fill the workspace, click the **Fit On Screen** button. To zoom the image to the approximate magnification it will be when you print it (based on the current image resolution), click the **Print Size** button.

4 Or Zoom with the Navigator Palette

Rather than switch from the tool you're using to the **Zoom** tool to zoom, use the **Navigator** palette: choose **Window, Navigator** if needed to display the palette. Select or type a zoom percentage in the box on the left side of the palette. You can also drag the slider on the **Navigator** palette to zoom. To zoom by a predetermined amount, click either of the **Zoom** buttons on the **Navigator** palette.

15

▶ TIPS

If you've zoomed in on an image, you can scroll to view hidden areas using the scroll bars, dragging the image with the **Hand** tool, or dragging the red rectangle on the **Navigator** palette. Hold down the **spacebar** to turn your pointer into the **Hand** tool for as long as you hold the **spacebar**.

When working with multiple images, you may want to use the **Navigator** palette to zoom, since the **Zoom** tool unarranges the windows.

---

16 Change Image Size or Resolution

→ SEE ALSO

3 Import and Separate Multiple Scanned Images
18 Increase the Canvas Area Around an Image
88 Prepare a Still for Video

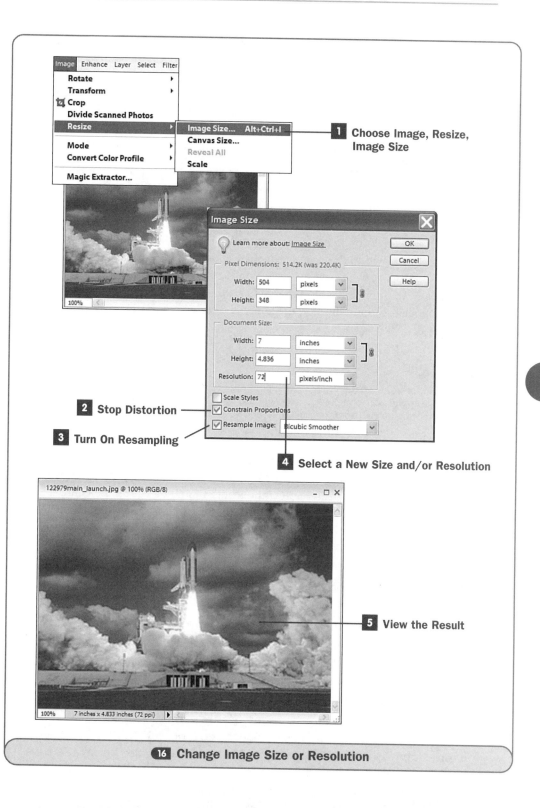

1 Choose Image, Resize, Image Size

2 Stop Distortion

3 Turn On Resampling

4 Select a New Size and/or Resolution

5 View the Result

16

16 Change Image Size or Resolution

An image's size is tied directly to the number of pixels in the image as well as the relative size of those pixels. When you create images with a digital camera or scan printed images with a scanner, you choose the resolution you want to use—for instance, 72 pixels per inch (ppi). The resolution you choose also determines the resulting print size. For example, an image that's 2048 pixels wide by 1536 pixels tall (the typical dimensions of an image taken with a 3-megapixel camera), whose resolution is 300 pixels per inch, will print at 6.827" by 5.120".

So what do you do if you want to print your image at a different size—larger or smaller—while maintaining or even increasing its resolution? Answer: You use *resampling*. When you resample to increase an image's print size and/or its resolution, new pixels are inserted between existing ones. The Editor determines the colors of the new pixels by sampling the color value of each surrounding pixel, calculating a value within the sample range, and assigning that value to that new pixel. Conversely, when you reduce an image's print size, resampling removes pixels from the image and then adjusts the colors of the pixels remaining in the image by approximating the blended color values of the pixels that were removed.

16

▶ **KEY TERM**

Resampling—The mathematical process applied during image resizing that evaluates the content of the pixels in the image to calculate the value of new pixels (when enlarging) or neighboring pixels (when reducing), and which re-interprets the result to minimize loss of detail.

Because resampling is based on best-guess estimation, using it to change an image's size or resolution by more than 20% often produces poor results. You can resize or change an image's resolution without resampling by telling the Editor that you want to turn resampling off, and therefore maintain the relationship between the size and the resolution. In this manner, you can double an image's print resolution by cutting its print size in half (the image contains as many pixels as it did before, but the pixels are smaller, and there are more of them per inch). Onscreen, you won't see any apparent change at all.

▶ **NOTE**

To display an image in its print size, click the **Zoom** tool on the **Toolbox** and then click the **Print Size** button on the **Options** bar.

1 Choose Image, Resize, Image Size

In the Editor, open the image you want to resize or whose resolution you want to change and save it in Photoshop (***.psd**) format. Then choose **Image, Resize, Image Size** from the menu bar. The **Image Size** dialog box appears.

To resize a group of images in one step, see **17** **Rename, Resize, Reformat, and Retouch a Group of Images**.

2 Stop Distortion

If you want to make sure that the image is not distorted during the resizing process, enable the **Constrain Proportions** check box.

If you've applied a layer style to the image and want the pattern of that style to be resized as the image is resized, enable the **Scale Styles** option as well. Note that the **Scale Styles** option does not affect the size of patterns formed by effects, so you might want to apply such embellishments after resizing the image.

3 Turn On Resampling

To have the Editor mathematically re-evaluate and re-render the content of the image when you change its print size or resolution, enable the **Resample Image** option and select a sampling formula from the list. Here's a brief description of the formulas:

- **Bicubic**—Estimates each new pixel's color value based on the values of the 16 pixels nearest to the new pixel's location relative to the original image, in a 4×4 array. This method is best used when enlarging an image.

- **Bicubic Smoother**—Similar to the **Bicubic** formula, except that the tendency of Bicubic resampling to create halos around highly contrasting edges is reduced. Best used when enlarging an image.

- **Bicubic Sharper**—Similar to the **Bicubic** formula, except the edges are sharper with even higher contrast. Best used when reducing the size of an image.

- **Bilinear**—Estimates each new pixel's color value based on the values of the four pixels nearest to the new pixel's location relative to the original image. This method is best used when reducing an image.

- **Nearest Neighbor**—Estimates each new pixel's color value based on the values of all the pixels that fall within a fixed proximity of the new pixel's location relative to the original image. Here, the pixel residing in the same proportionate location in the original image as that of the new pixel in the resized image is given the extra "weight" when estimating the new color value. This method is best used when reducing the size of an image, but only for those images with edges that have not been anti-aliased.

16

▶ **NOTES**

When you make your image larger or smaller, the rescaling process can introduce arti-facts or patterns that resampling can eliminate. However, in smoothing out any possible artifacts or unwanted patterns, resampling after you resize can result in loss of detail, especially in the background or in small areas. So limit the number of times you resam-ple an image to *once*; if you have detail in the background you don't want to risk losing, do not resample.

To avoid resampling an image, disable the **Resample Image** option and change either the **Height/Width** or **Resolution** values in the **Document Size** area. Just keep in mind that if you increase the **Resolution** without resampling, the image will be resized smaller.

If you want to print an image in some size other than its normal print size, you can "rescale" the image on the fly when you print it. If you print an image in a larger size than normal, however, the resolution is decreased proportionately to compensate (pixels are not added). If the resulting resolution falls below acceptable levels of quality, you'll see a warning so that you can choose a different print size. Regardless, with this method, the original resolution and print size of the image are left unchanged. If you get the warning, it's best to choose a smaller print size (or abandon printing and then resize and resample the image to the print size you want) by following the steps in this task.

16

4 **Select a New Size and/or Resolution**

If you know what size you want the final image to be, type a value in the **Document Size Width** box; the **Height** value changes proportionately (or vice versa).

You can also change an image's size by adding or removing pixels. When you add pixels while maintaining the same resolution, you make the image bigger. For example, if you want the image to be twice as big, in the frame marked **Pixel Dimensions**, for either **Width** or **Height**, type **200** in the text box, and from the adjacent drop-down list, choose **Percent**. This increases the number of pixels without affecting the size of the pixels (assuming that **Resample Image** is on).

To change the resolution, type a value in the **Resolution** box. Altering resolu-tion in this manner does not change the image's print size unless you entered new values for **Document Size** earlier. Click **OK**. The image's size/resolution is adjusted as selected.

5 **View the Result**

After you're satisfied with the result of the resizing process, make any other changes you want and then save the final image in JPEG, PNG, or non-layered TIFF format, leaving your PSD image with its layers (if any) intact so that you can return at a later time and make different adjustments if you want.

Even though I increased the size of this photo by quite a lot (from roughly 4" × 3" to 7" × 5"), the quality (resolution) was maintained because I selected **Bicubic Smoother** resampling.

Because resampling often leaves an image a bit fuzzy, it's best to follow up by applying an **Unsharp Mask**. See 62 **Sharpen an Image**.

17 Rename, Resize, Reformat, and Retouch a Group of Images

✔ BEFORE YOU BEGIN	→ SEE ALSO
39 Apply a Quick Fix	16 Change Image Size or Resolution

It's easier than you might think to collect hundreds, if not thousands, of digital photos before you realize it. Managing these photos can become a full-time job if you don't establish a routine for processing new images that includes copying the files to your computer, backing them up onto CD-R or similar media, and converting those files you want to work with to PSD format or some other lossless format, such as TIFF. You should follow a similar process for images you copy to the computer using your scanner.

Luckily, the Editor provides a method for easily converting a group of files from one format to another *all at once*. In addition, you can rename the files (which you might want to do if they use generic names such as **DSC01982.jpg**), resize them (and even increase their resolution), and automatically adjust their brightness, contrast, and saturation.

▶ **TIP**

If you are processing files that are already in the catalog, you will need to update their catalog information. After you've processed the files, in the Organizer, choose **File, Reconnect, All Missing Files**. See 4 **Locate Moved Files**.

1 In the editor, choose **File, Process Multiple Files** from the menu bar. The **Process Multiple Files** dialog box opens.

2 **Select Files to Process**

To import images from your scanner, digital camera, or a PDF document for processing, from the **Process Files From** list, choose **Import**. Then select the source you want to use from the **From** list.

To process all the files that are currently open in the Editor's workspace, from the **Process Files From** list, choose **Opened Files**.

17

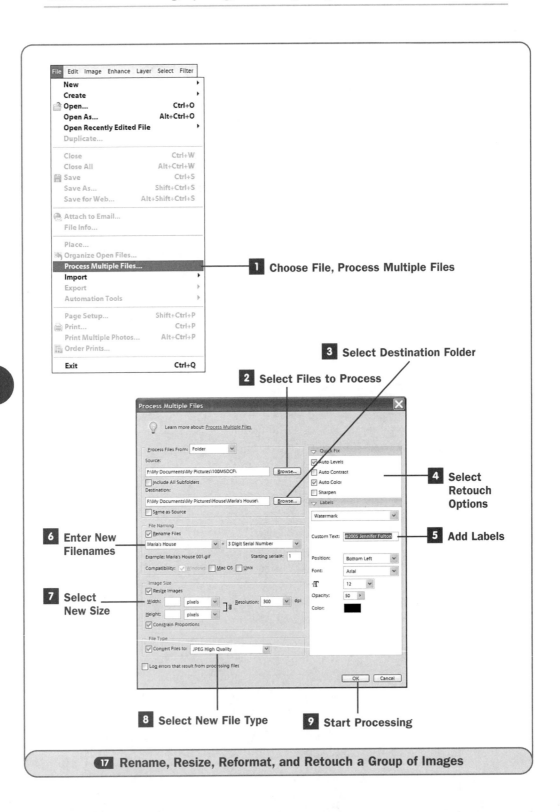

1 Choose File, Process Multiple Files

3 Select Destination Folder

2 Select Files to Process

4 Select Retouch Options

6 Enter New Filenames

5 Add Labels

7 Select New Size

8 Select New File Type

9 Start Processing

17 Rename, Resize, Reformat, and Retouch a Group of Images

To process all the images in a folder (and perhaps its subfolders), from the **Process Files From** list, choose **Folder**. Click the **Browse** button next to **Source**, select the folder that contains the files you want to process, and click **OK**. You're returned to the **Process Multiple Files** dialog box. If you want to include images stored in subfolders of the folder you selected, enable the **Include All Subfolders** option.

3 Select Destination Folder

If you want to save the processed files in the same folder in which they are now, enable the **Same as Source** option. If you choose this option, be sure to rename the files as well so that you don't overwrite your originals (see step 6). Otherwise, click the **Browse** button next to **Destination**, select the folder in which you want to save the converted files, and click **OK**.

4 Select Retouch Options

If you want to retouch the images automatically, select the adjustments you want to apply (such as **Auto Levels**) from the **Quick Fix** pane on the right side of the **Process Multiple Files** dialog box.

5 Add Labels

You can add a *watermark* or caption to identify your personal images and to protect them from being used without your permission. To create a watermark, select **Watermark** from the drop-down list at the top of the **Labels** pane. Enter the text you want to use in the **Custom Text** box. Adjust the font, size, position, opacity, and text color as desired.

▶ KEY TERM

Watermark—Slightly transparent text placed over a portion of an image, not only to identify its creator but also to protect the image from being used illegally.

To add a caption, select **Caption** from the drop-down list at the top of the **Labels** pane. Then select the text you want to include in the caption: **File Name**, **Description**, and/or **Date Modified**. You can choose as many of these text elements as you like—each appears on its own line in the image. The **Description**, by the way, is the same description you can enter on the **Description** page of the **File Info** dialog box or as an image caption in the Organizer. Select a **Position** for the caption (such as **Bottom Right**), and adjust the font, size, opacity, and text color as desired.

► **TIP**

To enter the copyright symbol into the **Custom Text** box, press and hold **Alt** as you type **0169** on the numeric keypad.

6 **Enter New Filenames**

To rename the files, enable the **Rename Files** check box. By selecting items from one or both of the lists, you can use the existing properties of an image to create a unique filename. For example, you can use an image's date as part or all of its new name. You can also combine your own text such as **Jan's Birthday** with a sequence number, creating a unique filename for each image—**Jan's Birthday 01**, **Jan's Birthday 02**, and so on.

Start by choosing a property you want to use from the first list box in the **File Naming** area. To enter your own text, simply type it into the first list box. Choose a second property (such as **2 digit serial number**) from the second list box if desired. If you plan to use the converted files on a computer with a different operating system, select that system in the **Compatibility** area. As you make your selections, a sample filename appears in the **Example** area.

17

► **NOTES**

If you're using a serial number as part of the filename, you can change the starting number by changing the value in the **Starting serial#** text box.

The **Document Name** property simply refers to the image's current filename. Selecting that property will enable you to use the existing filename and add something to it by selecting an additional property from the second list. This way, for instance, you can change the filename **DCX0304987.jpg** to **Walt and Saundra's Wedding - DCX0304987.jpg** if the original filename is important to you. Also, if you select **document name** from the list and the file is currently named **BBQ Party.jpg**, the file will be renamed **bbq party.jpg**; if you select **DOCUMENT NAME**, the file will be renamed **BBQ PARTY.JPG**, and so on.

7 **Select New Size**

If you want to resize these images or change their resolution, enable the **Resize Images** option. Then enter new **Width** and **Height** values. Resampling will take place during resizing. To make sure that the images are not distorted as they are resized, enable the **Constrain Proportions** option. Enter a new **Resolution** if desired. See **16 Change Image Size or Resolution** for more information.

8 Select New File Type

If you want to convert these images to a different file type (such as from GIF to PSD), enable the **Convert Files to** option, and then open the drop-down list and select the file type to which you want to convert the selected files.

9 Start Processing

When you're satisfied with your choices, click **OK**. Each image appears briefly in the Editor window as it is being processed. To save any error messages that appear during processing in a text file that you can review later, enable the **Log errors that result from processing files** option before clicking **OK**. This log file is saved to the destination folder you identified in step 3.

---

18   **Increase the Canvas Area Around an Image**

✔ BEFORE YOU BEGIN	→ SEE ALSO
40 Select a Color to Work With	**16** Change Image Size or Resolution

---

18

Each image has a *canvas*—essentially the image's background layer—that can be stretched to increase the size of the area on which you can paint, draw objects, and insert text. For a newly imported digital photo, the image fills the canvas. You can expand the background layer (the canvas) of an image such as a photograph, for example, to make room for a frame, and fill the new area with color and apply a filter, style, or effect. Or you might simply want to expand the canvas to create more room in which to add a clip from another image, an object, or some text.

▶ KEY TERM

Canvas—The working area of an image, as defined by the image's outer dimensions.

When you expand the canvas of an image, you add new pixels around its edges in a color you select. If an image has no background layer—for example, if you created the image using the **File**, **New** command and made the bottom layer transparent, or you converted the original **Background** layer to a regular layer using the **Layer**, **New**, **Layer from Background** command—then the new pixels are made transparent. Every layer above the base layer—whether it's a background layer or a regular layer—is expanded by the same amount.

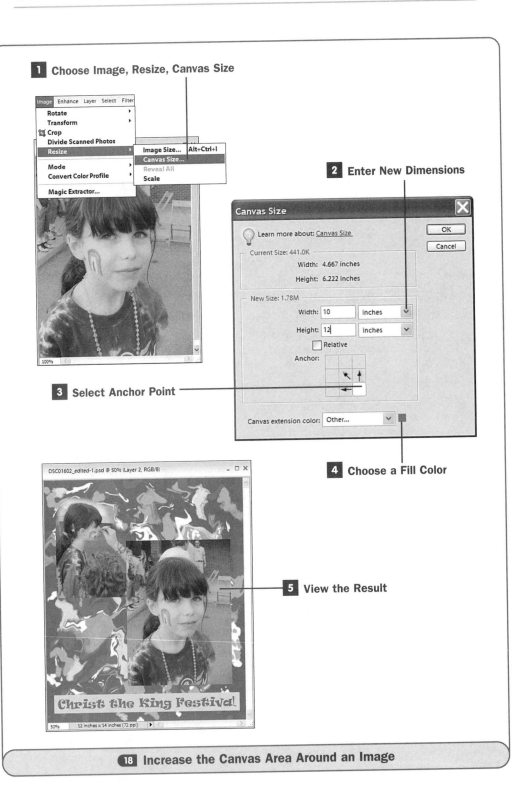

1 Choose Image, Resize, Canvas Size

2 Enter New Dimensions

3 Select Anchor Point

4 Choose a Fill Color

5 View the Result

18 Increase the Canvas Area Around an Image

▶ **NOTE**

You can reduce the canvas size of an image. If you do, although all the layers are reduced in size, data is not removed from the upper layers—it's just placed off the canvas where it is not seen in the final image. You can then use the **Move** tool to move the data on these non-background layers to display exactly the portion you want. Data from the bottom layer is clipped and cannot be retrieved. But if you increase the canvas size later on (even after saving and closing the image), you'll see that the data on upper layers is now visible again. See **32** **Move, Resize, Skew, or Distort a Layer or Selection**.

1 In the Editor, open the image whose canvas size you want to adjust and save it in Photoshop (*.psd*) format. Choose **Image, Resize, Canvas Size** from the menu bar. The **Canvas Size** dialog box is displayed.

2 **Enter New Dimensions**

The current dimensions of the image are displayed at the top of the **Canvas Size** dialog box. If you want to simply *add* a certain amount to the outer dimensions of the image, enable the **Relative** option. If the option is disabled, the dimensions you enter reflect the *total* width and height of the image.

In the **New Size** pane, select a unit of measure such as inches or pixels from one of the drop-down lists next to the **Width** and **Height** boxes (the other will change automatically). Then type values in the **Width** and **Height** boxes.

3 **Select Anchor Point**

Normally, the anchor point is in the center of the **Anchor** pad. This means that the added canvas is placed equally around the image. If you want to add canvas to just one side of the image, click the appropriate arrow on the **Anchor** pad.

4 **Choose a Fill Color**

If the bottom layer of the image is not a **Background** layer, the added canvas will be transparent. If the bottom layer is the **Background** layer, the added canvas will be set to the color you choose from the **Canvas extension color** list: **Background** (applies the current background color; **Other** displays the **Color Picker** with which you can choose a color. You can also click in the image to pick up that color with the dropper in the **Color Picker**. Click **OK**.

▶ **TIP**

To display the **Color Picker** without choosing **Other** from the **Canvas extension color** list, just click the box to the right of the list.

5 View the Result

After expanding the image canvas, make any other changes you want and then save the final image in JPEG, PNG, or non-layered TIFF format, leaving your PSD image with its layers (if any) intact so that you can return at a later time and make different adjustments if you want.

In the sample figure, the canvas was expanded above and to the left of the main image, text was added, and another image was pasted into the new space, creating a photo collage of a wonderful day spent at a local festival.

---

19   Change Color Mode

→ **SEE ALSO**

13 Create a New Image

18

One of the key factors affecting the size of an image file is the maximum number of colors it can include. If a file is theoretically capable of including a large number of colors—even though it may actually contain very few—the file's size will be large, just to ensure that capacity. If you're working on an image to be shared over the Internet, small file size is often a high priority. One way you can reduce a file's size is to change its color mode—the number of colors an image can contain, even if it doesn't actually contain that many. When you select certain file types that offer image compression, you'll be asked to make decisions on how to reduce the number of colors. You can also manually change to a different color mode, as explained in this task, and reduce the number of colors (and an image's file size) that way. Just keep in mind that reducing the number of colors in an image might lead to striation and patchiness in large areas of solid color.

Photographs typically use **RGB color mode**, which gives them access to all 16 million-plus colors that standard video cards support. **Indexed color mode**, used in GIF images, provides a limited color palette of only 256 colors, although these colors are selected from all the 16,777,216 hues the standard video card produces. If your image is black and white, or black and white plus gray, there are other modes you can use to make your image file even smaller. How perceptible the difference is, when changing to a lower color mode, depends on the image you're working with. For this reason, the Editor makes it possible for you to sample different color reduction modes, enabling you to choose the least detrimental mode for your image.

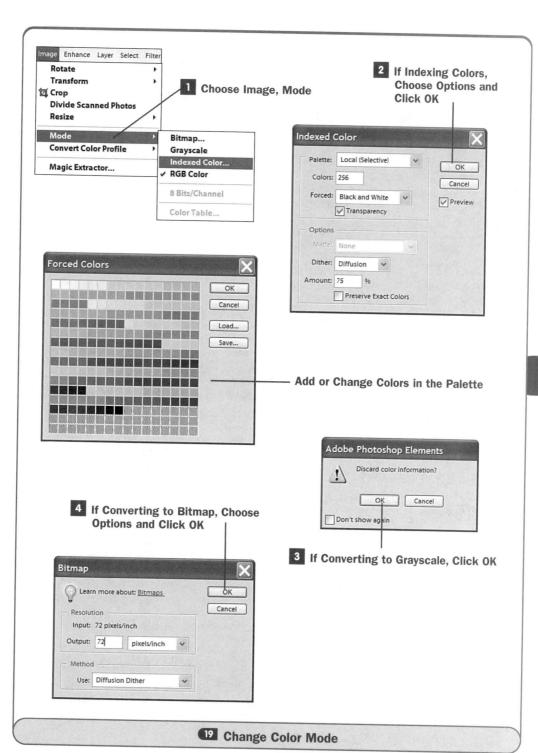

1 Choose Image, Mode

2 If Indexing Colors, Choose Options and Click OK

Add or Change Colors in the Palette

19

4 If Converting to Bitmap, Choose Options and Click OK

3 If Converting to Grayscale, Click OK

19 Change Color Mode

▶ **NOTES**

Because some commands are available only for images that use RGB or grayscale mode, you might sometimes find yourself temporarily increasing an image's color mode (from grayscale to RGB, for example). This won't, however, improve the resolution or quality of a low-resolution image—increasing an image's color palette simply makes more colors available for use; it does not tell the Editor where to use them in an image to boost detail and clarity.

The color mode of an image appears after its name, in the image window title bar.

1 Choose Image, Mode

In the Editor, open the image you want to convert, and save it in Photoshop (*.psd) format. Choose **Image, Mode** from the menu bar. Select the color mode you want to convert to from the submenu that appears:

- **Bitmap**—1-bit color in black and white; suitable for images in black and white only, with no gray tones.

- **Grayscale**—8-bit color in 256 shades of gray.

- **Indexed Color**—8 bits per pixel, in 256 colors, selected from the entire color gamut. Perfect for use with GIF images.

- **RGB**—24-bit color, with 8 bits per color channel, with more than 16 million colors available.

If you're increasing color depth, the image itself is not changed, but more colors become available for your use. If you're reducing color depth, a dialog box appears from which you must choose options. Continue to step 2, 3, or 4.

▶ **NOTE**

Technically speaking, the number of bits (binary digits) required for an image to encode the color value for one pixel is the base-2 logarithm of the maximum number of colors. In other words, 2 raised to that power equals the maximum number. It takes 8 bits to encode up to 256 values, and 24 bits to encode up to 16,777,216 values—thus the arithmetic behind the phrase *24-bit color*.

2 If Indexing Colors, Choose Options and Click OK

If you're reducing colors in an image with **Indexed Color** mode, select how you want the Editor to choose the colors for the palette by choosing from various options in the dialog box that appears. Before you begin making selections, enable the **Preview** option so that you can see how your selections affect the actual image. From the **Palette** list, choose one of the following options:

19

► **NOTE**

If the image already uses 256 colors or less, the **Palette** option is automatically set to **Exact**, which means that all colors in the image are added to the palette. You do not have to make a selection.

- **System (Mac OS)** uses the 256-color palette developed for the first color Macintosh computers. Select this palette to generate small files best displayed on Macs.

- **System (Windows)** uses the 256-color palette developed for Windows 3.0, which has been used as the backup palette for 8-bit color mode ever since.

- **Web** uses a 216-color palette (the last 40 index values are reserved), recommended for use in generating images for web pages because these are the 216 values that Mac and Windows machines have in common. Choosing this option ensures that the image will appear the same on both a Windows and a Mac computer.

- **Uniform** calculates 216 colors from equidistant positions in the RGB color gamut by rotating color index values from all-white to all-black. This setting ensures that your image uses colors sampled from throughout the image's color spectrum.

- The three **Local** options direct the Editor to create a palette based solely on the colors found in the currently open image.

- The three **Master** options instruct the Editor to create a palette based on the colors found in all the images currently open in the Editor.

  Among the **Local** and **Master** options, **Adaptive** instructs the Editor to select 256 colors that are mathematically most similar to the colors in the original image.

  Perceptual takes the 256 colors generated by the **Adaptive** algorithm and alters the selections slightly to favor colors that the human eye would tend to notice if they were changed—typically throwing away more colors in areas with the least amount of contrast, while favoring colors in areas with high contrast because the eye would notice that more.

  Selective takes the 256 colors refined by the **Perceptual** algorithm and then weights the values to more closely resemble the Web spectrum, while also favoring broad areas of color within the image.

- Select **Custom** to make changes to any colors in the palette that the Editor is currently preparing to adopt. When the **Color Table** dialog box appears (which looks similar to the **Forced Colors** dialog box shown here), double-click the color in the palette you want to change. Select a new color from

19

the **Color Picker** dialog box and click **OK**. To add a color to the palette, click an empty spot and then select a color to add. Repeat for any other palette colors you want to change or add, and click **OK** when finished. You're returned to the **Indexed Color** dialog box.

- Choose **Previous** to load the previously used custom color palette. Use **Previous** to convert a series of images to indexed color mode, using the same color palette.

▶ **TIP**

To reduce your file size even further, set **Colors** to a value less than 256 (to reduce file size *significantly*, select a value less than 128).

The options in the **Forced** list instruct the Editor to override some or all of its palette color choices and to include specific color values, some of which you can choose yourself from the **Forced Color** dialog box that appears. These "forced" choices may or may not be represented in the actual image, but they are included in the image's palette:

- **Black & White** forces the Editor to include pure black and pure white as two of the colors in the palette.

- **Primaries** forces the Editor to include the first eight colors of the old IBM Extended Graphics palette: red, green, blue, cyan, magenta, yellow, black and white. This allows a large measure of downward compatibility (if you really need it) with some of the first images ever produced for display on PCs.

- **Web** forces the Editor to include the entire 216-color Web palette (essentially the same as choosing **Web** from the **Palette** list).

- Choose **Custom** to enable you to change or add colors to the palette. Double-click a palette color. Select a new color from the **Color Picker** dialog box and click **OK**. To add a color, click an empty spot, select a color, and click **OK**. Repeat for any other palette colors you want to add or change and click **OK** when finished.

If the image has transparency but you don't want to retain it, disable the **Transparency** option. Then select from the **Matte** drop-down list a color to change the transparent pixels to. Semi-transparent pixels are blended with the color you choose to make them fully opaque. You can choose **Foreground Color**, **Background Color**, **White**, **Black**, **50% Gray**, or **Netscape Gray** (a lighter gray) from the list, or select your own color by choosing **Custom** from the **Matte** drop-down list and using the **Color Picker** that appears to select a color to use. To choose a color from the image, just click in the image with the **Eyedropper** tool.

If the image contains transparent pixels and you want to retain them, enable the **Transparency** option. If the image contains semi-transparent pixels, open the **Matte** list and choose a color to blend with them to make them fully opaque.

▶ NOTES

If you choose **None** from the **Matte** drop-down list, semi-transparent pixels are simply changed to fully opaque ones and are not blended with anything. Transparent pixels are made white.

Because it uses a mathematical formula, error diffusion (when used in images with a very limited color palette or large blocks of color, such as comics art) can sometimes generate artifacts in a color blended area, more so than if you use an ordered dither method such as **Pattern**.

To reduce the side effects caused by using a smaller number of colors than the original image contained, select the dither pattern you prefer from the **Dither** list:

- **Diffusion** instructs the Editor to apply an *error diffusion* algorithm to blend dissimilar colors by dividing the differences between them mathematically and spreading that difference to neighboring pixels, hiding the transition. When you make this choice, enter the relative percentage of error diffusion in the **Amount** text box. Enable the **Preserve Exact Colors** option to instruct the Editor not to dither any colors it encounters in the original image whose values exactly match any of those in the current reduction palette.

▶ KEY TERM

Error diffusion—Any of several mathematical techniques that attempt to compensate for large differences (errors) between the color of an original pixel and its replacement in a resampled image by dividing this difference into parts and distributing it to neighboring pixels, thus masking the obvious inaccuracy.

- **Pattern** applies a geometric dithering pattern, which might be noticeable in photographic images but is permissible in more patterned images such as original drawings.

- **Noise** scatters dithered pixels randomly.

- **None** turns off diffusion and causes the Editor to substitute the closest color in the palette for any color not in the palette.

To finalize your choices, click **OK**.

19

3 If Converting to Grayscale, Click OK

When you're converting a color image to various hues of gray (grayscale), click **OK**; if the image has multiple layers, you'll be asked whether you want to flatten all layers before proceeding. Click **Merge**.

▶ **NOTE**

If the color layers currently in the image use blend modes other than **Normal** to create its current appearance—especially if that appearance depends on how the color of one layer interacts with the colors of the layers beneath it—then these effects will probably be completely lost if the image is flattened while converting it to grayscale. To preserve the layers and their blend modes, click **Don't Merge** in step 3.

4 If Converting to Bitmap, Choose Options and Click OK

When converting an image to pure black-and-white (**Bitmap** mode), the Editor could simply make relatively dark pixels black and the relatively light ones white. However, the result might not be desirable, so you might want to apply dithering.

First, let the Editor convert your image to grayscale by clicking **OK**. It's easier for the Editor to convert grays to black-and-white than to convert colors directly to black and white. If there are multiple layers, the Editor warns you to flatten them first; click **OK** to have it do that and continue. In the **Bitmap** dialog box that appears, in the **Resolution** area, make sure that your image is set for the resolution of your output device. At first, this is set to the image's current resolution. To ensure best appearance, you might have to adjust resolution—and thus, its size—accordingly. For on-screen use, choose 72 PPI as a minimum; for printing, choose 200–300 ppi as a minimum. Altering this setting resizes the image, both in print and on-screen.

In the **Method** area, choose how you want the Editor to apply dithering. The **50% Threshold** option applies no dithering whatsoever—light pixels are made white, and dark ones are made black. The **Pattern Dither** option applies a geometric dithering pattern, which might be adequate if your original image is a simple drawing—such as a corporate logo—rather than a photograph. **Diffusion Dither** applies an error diffusion pattern, distributing vast differences in brightness value over wider areas—which is generally more appropriate for photographs.

To finalize your choices, click **OK**.

After changing the color mode of your image, make any other changes you want and then save the final image in JPEG, PNG, or non-layered TIFF format (or GIF, if you've converted to **Indexed color** mode), leaving your PSD image with its layers (if any) intact so that you can return at a later time and make different adjustments if you want.

5

Selecting a Portion of an Image

IN THIS CHAPTER:

Many of the modifications you make to an image in Photoshop Elements are applied to only a portion of the image. For example, you might want to delete an item from the background or change the color of part of the image. To make modifications to any portion of an image, you must first select the area to change. Selecting an area enables you to make modifications to only that portion of the image without affecting the rest of the image.

In this chapter, you will learn how to make selections using the different selection tools available in Photoshop Elements. You will see that the tool you choose to make selections is based on the type of selection you want to make. You will learn to select geometric portions of the image (such as a rectangle or an oval) or to select specific objects by tracing the object's borders (such as selecting only the light post in front of a house). You will also learn how to select specific portions of the image based on their color, such as selecting only the red balloons in a balloon bouquet. You'll learn how to save selections and then reuse those selections to edit the image. You'll see how selections can be used to create a new image or layer.

Regardless of how you select a portion of the image, after you've done that, all the editing commands you then make affect only that portion. So, you can change the color of only the red balloons to blue or use the **Dodge** tool on just the light post without affecting the house.

20 Select a Rectangular or Circular Area

→ **SEE ALSO**

21 Draw a Selection Freehand or By Tracing Its Edge

You can use the **Marquee Selection** tools to select any rectangular or elliptical area in an image. These are the most common selection tools in this or any other image editing program. But you might be wondering, now that you know you can select *just* the subject of your image or *just* some element you want to remove, why would you *want* to select something that's rectangular or elliptical? Rectangles are the most common shapes for *frames*, ovals the second most common. For example, to apply many of the frame effects on the **Styles and Effects** palette, you must make a selection first.

1 Select the Marquee Tool

Open an image in the Editor in **Standard Edit** mode and save it in Photoshop (*.psd**) format. In the **Layers** palette, click the layer that contains the data you want to select. Select the **Rectangular Marquee** or **Elliptical Marquee** tool on the **Toolbox**.

1 Select the Marquee Tool

New Selection Button

2 Set Options

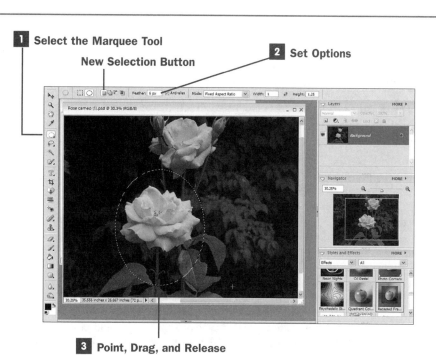

3 Point, Drag, and Release

20

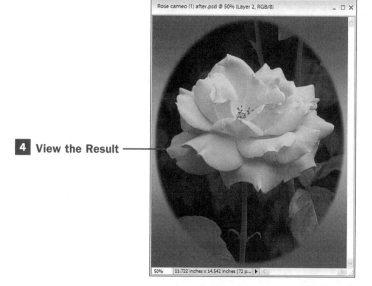

4 View the Result

2 Set Options

On the **Options** bar, click the **New Selection** button. Set other options as desired. For example, to soften the edge of your selection, adjust the **Feather** value and turn on the **Anti-aliased** option.

The default **Mode** setting is **Normal**, which means that you control the size of the selection yourself. If you want to specify the proportions of your selection, choose **Fixed Aspect Ratio**. To specify an exact size, choose **Fixed Size** instead. For the **Fixed Aspect Ratio** or **Fixed Size** option, enter the proportions or exact measurements you want (in pixels) in the **Width** and **Height** boxes.

3 Point, Drag, and Release

Drag to create the selection. If the **Mode** setting is **Fixed Size**, just click without dragging.

▶ TIPS

If you want to create a perfectly square or circular selection instead of a rectangular or elliptical selection, press and hold the **Shift** key as you drag to create the selection.

To create a circle from the center out, press **Alt+Shift** as you drag.

4 View the Result

Add to or subtract from the selection using the same **Marquee** tool or a different selection tool. Make changes to the area within the selection, copy or cut it to another image or layer, or delete the data. After you're satisfied with the result, make any other changes you want and then save the PSD file. Resave the result in JPEG, PNG, or non-layered TIFF format, leaving your PSD image with its layers (if any) intact so that you can return at a later time and make adjustments if you want.

Here, I've used the **Elliptical Marquee** tool with feathering set to **6**, to cut a rose out of one photo and paste it into this new, blank layer. I then added a layer painted with a gradient to create a frame for the rose.

---

21   Draw a Selection Freehand or By Tracing Its Edge

→ SEE ALSO

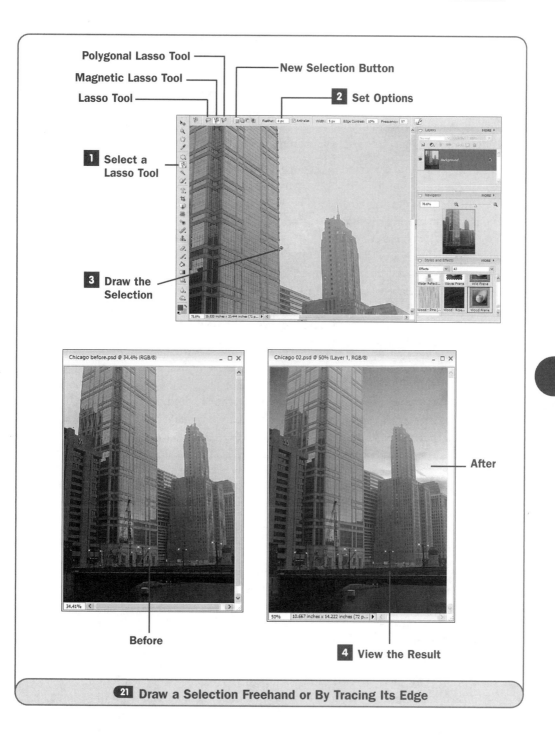

The principal reason you'd want to use one of the Editor's lasso tools is so you can select a region in your photograph whose shape does not fit within a rectangle, square, or circle, and also so that you don't select anything else in the photo except for that region. For example, you can use a lasso tool to designate the head of a person or an animal lying on the ground, or a naval destroyer, or even a respectable approximation of the edge of a dandelion puff-ball, while at the same time *excluding* the object's surroundings.

To use the standard **Lasso** tool, you drag it around the area you want to select as though you're drawing a chalk boundary around it. With patience, you can trace intricate shapes with the **Lasso** tool. However, in the case of objects whose color and shade are clearly distinguished from its surroundings—for example, a grey skyscraper against a clear blue sky—you can use the **Magnetic Lasso** tool. With this tool, the boundary you draw automatically snaps to the edges of objects you drag near. When you use the **Magnetic Lasso** tool, you must specify settings that help Photoshop Elements locate the edges of your object. For example, you can indicate a pixel **Width** value to define the width of the area near where you drag; Photoshop Elements looks in this area to locate the object edge. Photoshop Elements places the selection line along the edge it finds in that search area.

21

The **Polygonal Lasso** tool becomes most helpful in best-guess scenarios, such as selecting a fuzzball or a cloud or a stream of water, where exact edges won't be ascertained anyway, and it might not matter too much whether you end up selecting indetectably small swatches of sky or background. With the **Polygonal Lasso**, you mark points along the edge of the image that you want to select, and the Editor automatically connects those points with straight lines.

1 Select a Lasso Tool

Open an image in the Editor in **Standard Edit** mode and save it in Photoshop (***.psd**) format. In the **Layers** palette, click the layer that contains the data you want to select.

Select the desired lasso tool from the **Toolbox: Lasso, Magnetic Lasso,** or **Polygonal Lasso.** The icon for the last lasso tool you used is the one displayed in the **Toolbox.**

2 Set Options

Click the **New Selection** button. Set the desired options for the tool on the **Options** bar, such as **Feather** and **Anti-alias.** If you choose the **Magnetic Lasso** tool, adjust the **Width** (1 to 256 pixels) to the area you want the Editor to look within, in order to identify the edge of the object (pixels whose brightness contrast with their neighbors). The **Edge Contrast** option indicates the amount of contrast to look for, between **1%** and **100%**. If your object has low-contrast edges, use a higher value. The **Frequency** option indicates the rate at which you want the lasso to set the anchor points along the object's edge as you drag. Enter a frequency value between **0** and **100**. Use a higher value to have the Editor set border points more often.

▶ **TIP**

If you are using a pen and drawing tablet, select the **Pen Pressure** option. When this option is enabled, if you increase the pen pressure, the **Width** value increases for the selection.

3 Draw the Selection

The hotspot for each of the lasso tools is the tip of the little loop in the lower-left corner. For the **Lasso** tool, just drag to draw a freehand selection. Make sure that you draw your selection so that it ends at the same point you start-ed. When you release the mouse button, the Editor completes the selection by connecting the start and end of your selection.

For the **Magnetic Lasso** tool, click the location on the image where you want to start your selection. Continue holding down the left mouse button and drag the mouse pointer along the edge of the object to select. The Editor drops selection points along this edge, identifying the edge by looking for high con-trast within the **Width** area surrounding where you drag. You can drop a selection point yourself by just clicking. Double-click to connect a selection's starting and ending points.

For the **Polygonal Lasso** tool, click the location on the image where you want to start your selection, move the mouse pointer to where you want to create a corner in the selection, and click again. As you reposition the mouse pointer, a springy line extends between the last anchor point and the mouse pointer so that you can see how the selection line will lay against the area you are selecting. Continue to click to set corner points; double-click to close the selection.

▶ **TIP**

With the **Magic Lasso** or **Polygonal Lasso** tool, you can remove selection points as you drag by simply pressing the **Backspace** key as many times as necessary. Points are removed in reverse order. Removing points allows you to correct a bad selection; for example, if the Editor selected something far from the edge of the object.

21

4 View the Result

Add to or subtract from the selection using the same **Lasso** tool or a different selection tool. Make changes to the area within the selection, copy or cut it to another image or layer, or delete the data. When you are satisfied with the result, congratulate yourself, then make any other changes you want and save the PSD file. Resave the result in JPEG, PNG, or non-layered TIFF format, leaving your PSD image with its layers (if any) intact so that you can return at a later time and make adjustments if you want.

In this example, I used the **Magnetic Lasso** tool to draw the boundaries between these Chicago skyscrapers and the sky. I could have used the **Polygonal Lasso** tool, but I would have missed the faint ridges that make up the texture of the center building; the **Magnetic Lasso** tool found them automatically. Selecting this rather cloudy and, frankly, uninteresting sky enabled me to remove it and replace it with a more striking background.

21

22 Select Areas of Similar Color

→ **SEE ALSO**

21 Draw a Selection Freehand or by Tracing Its Edge
23 Paint a Selection

Despite its name, don't expect the **Magic Wand** tool to select exactly the region you want in an image with just one touch. The reason is because most things in a digital photograph are not often composed of a single color (although they may seem to be), but rather, several shades of a single color or closely matching colors. Although you might see a landscape composed of leaves, branches, sky, clouds, and water, how Photoshop Elements' Editor sees it is a cluster of pixels of various colors.

When you click a pixel in your image with the **Magic Wand** tool, the Editor evaluates neighboring pixels (or all the pixels in the image, if the **Contiguous** option is disabled) for color similarity, the degree of which is based on the **Tolerance** setting you specify in the **Options** bar. For example, if the **Tolerance** value is low, only pixels adjacent to the one you click, whose color values are very similar, are selected. Specify a higher **Tolerance** setting to widen the range of colors that are selected, such as the shadows in the petals of a red rose or variations in the green of the picnic grass. Sometimes you'll need to make these adjustments intermittently while you touch the image with the **Magic Wand** a handful of times, each time building onto the existing selection—or perhaps removing a small portion from it—until its final selection becomes something you can work with.

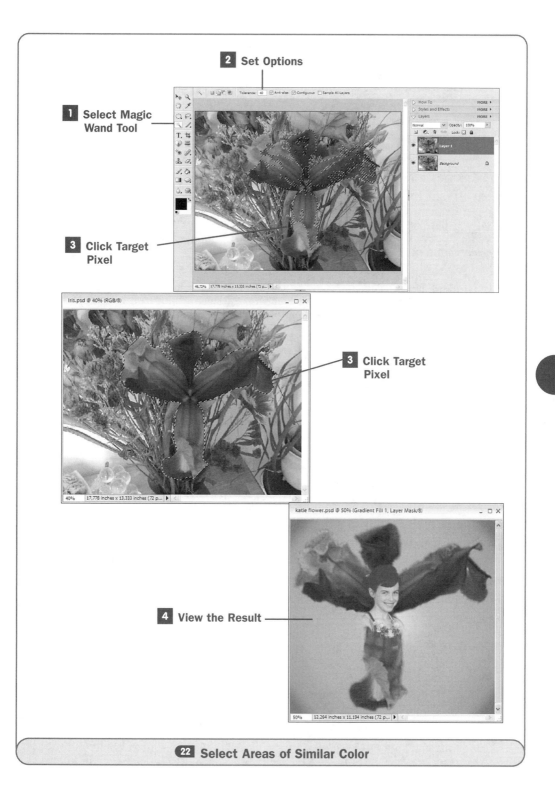

2 Set Options

1 Select Magic
Wand Tool

3 Click Target
Pixel

3 Click Target
Pixel

4 View the Result

1 Select Magic Wand Tool

Open an image in the Editor in **Standard Edit** mode and save it in Photoshop (***.psd**) format. In the **Layers** palette, select the layer that contains the data you want to select. Select the **Magic Wand** tool on the **Toolbox**.

2 Set Options

On the **Options** bar, click the **New Selection** button. Adjust the **Tolerance** value to fit the similarity of the pixels you want to select; with very similar pixels, you can set a low **Tolerance** and still select the area you want with just a few clicks. Set the other options, such as **Anti-aliased**, **Contiguous**, and **Sample All Layers**.

▶ **TIP**

You can select all pixels in a layer with an opacity of 50% or higher by pressing **Ctrl** and clicking the layer's thumbnail in the **Layers** palette. To select all pixels, regardless of their transparency, choose **Select**, **All** from the menu bar.

22

3 Click Target Pixel

In the image window, locate the point that best exemplifies the pixels you want to select, and click that point. The Editor selects similar pixels in accordance with your option settings.

▶ **TIP**

You cannot use the **Magic Wand** tool with an image that uses **Bitmap** or **Indexed Color** mode. If you want to use this tool, you must first choose **Image**, **Mode**, **Grayscale** or **RGB Color** from the menu bar to convert the image.

4 View the Result

Add to or subtract from the selection using the **Magic Wand** tool or a different selection tool. Make changes to the area within the selection, copy or cut it to another image or layer, or delete the data. When you're satisfied with the result, make any other changes you want and save the PSD file. Resave the result in JPEG, PNG, or non-layered TIFF format, leaving your PSD image with its layers (if any) intact so that you can return at a later time and make adjustments if you want.

In this example, I wanted to isolate the iris from the rest of the bouquet so that I could use it to frame a photo of my daughter. There are several regions of differing hues in this iris, obviously including the deep blues, but also incorporating the light lavenders (which contain a small hint of red tint, optically) and the bright yellows of the stamen. So even with a relatively loose

Tolerance setting of 40, I still had to select about eight different contiguous regions, and then trim the result using the **Lasso** tool in **Subtract from Selection** mode, especially for the purple daisies along the side that I wanted to exclude. But even this process was faster and less tedious than trying to draw around the perimeter of the iris with the **Magnetic Lasso** tool.

---

23 Paint a Selection

→ **SEE ALSO**

- **20** Select a Rectangular or Circular Area
- **21** Draw a Selection Freehand or by Tracing Its Edge
- **22** Select Areas of Similar Color

The Editor's selection brushes work in either of two ways: With the conventional **Selection Brush** tool, whatever your paintbrush touches becomes selected. With the new **Magic Selection Brush** tool, after you've applied your "paint" stroke, the selected region takes on the characteristics of the **Magic Wand** tool (explained in **22** **Select Areas of Similar Color**). All the pixels throughout the image whose color and brightness characteristics are similar to those you brushed are also selected. You could use this tool to select an oddly shaped object, such as a leaf set against the sky, by painting inside of it and then letting the Editor expand the painted region to encompass the entire leaf, right to the edges.

The **Selection Brush** tool can be rigged to work the opposite way, using what the Editor calls **Mask** mode. Here, you paint a mask, represented by a red overlay, over the areas of the image you *do not* want to select. You can switch between **Mask** and **Selection** modes by changing the **Mode** option on the **Options** bar. When the Editor is in **Mask** mode, the mask covers the unselected areas, and the "windows" left open by the red mask overlay reveal the parts of the image ready to be changed with a filter or other adjustment.

23

▶ **NOTE**

Although the process is similar, the **Mask** mode of the **Selection Brush** tool is not the same kind of mask you paint to protect lower layers from the effects of a fill or adjustment layer. The painted mask is also different from a clipping mask, which you can use to block parts of an upper layer from covering lower layers.

1 Choose the Selection Brush Tool

Open an image in the Editor in **Standard Edit** mode and save it in Photoshop (***.psd**) format. In the **Layers** palette, click the layer that contains the data you want to select. On the **Toolbox**, choose the **Selection Brush**.

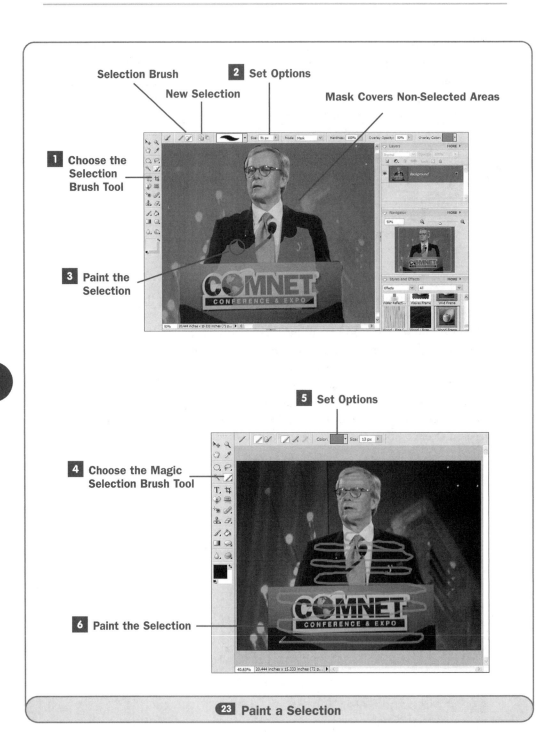

Selection Brush

New Selection

2 Set Options

Mask Covers Non-Selected Areas

1 Choose the
Selection
Brush Tool

3 Paint the
Selection

5 Set Options

4 Choose the Magic
Selection Brush Tool

6 Paint the Selection

23 Paint a Selection

23

Indicate
Foreground   Indicate
Background   **5** Set Options

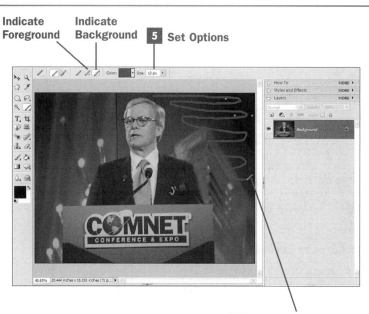

7 Refine the Selection

23

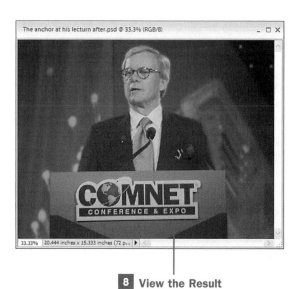

8 View the Result

23 Paint a Selection (continued)

2 Set Options

On the **Options** bar, choose a brush tip, **Size**, and **Hardness**. A soft round brush works well in most cases. To have the brush select everything you paint, in the **Mode** list, if you choose **Selection** then everything you paint with the brush is selected; to have the Editor deselect everything the brush paints, choose **Mask**.

▶ TIP

The mask overlay is usually red, but you can select a different mask color from the **Overlay Color** list in the **Options** bar. Typically, you select a color that will stand out against the image so that you can easily identify the masked area. You can also adjust the opacity of the mask with the **Overlay Opacity** value.

3 Paint the Selection

Assuming you're using the **Selection** mode, paint over the area you want to select. The selected area is surrounded by the marquee. If you're using **Mask** mode, paint the area you do *not* want to select; the area you paint is marked by the red mask overlay. You can change between the two modes as needed to select the area you want.

23

4 Choose the Magic Selection Brush Tool

On the **Toolbox**, choose the **Magic Selection Brush** tool.

5 Set Options

On the **Options** bar, you only need to select a brush **Size** because the only purpose the brush serves when you use this tool is to indicate *very roughly* the item or region you want selected. The only purpose for the **Color** setting (which, by default, is red) is to let you see what you're brushing; the color is never applied to the image or layer you're painting on.

6 Paint the Selection

Make sure that the **New Selection** is enabled on the **Options** bar. Then brush over the area you want to select, making sure that you brush over a good sampling of the pixels that comprise the region you want to select. The area you brush is marked in red; these marks are not permanent and do not affect the image. After you release the mouse button, the Editor analyzes the pixels you've marked, and selects similar, contiguous pixels. (Note there is no tolerance option here, as there is for the **Magic Wand** tool.)

7 Refine the Selection

To add to the pixels being sampled so that the Editor can make a broader approximation of the region you want selected, click the **Indicate Foreground** button on the **Options** bar (it is automatically selected after the first brush stroke), then brush another area of the image as you did before. You can remove regions from the current selection by clicking **Indicate Background**, and then brushing the area (this mark shows up in blue, by default) that represents the general color and variety of pixels you want *removed* from the current selection.

8 View the Result

Add to or subtract from the selection using the **Selection Brush** or a different selection tool. Make changes to the area within the selection, copy or cut it to another image or layer, or delete the data. When you're satisfied with the result, make any other changes you want and save the PSD file. Resave the result in JPEG, PNG, or non-layered TIFF format, leaving your PSD image with its layers (if any) intact so that you can return at a later time and make adjustments if you want.

In this example, I was never particularly pleased with this photo of a keynote speaker at a networking conference. If you're thinking, "Hey, that looks like Tom Brokaw," well, *it is*, but that's not the problem: The photo is a little fuzzy up front, and the background is too blue and distracting. After selecting Tom, I sharpened him. I then inverted the selection, blurred the background, and lowered the saturation, making the resulting background area much more tolerable.

24

24 Expand, Shrink, or Add Similar Areas to a Selection

→ SEE ALSO

25 Smooth and Soften a Selection

After you've made a selection with a lasso tool or the **Magic Wand** tool, adjusting that selection so that it encompasses a larger or smaller region is a simple matter. You can inflate or deflate a selection just like controlling the air in a balloon, using the **Select**, **Modify**, **Expand** and **Select**, **Modify**, **Contract** commands, respectively. For example, you might select a subject, expand the selection and fill it with color, then place the layer with the filled selection below the subject, creating a frame that perfectly traces the object's outline.

24

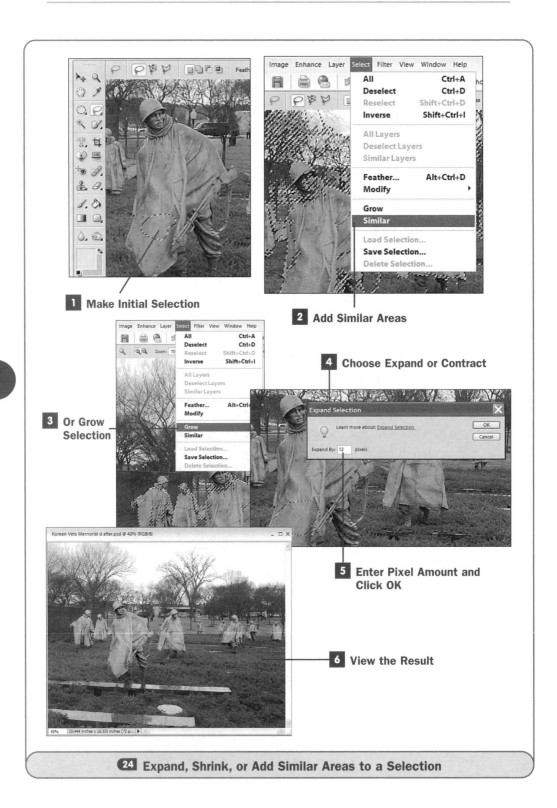

1 Make Initial Selection

2 Add Similar Areas

3 Or Grow Selection

4 Choose Expand or Contract

5 Enter Pixel Amount and Click OK

6 View the Result

24 Expand, Shrink, or Add Similar Areas to a Selection

Another technique that will come in handy when perfecting a selection is the ability for the Editor to select all the pixels in the image whose color values are close to those in the current selection. For this equally simple technique, you use the **Select**, **Similar** command. Suppose, for instance, that you have a photo of a troupe of costumed dancers, and you've selected just a portion of a single blue costume. The **Select**, **Similar** command selects not only the rest of the original blue costume, but all similarly colored blue costumes in the image. If you want to select only similarly shaded pixels adjacent to the current selection—for example, only the remainder of the single blue costume—choose the **Select**, **Grow** command instead.

1 Make Initial Selection

Open the image you want to select in the Editor in **Standard Edit** mode and save it in Photoshop (***.psd**) format. In the **Layers** palette, choose the layer that contains the data you want to select, and then use any selection tool to make the initial selection. The colors and tone in this selection will be used to find matching pixels in the image. In this example, I made a small selection in the front statue in this photo of the Korean War Memorial in Washington, D.C.

2 Add Similar Areas

Choose **Select**, **Similar** to select all areas in the image that are similar in color and tone to the area you selected in step 1. In my image, this command causes all of the medium-gray pixels to be selected, including the other statues, parts of the sky, and the marble "rice paddies."

▶ TIP

With both the **Grow** and **Similar** commands, you can control how closely pixels must match your original selection before being included in the expanded selection by simply adjusting the **Tolerance** value on the **Options** bar when the **Magic Wand** is selected. Seems strange, but true. So, select the **Magic Wand** tool, adjust the **Tolerance** to suit your needs, then apply the **Grow** or **Similar** command as explained here.

3 Or Grow Selection

Alternatively, choose **Select**, **Grow** to expand the current selection to include only neighboring pixels of similar color and tone. In my image, the command causes the selection to expand to include the rest of the soldier's cape I originally selected only partially, plus the capes of two neighboring soldiers whose pixels are contiguous to (happen to be touching) the original soldier.

24

4 Choose Expand or Contract

Choose **Selection**, **Modify**, **Expand** to expand the selection at all points by the same amount, or **Selection**, **Modify**, **Contract** to shrink it uniformly along all points. The **Expand Selection** or **Contract Selection** dialog box appears; both are remarkably similar.

5 Enter Pixel Amount and Click OK

In the **Expand Selection** or **Contract Selection** dialog box, enter the number of pixels you want to expand or contract by, and then click **OK**. The selection is immediately modified. With my original, small selection, I expanded it by 12 pixels; this adjustment simply made the small oval a little bigger.

▶ TIPS

You can refine a selection by adding to or subtracting from it, or by creating a new selection from the intersection of two selections, using the buttons on the **Options** bar for most of the selection tools (**Selection Brush** excluded): **Add to Selection**, **Subtract from Selection**, and **Intersect with Selection**. To build a selection, you can switch from selection tool to selection tool freely, using each tool to your advantage when trying to snag a particular area.

To select the outline of a selection, choose **Select**, **Modify**, **Border**. Enter the number of pixels on either side of the outline to include, then click **OK**. You might use this command to create a narrow frame around a selection. You can also use the **Stroke** command to create a frame: Create the selection first, then choose **Edit**, **Stroke (Outline) Selection**. Enter the **Width** for the frame and choose a **Color**. Select whether you want the frame created on the **Inside**, **Center**, or **Outside** of the selection border. Choose a blend mode and **Opacity**. To preserve the transparency within a selection and not stroke those pixels, choose **Preserve Transparency**. Click **OK**.

6 View the Result

Add to or subtract from your original selection using a combination of tools and commands. When you're satisfied with the selection, make changes to the area within the selection, copy or cut its data to another image or layer, or delete the data within the selection. Save the PSD file and then resave the file in JPEG, PNG, or non-layered TIFF format, leaving your PSD image with its layers (if any) intact so that you can return at a later time and make adjustments if you want.

Using the **Grow** command, I was able to expand my small selection to include almost all the closest soldiers. I saved this selection and then started over, growing a similar selection until I had selected all the soldiers on the right. Then I combined the two selections using the **Select**, **Save Selection** command. When I had all the soldiers selected, it was easy to lighten them a bit and adjust their color to restore their original greenish overcast.

25 Smooth and Soften a Selection

→ **SEE ALSO**

24 Expand, Shrink, or Add Similar Areas to a Selection

After you've used the **Magic Wand** tool to select a region from an image, there's a good chance the selection will have a number of pits and bumps. Photoshop Elements's **Smooth** command analyzes the color values of selected pixels and uses that information to decide how to adjust a selection border to smooth it visually. In this way, the **Smooth** command does not select pixels outside a selection that are obviously different in color. The goal of the **Smooth** command is to make a selection border less jagged. It's quite possible that, after smoothing, some portion you might have meant to exclude could end up being included, and other portions you meant to include could end up excluded. That's because the **Smooth** command actually changes the selection marquee here and there, smoothing out jagged ins and outs. The purpose of this kind of smoothing is not to create precise selection areas but more general ones—areas that appear more naturally cut out, especially when pasted into another image. The **Smooth** command can also be used to include previously non-included pixels within a selection that obviously should be included—for example, lighter green pixels in a leaf that were not included when you clicked with the **Magic Wand**.

Another common modification you might find yourself making to a selection is *feather* it, either when making the selection, or after the fact, with the **Feather** command. When you feather a selection, semitransparent pixels are added to the edge of the selection to soften it. Feathering a selection is often preferable when you intend to copy the selection and place it on a different background, or to fade the edge of a selection gradually to white or black, creating an old-fashioned photographic vignette. Feathering is also preferred when you intend to change the color or tone of the data within the selection, or apply a filter or effect, and you want the resulting data to blend into surrounding pixels. By feathering the edges of the selection, the edges seem softer and appear to fade into whatever background on which you place the object.

▶ **KEY TERM**

Feathering—The addition of partly selected pixels along the edge of a selection, often to help blend a relocated selection into its new surroundings.

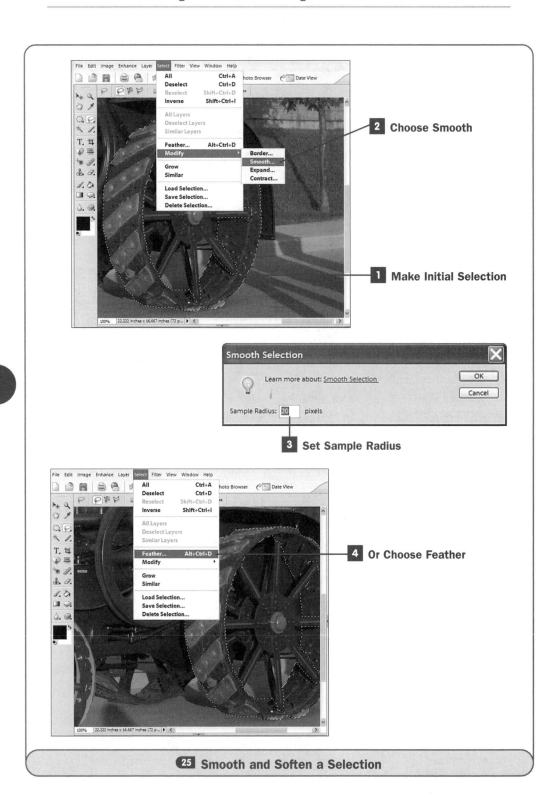

2 Choose Smooth

1 Make Initial Selection

3 Set Sample Radius

4 Or Choose Feather

25 Smooth and Soften a Selection

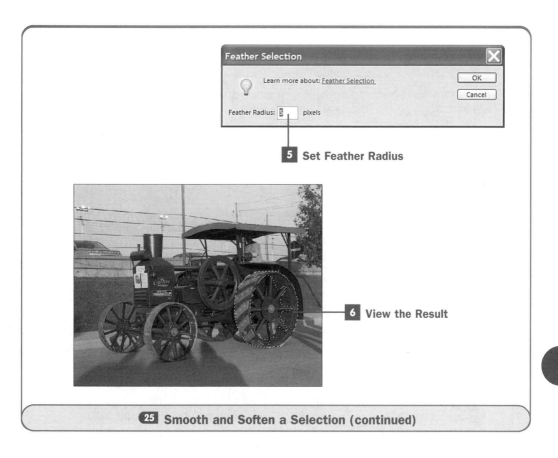

Feather Selection

Learn more about: Feather Selection

OK

Cancel

Feather Radius: [5] pixels

5 Set Feather Radius

6 View the Result

25

25 Smooth and Soften a Selection (continued)

▶ NOTES

Feathering occurs on both sides of the original selection marquee. When you feather the selection within your image, however, you will not see the feathering in the selection itself. For example, if you feather the edge of a selection by 10 pixels, the marquee will shrink by that amount to surround only the area of 50% or more selected pixels. If you copy or cut the data and then paste the selection into another image or onto another layer however, you'll notice that the copied data includes the partially selected pixels outside the marquee where the feathering occurred.

Although feathering, anti-aliasing, and smoothing might appear to be synonymous, each actually refers to a different concept. Feathering a selection's border enables pixels along the very rim to be partly selected, for a fuzzy border. This causes a regular change in opacity to the pixels along the entire border of a selection. Anti-aliasing adjusts the opacity of certain pixels only to help a selection look less jagged along the edges. Smoothing, like anti-aliasing, also makes a selection look less jagged by changing the border of a selection and not by partially selecting pixels.

1 Make Initial Selection

Open the image you want to work with in the Editor in **Standard Edit** mode and save it in Photoshop (***.psd**) format. In the **Layers** palette, choose the layer that contains the data you want to select and then use any selection tool to make the initial selection in the image.

2 Choose Smooth

To include the stray pixels around the current selection, choose **Select**, **Modify**, **Smooth** from the menu bar. The **Smooth Selection** dialog box displays.

3 Set Sample Radius

In the **Sample Radius** field, specify a number between **1** and **100** that indicates the maximum number of pixels that the Editor will add to or subtract from either side of the existing selection border to smooth out any jagged ins and outs it finds. This number represents how much change you'll allow to the existing selection perimeter. With a high value, your selected region could conceivably become much smaller. On the other hand, pockets of unselected pixels in the original region could become selected when smoothed because the **Smooth** command doesn't look just outside a selection for similar pixels, but inside as well. Also, because higher resolution images have pixels that are closer together (more dense), you might have to set the **Sample Radius** value higher than you would in a lower-resolution image to get the same result. Click **OK** to proceed.

25

4 Or Choose Feather

Choose **Select**, **Feather** from the menu bar to display the **Feather Selection** dialog box.

5 Set Feather Radius

In the **Feather Radius** field, type a value larger than **0** to indicate the number of pixels inside the marquee that will be used to create a fuzzy border around the selection. Click the **OK** button to close the **Feather Selection** dialog box.

▶ NOTES

Setting the **Feather** value in the **Options** bar when you make the initial selection with the **Lasso** or **Marquee** tools does the same thing as opening the **Feather Selection** dialog box after the selection has already been made. However, using the **Feather** command after the fact allows you the freedom to undo the feathering and adjust its value until you get the effect you want.

The **Magic Wand** and **Selection Brush** tools do not allow you to specify feathering on the **Options** bar, although the **Selection Brush** does enable you to lower the **Hardness** of its tip, which creates the same effect as feathering. For the **Magic Wand**, however, you must add feathering after the fact (if desired) by following the steps in this task.

6 View the Result

When you're satisfied with the selection, make changes to the area within the selection, copy or cut its data to another image or layer, or delete the data within the selection. Save the PSD image and then resave the file in JPEG, PNG, or non-layered TIFF format, leaving your PSD image with its layers (if any) intact so that you can return at a later time and make adjustments if you want.

In this example, I used the **Magnetic Lasso** to select the back wheel of a 1929 Rumely Oil-Pull farm tractor I photographed at a State Fair parade. The reason I did this was to adjust the lighting on this rubber-treaded steel wheel, which unfortunately caught too much shadow from the early evening sun. The **Magnetic Lasso** did a pretty good job, but the curves on the tractor wheels' edges looked like they'd been through a muddy pit. A quick smoothing, using the **Select**, **Modify**, **Smooth** command with **Sample Radius** set to 20, rounded out those curves easily.

26

26 Save and Reload a Selection

✔ BEFORE YOU BEGIN

20 Select a Rectangular or Circular Area
21 Draw a Selection Freehand or By Tracing Its Edge

Sometimes, image attaining the perfectly selected region is a hard-won victory. It's difficult to cast aside the fruits of that victory to work on some other region. For this reason, Photoshop Elements makes it easy for you to save the *pattern* of a selection. Note that you don't save the *contents* of the selected region, just the shape, in case you need to use that shape to select the same region—or a different region with the same shape—later. When you save a selection, the Editor records the exact position and shape of the selection marquee, and whether it had any feathering, anti-aliasing, or smoothing at its edges. That recording becomes part of the image's Photoshop .PSD file. Saved selections are also useful for creating masks, frames, or for making the same-shaped selection in several images.

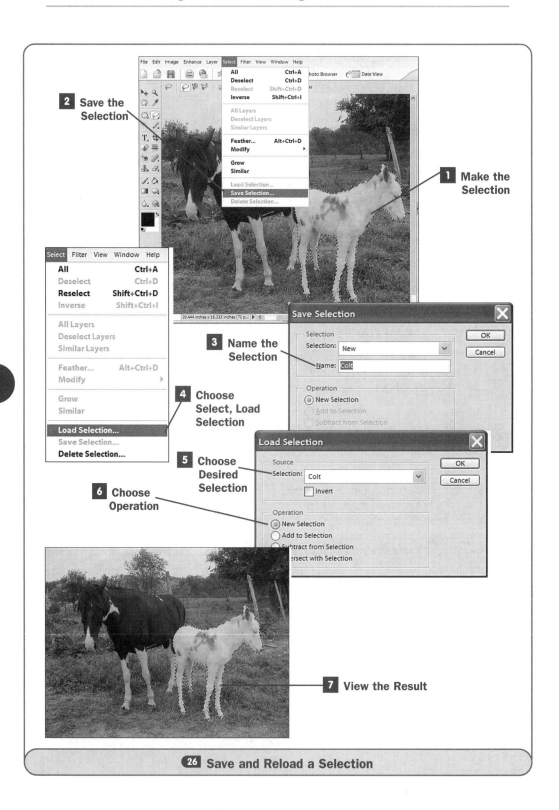

2 Save the Selection

1 Make the Selection

3 Name the Selection

4 Choose Select, Load Selection

5 Choose Desired Selection

6 Choose Operation

7 View the Result

26 Save and Reload a Selection

After you save a selection pattern, you can reload it at any time from within the image where you saved it. You can reload the saved selection to the same layer or to another layer. You can even add or subtract the saved selection from a current selection, creating a complex selection such as an oval frame. You build complex selections like these by making the outer selection, saving it, shrinking the selection, and subtracting this modified selection (the "hole") from the first selection ("the outer border"), leaving a selection "rim." When you reload a selection, pixels within its border are instantly selected, even if those pixels are different from the ones you originally selected when you saved the selection border.

■ Make the Selection

Open an in the Editor in **Standard Edit** mode and save it in Photoshop (***.psd**) format. Use any of the selection tools in any combination to create your selection.

② Save the Selection

Choose **Select**, **Save Selection** to display the **Save Selection** dialog box.

► NOTE

Selections can be saved only in PSD, JP2 (JPEG 2000), and TIFF files. So if you saved a selection in a file with one of these formats, and then resaved that image in a different format (such as JPEG), the selection is no longer contained in the JPEG file and you won't be able to reload it. The selection should still be in the original PSD, JP2, or TIFF file—assuming that you saved that file again after saving the selection.

③ Name the Selection

In the **Save Selection** dialog box, choose **New** from the **Selection** drop-down list. In the **Name** field, type the name you want to assign to the selection. You can use any combination of characters to name the selection, but the selection name cannot be longer than 32 characters. Click **OK** to save the selection to the image.

After you've saved the selection, you can keep on working as usual. For example, you could make changes to the area within the selection, copy or cut its data to another image or layer, or delete the data within the selection. You can make other changes and even make another selection without fear of losing the original saved selection, which can be recalled when needed. When you're satisfied with all your changes, save the PSD image. Resave the result in JPEG or TIFF format, leaving your PSD image with its layers (if any) and selections intact so that you can return at a later time and make adjustments if you want.

26

▶ **NOTE**

You can modify an existing saved selection by making a selection and redisplaying the **Save Selection** dialog box. Select the name of the previously saved selection from the **Selection** drop-down list and then select the desired type of modification from the **Operation** area and click **OK**. For example, if you choose the **Add to Selection** operation, the current selection is added to the saved selection you chose from the **Selection** list.

4 Choose Select, Load Selection

At a later point in time, you might want to recall this selection. For example, you might want to perform further adjustments to the object you originally selected. Perhaps you want to adjust everything *but* that object; if so, you can invert the selection as you load it.

When you're ready to reuse the stored selection, select the layer that contains the pixels you want selected, then choose **Select, Load Selection** from the menu bar. The **Load Selection** dialog box is displayed.

5 Choose Desired Selection

From the **Selection** drop-down list, choose the name of the previously saved selection you want to load. If the **Load Selection** command is grayed out on the **Select** menu, the current image does not contain any saved selections. If you want to load a pattern that includes everything *except* the saved selection, enable the **Invert** check box.

6 Choose Operation

If you made a selection in your image before step 4, then under **Operation**, choose one of the following:

- **New Selection**—Replaces any existing selection in the image with the pattern you choose.

- **Add to Selection**—Produces a selection in the image that joins the existing pattern with the one you choose.

- **Subtract from Selection**—Removes the pixels included in the selection you choose, from the pattern currently in the image.

- **Intersect with Selection**—Produces a selection that includes only the pixels that the existing pattern and the pattern you choose have in common.

To finalize your choice, click **OK**.

▶ TIPS

For a neat effect, create a text selection (using the **Horizontal** or **Vertical Type Mask** tool), save it, and then make a new selection to act as the text background, such as a rectangle or a freely drawn shape. When the background for the text is just as you like, reload the text selection with the **Subtract from Selection** option so that it cuts out of the second selection an area in the shape of the text. Fill this new selection with a color or pattern, and the result looks impressive and unusual.

To use your saved selection in another image, just reload the selection in the original image as explained here. Then open the other image in which you want to use the selection, choose any selection tool other than the **Selection Brushes**, enable the **New Selection** button, position it over the selection, and then drag the selection into the image and drop it.

7 View the Result

After loading the selection, make changes to the area within the selection, copy or cut its data to another image or layer, or delete the data within the selection. When you're satisfied with the result, make any other changes you want and save the PSD file. Resave the result in JPEG, PNG, or non-layered TIFF format, leaving your PSD image with its layers (if any) and selections intact so that you can return at a later time and make adjustments if you want.

This example has as many as five components: the two horses, the ground, the part of the image that's above the ground, and the tree in the upper-right corner. To make the most of this image, I selected and stored each of these parts separately. The benefit of storing patterns for the horses first is that it's easy to select the ground (everything from the horizon line down) and then subtract the already stored horses from that area to attain just the region that needs to be edited. Here you can see the **Colt** selection in its entirety.

27

---

27 | **Create a New Image or Layer from a Selection**

→ SEE ALSO

157 Create a Graphic with Transparent Areas in Photoshop Elements
159 Move Images Between Premiere Elements and Photoshop Elements

---

You can create new images in the Editor by using selections from other images. For example, you might want to create a new image that contains only a portion of the original image, such as the head and shoulders of a person taken from a full-length photo of that person. When you have copied the selection to the new image, you can make modifications to the new image without affecting the original image. In this task, you'll learn how to copy a selection and create an image from it.

27

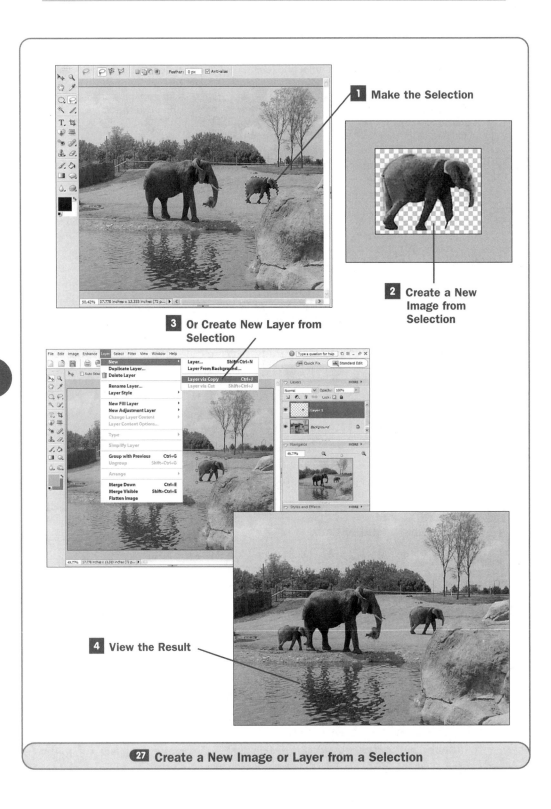

1 Make the Selection

2 Create a New
Image from
Selection

3 Or Create New Layer from
Selection

4 View the Result

27 Create a New Image or Layer from a Selection

You can also create a new layer with data you've copied from a selection instead of an entire image. When you use layers, you can isolate portions of an image and make changes to only that portion. If you create a selection of your family from a larger image taken in front of your house, you can create a new layer with just your family on it. Now you have two layers: your family on one layer and your house plus your family on another. The composite image still shows your family in front of your house because the copy of your family, when initially pasted to the new layer, is in exactly the same location on that layer as it was on the original layer—in effect, there are two copies of your family, one directly on top of the other. You can do a lot of things now. You can move the family on the top layer over to one side, and have two families show up in the photo. Because the family is isolated on its own layer, you can adjust the brightness and contrast of just the family; select a blend mode on the top layer that causes the families to blend in such a way that makes the family appear more saturated, darker, or artfully colored; blur the entire bottom layer and make the duplicate family (which remains sharp on its own layer) stand out better against the background; resize the top family and move it to one side so they appear as a miniature with themselves; or you can replace the layer containing your house with an image of the White House. Just that easily, you've taken your family on "vacation" to Washington, D.C. The tricks begin, however, by first selecting the family and transferring that selection onto another layer in the same image, which is one of the things you'll learn to do in this task.

27

▶ NOTE

When you're copying data from one image to another, you're using the Photoshop Elements clipboard. If you have enabled the **Export to Clipboard** option in the **Preferences** dialog box, data on this clipboard is also copied to the Windows Clipboard for use in other programs—the purpose of that option is to help you get data *out of Photoshop Elements*; thus, that option does not have to be on for this task to work, even if you want to create a new image from data copied from another program (the option has nothing to do with data coming *into* Photoshop Elements).

1 Make the Selection

Open the image from which you want to copy data in the Editor in **Standard Edit** mode. From the **Layers** palette, choose the layer whose contents you want to copy—in whole or part—into a new image. Make your selection using the tools of your choice.

2 Create a New Image from Selection

To create a new image from the selected data, select **Edit, Copy** from the menu bar to copy the selection to the Photoshop Elements clipboard. To copy all visible pixels within the selection, regardless of what layer they are on, choose **Edit, Copy Merged** instead.

Now that the data's on the clipboard, select **File**, **New**, **Image from Clipboard** to create a new image from the contents of the clipboard. The new image is sized to match the actual size of the data within the clipboard. In other words, if the selection was 400 × 400 pixels in size, that will be the size of the new image.

When you create a new image file, the existing image file from which you copied the selection remains open. (You can see the open files in the **Photo Bin** at the bottom of the screen.) The Editor indicates the selected image file by outlining it in blue.

▶ **TIP**

To create an image using data you capture from your computer screen, arrange the monitor display to show the programs or elements you want to capture and press the **Print Screen** key. Return to the Editor and select **File**, **New**, **Image from Clipboard** to create a file containing whatever data was displayed on your computer monitor.

3 **Or Create New Layer from Selection**

27

To create a new layer in the current image using the data you've selected, you do not have to copy it first. Instead, select **Layer**, **New**, **Layer via Copy** to copy the current selection to a new layer. This new layer appears above the current layer in the **Layers** palette. The selection appears in the same location on the new layer as it occupied in the original layer, but you can move it with the **Move** tool.

You can also select **Layer**, **New**, **Layer via Cut** to cut the current selection from its existing layer and paste it in a new layer. If used in this example, the selected baby elephant would be cut from the **Background** layer and pasted on the new layer. A hole would be left in the **Background** layer where the baby elephant was originally located, and that hole would be filled with the background color, or transparent pixels (if the background layer had been converted to a regular layer, such as **Layer 0**).

▶ **NOTE**

If your purpose is to copy data from one image to another, just select it and choose **Edit**, **Copy** or **Copy Merged**; then change to the other image and choose **Edit**, **Paste**. The data is pasted onto a new layer automatically, just above the current layer.

4 View the Result

Save the new image in Photoshop (***.psd***) format. Make any changes you want and save the PSD file again. Resave the final result in JPEG, PNG, or non-layered TIFF format, leaving your PSD image with its layers (if any) intact so that you can return at a later time and make adjustments if you want.

In this example, I used the **Magnetic Lasso** tool to select the walking baby elephant. I then used the **Layer via Copy** command to move just the baby elephant onto a new layer all to himself. I wanted to make the photo a bit more interesting by adding another elephant, but to disguise that fact, I resized him slightly and moved him closer to his mother. See **32 Move, Resize, Skew, or Distort a Layer or Selection**. I had to clone in the missing trunk and leg that was hidden behind the rock on the original elephant. See **52 Repair Minor Tears**. I still have some more work to do, adding a shadow and a reflection in the water, but even now the effect is pretty convincing.

27

6

Using Multiple Layers to Edit Images

IN THIS CHAPTER:

The use of layers to edit an image is the most powerful feature in Photoshop Elements. Using multiple layers, you can isolate each element of the image, in the same way a cartoonist isolates each element of a scene by placing them on sheets of clear acetate. You could put the sky and a roadway on the bottom layer, a sports car on the next layer, and your son on the top layer. Separating your image into layers gives you the ability to make adjustments to any one of the objects within the image—such as the location of the sports car or the sharpness, brightness, and tone of your son—without affecting the background or other objects on different layers. When elements in an image are separated, you can apply effects, filters, and layer styles to specific objects without applying them to the entire image.

In Chapter 1, "Start Here," you learned about the different layer types available: image layers, fill layers, and adjustment layers. In this chapter, you'll learn how to create them. You'll learn how to erase part of a layer to let the background show through, and how to erase the background layer so that you can place the graphic seamlessly on a Web page or your desktop. You'll learn how to move, resize, skew, and distort the data on a layer or in a selection so that it looks exactly how you want. You'll also learn how to mask a portion of a layer to create special effects such as picture frames or to insert fake backgrounds behind a subject.

28 Create a New Image Layer

✔ BEFORE YOU BEGIN	→ SEE ALSO
Just jump right in!	**29** Create a Layer Filled with a Color, Gradient, or Pattern
	30 Create an Adjustment Layer
	159 Move Images Between Premiere Elements and Photoshop Elements

You can add a new image *layer* to just about any image you have open in the Editor. Because an image layer can hold any type of raster data, you might insert an image layer so that you can paint or draw on it, make a selection on the new layer and copy data into that selection, create a clipping mask to partially block data on another layer, or fill the layer using a filter or effect, such as a rendering of clouds. However, you don't have to create an image layer if your plan is to copy data from some other layer or image into this image; the Editor will paste the data on a new layer automatically.

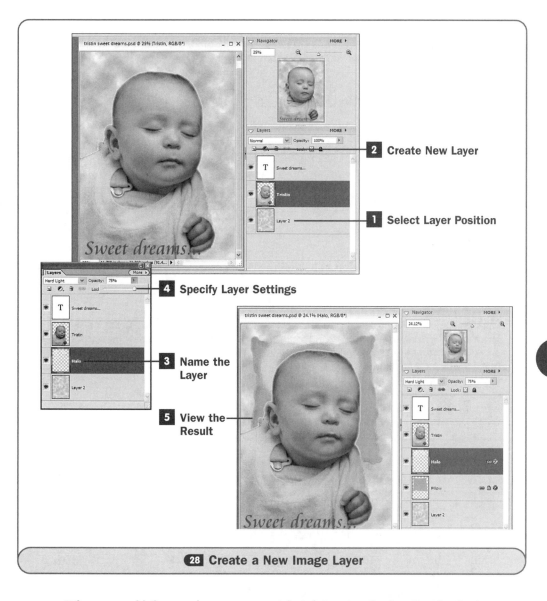

2 Create New Layer

1 Select Layer Position

4 Specify Layer Settings

3 Name the Layer

5 View the Result

28

28 Create a New Image Layer

When you add the new layer, you must first determine the location for the layer within the layer stack. To specify the layer location, select the layer *below* where you want the new layer (in other words, the new layer is added above the current layer). For example, to insert a new layer at the top of the layer stack, you select the top layer in the **Layers** palette. If the only layer is the **Background** layer, the new layer is always placed on top of the **Background** layer because you cannot place any layers below the **Background** layer—unless you first convert the **Background** layer to a regular layer by choosing **Layer**, **New**, **Layer from Background**.

▶ **NOTE**

You cannot add layers to images that are using bitmap or indexed color mode. To change color modes, see **19 Change Color Mode**.

1 Select Layer Position

Open an image in the Editor in **Standard Edit** mode and save it in Photoshop (***.psd**) format. In the **Layers** palette, select the layer you want to be below the new layer you are adding. Photoshop Elements will insert the new image layer directly above the selected layer.

2 Create New Layer

To create a new layer above the selected layer, click the **Create New Layer** button on the **Layers** palette. The new layer appears on the **Layers** palette above the layer you selected in step 1.

▶ **TIPS**

You can duplicate the contents of a layer by dragging that layer onto the **Create New Layer** button on the **Layers** palette. You can make a selection and create a new layer above the current layer by choosing **Layer**, **New**, **Layer Via Copy** from the menu bar. A new layer is created instantly, and the data in the selection is placed on that layer.

If you select an object from another layer and copy and paste it onto your new blank layer, the copied data is placed on that layer. In other words, unlike normal **Copy** and **Paste** operations in which new layers are created automatically, *a new layer is not created when data is pasted onto an empty layer.*

3 Name the Layer

In the **Layers** palette, double-click the default layer name and type a **Name** that describes the layer's content or purpose. Press **Enter**. I know that I want to create a halo on my new layer, so I'll name it **Halo**.

4 Specify Layer Settings

After you have created the layer, it is ready for you to add data to it. A new image layer is filled with transparent pixels so that, at least initially, it does not block any layers below it. However, as you add opaque pixels, they will block the data below (or blend with them, if you select a blend mode other than **Normal** as explained here). Paint or draw on the new layer, or copy data there.

28

Next, play with the blend mode and opacity of the layer to get the effect you want. Typically, I play with these settings as I work, making frequent changes. The *blend mode* of a layer specifies how the pixels on that layer mix with pixels in the layer(s) below. The blend mode for a new layer is set to **Normal** by default. To select a different blend mode, open the **Blend Mode** list at the top of the **Layers** palette and select the one you want to use. See the website for this book (start at www.samspublishing.com) for more information on blend modes.

The opacity of a new layer is set to 100% by default. To reduce the overall opacity of the new layer, adjust the **Opacity** value at the top of the **Layers** palette. The lower the **Opacity** setting, the more transparent that layer's pixels appear. If you add semi-transparent pixels to this new layer, the **Opacity** setting reduces their overall transparency even more.

5 View the Result

When you're satisfied with the image, save the PSD file. Then merge the layers together and resave the result in JPEG, PNG, or non-layered TIFF format, leaving your PSD image unflattened so that you can return at a later time and make adjustments if you want.

I started with a photo of my great-nephew sleeping peacefully. I added some text, and then inserted a new layer and used the **Clouds** filter to create a puffy cloud background. I moved this clouds layer (**Layer 2**) to the bottom of the layer stack so that it would be behind the baby and not on top of him. Next I inserted the **Halo** layer, on which I painted a yellow halo. I set the blend mode to **Hard Light** and set the **Opacity** to 75% so the halo would be semi-transparent. I added an **Outer Glow** *layer style* to complete the halo effect. I inserted a **Pillow** layer just above the **Cloud** layer and used the **Brush** tool to paint a pillow for the baby's head. I locked the transparency on this layer so that I could brush soft texture along the edges of the pillow, giving it some dimension.

---

29 Create a Layer Filled with a Color, Gradient, or Pattern

→ SEE ALSO

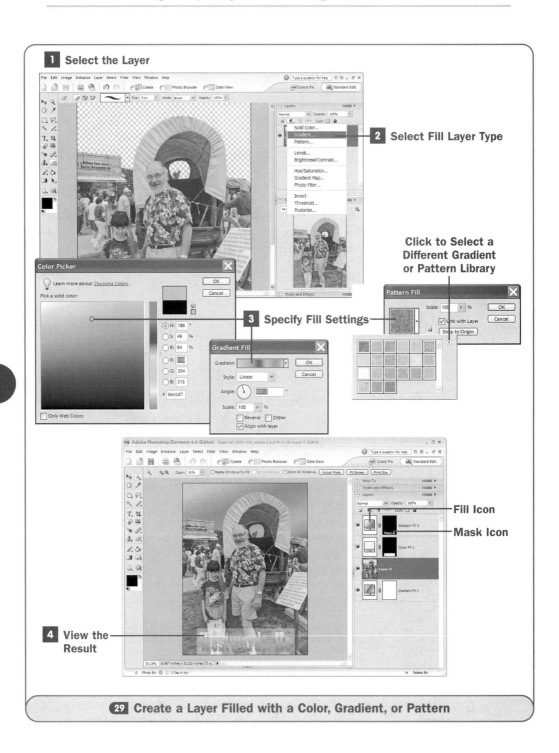

1 Select the Layer

2 Select Fill Layer Type

Click to Select a
Different Gradient
or Pattern Library

3 Specify Fill Settings

Fill Icon

Mask Icon

4 View the Result

29 Create a Layer Filled with a Color, Gradient, or Pattern

If you want to insert a layer completely filled with a color, pattern, or gradient, create a fill layer. True, you could insert an image layer and fill it with a color or pattern (using the **Paint Bucket** tool) or a gradient (using the **Gradient** tool), but you can accomplish things with a fill layer that you can't easily duplicate with an image layer. For example, you could erase the background around a subject, allowing a more interesting background created by a gradient or pattern fill layer to show through. See **56** **Remove Unwanted Objects from an Image**. You could mask out the center of a fill layer so the fill layer only shows through along the edges, creating a "frame" around the layer(s) below it. See **33** **Mask an Adjustment or Fill Layer**. And because you used a fill layer, you can change the fill type (from a pattern to a gradient, for example) until you find the right look for your frame.

You might place a pattern fill layer over another layer, lower its opacity, and use the pattern to give that layer a "texture." Or you could make a selection and instantly fill the selection with a color, gradient, or pattern. The selection in this case is not *actually* filled, but its shape is used on the fill layer's mask to block the layer's fill from appearing anywhere else but within the confines of your selection. Although you could use this technique to fill any selection shape with the contents of a fill layer, you can also fill text you created using the **Horizontal** or **Vertical Type Mask** tool with a pattern or a gradient—something you can't do using the ordinary text tools.

29

1 Select the Layer

Open an image in the Editor in **Standard Edit** mode and save it in Photoshop (***.psd**) format.

In the **Layers** palette, select the layer *below* where you want the new fill layer to be. The Editor will insert the fill layer directly above the selected layer. To create a fill layer that automatically fills only the area within a selection, select that portion of the layer now.

2 Select Fill Layer Type

Click the **Create Adjustment Layer** button on the **Layers** palette and select **Solid Color**, **Gradient**, or **Pattern** from the menu that appears.

3 Specify Fill Settings

A dialog box for the fill type you selected in step 2 appears. If you selected a **Solid Color** fill layer, choose a color from the color picker and click **OK**. See **40** **Select a Color to Work with**.

If you selected a **Gradient** fill layer, select a **Gradient** from the list box. Choose a gradient **Style** and adjust the **Angle**, which controls the direction in which the gradient transitions from one color to the next. By lowering the

Scale, you can have these transitions occur more often. Enable the **Reverse** option to reverse the colors in the gradient. Enable the **Dither** option to reduce jagged transitions, especially in lower-resolution images. Enable the **Align with Layer** option to use the layer's outer perimeter to calculate the gradient. Click **OK**. See **45 Fill an Area with a Gradient** for help.

If you selected a **Pattern** fill layer, select a pattern and adjust its **Scale**. Click the **Snap to Origin** button to reposition the pattern so that it's aligned with the image borders. Enable the **Link with Layer** option so that you can click in the image and move the pattern on the layer until you get its position just right for your purposes. Click **OK**.

▶ TIPS

To display a different set of gradients or patterns, click the triangle button to open the pop-up menu, and select the library of gradients or patterns to use.

Several gradient patterns use the current *foreground color*. Before creating a gradient fill layer, select the desired foreground color to make finding the right gradient colors easier. See **40 Select a Color to Work with** for more information on selecting the foreground color.

If you want to make modifications to a fill layer later on, double-click the fill thumbnail on the **Layers** palette. The corresponding dialog box reopens so that you can adjust the fill's settings.

4 View the Result

The new fill layer is created using the color, pattern, or gradient option you selected. If desired, you can change the layer's **Opacity** and **Blend Mode** using those options at the top of the **Layers** palette. Notice that in the **Layers** palette there are two icons for the layer: The first icon shows the type of fill that was added. For example, if you created a color fill, the icon contains the color that was used. The second icon shows the mask. It's white where the fill shows through to other layers and black where the fill is blocked. Unless you made a selection in step 1, you'll notice that the mask is initially white, meaning that the fill completely shows through at the moment, covering all data on the layer below. You'll learn how to edit the mask to block the effects of the fill in **33 Mask an Adjustment or Fill Layer**.

When you're satisfied with the image, save the PSD file. Then merge the layers together and resave the result in JPEG, PNG, or unlayered TIFF format, leaving your PSD image unflattened so that you can return at a later time and make adjustments if you want.

In this example, I removed the background around my subjects and added a gradient fill layer behind them to act as a new "sky." To add a gradient to the text, I added another gradient fill layer and masked it (so that only part of the gradient fill shows through) the text caption.

30 Create an Adjustment Layer

→ **SEE ALSO**

29 Create a Layer Filled with a Color, Gradient, or Pattern
33 Mask an Adjustment or Fill Layer

If you want to make adjustments to the color, contrast, brightness, or saturation of the *layers* in your image, you can add an *adjustment layer*. An adjustment layer changes the appearance of the layers below it in the layer stack without affecting the actual contents of those layers. Adjustment layers let you try out various adjustments without making any permanent changes to the image layer(s). If you don't like the result, you can open that adjustment dialog box again and make other changes, which is the same as if you had clicked **Undo** and had started over. However, in this case, you can change your mind at any time, even way down the editing process! You can also remove the adjustment layer and its effects completely.

30

▶ KEY TERM

Adjustment layer—A special layer that allows you to make a specific color or contrast adjustment to the layers underneath it.

There are several types of adjustment layers you can create:

- **Levels**—Allows you to adjust the highlight, midtone, and shadow values for a single color channel (the red, green, or blue channel) or the entire tonal range. You can also remove a color cast using **Levels**.

- **Brightness/Contrast**—Allows you to decrease or increase the general amount of brightness and contrast for all pixels on the affected layers. See 57 **Improve Brightness and Contrast**.

- **Hue/Saturation**—Allows you to adjust the hue, saturation, and lightness of all pixels on the affected layers. See 61 **Adjust Hue and Saturation Manually**.

- **Gradient Map**—Applies the colors in the gradient you select to the pixels in the affected layers, based on their brightness value.

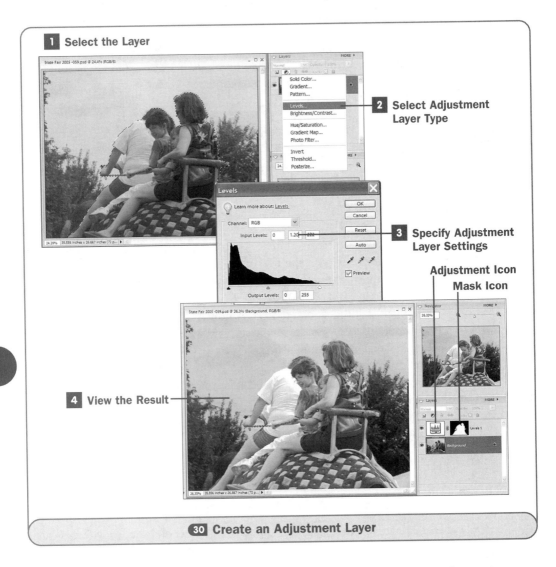

1 Select the Layer

2 Select Adjustment Layer Type

3 Specify Adjustment Layer Settings

Adjustment Icon
Mask Icon

4 View the Result

30

30 Create an Adjustment Layer

- **Photo Filter**—Allows you to apply an effect that simulates the use of a particular photo filter to the affected layers. For example, if you want your image to have a sepia appearance, apply the **Sepia** photo filter.

- **Invert**—Changes the pixels on the affected layers so they are reversed in color and tone.

- **Threshold**—Allows you to convert the pixels in the affected layers to either black or white. Light areas are converted to white and dark areas are converted to black, depending on the threshold you select.

- **Posterize**—Allows you to control the number of tones in the affected layers by specifying the number of brightness levels you want. The brightness of each pixel is then adjusted to fit within one of these tonal levels.

1 Select the Layer

Open an image in the Editor in **Standard Edit** mode and save it in Photoshop (*.**psd**) format. In the **Layers** palette, select a layer; all layers below the layer you choose will be affected by the adjustment layer. The adjustment layer will appear in the **Layers** palette above the layer you select and will affect all layers below. To create an adjustment layer that automatically adjusts only the area within a selection, select that portion of the image now.

2 Select Adjustment Layer Type

Click the **Create Adjustment Layer** button on the **Layers** palette and select the type of adjustment layer you want to create.

3 Specify Adjustment Layer Settings

Depending on the type of adjustment layer you create, a different dialog box displays. For example, if you select the **Levels** adjustment layer type, the **Levels** dialog box displays. Make your selections for the type of adjustment you want to make and click **OK** to apply the adjustment filter.

30

▶ TIPS

If you want to make modifications to an adjustment layer later, double-click the adjustment thumbnail on the **Layers** palette.

Because its effects are easy to change or remove, an adjustment layer is preferable to applying that same adjustment directly to a layer. In addition, by adding a mask, you can easily limit the adjustment to particular portions of the layers below, *and even change your mind on which portions* you want affected, any time you want. See **33** Mask an Adjustment or Fill Layer.

4 View the Result

The new adjustment layer is created using the adjustment settings you specified. If desired, you can change the layer's **Opacity** and **Blend Mode** using those options at the top of the **Layers** palette. Notice that in the **Layers** palette there are now two icons for the layer: The first icon shows the type of adjustment that was added. The second icon shows the mask. It's white where the adjustment is applied to other layers and black where the adjustment is blocked. Unless you made a selection in step 1, you'll notice that the mask is initially white, meaning that the adjustment is currently being applied to all layers below. You'll learn how to edit the mask to block the effects of the adjustment in **33** **Mask an Adjustment or Fill Layer**.

When you're satisfied with the image, save the PSD file. Then merge the layers together and resave the result in JPEG, PNG, or non-layered TIFF format, leaving your PSD image unflattened so that you can return at a later time and make adjustments if you want. In this example, I selected my subjects and inserted a **Levels** adjustment layer. I then changed the settings to make that area brighter, without losing the details in the shadows. Because the adjustment affected only the subjects, the background remained dull, drawing more attention to the subjects.

---

31   Erase Part of a Layer

→ **SEE ALSO**

34 **Mask an Image Layer**

30

One advantage of using layers is the ability to isolate changes to various elements in an image, such as applying a contrast adjustment to just the subject and not the entire image. Another advantage of using layers is that you can easily add and remove data from a layer without affecting the other layers in your image. In fact, when you erase data from a layer using one of the eraser tools, the pixels are changed to transparent ones, and the contents of the layers below become visible "through" the area you just deleted. If you attempt to "erase" data from a layer that has transparency locked (such as the **Background** layer), the pixels are not made transparent but are instead filled with the current background color. To erase the pixels on a background layer, convert it to a regular image layer by choosing **Layer, New, Layer from Background**.

To erase part of a layer, you use the eraser tools: the regular *Eraser*, the *Background Eraser*, and the *Magic Eraser*. The **Eraser** works just as you might expect, making transparent the pixels the brush passes over. The **Background Eraser** works a little differently. As you drag the **Background Eraser** tool, pixels under the brush that match the pixel in the center of the brush tip crosshair are made transparent. How closely these pixels must match before being erased is controlled by the tool's **Tolerance** level, which is set on the **Options** bar. With the **Magic Eraser** tool, you erase matching pixels by clicking a sample pixel. Pixels that match the sample you clicked are erased from the layer. Again, the **Tolerance** option controls how closely this match must be before pixels are erased (made transparent). These tools work well if there is a lot of difference between the pixels you want to erase and the portion you want to remain. The Magic Eraser is best at removing large areas of similar color. To remove a background with lots of different colors, it's easier to use the **Background Eraser** because you can drag and you do not have to click each color to remove.

▶ KEY TERMS

Eraser—A tool that erases (makes transparent) the pixels under its brush.

Background Eraser—A tool that erases pixels (makes transparent) that match the pixel under its crosshair as you drag.

Magic Eraser—A tool that erases (makes transparent) pixels that matches any pixel you click.

▶ TIPS

You can also erase data by making a selection and pressing the **Delete** key.

Another way you can erase the background from around a subject is to use the **Magic Extractor**, a dialog box with tools that allow you to select areas to erase, preview your changes, and make adjustments *before* the pixels are actually erased from the image. See **58** **Replace a Background with Something Else.**

31

1 Select Eraser Tool

Open an image in the Editor in **Standard Edit** mode and save it in Photoshop (***.psd**) format. On the **Toolbox**, select the **Eraser** tool.

2 Adjust Eraser Settings

On the **Options** bar, select the **Mode** (**Brush**, **Pencil**, or **Block**), which determines the shape of the brush tip. For the **Brush** and **Pencil** options, you can further refine the tip by selecting an option from the **Presets** list. Set the **Size** and **Opacity** for the brush. If you lower the **Opacity**, for example, the eraser only partially erases (it makes the pixels partially transparent instead of fully transparent).

▶ TIPS

When selecting a brush tip from the **Presets** list for any of the eraser tools, you can display a different set of brush tips by clicking the triangle button to open the pop-up menu and choosing a different library of brush tips.

Before using any of the eraser tools, you can make a selection to limit the erasure to that area so that you don't accidentally erase something you don't want to. For example, to erase the sky around a girl's face who also happens to be wearing a blue hat, draw the selection boundary omitting the hat so that it isn't mistaken for the background and isn't erased as you work at removing the background from around her face.

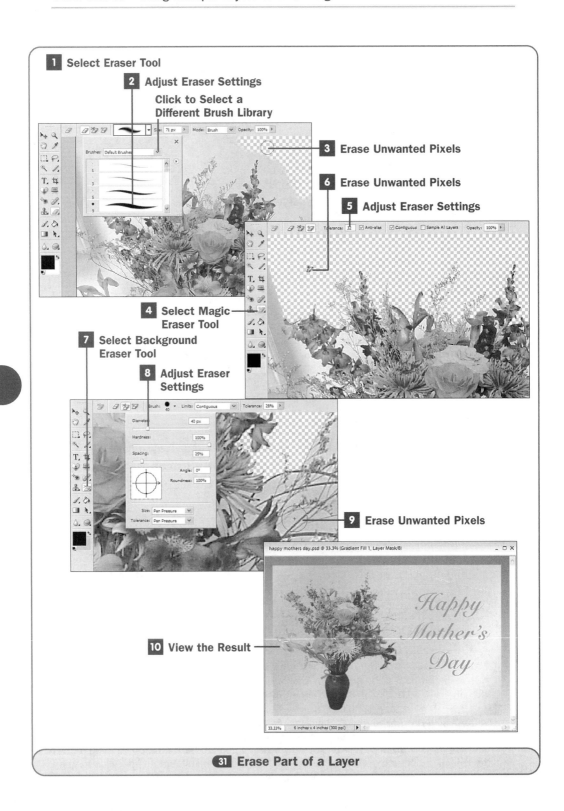

1 Select Eraser Tool

2 Adjust Eraser Settings

Click to Select a
Different Brush Library

3 Erase Unwanted Pixels

6 Erase Unwanted Pixels

5 Adjust Eraser Settings

4 Select Magic Eraser Tool

7 Select Background Eraser Tool

8 Adjust Eraser Settings

9 Erase Unwanted Pixels

10 View the Result

31

31 Erase Part of a Layer

3 Erase Unwanted Pixels

In the **Layers** palette, change to the layer you want to erase. If you want to erase pixels on the background layer using the **Eraser** tool, you'll need to convert it to a regular layer first by choosing **Layer**, **New**, **Layer from Background**. To preserve the data on the layer against possible mistakes you might make while erasing, consider duplicating the layer and erasing the new layer instead. To do that, choose **Layer**, **Duplicate Layer**.

In the image area, drag with the **Eraser** tool; pixels under the tip are erased (made transparent). I used the **Eraser** here to erase large areas of the background where I'm not afraid of accidentally erasing the subject—the flowers.

4 Select Magic Eraser Tool

Select the **Magic Eraser** on the **Toolbox** (if an eraser tool is already selected, just click the **Magic Eraser** icon in the **Options** bar).

5 Adjust Eraser Settings

Set the **Tolerance** to a value that tells the Editor how closely you want pixels to match the one you click before they are erased. A low **Tolerance** level indicates that only pixels that are very similar to the pixel you click will be erased. The higher the **Tolerance** value, the broader the range of pixels that will match.

Enable the **Anti-Aliased** check box to make sure that the edges are smooth around the area that is erased. Enable the **Contiguous** check box to erase only pixels that are adjacent to the pixel you click. If you clear the **Contiguous** check box, Photoshop Elements will find all the pixels in the layer or selection that match the pixel you click. Enable the **Sample All Layers** check box to remove pixels on the current layer, based on the blended color (from all layers) that you click. Adjust the **Opacity** value to only partially erase matching pixels.

6 Erase Unwanted Pixels

In the **Layers** palette, change to the layer you want to erase. If you choose the background layer, the **Magic Eraser** tool automatically converts the layer to a regular layer as soon as you begin erasing. To preserve the data on the layer against possible mistakes you might make while erasing, consider duplicating the layer and erasing the new layer instead. To do that, choose **Layer**, **Duplicate Layer**.

31

Click a pixel that matches the ones you want to erase. Pixels that match closely enough (based on the **Tolerance** setting) to the one you click are erased. Continue the process until you have removed the unwanted portion of the layer. Here I use the **Magic Eraser** to remove large sections of a background, especially where the background is mostly one color (as it is here) where it's a blend of colors from several layers (I can enable the **Sample All Layers** option).

7 Select Background Eraser Tool

Select the **Background Eraser** on the **Toolbox** (if an eraser tool is already selected, just click the **Background Eraser** icon in the **Options** bar).

8 Adjust Eraser Settings

On the **Options** bar, select the brush tip you want to use by clicking the arrow next to the brush tip and choosing a **Diameter** (size) and **Hardness**.

To control which pixels are similar enough to warrant erasure, adjust the tool's **Tolerance** and **Limits** options. When you set **Limits** to **Contiguous**, the **Background Eraser** tool samples the pixel under the *hotspot* (located at the center of the brush tip and marked by a crosshair) and erases similar pixels under the brush that touch the hotspot or another similarly colored pixel. When **Limits** is set to **Discontiguous**, the tool erases any and all similarly colored pixels under the brush tip, regardless of their position. By default, the **Limits** value is set to **Contiguous**, but this setting might make it difficult to erase the background if it peeks through your subject (as the sky does through tree branches). Use **Discontiguous** in such a case.

9 Erase Unwanted Pixels

In the **Layers** palette, change to the layer you want to erase. If you choose the background layer, the **Background Eraser** tool automatically converts it to a regular layer as soon as you begin erasing. To preserve the data on the layer against possible mistakes you might make while erasing, consider duplicating the layer and erasing the new layer instead. To do that, choose **Layer, Duplicate Layer**.

Click and drag with the **Background Eraser** tool. Pixels within the circular area of the brush tip, that are a relative match for the pixel under the hotspot, are erased.

10 View the Result

When you're satisfied with the image, save the PSD file. Then merge the layers together (if any) and resave the result in JPEG, PNG, or non-layered TIFF

31

format, leaving your PSD image unflattened so that you can return at a later time and make adjustments if you want.

In this example, I erased the background behind the floral bouquet, expanded the canvas, added a colorful background and some text, and created a nice Mother's Day greeting.

---

32 **Move, Resize, Skew, or Distort a Layer or Selection**

✔ BEFORE YOU BEGIN	→ SEE ALSO
28 Create a New Image Layer	**133** Make Your Clip Appear on an Object

---

One advantage of layers is that you can move, resize, *skew,* or *distort* the contents of each individual layer without affecting the data on other layers. For example, you might decide to reduce the size of a layer so that its contents fit better with the proportions of the contents of the other layers. This is common procedure after pasting data onto a new layer taken from a different image. For example, if you paste your dog into a family photo, you'll probably need to move and resize him so that he doesn't look out of proportion with the rest of the family members. You can skew or distort data to tilt or stretch it—sometimes just for fun, and sometimes to correct for perspective. For example, if you take a photo of a tall object while looking up, the base looks wider than the top, even if the object (such as a building) is the same size all the way up. By distorting the image, you can pull the base of the building inward, eliminating the illusion of a wide base.

32

▶ **KEY TERMS**

Skew—To tilt (slant) a layer right, left, up or down.

Distort—To stretch a corner of a layer in any one direction.

You can move, resize, skew, or distort a layer using the **Move** tool. You can also perform these same functions on a shape or text object or on a selection. When you move, resize, skew, or distort the data in a selection, however, the hole that is left by the selection's former location is filled with transparent pixels (if the layer supports transparency). For the **Background** layer, which does not allow transparency, the hole left by the altered selection is filled with the current background color. If you alter a selection surrounded by colored pixels on any other layer, the hole is filled with transparent pixels. You can then fill the hole by cloning the surrounding data.

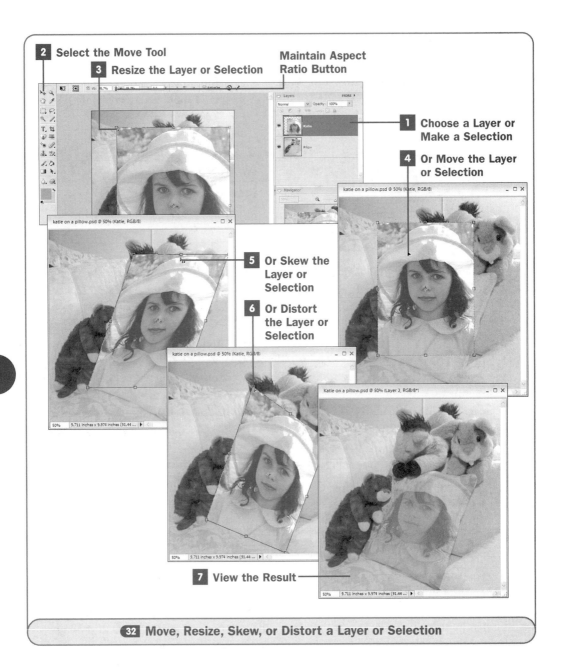

32

32 Move, Resize, Skew, or Distort a Layer or Selection

1 Choose a Layer or Make a Selection

Open an image in the Editor in **Standard Edit** mode and save it in Photoshop (***.psd**) format. In the **Layers** palette, select the layer you want to modify. To alter the entire **Background** layer, you must first convert it by choosing **Layer, New, Layer from Background**. If you want to alter a portion of the layer, make that selection now.

2 Select the Move Tool

On the **Toolbox**, select the **Move** tool. On the **Options** bar, enable the **Show Bounding Box** option. To automatically grab whatever object or layer under the mouse pointer is highest in the layer stack, enable the **Auto Select Layer** option as well. These two options disappear from the **Options** bar as soon as you start making adjustments, so be sure to set them before you continue.

The mouse pointer changes to a solid black arrow, and assuming that you have enabled the **Show Bounding Box** option, a bounding box appears around the edges of the selection or layer. If the layer is a shape or text layer, the bounding box appears around the edges of the shape or text object.

3 Resize the Layer or Selection

If you're altering an entire layer rather than a selection, maximize the image window and adjust the zoom so that the image is smaller than the window itself. This arrangement will give you the space you need to grab the layer handles properly.

To resize the contents of the layer or selection, position the mouse pointer over one of the handles on the edge of the bounding box until it changes to the **Resize** pointer (a straight line with arrows on each end). Drag to resize the layer or selection. Press **Shift** as you drag a corner handle to retain the proportions of the layer, selection, or object. If you begin resizing and then realize that the object is out of proportion, stop dragging and click the **Maintain Aspect Ratio** button that appears on the **Options** bar. The object's size is adjusted to fit its original proportions, and if you start dragging again, these proportions are maintained.

▶ NOTE

You can enter a percentage in the **W** and **H** boxes on the **Options** bar after beginning to drag. The selection, object, or layer is then instantly scaled by that amount, such as 50%.

4 Or Move the Layer or Selection

To move the layer or selection, click in the center of the bounding box and drag the layer or selection to the desired position. To move in one-pixel increments, press the arrow keys. To move in 10-pixel increments, hold down the **Shift** key while you press the arrow keys.

32

5   Or Skew the Layer or Selection

If you want to skew the layer or selection (tilt it horizontally or vertically in one direction), press **Ctrl+Shift** and then position the mouse pointer on a side (not a corner) handle. The mouse pointer changes to a gray arrow with a small double-headed arrow beneath it. Drag left or right to skew horizontally; drag up or down to skew vertically.

▶ TIPS

You can also skew by first clicking the **Skew** button on the **Options** bar (it might not be showing yet; it appears when you begin to resize, skew, or distort) or by selecting **Image, Transform, Skew** and then dragging any side handle in the direction you want to skew.

You can also distort by selecting **Image, Transform, Distort** and then dragging any handle in the direction you want to stretch.

6   Or Distort the Layer or Selection

If you want to distort the layer or selection (stretch one corner), hold down the **Ctrl** key and position the mouse pointer on a corner or side handle. The mouse pointer changes to a gray arrow. Drag the handle of the bounding box inward or outward.

7   View the Result

When you're satisfied with your changes, click the **Commit** button (the check mark) on the **Options** bar. To undo all changes made with the **Move** tool this session, click the **Cancel** button (the circle-with-a-slash icon) instead.

Make any other changes you want in the image and save the PSD file. Then merge the layers together (if any) and resave the result in JPEG, PNG, or non-layered TIFF format, leaving your PSD image unflattened so that you can return at a later time and make adjustments if you want.

In this example, I took a photo of a pillow surrounded by some much loved stuffed animals and combined it with a photo of my daughter, which I first resized and then skewed to the left. I then distorted the corners of the photo, positioning them exactly over the corners of the pillow. The result was a photo of my daughter that exactly matched the shape of the pillow below. It was then a simple matter to change the photo layer's blend mode to **Multiply** and set the **Opacity** to 62%, causing the photo of my daughter to blend into the pillow on the layer below, making it look as if her face was lightly painted on the pillow.

32

33 | Mask an Adjustment or Fill Layer

✔ BEFORE YOU BEGIN	→ SEE ALSO
29 Create a Layer Filled with a Color, Gradient, or Pattern **30** Create an Adjustment Layer	**34** Mask an Image Layer **42** Paint an Area of a Photo with a Brush

Unless you made a selection when you created an adjustment or fill layer, the fill or adjustment layer initially "flows through" to the layers below, affecting all of them. That's because the *mask* for the layer (the thing that controls what portions of the layers below are affected) is *all white*. White on a mask shows you where the pixels on a fill or adjustment layer affect the layers below.

▶ KEY TERM

Mask—The part of an adjustment or fill layer that acts as a filter, blocking the adjustment or fill from affecting the other layers that lie beneath it in the layer stack.

You might decide after inserting an adjustment or fill layer that you do not want its effect to be applied to your entire image. For example, if you created an adjustment layer and selected the **Brightness and Contrast** adjustment, you might want to apply the adjustment to just your subject and not to the entire image layer below. To prevent adjustment and fill layers from affecting areas of an image, you must edit the mask for that layer—basically painting parts of the mask black, which causes the mask to block the effect in that area of the layers below. If you use gray to paint on the mask, the effects of the adjustment or fill layer are only partially blocked. You can use any painting tool to accomplish this, such as the **Brush**, **Pencil**, or **Paint Bucket**. You can also apply a black-to-white gradient, for example, to fade the effect of the fill or adjustment layer in one direction. You can also apply any filter or effect that works on grayscale images to a mask, or use the **Text** or **Shape** tools to draw the area you want to block.

1 Select Layer

Open an image in the Editor in **Standard Edit** mode and save it in Photoshop (***.psd**) format. In the **Layers** palette, select the adjustment or fill layer whose mask you want to edit.

33

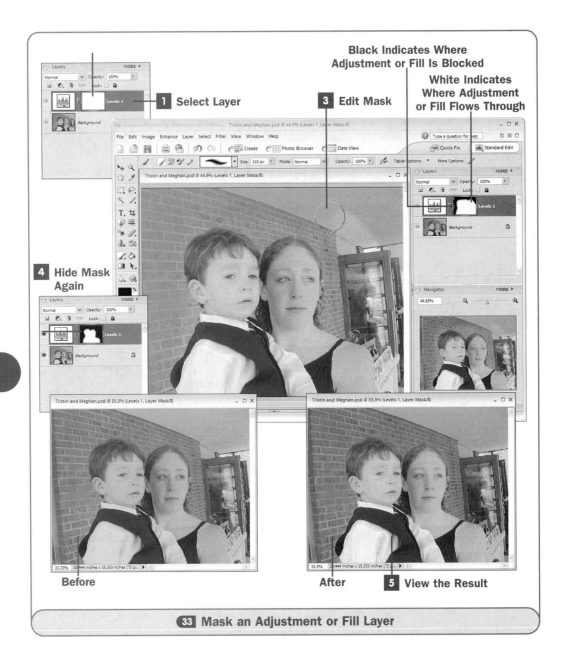

Black Indicates Where
Adjustment or Fill Is Blocked

White Indicates
Where Adjustment
or Fill Flows Through

1 Select Layer

3 Edit Mask

4 Hide Mask
Again

33

Before

After

5 View the Result

33 Mask an Adjustment or Fill Layer

2 Display the Mask

Press **Alt+Shift**, and on the **Layers** palette, click the mask thumbnail (the thumbnail on the right) for the adjustment or fill layer you want to change. This displays the mask in the image window as a red overlay (so that you can see the image through the mask). To display the mask in black and white (so that the mask covers the image), press **Alt** as you click instead. If you haven't edited the mask, the entire mask layer will be white (indicating that the adjustment or fill layer is affecting all the pixels on the layers below it in the layer stack).

3 Edit Mask

Click one of the painting tools in the **Toolbox**, set the foreground color to black, and paint on the mask in the area where you want to block the adjustment layer's effect. Paint with gray to partially block the layer's effects. Paint with white again to let the layer's effects flow through.

You can use any tool, filter, effect, or command that works with grayscale images to edit the mask, such as the **Gradient** tool, **Text** tool, **Shape** tool, **Paint Bucket** tool, **Brightness/Contrast** or **Levels** command, or **Posterize** filter.

▶ TIPS

After the mask is displayed, you can copy data onto it and use that data as your mask. For example, you could select a portion of your image or another image, and paste that onto the mask. The data appears in grayscale; the black pixels (represented by the darkest parts of the image you pasted) block the fill or adjustment layer, and the lighter gray pixels only partially block it.

If you need to reposition the mask on the fill or adjustment layer, you must unlink it first by clicking the link icon (the chain), located between the layer thumbnail and the mask thumbnail. Use the **Move** tool to reposition the mask, and then click the link icon again to re-link the mask to the fill/adjustment layer.

4 Hide Mask Again

To view the image again and hide the mask, press **Alt** and click the mask thumbnail on the **Layers** palette. Notice that the mask thumbnail has been updated to reflect your changes to the mask.

5 View the Result

When you're satisfied with the image, save the PSD file. Then merge the layers together (if any) and resave the result in JPEG, PNG, or non-layered TIFF format, leaving your PSD image unflattened so that you can return at a later time and make adjustments if you want.

▶ TIP

You can temporarily turn off a mask (and let the fill or adjustment flow through freely) by pressing **Shift** and clicking the mask thumbnail for the adjustment/fill layer on the **Layers** palette.

In this example, I first applied a **Levels** adjustment to improve the contrast in my niece and great-nephew's face. But I didn't like what it did to the background (it made it too bright and distracting). So, I displayed the mask by following steps 1 and 2 and then painted the background black (to stop the **Levels** adjustment). The result is a subtle yet striking difference.

34 Mask an Image Layer

→ **SEE ALSO**

33 Mask an Adjustment or Fill Layer

A mask blocks data on a layer from covering up data on the layers below it. Masks are automatically created when you insert an adjustment or fill layer. For an adjustment layer, the mask blocks the adjustment from affecting certain areas of the layers below. For a fill layer, the mask simply blocks the fill from appearing in particular areas of the layers below.

But what do you do if you want to mask an image layer rather than an adjustment or fill layer? For example, suppose you want a flag to appear within the contours of an American eagle? You could use the **Cookie Cutter** tool to cut the flag into an eagle shape (if it had an eagle shape to use, which it doesn't). But even if the **Cookie Cutter** tool had the shape you wanted, you couldn't reposition the flag image within the eagle shape after committing the change. The simplest way to create what you want is to use a *clipping mask* in the shape of an eagle to control what portions of the flag appear in the final image. Unlike an adjustment or fill mask, in which black is used to block data and white is used to allow data on upper layers to show through, in a clipping mask, opaque pixels (regardless of their color) allow data to show through, and transparent or partially transparent pixels block data fully or partially.

▶ **KEY TERM**

Clipping mask—Controls what portions of any upper layers grouped with the mask appear in the final image.

1 Add Clipping Mask Layer

Open the image you want to mask in the Editor in **Standard Edit** mode and save it in Photoshop (***.psd**) format. Insert a new layer for the clipping mask by clicking the **Create new layer** button on the **Layers** palette. Name this new layer **Clipping Mask**.

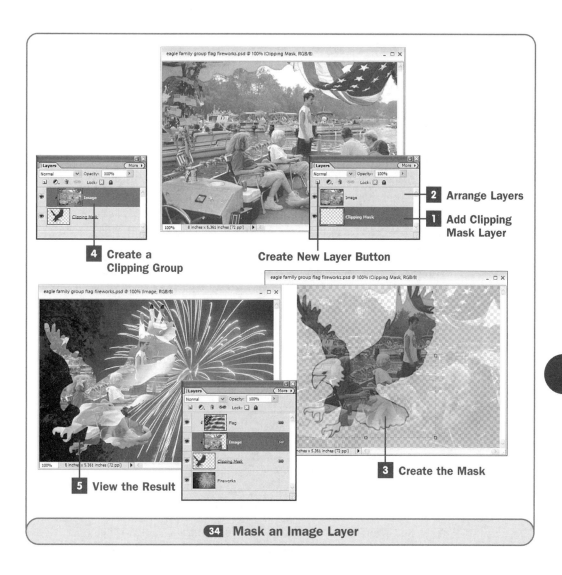

Create New Layer Button

2 Arrange Layers

1 Add Clipping Mask Layer

4 Create a Clipping Group

3 Create the Mask

5 View the Result

34 Mask an Image Layer

2 Arrange Layers

The **Clipping Mask** layer must go beneath the layer(s) you want to mask. So, if necessary, in the **Layers** palette, drag the **Clipping Mask** layer into position under the layer you want to mask.

▶ **NOTE**

To move the **Clipping Mask** layer below the background layer, you must first convert the background layer to a regular layer by choosing **Layer, New, Layer from Background**. In the **New Layer** dialog box that appears, you can name the converted layer **Image** if you like, so that you'll remember what it contains.

3 Create the Mask

On the **Layers** palette, select the **Clipping Mask** layer. Lower the **Opacity** of the **Image** layer so that you can see the data on the **Clipping Mask** layer more clearly as you work. To create a mask on this layer in the shape you want, you have the following choice of methods:

- Paint on the **Clipping Mask** layer with any color using the **Brush** tool, or draw with the **Pencil**. To create a feathered effect, select a soft brush to apply semi-transparent pixels to allow the upper layers to show partially through. Remember: Where you paint or draw, that portion of the image layer will show through in the final image. See **41** **Draw on a Photo with a Pencil** and **42** **Paint an Area of a Photo with a Brush**.

- Draw any shape you want onto the **Clipping Mask** layer, using any of the shape tools, such as the **Rectangle** tool or the **Custom Shape** tool. If you want more than one shape on the **Clipping Mask** layer, or if you want to create an object with a complex shape made up of several different shapes (such as a rectangle and two circles), draw your shapes with the **Add to Shape Area** button enabled on the **Options** bar. Again, the portion of the image layer that appears in the final image will be in the shape you draw. See **46** **Draw a Shape**.

- Fill the layer with a gradient, using the **Gradient** tool. The upper layers will be blocked only where the gradient is fully transparent, will show through partially where the gradient is partially opaque, and will show through fully where the gradient uses fully opaque pixels, so keep that in mind when selecting a gradient preset. See **45** **Fill an Area with a Gradient**. In a similar manner, you can fill the **Clipping Mask** layer with a *pattern*. See **44** **Fill an Area with a Color or Pattern**.

- Use the **Selection Brush** to create a selection in the shape you need, then fill the selection with any color using the **Paint Bucket** tool. The image layer will show through only in the area you fill. If you feather the edges of the selection, the upper layers will show through at the edges, but only partially. This might enable you to blend the masked area more smoothly into the layers below. See **23** **Paint a Selection**.

▶ **TIP**

You can create a clipping mask layer using any of the selection tools to select an object in another image that's in the shape you want to use and copying that object into your image, to a new layer below the image layer you want to clip. This process saves you from having to create a clipping mask layer manually because pasting data from a different image always results in a new layer. Skip step 1 here that creates a **Clipping Mask** layer, remove the **Clipping Mask** layer if you've already created one, or merge the layer you pasted into the image with the **Clipping Mask** layer so that there's just one layer.

34

- Type text, and then merge the text layer into the **Clipping Mask** layer by selecting the text layer in the **Layers** palette and choosing **Layer, Merge Down**. The upper masked layer(s) will then appear only within the outline of the text. See **47** **Add a Text Caption or Label**.

4 Create a Clipping Group

In the **Layers** palette, choose the **Image** layer. Group this layer with the **Clipping Mask** layer by choosing **Layer, Group with Previous**. On the **Layers** palette, the **Image** layer is indented, indicating that the upper layer is being clipped (masked) by the layer below. Data on the **Image** layer is now masked by the **Clipping Mask** layer and shows through only where the **Clipping Mask** layer is partially or entirely opaque.

You've just created a clipping group. Now, if you'd like to clip other layers as well, you can add those layer(s) just above the **Image** layer to the clipping group—there cannot be any other layers in between. In the **Layers** palette, select the layer above the **Image** layer and choose **Layers, Group with Previous** to group the layer with the clipping group. In this same manner, add as many other layers as you like to the clipping group.

5 View the Result

34

After you're satisfied with the result, make any other changes you want and then save the PSD file. Resave the result in JPEG, PNG, or non-layered TIFF format, leaving your PSD image with its layers intact so that you can return at a later time and make adjustments if you like.

To create this image, I used the shape of an eagle to mask two layers—one of my sister's family enjoying the Fourth of July on their pontoon boat, and another layer of an American flag. I blended these two layers together so that you can just see the ripple of the flag across the family photo, and the result was clipped by the eagle mask. On the bottom layer, I placed an image of the fireworks we enjoyed later that evening. By placing the fireworks layer on the bottom, its contents are obstructed by only the portion of the image layer that's clipped by the mask.

7

Making Quick Corrections to a Photograph

IN THIS CHAPTER:

Using the Editor, you can easily make adjustments to your photographs before printing them. For example, you might want to rotate or straighten an image, or crop it to remove distractions from around your subject. If the image is pretty good, you might want to give it only a quick fix (a series of simple, automated adjustments to an image's brightness, contrast, saturation, and sharpness), rather than a more complex, manual editing job. You'll learn how to perform all these simple, easy corrections in this chapter. For images that require a bit more work before you can print them, see upcoming chapters for help.

The Organizer provides a way for you to make automatic improvements to a selected image without invoking the Editor. The **Edit**, **Auto SmartFix** command makes automatic adjustments to color and tone *without any input from you*. However, you'll most likely prefer the results you get with the Editor's **Quick Fix** tool, which allows you to select not only the type but the amount of the automatic adjustment you want to apply. See **39 Apply a Quick Fix**. For full access to all adjustments and tools, choose **Standard Edit** mode in the Editor; see upcoming tasks for information on how to use the Editor's tools. Before editing on any image, however, you must adjust your monitor so that the colors you see onscreen will match the colors you get when you print an image. See **35 About Color Management**.

35 About Color Management

→ SEE ALSO

70 Print an Image

What you see onscreen when you view an image is often very different from what you get when you print an image on paper. Not only do your monitor, printer, and even your scanner use different methods to render color images, each device works with its own separate range of possible colors (also called a *gamut*). What this means is that, when representing an image onscreen, your monitor might display a grayish red for an area of an image, which is not reproducible by your printer as *an exact* match. The printer, in such a case, simply substitutes a *close* match to the grayish red from similar colors in its gamut. So, when the image is printed, you get something that's close to what it looked like onscreen, but not exactly. The best way you can deal with this messy situation is to create an environment that simulates onscreen (as nearly as possible) what an image will look like when it's finally printed. To do that, you use *color management*.

▶ **KEY TERMS**

Gamut—A palette comprised of all the individual colors that can be reproduced by a device. Your monitor, printer, scanner, and your digital camera each have separate gamuts, and sometimes colors within them might match closely but not precisely.

Color management—The process of coordinating the color gamut of your monitor with that of your scanner and printer so that the same colors are reproduced throughout your system.

Microsoft Windows has the unenviable task of translating colors from one device to another using specific ICM (Image Color Management) profiles for the devices involved. All devices that use color should have one of these profiles installed (specifically, your monitor, printer, scanner, and some digital cameras). Usually, the color profile for a device is located on the manufacturer's disc, and you install it at the time you install the device driver and other software for that device—monitor, printer, scanner, and digital camera. With a profile installed, Windows translates colors between devices, so that "rosy red" shows up as exactly that on your monitor, printer, and scanner. Sounds easy, but it isn't. For example, suppose you scan in an image. Windows translates the colors from the scanner's profile into a set of colors matching those in the monitor's profile. If there is no monitor profile installed, Windows translates the scanner colors into colors within its own standard color gamut. This result goes through a further translation by your video card, using its own methodology and driver. (For good reason, high-end video cards do not trust Windows's results, and so they typically tweak these colors before displaying them.) Photoshop Elements takes this one step further by making minor adjustments to these monitor colors with some help from a program called Adobe Gamma.

35

▶ **NOTES**

Adobe Gamma creates an ICC color profile of its own, using information provided by the video card through Windows. The resulting profile is what Photoshop Elements uses to represent colors onscreen.

Because paper plays a critical role in the quality of photos printed at home, manufacturers of paper for inkjet and photo printers are now releasing ICC color profiles for their various grades and bonds of paper. How you use one of these profiles depends on how your printer driver manages color. Newer printer drivers can incorporate separate paper profiles along with their existing printer profiles. Some printer manufacturers' brands of paper—for instance, HP and Epson—provide color profiles that override the existing profiles for their older models of printers (those that don't manage paper profiles separately), thus becoming combination "printer + paper" profiles.

Earlier, I mentioned that some digital cameras have color profiles you need to install. Most cameras, however embed their color profiles within recorded images and therefore, cameras of this type do not need to have a color profile "installed" on your system. The color gamut for an image is saved in the image's EXIF data, which you can view on the **Metadata** tab of the **Properties** pane in the

Organizer, and on the **Camera Data 2** page of the **File Info** dialog box in the Editor. For most digital cameras, the gamut saved in an image file is sRGB. If you turn color management on within the Editor, the gamut used by the digital camera (and included in an image's EXIF data) is used to translate the image to the screen. For images that don't have a gamut listed in their EXIF data (again assuming you turn on color management within Photoshop Elements), you can choose which gamut to use. Again, sRGB is the gamut typically used by most digital cameras, so it's a good choice for use in the Editor if you're prompted to make a choice when opening an image.

35

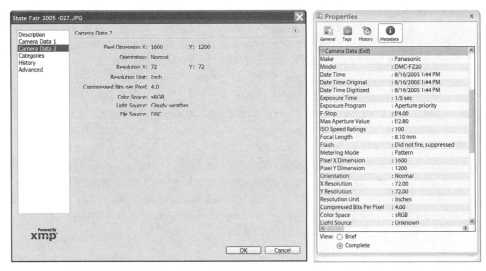

File Info Dialog Box in the Editor   Properties Pane in the Organizer

You can view the EXIF data attached to an image using the Editor or the Organizer.

▶ **NOTE**

Some cameras tag their images with the sRGB color space (gamut), even if that is not the actual gamut used by the camera. This causes a noticeable color cast in all images from that camera, when viewed in Photoshop Elements because the program assumes that sRGB was actually used, and uses that gamut to display the image onscreen. When your digital camera is pretending to use sRGB and it really isn't, you'll want to ignore the EXIF data when saving an image and have Adobe Gamma provide the color space data instead. Simply choose **Edit**, **Preferences**, **Saving Files** from the Editor menu, enable the **Ignore Camera Data (EXIF) Profiles** check box, and click **OK**.

Printing and Color Management

Now that you understand more clearly how an image is translated to the screen, let's take a closer look at the translation to the printer. When Photoshop Elements sends an image to the printer, Windows just passes it along, because when

Windows processes the image to display it on the screen, its Graphics Device Interface bases its color decisions partly on the current printer driver. If you have no printer installed, the GDI translates color information using Windows's generic printer driver. Which is why it's a really good idea to make sure that the printer you intend to use is selected in the **Printer** dialog box, before you go making a lot of changes to an image. (You can choose which printer to use from the **Page Setup** dialog box in the Editor; see **70** **Print an Image.**)

▶ **NOTE**

It's important to note that I'm talking about translation here—getting the image data from the file and onto the screen with some degree of accuracy, and then getting that data from the screen to the printer correctly. The data in an image file itself isn't changed at all during this translation process—neither by Windows nor by the printer. Image data can be changed by Photoshop Elements, of course, as you edit an image to make it ready for its final use. As you edit, however, it's important not to lose any image data that will help in printing the image, which is why you should be careful to protect the original EXIF information in your digital camera images.

After Windows passes the image data to the printer, most photo printers tweak it a bit using the EXIF data in the image file. The EXIF data helps the printer translate the image data into as accurate a reproduction of the onscreen image as possible. So it's important that you don't remove EXIF data from an image file, which will happen if you save the image in anything other than JPEG, TIFF, or PSD format. Some printers do not interpret EXIF data. Recently, Epson has engineered a system for its inkjet and photo printers that gives the printer the EXIF data for an image directly, by way of a bypass driver. Epson calls its system Print Image Management (PIM), and it enables its printers to see with a high degree of accuracy (albeit through two translators) what a PIM-enabled digital camera saw when it recorded an image, and to be able to print that image as accurately as possible. Essentially, PIM—and its successor, PIM II—ensure that both the Epson printer and the PIM-enabled digital camera interpret color and present EXIF data in the same way. If you plan to use the PIM feature of your printer as it was intended, you should purchase or use a digital camera that explicitly supports PIM as well—and thankfully, many do, but you *do* have to look. When PIM is involved, the color management scheme changes. Software called the *PIM plug-in* bypasses Windows color management and the ICC color profile, presenting EXIF data from an image directly to Photoshop Elements.

35

Setting Monitor Chromaticity

Assuming that you have a desktop monitor, or a newer notebook (post-2004, with 15" monitor or larger), you should calibrate your monitor, using a utility called Adobe Gamma. (Older or less expensive, newer notebooks cannot be easily calibrated because their colors change too much depending on the lighting and angle of viewing.) Keeping your monitor calibrated is the best way for you to ensure that the image you see onscreen is the same image you get when you print. Photoshop Elements includes a tool for calibrating your monitor called Adobe Gamma. Using Adobe Gamma, you should calibrate your monitor at least twice per year, plus every time you replace your video card or update your video drivers. Monitor calibration affects how data is displayed onscreen, not just in Photoshop Elements, but in all your Windows applications.

There are some technical terms you must understand to complete the steps, and the first one is called *monitor chromaticity*. Basically, every monitor has its own idea of how to display pure red, green, and blue, and that information is stored in the monitor's *ICC color profile*. If you have already installed a monitor profile, or if you're using the default sRGB color space that Windows provides when no profile is present, you'll have no problems in Adobe Gamma, because it will read values currently in use. However, you might still need to make changes to these values to enable the colors you *see* to more closely approximate the colors that the current profile would have you see. The sRGB color space is often inadequate for many brands of monitors—it makes a best-guess estimate of what colors you should see, and might be off-target.

35 ▶ KEY TERMS

Monitor chromaticity—A particular monitor's definition of pure red, green, and blue. A monitor's chromaticity is stored in its ICC color profile.

ICC color profile—Also known as an ICM profile. Each imaging device should have its own color profile installed; the file is used to translate image data from one device (such as a monitor) to another (such as a printer), so that the colors delivered by both devices match up as much as possible.

36 Crop a Portion of an Image

→ SEE ALSO

16 Change Image Size or Resolution

To ensure a quality photograph that uses good composition, it's important to properly frame a photograph before you shoot. Whenever possible, you should crop in the lens, when taking the photo. Doing so prevents the loss of quality (resolution) that occurs when you have to manually crop an image after the fact. However, even with careful planning, unwanted objects sometimes appear along the border of otherwise perfect images. In such cases, careful cropping after the fact can help eliminate the unwanted distractions. Cropping, by the way, is a process that cuts away the outer portions of an image that you no longer want to keep. Cropping not only eliminates distractions from your subject, it can also create a stronger composition by concentrating the image on your subject rather than the background.

Using the Editor, you can crop an image to any size you want. However, if you intend to print the image, you might prefer to crop the image to a particular print size, such as 4" × 6". To ensure that you maintain proper quality after cropping, you can also specify the resolution you want to use. If necessary, the Editor automatically generates extra pixels through resampling so that the final image matches the desired resolution. As you crop, a rectangle appears on the image; portions of the image outside this rectangle are discarded when the cropping is complete.

▶ TIPS

With the **Cookie Cutter** tool, you can crop a single layer of an image using a shaped border (such as a heart or an arrow) rather than a rectangular-shaped border.

If you want to crop the image to the same dimensions as another image, open that image, click the **Crop** tool, and then select **Use Photo Ratio** from the **Aspect Ratio** list on the **Options** bar. The dimensions of the current image appear in the **Width**, **Height**, and **Resolution** boxes. Change back to the image you want to crop, and continue to step 3.

You can crop to the rectangular area surrounding a selection by choosing **Image**, **Crop** from the menu bar.

36

■ Click Crop Tool

Open the image you want to crop in the Editor in **Standard Edit** mode and save it in Photoshop (***.psd**) format. Then click the **Crop** tool in the **Toolbox**.

② Set Crop Dimensions

You can crop the image to any specific size you want by selecting that size beforehand. Open the **Aspect Ratio** list on the **Options** bar and select a size. To flip the dimensions (to specify 4" × 6" for example instead of 6" × 4") click the **Swap** button on the **Options** bar. To retain the photo's original aspect ratio, choose **Use Photo Ratio**. If you can't find a preset that matches the exact size you want to crop the image to, choose **Custom** and enter the dimensions you want to use in the **Width** and **Height** boxes. If you want to draw the exact cropping area yourself, choose **No Restriction**.

Enter the **Resolution** you want to use. For images you intend to print (photo prints), use a resolution setting of 200 to 300 PPI; for images meant to be seen on-screen only (for instance, in web pages), use a resolution of 72 PPI.

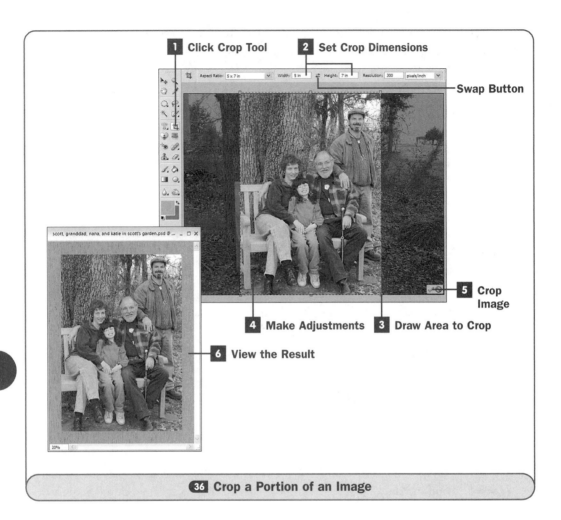

1 Click Crop Tool   **2** Set Crop Dimensions

Swap Button

5 Crop Image

4 Make Adjustments   **3** Draw Area to Crop

6 View the Result

36

36 Crop a Portion of an Image

3 Draw Area to Crop

Click on the image in the upper-left corner of the area you want to keep. Drag downward and to the right to draw the cropping rectangle. The portions of the image within this rectangle are kept, and portions outside the rectangle (shown in a darkened color) are discarded.

4 Make Adjustments

To move the cropping rectangle around the image, click inside the rectangle and drag. To resize the rectangle while maintaining the same dimensions you specified in step 2, drag a corner handle inward to make the rectangle smaller or outward to make it bigger.

To rotate the rectangle (place the rectangle at an angle), move the mouse pointer a slight distance from any outer edge of the rectangle, until the mouse pointer changes to a curved two-headed arrow. Then drag in a clockwise or counter-clockwise direction to rotate the rectangle.

5 Crop Image

When the cropping rectangle is positioned as desired, click the **Commit** (the check mark) button to crop the image. The outer portions of the image are cropped. If the image contains layers, all the layers are cropped to this same size. To cancel the cropping operation, click the **Cancel** button (the slashed circle) instead.

6 View the Result

After you're satisfied with the image, save the PSD file. Then resave the result in JPEG, PNG, or non-layered TIFF format, leaving your PSD image unflattened so that you can return at a later time and make adjustments if you want.

Cropping this informal portrait of my husband and his family improved its composition. I then added a blue-gray wooden frame using a technique discussed in **69** **Frame a Photograph**.

37

37 Straighten an Image

→ SEE ALSO

36 Crop a Portion of an Image
52 Repair Minor Tears

Straightening an image is the process of rotating it by just a few degrees. The main reason for straightening an image is to draw the viewer's attention away from distractions such as a sidewalk running downhill, a slanting horizon, a pole that's leaning to one side, and so on. You might also use this technique to deliberately place an image on a slant to make it more interesting for use on a greeting card, Web page, scrapbook page, and so on.

Unfortunately, although the Editor provides you with both the **Image, Rotate, Straighten Image** and an **Image, Rotate, Straighten and Crop Image** command, neither one seems to make the same automatic choices that you would have made. So, to straighten a crooked image, you should use the **Straighten** tool. With the **Straighten** tool, you draw a horizontal or vertical line to mark the alignment of the horizon or the vertical edge.

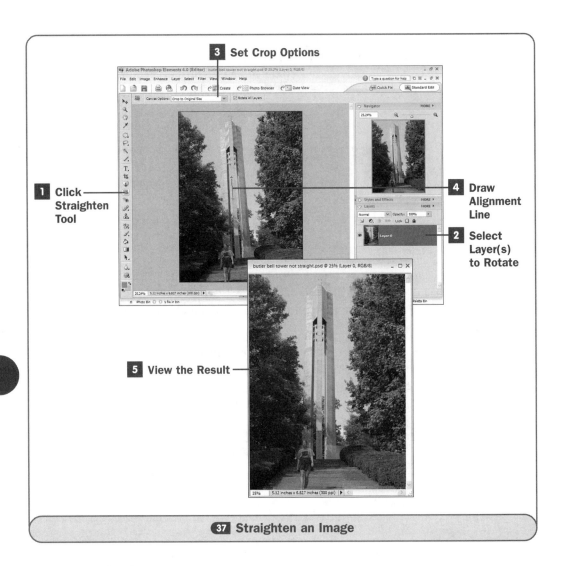

3 Set Crop Options

1 Click Straighten Tool

4 Draw Alignment Line

2 Select Layer(s) to Rotate

5 View the Result

37

37 Straighten an Image

1 Click Straighten Tool

Open the image you want to straighten in the Editor in **Standard Edit** mode and save it in Photoshop (***.psd**) format. Click the **Straighten** tool on the **Toolbox**.

2 Select Layer(s) to Rotate

If the image contains more than one layer, select the layer you want to straighten from the **Layers** palette. If this layer is the background layer, convert it to a regular layer by choosing **Layer, New, Layer From Background,** type a **Name** for the layer, and click **OK**. (If you don't convert the layer, open areas created by the straightening will be filled with the current background color.) To straighten all layers, select **Rotate All Layers** on the **Options** bar.

▶ **TIP**

Suppose that you have a photo in which the subject appears crooked but the background seems straight, or vice versa. Using selection tools, you can separate the elements into different layers and then use these steps to straighten just one layer and leave the other as it is. See **27** Create a New Image or Layer from a Selection.

3 Set Crop Options

Normally, when you straighten an image, one pair of opposite corners of the image will extend past the edges of the canvas. From the **Canvas Options** menu on the **Options** bar, select how you want holes created along the sides of the image during the straightening process to be handled:

• **Grow Canvas to Fit**—After straightening, this option changes the size of the image canvas to include all image data so that no data is lost.

• **Crop to Remove Background**—This option crops the image to remove empty areas created by the straightening, causing some data loss.

• **Crop to Original Size**—This option crops the image to its original size, removing data outside that area. Some blank areas will still exist with this option, but the result is less data loss than **Crop to Remove Background**, but more than **Grow Canvas to Fit**.

4 Draw Alignment Line

Drag to draw a line against something in the image that you want to be perfectly horizontal. The line doesn't have to touch anything, but tracing an object you know isn't straight will help you indicate clearly what needs to be straightened. To draw a vertical alignment line instead, press **Ctrl** as you drag. As soon as you release the mouse button, Photoshop Elements uses the line you drew to straighten the image.

5 View the Result

When you're satisfied with the image, save the PSD file. Then resave the result in JPEG, PNG, or non-layered TIFF format, leaving your PSD image unflattened so that you can return at a later time and make adjustments if you want.

37

After straightening and cropping, this image of a bell tower at a local college had some gaps on either side. I quickly filled the small gap in the lower left corner using the **Clone Stamp** tool, as described in **52** **Repair Minor Tears**. For the larger gap in the upper-right corner, I used the technique described in **53** **Repair Large Holes, Tears, and Missing Portions of a Photo**.

38 Correct Red Eye

→ SEE ALSO

67 Awaken Tired Eyes

When used properly, a camera flash can help lighten shadows and illuminate an otherwise dark image. Unfortunately, using a flash might sometimes have unintended effects, such as *red eye*. In nonhuman subjects such as dogs or cats, the result might be "glassy eye" rather than red eye. You have several options when dealing with photos that contain red eye. For example, you can have Photoshop Elements automatically remove red eye from photos as you import them into the Organizer catalog (see **1** **Import Media from a Folder, CD-ROM, or DVD** and **2** **Import Images from a Digital Camera**). You can also remove red eye automatically from selected photos already in the catalog, by choosing **Edit, Auto Red Eye Fix**. For an equally easy and yet still hands-on approach, you can use the Editor's **Red Eye Removal** tool as explained in this task.

▶ **KEY TERM**

Red eye—A reddening of the pupil caused by a reflection of the intense light from a camera flash against the retina in the back of the subject's eyes.

▶ **TIPS**

When you're shooting your photograph, you can avoid giving your subjects red eye by separating the flash unit from the camera (if possible), or by telling your subjects to not look directly at the camera.

Some cameras have a red-eye reduction feature, which causes the flash to go off several times. The first series of flashes at lower intensity cause the pupil to contract, thus blocking the reflection, while the final flash at full intensity illuminates the subject for the picture. Just be sure to warn your subject not to move until the second flash goes off.

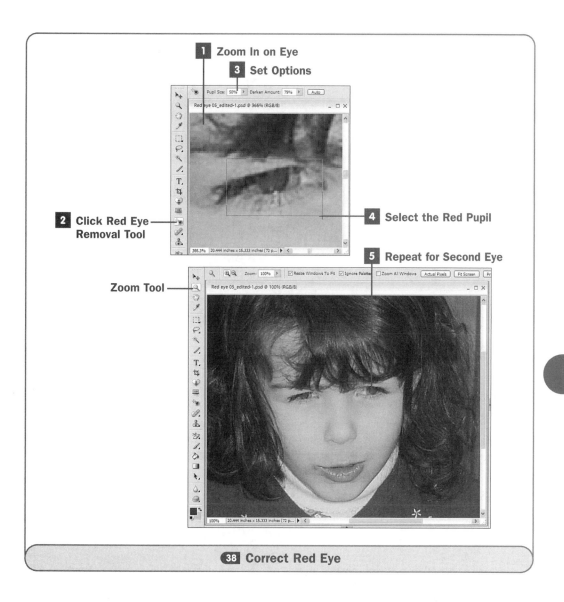

38 Correct Red Eye

1 Zoom In on Eye

Open an image in the Editor in either **Quick Fix** or **Standard Edit** mode and save it in Photoshop (***.psd**) format. Zoom in on the first eye you want to correct so that you can see it better. To zoom in, click the **Zoom** tool in the **Toolbox**. Then click on the image to zoom in, or drag a rectangle within the image around the eye you want to see more closely.

2 Click Red Eye Removal Tool

Click the **Red Eye Removal** tool in the **Toolbox**.

3 Set Options

If the *pupil* of the eye you want to correct is larger in area than 50% of the *iris*, change the **Pupil Size** setting on the **Options** bar to the correct ratio. If the **Pupil Size** ratio is way off, the Editor might not remove all the red eye, or it might paint in too much of the iris color, making the iris larger than it should be.

Typically, you won't have to adjust the **Darken Amount** on the **Options** bar. However, if the pupil is not darkened enough after you apply the **Red Eye Removal** tool, you can try the tool again after increasing the **Darken Amount**.

▶ KEY TERMS

Pupil—The black center of the eye that adjusts in size based on the amount of ambient light.

Iris—The colored part of the eye; typically brown, blue, or green.

4 Select the Red Pupil

Drag the **Red Eye Removal** tool to select the eye—iris, pupil, and all. You don't have to be terribly precise because the Editor is looking for a large group of contiguous red pixels within the selected area. After you drag, those red pixels are changed to black or the iris color, depending on the **Pupil Size** you've set.

5 Repeat for Second Eye

Scroll the image if necessary so that you can see the second eye. Drag again to select the red area. The red pixels within that area are changed to black.

▶ TIPS

Instead of dragging to select the area to change, you can click anywhere within the red area of the pupil. Red pixels contiguous to the pixel you clicked are changed to black. If one method doesn't work for you, try the other and you might get better results.

Sometimes, when photographing a pet, you'll get red eye that can easily be removed by following these steps. Other times, you'll get yellow glassy eye. To remove it, use the **Magic Wand** to select the glassy area. Feather the selection to soften the effect, then use the **Paint Bucket** to fill the selection with black to restore the pupil that was washed out by the camera flash.

After you're satisfied with the result, make any other changes you want to the PSD image then save it. Resave the result in JPEG, PNG, or non-layered TIFF format, leaving your PSD image with its layers (if any) intact so that you can return at a later time and make adjustments if you want.

39 Apply a Quick Fix

→ **SEE ALSO**

57 Improve Brightness and Contrast

61 Adjust Hue and Saturation Manually

62 Sharpen an Image

158 Create a Still Image from Video and Save it to Photoshop Elements

The strategies for making a particular image more pleasing to the eye are frequently the same for most images. Using the Editor's **Quick Fix** tools, you can make the most common image corrections easily, without messing around with a lot of separate dialog boxes. In the **Quick Fix** pane, you can rotate an image, improve its contrast, remove a color cast, reduce or increase saturation, remove red eye, or sharpen a fuzzy image. Quick Fix might not help you fix every photo, but it can save you from engaging the **Standard Edit** mode in the Editor in an attempt at a more complex solution.

Two of the **Quick Fix** tools are similar in purpose: **Auto Levels** and **Auto Contrast**. With both **Auto Levels** and **Auto Contrast**, the darkest darks and the lightest lights are adjusted while the medium tones are not affected. Because of the way **Auto Levels** goes about this process, however, its result might introduce a color cast in some images. **Auto Levels** balances the range of light to dark pixels in each of the three color channels—red, green, and blue. **Auto Contrast** balances the range of light to dark pixels by darkening the darks and lightening the lights in the final image rather than within each color channel. If you're not sure which option to pick, try one, undo it, and then try the other and pick the result that works best for the image you are attempting to fix.

39

▶ **NOTE**

The automatic commands discussed in this task can also be activated by selecting that command from the **Enhance** menu. For example, selecting **Enhance, Auto Levels** is the same as clicking the **Auto** button in the **Levels** area on the **Quick Fix** pane. (There is, however, no "auto sharpen" menu command, so to sharpen an image automatically, you *must* use **Quick Fix**.)

1 Open Image in Quick Fix

In the Organizer, click the thumbnail of the image you want to change. Then click the **Edit** button on the **Shortcuts** bar and, from the menu, select **Go to Quick Fix** to send the image to the Editor. Save the image in Photoshop (*****.psd**) format.

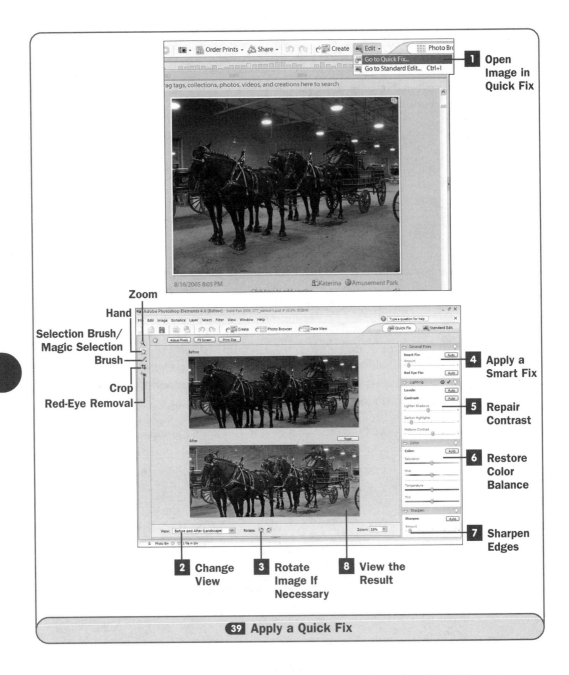

39

1 Open Image in Quick Fix

Zoom

Hand

Selection Brush/ Magic Selection Brush

Crop

Red-Eye Removal

4 Apply a Smart Fix

5 Repair Contrast

6 Restore Color Balance

7 Sharpen Edges

2 Change View

3 Rotate Image If Necessary

8 View the Result

39 Apply a Quick Fix

If the image is already open in the Editor, save it in Photoshop (***.psd**) format and then if needed, click the **Quick Fix** button on the **Shortcuts** bar to change to **Quick Fix** mode. If your image has multiple layers, click the layer you want to edit in the **Layers** palette before changing to **Quick Fix** mode. To work on the image as a whole, select **Layer**, **Flatten Image** before changing to **Quick Fix** mode to reduce your image to a single layer.

2 Change View

In **Quick Fix** mode, only a limited set of tools appear on the left. On the right is the **Quick Fix** pane; you'll make your choices here to adjust the image. You can apply any or all of these options as you see fit. Initially, only the **After** image is shown; to compare your selections to the original image, choose **Before and After (Portrait)** or **Before and After (Landscape)** from the **View** list.

▶ **NOTE**

For help in using the **Zoom** and **Hand** tools, see **15** Zoom In and Out; for help with the selection brush tools, see **23** Paint a Selection; for help with the **Crop** tool, see **36** Crop a Portion of an Image; for help with the **Red-Eye Removal** tool, see **38** Correct Red Eye.

3 Rotate Image If Necessary

If needed, click either the **Rotate photo 90° clockwise (right)** or **Rotate photo 90° counterclockwise (left)** button at the bottom of the **Quick Fix** window to rotate the image.

4 Apply a Smart Fix

Instead of applying individual changes to an image's color, contrast, and sharpness, apply a **Smart Fix**. To apply an automatic **Smart Fix**, click the **Smart Fix Auto** button. To adjust how obvious or how drastic you want the **Smart Fix** change to be, drag the **Amount** slider left for less or right for more, then click the **Commit** button (the check mark) to make the change.

5 Repair Contrast

To have the Editor automatically adjust the contrast within each color channel individually, click the **Levels Auto** button. If you prefer to automatically adjust the image's total contrast (rather than the contrast within each color channel), click the **Auto** button next to **Contrast** instead.

You can make manual adjustments to an image's contrast if you prefer. To lighten the darkest pixels, increase the **Lighten Shadows** value. To darken the lightest pixels, increase the **Darken Highlights** value. Finally, to lighten the midtones, drag the **Midtone Contrast** slider to the left. To darken the midtones, drag the slider to the right instead. Then click the **Commit** button (the check mark) to make the change.

39

6 Restore Color Balance

To normalize the colors throughout the image so that any unnatural color cast is removed or so that any over- or under-saturation is compensated for, click the **Color Auto** button.

You can make manual adjustments to color if you like. To desaturate the image, drag the **Saturation** slider to the left; to add more saturation, drag it to the right. To shift the colors along the color wheel, drag the **Hue** slider to the left (toward teal) or to the right (toward green). To make an image cooler (more bluish), drag the **Temperature** slider to the left; to make the image warmer (more reddish), drag the slider to the right. To add more green to an image (and possibly remove a color cast), drag the **Tint** slider to the left; to add magenta instead, drag the slider to the right. Then click the **Commit** button (the check mark) to make the change.

7 Sharpen Edges

To sharpen the image automatically, click the **Sharpen Auto** button. You might also notice, especially in large areas of primarily one shade, an increase in graininess and the possible inclusion of spots. You can click the **Auto** button more than once to increase the contrast along the edges of objects in a photo.

To manually select the amount of sharpening applied to the image, drag the **Amount** slider to the right to strengthen it or to the left to reduce it. Then click the **Commit** button (the check mark) to make the change.

39

▶ NOTES

To sharpen an image, **Quick Fix** increases the contrast along the edges of objects in a photo. To determine where the edges are, **Quick Fix** looks for significant differences in lightness between adjacent pixels and then makes those differences greater. The **Sharpen** option cannot fix a photo that is really fuzzy or out of focus.

At any time, you can undo all changes made to an image using **Quick Fix** by clicking the **Reset** button.

8 View the Result

When you're satisfied with the image, save the PSD file. Then resave the result in JPEG, PNG, or non-layered TIFF format, leaving your PSD image unflattened so that you can return at a later time and make adjustments if you want. To display just the after image, select **After Only** from the **View** list. If you want to return to regular editing, click the **Standard Edit** button.

For this photo I took of a competitive Clydesdale team, I increased the **Temperature** setting and adjusted the **Tint** to remove a bluish cast to the image that was making it look cold. I then lightened the shadows to bring out the details in the black horses and darkened the highlights to make the lights above them less prominent.

39

8

Retouching Photos with Tools

IN THIS CHAPTER:

Sometimes you might have to repair a damaged photograph or reinvigorate one that is old and faded. But often you'll just want to retouch an image that is not too bad but still could be better. The Editor has several tools you can apply to retouch an image. Naturally enough, you'll find many of them on the **Toolbox**: brushes, pens and pencils, and the means to add patterns, shapes, and *gradients* to your images. Each tool comes with an assortment of options that you choose from the **Options** bar. For example, the **Brush** tool lets you select from an assortment of brush sizes and stroke patterns. In this chapter, you'll learn how to use a variety of tools to add shapes and text to your images.

▶ **NOTE**

If you want to apply a filter to a shape or a bit of text, you'll need to convert the shape/text to raster data by choosing **Layer**, **Simplify Layer**.

---

40 **Select a Color to Work With**

→ **SEE ALSO**

🔟 Change Color Mode

At the bottom of the **Toolbox** you'll find the foreground/background color swatches. The *foreground color* is applied with the **Brush**, **Pencil**, and **Paint Bucket** tools; it's also the color that initially appears on the **Options** bar for the **Text** and **Shape** tools (although you can change it to a different color without affecting the foreground color on the **Toolbox**). The *background color* is applied by the **Eraser** when you erase pixels on the background layer. These colors are also used jointly by the **Gradient** tool as well as by some filters such as the **Clouds** filter. By default, the foreground color (the upper swatch) is black and the background color (the lower swatch) is white. You can select a new foreground or background color from the **Color Picker** or the **Color Swatches** palette. You can also pick up the color to use from the image by using the **Eyedropper** tool.

▶ **KEY TERMS**

Foreground color—The color that's applied through the **Brush**, **Pencil**, **Paint Bucket**, **Text**, and **Shape** tools.

Background color—The color that's applied when you erase the background layer with the **Eraser** tool.

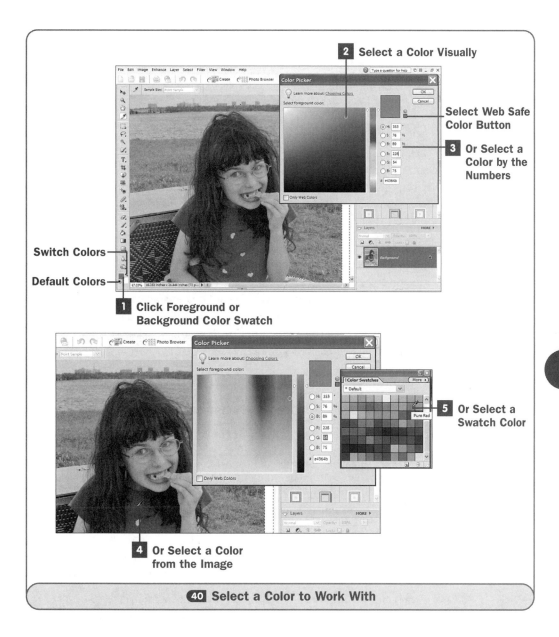

2 Select a Color Visually

Select Web Safe Color Button

3 Or Select a Color by the Numbers

Switch Colors

Default Colors

1 Click Foreground or Background Color Swatch

5 Or Select a Swatch Color

4 Or Select a Color from the Image

40 Select a Color to Work With

1 Click Foreground or Background Color Swatch

Select a tool from the **Toolbox** that uses the foreground or background color. Click the foreground color swatch or the background color swatch at the bottom of the **Toolbox**. The **Color Picker** opens.

▶ **NOTE**

To return the foreground and background swatches on the **Toolbox** back to black and white, click the **Default Colors** button or press **D**. To swap the foreground and background colors, click the **Switch Colors** button or press **X**.

2 Select a Color Visually

If needed, click the **H** (hue) radio button. Click in the large color field to choose a color, or drag the vertical color slider. Click the **S** (saturation) radio button and drag the color slider to adjust the amount of saturation (the amount of white) in the selected color. Click the **B** (brightness) radio button and drag the color slider to adjust the lightness (the amount of black) in the selected color.

The new color appears on the right in the upper box; the original color appears in the lower box. You might see an alert cube next to the original color box; this tells you that the chosen color is not a web-safe color (is not one of the 216 colors both Macs and PCs use). To adjust your chosen color so that it is web safe, click the **Select Web Safe Color** button. The Editor then changes your chosen color to a web-safe color.

40

▶ **NOTES**

To limit the color field to display only web-safe colors so you won't accidentally choose a non-web color, enable the **Only Web Colors** check box in the lower-left corner of the **Color Picker**.

The number of colors in the **Color Picker** is limited by the number of colors allowed in the image, which is based on the color mode the image is using. To change color modes—and the number of colors allowed in an image—see **19** Change Color Mode.

3 Or Select a Color by the Numbers

Instead of clicking the color you want in the large color field, you can specify an exact color by entering its numeric value using one of three color systems:

- **RGB**—Enter the values of red, green, and blue that make up the color you want, using a scale of 0 to 255 for each component. For example, a medium orange is R254, G147, B41.

- **HSB**—Enter the color's hue, saturation, and brightness. The hue indicates a color's position on the color wheel; saturation and brightness values indicate a color's percentage of white and black. On this scale, medium orange is H30, S84, B99.

- **HTML**—Enter the HTML color code for the desired color. This is a single value, using six digits preceded by a pound sign. The digits express the RGB values on a hexadecimal scale. The first two digits contain the red value, the second two the green value, and the final two the blue value. In this notation, medium orange is #FE9329.

4 Or Select a Color from the Image

In the **Color Picker**, you can pick up a color from the image rather than selecting that color visually or by the numbers. Simply move the mouse pointer over the image; it changes to an eyedropper. Click anywhere on the image to choose that color.

To finalize your color choice and close the **Color Picker**, click **OK**.

5 Or Select a Swatch Color

Instead of using the **Color Picker** to select a color to work with, you can choose a color from those saved to the **Color Swatches** palette. Choose **Windows, Color Swatches** to display the palette. From the list at the top of the palette, select the library of swatches you want to use, such as **Default** or **Web Safe Colors**. Move the mouse pointer over a swatch, and the pointer turns into an **Eyedropper** icon. To set the foreground color, click a swatch; to set the background color, **Ctrl+click** a swatch.

▶ TIPS

To save the current foreground color as a swatch on the **Color Swatches** palette, move the mouse pointer over an empty area of the palette; the pointer turns into the **Paint Bucket** icon. Click, and in the dialog box that appears, type a **Name** for the color and click **OK**. The color is added to the **Color Swatches** palette.

You can pick up a color from the image at any time, without opening the **Color Picker**: Click the **Eyedropper** tool in the **Toolbox** and click the image to set the foreground color; **Alt+click** the image to set the background color. To get an average color within an area, set the **Sample Size** value on the **Options** bar before clicking.

41 Draw on a Photo with a Pencil

✔ BEFORE YOU BEGIN	→ SEE ALSO
40 Select a Color to Work With	42 Paint an Area of a Photo with a Brush

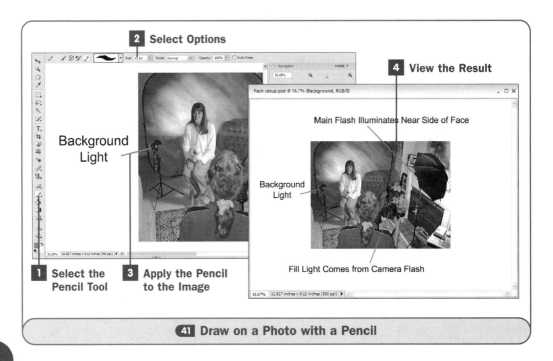

2 Select Options

4 View the Result

Background Light

Main Flash Illuminates Near Side of Face

Background Light

Fill Light Comes from Camera Flash

1 Select the Pencil Tool   **3 Apply the Pencil to the Image**

41 Draw on a Photo with a Pencil

41

The **Pencil** and **Brush** tools are close cousins; you can use either to draw on a picture. The main difference is that the **Brush** tool is intended to create often fluffy strokes of color; the **Pencil** is designed to create hard-edged lines. You might use the **Brush** to add a decorative swath of color or pattern to an image, or to paint in missing detail on a badly damaged photo. A typical use of the **Pencil** is to call out various elements of a diagram or photo.

1 Select the Pencil Tool

Open the image you want to modify in the Editor in **Standard Edit** mode and save it in Photoshop (*.**psd**) format. In the **Layers** palette, select the layer on which you want to draw. In the **Toolbox**, select the **Pencil** tool.

2 Select Options

Set the foreground color to the color you want to use for the pencil line. See **40 Select a Color to Work With**. Select a brush tip from the **Brushes** list. Adjust the **Size** of the brush tip in the **Options** bar as well.

You also can select a blend **Mode** and adjust the **Opacity** of the line you will draw.

▶ NOTES

The **Brushes** list includes brush tips that are soft and fuzzy (feathered); when these kinds of brush tips are applied to the **Pencil** tool, the brush shape is retained, but not its softness. After selecting such a brush tip, notice the preview of an unfeathered version of that tip that appears in the **Options** bar so there's no confusion of what you'll get when you use that brush tip with the **Pencil**.

If you enable the **Auto Erase** option, the **Pencil** paints with the background color if you start your stroke over pixels of the foreground color. If you start your stroke over pixels of any other color, the **Pencil** paints with the foreground color. See **40** Select a Color to Work With.

3 Apply the Pencil to the Image

Drag with the **Pencil** tool to draw. To draw a straight line, click to mark the starting point, press **Shift**, and then click to mark the ending point.

4 View the Result

After you're satisfied with the result, make any other changes you want, then save the PSD image. Resave the result in JPEG, PNG, or non-layered TIFF format, leaving your PSD image with its layers (if any) intact so that you can return at a later time and make adjustments if you want.

Here, I used the **Pencil** and **Type** tools to help create some basic callouts for a photo illustrating the flash setup for shooting a portrait at home.

42

42 Paint an Area of a Photo with a Brush	
✔ **BEFORE YOU BEGIN**	→ **SEE ALSO**
40 Select a Color to Work With	**41** Draw on a Photo with a Pencil
	160 Move a Video Filmstrip Between Premiere Elements and Photoshop Elements

The **Pencil** draws lines; the **Brush** works in smoother, softer, and more variable strokes. For that and many other reasons, you probably will find the **Brush** a much more versatile tool than the **Pencil**. You can use it to fix someone's hair or darken their eyelashes; or paint a flowery or leafy border around an image.

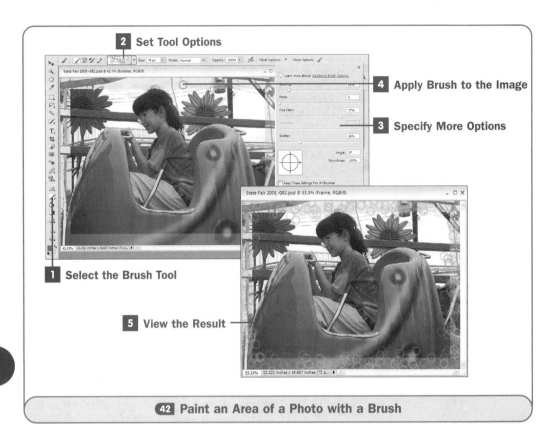

2 Set Tool Options

4 Apply Brush to the Image

3 Specify More Options

1 Select the Brush Tool

5 View the Result

42

42 Paint an Area of a Photo with a Brush

The **Brush** tool offers a set of brush dynamics options through its **More Options** button. These brush settings are not critical, but they are nice to use when you want to have fun making a unique brush that you might even save and use later. Among the dynamics options are settings for the rate at which a brush stroke fades out, and the rate at which patterns repeat themselves or change color.

1 **Select the Brush Tool**

Open an image in the Editor in **Standard Edit** mode and save it in Photoshop (*.psd) format. In the **Layers** palette, select the layer you want to paint on. Select the **Brush** tool in the **Toolbox**.

2 **Set Tool Options**

Select a brush tip, adjust its **Size**, and set other options such as **Mode** and **Opacity** as desired. Set the foreground color swatch at the bottom of the **Toolbox** to the color you want to apply with the brush.

3 Specify More Options

To set brush dynamics, click the **More Options** button on the **Options** bar and adjust the desired settings. As you do, the brush thumbnail on the **Options** bar changes to reflect your choices:

- **Spacing**—The distance between deposits of color, measured from the center of one deposit to the center of the next. Spacing is expressed as a percentage of the brush's current size. At 100%, each deposit just touches the next. At 200%, the gap between deposits is equal to the width of the brush; this seems weird, but if you measure the distance between centers of those two deposits, you'll see that it is 2 times the width of the brush. You might use this setting to create a dotted line or a string of cloud puffs.

- **Fade**—This setting enables a brushstroke to run out of paint gradually (the stroke gradually grows more transparent). It is expressed as the number of *steps* (deposits of paint) before the brush runs out of paint. So if you're using a high **Spacing** value and thus are dropping deposits of paint far apart, set **Fade** low if you want to run out of paint quickly. You could use this setting to re-create the look of a real paint brush.

- **Hue Jitter**—This setting enables the brush to switch within the range of colors between the foreground and background colors with each deposit of paint (step). At 100%, the color changes with each step, with the color selected from the range of colors between the foreground and background colors. You could use this setting to paint delicate repairs in a background area on a photo, re-creating the subtle color changes nature makes.

- **Hardness**—Sets the size of the hard center of a brush, the part with pure color. The **Hardness** value is relative to the brush tip size; at 50%, the hard center is half the size of the brush tip. With a feathered brush, **Hardness** is initially set to 0%, so increasing the **Hardness** setting increases the area of pure color.

- **Scatter**—Scatter causes each deposit (step) to be placed "off center" from the line you drag, by the amount you specify. Set this to a high value, and steps are placed within a wide area from the line you drag. With an unusual brush tip pattern, such as stars, balloons, or blades of grass, a high **Scatter** setting lets you create instant pointillism and frivolity.

- **Angle**—This setting governs the tilt of the brush tip by the number of degrees you specify. Its range is –180° to +180°, with a positive setting twisting the brush tip counter-clockwise from straight east. With a

42

round brush tip, this setting is inconsequential. For a wedged tip, how-ever, the **Angle** setting enables you to rotate the brush the way you'd tip the nib of a calligraphy pen, enabling such effects as thin side-to-side strokes and thick downstrokes.

- **Roundness**—Allows you to set how round or flat a brush tip is. At 50%, a brush is half as tall as it is wide.

▶ TIPS

If you're using the **Brush** tool with a pen tablet, you can select specific tool settings that are controlled by the pressure of the pen on the tablet. On the **Options** bar, click the **Tablet Options** button to display a palette of settings. Enable any settings you want to control with the tablet, such as **Size**, **Opacity**, **Hue Jitter**, **Scatter**, and **Roundness**. Then press harder with the pen to increase the chosen settings; press lighter to decrease them. For example, if you enable the **Size** and **Opacity** settings, when you press down with the pen, the brush tip size and opacity gradually increases until it reaches the limit set on the **Options** bar.

The changes you make to the dynamics of any brush tip are *not* permanent; if you choose a different preset from the **Brushes** list, the brush dynamics are reset. To use the same dynamics settings for any new brush tip you choose, enable the **Keep These Settings for All Brushes** check box.

42

4 Apply Brush to the Image

Click and drag to paint with the brush. To paint a straight line, press **Shift** and then drag, or click to mark the starting point, press **Shift**, and click to mark the ending point.

5 View the Result

After you're satisfied with the result, make any other changes you want, then save the result in JPEG, PNG, or non-layered TIFF format, leaving your PSD image with its layers (if any) intact so that you can return at a later time and make adjustments if you want.

For this photo, I drew a rectangular selection in the center of the photo and inverted it to select the outer area for a frame. I filled the frame area with a bright blue and used the **Hard Light** blend mode to make the "frame" semi-transparent. To dress up the frame, I chose a brush with a circular tip to pick up the dot motif on the amusement car. I chose a dark blue and a lime green (colors picked up from the photo) as my foreground and background colors, set the brush dynamics to scatter the paint and to jitter between the two colors, and then used my customized brush to paint dots along the frame.

▶ **TIP**

For a special effect, try the **Impressionist Brush**; just drag the brush over an image to remix existing pixels, creating a simulation of an Impressionist painting.

---

43 | **Paint an Area of a Photo with the Airbrush**

✔ BEFORE YOU BEGIN	→ SEE ALSO
40 Select a Color to Work With	**42** Paint an Area of a Photo with a Brush

---

Without the **Airbrush** option, the **Brush** tool applies paint to an image *as you move the mouse pointer*. With the **Airbrush** option turned on, the **Brush** tool applies paint to an image *as long as you hold the mouse button down, whether you move the mouse or not*. If you hold the brush still, the **Airbrush** continues to flow paint onto the layer until it fills the brush tip and little bit beyond. At that point, the paint flow stops, even if you continue to hold the mouse button down and the keep the brush still. It's also important to note that although the paint will flow outward if you hold the brush still, the paint will not accumulate; in other words, the paint will retain its opacity and will not "increase in thickness" or "build up." You can, of course, accumulate paint over an area by making multiple strokes of the **Airbrush** at low opacity. But you can do that with the **Brush** tool as well.

43

1 **Select the Brush Tool**

Open an image in the Editor in **Standard Edit** mode and save it in Photoshop (*.psd*) format. In the **Layers** palette, select the layer you want to paint. Select the **Brush** tool from the **Toolbox**.

2 **Enable the Airbrush Option**

Click the **Airbrush** icon on the right side of the **Options** bar.

3 **Set Options**

Select a brush tip, adjust its **Size**, and set other options such as **Mode** and **Opacity** as desired. No single stroke of the **Airbrush** can build up paint beyond the amount specified in the **Opacity** setting; single **Airbrush** strokes are not cumulative within themselves, although multiple passes with a less-than-fully opaque airbrush *do* accumulate paint. Set the foreground color swatch at the bottom of the **Toolbox** to the color you want to apply.

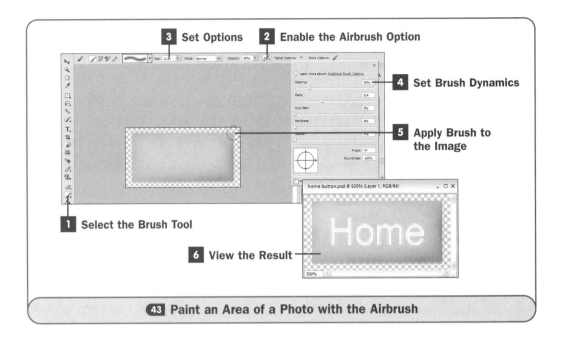

43 Paint an Area of a Photo with the Airbrush

43

4 Set Brush Dynamics

To set brush dynamics options, click the **More Options** button on the **Options** bar. Descriptions for the brush dynamics settings appear in **42** **Paint an Area of a Photo with a Brush**.

▶ **NOTE**

The **Airbrush** option of the **Brush** tool changes the meaning of the **Spacing** dynamics setting. Instead of measuring the distance between deposits, the **Spacing** option for the **Airbrush** controls *how long* to wait between deposits.

5 Apply Brush to the Image

Click and drag to paint with the brush. If you hold the mouse pointer over an area with the mouse button still pressed, paint spills outward from the tip. To paint a straight line, press **Shift** and then drag, or click to mark the starting point, press **Shift**, and click to mark the ending point.

6 View the Result

After you're satisfied with the result, make any other changes you want and save the result in JPEG, PNG, TIFF format, leaving your PSD image with its layers (if any) intact so that you can return at a later time and make adjustments if you want.

In this example, I used the **Airbrush** to softly paint shadows on the sides of this web button to make it look more three-dimensional. To make sure that I sprayed only the sides of the button and not the transparent area around it, I locked the transparency on that layer. I then added a layer and used the **Airbrush** to paint a soft white highlight in the upper-left corner of the button. To soften the effect even further, I added a **Gaussian Blur** to the highlight layer.

44 Fill an Area with a Color or Pattern

→ SEE ALSO

45 Fill an Area with a Gradient

Using the **Paint Bucket** is like throwing a bucket of paint at the side of a barn. It fills large areas with a color or *pattern*, and does it with a single click. Actually, the **Paint Bucket** identifies the color of the pixel you click and throws paint on pixels of a similar color. You use the **Tolerance** setting on the **Options** bar to control how similar a pixel must be to "match" the pixel you click. If the **Tolerance** is set low, then pixels must match pretty closely to be changed. If **Tolerance** is set high, the matches won't be that exact. The **Contiguous** setting can also be used to control the **Paint Bucket**'s effects. When you enable this option, the **Paint Bucket** changes only neighboring pixels of similar color to those it has already changed. If this option is disabled, the **Paint Bucket** searches the entire layer for similar colors and changes every instance it finds. The results are unpredictable.

▶ **KEY TERM**

Pattern—A design that repeats at regular intervals, like wallpaper.

■ Select the Paint Bucket Tool

Open an image in the Editor in **Standard Edit** mode and save it in Photoshop (***.psd**) format. In the **Layers** palette, select the layer you want to fill. Click the **Paint Bucket** tool on the **Toolbox**.

▶ **TIP**

To prevent transparent pixels from being filled, lock the layer's transparency by selecting the layer in the **Layers** palette and then clicking the **Lock transparent pixels** button at the top of the palette.

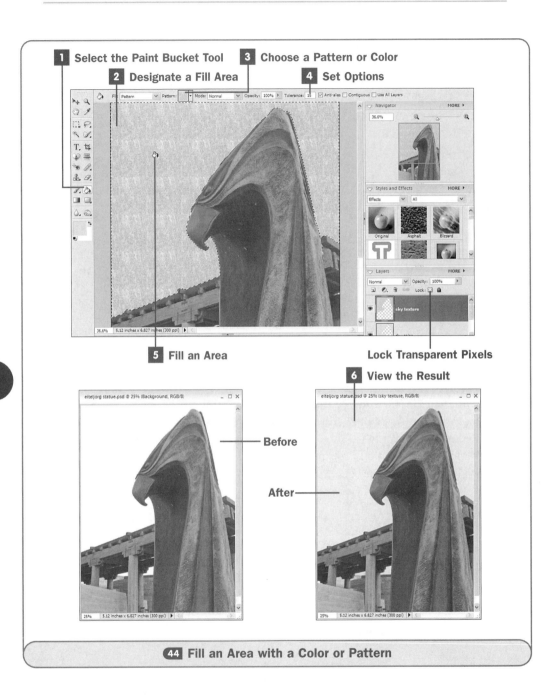

1 Select the Paint Bucket Tool   **3** Choose a Pattern or Color

2 Designate a Fill Area   **4** Set Options

5 Fill an Area   Lock Transparent Pixels

6 View the Result

Before

After

44 Fill an Area with a Color or Pattern

2 Designate a Fill Area

To limit the area that might be filled by the **Paint Bucket**, select a portion of the layer using any selection tool.

3 Choose a Pattern or Color

On the **Options** bar, select **Foreground** or **Pattern** from the **Fill** drop-down list. If you choose **Foreground**, be sure to set the foreground color swatch at the bottom of the **Toolbox** to the color you want to use for the fill. If you choose **Pattern**, open the **Pattern** drop-down list and select the pattern to use for the fill.

4 Set Options

On the **Options** bar, set the **Mode**, **Opacity**, and **Tolerance** you want. The **Tolerance** value controls how similar pixels must be to the one you click in order to also be filled. Enable the **Anti-alias**, **Contiguous**, and **Use All Layers** options as desired.

5 Fill an Area

In the layer, click a pixel in the area you want to fill. The **Paint Bucket** fills similar pixels with the color or pattern you chose based on the options you set in step 4.

▶ NOTES

44

You can define your own patterns and add them to the pattern libraries. Create a pattern with the tools, filters, effects, or layer styles, or pick one up from an image (make a rectangular selection of the pattern with no feathering). Then choose **Edit**, **Define Pattern from Selection**. Name the pattern and click **OK** to add the pattern to the current library.

With the **Pattern Stamp** tool, you can stamp a pattern onto a layer, rather than pouring it on with the **Paint Bucket**. The tool has one unique option, **Impressionist**, which paints the pattern you select using blurry daubs of color, rather than as a sharply textured pattern. The **Healing Brush** tool also uses patterns, not to help you paint patterns all over an image, but rather to help you hide your repair work as you copy pixels from one area to another. See **51** Remove Specks, Spots, and Scratches.

6 View the Result

After you're satisfied with the result, make any other changes you want and save the result in JPEG, PNG, or non-layered TIFF format, leaving your PSD image with its layers (if any) intact so that you can return at a later time and make adjustments if you want.

This photo of a lovely statue outside a local museum was almost overshadowed by the overly white sky. Fortunately, this deficit was easy to fix: First, I selected the white sky areas using the **Magic Wand**. Then I inserted a new layer and used the **Paint Bucket** to fill the selection with a light gray blue.

By placing the sky color on its own layer, I can better control the effect; for example I lowered the **Opacity** of the sky layer. Because the original sky was so white and textureless, I added a second layer and filled the same selected areas with a **Textured Tile** texture (although there is a **Clouds** texture available, it seemed too rough for my photo). I applied the **Soft Light** blend mode to blend the texture with the sky color and the original photo layers.

45   Fill an Area with a Gradient

→ **SEE ALSO**
_____

44 Fill an Area with a Color or Pattern

A *gradient* is a transition from one color to another—often between several colors. You might use a gradient as a backdrop for an image or to fill a frame around an image. The simplest gradient is one that gradually fades in linear fashion from the foreground color to the background color. More complex gradients make the transition outward from the center, at angles, and across multiple colors. There are many preset gradients you can choose from with the **Gradient** tool. If you don't find what you want, click the **Edit** button on the **Options** bar to create your own gradient.

44

▶ KEY TERM

Gradient—A gradual transition between two colors, sometimes by way of a third (or more) color.

1   Select Gradient Tool

Open an image in the Editor in **Standard Edit** mode and save it in Photoshop (*.psd) format. In the **Layers** palette, select the layer you want to change. To put the gradient on a new layer, create the layer by clicking the **Create a new layer** button on the **Layers** palette. To limit the gradient to a specific area of a layer, make a selection now. To limit the gradient to non-transparent areas of the layer, lock the transparency by clicking the **Lock Transparent Pixels** button on the **Layers** palette.

Because a lot of gradients use the foreground and background colors, set the foreground and background colors to the colors you want to use, as explained in **40** **Select a Color to Work With**. Click the **Gradient** tool on the **Toolbox**.

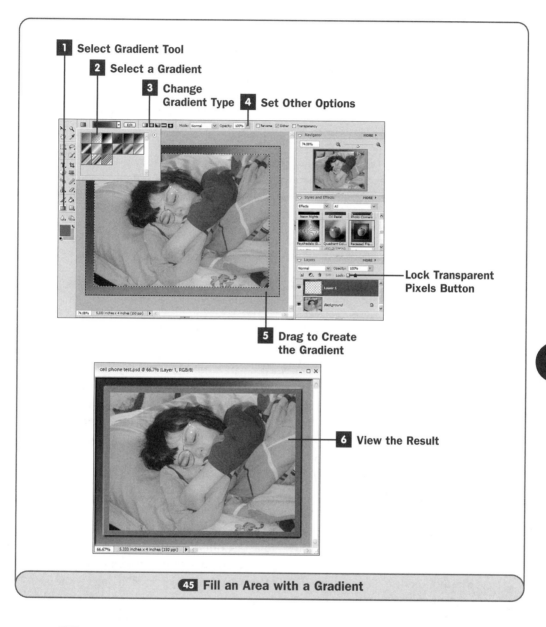

1 Select Gradient Tool

2 Select a Gradient

3 Change Gradient Type **4** Set Other Options

Lock Transparent Pixels Button

5 Drag to Create the Gradient

45

6 View the Result

45 Fill an Area with a Gradient

2 Select a Gradient

On the **Options** bar, open the **Gradient Picker** drop-down list and select a gradient. To change to a different library of gradient styles, click the **Palette Menu** button (right arrow) on the palette and choose a gradient set from those listed at the bottom of the menu that appears.

3 Change Gradient Type

Make a selection from one of the five gradient styles displayed on the **Options** bar. The gradient styles define how the gradient will fill the area you select:

- **Linear** applies a straight-line gradient from one color to the next.

- **Radial** applies the gradient outward in all directions from the center of the selected area.

- **Angle** applies the gradient in a 360° sweep starting at a designated angle, resulting in an effect that looks like an old air traffic control radar.

- **Reflected** applies the gradient in bands on either side of the center of the selected area.

- **Diamond** applies the gradient in a diamond shape, radiating from the point where you click to begin the gradient.

4 Set Other Options

45

Set the **Mode** and **Opacity** as desired. You can reverse the order of the colors in the gradient by enabling the **Reverse** option. To reduce a possible banding effect where colors blend when the gradient is printed, enable the **Dither** option. To retain transparent areas of a gradient, enable the **Transparency** option. If you turn this option off (or if you use the gradient on the **Background** layer which does not support transparency), then the transparent areas are filled with the colors from the gradient.

5 Drag to Create the Gradient

Click and drag across the area you want to fill with the gradient in the direction you want the gradient to transition. For example, drag from the upper-left corner of the layer to its lower-right corner to have the gradient's colors transition in that direction. If you made a selection, you can drag outside the area of the selection, but the gradient is applied only to the selected area. If you didn't make a selection in step 1, the gradient is applied to the entire layer (assuming that the transparency for the layer is not locked; if it is, then the gradient is applied to only the non-transparent pixels).

▶ NOTES

When you drag to create the gradient, keep in mind that the gradient bands of color often appear in the opposite direction. For example, if you drag from upper-left to lower-right to create a **Linear** gradient, the color bands appear in diagonals that bend from the lower-left to the upper-right. The color in the gradient bands, however, changes as it moves from upper-left to lower-right.

To create a gradient with an angle that's an exact multiple of 45 degrees, press and hold **Shift** as you drag to create the gradient.

6 View the Result

After you're satisfied with the gradient, make any other changes you want and save the result in JPEG, PNG, or non-layered TIFF format, leaving your PSD image with its layers (if any) intact so that you can return at a later time and make different adjustments if you want.

To create a frame for this photo of a sleeping child, I made a rectangular selection then inverted it to select the frame area. I then selected a gradient that happened to use colors present in the photo, and filled the selection with the gradient. I expanded the selection to create an inner frame, and on another layer, filled that second selection with a complementary gradient created with the foreground and background colors. Finally, I returned to the layer with the first (outer) gradient, and applied a bevel layer style to give the outer frame more dimension.

46

46 Draw a Shape

SEE ALSO

40 Select a Color to Work With

With the **Shape** tool, you can add to an image shapes such as a rectangle, circle, or a line. With the **Custom Shape** tool, you can draw a variety of irregular shapes such as a heart, star, flower, butterfly, or pawprint. You might add a circle, for example, to frame some text, or a star to adorn a favorite photo of your son. Shapes are placed on special shape layers; typically, you'll find only one shape on a layer, although you can draw more than one shape on a shape layer if you like. You might place multiple shapes on the same layer to build a larger shape, or to easily format those shapes the same way. Shapes are vector objects, so they can be easily edited and reedited. For example, you can change the color, size, and rotation of a shape after you've drawn it.

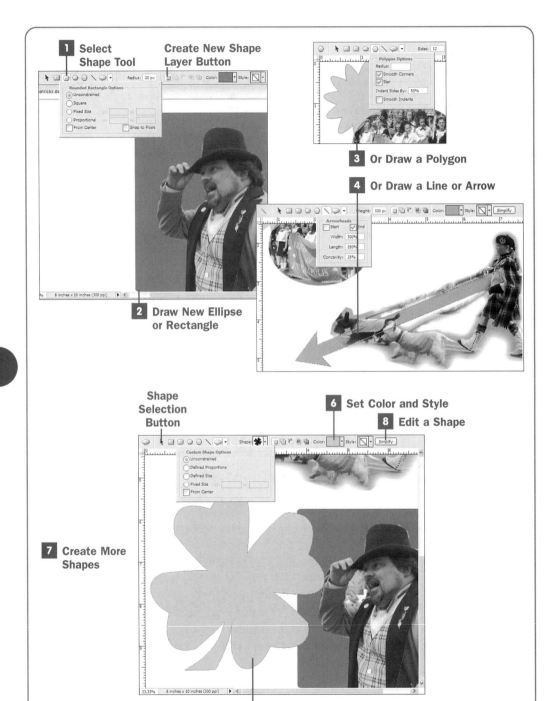

1 Select Shape Tool

Create New Shape Layer Button

3 Or Draw a Polygon

4 Or Draw a Line or Arrow

2 Draw New Ellipse or Rectangle

Shape Selection Button

6 Set Color and Style

8 Edit a Shape

7 Create More Shapes

5 Draw a Custom Shape

46

1 Select Shape Tool

Open an image in the Editor in **Standard Edit** mode and save it in Photoshop (***.psd**) format. In the **Layers** palette, select the layer above which you want the object to appear. (The shape will appear on a shape layer above the layer you select.) Click the **Shape** tool on the **Toolbox**. Don't worry about what shape is shown on the button; you'll select the actual shape you want to draw in upcoming steps.

2 Draw New Ellipse or Rectangle

At the left end of the **Options** bar, in the shapes section, click the button for the shape you want to draw: **Rectangle**, **Rounded Rectangle**, or **Ellipse**. Click the **Create New Shape Layer** button on the **Options** bar.

Click the arrow at the right end of the shapes section to display the **Geometry Options** palette, and then select the size you want: **Square** (creates a square with the **Rectangle** or **Rounded Rectangle** tools), **Circle** (creates a circle with the **Ellipse** tool), **Fixed Size** (draws the shape in the exact size you specify in the **Width** and **Height** boxes that appear), **Proportional** (draws the shape using the aspect ratio indicated by the **Width** and **Height** values), or **Unconstrained** (draws a shape in the size you designate by dragging).

On the **Geometry Options** palette, set how you want to draw the shape, choosing as many options that apply: **From Center** (draws the shape from the center out) or **Snap to Pixels** (snaps the edges of the shape to the nearest pixel). On the **Options** bar, adjust the **Radius** to adjust the roundness of corners on a rounded rectangle.

Click on the layer and drag to draw the shape. The shape is placed on its own layer, and is restricted in size or proportion as specified.

3 Or Draw a Polygon

On the **Options** bar, in the shapes section, click the **Polygon** button. Set the number of **Sides** you want in your polygon. Click the **Create New Shape Layer** button.

Click the arrow at the right end of the shapes section to display the **Geometry Options** palette, and set other options: **Radius** (sets the exact size of the polygon by limiting the distance from the center of a polygon to one of its outer points, in inches), **Smooth Corners** (smoothes the corners of the polygon, in most non-star polygons, this option creates a circle), or **Star** (creates a star). If you chose **Star**, set other options as desired: **Indent Sides By** (sets the depth of a star's indentation) and **Smooth Indents** (rounds a star's indents).

Click on the layer and drag to draw the polygon. The polygon is restricted in size (radius) and number of sides as specified.

4 Or Draw a Line or Arrow

On the **Options** bar, in the shapes section, select the **Line** button. Set the line thickness (**Weight**). Click the **Create New Shape Layer** button.

If you want to create an arrow, click the arrow at the right end of the shapes section to display the **Geometry Options** palette, and indicate whether you want to add an arrowhead at the **Start** and/or **End** of the line. Set the size of the arrowheads: **Width** (sets the width of arrowhead, as a percentage of the line weight, from 10%–1000%), **Length** (sets the length of the arrowhead, as a proportion of the line weight, from 10%–5000%), and **Concavity** (sets the curvature of the back of the arrowhead, where it touches the line, as a percentage of the arrowhead length; this ranges from 50% to –50%, 0% being flat, and negative values curving back toward the line rather than toward the point).

Click on the layer and drag to draw the line. Press **Shift** as you drag to restrict the angle of the line in 45° increments from the starting point. The line is placed on its own layer, and the line and its arrowheads (if any) are restricted in thickness and size as specified.

46

5 Draw a Custom Shape

On the **Options** bar, in the shapes section, click the **Custom Shape** button. Open the **Shape** list and select a shape from the palette. Some of the shapes have an open center, and create a natural frame around an image, which is a nice effect. To display a different library of shapes, click the **Palette Menu** button (the right arrow) on the **Shapes** palette and select a library from the menu that appears.On the **Options** bar, click the **Create New Shape Layer** button.

Click the arrow at the right end of the shapes section to display the **Geometry Options** palette, and select the size you want: **Defined Proportions** (draws shape using the proportions defined in its style), **Defined Size** (draws shape in the size defined in its style), **Fixed Size** (draws the shape in the exact size you specify in the **Width** and **Height** boxes), or **Unconstrained** (draws a shape in the size you designate by dragging). To draw the shape from the center out, select **From Center**.

Click on the layer and drag to draw the custom shape. The shape is placed on its own layer and is restricted in size and proportion as specified.

6 Set Color and Style

Select a **Color** and a layer style (**Style**) for the new shape. To remove a layer style applied in error, choose **Layer, Layer Style, Clear Layer Style**.

▶ **NOTE**

Although you can select a **Color** and **Style** for a shape before you draw it, if the current layer is also a shape layer, your selections will change the current shape layer as well. So it's typically better to select a shape color and style *after* it's drawn.

7 Create More Shapes

Repeat steps 1–6 to create new shapes on their own layer. You can modify an existing shape by indicating how you want the new shape to interact with the existing shape: on the **Options** bar, click **Add** to add the area defined by the new shape to the existing shape; click **Subtract** to subtract the new shape's area from the existing shape where they overlap; click **Intersect** to create a shape defined by where the two shapes overlap; or click **Exclude** to combine the two shapes, removing the area where they overlap.

8 Edit a Shape

Click the **Shape** tool on the **Toolbox** (if needed), and then on the **Options** bar, in the shapes section, click the **Shape Selection** button. Click a shape in the image; *handles* appear around the perimeter of the shape's *bounding box*. Resize a shape by dragging a handle inward (to make the shape smaller) or outward (to make it bigger). To move the shape, drag it from the center. You can skew or distort an object in the same way you can a layer; see **32 Move, Resize, Skew, or Distort a Layer or Selection**. You can rotate a shape in the same way you rotate a layer.

To recolor a shape, double-click its layer thumbnail on the **Layers** palette. To apply a filter or effect to the shape, the shape must be simplified first (that is, converted to raster data). Click the **Simplify** button on the **Options** bar.

▶ **KEY TERMS**

Bounding box—A rectangle that describes the boundaries of a drawn object, cropping border, or the data on a layer.

Handles—Small squares that appear along the perimeter of the bounding box surrounding a drawn object, layer or cropping border. By dragging these handles, you can resize the object, layer data, or cropping border.

After you're satisfied with the result, make any other changes you want and save the result in JPEG, PNG, non-layered TIFF format, leaving your PSD image with its *layers* (if any) intact so that you can return at a later time and make adjustments if you want.

In this example, I used a variety of shapes to frame a collage of images taken at a St. Patrick's Day parade.

47   Add a Text Caption or Label

→ **SEE ALSO**

50 Fill Text with an Image

In the Editor, you add a text label or caption to an image using the **Type** tool on the **Toolbox**. When you select the **Type** tool, you can customize how the text will look by selecting the appropriate options such as font, size, and color on the **Options** bar. There are actually four **Type** tools. You use the **Horizontal Type** tool to type horizontal (left to right) text, and the **Vertical Type** tool to type vertical (up and down) text. Even so, because text is a vector object, you can rotate, skew, or distort it after the fact by using the **Move** tool (see **32** **Move, Resize, Skew, or Distort a Layer or Selection**). You can also type text as a selection you can fill, modify, and use just like any other selection, using the **Horizontal Type Mask** and the **Vertical Type Mask** tools. See **50** **Fill Text with an Image**.

▶ **NOTE**

The type of text label/caption you'll learn to add in this task is different from a caption you might add through the Organizer: in the Editor, the text caption/label becomes a part of the image itself, while in the Organizer, any caption you add becomes part of the image's EXIF data, but does not appear on the image itself.

1 Select Type Tool

Open an image in the Editor in **Standard Edit** mode and save it in Photoshop (***.psd**) format. On the **Layers** palette, select the layer above which you want the text layer to appear. The text layer will be inserted above the layer you choose. Select the **Type** tool on the **Toolbox**.

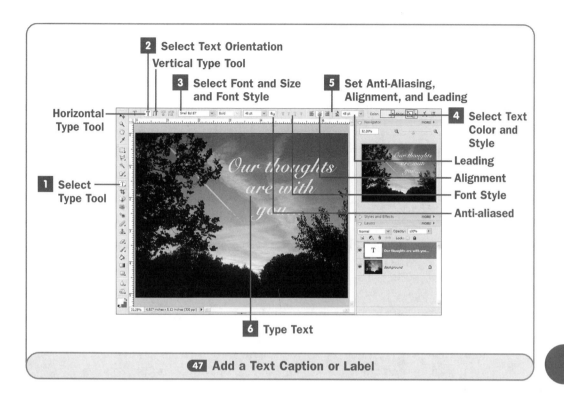

2 **Select Text Orientation**
Vertical Type Tool

3 **Select Font and Size and Font Style**

5 **Set Anti-Aliasing, Alignment, and Leading**

Horizontal Type Tool

4 **Select Text Color and Style**

Leading

Alignment

Font Style

Anti-aliased

1 **Select Type Tool**

6 **Type Text**

47 Add a Text Caption or Label

47

2 Select Text Orientation

In the **Options** bar, click the **Horizontal Type** or **Vertical Type** tool. Because a lot of formatting options are not available on the **Options** bar until you set the cursor, click in the image where you want to align the text. *To make formatting the text easier, however, do not type the text until after you select the formatting options you want in the upcoming steps.*

3 Select Font and Size and Font Style

Click the arrow next to the **Font** drop-down list box and select the font you want to use for your text label or caption. Open the **Font Style** list and select a font style if desired, such as bold. If the font you've chosen does not offer the font style you want, you can click the **Faux Bold**, **Faux Italic**, **Underline**, or **Strikethrough** buttons located to the right of the **Font Style** list. Select or type a font **Size** (in points).

▶ **NOTES**

Normally, when choosing fonts to use in a file that you intend to share with other people, you should select a font you know they also have, or risk having your text re-rendered in an alternative font. However, unless you're going to share your actual PSD working file, you can use any font you like because the vector text will be converted to raster when you flatten the image to save it in a single layer format such as non-layered TIFF, JPEG, or GIF.

After you type text, you can select portions of text by dragging over it and apply formats such as bold to just those selected characters.

4 Select Text Color and Style

Open the **Color** list and select a color from the **Color Swatch** palette. To pick a color using the **Color Picker**, click the **More Colors** button. The color you choose is added to the swatch palette. You can also apply a layer style (**Style**) to the text layer if desired.

5 Set Anti-Aliasing, Alignment, and Leading

Click the **Anti-aliased** button to soften jagged curves by adding semi-transparent pixels. Choose a text **Alignment**, such as center or left-align. If you plan on typing more than one line of text, adjust the spacing between lines by setting a **Leading** value (in points) or choose **Auto** (to allow Photoshop Elements to adjust the leading based on the text's font size).

6 Type Text

Type your text. Press **Enter** to begin a second line of text. Click the **Commit** button (the check mark) to finalize the text, or click **Cancel** (the circle with slash) to abort. The text is added to your image on a new text layer, which is named using the text you wrote. The text layer is marked in the **Layers** palette with a large *T* on its layer thumbnail.

Make additional changes to the image. When you're satisfied with the image, save the PSD file. Then merge the layers together and resave the result in JPEG, PNG, or non-layered TIFF format, leaving your PSD image unflattened so that you can return at a later time and make adjustments if you want.

47

▶ TIPS

To change text after committing it, click the text layer on the **Layers** palette and then choose a **Type** tool or double-click the text layer's thumbnail. Select the text and then make any desired changes to the settings on the **Options** bar. To change horizontal text to vertical text or vice versa, select the text and click the **Change the Text Orientation** button (at the right end of the **Options** bar). Notice that the **Style** option doesn't appear when you're editing text; to add a layer style to the text, select the style from the **Styles and Effects** palette.

If you do not like the positioning of the text after committing it, select the text layer in the **Layers** palette and click the **Move** tool on the **Toolbox**. A bounding box appears around the text object. Click within this box and drag the text to the desired location on the layer.

If you are adding text to create a copyright for an image, you might want to add the **Emboss** filter and apply the **Hard Light** blend mode to make the copyright text more subtle. Merge all layers and then resave the file in its final format for distribution. To apply the filter, you'll need to convert the layer to raster data (simplify the layer, which makes it uneditable). Luckily Photoshop Elements automatically prompts you to simplify the layer when you add the filter; to simplify a layer manually, choose **Layer**, **Simplify Layer**.

48	**Create Metallic Text**		**48**
	✔ **BEFORE YOU BEGIN**	→ **SEE ALSO**	
	47 Add a Text Caption or Label	**49** Create Text That Glows	

Sometimes, plain text is just not what you are looking for to set off an image. Photoshop Elements provides several different effects, filters, and layer styles you can use to create metallic text. You'll find these effects and filters on the **Styles and Effects** palette, which you can display if needed by selecting **Window**, **Styles and Effects**. To apply some of the effects and filters, you might have to simplify the text first (convert it to raster data), which means that the text won't be editable after that. Simplifying text is usually done automatically for you after you select the style you want to apply; to simplify text manually, choose **Layer**, **Simplify Layer**. So be sure to make your edits to the text *before* attempting this task.

1 Add Text

Open an image in the Editor in **Standard Edit** mode and save it in Photoshop (***.psd**) format. On the **Layers** palette, select the layer above which you want the text layer to appear. The text layer is inserted above the layer you choose.

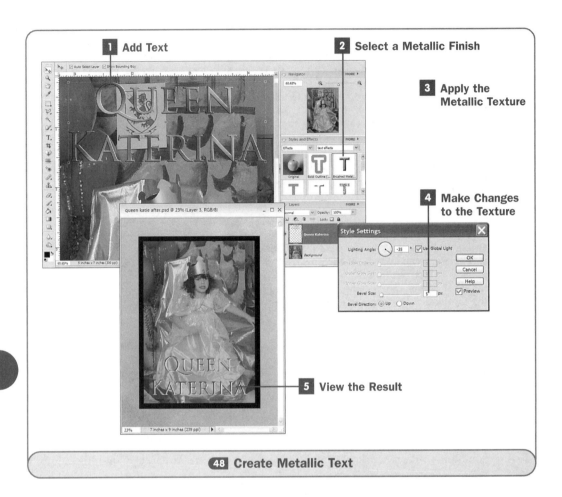

1 Add Text

2 Select a Metallic Finish

3 Apply the Metallic Texture

4 Make Changes to the Texture

5 View the Result

48 Create Metallic Text

48

Select the **Type** tool from the **Toolbox** and add text to your image. It usually doesn't matter what color you use to create the text; the filters, effects, and layer styles usually replace the color with the metallic finish. You might want to use a font with enough size and body, however, so that you can see that the text is metallic. See **47** **Add a Text Caption or Label** for more information on adding text.

2 **Select a Metallic Finish**

In the **Styles and Effects** palette, select the metallic finish you want to use. Layer styles leave your text editable, while filters and effects do not. First, select **Layer Styles**, **Filters**, or **Effects** from the first list on the **Styles and Effects** palette. Then choose a category from the second list, such as **text effects**. Here's a listing of metallic finishes you might want to try:

- **Chrome** (sketch filter)

- **Brushed Metal** (text effect)

- **Gold Sprinkles** (textures effect)

- **Rusted Metal** (textures effect)

- **Brushed Metal** (patterns layer style)

- **Copper** (patterns layer style)

- **Chrome Fat** (complex layer style)

- **Diamond Plate** (patterns/complex layer style)

- **Molten Gold** (complex layer style)

- **Rivet** (complex layer style)

- **Wow Chrome** (Wow Chrome layer style)—A collection of five different chrome layer styles

③ Apply the Metallic Texture

To apply the two textures effects (**Gold Sprinkles** and **Rusted Metal**), you must select the text first by clicking it with the **Magic Wand** tool; otherwise, the effect will be applied to the entire layer.

To apply the chosen metallic texture, in the **Styles and Effects** palette, double-click the thumbnail of the filter, effect, or layer style you want to apply. If prompted to flatten the image or to simplify the layer, click **OK** to continue.

④ Make Changes to the Texture

If you applied an effect or layer style, you can customize the metallic texture somewhat. In the **Layers** palette, double-click the **f** icon next to that layer's name. The **Style Settings** dialog box appears. Change options as desired (some options are not available with every texture.)

Adjust the **Lighting Angle** by typing a value in the field or twisting the **Lighting Angle** knob. To ensure that the text is given the same lighting angle as all other 3D effects in the image, enable the **Use Global Light** check box. Adjust the amount of shadow with the **Shadow Distance** value. Change the amount of glow with the **Outer Glow Size** and **Inner Glow Size** values. Adjust the bevel size by dragging the **Bevel Size** slider or by typing a value. The **Bevel Direction** option designates whether the appearance of the metal bevel is raised (**Up**) or lowered (**Down**). Click **OK**.

48

You can remove an effect or layer style from your text by right-clicking the layer in the **Layers** palette and selecting the **Clear Layer Style** option from the context menu that appears.

▶ **TIP**

To create your own style of gold text, apply one of the chrome or silvery metallic textures, then group it with a **Hue/Saturation** adjustment layer (by choosing **Layer, New Adjustment Layer, Hue/Saturation** and enabling the **Group With Previous Layer** option) that you use to colorize the text with a **Hue** of **59**, **Saturation** of **58**, and **Lightness** of **–26**, and enabling the **Colorize** option. For bronze text, try a **Hue** of **31**, **Saturation** of **58**, and a **Lightness** of **18**.

5 **View the Result**

When you're satisfied with the image, save the PSD file. Then merge the layers together and resave the result in JPEG, PNG, or non-layered TIFF format, leaving your PSD image unflattened so that you can return at a later time and make adjustments if you want.

In this example, I applied the **Brushed Metal** text effect, then recolored it with a **Hue/Saturation** adjustment layer so it would look golden. For the text to more closely match the color of the gold in the girl's crown and the throne, I used the **Colorize** settings of **Hue 43**, **Saturation 58**, and **Lightness 28**. I decided the text looked better at the bottom of the photo, so I moved it there and added a backscreen rectangle of light blue behind it to make it more readable. Next, I cropped the photo to remove some of the busy background. I expanded the canvas and created a gold frame by applying the **Gold Sprinkles** layer style to a new layer. I then made a selection around the photo and filled with it with black to create an inner mat.

49 | **Create Text That Glows**

✔ BEFORE YOU BEGIN	→ SEE ALSO
26 Save and Reload a Selection	**48** Create Metallic Text
47 Add a Text Caption or Label	**50** Fill Text with an Image

When I think of the term *glowing*, I infer from it the concept of emitting light. The best way I know to suggest that something gives off light is to show something that the light is reflecting off. Surprisingly, the Editor's **Outer Glows** layer styles are not too convincing. Its **Wow Neon** layer styles are better at achieving a convincing glow effect, but what I prefer is an effect that looks like one of those shadow-box neon signs, where light is emitted from the *back* of the letter blocks and bounces off the back plate, illuminating the area *around* the letters. This task shows a homemade version of that glowing text style.

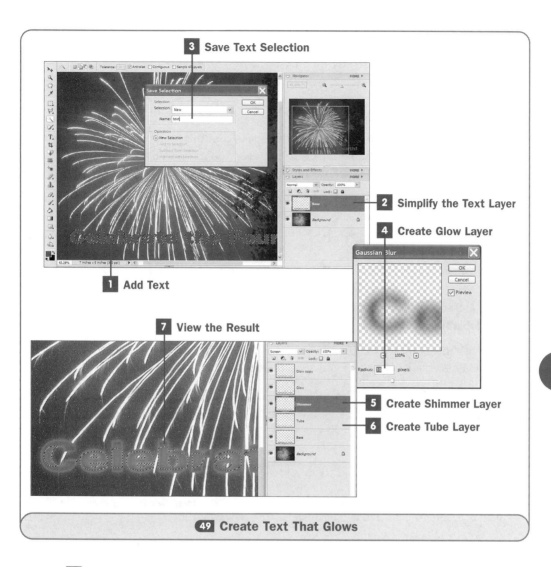

49 Create Text That Glows

1 Add Text

Open an image in the Editor in **Standard Edit** mode and save it in Photoshop (***.psd**) format. On the **Layers** palette, select the layer above which you want the text layer to appear. The text layer is inserted above the layer you choose.

Select the **Type** tool from the **Toolbox** and add text to your image. Choose a well-saturated color with a brightness of about 50 to 60, since the brightness of your final text will increase significantly with this technique. Choose a large fat font or add bold to make the glowing text effect more apparent. See **47** Add a Text Caption or Label.

2 Simplify the Text Layer

When the text looks exactly the way you want, select **Layer**, **Simplify Layer** to convert the layer to raster data. Name this new layer **Base**.

3 Save Text Selection

In the **Layers** palette, choose the **Base** layer. From the **Toolbox**, click the **Magic Wand** tool, disable the **Contiguous** option on the **Options** bar, and click the text to select the individual letters.

You'll be using this selection pattern more than once in this task, so choose **Select**, **Save Selection** to save it. In the **Save Selection** dialog box, enter **Text** as the selection's name and click **OK**. See **26** **Save and Reload a Selection**.

4 Create Glow Layer

Choose **Select**, **Deselect** to remove the selection marquee from the text. With the **Base** layer still chosen, select **Layer**, **Duplicate Layer** to make a copy of it. Name the new layer **Glow** and click **OK**.

With the **Glow** layer chosen, select **Filter**, **Blur**, **Gaussian Blur**. For the blur effect to be effective in creating a glow, set **Radius** to **10.0** or higher. Click **OK**.

In the **Layers** palette, set the blend mode for the **Glow** layer to **Screen**. If you like what you see, *you can stop here* and save your results. The next steps reproduce a neon glow effect.

▶ **NOTE**

To increase the glow effect, duplicate the **Glow** layer (select **Layer**, **Duplicate Layer**). The **Glow copy** layer will dramatically brighten the glow effect.

5 Create Shimmer Layer

To reload the selection you saved in step 3, choose **Select**, **Load Selection**, choose **Text** from the **Selection** list, and click **OK**.

Choose **Select**, **Feather**. For text above 72 points in size, enter a large **Feather Radius** amount such as **20**; for 72 points and smaller, enter a smaller feather value. Click **OK**. The effect you're going for is to reduce the selection to a series of blobs inside the letters, as shown. The area you select will be copied to a new layer and will create an inner glow like the inside of a neon bulb, so be sure the part of each letter you want to glow is selected.

In the **Layers** palette, choose the **Base** layer. Then select **Layer**, **New**, **Layer via Copy** from the menu bar. Rename the layer **Shimmer**. Change its blend mode to **Screen**. To see what you've made, turn off visibility for the **Base**, **Glow**, and **Glow copy** layers for a moment. Each letter should look very faint, like a ghost of the text layer.

6 Create Tube Layer

On a neon sign, the inner neon tube is always visible, even if the sign glows brightly. In this step, you'll create the neon tube. In the **Layers** palette, make the layers visible. With the **Base** layer chosen, load the **Text** selection again. Then choose **Select**, **Modify**, **Contract** from the menu bar, and enter a value about one-fourth the amount you entered in step 5. Click **OK**. You'll end up with a selection that's shaped like the text, but smaller.

Choose **Select**, **Modify**, **Feather** and enter a small value such as **2**. Click **OK**. The feathering will soften the edges of the selection, softening the effect. You'll use this selection to create the neon tube inside your glowing text.

With the **Base** layer still chosen, select **Layer**, **New**, **Layer via Copy**. Name the new layer **Tube**. Then set its blend mode to **Difference**. Restore the visibility of all layers. Now your letters have a glowing rim and a second tier of glow on the inside.

7 View the Result

When you're satisfied with the image, save the PSD file. Then merge the layers together and resave the result in JPEG, PNG, or non-layered TIFF format, leaving your PSD image unflattened so that you can return at a later time and make adjustments if you want.

▶ TIP

One of my favorite twists on this technique is to pick one letter and eliminate the selection for that letter before creating the **Shimmer** layer, thus making it look like the light has burned out on one of the letters.

50 Fill Text with an Image

✔ BEFORE YOU BEGIN	→ SEE ALSO
47 Add a Text Caption or Label	**48** Create Metallic Text
	49 Create Text That Glows

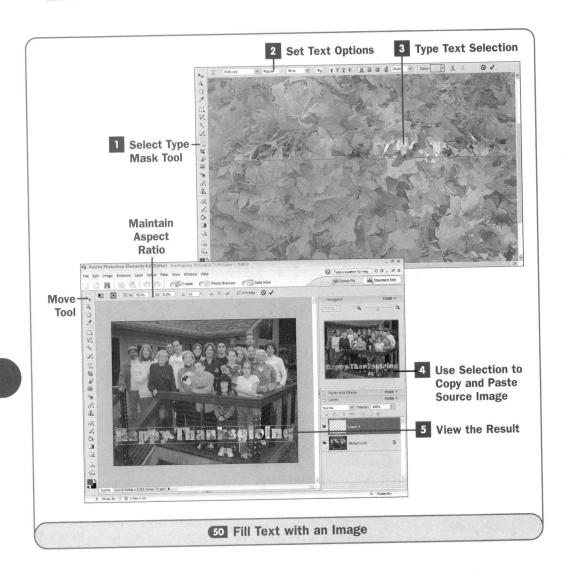

50

50 Fill Text with an Image

You can make your text more interesting by filling it with another image rather than a color. When you do this, the image is visible only inside the letters of the text—in effect, framing the image. To create this magic, you use either the **Horizontal** or **Vertical Type Mask** tool to create a type-shaped selection. You can do anything you want with this text selection, including making modifications to it using any of the selection tools (such as the **Selection Brush**), filling it with a gradient or pattern using the **Paint Bucket** or **Gradient** tools, and even saving it for reuse.

You can fill a text selection using one of two methods: First, you could paste all or part of an image into the selection. The problem with the first method is that you have little control over what portion of the image shows up within the text "frame"; and manipulating the image so that the exact portion you want to see shows through is difficult because you can't see the image as you make your adjustments.

As explained in this task, the second method you can use to fill a text selection is to maneuver the selection itself over the image and copy exactly the data you want. If the image doesn't fill the selection adequately no matter where you move it, you can change the selection text's size or font to find a better fit.

■ Select Type Mask Tool

In the Editor, in **Standard Edit** mode, open the source image you want to use for the interior of your text. On the **Layers** palette, select the layer that contains the data you want to appear within your text. Click the **Horizontal Type Mask** tool or the **Vertical Type Mask** tool on the **Toolbox**.

▶ TIP

For my source image, I typically pick something that's dense with texture or color, because you're probably not going to be able to make out a lot of individual detail within the text.

50

■ Set Text Options

On the **Options** bar, select a fairly wide **Font** and a large **Size**. Set other options as desired, such as **Anti-aliased** (which helps soften any jagged curves in the text selection).

■ Type Text Selection

Click on the image in the area you want to use to fill your text and type the text. A red mask appears over your image, and the text is revealed as you type. This red screen (the mask) helps you see how the image below will fill the text.

Edit the text if needed; because this is a selection and not actual text, you won't be able to go back later and make changes to it after you commit (although you will be able to reposition the selection; see the following **Note**). When you have created a text selection that's the size and shape you need, click the **Commit** button (check mark) on the **Options** bar.

▶ **NOTE**

If the text-shaped selection is not positioned to select the exact area of the image you want to use, move the selection after committing it by clicking any selection tool (but not the **Selection Brush**), enabling the **New Selection** option on the **Options** bar, and dragging the selection marquee.

▣ Use Selection to Copy and Paste Source Image

Select **Edit, Copy** to copy the data within the text selection. Select **Edit, Copy Merged** instead if you want to select all visible pixels within the selection and not just those on the current layer.

Open the image in which you want the text to appear and save it in Photoshop (*.psd) format. On the **Layers** palette, select the layer above which you want the filled text to appear. Select **Edit, Paste**. The filled text appears on its own layer within the image, above the layer you selected.

▶ **TIP**

You can move and resize the filled text if needed; see ㉜ Move, Resize, Skew, or Distort a Layer or Selection. If you're resizing, be sure to enable the **Maintain Aspect Ratio** option. You can also rotate the filled text layer if you like.

▣ View the Result

When you're satisfied with the image, save the PSD file. Then merge the layers together and resave the result in JPEG, PNG, or non-layered TIFF format, leaving your PSD image unflattened so that you can return at a later time and make adjustments if you want.

In this example, I started with a photograph of some fall leaves. I used the **Horizontal Type Mask** tool to copy the leaves in a text shape into an image of my family enjoying a nice Thanksgiving. I then used the **Move** tool to resize the text and to position it in the lower portion of the photo.

9

Repairing and Improving Photographs

IN THIS CHAPTER:

When people suffer a disaster, what are some of the first things they try to protect or recover? Family pictures. No doubt more than once you've seen heartbreaking stories on the news of people searching through the wreckage of their homes, looking for pictures that were dear to them. Even without natural disasters, the pictures from your past face a formidable hazard: old age. Even if you store them carefully in albums, your cherished images tend to fade, bend, and decay.

Recognizing this, the makers of Photoshop Elements have packed up an extensive kit of tools to help restore old photographs. In this chapter, you'll learn how to remove scratches and specks and to repair tears, stains, and even holes. You'll also learn how to quickly restore color and contrast to an old photograph, and to repair any loss of quality when you scanned in the photograph. When you're finished, you might look at the results and decide the old homestead never looked better and that Uncle Ben was a surprisingly handsome guy.

51 Remove Specks, Spots, and Scratches

→ **SEE ALSO**

52 Repair Minor Tears
87 Grab a Still From Video

This small photo has been around since the 1940s and has had plenty of opportunity to acquire small specks, dust spots, and scratches. Such a picture is a good candidate for a progressive approach: Start with a tool such as the **Dust & Scratches** filter to remove thin, short scratches and scattered dust spots in a small area. Then, move up to the **Healing Brush** or the **Spot Healing Brush** to remove longer and wider scratches. The **Healing Brush** works like the **Clone Stamp**, copying pixels from another area of a photo to make a repair. Unlike the **Clone Stamp**, the **Healing Brush** *blends* copied pixels with existing pixels, creating a softer, less visible, repair—this makes the **Healing Brush** perfect for repairing large areas of a photograph in which detail is not critical, such as a background area. The **Spot Healing Brush** is great for repairing small, isolated spots or scratches, because it copies pixels from the outer edges of the brush tip to the area under the tip to make its repair.

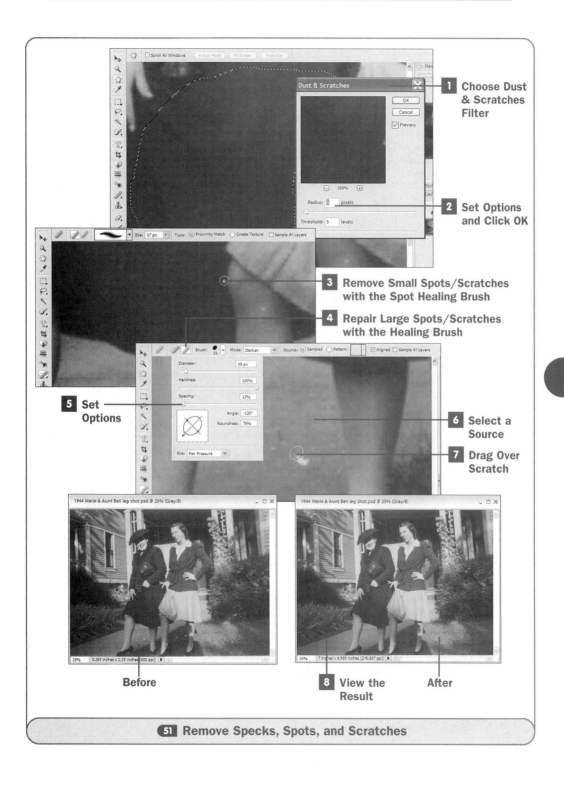

1 Choose Dust & Scratches Filter

2 Set Options and Click OK

3 Remove Small Spots/Scratches with the Spot Healing Brush

4 Repair Large Spots/Scratches with the Healing Brush

5 Set Options

6 Select a Source

7 Drag Over Scratch

51

Before

8 View the Result

After

▶ **NOTE**

Dust specks, scratches, and other "age spots" aren't the only kinds of damage a picture can suffer. Digital cameras and cell phone cameras might add *noise* to an image, if you take a long exposure in low light, overextend the digital zoom, or use an ISO setting above 100. Noise can also appear in scans of printed newspaper or magazine photos or in still images captured from video. You can use one of three noise filters to eliminate these specks from an image: The **Median** filter changes pixels to the same average brightness as their neighbors, making it a good choice to remove general, high-contrast noise. The **Despeckle** filter blurs pixels to smooth out areas of low contrast, leaving areas of high contrast (which are typically the edges of objects in a photo) untouched, making it good at removing low-contrast noise in a large area while preserving your edges. The **Reduce Noise** filter, like the **Median** filter, changes the brightness of pixels that are much brighter than their neighbors; the filter also evens out color by averaging the hue of each pixel with that of its neighbors. And like **Despeckle**, the **Reduce Noise** filter preserves the contrast along edges in your photo.

▶ **KEY TERM**

Noise—A random pattern of pixels over the entire surface of an image, giving it a grainy texture.

51

1 Choose Dust & Scratches Filter

Open an image in the Editor in **Standard Edit** mode and save it in Photoshop (***.psd**) format. Zoom in on an area of dust spots—it's easier to work with an enlarged view.

To limit the effect of the filter (and prevent it from removing detail you want to keep), use any of the selection tools to select an area that contains thin scratches or dust spots. Choose **Filter**, **Noise**, **Dust & Scratches**. The **Dust & Scratches** dialog box appears.

2 Set Options and Click OK

The **Dust & Scratches** filter searches for pixels that contrast greatly with their neighbors and reduces this contrast to remove high-contrast dust spots and very small scratches. The larger the **Radius**, the larger the area examined for brightness differences, and the larger the spots the filter can remove. Ideally, you want to set the **Radius** to roughly the same size as the scratches or spots you're trying to get rid of.

If **Threshold** is set to a low value, the spot or scratch must contrast a lot with neighboring pixels before it will be removed. As you raise the **Threshold** little by little, you'll remove more spots at the risk of possibly losing some detail in the selected area. When you find the right balance between the settings, click **OK** to apply them.

► **TIP**

Repeat steps 1 and 2 to remove the next set of spots and scratches. To reapply the last filter you used, with the exact same settings, press **Ctrl+F**, or choose that filter from the very top of the **Filter** menu, where it will continue to appear until you use a different filter.

3 **Remove Small Spots/Scratches with the Spot Healing Brush**

The **Dust & Scratches** filter does a wonderful job of removing tiny spots, especially when they are grouped together, but you must be careful to apply the filter to a small area or you'll lose detail. To remove spots that are isolated or larger than a small dot, use the **Spot Healing Brush**.

You don't have to make a selection first; the effect is controlled by the size of your brush tip. Zoom in so that you can see the spot you want to remove, and then select the **Spot Healing Brush** on the **Toolbox**. On the **Options** bar, select a brush tip and adjust its **Size** to something slightly larger than the size of the spot you want to repair. Set the **Type** option to **Proximity Match**. This option analyzes the pixels around the edges of the brush to create a patch for the repair. Click the spot to remove it.

► **TIP**

If the area the spot is in has a definite texture, you can replicate that texture to a degree by enabling the **Create Texture** option on the **Options** bar. This option analyzes all the pixels under the brush tip for both color and tone, and then uses that sampling to create a similar pattern.

4 **Repair Large Spots/Scratches with the Healing Brush**

To remove wider spots or longer scratches, select the **Healing Brush** tool. You'll use the tool to copy pixels from an undamaged area of the image, in a manner similar to the **Clone Stamp** tool. The **Healing Brush**, however, blends these copied pixels with existing pixels at the site, creating a more invisible repair than you could achieve by using the **Clone Stamp** tool.

5 **Set Options**

On the **Options** bar, open the **Brush** palette and adjust the brush **Diameter** to the size of the scratch or spot you're trying to repair. For a scratch, try reducing the **Roundness** setting to flatten the brush tip and adjusting the tip **Angle** to match the angle of the scratch. Enable the **Sampled** option. Because the scratch is lighter than the pixels you'll be copying from an undamaged area of the image, select **Darken** from the blend **Mode** list. Set any other options as desired, such as **Aligned**.

51

6 Select a Source

Press **Alt** and click the image to establish the source for the repair. Be sure to select a source area from an undamaged part of the image. I typically click very near the scratch so that the cloned pixels will match the repair area closely.

7 Drag Over Scratch

Drag the brush over the scratch to remove it. The source point (the crosshair) moves along with you, showing you exactly which pixels are being copied. If you did not enable the **Aligned** option, then as you begin each stroke, the source point (the crosshair) moves back to the original source point (the original point you clicked in step 6). If you *did* enable the **Aligned** option, the source point when you begin a new stroke is placed relative to the original source point and the place where you click to begin the stroke. In other words, assume that you selected a source point and then clicked to begin the first stroke just to the left of that point (the source is located on the right). If the **Aligned** option is enabled, then when you begin a second stroke, the source point is located just to the right of that stroke.

Pixels are copied from the source and blended with existing pixels, completing the repair. Because you selected the **Darken** blend mode, the cloned pixels replace the source pixels completely if they are darker than the scratch. Repeat steps 4 to 7 to repair any remaining scratches.

8 View the Result

After removing the scratches and spots on your photo, make any other changes you want and save the PSD file. Then resave the file in JPEG, PNG, or non-layered TIFF format, leaving your PSD image with its layers (if any) intact so that you can return at a later time and make adjustments if you want.

After less than five minutes, and with the help of the **Dust & Scratches** filter, **Spot Healing Brush**, and the **Healing Brush**, I have easily removed the majority of the specks, spots, and faint scratches on this old photo.

52 Repair Minor Tears

→ **SEE ALSO**

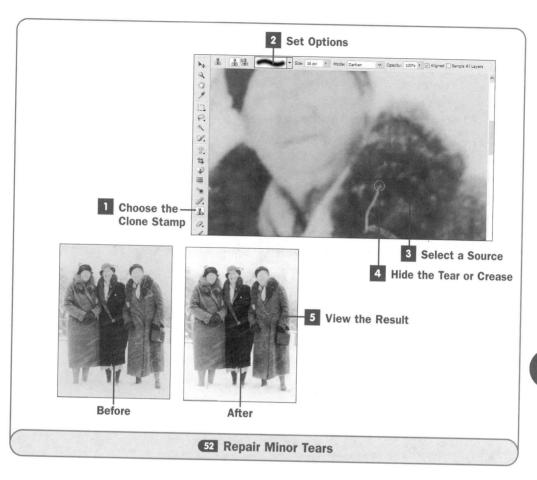

2 Set Options

1 Choose the Clone Stamp

3 Select a Source

4 Hide the Tear or Crease

5 View the Result

Before

After

52 Repair Minor Tears

Even cute pictures from the past are vulnerable to damage. Sometimes the damage is minor but annoying, such as a thin crease, small tear, scratch, spot, or stain. As you learned in **61 Remove Specks, Spots, and Scratches**, you can use the **Dust & Scratches** filter to remove tiny specks grouped in the same area, the **Spot Healing Brush** to remove small spots and scratches by blending them with surrounding pixels, and the **Healing Brush** to remove larger scratches and specks.

Sometimes the damage to the image is too much for the **Healing Brush** to correct. Although the **Healing Brush** works in a manner similar to the **Clone Stamp**, it *blends* copied pixels with those in the area you're repairing, and sometimes, blending is not what you want. For example, if you're repairing a tear that's fairly white, the **Healing Brush** blends the copied pixels (taken from an intact part of the picture) with the whiteness of the tear, creating an almost ghost-like effect. The same thing happens if you use the **Healing Brush** to repair a large hole; the whiteness of the hole will interfere with the cover-up job you're trying to achieve. In this task, you'll learn how to use the **Clone Stamp** to clone missing data back into a photo. In 🔲 **Repair Large Holes, Tears, and Missing Portions of a Photo**, you'll learn an alternative technique that's quick and effective at filling in missing information.

1 Choose the Clone Stamp

Open an image in the Editor in **Standard Edit** mode and save it in Photoshop (*.psd) format. Select the **Clone Stamp** tool from the **Toolbox**.

2 Set Options

Select a soft brush tip and set the **Size** just a bit larger than the flaw you want to repair. Because tears and creases are lighter than surrounding pixels, select the **Darken** blend **Mode**. Enable the **Aligned** option, and set **Opacity** to 100% to fully replace the tear.

3 Select a Source

Press and hold the **Alt** key. Click in the image near the crease or tear to specify the source point—the "good pixels" you want the tool to clone to fix the flaw.

52

▶ TIPS

The source point (the crosshair) moves along with you as you drag the **Clone Stamp** tool, showing you exactly which pixels are being copied. If you do not enable the **Aligned** option, then as you begin each stroke, the source point (the crosshair) moves back to the original source point (the original source point you click in step 3). If you *do* enable the **Aligned** option, then the source point when you begin a new stroke is placed relative to the original source point and the place where you click to begin the stroke. In other words, assume that you select a source point and then click to begin the first stroke just to the left of that point (the source is located on the right). If the **Aligned** option is enabled, then when you begin a second stroke, no matter where you click, the source point is located just to the right of that stroke.

The disadvantage in using the **Clone Stamp** tool is that it copies flaws along with good pixels. This is why selecting your source point is important. As a rule, select the source as physically close to the flaw as you can. As the tear or crease changes direction, adjust the source point as well (by pressing **Alt** and clicking the image again) so that you can continue to match objects perfectly, without picking up any flaws near the tear you're repairing.

4 Hide the Tear or Crease

Click at the beginning of the tear or crease and drag slowly down the crease. The pixels you sampled in step 3 are copied over the flaw as you drag. As you work, the source point (marked by a crosshair) moves with the brush tip.

5 **View the Result**

This photo of three elderly aunts braving a snow storm was apparently stored in someone's pocket. It has many creases, spots, specks, and a few water stains. It took a little while to repair the damage, but as you can see, the result is a great improvement. After making the repairs, I adjusted the contrast to bring the portrait back to life.

---

53 Repair Large Holes, Tears, and Missing Portions of a Photo

✔ BEFORE YOU BEGIN	→ SEE ALSO
28 Create a New Image Layer	**52** Repair Minor Tears
31 Erase Part of a Layer	

Photoshop Elements has retouching tools that can take care of most of the small defects in an old photo. They will even take care of some of the larger ones. But once in a while, a picture might be missing a corner or have holes in it from being mounted on a bulletin board. Repairing this kind of damage has the same purpose as using the **Clone Stamp** or the **Healing Brush** to repair smaller areas: The goal is to replace the bad section of a photo with a good section of the photo. However, when you must repair a large damaged area, using the **Clone Stamp** or **Healing Brush** to copy data is not only tedious (you have to move the source often to hide what you're doing) but often leads to poor results despite your best efforts. In this task, I show you a slick approach to filling in big gaps in your photo.

1 **Copy Bottom Layer**

Open an image in the Editor in **Standard Edit** mode and save it in Photoshop (*.psd) format. On the **Layers** palette, drag the layer onto the **Create a New Layer** button or select **Layer, Duplicate** to create a duplicate of the original **Background** layer. Rename this new layer **Shifted.**

▶ **TIP**

If the good information you want to use to repair the hole or tear is located in another image, open that image and adjust its size and resolution to match the image you want to repair. See **16** Change Image Size or Resolution. Then, instead of duplicating the **Background** layer as instructed in step 1, choose **Select, All** to select the entire good image, and then choose **Edit, Copy** to copy the good image. Change to the image you want to repair and choose **Edit, Paste** to paste the image with the good data onto a new layer. Rename this new layer **Shifted.**

53

53

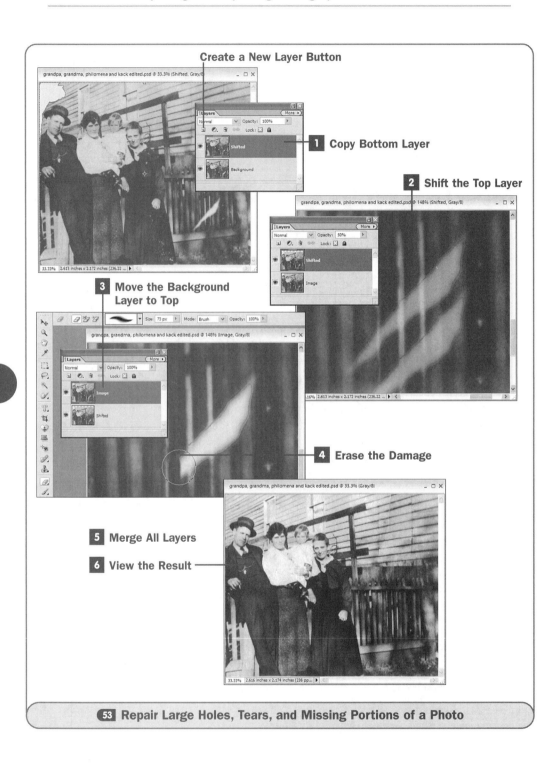

Create a New Layer Button

1 Copy Bottom Layer

2 Shift the Top Layer

3 Move the Background Layer to Top

4 Erase the Damage

5 Merge All Layers

6 View the Result

53 Repair Large Holes, Tears, and Missing Portions of a Photo

2 Shift the Top Layer

On the **Layers** palette, change the **Opacity** of the **Shifted** layer to **50%**. This setting lets you see the **Background** layer as you shift the top layer. You're going to use good pieces of the **Shifted** layer to cover the holes and tears in the **Background** layer.

Click the **Move** tool on the **Toolbox**. Click the **Shifted** layer in the image and slowly move it left, right, up, or down until its good portion covers up the area on the **Background** layer that you want to fill in.

3 Move the Background Layer to Top

In the **Layers** palette, reset the **Opacity** of the **Shifted** layer to 100%. Convert the **Background** layer to a regular layer (a process also known as "simplifying") by choosing the **Background** layer in the **Layers** palette and choosing **Layer, New, Layer from Background**. Name the converted layer **Image**. Simplifying the background layer allows you to move its position in the layer stack.

Click the newly created **Image** layer in the **Layers** palette and drag it above the **Shifted** layer. The **Shifted** layer is now on the bottom, with the **Image** layer on top. Notice that the hole in the original image is noticeable once again.

53

4 Erase the Damage

On the **Layers** palette, select the **Image** layer. In the **Toolbox**, select the **Eraser** tool. In the **Options** bar, set the **Mode** option to **Brush**, select a soft-edged brush, and adjust its **Size** to fit the size of the hole or tear. Set **Opacity** to **100%**.

Start brushing over the damaged area, erasing the top image layer to reveal the undamaged area of the **Shifted** layer under it.

5 Merge All Layers

If the shifted data happens to line up with another hole or tear, you can repeat step 4 to repair that damage as well. If not, you'll need to merge the layers, and then repeat steps 1 to 4 to repair any other damaged areas. To merge the layers, choose **Layer, Flatten Image**.

6 View the Result

After you've made all necessary repairs to the holes and tears, make any other changes you want, such as removing small spots and creases. Save the PSD file, and then resave the file in JPEG, PNG, or non-layered TIFF format, leaving your PSD image with its layers (if any) intact so that you can return at a later time and make different adjustments if you want.

This old photo of my grandparents, great-grandmother, and aunt (as a baby) has been through a lot, as you can see. There was a tear in the middle and in one corner; small specks and spots adorned various areas, and it had lost its tone. To repair the damage, I borrowed a good spot in the fence and, following the steps in this task, repaired it. I repeated the process to fix the missing section in the upper-left corner. After merging all layers, I adjusted the contrast and used the **Spot Healing Brush** on the specks. The result, as you can see, is much improved.

54   Restore Color and Tone to an Old Photograph

→ SEE ALSO

57 Improve Brightness and Contrast
61 Adjust Hue and Saturation Manually

53

The colors in this picture are a clue to the picture's age. As photos age, their colors fade at different rates, causing not only a loss in saturation, but a color shift as well. The Editor has several automatic tools on the **Enhance** menu to correct the color balance and tone of photos like this one, but they aren't always as precise as you might like. In the case of this picture, using **Enhance**, **Auto Levels** or **Enhance**, **Auto Color Correction** was like using a sledgehammer when the situation called for a scalpel.

In this task, I'll explain how to manually adjust the color saturation and tones in your image to improve its overall appeal. In most old photos, the overall tone is medium and the contrast is not as sharp as it should be; when you display a histogram for the image, the graph doesn't meet either end of the scale. The first step in restoring an old photograph is to find the brightest and darkest points in the picture and place them at each end of the histogram to balance the overall tone. You'll accomplish that task with the **Levels** dialog box. To help you make precise adjustments, you'll display the **Info** palette and use its information to help you locate the lightest and darkest pixels in the image so that the various levels of brightness can be evenly distributed throughout the image. This process also helps to balance the color in an image, removing any color cast. Finally, to restore your old photo to its former brilliance, you'll increase the saturation as needed.

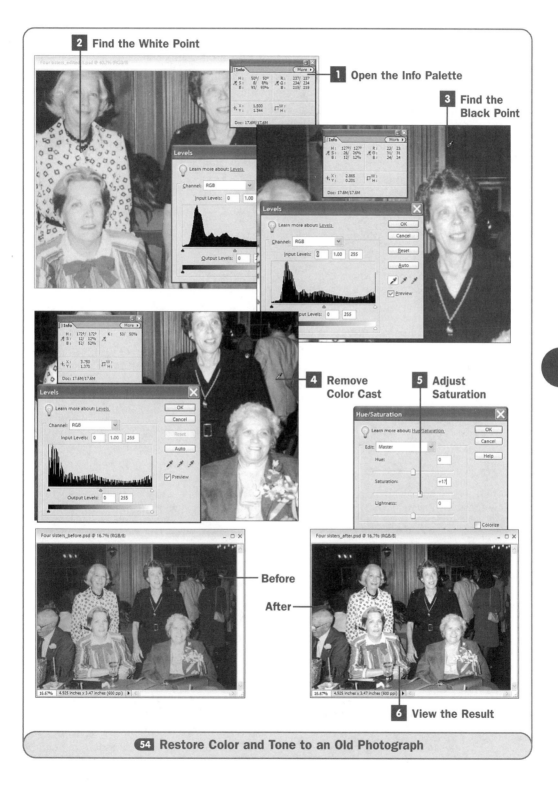

2 Find the White Point

1 Open the Info Palette

3 Find the Black Point

4 Remove Color Cast

5 Adjust Saturation

Before

After

6 View the Result

54

1 Open the Info Palette

Open an image in the Editor in **Standard Edit** mode and save it in Photoshop (***.psd**) format. Open the **Info** palette by choosing **Window, Info** from the menu bar. The **Info** palette provides data about whichever pixel is currently under the mouse pointer; you'll use this information to select the darkest and lightest points in the image. To make the **Info** palette show the HSB (hue, saturation, and brightness) values you'll need to complete this task, click the **Eyedropper** icon in the first pane and select **HSB Color** from the context menu.

2 Find the White Point

Choose **Enhance, Adjust Lighting, Levels** from the menu bar. The **Levels** dialog box appears. To locate the lightest point in the image, press **Alt** and click the white slider just below the right end of the histogram. The image changes to display the lightest points. Memorize the general area of one of these points.

Select the white eyedropper in the **Levels** dialog box. Move the dropper over the area you identified earlier as containing the lightest spot. Look for the highest **B:** reading in the **Info** palette. When you find the lightest pixel, click it. The picture brightens considerably because the **Levels** dialog box uses the white point you just specified to adjust its histogram. The point you clicked becomes "absolute white" in the image, and the brightness of the rest of the pixels in the image are adjusted to accommodate this shift.

54

▶ TIP

When selecting the whitest point in the image, ignore reflections. Extreme bright spots like these are called *specular highlights* and should not be considered when finding the true white point in an image.

3 Find the Black Point

Press **Alt** and click the slider below the left end of the histogram in the **Levels** dialog box, and make note of the darkest points in the image. Select the black eyedropper in the **Levels** dialog box. As you move the mouse pointer over the image, look for the lowest **B:** value on the **Info** palette. When you find the darkest point in the image, click it.

4 Remove Color Cast

Assuming there's something in your photograph that should look medium gray (but it's not shown in its true color right now), you can use the gray eyedropper in the **Levels** dialog box to remove any color cast in the image.

Otherwise, remove any color cast by choosing **Enhance**, **Adjust Color**, **Remove Color Cast** and clicking a point in the image that should be true white or true black.

Click the gray eyedropper in the **Levels** dialog box. Click a pixel in the image that you think should look medium gray—for example, concrete or stone, a light shadow on a white wall, or a gray hair. The colors in the image shift; assuming that you've clicked a pixel that should be medium gray, any color cast is removed. (If you select an incorrect pixel, the colors still shift, but in that case, you'll actually *create* a color cast.) Click **OK** to close the **Levels** dialog box and accept the changes.

5 Adjust Saturation

Choose **Enhance**, **Adjust Color**, **Hue/Saturation** from the menu bar to display the **Hue/Saturation** dialog box. Drag the **Saturation** slider to the right to increase the intensity of the colors in a faded image. (For more information about the **Hue/Saturation** dialog box, see **61** **Adjust Hue and Saturation Manually**.) Click **OK** to save your changes.

▶ TIPS

54

Sometimes the color in a photograph fades unevenly. You can increase the saturation in selected parts of an image using the **Sponge** tool. Click the **Sponge** tool on the **Toolbox**, set the **Mode** to **Saturate**, adjust the **Flow** as desired, and then drag the tool over the area you want to saturate.

You can also increase the saturation in an old photo by duplicating the image on another layer and setting the duplicate layer's blend mode to **Multiply**.

6 View the Result

When you're satisfied with the color and tone of the image, make any other changes you want and save the PSD file. Then resave the file in JPEG, PNG, or non-layered TIFF format, leaving your PSD image with its layers (if any) intact so that you can return at a later time and make adjustments if you want.

After improving the contrast and saturation in this old photo and removing a color cast that seemed to make everything greenish, the final result is a much improved treasure.

55   Restore Quality to a Scanned Photograph

✔ BEFORE YOU BEGIN	→ SEE ALSO
3 Import and Separate Multiple Scanned Images	51 Remove Specks, Spots, and Scratches
	57 Improve Brightness and Contrast
	62 Sharpen an Image
	88 Prepare a Still for Video
	170 Make an Instant Slideshow in Premiere Elements

Even if the original photograph is sharp and vibrant, these subtle qualities some-times can be lost when you scan the picture. To improve your chances of getting a good scan, you might want to scan at double the image resolution you're going to need for printing—600 PPI. After making the adjustments shown in this task, you can resize the image downward as a last step, a process that increases the quality of the scan by making the pixels in an image even smaller.

The worst type of photo to scan is a halftone photograph common to newspapers and some magazines. In fact, scanning any type of printed material often results in a poor-quality digital image. If your scanner has a **Descreen** option, turn it on when scanning such photos; it can help remove the *moiré pattern* that often occurs. If your scanner does not have a **Descreen** option, you can use the filters in Photoshop Elements to remove a moiré pattern.

▶ KEY TERM

Moiré pattern—The pattern that appears when one regular geometric pattern—such as a grid made up of dots—overlays another or similar pattern when placed slightly askew. For example, two window screens placed on top of each other at an angle form a moiré effect.

1 Remove Moiré Pattern and Noise

Open an image in the Editor in **Standard Edit** mode and save it in Photoshop (*.**psd**) format. If your scan is of a halftone image, it might have a moiré pattern. Even if a scan is of a regular photograph, the scanning process might have introduced some noise that's more easily seen when the image is zoomed in.

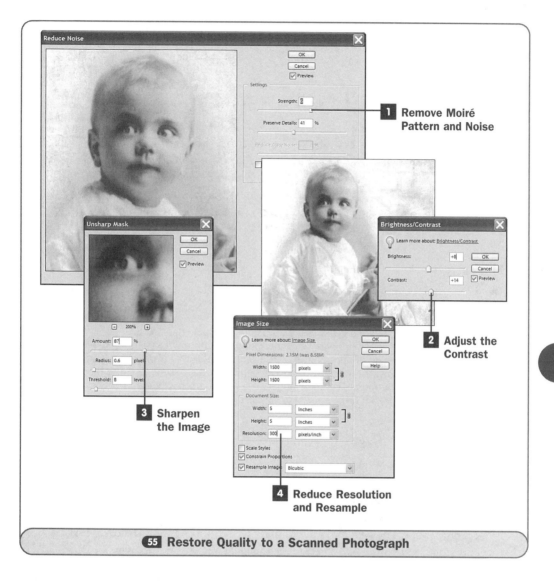

1 Remove Moiré Pattern and Noise

2 Adjust the Contrast

3 Sharpen the Image

4 Reduce Resolution and Resample

55 Restore Quality to a Scanned Photograph

55

In **51** **Remove Specks, Spots, and Scratches,** you learned about the various filters Photoshop Elements provides for removing noise from an image. Because it combines the best of both the **Despeckle** and **Median** filters, the **Reduce Noise** filter is often a very good choice: choose **Filter, Noise, Reduce Noise.** Increase the **Preserve Details** setting to preserve as much sharpness along the edges of objects in the photo as you can; at the same time, increase the **Strength** until you notice that a sufficient amount of noise has been reduced, without losing the natural texture of elements such as skin or fabric. For color scans, adjust **Reduce Color Noise** as needed to remove the color dotted noise. When you're satisfied, click **OK.**

▶ **TIP**

For persistent noise, you might have to blur the image while preserving the edge contrast (sharpness). See 🔢 **Blur an Image to Remove Noise**.

2️⃣ Adjust the Contrast

Next, you should improve the scan's contrast and tone. There are various ways you can do that, but the easiest method is to use the **Brightness/Contrast** command, described in 🔢 **Improve Brightness and Contrast**. Select **Enhance, Adjust Lighting, Brightness/Contrast**. The **Brightness/Contrast** dialog box appears. Drag the **Brightness** or **Contrast** slider to the right to increase it, or drag to the left to decrease it. When you're satisfied, click **OK**.

▶ **NOTES**

The techniques illustrated in 🔢 **Restore Color and Tone to an Old Photograph** might also help restore contrast and saturation to your scan.

One way to quickly improve contrast in a dark scan is to apply the **Equalize** filter. Choose **Filter, Adjustments, Equalize** from the menu. The filter works automatically to create an even distribution of light and dark pixels throughout the image. You can also improve the contrast in most scanned images by dragging the outer white and black level markers inward to match the outer edges of the histogram (these markers are located just below the histogram) in the **Levels** dialog box.

3️⃣ Sharpen the Image

When making multiple changes to an image, it's generally recommended that you not do any sharpening until the final step because sharpening is really a process that adjusts the contrast between pixels. If you sharpen too early in the process, other changes you make can sometimes undo the effects of sharpening. The best tool for sharpening an image is the **Unsharp Mask**, explained in detail in 🔢 **Sharpen an Image**. Select **Filter, Sharpen, Unsharp Mask**. The **Unsharp Mask** dialog box opens. Adjust the **Radius** to set the size of the area around each pixel to be examined for contrast, and set the **Threshold** to a value that tells the filter what level of contrast must exist before a pixel is changed. Finally, set the **Amount** to the amount of contrast by which you want to increase qualifying pixels. When you're happy with the results, click **OK**.

4 Reduce Resolution and Resample

If you scanned the image at 600 PPI or higher, you can reduce the resolution without changing the image's print size. Although you might think the fatter pixels that would result would also leave you with a less clear image, for many scanned images—especially those scanned from newspapers—the resampling process that takes place when you reduce the resolution can also average out the contrasting areas that cause moiré patterns. The result is an image that looks clearer *to your own eyes*, which is where it really counts anyway.

Save the PSD file and then resave the file in JPEG, PNG, or non-layered TIFF format, leaving your PSD image with its layers (if any) intact so that you can return at a later time and make adjustments if you want. Starting with a flattened image speeds up the process of resampling, while preserving the resolution of your original scan.

Choose **Image**, **Resize**, **Image Size** from the menu. The **Image Size** dialog box appears. Enable the **Resample Image** option, and from the drop-down list beside it, choose **Bicubic Sharper**, which is the resampling mode most preferred for downsizing. Next, type a value that's half the image's current resolution in the **Resolution** box. To finalize your choices, click **OK**. See **16** Change Image Size or Resolution.

56

▶ NOTE

Scanning your original photo at very high resolution—especially higher than what you intend to print—and then resizing downward and resampling, is not a solution for every photograph, but it *does* work for any image in which the scanning process generates geometric patterns that don't belong to the image. If you don't have to remove moiré patterns from a scan, you can leave the image in its higher resolution and skip step **4**.

---

56 Remove Unwanted Objects from an Image

→ SEE ALSO

52 Repair Minor Tears

56

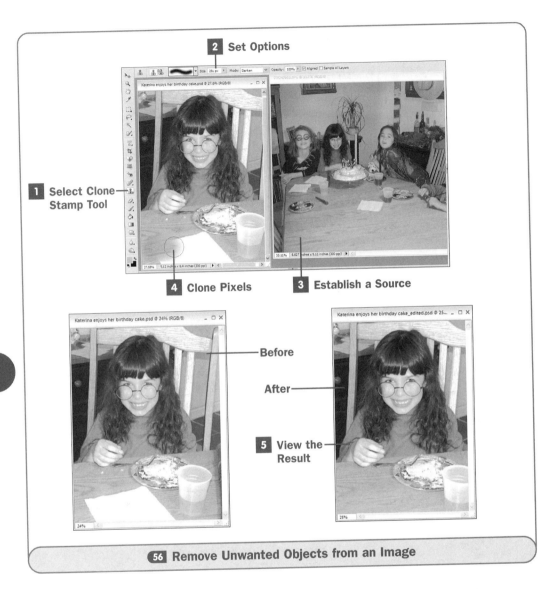

2 Set Options

1 Select Clone Stamp Tool

4 Clone Pixels

3 Establish a Source

Before

After

5 View the Result

56 Remove Unwanted Objects from an Image

Using the **Clone Stamp** tool, you can easily remove from an image unwanted objects such as telephone poles, wires, trash cans, a thumb that wandered in front of the lens, or a few stray hairs blown in the wind simply by copying over these distractions with pixels located somewhere else in the image (or in another image). To use the **Clone Stamp**, you first indicate the source area, and then you drag to paint with pixels copied from the source. Be sure to "cover your tracks" and avoid creating a noticeable pattern as you copy. The best ways to do that are to lower the **Opacity** of the **Clone Stamp** tool, to select a blend mode so that the pixels you clone blend with existing pixels, to paint with single clicks or very short strokes, to use a large brush to avoid copying multiple times to the same area (but a small-enough brush that you don't copy things you don't want), and to vary the source area from which you're copying by re-establishing a new source point every so often. The source you select for the **Clone Stamp** can be located within a different image, on a different layer, or on the same layer. For example, you might clone some hair from one side of a photo to repair a small rip or a bad hair day. Or, you might clone a squirrel from one photo onto the head of your brother in another photo to create a comic image.

▶ TIPS

You might also be able to remove objects from an image in the same way you repair tears and holes. See **53** Repair Large Holes, Tears, and Missing Portions of a Photo.

You can remove small objects with the **Spot Healing Brush** or **Healing Brush** by covering them up with pixels copied from the surrounding area. See **51** Remove Specks, Spots, and Scratches.

1 Select Clone Stamp Tool

Open an image in the Editor in **Standard Edit** mode, and save it in Photoshop (*.psd) format. Click the **Clone Stamp** tool on the **Toolbox**.

56

2 Set Options

On the **Options** bar, select a brush tip and brush **Size** and enable the **Aligned** check box. Set other options as desired.

3 Establish a Source

If you're cloning a region from another image, open that image in the Editor. On the **Layers** palette, choose the layer containing the data you want to copy. If the image has multiple layers, enable the **Sample All Layers** option to copy data from all visible layers.

Finally, press **Alt** and click on the image layer to establish the source point. Be careful not to click too close to objects you don't want to clone.

▶ TIPS

If you're cloning data from one image into another, it might be easier if you tile the images so that you can see them both at the same time, but you don't have to. The source point is maintained as you clone, even if you can't see the source image. To tile all the open images, choose **Window**, **Images**, **Tile** from the menu.

To hide your clone tracks (if you're cloning a texture such as skin rather than a specific object such as a nose), change the source often by pressing **Alt** and clicking a different source point.

4 Clone Pixels

If needed, change to the image to which you want to copy the source data. On the **Layers** palette, change to the layer on which you want to copy the data.

To begin copying pixels, click on the layer or drag with short strokes to sample pixels from the source and paint them under the brush tip. Note that a crosshatch pointer shows you the location of the source point, and that it moves as your painting point moves. Don't confuse one point with the other. Repeat until the repair has been made or until the undesirable object has been painted over.

5 View the Result

After you're satisfied with the result, make any other changes you want and save the PSD file. Then resave the file in JPEG, PNG, or non-layered TIFF format, leaving your PSD image with its layers (if any) intact so that you can return at a later time and make adjustments if you want.

I liked this photo of my daughter's seventh birthday, but the more I looked at it, the more distracting the large white napkin in the foreground became. And no matter how I cropped the photo, that napkin still seemed to draw attention to itself. So, I cloned a bit of the same table from another photo taken at that same time and with the same lighting conditions, over top of the napkin, essentially removing the napkin from the photo. I used the **Clone Stamp** and not the **Healing Brush**, even though it does a very nice job of cloning, because the **Healing Brush** also *blends* the cloned pixels with the existing pixels. If I had used the **Healing Brush**, it would have blended the table pixels with the white napkin pixels, creating a "ghostly napkin" effect.

56

10

Correcting Brightness, Contrast, Color, and Sharpness

IN THIS CHAPTER:

This chapter is about how you can address the attributes of a photograph that affect its perceived quality. One of the easiest problems to overcome is poor exposure. Your picture might be overexposed (too light) or underexposed (too dark). It might have too little contrast (flat) or too much contrast (harsh shadows). Color balance is another characteristic that can ruin a good photo, and when it's off, you'll know it because the colors will just look "wrong." Perhaps someone's skin tone looks too red or too green, or perhaps Uncle John's favorite blue sweater is just not the color you remember it to be. Removing a color cast (a bias towards one color, such as red) will fix all the colors in an image, making the photo instantly "right."

Sharpness is the final critical factor in creating a great photograph. Digitally, sharpness is increased or decreased by changing the level of contrast along the edges of objects. Unfortunately, you will not be able to sharpen an out-of-focus image and make it look right, but if an image is only slightly off, you can gently sharpen it and improve its appearance. You can also blur portions of an image, which you might do in order to get a subject to stand out more against a busy background. In this chapter, you'll learn how to improve the brightness, color, and sharpness of your images.

57 Improve Brightness and Contrast

→ SEE ALSO

87 Grab a Still from Video

88 Prepare a Still for Video

If you grew up using a television set that had an old style of operating control called *knobs*, you'll recall there were two such gadgets, generally labeled *Brightness* and *Contrast*. And if you ever played with these knobs as a child—and survived with your wrists unscathed—you remember that Brightness made your picture *whiter* while Contrast made the blacks and whites in your picture stand out.

▶ **NOTE**

With the **Brightness/Contrast** command, brightness is added to an image (or to a layer or selection) by adding equal amounts to, or subtracting from, the **Brightness** component of *every pixel in the image*. So, although you might be restoring the natural brightness level of the midtones, natural darks might be washed out. By comparison, a contrast adjustment mathematically redistributes brightness across the entire image, flattening the image's histogram and reducing its peaks. However, the same danger of losing bright and dark values remains valid with contrast adjustment, except on both sides of the histogram instead of one.

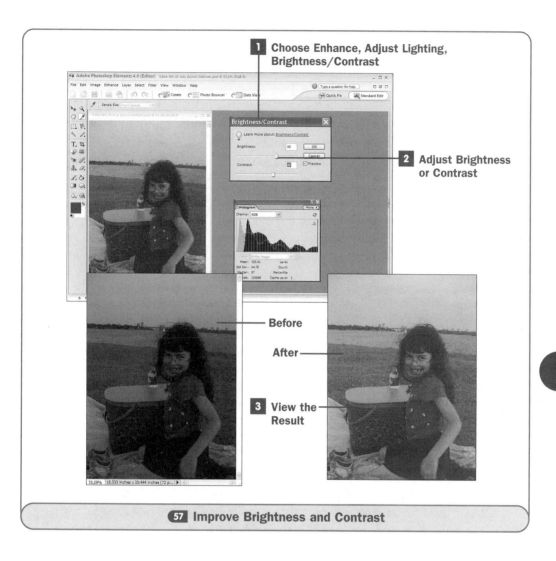

1 Choose Enhance, Adjust Lighting, Brightness/Contrast

2 Adjust Brightness or Contrast

Before

After

3 View the Result

57 Improve Brightness and Contrast

With all due respect to Philco-Ford, Admiral, Magnavox, and the other great manufacturers of the past century, I'm going to show you here how to use Photoshop Elements's equivalent of the Brightness and Contrast knobs. And then I'm going to rap you on the wrists if you use them too much. Actually, I'm not kidding this time: Although it does help in some circumstances to restore a more natural appearance to an image, the **Brightness/Contrast** command, when used too liberally, can result in a washed-out look (too bright), a washed-*down* look (too dark), or an underexposed look (too much contrast). More importantly, because pixels cannot have a brightness value of greater than 255 or less than 0, when you brighten or darken pixels *too much*, you lose the distinguishing contrasts between the brightest or darkest pixels among them. Then when you try to get those contrasts back with a **Levels** adjustment, you can't. With the technique demonstrated here, you can use the **Brightness/Contrast** command effectively and safely, without losing information in your image.

1 Choose Enhance, Adjust Lighting, Brightness/Contrast

Open the image you want to adjust in the Editor in **Standard Edit** mode and save it in Photoshop (*.psd) format. To display the **Histogram** palette if it is not already showing, select **Window, Histogram**. From the palette's **Channel** drop-down list, choose **RGB**. If there is more than one layer in the image, choose the layer you want to adjust in the **Layers** palette. If you want to limit your adjustment to a region of the image, use a selection tool to select that region.

Choose **Enhance, Adjust Lighting, Brightness/Contrast** from the menu bar. The **Brightness/Contrast** dialog box opens. Enable the **Preview** check box so that you can see the results of the adjustments you're making in the actual image.

In this example, the photo was taken at dusk without a flash. Although it does capture the moment, it's the worst time of day to take a digital photo for many cameras. If the flash had been turned on, the subject would have been well lit, but the sky would no longer be a dreamy blue but a dreary clay color. My goal here, for now, is to make the subject matter clearly visible while losing as little of the original color scheme as possible.

2 Adjust Brightness or Contrast

To add brightness to all the pixels in the designated region, slide the **Brightness** slider to the right, or enter a positive value in the **Brightness** text box. To reduce brightness in all the pixels in the designated region, slide the **Brightness** slider to the left, or enter a negative value in the **Brightness** text box.

▶ NOTE

As you increase contrast for an image, you might notice that the black curve in the **Histogram** palette has "teeth" in it—specifically, evenly spaced vertical stripes. This is natural, and is an accurate depiction of the brightness values in an adjusted image. For the sake of argument, suppose that there were only 10 levels of brightness in a given image, ranging in value from 10 to 20. After the adjustment, suppose that they now ranged in value from 5 to 25. Because all pixels were adjusted—none are left behind—*there are still only 10 levels of brightness.* They've just been broken up, such that there are pixels with brightness of 5, 7, 9, and so on, but none with 6, 8, 10, and so on. Notice in the example how the contrast-adjusted image looks spotty, noisy, and unsmooth. What your eyes see is verified by the "teeth" in the contrast-adjusted histogram.

57

▶ **TIP**

If you press the **Alt** key on your keyboard, the **Cancel** button changes to read **Reset**. Click that button to erase your changes to the image, leaving the dialog box open so that you can try again.

To add contrast between pixels in the designated region (making light pixels lighter and darks darker), slide the **Contrast** slider to the right, or enter a positive value in the **Contrast** text box. To reduce contrast between pixels in the designated region (bringing all brightness values together toward a middle gray tone), slide the **Contrast** slider to the left, or enter a negative value in the **Contrast** text box.

As you make adjustments, notice the instant change to the **Histogram** palette. The gray curve with the bright tip represents the image's existing histogram; the black curve represents the adjusted state as you see it in the preview. With a brightness change, the entire "mountain" of the graph shifts to the left or right. With a contrast change, the entire "mountain" is flattened, as if eroded by a rising tide. While you're making these changes, watch the **Histogram** palette, being mindful of two things:

- Don't adjust the image so much that pixels on either or both sides of the histogram fall off the edge. When that happens, you're losing vital information which, when saved, cannot be retrieved.

- In the interest of restoring one of the image's qualities to a natural or pleasing appearance—for example, distinguishing a little girl from her picnic basket—don't introduce negative qualities on the opposite end of the scale, such as a washed-out tone for the grass, or water that appears to glow as if it were emanating from a nuclear facility.

To finalize your adjustments, click **OK**.

3 View the Result

When you're satisfied with the result, make any other changes you want and save the PSD file. Then resave the result in JPEG, PNG, or non-layered TIFF format, leaving your PSD image with its layers intact so that you can return at a later time to make new adjustments.

In the example, after adding **+30** to brightness and **+20** to contrast, the range of color now looks more natural. But the image has far to go before it's fixed. In the adjustment, I did lose some of the distinguishing bright values along the right side of the histogram, although not many.

57

58   Lighten a Subject on a Snowy Background

→ SEE ALSO

57 Improve Brightness and Contrast

Typically, the sheer brightness of snow changes the way your camera handles light from darker objects—and on a snowy day, almost everything is darker than snow. Digital cameras are especially sensitive to bright light reflecting off snow, bleaching out the rest of the scene and causing subjects in the foreground, including people, to appear muted and dark. Furthermore, because many digital cameras tend to normalize their light input on-the-fly, even though the snow is the brightest thing in the image, the camera makes it gray, making your foreground subjects even darker to compensate.

In remedying an image that suffers from this problem, you could start by invoking the **Levels** command, but you know already that your bright whites are going to command the right edge of the graph for the **RGB** channel. Besides, you might not want to change your *snow* at all, especially if it's bright enough. The technique you're about to see helps you easily separate your foreground subject from your background snow (which is, after all, mostly the same shade), so that you can restore the foreground despite the snow.

58

▶ **NOTE**

If your digital camera includes a scene mode such as **Snow** or **Beach**, use it when taking a photo with a bright background, and your subject will not appear so dark in the resulting photograph.

1   Duplicate the Background Layer

Open the image you want to adjust in the Editor in **Standard Edit** mode and save it in Photoshop (***.psd**) format. To display the **Histogram** palette if it is not already showing, select **Window, Histogram**. From the **Channel** drop-down list, choose **Luminosity**.

In the **Layers** palette, choose the **Background** layer. From the menu bar, select **Layer, Duplicate Layer**. Name the new layer **Threshold**.

2   Blacken the Subject Using Threshold

With the **Threshold** layer chosen, from the menu bar, select **Filter, Adjustments, Threshold**. In the **Threshold** dialog box, adjust the **Threshold Level** setting until the black area just covers your subject. You'll probably also blacken *some* of the shadows your subject is casting on the snow; don't worry, that's okay. Click **OK**.

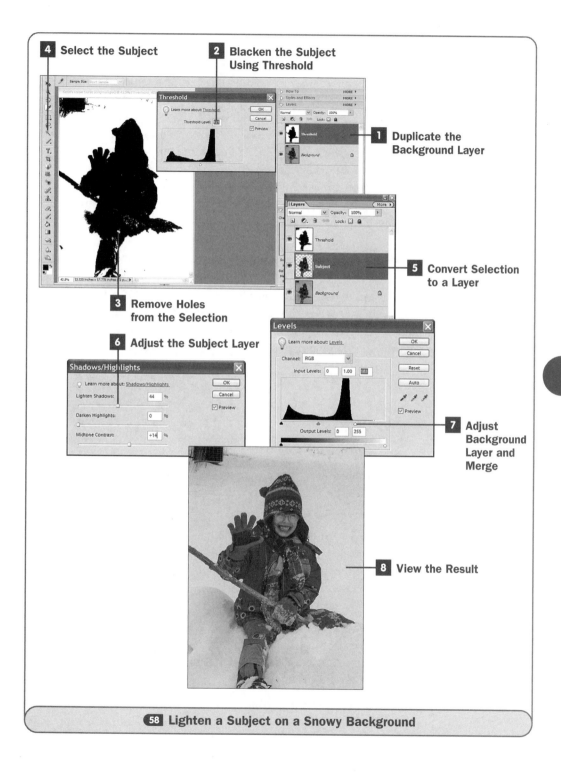

4 Select the Subject

2 Blacken the Subject Using Threshold

1 Duplicate the Background Layer

5 Convert Selection to a Layer

3 Remove Holes from the Selection

6 Adjust the Subject Layer

7 Adjust Background Layer and Merge

8 View the Result

58

58 Lighten a Subject on a Snowy Background

3 Remove Holes from the Selection

Your subject should now be black and the background white, but that's only temporary. At this moment, your selection probably includes some specks of snow on your subject—especially if she's recently been in a snowball fight. These beads of snow will produce holes in your black subject area. The simplest way to remove them is using the **Brush** tool. In the **Toolbox**, click the **Brush** tool, and then click the **Default Colors** button in-between the foreground color and background color boxes. Choose a five-pixel-wide brush tip from the **Options** bar and apply that brush tip to the small holes in the black image. Choose a larger brush tip and sweep away the larger areas of dustier snow from the subject.

4 Select the Subject

From the **Toolbox**, click the **Magic Wand** tool. In the image, use the tool to select the subject. In this example, the selection included the girl, the big stick she was holding, and a portion of the shadow behind her back. It did not include the shadow of the air conditioning unit in the upper-left corner. Use of the **Magic Wand** tool is explained in 22 **Select Areas of Similar Color**.

58

5 Convert Selection to a Layer

In the **Layers** palette, change to the **Background** layer, and select **Layer, New, Layer via Copy** from the menu bar. Right-click **Layer 1** in the **Layers** palette, and from the context menu, select **Rename Layer**. In the dialog box, type **Subject** and click **OK**. Your subject is now isolated on its own layer, where you can make adjustments that bring out its own details without disturbing the snowy background. You can also adjust the snowy background by brightening it significantly, without in turn over-brightening the subject.

You no longer need the **Threshold** layer. In the **Layers** palette, choose the **Threshold** layer and select **Layer, Delete Layer** from the menu bar. Click **Yes** to confirm. For now, your image looks exactly as it did before.

6 Adjust the Subject Layer

In the **Layers** palette, choose the **Subject** layer. From the menu bar, select **Enhance, Adjust Lighting, Shadows/Highlights**. The **Shadows/Highlights** dialog box appears. You might have to reposition it to get a clear view of both your image and the **Histogram** palette.

With the **Histogram** palette open and visible, it's easy to get a clear read of what the **Shadows/Highlights** command does, and what your limits are with regard to safely using it. Sliding the **Lighten Shadows** setting forward clearly bunches up the histogram from the left side against the right edge. You gain brightness, but at the expense of contrast, so be careful not to trade off too much. Similarly, sliding the **Darken Highlights** setting forward bunches up the histogram from the right side against the left edge.

Sliding the **Midtone Contrast** to the left bunches up tones in the histogram toward the middle of the chart, whereas sliding it to the right splits tones into two humps. The simple rules of shaping a histogram (don't push tones off the edges; evenly distribute them whenever possible; don't segment tones into two equal humps like a camel's back) and the rules of adjusting an image (don't overcorrect for brightness; balance your lights, darks, and midtones whenever possible; don't sacrifice your midtones for darks and lights) correspond to one another. You'll be surprised how many corrections you can make "flying on instrumentation alone"—trusting the histogram to tell you how far to go, and when you're in danger of going too far.

For this example, the highlights were dark enough already. I needed to lighten the shadowy areas to give the picture more punch—especially to bring Katerina's bright red glove toward you (because vivid colors tend to convey the illusion of dimension better). I adjusted **Lighten Shadows** significantly higher, and then added a little to **Midtone Contrast** to compensate.

To finalize your adjustments, click **OK**.

7 Adjust Background Layer and Merge

On the **Layers** palette, choose the **Background** layer. From the menu bar, select **Enhance, Adjust Lighting, Levels**. Reduce the white point until you've restored your snowy whites. Your subject will be unaffected. With this method, I significantly lowered the white point from 255 all the way down to 186 without losing any information about the crisp, clear, fresh snow.

8 View the Result

When you're satisfied with the result, make any other changes you want and save the PSD file. Resave the image in JPEG, PNG, or non-layered TIFF format, leaving your PSD image with its layers intact so that you can return at a later time to make new adjustments.

My original photo suffered from a phenomenon common to digital cameras: The brightness of the snow overwhelmed the light detectors, even when the camera was set for bright outdoors. As a result, Katerina's colors were muted and dull. I made **Shadows/Highlights** adjustments to brighten her clothes, but had my image been one undivided layer, the same changes I made to her clothes and skin tones would have made the snow pink. By separating the snow from the foreground, I was able to shield the snow from the changes I made to the color channels, and then applied color-safe changes to the snow.

58

59 Lighten or Darken Part of an Image

→ **SEE ALSO**

57 **Improve Brightness and Contrast**

To make a photographic print, the classic development technique is to project an image of the negative onto sensitized printing paper. To lighten an area, the developer can *dodge* it by placing an object, usually a small paddle, in the projected light. To darken an area, he would *burn* it by forming a sort of donut hole with his hands and directing extra exposure light to the target area.

The **Dodge** and **Burn** tool icons in Photoshop Elements depict these traditional tools. Their jobs are, in essence, to lighten a spot and to blacken a spot, respectively. But they don't do this by painting white and black; you could do that with a **Brush** tool. Instead, the **Burn** tool reduces the brightness of whatever it touches, while the **Dodge** tool increases brightness. It's like taking the portion of the image you touch and moving its **Luminosity** values on the histogram down (**Burn**) or up (**Dodge**). Along the way, both contrast and saturation in the areas you touch is generally reduced with both tools. Because you apply these tools to your image using an adjustable brush tip, you can pinpoint your changes to a few pixels or make changes to broader areas of the image. The effect much more closely resembles the old darkroom technique.

59

▶ **NOTE**

Both the **Dodge** and **Burn** tools have the side effect of desaturating what they touch. But they're not to be confused with another tool specifically designed for desaturation (or resaturation): the **Sponge** tool. The **Sponge** could conceivably darken an area by compounding its native color. And when desaturating a spot, the **Sponge** doesn't lighten it; instead, it removes the colored hue, shifting it more toward grayscale.

1 Click Dodge or Burn Tool

Open the image you want to adjust in the Editor in **Standard Edit** mode and save it in Photoshop (***.psd**) format. If there's more than one layer in the image, from the **Layers** palette, choose the layer containing the contents you want to modify. To protect parts of the image, select the region containing the spot you want to correct.

In the **Toolbox**, click the **Dodge** tool if you want to lighten an area; click the **Burn** tool if you want to darken an area.

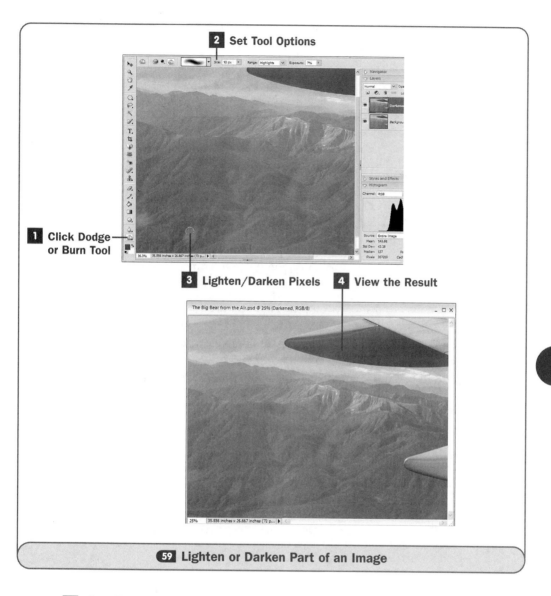

2 Set Tool Options

1 Click Dodge or Burn Tool

3 Lighten/Darken Pixels   **4** View the Result

59

59 Lighten or Darken Part of an Image

2 Set Tool Options

The **Options** bar offers several options that control the brush you'll use to apply the burn to the image. Open the brush presets drop-down list and select the type of brush you want to use. One with a feathered edge works best with these tools; hard-edged brushes can result in unnatural effects. In the **Size** text box, enter a brush size in pixels or select one using the slider. You can check the relative size by passing the tool over the picture without clicking; a circle shows the brush area that will be used.

From the **Range** drop-down list, select whether to alter shadows, midrange tones, or highlights. This is an extremely important setting because it enables you to further protect those elements of your image that don't need correcting. For instance, you might not want to indiscriminately darken *everything* the **Burn** tool touches, so you might consider setting its **Range** to **Midtones**. Likewise, using the **Dodge** tool, you might not want to lighten the lightest tones, but only the **Shadows**. Choose the **Range** you want to change.

The **Exposure** scale enables you to set the strength of the effect. In general, stick to the standard **Exposure** setting of 50% or less. That way, you can make multiple passes that change the picture in small increments.

3 Lighten/Darken Pixels

Begin applying the tool by clicking and holding the mouse button where you want to start. For a pen tablet, position the pointer by hovering the pen, and then tap and hold the pen where you want the stroke to begin.

To draw a freehand stroke, continue holding the button down as you drag the mouse. The mark you draw will follow your pointer. As you continue applying the tool to an area, its effects are cumulative—which means you can continue applying the **Dodge** tool to the same area within the same stroke, and it will continue to lighten the area. The tool's effect within the same stroke are limited, however, to the extent of the **Exposure** setting.

To draw a straight horizontal or vertical line, press **Shift** now and continue dragging the mouse. The Editor senses whether you intend for the line to move up, right, left, or down, by the general direction in which you're moving the mouse—it doesn't have to be exact.

▶ **TIP**

To change brush tips for the **Burn** or **Dodge** tool at any time, right-click the image. The **Brush Presets** palette appears. Choose a new tip from the **Brushes** list, and then click the **X** button to dismiss the palette.

To draw a straight line between points, release the mouse button. For a pen tablet, lift the pen. Move the pointer to where you want the end of the line (or, to be geometrically accurate, the *line segment*) to appear. Press **Shift** and click this point. The line will be an application of the tool over the distance between the start and end points, relative to the tool's current **Exposure** setting. You can continue drawing from here—either a freehand mark or another straight line segment.

4 View the Result

When you're satisfied with the result, make any other changes you want and save the PSD file. Then resave the result in JPEG, PNG, or non-layer TIFF format, leaving your PSD image with its layers intact so that you can return at a later time to make new adjustments.

This sample image is a natural candidate for dodging and burning. The key problem with taking aerial shots from a commercial aircraft is never really having control of how clean the window is, or how much glare you'll have to put up with. There are a number of possible ways to correct this image, one of which is to restore some of the natural shadows in select areas using the **Burn** tool. The advantage of this method over a **Levels** adjustment, for this image, is that you're able to apply small changes to the areas that need it. For example, I used the **Burn** tool to darken the water droplets and remove them from the left side of the image, and to deepen the shadows in the mountain top. I also used the **Dodge** tool to lighten the snow and the top edge of the mountain to make it more of a focus for the image.

---

60   Correct Color, Contrast, and Saturation in One Step   **60**

→ **SEE ALSO**

61 Adjust Hue and Saturation Manually
88 Prepare a Still for Video

You can quickly correct the color, contrast, and saturation in a photo using the **Color Variations** command. With this command, you select the color correction for the image by simply clicking a thumbnail variation of the image. For example, if you want to reduce the red in your image, you click the **Decrease Red** thumbnail.

You can adjust the color variations within your image for the **Midtones**, **Shadows**, and **Highlights** tonal areas. The **Shadows** adjustments affect all the darker areas in the image. The **Highlights** adjustments affect the lighter areas, and the **Midtones** adjustments affect the middle values in the image.

You can also control the saturation of the colors in the image by selecting the **Saturation** option. Then you can click either the **Less Saturation** thumbnail to decrease saturation (making the color more muted) or the **More Saturation** thumbnail to increase it (making the color more vivid).

As you make changes to the color, contrast, and saturation of the image, the before and after previews display at the top of the **Color Variations** dialog box. These views of your image enable you to see your progress. At any time, you can restart the process by clicking the **Reset Image** button.

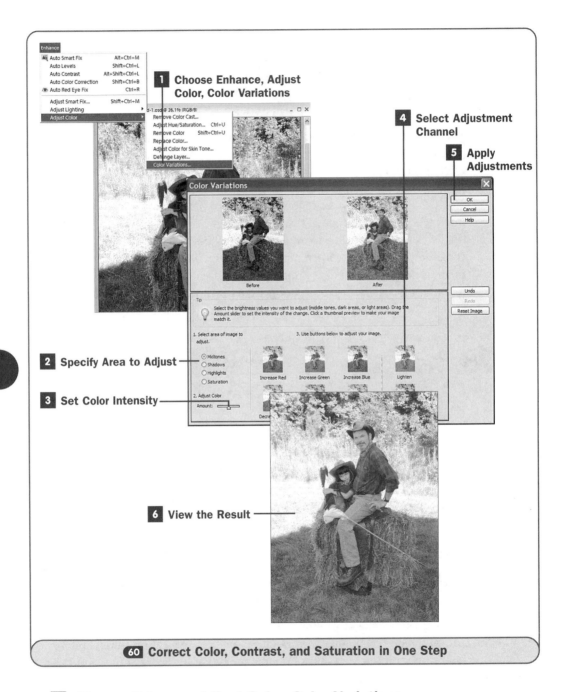

60

60 Correct Color, Contrast, and Saturation in One Step

1 Choose Enhance, Adjust Color, Color Variations

Open the image you want to correct in the Editor in **Standard Edit** mode and save it in Photoshop (*.psd) format. In the **Layers** palette, choose the layer you want to correct.

From the menu bar, select **Enhance**, **Adjust Color**, **Color Variations** from the menu. The **Color Variations** dialog box appears.

2 Specify Area to Adjust

Select the radio button that corresponds to the tonal area of the image you want to adjust. For example, to adjust the middle range of colors, select the **Midtone** radio button.

3 Set Color Intensity

Set the color intensity for the adjustment by dragging the **Adjust Color Amount** slider to the left to decrease the intensity or to the right to increase it. As you drag the slider, you will see the color intensity adjusted for the thumbnail images.

▶ TIP

If you select the **Saturation** option, buttons appear to adjust the saturation. Click the **Less Saturation** button to reduce the saturation or the **More Saturation** button to increase it.

4 Select Adjustment Channel

60

Click the thumbnail image that corresponds to the type of color adjustment you want to make. For the **Midtones**, **Shadows**, and **Highlights** adjustment areas, the top row of thumbnails is devoted to *increases*, the bottom row to *decreases*. The group of adjustments on the left is devoted to individual color channels (red, green, and blue); on the right, **Lighten** and **Darken** apply changes to all three channels simultaneously. When you click a thumbnail, the changes are applied to the image in the right preview widow at the top of the dialog box. In addition, the thumbnail images at the bottom of the dialog box update to reflect the changes you just applied.

Repeat steps 2 through 4 to make adjustments for other areas of the image. As the adjustments are made to the image, you can view the result in the **After** preview window on the top-right of the **Color Variations** dialog box.

▶ **TIPS**

If you do not like the corrections selected, click the **Reset Image** button to switch back to the original version of the image.

To quickly correct an image in which a person's skin tone is off (typically because of a color cast), choose **Enhance**, **Adjust Color**, **Adjust Color for Skin Tone**. After the dialog box appears, click any area of someone's skin whose color seems wrong to you, and the colors in the image are instantly adjusted. If the result is still "off," you can adjust the **Tan** and **Blush** values. You can also adjust the **Ambient Light** temperature to change the skin tone—push the slider toward blue to cool a picture and remove a warm orange or reddish color cast; push it toward red to remove a cool blue or greenish color cast. Click **OK**. This adjustment, however, does not correct saturation or brightness problems; it only removes a color cast.

5 Apply Adjustments

When you have made the desired adjustments, click the **OK** button to close the dialog box and apply the color variation selections to the image.

6 View the Result

When you close the dialog box, Photoshop Elements applies the selections to your image. This process might take a few seconds. When you're satisfied with the results, make any other changes you want and save the PSD file. Resave the result in JPEG, PNG, or non-layered TIFF format, leaving your PSD image with its layers (if any) intact so that you can return at a later time and make different adjustments if you want.

For this example, we didn't exactly pick the best location or time of day to shoot this photo. It was mid-morning on the West side of the house; as a result, we appeared in shadow. To compensate for this, I needed to bring back some of the richer colors that match the leafy greens in the background. So I added a few "shots" of green, if you will, and quite a bit of red—almost too much, but the slightly rustic look that resulted is in keeping with our costumes.

61 Adjust Hue and Saturation Manually

→ **SEE ALSO**

60 Correct Color, Contrast, and Saturation in One Step
87 Grab a Still from Video

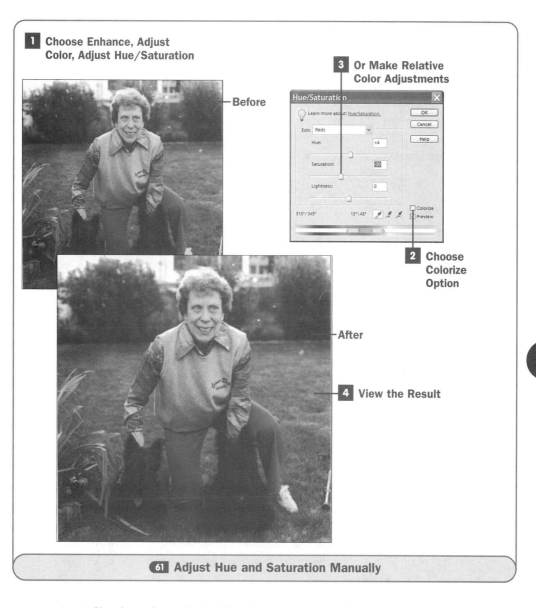

1 Choose Enhance, Adjust Color, Adjust Hue/Saturation

3 Or Make Relative Color Adjustments

Before

After

2 Choose Colorize Option

4 View the Result

61 Adjust Hue and Saturation Manually

A pixel's color value is defined by three components: hue, *saturation*, and lightness (or *luminance*, or *luminosity*). A pixel's hue represents its location on the color wheel, which is the entire spectrum of colors in the computer's gamut or colorspace. Saturation defines the relative power of that hue within a pixel—quantifying, for instance, the range between a clear red (full saturation) to a colorless gray (no saturation). Lightness defines the amount of white in a pixel, from black (no light) to white (all light) to somewhere in-between (light pink). To make individual adjustments to these components of pixels within a given region, use the **Adjust Hue/Saturation** command. For example, many images taken with digital cameras seem to lack saturation. A boost of saturation by even a few degrees can revive an otherwise dull image, infusing it with excitement and drama.

By reducing the saturation in a color image, you can create a black-and-white photo—often with better results than simply converting the image to grayscale. By adjusting the hue of a selected object, you can change its color from red to green, for example. By reducing the lightness of an image's background, you can make it fade into the distance—placing more importance on the subject of your image.

▶ **KEY TERM**

Saturation—The amount of a particular hue present in a pixel. A fully saturated red pixel is bright red; a less saturated red pixel has more gray and its reddish tone is more subtle.

1 Choose Enhance, Adjust Color, Adjust Hue/Saturation

Open the image you want to correct in the Editor in **Standard Edit** mode and save it in Photoshop (**.psd*) format. In the **Layers** palette, choose the layer you want to adjust. To restrict your adjustment to a given region of the chosen layer, use a selection tool to select that region.

From the menu bar, select **Enhance, Adjust Color, Adjust Hue/Saturation** to display the **Hue/Saturation** dialog box. Enable the **Preview** check box to see examples of your choices in the image before making them final.

2 Choose Colorize Option

This dialog box has two purposes: The *second* of these purposes is to give you a way to apply a single hue to the designated region. *Colorizing* a region in this way eliminates all the area's original color information, replacing it with the values designated by the **Hue** and **Saturation** settings. To colorize the designated region and *replace* color values rather than simply *adjust* them, enable the **Colorize** check box. When you do this, the meanings of the sliders change. The **Hue** slider represents an angle on the color wheel between **0°** and **360°**, theoretically encompassing all the colors of the rainbow. **Saturation** is a percentage representing how much of the chosen **Hue** to apply to the region, while **Lightness** remains a relative setting between **–100** and **+100**, governing how much white is added or removed. (Technically, sliding **Lightness** in either direction should remove saturation, but in this case, the **Saturation** slider remains stable.)

61

If you're colorizing the designated region, make your adjustment choices from these sliders and click **OK** to exit the dialog box and skip to step 4. Otherwise, continue to step 3.

▶ **TIP**

Whereas the **Adjust Hue/Saturation** command applies changes to all or part of a layer, you can create an adjustment layer that applies a saturation adjustment to several underlying layers in an image. See **30** Create an Adjustment Layer for details.

3 Or Make Relative Color Adjustments

With the **Colorize** option disabled, the purpose of the **Hue/Saturation** dialog box is to make *relative* adjustments to one, two, or all three of the color channels in the designated region.

From the **Edit** drop-down list, select the color channels you want to adjust. The **Master** option refers to all three (red, green, and blue) in combination. The primary channels (**Reds**, **Greens**, and **Blues**) are represented on this list, as well as the secondary colors (**Yellows**, **Cyans**, and **Magentas**). **Yellows** refers to the red and green channel, **Cyans** to the green and blue channel, and **Magentas** to the blue and red channel.

At this point, the **Hue** slider represents an angle of adjustment between –180° and +180°. When you adjust this setting, the **Hue** component values of all pixels in the selected region are adjusted by that amount on the color wheel. For example, a yellow pixel when increased 180 degrees becomes blue.

The **Saturation** slider represents a percentage of adjustment between –100 and +100. Any non-zero setting represents a degree of increase or decrease of color in the chosen channels. Drag the **Saturation** slider to the right to increase the saturation of the designated region or to the left to decrease the saturation.

The **Lightness** slider represents a percentage of adjustment between –100 and +100. Any non-zero setting represents a degree of increase or decrease of *whiteness* in the chosen channels. Drag the **Lightness** slider to the right to increase the lightness of the selected color range or to the left to decrease the lightness. If you've chosen **Blues**, for instance, setting **Lightness** above zero adds *white* to the blues in the selected region.

Click the **OK** button to close the dialog box and apply the adjustments to your image.

61

4 View the Result

When you're satisfied with the results, make any other changes you want and save the PSD file. Resave the result in JPEG, PNG, or non-layered TIFF format, leaving your PSD image with its layers (if any) intact so that you can return at a later time and make adjustments if you want.

This example featured a scanned photograph that was damaged from exposure to sunlight for several years, probably clinging to the front door of the refrigerator. My first objective was to restore some of the warm skin tones to Aunt Betty's face. I did this by choosing the **Reds** channel, moving the **Hue** setting to **+4** to restore some of the yellows that had faded (yellows always fade first from exposure to sunlight), and set **Saturation** to **–20** to help balance her skin tones.

Next, I restored the radiant sunlight on the edges of Betty's sweater and hair by choosing the **Yellows** channel, setting **Hue** to **+9**, **Saturation** to a relatively high **+41**, and **Lightness** to a quite high **+63**. Now the subject matter looks bright and in the center of the picture once again. I used the **Magentas** channel as an opportunity to bring back contrast to Betty's face because the print was using magenta tones in the shadows. With the **Magentas** channel chosen, I set **Hue** to **+11** (taking it more toward the red), **Saturation** to **+9**, and **Lightness** way down to **–25**. Now Betty's face truly is in the center of the picture.

These adjustments were far from enough to fix the overall picture. I tried to add saturation to the **Greens** channel, for instance, but the problem with this faded print is that too much of the grass and shrubbery color is made up of elements from the **Blues** channel. I'll need to make spot adjustments to the garden, perhaps with the **Color Replacement** tool. And nothing I do with the **Hue/Saturation** dialog box will help me restore contrast to Betty's two jet-black Scottie dogs. And now, I have Betty's warm, radiant face smiling at me again, and that's a very good start. Look for this image in the Color Gallery.

▶ **TIP**

It is extremely difficult to demonstrate in black-and-white what the color adjustment does for this photo—when you put the two side by side *in monochrome*, there's almost no difference. In a way, that's what you want. This shows that we've retained the natural brightness values while adjusting the color fade.

62 Sharpen an Image

✔ BEFORE YOU BEGIN	SEE ALSO
Just jump right in!	**25** Smooth and Soften a Selection **34** Mask an Image Layer **63** Blur an Image to Remove Noise

Virtually every image you create will have a particular point on which you want the viewer to focus. This focal point is often referred to as the *subject* of the image. When the subject of your photo stands out sharply from the background, it helps the viewer to maintain the illusion of depth and focus. One tool that works well for sharpening an image is the **Unsharp Mask** filter. When you apply this filter to your image, it locates the pixels in the image that differ from the surrounding pixels and increases the contrast between those pixels. When you use this filter, you control the sharpening effect by specifying the amount of contrast, the number of pixels to sharpen around the edges, and the **Threshold**, or how different the target pixels need to be from the surrounding pixels.

You can apply the **Unsharp Mask** to an entire layer or to a selection. Keep in mind that everything within the selection will be affected by the filter. If you don't select a portion of the image, the entire active layer is sharpened. You might want to sharpen only the subject of the image, leaving its surrounding elements as they are so that the subject stands out even more. To accomplish this, select that subject using one of the selection tools and then apply the **Unsharp Mask** filter. If you want to have more control over how the **Unsharp Mask** filter affects the final image, you can use an *edge mask* to apply the filter as explained in this task. In creating an edge mask, you sharpen an image so that the edges of its subject matter are well pronounced. You can then mask the image so that only the edges you select are actually visible to the viewer.

▶ **NOTE**

Although Photoshop Elements allows you to create masking effects, you cannot create and save masks as you can with other photo editing software packages such as Adobe Photoshop. Masking works well for hiding portions of an image you don't want to be visible. See **34** Mask an Image Layer for more information on masking portions of an image.

▶ **KEY TERM**

Edge mask—A selection that encompasses only the edge pixels in an image, thus preventing unwanted sharpening to everything else.

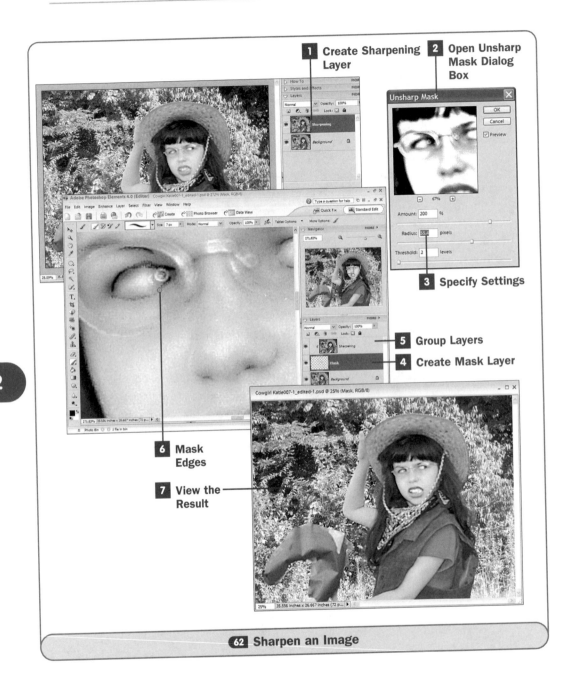

1 Create Sharpening Layer

2 Open Unsharp Mask Dialog Box

3 Specify Settings

5 Group Layers

4 Create Mask Layer

6 Mask Edges

7 View the Result

62

62 Sharpen an Image

1 Create Sharpening Layer

Open the image you want to adjust in the Editor in **Standard Edit** mode and save it in Photoshop (***.psd**) format. If it's not already showing, display the **Layers** palette by selecting **Window, Layers**. In the **Layers** palette, click to select the **Background** layer and choose **Layer, Duplicate Layer** from the menu bar to duplicate the background layer. On the **Duplicate Layer** dialog box, specify a name for the duplicate layer, such as **Sharpening**. The layer you are creating is where you will apply the **Unsharp Mask** filter. You want to create a separate sharpening layer so that you can mask out the edges you want visible in the image.

2 Open Unsharp Mask Dialog Box

With the **Sharpening** layer chosen in the **Layers** palette, select **Filter, Sharpen, Unsharp Mask**. The **Unsharp Mask** dialog box opens. Enable the **Preview** check box.

▶ TIPS

Don't worry about oversharpening the background. You are going to use a mask to display only the desired sharpened edges of the subject.

Use the – and + buttons to change the size of the image that displays in the preview window.

If you plan to print the image, you'll want the sharpening effects to be more dramatic. Images from printers are not as sharp as they appear on the screen.

62

3 Specify Settings

In the **Amount** field, specify a value representing the amount by which you want to increase the contrast between the pixels. For these purposes, you'll want to choose a much higher value than you'd want for a layer you actually intend to keep, such as **200%** or higher.

In the **Radius** field, specify a value that indicates how many pixels around the vicinity of each pixel play a role in adjusting the color to appear sharper. The larger the number, the wider the band of pixels that are evaluated when sharpening each one.

The **Unsharp Mask** filter adjusts every pixel to some extent based on its evaluation of the color values of its neighboring pixels. The **Radius** setting determines how many neighboring pixels to evaluate for each pixel being evaluated. **Threshold** is a relative setting designating how much of a brightness difference between neighboring pixels constitutes a *meaningful* difference—in other words, how much contrast is a contrast that *matters*. Material contrasts are the ones that are enhanced, so a lower **Threshold** setting means that more contrasts (by lesser differences) are enhanced.

For the purposes of this task, you want to turn up the contrast along the edges of objects as much as possible. This generally means you should set **Radius** to a high value (above **50**) and **Threshold** to a low value to compensate, such as **2**. Take a good look at the preview and remember that you're looking for edges to be *overemphasized*. Click the **OK** button to finalize your choices.

4 Create Mask Layer

In the **Layers** palette, click the **Background** layer and then choose **Layer, New, Layer** from the menu bar to create a new blank layer. Name this layer **Mask** because it is the layer where you will mask the sharpened edges of the image. You are going to create a mask that includes just the sharper edges of the image.

5 Group Layers

In the **Layers** palette, choose the **Sharpening** layer. Select **Layer, Group with Previous** from the menu bar to group the **Sharpen** layer with your new **Mask** layer. The **Mask** layer is indented under the **Sharpening** layer on the **Layers** palette to indicate that the **Mask** layer is masking the contents of the **Sharpening** layer (controlling what portion of the **Sharpening** layer shows through).

62

▶ TIP

If you don't want some of the edges to appear as sharp, you can reduce the **Opacity** setting for the **Brush** tool in the **Options** bar before painting those edges.

Notice that the sharpening effects are no longer visible—now the image looks as it did in step 1. When you group layers, the top layer (in this case, the **Sharpening** layer) shows through only where there is *content* in the bottom layer (in this case, the as-yet empty **Mask** layer). When you paint on the **Mask** layer in the next step, however, you will allow only selected areas of the **Sharpening** layer to appear.

6 Mask Edges

The next thing to do is to add content to the **Mask** layer where you want the edges of the image to appear sharpened. To accomplish this, you use the **Brush** tool.

In the **Layers** palette, choose the **Mask** layer, and then select the **Brush** tool from the **Toolbox**. On the **Options** bar, select a soft brush style and a brush size that matches the width of the edge you want to sharpen. Make sure that the **Opacity** setting is **100%**, and that **Mode** is set to **Normal**. It actually does not matter what you use for your foreground color, although you might want to choose black simply because your marks become more visible in the thumbnail for the **Mask** layer in the **Layers** palette.

In the image, paint along the edges of the subject where you want to sharpen. As you paint, the sharpened edges from the **Sharpen** layer will become visible.

▶ NOTE

Because this task involves the use of the **Unsharp Mask** filter as well as *masks* (a principal feature of Photoshop CS2), you might be wondering what the connection is. Despite their labels, they're two different types of masks entirely. It would be less confusing, I admit, if they had different names.

To remove part of a sharpened edge, select the **Mask** layer and, using an eraser tool, remove the portion you do not want visible. You can also use any of the selection tools to delete part of the mask. For example, you can use the **Lasso** tool to select part of the mask, and then press the **Delete** key to remove the selection.

7 View Results

When you're satisfied with the result, make any other changes you want and save the PSD file. Then resave the result in JPEG, PNG, or non-layered TIFF format, leaving your PSD image with its layers intact so that you can return at a later time to make changes or additions.

The **Unsharp Mask** filter makes a number of positive corrections to the sharpness of a layer, along with a wide array of really wild and unwanted changes. But with masking, you can paint directly on top of those areas that reflect the **Unsharp Mask** changes you do want, and leave behind those areas of changes you don't want.

You should never put too much faith in the autofocus of your digital camera. Luckily, I took several shots of Katie on her hay-horse during her birthday, but I wanted to try to save this shot, for which the autofocus centered in on the background foliage and not the subject. Separating the unsharp mask layer from the background layer, and then using the mask to bring in just the distinctions between Katie—or Katie's hat—and her background, enabled me to remove most of the shimmering halo between the foreground subject and the greenery in the background. Later, I could blur the greenery to help create the illusion of depth of field.

62

---

63 Blur an Image to Remove Noise

→ SEE ALSO

62 Sharpen an Image
87 Grab a Still from Video

63

If you have a grainy-looking image such as an old photograph you scanned in, you can blur portions of it to remove the graininess (noise). You might also need to remove noise caused by taking a digital image with too little light. Unfortunately, removing noise by blurring pixels often removes any sharpness the image may have had. You can, of course, opt to blur selected areas of an image, creating the *perception* of sharpening the subject of the image by blurring the surrounding background. But this approach won't solve the problem of any graininess that remains in the subject itself. You can approach this problem by blurring a copy of the image, and then erasing the blurred edges to reveal the sharp edges in the original layer beneath. See **62** **Sharpen an Image** for a task that uses this approach.

When you blur an image or portion of the image, the pixels along color edges are blended with one another—sometimes using averaging—to create a softer edge. This averaging and blending of colors creates smoother transitions between different colored sections of the image, thus eliminating the appearance of tiny spots, often called noise, from the image. With the **Blur** filter, noise is eliminated from the photo by averaging the color values of the pixels where transitions occur to create hard lines or shaded areas. The **Blur More** filter performs the same steps as the **Blur** filter, but the effect is much stronger. Neither filter is really the best to use when removing noise, however, because you'll lose sharpness in your image. You can use the **Blur** tool if you like, to selectively blur areas of an image, but to remove noise from an image requires an all-over blur, and such an approach would be tedious at best.

To remove noise effectively while retaining sharpness, you have two choices: **Smart Blur** or **Reduce Noise**. You can try both and compare the results. The **Smart Blur** dialog box enables you to specify custom **Radius** and **Threshold** settings. By specifying a **Radius** value, you indicate how far to search for pixels that don't match. You indicate the **Threshold** value to specify how different the pixels must be before they are blurred. This filter also enables you to select the blur quality and indicate the blur mode. The **Reduce Noise** filter works by combining the best of the **Despeckle** and **Median** filters (see **51** **Remove Specks, Spots, and Scratches**). Like the **Median** filter, the **Reduce Noise** filter looks for pixels that contrast a lot with the ones around it and then reduces that contrast. Like the **Despeckle** filter, the **Median** filter preserves the contrast only along an object's edges. With this filter, you indicate the relative strength of the blur and the amount of detail you want to preserve. You can also reduce color noise (pixels whose colors vary greatly from those around them) and JPEG artifacts, which can creep in with noise when you save an image in a low-quality JPEG format.

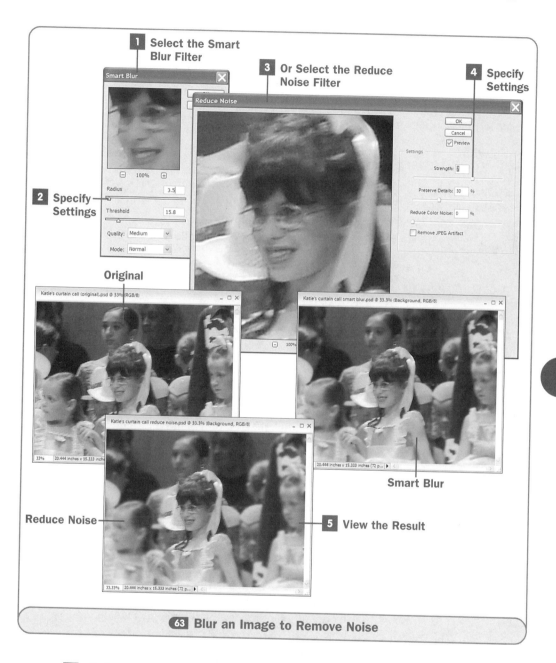

1 Select the Smart Blur Filter

2 Specify Settings

3 Or Select the Reduce Noise Filter

4 Specify Settings

Original

Reduce Noise

Smart Blur

5 View the Result

63 Blur an Image to Remove Noise

1 Select the Smart Blur Filter

Open the image you want to adjust in the Editor in **Standard Edit** mode and save it in Photoshop (***.psd**) format. If it's not already showing, display the **Layers** palette by selecting **Window, Layers**. In the **Layers** palette, click the layer you want to sharpen by blurring its graininess and select **Filter, Blur, Smart Blur**.

▶ **NOTE**

See **62** Sharpen an Image for a technique that describes how to apply the filter to a duplicate layer and then reveal the sharp edges in the original layer using a clipping mask. If your original image doesn't have sharp edges worth protecting, you can apply the blur filter to the original layer and use the technique described in the task to generate sharp edges on a duplicate layer.

2 Specify Settings

In the **Smart Blur** dialog box, specify the settings for blurring your image. You can view a sample of how the image will be blurred in the preview window at the top of the dialog box. In the **Radius** field, specify a value that indicates the number of pixels around each pixel that the **Smart Blur** filter will search for dissimilar pixels to blur.

▶ **TIPS**

Use the – and + buttons to adjust the zoom size of the preview window. As you point to the preview, the mouse pointer becomes the **Hand** tool. Use this tool to drag the image to see another portion.

Click and hold the preview window to toggle the effect off, and release to turn it back on. This trick enables you to compare the look of the image before and after the effect is applied.

In the **Threshold** field, specify a value between **0** and **100** that indicates, relatively, how different the pixels must be in tonal difference before they are blurred. The higher the **Threshold** level, the more pixels are blurred in your image.

In the **Quality** drop-down list box, specify the desired blur quality for the image. You can select from **Low**, **Medium**, or **High** quality. The higher the quality setting, the longer it takes to apply the filter, although a **Quality** setting of **High** produces the smoothest results. However, the higher the **Quality** setting, the more likely you will have banding when you print or view the image.

The **Mode** list box presents the different modes the filter uses to create the blur. The default selection, **Normal**, blurs the entire selection. Select **Edge Only** if you want to create pure white edges on a pure black background, like sketches made with a thin stylus on a blackboard. Select **Overlay Edge** to combine this white edge with the existing image contents for a special effect that divides contrasting regions of the image by a thin white boundary.

When the preview appears as you intend, click **OK**.

63

3 Or Select the Reduce Noise Filter

In the **Layers** palette, click the layer you want to sharpen by blurring its graininess and select **Filter, Noise, Reduce Noise**.

4 Specify Settings

In the Reduce Noise dialog box, start by lowering the Preserve Details value so that you can see the effect. This value controls how much contrast a pixel must have with its neighbor before its brightness is lowered to bring it more in line with the "neighborhood average." Slowly increase this value to preserve your edges, lower it as needed to reduce noise even more. Strength controls how much a pixel's brightness can be changed.

To change pixel colors in a manner similar to the way Strength affects the brightness of discordant pixels, adjust the Reduce Color Noise value. To remove artifacts caused by low JPEG quality, enable the Remove JPEG Artifact option. Click OK.

5 View the Result

When you're satisfied with the result, make any other changes you want and save the PSD file. Then resave the result in JPEG, PNG, or non-layered TIFF format, leaving your PSD image with its layers intact so that you can return at a later time to make changes or additions.

This example features a digital photo of a ballet curtain call that suffers from many of the same problems faced by digital video photographers: It was taken at high digital zoom, using no tripod. So, the shakiness of the photographer's hand (mine), coupled with noise introduced by the digital zoom, resulted in a nice moment confounded by the problems of modern technology.

Neither sharpening nor blurring restores focus to an image, but it can restore some sense of *composition*...or, at least, cover up some of my mistakes. This example actually shows two types of blurs at work: Along the edge of the photo, I used the **Elliptical Marquee** tool to create a feathered, vignette-shaped selection around my daughter, inverted the selection, and then applied a mild **Gaussian Blur**. For the **Background** layer, I used the **Smart Blur** filter described here. I set **Radius** to a low value of **3.5** to preserve the shading of Katerina's face and to prevent posterization. I then set **Threshold** to **15.8**, which was a nice balance between blurring and losing her face altogether (higher) and returning to the original spottiness (lower).

63

The result shows how **Smart Blur** reconstructed an even tone to the subject of the image, thus restoring the illusion of sharpness; the **Gaussian Blur** technique compounded the illusion by taking the viewer's focus away from the edges and corners, without disrespecting the other fine performers in the production.

The second example shows the same technique but using the **Reduce Noise** filter instead. I think that the **Smart Blur** filter did a slightly better job at removing noise while preserving edges in this particular image, but you can judge for yourself.

63

11

Improving Portraits

IN THIS CHAPTER:

Although a photograph is an accurate record of a specific moment in time, there's no particular reason why you have to "remember" the flaws your camera captured as well: the slightly yellow teeth, the blotchy skin, the wrinkles, and the wind that blew everyone's hair out of place. Using the Editor's tools, you can erase these flaws or simply make them less noticeable. For example, you can erase freckles and blemishes, lighten the skin under someone's eyes, and remove an annoying glare from their eyeglasses. You can even add a soft glow around your subject to soften an otherwise harsh appearance, or to project a sense of innocence. In this chapter, you'll learn how to perform these and other digital tricks while maintaining the essential loveliness and inner beauty of your subjects.

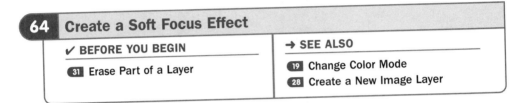

64 Create a Soft Focus Effect

✔ BEFORE YOU BEGIN	→ SEE ALSO
31 Erase Part of a Layer	**19** Change Color Mode
	28 Create a New Image Layer

To apply a soft, romantic look to an image, you can use the **Gaussian Blur** filter. This filter applies a soft blur to the entire layer or selection and is easy to use. The filter has only one option—the radius, which controls the amount of blur. The larger the radius, the greater number of pixels blurred together, and the more detail you lose. I like to control the effect somewhat by using it on a duplicate layer and then softly sharpening important features such as a person's eyes, nostrils, and mouth. In this task, you'll learn how to perform this same trick.

1 Duplicate the Image

Open the image in the Editor in **Standard Edit** mode and save it in Photoshop (*.**psd**) format. If the image isn't already in grayscale or RGB color mode, then you must convert it by selecting either option from the **Image**, **Mode** menu.

If the image has more than one layer, select the layer you want to soften from the **Layers** palette. Then drag the layer you want to blur onto the **Create a new layer** button on the **Layers** palette to create a copy of it, or select **Layer**, **Duplicate Layer**. Name the new layer **Blurred**.

2 Select Gaussian Blur Filter

With the **Blurred** layer selected, select **Filter**, **Blur**, **Gaussian Blur** from the main menu or double-click the **Gaussian Blur** icon on the **Filters** list of the **Styles and Effects** palette. The **Gaussian Blur** dialog box appears.

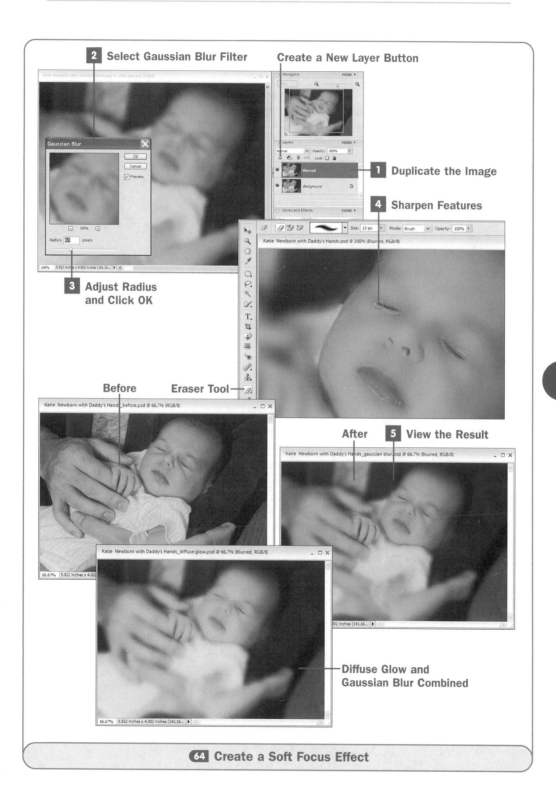

2 Select Gaussian Blur Filter

Create a New Layer Button

1 Duplicate the Image

4 Sharpen Features

3 Adjust Radius and Click OK

Before

Eraser Tool

After **5** View the Result

Diffuse Glow and Gaussian Blur Combined

64 Create a Soft Focus Effect

64

▶ TIPS

The Editor comes with a **Soft Focus** effect you can try if you like, but the result is very, very subtle and produces a very soft overall blurring of the current layer.

Another way to create a soft glow in a photograph is to apply the **Diffuse Glow** filter (choose **Filter, Distort, Diffuse Glow**). This filter uses the current background color, so be sure to reset it to white or a very light color before beginning. Set the **Graininess** value to **0**, the **Clear Amount** to **10** or more (to control the amount of the background color that shows through the glow), and the **Glow Amount** to **2** or so. If you want to combine the **Diffuse Glow** filter with the technique discussed here, apply it to the **Background** layer before copying it. The result of applying both filters is shown in the second example.

3 Adjust Radius and Click OK

Adjust the **Radius** setting in the **Gaussian Blur** dialog box to a value that blurs the image enough to soften it, typically somewhere between **4** and **9**. You'll be unblurring any areas you want to remain sharp (such as your subject's features) in step 4, so don't worry about getting the image too blurry. Click **OK**.

4 Sharpen Features

64

The **Gaussian Blur** filter blurs everything on the current layer, including the features of your subject's face. This causes the image to lose impact because the viewer's eye depends on sharp features to distinguish a person. Select the **Eraser** tool from the **Toolbox**. On the **Options** bar, select a soft, small brush from the **Brushes** drop-down list. Lightly brush over the eyes, nostrils, and mouth areas of your subject. This action reveals the original, sharp layer underneath, bringing those features back into focus.

▶ TIP

You can further lessen the effect of the blur by lowering the **Opacity** of the **Blurred** layer on the **Layers** palette.

5 View the Result

After you're satisfied with the image, save the result in the PSD file. Then resave the image in JPEG, PNG, or non-layered TIFF format, leaving your PSD image unflattened so that you can return at a later time and make different adjustments if you want.

I've always loved this photo of my daughter, lying contentedly in her daddy's arms on the day she was born. But I thought a bit of soft focus might improve the image. So, I applied a Gaussian blur using a radius of 6.1 to blur the image. Then I sharpened her features just a bit, placing the focus clearly on her peaceful face. I also sharpened her hand because I considered it an intimate part of the photograph. Having just her hand in sharp focus made her father's hand look strange because it was blurred. But I didn't want to sharpen it because I didn't want her father's hand to dominate the photo (which it could have because his hand was so much larger than she was at that time). So, I sharpened along the edges of two fingers only, using the **Eraser** set to half opacity.

---

65 **Remove Wrinkles, Freckles, and Minor Blemishes**

✔ BEFORE YOU BEGIN	→ SEE ALSO
28 Create a New Image Layer	**66** Whiten Teeth
	67 Awaken Tired Eyes

Almost everyone has certain…er…cosmetic distinctions that help identify and even glamorize a person. However, if they're the temporary kind, you might not want a permanent record of them. Sometimes a perfectly good photograph is marred by minor distractions such as a few blemishes, a mole, a cold sore, or a few wrinkles just beginning to show. Is it vain to want to fix nature? Perhaps, but don't let that stop you—especially when it's so easy to eliminate imperfections you don't want to show.

65

As explained in **56** **Remove Unwanted Objects from an Image**, you can use the **Clone Stamp** tool to paint away minor defects in a photograph by copying good pixels from some other area. For some very minor problem areas, you might try the **Healing Brush** or the **Spot Healing Brush** discussed in **51** **Remove Specks, Spots, and Scratches** and an upcoming tip. But in either case, the process is tedious and often easily detectable unless the tools are used sparingly. In this task, you'll use a quicker method that involves one of the blur filters.

1 **Duplicate Background Layer**

Open an image in the Editor in **Standard Edit** mode and save it in Photoshop (***.psd**) format. Then drag the Background layer onto the **Create a New Layer** button on the **Layers** palette to create a copy of it or select **Layer**, **Duplicate Layer**. Name the new layer **Unblurred**.

2 **Blur Background Layer**

Change to the **Background** layer and select **Filter**, **Blur**, **Blur More** from the menu or double-click the **Blur More** icon on the **Filters** list of the **Styles and Effects** palette. The **Background** layer is blurred just a bit.

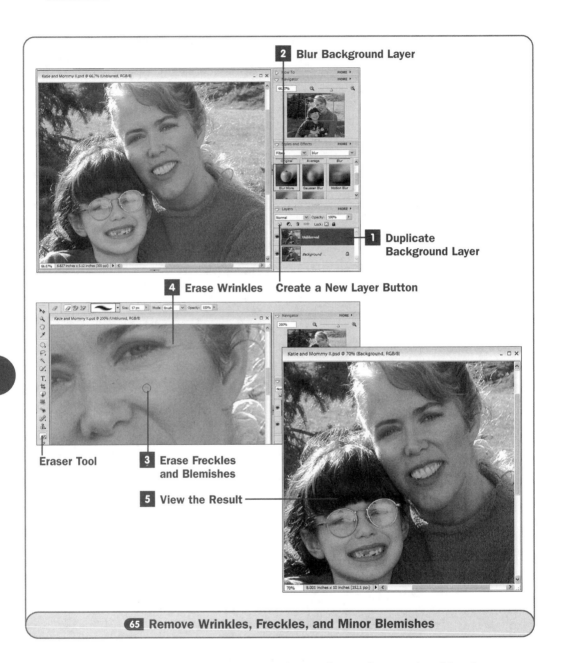

2 Blur Background Layer

1 Duplicate Background Layer

4 Erase Wrinkles   Create a New Layer Button

Eraser Tool

3 Erase Freckles and Blemishes

5 View the Result

65 Remove Wrinkles, Freckles, and Minor Blemishes

For very large images, the **Blur More** filter might not do enough to blur the layer. In such cases, try the **Gaussian Blur** filter (choose **Filter, Blur, Gaussian Blur**) or double-click the **Gaussian Blur** icon in the **Filters** list of the **Styles and Effects** palette. Increase the **Radius** until the imperfections are blurred, and click **OK**.

▶ **TIP**

To see if the **Background** layer is blurred enough, hide the **Unblurred** layer temporarily by clicking its eye icon on the **Layers** palette. Redisplay the layer when you're done.

3 Erase Freckles and Blemishes

On the **Layers** palette, change to the **Unblurred** layer. Click the **Eraser** tool on the **Toolbox**. On the **Options** bar, select a soft round brush. Adjust the **Size** value so that the eraser is slightly bigger than the blemish you want to remove. Click the freckle or blemish with the eraser, which erases that spot, revealing the blurred layer beneath.

4 Erase Wrinkles

Change the **Size** value on the **Options** bar to resize the **Eraser** tool so that it's just wider than the wrinkles you want to remove. Then drag the **Eraser** over any wrinkles to erase the wrinkle, revealing the blurred wrinkle on the **Background** layer.

▶ **TIP**

Another way you can remove blemishes and freckles quickly is to blend them away with the **Spot Healing Brush** tool. Set the **Size** so that the brush includes the clean area of skin around the blemish or freckle, set **Type** to **Proximity Match**, position the pointer over the blemish or freckle, and click to blend it away.

65

5 View the Result

After you're satisfied with the image, save it in its PSD format. Then save the result in JPEG, PNG, or non-layered TIFF format, leaving your PSD image unflattened so that you can return at a later time and make different adjustments if you want.

This photo of me and my daughter is just wonderful, but the small blemish and the wrinkles just beginning to show around my eyes made the photo less than perfect for me. A bit of blur and a few minutes with the **Eraser**, and I'm the person I see when I look in the mirror. Add a bit of judicious cropping and some work at removing the reflections from my daughter's glasses as described in **68 Remove Glare from Eyeglasses**, and I have a portrait worthy of my living room wall.

66   Whiten Teeth

→ **SEE ALSO**

65 Remove Wrinkles, Freckles, and Minor Blemishes

67 Awaken Tired Eyes

There are many products on the market you can use to whiten your teeth—gels, toothpastes, whitening strips, and bleaches—but none work as fast and as effectively as digital editing. It's not vanity to want to improve Mother Nature; in our culture today, a great importance is placed on having clean, white teeth, and if a photo will be used in a resume or to advertise a product, you'll want to give the best impression you can by making sure that your subject looks his or her best.

Whitening teeth is tricky, however; you don't want the effect to look obvious and artificial. You'll want to avoid the temptation to use pure white to paint over all your teeth, which results in a picket-fence effect that can look genuinely scary. The technique explained here uses the **Dodge** tool, which selectively lightens the brightness of the pixels over which it passes. You must be cautious, however, so that you don't burn out the color and create a fake whiteness.

66

▶ **NOTE**

I always get good results with the **Dodge** tool, but if you don't like its effects, try selecting the teeth, choosing **Enhance**, **Adjust Color**, **Color Variations**, choosing **Highlights**, and clicking the **Increase Blue** and **Lighten** buttons. See 60 Correct Color, Contrast, and Saturation in One Step. You can also try choosing **Enhance**, **Adjust Color**, **Adjust Hue/Saturation**, and then increasing the lightness in the **Master** channel and decreasing the saturation in the **Yellow** channel. See 61 Adjust Hue and Saturation Manually.

1 Select the Dodge Tool

Open an image in the Editor in **Standard Edit** mode and save it in Photoshop (***.psd**) format. Zoom in on the teeth so that you can see them clearly, and then select the **Dodge** tool in the **Toolbox**.

2 Set Options

On the **Options** bar, choose a soft round brush. Adjust the **Size** of the **Dodge** tool so that the brush tip is about the size of one tooth. Set the **Range** to **Midtones** so that you affect only the midtones, and set **Exposure** to about **20%** so that you don't lighten the teeth too fast and accidentally burn out the color.

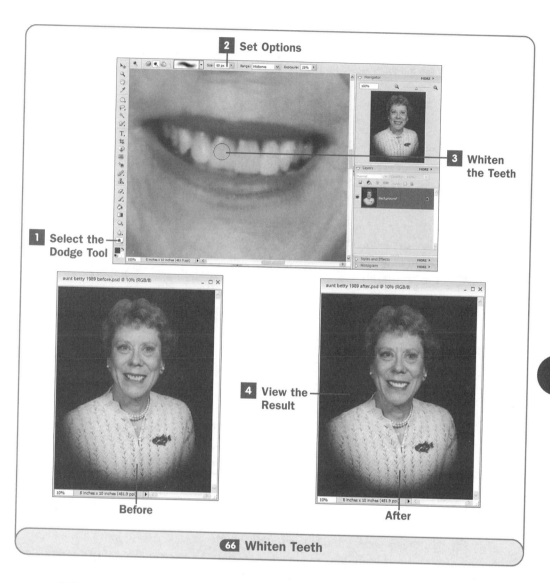

2 Set Options

3 Whiten the Teeth

1 Select the Dodge Tool

4 View the Result

Before

After

66

66 Whiten Teeth

3 Whiten the Teeth

Position the brush tip over the first tooth and click once. The tooth should get just a bit lighter. Click again to lighten a bit more, or move to the next tooth. Repeat until all the teeth are whiter. You can also drag the brush over the teeth.

Remove any remaining imperfections (such as uneven color or spots on the teeth) with the **Clone Stamp** tool. See 56 **Remove Unwanted Objects from an Image**.

▶ **TIP**

To isolate the effects of the **Dodge** tool, select the teeth before beginning. You might want to select the gums as well (if they are reddish and irritated) so that you can lighten them, too.

4 View the Result

When you're satisfied with the result, make any other changes you want and save the PSD file. Resave the result in JPEG, PNG, or non-layered TIFF format, leaving your PSD image with its layers (if any) intact so that you can return at a later time and make additional adjustments if you want.

My Aunt Betty prided herself on her appearance, so I know she'd be horrified to learn that her teeth were not perfectly white when she sat for this otherwise impeccable portrait. (Frankly, I suspect the culprit was her lipstick.) In any case, a few minutes with the **Dodge** tool fixed that easily. Compare the original to the whitened version; you can see that the teeth look better, and yet still natural. The last things to address are the circles under her eyes, an unfortunate family trait, emphasized by the type of lighting being used. To fix that problem, I'll follow the steps in the next task, **67** Awaken Tired Eyes.

66

> ### 67 Awaken Tired Eyes
>
> → SEE ALSO
>
> **38** Correct Red Eye
> **59** Lighten or Darken Part of an Image
> **65** Remove Wrinkles, Freckles, and Minor Blemishes
> **66** Whiten Teeth

They say that the eyes are the window to the soul. It must be true because if a woman has dark circles under her eyes, we think she looks tired (even if the dark circles are a natural skin condition). By slightly lightening the skin under the eyes, you can take years off a face and brighten a person's outlook. And it's simple to do, using the **Dodge** tool.

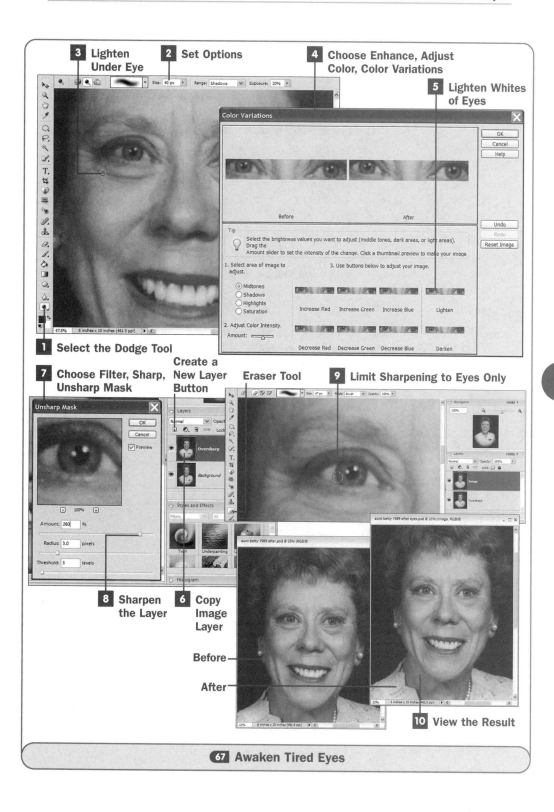

3 Lighten Under Eye

2 Set Options

4 Choose Enhance, Adjust Color, Color Variations

5 Lighten Whites of Eyes

1 Select the Dodge Tool

7 Choose Filter, Sharp, Unsharp Mask

Create a New Layer Button

Eraser Tool

9 Limit Sharpening to Eyes Only

8 Sharpen the Layer

6 Copy Image Layer

Before

After

10 View the Result

67

Redness in the whites of the eyes caused by chlorine in swimming pools or lack of sleep can also make your subject look tired. To whiten the eyes, you'll remove the redness gradually and lighten them a little using the **Color Variations** command. One final thing that can make eyes look tired is a lack of sharpness. Eyes that are in sharp focus have a distinctive twinkle that makes their owner look alert, interesting, and beautiful. Eyes such as these invite a viewer to look a moment longer at the subject. To fix a problem with slightly out-of-focus eyes, you'll over-sharpen a copy of the image on a new layer and use the **Eraser** to reveal only the sharpened eyes.

1 Select the Dodge Tool

Open an image in the Editor in **Standard Edit** mode and save it in Photoshop (***.psd**) format. Zoom in on the eyes so that you can see them clearly, and then select the **Dodge** tool in the **Toolbox**.

▶ TIP

If you'd like more control over the **Dodge** tool, try duplicating the image layer and performing your lightening on the copy layer. You can then adjust the **Opacity** of the copy layer to lower the effect of the lightening if you accidentally apply too much.

67

2 Set Options

On the **Options** bar, choose a soft round brush. Adjust the **Size** of the **Dodge** tool so that the brush tip is about the size of the area you want to lighten. In this case, I adjusted the size so that the brush was the same size as the crease under one eye.

Set the **Range** to **Shadows**, and **Exposure** to about **20%** so that you don't lighten the under-eye area too fast and accidentally burn out the color.

3 Lighten Under Eye

Drag the brush over the area you want to lighten. In my case, I dragged the brush carefully over the under-eye crease. Repeat this step for the second eye.

4 Choose Enhance, Adjust Color, Color Variations

If your subject's eyes are red or tired looking, select the white area of both eyes using your favorite selection tool. (I used the **Magic Wand** tool to select the whites of each eye, and the **Lasso** to snag any parts that didn't get selected.)

Choose **Enhance, Adjust Color, Color Variations**. The **Color Variations** dialog box appears.

5 Lighten Whites of Eyes

Select the **Midtones** option in the lower-left corner of the dialog box so that you affect only the midtones in the image, and then click the **Decrease Red** button to remove the redness from the eye area. Click the **Lighten** button to make the whites a little whiter. The **After** image at the top of the dialog box reflects the changes you're making. When you're through, click **OK**.

▶ **NOTE**

You can click the buttons in the **Color Variations** dialog box more than once to apply the same change multiple times. For example, you could click the **Decrease Red** button twice if your subject's eyes are particularly reddish.

6 Copy Image Layer

To sharpen the eyes of your subject, drag the image layer onto the **Create a New Layer** button on the **Layers** palette to create a copy of it or select **Layer**, **Duplicate Layer**. Name the new layer **Oversharp**.

7 Choose Filter, Sharp, Unsharp Mask

With the **Oversharp** layer selected, choose **Filter**, **Sharpen**, **Unsharp Mask** from the menu or double-click the **Unsharp Mask** icon on the **Filters** list of the **Styles and Effects** palette. The **Unsharp Mask** dialog box appears.

67

8 Sharpen the Layer

In the **Unsharp Mask** dialog box, zoom in on one of the eyes and then adjust the settings for the filter until the eye is sharp and crisp. I typically leave the **Threshold** at a low value, set the **Radius** to somewhere between 1 and 3, and then play with the **Amount** until I get the effect I want. See **62** **Sharpen an Image** for more help. Check the other eye in the preview window of the dialog box (by dragging the image in the preview), and when you're satisfied with the look, click **OK**.

To make the eyes really sharp, reapply the **Unsharp Mask** settings one or two more times by choosing **Filter**, **Unsharp Mask**.

9 Limit Sharpening to Eyes Only

The effect right now is a too-sharp image, and we wanted to limit the effect to just the eyes. First, if the image is on the background layer, convert it to a regular layer by choosing **Layer**, **New**, **Layer from Background**. Rename this layer **Image**. Drag the **Oversharp** layer below the **Image** layer.

The sharpness will appear to go away, but really it's just hidden by the image layer above it. To reveal the sharpened eyes, click the **Eraser** tool on the **Toolbox**. On the **Options** bar, select a small, soft brush. On the **Layers** palette, select the **Image** layer. Then erase just the eyes, revealing the over-sharpened layer below.

▶ **NOTE**

Because the **Oversharp** layer is below the **Image** layer, you won't see the effects of the sharpening on your actual image at first. To view the sharpening, on the **Layers** palette, click the eye icon on the **Image** layer to hide that layer temporarily.

[10] View the Result

After you're satisfied with the result, make any other changes you want and save the PSD file. Resave the result in JPEG, PNG, or non-layered TIFF format, leaving your PSD image with its layers (if any) intact so that you can return at a later time and make additional adjustments if you want.

Although I had brightened Aunt Betty's teeth, the circles under her eyes and their tired look still bothered me. So I lightened the creases under her eyes just a little; the goal was not to make her look half her age, but the way in which I remember her—a happy, beautiful woman. I also whitened her eyes just a bit, and then sharpened them, which helps me to feel like Aunt Betty is looking more directly at me, making this a more engaging portrait of my aunt.

67

---

68   Remove Glare from Eyeglasses

✔ BEFORE YOU BEGIN	→ SEE ALSO
21 Draw a Selection Freehand or by Tracing Its Edge	**59** Lighten or Darken Part of an Image
29 Create a Layer Filled with a Color, Gradient, or Pattern	**67** Awaken Tired Eyes

Probably the most difficult photographic repair you will ever attempt is to remove glare from a person's eyeglasses. What makes this repair so difficult is that no one method works every time. In this task, you'll learn a variety of techniques, one or two of which should work on your photograph.

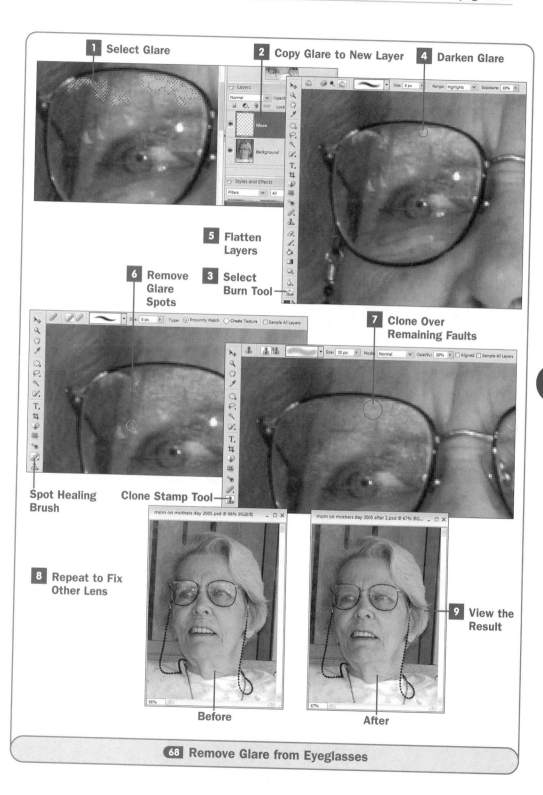

1 Select Glare

2 Copy Glare to New Layer

4 Darken Glare

5 Flatten Layers

6 Remove Glare Spots

3 Select Burn Tool

7 Clone Over Remaining Faults

Spot Healing Brush

Clone Stamp Tool

8 Repeat to Fix Other Lens

9 View the Result

Before

After

68

Because glare is difficult to remove, it's best to try to eliminate it while taking the photograph. One way to remove glare is to use a polarizing filter—a special filter that you twist to allow light polarized in one direction only to enter the lens, eliminating glare. If you don't happen to have a polarizing filter with you, try moving your subject so that the light is coming at him or her from a different angle, moving your own position in relation to the subject, or simply having your subject remove his or her eyeglasses or look off to one side or slightly downward.

▶ **TIP**

If you wear eyeglasses, you can keep an old pair of frames (minus the lenses) on hand for picture-taking time. Without the lenses, you obviously won't get the glare, and the empty frames will help your face look more natural.

1 Select Glare

Open an image in the Editor in **Standard Edit** mode and save it in Photoshop (*.psd*) format.

Because each eyeglass lens typically needs a slightly different adjustment, it's best to work on one eye at a time. It's also best to isolate what you're doing on another layer so that you can easily start over (by deleting the layer) if need be. Zoom in and then, using either the **Lasso** or **Magic Wand** tool, select the area of glare on the first lens. You'll copy this area to another layer before making changes to it.

2 Copy Glare to New Layer

To copy the selected area, choose **Edit, Copy** from the menu. To place the copy on a new layer, choose **Layer, New, Layer via Copy**. Name the new layer **Glare**.

▶ **TIP**

If only one eyeglass lens has glare, you can try another method to remove it. Try copying the good eye to another layer, flipping it, and skewing it to conform to the other eye space. Then flatten the layers and use the **Clone Stamp** tool to blend the eye into its new surroundings. You can also try copying an eye from a similar photograph that does not have any glare.

3 Select Burn Tool

Click the **Burn** tool on the **Toolbox**. On the **Options** bar, choose a soft round brush. Adjust the **Size** of the **Burn** tool so that the brush tip is about the size of the area you want to darken. Set the **Range** to **Highlights** so that you affect only the lightest areas of the image, and set the **Exposure** to a small

68

value such as **10%** so that each stroke over the area darkens the pixels only slightly. These settings enable you to work slowly to remove the glare.

4 Darken Glare

Make sure that the **Glare** layer is selected on the **Layers** palette. Brush the **Burn** tool over the glare to darken it so that it better matches the surrounding area. If necessary, darken the midtones as well by setting the **Range** to **Midtones** in the **Options** bar. You might not be able to remove the glare entirely; your goal here is to bring out the detail of the face behind the glare.

5 Flatten Layers

Before you can perform the next step, which involves using the **Spot Healing Brush** to blend pixels to remove remaining trouble spots, you'll want to flatten the image so that you can use the repairs you've made so far in the blending process. You might want to save the PSD image at this point, before merging layers. Before you merge the layers, however, you might want to increase the saturation in the glare area because it might have been desaturated by the **Burn** tool. Select the **Sponge** tool from the **Toolbox**, set the **Mode** to **Saturate**, adjust the **Size** and **Flow** settings, and drag over the area to bring its colors back.

When you're satisfied that you've done all you can with the **Burn** tool, choose **Layer**, **Flatten Image** to merge the layers together.

68

6 Remove Glare Spots

After merging the layers, if there are any sharp points of glare (as opposed to larger glare patches), you can remove them with the **Spot Healing Brush**. Click the **Spot Healing Brush** on the **Toolbox**. Set the **Type** to **Proximity Match** and adjust the **Size** so that the brush is slightly larger than the glare spot you want to remove. Then click the spot to remove it. Repeat this process as needed to remove any other glare spots. You can also use the **Spot Healing Brush** to blend good pixels with pixels you darkened in step 5, making your repairs less noticeable.

7 Clone Over Remaining Faults

To fix the remaining problem areas, click the **Clone Stamp** tool on the **Toolbox**. On the **Options** bar, select a soft round brush, adjust the **Size**, and set the **Mode** to **Normal**. You might want to lower the **Opacity** as well to help disguise what you're doing. Press **Alt** and click the area you want to clone, and then drag the brush over the glare area to transfer the **Alt**-selected pixels to the new area. Repeat to repair any other flaws.

▶ **TIP**

To clone a skin color from another portion of the face, you might want to turn off the **Aligned** option for the **Clone Stamp** tool in the **Options** bar so that you don't clone anything but that small area, and not the objects in that same vicinity.

8 Repeat to Fix Other Lens

After you're satisfied with the way in which the first eyeglass lens looks, repeat steps 1–7 to remove the glare from the second lens (if any).

9 View the Result

After you're satisfied with your changes, save the PSD image. Then resave the result in JPEG, PNG, or non-layered TIFF format, leaving your PSD image with its layers (if any) intact so that you can return at a later time and make additional adjustments if you want.

Even though this portrait of my mother was taken in the shade of a covered porch, the glare of the sunlight still caught her eyeglasses. After removing the glare, her wonderful eyes are now much more apparent.

68

69 Frame a Photograph

✔ **BEFORE YOU BEGIN**

16 Change Image Size or Resolution

29 Create a Layer Filled with a Color, Gradient, or Pattern

34 Mask an Image Layer

→ **SEE ALSO**

134 Frame Your Video with an Image

88 Prepare a Still for Video

After spending lots of time creating the perfect image, why not frame it? With the Editor, it's easy to add a frame—brushed aluminum, rough wood, and other styles—simply by applying a frame effect. Some frame effects require you to make a selection first, and then the frame is placed around this selection. One frame effect creates a simple frame using the current foreground color. Although applying a frame effect is quick and easy, it allows you° no artistic freedom whatsoever. In this task, I'll show you how to create your own frame and mat.

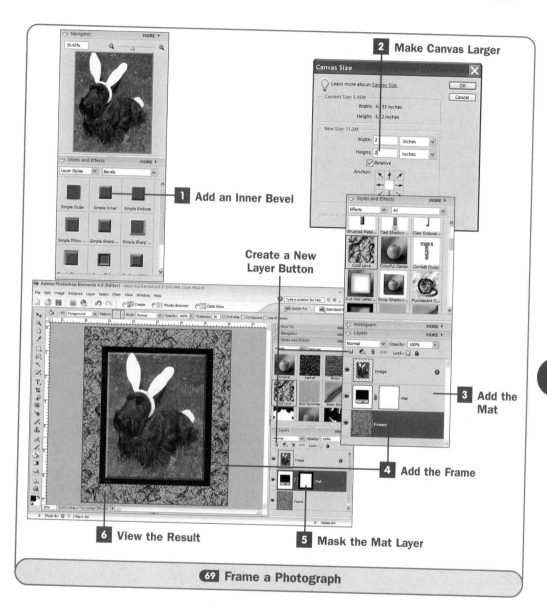

2 Make Canvas Larger

1 Add an Inner Bevel

Create a New
Layer Button

3 Add the Mat

4 Add the Frame

69

6 View the Result

5 Mask the Mat Layer

69 Frame a Photograph

▶ NOTES

Obviously, you wouldn't take the trouble to add a graphic "frame" around an image that you intend to print and frame yourself, but you might add a digital frame to an image destined for a card, scrapbook, or web page.

To apply a frame effect, select **Effects** from the first drop-down list on the **Styles and Effects** palette, and select **Frames** from the second list. Then, double-click any effect thumbnail to apply it to your image. You might be asked to flatten the image first; click **OK** to continue. If an effect's name contains the {**selection**} notation, you must make a selection first before applying that effect to the image.

1 Add an Inner Bevel

Open an image in the Editor in **Standard Edit** mode and save it in Photoshop (***.psd**) format. If your image contains more than one layer, flatten the image by selecting **Layer, Flatten Image** from the menu bar so that it will be easier to add a frame and a mat.

Add an inner bevel to the image to simulate the bevel normally found along the inner edge of a photographic mat. On the **Styles and Effects** palette, select **Layer Styles** from the first drop-down list, and select **Bevels** from the second list. Double-click the **Simple Inner** or **Simple Sharp Inner** thumbnail to apply that style to the image. You might be asked if you want to convert the Background layer into a full layer. Click **OK** and name the new layer **Image**.

▶ **NOTE**

The bevel Photoshop Elements applies is slanted up; if you want your bevel to slant down (so that the image seems to be *below* the mat and frame), double-click the layer style icon on the **Layers** palette for the image layer and select **Down** at the bottom of the **Style Settings** dialog box. You can also change the direction of the light on the bevel and the size of the bevel in this dialog box.

69

2 Make Canvas Larger

Increase the canvas size to make room for the mat and the frame. Choose **Image, Resize, Canvas Size** from the menu. Enable the **Relative** option and click the center box in the **Anchor** pane. Type the same amount in the **Width** and **Height** boxes, and click **OK**. I usually add an amount that's roughly 1/2 the smallest dimension of the original image. For example, if your image is roughly 4" × 5" like mine, add 2" to the width and height.

3 Add the Mat

To add the mat, insert a fill layer below the **Image** layer. To create this new layer, choose **Layer, New Fill Layer, Solid Color** from the menu bar. Name the new layer **Mat**. *Do not enable the **Group with Previous Layer** option.* Click **OK**, then choose the color you want for the mat from the **Color Picker**. Click **OK** to finalize your color choice. Then on the **Layers** palette, drag the **Mat** layer below the **Image** layer.

▶ **TIPS**

Add a texture to your mat by applying a texture filter or effect using the **Styles and Effects** palette.

4 Add the Frame

To create the frame, do any of the following:

- Add a new fill layer and fill it with any color you want. (You're not going to actually see this color when you're finished; you're using the color only to make the layer opaque.) Name this new layer **Frame**. On the **Layers** palette, drag the **Frame** layer to the bottom of the layer stack. Then apply a layer style that compliments your photo; the layer style replaces the color you chose earlier and fills the layer. On the **Styles and Effects** palette, with **Layer Styles** still selected in the first drop-down list, select **Patterns** from the second list. Then, double-click the thumb-nail of the pattern you want to use for your frame. For example, you might choose **Batik, Manhole, Oak,** or **Dry Mud**. There are some options on the **Complex** list you might like, such as **Diamond Plate, Molten Gold, White Grid on Orange,** or **Red, White, and Blue Contrast**. Experiment until you find the perfect compliment to your photograph.

- Insert a new layer by clicking the **Create a New Layer** button on the **Layers** palette or choosing **Layer, New, Layer**. Name this new layer **Frame**. On the **Layers** palette, drag the new layer to the bottom of the layer stack. Then, fill the new layer with a color or gradient, or simply paint or stamp a pattern on it with various colors taken from the pho-tograph. You also could draw shapes using the **Custom Shape** tool, such as a paw print or a butterfly. (After using the **Custom Shape** tool, merge the shape layers with the **Frame** layer by turning off the visibili-ty of *all of the other layers*, and then choosing **Layer, Merge Visible**.) If you like, add a filter to mix the colors to create a pattern or texture or to achieve an artsy look.

▶ **TIP**

Instead of creating a mat and frame, you can create a decorative edge for a photo by simply painting on a layer below your image layer (lower the opacity of the image layer to aid your work), and then creating a clipping mask using that layer. See **34** Mask an Image Layer.

- Choose an effect to create your frame. Because effects automatically add a layer to your image, you don't have to create the frame layer first. On the **Styles and Effects** palette, select **Effects** from the first drop-down list. Select **Textures** from the second list, and then double-click the thumbnail of a texture that complements your image. Drag the new layer to the bottom of the layer stack of the **Layers** palette. From there, you can rename this new layer **Frame**.

5 Mask the Mat Layer

Right now, with the **Frame** layer at the bottom of the layer stack, you can't see the frame at all because the **Mat** layer is covering it up. So, you need to mask the **Mat** layer so that only part of it shows through.

Turn on the rulers to guide you by choosing **View**, **Rulers**. Click the **Rectangular Marquee** tool and drag to create a selection around the image by the amount you want the mat to show, roughly 1/4 the size of the frame. Invert this selection by choosing **Select**, **Inverse**. The portion of the image you want the frame to fill is now selected. On the **Layers** palette, select the **Mat** layer, and fill the selection with black, using the **Paint Bucket** tool. This action fills the selected area of the mask for the **Mat** layer with black, which causes the mask to block the mat in that area (preventing that portion of the mat from showing through). The **Frame** layer below, which is no longer blocked by the **Mat** layer in that area, now shows through.

69

▶ NOTE

If you want, you can add an inner bevel to help the **Mat** layer look more like a mat. Select the **Mat** layer on the **Layers** palette. Using the **Magic Wand** tool, click the center of the image to select the white portion of the **Mat** layer. Then repeat step 1 to add the inner bevel.

6 View the Result

After you're satisfied with the result, make any other changes you want and save the PSD file. Resave the result in JPEG, PNG, or non-layered TIFF format, leaving your PSD image with its layers (if any) intact so that you can return at a later time and make adjustments if you want.

I wanted to frame this photo of Hattie, my Aunt Betty's Scottie dog, for use on a greeting card. I used a black mat and a frame created with the **Cold Lava** texture effect. I added a border outside the frame by **Ctrl**+clicking the thumbnail for the **Frame** layer on the **Layers** palette (which selected the **Frame** layer), choosing **Select**, **Modify**, **Border** and expanding the border selection by 25 pixels, and filling the selection with black using the **Paint Bucket** tool.

12

Printing and Emailing Images

IN THIS CHAPTER:

In Photoshop Elements, printing is the final step you take in rendering a picture, a group of pictures, or a printed creation. As a first step before you do any editing of an image, you should calibrate your monitor so that what you see onscreen in Photoshop Elements is similar to what you should expect when you print. If you haven't calibrated your monitor, do that now. Then preview the images you want to print, using the newly calibrated monitor, and make any further adjustments to the images as needed before printing.

▶ **TIP**

If you use more than one printer, select that printer before you edit, so that what you see onscreen is coordinated with the printer you intend to use. To select a printer for editing, choose **File**, **Page Setup** from the Editor or the Organizer. Select a paper **Size** and **Source** from the first **Page Setup** dialog box and click **OK**. In the second **Page Setup** dialog box that appears next, choose your printer from the **Name** list and click **OK**.

You can print single images from the Editor or multiple images the Organizer. Just before printing, you can adjust the printer options to change the print quality to **Best** and the paper type to photo paper or heavy bond paper (if you're printing a card, for example). And then, if you're printing photos, there are the endless choices you can make about what to print: multiple copies of the same image, single prints from a group of images, a set of prints in standard photo sizes, photo labels, or small thumbnails of each image you can use as a reference. You can also reverse the image on-the-fly when printing onto iron-on transfer paper. As a final option, you might choose not to print your images at all, but to upload them to an Internet printing service instead. In this chapter, you'll learn how to complete all these tasks.

You'll also learn how to share your photos. Photoshop Elements is not an email program, but it can work in close partnership with the email software you *do* have, allowing you to easily send photos via email whenever you like. In addition to individual pictures, you can email creations such as slide shows, photo albums, postcards, and calendars. You also can include sound and video files, but not automatically. You must manually attach them to the email message. If your friends and relatives have a slow connection to the Internet, you can share images using an online service. Not only does this make it quicker and easier for Grandma to view the latest photos of your daughter's birthday party, she can select the ones she wants to have copies of and have the service print and mail them directly to her. Of course, Adobe's online service, Adobe Photoshop Services, comes with built-in security so that you don't have to worry about someone viewing your photos if you didn't invite them to.

70 Print an Image

→ **SEE ALSO**

71 Print Images Using an Online Service

▶ **NOTE**

You can print an existing creation from the Organizer by selecting it and clicking the **Print** button on the **Shortcuts** bar and then selecting a printer and clicking **Print** from the **Print** dialog box that appears. You can also print a creation just after creating or editing it by clicking the **Print** button on the **Step 5: Share** page of the **Creation** wizard. See **11** **Make a Creation**.

After you're through making changes, you can print an image from the Editor. (To print multiple copies of an image or multiple images, use the Organizer. Although you can scale the image to fit a particular size (such as 5" × 7") the process may result in portions of the image being cropped (not printed). In addition, scaling the size of an image within the **Print Preview** dialog box may also reduce image resolution (and thus, in turn, quality), so in most cases, you should resize the image using the steps in **16** **Change Image Size or Resolution**. For prints that are smaller than the paper you're using, you can adjust *where* the photo prints on the paper (which may help you trim the print). You'll be able to add a colored border around the image, print the image filename and text caption, and select the specific ICC printer profile you want to use. Before printing, you can preview your selections to see how your image will look.

70

▶ **NOTE**

Printing low-resolution images in a large size results in poor quality (grainy) photos. If you took the photos using a low-resolution setting on your digital camera (or scanned them using a low-resolution setting), choose a small print size for best print results.

1 Click Print

Open the image you want to print in the Editor and save it in Photoshop (*.psd) format. Calibrate your monitor if needed, make any changes you want, including resizing the image to fit the print size you need, then save the result in JPEG, PNG, or non-layered TIFF format, leaving your PSD image with its layers intact so that you can return at a later time and make different adjustments if you want.

Click the **Print** button on the **Shortcuts** bar, or select **File**, **Print** from the menu. The **Print Preview** dialog box appears.

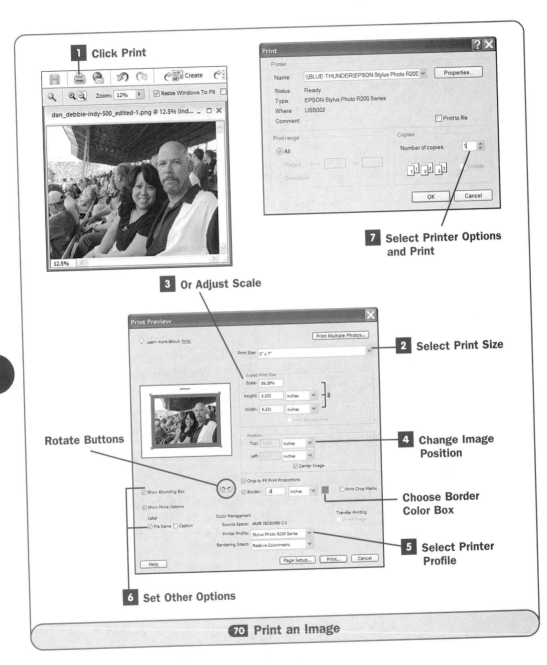

1 Click Print

7 Select Printer Options and Print

3 Or Adjust Scale

2 Select Print Size

Rotate Buttons

4 Change Image Position

Choose Border Color Box

5 Select Printer Profile

6 Set Other Options

70 Print an Image

2 Select Print Size

If you need to change the paper size, orientation, or paper type for this print job, click the **Page Setup** button to display the **Page Setup** dialog box. Select the paper **Size** and orientation; click the **Printer** button, select the printer to use, and then click **Properties** to display your printer's **Properties** dialog box where you can set the paper type.

The photo normally prints at its actual size (image size in pixels, divided by its image resolution or PPI). One way to scale the photo to print at a different size is to open the **Print Size** list and select the photo size, such as 5" × 7". The **Fit to Page** option from this list makes the photo as large as possible, while still fitting the paper size you chose. As noted earlier, scaling in this way could affect print quality. To resize correctly, see **16 Change Image Size or Resolution**.

To adjust the photo to fit the print size you select (if not **Actual Size**), the Editor may crop portions of the image. To prevent cropping, disable the **Crop to Fit Print Proportions** option, and then the image will print at the largest size possible within the **Print Size** dimensions you've chosen.

After you select a photo size from the **Print Size** list, the Editor adjusts the photo as best it can to fit that size. Still, you can fine-tune the **Height** and **Width** values as desired.

▶ NOTES

For best results, change the **Print Size** only when the size you select is smaller than the actual print size. To print in a size larger than the image's actual print size, resize the image as described in **16 Change Image Size or Resolution**.

You can print a photo in a custom size by selecting the **Custom Size** option from the **Print Size** drop-down list and entering the **Height** and **Width** dimensions. Alternatively, if the **Show Bounding Box** option is enabled, you can resize the image by dragging the corners of the bounding box that surrounds the image in the preview window.

3 Or Adjust Scale

You can also set the print size on an image as a percentage of the actual print size by entering a value in the **Scale** box. It's best to choose percentages that make for less awkward fractions. For example, 50% (1/2) or 75% (3/4) scale produces less degradation in the image than 95% (19/20) or 98% (49/50).

▶ NOTE

If you make a rectangular selection (with no feathering) before printing an image, you can enable the **Print Selected Area** option in the **Scaled Print Size** frame to print just the selected area. See **20 Select a Rectangular or Circular Area**.

4 Change Image Position

Typically, the photo prints in the center of the page. To position the photo along the side (so that you can easily cut it) or anywhere else on the paper, disable the **Center Image** option and enter values in the **Position** frame that place the image relative to the **Top** and upper **Left** corner of the paper. A 1-inch **Top** value, for example, places the image 1" from the top of the page; −.5 places the image 1/2" above the top of the page, essentially cropping off the top of the image and not printing it.

▶ **TIP**

You can also reposition the image on the page by disabling the **Center Image** option and then dragging the image inside the preview area.

5 Select Printer Profile

Assuming that you've calibrated your monitor, you've done half of what you need to do to ensure that the image you see onscreen is what you get when you print. To print properly, Photoshop Elements needs to know which printer profile you want to use, so it can match up the colors in your monitor profile with those in the printer profile you select from the **Printer Profile** list. To see this list, make sure that the **Show More Options** check box is enabled.

For best results, choose your printer's specific ICC color profile, or a profile designed for the photo paper you're using, *and* disable printer color management through the printer driver, whose icon is located in the Windows **Control Panel**.

In the absence of a printer color profile, your next best bet is choosing **Printer Color Management**, which assumes that your printer driver has its own color management routine (most photo printers do) and that *it's turned on*. If you don't like these results, try choosing **Adobe RGB**, with the printer driver's color management *turned off*. When you can't specify a specific printer profile to use, you can determine the methodology suited for approximating colors that don't exist in the printer's color space by choosing that methodology from the **Rendering Intent** list.

▶ **NOTE**

Whatever you do, *do not* choose your monitor's color profile from the **Printer Profile** list because you are trying to select the color spectrum intended for your *printer* and not for your monitor.

6 Set Other Options

Enable the **Show More Options** check box to display all options related to printing, then select from among these additional options:

- Add a border around your image by enabling the **Border** option, setting the size, and then clicking the **Choose border color** box to select a color using the **Color Picker**.

▶ NOTE

When you change the width of the **Border** option to any value above **0**, the Editor scales the print size *down* to compensate. This can result in loss of print quality. You can adjust **Scale** back to 100%, but if you're working with a large image or with small paper, you could conceivably push the border off the edge of the page. Be sure to check the preview in the **Print Preview** dialog box to make sure that your image size is what you intend and that your bounding box falls completely within the page edges.

- To print crop marks (tiny **Xs** at the corners) that can help you trim the image after it's printed, enable the **Print Crop Marks** check box.

- Print the image **File Name** or text **Caption** just below the photo by selecting the corresponding options. See **10** Add a Text Caption or Note.

- To flip the image so that you can print it backward onto iron-on transfer paper, enable the **Invert Image** option in the **Transfer Printing** frame. This way, when you iron the image onto your t-shirt, sweatshirt, or other material, the image will look correct.

- To rotate the image on the paper, click the **Rotate 90° Left** or **Rotate 90° Right** button below the preview window. When you do this, even though the upper-left corner of the image might be shifted to a different corner, the **Position** of the image remains relative to the upper-left corner of the area being printed.

7 Select Printer Options and Print

Click the **Print** button to display the **Print** dialog box. Because you selected your printer, paper type and page size in step 2, click **OK** to print the image.

71 **Print Images Using an Online Service**

→ SEE ALSO

72 Share Images Using Email
73 Share Images Using an Online Service

71

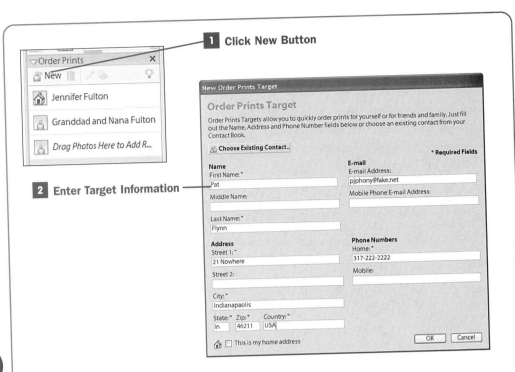

1 **Click New Button**

2 **Enter Target Information**

View Photos in Order Button

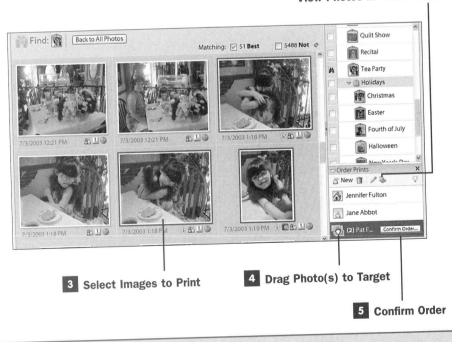

3 **Select Images to Print**

4 **Drag Photo(s) to Target**

5 **Confirm Order**

71 **Print Images Using an Online Service**

If you don't have a photo printer or a printer capable of printing on photo paper, or you're looking for professional results, you can link directly from the Organizer or the Editor to Adobe Photoshop Services (an online service), upload your images, have the service print the images (perhaps with professional corrections), and ship you the results—in some cases, by next-day air!

Before printing, however, you should prepare your images properly: Select each image in the Organizer, send it to the Editor, save the file in PSD format, and make any necessary improvements to the image's color, contrast, saturation, and sharpness. Resize the image as needed to ensure that its print size matches the size you want to use when printing, and that it has a high-enough resolution to produce a good quality print. See **16 Change Image Size or Resolution** for help. Finally, save a copy of your image in a shareable format you can upload to an online service, such as TIFF or JPEG.

The simplest way to order prints from an online service is to use the **Order Prints** palette. There, you set up various *targets* (people to whom you want to ship the finished prints), and then simply drag and drop photos from the Organizer catalog onto a target—so that most of the order information is already completed for you!

1 Click New Button

If you have not set up a target for the person to whom you want the photos sent, do that now. On the **Order Prints** palette, click the **New** button. (To display the palette, choose **Window, Order Prints**.) The **New Order Prints Target** dialog box appears.

2 Enter Target Information

Enter information for the chosen target, completing at least all the required fields (those marked with an asterisk). If you enter other information such as an email address or mobile phone email, this data is added to the **Contact Book** so that you can use it to email photos at a later time.

If this person is already in your **Contact Book**, click **Choose Existing Contact**, select a contact, and click **OK** to copy the contact's information into the dialog box. Click **OK** to save the target. The target appears alphabetically with those listed in the **Order Prints** palette.

▶ TIPS

If you're setting up yourself as a target, enable the **This is my home address** option, which causes your name to appear with a special house icon at the top of the **Order Prints** palette instead of alphabetically by last name. If you enable this option for more than one target, the targets will appear at the top of the palette, listed alphabetically by last name.

To change a target's information, select the target in the **Order Prints** palette and click the **Edit** button (the pencil icon).

71

3 Select Images to Print

After you've prepared each image for printing, in the Organizer, press **Shift** and click the first image in the group you want to upload for printing, and then click the last image in the contiguous group. Alternatively, click the first image, press **Ctrl**, and click each additional image you want to upload for printing.

4 Drag Photo(s) to Target

Drag the selected photo(s) to the **Order Prints** palette, and drop them on the icon for the target to which you want them shipped. You can select other photos, and then drag and drop them to the target as needed.

5 Confirm Order

When you're ready to send the selected photos to the online service, click the **Confirm Order** button next to the target on the **Order Prints** palette. You'll be asked to register for the service, providing your email address and password to use. After you register, you can log on to the online service, then select the print sizes you want for each photo, enter your billing and shipping information, and place the order.

After the images are uploaded, a confirmation screen appears, displaying your order number and an order summary. You'll also receive an email message confirming your order and providing a delivery date. Now simply wait for your selected delivery service to deliver your prints!

71

▶ TIPS

To preview the photos you've collected before you confirm your order, select the target in the **Order Prints** palette and click the **View Photos in Order** button.

You can also order prints by selecting images in the Organizer (or opening images in the Editor) and choosing **File, Order Prints** or (in the Organizer) clicking the **Order Prints** button on the **Shortcuts** bar.

You can print an existing creation using an online service by clicking the **Order Prints** button. Send a new creation to Adobe Photoshop Services by clicking the **Order Online** button on the **Step 5: Share** page of the **Creation Wizard**. Certain creation types (such as a slide show) cannot be uploaded to an online service for printing.

72 **Share Images Using Email**

→ **SEE ALSO**

73 Share Images Using an Online Service
169 Export Your Slideshow

If you have selected your preferred email client in the **Preferences** dialog box, you can send anything you create in Photoshop Elements to anyone who has an email address. Just select what you want to send from the Organizer catalog or open an image in the Editor, decide who to send it to, add a message, and give the order to **Send**. And you can do all this without shutting down or minimizing the Editor or the Organizer window and switching to your email program. You do all the work in Photoshop Elements, and the application then hands off the message to your email client to process and send.

When you send images, tags are sent as well (with the exception of **Hidden** and **Favorites** tags), so if the recipient uses Photoshop Elements, the images will already be tagged when they import them into their catalogs. In addition to individual pictures, you can send creations such as slide shows, photo albums, postcards, and calendars. You also can include sound and video files with your photos, but not in the same email message as you send creations: Only one creation can be included in an email message, and you can't send it with any other item type.

1 **Select Items to Send**

In the Organizer catalog, select one or more items to send. To select contiguous items, click the first item, press and hold the **Shift** key, and click the last item in the group. To select noncontiguous items, click the first item, hold the **Ctrl** key, and click each additional item.

▶ **TIPS**

If no items are selected, all displayed items are included in the email. To send a group of related images, such as the photos of a recent family outing, use the **Find** feature to display them in the catalog. If the catalog is sorted by batch or folder, click the gray bar above a group to select every item in a group.

You can send an image from within the Editor by saving it first and then choosing **File**, **Attach to Email**. The **Attach to E-mail** dialog box appears.

72

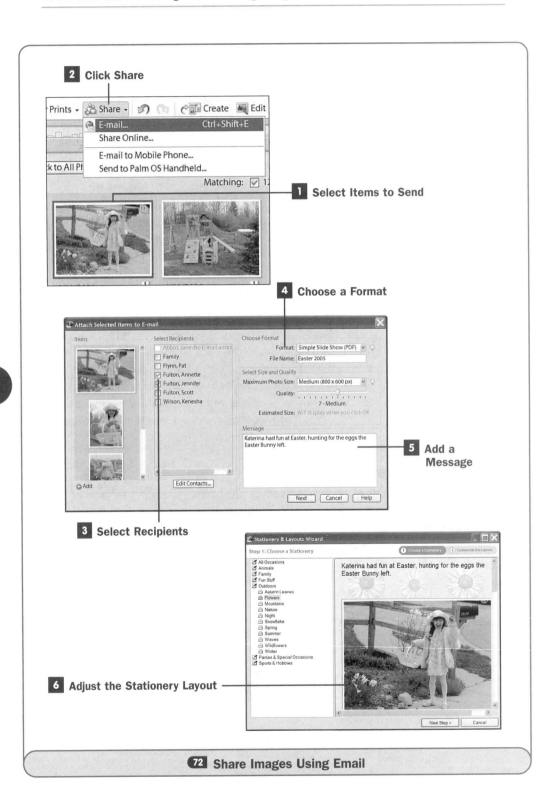

2 Click Share

1 Select Items to Send

4 Choose a Format

5 Add a Message

3 Select Recipients

6 Adjust the Stationery Layout

72 Share Images Using Email

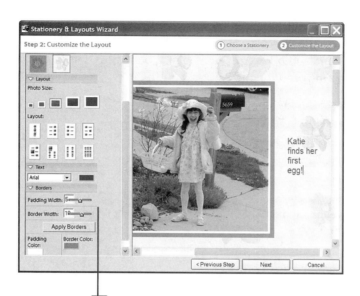

6 Adjust the Stationery Layout

7 Send the Email

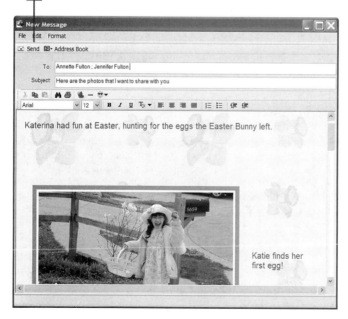

2 **Click Share**

Click the **Share** button on the **Shortcuts** bar. From the menu that opens, select **Email** or **Email to Mobile Phone**. The **Attach Selected Items to E-mail** or **Send to Mobile Phone** dialog box opens. The items you selected to send are displayed on the left.

To email open images from the Editor, choose **File, Attach to E-Mail** or click the **Attach to E-Mail** button on the **Shortcuts** bar. If this is your first time emailing photos, you'll be asked to confirm your choice of email client. Do so and click OK.

▶ **TIP**

To send a creation immediately after making it, click the **Email** button in the last step of the **Creations Wizard**.

3 **Select Recipients**

In the **Select Recipients** section of the dialog box, check one or more of the names in your **Contact Book** to identify those you want to receive the message.

If a recipient's name doesn't appear on this list, click the **Edit Contacts** button to add the name to your **Contact Book**.

▶ **TIPS**

You do not have to designate recipients at this stage. If you are using Outlook or Outlook Express, you can add recipients using the address book of your email client in step 7.

If you forgot an item you wanted to send, click the **Add** button at the bottom left. Select the items to add and click **OK**.

If you've set up Photoshop Elements *not* to use an email client (such as Outlook) but to instead save email attachments directly to the hard disk (choose **Edit, Preferences, Sharing, E-mail Settings** to access these options), then skip step 3. One reason you'd do this is because you want to use your web mail client (such as YahooMail or GMail) or AOL, and not Adobe, Outlook, or Outlook Express. In step 4, you can choose a slide show or file attachments, and set the quality (photo size) you want. The images or PDF file is then prepared and placed in the folder you designated in your preferences.

4 **Choose a Format**

If you are sending a creation, it will be converted to PDF format before sending. Enter a **File Name** for the resulting file and select a **Size and Quality** option.

If you're emailing to a mobile phone, the images are converted to JPEG and attached as individual files in the **Maximum Photo Size** you set. You can choose a similar option when sending to a regular email address by selecting **Individual Attachments** from the **Format** list. Enable the **Convert Photos to JPEGs** option to have the Organizer compress the attachments using JPEG compression and the **Maximum Photo Size** and **Quality** you choose. If you don't convert the images, they are attached to the email as is. Because some email systems place limits on the file sizes they will handle, try to send small files whenever possible so that you do not exceed that limit.

If you're sending images, audio files, or video files to a regular email address (no creations), you can embed them in a fancy background. Open the **Format** list and choose **Photo Mail (HTML)**. To include captions from the catalog, select **Include Captions**.

▶ **NOTE**

Aware that viruses are often planted with embedded graphics, some email systems strip the illustrations from HTML mail and send them as attachments instead.

If you're sending just images to a regular email address, you can combine that can be played on the recipient's computer using Adobe Reader. Select **Simple Slideshow (PDF)**. Type a **File Name** for the file. Adjust the quality of the resulting slide show by selecting a **Maximum Photo Size** and **Quality**.

5 **Add a Message**

If you want to include a message to the people who are receiving the selected items, type it in the **Message** text box. Click **Next**.

6 **Adjust the Stationery Layout**

If you are using the **Photo Mail** format, the message appears in the **Stationery & Layouts Wizard**. Select the stationery to use from those listed on the left. Click **Next Step**, and set options to customize the stationery (such as text font, background color, borders, and layout). For images that don't have a caption, click **Enter caption here** under the image and type a description. These captions are saved to the catalog if you set that option in the **Preferences** dialog box. Click **Next**.

7 **Send the Email**

Organizer prepares the images, creates the message, and hands the result to your email client. At this point, you can do anything the email program allows, including adding or subtracting recipients and editing the message text. Click **Send** to send the email.

72

▶ **NOTES**

Photoshop. You might want to take this opportunity to replace it with something more personal.

If any items you selected were not embedded in the email message or attached for you, you can attach them yourself. Follow the steps for adding attachments using your particular email client. For example, both of the Outlook programs have an **Attach** button. Click it to select the files to attach.

73 Share Images Using an Online Service

→ **SEE ALSO**

71 Print Images Using an Online Service
72 Share Images Using Email

72

As you learned in **72** **Share Images Using Email**, you can use email to quickly send photos to friends and family members, as long as the photos are small enough to travel through the Internet mail system without being rejected by an email server. Small files, particularly if they're compressed for transmission, often leave much to be desired in terms of quality. An additional problem with email is that not everyone has an email connection at home, and many people rely on the service they have available at work. Receiving your pictures on office email systems does not always go over well with employers.

An alternative is to post your pictures on the World Wide Web using Adobe Photoshop Services with Kodak EasyShare Gallery. There, you can display pictures in larger sizes and at higher resolution. Your recipients can check out your images at times convenient to them; using a web browser to view images is much easier for most people than dealing with an email client. Your photos are secure because you decide with whom to share them. If they want, visitors can select images for printing by Kodak.

▶ **NOTES**

Rather than upload your images to Kodak's EasyShare Gallery to share them, you can create an **HTML Photo Gallery**. Most web service providers will let you have a bit of free space for storing files to share. An **HTML Photo Gallery** creation will take your images and build a series of interlinked web pages for you, featuring thumbnails of your images, with links to larger versions. If you don't want to post the pages on the Web or you're not sure how, you can always copy the web pages and supporting folders to a CD instead. The pages will make it easy for even a novice to browse through the images on the CD, using his web browser. See **11** **Make a Creation**.

Another way to share images is with a slideshow, which can also be copied to a CD for sharing. If you create a series of slideshows, you can organize them all on a VCD, which is playable on a DVD player.

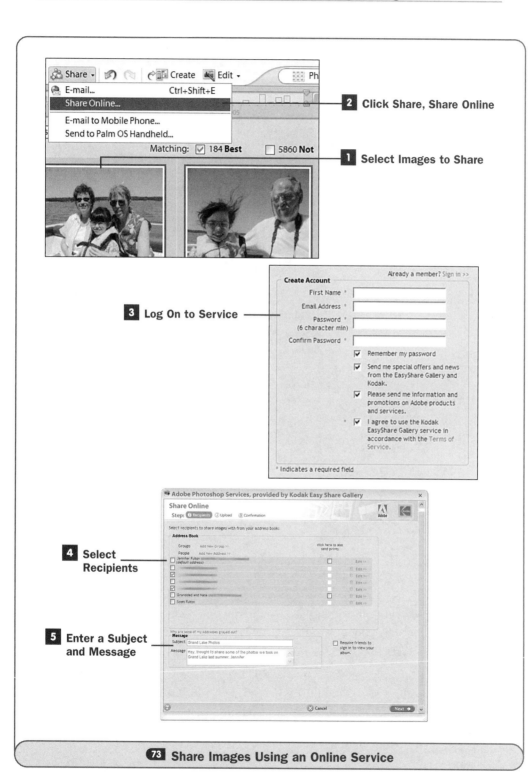

2 Click Share, Share Online

1 Select Images to Share

3 Log On to Service

4 Select Recipients

5 Enter a Subject and Message

73 Share Images Using an Online Service

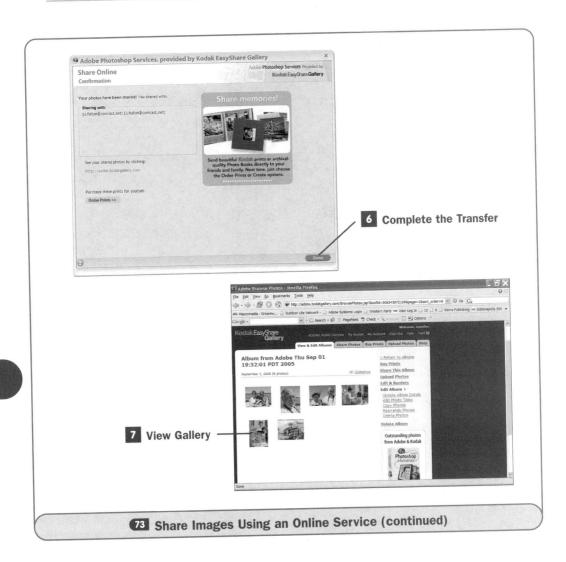

6 Complete the Transfer

7 View Gallery

73

73 Share Images Using an Online Service (continued)

1 Select Images to Share

In the Organizer, review the images you want to share and edit them as needed so that they look their best. You might also want to give each image a text caption to help identify and explain it when people visit your online gallery (see 10 **Add a Text Caption or Note**).

When you're ready, select the images you want to share. To select a single image, click it. To select multiple images, click the first one, press and hold the **Ctrl** key, and click each additional thumbnail. To select a range of contiguous images, click the first image, press and hold the **Shift** key, and then click the last image of the group.

► **TIP**

If the catalog is sorted by batch or folder, you can click the gray bar above a group to select all the items in that group. To display a group of related images, such as all the images of your son or daughter, use the **Find** bar.

2 **Click Share, Share Online**

On the **Shortcuts** bar, click **Share**. From the menu that opens, select **Share Online**. The **Adobe Photoshop Services Kodak EasyShare** dialog box appears.

3 **Log On to Service**

If this is your first time using the service, you'll be asked to set up an account. Enter the required information and select additional options (such as automatic notification of sales and other offers). Read the **Terms of Service** by clicking its link, and enable the check box to indicate that you agree with the terms. Enable the **Remember my password** check box to have the Organizer log you in automatically the next time you use this service.

If you're already a Kodak EasyShare member and you asked that your password be remembered, click **Next**. Otherwise, enter your email address and password, and then click **Next**.

73

► **NOTES**

If you want your password remembered and you forgot to indicate that initially, select the **Remember my password** option when you log in.

Currently, Kodak doesn't charge its customers for sharing pictures through EasyShare. The company makes money on producing photo prints, as well as packages and gift sets based on those prints. Still, you may want to investigate EasyShare's policies and pricing through its website (http://www.easyshare.com) before registering.

4 **Select Recipients**

On the **Step 1 Recipients** screen, a list of people in your **Contact Book** appears on the left. Enable the check boxes in front of the persons with whom you want to share these photos. You can also order prints of the shared photos for each person you selected (assuming that you've also entered street addresses for those contacts)—just click the **click here to also send prints** check box to the right of their names. If you chose this option, a few extra pages in the wizard appear so that you can select the number of prints and their sizes.

▶ TIPS

To add a new address to the **Contact Book**, click the **Add New Address** link, enter the address data, and click **Next** to return to this screen. If a person's name is grayed out, you must complete her information by clicking **Edit** to the right of her name, entering the rest of the email and address data, and clicking **Next** to return.

5 Enter a Subject and Message

Type a **Subject** and **Message** in the email notification form near the bottom of the dialog box. Click **Next**.

6 Complete the Transfer

To make each invitee join Kodak EasyShare and sign in to view the images, enable the **Require friends to sign in to view your album** option. Without this option, anyone who knows the link to the album web page can view your photos. Click **Next** to upload the images.

After the images are uploaded, the **Confirmation** screen appears, displaying the list of names with whom you shared the photos, and a link to the website.

If you ordered prints, the **Confirmation** screen will include an order summary. Click the **Print this Confirmation** button to print a copy of this page.

Click **Done**. The wizard closes, and you return to the catalog. Recipients will receive email invitations to look at your images.

7 View Gallery

You should receive an email confirming the location of the gallery. Open the email and click the **View Photos** link. Your web browser opens; you're taken to the EasyShare Gallery website. Log in to your account using your email address and password and view a slideshow of the image you just uploaded. You can mark images for printing while reviewing the show if you like.

73

When you're through, click the **View & Edit Albums** tab to review other galleries you've shared. Albums appear as icons; click one to view its images. From there, you can rearrange photos, delete photos, and perform other maintenance tasks including, deleting the album totally.

73

PART II

Working with Premiere Elements

IN THIS PART:

13

Getting to Know the Workspace

IN THIS CHAPTER:

Now that you have covered the need-to-know items in Chapter 1, "Start Here," it is time to get started on your first masterpiece. But, before you can get down to the business of creating your movie, you will need a little more help navigating through Premiere Elements.

74   Start a New Project

→ SEE ALSO

75 Customize Your Workspace

76 Nest Your Panels to Save Desktop Space

84 Add Media with the Adobe Media Downloader

Chapter 1 provided enough information for you to start a video project. You might want to get together all the images and clips you will be using to create your video masterpiece. It never hurts to be organized. The more organized you are for a project, the more time you will have to spend on future projects (or other things). In this task, you'll learn how to start a new project in Premiere Elements and give it a name and storage location on your computer.

▶ TIPS

Put together a storyboard, just like the pros. You can download free storyboards and get tips on how to use them; just search for *storyboard* on the Internet. A storyboard is a panel, or series of panels, on which a set of sketches is consecutively arranged depicting the important changes of scene and action in a series of shots (as for a film, television show, or commercial).

Put together a list of images, video clips, and tapes to capture (and place them in their own folder on your computer, with a label such as Next Project). Add thoughts on transitions that you might like to use and what menu might look good for this project. The more you do on the front end, the easier it will be when you start putting your video project together in Premiere Elements.

1 Start Premiere Elements

Double-click the **Premiere Elements** shortcut icon on your desktop or go to the **Start** menu and choose **Premiere Elements**. Premiere Elements launches and the splash screen appears.

2 Select New Project

From the splash screen, click the **New Project** icon. The **New Project** dialog opens.

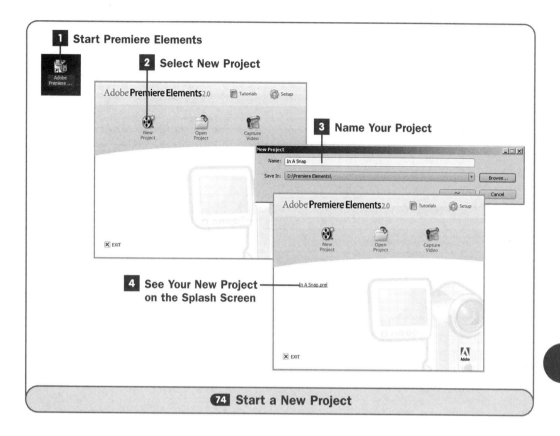

1 Start Premiere Elements

2 Select New Project

3 Name Your Project

4 See Your New Project on the Splash Screen

74

3 **Name Your Project**

In the dialog box that appears, you can either enter a new name or leave the default name **untitled**. You also want to specify an appropriate **Save In** location—this is where Premiere Elements will save the files for this project.

▶ **TIP**

Provide a project name that is descriptive and meaningful for your new project. If you have a second internal hard drive or an external USB 2.0 drive, it is best to use it for storing all your video and project files. If you can designate a second drive solely for video, you will speed up the processes and make your life a whole lot easier. Whatever drive you use, be sure to run the Windows Defragmentation utility on a regular basis. Digital video production software of all kinds runs best on a clean, well-organized drive.

When you've provided a project name and specified a storage location, click **OK**. The Premiere Elements workspace appears, with the new, blank project loaded.

4 See Your New Project on the Splash Screen

The next time you visit the splash screen (when you launch Premiere Elements), your new project will appear in the list of recent projects.

▶ **NOTE**

If you've already launched Premiere Elements, you can still access your existing projects. From the main menu, select **File, Open Project** or **File, Open Recent Project**. You can also return to the splash screen by selecting **File, Close**.

---

75 Customize Your Workspaces

✔BEFORE YOU BEGIN	→ SEE ALSO
74 Start a New Project	76 Nest Your Panels to Save Desktop Space

---

74

Premiere Elements is a task-oriented tool. Many capabilities have been added to the program to allow users to create workspaces that suit their needs. At times, some of the panels and various screens can get in the way of getting the job done. For this reason, the workspaces in Premiere Elements can be changed to each user's requirements.

Many options exist to help you get and stay organized, as well as to help create a smooth workflow. Changing defaults, creating label colors, and shrinking panels can all help make Premiere Elements a versatile tool.

1 Adjust Interface Brightness

From the main menu, choose **Edit, Preferences**. When the **Preferences** dialog box opens, click the **User Interface (UI)** option at the bottom of the list on the left side to open the dialog box to the **User Interface** page. Drag the slider to set the darkness and brightness of the application's user interface. This setting does not affect the way video or any images appear on the screen; only the workspace windows and panels are affected by the changes you make here. You can also specify that you want Premiere Elements to use the Windows background color as its own background color. The best way to see what type of effect this has on your workspace is to change the settings and look at the difference. Moving the slider to the left darkens the UI; moving it to the right lightens the UI. You always have the option to return the UI to the default setting by clicking the **Default Brightness** button.

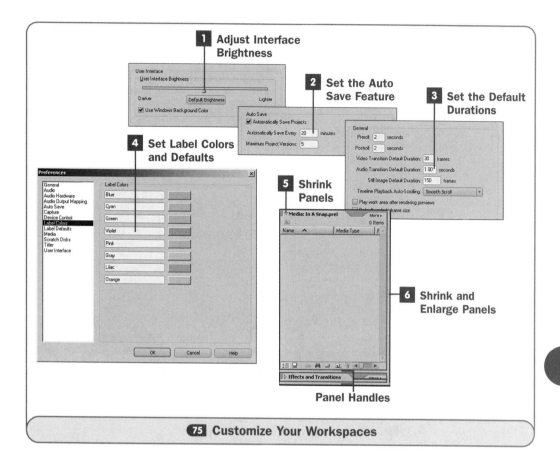

1 Adjust Interface Brightness

2 Set the Auto Save Feature

3 Set the Default Durations

4 Set Label Colors and Defaults

5 Shrink Panels

6 Shrink and Enlarge Panels

Panel Handles

75 Customize Your Workspaces

2 Set the Auto Save Feature

To get to the Auto Save settings, choose **Edit**, **Preferences**, **Auto Save** (if the **Preferences** dialog box is still open from step 1, click **Auto Save** in the list of categories on the left). You use the **Auto Save** feature to save copies of your project at regular intervals. This function saves you tons of time if something bad should ever happen to your computer while you're working on a project. To activate the **Auto Save** feature, check the **Automatically Save Projects** check box (it should already be checked by default). By default the **Automatically Save Every** field is set to **20** minutes and the **Maximum Project Versions** is set to **5**. Changes to these numbers take effect immediately. The **Auto Save** message pops up for a second or two at the set intervals. Because this message can be annoying when you're working on a project, make sure that the setting is low enough to save your work frequently, but not so short that you are constantly being interrupted by it.

▶ **NOTE**

The **Auto Save** feature is not activated until you save your project manually at least one time. After saving manually, the **Auto Save** feature kicks in and saves your project at the intervals set in the **Preferences** dialog box. The project versions are saved to the **Adobe Premiere Elements Auto Save** folder. The saved projects can be used to recover your project after a crash or to start your project over from a specific point. If you select five project versions (the default), five versions of each project are saved. These project files take up very little space, so for safety, more is better.

3 Set the Default Durations

Chances are you will want to change the duration of certain transitions or images at some point in your editing career. These durations can be changed easily under the **General** category in the **Preferences** dialog box. From the main menu at the top of your screen, select **Edit**, **Preferences**, **General** to open the **General Preferences** dialog box.

▶ **NOTE**

Changes to the duration settings are not applied to any items already on the **Timeline** in any project. If you already have all your images and transitions on the **Timeline** and decide the durations are too short or long, there are two options: You can change all the transition and image durations manually (see **90** Set Still Image Duration). This can be quite a time-consuming procedure, as you can imagine. Alternatively, you can remove all the transitions and images from the **Timeline**, change the default durations in the **Preferences** dialog box, and then put the images and transitions back on the **Timeline**. This can also be quite time consuming. The best practice is to think ahead; make sure your defaults will work with your project before you start.

Video transitions, by default, are set to 30 frames because you are working with the NTSC format (that PAL format has a 25-frame transition default). Your video is captured at 30 frames per second, so a 30-frame transition lasts for a total of one second. If your transition is between two clips or images, one-half second would be over the first clip and another one-half second over the second clip. This might or might not work for your project at any given time. It is not difficult to change the duration of transitions manually if there are only a few.

▶ **TIP**

To change the duration of a single clip on the **Timeline**, drag either end of the clip to the right or left. Be careful if there is a clip on either side because dragging over the adjacent clip could overlay the video. If you *want* to overlay the video, just drag the edge of the clip over the adjacent clip and drop it there. If you *do not want* to overlay, press and hold the **Ctrl** key while dragging the clip to move the other clips over to make room for the current clip's new duration. You can use this technique to make clips longer or shorter.

But if you are going to add many images and many transitions, make sure that the default is set where you need it before adding items to the **Timeline**. When changing the duration, remember that you set the value in frames, 30 frames per second for NTSC, 25 frames per second for PAL.

Audio transitions, like video transitions, last for one second by default. Changes you make to the **Preferences** dialog box do not affect any audio files already on the **Timeline**. This setting is given in seconds of audio.

As you drag **still images** from the **Media** panel to the **Timeline**, Premiere Elements needs to determine how long that image will be displayed in your movie. By default, the still image duration is 150 frames. 150 frames divided by 30 frames per second equals a 5-second duration (for PAL, the default still image duration is 125 frames). Again, manually changing the duration of a few still images is not hard or time consuming; changing the duration for hundreds of images is. Think ahead before adding groups of stills to the **Timeline**; is the default duration going to be too long or short? For information about changing the duration of individual still images, see **90** **Set Still Image Duration**.

4 Set Label Colors and Defaults

75

Open the **Preferences** dialog box if it is not already open and click the **Label Colors** category on the left. This page of the dialog box shows the default label colors available. Click the button next to the color name to open a panel that enables you to choose a color. Then click in the box with the color name and change the name to best describe the color you just selected (you can type whatever you like in this text box). After you have chosen and named up to eight colors, it is time to apply them to the various available items.

Click **Label Defaults** in the category list on the left side of the **Preferences** dialog box to see a list of the items to which you can apply the colors you just selected: Folders, Timeline, Video, Audio, Movie (audio and video), Still, and Adobe Dynamic Link. For each of the items listed, choose a color from the drop-down list next to the item. Play around with assigning colors to the items until you have everything the way you like it, just like doing some interior designing. The colors visually separate one type of item from another when you are working on a project to help you achieve a well-organized project.

5 Shrink Panels

Sometimes the panels get in the way of the work you're doing on a project. By clicking the little blue triangle in the top-left corner of a panel, you can shrink, or collapse, the panel. Click the arrow again (it faces right when the panel is collapsed) to open the panel again.

6 Shrink and Enlarge Panels

In **76** Nest Your Panels to Save Desktop Space, you learn to move the panels to make more room in the workspace. Here is another means of creating some extra room in the work area when you need it.

Click and hold on one of the panel sides to drag the panel up and down or right and left. Changing the size of the panel will be a big help when, for example, you need your **Monitor** panel to be a little larger.

---

76 Nest Your Panels to Save Desktop Space

✔ **BEFORE YOU BEGIN**

74 Start a New Project
75 Customize Your Workspaces

75

As you have seen, there are many panels, windows, dialog boxes, and workspaces. With all of that going on in one screen, it can be hard to keep track of where everything is. For this reason, Premiere Elements helps you create the perfect working environment, just for you. The panels can be moved anywhere on the screen. The panels can be nested in with other panels and can also be free floating. In this task, you see how easy it is to customize you own workspace according to your workflow needs.

▶ **NOTE**

After moving or nesting panels, the workspace remains that way until you either make another change or restore the workspace to its default. The panel arrangement remains as you left it even after closing and re-opening the program or opening another project.

1 Drag a Panel

Simply click the tab at the top of the panel and hold down the left mouse button to drag and drop the panel wherever you want it to be. As you drag the panel, notice that three-dimensional boxes appear to show you what space is available for your panel and what it would look like if it were dropped at that location. You can drop the panel in a whole new panel, or drop it in a panel that already contains other panels (this is where the space savings comes in). You can nest all the panels in one panel if you like—the possibilities are pretty much endless. It just depends on what is best for the way you work and what panels you tend to need most often, as well as what panels you don't use. Even the **Timeline** can be nested with other panels. Try moving a few panels to get a good idea of how the process works. Don't worry if things get a little messed up; at the end of this task, we will show you how to restore your workspace.

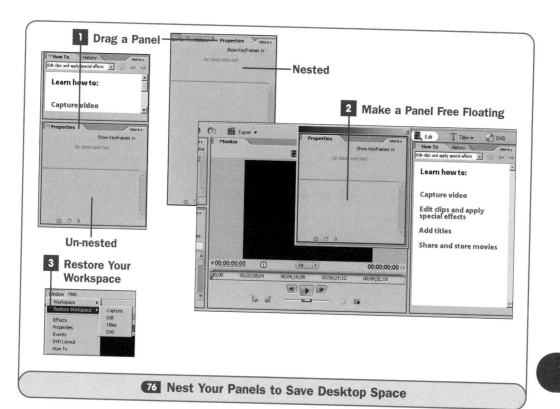

76 Nest Your Panels to Save Desktop Space

2 Make a Panel Free Floating

If you want to have a particular panel floating rather than in another panel, Premiere Elements allows you to do that also. Drag the panel, as described in step 1, to the top of your screen (the taskbar area) and drop it there. That's all there is to it. Now you have a free-floating panel you can move anywhere on the screen. Just be careful where you drop it, or you will nest it within another panel.

3 Restore Your Workspace

The ability to restore your workspace will come in handy on more than one occasion, I'm afraid. As you start moving things around, panels begin to hide themselves or end up in places other than where you want them. In that case, you can always restore the workspace to its default appearance. Choose **Window, Restore Workspace** and then click the workspace you want to restore (**Capture, Edit, Titles,** or **DVD**).

▶ **NOTE**

After you restore a workspace, it remains that way until you again make changes. Changes made to the workspace are not kept in the **History** panel, and there is no way to restore to a custom workspace; you can only restore a workspace to its default configuration.

In its seemingly unlimited ways to customize the application to your needs, Premiere Elements has gone all out with these types of features. Features that allow you to be in control of your own workspace and workflow are very important in the world of video editing, something that Adobe knows a lot about.

76

14

Get the Picture: Capturing Video

IN THIS CHAPTER:

Before you can edit your video, you need to somehow get it into your computer—a process known as *capturing*. (There are means of getting media into your computer other than traditional capture, however. See **84 Add Media with the Adobe Media Downloader.**)

In this chapter, you'll see the ways Premiere Elements can turn the video in your camcorder into video files on your computer. And then you'll learn how to troubleshoot problems when things don't go quite as smoothly as they should.

77   Capture Digital Video Using FireWire

✔ BEFORE YOU BEGIN	→ SEE ALSO
79 Control Your DV Camcorder During Capture	**81** Capture to the Timeline or Media Panel
	82 View Captured Clips
	83 About Troubleshooting Capture Problems

Initially an Apple brand name, the word *FireWire* has become standard shorthand for an OHCI-Compliant IEEE-1394 high-speed data connection. (Sony calls their IEEE-1394 port iLink.)

FireWire connections are fast and, what's more, they're consistently fast. In fact, when it comes to capturing, outputting, or otherwise exchanging data between your camcorder and your computer, there's almost no substitute (with the possible exception of the new USB video standard).

Capturing video into your computer and outputting data from your computer to your camcorder are two of the most processor-intensive tasks a computer can do, and you need a fast, consistent, uninterrupted data flow or it's not going to work.

This is why an IEEE-1394 cable and port is the preferred method for getting digital video, or DV, from your camcorder and back again. (In fact, even when digitizing analog video with a piece of third-party software, FireWire is the preferred method for connecting the digitizer to the computer. (See **80 Capture Analog Video.**)

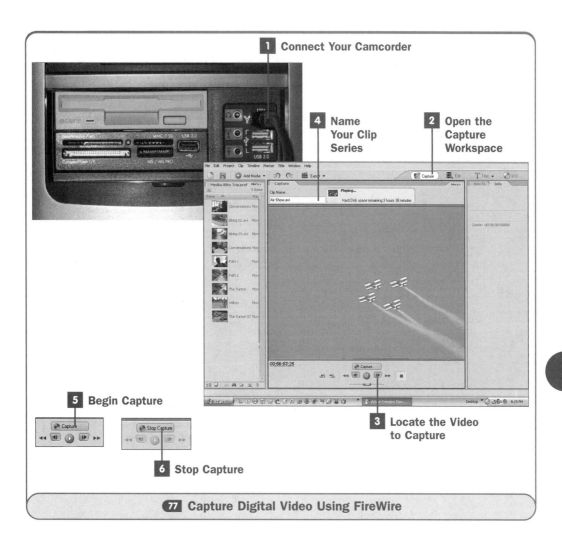

77 Capture Digital Video Using FireWire

1 Connect Your Camcorder

All MiniDV and Digital8 camcorders have a FireWire connection, even if an IEEE-1394 cable wasn't included with the camcorder when you bought it.

Although the risk of a surge damaging your equipment is low, it's best to turn off your camcorder when you connect the cable between your camcorder and your computer. After the two devices are connected, however, set your camcorder to the VTR mode. Windows registers the connection, usually with a sound effect. A connection icon also appears in the lower-right corner of your Windows taskbar. (See **83** About Troubleshooting Capture Problems.)

▶ **NOTES**

If your computer doesn't have a FireWire port and you plan to do any serious video editing, particularly with digital video, a FireWire card is one of the best investments you can make. Virtually any OHCI-Compliant IEEE-1394 card will work. Some even come with a free FireWire cable.

A display at the top of the **Capture Monitor** panel estimates how much room you have to store captured video on your hard drive. It's important to note, however, that it's impossible to fill a hard drive. When free space on your drive gets pretty low, you probably won't be able to continue to capture video.

▶ **TIP**

Windows might not be able to detect a connected camcorder unless the camcorder is also connected with an AC adaptor to a power source.

2 Open the Capture Workspace

Often, simply connecting your camcorder automatically opens the **Capture** workspace. Otherwise, clicking the **Capture** button in the upper-right corner of any Premiere Elements workspace will open it.

3 Locate the Video to Capture

By using Premiere Elements' playback and shuttle controls to operate your camcorder (see **79 Control Your DV Camcorder During Capture**), locate a scene on your videotape you want to capture to your computer. Pause the video where you want to begin capture.

▶ **TIP**

Ideally, capturing video, as well as outputting video back to your camcorder, is a simple process. However, occasionally it doesn't go as smoothly as it should. If you're having problems, such as dropped frames or interruptions, or you simply can't get Premiere Elements to connect to your camcorder, see **83 About Troubleshooting Capture Problems**.

4 Name Your Clip Series

In the **Clip Name** space at the upper-left corner of the **Monitor** panel, drag to select the name (which defaults to the name of your video project) and give it a name.

As Premiere Elements breaks this captured sequence into short clips, these clips are automatically given the names you specify here followed by a numerical sequence beginning with **01**, then **02**, and so on.

77

▶ **NOTE**

By default, Premiere Elements breaks your captured video into clips, based on points at which your camcorder was started and stopped when you initially shot your video. If you'd like to turn off (or on) this feature, click the **More** button in the **Monitor** panel and uncheck (or check) the **Scene Detect** option.

5 **Begin Capture**

Above the playback controls at the bottom center of the **Capture** workspace is the **Capture** button. Click the **Capture** button while your video is paused, and capture begins as your video plays in the **Monitor**.

It's also possible to simply click the **Capture** button while your camcorder video is playing. However, the capture process takes a few seconds to start up, and you might miss a key moment. To ensure that your capture is beginning where you want it to begin, it's best to always begin your capture from the video's paused state.

6 **Stop Capture**

Click the **Stop Capture** button when you want your capture to stop. Your camcorder returns to pause mode and your clip or clips are automatically added to the **Media** panel. To review your captured clips, see **82** **View Captured Clips**.

For custom captures, see **81** **Capture to the Timeline or Media Panel**.

---

78 | **Capture Digital Video Using USB**

✔ BEFORE YOU BEGIN	→ SEE ALSO
79 Control Your DV Camcorder During Capture	**81** Capture to the Timeline or Media Panel
	82 View Captured Clips
	83 About Troubleshooting Capture Problems

78

Several models in a newer class of DV camcorders are capable of transferring digital video to your computer by way of the recently developed USB Video Class 1.0, an extremely fast delivery system for streaming data over a USB 2.0 connection. A powerful new feature of Premiere Elements 2.0 is its capability to connect to these camcorders and then capture their video files at least as effectively as it can capture over FireWire.

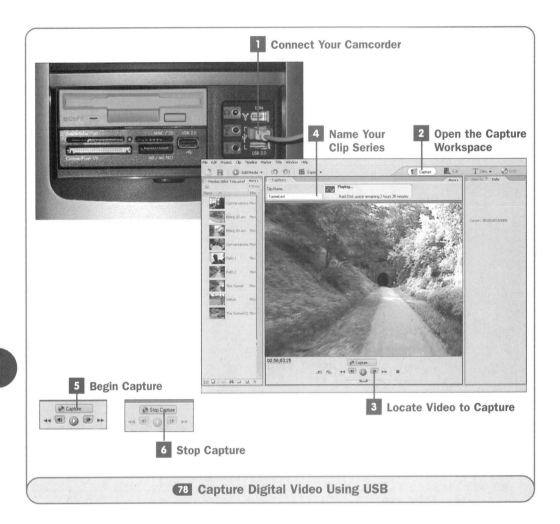

1 Connect Your Camcorder

4 Name Your Clip Series

2 Open the Capture Workspace

5 Begin Capture

6 Stop Capture

3 Locate Video to Capture

78 Capture Digital Video Using USB

It's important to note, however, that the Premiere Elements USB capture system is designed to work only with this still relatively rare class of camcorder. Other USB-connected devices, including MicroMV and DVD camcorders, digital still cameras, picture phones, or other non-DV media should load their files using Premiere Elements's **Media Downloader**. (See **84 Add Media with the Adobe Media Downloader**.)

▶ **NOTE**

Your Windows XP operating system must include Service Pack 2 in order to interface with a USB Video Class device.

■ Connect Your Camcorder

Although the risk of a surge damaging your equipment is low, it's best to turn off your camcorder when you connect the cable between your camcorder and your computer. After the two devices are connected, turn on your camcorder and put it in VTR mode. Windows registers the connection, usually with a sound effect. A connection icon also appears in the lower-right corner of your Windows taskbar.

▶ TIPS

Windows might not be able to recognize a connected camcorder unless it is also connected with an AC adaptor to a power source.

Premiere Elements should recognize your USB Video Class 1.0 camcorder after a connection has been made. However, if Premiere Elements does not recognize your camcorder, click the **More** button in the upper-right corner of the **Capture Monitor** panel, select **Device Control** and, from the **Devices** drop-down list, select **USB Video Class 1.0**. It might also be helpful to click on the **Options** button on this screen and specify the driver for your model of camcorder. (See **83** About Troubleshooting Capture Problems.)

■ Open the Capture Workspace

Often, simply connecting your camcorder automatically opens the **Capture** workspace. Otherwise, click the **Capture** button in the upper-right corner of any Premiere Elements workspace to open it.

78

▶ NOTE

No preview image appears in the **Monitor** panel until you play your first clip of video. After playback has begun, the clip continues to be displayed, even while in the pause mode. When you stop the camcorder, the **Monitor** again displays black.

■ Locate Video to Capture

By using the playback and shuttle controls at the bottom center of the **Capture** workspace to operate your camcorder (see **79** Control Your DV Camcorder During Capture), locate a scene on your videotape that you want to capture to your computer. Pause your video where you want to begin capture.

▶ TIP

Ideally, capturing video and outputting video back to your camcorder is a simple process. However, occasionally it doesn't go as smoothly as it should. If you're having problems, such as dropped frames or interruptions, or you simply can't get Premiere Elements to connect to your camcorder, see **83** About Troubleshooting Capture Problems.

4 Name Your Clip Series

In the **Clip Name** window at the upper-left of the **Monitor** panel, drag to select the name (which defaults to the name of your video project) and then type the name you'd like to give this clip.

As your footage is captured, your clips are automatically named with the name you supply here as well as a sequential number, as in **My Movie 01**, **My Movie 02**, and so on.

5 Begin Capture

Click the **Capture** button just above the playback controls while your video is paused; capture begins as your playback is displayed in the **Monitor** panel.

It's also possible to begin capture by simply clicking the **Capture** button while your video is playing. However, the capture process takes a second or two to start up, and you might miss a key moment. To ensure that your capture begins where you want it to begin, it's best to always start your capture from the video's paused state.

6 Stop Capture

Click the **Stop Capture** button when you want your capture to stop. Your camcorder goes to pause mode and your clip or clips are automatically added to the **Media** panel. To review your captured clips, see **82** **View Captured Clips**. For custom captures, see **81** **Capture to the Timeline or Media Panel**.

---

79 Control Your DV Camcorder During Capture

✔ BEFORE YOU BEGIN	→ SEE ALSO
77 Capture Digital Video Using FireWire	**81** Capture to the Timeline or Media Panel
78 Capture Digital Video Using USB	**82** View Captured Clips
	83 About Troubleshooting Capture Problems

After you've connected your camcorder to your computer and Premiere Elements using a FireWire or USB Video Class 1.0 connection, you can operate the camcorder using the controls in the **Capture** workspace.

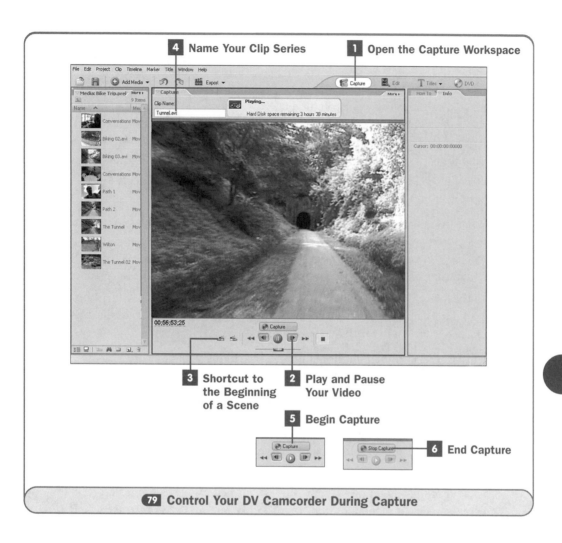

4 Name Your Clip Series

1 Open the Capture Workspace

3 Shortcut to the Beginning of a Scene

2 Play and Pause Your Video

5 Begin Capture

6 End Capture

79 Control Your DV Camcorder During Capture

1 Open the Capture Workspace

Your **Capture** workspace might open automatically when you connect your camcorder. (See **83** About Troubleshooting Capture Problems.) Otherwise, you can jump to it by clicking the **Capture** button in the upper-right corner of any Premiere Elements workspace.

If your camcorder is properly connected to the program, this condition is indicated in the status bar at the top of the **Monitor** panel. The status bar also estimates how much capture time is left on your hard drive.

No preview image appears in the **Monitor** panel until you play your first clip of video. After you play your first clip, the digital time code on the lower-left of the **Monitor** panel tracks along with your camcorder's time code.

The basic playback controls are intuitive and exactly like those in the **Edit** workspace's **Monitor** panel except that here they control your *camcorder* rather than your **Timeline** playback. The slider below the playback controls can be used to shuttle through your video at various speeds, depending on how far to the left or right you drag it.

2 Play and Pause Your Video

Click the **Play** button to start playback on your camcorder and display the video in the **Monitor**. During playback, the **Play** button becomes a **Pause** button.

When you pause the video, the **Monitor** continues to display the paused video until you click the **Stop** button or jump to a new workspace.

3 Shortcut to the Beginning of a Scene

To the left of the playback controls are two shortcut buttons. Click the shortcut button on the left to shuttle your camcorder to the beginning of the current scene on your video.

Likewise, click the second shortcut button to shuttle your camcorder to the beginning of the next scene.

4 Name Your Clip Series

Type the name you'd like to give your clip series in the space in the upper-left corner of the **Monitor** panel (which, by default, is the name of your video project).

As your footage is captured, your clips are named using the name you type here as well as a sequential number, as in **My Movie 01**, **My Movie 02**, and so on.

5 Begin Capture

To begin capture, click the **Capture** button.

It's always best to start a capture from the paused tape position because it takes a second or two for the capture to kick in. Clicking the **Capture** button while the tape is moving can mean missing a key moment in your clip. Starting your capture from the paused state ensures that the capture begins at the exact point in the tape where you want it to begin.

79

6 End Capture

To end capture, click the **Stop Capture** button. Your camcorder automatically shifts back into pause mode as the capture footage is added to your **Media** panel.

Playback automatically stops if you jump to another workspace. When you leave the **Capture** workspace or view your clips, be sure to disconnect or turn off your camcorder (See **82** **View Captured Clips.**)

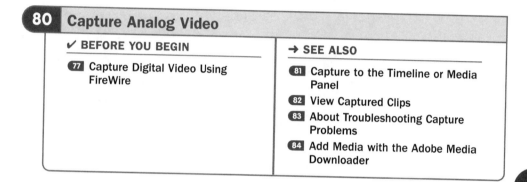

80 | **Capture Analog Video**

✔ BEFORE YOU BEGIN	→ SEE ALSO
77 Capture Digital Video Using FireWire	**81** Capture to the Timeline or Media Panel
	82 View Captured Clips
	83 About Troubleshooting Capture Problems
	84 Add Media with the Adobe Media Downloader

80

Analog video includes most of the video systems consumers have been using for the past couple of decades: VHS, VHS-C, 8 millimeter, Hi-8, and S-VHS.

Capturing analog video can present some unique challenges. Chief among them is that fact that, because computers must store files in digital code to be able to work with them, the video information from an analog camcorder or VCR must be converted, or digitized, as it is streamed in to your computer. Whatever hardware device or set-up you choose to use to capture your video, it is best to do your capturing with Premiere Elements over a FireWire connection.

Although you don't necessarily need a compatible driver to connect a digitizing device, or *DV bridge*, to your computer, Premiere Elements 2.0 comes loaded with drivers for most digitizing devices capable of converting your analog video to DV-AVIs, the preferred digital file format for editing on a PC. If you don't have a bridge but do own both a digital and an analog camcorder, this task offers an alternative method for analog capture, commonly called a *passthrough*.

▶ KEY TERMS

DV bridge—A hardware device that connects an analog camcorder to a computer for the purpose of converting the analog video stream into digital video files.

Passthrough—A method of digitizing analog video by connecting an analog camcorder to a computer through a digital camcorder.

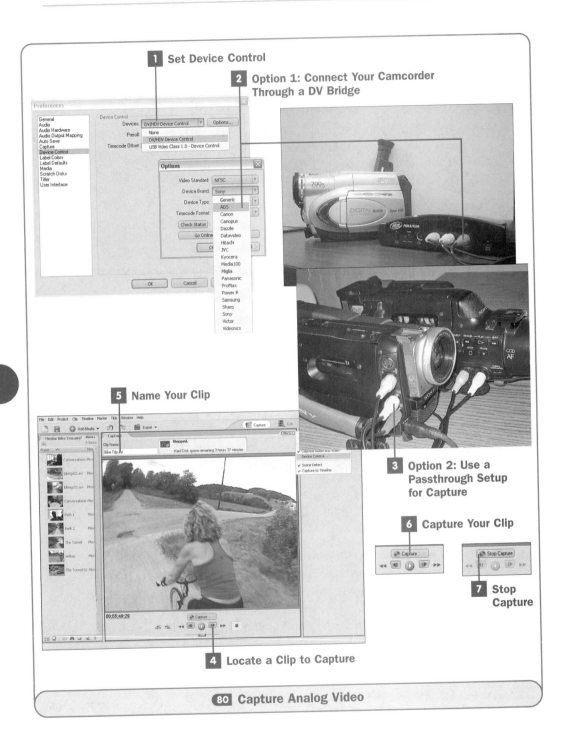

1 Set Device Control

2 Option 1: Connect Your Camcorder Through a DV Bridge

5 Name Your Clip

3 Option 2: Use a Passthrough Setup for Capture

6 Capture Your Clip

7 Stop Capture

4 Locate a Clip to Capture

80 Capture Analog Video

▶ NOTES

Premiere Elements marries nicely with virtually all of the top brands of DV bridges, including many higher-end pieces that can cost more than the average home computer! When searching for a DV bridge, your priority should be to choose one that can convert your analog video files to DV-AVIs, the preferred file format for PC-based video editing.

The two most popular and affordable analog capture devices are the **ADS Pyro AV Link** and the **Canopus ADVC** series, both of which connect easily to your computer with a FireWire connection and produce excellent quality digital files.

▌1▐ Set Device Control

The only real inconvenience in a properly set up analog capture is that you are not able to control your camcorder with Premiere Elements, as you can during DV capture.

With Premiere Elements in the **Capture** workspace, click the **More** button in the **Capture Monitor** panel and select **Device Control**. If you are using a DV bridge, as described in step 2, set **Device Control** to **None** and then click the **Option** button. From the **Device Brand** and **Device Type** drop-down lists, select the device driver you are using for your capture.

If you are using a DV camcorder as a passthrough as described in step 3, set up your DV connection and device control as you normally would.

80

▌2▐ Option 1: Connect Your Camcorder Through a DV Bridge

Premiere Elements 2.0 is capable of creating a custom connection with all major digitizing devices capable of producing DV-AVIs. These devices have standard *AV inputs* for connecting to your camcorder or VCR, and an output port that you can plug into your computer's FireWire port.

▶ KEY TERM

AV inputs—The usually red, white, and yellow (white and yellow only on a monaural unit) RCA-style jacks used for connecting an analog camcorder to a television or other playback device.

After the cabling is connected and your camcorder or VCR is powered on, click the **Capture** button in the upper-right corner of any workspace to open the **Capture** workspace. Click the **More** button in the **Capture Monitor** panel and select **Device Control** to display the **Device Control** page of the **Preferences** dialog box.

Click the **Options** button to display the **Options** dialog box; from the **Device Brand** drop-down, choose your digitizing device brand. From the **Device**

Type drop-down, choose the model number, if possible, or one of the standard or alternative options. (You might have to experiment to find the best generic driver for your device.)

Click the **Check Status** button if your device is listed as being **Offline**. If your device is still listed as being **Offline**, recheck your connections and setup or go to **83** **About Troubleshooting Capture Problems**.

▶ **NOTE**

The **Scene Detect** feature in Premiere Elements is available only for DV capture using IEEE-1394 FireWire or USB Video Class 1.0. You can break your analog footage into clips based on content or timing, if you'd prefer, by using a third-party program called Scenalyzer (available at www.scenalyzer.com) to run your capture. Because the files captured using Scenalyzer are still DV-AVIs when the software is used with one of the digitizing methods recommended here, they can be easily imported and used in your Premiere Elements video project.

3 **Option 2: Use a Passthrough Setup for Capture**

A passthrough setup can be a very effective alternative to using a DV bridge to capture your analog video.

To set up a passthrough, connect your analog camcorder's AV inputs to the AV inputs of a DV camcorder connected to Premiere Elements by FireWire or USB Video Class 1.0. (See **77** **Capture Digital Video Using FireWire** or **78** **Capture Digital Video Using USB** for instructions on setting up your DV connection.)

Ensure that there is no tape in the DV camcorder and set it to VTR mode.

Your analog tape is played through the DV camcorder and across the cable connection to your computer, where Premiere Elements saves it as a DV-AVI. (You are not able, of course, to operate your camcorder with Premiere Elements's playback controls.)

Although this setup usually works quite effectively, every DV camcorder has its quirks, and you might have to do some additional setup, such as ensuring that your DV camcorder's AV inputs are set to receive the incoming signal. Also note that some DV camcorders allow for AV output but not AV input. Naturally, these camcorders are not capable of functioning as a passthrough.

4 **Locate a Clip to Capture**

Operating your analog camcorder with the camcorder's physical playback controls, locate the clip you want to capture.

5 Name Your Clip

Type the name you'd like to give your clip in the space in the upper-left corner of the **Monitor** panel. By default, your clip is given your project's name.

▶ **NOTE**

During analog capture, Premiere Elements will sometimes give you warnings of dropped frames or even abort your capture completely. This is because the program has become confused by the nonstandard connection. If you're receiving these warnings but your clips look fine on playback, you can turn off the warnings and the **Abort on Dropped Frames** option as explained in **83** About Troubleshooting Capture Problems.

6 Capture Your Clip

Start your analog tape rolling at least five seconds before you want to begin capture and immediately click the **Capture** button in the **Monitor** panel. (It takes a few seconds for capture to kick in, so a little extra start-up time is better than too little.)

Your video should play in the **Monitor**, and the **Capture** button becomes a **Stop Capture** button.

7 Stop Capture

Click the **Stop Capture** button to stop your capture. Your new clip is added to the **Media** panel. To review your captured clips, see **82** View Captured Clips.

Stop your video playback with your camcorder's VTR controls or set up for your next clip capture.

---

81 Capture to the Timeline or Media Panel

✔ **BEFORE YOU BEGIN**	→ **SEE ALSO**
77 Capture Digital Video Using FireWire	**82** View Captured Clips
78 Capture Digital Video Using USB	**83** About Troubleshooting Capture Problems
79 Control Your DV Camcorder During Capture	
80 Capture Analog Video	

By default, Premiere Elements captures your video directly to your **Timeline**, a very convenient feature if you plan to simply capture, adjust your clips, and output.

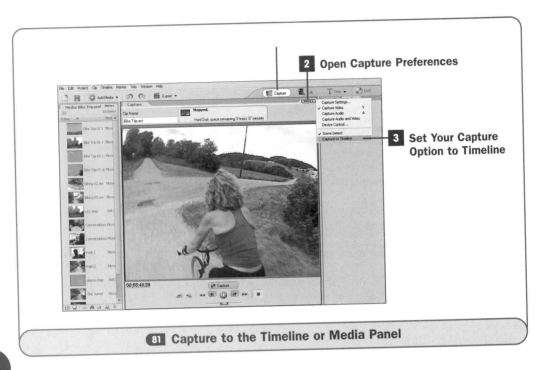

2 Open Capture Preferences

3 Set Your Capture Option to Timeline

81 Capture to the Timeline or Media Panel

81

However, many editors prefer to capture to the **Media** panel only, trimming and ordering their clips before assembling them on the **Timeline**.

Whatever your preference, you can easily change this default setting.

1 Open the Capture Workspace

To open the **Capture** workspace, click the **Capture** button in the upper-right corner of any workspace.

2 Open Capture Preferences

Click the **More** button in the **Capture Monitor** panel.

3 Set Your Capture Option to Timeline

Check or uncheck the **Capture to Timeline** option. Continue the process of capturing your audio or video, as described in the preceding tasks.

82 | View Captured Clips

After you've captured your clips, you can view them right in your **Capture** workspace to ensure that your captures have been successful.

1 Disconnect Your Camcorder

Disconnect or simply turn off the camcorder. This might seem like a superfluous step but, because of the way Premiere Elements diverts resources during capture and output to tape, it can make a real difference in playback. If you leave your camcorder plugged in when you view your captured clips, the video playback often appears jumpy and uneven.

2 Select a Clip

While still in the **Capture** workspace, double-click the clip you want to review in the **Media** panel. This action opens the **Edit Monitor** panel. If your clip doesn't immediately appear in the **Monitor**, double-click it again or click the **Clip View** button at the top of the panel.

3 Play the Clip

Use the playback controls and the shuttle slider in the **Monitor** panel to play the selected clip in the **Edit Monitor** panel.

To keep your workspace from becoming cluttered, you can close the **Edit Monitor** panel.

82

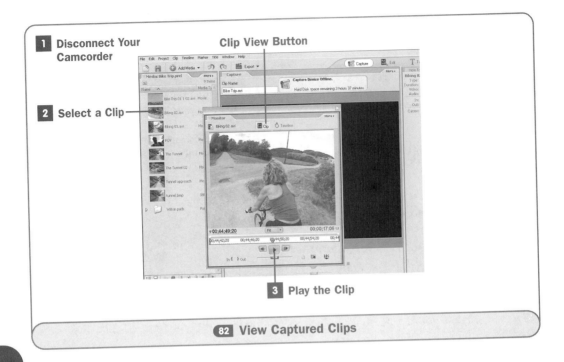

1 Disconnect Your Camcorder

Clip View Button

2 Select a Clip

3 Play the Clip

82 View Captured Clips

82

83   About Troubleshooting Capture Problems

Capture is a vital part of a video editor's workflow. And there are few things as frustrating as not being able to start a project because you can't get your video into your computer.

Unfortunately, capture, along with its companion process of output to tape, is one of the processes most prone to technical challenges—some are related to the amount of power it demands and some are related to the way the operating system's drivers conflict or corrupt as they are affected by other programs installed on your computer.

If you're experiencing challenges connecting your camcorder to Premiere Elements or capturing to the program, here are some troubleshooting suggestions.

Your Camcorder Won't Connect to Windows

If a connection is being made between your camcorder and computer, you'll hear a tone or sound of some sort from your computer registering the connection. Your camcorder will also appear as an icon on the right side of the taskbar at the bottom of the screen. If your computer isn't registering your connection, a closer look at your system can yield some clues as to why not.

With your camcorder plugged in to your computer and turned on, right-click the **My Computer** icon on your desktop, select **Properties** from the context menu, click the **Hardware** tab at the top of the System Properties dialog box, and click the **Device Manager** button to open the **Device Manager** dialog box. Under the **Imaging Devices** category, you should see your camcorder listed.

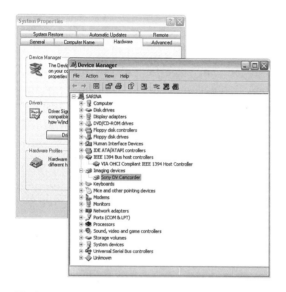

The Windows Device Manager lists your camcorder.

If your device does not appear, you are not making a proper connection—quite possibly the result of a defective or improperly installed USB, USB Video Class 1.0 or IEEE-1394 (FireWire) device. If an unfamiliar driver name appears, your capture driver might have been overwritten or customized by another piece of capture software.

If you suspect that your drivers might be corrupted, there's an undocumented method for refreshing your drivers that, at the very least, won't do your computer or your operating system any harm. With your device connected and turned on, right-click on your device's listing in the **Imaging Devices** section of the **Device Manager** listing and select **Uninstall**. Your device listing temporarily disappears; a few moments later, Windows recognizes your device and installs fresh drivers for it. (If your camcorder or digitizing device came with a CD of its own driver software, be sure to install that software before refreshing your drivers. The hardware's website might provide even more recent driver updates.)

If you are connecting your computer and camcorder using FireWire, check under the listing for **IEEE-1394 Bus Host Controller** to ensure that it is listed as an **OHCI-Compliant IEEE-1394 Host Controller**. Only OHCI-compliant IEEE-1394 FireWire units can be guaranteed to work with Premiere Elements.

▶ **NOTES**

USB Video Class 1.0 connections require Windows XP with Service Pack 2.

Windows is only as good as the drivers it has in its library. Keep your drivers updated by installing any driver software that came with your camcorder or other digitizing device and regularly check the product's website for updates.

Your Camcorder Connects to Windows but Premiere Elements Doesn't Show It As Connected

Unfortunately, programs installed on your computer don't like to share. Video-editing programs are particularly greedy, each one vying for control over your video capture driver. If you have more than one video-editing program installed on your computer (particularly if you're running another version of Adobe Premiere), you might be experiencing a conflict.

In most cases, the most recently installed editing program takes control of the capture drivers. However, sometimes the simple act of opening another editing program transfers control of those drivers back to the other editing program.

83

▶ **NOTES**

Unlike most video-editing programs, Windows MovieMaker seems to freely share capture drivers with other editing programs and virtually never causes a programming conflict. In fact, a good test to find out whether Windows is connecting to your camcorder is to attempt to capture your video in MovieMaker.

Running a version of Adobe Premiere, especially an older version, on the same computer as you're running Premiere Elements has been known to cause capture problems. It's best to uninstall all but your current or preferred version of the software.

If this seems to be your situation, try re-installing Premiere Elements. You can also try re-installing Premiere Elements without uninstalling it, which will give you the option of running the repair utility. If this doesn't solve your problem, you might have to uninstall the conflicting program(s), refresh your drivers (as described in the preceding section), and re-install Premiere Elements as your only DV-AVI editing program.

It might also be worth your while to make sure that all is well in your **Device Manager**, as described in "Your Camcorder Won't Connect to Windows" earlier in this task. Also refer to the "You Can't Control Your Camcorder in Premiere Elements" section, later in this task.

Your Digitizing Device Doesn't Operate with Premiere Elements

Most third-party digitizing devices, particularly those sold to capture footage for export directly to DVDs, do not capture directly into Premiere Elements. These devices usually come with proprietary software and work ideally with that software. In most cases, the files (usually MPEGs) produced by these devices can then be imported into Premiere Elements using the **Media Downloader**.

However, only digitizing devices capable of saving video as DV-AVIs capture directly into Premiere Elements. (See **80** Capture Analog Video.)

On the other hand, many USB-connected digitizing devices work with the **Media Downloader**. (See **84** Add Media with the Adobe Media Downloader.)

To ensure your device is properly set up in Premiere Elements, see the following section.

You Can't Control Your Camcorder from Premiere Elements

Only camcorders connected directly to Premiere Elements by a FireWire or USB Video Class 1.0 connection can be controlled by the program.

If your camcorder is connected to Windows but you aren't making a proper connection with Premiere Elements, go to the **Capture** workspace (click the **Capture** button in the upper-right corner of any workspace) and, in the **Monitor** panel, click the **More** button and select **Device Control**.

Check the **Devices** drop-down menu to make sure that your connection method (**DV/HDV Device Control** or **USB Video Class 1.0 - Device Control**) is selected. If so, click the **Options** button to open the **Options** dialog box.

From the **Device Brand** drop-down list, choose your camcorder or digitizing device. If the specific brand is not listed, select **Generic**. Then open the **Device Type** drop-down list and, if available, choose the model number of your device. If you are using **Generic** or **Alternative** drivers, you might have to experiment with different settings from this second menu.

83

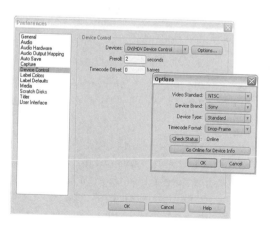

*Check the **Device Control** page of the Premiere Elements **Preferences** dialog box to make sure that the correct capture device is selected.*

If your device is turned on, Windows is registering it as being connected, but its status in this menu is still listed as **Offline**, click the **Check Status** button. If your device is still listed as being **Offline**, check to ensure that you have a proper connection as described in "Your Camcorder Won't Connect to Windows," earlier in this task.

Premiere Elements Doesn't Break Your Footage into Clips During Capture

Premiere Elements breaks your captured footage into clips based on points at which your camcorder was paused during recording. It is a time code–based process, and only works with DV that was captured using a FireWire or USB Video Class 1.0 connection.

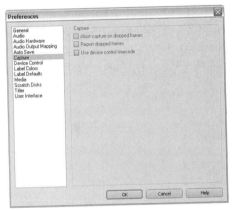

*Capture options in the Premiere Elements **Preferences** dialog box.*

In the **Capture Monitor** panel, click the **More** button and ensure that the **Scene Detect** option is enabled.

Capture Continually Aborts

Your capture aborts for one of three reasons: The data flow cannot be sustained, a process has interrupted the data flow, or Premiere Elements believes you are dropping frames.

Your system might not be able to sustain the necessary data flow for video capture for a variety of reasons, all related to hardware. If your hard drive is too full (if it has less than 10–20GB of free space, for instance), the program has likely run out of space to write its relatively large video files. If this is the case, you might have to clear considerable data off your hard drive or add a larger drive for your captures. (See the "You Receive a Disk Full Error" section, later in this task.)

83

Processes interrupting your data flow can be more challenging. Most new computers can handle the intensive data flow required for video capture. However, computers operating at less than 2GHz or without enough RAM might find background processes and even spyware choking their captures.

Your capture might also abort because of an indication of dropped frames. To override this, use the steps described in the following section.

Capture Continually Shows Dropped Frames Warning

Dropped frames can occur when a process or some other stoppage interrupts your capture. But you can also get a dropped frames warning when the program just can't quite figure out what's going on with your capture. These warnings are quite common when you're trying to capture analog video using a passthrough or DV bridge (See **80** **Capture Analog Video**). They don't always mean, however, that your captured video will be unusable.

Play back your captured video (see **82** **View Captured Clips**). If you find that the video is full of dropped frames and is unacceptable in terms of quality, you might want to turn off some background processes and/or increase your hardware resources.

If you find that your captured video looks acceptable despite these warnings, you can turn off the dropped frame warning by clicking the **More** button in the **Capture Monitor** panel and selecting **Device Control**. In the **Preferences** dialog box that opens, click the **Capture** category in the list on the left side and disable both the **Abort Capture on Dropped Frames** and **Report Dropped Frames** options.

83

You Cannot Capture to an Internally Installed Second Hard Drive

A second drive, one dedicated to your video files, can greatly improve your performance, especially during capture and output to tape. But if you're continually finding your captures aborted or if your captured files look corrupted, your drive is likely set up improperly.

There is some debate about whether it is better to install your second hard drive as a slave channel with your C drive as the master, or whether you should install your second drive as the master on a second channel with your DVD burner as the slave. In our experience, either is acceptable and both should provide for an easy data flow during capture and output to tape.

Of greater importance is that your second drive is properly installed in your BIOS. In most cases in which capture to a second internal drive is problematic, an improper installation in the BIOS is the problem.

When you first boot up your computer, follow the instructions at your logo screen, before Windows starts up, to access your BIOS setup. (Usually you press the **Esc** or **F1** key.) If your drives are set up properly, you should see them listed as drives in this setup area. Otherwise, follow the necessary steps to set up your hardware. Remember that your hardware must be set up here—regardless of whether it is set up in your operating system—for it to function properly.

You Cannot Capture to an External Hard Drive

The challenges of capturing to an externally connected drive usually have to do with the limitations of the connection. An external drive that is connected to your computer with a FireWire connection might have problems maintaining the data flow of a video capture because it is sharing the line with your camcorder's incoming video data. This is definitely the case if you are using a router of some sort so you can have both devices attached to the same FireWire card at the same time. As a rule, it's not a good idea to have both your camcorder and an external drive attached to your computer by FireWire.

You might be able to capture your camcorder's video over a FireWire connection to an external drive connected to your computer by USB 2.0. A USB 1.0 connection for your external drive, however, is not able to handle the necessary throughput to accept video files as they are being captured.

83

You Receive a Disk Full Error

Although you might believe you still have room on your hard drive, it's technically impossible to literally fill a disk. Your operating system and other programs are continually writing temporary files to and reading temporary files from your disk. And huge files, such as video captures, often require large, contiguous blocks of space.

Try to keep at least 10–20GB of space available on your hard drive to ensure smooth operation of your system. (Encoding for DVD output can require much, much more.

In short, the less free space you have on your hard drive, the more likely you are to run into processing errors. If you find the free space on your disk getting a bit lean, move or delete some of your files to make more room or install a larger hard drive. Giving your programs and your operating system lots of breathing room, especially when working with extremely large files, will definitely save you a lot of heartache in the long run.

15

Adding Media

IN THIS CHAPTER:

Being able to capture and edit your video is great; but what if you would like to add more? This chapter covers all the other types of media you can add to your project. It also discusses how to perform some simple edits on the front end, before your clips are actually on the **Timeline**.

You might want to add many file types to your movie. Sometimes you might find short clips on the Internet you would like to download and use.

http://www.archive.org/details/prelinger
The Prelinger Archives have many videos that can be downloaded. Some of these date back to the early 1900s. Many of the clips are available in a number of formats and are in the public domain. This can be a fun place to search for clips that will add a special touch to your movie.

One creative way of enhancing your movie is to add still images along with the video. To do that, you have to import still image files from your hard drive. Whether the original source was from a digital camera, a scanner, or the Internet, you can add those still images to your movie. Another fun addition covered in this chapter is the Counting Leader (you know, the little countdown before the movie starts).

You will also learn how to extract video from a non-copy-protected DVD. This way, you can get clips from previous projects into new ones, even if you don't have the original files anymore. You can also download still images directly from your digital camera. So let's see what the **Media** panel is all about.

84   Add Media with the Adobe Media Downloader

→ **SEE ALSO**

170 Make an Instant Slideshow in Premiere Elements
159 Move Images Between Premiere Elements and Photoshop Elements

You can add media from a various number of sources: DVDs, images and video from your hard drive, images stored on removable drives, or images from a digital camera. Premiere Elements makes it very simple to add image and video files to your projects with the Adobe **Media Downloader** and the **Add Media** button.

1 Select Add Media from Files or Folders

Click the **Add Media** button in the taskbar and select **From Files or Folders**. The **Add Media** dialog box opens.

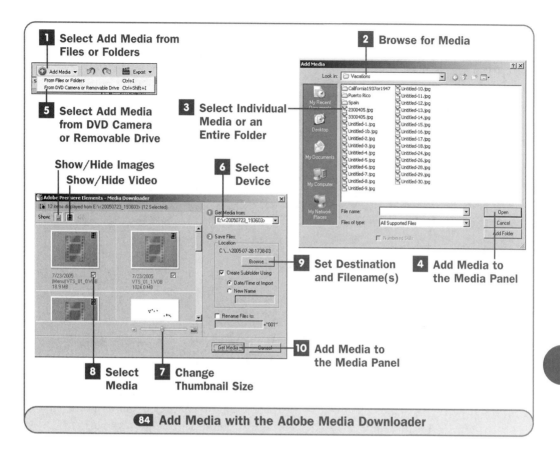

1 Select Add Media from Files or Folders

2 Browse for Media

5 Select Add Media from DVD Camera or Removable Drive

3 Select Individual Media or an Entire Folder

Show/Hide Images
Show/Hide Video

6 Select Device

9 Set Destination and Filename(s)

4 Add Media to the Media Panel

10 Add Media to the Media Panel

8 Select Media

7 Change Thumbnail Size

84 Add Media with the Adobe Media Downloader

2 Browse for Media

In the **Add Media** dialog box, you can go browsing for images or video that you want to use in your project. From the **Look in** drop-down list, choose the drive or main folder in which you want to look for media.

3 Select Individual Media or an Entire Folder

To select multiple media files, press the **Ctrl** key and click the images you want to bring into your project. Alternatively, click to select an image, press the **Shift** key, and use the down-arrow key to select consecutive images. If you want to add all the images in a folder to the **Media** panel, just click to select the folder.

4 Add Media to the Media Panel

If you have selected a number of images inside a folder, click the **Open** button to add those images to the **Media** panel. If you selected an entire folder, click the **Add Folder** button.

▶ **NOTE**

After adding an audio file or a video file that contains audio, Premiere Elements performs a scan of the audio. At the bottom-right side of the screen you might see the message "Conforming audio" or "Generating peak file." This process is normal and is needed
for Premiere Elements to play back the audio properly. Depending on the size of your file
and the speed of your computer, this process can take anywhere from a few seconds to
more than 10 minutes.

5 Select Add Media from DVD Camera or Removable Drive

To add media that's located on a DVD, digital camera, or a removable drive,
click the **Add Media** button and select **From DVD Camera or Removable
Drive**. This command takes you to the **Adobe Media Downloader** dialog box.

6 Select Device

When the **Media Downloader** first opens, the center area, where the media is
displayed, is empty. You see a message in that area that says, "Please select a
device to get media."

The **Get media from** drop-down list at the top-right side of the screen is where
you select the device from which you want to retrieve the media. If you have
only one device (such as a digital camera) connected to your computer, that
device is the only option in this list. If, however, you have multiple DVD drives
and have inserted a DVD in each one, plus you have connected your digital
camera, you can select any of these devices from the **Get media from** list.

The combo box displays the message "Select a Device;" click the down arrow
and select the device that holds the media you want to add to the **Media**
panel. After the device is selected, the images appear automatically in the
Media Downloader's importable files area.

7 Change Thumbnail Size

At the bottom center of the screen there is a slider. Move the slider to the
right to make the images in the center part of the screen larger; move the
slider to the left to make the images smaller.

▶ **NOTE**

The **Adobe Media Downloader** dialog box can be resized by dragging the sides of the
dialog box in or out. The dialog box does have a minimum size, however, and will not let
you make it smaller than that minimum.

8 Select Media

Each media item shown in the center of the box has a filename and check box. The filename tells you something about the file and its size. Click to place a check in the box under each file that you want to download into the **Media** panel for the current project. There are two buttons at the top of the **Media Downloader**: One is a small framed picture icon and is used to show or hide the images in the importable files area. The other is a small film icon that is used to show or hide the video in the importable files area.

9 Set Destination and Filename(s)

On the right side of the screen are various **Save Files** options for the destination and name of the files you are going to download. You can browse for a destination folder for the files. You can also have the **Media Downloader** create a subfolder for you with options of date/time and name. You can even give each file a name of your choice, followed by an incrementing number starting with 001 (such as **MyMediaFile001**, **MyMediaFile002**, and so on).

10 Add Media to the Media Panel

Now that you have selected the media files to be downloaded and specified where you want these files stored on your computer, click the **Get Media** button. The files are added to the **Media** panel and saved in the location you selected. The default location is **My Documents**, **My Videos**, **Adobe**, in a new subfolder named with the date and time.

85

---

85 Add Special Media Clips

→ SEE ALSO

95 Trim a Clip on the Timeline

121 Control a Video Track's Opacity over Time

Premiere Elements comes with four clips that will become quite valuable to you and your movies. The clips include Bars and Tone, Black Video, Color Matte, and a Universal Counting Leader.

1 Open the Context Menu and Choose New Item

Find an empty area in the **Media** panel and right-click it. This action brings up a context menu with various options; the third item down is **New Item**.

Move your mouse to highlight the **New Item** selection; another menu drops down. This submenu holds all the special media clip choices.

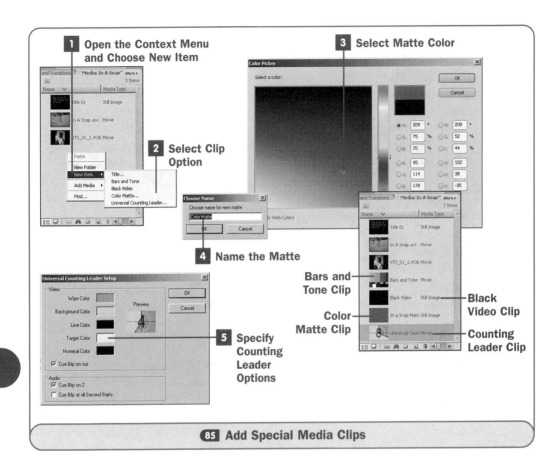

85 Add Special Media Clips

2 Select Clip Option

From the **New Item** submenu, select the name of the clip you want to add to the **Media** panel (and eventually to the **Timeline** and your movie).

You might have seen something similar to a **Bars and Tone** clip come up on your television set from time to time. (This kind of clip is also known as a *test pattern* or *test screen*.) The special clip in the **New Item** submenu is called **Bars and Tone** because that is what you see and hear: There are colored bars that appear on the screen and a very audible tone to go along with it. To add the **Bars and Tone** clip to the **Media** panel, select that option.

▶ **TIP**

Use the **Bars and Tone** clip at the end of your movie to remind you when the movie ends. That way you will never have to wait and wonder if there is another clip coming up.

The **Black Video** clip is just what it says, a clip of nothing but black. To add the **Black Video** clip to the **Media** panel, select that menu option.

▶ **TIP**

The **Black Video** clip is great for separating clips and for using as a background for text-only titles.

Another clip option is the **Color Matte**. Similar to the **Black Video** clip, the **Color Matte** clip allows you to choose from millions of colors. This is an excellent tool for adding color background to your slideshows along with many other uses. The **Color Matte** clip also gives you the ability to add a White Video, which works well as a background for a title with black or dark-colored text. The **Color Matte** clip has many uses, and in time you will probably think of them all. If you select the **Color Matte** option, you will be taken to the **Color Picker** dialog box (continue with step 3).

▶ **TIP**

You can export the **Color Matte** clip, add a cutout to the matte in Photoshop Elements, and import the clip back into Premiere Elements. Then you can use the edited matte as an overlay for a title or intro clip.

The next clip option is the **Universal Counting Leader**. Leaders are used to mark the beginning of a roll of film. You sometimes see them at the start of a movie, counting down from 10 to 1 with a few beeps thrown in. Many people like to have the countdown at the beginning of their movies, and it is a very popular addition. Premiere Elements gives you one counting leader clip option, but many ways to enhance and customize it.

85

▶ **TIP**

Be sure to give your **Color Matte** a pertinent name. Use a name that will help remind you of its purpose, and where it will be used (such as **pink matte for baby video**).

3 Select Matte Color

In the **Color Picker** dialog box, choose a color for your matte. You can choose from millions of colors, or from a more limited selection of web-safe colors. Simply pick the color you want the matte to be and click **OK**.

4 Name the Matte

After you have chosen the color for your **Color Matte** clip and clicked the **OK** button, you are asked to name your matte. Simply type the new name for the matte in the text box and click **OK**. Your new **Color Matte** clip is added to the **Media** panel.

5 Specify Counting Leader Options

If you select the **Universal Counting Leader** option from the **New Item** submenu, the **Universal Counting Leader Setup** dialog box opens.

You can change the color of any object on the counting leader screen—from the target to the number and the wipe. To select a new color for that object, click the color box next to the object's name. The **Color Picker** appears, offering you a choice of millions of colors. Because you can select a different color for each of the objects (**Wipe Color, Background Color, Line Color, Target Color,** and **Numeral Color**), the combinations are limitless. You can also set the audio cue blips—the little *blip* noises you hear during the countdown. The options are **Cue Blip on Out, Cue Blip on 2,** and **Cue Blip on all Second Starts**. The counting leader clip is a fun clip to play around with.

After you have set your sound options and colors for the counting leader, click the **OK** button to add the **Universal Counting Leader** clip to the **Media** panel.

85

86 Trim Clips in the Media Panel

✔ BEFORE YOU BEGIN	→ SEE ALSO
84 Add Media with the Adobe Media Downloader	**95** Trim a Clip on the Timeline
	98 Remove a Section of a Clip
	100 Remove Audio and Video from a Clip

You can perform some simple edits before moving your clips to the **Timeline**. The **Timeline** is where you do your precise editing—adding effects and transitions—on the way to your finished product. If you are like most videographers, you end up capturing more video than you can use in the final movie project. Sometimes you have no choice but to add an entire clip when all you want is a small piece of it. This task explains how to trim those clips down to just the size you need while the clip is still in the **Media** panel. One of the great things about Premiere Elements is that it is a nonlinear editing system, which means that any clips you happen to trim or cut into pieces actually remain intact. The process of editing the clips on the **Timeline** never harms the original file in any way. You can add that original file to other projects over and over—in its original state. All information about the clips and what has been done to edit them is stored in the Premiere Elements project files.

Even if you have already dropped the clip on the **Timeline**, you can extract a small piece to be used again, without having to drop the whole clip onto the **Timeline** a second time.

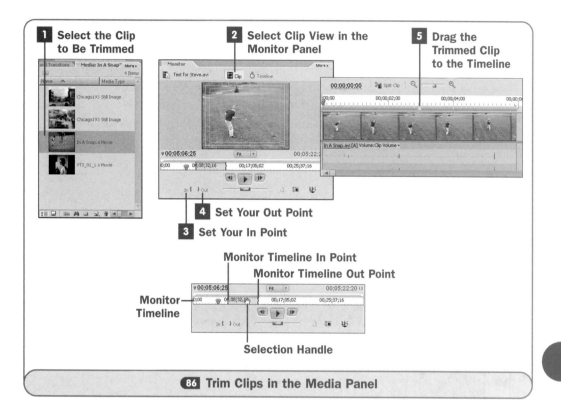

1 Select the Clip to Be Trimmed

2 Select Clip View in the Monitor Panel

5 Drag the Trimmed Clip to the Timeline

4 Set Your Out Point

3 Set Your In Point

Monitor Timeline In Point

Monitor Timeline Out Point

Monitor Timeline

Selection Handle

86 Trim Clips in the Media Panel

86

▶ **NOTE**

Before you begin this task, make sure that you have at least one video clip added to the **Media** panel.

1 **Select the Clip to Be Trimmed**

Click the clip in the **Media** panel that you want to trim. This action highlights the clip. Double-clicking the clip in the panel also works; the clip opens in the **Monitor** panel. You can also drag the clip to the **Monitor** panel and drop it there. (If you double-click or drag and drop the clip, continue with step 3.)

2 **Select Clip View in the Monitor Panel**

With your clip highlighted, click the **Clip View** button in the **Monitor** panel. This action opens the selected clip in the **Monitor**. If you double-clicked the clip in step 1, the clip should already be visible and the **Clip View** button already engaged.

3 Set Your In Point

First find the scene you want to add to your project. Use the shuttle and VCR controls or drag the CTI along the timeline in the **Monitor** panel to find the beginning of the scene you want to keep from the current clip. When you have the beginning frame of your scene in the **Monitor**, click the **In** button to set your *In point*. You have just marked the beginning point of your video clip that will be added to the **Timeline** later.

▶ **TIP**

With Premiere Elements, you can choose to trim audio and video together, audio only, or video only by clicking the **Audio/Video Toggle** button.

▶ **NOTE**

The shuttle is a great tool and can show the video at fast or slow speeds in the **Monitor** panel. The VCR controls can be used to play the video at normal speed; use the **Step Forward** button to advance one frame at a time; use the **Step Back** button to reverse through the video one frame at a time. These controls give you the ability to set precise **In** and **Out** points. Your **In** and **Out** points can be as close together or as far apart as you like.

86

4 Set Your Out Point

Just as you located the beginning of the scene to set the **In** point, use the controls to advance the video to find your ending or **Out** point. When you find the place where you want the scene to end, click the **Out** button.

As you set your initial **In** and **Out** points, the selected area appears in the **Monitor Timeline**. You can also grab the **In** and **Out** points on the **Monitor Timeline** and drag to the right or left to set new **In** and **Out** points. You can also grab the selection handle and drag all of the selected area right or left along the **Monitor Timeline**.

5 Drag the Trimmed Clip to the Timeline

You have just created one small clip out of the larger clip. The **In** point you set is the beginning and the **Out** point is the end of your new subclip. Click the clip in the preview window (any area that shows your clip will do) in the **Monitor** panel, drag it to the **Timeline**, and drop it there. Only the trimmed section of the original video clip is now on the **Timeline**. The entire clip still remains in the **Media** panel to be used again.

For example, you can go back to the **Monitor** panel and set new **In** and **Out** points for the original video clip to create a different subclip. You can then drag that new trimmed clip to the **Timeline** as well.

▶ **NOTE**

You can set only one **In** and one **Out** point each time you trim a clip.

---

87 | **Grab a Still from Video**

✔ BEFORE YOU BEGIN	→ SEE ALSO
84 Add Media with the Adobe Media Downloader	**89** Scale and Position a Still
86 Trim Clips in the Media Panel	**148** Customize an Image as a Chapter Marker
	150 Customize a Menu with Any Background
	150 Apply a Quick Fix

Eventually, you will look at captured video and decide it would be nice to grab a still image from the video footage. Sometimes you get a great shot with your camcorder and wish you would have used a camera. These great shots *can* be exported as still images with Premiere Elements in a few simple steps. The stills you capture from your video footage can be added to your project automatically and also saved to your hard drive.

▶ **NOTE**

The still is saved as an interlaced 720×480 pixel image in the format you select in step 4. The quality of video stills is a bit low for printing—although a 4"×6" photo print might be satisfactory. The resolution of the extracted still image also depends on the source of the clip (analog video from a VHS tape or video from a DV camcorder). If you want to print your still image, you might have to de-interlace it in Premiere Elements or with Photoshop Elements. If you use the image in your project and burn it to a DVD, the interlaced image will look just fine when viewed on a TV screen. For computer viewing, just as with printing, the still image must be de-interlaced to get a clearer image.

1 **Place a Clip in the Monitor View**

Select the clip from which you want to grab the still image. You can select a clip from the **Media** panel or one from the **Timeline**. Select the clip and click the **Clip View** button at the top of the **Monitor**, or simply double-click the clip. The clip appears in the **Monitor** view. Scrub through the clip to locate that one frame that is a keeper by using the VCR and shuttle controls. When the image you want to grab appears in the **Monitor** view, continue with step 2.

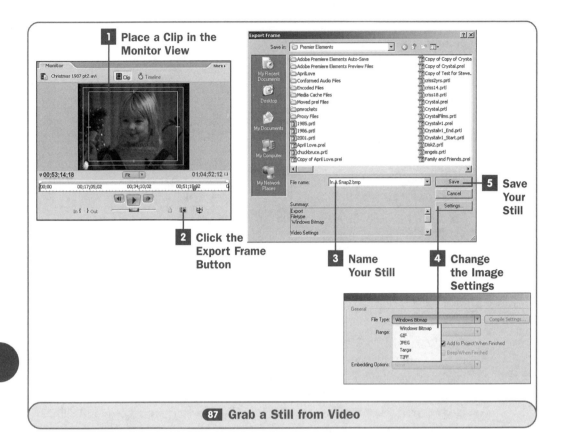

1 Place a Clip in the Monitor View

2 Click the Export Frame Button

3 Name Your Still

4 Change the Image Settings

5 Save Your Still

87

87 Grab a Still from Video

2 Click the Export Frame Button

The image you see in the **Monitor** view is the image that will become your still. To grab this still, click the **Export Frame** button (the camera icon). The **Export Frame** dialog box appears.

▶ **TIP**

Your video is a mass of frames; 30 frames per second to be exact. With 30 frames per second to choose from, there must be one that is "just right." Use the **Step Forward** and **Step Back** buttons in the VCR controls to move the clip one frame at a time until you find just the right one.

3 Name Your Still

Decide on a name for your clip and type it in the **File name** text box. You can also select the directory where you would like the image to be placed from the **Save in** drop-down list at the top of the dialog box.

4 Change the Image Settings

Click the **Settings** button to open the **Export Frame Settings** dialog box. From the **File Type** drop-down list, select the format in which you want to save the still image: **Windows Bitmap**, **GIF**, **JPEG**, **Targa**, or **TIFF**. Depending on your selection, other options become available.

▶ **TIP**

If you save your image as a GIF, you will have the option of a transparent background. However, many videographers choose the TIFF format because it has less compression and holds its quality better after editing and copying.

5 Save Your Still

After you have made any desired changes in the **Export Frame Settings** dialog box, click the **OK** button and click the **Save** button in the **Export Frame** dialog box. Now your still image is preserved on your hard drive for this project (and possibly for future projects) as well as being added to the **Media** panel for this project.

▶ **TIP**

Still images grabbed from video clips and used in your project make great backgrounds for titles and DVD menus.

87

16

Working with Stills and Graphics

IN THIS CHAPTER:

Chances are you'll regularly use still photos and graphics in your video projects. They're a great way to compliment your video footage and, when properly used, a still can be every bit as exciting and full of movement as a video clip. (See ⑪⑧ **Add Motion to a Still** and ⑪⑨ **Pan and Zoom Still Images a la Ken Burns** for ways to bring your still photos and graphics to life.)

Premiere Elements offers many features that help you make the most of your stills and graphics, including some powerful automatic features (see ⑰⑩ **Make an Instant Slideshow** and ⑰① **Change Slides to the Beat of Music**).

Before you bring a photo or graphic into Premiere Elements, however, you'll need to make sure it's properly formatted and prepared. In ⑧⑧ **Prepare a Still for Video**, you learn how to ensure that the graphic or photo you put in looks great when you output it as video.

---

88 Prepare a Still for Video

✔ BEFORE YOU BEGIN	→ SEE ALSO
⑧④ Add Media with the Adobe Media Downloader	⑧⑨ Scale and Position a Still
⑧⑦ Grab a Still from Video	⑨⑩ Set a Still Image Duration
	⑪⑨ Pan and Zoom Still Images a la Ken Burns
	①⑥ Change Image Size or Resolution

Although they share many basic features, a digitized photo and digitized video are two very different media. Although Premiere Elements does its best to render your photo into a video format, an improperly prepared photo can often produce some unfortunate results in your project, and photos with unnecessarily high resolution can cause extremely long rendering times and even complete system lockups.

Premiere Elements accepts a wide variety of graphics file formats including TIFs, BMPs, JPGs, PNGs, GIFs, PDFs, EPSs, and even native Photoshop (PSD) and PhotoDeluxe (PDD) files. Your choice of graphic format will often be a matter of convenience. However, there are definite advantages (and disadvantages) to each format type.

There are two prime considerations when selecting a format for your graphic. First, consider the amount and type of compression the file format uses. JPEGs, for instance, are relatively small graphics files. However, they also use a compression system that, at higher levels, can actually change or even damage the details of your graphic. Whether the effect this type of compression has on your file is at an acceptable level and worth the trade-off for a smaller file depends on your personal feelings and how you plan to ultimately use this graphic.

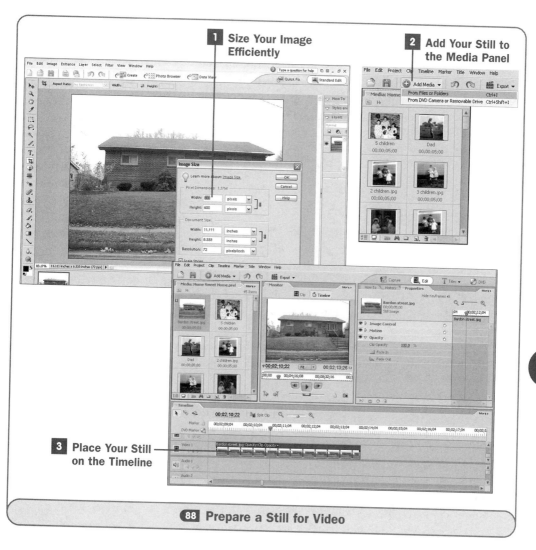

1 Size Your Image Efficiently

2 Add Your Still to the Media Panel

3 Place Your Still on the Timeline

88

88 Prepare a Still for Video

The second consideration in selecting the ideal format for your graphic has to do with the file's capability to carry an alpha channel. Alpha channels can be a powerful aspect of your graphics workflow, as you can see in **134** Frame Your Video with an Image.

Tagged Image Format (TIF or TIFF) files are one of the most commonly used image formats. Because they are relatively uncompressed, they are the preferred format of professional designers. A TIF can be opened, modified, and resaved indefinitely without any loss or damage to the image data (unlike more compressed file formats such as JPEGs), and they are far and away the most hardy digital image format in use today.

An added advantage of TIFs is that they can also save layers of images. This means that if you've created an image sized or shaped differently than your canvas in Photoshop Elements and you leave your background layer blank, your image is displayed in Premiere Elements with the transparent background carried as an alpha channel, displaying as transparent in Premiere Elements. (Technically, this is because Premiere Elements reads the transparent areas as an alpha channel. See 134 **Frame Your Video with an Image**.)

The *PSD* format is a native Photoshop file. PSD files can be imported into Premiere Elements with their alpha channels, or transparent areas, displayed as transparent. Additionally, Premiere Elements and Photoshop Elements are designed to work hand in hand; for a variety of reasons, PSD is an ideal format for bringing Photoshop and Photoshop Elements graphics into Premiere Elements.

Bitmap (BMP) is an older file format created by Microsoft in the early days of personal computers. Although BMPs are not the most efficient size-wise, they are a perfectly acceptable graphics format in which to save your video graphics.

Named for the Joint Photographic Experts Group, *JPGs* (also known as *JPEGs*) are perhaps the most common graphics format used by consumers. Most digital still cameras save their photos as JPEGs because the format allows for a high compression of the image data and a much smaller file size than TIFs. Unfortunately, the smaller file size comes with a price. Repeated saving of JPEGs, especially at higher compression levels, can damage the image data, resulting in corrupted pixels, particularly in the finer details of your photo and at color breaks.

In most cases, however, a first- or second-generation JPEG file is perfectly acceptable for your video—the exception being in situations in which the finer details of your graphic are going to be scrutinized (as when you're applying a major scaling effect), when you are planning to use the Chromakey effect on your photo, or you are applying a color substitution. Because JPEGs use a compression system that averages the color values of pixels near color breaks, any precise effect applied to a color might appear with ragged edges. In these cases, a TIF or BMP might be a better graphic format choice.

Portable Network Graphics (PNG, and pronounced *ping)* files were initially developed for the Internet. For Premiere Elements's needs, the chief advantage of this format is that it can be created with transparent areas that remain transparent when the image is placed in your video timeline.

The *Graphic Interchange Format (GIF)* was developed by CompuServe and is correctly pronounced *jiff*. This format was initially developed for the Internet and has advantages related to its color management properties that are relevant to web design. For Premiere Elements's needs, the chief advantage of this format is that it can be created with transparent areas that remain transparent when the image is placed in your video timeline.

88

The *Portable Document File (PDF)* format was created by Adobe, which has long promoted the format's use as a lightweight, universal way to transfer text and graphics files between programs.

Encapsulated Post Script (EPS) files are unique in that they are usually a vector rather than raster format. The difference between these two formats is that raster images are composed of blocks of pixels while vector images are defined by a series of outline points that designate fields of color (a square, for instance, is defined only by its four corners). The main advantage to using a vector graphic is that, unlike raster images, you do not need to worry about *resolution*. Because a vector image is defined by outline points rather than being painted with blocks of color, it can be scaled to any size without becoming pixilated. This advantage is somewhat nullified by the fact that after a vector EPS is added to the **Timeline** of your video, it becomes a piece of raster art by nature of the medium. Therefore, you still need to concern yourself with issues such as resolution and the dangers of over-scaling your image.

▶ **NOTE**

Although EPS files are presumed to be vector art, programs such as Photoshop can produce raster EPS files. Only EPS files created in a vector art program, such as Adobe Illustrator, will produce true vector EPS files.

▶ **KEY TERM**

Resolution—The pixel density of an image. Print images require a much higher resolution (200–300 pixels per inch) than onscreen images (about 72 pixels per inch), but too little resolution in any medium reveals the pixels that make up the image, making the picture look jagged.

1 Size Your Image Efficiently

The primary issue for you to consider when working with any still image you plan to use in your video is the image's resolution. If you use a still image straight from your digital camera (today's 3.5 megapixel digital cameras produce images at 2048×1536 pixels, nearly 10 times the size of a video frame), the still file is too large to be handled efficiently by Premiere Elements. On the other hand, if the still image doesn't contain enough pixels, you won't be able to zoom in on or pan the image in the video project without the image becoming pixelated. See **119** Pan and Zoom Still Images a la Ken Burns.

Unlike most digital imagery, video is composed of non-square pixels. NTSC video (a frame made up of 720×480 pixels) uses pixels that are about 90% as wide as they are tall to produce standard 4:3 video and 120% wider than they are tall to produce a 16:9 widescreen video. The PAL system (a frame of

786×576 pixels) uses pixels that are 106% wider than they are tall for standard video and 142% wider than they are tall for widescreen. Fortunately, you won't need to reshape the pixels in your stills before placing them in your video. Premiere Elements converts standard, square-pixel images to their non-square pixel equivalents automatically.

▶ NOTES

Because a video frame is made up of non-square pixels and most digital images are made up of square pixels, the pixel dimensions for a full-screen image are different for stills and photos than they are for video. Here are approximate dimensions for full-screen graphics in each video system:

- NTSC's 720×480 non-square video pixel TV screen is approximately equal in size to a graphic that measures 720×535 square pixels.

- PAL's 786×576 non-square video pixel TV screen is approximately equal in size to a graphic that measures 835×576 square pixels.

Don't worry that your graphics are composed of square pixels and video is composed of non-square pixels. Premiere Elements renders your graphics to a full screen of video as long as you use the dimensions given here.

Should you work in widescreen video, the following dimensions will work for your graphics (oddly, for widescreen video, only the non-square pixel shapes change—they're much wider—the actual number of video pixels are the same as for standard video):

- NTSC's 720×480 non-square video pixel widescreen is approximately equal in size to a graphic that measures 865×480 square pixels.

- PAL's 786×576 non-square video pixel widescreen is approximately equal in size to a graphic that measures 1220×576 square pixels.

88

The goal is to find a balance between too much and too little resolution for your stills. Assume that you're going to load your photo into a standard NTSC 720×480 video and that you plan to zoom in to a spot about a fourth of the area of the image. (In other words, you're going to scale the image to four times the area of the screen.) What does the resolution of the original still image file have to be?

A 720×480 NTSC screen has an area of about 345,000 pixels. Four times that size is about 1,380,000 square pixels, or approximately 1440×960—about twice the width and twice the height.

Too much math? Don't worry about it. A rough estimation is usually more than adequate. If you plan to scale your image to 2 or 3 times the screen size, use an image about 1 and a half times each dimension; if you plan to scale your image to 4 times the screen size, double each dimension, and so on. A little extra resolution doesn't hurt, but a lot extra does. And it's unlikely that you'll ever need an image with more than 2,500 pixels in either dimension.

▶ **TIP**

If you have a 1–4 megapixel still camera, you can generally import an image file from the camera straight into Premiere Elements. Premiere Elements resizes the image as needed, and you should have enough extra resolution to zoom and pan if you chose to do that.

If you need to resize a super-high-resolution image file before importing it into Premiere Elements, you must size it using an outside graphics program such as Photoshop Elements or Paint Shop Pro. After the image is sized to the necessary video dimensions, you'll be able to easily work with it in Premiere Elements.

2 Add Your Still to the Media Panel

Click the **Add Media** button in the shortcuts bar and select **From Files and Folders**. Browse and select the (resized) photo or photos you want to add to your project. (See **84** **Add Media with the Adobe Media Downloader**.) You might find it helpful to create a new folder in your **Media** panel for your still images to better organize your media.

89

3 Place Your Still on the Timeline

When you add the still to the project **Timeline**, it becomes a clip at the default duration, initially 5 seconds (see **90** **Set Still Image Duration** for information on how to change this default setting) and, by default, is sized to the video frame (see **89** **Scale and Position a Still** for information on how to change this default setting).

▶ **NOTE**

Although Premiere Elements accepts most major graphics formats, including TIFs, it does not accept 16-bit TIFs or images in any format saved in CMYK color mode.

89 Scale and Position a Still

✔ BEFORE YOU BEGIN	→ SEE ALSO
88 Prepare a Still for Video	**90** Set Still Image Duration
	118 Add Motion to a Still
	119 Pan and Zoom Still Images a la Ken Burns

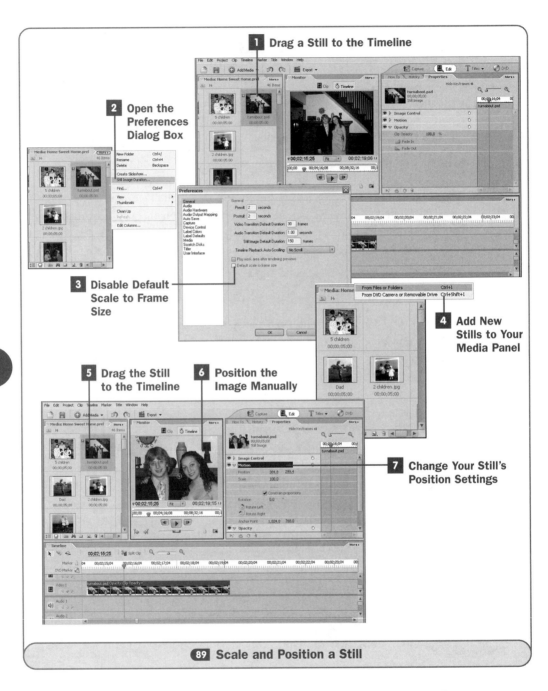

1 Drag a Still to the Timeline

2 Open the Preferences Dialog Box

3 Disable Default Scale to Frame Size

4 Add New Stills to Your Media Panel

5 Drag the Still to the Timeline

6 Position the Image Manually

7 Change Your Still's Position Settings

89 Scale and Position a Still

Premiere Elements has a number of settings that determine how your still images will behave by default when placed on the **Timeline**. Depending on your needs and preferences, you might decide to position your stills manually or change the default settings so your image lands in your preferred position automatically.

1 Drag a Still to the Timeline

By default, Premiere Elements automatically scales the image you drop on the **Timeline** to the size of the video frame.

▶ **NOTE**

Although Premiere Elements automatically scales your image to the size of the video frame when you place it on the **Timeline**, this scaling does not affect the aspect ratio of your image. In other words, if your graphic is not the same shape as your video frame, Premiere Elements does not stretch it in either dimension to fill the frame (which is preferable, of course) and the video frame might be wider or taller than your image, resulting in black bars along the sides of the image.

2 Open the Preferences Dialog Box

Click the **More** button in the **Media** panel. From the drop-down menu, select **Still Image Duration** to open the **Preferences** dialog box to the **General** category page. Alternatively, open the **Preferences** dialog box to this page by choosing **Edit, Preferences, General**.

If you want, you can change the default duration of your stills (see **90** Set **Still Image Duration**).

3 Disable Default Scale to Frame Size

Uncheck the **Default scale to frame size** option to disable Premiere Elements's automatic scaling feature. With this feature disabled, new stills or graphics placed on the **Timeline** appear at their actual size rather than automatically being scaled to the video frame size.

Click **OK** to close the **Preferences** dialog box.

▶ **NOTE**

If you change the default settings for still duration or scale, this does not affect stills already in the **Media** panel. Only stills added to the **Media** panel after the settings have been changed are affected by the changes (see **90** Set Still Image Duration).

4 Add New Stills to Your Media Panel

Click the **Add Media** button, select **From Files or Folders**, and browse to select the images you want to add to the **Timeline** at this new setting.

If you already have a photo in your **Media** panel with which you want to use the new default settings you just established, you must re-import the image to the **Media** panel: Right-click the image in the **Media** panel and select **Clear** to remove it from the panel. (This action does not erase the file from your hard drive.) Then click the **Add Media** button, select **From Files or Folders**, and browse to add the image to your **Media** panel again. The new default setting is applied to this still image.

▶ **TIP**

You can also change the **Scale to Frame** option for a clip on the fly. Right-click on the clip on the **Timeline** and uncheck **Scale to Frame**. The clip reverts to its actual pixel dimensions in the video frame.

5 Drag the Still to the Timeline

Drag the still (with its new scale settings) to the **Timeline**. The still is added at its actual size rather than at the enforced size of the video frame. In the case of my example, the image is now much larger than the video frame, and only a portion of the image is displayed in the **Monitor**.

If you plan to add motion to your stills by panning and zooming around them (see ⑪⑨ **Pan and Zoom Still Images a la Ken Burns**), you might find it easier to work with your still at its actual size as it appears in the example, rather than automatically scaling it to the video frame size. When it is displayed at its actual size, you'll have a much better idea of how much scaling the still's size and resolution will allow for. But this is purely a matter of personal preference. Choose the default setting that best fits your personal workflow.

6 Position the Image Manually

You can reposition your still in this frame of the video by clicking the image in the **Monitor** panel and dragging it into whatever position you'd like.

7 Change Your Still's Position Settings

Alternatively, you can position your still using the **Position** settings in the **Properties** panel. With your still selected on the **Timeline**, click the triangle to the left of **Motion** in the **Properties** panel to reveal the **Motion** property's details, including **Position** and **Scale**. The first number represents the horizontal position (in pixels) *of the center of your image* in the video frame. The second number represents its vertical position. By changing one or both of these numbers, you can adjust the still's placement in the video frame. You can also change these numbers more fluidly by moving your mouse over numbers until the settings icon appears, and then dragging across the numbers to raise or lower the settings.

You can also resize the image in the video frame by changing the **Scale** settings in the **Motion** panel.

90   Set Still Image Duration

✔ BEFORE YOU BEGIN	→ SEE ALSO
88 Prepare a Still for Video	**84** Add Media with the Adobe Media Downloader
	89 Scale and Position a Still
	171 Change Slides to the Beat of Music

By default, any still image or graphic you add to the Premiere Elements **Timeline** comes in with a duration of 5 seconds. (The exception is when you create a slideshow set to unnumbered timeline markers, as described in **171** **Change Slides to the Beat of Music**.) However, this default setting can be changed very easily.

1   Open General Preferences

Click the **More** button in the **Media** panel and select **Still Image Duration**. The **Preferences** dialog box opens to the **General** page.

Among the **General Preferences** are options for setting stills to default to the video frame size when imported into your project (See **89** **Scale and Position a Still**.)

▶ **NOTE**

You can also access the **Preferences** dialog box from the **Edit** drop-down menu. The **Preferences** dialog box offers several pages of settings that can be helpful in troubleshooting functional and hardware problems.

2   Change the Still Image Default Duration

Time, in terms of duration in video, can be set in seconds or in frames. In the NTSC system, video has approximately 30 frames per second. The NTSC factory default of a 5-second duration for stills is therefore listed as 150 frames. In the PAL system, video runs at 25 frames per second, and therefore 5 seconds is represented as 125 frames.

▶ **NOTE**

In reality, NTSC video runs at 29.97 frames per second rather than 30. However, because the drop-frame system employed by Premiere Elements makes that fractional difference invisible, we can safely use the more manageable rate of 30 frames per second for any calculations.

Type the number of frames you'd like to be the default for your still image duration. Click **OK**.

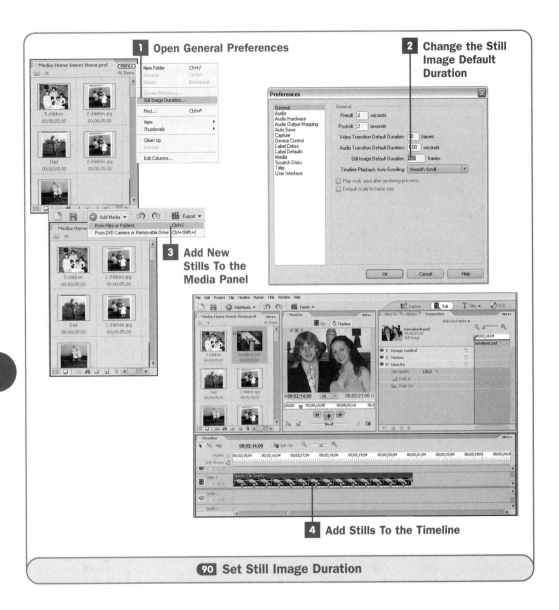

1 Open General Preferences

2 Change the Still Image Default Duration

3 Add New Stills To the Media Panel

4 Add Stills To the Timeline

90 Set Still Image Duration

▶ **NOTE**

Changed default settings for still duration or still size do not affect stills already in the **Media** panel. Only stills added *after* the settings have been changed are affected by the changes. (See also **89** Scale and Position a Still.)

3 Add New Stills To the Media Panel

Click the **Add Media** button, select **From Files or Folders**, and browse to select the pictures you want to add to the **Timeline** at this new setting. (See also **84** **Add Media with the Adobe Media Downloader**.)

If you already have a photo in your **Media** panel with which you want to use the new default settings you just established, you must re-import the image to the **Media** panel: Right-click the image in the **Media** panel and select **Clear** to remove it from the panel. (This action does not erase the file from your hard drive.) Then click the **Add Media** button, select **From Files or Folders**, and browse to add the image to your **Media** panel again. The new default setting is applied to this still image.

4 Add Your Stills To the Timeline

Drag the still image from the **Media** panel to the location you want it to occupy in the **Timeline**. The still has a default duration equal to the new setting.

After you've place the still on the **Timeline**, you can increase or decrease the clip's duration by dragging the ends of the clip out or in as described in **95** **Trim a Clip on the Timeline**.

90

17

Editing on the Timeline

IN THIS CHAPTER:

The **Timeline**: What a concept. Although this is the computer age, the concept of the **Timeline** was taken from the real-life video editing of the past. The best of applications take a manual process and automate it. That is exactly what Adobe has done with Premiere Elements. By using a digital timeline, tasks that weren't possible or even attempted in the past because of their difficulty or the time they took can now be accomplished in a very short and simple fashion. Digital video editing has shortened the amount of time it takes to edit a film, but the overall process has increased because of the unlimited number of things you can do with the video after it is on your computer. There was a time when it was very difficult to get film from several cameras or sources together into one movie. That is no longer the case; and you can do more today with Premiere Elements than the professionals did 20 years ago. Much of this is because of the ability to add many video and audio tracks to your movie.

Many video-editing software applications have some form of Timeline. Some of those even have multiple video and audio tracks. However, very few consumer editing applications can add unlimited numbers of video and audio tracks, like Premiere Elements can do. This is one of the features that helps provide professional results and functions without the cost of professional software.

For you, the video artist, the **Timeline** is your canvas. This is where you do the majority of your editing, add effects and transitions, and perform all of the tasks necessary to produce your movie.

In this chapter, we will cover everything from getting media from the **Media** panel onto the **Timeline** to editing and rendering your clips. We will introduce you to *video tracks* (sometimes called *layers*), and show you how to use them. You will learn how to prepare your clips for transitions, remove unwanted scenes, and do a few things just like they do in Hollywood.

As you begin your video-editing adventure, you will most likely return to this chapter repeatedly. This chapter and Chapter 19, "Advanced Timeline Video and Audio Editing," explain all the features available to you from the **Timeline**. Considering this is where you will spend well over 50% of the your time creating your movie, the information in these two chapters will become second nature to you. Before you know it, you will be creating L-cuts and J-cuts just like the pros.

91   Add, Delete, and Size Tracks

✔ BEFORE YOU BEGIN	→ SEE ALSO
84 Add Media with the Adobe Media Downloader	125 Create a Picture-in-Picture Effect 136 Create a Title Overlay for Your Video

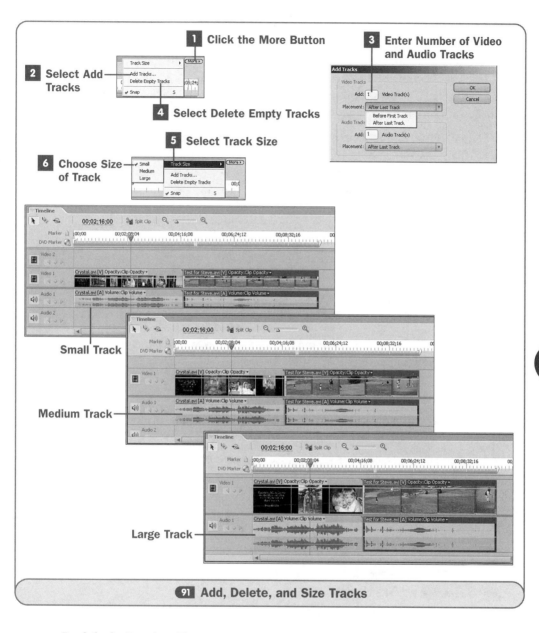

1 **Click the More Button**

2 **Select Add Tracks**

3 **Enter Number of Video and Audio Tracks**

4 **Select Delete Empty Tracks**

5 **Select Track Size**

6 **Choose Size of Track**

Small Track

Medium Track

Large Track

91 Add, Delete, and Size Tracks

By default, Premiere Elements gives you two video and two audio tracks with which to work. You have the ability to add additional video and audio tracks at any time. You'll need additional tracks for special effects such as picture-in-picture (showing multiple images at the same time), adding background images, titles, and text. Each still image also needs its own track; therefore, the more images you want to display simultaneously, the more tracks you need.

Tracks are prioritized from top to bottom (or layered in visibility); the bottom track being track number 1. The higher the track number, the higher the priority. When adding an image to track 1, with nothing above it, the image on track 1 is clearly visible in the **Monitor**. If you add an image to track 2, directly above the track 1 image, all you see in the **Monitor** is the track 2 image because the higher track has priority.

This all becomes more understandable when you resize and position the images, lower their opacity, or make parts of the tracks transparent. When those effects are applied to higher tracks, parts (or all) of the lower tracks become visible. One of the best examples of this is seen in the famous *Brady Bunch* introduction. Each image in the intro is on a separate track, scaled and positioned so all the images are visible in the same screen. Keep **Track Priority** in mind as you add clips to the **Timeline**. Make sure what you want to see is on the proper track; and that there are no clips on tracks above it that don't belong there.

After adding additional tracks, you might need to delete some empty tracks. That can easily be accomplished with a few keystrokes.

Premiere Elements also enables you to set the size of the tracks. Changing the track size also enlarges the thumbnail images you see on the **Timeline**, making it easier to see the audio and video detail.

91

▶ **NOTE**

To change the default number of tracks displayed in the **Timeline**, choose **Project, Project Settings, Default Timeline** from the main menu at the top of your screen. There, you can set the default number of tracks (for both video and audio tracks) for all your future projects. Changing the default does not alter the number of tracks in any projects created before this change.

1 Click the More Button

Click the **More** button in the top-right corner of the **Timeline** to open the **More** menu.

2 Select Add Tracks

To add tracks to the **Timeline**, select the **Add Tracks** option. The **Add Tracks** dialog box opens.

3 Enter Number of Video and Audio Tracks

In the **Add Tracks** dialog box, you see separate entries for **Video Tracks** and **Audio Tracks**. With these settings, you can add only video tracks or only audio tracks if that is what you require. Enter the number of additional tracks in the boxes and select the **Placement** of the new tracks. You can place the new tracks before the first track or after the last track. When you are finished, click the **OK** button to add those tracks to the **Timeline**.

4 Select Delete Empty Tracks

To clean up the **Timeline** and remove unused tracks (audio or video tracks that contain no images or clips), open the **More** menu and choose **Delete Empty Tracks**. All unused audio and video tracks are deleted.

▶ **NOTE**

When deleting empty tracks, Premiere Elements does not show a confirmation dialog box asking, "Are sure you want to delete these tracks?" After you select **Delete Empty Tracks**, the tracks just disappear.

5 Select Track Size

You can change the size of the tracks in the **Timeline**. To do so, open the **More** menu and select **Track Size**. A submenu with three choices opens.

6 Choose Size of Track

For the size of the track, you have the choice of **Small**, **Medium**, or **Large**. Change the setting and notice the difference in the size of the tracks. Changing the track size also enlarges or reduces the images and clips on the **Timeline**. When you need to see more tracks and less detail, choose **Small** (the default). When you need to see a single track and a lot of detail, choose **Large**. **Medium** is a good setting for average editing tasks.

92

---

92 Set Video and Audio Track Display

✔ **BEFORE YOU BEGIN**

91 Add, Delete, and Size Tracks

To the far left of each video track you see a film reel icon; this is the **Video Track Display** toggle. To the far left of each audio track you see a speaker icon; this is the **Audio Track Display** toggle. Depending on your workflow, current task, or personal preference, you can have different display settings for each video and audio track.

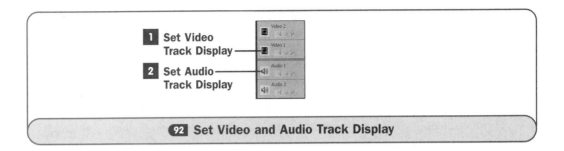

1 Set Video Track Display

2 Set Audio Track Display

92 Set Video and Audio Track Display

1 Set Video Track Display

The video track display can be toggled to different views by clicking the film reel icon at the left end of the video track. Clicking this icon switches between four views; keep clicking the icon until you see the view you want:

- Thumbnails across the entire track

- Thumbnails at the beginning of the clip

- Thumbnails at the beginning and end of the clip

- Hide the thumbnails on the track

▶ **TIP**

To make the keyframe markers more visible, choose the view that hides the thumbnails. The keyframe markers and line will be clearly visible on the **Timeline**.

2 Set Audio Track Display

The audio track display can also be toggled to different views by clicking the speaker icon at the far left of the audio track. Click this icon to switch between two views:

- Audio waveform shown across the entire track

- Hide the audio waveform on the track

93 Define the Beginning and End of Your Project

The work area bar is located at the top of the track view, below the **Timeline** where the CTI is located. This bar helps to determine the beginning and end of your project for certain tasks. During the rendering, viewing, playing, and export- ing of your project, the work area bar sets the start and end points. You can adjust the start and end points when you are interested in working with only a particular section of your project.

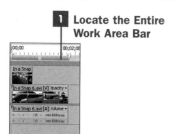

1 Locate the Entire
Work Area Bar

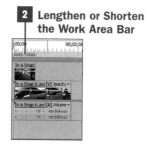

2 Lengthen or Shorten
the Work Area Bar

93 Define the Beginning and End of Your Project

1 Locate the Entire Work Area Bar

Under normal circumstances, the work area bar covers your entire project.

Hover the mouse pointer over the work area bar to display the start timecode, end timecode, and duration of the portion of the movie contained under the work area bar.

2 Lengthen or Shorten the Work Area Bar

93

When the need arises, you can drag either end of the work area bar to shorten or lengthen it. Simply drag the handles at each end of the bar in or out.

You can click the center of the work area bar and drag the entire bar to another section of the **Timeline**. This action effectively moves the currently active section of the project to encompass a new group of clips in the **Timeline**.

The ability to move, lengthen, and shorten the work area bar comes in useful when outputting your video (see **141** **Output to an AVI Movie**). When outputting, you will have options to output the entire **Timeline** or what is covered by the work area bar only. Using the work area bar, you can output just portions of your video and create new clips. When adjusting the work area bar, all of your project is still visible on the **Timeline**, and you can play the entire **Timeline** in the **Monitor**. Also, timeline rendering ignores any area not covered by the work area bar: If there is a red line above one of your clips and you want to render only that part of the **Timeline**, make sure that the work area bar is covering that area before you render.

▶ **TIP**

Double-clicking the work area bar stretches or moves it the length of what you see in the **Timeline**. If you see 20 frames, the work area bar will extend over those 20 frames. If you see the entire project, the work area bar will extend over the entire project. Zooming out until your complete project is in view and then double-clicking the work area bar is the best way to ensure that the bar covers your whole project.

You might want to adjust the work area bar before you render a portion of the movie. To render just a portion of the movie in the **Timeline**, position the work area bar over the section of the **Timeline** you want to render and press **Enter**. Even if the whole **Timeline** needs to be rendered, just the portion below the work area bar is rendered at this time. If you're trying to render a section of the **Time-line** but the entire section will not render, double-check the position and length of the work area bar. The work area bar should cover the entire section you want to render.

▶ **TIP**

If you cannot render or export your entire movie, double-check the position and length of the work area bar. To render or export the entire movie, the work area bar should extend to contain all the project's clips.

93

94 **Add or Move a Clip on the Timeline**

✔ BEFORE YOU BEGIN	→ SEE ALSO
81 Capture to the Timeline or Media Panel	**96** Delete and Close Gaps in the Timeline
84 Add Media with the Adobe Media Downloader	

Now it's time to really get down to business: getting clips onto the **Timeline**. Although you can trim clips while they are still in the **Media** panel (as explained in **86** **Trim Clips in the Media Panel**), you can do nothing beyond that without getting those clips onto the **Timeline**, where editing begins (and when you're finished editing, what is on the **Timeline** is what gets burned to DVD). Before we begin this task, you must have a few clips in the **Media** panel that can be added to the **Timeline** (see **84** **Add Media with the Adobe Media Downloader**). Of course, if you have captured your clips and used the default **Capture to Timeline** option, your clips are already there. The sooner you get the clips down there, the sooner you can start your editing process and burn that DVD. Note that there are two ways a clip can be added to the **Timeline**: with the **Insert** or **Overlay** option.

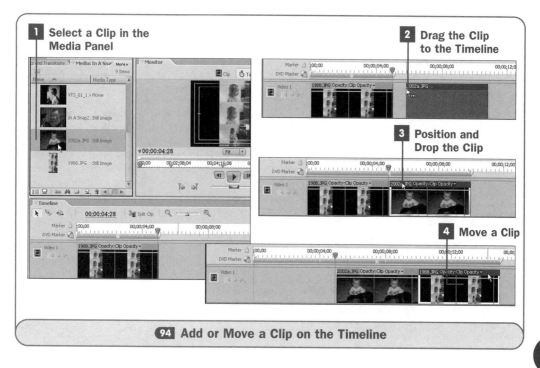

94 Add or Move a Clip on the Timeline

The **Insert** option places the new clip on the **Timeline**, splitting an existing clip, or (if positioned at the beginning, end, or *between* video clips), inserting the new clip and moving all clips to the right to make room for the new clip. The **Overlay** option places the new video over existing video, removing any of the existing video it is placed over.

▶ **NOTE**

You can capture clips directly to the Timeline as explained in **81** Capture to the Timeline or Media Panel.

1 **Select a Clip in the Media Panel**

Click the clip thumbnail in the **Media** panel that you want to add to the **Timeline** and to your project. The clip is selected and appears highlighted.

2 **Drag the Clip to the Timeline**

Drag the clip thumbnail to the **Timeline**.

▶ **TIP**

Instead of dragging the clip to the **Timeline**, you can right-click the clip in the **Media** panel to open the context menu and choose the **Insert to Timeline** option to insert the selected clip on the **Timeline** at the CTI. If the CTI is positioned in the middle of a clip, the clip on the **Timeline** is split and the new clip is inserted at that point.

3 Position and Drop the Clip

Position the clip where you want it to be on the **Timeline** and release the mouse button to drop the clip.

▶ **NOTE**

If you have selected the **Snap** option from the **Timeline's More** menu, the clip snaps to the beginning of the **Timeline** (if there are no other clips present on the **Timeline**). If there are other clips on the **Timeline**, the current clip snaps to an adjacent clip. With the **Snap** option enabled, you don't need to be perfect when you drop your clips, just close. The **Snap** option also prevents you from overlaying or splitting a clip already on the **Timeline** by accident.

4 Move a Clip

If, by chance, you don't hit your mark when you drop your clip on the **Timeline**, don't worry. Simply grab the clip on the **Timeline** and drag and drop it to a new position.

94

95 Trim a Clip on the Timeline	
✔ BEFORE YOU BEGIN	→ SEE ALSO
94 Add or Move a Clip on the Timeline	**97** Split a Clip **98** Remove a Section of a Clip **100** Remove Audio or Video from a Clip

As you start your editing experience, you will need to recognize the **Trim** icons. Move the mouse pointer over the edge of a clip and notice that one of these **Trim** icons appears. The only way you can trim your clip is when one of these icons is visible.

There is more than one way to trim a clip, and this is one of them. Later in this chapter you will be instructed in other trimming methods. The trimming method described in this task is not intended for fine, detailed editing, but it *is* a good way to quickly remove unwanted scenes or footage from a clip. As you trim your clip, you can see the corresponding frame in the **Monitor** to help you keep track of where you are and what you are trimming.

1 Drag the Right Edge to Extend the Duration of a Still

Drag a still image from the **Media** panel to the beginning of the **Timeline**. If the default **Still Image Duration** has not been changed, the image will have a duration of 5 seconds on the **Timeline**. If you need to extend the duration of a single clip without changing the default setting for still-image duration, you can drag out some additional time for this specific still image.

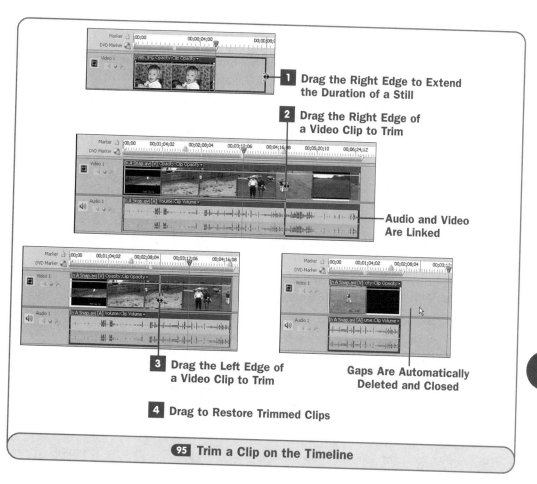

1 Drag the Right Edge to Extend the Duration of a Still

2 Drag the Right Edge of a Video Clip to Trim

Audio and Video Are Linked

3 Drag the Left Edge of a Video Clip to Trim

Gaps Are Automatically Deleted and Closed

4 Drag to Restore Trimmed Clips

95 Trim a Clip on the Timeline

95

▶ NOTE

To change the default **Still Image Duration**, select **Edit, Preferences, General** from the menu at the top of your screen. The default duration for a still image is 150 frames (30 frames per second times 5 seconds). Change this value and click **OK** to change the default duration for still images.

Click the left mouse button over the right edge of the still image clip in the **Timeline**. Make sure that you can see the **Right Trim** icon before clicking. Drag the edge to the right until the CTI gets to the 8-second mark. Release the mouse button; this single still image clip now has an 8-second duration. All other still images maintain the default duration set in the **Preferences** dialog box.

▶ **NOTES**

If you drag the mouse to the left, you will decrease the duration of the still. When trimming or extending a still image, you are adding or removing identical frames. The only change trimming makes to a still image is to its duration on the **Timeline**.

When you release the mouse button after extending or decreasing the duration of a still image on the **Timeline**, the work area bar adjusts to the new image length. This works as long as you have not manually made adjustments to the position of the bar.

Now right-click the still image in the **Timeline** and select **Clear** from the context menu to delete this practice still from the **Timeline**. Alternatively, select the clip and press the **Delete** key to delete the clip.

2 **Drag the Right Edge of a Video Clip to Trim**

Drag a video clip from the **Media** panel and drop if at the beginning of the **Timeline**. Click the right edge of the video clip, making sure that you see the **Right Trim** icon before clicking the mouse button.

If you are working with a still image, you can always drag the trimmer to the right; Premiere Elements adds as many additional frames as needed. However, if you are working with video- or audio-only clips, you can only extend to the end of the clip; Premiere Elements will not add or repeat frames in this case. You can grab a still of the last image in the clip and drag that out farther if that is your goal (see **87** **Grab a Still from Video**).

▶ **NOTE**

As you drag the **Right Trim** icon, watch the **Monitor**; it will give you a view of what you are trimming from your clip.

Drag the edge of the clip to the left 10 seconds. As you drag, notice that both the video and audio tracks are being trimmed. Release the mouse button, and your trimmed clip will be 10 seconds shorter than it originally was.

To trim only the video or the audio, right-click the clip and select **Unlink Audio and Video** from the context menu. To trim only the audio, position the mouse pointer over the edge of the audio track and drag without affecting the video track; to trim only the video, position the mouse pointer over the edge of the video track and drag without affecting the audio track.

▶ **TIP**

If you are trimming your clip to be used in an L-cut or a J-cut, see **99** **Create an L-Cut or a J-Cut.**

3 Drag the Left Edge of a Video Clip to Trim

Now move to the beginning of the clip, the left side. Click the left edge of the clip, making sure that you see the **Left Trim** icon before clicking.

Drag the edge to the right 10 seconds and release the mouse button. The clip will now be 20 seconds shorter than the original—you've trimmed 10 seconds off each end of the clip. You can trim as much or as little as necessary; it is totally up to you. Don't be afraid to experiment because the original clip on the hard drive is not altered during the nonlinear editing process.

▶ NOTE

As you trim your clips, the clips automatically move to the left on the **Timeline** to close any space or gaps. (see **96** Delete and Close Gaps in the Timeline).

If your trimming has left gaps in the **Timeline**, Premiere Elements automatically deletes and closes any gaps. In the example you just completed, the clip was moved back to the beginning of the **Timeline**, even though you trimmed 10 seconds from that end.

▶ TIP

If you would rather the clip did not move to the left and fill in any gaps in the **Timeline**, hold the **Ctrl** key while you drag the **Trim** icon. Be sure to release the mouse button before releasing the **Ctrl** key. As you hold the mouse pointer over a clip and press the **Ctrl** key or the **Shift** key, notice the messages under the **Timeline**. These messages let you know what will happen when you drag or drop with one of these keys pressed.

4 Drag to Restore Trimmed Clips

If you accidentally trim too much from a clip, move the **Trim** icon in the opposite direction to get the trimmed parts back. The trimmed scenes are never deleted from the actual footage, so the trimmed frames are always available to be added to your project.

96 Delete and Close Gaps in the Timeline

✔ BEFORE YOU BEGIN	→ SEE ALSO
94 Add or Move a Clip on the Timeline	**97** Split a Clip

96

If you encounter unwanted gaps in your **Timeline**, there is a quick fix to help you remove them.

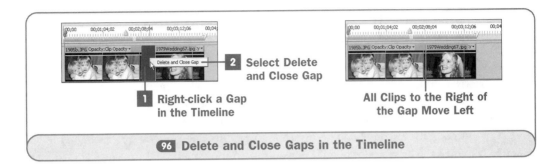

2 Select Delete and Close Gap

1 Right-click a Gap in the Timeline

All Clips to the Right of the Gap Move Left

96 Delete and Close Gaps in the Timeline

96

1 Right-click a Gap in the Timeline

Right-click a gap in the **Timeline** to display the context menu. If you have more than one gap in the Timeline, you will have to manually close them one at a time.

2 Select Delete and Close Gap

The context menu offers only one option to choose: **Delete and Close Gap**. If the gap cannot be deleted and closed (if there are audio or video clips on other tracks in the same position of the **Timeline**), the context menu option is not available. In this case, you can manually drag the clip to close the gap.

After selecting the **Delete and Close Gap** option, the gap is removed from between the clips. All clips to the right of the gap move to the left to fill in the gap.

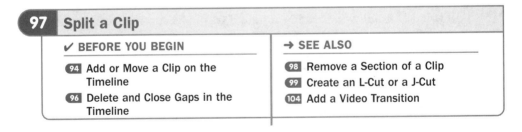

97 Split a Clip

✔ BEFORE YOU BEGIN	→ SEE ALSO
94 Add or Move a Clip on the Timeline	**98** Remove a Section of a Clip
	99 Create an L-Cut or a J-Cut
96 Delete and Close Gaps in the Timeline	**104** Add a Video Transition

One method of splitting or cutting a clip is by using the **Split Clip** button, located just above the timecode bar in the **Timeline**. You can use this button to do some very detailed trimming of your clips. You can zoom in on the **Timeline** to see individual frames in the video clip, position the CTI on the **Timeline**, and then click the **Split Clip** button to split the clip at the CTI position.

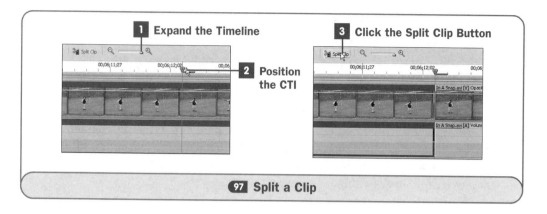

You might use the **Split Clip** feature when you want to add a transition *inside* a clip. As you know, you cannot place a transition in the middle of a clip, only to the beginning, end, or between two clips. You can use the **Split Clip** feature to create two clips so you can place the transition between them. You might want to move a section of a clip to another part of the **Timeline**. By creating two splits in a clip, you create three separate clips, and any of the three can be moved anywhere on the **Timeline**. A clip can be split between every frame, making it possible to have as many as 29 splits in one second of video (creating 30 separate clips of one frame each).

1 Expand the Timeline

Find the general area of your clip where you would like the split to occur. Move the CTI to that location on the **Timeline**.

Use the **Timeline Magnifier** to expand (or zoom into) the **Timeline** as far as you can to get a view of each individual frame in the video clip. This type of split, or cut, is a very precise and detailed edit. You want to make sure you can see all the detail you can so you are sure you are splitting the clip between the correct frames. When splitting audio clips, you want to split at a precise point in the waveform. Zoom into the **Timeline** to make this possible by providing very clear detail of the audio waveform.

2 Position the CTI

Locate the frames between which you want to create the split, and position the CTI between the two frames.

▶ TIP

If the CTI is not visible, click the **Timeline** anywhere above the work area bar. The CTI moves to that position.

3 Click the Split Clip Button

When you have the CTI positioned between the two frames where you want the split created, click the **Split Clip** button. The clip is divided at the CTI location, creating two clips out of the original one. You can now delete, add a transition between, or move either clip—they are totally separate clips now. Notice that the two clips share the same name because they are still parts of the original still on your hard drive as one complete clip. If the clips remain adjacent to each other, there will be no noticeable difference when playing the clips because playback will ignore the split. You can undo the split by clicking the **Undo** button or by pressing **Ctrl+Z**.

▶ **TIP**

If you select multiple clips on multiple tracks, the **Split Clip** button will split *all* the selected clips at the CTI, not just one.

▶ **NOTE**

Notice that both the video and audio tracks are split. To split only the video or the audio track, right-click the original clip and select **Unlink Audio and Video** from the context menu. Select either the video or the audio track portion of the clip by clicking it and then click the **Split Clip** button; only the selected track is split.

You can also cut and split clips using the **Razor** tool, as explained in **98** **Remove a Section of a Clip**. When you use the **Razor** tool, the clips are cut at the mouse pointer, not at the CTI position.

98	Remove a Section of a Clip
✔ **BEFORE YOU BEGIN**	→ **SEE ALSO**
94 Add or Move a Clip on the Timeline	**95** Trim a Clip on the Timeline
	99 Create an L-Cut or a J-Cut
	100 Remove Audio or Video from a Clip

People generally capture way more video than they will use in a movie. Just like in Hollywood, the more footage you have, the better the possibility of creating a great scene. Because you have all this extra footage, you usually need to remove sections from the middle of a clip. Even after trimming a clip in the **Media** panel or on the **Timeline**, you will still have sections you want to remove. This is where the **Razor** tool becomes a valuable feature.

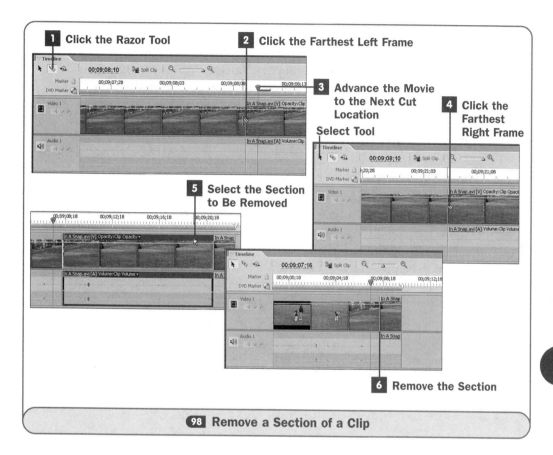

1 Click the Razor Tool   **2** Click the Farthest Left Frame

3 Advance the Movie to the Next Cut Location
Select Tool

4 Click the Farthest Right Frame

5 Select the Section to Be Removed

6 Remove the Section

98 Remove a Section of a Clip

To use the **Razor** tool, you must locate an area of a clip that you want to remove. You make two cuts in the clip, one at the beginning of the section to be removed and one at the end. Selecting the footage to remove requires detailed editing, and you will zoom in and out of your clip, possibly a few times, to get the exact location of each cut. While searching for the section to be removed, look for a place on the clip where two frames meet. One frame is a frame you want to keep, the other is a frame you want to remove. All the frames between the two cuts are turned into a new clip and can be deleted or just moved to another location on the **Timeline**.

▶ **NOTE**

When cutting a clip with the **Razor** tool, both the video and audio tracks are cut. If you do not want the audio cut along with the video (or vice-versa), see **100** Remove Audio or Video from a Clip; alternatively, you can unlink the audio and video tracks as explained in **97** Split a Clip.

1 Click the Razor Tool

Locate a section of a clip that you want to remove. You can zoom out on the Timeline to get a wider view by using the **Timeline Magnifier**. After you have located the section of the clip you want to remove, zoom in on the Timeline as far as you can to see individual frames, 30 frames per second. When you have located the first frame of the section you want to remove, click the **Razor** tool.

2 Click the Farthest Left Frame

As you move the mouse pointer to the clip in the **Timeline**, notice that the pointer turns into a razor blade. The line to the left of the **Razor** tool is where the cut occurs. Also notice that the **Razor** position moves along the **Timeline** where the CTI is located. Move the **Razor** tool to the farthest left frame that you want to remove (the first frame of the footage you want to remove) and click. A cut, or split, is placed at the frame where the **Razor** tool was located. If you missed your mark, undo the cut and try again.

▶ NOTE

You cannot cut a clip in the middle of a frame. The **Razor** tool and the **Split Clip** feature always cut the clip between two frames.

98

3 Advance the Movie to the Next Cut Location

Using the shuttle in the **Monitor** panel or the CTI, find the last frame in the section you want to remove. This is clearly visible when you zoom in to the **Timeline** as far as possible. The tick marks at the top of the **Timeline** show where each frame starts and stops. The current frame is indicated by a marker at the top of the CTI that covers the frame to the right of it.

▶ TIP

If you make a mistake and cut the clip at the wrong location, press **Ctrl+Z** to undo the last action. You can then find the correct position and cut again.

4 Click the Farthest Right Frame

When you have identified the last frame of the section you want to cut, click the **Razor** tool on the last frame (the farthest right frame in the section being removed). This action creates another cut at the position of the **Razor** tool.

5 Select the Section to Be Removed

Now you have successfully turned one clip into three, the middle section being the section you want to remove. If you zoom out on the **Timeline**, you will be able to clearly see the two cut points.

Click the **Select** tool and then click the section of clip you want to remove. This action highlights that clip only.

▶ **TIP**

You can click the **Selection** tool, grab the clip, and drag to move it to another location on the **Timeline**.

6 Remove the Section

With the section of the original clip highlighted, press the **Delete** key to remove it from the **Timeline**.

---

99 **Create an L-Cut or a J-Cut**

✔ BEFORE YOU BEGIN	→ SEE ALSO
86 Trim Clips in the Media Panel	**98** Remove a Section of a Clip
94 Add or Move a Clip on the Timeline	**100** Remove Audio or Video from a Clip
95 Trim a Clip on the Timeline	**109** Add Narration to Your Movie

99

The two most common and most used transitions in film are the L-Cut and the J-Cut. Both are cutaways and move from one video scene to another, with the same underlying audio track for both.

Here's an example of an L-Cut: Start the scene with a clip showing two people talking. Cut away to a clip of the surrounding area, without the two people in the frame; keeping the audio of the conversation going.

Here's an example of a J-Cut: Start the scene with a clip that shows the surrounding area and the audio of two people talking, without the two people in the frame. Then cut away to the clip showing the two people holding the conversation.

For this task you will need two clips in the **Media** panel, one clip should be longer than the other. You can trim one of the clips in the **Media** panel as explained in **86** **Trim Clips in the Media Panel**, or you can trim the clip after you drop it on the **Timeline** as explained in **95** **Trim a Clip on the Timeline**. The longer clip will be the Track 1 clip, and the shorter clip will be the Track 2 clip in the steps that follow.

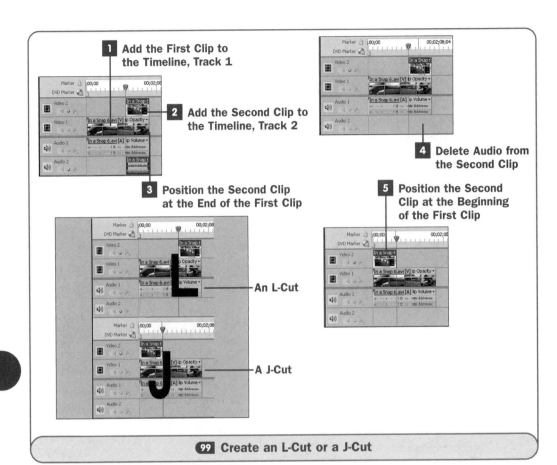

99 Create an L-Cut or a J-Cut

▶ **TIP**

There are various ways to trim a clip: You can set in and out points in the **Monitor** and drag the trimmed clip to the **Timeline** (see **86** Trim Clips in the Media Panel), you can razor the clip and delete the part you don't need (see **98** Remove a Section of a Clip), you can split the clip and delete the part you don't need (see **97** Split a Clip), or you can drag either end of the clip to trim it (see **95** Trim a Clip on the Timeline).

1 Add the First Clip to the Timeline, Track 1

Drag and drop the first (the longer) clip on Track 1, at the beginning of the Timeline.

2 Add the Second Clip to the Timeline, Track 2

Drag and drop the second (the shorter) clip to Track 2 of the **Timeline**.

3 Position the Second Clip at the End of the First Clip

Move the second clip—the one on Track 2—so that its right edge lines up with the right edge of the clip on Track 1.

4 Delete Audio from the Second Clip

Because this transition effect runs the audio from the first clip over the video of the second clip, you will likely want to remove the audio from the second clip so the audio from the first clip can be heard. Right-click the second clip (the one on Track 2) to open the clip's context menu and select **Delete Audio**.

With the clips as they are currently arranged on the **Timeline**, the scene starts with the video and audio from the Track 1 clip and ends with the video from Track 2. This is the L-Cut.

5 Position the Second Clip at the Beginning of the First Clip

Creating a J-Cut after you've arranged the L-Cut is a simple matter of moving the Track 2 clip. Drag the Track 2 clip from the end of the Track 1 clip to the beginning of the Track 1 clip. Now the scene will start with the video from Track 2 but the audio from Track 1. The scene then cuts away to the video from Track 1, where the audio originates. This is the J-Cut.

100

---

100 **Remove Audio or Video from a Clip**

✔ BEFORE YOU BEGIN	→ SEE ALSO
94 Add or Move a Clip on the Timeline	**99** Create an L-Cut or a J-Cut
96 Delete and Close Gaps in the Timeline	**109** Add Narration to Your Movie
	168 Add Graphics, Text, and Narration to Your Slideshow

There are two ways to remove audio or video from your clips. Both are important depending on your task and workflow, so we will cover them both here. For purposes of creating an L-Cut, J-Cut, a silent movie, or when adding narration or music, you will need to remove the audio or video portion of a clip.

1 Select a Clip in the Timeline

Add a clip to the **Timeline** that contains both audio and video. When you click the clip's audio or video track, notice that both the audio and video tracks become highlighted. This is because the two tracks are linked together. Before you can delete either the audio or video, you must first unlink the tracks.

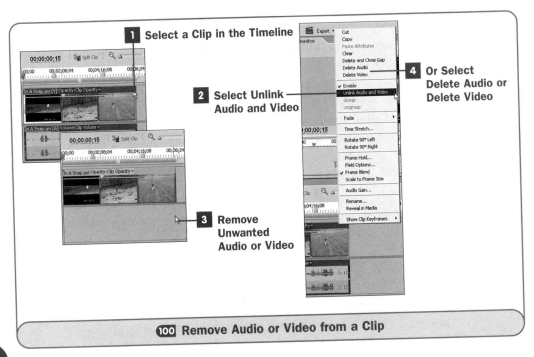

100 Remove Audio or Video from a Clip

2 Select Unlink Audio and Video

Right-click the clip—either the audio or video track will do. The clip's context menu opens. Select **Unlink Audio and Video**.

▶ **TIP**

You can link audio and video in the same way you unlink them: Select the audio and video clips you want to link and right-click one of them. From the context menu, choose **Link Audio and Video**.

3 Remove the Unwanted Audio or Video Portion

The audio and video tracks are now unlinked. Notice that when you click the video track now, the audio track is not highlighted (and vice-versa). To remove the video portion of the clip, click the clip's video track and press the **Delete** key. To instead delete the audio portion of the clip, click the clip's audio track and press the **Delete** key. Simple isn't it? Well, if all you wanted to do was delete the audio or video there is an easier way to do this.

▶ **TIP**

By unlinking the audio and video tracks, you are now free to move the audio and video clips separately. If your audio is slightly out of sync, unlinking the audio and video gives you the ability to move the audio portion of the clip into sync with the video.

4 Or Select Delete Audio or Delete Video

An alternative approach to deleting the audio or video portion of a video clip saves you the step of unlinking the tracks. To practice this alternative method, add another video clip to the **Timeline**, undo the **Unlink** operation, or relink the audio and video for the current clip. In effect, start this step with a video clip that has both the audio and video tracks present and linked.

Right-click the clip's audio or video track to open the clip's context menu. Select **Delete Audio** or **Delete Video** to delete one or the other track.

---

101 Slow/Speed/Reverse Audio/Video

→ **SEE ALSO**

107 Freeze a Frame

If you've ever thought about doing some slow-motion instant replays, speeding up a clip to look like a silent movie, or playing your clip in reverse, the **Time Stretch** tool is for you. You can use the **Time Stretch** feature two ways: The first is a button on the **Timeline** that enables you to speed up or slow down a clip by simply dragging. The second option is found in the clip context menu and allows you to fine tune the speed, duration, reverse speed, and audio pitch of the selected clip. Using the **Time Stretch** tool, you can have multiple copies of a clip on the **Timeline**, play the first copy at normal speed, then show the slow-motion instant replay, then show the clip again in reverse, and finally play it in fast motion—all in the same movie.

1 Select the Time Stretch Tool

Make sure you have a video clip on the **Timeline**. At the top-left side of the **Timeline** is the **Time Stretch** button. Click this button and move the mouse pointer over the edge of your video clip. Notice that the pointer changes to the **Time Stretch** icon.

2 Drag the Outer Edge of a Clip

Click the outer edge (either the left or the right edge) of the video clip and drag the edge. Drag to the right to produce a slow-speed effect; drag to the left to produce a fast-speed effect. What you are actually doing is shortening or lengthening the duration of the clip. Slowing the clip down requires Premiere Elements to repeat frames, speeding it up requires Premiere Elements to remove frames.

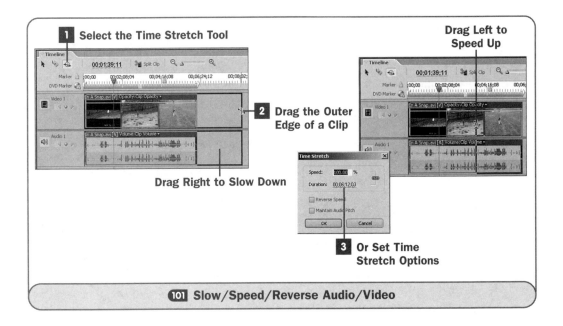

1 Select the Time Stretch Tool

Drag Left to Speed Up

2 Drag the Outer Edge of a Clip

Drag Right to Slow Down

3 Or Set Time Stretch Options

101 Slow/Speed/Reverse Audio/Video

101

3 Or Set Time Stretch Options

If you want finer control over the speed of your video clip, you can get it using the **Time Stretch** dialog box. Undo the drag-and-drop changes you made to the video in steps 1 and 2, and then right-click the clip to open the clip context menu. Select the **Time Stretch** option to open the **Time Stretch** dialog box.

Here you have a bit more control over what happens to your clip. You can set the precise percent of increase or decrease in speed (a value less than 100% slows down the clip, a value over 100% speeds up the clip), change the speed by setting the duration of the clip (a shorter duration than the original speeds up the clip, a longer duration slows down the clip), choose to play the clip in reverse, and maintain the audio pitch (keeping the pitch of the audio portion of the clip unchanged).

▶ TIP

The **Duration** setting in the **Time Stretch** dialog box comes in very handy for music tracks. If your music is a little too short or a little too long, you can set the duration of the audio clip to match the duration of the video on the **Timeline**. A small difference in the duration audio clip is not noticed when you're watching the movie. This happens in television quite often, to fit a 32-minute program into 30 minutes or a 2-hour movie into 1 hour and 55 minutes. That is what makes room for all of those commercials.

After you have made the necessary modifications, click **OK**. These settings are applied to your clip.

▶ **TIP**

You can apply the **Time Stretch** feature to clips not yet on the **Timeline**; just right-click the clip in the **Media** panel and choose **Time Stretch** from the context menu.

102 **Group Clips**

✔ **BEFORE YOU BEGIN**

94 Add or Move a Clip on the Timeline

Another means of manipulating or moving multiple clips is by grouping them. Officially grouped clips stay together. In the previous task, lassoing or selecting multiple clips groups the clips only until you click something else. When you group clips, they stay grouped—at least until you ungroup them. If you know you will be moving or copying several clips together on a consistent basis, consider grouping them.

1 Select Clips to Be Grouped

Drag across multiple clips to lasso the adjacent clips you want to group together. Alternatively, hold the **Shift** key and click to select multiple disparate clips.

102

2 Right-click One of the Selected Clips

Right-click any one of the selected clips to open the clip context menu.

3 Choose Group

From the context menu, choose **Group**. From that point on, whenever you click one of the grouped clips, all the clips in the group are selected.

▶ **TIP**

If you rotate one clip in a group, all the clips in the group rotate. Basically, anything you do to one of the clips in the group is applied to all the clips—with the exception of transitions or effects.

4 Ungroup Clips

You ungroup clips in the same way you group them: Right-click any one of the grouped clips and choose **Ungroup** from the context menu. All the clips in that group return to being separate clips.

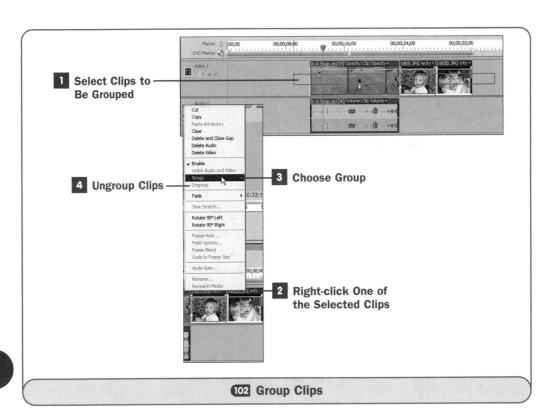

1 Select Clips to Be Grouped

4 Ungroup Clips

3 Choose Group

2 Right-click One of the Selected Clips

102 Group Clips

18

Using Transitions

IN THIS CHAPTER:

One thing that can really make your video appealing is the way you transition, or move, from one clip to the next. If you haven't already done so, start paying attention to your favorite movies and TV shows. They will not only give you some ideas on how to transition from scene to scene, but what kinds of transitions to use where. I love to watch documentaries (this was not the case before I embarked on the video-editing trail) and see how professionals such as Ken Burns do their thing. When you think about it, a home movie is very much like a documentary.

In this chapter, you will be using two basic types of transitions: single-sided and double-sided. A single-sided transition is used when there is no clip to transition from or to or when the clips are on different tracks. A double-sided transition is used between two clips. In both cases, the transition helps create a smooth flow into or out of a clip.

Premiere Elements comes with more than 70 transitions. You can customize each one and add effects, making the effective list of transitions virtually infinite. Transitions, much like the right soundtrack, are a great way to keep the audience interested in your movie. They can be a lot of fun to play with, and they add a real professional touch. But let me warn you: Too many transitions will make your viewers' heads spin and ruin even the best production, so use them sparingly.

103

103	**Fade In or Out of a Video Clip**

✔ **BEFORE YOU BEGIN**	→ **SEE ALSO**
92 Set Video and Audio Track Display	**106** Save a Custom-Designed Transition
	121 Control a Video Track's Opacity over Time
	123 Control a Video Effect with Keyframes

In this task, you will begin by adding a quick and easy transition between two video clips. Premiere Elements enables you to fade in or out of a clip with a few keystrokes. The Fade In and Fade Out effect is a very effective transition and is probably the second most used—next to the straight cut (and you can certainly argue whether the straight cut is actually a transition).

If you have two clips side by side on the **Timeline** with no transition, you have a straight cut. Cutting directly from one clip to the next is the most commonly used method for moving from one clip to the next. No frills or twirls. If you place still images on the **Timeline** and do not add transitions between the stills, you will have room to apply Ken Burns-type effects such as Pan and Zoom.

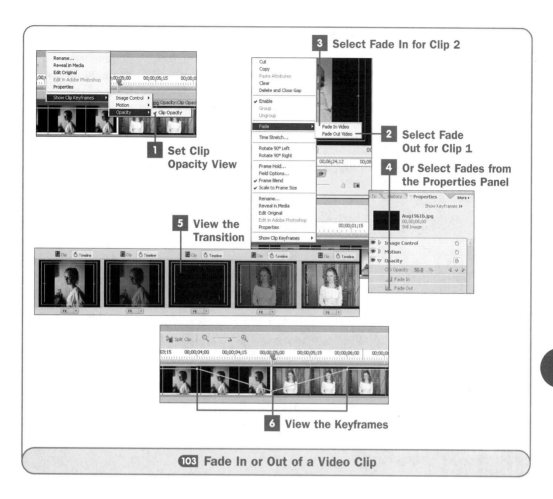

3 Select Fade In for Clip 2

1 Set Clip Opacity View

2 Select Fade Out for Clip 1

4 Or Select Fades from the Properties Panel

5 View the Transition

6 View the Keyframes

However, there are many cases where a pan, zoom, or a straight cut just doesn't work. You need something not too flashy or dramatic, just a nice little transition from one image to the next. That is were the **Fade In** and **Fade Out** effect comes in handy.

1 Set Clip Opacity View

Make sure you have two clips side by side on the same track on the **Timeline**. Right-click each of these clips and make sure the **Clip Opacity** option is checked in the clip's context menu. This is the default setting, so if you haven't changed from the default, this option should already be checked. If it is not, select it by simply clicking **Clip Opacity**. In doing this, you can later see the modifications Premiere Elements has made to your clip's opacity. *Opacity* is another word for transparency; if a clip has 0% opacity, it is 100% transparent and therefore is invisible; at 100% opacity, it is 0% transparent.

2 **Select Fade Out for Clip 1**

To create the transition, you want the last frames of the first clip to fade out into black and the first frames of the second clip to fade in from black. Right-click the first video clip on the **Timeline** and select **Fade Out Video** from the context menu.

▶ **NOTE**

If you right-click an audio clip instead of a video clip, you have the option of selecting **Fade In Audio** or **Fade Out Audio**.

3 **Select Fade In for Clip 2**

Right-click the second video clip on the **Timeline** (the clip you want to fade in to) and select **Fade In Video** from the context menu.

4 **Or Select Fades from the Properties Panel**

If you don't like working with context menus, you can apply the **Fade Out** and **Fade In** effects to the two clips by using the **Properties** panel. Click to select the first clip and open it in the **Properties** panel. Click the triangle to the left of the **Opacity** section to open the **Opacity** properties for the selected clip. Notice the two options: **Fade In** and **Fade Out** (each has a triangle icon to give you a visual indication of how the effect works). Click to apply the appropriate **Fade In** or **Fade Out** effect to the selected clip.

5 **View the Transition**

Move the CTI back to a point before the **Fade Out** effect starts for the first clip. Click the **Play** button on the **Monitor** panel to start the movie rolling. Observe how clip 1 fades out into black and clip 2 fades in from black.

6 **View the Keyframes**

Looking at the **Timeline**, you can see that applying a fade sets a keyframe marker at the Fade In and Fade Out points. The small diamond shape along the line over the frames of the clip is a keyframe marker, or keyframe point. You can adjust the start, duration, and end of the fade by dragging the markers with your mouse. As your mouse pointer is over a keyframe marker, notice that the mouse pointer changes: It has a small dot at the bottom of the arrow. The markers can be moved anywhere along your clip and allow you to customize the length of your fades. If you're pleased with the resultant fade effect, you can save this customized transition as discussed in **106** **Save a Custom-Designed Transition**. For information on how to transition audio clips, see **105** **Add an Audio Transition**.

104 Add a Video Transition

✔ **BEFORE YOU BEGIN**

92 Set Video and Audio Track Display

Adding a transition to the start of a clip, the end of a clip, or between two clips is easy. Simply drag the desired transition from the **Effects and Transitions** panel to the clip in the **Timeline**. When the transition is over an area where it can be placed, the clip becomes highlighted. Drop the transition by releasing the mouse button.

1 Select the Transition

Make sure you have two clips side by side on the same track on the **Timeline**. For this task, you will be using the **Cross Dissolve** transition, located in the **Dissolve** category of the **Video Transitions**. To apply this transition, drag from the **Effects and Transitions** panel to the appropriate clip(s) in the **Timeline**.

2 Drop the Transition at the Beginning of a Clip, at the End of a Clip, or Between Two Clips

As you drag the transition over the clips in the Timeline, notice that different parts of the clips are highlighted. Also look for a small icon next to the mouse pointer that shows you the direction in which the transition will be applied (right, left, or middle). You can apply the transition to the end of a clip, between two clips, or at the beginning of a clip. For this example, drop the **Cross Dissolve** transition between the two clips.

After dropping the transition on the desired clip, notice a rectangle at the top of the clip with the transition name inside. This rectangle shows where the transition starts and stops.

104

▶ **NOTES**

Right-click the transition rectangle and choose **Clear** from the context menu to remove the transition from the clip.

Drag the beginning or end of the transition rectangle to make the duration of the transition longer or shorter.

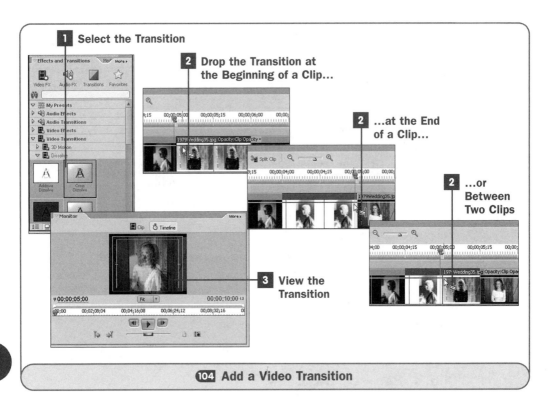

104 Add a Video Transition

3 View the Transition

View the transition by moving the CTI to a point before the transition begins and clicking the **Play** button in the **Monitor** panel. Alternatively, scrub the CTI over the transition on the **Timeline**.

▶ **TIP**

If, after viewing the transition, you change your mind about its appropriateness, don't worry. Just choose another transition and drop it over the old one to replace the old transition with your new selection. There is no need to undo the first transition, unless you decide not to transition at all.

After the transition is placed on the **Timeline**, a number of controls become available in the **Properties** panel. For most transitions, you can use these controls to set the duration and the center of the transition, and to reverse the motion of the transition. Simply click the transition rectangle, located above the clip on the **Timeline**, and the transition opens in the **Properties** panel. Make adjustments there as appropriate.

105 Add an Audio Transition

✔ BEFORE YOU BEGIN	→ SEE ALSO
92 Set Video and Audio Track Display	**111** Raise, Lower, and Normalize Sound Volume
104 Add a Video Transition	

In addition to the video transitions on the **Effects and Transitions** panel, you also find audio transitions. Audio transitions have the same purpose as their video counterparts: to move smoothly between clips. Audio transitions are applied the same way as video transitions and have many of the same options available.

◼ Select an Audio Transition

Located in the **Effects and Transitions** panel in the **Audio Transitions, Crossfade** category, the two audio transitions can be added to clips on the audio tracks in the **Timeline**. Both transition effects similarly dissolve sound between two clips. The **Constant Gain** transition, however, fades sound out on one clip and in on the other in a linear pattern; the result sometimes sounds rather abrupt. The **Constant Power** transition, on the other hand, curves the sound transitions, offering a smoother dissolve. **Constant Power** is probably the preferred audio transition of the two.

◼ Drop the Transition on the Audio Clips

Drag and drop the transition from the **Effects and Transitions** panel on the audio clips in the audio tracks in the **Timeline**, just as you would a video transition. The **Constant Gain** transition can be dropped at the beginning or end of a clip; the **Constant Power** transition can be dropped at the beginning of a clip, between two clips, or at the end of a clip.

◼ Listen to the Transition

Scrub the CTI over the audio transition area of the **Timeline**. Alternatively, place the CTI in front of the transition on the **Timeline** and click the **Play** button on the **Monitor**. If you don't like what you hear, continue on.

105

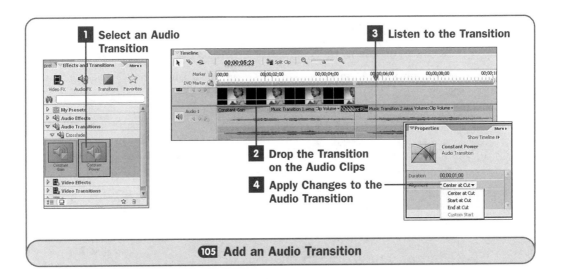

1 Select an Audio Transition

3 Listen to the Transition

2 Drop the Transition on the Audio Clips

4 Apply Changes to the Audio Transition

105 Add an Audio Transition

4 Apply Changes to the Audio Transition

Both transitions can be manipulated to some extent in the **Properties** panel. You play with audio transitions in the same way you do video transitions: Click the transition rectangle above the audio clip to open the transition in the **Properties** panel. You can also drag the left edge of the transition rectangle to lengthen the transition. For the **Constant Gain** transition, the adjustments are limited to changing the **Duration**. For the **Constant Power** transition, you can also choose to place the transition at the beginning, end, or between two audio clips.

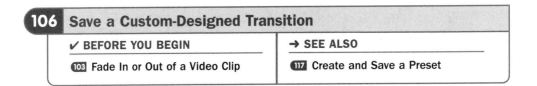

106 Save a Custom-Designed Transition

✔ BEFORE YOU BEGIN	→ SEE ALSO
103 Fade In or Out of a Video Clip	117 Create and Save a Preset

Any of the transitions that allow you to customize its motion (that is, where you can specify **Scale** and **Position** values), opacity, or Image Control can be saved for later use. Because there is no preset transition that fades in and out on a clip, you will save that customized transition effect for reuse later. If you worked through 103 **Fade In or Out of a Video Clip**, you can create it once, save it, and use it over and over.

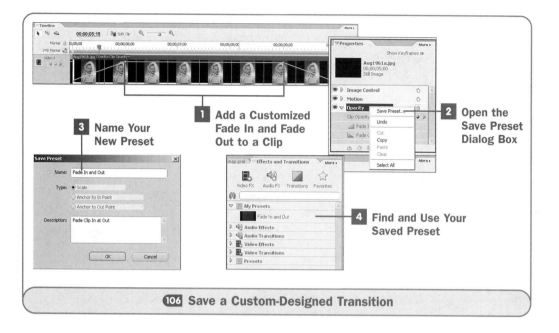

106 Save a Custom-Designed Transition

1 Add a Customized Fade In and Fade Out to a Clip

Make sure you have one clip that's 5 seconds long or 150 frames (NTSC), with no effects or transitions applied, on the **Timeline**. Follow the instructions in **103 Fade In or Out of a Video Clip**. Apply the **Fade In** effect to the beginning of the clip and the **Fade Out** effect to the end of the clip. As you can see by the keyframe markers on the **Timeline**, the default duration of each effect is 30 frames or 1 second. The first second of the clip shows the Opacity line going up (the **Fade In** effect) and the last second of the clip going down (the **Fade Out** effect). You can change the duration of these effects by moving the keyframe markers until you get the effect for which you are looking.

▶ NOTE

After this transition is saved, whenever you apply it to a 5-second clip, the transition will fade the clip in for 1 second, show 3 seconds of the clip, and end with a 1-second fade out.

2 Open the Save Preset Dialog Box

To save your new, customized transition, click the clip to which you've applied the **Fade In** and **Fade Out** effects. This action highlights the clip and opens it in the **Properties** panel. In this case, you have created a transition that affects the **Opacity** of a clip; therefore, the settings and keyframes are

106

under the **Opacity** property in the **Properties** panel. Right-click the **Opacity** heading and choose **Save Preset** from the context menu. The **Save Preset** dialog box opens.

▶ **TIP**

Saving a customized effect is discussed in detail in ⟨117⟩ **Create and Save a Preset.**

3 Name Your New Preset

In this dialog box, name the customized transition and select the **Type** of preset it is. For this example, leave the **Type** option set at the default setting **Scale**, and type a description to remind you of what the preset does. Click **OK** to save the custom transition or click **Cancel** if you decide not to save it now.

When creating a preset, you have three options: **Scale**, **Anchor to In Point**, and **Anchor to Out Point**:

- The **Scale** option scales the keyframes markers proportionally to the length of the clip to which it will be applied. Applying this preset also deletes any existing keyframes on the applied clip.

- The **Anchor to In Point** option places the first keyframe marker the same distance from the first frame in the applied clip as it was from the original clip's first frame. This option does not do any scaling.

- The **Anchor to Out Point** option places the last keyframe marker at the same distance from the last frame in the applied clip as it was from the original clip's last frame. This option does not do any scaling.

▶ **TIP**

Use preset names that will easily remind you, at a glance, what that saved preset does.

4 Find and Use Your Saved Preset

The new transition is added to the **My Presets** category in the **Effects and Transitions** panel. You can now drag and drop your customized transition onto any clip on the **Timeline**.

19

Advanced Timeline Video and Audio Editing

IN THIS CHAPTER:

This chapter continues where Chapter 17, "Editing on the Timeline," left off. Advanced editing gives you the ability to change video field properties, freeze a frame and change clip opacity, add narration, enhance and control audio, add interactive content for Web use, and combine multiple projects into one.

This chapter is considered advanced because it takes you beyond the simple cutting of clips. You will look at the opacity, or the transparency, of a clip, and see how simple it can be to make your clip semi-transparent. When you are ready to create your first major documentary, narration will be important, so you will learn how to add that to your movie project. Audio is a major part of most projects and can sometimes need a little tweaking. You will see where the options are that allow you to control how your audio sounds, and make sure that the audio you use is of the best possible quality and balance.

Video is widely used on the Internet these days. Many websites have video introductions that start when you enter the site. You will learn how to create an interactive video that you can use on a website and that will allow your video to interact with other sites, pages, or images on the Internet.

Lastly, you will discover the ease of copying your **Timeline**, or parts of it, from one project to another. This might not seem like a big deal right now, but you will probably need to do this at some time.

107

107 | Freeze a Frame

✔ BEFORE YOU BEGIN	→ SEE ALSO
171 Change Slides to the Beat of Music	**87** Grab a Still from Video
	101 Slow/Speed/Reverse Audio/Video

Frame Hold, or freeze frame, is one of the fun video tricks you can use in your movies. This option allows the audio to continue rolling while the video stays put on a single frame. I imagine that at some time during the editing of your movies that you will come up with that one frame in a clip that just needs to be frozen in time.

The frame you choose as the freeze frame will appear and freeze from the beginning (the In Point) to the end (the Out Point) of the clip. Take this into consideration to determine whether your clip needs to be split to better isolate the freeze frame; that way you are not freezing a frame for an entire 45-minute movie.

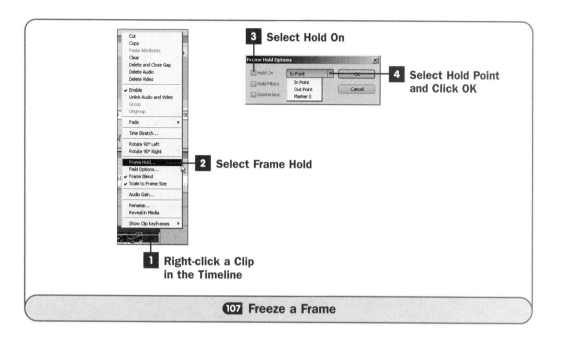

107

■ Right-click a Clip in the Timeline

Right-click the clip in the **Timeline** that contains the frame you want to freeze. The clip is selected and the clip's context menu opens.

■ Select Frame Hold

Select **Frame Hold** to open the **Frame Hold Options** dialog box.

■ Select Hold On

Enable the check box in front of the **Hold On** option. This option selects and applies the freeze frame option to the selected clip.

▶ NOTES

The **Hold Filters** option, also in the **Frame Hold Options** dialog box, prevents any keyframed effects that were applied to the clip from taking place.

The **Deinterlace** option removes one field from an interlaced clip and doubles the remaining field. This option removes interlace artifacts from the freeze frame, if they exist.

4 Select Hold Point and Click OK

You must identify the frame in the clip you want to freeze. The frame you want to freeze is called the *hold point*, and Premiere Elements offers three options for the identifying the hold point in your clip: **In Point**, **Out Point**, and **Marker 0**:

- **In Point**—The hold point is the very first frame of your clip as it appears on the **Timeline**. When you choose this option, the very first frame of the clip is frozen for the entire clip.

- **Out Point**—The hold point is the very last frame in your clip. When you choose this option, the very last frame of the clip is frozen for the entire clip.

- **Marker 0**—This option requires that you set an other numbered clip marker and specify 0 (zero). The marker indicates the frame you want to freeze; that frame is frozen for the entire clip.

▶ **TIP**

107

To set an other numbered clip marker, zoom in on the clip so you can see the individual frames and position the CTI so the frame you want to freeze is selected. From the menu at the top of the screen, choose **Marker, Set Clip Marker, Other Numbered**. A dialog box opens with the option to enter a number; be sure that the marker's number is 0 (zero), and then press OK. The marker is applied to the current frame marked by the CTI.

When selecting the hold point option, remember that when you choose **In Point** or **Out Point**, later changing the In or Out point (as described in **86 Trim Clips in the Media Panel**) does not change the freeze frame. When you choose the **Marker 0** option, however, changing the position of the marker *does* change the freeze frame.

When you are finished setting your options, click the **OK** button. You can then view the results of your freeze frame by scrubbing over the clip in the **Timeline**. The audio from the clip plays as usual, but the video freezes on the frame you selected as your hold point.

108 Make a Clip Semi-Transparent

✔ BEFORE YOU BEGIN	→ SEE ALSO
91 Add, Delete, and Size Tracks	**121** Control a Video Track's Opacity over Time
92 Set Video and Audio Track Display	**136** Create a Title Overlay for Your Video
94 Add or Move a Clip on the Timeline	

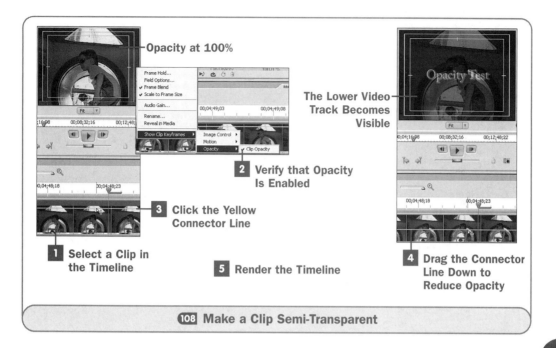

Opacity at 100%

The Lower Video Track Becomes Visible

2 Verify that Opacity Is Enabled

3 Click the Yellow Connector Line

1 Select a Clip in the Timeline

5 Render the Timeline

4 Drag the Connector Line Down to Reduce Opacity

108 Make a Clip Semi-Transparent

108

Opacity is the opposite of transparency. So when we talk about a clip's opacity, we are talking about how transparent it is. There are many reasons for making a clip semi-transparent: You can lower the opacity of a clip to create a ghost-type effect or to allow clips on tracks below the current track to become visible. This task explains the quick and easy way to change the opacity of an entire clip.

1 Select a Clip in the Timeline

Make sure you have one clip on video track 1 and another clip on video track 2, directly above the track 1 clip. Click any clip in the **Timeline** to select it. Zoom in to the clip so you can see the individual frames in the clip.

2 Verify that Opacity Is Enabled

At the top of the selected clip you will see a yellow line; this line is the **Keyframe Connector**. Use this line to adjust the opacity of the clip. To ensure that the **Opacity** feature of the **Keyframe Connector** is enabled, right-click the clip to open the context menu. Select **Show Clip Keyframes**, **Opacity** and make sure that there is a check mark in front of the **Clip Opacity** option. This option specifies that the yellow connector will be used to control the opacity of the clip.

3 Click the Yellow Connector Line

When the yellow connector line is at the top of the frame, the frame is showing at 100% opacity (that is, it has no transparency). To adjust the clip's opacity, click and hold the mouse pointer on the yellow connector line.

4 Drag the Connector Line Down to Reduce Opacity

Drag the line down about half way, decreasing the opacity of the selected clip to 50%. You can set the opacity at whatever percent you desire. Notice that you do not see the opacity of the clip change in the **Monitor** panel until you release the mouse button. By lowering the opacity, you are making the lower clip (in this case, a title) visible. The lower the opacity of the track 2 clip, the more visible the clip on the lower track becomes.

5 Render the Timeline

After changing the opacity of a clip, you should render that area of your **Timeline**. To do so, press **Enter**.

108   109 Add Narration to Your Movie

✔ BEFORE YOU BEGIN	→ SEE ALSO
84 Add Media with the Adobe Media Downloader	**111** Raise, Lower, and Normalize Sound Volume
	153 Add Audio to a Menu
	168 Add Graphics, Text, and Narration to Your Slideshow

Normally, we would not add a task for something that Premiere Elements doesn't do. This case, however, is an exception. *Narration* is a very important part of many home movies and independent films, especially documentaries. Even though Premiere Elements cannot *record* your narration, it can capture the audio narration file and sync it to the video on the **Timeline**. You can do this by recording audio onto your camcorder and using Premiere Elements to capture just the audio narration you recorded. Then move the audio clip to the **Timeline** and sync it with your video. This approach to narration is particularly useful for slideshows and documentary-type movies.

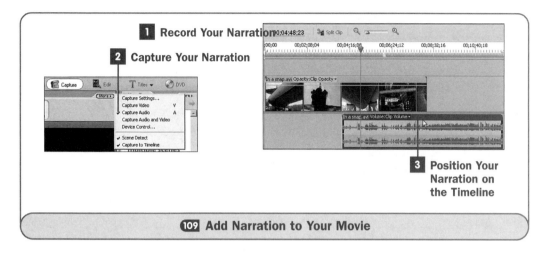

1 **Record Your Narration**

2 **Capture Your Narration**

3 **Position Your Narration on the Timeline**

109 Add Narration to Your Movie

1 Record Your Narration

The first step in adding narration to a movie project is to record the narration on tape. You can do this by simply talking into your camcorder while you watch the video on your computer. It is best to have some sort of script to refer to or read from, otherwise you might be doing more takes than necessary.

2 Capture Your Narration

After you have your narration on tape, capture the audio in Premiere Elements just like you would any other clip from your camcorder. To capture just the audio track from the camcorder, open the **More** menu in the **Capture** workspace and select the **Capture Audio** option. You might also want to make sure that the **Capture to Timeline** option is selected in the **More** menu so the audio track is added to both the **Media** panel *and* the **Timeline**.

▶ TIP

When recording your narration, record a loud noise, such as a hand clap, at the beginning of every scene change. This makes it much easier to line up the audio with the video later on. You can edit out the clap (use the **Razor** tool to do this) after you have the narration in sync with the video.

3 Position Your Narration on the Timeline

If you started your narration with a noise to reference the start of the first scene, line that noise up with the first frame of the scene. The noise is displayed by a high, sharp peak in the audio waveform and can be clearly heard through the speakers. Play the **Timeline** to determine whether the narration is in sync with the video. If not, make minor adjustments by dragging the narration clip on the **Timeline**, a little at a time, until the narration comes into sync with the video.

110	Track Audio Volume

✔ BEFORE YOU BEGIN	→ SEE ALSO
94 Add or Move a Clip on the Timeline	111 Raise, Lower, and Normalize Sound Volume
	112 Balance Sound over Left and Right Channels

If you don't keep an eye on the audio levels in your movie project, you might have a surprise after you view the DVD on a television. Even though the audio might sound okay on your computer speakers, it might not sound that way after putting it onto a DVD or exporting the movie project. One of the ways to avoid audio volume issues in a pro-active way is by using the **Audio Meters** feature.

109

The **Audio Meters** window helps you determine whether any portions, or possibly all, of your audio clips are over (or under) the recommended levels. To monitor your audio levels, open the **Audio Meters** window and play your clip while watching what the meters do.

1 Choose Windows, Audio Meters

From the menu at the top of your screen, choose **Windows**, **Audio Meters** to open the **Audio Meters** window.

2 Play the Clip

With the **Audio Meters** window open on your screen, click the **Play** button in the **Monitor** panel to play your clip. If you have the time, you can play the entire movie.

▶ **NOTE**

It is not necessary to view the **Audio Meters** for the entire clip unless you have good reason to do so. You can spot check the clip by scrubbing through the clip, primarily checking the louder portions. You just want to make sure that the audio is not off the scale anywhere. At some point, however, you are going to have to listen to the entire movie, making sure that the audio is at reasonable levels. You wouldn't want your viewers to get a big surprise when they watch your movie.

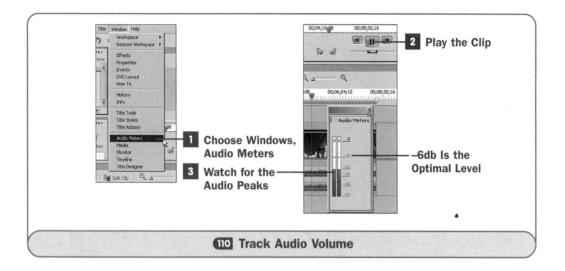

1 Choose Windows, Audio Meters

2 Play the Clip

3 Watch for the Audio Peaks

−6db Is the Optimal Level

110 Track Audio Volume

3 Watch for the Audio Peaks

Watch to see where the peaks are in the audio track of the clip. Peaks of −6db or above (between −6 and 0) should be adjusted; peaks of 0 or more (constant red in the audio monitor) must be adjusted or the output will be poor. The tasks that follow show you how to adjust the volume and other audio properties.

▶ **TIP**

Watch for levels that get above −6db (between −6 and 0) and adjust the volume accordingly. Constant levels of between −12db and −6db, with the peaks below 0db, are the best. An average level of −6db is optimal.

111 Raise, Lower, and Normalize Sound Volume	
✔ **BEFORE YOU BEGIN**	→ **SEE ALSO**
110 Track Audio Volume	**112** Balance Sound over Left and Right Channels

Volume levels are important to the overall quality of your production. There is nothing worse that having the volume increase by 20db just as a cannon is being shot off in the video clip. Poor audio levels can really put a damper on the whole video experience. With Premiere Elements, you can control the volume level for each clip individually. You can even split a clip and then control the volume for each piece individually, if you need that kind of control. You can also normalize the sound over an entire clip, making the audio volume levels more consistent over the length of the clip and the project.

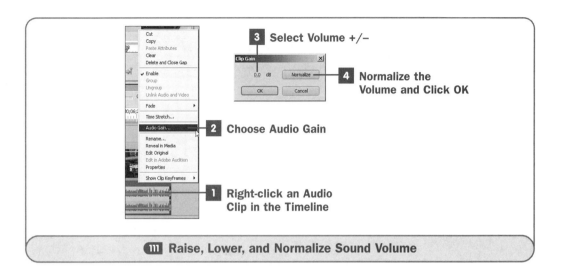

111 Raise, Lower, and Normalize Sound Volume

1 Right-click an Audio Clip in the Timeline

Right-click an audio clip in the **Timeline** to select it and open the clip's context menu.

2 Choose Audio Gain

From the context menu, select **Audio Gain** to open the **Clip Gain** dialog box.

3 Select Volume +/−

To change the clip's volume, position the mouse pointer over the **0.0** area. Click and drag to the right or left: Drag left to decrease the number and the volume; drag right to increase the number and the volume. Alternatively, click the **0.0** value and type a specific number, rather than dragging. The **0.0** value is the clip's volume at the point before you make any changes. Entering a positive number increases the volume by that many decibels; entering a negative number lowers the volume by that many decibels.

▶ NOTE

When adjusting the volume, remember that **0.0db** is the clip's original volume level. Any positive value is an increase in the original volume, and any negative value is a decrease in the original volume.

4 Normalize the Volume and Click OK

After you have made any volume changes necessary, you can normalize the audio levels. By selecting this option, the audio levels of the clip are automatically adjusted. Levels that are too high are reduced and levels that are too low are increased to create a more even volume across the entire clip. If there are certain places in the audio clip where you want the levels higher or lower on purpose, normalizing might do more harm than good. Listen to the normalized clip to ensure you get the desired result.

After you have made any volume changes and normalized the audio levels for the clip, click the **OK** button. Play your adjusted clip to see whether the changes made accomplished your goal of adjusting the clip's volume. If not, open the **Clip Gain** dialog box again and make finer adjustments. Don't forget you can always undo your changes!

---

112 **Balance Sound over Left and Right Channels**

✔ BEFORE YOU BEGIN	→ SEE ALSO
94 Add or Move a Clip on the Timeline	**109** Add Narration to Your Movie
	111 Raise, Lower, and Normalize Sound Volume

The **Balance** audio effect lets you control the volumes of the left and right channels in the audio track for a particular clip. If your audio clip is in stereo, you will see two audio waveforms for each clip—the left stereo channel (on top) and right stereo channel (on the bottom); a mono clip shows only one waveform.

112

1 **Open the Effects and Transitions Panel**

To gain access to the **Balance** audio effect, you must add that effect to an audio clip. First, open the **Effects and Transitions** panel by choosing **Window, Effects**. When the panel opens, click the **Audio FX** button at the top of the panel to view the audio effects.

2 **Expand the Audio Effects Group**

Open the **Audio Effects** group by clicking the arrow to the left of the group's name and locate the **Balance** effect in the list.

3 **Drag the Balance Effect to an Audio Clip in the Timeline**

After locating the **Balance** effect in the **Audio Effects** group, drag it to the audio clip you want to modify on the **Timeline** and drop it on the clip.

4 **Open the Balance Properties**

Open the **Properties** panel for the targeted audio clip and click the **Balance** effect. The effect provides options to adjust the audio balance between the left and right channels.

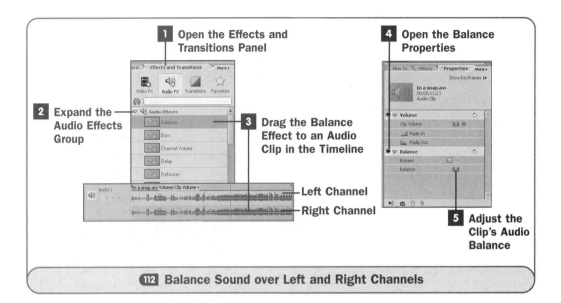

5 Adjust the Clip's Audio Balance

Click the **Balance** number indicator and type positive or negative values. Positive values increase the proportion of volume for the right channel; negative values increase the proportion of volume for the left channel. Alternatively, drag the indicator to the left to adjust the volume for the left channel; drag to the right to adjust the volume for the right channel. Play back the audio clip to test your results. You can use the **Bypass** check box to hear the sound before and after. Checking the box ignores the effect, unchecking the box applies the effect.

20

Adding Spice to Your Video

IN THIS CHAPTER:

One of the most interesting aspects of Premiere Elements is that it is accessible by editors with many levels of technical skill and experience. For the hobbyist or the novice user, it offers many automatic and preset features. Yet most experienced users are pleasantly surprised to find how deep this program goes and how customizable nearly all its features are.

In this chapter, we'll look at some of the tools Premiere Elements offers to affect your video and audio qualities. Many of these are automatic or preset effects—but even the more advanced tools are remarkably intuitive and easy to use, and it's likely you'll quickly become very comfortable using them on a regular basis.

---

113   Adjust Color and Brightness

→ **SEE ALSO**

123 Control a Video Effect with Keyframes

113

Because you often need to correct the color, brightness, or contrast for a clip or still, Premiere Elements places controls for these settings conveniently in the **Properties** panel by default. You can also access these settings directly from the clip in the **Timeline**.

1   Select a Clip on the Timeline

Click a clip on the **Timeline** to select it. By default, four categories of properties for the selected clip appear in the **Properties** panel: **Image Control**, **Motion**, **Opacity**, and **Volume**. Naturally, these properties appear only if they're applicable to the clip. Stills, for instance, do not have **Volume** properties, and audio clips do not have image properties.

2   Change Settings in the Properties Panel

Click the triangle to the left of **Image Control** to expand this property's details. A control panel for setting **Brightness**, **Contrast**, **Hue**, and **Saturation** becomes available.

- The **Brightness** setting, which controls the tonal values of the image, defaults at 0% and can be adjusted from –100% to 100%.

- The **Contrast** setting, which sharpens the image's tonal qualities by emphasizing the difference between dark and light areas, defaults at 100% and can be adjusted from 0% to 200%.

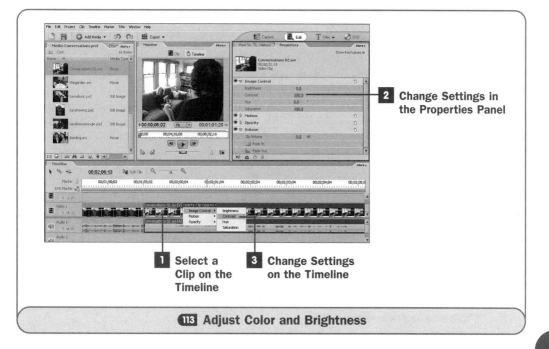

2 Change Settings in the Properties Panel

1 Select a Clip on the Timeline

3 Change Settings on the Timeline

113 Adjust Color and Brightness

113

- The **Hue** option is set in degrees as on a color wheel, with different degree settings changing the color tone of the image. It defaults at **0.0** (which is the basic color tone of the original image). Changing this setting 180° sets color tone to the opposite, or complementary, color; other settings move the image's color tone through variations of red, green, and blue.

- The **Saturation** setting defaults to 100%. Change this value to 0% to remove all color, leaving you with a black-and-white image. Change it to 200% to double the amount of all color applied to your image. Values in between produce variations on these results.

These values can either be set numerically by typing in new values, or by sliding the values across settings. To slide the values, mouse over the settings until the mouse pointer changes to a hand with an arrow on either side, and then click and drag. The numbers increase or decrease fluidly, and the results of the new settings are displayed in the **Monitor** panel.

▶ **NOTE**

Hue, **Saturation**, and **Brightness** form the three dimensions of color. The range of hues is usually illustrated as a wheel of color ranging from red through green through blue and back to red. Saturation is the density of hue in a given color, whereas brightness is the amount of lightness or whiteness in the color.

3 Change Settings on the Timeline

An alternative way to change these settings is to right-click the clip on the Timeline and, from the context menu that appears, choose **Show Clip Keyframe** and then choose one of the submenus for **Hue**, **Saturation**, or **Brightness**.

Select a property detail. This detail now appears on the clip's title bar where the words **Motion: Position** initially were. Raise or lower the horizontal yellow line that appears in the clip to adjust the settings for that property detail.

▶ **NOTE**

Properties, as well as nearly all effects, when applied to a clip can also be set to change or move over time with keyframes. See **123** Control a Video Effect with Keyframes.

---

114 **Add and Customize an Effect**

→ SEE ALSO

117 Create and Save a Preset
123 Control a Video Effect with Keyframes

113

Every one of Premiere Elements's effects, whether it's a preset, a motion effect, or a transition, can be tweaked and customized until you achieve precisely the effect for which you're looking. (And after you've changed the settings for an effect, you can save the modified effect as your own personal preset; see **117** **Create and Save a Preset**.)

In fact, it's often more effective, and more fun, to think of preset effects as merely starting points for more elaborate effects.

1 Select the Clip to Be Affected

Click the clip you want to modify on your **Timeline**. A default list of the clip's properties appears in the **Properties** panel, including **Image Control**, **Motion**, **Opacity**, and **Volume** (as applicable to the clip).

2 Apply the Effect

Locate an effect in the **Effects and Transitions** panel and drag and drop it on the clip in the **Timeline**.

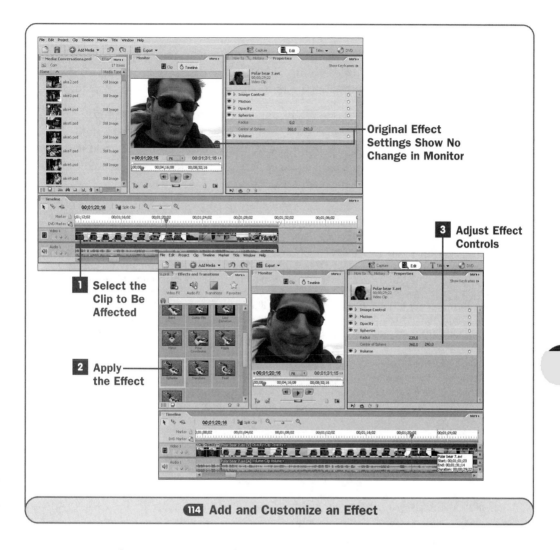

Original Effect Settings Show No Change in Monitor

3 Adjust Effect Controls

1 Select the Clip to Be Affected

2 Apply the Effect

114 Add and Customize an Effect

For this example, I used the **Spherize** effect, which can be found in the **Video FX** collection in the **Distort** category. The **Spherize** effect, which ultimately produces a fish-eye distortion, is one of many effects that doesn't display an immediate change when applied to the clip. Adding the effect gives you access to a control panel for the effect rather than producing an immediate change. After you change a few settings, you'll see the effect at work.

▶ NOTE

The center of your video frame is presented as a measurement in pixels, half the width and half the height of a video frame. In other words, in the NTSC system, the center point of your screen image is 360/240. In the PAL system, the center of the frame is 393/288.

3   Adjust Effect Controls

Click the triangle next to your effect in the **Properties** panel to reveal the control panel for that effect's details. The **Spherize** effect offers controls for designating the radius of the sphere (in pixels) and the sphere's center point.

Type new numbers into these settings and view the results in the **Monitor** panel. As an alternative, you can mouse over either setting's numbers until your mouse pointer looks like a hand with a double-headed arrow, and then click and drag left or right to increase or decrease the numbers more fluidly. The results are displayed in your **Monitor** panel.

▶ TIP

After you begin applying effects to your clip, you'll notice that the quality of the image played back in the **Monitor** has apparently deteriorated. On slower computers, playback might even seem jumpy or irregular. This is because you are looking at a soft render of your clip—drawn on the fly by your computer as you play the affected clip. (A clip that should be hard rendered is indicated by a red line above the clip on the **Timeline**.) To see a better example of what your clip will look like on final output, press **Enter** to render the **Timeline**. The red line above the clip turns green when rendering is complete, and the quality of your playback will be an accurate representation of what your final output will look like.

114

---

115   **Rotate or Flip a Clip**

→ SEE ALSO

   117 Create and Save a Preset
   123 Control a Video Effect with Keyframes

Premiere Elements offers a variety of effects for distorting your screen image—both in two-dimensional and three-dimensional space (see **128** **Rotate a Clip in 3D**). What's more, by adding keyframes (see **118** **Add Motion to Still**), you can even animate these distortions, saving your result as your own, custom preset (see **117** **Create and Save a Preset**).

1   Select the Clip to Be Affected

Click the clip you want to modify on your **Timeline**. A default list of the clip's properties appears in the **Properties** panel, including **Image Control**, **Motion**, **Opacity**, and **Volume** (as applicable to the clip).

Click the triangle to the left of the **Image Control** property to reveal the detail settings.

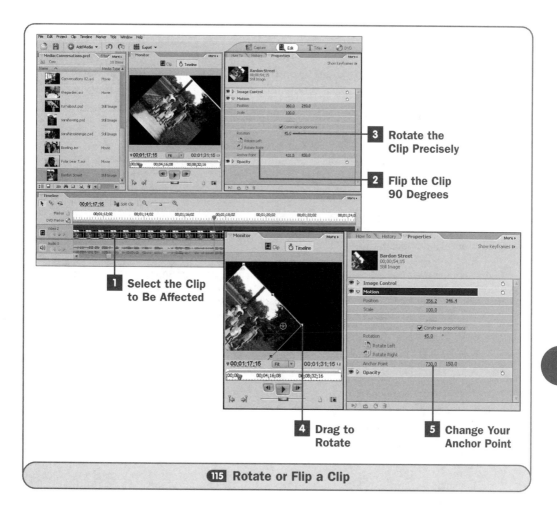

3 Rotate the Clip Precisely

2 Flip the Clip 90 Degrees

1 Select the Clip to Be Affected

4 Drag to Rotate

5 Change Your Anchor Point

115

115 Rotate or Flip a Clip

▶ **NOTE**

As you can do with all the effects that change the screen image's scale, dimensions, or shape, you can rotate your screen image by clicking the image in the **Monitor** panel and manipulate it by dragging the control handles that appear on the image's corners.

2 **Flip the Clip 90 Degrees**

The **Properties** panel has two one-click **Rotate** settings that flip your clip 90° to the right or left. Click the **Rotate Left** or **Rotate Right** button to change the orientation of the image.

3 Rotate the Clip Precisely

You can rotate your clip by an arbitrary amount by typing the number of degrees you want to turn your clip in the numerical settings area. You can also change the settings more fluidly by mousing over the numbers until the mouse pointer turns into a little hand with a two-headed arrow. Click and drag left or right over the settings to roll the numbers up or down. The changes are displayed in the **Monitor** panel. You can also rotate your clip in 3D or make it appear to tumble through space (see **128 Rotate a Clip in 3D**).

▶ NOTES

You can easily flip your clip, horizontally or vertically, in a single move by dragging it onto the **Horizontal Flip** or **Vertical Flip** effects found in the **Transform** collection in the **Effects and Transitions** panel.

When many of the effects are applied to a clip, the clip's position on the **Timeline** can affect what the resulting video will look like. Many distortions, for instance, pull the image in from the sides of the video frame, resulting in the clip appearing against a black background (if the clip is on an upper video track, the background reveals the clip on the video track below it).

115

4 Drag to Rotate

Alternatively, you can change your image's position, scale, rotation, and other settings by clicking the screen image in the **Monitor** panel and dragging the clip around by the center and corner handles that appear.

5 Change the Anchor Point

The anchor point is the point around which the clip pivots when you rotate it. By default, this point is the center of the clip.

Change the **Anchor Point** settings in the **Properties** panel and click the screen image in the **Monitor** panel. Note that the image has shifted to one side and that the circled cross, representing the anchor point, is no longer in the center. Even if you drag the screen image back into the center of the frame, the anchor point remains in this new position.

Now type a new **Rotate** value. The image seems to hook around the point rather than spin around its center.

If you'd like, you can use keyframing to set waypoints for the **Rotate** positions, creating an animated spin effect for your clip (see **123 Control a Video Effect with Keyframes**).

▶ **NOTE**

If your image is smaller than your video frame—as can be the case with a logo or other graphic—you can set the anchor point for your rotation outside the image, using negative numbers if necessary. By using keyframes to create a motion path, you can animate your graphic to move around a circular path.

---

116 Reset or Remove an Effect

✔ **BEFORE YOU BEGIN**	→ **SEE ALSO**
114 Add and Customize an Effect	**115** Rotate or Flip a Clip
	117 Create and Save a Preset
	123 Control a Video Effect with Keyframes

No change is permanent in nonlinear editing. This is why computer-based, nonlinear editing is often referred to as a nondestructive editing process. Everything, short of overwriting your original files, can be undone.

So feel free to experiment with effects on your clips. And if you want to compare how the clip looked before and after you applied the effect, you can do so with a single click of the mouse.

116

1 Apply an Effect to a Clip

Browse the **Effects and Transitions** panel for an effect. As you open each collection, look at the thumbnails to see a sample of each effect. If you click to select a **Motion** or **Transitional** effect, the thumbnail displays an animated preview.

When you've found an effect you want to use, drag it onto a clip on the **Timeline**.

▶ **NOTE**

You can apply as many effects as you want to a single clip. As you do, the effects are added to the clip's properties in the **Properties** panel. Premiere Elements applies these effects in the order they appear in the **Properties** panel, so rearranging their order can often produce significantly different results.

2 Adjust the Effect

When an effect is applied to a clip and the clip is selected on the **Timeline**, the effect is listed in the clip's **Properties** panel. Click the triangle to the left of the effect name to open the detail controls.

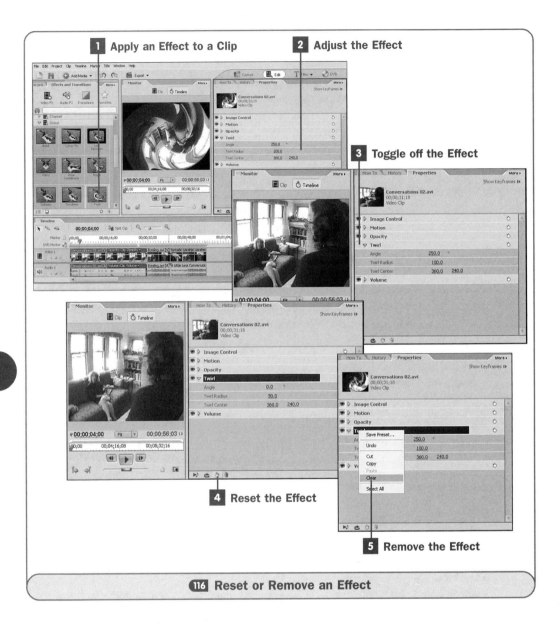

116   Reset or Remove an Effect

Adjust the controls to affect your screen image (see **114** **Add and Customize an Effect** and **115** **Rotate or Flip a Clip**). Your changes are displayed in the **Monitor** panel.

3   Toggle off the Effect

To compare the before and after of your applied effect, click the eye icon to the left of the effect's name in the **Properties** panel. This action turns on and off the effect and all its current settings.

If you have more than one effect applied to your clip, you can toggle each effect individually.

4 Reset the Effect

Occasionally, especially with preset or automatic effects, you might find that your adjustments to the settings have taken your image some place you really didn't want to go. If so, you can easily reset the effect to its initial settings—without affecting any other changes you've made to other effects for the clip.

With the name of the effect you want to reset selected in the **Properties** panel, click the little stopwatch icon at the bottom of the panel. The effect reverts to its default settings.

5 Remove the Effect

If you decide you don't want any or all of your effects, you can easily remove them from the clip.

To remove an effect, right-click the name of the effect in the **Properties** panel and, from the context menu that appears, select **Clear**.

▶ **NOTE**

To remove all the effects you added to a clip in one move, click the **Properties** panel's **More** button and select **Delete All Effects from Clip**.

---

117 **Create and Save a Preset**

✔ BEFORE YOU BEGIN	→ SEE ALSO
114 Add and Customize an Effect	**118** Add Motion to a Still
	119 Pan and Zoom Still Images a la Ken Burns
	123 Control a Video Effect with Keyframes

If you like the effects and motions you've applied to a clip, you can save each effect as your own, custom preset, so you can easily recall it in this and future projects.

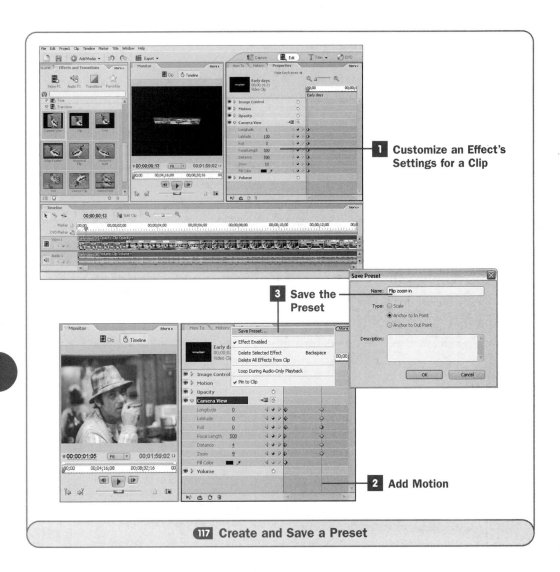

1 Customize an Effect's Settings for a Clip

3 Save the Preset

2 Add Motion

117 Create and Save a Preset

1 Customize an Effect's Settings on a Clip

Browse the **Effects and Transitions** panel for an effect. As you open each collection, look at the thumbnails to see a sample of each effect. If you click to select a **Motion** or **Transitional** effect, the thumbnail displays an animated preview.

When you've found an effect you want to use, drag it onto a clip on the **Timeline**.

▶ **NOTE**

Although you can add as many effects as you'd like to any clip, you can save a preset for only one effect or motion at a time.

With the clip selected on the **Timeline**, customize the effect you've applied in the **Properties** panel as described in **114 Add and Customize an Effect**.

For this example, I applied the **Camera View** effect (from the **Video FX Transform** collection). I set the **Focal Length** to **500**, the **Distance** to **500**, and **Latitude** to **100**—essentially making my initial screen image appear to be rotated facing down in three-dimensional space, a long distance from the camera.

2 Add Motion

If you'd like, you can add keyframed motion to your effect either by starting from a preset motion effect or by creating custom movement from scratch (as described in **118 Add Motion to a Still** and **119 Pan and Zoom Still Images a la Ken Burns**).

In my example, I clicked the **Show Keyframes** button at the top of the **Properties** panel and then clicked the stopwatch icon to the right of the **Camera View** listing in the **Properties** panel, which set my first set of keyframes. Then I moved the current time indicator (CTI) in the **Properties** panel one second to the right and changed my effect's **Longitude**, **Latitude**, **Distance**, and **Zoom** settings so the image filled the screen—automatically creating a new set of keyframe points in which my screen image is now a normal, full-screen clip.

Move the CTI back to the beginning of your clip and render the affected clip by pressing the **Enter** key.

▶ **NOTE**

After you apply an effect to a clip, press the **Enter** key to render it. Rendering creates a clean-looking, final version of the modified clip and motion path, improving your play-back quality immensely and saving your computer the taxing work of having to re-create a preview of your affected clip on the fly.

In my example, the image zooms into full screen as it appears to rotate up in three-dimensional space toward the camera.

3 Save the Preset

Click the effect in the **Properties** panel whose settings or motion path you'd like to save (in this case, the **Camera View** effect) and then click the **More**

117

button. From the menu, select **Save Preset**. The **Save Preset** dialog box opens.

You'll be asked to name your preset. You'll also have the option of beginning any change in the effect or motion path at the clip's In or Out point.

Your new preset is added to the **My Presets** collection in the **Effects and Transitions** panel. You can apply it to any other clips in the current project—or to clips in any other project—by dragging it from the **Effects and Transitions** panel and dropping it on the desired clip, just as you would any of Premiere Elements' standard presets.

If you later decide you want to remove this custom preset from your collection, right-click it in the **Effects and Transitions** panel and select the **Clear** option from the context menu.

117

21

The Power of Keyframing

IN THIS CHAPTER:

Keyframing is one of the most powerful tools in Premiere Elements. Its methodology might seem a bit challenging at first. But, when you master it, you'll find the true power of this program unleashed.

The principle is simple: For any effect, you designate points on your still's, your audio clip's, or your video clip's **Timeline** where you want the effect to occur or change—then Premiere Elements automatically creates the motion path or transition between those points.

The beauty of this system is that these points, or keyframes, can be easily added, moved, changed, and rearranged indefinitely until your video project produces exactly the effect you're trying to achieve. Again, this system might seem a bit challenging at first. However, when you see what's happening, you'll find keyframes a very natural and intuitive way to create movement and effects.

It's also worth noting that many of the movements and presets built into Premiere Elements's video and audio effects are, in reality, composed of or created with keyframes. And, in fact, after you apply these effects to your clips, you can easily manipulate the keyframe points and customize the effects to whatever degree you see fit.

▶ KEY TERM

Keyframing—The method used by Premiere Elements (as well as Premiere Pro and After Effects) for creating motion paths and transitioning effects. Points representing precise settings for effects or positions are placed on the **Timeline**, and the program automatically creates a movement or transition between those points.

---

118   Add Motion to a Still

✔ BEFORE YOU BEGIN	→ SEE ALSO
88 Prepare a Still for Video	**117** Create and Save a Preset
	119 Pan and Zoom Still Images a la Ken Burns
	120 Make a Variable-Speed Pan and Zoom

It's the first principle of great movie making: Movies move.

Adding motion to a still photo or graphic in your video gives the still image life. It's the difference between merely running a slideshow and telling a story with pictures. Motion directs your audience's attention to certain elements of your image. It isolates an area and then reveals its context. Motion makes the static dynamic.

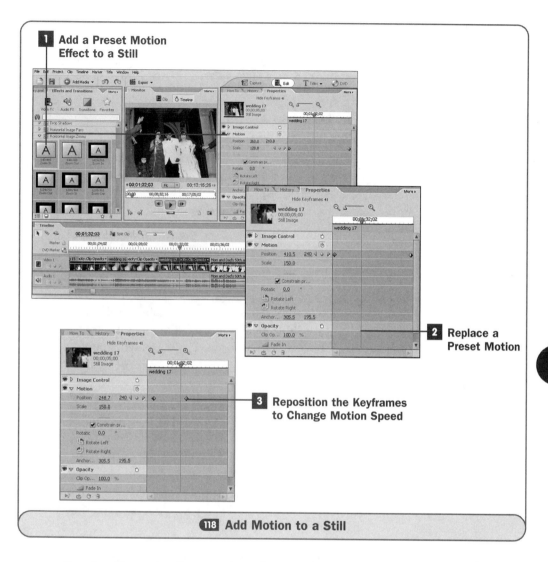

1 Add a Preset Motion Effect to a Still

2 Replace a Preset Motion

3 Reposition the Keyframes to Change Motion Speed

118

118 Add Motion to a Still

Premiere Elements offers a variety of presets that allow you to simply drag and drop horizontal and vertical pans and in and out zooms onto your clips. These presets add the motion you want, and offer you some control over the way the motion works. As you know, creating and customizing such motion is easy using the keyframing tool in Premiere Elements. After you establish the points at which you want your scale and position to change, Premiere Elements fills in the movement between those points, creating a smooth motion from one keyframe point to the next.

▶ **NOTE**

After you've created or customized your keyframed movement or effect, you can save it as a permanent preset, and it will be automatically added to your preset collection. Just select **Save Preset** from the **Properties** panel's **More** menu.

1 Add a Preset Motion Effect to a Still

The preset motions you can add to a still image are limited to panning over the still or zooming in or away from the image. Open the **Effects and Transitions** panel and click the **Video FX** button at the top of the panel. Scroll through the list of preset effects and look for the **Horizontal** or **Vertical Image Pans** or the **Horizontal** or **Vertical Image Zooms**.

Drag a preset pan or zoom onto a still on the **Timeline**. The motion of the selected pan or zoom is automatically timed to the duration of the still. Play the clip and watch how the preset affects the clip.

Unless the size of your image has the same dimensions as those listed in the name of the preset (for example, 640×480 pixels), it's possible that the preset you selected will either show too little of your image or the motion will extend beyond the edges of the clip. If so, you can customize the motion.

118

2 Replace a Preset Motion

Because all preset motions are based on the **Motion** property, dragging another motion or zoom preset onto your clip will overwrite the previous effect.

3 Reposition the Keyframes to Change Motion Speed

The motion path is set to the keyframe points on the **Properties** timeline. By moving these points, you can control the speed of the transition or motion path between the points.

If you lengthen the duration of the clip, the keyframes remain in their original places, ending the motion path at the final keyframe point and holding that position until the end of the clip. Repositioning the keyframe point to the end of the clip results in a steady motion from beginning to end.

Finally, you can save the new positions you've created as a custom preset as explained in **117** **Create and Save a Preset**.

119 Pan and Zoom Still Images a la Ken Burns

✔ BEFORE YOU BEGIN	→ SEE ALSO
88 Prepare a Still for Video	**117** Create and Save a Preset
118 Add Motion to a Still	**120** Make a Variable-Speed Pan and Zoom
	122 Control Volume at Specific Points

Although filmmaker Ken Burns (notable for such epic PBS documentaries as *Jazz*, *Baseball*, and *The Civil War*) didn't invent the technique of slowly moving in and around a photo to make it seem to come to life, he has used it so extensively and so effectively that it has become forever linked to his name—the Ken Burns Effect. By carefully and creatively isolating areas of photos and then revealing a wider context by moving across them, Burns has managed to bring action, suspense, and drama to stills and paintings, giving them a dynamic, intriguing, almost movie-like quality.

By controlling the **Scale** and **Position** settings for your stills over time, Premiere Elements's keyframing tool gives you the ability to produce the very same effects. But, even greater, the nature of the keyframing tool is that it also allows for easy revision and customization, making it simple for you to match the motions you create to music, sound effects, and narration.

By controlling motion, you decide how your audience experiences a photo. You show them what to focus on. You decide how the photo is revealed to them; you control their eye movement through the scene. In doing so, you give your audience not merely a picture to look at but a story to experience.

Before you begin, remember that whenever you change the scale of a still or any raster image, there are resolution issues to consider. **88** **Prepare a Still for Video** discusses how best to ensure that your image quality is maintained throughout this effect.

1 Drag to Set the Photo's Duration

Stretch the photo or clip you want to pan and zoom down the main **Timeline** until it's your desired duration.

You can extend or trim the clip later, and it won't affect the positions of the keyframes.

119

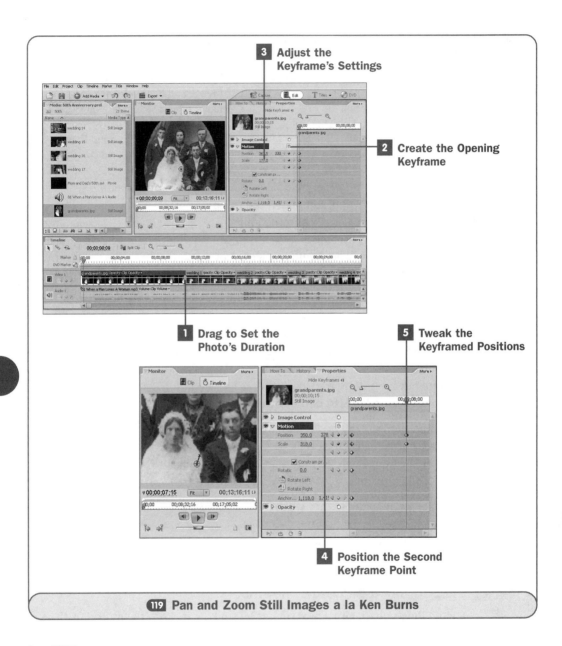

3 Adjust the Keyframe's Settings

2 Create the Opening Keyframe

1 Drag to Set the Photo's Duration

5 Tweak the Keyframed Positions

4 Position the Second Keyframe Point

119 Pan and Zoom Still Images a la Ken Burns

▶ **TIP**

When you start changing the positions and scale of your clips and adding effects, you'll find that the playback becomes irregular or that the video image seems degraded. This is because you're actually looking at a *preview* of the affected clip, which the program is creating on-the-fly. (You'll also notice that a red line has appeared on the **Timeline** above the clip.) To see a more true representation of what your final clip will look like, render the clip by pressing the **Enter** key. (When your clip is rendered, the red line above it becomes a green line.)

2 Create the Opening Keyframes

Make sure that the photo to which you want to apply the Ken Burns effect is selected on the **Timeline**. If the **Properties** panel timeline is not already visible, click the **Show Keyframes** button at the top of the panel. Also click the triangle to the left of the **Motion** property to reveal the motion details control panel. Move the current time indicator (CTI) on the **Properties** timeline to approximately the point you want your motion path to begin.

Click the stopwatch icon to the right of the **Motion** property title. A column of small diamonds appears on the timeline to the right of the **Motion** details. These are the opening keyframes for your motion path.

3 Adjust the Keyframe's Settings

As long as the CTI remains at the position of the newly created keyframe points, you can continue to tweak their settings.

You can change the **Position** and **Scale** settings several ways:

- Type new coordinates or percentages

- Drag across the numerical settings so they increase or decrease; watch the effect in the **Monitor** panel

- Click the image in the **Monitor** panel and drag it to a new position or resize it by pulling the corner handles

In this example, I began with a wider shot of the wedding photo, using **Position** settings of **367×330** and a **Scale** of **177%**. (Naturally, I made sure that my photo had enough resolution to allow for this much scaling.)

4 Position the Second Keyframe Points

Move the CTI to the approximate position where you'd like your motion path to change directions.

Change the **Position** and/or **Scale** settings. As you do, new keyframe points are automatically created for those settings at the CTI's current position.

In this example, I set the second set of keyframes to a **Position** of **350×378** and a **Scale** of **318%**—a close-up of the bride and groom's faces.

Premiere Elements will create a smooth path between these two keyframe points. In this example, the clip begins with a wide shot of the entire wedding party and then slowly zooms into a tight shot of just the bride and groom.

119

▶ **NOTE**

As long as the current time indicator (CTI) remains in position, you can tweak your newly created keyframe point's settings. It's only after the CTI is repositioned that the settings become permanently locked to that keyframe point. To change the settings for the keyframe point after moving the CTI, click the left or right arrows to the right of the property in the **Properties** panel. The CTI jumps to the next or previous keyframe point, at which point you can tweak the point's settings.

Just as you can set **Position** values either by changing the property's numerical settings or manipulating the image in the **Monitor** panel, you can set **Scale** and **Rotation** numerically or by clicking the image in the **Monitor** panel and resize or rotate it by dragging the corner handles.

▶ **TIP**

Keyframe points are added only as settings for each individual property changes. It's quite possible for a motion to be created in which one property has several keyframe points while another has one or no keyframe points at all.

119

5 **Tweak the Keyframed Positions**

There's no need to create your keyframes in the exact timeline positions you ultimately want them. Positioning them farther apart slows the transition between them. Positioning them closer together speeds the transition. (Also see **120** **Make a Variable-Speed Pan and Zoom**.)

Using the same process you used to create the second keyframe, continue to add a virtually unlimited number of keyframes to a clip, creating custom motion paths or controlling effects as precisely as you desire.

Remember, nothing is permanent in keyframing. And changing a transition or motion path's speed, keyframe points, or even eliminating the keyframe points completely is as simple as moving, revising, or deleting a keyframe point.

120 | **Make a Variable-Speed Pan and Zoom**

✔ BEFORE YOU BEGIN	→ SEE ALSO
88 Prepare a Still for Video	**118** Add Motion to a Still
	119 Pan and Zoom Still Images a la Ken Burns
	122 Control Volume at Specific Points

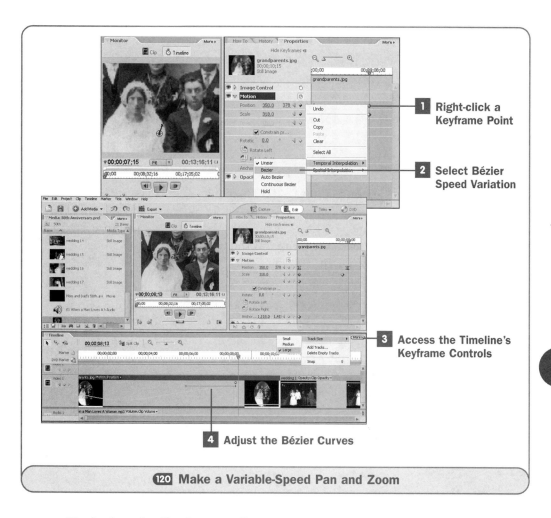

1 **Right-click a Keyframe Point**

2 **Select Bézier Speed Variation**

3 **Access the Timeline's Keyframe Controls**

120

4 **Adjust the Bézier Curves**

120 **Make a Variable-Speed Pan and Zoom**

The basic tools of keyframing allow you to create a simple path of motion around your still photos and graphics. However, there are times when you also want to vary the speed of that motion. Premiere Elements provides several options for varying speed of motion along a path.

You'll find instructions for creating a simple motion using presets in 118 **Add Motion to a Still** or a more complicated motion path using your own keyframe points in 119 **Pan and Zoom Still Images a la Ken Burns**.

After you've clicked to select the clip in the main **Timeline**, open the **Properties** panel and, if the **Properties** timeline is hidden, click the **Show Keyframes** button at the top of the panel. Now you're ready to create a panning or zooming motion that varies its speed across the duration of the clip.

1 Right-click a Keyframe Point

Right-click a keyframe point to open the keyframe general context menu.

By default, the speed of motion from one keyframe point to the next is **Linear**, or constant. In other words, if you were move the CTI to a point halfway between two **Linear** keyframes, you would find that the effect at this point is 50% completed.

2 Select Bézier Speed Variation

The **Spatial Interpolation** options affect the motion of the effect on your image through space. The **Temporal Interpolation** options affect the motion of the effect on your image through time. To change the pan or zoom effect so it varies over time, select the **Temporal Interpolation** option from the context menu you opened in step 1. A submenu of time-based options appears.

The **Linear** option makes the speed of the motion constant; **Ease In** is a *Bézier* preset in which the motion begins slowly and speeds up as it approaches the next keyframe; **Ease Out** is a Bézier preset that begins quickly but slows as it approaches the next keyframe; the **Hold** option holds the keyframe's position until the next keyframe; the **Auto Bézier**, **Bézier**, and **Continuous Bézier** options allow you to manipulate curves to control speed throughout the path or transition.

Choose the **Bézier** motion option and notice that the shape of the keyframe in the main **Timeline** changes from a straight line into a curved figure.

▶ KEY TERM

Bézier—A system for controlling a curve's shape by manipulating handles at the end points of the curve.

3 Access the Timeline's Keyframe Controls

Click the **More** button in the **Timeline** panel and select **Track Size/Large** to give yourself better access to the keyframe controls.

Right-click the clip on the **Timeline** and, from the context menu that appears, choose **Show Clip Keyframes** and then choose the effect whose keyframes you want to control (in this case, **Motion: Position**).

4 Adjust the Bézier Curves

By manipulating the control handles on the Bézier curve in the **Timeline**, adjust the curve of motion or transition to your preference. The shape of the curve represents the variations of the speed of the motion between the

120

keyframes, with the lowest portions of the curve representing slowest motion and the highest portions of the curve representing the fastest motion.

The **Bézier** curve in this example produces a movement between my **Position** settings that is slow in movement to about the three-second point, then increases in speed as it approached the second keyframe. (**Bézier** settings are a rather high-level concept, so you might want to experiment to develop a feel for how the various settings affect the results.)

---

121 Control a Video Track's Opacity over Time

→ SEE ALSO

118 Add Motion to a Still
119 Pan and Zoom Still Images a la Ken Burns
122 Control Volume at Specific Points

Just as you can map motion to specific points in a clip using keyframing, you can map other effects and properties (such as **Image Control** and **Opacity**) to specific points in a clip.

The automatic video **Fade In** and **Fade Out** effects are actually keyframed effects. Creating such an effect from scratch is also easy, the result being the video equivalent of the audio fade effect created in **122** **Control Volume at Specific Points**.

1 Select a Clip on the Timeline

Click to select a video clip on the main **Timeline**. If you have clips on more than one track and you want to adjust the opacity for one clip so another clip shows through the first clip, arrange the clips in the tracks so the clip to adjust is on an upper track and the clip you want to show through is on a lower track.

The **Properties** panel shows the standard properties of **Image Control**, **Motion**, and **Opacity**. If the **Properties** panel timeline isn't visible, click the **Show Keyframes** button at the top of the panel to reveal the timeline. Also click the triangle to the left of the **Opacity** property to reveal its detail settings.

▶ NOTE

The **Opacity** settings affect the transparency of a clip in your **Timeline**. If nothing is on the video track below the affected clip, making your clip transparent reveals the black background. If a clip does exist on the video track below the clip you're affecting, reducing the clip's **Opacity** reveals the clip on the track below.

121

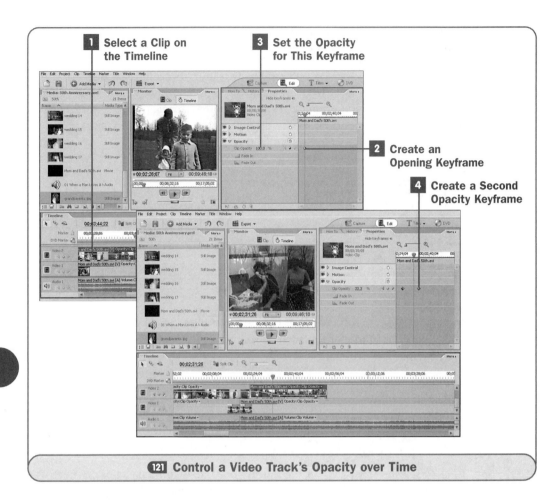

121 Control a Video Track's Opacity over Time

2 Create an Opening Keyframe

Move the current time indicator (CTI) on the **Properties** timeline to the beginning of the timeline and click the stopwatch icon to the right of the **Opacity** label. A second hand appears on the stopwatch icon, indicating that the property is keyframed, and a keyframe point for the **Opacity** setting appears at the CTI on the timeline.

3 Set the Opacity for This Keyframe

As long as the CTI remains in position, you can adjust the settings for the current keyframe points. (Move the CTI to apply the current settings and create another set of keyframe points.) Set the **Opacity** value for the first keyframe point to 100%. The selected clip (for example, the clip on the Video 2 track), is displayed in the **Monitor** panel and the clip on the Video 1 track (the lower track) is not visible.

4 Create a Second Opacity Keyframe

Move the CTI to the right some distance and set the **Opacity** value for this point to **0%**. A keyframe point is automatically added at the CTI as you change the **Opacity** settings for this clip. (You can reposition the keyframe point on the **Properties** panel timeline if you later decide to do so.)

In the **Monitor** panel, you'll see that the clip has become transparent, revealing the clip on the Video 1 track. (If there is no clip on a lower track, the black background shows through the selected clip.) As you scrub between the two points or play the clip, notice that Premiere Elements has filled in the transitional frames, creating essentially a dissolve from the clip on Video 2 to the clip on Video 1.

Creating additional keyframe points, you can continue to control the opacity of the clip at various points.

Any audio or video property can be keyframed to transition in this way. And, just as you can add motion to a still image by setting keyframe points (see **119 Pan and Zoom Still Images a la Ken Burns**), you can morph nearly all the effects and image adjustments by modifying the effect's keyframe settings.

122

122 Control Volume at Specific Points

✔ BEFORE YOU BEGIN	→ SEE ALSO
105 Add an Audio Transition	**119** Pan and Zoom Still Images a la Ken Burns

Unfortunately, some people speak too quietly on camera, and you need to bring up the audio on your video so you can hear them. Others speak louder than anyone else in the scene, and you need to bring down their audio to make the sound levels more even. And sometimes you just want to lower or completely mute the volume on a clip so an alternate track of music or narration can dominate. Fortunately, Premiere Elements's keyframing tool allows you to easily set the audio levels at specific points on your **Timeline**—points you can also easily revise, move, or remove. (Note that the effect described in **105 Add an Audio Transition** is essentially a keyframed preset that fades the audio in or out.)

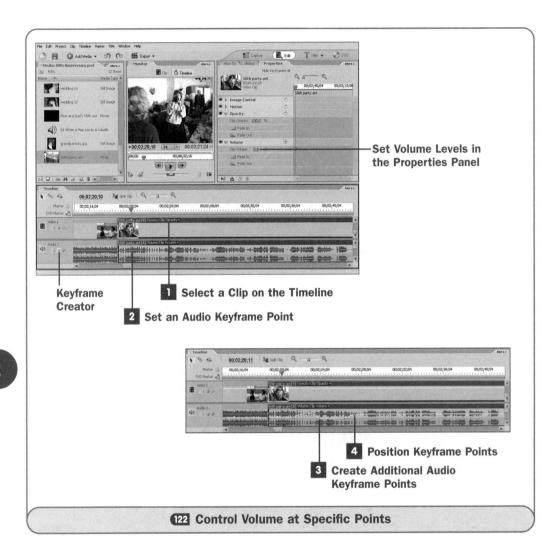

Set Volume Levels in the Properties Panel

Keyframe Creator

1 Select a Clip on the Timeline

2 Set an Audio Keyframe Point

4 Position Keyframe Points

3 Create Additional Audio Keyframe Points

122 Control Volume at Specific Points

1 Select a Clip on the Timeline

Click an audio or a video clip on the main **Timeline**. In the **Properties** panel, you'll see the standard properties of **Image Control**, **Motion**, **Opacity**, and **Volume** if you selected a video clip; if you selected an audio clip, the only property in the **Properties** panel is **Volume**. For this task, we will be concerned with only the **Volume** property of the clip you've selected.

When using keyframing in audio, it's worth noting that the same principles apply to audio keyframing as apply to video keyframing—namely that you set specific points on the timeline at which you want certain effects to occur. With audio levels, however, your main concern is not so much setting up keyframes for effects (although that is also possible) but with setting your audio volume to raise or lower at specific points.

2 Set an Audio Keyframe Point

Although you can set your keyframe points in the **Properties** panel, as you would with a video effect or movement, it is usually easier, and more intuitive, to set audio keyframe points right in the audio track on the main **Timeline**.

After you've selected a video clip with an audio track, the keyframe creator (the little diamond next to the audio track's name on the left end of the **Timeline**) becomes activated. Click the little diamond in this control panel and a keyframe point appears on the yellow line that runs horizontally through the audio track of your clip at the position of the current time indicator (CTI).

This yellow line represents the clip's audio level. By raising and lowering it, you can raise or lower the audio level of the clip. By placing keyframe points on this line, you can raise or lower the levels of *specific points* on the clip.

For this example, I wanted the audio for the clip to start at its default level (the level I recorded when I shot the video with my camcorder) and then increase slightly for about three seconds to compensate for some dialog recorded at a low volume before tapering off again for another four seconds when the sound level on my audio track gets louder than I'd prefer. About 9 seconds into the video clip, I want the volume level to again return to the default level. I'll set keyframe points at roughly the 3-second, 7-second, and 9-second positions on the **Timeline**.

122

▶ NOTE

The yellow, horizontal line that runs through every audio clip is, by default, a volume level control. Without a keyframe point, you can raise or lower the volume of an entire clip by raising or lowering this line in the track.

3 Create Additional Audio Keyframe Points

To create another audio keyframe point, move the CTI on the main **Timeline** to the right and click the audio keyframe creator (the little diamond on the left end of the audio track) again.

You need not create your keyframe points at the exact positions you want them. You can move them around and adjust their levels later as needed.

▶ **NOTE**

Although most people find it easier to set audio keyframe points right in the **Timeline** panel, you can also do so on the **Properties** panel timeline, where volume levels for each keyframe point can be set numerically or by using the slider control.

4 Position Keyframe Points

Drag the CTI back to the beginning of your clip and click the Play button on the **Monitor** panel. Listen to your clip or, better yet, open the **Audio Meters** panel (choose **Window, Audio Meters** to display it) and watch the audio levels. Pause your playback when you reach a spot where you want to raise or lower the audio level for the clip.

The higher you drag the keyframe point, the louder the track plays. The lower you drag the keyframe point, the lower the track plays. To sustain an increased or decreased level, position a keyframe at the beginning and end of the section you want to affect and make sure that the keyframe points are exactly opposite each other on the yellow volume control line (at the level you want to sustain).

Continue to add and position keyframes as necessary to vary the clip's volume as desired.

122

▶ **NOTES**

You might find it easier to position the keyframed audio levels if you expand the height of the audio track. To do this, mouse over the seam between two audio tracks on the left side of the **Timeline** panel until the mouse pointer becomes a double-horizontal line. Click and drag the audio track to whatever height with which you find it easiest to work.

You can also set the height of the tracks on the **Timeline** by clicking the **Timeline** panel's **More** button and choosing the track size from the menu.

22

Special Effects

IN THIS CHAPTER:

Adding special effects to your video project is both fun and easy using Premiere Elements. Premiere Elements offers a variety of professional-level effects for adjusting your image and sound as well as a variety of cool, instant effects for adding lightning bolts, lens flare, and picture-in-picture effects, each one infinitely customizable.

123   Control a Video Effect with Keyframes

✔ BEFORE YOU BEGIN	→ SEE ALSO
94 Add or Move a Clip on the Timeline	**116** Reset or Remove an Effect
114 Add and Customize an Effect	**117** Create and Save a Preset
	120 Make a Variable-Speed Pan and Zoom

When you first apply an effect to a clip, the effect applies to the entire clip at the same level. By using keyframing, however, you can control how the effect is applied and when it is applied at what level. With keyframing, you lock the effect's settings to various points on the **Timeline**, and Premiere Elements creates the transition between the points.

1 Select an Effect

Select an effect from the **Effects and Transitions** panel. As you browse each collection (**Video FX**, **Audio FX**, and **Transitions**) and the categories within each collection, notice that each effect is displayed as a thumbnail preview.

2 Apply an Effect to a Clip

Drag the effect you want to apply from the **Effects and Transitions** panel onto a clip on the **Timeline**. The effect also appears in the **Properties** panel, where you can control the settings for the effect.

With many effects, a change in the clip is not immediately apparent until you adjust the effect's properties.

3 Set an Opening Keyframe

With the clip selected, click the triangle to the left of the effect name in the **Properties** panel to display the details of that effect. If the **Properties** panel timeline is not visible, click the **Show Keyframes** button at the top of the panel.

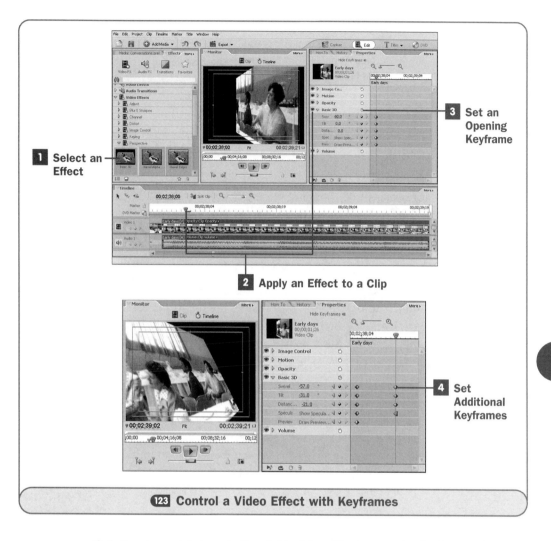

1 Select an Effect

3 Set an Opening Keyframe

2 Apply an Effect to a Clip

4 Set Additional Keyframes

123

123 Control a Video Effect with Keyframes

Click the stopwatch icon to the right of the effect's name in the **Properties** panel. A column of diamonds appears next to each of the effect's controls at the current position of the CTI. These are the opening keyframes of your effect.

As long as the CTI remains in its current position, you can adjust and tweak the settings for the keyframe points. The results of your settings are displayed in the **Monitor** panel.

In this example of the **Basic 3D** effect, I adjusted the **Swivel** setting to **60** degrees to make my clip appear as if it were being viewed in three-dimensional space from the side. I also could have tilted it, made it appear to be farther away, or even added a **Specular Highlight** to it.

▶ **NOTE**

Keyframe points don't have to be created in their final positions. After you set them, you can slide the keyframe points to different positions on the **Properties** panel timeline to achieve the effect you're going for.

4 **Set Additional Keyframes**

Move the CTI down the **Properties** panel timeline and adjust the settings for this new position. Keyframe points are automatically created along the CTI when you change any of the settings.

For this example, I made changes to virtually every **Basic 3D** setting including **Swivel**, **Tilt**, and **Distance**, and I even added a **Specular Highlight** to make it appear that a light source was passing over the clip. The result, after Premiere Elements generates the frames between these keyframes, will be as though my screen image is floating and turning through space.

Continue creating keyframe points as needed to continue the movement or transition. Adjusting the position of the keyframe points on the **Properties** timeline controls the speed of the transition between keyframes. You can also *vary* the speed of the transition between the keyframes using Bézier curves, as explained in **120** **Make a Variable-Speed Pan and Zoom.**

As you add effects to a clip, you might notice that playback seems stilted or the quality of the image seems to have deteriorated. Also notice that a red bar appears on the **Timeline** above the affected clip. This lower-quality playback happens because your computer performs a soft render of the effect, created on-the-fly as you play your clip. To see a better representation of what your clip will ultimately look like, render it by pressing the **Enter** key. After your clip is rendered, the red bar above the clip turns green.

---

124 **Make an Area of a Clip Transparent**

✔ BEFORE YOU BEGIN	→ SEE ALSO
88 Prepare a Still for Video	**116** Reset or Remove an Effect
	132 Make a Person Appear with a Different Background
	131 Make a Line Move Across a Map

Keying means making an area of a clip transparent based on its color values. **Chroma Key** is a more general version of the same effect that appears as the **Blue Screen Key**, the **Green Screen Key**, and the **Non-Red Key** effects (the latter effects are preset to certain commonly used key colors, while the **Chroma Key** effect can be set to *any* color).

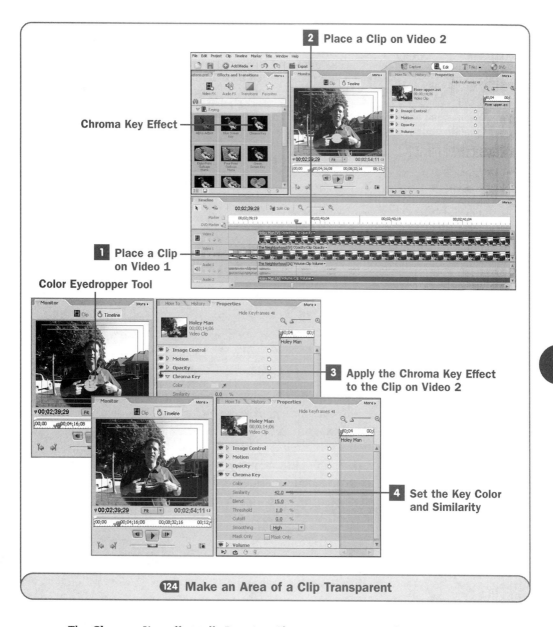

2 Place a Clip on Video 2

Chroma Key Effect

1 Place a Clip on Video 1

Color Eyedropper Tool

3 Apply the Chroma Key Effect to the Clip on Video 2

4 Set the Key Color and Similarity

124

124 Make an Area of a Clip Transparent

The **Chroma Key** effect tells Premiere Elements to treat a color or a range of colors in your clip as transparent, revealing a clip or clips on the tracks below through the transparent area.

▶ **NOTE**

The **Chroma Key** effect is the most general of several Key effects, all of which accomplish the task of designating a color or range of colors on a clip as transparent. The **Green Screen Key**, **Blue Screen Key**, and **Non-Red Screen Key** effects are basically the same as the **Chroma Key** effect, although the former effects are prekeyed to certain commonly used color ranges. Green and blue are the most commonly used Key colors—they are used in virtually all television and feature film effects shots—because they are not found in human flesh tones and therefore their effect can be isolated to certain intentionally colored areas of the screen image.

1 Place a Clip on Video 1

Place a clip on the Video 1 track. Because this clip appears on the lower track, it is the clip that will be revealed through the transparent areas of the clip on Video 2. The clip you place on Video 2 should include the background you want to show through your keyed clip.

2 Place a Clip on Video 2

Because of the way the **Chroma Key** effect works, it's best to select as your foreground video a clip that has an area of flat color—such as a blue or green screen or the purple side of a barn, or a red velvet curtain—and this color should appear only in the area you want to make transparent.

In this example, I posed the man in my video clip holding a bright-green circle against his chest. I was careful to choose the material for this circle (a smoothly-colored piece of paper) in a shade of green that did not appear anywhere else in the shot. My intent is to key the green circle so a video clip on a lower track can show through it, making it look as though the man is holding a moving picture between his fingers.

Place this clip on the Video 2 track, directly above the clip you placed on the Timeline in step 1.

3 Apply the Chroma Key Effect to the Clip on Video 2

Open the **Effects and Transitions** panel and click the **Video FX** button. Scroll to find the **Keying** category and look for the **Chroma Key** effect.

Drag this effect to the clip on Video 2. The **Chroma Key** effect is added to the list in the clip's **Properties** panel. Click the triangle to the left of the **Chroma Key** name in the **Properties** panel to open the effect's control panel.

4 Set the Key Color and Similarity

Although you can set the Key color using the color panel, it's usually easier to use your screen image to designate the Key color. Click the **Color** eyedropper icon in the Properties panel; the mouse pointer becomes an eyedropper. Now

124

click the color in the image in the **Monitor** panel that you want to designate as transparent. In this example, I clicked the green circle held against the man's chest.

You'll see an effect immediately: The clip on Video 1 is revealed through the area of the clip on Video 2 that you just keyed. Unless your clip has an absolutely flat area of color with no color variations (as was the case in this example), you'll probably have to adjust the **Similarity** setting (which widens the range of color to be affected) to get a good, clean, transparent area. For example, if you have a video of a man wearing a yellow shirt, and want to make the shirt transparent to reveal a video of a woman and child (so that it looks as if the shirt is made of a moving video), adjust the **Similarity** setting in the **Properties** panel to select all of the varieties of yellow in the man's shirt. The higher the **Similarity** setting, the more shades of yellow will be selected.

The **Blend, Threshold, Cutoff,** and **Smoothing** settings in the Properties panel also help you control transparency and the softness of the transparent area's edge.

When adjusting your key settings, you might find it helpful to turn on the **Mask Only** option. This option temporarily masks the areas that will *not* be keyed out, revealing only the transparent portions of your screen image. When you have a good, clean **Chroma Key** set up, uncheck the **Mask Only** option to return to normal view.

The end result, in my example, is that you can now see the clip which was on a lower video track through this keyed, or transparent, area. And because the clip on the lower track was of the scenery behind the man in my shot, the illusion is that you can actually see through a round hole in the man's chest!

▶ **TIP**

For some illusions, you might want to resize or reposition the clip on the lower track so that it "fits" in the keyed area of the top track. See **89** Scale and Position a Still for more information.

---

125 | **Create a Picture-in-Picture Effect**

✔ **BEFORE YOU BEGIN**

94 Add or Move a Clip on the Timeline
114 Add and Customize an Effect

→ **SEE ALSO**

116 Reset or Remove an Effect
117 Create and Save a Preset
120 Make a Variable-Speed Pan and Zoom
123 Control a Video Effect with Keyframes

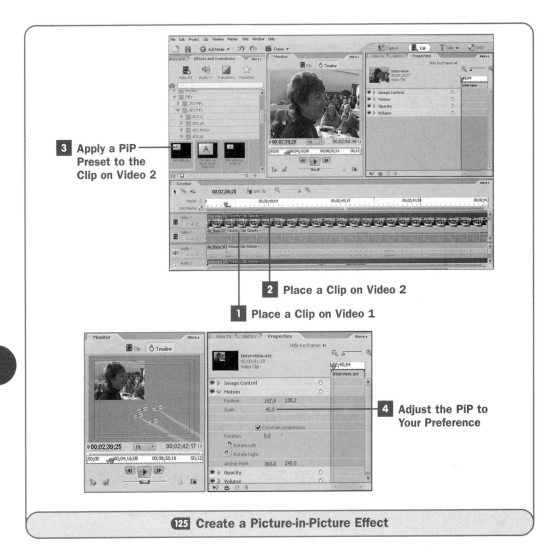

3 Apply a PiP Preset to the Clip on Video 2

2 Place a Clip on Video 2

1 Place a Clip on Video 1

4 Adjust the PiP to Your Preference

125   **125** Create a Picture-in-Picture Effect

Although you can manually create a picture-in-picture effect by scaling one clip to a portion of your video frame to reveal a second clip on the video track below it, Premiere Elements offers a large variety of Picture-in-Picture (or **PiP**) presets that you can easily apply and adjust as needed.

Technically, PiPs are not effects unto themselves. That's why they show up in the **Presets** collection rather than among the **Video FX**. They are, in fact, presets for **Scale** and **Position** (sometimes the effect applies itself to more than one video track at the same time). If you select a clip that has had a **PiP** preset applied to it, you will not see **PiP** listed in the **Properties** panel. To see the settings for the PiP, open the control panel for the **Motion** property.

1 Place a Clip on Video 1

Video 1 is the bottom video track, so the clip you place on this track should be the clip you plan to use as your full-screen, background video.

2 Place a Clip on Video 2

Place a second clip—the one that will serve as your picture-in-picture—on the Video 2 track, directly above the clip you've placed on Video 1.

3 Apply a PiP Preset to the Clip on Video 2

The **PiP** category is located in the **Effects and Transitions** panel in the **Video FX** collection. The **PiP** category contains 180 picture-in-picture variations, divided into two subcategories: **25% PiPs** (in which the picture-in-picture is 25% of the size of the video frame), and **40% PiPs**, in which the picture-in-picture is 40% of the size of the video frame. Each of these subcategories is further divided into groupings based on the quadrant in which the effect appears in the video frame: upper-left (**UL**), lower-left (**LL**), upper-right (**UR**), and lower-right (**LR**). Also included is a **Motion** group, in which the picture-in-picture migrates around the video frame. Each of these quadrant groupings offers both a stationary position and several transitional or moving versions.

The **PiPs**, like all effects and transitions in the panel, are displayed as thumbnails. Click any effect to see an animated preview of its movement.

Drag the PiP you want to apply—or one that is close to what you'd like—onto the clip on Video 2. Immediately, you'll see the result displayed in the **Monitor** panel.

125

4 Adjust the PiP to Your Preference

If the PiP preset isn't quite what you'd like, you can easily tweak it. With the affected clip selected, click the triangle to the left of the **Motion** property in the **Properties** panel to reveal the detail settings for that property. Adjust the **Scale** and **Position** settings as needed.

For best results, turn on your **Safe Margins** (click the **More** button in the **Monitor** panel), to ensure that you don't position your picture-in-picture too close to the edge of the TV screen.

▶ **TIP**

After you begin applying effects to your clip, you'll find that the quality of the image in your playback has apparently deteriorated. On slower computers, playback might even seem jumpy or irregular. This is because your computer is creating a soft render of the clip on the fly. Also notice that the affected clip is marked by a red line above the clip on the **Timeline**. To see a better example of what your clip will look like on final output, press **Enter** to render the **Timeline**. The red line above the clip turns green when rendering is complete, and the quality of your playback will be an accurate representation of what your final output will look like.

---

126 **Add a Lens Flare**

✔ BEFORE YOU BEGIN	→ SEE ALSO
94 Add or Move a Clip on the Timeline	**116** Reset or Remove an Effect
114 Add and Customize an Effect	

The **Lens Flare** effect can add interest to a video clip, particularly when used in conjunction with another effect. Keyframing a lens flare can add excitement to a 3D movement, such as the **Camera View** effect—the flare can appear as a brief highlight on a rotating graphic or can track with another effect's motion. The **Lens Flare** effect can also be used to highlight, or draw attention to, an area of your clip, like the sparkle of a shiny object or the flash of a knife blade.

▶ **TIP**

To make the **Lens Flare** effect appear for only a moment, zoom into the **Timeline** (press the + key) and use the **Split Clip** tool described in **97** **Split a Clip** to slice your clip. Nudge the CTI about five frames to the right and slice the clip again, creating a tiny, isolated segment of the original clip. Apply the **Lens Flare** effect to this segment. Your clip will still play seamless over the slices, but the flash of light will appear for only those few, isolated frames. (Unfortunately, although you can use keyframes to move or temporarily brighten a **Lens Flare** effect, you can't use them to make the **Lens Flare** suddenly appear and then disappear; for that, you must split the clip.)

The **Lens Flare** effect is one of three effects categorized as **Render** effects. This means that, rather than merely affecting the screen image, they actually render, or add, something to the screen image that wasn't there before (see **127** **Add a Lightning Bolt Effect**).

You can add several copies of the **Lens Flare** effect to a clip, by the way, with the result being as if many lights or stars were shining into the camera lens while you were filming.

125

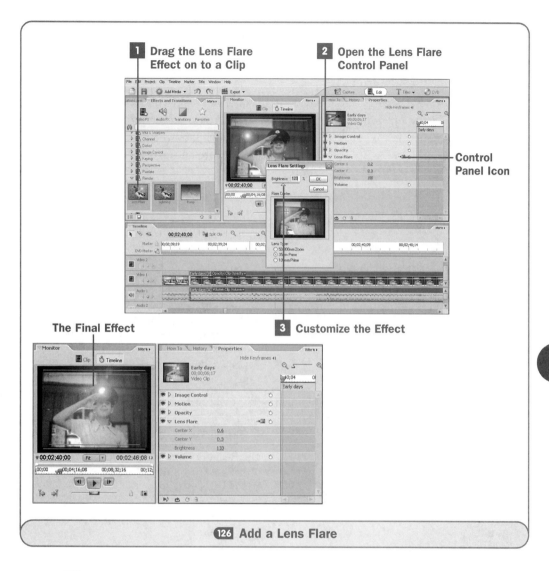

1 Drag the Lens Flare Effect on to a Clip

2 Open the Lens Flare Control Panel

Control Panel Icon

The Final Effect

3 Customize the Effect

126 Add a Lens Flare

1 Drag the Lens Flare Effect on to a Clip

The **Lens Flare** effect is located on the **Effects and Transitions** panel in the **Render** category of the **Video FX** collection. The flare appears in a default position on the screen image in the **Monitor** panel. Drag the effect from the **Effects and Transitions** panel to the clip in the **Timeline**.

2 Open the Lens Flare Control Panel

With the clip selected, click the triangle to the left of the **Lens Flare** listing in the **Properties** panel to access the control panel for the effect.

Click the control panel icon to the right of the effect's name to open a dialog box that offers several settings and a preview of your affected screen image.

3 Customize the Effect

Different lens settings create a wider and softer or smaller and more intense flare. Experiment with the settings to see which combination provides the best visual effect for your clip. To position the lens flare where you want it in the clip, click in the preview pane in the **Lens Flare Settings** dialog box and drag the flare to whatever position you'd prefer.

You can also keyframe the lens flare effect to track with an image, as explained in **123 Control a Video Effect with Keyframes**.

▶ **TIP**

After you begin applying effects to your clip, you'll find that the quality of the image in your playback has apparently deteriorated. On slower computers, playback might even seem jumpy or irregular. This is because your computer is creating a soft render of the clip on-the-fly. Also notice that the affected clip is marked by a red line above the clip on the **Timeline**. To see a better example of what your clip will look like on final output, press **Enter** to render the **Timeline**. The red line above the clip turns green when rendering is complete, and the quality of your playback will be an accurate representation of what your final output will look like.

126

---

127 Add a Lightning Bolt Effect

✔ BEFORE YOU BEGIN	→ SEE ALSO
94 Add or Move a Clip on the Timeline	**116** Reset or Remove an Effect
114 Add and Customize an Effect	**117** Create and Save a Preset
	120 Make a Variable-Speed Pan and Zoom
	123 Control a Video Effect with Keyframes

The infinitely customizable **Lightning** effect is one of the coolest in the Premiere Elements **Video FX** collection. By adjusting its settings, you can make the effect appear as anything from a single bolt to an elaborate plasma array of Tesla lightning.

You can also use the effect with keyframing to track the endpoints of the lightning with a moving object on screen. For example, you can follow an object as the camera angle changes, show one end of a lightning bolt following a path (as if it were "writing" text in wood, for instance), or even creating the illusion that a person or object is actually carrying the lightning bolts.

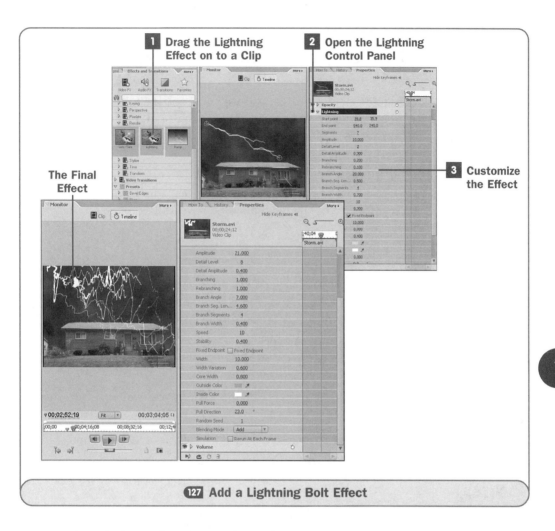

1 Drag the Lightning Effect on to a Clip

2 Open the Lightning Control Panel

3 Customize the Effect

The Final Effect

127

127 Add a Lightning Bolt Effect

The only downside is that it's definitely a resource-intensive effect, and even state-of-the-art computers might have trouble rendering previews on-the-fly. But be patient. The results are well worth it. In fact, it's worth your time to render the clip as you experiment with its settings (press **Enter** to render) so you can see this effect in all its glory as you work.

▶ **TIP**

To make a lightning bolt appear briefly, as if it were a lightning strike, zoom into the **Timeline** (press the + key) and use the **Split Clip** tool as described in 🔟 Split a Clip to slice your clip at the point at which you want the lightning bolt to begin. Nudge the CTI about half a second to the right and slice the clip again, creating a tiny, isolated segment of the original clip. Apply the **Lightning** effect to this short segment. The clips will still play seamlessly over the slices, but the dancing bolt of lightning will appear for only those few, isolated frames. Add a sound from your own collection to complete the effect!

1 **Drag the Lightning Effect on to a Clip**

The **Lightning** effect is found on the **Effects and Transitions** panel, in the **Render** category of the **Video FX** collection.

Drag the clip from the **Effects and Transitions** panel and drop it on a clip in the **Timeline**. Applying the effect to a clip generates a default lightning array, as you can see in the **Monitor** panel.

2 **Open the Lightning Control Panel**

With the clip selected, click the triangle to the left of the **Lightning** listing in the **Properties** panel to reveal one of the most powerful control panels in the **Video FX** library.

3 **Customize the Effect**

The **Lightning** control panel allows you to set the locations of the beginning and end points of the lightning bolt; the number of branches and rebranches; the angle of the branches; the length, width, and flickering speed of the branches; plus options to set a free form (random) endpoint, choose the colors of the lightning branches, specify the pull direction, and choose to have the flickering branches repeat their movements or randomize them.

127

Experiment with these options to get the lightning effect you're after—or discover an effect you didn't know existed!

You can apply keyframes to the effect to vary the locations of the **Start** and **End Points** over the course of your clip.

▶ **TIP**

After you begin applying effects to your clip, you'll find that the quality of the image in your playback has apparently deteriorated. On slower computers, playback might even seem jumpy or irregular. This is because your computer is creating a soft render of the clip on-the-fly. Also notice that the affected clip is marked by a red line above the clip on the **Timeline**. To see a better example of what your clip will look like on final output, press **Enter** to render the **Timeline**. The red line above the clip turns green when rendering is complete, and the quality of your playback will be an accurate representation of what your final output will look like.

128 Rotate a Clip in 3D

✔ BEFORE YOU BEGIN	→ SEE ALSO
94 Add or Move a Clip on the Timeline **114** Add and Customize an Effect	**116** Reset or Remove an Effect **120** Make a Variable-Speed Pan and Zoom **123** Control a Video Effect with Keyframes

The **Camera View** effect enables you to treat your screen image as if it were on a flat screen; by controlling its longitude, latitude, and distance, you can make this flat screen appear to rotate in three-dimensional space.

1 Drag the Camera View Effect on to a Clip

The **Camera View** effect is found on the **Effects and Transitions** panel, in the **Transform** category of the **Video FX** collection. Drag the effect from the **Effects and Transitions** panel and drop it on a clip in the **Timeline**. You will not see an immediate change in your clip.

2 Open the Camera View Control Panel

With the clip selected, click the triangle to the left of the **Camera View** listing in the **Properties** panel to reveal the effect's control panel.

You can also access this effect's controls by clicking the control panel icon to the right of the **Camera View** listing in this panel. The **Camera View Settings** dialog box opens. The controls are exactly the same in the dialog box and the **Properties** panel; only the interface is different. The **Properties** panel settings change numerically while the dialog box settings change with sliders.

▶ TIP

Using the **Camera View Settings** dialog box has one advantage over changing the settings in the **Properties** panel—the dialog box allows for the option of filling the alpha channel. With the alpha channel filled, you can designate a color for the background that's revealed as the image rotates. Leaving the alpha channel unfilled makes the background area transparent, revealing whatever clip is on the video track below the effected clip.

128

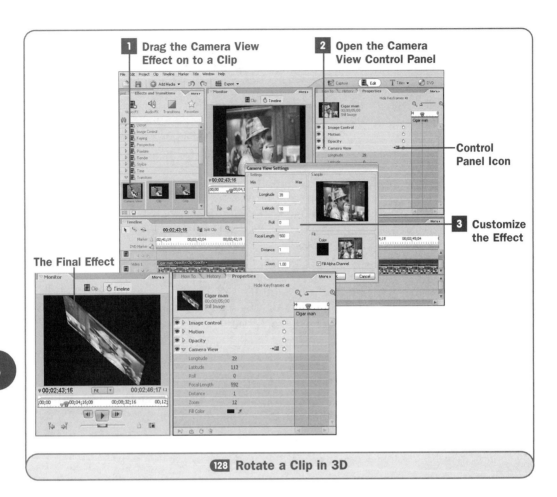

1 Drag the Camera View Effect on to a Clip

2 Open the Camera View Control Panel

Control Panel Icon

3 Customize the Effect

The Final Effect

128 Rotate a Clip in 3D

3 **Customize the Effect**

Changing the **Longitude** and **Latitude** settings turns the screen image to the left or right or leans the image forward or backward in space while **Roll** rotates the clip from side to side. The **Focal Length** and **Distance** settings add to the illusion of 3D space by exaggerating the distance between the near and far areas of the screen image; the **Zoom** setting scales your screen image to make it appear nearer or farther away.

In the **Fill** area of the **Camera View Settings** dialog box, enable the **Fill Alpha Channel** check box and click the **Color** swatch to designate a color for the background that's revealed as the image rotates. If you want to make the background transparent so a clip on the video track below is revealed as the image changes shape, disable the **Fill Alpha Channel** check box.

The **Camera View** effect lends itself particularly well to keyframing; setting various positions with keyframes can make your clip appear to tumble through space, as demonstrated in **117 Create and Save a Preset**. A version of it shows up as the **Tumble Away** transition in the **Effects and Transitions** panel, in the **Transitions** collection.

▶ **TIP**

Similar to the **Camera View** effect is the **Basic 3D** effect in the **Perspective** category. Although both effects allow you to spin or rotate your clip completely, you might find that the simpler **Basic 3D** effect is much easier to control than the **Camera View** effect.

---

129 Replace a Color

✔ BEFORE YOU BEGIN	→ SEE ALSO
94 Add or Move a Clip on the Timeline	**116** Reset or Remove an Effect
114 Add and Customize an Effect	**117** Create and Save a Preset
	120 Make a Variable-Speed Pan and Zoom
	123 Control a Video Effect with Keyframes

129

The **Color Replace** effect allows you to select a color or range of colors in your screen image and replace it with a new color you designate—replacing, for instance, a blue area with a red area.

The results of the **Color Replace** effect, however, tend to look rather flat and artificial. For this reason, it is more effective on flat-colored graphics such as company logos and less effective on continuous gradations of color, such as video or photos. If you applied **Color Replace** to a person's shirt, for instance, the result would be that the shirt, with its depth, wrinkles, and shadows, would be replaced with a flat block of color that would look nothing like a shirt.

▶ **TIP**

You can use keyframing, setting points for various replacement colors, to create an interesting effect by having an object's color dissolve into several replacement colors over the course of a clip.

1 Drag the Color Replace Effect on to a Clip

The **Color Replace** effect is located on the **Effects and Transitions** panel, in the **Image Control** category of the **Video FX** collection. Drag the effect from the **Effects and Transitions** panel and drop it on a clip in the **Timeline**. You will not see any immediate change to the clip in the **Monitor** panel.

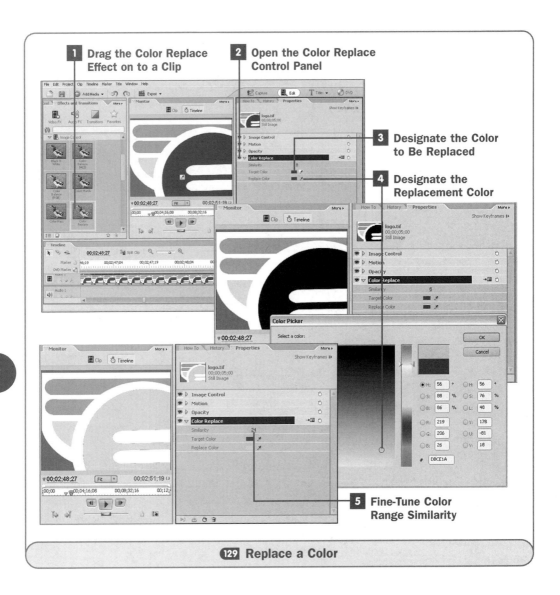

1 Drag the Color Replace Effect on to a Clip

2 Open the Color Replace Control Panel

3 Designate the Color to Be Replaced

4 Designate the Replacement Color

5 Fine-Tune Color Range Similarity

129 Replace a Color

2 Open the Color Replace Control Panel

With the clip selected, click the triangle to the left of the **Color Replace** listing in the **Properties** panel to reveal the effect's control panel.

3 Designate the Color to Be Replaced

The **Target Color** setting designates which color is to be replaced. Click the eyedropper next to this control; the mouse pointer becomes an eyedropper. Use this eyedropper to click a sample of the color you want to replace in the screen image in the **Monitor** panel.

4 **Designate the Replacement Color**

Click the eyedropper next to the **Replace Color** setting and click in the image in the **Monitor** to select the replacement color. Alternatively, click the white swatch next to the **Replace Color** setting to open the **Color Picker**; select a color from those displayed and click **OK** to designate your replacement color.

5 **Fine-Tune Color Range Similarity**

By tweaking the **Similarity** setting, you can widen or narrow the **Target Color**'s range of similar colors until you achieve your desired results.

129

23

Cool Tricks

Premiere Elements offers many easy-to-use effects that do a host of cool tricks right out of the box. But sometimes the most obvious use for an effect is only the beginning. With a little creativity, you'll be amazed at what you can do!

This chapter offers some not-quite-so-obvious but oft-requested tricks you can perform with the Premiere Elements's **Video FX** collection.

How *do* you make a line move across a map anyway?

130 Create a Split-Screen Effect

✔ BEFORE YOU BEGIN	→ SEE ALSO
94 Add or Move a Clip on the Timeline	**116** Reset or Remove an Effect
114 Add and Customize an Effect	**120** Make a Variable-Speed Pan and Zoom
	125 Create a Picture-In-Picture Effect

It's easy to create a Picture-In-Picture effect, as explained in **125** **Create a Picture-in-Picture Effect**. But what happens when you want to balance the images in your video frame more evenly—or you want two or more clips to share the screen at once?

With a combination of Premiere Elements's **Crop** and **Motion** effects, it's easy to shape and position any number of clips on your screen.

1 Place Clip A on Video 1

Drag one clip from the **Media** panel to the **Video 1** track on the **Timeline**. (See **94** **Add or Move a Clip on the Timeline**.)

2 Place Clip B on Video 2

Drag another clip from the **Media** panel to the **Video 2** track, directly above clip A.

▶ **TIP**

When positioning your clips on the **Timeline**, view them in the **Monitor**. Be sure you have the safe margins turned on (click the **More** button in the **Monitor** panel to access the margin guides). The safe margins indicate both the possible and likely edges of your video frame that will be cut off by a typical television. Stay within these margins to ensure that you don't position the clip offscreen!

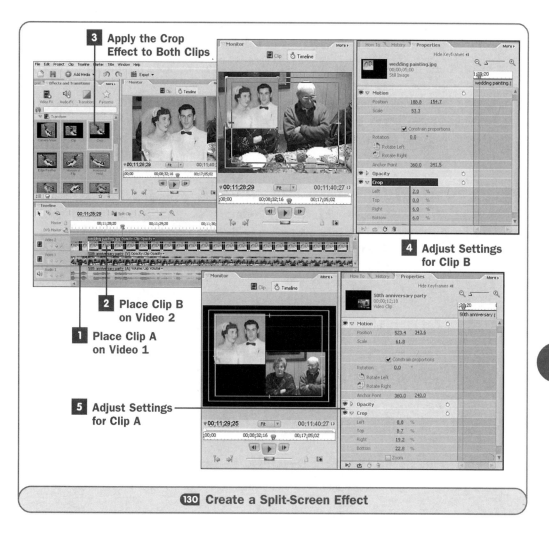

3 Apply the Crop Effect to Both Clips

2 Place Clip B on Video 2

1 Place Clip A on Video 1

4 Adjust Settings for Clip B

5 Adjust Settings for Clip A

130

130 Create a Split-Screen Effect

3 Apply the Crop Effect to Both Clips

The **Crop** effect is located on the **Effects and Transitions** panel, in the **Video FX** collection, in the **Transform** category.

Drag this effect to the clip on **Video 1** and drag it again to the clip on **Video 2**. The effect initially shows no change to either clip.

4 Adjust Settings for Clip B

With clip B selected, click the triangle to the left of the **Crop** listing in the **Properties** panel as well as the triangle to the left of the **Motion** listing to open each effect's control panel.

Use the **Position**, **Scale**, and **Crop** settings in the **Motion** control panel to position, size, and shape your clip. (See ⑪⑭ **Add and Customize an Effect**.)

To change the settings for either effect, you can type in new coordinates or percentages for each setting; you can drag across the numerical settings so they increase or decrease, watching the results of the changes in the **Monitor** panel; or you can click the image in the **Monitor** panel and drag the sides in or position the image manually. Use the method that makes the most sense for you.

When you make adjustments by dragging the clip in the **Monitor**, make sure that the effect you want to adjust at the time is selected in the **Properties** panel. In other words, by clicking the **Motion** listing, you can change your clip's **Position** and **Scale** in the **Monitor** by dragging it and manipulating its corner handles. When you have the **Crop** effect selected, however, dragging the corner handles will crop your image instead of resizing it.

⑤ Adjust Settings for Clip A

As you did with clip B, crop and position the image on **Video 1**.

Repeats steps 2–4 with as many clips on as many separate video tracks as you'd like.

You can even use keyframing for either or both effects so your clips keep moving and changing shape throughout the sequence.

▶ **TIP**

As you know, virtually any time you apply an effect, the clip does not have to remain in one position, at one **Crop** setting, throughout its duration. Using the keyframing feature, you can keep the clips in your split screen in constantly changing shape and position.

---

131 | **Make a Line Move Across a Map**

✔ BEFORE YOU BEGIN	→ SEE ALSO
88 Prepare a Still for Video	120 Make a Variable-Speed Pan and Zoom
16 Change Image Size or Resolution	134 Frame Your Video with an Image
119 Pan and Zoom Still Images a la Ken Burns	

Making a line move across a map is a great way to show your audience where your travels have taken you.

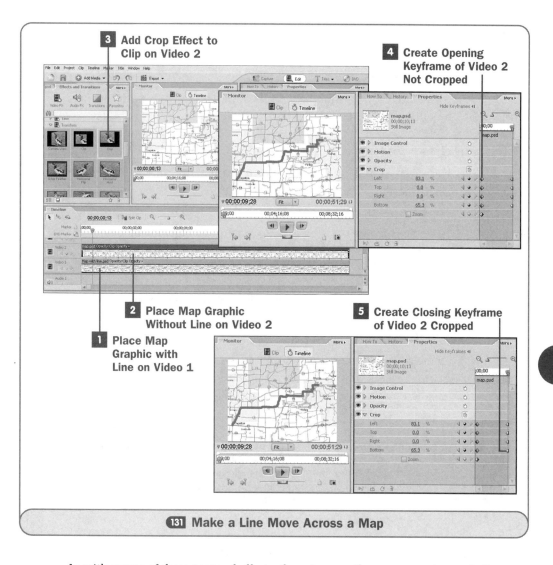

3 Add Crop Effect to Clip on Video 2

4 Create Opening Keyframe of Video 2 Not Cropped

2 Place Map Graphic Without Line on Video 2

1 Place Map Graphic with Line on Video 1

5 Create Closing Keyframe of Video 2 Cropped

131 Make a Line Move Across a Map

As with many of these types of effects, there is more than one way to create it. The method shown in this task is one of the simplest; when combined with keyframing, it's also one of the most effective.

1 Place Map Graphic with Line on Video 1

You'll want two otherwise identical map clips—one plain and one with your route drawn as a dark line using Photoshop Elements. See **41** **Draw on a Photo with a Pencil** or **42** **Paint an Area of a Photo with a Brush**.

Drag the map clip with the line onto the **Video 1** track.

2 Place Map Graphic Without Line on Video 2

Drag the plain map clip to the **Video 2** track, directly above the clip showing the map with the line. Set the two clips to exactly the same duration.

You can see only the plain map clip in the **Monitor**; the map with the line is hidden underneath the plain map clip.

3 Add Crop Effect to Clip on Video 2

The **Crop** effect is found on the **Effects and Transitions** panel, in the **Video FX** collection, in the **Transform** category. Drag this effect onto the plain map clip on **Video 2**.

4 Create Opening Keyframe of Video 2 Not Cropped

With the clip on **Video 2** selected, click the triangle to the left of the **Crop** listing in the **Properties** panel to open the effect's control panel. If the **Properties** panel timeline is not visible, click the **Show Keyframes** button at the top of the panel. Move the **Properties** panel timeline's CTI to the beginning of the clip.

With all the controls at their default settings (no crop is applied to the clip), click the stopwatch icon to the right of the **Motion** listing. A column of little keyframe diamonds appears on the timeline adjacent to each **Crop** setting.

▶ **TIP**

For added effect, add synchronized motion to your two map clips. Before you apply the **Crop** effect, create a motion path by increasing the plain map's scale to zoom in to one area and then panning across the route of travel. Right-click the plain map clip in **Video 2**, select **Copy**, and then right-click the map clip with the line on **Video 1** and select **Paste Attributes**. The motion path from the clip in **Video 2** is copied to the clip in **Video 1**.

5 Create Closing Keyframe of Video 2 Cropped

Move the CTI to the end of the **Properties** timeline for the plain map clip and adjust the **Crop** settings for two adjacent sides so the map with a line clip is completely revealed. (See **130** **Create a Split-Screen Effect**.) Your changed settings should crop the sides of the plain map clip to reveal the map with the line as you'd like it to be revealed in the final animation.

There are a number of ways to change the settings for the plain map clip: You can type new coordinates for each corner point; you can drag across the numerical settings so they increase or decrease, watching the effect as it changes in the **Monitor** panel; or you can click the image in the **Monitor** panel and crop it by dragging the side handles. Use the method that makes the most sense for you.

After you have the opening and closing keyframes in place, Premiere Elements creates the motion frames in between.

When you play this segment, you'll see the side of the plain map clip on **Video 2** crop back to reveal the map with a line on **Video 1**—but the effect is as if the line were being drawn on the screen as the sequence plays.

If you'd like to control the movement of the **Crop** effect throughout the movie segment—such as to reveal the line moving as it changes directions from east to north—add additional keyframes.

▶ TIP

By creating additional keyframe points, you can vary the direction and speed of the line's movement across the map—even stopping its motion completely if you'd like. Because you can add an indefinite number of keyframes, you can precisely control how and how fast the map, or any object, moves.

132 Make a Person Appear with a Different Background

132

✔ BEFORE YOU BEGIN	→ SEE ALSO
94 Add or Move a Clip on the Timeline	**88** Prepare a Still for Video
124 Make an Area of a Clip Transparent	**91** Add, Delete, and Size Tracks
	120 Make a Variable-Speed Pan and Zoom
	16 Change Image Size or Resolution

Here's a very simple and very commonly used application of the **Chroma Key** effect. It's so commonly used, in fact, that you can see it every night on the local news—as the weatherperson, standing in front of a green screen, appears to actually be standing in front of a moving weather map.

1 Place a Background Clip on Video 1

Drag the background clip onto the **Timeline**. The background clip need not be animated. You can use a still or even a drawing. But video, with action and movement, can make the effect seem even more realistic.

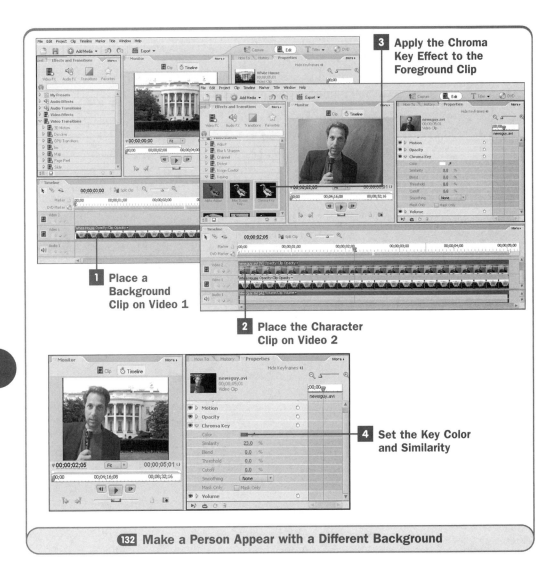

3 Apply the Chroma Key Effect to the Foreground Clip

1 Place a Background Clip on Video 1

2 Place the Character Clip on Video 2

4 Set the Key Color and Similarity

132 Make a Person Appear with a Different Background

2 Place the Character Clip on Video 2

Preparation means everything for the character clip. Shoot your character against a flat-colored background—ideally blue, green, or some color not likely to be in the person's flesh tones or clothing. Lighting the background evenly is very important, too. The smoother the color of the background, the easier it is to key out.

▶ **TIP**

You can key out the background behind the person or character much more easily if the background is a smooth, consistent color. For this reason, it's much better to use a drape made of a soft fabric or cloth than a shiny surface such as plastic.

Place the character clip on the **Timeline**, directly above the background clip.

3 **Apply the Chroma Key Effect to the Foreground Clip**

The **Chroma Key** effect is located on the **Effects and Transitions** panel, in the **Video FX** collection, in the **Keying** category. Drag the effect to the clip on **Video 2**. When the clip in **Video 2** is selected, you will see the **Chroma Key** effect listed in the **Properties** panel.

▶ **NOTE**

If your background moves or if you're using a background video clip that pans, you can use keyframing to synchronize the movement of your foreground clip to match the motion of the background.

4 **Set the Key Color and Similarity**

Click the triangle to the left of the **Chroma Key** listing in the **Properties** panel to open the effect's control panel. Although you can set the color manually using the color panel, it's usually easier to use the screen image to designate the **Key** color. Click the eyedropper icon to the right of the color swatch in the **Chroma Key** control panel. The mouse pointer becomes an eyedropper. Click the color in the screen image in **Video 2** (the background behind the person or character) that you want to designate as transparent.

You'll see an effect immediately, as the clip on **Video 1** replaces the plain-color background of the character clip on **Video 2**. You'll probably have to adjust the **Similarity** setting in the **Properties** panel, widening the range of color to be affected, to get a good, clean transparent area. The **Blend**, **Threshold**, **Cutoff**, and **Smoothing** settings can also help control the transparency and the softness of the transparent area's edge.

▶ **NOTE**

Occasionally, when you scale a clip that has been modified with the **Chroma Key** effect, an edge line shows. You can remove this easily by adding and adjusting the **Crop** effect to the clip. (As you know, you can apply multiple effects to a clip.)

132

133 **Make Your Clip Appear on an Object**

✔ BEFORE YOU BEGIN	→ SEE ALSO
114 Add and Customize an Effect	**88** Prepare a Still for Video
	91 Add, Delete, and Size Tracks
	120 Make a Variable-Speed Pan and Zoom
	16 Change Image Size or Resolution

Although you can pin your clip onto any object, large or small, it's especially impressive to make your clip appear to be projected onto the side of a tall building above a crowded street—sort of the Big Brother effect. In this task, you learn to "project" a video clip onto an object in another clip or a still image. Using the **Corner Pin** effect, you can distort your video clip so it truly looks as if it is part of the background clip or still.

1 Place a Background Clip on Video 1

A background clip with recognizable scenery, such as the Times Square Jumbotron or the side of a well-known building, can be particularly effective. Other objects that can be fun to project a clip onto are a drive-in movie screen (if you can still find one!) or a billboard.

Although you can use keyframing to track the motion of an object, it's often easier—and just as effective—to use a stable, tripod-steady shot of a scene or object as the background clip for this effect. Drag the background clip from the **Media** panel to the **Video 1** track on the **Timeline**.

2 Place a Video Clip on Video 2

The second clip is the video clip you'll be projecting onto the scenery or object in the background clip on **Video 1**.

When you first place the video clip on the **Timeline** on the **Video 2** track, directly above the background clip in **Video 1**, you won't be able to see the background in the **Monitor** panel.

3 Apply the Corner Pin Effect to the Clip on Video 2

The **Corner Pin** effect is located on the **Effects and Transitions** panel, in the **Video FX** collection, in the **Distort** category.

Drag the effect onto the video clip on **Video 2**. When the video clip is selected, the **Corner Pin** effect is listed in the **Properties** panel.

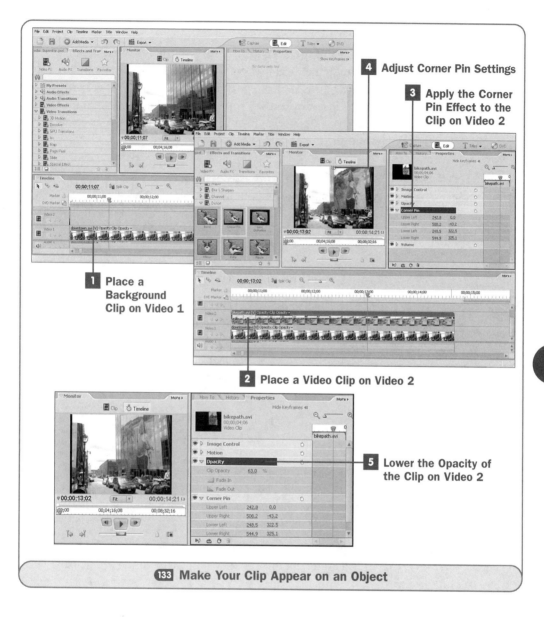

4 Adjust Corner Pin Settings

3 Apply the Corner Pin Effect to the Clip on Video 2

1 Place a Background Clip on Video 1

2 Place a Video Clip on Video 2

5 Lower the Opacity of the Clip on Video 2

133 Make Your Clip Appear on an Object

▶ **TIP**

To shape your clip to fit the shape of the area you are projecting it onto, you can also combine the **Corner Pin** effect with the **Crop** effect or even with one of the **Garbage Mattes**. You can combine as many effects as you'd like on a single clip.

4 **Adjust the Corner Pin Settings**

Click the triangle to the left of the **Corner Pin** listing in the **Properties** panel to open the effect's control panel. You can adjust the corners of the clip by changing the coordinates in this control panel, but you might find it easier to simply click the **Corner Pin** listing in the **Properties** panel and then manipulate the clip by dragging the four corner control handles that appear as encircled crosses in the **Monitor**.

5 **Lower the Opacity of the Clip on Video 2**

To blend your clip into the background—to make the video clip appear to be projected onto an object or building—lower the **Opacity** setting of the clip on **Video 2** until some of the object's or building's texture shows through the video clip.

---

134   **Frame Your Video with an Image**

✔ BEFORE YOU BEGIN	→ SEE ALSO
88 Prepare a Still for Video	**94** Add or Move a Clip on the Timeline
89 Scale and Position a Still	**16** Change Image Size or Resolution
28 Create a New Image Layer	
159 Move Images Between Premiere Elements and Photoshop Elements	

133

The alpha channel travels, usually invisibly, along with the red, green, and blue color channels in a graphic or video clip. However, unlike the color channels, the alpha channel designates transparency, communicating which areas of a clip are transparent and which areas are opaque.

A layered Photoshop document (PSD), or a PDF or TIF document that has no background layer and in which the graphics do not completely fill the frame, carries its non-filled areas as an alpha channel. When you place these types of graphic files into Premiere Elements, the alpha channel remains intact, and these unfilled areas are read as transparent, revealing the clip or clips on the video tracks below.

▶ **NOTE**

The graphics that make up many of the Title templates and DVD templates and menus are, in fact, layered Photoshop documents with no backgrounds and their transparency areas are carried as alpha channels.

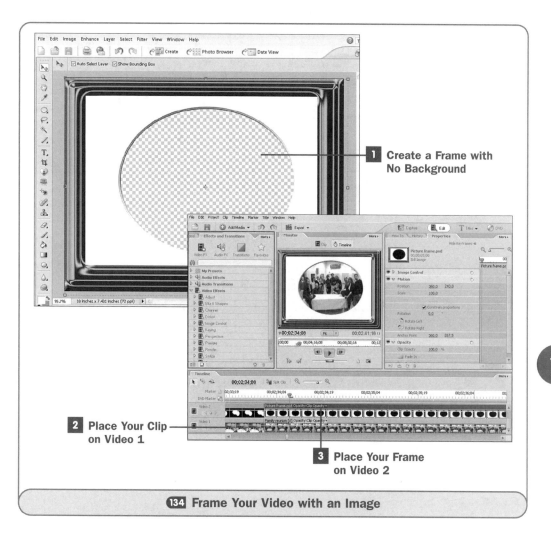

134 Frame Your Video with an Image

Any graphic or photo with the alpha channel enabled can be used as a frame for your video clips.

1 Create a Frame with No Background

With Photoshop Elements, create a multi-layered graphic. In Photoshop Elements, double-click the **Background** layer in the **Layers** panel to turn the background into a layer that can be deleted, leaving you with a transparent canvas. See 159 **Move Images Between Premiere Elements and Photoshop Elements**.

Create a graphic with a window cut through it. This window should be completely transparent, showing whatever your graphics program uses to indicate no background behind it (in this example from Photoshop Elements, the transparent background is indicated by a gray-and-white checkerboard pattern).

Save your frame as a Photoshop (PSD), PDF, or a TIF document with layers enabled. The transparent background travels with these file formats as an alpha channel.

2 Place Your Clip on Video 1

Add the video clip you want to frame on a lower video track (such as **Video 1**) on the **Timeline**.

3 Place Your Frame on Video 2

Add your frame graphic to the **Media** panel using the **Add Media** button and then drag the graphic to the **Timeline** and place it on the video track directly above the clip you want to frame (on **Video 2** in this example). Your clip is visible through the transparent area of the frame graphic.

134

Depending on how much of your screen your frame graphic covers, you might have to adjust the **Scale** setting in the **Properties** panel for the clip on **Video 1** to keep too much of it from being covered.

24

Adding Text, Creating Titles, Making Credits

IN THIS CHAPTER:

If the workspaces you spent the most time in were put on a top-four list, **Titles** would be number two, right behind the **Edit** workspace. *Titles* make your movie unique and give it that professional look. Premiere Elements gives you 10 categories of predesigned title templates; with more than 60 titles and an average of four variations of each title, that's more than 240 title templates.

▶ **KEY TERM**

Title—An image used to display credits, the name of a movie, identify people or places when they appear in a movie, or to superimpose text.

Some of the uses for titles are rolling credits, movie intros, lists, framing a scene or still, track mattes, and lower thirds. Every time you watch a television show or go to a movie, you see titles. The intro is a title, the credits are a title, breaks before commercials are titles, and any time text or a shape is shown over video (or a video is shown through the text or shape), you're seeing a title. You see lower-third titles whenever you watch the news—they are the titles at the bottom of the screen with the reporters' names. Track mattes are used to make text move across a screen with video behind the text remaining stationary, or to have text remaining stationary with video behind the text moving.

With Premiere Elements, titles are easy to create; the program gives you many templates to help you get started. You can use the templates as they are, or you can customize them to suit your particular project. You can even start from scratch with a blank canvas and make your very own creation. It doesn't matter if you use or customize the templates or create titles from scratch—titles are a lot of fun.

135 | **Use and Customize a Title Template**

→ **SEE ALSO**

134 Frame Your Video with an Image
140 Create a Title from Scratch

This task guides you through the selection, use, and customization of one of the many title templates available in Premiere Elements. Considering that the titles are already predesigned, all you really have to do is select the proper template and change the text. Doing so gives you a very nice, easily created title. The hardest part is trying to decide which template to use!

1 **Click the Titles Button**

In the main taskbar at the top of the screen, click the **Titles** button to open the **Title Templates** dialog box.

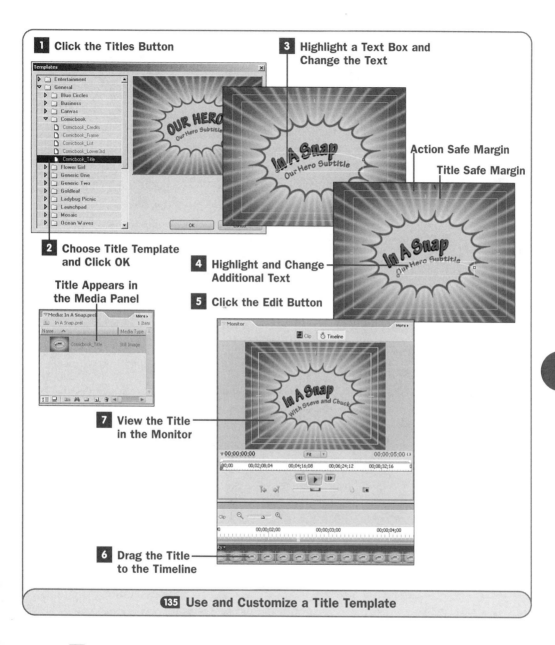

1 Click the Titles Button

3 Highlight a Text Box and Change the Text

Action Safe Margin

Title Safe Margin

2 Choose Title Template and Click OK

Title Appears in the Media Panel

4 Highlight and Change Additional Text

5 Click the Edit Button

7 View the Title in the Monitor

6 Drag the Title to the Timeline

135

135 Use and Customize a Title Template

2 Choose Title Template and Click OK

The **Title Templates** dialog box has a list of title categories, title names, and title types on the left; click a title and view the selected title in the preview screen on the right. Click the arrow to the left of a category name to see a list of title names for that category. The title names also have an arrow in front of them; click that arrow to see a list of title types. For this example, I used a title type from the **General** category, with the title name **Comicbook**, and with the title type **Comicbook_title**. When you click the **Comicbook_title** selection, the title appears in the preview on the right side of the dialog box. You can choose any other category of titles and look for title types that end in **_title** to achieve similar results.

When you're satisfied with the title you've selected, click **OK**. The **Titles** workspace opens with the selected title in the work area.

3 Highlight a Text Box and Change the Text

By default the **Type** tool is selected when you enter the **Titles** workspace. To edit the placeholder text in the title, simply click the main title text (in this example, *Our Hero*) and either press **Delete** or use the **Backspace** key to delete all the existing text. Either action empties the text box and allows you to enter new text into the area. Now just type the main title for your movie.

4 Highlight and Change Additional Text

Most title templates also have another text area you can edit. For the **Comicbook_title** template, click in the text box that says *Our Hero Subtitle* and clear out the text box; you can leave it blank or enter new text here just as you did in step 3.

135

5 Click the Edit Button

When you are finished making text changes in the title, click the **Edit** button in the taskbar at the top-right corner of the screen.

Locate the **Media** panel and notice that the title has been added to the list of clips automatically. This happens every time you create a new title or open a title template.

6 Drag the Title to the Timeline

Simply drag the title clip from the **Media** panel to the **Timeline** to use it in your project. You can place the title anywhere on the **Timeline**, on any video track. Just remember that a main title does not have any transparent areas and will cover any images on tracks below it.

7 View the Title in the Monitor

Position the CTI in the **Timeline** over your title clip and click **Play** to see what the title looks like in the **Monitor**. After a title is on the **Timeline**, it behaves just like any other clip of a still image. You can add transitions and effects, change the duration, or anything else that you can do with a regular still-image clip.

136 Create a Title Overlay for Your Video

✔ BEFORE YOU BEGIN	→ SEE ALSO
135 Use and Customize a Title Template	**159** Move Images Between Premiere Elements and Photoshop Elements

One of the most used title types is a *title overlay*. You see this often in newscasts, sportscasts, movie intros, and almost every television show imaginable. In this task you will create two very common title overlays: the frame and the lower third.

▶ KEY TERM

Title overlay—The use of a title, containing transparent areas, to overlay a clip so the clip shows through the title. The title can contain text, shapes, or graphics in any combination.

■ 1 Click the Titles Button

From the main taskbar at the top of your screen, click the **Titles** button to open the **Title Template** dialog box.

■ 2 Choose a Frame Template and Click OK

For this example, I used the title type **Launchpad_frame**, located in the **General, Launchpad** selections. Click this frame to select it and look at the frame title in the preview window on the right side of the dialog box. You can choose any other category of titles and look for title types that end in **_frame** to achieve similar results.

When you've selected a frame you like, open it in the **Titles** workspace by clicking the **OK** button.

■ 3 Click More and Choose Show Video

After clicking the **OK** button, the **Titles** workspace opens with your template in the **Titler** panel. Make sure that the CTI is over a video or a still clip on the **Timeline**. Click the **More** button at the top-right corner of the **Titler** panel. From the **More** menu, ensure that the Show Video option is selected.

▶ TIP

By moving the CTI over different clips, you can see what will look best behind your new title.

136

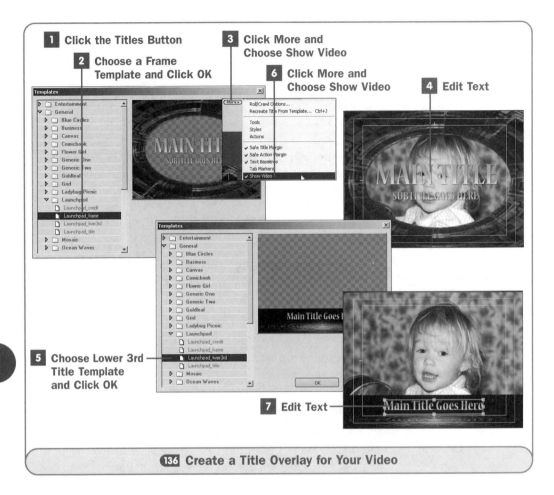

136 Create a Title Overlay for Your Video

4 Edit Text

You should see the frame overlaying the current video clip on the **Timeline**. To make changes to the title text, click the text area and type to make your changes. When you're satisfied with the text, your frame title is ready and is placed in the **Media** panel, ready to be used in your movie.

Drag the title to the **Timeline** and place it on a track above the clip you want to overlay. Position the title by moving it up and down the **Timeline** and watching the **Monitor**, making sure that you place the title in just the right spot. To save your title for use in another project see **139** Save Your Title.

5 Select a Lower 3rd Title Template and Click OK

Creating a title frame was just as easy as you'd expect it to be in Premiere Elements. A similar kind of title that lets a video clip show is the lower-third title—the title graphic appears in the lower third of the video screen with the video clip playing behind the title. Now let's create a lower-third title.

Without doing anything to your current workspace, click the **Titles** button in the top-right corner of the screen to launch the **Title Template** dialog box. For this example, I chose the **Launchpad_lwer3rd** type and clicked **OK**. You can choose any other category of titles and look for title types that end in **_lwer3rd** to achieve similar results.

When you're satisfied with the title you've selected, click the **OK** button.

6 Click More and Choose Show Video

Click the **OK** button to open the new title template in the **Titler** panel. Again, make sure that you have a video or still clip on the **Timeline** and that the CTI is positioned over that clip. Click the **More** button in the **Titler** panel and make sure that the **Show Video** option is selected.

7 Edit Text

Make any changes to the text; the title is automatically added to the **Media** panel, ready to be added to your movie.

Drag the title to the **Timeline** and place it on a track above the clip you want to overlay. Position the title by moving it up and down the **Timeline** and watching the **Monitor**, making sure that you place the title in just the right spot. To save the title for use in another project, see **139** **Save Your Title**.

137

---

137   Create Rolling and Moving Credits

✔ BEFORE YOU BEGIN	→ SEE ALSO
135 Use and Customize a Title Template	**140** Create a Title from Scratch

---

Just like in Hollywood, you can create rolling credits for your movie. I can't even think of a movie that doesn't have rolling credits—it's an unwritten law that you have to have them!

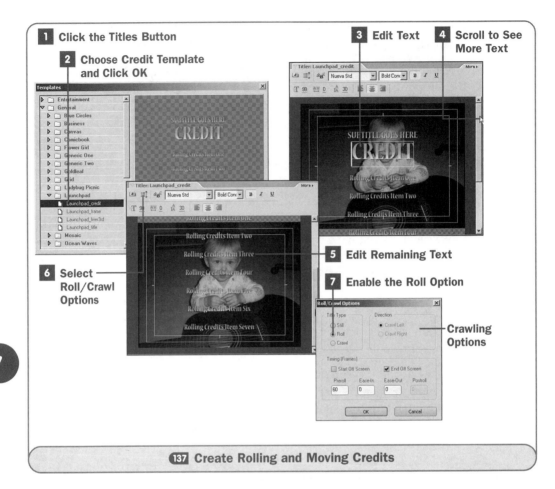

137 Create Rolling and Moving Credits

▶ **NOTE**

Moving panoramas have been in use since the days of Lewis and Clark. The moving panorama, or diorama, consists of a series of paintings on canvas which were then joined together to form one very long canvas sheet. This sheet was wound onto a vertical roller and moved across the stage and wound up on a similar roller on the other side. The canvas could be lighted from behind, front, or both, using oil or gas lamps. Smaller panoramas were placed in a box that someone could look into. If these dioramas had stationary objects inside the box while the canvas moved from behind, the result was a kind of modern video effect. In those days, moving panoramas were used primarily for advertising, but the same principle is still with us today in rolling credits.

Obviously, rolling credits are a good way to display a lot of information in a little space. I say "obviously" because the idea has spanned decades of film and is used constantly by the film industry. Seeing that this type of title has stood the test of time and that no one has seemingly come up with a better idea, I am sure that you will find a need to use rolling credits in your projects at some time.

With Premiere Elements, you can not only roll your title, you can also crawl your title. *Crawling* moves the title across the screen from right to left or from left to right. *Rolling* moves the title from the bottom of the screen to the top. No matter what type of motion you use, rolling or crawling, I am sure that you will find dozens of uses for this type of title. This type of title always has a transparent background so you can view the title over a color matte, a clip, a still image, or just a black background.

▶ **TIP**

To run your title over a color background instead of black, use a color matte. You can add a color matte to a track from the **Media** panel by clicking the **New Item** icon and selecting **Color Matte**. After the matte is created, you can drop it on a track below your title. For more details on color mattes, see **85** **Add Special Media Clips**.

1 Click the Titles Button

In the main taskbar, click the **Titles** button to open the **Title Templates** dialog box.

2 Choose Credit Template and Click OK

For this example, I used the title type **Launchpad_credit**, found in the **General, Launchpad** category. You can choose any other category of titles and look for title types that end in **_credit** to achieve similar results.

When you have selected the credit title you want to use, click **OK** to open the title in the **Titles** workspace.

▶ **TIP**

You can have your title move over a black background, a color background, a still image or video clip. Click the **More** button and select **Show Video**; the CTI controls what video is visible behind the title. You can view the image behind the title exactly as it will appear if, when finished, you place your title on a video track above the selected image on the **Timeline**.

3 Edit Text

This particular credit title template provides you with many lines of text. The text even continues below what you see in the **Titler** window. Click each section of text and make the appropriate changes to create a meaningful credit list for your movie project.

4 Scroll to See More Text

When you have edited all the lines of text you can see in the **Titler** panel, drag the scrollbar on the right side of the **Titler** panel to reveal additional text boxes.

5 Edit Remaining Text

Make changes to the remaining text. If there are more text lines than you need, you can delete the text boxes altogether: Click in the text area and press **Backspace** or **Delete** to clear the existing text. If you don't have enough lines of text, you can add more text by clicking the Type tool (see **95 About Titles**) and then clicking the space in the title where you want the text to be. This action creates a text box into which you can enter your additional text. You can also add additional text to an existing text box. Using the **Type** tool, select the text box you want to add text to and then position the cursor where you want to start typing. When you get to the end of a line, press the **Enter** key to create a new line.

6 Select Roll/Crawl Options

137

Click the **Roll/Crawl Options** button at the top of the **Titler** panel to open the **Roll/Crawl Options** dialog box.

7 Enable the Roll Option

Considering that in this example we have chosen a credit type title, the **Roll** option should already be selected. If you want your title to crawl horizontally across the screen instead of roll from top to bottom, enable the **Crawl** option.

▶ TIP

If you chose the **Crawl** option in step 7, the **Direction** options become available. Choose **Crawl Left** to make the text move from the right side of the screen and off the left side; choose **Crawl Right** to make the text start on the left side of the screen and move off the right side.

This dialog box also offers options under the **Timing (Frames)** section:

- **Start Off Screen**—The title starts rolling or crawling from off the screen. If it is a rolling title, the title appears first at the very bottom of the screen.

- **End Off Screen**—The title continues moving off the screen until it disappears from view. If it is a rolling title, the title disappears off the top of the screen.

If neither of these options is selected, the title will not roll or crawl. To start a title somewhere other than off screen, position the title where you want it to start and select only the **End Off Screen** option. To end your title somewhere other than off the screen, position your title where you want it to end and select only the **Start Off Screen** option.

- **Preroll**—The number of frames that will play before the roll or crawl begins. Only available if the **Start Off Screen** option is not checked.

- **Ease-In**—The number of frames to move at a slowly increasing speed at the beginning of the roll or crawl, increasing to the normal crawl or roll speed.

- **Ease-Out**—The number of frames to move at a slowly decreasing speed at the end of the roll or crawl, decreasing from the normal crawl or roll speed.

- **Postroll**—The number of frames that will play after the title has finished its roll or crawl. Only available if the **End Off Screen** option is not checked.

Make any changes you want to the settings in the **Roll/Crawl Options** dialog box and click the **OK** button. The rolling title has already been added to the **Media** panel for use in your movie.

138

To use the credit clip as either opening or closing credits in your movie project, drag the credit title clip off the **Media** panel and drop it on an upper video track on the **Timeline**. Position the clip so it aligns with the clip you want to show through the transparent background of the credit title clip.

---

138 | **Create Custom Motion for Text**

✔ BEFORE YOU BEGIN	→ SEE ALSO
118 Add Motion to a Still	**140** Create a Title from Scratch
	134 Frame Your Video with an Image

Sometimes you want something more than a simple rolling or crawling title. You might want the title to move like an old Pong game, or maybe you want the text to move diagonally. Premiere Elements gives you the tools you need to accomplish this task. Using keyframes, you can make a title change size or direction easily. By adjusting title size and movement, and adding additional effects, the number of title possibilities is unlimited.

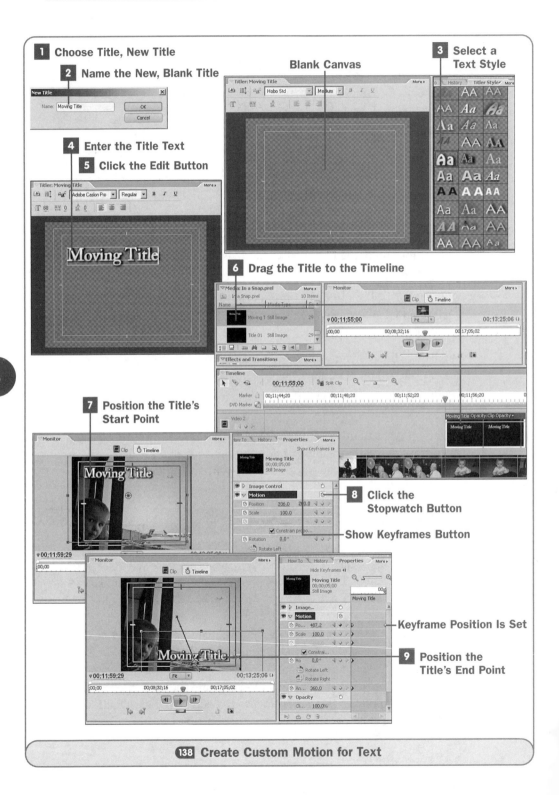

1 Choose Title, New Title

2 Name the New, Blank Title

Blank Canvas

3 Select a Text Style

4 Enter the Title Text

5 Click the Edit Button

6 Drag the Title to the Timeline

7 Position the Title's Start Point

8 Click the Stopwatch Button

Show Keyframes Button

Keyframe Position Is Set

9 Position the Title's End Point

138

138 Create Custom Motion for Text

1 Choose Title, New Title

From the menu bar at the top of the screen, choose **Title, New Title**, and then select your title type (**Default Still, Default Roll,** or **Default Crawl**) to open the **New Title** dialog box. For this task, I selected the **Default Still Title**; we will add the motion later.

▶ NOTES

Alternatively, you can access the **New Title** dialog box in a more roundabout fashion: In the main taskbar at the top of your screen, click the **Titles** button to open the **Title Templates** dialog box. Click the **Cancel** button to dismiss the **Templates** dialog box and instead open the **New Title** dialog box.

Alternatively, you can click and hold the **Titles** button to access a submenu with an option for a **New Title**.

2 Name the New, Blank Title

In the **New Title** dialog box, give your title a name. Click the **OK** button; the **Titles** workspace opens with a completely blank title in the **Titler** panel.

3 Select a Text Style

From the **Titler Styles** panel, select the text style you want to use for the title by clicking it.

4 Enter the Title Text

Click the location in the **Titler** panel where you want to add the text. This action opens a text box to hold the text you are typing. For this example, I added text to the upper-left area in the **Titler**. Be sure to keep your text within the safe title margin.

In most cases, you want to limit your text to a single line or even a single word. With the text moving around, you don't want to make it difficult for your audience to read.

5 Click the Edit Button

When are done entering your text, click the **Edit** button on the main taskbar at the top of your screen. The **Edit** workspace opens, where you can start to put motion to your title.

138

▶ **NOTE**

It is possible to complete this task from within the **Titles** workspace. The **Effects and Transitions** panel, along with the **Timeline** and **Monitor**, are visible in the Titles workspace. And the **Properties** panel can be opened as a free-floating window by choosing **Window, Properties** from the main menu. The only problem with working from the **Titles** workspace is that space gets even more limited than normal. With video editing, space is very important, and the **Edit** workspace is designed for just that: editing.

6 Drag the Title to the Timeline

The title you just created has been automatically added to the **Media** panel. To add the title to your current project, just drag the title from the **Media** panel and drop it on the **Timeline**. This particular title, as well as many others, has a transparent background. Video shows through the title when it is placed on a track above an image or clip on the **Timeline**. If the title is placed on **Video 1**, the background is black.

7 Position the Title's Start Point

Position the CTI at the first frame of your title. You might have to zoom way in on the **Timeline** to make sure you get the very first frame; view the title in the **Monitor**. Make sure that the title is still selected on the **Timeline** and look at the **Properties** panel.

138

8 Click the Stopwatch Button

In the **Properties** panel, click the arrow in front of the **Motion** listing to open up the control panel for that property. For this moving-title effect, you are interested in the title's opening **Position** and **Scale** keyframe options. In the **Monitor**, drag the title to the position where you want it to appear when the title clip starts playing. When the title text is where you want it, click the stopwatch icon next to the **Motion** listing in the **Properties** panel to set the keyframe markers.

▶ **NOTE**

If you don't see the timeline in the **Properties** panel, click the **Show Keyframes** button at the top of the panel to display it.

9 Position the Title's End Point

Position the CTI in the main **Timeline** at the very last frame of the title. You might have to zoom out and back in on the **Timeline** to ensure that you have selected the last frame of the title. You should still be able to see the title in the **Monitor**.

Click the title in the **Monitor** and drag it to the position you want it to be at the end of its movement. Because you have already set keyframe markers for this clip in step 8, the markers for this new position are set for you automatically.

The only thing left to do is render the **Timeline** and play the title. If you don't quite like the movement, go back to the first frame of the title clip and make adjustments; then make adjustments to the final frame of the title clip. Continue tweaking the positions of the title until you have the exact movement for which you are looking.

▶ **TIP**

Use the **Scale** option in the **Properties** panel to make your title shrink or grow as it moves. Simply adjust the scale up (more than 100) to make it larger, or down (less than 100) to make it smaller. Try setting it very small on the first frame and very large on the last frame. Not only will the title text move across the screen as you've plotted it, it will grow in size as it does.

139 Save Your Title	
✔ **BEFORE YOU BEGIN**	→ **SEE ALSO**
135 Use and Customize a Title Template	**140** Create a Title from Scratch

139

As you know, after you create and edit a title, it is automatically added to the **Media** panel. You can use that title again in the project in which it resides. But what if you want to use that same title in another project?

A simple process allows you to save any title for use in any project. After you save a title, it is as easy to add it to a project as it is to add any other media to your project. When you have created a few different titles (as described in the previous tasks), let's learn how to save a title to use again.

1 **Select the Title to Be Saved**

In the **Media** panel, highlight the title you want to save as a template for use in other projects.

2 **Choose File, Export, Title**

From the main menu bar, select **File**, **Export**, **Title**. The **Save Title** dialog box opens.

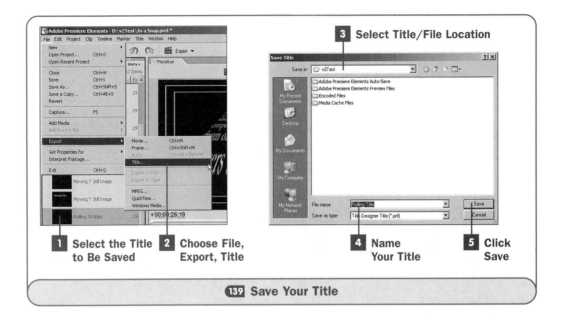

3 Select Title/File Location

1 Select the Title to Be Saved   **2** Choose File, Export, Title   **4** Name Your Title   **5** Click Save

139 Save Your Title

139

3 Select Title/File Location

In the **Save in** text box, select the location where you want to save the title. You can use the default location or browse to another folder or directory.

4 Name the Title

In the **File name** text box, type a name for your title. Be sure to give it a name that will help you remember what type of title it is and what it would be used for.

5 Click Save

Click **Save**, and the title is saved in the selected destination. It will have the filename you entered followed by a **.prtl** extension.

▶ **TIP**

Titles are saved with a **.prtl** extension. If you want to use this particular title in another project, use the **Add Media** button to add the title file to the **Media** panel, just as you would to add any other type of media to your project (see **84** **Add Media with the Adobe Media Downloader**). When browsing for the file, look for the filename you gave the title and the **.prtl** extension at the end.

140 Create a Title from Scratch

✔ BEFORE YOU BEGIN	→ SEE ALSO
137 Create Rolling and Moving Credits	**139** Save Your Title

Even though Premiere Elements comes with hundreds of title templates, sometimes you just can't find a template that will accomplish what you want. What do you do then?

That's what this task is all about. Here we will provide the instruction you need to successfully create a title from scratch. With virtually unlimited fonts, styles, colors, backgrounds, and various other options, I doubt there is a limit to what you can do. You can even create your own unique background in Photoshop Elements and use that as your title.

1 Choose Title, New Title, Default Still

From the main menu, choose **Title, New Title, Default Still**. The **New Title** dialog box opens, where you can name your new title.

2 Name the Title

In the **New Title** dialog box, type a name for your title and click **OK**. The **Titles** workspace opens.

In the **Titles** workspace, you will see a blank canvas to work with. Now it is up to you and your imagination. For this task, you will add a shape, horizontal and vertical text, and an image, just to get your creative juices flowing.

3 Add a Rectangle-Shaped Background

Click the **Rectangle** tool, and then click in a corner of the **Titler** panel. Drag the mouse to create a rectangle to cover the inside margin box (the Title Safe Margin). After you have the rectangle the correct size, open the **Color Properties** dialog box by clicking the **Color Properties** button. Select a four-color gradient, your colors, and a drop shadow.

140

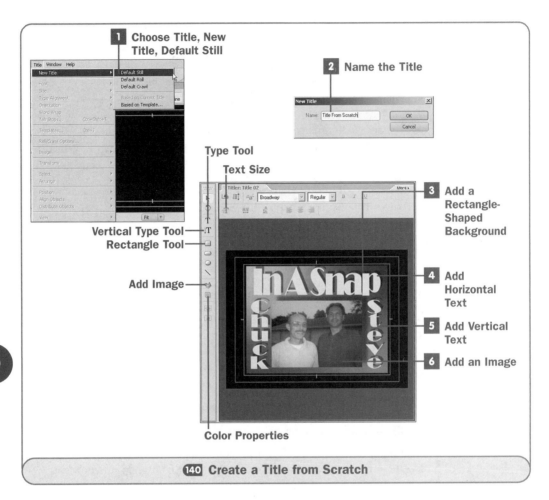

1 Choose Title, New Title, Default Still

2 Name the Title

Type Tool

Text Size

Vertical Type Tool

Rectangle Tool

Add Image

3 Add a Rectangle-Shaped Background

4 Add Horizontal Text

5 Add Vertical Text

6 Add an Image

Color Properties

140

140 Create a Title from Scratch

4 Add Horizontal Text

Click the **Type** tool and then click on the area of the **Titler** panel where you want the text to appear. Before you start typing, select the font you want to use by clicking the **Font** selection; a drop-down menu shows all the available fonts. Pick a font. To the right of the **Font** drop-down list are font attributes (bold, italic, and underlined). Use these options the same as you do in most word-processing applications such as Microsoft Word. To change the size of the text, click the **Text Size** button and drag the mouse to the right to make the text larger, or to the left to make the text smaller.

▶ **TIP**

To center your text vertically or horizontally, use the centering tools in the **Title** toolbar, located below the **Color Properties**.

5 Add Vertical Text

Add vertical text by clicking the **Vertical Type** tool and then clicking the area of the **Titler** panel where you want the text to be placed. The same options mentioned in step 4 are available to change the font and the text characteristics.

6 Add an Image

Click the **Add Image** button to open a browse dialog box that will allow you to find an image for your title. Select the image you want to use and click **OK** to open that image in the **Titler** panel. To resize the image to fit in the available space, right-click the image and choose **Transform**, **Scale** from the context menu. In the **Scale** dialog box that opens, enter a number greater than or less than 100%. Entering a number greater than 100% makes the image larger; entering a number less than 100% makes the image smaller.

▶ TIPS

To add an image to your title, use the **Add Image** button or choose **Image**, **Add Image** from the main menu bar or a context menu. You cannot drag an image clip from the **Media** panel to the **Titler** panel.

If you have photo-editing software such as Photoshop Elements, you can use that to create a unique background for your title. The image you create can have transparent areas that video can show through, or you can create transparent cookie-cutter shapes. Premiere Elements works very well with Photoshop Elements; all the images you create in Photoshop Elements can easily be imported into Premiere Elements, retaining all the image characteristics and properties.

▶ NOTE

At any time, you can click the **Selection** tool and then click any item in the **Titler** panel to drag, reposition, or resize the item.

140

25

Outputting Your Video

IN THIS CHAPTER:

Not only can you burn your finished movie to a DVD, you can also output your project file in four formats. You can even output your movie back to your camcorder or, with the proper mechanical setup, to a VHS tape. All the tasks in this chapter dealing with outputting your video start in the same place: the **File**, **Export** submenu on the taskbar at the top of your screen. You can export a clip from the **Media** panel, a portion of the **Timeline**, or the entire **Timeline**. This submenu contains the following output, or export, options:

- The **Movie** option creates your movie as a Microsoft DV-AVI file, or as other formats if you use the **Advanced** features.

- The **Frame** option grabs a still from your video. For details on how to capture a still image from your video clip, see **87** **Grab a Still from Video**.

- The **Audio** option exports only the audio from a video clip.

- The **Title** option exports a selected title.

- Selecting the **Export to DVD** option opens the **Burn DVD** dialog box.

- The **MPEG** option outputs your movie as an MPEG file, as explained in **143** **Output an MPEG File**.

- The **QuickTime** option outputs your movie as a QuickTime MOV file.

- The **Windows Media** option outputs your movie as a Windows Media WMV file, as explained in **142** **Output a Windows Media (WMV) File**.

These output options are necessary if you would like to put your movie on a CD, send your movie as an email attachment, or upload your movie to be viewed on a website.

The **MPEG**, **Windows Media (MWV)**, and **QuickTime** file outputs all have settings you can change. These settings control the viewable size, the choice of codec, various audio properties, and the choice of template suitable for web viewing. The templates are based on the viewer's Internet connection speed. For example, the DSL template creates a larger file and viewable image than the mobile phone template does.

▶ WEB RESOURCES

www.apple.com/quicktime

www.real.com

MPEG files play in a variety of media players, WMV files play in Windows Media Player, and QuickTime files play in the QuickTime Player. Many of these files can also be played in RealPlayer. QuickTime Player and RealPlayer are available free at their respective websites.

▶ **NOTE**

Make sure you have a clip highlighted in the **Media** panel or on the **Timeline** before you choose an option from the **File, Export** submenu. If not, the **Export** option is not available.

When outputting to the various formats in this chapter, we will talk briefly about the advanced settings. Although the advanced settings are illustrated in the tasks, I recommend that you leave them at their defaults. If you are already—or when you become—an advanced user, the basic information in these tasks can help you find the advanced settings you need.

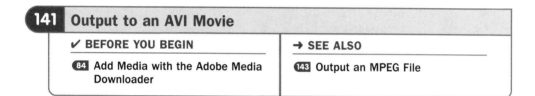

141 Output to an AVI Movie

✔ BEFORE YOU BEGIN	→ SEE ALSO
84 Add Media with the Adobe Media Downloader	143 Output an MPEG File

Audio Video Interleaved (AVI) is a container format for video with synchronized audio. An AVI file can contain different compressed video and audio streams. AVI files can be played on most computers using software such as Windows Media Player. The AVI format has less compression than formats such as MPEG2 and therefore creates larger files. Although the lesser-compressed files produce better quality video, they are not very useful for the Internet. The most common use for AVI files with Premiere Elements is for combining projects. You can export multiple projects as AVI files and then add them all to a single project using the **Add Media** feature. The AVI files created can also be opened in many third-party editing and DVD authoring applications.

1 Open the Export Movie Dialog Box and Name Your File

To get started outputting your movie as an AVI file, choose **File, Export, Movie** from the menu bar at the top of the screen. Choose a name for your AVI file and type it in the **File name** box.

2 Change General Settings

If you want to change the settings for your AVI file, click the **Settings** button; otherwise jump ahead to step 6.

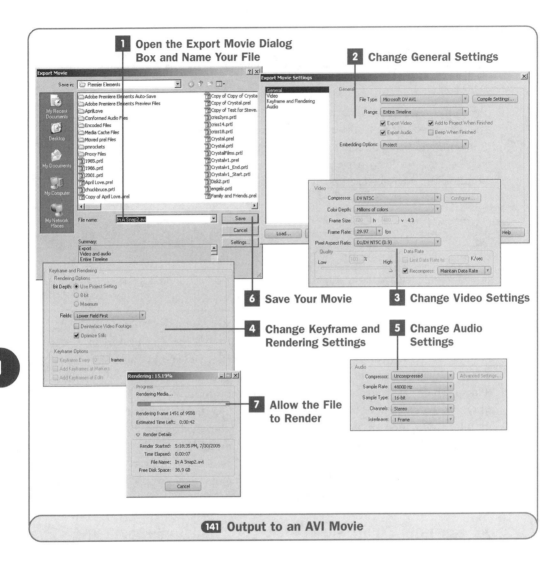

1 Open the Export Movie Dialog Box and Name Your File

2 Change General Settings

6 Save Your Movie

3 Change Video Settings

4 Change Keyframe and Rendering Settings

5 Change Audio Settings

7 Allow the File to Render

141 Output to an AVI Movie

141

In the **Export Movie Settings** dialog box that appears, click a category name in the left pane to switch between the various kinds of settings (**General, Video, Keyframe and Rendering,** and **Audio**). In the **General** settings, you can change the following options:

▶ **TIP**

For more information about all the settings available when exporting to any of the file formats (AVI, WMV, MPEG, or QuickTime), see the Adobe Premiere Elements Help files. Simply enter the setting name in the search box to get a detailed description of what that setting does. You can also search the Internet using your favorite search engine to come up with even more detailed information on various settings.

- **File Type**—Allows you to select from various codecs and file types such as Microsoft AVI, Microsoft DV-AVI, and various image formats, as well as filmstrip. The filmstrip option exports a video as a number of still images. The default is Microsoft DV-AVI.

- **Compile Settings**—These options vary depending on the file type you choose.

- **Range**—Specifies the range to export (**Entire Timeline** or **Work Area Bar**). The **Work Area Bar** option exports the range covered by the work area bar. The default is **Entire Timeline**.

- **Export Video**—When this option is selected, the video tracks are exported. Do not select this option if you do not want to export the video tracks.

- **Export Audio**—When this option is selected, the audio tracks are exported. Do not select this option if you do not want to export the audio tracks.

- **Add to Project When Finished**—Selecting this option adds the resulting file to the **Media** panel.

- **Beep When Finished**—When this option is selected, your computer will beep when it has finished creating the file.

141

- **Embedding Options**—Includes in the exported file the information needed to use the **Edit Original** command. When this information is available in your file, you will be able to open and edit the original project from any application that supports the **Edit Original** command. This option is on by default.

When you have made the changes you want to these settings, click the **Video** option in the left pane to move to the **Video** settings.

3 Change Video Settings

On the **Video** page of the **Export Movie Settings** dialog box, the following options are available:

- **Compressor**—Selections vary depending on the file type. For Microsoft DV-AVI, the options are **DV NTSC** and **DV PAL**.

- **Color Depth**—Selections vary depending on the file type. In most cases, the only choice is **Millions+** of colors.

- **Frame Size**—Enter the horizontal and vertical size in pixels. The default for NTSC is **720×480**. Depending on your use, you might want to make changes to the frame size such as 800×600 or 1024×768.

- **Frame Rate**—Selections vary depending on the file type. For Microsoft DV-AVI, you can choose a frame rate between 1 frame per second and 60 frames per second. The default for NTSC is 29.97 frames per second.

- **Pixel Aspect Ratio**—Selection varies depending on the file type. For Microsoft DV-AVI and NTSC, there are various options such as 2:1 or 16:9 (widescreen). The default is **D1/DV NTSC (.09)**.

- **Quality**—This slider can range from 1% to 100%. This option is not available for all codecs.

- **Data Rate**—Allows you to change the data rate in kb/second and also enables you to choose whether to recompress the video.

When you have made the changes you want to these settings, click the **Keyframe and Rendering** option in the left pane to move to the **Keyframe and Rendering** settings.

141

4 Change Keyframe and Rendering Settings

On the **Keyframe and Rendering** page of the **Export Movie Settings** dialog box, the following **Rendering** options are available:

- **Bit Depth**—Choose from **Use Project Setting**, **8 bit**, or **Maximum**.

- **Fields**—Choose from **Progressive Scan, Lower Field First**, or **Upper Field First**. The default is **Lower Field First**. You also have the option to select **Deinterlace Video Footage** and **Optimize Stills**.

- **Keyframe Options**—Select from **Keyframe Every XX frames, Add Keyframes at Markers**, or **Add Keyframes at Edits**. These options are not enabled with all file types.

When you have made the changes you want to these settings, click the **Audio** option in the left pane to move to the **Audio** settings.

5 Change Audio Settings

On the **Audio** page of the **Export Movie Settings** dialog box, you can change the following options:

- **Compressor**—Allows you to select the type of codec used for compression of the audio portion of the file. The default is **Uncompressed** and is usually the only option.

- **Sample Rate**—Allows you to select a rate in Hz (32000, 44100, or 48000); the default is 48000Hz. CD quality is 44.1kHz. Resampling (setting a different rate than the original audio) also requires additional processing time; avoid resampling by capturing audio at the final rate.

- **Sample Type**—Choose from 8 bit or 16 bit. In most cases, the only option is the default of 16 bit. Choose a higher bit depth and **Stereo** for better quality, or choose a lower bit depth and **Mono** to reduce processing time and disk-space requirements. CD quality is 16-bit stereo.

- **Channels**—Choose between **Mono** and **Stereo**. **Stereo** provides two channels of audio; **Mono** provides one channel. If you choose to export a stereo track as mono, the audio will be downmixed.

- **Interleave**—This setting deals with audio processing. Higher values store longer audio segments and require less frequent processing. Higher values also require more RAM. The default is 1 Frame.

When you are finished making changes to any of the settings in the **Export Movie Settings** dialog box, click **OK** to go back to the **Export Movie** dialog box.

6 Save Your Movie

When you finish naming the AVI file and changing any necessary settings, click the **Save** button. Premiere Elements starts exporting your movie and opens the **Rendering** dialog box.

7 Allow the File to Render

Before Premiere Elements can save your movie, it must render the current video. How long this takes depends on the size of the video and the speed of your computer. You can watch the progress bar, see the number of frames rendered so far and the total number of frames, as well as the estimated time left. If, for some reason, you change your mind and don't want to save the AVI file with the settings you supplied, click the **Cancel** button to stop the rendering.

▶ **NOTE**

If you cancel the rendering of your movie, the AVI file is not saved.

If you selected the **Add to Project** option, your new AVI file is now in the **Media** panel. You can also import your AVI file into another project, combining multiple projects together. The resulting file can also be opened in Windows Media Player and other video-editing programs.

141

142 Output a Windows Media (WMV) File

✔ BEFORE YOU BEGIN	→ SEE ALSO
84 Add Media with the Adobe Media Downloader	**141** Output to an AVI File

Windows Media Video (WMV) is a popular format primarily because it plays well in Windows Media Player, a free media player that comes with the Microsoft Windows XP operating system. The WMV file format can also be compressed small enough to make it a great choice for email or websites, and the quality can be rather good. If bandwidth is an issue, this is a good option. A WMV file can be scaled to allow streaming over dialup and DSL connections and even for portable devices. If any of these options is your goal, consider outputting your Premiere Elements movie project as a WMV file.

142

1 Open the Export Windows Media Dialog Box and Choose Export Preset

Choose **File**, **Export**, **Windows Media** from the menu bar at the top of your screen to open the **Export Windows Media** dialog box.

If you want to output an DV-AVI file (as explained in **141 Output to an AVI Movie**), you know that DV-AVI files are much too large for email or website use; therefore, the output process does not ask you to make choices to establish the size (or compression and quality) of the output file. WMV, MPEG, and QuickTime formats, however, all provide you the ability to choose how the file will be viewed most often; you make a selection by choosing a preset.

When you choose one of the presets in the **Export Windows Media** dialog box, Premiere Elements automatically sets all the default settings based on that preset. The preset options are, broadly, **For Broadband**, **For Dialup**, and **For Wireless**. Each preset has an additional number of options based on the speed of the viewer's connection.

Select a preset option from the pane on the left side of the **Export Windows Media** dialog box; look at the description of the selection on the left.

After you have selected an output format, continue with step 2 to set more advanced options; if you do not need to make any advanced settings changes, skip ahead to step 6.

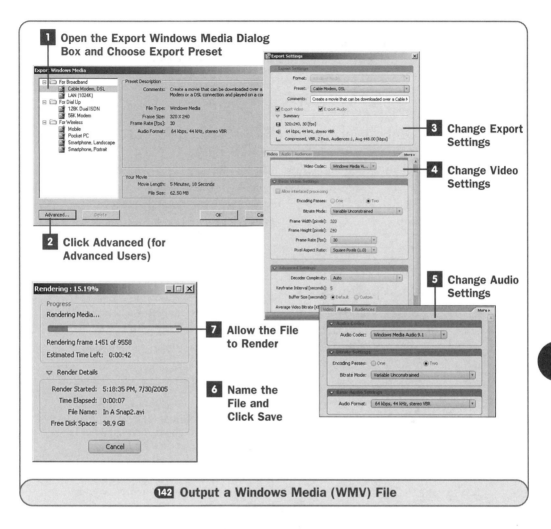

1 Open the Export Windows Media Dialog Box and Choose Export Preset

2 Click Advanced (for Advanced Users)

3 Change Export Settings

4 Change Video Settings

5 Change Audio Settings

6 Name the File and Click Save

7 Allow the File to Render

142 Output a Windows Media (WMV) File

2 Click Advanced (for Advanced Users)

If you have a need to change your output settings, click the **Advanced** button at the bottom of the **Export Windows Media** dialog box to open the **Export Settings** dialog box.

3 Change Export Settings

The **Export Settings** dialog box has four sections that allow you to change various properties of your output file. The **Export Settings** section includes the file **Format** (not changeable) to which you are outputting, the **Preset** (which you selected in step 1), and **Comments** (type a brief description of the settings you are creating). Enable the **Export Video** option to export the video tracks; deselect this option to prevent exporting video tracks. Enable the **Export Audio** option to export the audio tracks; deselect this option to prevent exporting audio. The **Summary** section summarizes the current property settings.

4 Change Video Settings

The **Video Settings** appear on a tab just below the **Export Settings** in the **Export Settings** dialog box. In this section are three tabs you can navigate between. The changeable properties on the **Video** tab are **Video Codec, Allow interlaced processing, Encoding Passes, Bitrate Mode, Frame Width [pixels], Frame Height [pixels], Frame Rate [fps], Pixel Aspect Ratio, Decoder Complexity, Keyframe Interval [seconds], Buffer Size [seconds],** and **Average Video Bitrate [Kbps]**. For additional information on most of these settings, see **141 Output to an AVI Movie**.

5 Change Audio Settings

By clicking on the **Audio** tab, you open a panel of audio settings. The available **Audio** settings are **Audio Codec, Encoding Passes, Bitrate Mode,** and **Audio Format**. For additional information on these settings, see **141 Output to an AVI Movie**.

142

▶ **TIP**

Click the **Audiences** tab to choose between **Compressed** and **Uncompressed**. The audience you are concerned about is mainly related to the Internet connection speed. If the people viewing the file have a dialup connection, you want a compressed file; if your audience uses a DSL connection, an uncompressed file might be best.

If you have made changes to the advanced settings that you want to save, click the **Save** button at the bottom of the **Export Settings** dialog box. If you have not made any changes or do not want to save the changes you have made, click **Cancel**.

6 Name the File and Click Save

After clicking **Save** or **Cancel**, you return to the **Export Windows Media** dialog box (back where you selected the preset). Click the **OK** button to open the **Save File** dialog box. Choose the destination location for the file, type the name of the file, and choose the **Export Range**. Here you have the option to export the **Entire Sequence (project)** or just what is under the **Work Area Bar**.

Click the **Save** button to begin saving your movie as a WMV file. After you click the **Save** button, the **Rendering** dialog box opens.

7 Allow the File to Render

The file must be rendered, just as if you were burning it to a DVD. The rendering process varies in time depending on the size of your project and the speed of your computer. The **Rendering** dialog box shows you the progress and estimated time remaining. If you decide not to continue rendering the file and click **Cancel**, the WMV file will not be created.

Now you have a file that can be used on a web page, emailed to a friend, or possibly even put onto a CD (size permitting). The file can also be viewed in Windows Media Player and even imported into Windows Movie Maker.

143 Output an MPEG File

✔ BEFORE YOU BEGIN	→ SEE ALSO
84 Add Media with the Adobe Media Downloader	**142** Output a Windows Media (WMV) File
	144 Archive Your Project

143

▶ **WEB RESOURCE**
www.chiariglione.org/mpeg

This is the homepage for the **Moving Picture Experts Group**, which can provide information about the MPEG file format.

The Moving Picture Experts Group (MPEG) format is available in a number of flavors: MPEG-1, MPEG-2, and MPEG-4. MPEG files are more compressed than DV-AVI files and cannot be edited as easily in Premiere Elements. Depending on the codec used to encode the MPEG, Premiere Elements might not be able to edit these files at all. By default, Premiere Elements uses the MainConcept MPEG codec for encoding and decoding MPEG files.

Premiere Elements can export your movie as either an MPEG-1 or MPEG-2 file. For the best quality, choose the MPEG-2 format. If you want to put your movie onto a CD so people can view it on computers and some DVD players, this is the format you should choose. These CDs are called VCD (Video Compact Disc, MPEG-1) and SVCD (Super Video Compact Disc, MPEG-2).

▶ **WEB RESOURCE**
www.videohelp.com/vcd

www.videohelp.com/svcd

If you want to learn more about VCDs and SVCDs, check out the resources at www.videohelp.com.

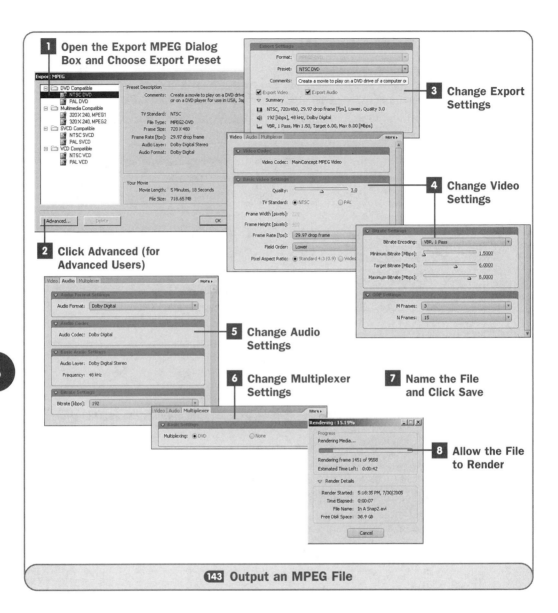

1 Open the Export MPEG Dialog Box and Choose Export Preset

2 Click Advanced (for Advanced Users)

3 Change Export Settings

4 Change Video Settings

5 Change Audio Settings

6 Change Multiplexer Settings

7 Name the File and Click Save

8 Allow the File to Render

143 Output an MPEG File

1 Open the Export MPEG Dialog Box and Choose Export Preset

Choose **File**, **Export**, **MPEG** from the menu bar at the top of your screen. If you want to output an AVI file (as explained in **141 Output to an AVI Movie**), you know that AVI files are much too large for email or website use; therefore, the output process does not ask you to make choices to establish the size (or compression and quality) of the output file. WMV, MPEG, and QuickTime formats, however, all provide you the ability to choose how the file will be viewed most often; you make a selection by choosing a preset.

When you choose one of the presets in the left pane of the **Export MPEG** dialog box, Premiere Elements automatically sets all the defaults based on that preset. The preset options are, broadly, **DVD Compatible**, **Multimedia Compatible**, **SVCD Compatible**, and **VCD Compatible**. Each preset has an additional number of options based on NTSC and PAL or on MPEG1 and MPEG2.

After you choose a preset, continue with step 2 to change the advanced options. If you do not need to make any changes to the advanced settings, skip ahead to step 7.

2 Click Advanced (for Advanced Users)

If you have a need to change your output settings, click the **Advanced** button at the bottom of the **Export MPEG** dialog box to open the **Export MPEG Settings** dialog box.

3 Change Export Settings

MPEGs have the most modifiable settings of all four output file types. The **Export Settings** options include the **Format** (not changeable) of the file you are exporting, the **Preset** (which you chose in step 1), **Comments** (type a note explaining what purpose you plan to use these settings for), **Export Video** (exports the video tracks; deselect this option to prevent exporting video tracks), **Export Audio** (exports the audio tracks; deselect this option to prevent exporting audio tracks), and a summary of the current format settings.

143

4 Change Video Settings

Under the **Export Settings** area in the dialog box are three tabs, **Video**, **Audio**, and **Multiplexer**. The **Video** options you can change are **Video Codec**, **Quality**, **TV Standard** (NTSC or PAL), **Frame Width in Pixels**, **Frame Height in Pixels**, **Frame Rate**, **Field Order**, **Pixel Aspect Ratio** (4:3 or 16:9), **Bitrate Encoding**, **Minimum Bitrate**, **Target Bitrate**, **Maximum Bitrate**, **M Frames**, and **N Frames**. For additional information on most of these settings, see **141** Output to an AVI Movie.

5 Change Audio Settings

Click the **Audio** tab to change the following options: **Audio Format**, **Audio Codec**, **Audio Layer**, **Frequency**, and **Bitrate in kbps**. For additional information on most of these settings, see **141** Output to an AVI Movie. The default audio option is **Dolby Digital**. You can take advantage of **Dolby Stereo** and

AC-3 support when importing and exporting video; these options give you full quality sound and leave more space on your DVD for the high-quality video.

6 Change Multiplexer Settings

Click the **Multiplexer** tab to choose either the **DVD** or **None** option. The **DVD** option creates one MPG file that contains both video and audio; such a file is known as a *program stream*. Selecting the **None** option creates separate video (.**m2v**) and audio (.**ac3**) files; such files are known as *elementary streams*. Use the **None** option if you are going to author a DVD from the resulting MPEG files. Some authoring programs prefer program streams while others prefer elementary streams. If you plan to use the MPEG files in a third-party DVD authoring application, consult your DVD authoring software documentation to determine the proper settings.

If you have made changes to the advanced settings that you want to save, click the **Save** button at the bottom of the **Export MPEG Settings** dialog box. If you have not made any changes or do not want to save the changes you have made, click **Cancel**.

143

7 Name the File and Click Save

After clicking **Save** or **Cancel**, you return to the **Export MPEG** dialog box (back where you selected the preset). Click the **OK** button. The **Save File** dialog box opens. Choose the destination location for the file, type the name of your file, and choose the **Export Range**. You can choose to export the **Entire Sequence (project)** or just what is under the **Work Area Bar**.

Click the **Save** button to begin saving your movie as an MPEG file. After you click the **Save** button, the **Rendering** dialog box opens.

8 Allow the File to Render

The file must be rendered, just as if you were burning it to a DVD. The rendering process varies in time depending on the size of your project and the speed of your computer. The **Rendering** dialog box shows you the progress and estimated time remaining. If you decide not to continue rendering the file, click **Cancel**; the MPEG file will not be created.

The resulting MPEG file can be put onto a CD (size permitting), used on a website, or even emailed to friends and family. The MPEG file can also be played in most media players and imported into third-party editing and DVD authoring software.

144 Archive Your Project

✔ **BEFORE YOU BEGIN**

74 Start a New Project
84 Add Media with the Adobe Media Downloader

The **Project Archiver** lets you save your project under a separate name and even on a separate hard drive. Archiving a project (making backups) is always a good idea to ensure their safe keeping.

The **Project Archiver** gives you two methods of archiving: **Archive** and **Copy**. The **Archive** option saves your project using only the media used on the **Timeline**, taking out all of the edits and anything not used that is still in the **Media** panel. The **Copy** option copies the *entire* project and *all* of the media, resulting in a file as large as the current project. The **Copy** option does not save disk space as the **Archive** option does.

1 Choose Project, Project Archiver

From the taskbar menu at the top of your screen, choose **Project, Project Archiver** to open the **Project Archiver** dialog box.

2 Select Archive or Copy

Select the **Archive Project** or **Copy Project** option, whichever you prefer.

3 Select Location

The default location is the same as your project. Alternatively, you can browse to a new location. You can even choose to store the archive or copy onto an external hard drive as a backup. Just make sure that whatever location you archive to has enough space for all the files.

4 Archive or Copy Your Project

After making your selections, click the **OK** button. A dialog box appears, showing you the progress of the archive or copy. When it is finished, you can open the copied or archived project at any time by browsing to the directory location you specified in step 3.

144

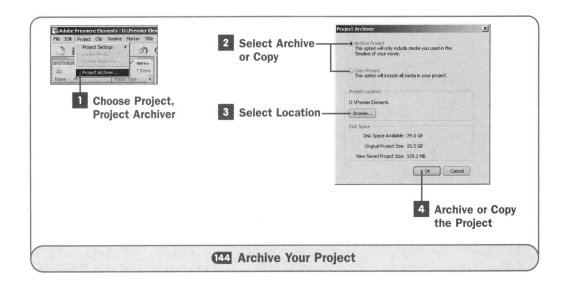

2 Select Archive or Copy

1 Choose Project, Project Archiver

3 Select Location

4 Archive or Copy the Project

144 Archive Your Project

26

DVD Authoring

IN THIS CHAPTER:

Those who've been with Premiere Elements since version 1.0 should be very pleased with the new features in the **DVD** authoring workspace in version 2.0.

Adobe has made several improvements to this workspace, including options for customizing fonts and the placement of navigation controls as well as the ability to add motion, video, and audio backgrounds to DVD menus. In addition, it has added several attractive, new menu templates.

With these improvements, Premiere Elements now has both the advantages of an integrated DVD program and most of the features of a quality, standalone DVD authoring application.

---

145 Create an Auto-Play DVD

✔ BEFORE YOU BEGIN	→ SEE ALSO
149 Customize a DVD Menu Screen Template	154 Preview and Test Drive a DVD Movie
	155 Burn Multiple Copies of a DVD
	172 About DVD Menus and the DVD Template Editor

An *auto-play DVD* is simply a no-frills, drop-it-in-and-play DVD movie. No menus. No colorful splash screen. Just your video on a shiny, little disc. Naturally, they're the simplest of all DVDs to create.

▶ KEY TERM

Auto-play DVD—A DVD in which the video automatically begins to play when it is loaded into a DVD player without first launching a splash screen or menu.

1 Open the DVD Templates

Use the instructions in the tasks in the first part of this book to create a movie project that you want to burn to a DVD. Make sure that that project is open and visible on the **Timeline**.

If you aren't already in the **DVD** workspace, click the **DVD** button in the upper-right corner of any workspace.

If you haven't already selected a DVD menu template for your project, simply jumping to this workspace will open the **DVD Template** library. To access the library otherwise, click the **Change Template** button in the **DVD Layout** panel. The **DVD Templates** dialog box opens.

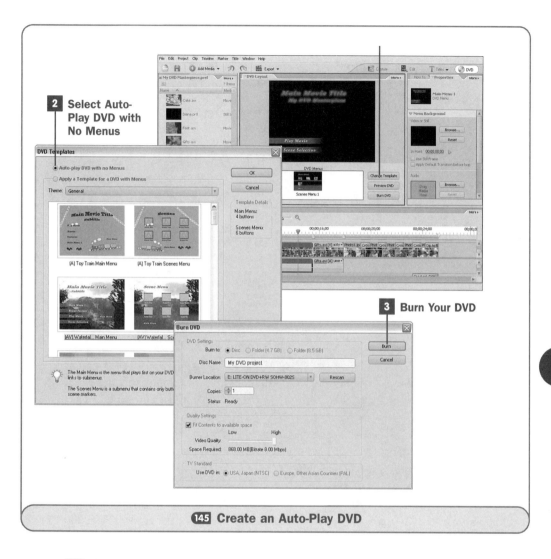

145

145 Create an Auto-Play DVD

2 Select Auto-Play DVD with No Menus

Select the option to create an **Auto-Play DVD with no Menus** at the top of the **DVD Templates** dialog box. Click **OK**. (For information on menu templates and their themes, see 149 **Customize a DVD Menu Screen Template**.)

3 Burn Your DVD

Back in the **DVD Layout** panel, click the **Burn DVD** button. In the **Burn DVD** dialog box that opens, you'll have the option of burning directly to a DVD or burning to a folder on your hard drive (See 155 **Burn Multiple Copies of a DVD**) as well as the option to burn to a different TV format.

If you're trying to fit a long movie onto a DVD, you can adjust the **Video Quality** slider or enable the **Fit Contents to available space** check box. Watch the **Space Required** area to make sure that the movie is small enough to fit onto a single-layer DVD (less than 4.7GB) or a dual-layer DVD (less than 8.5GB).

When you've selected the appropriate options, click the **Burn** button to burn your DVD.

---

146 Set DVD Chapter Markers

✔ BEFORE YOU BEGIN	→ SEE ALSO
149 Customize a DVD Menu Screen Template	**147** Auto-Generate Scene Markers
	148 Customize an Image As a Chapter Marker
	151 Create a Motion Menu
	154 Preview and Test Drive a DVD Movie
	155 Burn Multiple Copies of a DVD

145

One of the advantages to having an integrated DVD authoring application such as Premiere Elements is that you can use your standard editing **Timeline** to set your DVD *chapter markers*. Links to these DVD chapter markers are then automatically generated when you select your DVD menu template. With a single click on a link in the DVD menu, your viewer can jump to a point you've specified as a chapter marker in your video.

▶ **KEY TERM**

Chapter markers—Designated points in a video that the viewer can quickly jumped to by following links from a DVD menu.

1 Locate a Position on Your Timeline

You can access the **Timeline** in either the **Edit** or **DVD** workspace.

Position the CTI at the point you'd like to place a marker. This doesn't have to be an exact position. You can reposition the chapter marker later.

▶ **NOTE**

Although you can reposition your DVD markers at any point in the editing process, it should be pointed out that the marker positions are relative to the **Timeline** itself, not to your video project. In other words, if you lengthen, shorten, or change the positions of your clips, the markers remain in position relative to the **Timeline** itself, and not the clips, until you manually move the markers.

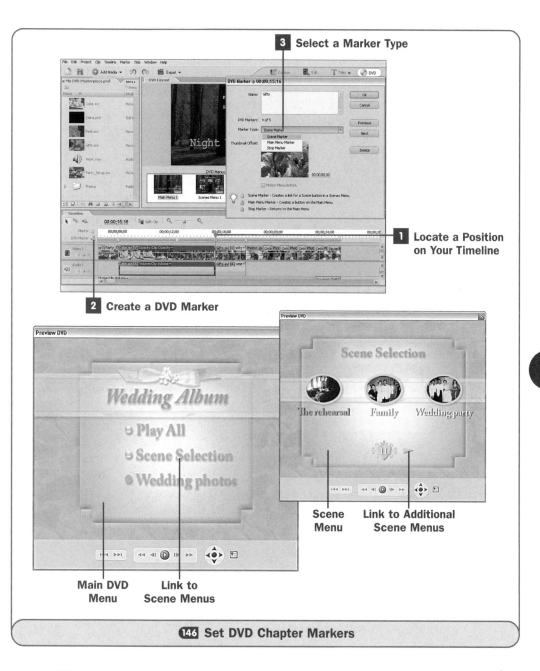

3 Select a Marker Type

1 Locate a Position on Your Timeline

2 Create a DVD Marker

Scene Menu   Link to Additional Scene Menus

Main DVD Menu   Link to Scene Menus

146 Set DVD Chapter Markers

2 Create a DVD Marker

Click the **DVD Marker** creator button at the top-left corner of the **Timeline**. A green marker appears on the **Timeline** at the point where the CTI is positioned, and the **DVD Marker** dialog box opens.

3 Select a Marker Type

The **DVD Marker** dialog box is where you designate your marker type as well as customize the appearance of the chapter marker (see ⟨148⟩ **Customize an Image As a Chapter Marker**.)

Select the type of DVD chapter marker you want to create from the **Marker Type** drop-down menu. A DVD chapter marker can serve one of three purposes:

- A **Main Menu Marker** creates a link to the main (opening) menu on your DVD. This main menu is the menu that appears when the viewer initially launches the DVD.

- A **Scene Marker** creates a link to the secondary (scene) menu on your DVD. (The viewer accesses the scene menu from a link on the main menu.) Links are automatically generated in this menu as you create them on the **Timeline**, and additional pages of scene menus are automatically added as needed to accommodate any number of scene markers; links to those additional scene menu pages are automatically generated.

- A **Stop Marker** stops DVD play and returns the viewer to the main menu. A **Scene Marker** followed by a **Stop Marker** can isolate a sequence for playback from the menus.

After you've selected a **Marker Type**, type the name you want to give the marker in the space at the top of the dialog box. Scene markers and main menu markers automatically generate links to your menus after you select a DVD template. The name you've given your DVD marker appears as this link, along with the Thumbnail Offset image, in the menu.

DVD markers can be repositioned at any time; when you move the markers, the links from the appropriate menu to these new points in the movie are automatically updated.

For information on creating an animated thumbnail, see ⟨151⟩ **Create a Motion Menu**.

147 | **Auto-Generate Scene Markers**

✔ BEFORE YOU BEGIN	→ SEE ALSO
146 Set DVD Chapter Markers	**148** Customize an Image As a
149 Customize a DVD Menu Screen	Chapter Marker
Template	**151** Create a Motion Menu
	154 Preview and Test Drive a DVD Movie
	155 Burn Multiple Copies of a DVD

Scene markers are DVD chapter markers used to create menu links to give your viewer quick, easy access to scenes in your video. You can set up your own scene markers as explained in **146** **Set DVD Chapter Markers**, or you can have Premiere Elements set them up for you, according to your criteria, as explained in this task.

► **KEY TERM**

Scene marker—A type of DVD chapter marker that links from the scenes menu to a designated point in the video.

147

1 **Open the Auto-Generate DVD Markers Menu**

Open the movie project for which you want to create scene markers. Make sure that you can see the project in the **Timeline**.

If you aren't already in the **DVD** workspace, click the **DVD** button in the upper-left corner of any workspace.

Click the **More** menu in the **DVD Layout** panel and select **Auto-Generate DVD Markers**. The **Automatically Set DVD Scene Markers** dialog box opens.

2 **Set the Criteria for Your Scene Markers**

Enable the **At Each Scene** option if you want to place a DVD scene marker at the beginning of each clip on your **Timeline**.

Enable the **Minutes** option if you want to place a scene marker at the time intervals you designate. In the text box that follows the option, type the time interval in **mm:ss** format at which you want to place markers.

The **Total Markers** option places the number of scene markers you indicate at evenly spaced intervals throughout your movie project.

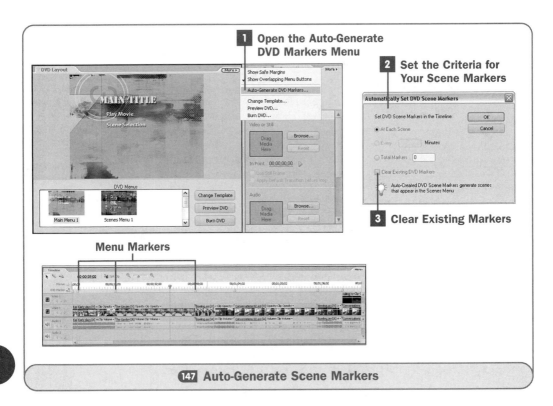

1 Open the Auto-Generate DVD Markers Menu

2 Set the Criteria for Your Scene Markers

Menu Markers

3 Clear Existing Markers

147 Auto-Generate Scene Markers

147

3 Clear Existing Markers

Enable the **Clear Existing DVD Markers** to clear all previously set scene markers as your new markers are generated.

When you've made your selections, click **OK** to close the **Automatically Set DVD Scene Markers** dialog box and generate the markers you've defined.

As with any DVD chapter marker, after the automatically-generated DVD scene markers appear on the **Timeline**, they can be positioned or customized as needed (see **148** **Customize an Image As a Chapter Marker**). Automatically generated DVD scene markers appear in the scenes menu with rather generic names, such as *Scene 1, Scene 2,* and so on. You can rename them by double-clicking the text in the menu template itself (see **149** **Customize a DVD Menu Screen Template**) or by double-clicking the DVD chapter marker on the **Timeline**.

148 Customize an Image As a Chapter Marker

✔ BEFORE YOU BEGIN	→ SEE ALSO
146 Set DVD Chapter Markers	149 Customize a DVD Menu Screen Template
147 Auto-Generate Scene Markers	151 Create a Motion Menu
	154 Preview and Test Drive a DVD Movie
	155 Burn Multiple Copies of a DVD

Scene buttons, which are automatically generated by Premiere Elements and linked to your DVD scene markers, appear on your scenes menu as visual indicators of where the links will take the viewer in the DVD movie project. (For information on how to select and create a DVD menu, see **149 Customize a DVD Menu Screen Template**.)

By default, these markers include a thumbnail showing the frame of the video at which you placed your DVD scene marker. You can customize the image that appears as the thumbnail without changing the location of the marker.

1 Select the Scenes Menu

In the **DVD Menus** list box at the bottom of the **DVD Layout** panel, click the **Scenes Menu** that contains the chapter marker you want to customize. The selected menu screen appears in the **DVD Layout** panel.

2 Select the Scene Marker to Customize

In the **DVD Layout** panel's monitor, click the DVD menu button (the scene marker thumbnail) you want to customize. The **Properties** panel displays the picture and text options for this item.

3 Edit the Scene Marker

Double-click the **Edit** button in the **Menus** listing in the **Properties** panel. The **DVD Marker** dialog box for that marker opens.

The space adjacent to the word **Name** at the top of this dialog box is where you name or rename your DVD marker. The text you type in this box is the text that appears with the chapter marker on the scenes menu of your DVD menu.

148

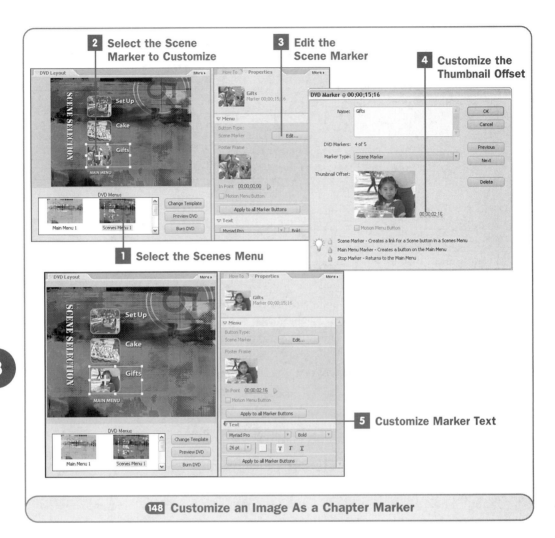

2 Select the Scene Marker to Customize

3 Edit the Scene Marker

4 Customize the Thumbnail Offset

1 Select the Scenes Menu

5 Customize Marker Text

148 Customize an Image As a Chapter Marker

4 **Customize the Thumbnail Offset**

The **Thumbnail Offset** is the icon that appears on the scene menu (or the main menu, in the case of a main menu marker) as a visual indicator of the scene to which the menu button links.

To change the image that appears on the DVD menu button, change the timecode counter to the right of the current **Thumbnail Offset** image.

The **00;00;00;00** timecode means that the current thumbnail is the exact frame at which the DVD chapter marker is located. You can manually change these numbers, but it's more intuitive to drag your mouse across them. As you do, the numbers scroll up and down, and the video frames will advance or retreat. Note that changing the thumbnail image doesn't affect the location of the marker—only the frame that is displayed on the menu button.

After you have selected the frame that you want displayed, click **OK** to close the dialog box. To create an animated icon, see **151** **Create a Motion Menu**.

5 Customize Marker Text

The **Text** customization area of the **Properties** panel enables you to select the font, font size, font color, and font style for the text on the menu button. Choose from the drop-down menus to apply these text attributes to the text associated with the currently selected menu button.

Click the **Apply to All Markers** buttons to apply the picture (the frame) or text settings for this button to all the menu buttons in the currently selected menu.

---

149 **Customize a DVD Menu Screen Template**

✔ BEFORE YOU BEGIN	→ SEE ALSO
146 Set DVD Chapter Markers **147** Auto-Generate Scene Markers	**150** Customize a Menu with Any Background **152** Add Video to a Menu Background **153** Add Audio to a Menu **154** Preview and Test Drive a DVD Movie **174** Create a DVD Menu Template from Scratch

149

Although you can't create a DVD menu from scratch in Premiere Elements, your ability to customize the existing templates in Premiere Elements 2.0 is light years ahead of where it was in version 1.0.

Premiere Elements 2.0 offers more than 70 DVD menu templates grouped in categories such as **Entertainment**, **General**, **Birthday**, **New Baby**, **Party Celebrations**, **Seasons**, **Sports**, **Travel**, and **Wedding**. Several of these templates include a default video background loop (these templates are marked with a **(V)**), an audio background loop (these templates are marked with an **(A)**) or both, and all can be modified to include a custom still background (see **150** **Customize a Menu with Any Background**), a custom video background (see **152** **Add Video to a Menu Background**), or a custom audio background (see **153** **Add Audio to a Menu**). Fonts, positions, and content of the navigation text can also be customized, and the thumbnail graphics for the scene markers can be customized and even animated.

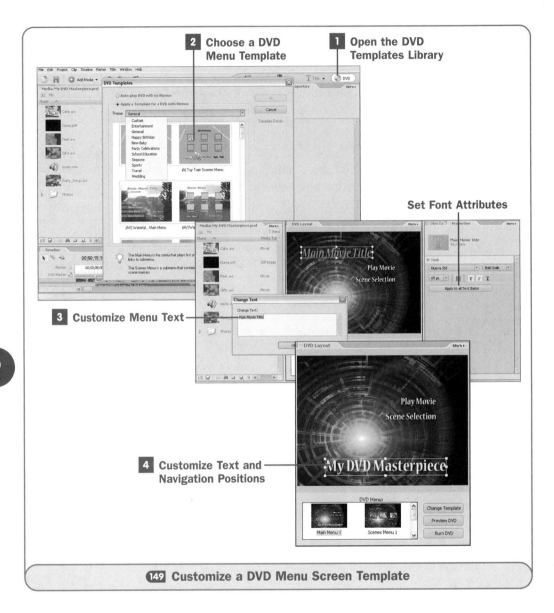

2 Choose a DVD Menu Template

1 Open the DVD Templates Library

Set Font Attributes

3 Customize Menu Text

4 Customize Text and Navigation Positions

149 Customize a DVD Menu Screen Template

▶ **NOTE**

Although Premiere Elements 2.0 allows you to customize existing DVD menu templates, it still doesn't allow you to create a template from scratch. Premiere Elements's companion program, Photoshop Elements 4.0, however, *does* include features for creating DVD templates as well as modifying existing ones. The new DVD templates you create in Photoshop Elements are automatically added to Premiere Elements's **DVD Templates** collection.

1 **Open the DVD Templates Library**

Open the movie project for which you want to modify a DVD menu. If you aren't already in the **DVD** workspace, click the **DVD** button in the upper-right corner of any workspace.

If you haven't already selected a DVD menu template for the current project, simply jumping to this space opens the **DVD Template** library. Otherwise click on the **Change Template** button in the **DVD Layout** panel.

2 **Choose a DVD Menu Template**

The **Theme** drop-down list gives you options for several collections of DVD menu templates. The most easily customized templates—and the templates with the least extraneous graphical elements—are the **Generic** and **Standard** templates in the **General** collection. Select a template collection from the **Theme** drop-down list to see a list of DVD menu templates within that collection.

Templates with a **(V)** in front of their names have animated video back-grounds. Templates with an **(A)** have an audio track. Those with an **(AV)** have both video backgrounds and an audio track. All templates can poten-tially have a still or video background and/or audio track added. (See **150** Customize a Menu with Any Background, **152** Add Video to a Menu Background, and **153** Add Audio to a Menu.)

Note that all DVD menu templates have a main menu that includes a **Play** button; most also have a scenes menu that allows for links up to the number of scenes or chapters indicated. If the number of scene markers included with your project exceeds the number indicated for that menu template, Premiere Elements automatically generates additional scenes menu screens with links between the menus.

When you have selected the DVD menu template you want to use for the cur-rent movie project, click **OK**.

3 **Customize Menu Text**

Double-click any text block to open a **Change Text** dialog box where you can replace the generic template text with your custom text.

When a text box is selected, the **Properties** panel indicates the customizable text properties including font, size, and color. You can also adjust the font size and shape by dragging the sides or corner handles of the text box.

149

Note, however, that some aspects of the text block are inherent in the template and are not customizable—most notably drop-shadows and stroking.

Click the **Apply to All Text Items** button to apply the text styles and colors you've set up for one text block to all text blocks in the current menu.

4 Customize Text and Navigation Positions

Drag the text and navigational graphics to any positions you'd like in the menu screen. To customize the chapter icons, see **148** **Customize an Image As a Chapter Marker**.

---

150 Customize a Menu with Any Background

✔ BEFORE YOU BEGIN	→ SEE ALSO
146 Set DVD Chapter Markers	**151** Create a Motion Menu
147 Auto-Generate Scene Markers	**152** Add Video to a Menu Background
149 Customize a DVD Menu Screen Template	**153** Add Audio to a Menu
	154 Preview and Test Drive a DVD Movie
	173 Modify an Existing DVD Menu Template

149

A nice new feature of the DVD menu templates in Premiere Elements 2.0 is that they all offer the option of replacing or customizing the menu backgrounds. (You can even replace the background with a video clip, as explained in **152** **Add Video to a Menu Background**.) Any graphic, photo, or video clip that can be used in a Premiere Elements project can be used as a DVD menu background.

1 Select a DVD Menu Template

With your movie project open, select a DVD menu template as described in **149** **Customize a DVD Menu Screen Template**.

Note that nearly all DVD menu templates contain foreground graphic elements in addition to the background image. In some cases, these graphics frame the background image. In other cases, the graphics appear over it. (For this example, I have selected a template with no foreground graphics. You can see an example of a template with foreground graphics in **152** **Add Video to a Menu Background**.)

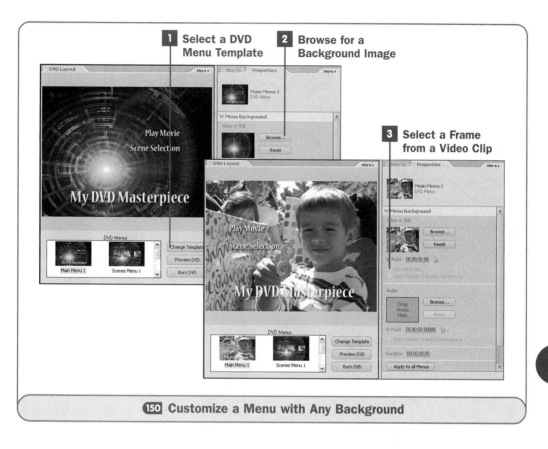

150 Customize a Menu with Any Background

Click the **Change Template** button in the **DVD Layout** panel and choose a template collection. From the list of individual templates that appears, select the one you want to use; it appears in the monitor. If you'd prefer minimal interference from these permanent graphics, choose the **Standard** template or one of the **Generic** templates from the **General** collection, as I have done in my example.

2 Browse for a Background Image

When you have selected a template, the option for changing the background image appears in the **Properties** panel.

Click on the **Browse** button in the **Menu Background Video or Still** section of the **Properties** panel and browse to the image of your choice. Note that this image does not have to have been imported into your video project. You can select it from anywhere on your hard drive. (For an explanation of how to create a video background for your menu, see **152 Add Video to a Menu Background**.)

▶ NOTE

Photoshop Elements 4.0 has a custom work area, specifically designed for working with Premiere Elements's DVD menu templates. This work area allows for easy revision of existing templates, including removing extraneous graphic elements, as well as the ability to create new DVD menu templates from scratch.

3 Select a Frame from a Video Clip

Although you can use a still image for your menu background, you can also designate that a frame from a video clip be used. Click in the **Timeline** to select an existing clip from which you want to select a frame.

After you have selected a clip, click the green arrow in the **Properties** panel to play the clip, or drag across the timecode to scrub through the clip until you locate the frame you'd like to use as the background image for the DVD menu.

Enable the **Use Still Frame** check box.

150

151 Create a Motion Menu	
✔ **BEFORE YOU BEGIN**	→ **SEE ALSO**
146 Set DVD Chapter Markers **147** Auto-Generate Scene Markers	**149** Customize a DVD Menu Screen Template **150** Customize a Menu with Any Background **152** Add Video to a Menu Background **153** Add Audio to a Menu **154** Preview and Test Drive a DVD Movie

---

Although Premiere Elements 1.0 gave you the ability to use a still frame from your video as a scene marker, Premiere Elements 2.0 gives you the ability to use a portion of a clip from your video project to create an animated, motion menu scene marker.

1 Select the Scenes Menu

Click the **Scenes Menu** thumbnail in the **DVD Layout** panel that contains the scene marker you want to customize. The scenes menu appears in the monitor in the **DVD Layout** panel.

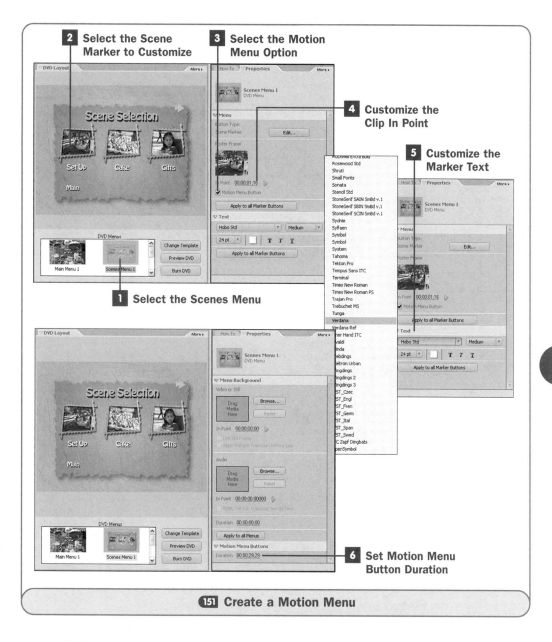

2 Select the Scene Marker to Customize

3 Select the Motion Menu Option

4 Customize the Clip In Point

5 Customize the Marker Text

1 Select the Scenes Menu

6 Set Motion Menu Button Duration

151 Create a Motion Menu

151

2 Select the Scene Marker to Customize

In the **DVD Layout** panel, click the scene marker you want to customize. The **Properties** panel displays the current video frame being used as this scene's marker as well as the options for customizing the text for this marker.

▣ Select the Motion Menu Option

In the **Properties** panel, enable the **Motion Menu Button** check box.

When the scene menu is displayed, the clip will play as a thumbnail, and then loop and repeat indefinitely.

▣ Customize the Clip In Point

To change the point in the clip at which the motion menu begins, click the green play button or change the timecode.

You can manually change the timecode numbers, but it's more intuitive to drag the mouse across them. As you do, the numbers scroll up and down and the video advances or retreats. Note that this adjustment doesn't affect the actual location of the scene marker on the **Timeline**. The scene marker still links to the spot in your movie where the marker is positioned. This adjustment only changes the image that is displayed as the scene marker button in your DVD menu.

▶ TIP

151

If you are locating the In Point by playing through the clip, click the yellow pause button when you've reached your desired In Point.

▣ Customize the Marker Text

The **Text** customization area of the **Properties** panel enables you to select the font, font size, font color, and font style for the scene marker button text.

Click the **Apply to All Marker Buttons** button to apply the picture and/or text attributes you've just set for this menu button to all the menu buttons in the scene menu.

▣ Set Motion Menu Button Duration

In the **DVD Layout** monitor, click the background of the scene menu (anywhere behind the DVD menu buttons). The **Menu Background** options appear in the **Properties** panel.

At the bottom of the **Menu Background** options are settings for the **Motion Menu Buttons Duration**, listed as a timecode.

The time period you designate here will set the duration of the video loops for all motion menu buttons.

▶ **NOTE**

In the timecode listed as **00;00;00;00**, the first set of numbers represents hours and the second set of numbers represents minutes (both pretty unlikely settings for a loop that plays on a menu button). The third set of numbers represents seconds, and the last set represents frames (25 frames per second of time in PAL and approximately 30 frames per second in NTSC).

---

152 Add Video to a Menu Background

✔ BEFORE YOU BEGIN	→ SEE ALSO
146 Set DVD Chapter Markers	153 Add Audio to a Menu
147 Auto-Generate Scene Markers	154 Preview and Test Drive a DVD Movie
149 Customize a DVD Menu Screen Template	155 Burn Multiple Copies of a DVD
150 Customize a Menu with Any Background	174 Create a DVD Menu Template from Scratch

A welcome feature in Premiere Elements 2.0 is the ability to use a loop of video as the background for a DVD menu template. (You can also replace the background with a still image, as explained in 150 **Customize a Menu with Any Background**.)

152

1 Select a DVD Menu Template

Open the movie project for which you want to customize the DVD menu. Select a DVD menu template as described in 149 **Customize a DVD Menu Screen Template**.

Note that nearly all DVD menu templates contain foreground graphic elements in addition to the background image. In some cases, these graphics frame your background image. In other cases, they appear over it. In this example, the stars and streamers across the top of the template are foreground graphics. As you will see, even after you replace the background imagery for this DVD menu, these graphic elements remain. Premiere Elements does not give you the ability to remove these graphics. (They can be easily removed, however, with the Photoshop Elements 4.0 DVD Template Editor.)

Click the **Change Template** button in the **DVD Layout** panel and choose a template collection. From the list of individual templates that appears, select the one you want to use; it appears in the monitor. If you'd prefer an easily customizable template that is free from foreground graphics, choose the **Standard** template or one of the **Generic** templates located in the **General** collection.

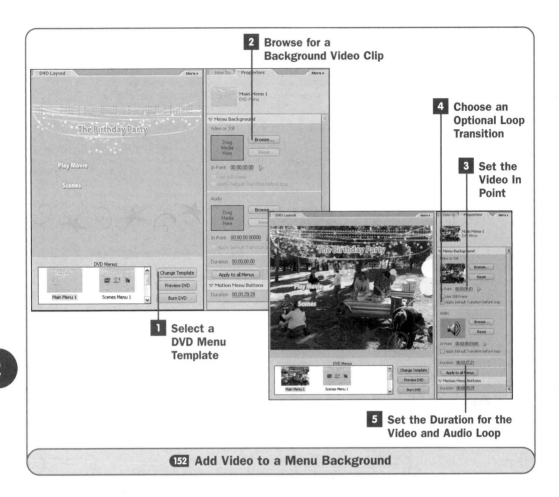

2 Browse for a Background Video Clip

4 Choose an Optional Loop Transition

3 Set the Video In Point

1 Select a DVD Menu Template

5 Set the Duration for the Video and Audio Loop

152 Add Video to a Menu Background

2 Browse for a Background Video Clip

When a template is selected, the **Menu Background** listing and its options appear in the **Properties** panel.

Click the **Browse** button and browse to the video clip you want to use as the background image for this DVD menu. Note that this clip does not actually have to be a part of your current video project and can exist any place on your hard drive.

▶ **NOTE**

Photoshop Elements 4.0 has a custom work area, specifically designed for working with Premiere Elements's DVD menu templates. This work area allows for easy revision of existing templates, including removing extraneous graphic elements, as well as the ability to create new DVD menu templates from scratch.

3 Set the Video In Point

To change the point in the clip at which the menu background video loop begins, click the green arrow play button or change the timecode for the In Point.

You can manually change these numbers, but it's more intuitive to drag the mouse across them. As you do, the numbers scroll up and down and the video advances or retreats.

If you are locating the In Point by playing the video, click the yellow pause button when you reach the desired In Point.

4 Choose an Optional Loop Transition

Enable the **Apply Default Transition before loop** check box to apply the default transition between the end of the video clip and the frame at which it restarts.

▶ TIP

To change the default transition, select any transition from the **Transitions and Effects** panel, click the **More** button at the top of that panel, and select **Set As Default Transition**.

152

5 Set the Duration for the Video and Audio Loop

At the bottom of the **Menu Background** options in the **Properties** panel are the settings for the duration of the loop, listed as a timecode. The time you set here determines how long the background video clip plays before it restarts.

In the timecode **00;00;00;00**, the first set of numbers represents hours, and the second set of numbers represents minutes (both pretty unlikely settings for a background video loop). The third set of numbers represents seconds, and the last set represents frames (25 frames per second of time in PAL and approximately 30 frames per second in NTSC). The **Duration** setting you specify applies to both the video and audio tracks in the background video for this menu.

The **Apply to All Menus** button applies these duration settings to all looping menu backgrounds for this project.

153 Add Audio to a Menu

✔ **BEFORE YOU BEGIN**

146 Set DVD Chapter Markers
147 Auto-Generate Scene Markers
149 Customize a DVD Menu Screen Template
150 Customize a Menu with Any Background

✔ **SEE ALSO**

152 Add Video to a Menu Background
154 Preview and Test Drive a DVD Movie
155 Burn Multiple Copies of a DVD

In addition to being able to customize the background of your DVD menu template (as explained in **150** **Customize a Menu with Any Background** and **152** **Add Video to a Menu Background**), Premiere Elements 2.0 gives you the option of adding your own custom audio loop. (Note that some templates—those marked with an **(A)** or a **(AV)**—have default audio loops. These templates, nonetheless, give you the option of replacing the default audio with a custom audio clip.)

1 Select a DVD Menu Template

Open a movie project that contains a DVD menu you want to customize. Select a DVD menu template for the project as explained in **149** **Customize a DVD Menu Screen Template**.

▶ **TIP**

The order in which you customize the DVD menu background video and audio affects how the template is ultimately customized. In other words, if you add a video background *after* you add customized audio, the audio from the video clip overwrites the audio selection. To override this effect, select or reselect your audio loop after you've selected your video background.

2 Browse for an Audio Clip

After you select a template, the **Menu Background** listing appears in the **Properties** panel, offering an option for changing or adding an audio clip.

Click the **Browse** button in the **Audio** section of the properties panel and browse to the audio clip of your choice.

3 Set the Audio In Point

To change the point in the audio clip at which the menu background audio begins, click the green arrow (play) button or change the timecode.

You can manually change the timecode numbers, but it's more intuitive to drag the mouse across them. As you do, the numbers scroll up and down and the audio clip advances or retreats.

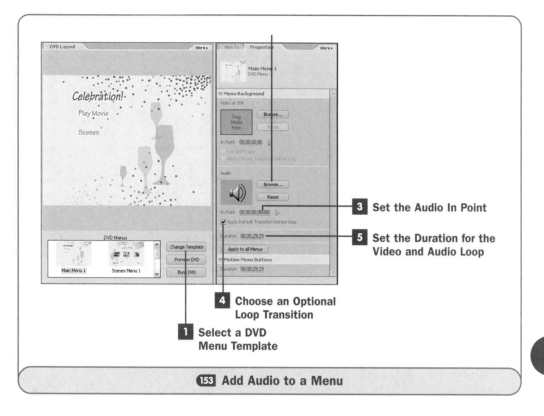

3 Set the Audio In Point

5 Set the Duration for the Video and Audio Loop

4 Choose an Optional Loop Transition

1 Select a DVD Menu Template

153

153 Add Audio to a Menu

In the audio timecode **00;00;00;00000**, the first set of numbers represents hours and the second set of numbers represents minutes (both pretty unlikely settings for your audio loop). The third set of numbers represents seconds, and the last set of numbers represents audio samplings—a standard 48,000 per second.

If you are locating the In Point by playing the audio clip, click the yellow pause button when you reach the desired In Point.

4 Choose an Optional Loop Transition

Enable the **Apply Default Transition Before Loop** check box option to apply the audio dissolve transition between your loop's end and its restart.

5 Set the Duration for the Video and Audio Loop

At the bottom of the **Menu Background** options in the **Properties** panel are the settings for the duration of the audio loop, listed as a video timecode. The time you set here determines how long the audio clip plays before it restarts.

In the video timecode **00;00;00;00**, the first set of numbers represents hours, and the second set of numbers represents minutes (both pretty unlikely settings for a background audio loop). The third set of numbers represents seconds, and the last set represents frames (25 frames per second of time in PAL and approximately 30 frames per second in NTSC). This setting applies to *both video and audio background loops* for this menu.

---

154 **Preview and Test Drive a DVD Movie**

✔ BEFORE YOU BEGIN	→ SEE ALSO
145 Create an Auto-Play DVD 149 Customize a DVD Menu Screen Template	148 Customize an Image As a Chapter Marker 150 Customize a Menu with Any Background 152 Add Video to a Menu Background 155 Burn Multiple Copies of a DVD 172 About DVD Menus and the DVD Template Editor

---

153

After you've set up and customized your DVD menus, you'll want to give them a good test drive to make sure that everything works as it should before you burn it to DVD or otherwise export the project.

Note, however, that animating menu backgrounds and menu buttons can be taxing on your computer system. Unless you have a very fast computer, the preview video might seem a bit sluggish or jumpy. Don't be concerned. The important thing is that everything appears as it should and that what you want animated is indeed animated.

1 Start the DVD Preview

Click the **DVD Preview** button in the **DVD Layout** panel. This should open a full-sized window **Preview DVD** window displaying your main menu.

2 Test the Play Button

Click the **Play** button.

Ensure that the video starts at the point you're expecting it to start. If not, check your work area settings. (See **93** **Define the Beginning and End of Your Project**.)

To return to the main menu from any point in the movie, click the **Menu** icon on the play window's control panel.

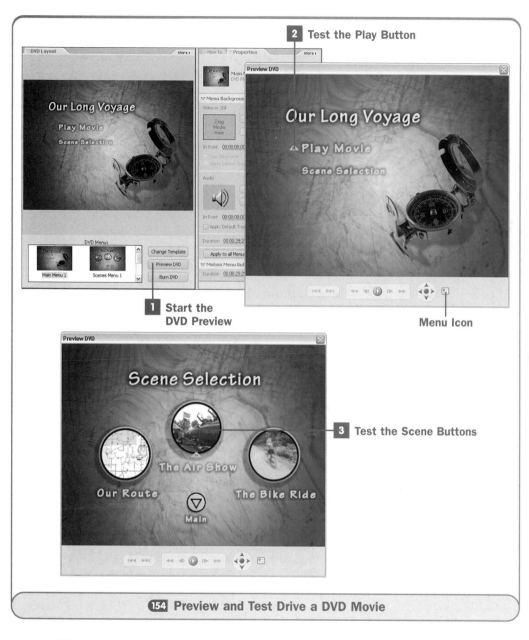

2 Test the Play Button

1 Start the DVD Preview

Menu Icon

3 Test the Scene Buttons

3 Test the Scene Buttons

In the main menu, click the link to the scene menu(s). Depending on the template or customizations you've made to the template, this link might be labeled **Scene Selections** or something similar.

Click each chapter marker icon to ensure that each button begins playback at the correct In Point and, if applicable, returns to the main menu at the Out Point you've designated with a stop marker. (For information on setting a chapter marker as a stop marker, see **146** **Set DVD Chapter Markers.**)

If you're happy with the preview, close the window and click the **Burn DVD** button back in the **DVD Layout** panel.

---

155   Burn Multiple Copies of a DVD

✔ BEFORE YOU BEGIN	→ SEE ALSO
145 Create an Auto-Play DVD **149** Customize a DVD Menu Screen Template	**154** Preview and Test Drive a DVD Movie

---

Although this task creates a set of DVD files on your hard drive that ostensibly you can use and re-use to burn several DVD copies, it's often the preferred way to produce even one copy of a DVD.

154

DVD burning actually combines several process—rendering and encoding, creating and linking menus, and the actual burning of the disc. Of these, the step most prone to problems is the burning of the DVD itself (an issue related to driver compatibility). Burning to a folder rather than directly to a disc removes one potentially problematic step, increasing the likelihood of producing a successful DVD.

1 Click Burn DVD

If you aren't already in the **DVD** workspace, click the **DVD** button in the upper-right corner of any workspace. Open the project you want to burn to multiple DVDs.

After you've selected and customized your menu screens (see **149** **Customize a DVD Menu Screen Template**) or chosen the option to create an auto-play DVD (see **145** **Create an Auto-Play DVD**), click the **Burn DVD** button in the **DVD Layout** panel. The **Burn DVD** dialog box opens.

2 Select the Burn to Folder Option

In the **Burn DVD** dialog box, you'll have the option to burn directly to a DVD or to burn to a folder. At the bottom of the dialog box, you can choose which TV format you plan to play the disc in—NTSC or PAL.

You have a choice between saving your files for a standard 4.7BG DVD or an 8.5GB dual-layer disc. Select the **Burn to Folder** option that is compatible with your DVD burner and media.

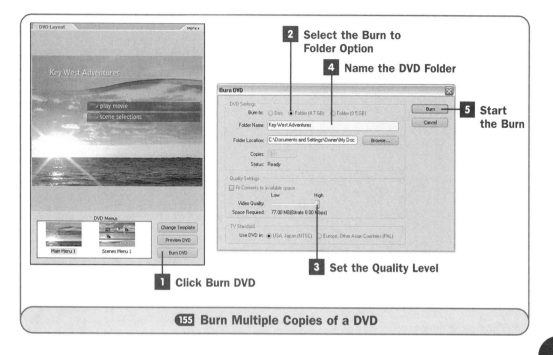

2 Select the Burn to Folder Option

4 Name the DVD Folder

5 Start the Burn

3 Set the Quality Level

1 Click Burn DVD

155 Burn Multiple Copies of a DVD

155

3 Select the Quality Level

The **Burn DVD** dialog box also indicates the approximate size of your final DVD output in the **Space Required** area in the middle of the dialog box.

A 4.7GB DVD can hold approximately one hour of standard-quality video. If the estimated output size is greater than your disc capacity, you can reduce the quality level of your video to accommodate the video.

Enable the **Fit Contents to Available Space** check box to force your movie project to fit on the selected media type.

4 Name the DVD Folder

Type a name for your DVD folder and browse to the folder location to which you want to save your video files. If you don't name your folder, the program automatically generates a default name based on the date and time of your burn.

5 Start the Burn

Click the **Burn** button. The program will render and encode your video project and save the menu and video files in two subfolders within the folder you specified in step 4.

To produce a DVD, use the software that came with your DVD burner or your system to burn the two subfolders and all their contents to a disc.

PART III

Putting It All Together: Working with Photoshop Elements and Premiere Elements

IN THIS PART:

27

Sharing Files Between Photoshop Elements and Premiere Elements

IN THIS CHAPTER:

You know that Photoshop Elements and Premiere Elements are made to work together. In this chapter, we will get down to showing you how that is accomplished and what you can do when using these two exciting programs together. In most of the tasks in this chapter, both programs must be open at the same time. It will be most beneficial if you already have images in your Photoshop Elements Organizer (see **❶ Import Media from a Folder, CD-ROM, or DVD** and **❷ Import Images from a Digital Camera** for information about getting files into the Organizer), and you should have a project started in Premiere Elements (see **❼❹ Start a New Project**).

In this chapter, you will learn various techniques for using both applications most efficiently. You will see how sending files back and forth between Premiere Elements and Photoshop Elements can save you time and give you the ability to add extra touches to your video. In Photoshop Elements, you can create exciting graphics that you can use in Premiere Elements as titles for scene introductions, DVD menu backgrounds, intermission clips, and much more. You can also create a still image from a video clip that you can then use in a title or DVD menu background, and you can prepare a clip for frame editing using a filmstrip file. You can use a filmstrip file to create a lightsaber effect, just like in the movie *Star Wars*.

156 About Sharing Files

✔ BEFORE YOU BEGIN

❶ Import Media from a Folder, CD-ROM, or DVD

❷ Import Images from a Digital Camera

❽❹ Add Media with the Adobe Media Downloader

❽❼ Grab a Still from Video

❶❹❶ Output to an AVI Movie

→ SEE ALSO

❶❺❾ Move Images Between Premiere Elements and Photoshop Elements

❶❻⓿ Move a Video Filmstrip Between Premiere Elements and Photoshop Elements

❶❻❾ Export Your Slideshow

❶❼❷ About DVD Menus and the DVD Template Editor

Graphics files, video files, and audio files all have what seem to be an unlimited number of file types. Some of the various graphics file types are GIF, TIF, and JPEG; video file types include AVI, WMV, and MOV; and audio file types include WAV and MP3. There are very few, if any, software programs that can handle all of the many media file types. Premiere Elements and Photoshop Elements, like many other programs, have their limits where file types are concerned.

Following is a list of all the file types you can import or export from each program. You can use this list as a cross-reference to see whether a particular file, when exported from one program, will be compatible with the other program. The list will also help you determine what file type to export from one program if you want it to be compatible with the other program.

Photoshop Elements Compatible File Types

Import (Photo/Image):	Photoshop (PSD, PDD)
	BMP (BMP, RLE, DIB)
	Camera Raw (CRW, NEF, RAF, ORF)
	Compuserve GIF (GIF)
	Photoshop EPS (EPS)
	Filmstrip File (FLM)
	JPEG (JPG, JPEG, JPE)
	JPEG2000 (JPF, JPX, JP2, J2C, J2K, JPC)
	Generic EPS (AI3, AI4, AI5, AI6, AI7, AI8)
	PCX (PCX)
	Photoshop PDF (PDF, PDP)
	Photo CD (PCD)
	Photoshop Raw (RAW)
	PICT File (PCT, PICT)
	Pixar (PXR)
	PNG (PNG)
	Scitex CT (SCT)
	Targa (TGA, VDA, ICB, VST)
	TIFF (TIF, TIFF)
	Wireless Bitmap (WBM, WBMP)
Import (Video):	AVI (only partially supported)
	MPEG (MPEG, MPG, MPE)
	Windows Media (WMV)
Export (Image):	BMP, GIF, JPEG, JPX, PSD, PCX, PDF, EPS, PICT, PXR, PNG, RAW, SCT, TGA, TIFF
Export (Video):	WMV

156

Premiere Elements Compatible File Types

Import (Video):	AVI Movie (AVI)
	Filmstrip (FLM)
	MPEG Movie (MPEG, VOB, MOD, MPE, MPG, M2V, MP2, MPV, M2P, M2T)
	Windows Media (WMV, ASF)
	QuickTime Movie (MOV, 3GP, 3G2, MP4, M4A, M4V)
Import (Audio):	Dolby AC-3 (AC3)

Premiere Elements Compatible File Types   (Continued)

	Macintosh Audio AIFF (AIF, AIFF)
	MP3 Audio (MP3)
	MPEG Audio (MPEG, MPG, MPA, MPE, M2A)
	QuickTime (MOV, M4A)
	Windows Media (WMA)
	Windows WAVE (WAV)
Import (Still Image):	Adobe Illustrator Art (AI)
	Adobe Title Designer (PRTL)
	Bitmap (BMP, DIB, RLE)
	Compuserve GIF (GIF)
	Encapsulated Postscript (EPS)
	Icon (ICO)
	JPEG (JPG, JPE, JPEG, JFIF)
	Macintosh PICT (PCT, PIC, PICT)
	PCX (PCX)
	Photoshop (PSD)
	Portable Network Graphic (PNG)
	TIFF (TIF, TIFF)
	Truvision Targa (TGA, ICB, VST, VDA)
Export (Video):	DVD (VOB), VCD (MPEG-1), SVCD (MPEG-2), MPEG-2 DVD Compatible, Tape (miniDV, Digital8, VHS), Filmstrip (FLM), Animated GIF, AVI, MOV, WMV
Export (Audio):	AVI, DV-AVI, WAV
Export (Image):	PRTL, GIF, JPEG, TIFF, TGA, BMP
Export (Sequence File Types):	GIF, JPEG, TGA, TIFF, BMP

156

Some of the file types that are supported by Photoshop Elements but not by Premiere Elements include RAW, PDF, JPEG2000, and TIFF with LZW Compression.

Some of the file types that are supported by Premiere Elements but not by Photoshop Elements include DVD (.VOB), ASF, MOD, AIFF, AVI (only partially supported), AC3, EPS, and AI.

Now that you know what files you can use in each of the programs, and what file types you can export from one program and import to the other, let's move on.

Sharing files between these two programs is as simple as saving a file in one and importing into the other. However, Adobe has integrated the two applications and made the transfer process much simpler in many ways. You can always use the **File**, **Open** command in Photoshop Elements to find what you are looking for, or you can use the **Add Media** button in Premiere Elements to find files. Sometimes these basic access methods are the easiest way to get your files from one program to the other. But there are added bonuses when you use these two programs together, in that you have the ability to send an image right to your Premiere Elements project from Photoshop. You can also create a new Photoshop image and add it to your Premiere Elements project in just a few simple steps; the remaining tasks in this chapter show you just how to do it.

---

157   Create a Graphic with Transparent Areas in Photoshop Elements

✔ BEFORE YOU BEGIN	→ SEE ALSO
28 Create a New Image Layer	**29** Create a Layer Filled with a Color, Gradient, or Pattern
84 Add Media with the Adobe Media Downloader	**34** Mask an Image Layer
156 About Sharing Files	**140** Create a Title from Scratch
158 Create a Still Image from Video and Save It to Photoshop Elements	**159** Move Images Between Premiere Elements and Photoshop Elements

157

Now it is time to get creative and learn the ways that Photoshop Elements and Premiere Elements can complement each other. In this task, you will see how you can create an image with a transparent background in Photoshop Elements and use that image in a Premiere Elements project. This is one way to make someone appear to be anywhere in the world, even though the photo of the person was taken in your living room.

Before you begin this task, open a Premiere Elements project and create a still image from a video clip as explained in **158** Create a Still Image from Video and Save It to Photoshop Elements or you can choose an existing still-image file. Now open Photoshop Elements and from the splash screen, choose **Start from Scratch** to open the Editor. Select the still image you created in Premiere Elements; alternatively, select any image you choose. Now let's get started!

1 Select and Copy an Area of the Image

In the Photoshop Elements Editor, with your image file open, select the **Magnetic Lasso** tool from the toolbar. Use the **Magnetic Lasso** tool to trace the part of the image you want to save with a transparent background. Copy the selected area by choosing **Edit**, **Copy** from the main menu (or use the **Ctrl+C** keyboard shortcut).

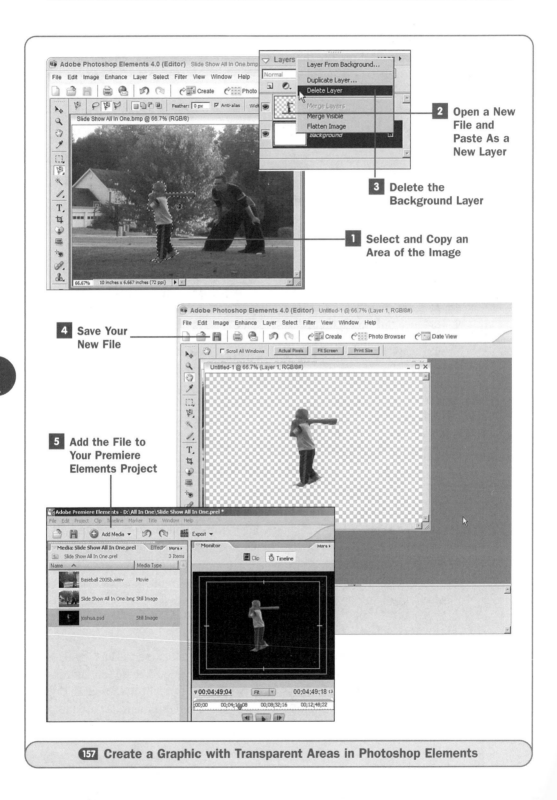

2 Open a New File and Paste As a New Layer

3 Delete the Background Layer

1 Select and Copy an Area of the Image

4 Save Your New File

5 Add the File to Your Premiere Elements Project

157

157 Create a Graphic with Transparent Areas in Photoshop Elements

2 Open a New File and Paste As a New Layer

Click the **New File** button to open a new image file. In the **New** dialog box that opens, name your image file and set the height to 720 pixels and the width to 480 pixels (the proper size for a full frame of NTSC video; if you are using PAL format, use a height of 720 pixels and a width of 576 pixels), then click **OK**.

Add a new *layer* to your new image. From the main menu, choose **Layer**, **New**, **Layer** (or use the **Shift+Ctrl+N** keyboard shortcut). The **New Layer** dialog box opens. No changes are necessary; just click **OK** to accept the default values.

Paste the portion of the original image you copied in step 1 onto the new layer of the new image file by choosing **Edit**, **Paste** (or use the **Ctrl+V** keyboard shortcut).

3 Delete the Background Layer

To create the transparent background for your image, select the *background layer* at the bottom of the **Layers** panel and drag it to the trash can at the top of the **Layers** panel. Alternatively, right-click the background layer, choose **Delete Layer**, and click **Yes** when asked to confirm the deletion of the layer. Now you have a new image with just the copied area and a transparent background.

4 Save Your New File

Click the **Save** button in the main toolbar. When the **Save As** dialog box opens, select the location for your new image file and change the filename if you did not name the file in step 2.

5 Add the File to Your Premiere Elements Project

Open your Premiere Elements project, click the **Add Media** button in the main toolbar, and browse for the new image file you just created. Add the image to your project's **Media** panel. Now the image is ready to be used in your movie.

▶ **TIP**

Let your creative juices flow; just think of the possibilities. That great video of Mount Rushmore or Stone Mountain could have *your* image on it. You could be standing on top of the Eiffel Tower; there are really no limitations to what you can do. For more information on how to accomplish these effects, **132** Make a Person Appear with a Different Background and **133** Make Your Clip Appear on an Object.

157

158   Create a Still Image from Video and Save It to Photoshop Elements

✔ BEFORE YOU BEGIN	→ SEE ALSO
77 Capture Digital Video Using FireWire	**49** Create Text That Glows
80 Capture Analog Video	**50** Fill Text with an Image
87 Grab a Still from Video	**62** Sharpen an Image
156 About Sharing Files	**140** Create a Title from Scratch
	157 Create a Graphic with Transparent Areas in Photoshop Elements
	162 Create a Slideshow in Photoshop Elements

Still images from video are wonderful in many ways. There always seems to be that one priceless frame that you want to save. You can use Premiere Elements to do just that, and then use Photoshop Elements to make the still image look a little bit better.

158

The quality of a still image taken from a video file will never be anything you would want to print as an 8×10 glossy and hang in your living room. But a still image grabbed from a video works great for video slideshows—and you might be able to get a decent 4×6 print. The pixel size and resolution of a frame of video saved as a still image is just too low to print the image much larger and retain good quality. Still, you can make some improvements by working with the image in Photoshop Elements. To do that, you must find that priceless frame of video, save it, and then import the still image file into Photoshop Elements.

Before we get started, open the Photoshop Elements Organizer and a Premiere Elements project.

1 Select a Video Clip

With your Premiere Elements project open, select a video clip in the **Media** panel or on the **Timeline** by double-clicking it. This action opens the clip in the **Monitor**.

2 Find a Frame and Click the Camera Icon

Using the VCR controls, the shuttle, and the CTI in the **Monitor**, locate the frame of the video clip that you want to save as a still image. With the frame of video you want to save showing in the **Monitor**, click the **Camera** icon. The **Export Frame** dialog box opens.

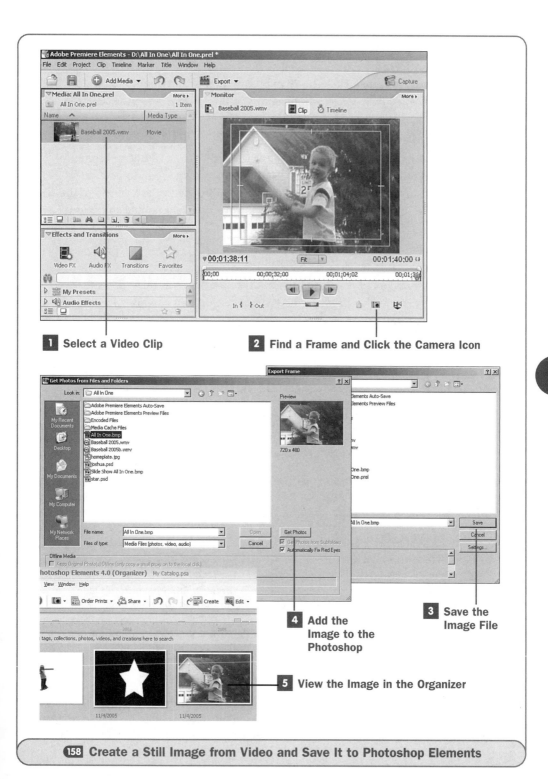

1 Select a Video Clip

2 Find a Frame and Click the Camera Icon

3 Save the Image File

4 Add the Image to the Photoshop

5 View the Image in the Organizer

158 Create a Still Image from Video and Save It to Photoshop Elements

3 Save the Image File

In the **Export Frame** dialog box, select the location for your still image, give it a filename, and then click the **Save** button. Remember your file's name and where you saved it; you will need this information in the next step.

4 Add the Image to the Photoshop Elements Organizer

Open the Photoshop Elements Organizer. Choose **File**, **Get Photos**, **From Files and Folders** (or use the **Ctrl+Shift+G** keyboard shortcut) to open the **Get Photos from Files and Folders** dialog box. Browse to the location of the file you saved in step 3. When you have located and selected the still image, click the **Get Photos** button.

5 View Your Image in the Organizer

The image appears in your Organizer workspace. You can now edit, enhance, resize, or do anything else with this still image that you can do with any other photograph.

▶ **NOTE**

158

Now that you have the still image in Photoshop Elements, see **51** Remove Specks, Spots, and Scratches; **57** Improve Brightness and Contrast; and **62** Sharpen an Image for some ideas of how you can make the still image look even better. Any corrections or changes you make to the file in Photoshop Elements will be automatically updated in your Premiere Elements project also. You can add the edited image to any other Premiere Elements project by using the **Add Media** button.

---

159 **Move Images Between Premiere Elements and Photoshop Elements**

✔ BEFORE YOU BEGIN	→ SEE ALSO
28 Create a New Image Layer	**49** Create Text That Glows
156 About Sharing Files	**50** Fill Text with an Image
157 Create a Graphic with Transparent Areas in Photoshop Elements	**158** Create a Still Image from Video and Save It to Photoshop Elements
	160 Move a Video Film Strip Between Premiere Elements and Photoshop Elements
	162 Create a Slideshow in Photoshop Elements
	175 Use Your DVD Menu Templates in Premiere Elements

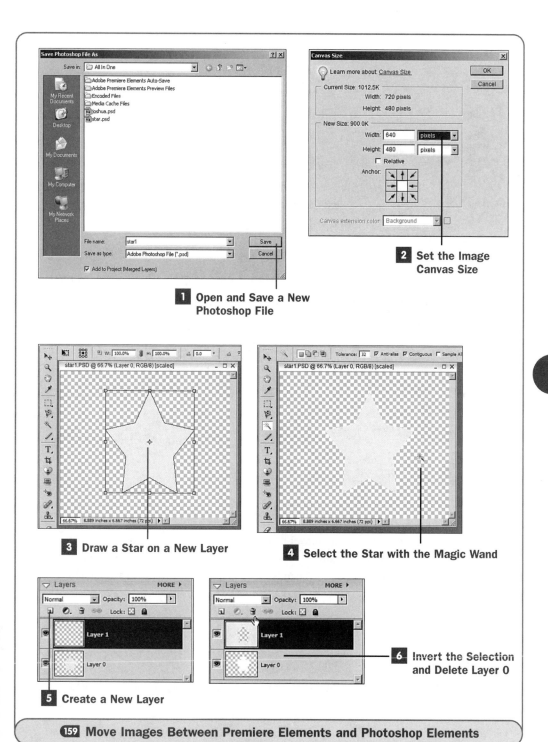

1 Open and Save a New Photoshop File

2 Set the Image Canvas Size

3 Draw a Star on a New Layer

4 Select the Star with the Magic Wand

5 Create a New Layer

6 Invert the Selection and Delete Layer 0

159 Move Images Between Premiere Elements and Photoshop Elements

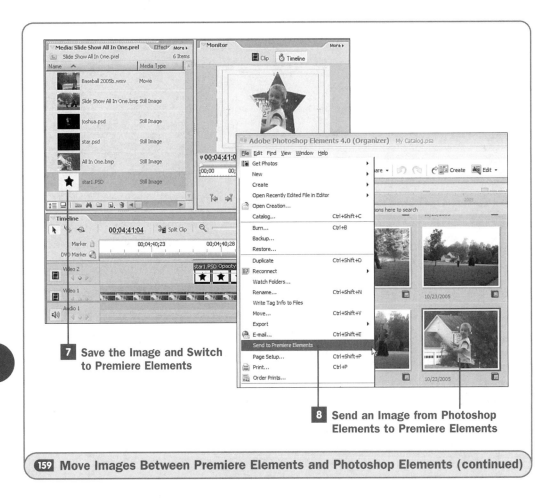

7 Save the Image and Switch to Premiere Elements

8 Send an Image from Photoshop Elements to Premiere Elements

159 Move Images Between Premiere Elements and Photoshop Elements (continued)

Of all the creative techniques included in this book, this is one of my very favorites. Images that have transparent areas are very useful in Premiere Elements (for example, many title templates have transparent areas in them). This task explains how to create an image with a transparent area in Photoshop Elements and also how to send an image from Photoshop Elements directly to your Premiere Elements project.

The image you create in this task is just one possibility. We will create an image with a transparent star shape that can be used as a *title* or even a *track matte*. When you get the hang of creating transparent shapes, you will be able to do the same with text. The Premiere Elements titler is very versatile, but this task gives you even more control over your creation.

1 Open and Save a New Photoshop File

Open the Photoshop Elements Editor, the Organizer, and a Premiere Elements project. From the main menu in your Premiere Elements project, select **File**, **New**, **Photoshop File**. The **Save Photoshop File As** dialog box opens. Select the location for the file, give it a filename, and click the **Save** button. The Photoshop Elements Editor opens, and you will see a new blank Photoshop image file.

2 Set the Image Canvas Size

For this image to be used correctly in Premiere Elements, we must ensure that the canvas size is of the proper proportions. From the main Photoshop menu, select **Image**, **Resize**, **Canvas Size**. In the **Canvas Size** dialog box, change the **Width** to **640** pixels and the **Height** to **480** pixels (these dimensions result in the standard 4:3 ratio for full screen; use a 16:9 ratio for widescreen) and click **OK**.

3 Draw a Star on a New Layer

Select **Layer**, **New**, **Background From Layer** to create the background layer on which you will draw your shape. From the toolbar on the left side of the screen, click the **Cookie Cutter** tool and choose a shape from the **Shape** drop-down list at the top of the image viewer. For this task, I selected the **Star** shape.

Click and hold the left mouse button on the blank image and drag the mouse. You will see the star taking shape over your image area. Release the left mouse button to drop the star shape onto the blank image; now you can use the handles to resize and rotate the shape. You can always draw your star again by clicking the **Undo** button and starting over.

Press the **Enter** key to cut the shape into your image. If you do not press the **Enter** key now, you can cut the shape after starting step 4. The objective is to create a shape that we will use to view our video through later.

4 Select the Star with the Magic Wand

Select the **Magic Wand** tool from the toolbar on the right side of your screen. If you did not press the **Enter** key to cut the shape in step 3, a dialog box opens after you click the **Magic Wand** button. This dialog box allows you to choose from the **Cut Shape**, **Cancel**, or **Don't Cut Shape** options; choose **Cut Shape**.

Click with the **Magic Wand** anywhere on your image outside the star shape. Everything except the star is selected. As you can see, the star is not transparent at this time, but the background is. The next steps change that.

159

5 Create a New Layer

Now it is time to create a new layer. We'll use this layer to invert our selection so that we can make our star shape transparent (instead of the background being transparent) by creating an *alpha channel*. In the **Layers** panel, click the **Create Layer** icon.

6 Invert the Selection and Delete Layer 0

Press **Alt+Backspace** to invert the selection—everything except the background is now selected.

Look at the two layers in the **Layers** panel; notice that **Layer 0** is a star with a transparent background, and **Layer 1** is a transparent star with a colored background. Drag **Layer 0** (the opaque star) to the trash can icon at the top of the **Layers** panel to delete **Layer 0** from your image, leaving you with just the transparent star image.

7 Save the Image and Switch to Premiere Elements

159

Click the **Save File** icon in the main toolbar to save your image. Open the Premiere Elements project we started in. Notice that the star image you just created in Photoshop Elements is now in the Premiere Elements **Media** panel, waiting to be used in your project. If you drop the transparent star image on a track above another image or video clip, you will see the lower track image through the transparent star shape.

▶ TIP

You can create your image with a colored background by setting the background color in step 3 or by using the color tools available in Photoshop Elements (see **29** Create a Layer Filled with a Color, Gradient, or Pattern).

8 Send an Image from Photoshop Elements to Premiere Elements

Open the Photoshop Elements Organizer and select an image; alternatively, **Shift+click** or **Ctrl+click** to select multiple images.

From the main Photoshop Elements menu, select **File**, **Send to Premiere Elements**. All the selected files are placed in the **Media** panel of your open Premiere Elements project.

160 Move a Video Filmstrip Between Premiere Elements and Photoshop Elements

✔ **BEFORE YOU BEGIN**

86 Trim Clips in the Media Panel
141 Output to an AVI Movie
156 About Sharing Files

→ **SEE ALSO**

158 Create a Still Image from Video and Save It to Photoshop Elements
159 Move Images Between Premiere Elements and Photoshop Elements

When you want to edit a video clip in Photoshop Elements, you can use the **Filmstrip** format. This format was specifically created for the purpose of editing video clips in graphics software. The **Filmstrip** format is useful when you want to paint directly on video frames, a process known as **rotoscoping**. You can export an entire video clip or just a portion of the **Timeline** as a filmstrip. Exporting a video file as a filmstrip file results in a single, still image file that contains all the frames of the clip.

▶ **KEY TERM**

Rotoscoping— Rotoscoping is used to create special visual effects (such as a glow) by actually painting on a filmstrip file in photo editing software. Then the "painted" filmstrip file is imported back into the video, replacing the original file. One use of traditional rotoscoping was in the original *Star Wars* films, where it was used to create the glowing lightsaber effect. The actors held sticks and the lightsaber effect was painted over the sticks on a filmstrip file, and then that "painted" file replaced the actual video footage. It is a very detailed process, but you can accomplish it with Premiere Elements and Photoshop Elements.

▶ **NOTE**

When working with Filmstrip files in Photoshop Elements, you should never resize or crop them. If you do, the file will no longer be usable in a Premiere Elements project.

If you have ever seen the original *Star Wars* movie, you have seen the effects of rotoscoping. This very old, yet effective, method was used for many years (even before *Star Wars* was made). The technique of painting on film or tracing live action movement, frame by frame, for use in animation, was used in some old *Dracula* movies to transform Dracula into a bat! In *Star Wars*, the technique was used to create the great lightsaber effect. Hollywood has moved on to higher technology now, but in its day, rotoscoping was the way to go. Although it is a very tedious and time-consuming process, it is also very rewarding. Using Photoshop Elements and Premiere Elements, you can do what took Hollywood many thousands of dollars to produce.

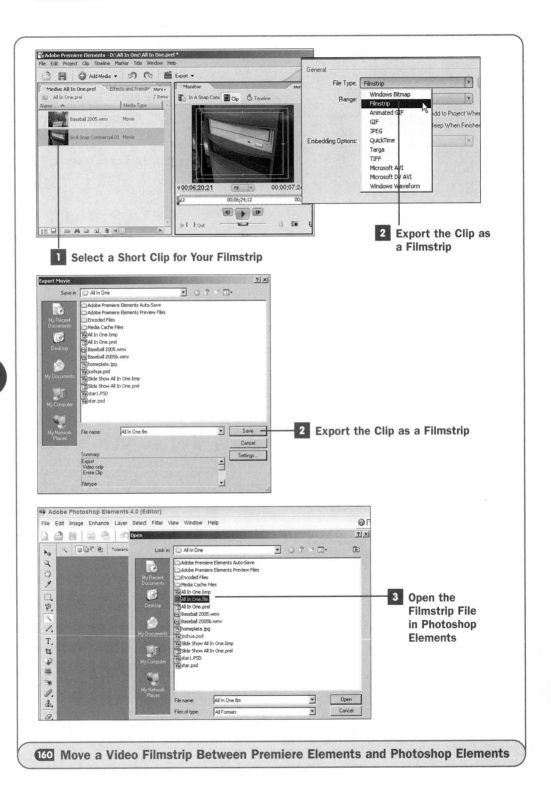

2 Export the Clip as a Filmstrip

1 Select a Short Clip for Your Filmstrip

2 Export the Clip as a Filmstrip

3 Open the Filmstrip File in Photoshop Elements

160 Move a Video Filmstrip Between Premiere Elements and Photoshop Elements

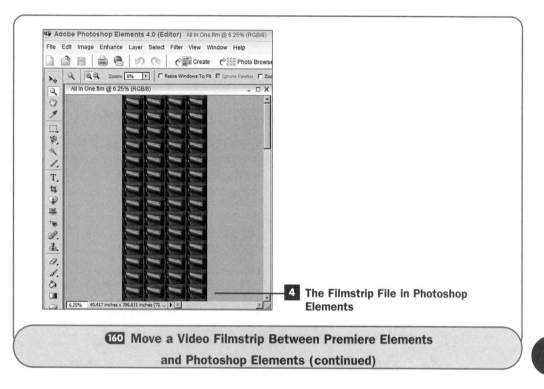

4 The Filmstrip File in Photoshop Elements

160 Move a Video Filmstrip Between Premiere Elements and Photoshop Elements (continued)

160

▶ **WEB RESOURCE**

http://designer.pri.ee/after_effects/1_27_20_0.html

http://www.alienryderflex.com/rotoscope/

These sites are great resources for rotoscoping and using filmstrip files.

1 Select a Short Clip for Your Filmstrip

Open the Photoshop Elements Editor and a Premiere Elements project that includes a video clip. In your Premiere Elements project, select a clip from the **Media** panel that you want to create a filmstrip file of. After the filmstrip file is created, you can open it in Photoshop Elements, paint on it, and use it in your Premiere Elements project along with the original footage.

▶ **TIP**

To get a short-enough clip, it might be necessary to trim a longer clip. To learn about trimming clips in the **Media** panel and setting the in and out points, see **86** Trim Clips in the Media Panel. When rotoscoping, you will be manually editing each frame of your video clip. At 30 frames per second, 5 seconds of video is 150 frames that you will have to manually add an effect to. The shorter the video clip, the fewer frames you will have to edit. Although rotoscoping involves a lot of work, the outcome can be amazing.

2 Export the Clip as a Filmstrip

If necessary, trim the video clip by setting new in and out points in the **Monitor** panel to make the clip shorter. At 30 frames per second, you probably don't want to do more than a few seconds' worth of video at a time. When you edit the filmstrip file in Photoshop Elements, you will be working on each individual frame, so make the video clip as short as possible.

From the Premiere Elements main menu, select **File**, **Export**, **Movie** to open the **Export Movie** dialog box. Click the **Settings** button to open the **Export Movie Settings** dialog box, where you will make selections for the filmstrip file you are about to save.

In the **General** category, open the **File Type** drop-down list and choose **Filmstrip** as the type of file you want to export. From the **Range** drop-down list, choose either **Entire Clip** or **In to Out** (if you have set the in and out points in the **Monitor** panel). After making these setting changes, click the **OK** button to return to the **Export Movie** dialog box. Select the location for your filmstrip file, give it a filename, and then click the **Save** button.

3 Open the Filmstrip File in Photoshop Elements

160

Open the Photoshop Elements Editor and chose **File**, **Open** from the main menu or click the **Open** button in the main toolbar. The **Open** dialog box appears; browse to the location of the filmstrip file you saved in step 2. When you have located and selected the file, click the **Open** button. The filmstrip file opens in the Photoshop Elements Editor, ready for editing. Now you can add any effect available to you in Photoshop Elements. In this example, I used a glow effect that could be added to the video file. Alternatively, we could add a blur to the DVD drawer, or we could make it look like the drive was on fire. You can use this technique to blur a face or license plate, make a flame burn a little brighter...the possibilities are limitless.

▶ TIP

Rotoscoping is a tedious and time-consuming process. The results are great, but getting there is sometimes a long road. You will find the process a lot easier if you break up your original video clip into very small filmstrip files. Start with just a few seconds and practice the technique first—don't attempt a 10-minute lightsaber battle on your first try. The people who used to do this in Hollywood were seasoned professionals; it took them years of practice to get the results you see in the movies. With the tools available to you in Photoshop Elements and Premiere Elements, you are already way ahead of them. Happy rotoscoping!

28

Creating Slideshows

IN THIS CHAPTER:

Slideshows have seemingly been around forever. My wife's grandfather, Ray, now 100 years old, has always had a slide projector. He has taken more pictures with slide film than with 35mm film, and we now have all 2,000+ of them. Setting up the projector and screen and then getting out the slides was great fun in those days, but it was quite a project in itself. Ray just loved dragging everything out and showing off the slides of his and his wife's vacations and their granddaughter.

Slideshows can also be called mini-documentaries. They generally tell a story about an event, a person, or a group of people (such as your family). Slideshows let you not only tell your story, but also add music and special effects. Slideshows don't require any video, so even if you only have a still camera, you can still create a great video slideshow.

With Photoshop Elements and Premiere Elements, you can create a simple slideshow or an elaborate one. You can add graphics, titles, and music and even put the finished product in an email, on the Internet, or on a CD or DVD. This chapter starts with tasks that create a slideshow in Photoshop Elements, the simpler approach; later tasks take you into Premiere Elements to create a slideshow masterpiece.

Before you begin any of the tasks in this chapter, get all your images, slides, graphics, music, and anything else you might need together. Now get ready to create some slideshows.

---

161 About Slideshows

✔ BEFORE YOU BEGIN	→ SEE ALSO
81 Capture to the Timeline or Media Panel	**173** Modify an Existing DVD Menu Template
156 About Sharing Files	**172** About DVD Menus and the DVD Template Editor

---

The first thing we need to do is get you into and help you navigate through the Photoshop Elements Slideshow Editor.

To open the Photoshop Elements Slideshow Editor, start Photoshop Elements by double-clicking the desktop icon. At the splash screen, choose either **View and Organize Photos** or **Make Photo Creations**. The Photoshop Elements Organizer opens. From the main menu, select **File, Create, Slideshow**. The **Slideshow Preferences** dialog box opens; click the **OK** button to enter the **Slideshow Editor** workspace.

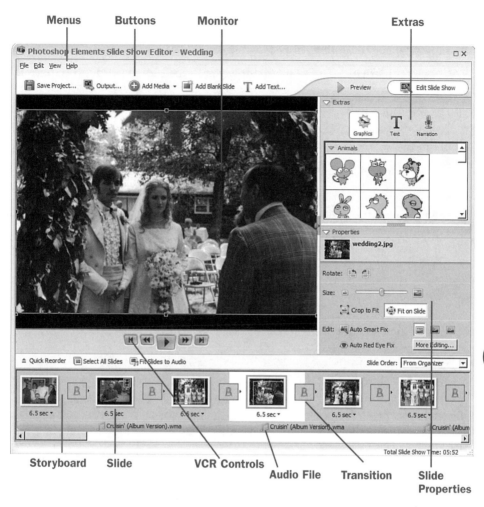

Get familiar with the Photoshop Elements Slideshow Editor and the common terms used there.

At the top of the screen is the main menu bar that includes drop-down menus for the various options, such as **File**, **Edit**, **View**, and **Help**.

Below the menu bar are buttons that perform various functions (these buttons are also shortcuts to items in the main menu):

- **Save Project**—This button saves your slideshow in its current state.

- **Output**—This button opens the **Output Slideshow** dialog box.

- **Add Media**—This button is used when adding images, music, and graphics to your slideshow.

- **Add Blank Slide**—This button adds a blank slide to your slideshow.

- **Add Text**—This button allows you to add text to a slide in your slideshow.

- **Preview**—This button starts playing your slideshow in a new, larger window.

- **Edit Slideshow**—This button returns you to the slideshow edit workspace.

The **Monitor** window is where all the action happens. In the **Monitor**, you adjust your slides, create pans and zooms, add text and graphics, and view your work in progress.

Below the **Monitor** window are the **VCR controls**, which work just like the buttons on a VCR: **Play, Next Slide, Previous Slide, Start, End,** and **Pause.**

Under the **Monitor** panel and the **VCR controls** is the *storyboard.* The storyboard is where all your video clips, images, and music are kept. The still images and video are kept in the main area of the storyboard, while music is kept just below that in the storyboard's **audio** section.

▶ **TIP**

Put together a storyboard just like the pros do. You can download free storyboards and get tips on how to use them—just search for *storyboard* on the Internet.

161

▶ **KEY TERM**

Storyboard—A panel or series of panels on which a set of sketches is arranged depicting the important changes of scene and action in a consecutive series of shots (as for film, a television show, a commercial, or a slideshow).

On the storyboard, you will notice that there is one thumbnail for each image, no matter how long that image is displayed onscreen. This image is called a *slide.* Between the slides are small square graphics; these icons indicate the transition between the two images on either side.

To the right of the **Monitor** is the currently selected slide's **Properties** panel; here is where you adjust the size and rotation of the selected slide. Above the **Properties** panel is the **Extras** panel; this is where you can add a range of graphic images to your slides, add text, and add narration to your slideshow.

Now that you're familiar with the Photoshop Elements Slideshow Editor, let's run through the Premiere Elements workspace. You can create an identical slideshow using both programs—use whichever program you prefer to accomplish the end result. The Photoshop Elements slideshows are a bit easier to create but have some limitations; the Premiere Elements slideshows are a bit more difficult to create but have very few limitations. After you graduate to creating slideshows with Premiere Elements Slideshow, you probably will not go back to Photoshop

Elements, except for the occasional time when you need something done in a hurry.

Many of the functions and options are the same in Premiere Elements as they are in Photoshop Elements Slideshow: Both have a main menu with various options and both have buttons and a **Monitor** window. The following list reviews the key elements to give you a head start when you are ready to use Premiere Elements to create a slideshow or are ready to burn your slideshow from Photoshop Elements to DVD:

- **Add Media**—This button adds video clips, images, and music to your slideshow. In Premiere Elements, you also have the option of downloading video from an existing DVD and capturing video from a digital camcorder or converter.

- **Media Panel**—This is where all the images and clips in your project are stored.

- **Video tracks and audio tracks**—To create your slideshow, the clips from the **Media** panel are placed on the **video tracks** and **audio tracks**. The clips on these tracks make up what will eventually become your slideshow.

- **Timeline**—The video and audio tracks are on what is called the **Timeline**, which is the counterpart to the **storyboard** in the Photoshop Elements Slideshow Editor. On the **Timeline**, you see various *clips*, both audio and video.

- **Properties panel**—Use the clip's **Properties** panel to adjust the various properties of a clip. In the **Properties** panel, you can change many characteristics of a clip, including its opacity, size, and position. The **Properties** panel also allows you to change the characteristics of various effects and transitions.

- **Buttons**—At the upper right of the screen are various buttons (**Capture**, **Edit**, **Title**, and **DVD**); click a button to go to that named workspace in Premiere Elements. When importing slideshows from Photoshop Elements, you are taken directly into the **DVD** workspace (see **169** **Export Your Slideshow**).

▶ WEB RESOURCE

http://www.videoinasnap.com

http://www.chuckengels.com

http://www.adobeforums.com/cgi-bin/webx?14@@.3bb574e6

These three sites are good resources for helping you create a great slideshow. They are also very helpful with Premiere Elements in general. (Note that the Adobe site requires free registration.)

162 Create a Slideshow in Photoshop Elements

✔ BEFORE YOU BEGIN

1 Import Media from a Folder, CD-ROM, or DVD

4 Locate Moved Files

6 Review Images

141 Output to an AVI Movie

→ SEE ALSO

8 Create a Collection

36 Crop a Portion of an Image

51 Remove Specks, Spots, and Scratches

57 Improve Brightness and Contrast

87 Grab a Still from Video

This task explains how to create a simple slideshow with the Photoshop Elements Slideshow Editor. If you haven't done so already, get together whatever images and photos you would like to put into your slideshow. If you have a shoebox full of photos, start scanning. If your photos are already on your computer, place a copy of the ones you want to use (or move them) into a new folder specifically for this project, or create a *collection* in Photoshop Elements. Placing all your media elements in the same folder or in a collection makes everything a bit easier; refer to 8 **Create a Collection**.

162

1 Open the Photoshop Elements Organizer and Create a Slideshow

From the Photoshop Elements Splash screen, click the **View and Organize Photos** icon to open the **Organizer** workspace.

▶ TIP

If you select any images in the **Organizer** or select a collection before creating your slideshow, the selected images are automatically added at the time the slideshow is created.

From the main menu, choose **File, Create, Slideshow**. The **Slideshow Preferences** dialog box opens.

2 Set Slideshow Preferences

The **Slideshow Preferences** dialog box allows you to set some of the various functions of the slideshow now. You can change any of these options later, and there is no need to make any changes to the default settings except for one: Disable the **Apply Pan and Zoom to All Slides** check box; we will cover this option in 164 **Pan and Zoom an Image in Your Slideshow**. Other settings you can change are

- **Static Duration**—The length of time each slide is displayed onscreen.

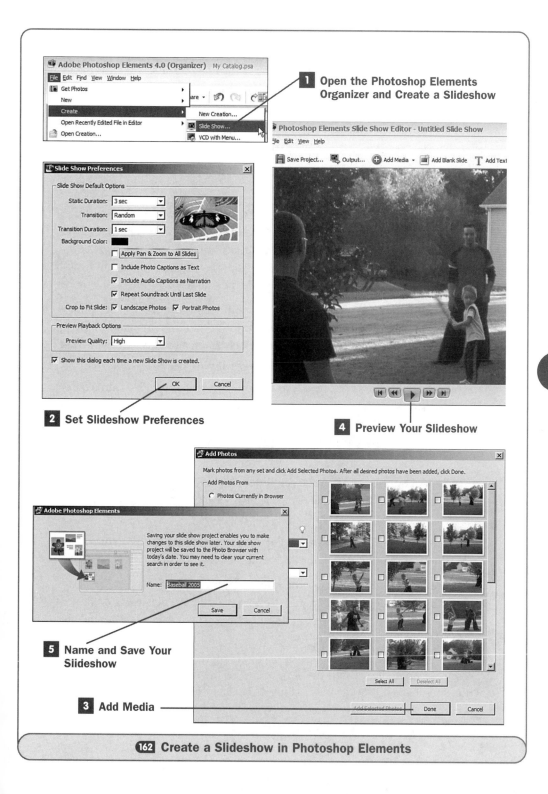

1 Open the Photoshop Elements Organizer and Create a Slideshow

2 Set Slideshow Preferences

4 Preview Your Slideshow

5 Name and Save Your Slideshow

3 Add Media

162

162 Create a Slideshow in Photoshop Elements

- **Transition**—The kind of action that takes place when one slide changes into the next. The choice you make here is the default transition used in your slideshow. Some of the choices include **Dissolve, Clock Wipe, Barn Doors**, and **Random**. You will have the opportunity to change transitions later, if you like.

- **Transition Duration**—The length of time it takes for the transition effect to occur.

- **Background Color**—The color you see if the slide does not fill the entire viewing area.

- **Apply Pan & Zoom to All Slides**— Motion (pan) and zoom are added to all the slides when this option is selected. Adding the pan and zoom features to all the slides might make the slideshow too active and can distract from the images themselves. You can add pan and zoom features to individual images from inside the Editor.

- **Include Photo Captions as Text**—If you added captions to your photos in the Photoshop Elements Organizer, those captions show up as text on your images when this option is selected. The text can be changed after you're inside the **Slideshow Editor** workspace.

- **Include Audio Captions as Narration**—If you have added audio captions to your photos in the Organizer, those captions are used as narration when this option is selected. You will have the opportunity to change the audio or remove it after you're inside the **Slideshow Editor** workspace.

- **Repeat Soundtrack Until Last Slide**—Select this option if the slideshow will be longer than the music you have selected for it. With this option enabled, the music repeats until the slideshow ends.

- **Crop to Fit Slide**—Enable the **Landscape Photos** or the **Portrait Photos** option to crop your images to fit the slide area.

- **Preview Quality**—Choose the quality of the preview; you can be set this option from low to high. If you notice that the preview is a bit jerky, change this option to a lower setting. The preview quality has no effect on the slideshow output.

When you have the settings the way you want them, click **OK** to open the Photoshop Elements **Slideshow Editor**, the place where everything happens.

162

3 Add Media

If you selected images before selecting the **File**, **Create**, **Slideshow** command in step 1, the images should already be on the *storyboard*. To add more images (or the first images to a blank storyboard), click the **Add Media** button at the top of the screen and choose the **Photos and Videos from Organizer** option. The **Add Photos** dialog box opens. Use this dialog box to select any of the images that are stored in the **Organizer**.

Select any of the radio buttons to limit your search to a specific *collection* or *tag*. Enable the check box under each of the images you want to add to your slideshow. When you have selected all the images for your slideshow, click the **Done** button. All the selected images now appear on the storyboard.

4 Preview Your Slideshow

Click the **Preview** button in the upper-right corned of the workspace to see how your slideshow looks so far. There may be more you want to do with it, and many of those things are covered in the upcoming tasks. For now, use the **VCR control** buttons located under the viewing area to advance through the basic slideshow. Now let's save what we have.

5 Name and Save Your Slideshow

From the main menu, select **File**, **Save As**. A dialog box opens in which you can name your slideshow. Type a name for the file and click **Save**.

163

---

163 Rotate, Size, and Edit Your Images

✔ BEFORE YOU BEGIN	→ SEE ALSO
162 Create a Slideshow in Photoshop Elements	16 Change Image Size or Resolution
	56 Remove Unwanted Objects from an Image
	60 Correct Color, Contrast, and Saturation in One Step

In 162 **Create a Slideshow in Photoshop Elements**, you created a basic slideshow. As expected, you can make some modifications to the images you've selected for your Photoshop Elements slideshow. Sometimes images don't come in quite the way we like, which requires you to have some tools available to quickly fix problems like size, rotation, and basic image problems. This task explains how to manipulate the images in your slideshow in these basic ways.

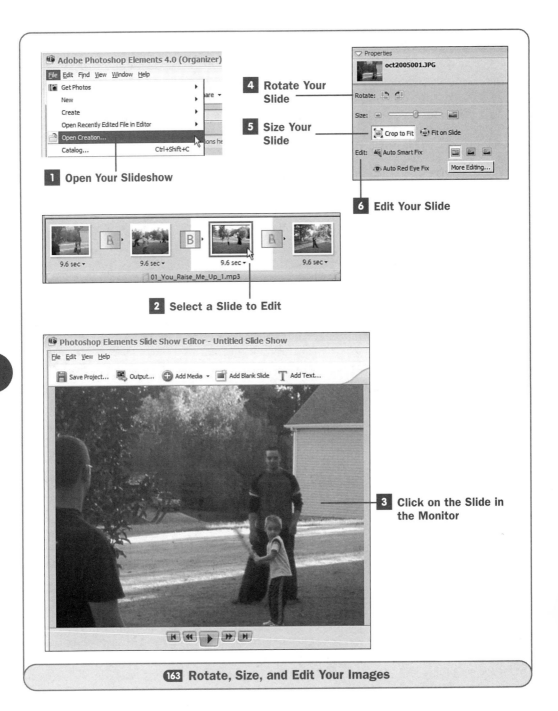

1 Open Your Slideshow

2 Select a Slide to Edit

3 Click on the Slide in the Monitor

4 Rotate Your Slide

5 Size Your Slide

6 Edit Your Slide

163 Rotate, Size, and Edit Your Images

1 Open Your Slideshow

If you have closed your slideshow, you can open it again from the Photoshop Elements **Organizer** by selecting **File, Open Creation** from the main menu. The **Open Creation** dialog box appears. If more than one option is listed in the **Open Creation** dialog box, choose the slideshow you created in the last task.

▶ **TIP**

You can open the Slideshow Editor only from the Photoshop Elements **Organizer**, not from the **Editor**.

2 Select a Slide to Edit

Select a slide in your slideshow storyboard by clicking it with the left mouse button. That slide appears in the **Monitor** window (also called the slide viewer).

3 Click the Slide in the Monitor

When the slide you need to correct (or any slide for that matter) is in the **Monitor** window, click the image. This action ensures that the **Properties** panel for that slide opens in the bottom-right corner of the screen. This panel offers several options for making modifications to your slides.

163

4 Rotate Your Slide

At the top of the **Properties** panel are the **Rotate** selections. Click the buttons to rotate the slide 90° at a time to the right or left.

5 Size Your Slide

In the **Size** area of the **Properties** panel, you can adjust the size of your slide. Clicking your slide in the **Monitor** window in step 3 displayed the sizing handles, which you can drag to adjust the image size, but the slider in the **Properties** panel is faster and easier to use. Simply drag the slider to the left to decrease the size of the image; drag to the right to increase the size of your slide. You can also choose **Crop to Fit** to remove parts of your image so that it fits in the **Monitor** window or **Fit on Slide** to shrink the image to fit in the available space.

6 Edit Your Slide

The **Edit** area of the **Properties** panel offers several options that can improve the quality of the image in the slideshow. Click the Photoshop Elements **Auto**

Smart Fix button to automatically adjust your image (see **39** **Apply a Quick Fix**). Click the **Auto Red Eye Fix** button to correct the red-eye effect that sometimes occurs in photos of people when you use a flash. Click one of the three buttons above the **More Editing** button to change the image from color to black-and-white or from color to sepia tone and back to color. Under extreme circumstances, you can click the **More Editing** button to open the image in the Photoshop Elements **Editor**.

Repeats steps 3–6 to fix all the images in your storyboard so that you are ready for the next task and that much closer to finishing your slideshow.

---

164 **Pan and Zoom an Image in Your Slideshow**

✔ BEFORE YOU BEGIN	→ SEE ALSO
162 Create a Slideshow in Photoshop Elements	**170** Make an Instant Slideshow in Premiere Elements
	119 Pan and Zoom a Photo a la Ken Burns
	120 Make a Variable-Speed Pan and Zoom

163

This task starts with a new slideshow and explains how to pan and zoom the images. Although the pan and zoom effects are much more customizable in Premiere Elements than they are in Photoshop Elements, this task explains how to create a nice look in a simple slideshow.

▶ **TIP**

The art of panning and zooming images was mastered by Ken Burns, a documentary director and producer who has created some of the greatest films in history, about history. It is worth the purchase price of one of his DVDs just for what you will learn—aside from the entertainment value.

The ability to pan and zoom images gives your slideshow the appearance of video, even though you are using still images. The art is in making the slides actually look like they are moving. Slow and steady is the key to creating the moving picture effect. *Pan* = motion and *zoom* = scale; when you pan a still image, you are moving horizontally, vertically, or diagonally across the image. When you zoom, you are changing the scale or size of the image, zooming in for a tighter shot or zooming out for a distance shot. A zoom can start up close on a specific object in the photo and then move out to view the whole image, or it can start far off and zoom in to a specific object. If you have the chance, catch one of Ken Burns's films on PBS; you won't be disappointed.

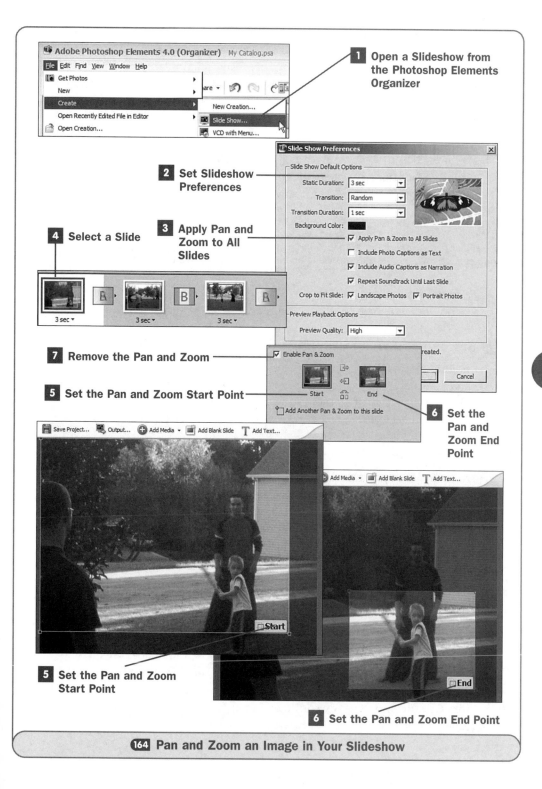

1 Open a Slideshow from the Photoshop Elements Organizer

2 Set Slideshow Preferences

3 Apply Pan and Zoom to All Slides

4 Select a Slide

7 Remove the Pan and Zoom

5 Set the Pan and Zoom Start Point

6 Set the Pan and Zoom End Point

5 Set the Pan and Zoom Start Point

6 Set the Pan and Zoom End Point

164 Pan and Zoom an Image in Your Slideshow

Depending on where you plan to view the finished slideshow (on the television or on the computer), you might need to resize your images. Panning is not generally a problem, but zooming in on images can be. If you magnify an image in Photoshop, at some point you will be able to see individual pixels—and I doubt you want that to happen in your slideshow. For more information about preparing images, see **88** **Prepare a Still for Video.**

1 Open a Slideshow from the Photoshop Elements Organizer

From the Photoshop Elements splash screen, click the **View and Organize Photos** icon to open the **Organizer** workspace.

▶ **TIP**

If you select any images or a collection in the **Organizer** before creating your slideshow, the selected images are automatically added to the slideshow at the time it is created.

From the main menu, choose **File**, **Create**, **Slideshow** to open the **Slideshow Preferences** dialog box.

2 Set Slideshow Preferences

The **Preferences** dialog box offers the option of setting many of the slideshow characteristics, such as the slide duration, background color, transition type, transition duration, and others. For a more detailed look at the slideshow preferences, see **162** **Create a Slideshow in Photoshop Elements.**

3 Apply Pan and Zoom to All Slides

To enable panning and zooming in your slideshow, ensure that the **Apply Pan & Zoom to All Slides** option is checked. This option applies the pan and zoom effects to all your images automatically, a good place to start. You can also disable this check box and add the pan and zoom features to individual slides once you're inside the **Slideshow Editor.** If you choose to apply the pan and zoom features automatically, you can remove them from any slide at any time when you're inside the **Slideshow Editor.** When you are ready click the **OK** button.

4 Select a Slide

If you selected images before creating the slideshow, the images are already on the storyboard. If you want to add images to the storyboard, click the **Add Media** button at the top of the screen and choose the **Photos and Videos from Organizer** option. To learn more about adding media to a slideshow, see **162** **Create a Slideshow in Photoshop Elements.**

164

Select a slide in your slideshow storyboard by clicking it once with the left mouse button. The slide appears in the **Monitor** window (also called the slide viewer).

5 Set the Pan and Zoom Start Point

Notice that all the slides in the storyboard have red and green boxes in them. The green box is the pan and zoom start point, and the red box is the end point. In the bottom-right corner of the screen is the slide's **Properties** panel; this panel now includes a **Pan and Zoom** control panel.

The **Enable Pan & Zoom** check box is enabled for this slide because you selected the **Apply Pan & Zoom to All Slides** option in step 2. Also on the **Pan and Zoom** control panel are two thumbnails; one is labeled **Start** and the other is labeled **End**. In between are three buttons—the top button copies the start point to the end point, making them the same; the middle button copies the end point to the start point, making them the same; and the bottom button does a start point/end point switch, where the end point becomes the start point and the start point becomes the end point. This last button is useful if you decide you would rather zoom in than out on an image; rather than redoing the whole thing, you can just switch the start and end points.

For now, we are concerned about where this slide starts—that is, where it appears onscreen when it is first displayed. Click the **Start** thumbnail. The green box appears on the slide in the **Monitor** window with the word **Start** in the bottom-right corner. At each corner of the image is a handle to allow you to resize the start point. Drag the handle to adjust the "clear" area over the image; click and drag the whole box to place it where ever you like. The clear area is all that will be seen; the grayed out area will not be visible. The clear area will be enlarged to cover the whole screen when viewed. When you are finished, the clear area should cover the portion of the image you want to appear when the slide first appears onscreen during the slideshow. This is the starting point of your pan and zoom.

6 Set the Pan and Zoom End Point

Click the **End** thumbnail in the **Pan and Zoom** control panel to display the red box in the **Monitor** window. Set the end point just as you did the start point in step 5. With your start and end points positioned, preview the slideshow and see how you like the look; you can always reposition the start and end points or turn off the pan and zoom feature if you don't like it. The most tedious process is manually changing every slide, which is the way you do it in Premiere Elements. Photoshop Elements provides an automatic pan and zoom applied to all your images; Premiere Elements does not have this

164

feature. If you don't like the way the automatic pan and zoom looks, the only way to change it is one image at a time, in either program.

With the start and end points set in this example, the image starts with only the area inside the green box covering the entire screen when viewed. Then the image zooms in and pans to a shot of just the boy batting, until the area inside the red box fills the entire screen.

7 Remove the Pan and Zoom

To remove the pan and zoom feature from an individual slide (that is, to display the slide at its full size without any implied motion), simply disable the **Enable Pan and Zoom** check box in the **Pan and Zoom** control panel.

---

165 **Add Music to Your Slideshow**

✔ **BEFORE YOU BEGIN**	→ **SEE ALSO**
1 Import Media from a Folder, CD-ROM, or DVD	**100** Remove Audio and Video from a Clip
156 About Sharing Files	**167** Trim Slideshow Audio and Control Volume
	168 Add Graphics, Text, and Narration to Your Slideshow

164

The ability to add music to slideshows is just short of fabulous. It creates a very special feeling to the whole show and sometimes can bring tears to your eyes. Just think of all those great songs you love and how you could incorporate them into a fantastic slideshow. You probably have at least a half dozen ideas already!

For a small amount of money, you can download a song from a website. During your video career, you will probably have the need to do that at some point. The problem is that the file you download cannot be used in your slideshow in its original format. The music files are licensed and have built-in security, making them unusable except in Media Player, QuickTime, or RealPlayer. There is a workaround for this file format problem that will get those songs into your project with little effort.

After downloading your song to the computer, use your CD-burning software to burn the song to a CD-ROM. Then rip the music back to your computer. That resulting music file can be easily imported into your slideshow.

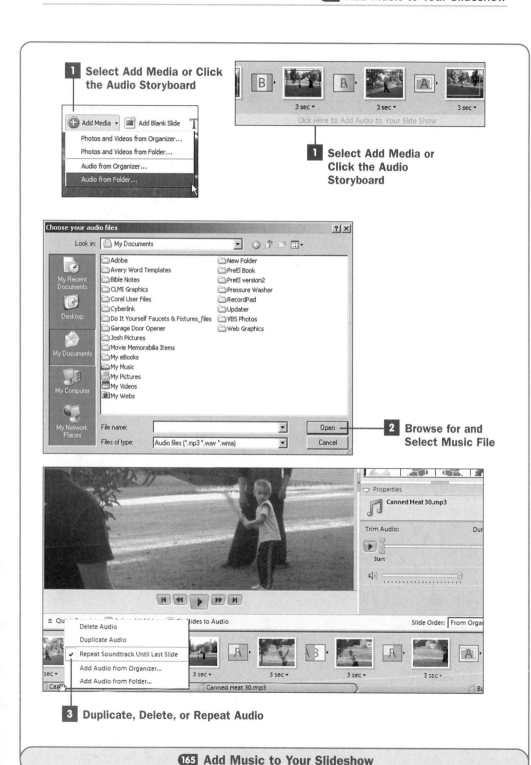

1 Select Add Media or Click the Audio Storyboard

Add Media ▾   Add Blank Slide
Photos and Videos from Organizer...
Photos and Videos from Folder...
Audio from Organizer...
Audio from Folder...

B · [ ] · B · [ ] · A · [ ]
3 sec ▾   3 sec ▾   3 sec ▾
Click Here to Add Audio to Your Slide Show

1 Select Add Media or Click the Audio Storyboard

Choose your audio files   ? ✕

Look in: My Documents

My Recent Documents
Desktop
My Documents
My Computer
My Network Places

Adobe   New Folder
Avery Word Templates   PreEl Book
Bible Notes   PreEl version2
CLMI Graphics   Pressure Washer
Corel User Files   RecordPad
Cyberlink   Updater
Do It Yourself Faucets & Fixtures_files   VBS Photos
Garage Door Opener   Web Graphics
Josh Pictures
Movie Memorabilia Items
My eBooks
My Music
My Pictures
My Videos
My Webs

File name: Open   ─── **2** Browse for and Select Music File
Files of type: Audio files (*.mp3 *.wav *.wma)   Cancel

▽ Properties
Canned Heat 30.mp3

Trim Audio: Dur
▶
Start
🔊 ....

⌃ Qu...   ...ides to Audio   Slide Order: From Orga

Delete Audio
Duplicate Audio
✓ Repeat Soundtrack Until Last Slide
Add Audio from Organizer...
Add Audio from Folder...

A · [ ] B · [ ] A · [ ] A · [ ]
3 sec ▾   3 sec ▾   3 sec ▾   3 sec ▾

sec ▾   3 sec ▾
Ca...   Canned Heat 30.mp3   B...

3 Duplicate, Delete, or Repeat Audio

165

165 Add Music to Your Slideshow

▶ **TIP**

When you rip the music back to your hard drive, save the file in the WMA, MP3, WAV, or PCM format. These file formats work best with Premiere Elements and Photoshop Elements. Windows Media Player 10 does an excellent job of burning and ripping—and best of all, it came free with your computer.

With all of what you just read in mind, make sure you have at least one music file on your computer so that you can add it to your slideshow. If you don't have a music file, rip one from a CD or download a song from one of the many music download sites on the Internet. After you have your music file on your hard drive (you can even add it to the Photoshop Elements Organizer), open a slideshow in the Photoshop Elements Slideshow Editor and begin this task.

▶ **WEB RESOURCE**

http://www.freeplaymusic.com

This website has a huge volume of free instrumental music in many genres and styles. The songs can be downloaded in various lengths in two formats, so be sure to use the MP3 format. The songs make great background music and can also be used as a soundtrack for videos in Premiere Elements. Not only is the music free, it sounds fantastic as well. Be sure to read the "Terms of Use" section to ensure that you are using the music legally.

165

1 **Select Add Media or Click the Audio Storyboard**

The audio portion of the storyboard, when it has no audio tracks, says **Click Here to Add Audio to Your Slideshow**. Clicking this link opens the **Choose your audio files** dialog box, where you can browse for your music file. Alternatively, click the **Add Media** button at the top of the Photoshop Elements workspace and select **Audio from Organizer** or **Audio from Folder**, depending on whether you have imported the music file into the **Organizer**.

2 **Browse for and Select Music File**

In the **Choose your audio files** dialog box, browse for the music file you want to use with this slideshow and select it. Then click **Open**. The selected music file(s) is added to the audio portion of the storyboard.

3 **Duplicate, Delete, or Repeat Audio**

Right-click one of the audio clips to open a context menu. From this menu, you have the following options:

- **Delete Audio**—This option deletes the selected audio clip.
- **Duplicate Audio**—This option duplicates the selected audio clip. The duplicated clip appears after the last music clip in your slideshow.

- **Repeat Soundtrack Until Last Slide**—Select this option to repeat the selected audio clip in a continuous loop until the slideshow ends. This is useful if your slides are longer than your music and you don't want to add more audio to the slideshow.

You can also choose to add more audio clips to your slideshow by selecting **Add Audio from Organizer** or **Add Audio from Folder**.

---

166 Fit Slides to Audio

✔ BEFORE YOU BEGIN	→ SEE ALSO
162 Create a Slideshow in Photoshop Elements	**170** Make an Instant Slideshow
165 Add Music to Your Slideshow	**171** Change Slides to the Beat of Music
	168 Add Graphics, Text, and Narration to Your Slideshow

This might seem like a simple task, but putting a feature into the Photoshop Elements Slide Show Editor that can fit all your slides to the length of an audio file is amazing. Without this feature, you might as well be a math professor trying to figure out the duration of each slide—just imagine a song that is 3 minutes and 23 seconds long during which you want to show the 87 photos in your slideshow. Quick, how many seconds should each slide duration be? Good question, and you don't need to know the answer because Photoshop Elements does the math for you. Be sure the slideshow you created in **165 Add Music to Your Slideshow** (or any slideshow with a music track) is open, and let's get the slides to match the length of the audio on the storyboard.

1 Click Fit Slides to Audio

With the previous task's slideshow open in the Photoshop Elements Slideshow Editor, click the **Fit Slides to Audio** button just below the **Monitor** window's **VCR controls**. This action determines the exact length each slide must be to fit the slides in the storyboard to the complete length of the audio track. If the audio is too long, Photoshop Elements extends the duration of each slide; if the audio is too short for the currently specified slide duration (which you might have specified in **162 Create a Slideshow in Photoshop Elements**), Photoshop Elements shortens the duration of each slide. Of course, this can cause some problems, such as the slide duration can become too long and drawn out or it might be so short that the slides flip by so quickly that you can't even see them. For that, there is a quick fix.

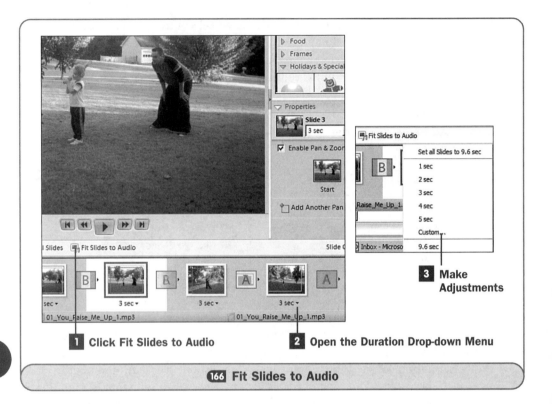

1 Click Fit Slides to Audio

2 Open the Duration Drop-down Menu

3 Make Adjustments

166 Fit Slides to Audio

2 Open the Duration Drop-down Menu

In the storyboard, click the little down arrow under a slide, next to the slide duration, to open the duration drop-down menu.

3 Make Adjustments

From the duration drop-down list, choose a new duration for the selected slide. The first option in the list changes the duration of all the slides in the slideshow. If the **Fit to Audio** option doesn't do what you need, you might need to find another song with a more appropriate duration, to edit the current song by making it longer or shorter (as explained in **86** **Trim Clips in the Media Panel** and **167** **Trim Slideshow Audio and Control Volume**), or to add audio to your slideshow and try the **Fit to Audio** feature again.

167 Trim Slideshow Audio and Control Volume

✔ BEFORE YOU BEGIN

162 Create a Slideshow in Photoshop Elements
165 Add Music to Your Slideshow
166 Fit Slides to Audio

→ SEE ALSO

170 Make an Instant Slideshow
171 Change Slides to the Beat of Music

Sometimes, the audio file you want to use with your slideshow just won't fit, or it is too loud or too soft. A feature in Photoshop Elements corrects these problems. If you read 166 Fit Slides to Audio, you know you can have too many slides and not enough audio, or just the opposite. The Fit Slides to Audio option adjusts the slides to fit the audio, no matter how long or short the sound file is. Because that option might not always provide the desired results, Photoshop Elements lets you add the same audio clip to a slideshow multiple times. You can then trim each of the audio clips to sync the two together—kind of like a disc jockey would do to make a smooth transition or to extend the length of a song.

▶ TIP

If trimming the audio in the Photoshop Elements Slideshow Editor is not producing the results you require, try doing some surgery on the audio clip in Premiere Elements. You can trim the audio file; add some effects if you like; and even add a fade in, fade out, or both. Then you can export the audio and add it to your slideshow in Photoshop Elements. For instructions on how to do audio editing in Premiere Elements, see 86 Trim Clips in the Media Panel, 111 Raise, Lower, and Normalize Sound Volume, and 142 Output a WMV File.

167

1 Select an Audio Clip

Select an audio clip on the storyboard by clicking it. This action opens the audio properties in the **Properties** panel in the bottom-right corner of the screen.

2 Set the Trim Audio Start Point

To trim the audio file, you must set a start point and an end point. At the upper-right corner of the **Properties** panel you can see the clip duration, which helps give you an idea of how much you need to cut. Set the start point of the audio clip by moving the slider to the right, which removes a section from the beginning of the song. You don't need to set a new start point; you can leave the start point at the beginning of the song and just set a new end point.

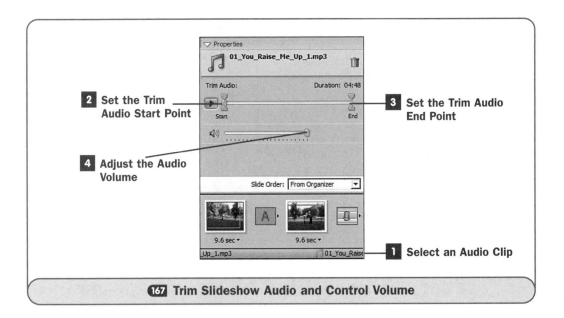

167 Trim Slideshow Audio and Control Volume

3 Set the Trim Audio End Point

Set the end point just like you set the start point, by dragging the slider. Drag the end point slider to the left, shortening the song and removing a section from the end of the clip. This might be your best option for trimming an audio clip, at least to start with. Most songs have a lot of very quiet, if not dead, space at the end of the clip. You can easily trim a few seconds from the end of most audio clips without even noticing a difference.

After you have set your new start and end points, click the little **play** button to the left of the start point to listen to your trimmed clip. You can adjust the start and end points repeatedly until you get it just right.

4 Adjust the Audio Volume

Just below the **Trim Audio** section of the **Properties** panel is the clip's **Volume** control. This is a simple slider; moving it to the right makes the audio louder, whereas moving it to the left makes the audio quieter.

168 Add Graphics, Text, and Narration to Your Slideshow

✔ **BEFORE YOU BEGIN**

162 Create a Slideshow in Photoshop Elements

163 Rotate, Size, and Edit Your Images

→ **SEE ALSO**

87 Grab a Still from Video

109 Add Narration to Your Movie

135 Use and Customize a Title Template

140 Create a Title from Scratch

156 About Sharing Files

Because Photoshop Elements primarily deals with graphics, you would expect it to have a little extra in the graphics department—and it does. There is a long list of graphics you can add to your slides, from animals to ornaments and more. The list of graphics categories is quite extensive.

The ability to add text in various fonts, sizes, styles, and colors is another great feature of Photoshop Elements. Adding text can create a whole new dimension to your slideshows.

Graphics and text are added on a slide-by-slide basis and last for the duration of that slide only.

One thing that really surprises me is that Photoshop Elements lets you add narration to your slideshows (a feature that doesn't yet exist in Premiere Elements). Adding narration to your slideshows is a real bonus and is easy to use. You'll need a computer microphone for the narration part of this task; if you have one, set it up. If you don't have a microphone, you can purchase one for as little as $10 at a local department or computer store.

▶ **NOTE**

You can create a narration for Premiere Elements using the narration feature in Photoshop Elements. In Photoshop Elements, create a small slideshow (you need only one image) and record your narration. Then export your slideshow as a Windows Media file (as explained in 169 Export Your Slideshow). In Premiere Elements, import the WMV file you created and remove the video portion, as explained in 100 Remove Audio and Video from a Clip; you have just created a narration audio file for use in Premiere Elements.

1 Select Graphics

To add a graphic to a slide, click the **Graphics** button in the upper-right corner of the **Extras** panel, below the **Preview** button. This action opens a list of graphics categories from which you can select many graphic images. To get an idea of what there is to choose from, open the individual categories by clicking the little arrow to the right of each category title. When you are finished browsing, move on to step 2.

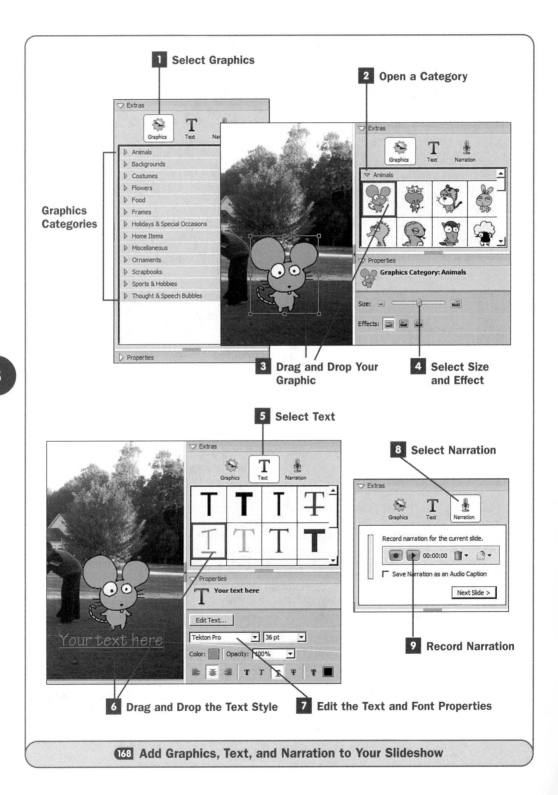

168 Add Graphics, Text, and Narration to Your Slideshow

2 Open a Category

Open one of the **Graphics** categories (such as the **Animals** category) by clicking the small arrow just to the right of the category name. All the images in that category are now available to be placed on the current slide in the **Monitor** window.

3 Drag and Drop Your Graphic

In this example, I selected the mouse graphic in the **Animals** category; take your pick—there are many to choose from. After you have found a suitable image, drag it from the **Extras** panel and drop the image on your slide in the **Monitor** window.

4 Select Size and Effect

After dropping the graphic on the slide, notice the eight sizing handles around the image. You can drag these handles to make the image larger or smaller. If you click the center of the image, you can drag the it to any area of the slide.

Take a look at the versatile **Properties** panel; now it has graphics properties for you to adjust. You can resize the graphic image by using the **Size** slider: Drag to the right to make the image larger; drag to the left to make the image smaller. You can also select one of three color **Effects** for your graphic: **Color**, **Black and White**, or **Sepia**.

168

5 Select Text

To add text to the slide in the **Monitor** window, click the **Text** button just to the right of the **Graphics** button in the **Extras** panel. This action opens a list of available text styles from which you can choose.

6 Drag and Drop the Text Style

Select a text style you like, drag it to the slide in the **Monitor** window, and drop it there. The sizing handles become available so you can resize the text right in the **Monitor**. If you click the center of the text area, you can drag the text box to a new location on the slide.

7 Edit the Text and Font Properties

Notice that the **Properties** panel holds the text properties. From the **Properties** panel, you can click the **Edit Text** button to display a dialog box in which you can edit the text that appears on the slide. From the drop-down lists, you can select a new font or specify a new point size for the text. You can choose a new color for the text by clicking the **Color** box, and you can even specify the **Opacity** of the text—for example, you might want the text to appear like it's fading into the image by setting the **Opacity** to something less than 100%. Set the **Text Justification** by clicking one of the three alignment buttons, and set the attributes of the text by clicking the **Bold**, **Italics**, **Underline**, and **Strikethrough** buttons as desired. If you want to give your text a **Drop Shadow**, click the **T** button that's second the right and choose the **Color** of the drop shadow by clicking the last button at the bottom of the **Properties** panel.

8 Select Narration

You can add narration to your slideshow; just imagine your voice or the voice of another person explaining what's happening on the current slide. Click the **Narration** button just to the right of the **Text** button at the top of the **Extras** panel. The **Record Narration** panel opens. It includes a vertical **Audio Meter** to watch so that the voice isn't too loud or too soft, a **Record button** (which becomes a **Stop** button after you click it), a **Play** button so you can listen to your narration, the **Recorded Narration Time**, a **Trash Can** so you can delete your recorded narration, a **File Folder** that opens an existing narration file and audio captions, and a **Save your Narration as an Audio Caption** check box. Click the **Next Slide** button so you can continue to add narration to the various slides in your slideshow, one slide at a time.

168

▶ **TIP**

It is usually best to write a script before attempting to record your narration. Even a few notes is better than nothing because the more prepared you are, the fewer times you will have to delete the narration and start over. Rehearsing your narration a few times before you actually start recording also can save you some time and aggravation.

9 Record Narration

To record your slide narration, you need a microphone. Connect your microphone to the computer and place it somewhere close by. It is best not to hold the microphone if you can help it; doing so just adds unwanted noise to your narration. When you are all set, click the red **Record** button and talk away.

▶ **NOTE**

Narration can be recorded for only one slide at a time. The length of your narration determines the length of the slide. If you have a slide duration of 5 seconds and record a 10-second narration, the slide duration is automatically increased to 10 seconds. If you have a 10-second slide duration and record a 5-second narration, however, the duration of the slide does not change.

169 Export Your Slideshow

✔ BEFORE YOU BEGIN

145 Create an Auto-Play DVD
156 About Sharing Files
162 Create a Slideshow in Photoshop Elements

→ SEE ALSO

142 Output a Windows Media (WMV) File
143 Output an MPEG File
172 About DVD Menus and the Template Editor

After you've finished creating your slideshow in Photoshop Elements, you can output the slideshow and share it with family and friends, or maybe just watch it yourself. This final step of the slideshow is where you get to see all the hard work and creativity you have put into your slideshow.

Photoshop Elements lets you output your slideshow in various file formats: Windows Media File (WMV) or Photoshop PDF, or (if you have a Windows Media Center PC) right to your television from your computer.

▶ **NOTE**

A Windows Media Center PC is a computer equipped with the Windows XP Media Center Edition operating system. Most of these PCs come with hardware and software enhancements for playing audio and video, such as surround sound audio cards and TV tuner/capture cards.

▶ **TIP**

Before outputting your slideshow, be sure to preview it using the **Preview** button. You want to catch any problems now before you post it on the Internet, send it in an email, or burn it to a CD or DVD.

1 Click the Output Button

Open your slideshow in the Photoshop Elements Slideshow Editor and click the **Output** button, located just above the **Monitor** window next to the **Add Media** button. The **Slideshow Output** dialog box opens. From there, you have four choices for what you can do with the slideshow:

- Save As a File
- Burn to Disc
- Email Slideshow
- Send to TV

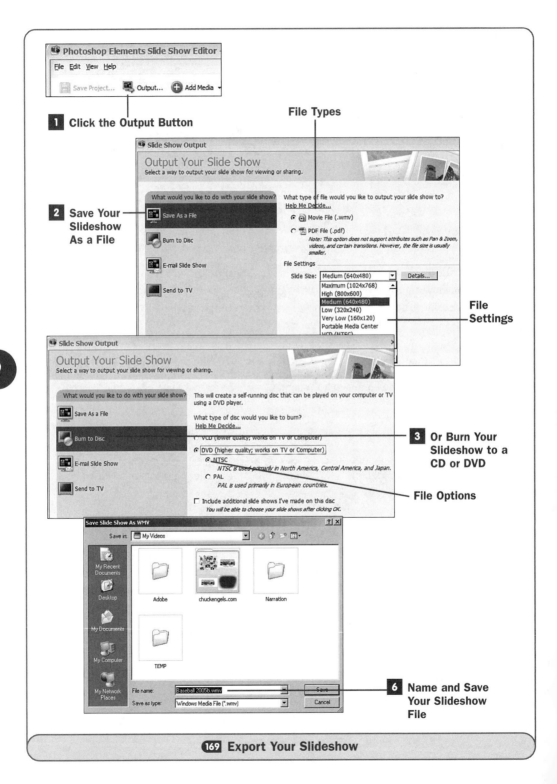

1 Click the Output Button

File Types

2 Save Your Slideshow As a File

File Settings

3 Or Burn Your Slideshow to a CD or DVD

File Options

6 Name and Save Your Slideshow File

169 Export Your Slideshow

169

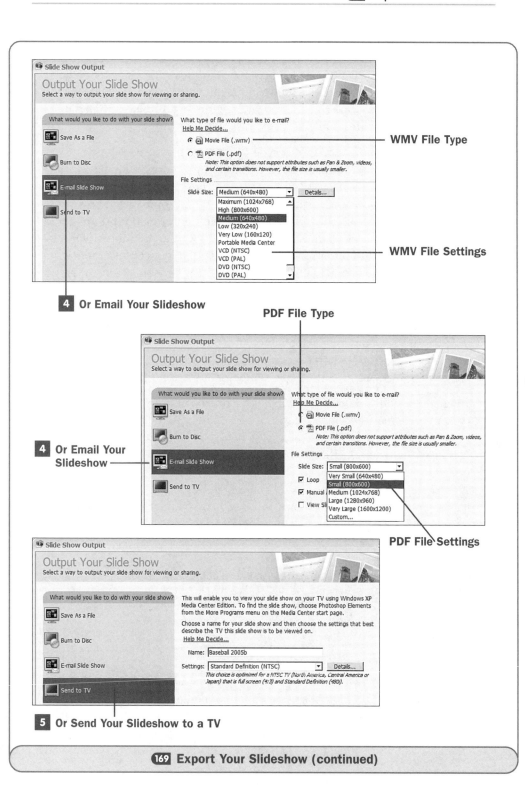

WMV File Type

WMV File Settings

4 Or Email Your Slideshow

PDF File Type

4 Or Email Your Slideshow

PDF File Settings

5 Or Send Your Slideshow to a TV

2 Save Your Slideshow As a File

From the **Slideshow Output** dialog box, select the **Save As a File** option if you want to save the slideshow as a Windows movie file or a PDF file that you can store on your computer or do what with. The file option properties open on the right side of the screen.

If you save the file in WMV format, you can import the file into Premiere Elements, burn it to a CD (if it does not exceed the maximum file size of 700MB, depending on the CD), or play it on a computer with Windows Media Player. You have various size and quality choices that come with the WMV file. The file size can range from **Portable Media Center** to **Maximum**, and from **DVD** to **VCD** in **PAL** (most of Europe) or **NTSC** (USA and Japan) formats. The **Maximum** setting creates a larger file than does the **Portable Media Center** setting, and the **DVD** options create a larger file than do the VCD setting. Just remember, the better the quality and the larger the slide image, the more space the file will take up on your computer or on a disc. You probably wouldn't want to email a 30-minute slideshow at maximum quality because the file would be way too large. After selecting a quality and size setting, click the **Details** button to get a good idea of what the resulting file will be good for and some technical information about how it will be created.

The other option you have for saving your slideshow as a file is PDF. The resulting PDF file can be opened with the free Adobe Acrobat Reader. Again, when you choose the **PDF File** option, you have various options as to quality and size—the larger the slideshow image and quality, the larger the resulting PDF file will be. If you choose a very small setting (such as **640 × 480**) for a short slideshow, the resulting PDF file might be small enough to email. PDF files can also be put on a DVD or CD and be viewed on a computer that has a compatible drive and the Adobe Acrobat Reader software.

▶ NOTE

Some slideshow features are not supported when you output a slideshow as a PDF file. Pan and zoom effects do not appear, video clips in your slideshow do not appear, and some transitions (such as the **Center Shape** and **Clock Wipe** transitions) are converted to the **Fade** transition.

3 Or Burn Your Slideshow to a CD or DVD

From the **Slideshow Output** dialog box, select the **Burn to Disc** option if you want to create a CD or DVD. The file option properties on the right side of the dialog box change to show VCD (video CD) and DVD options. Select the **VCD** option to create a file that will be burned to a CD directly from Photoshop Elements. The **Burn VCD** dialog box opens, and you can select the device you

169

want to burn to and the speed at which you want to write to the CD; then you can burn your VCD. The resulting CD can be played on most computers and some DVD players. The size of the resulting video file is smaller than that of the same video burned to a DVD. And because the file is smaller, the quality is also lower.

Select the **DVD** option if you want to create a high-quality WMV file in either **PAL** (for Europe) or **NTSC** (for North America, Central America, and Japan) format. After the WMV file is created, it is placed in the current, open Premiere Elements project; the slideshow is placed on the Timeline; and the DVD workspace is opened. From there, you can create menus and author the DVD See **145 Create an Auto-Play DVD** and **146 Set DVD Chapter Markers**.

4 Or Email Your Slideshow

From the **Slideshow Output** dialog box, select the **Email Slideshow** option if you want to create a file you can email to your family and friends. Photoshop Elements includes a contact list in which you can save your contact information so you can email family and friends without leaving the program. When you create a file to email, you can choose to create either a WMV or a PDF file and choose from various images sizes and quality settings. After you make your selections, the file is created and the Photoshop Elements **Attach Selected Items to Email** dialog box opens. There, you can select or add a contact, write a message, add photos, and open your email program with everything filled out and the slideshow file already identified as an attachment.

5 Or Send Your Slideshow to a TV

The final way you can choose to output your slideshow from Photoshop Elements is as a Windows XP Media Center file. If you have Windows Media Center, you can select the **Send to TV** option from the **Slideshow Output** dialog box. This option opens a set of property options where you give the slideshow a name and select the type of TV on which the slideshow will be displayed. For help determining the TV settings to choose, click the **Help Me Decide** link.

6 Name and Save Your Slideshow File

When you save your slideshow as a WMV file, you must give it a name and select the location where it will be stored. You do that in the **Save Slideshow as WMV** dialog box. Select the location for the file, give it a name, and click the **Save** button. Your file is saved to the selected location.

170 Make an Instant Slideshow in Premiere Elements

✔ BEFORE YOU BEGIN

- **84** Add Media with the Adobe Media Downloader
- **88** Prepare a Still for Video
- **89** Scale and Position a Still
- **161** About Slideshows

→ SEE ALSO

- **86** Trim Clips in the Media Panel
- **104** Add a Video Transition
- **162** Create a Slideshow in Photoshop Elements
- **171** Change Slides to the Beat of Music

If you have a selection of still images, Premiere Elements can automatically turn them into a slideshow on your **Timeline**. In addition, this feature gives you the option of customizing several of the slideshow's characteristics.

▶ **NOTE**

Although we usually think of slides as still images, the Premiere Elements **Create Slideshow** feature can also be used to load video clips, which will play at the intervals you designate in the **Still Image Duration** setting.

170

1 Arrange the Order of the Stills

A convenient feature of the Premiere Elements **Create Slideshow** tool is that it can add stills to the **Timeline** in the order they appear in the **Media** panel—this is usually much easier than rearranging the order of the slides after the stills have been placed on the **Timeline**. In the **Media** panel, arrange your stills in the order you want them to appear in the final slideshow. To do so, click the **Media** panel's **More** button and select the **Icon View**. You can then arrange your clips in any order by simply dragging them around within the panel.

You might find it helpful to create a separate folder in the **Media** panel for the still images, separating your stills from the rest of your project's media.

▶ **NOTE**

As an alternative to presorting your stills before creating the slideshow, you can select the slides in the order you want them arranged on the **Timeline**. To do so, hold down the **Ctrl** key and click to select the stills or clips one at a time in the **Media** panel. After you've gathered your slides and chosen **More**, **Create Slideshow**, set the **Ordering** option to **Selection Order**.

An alternative method of arranging your photos in the **Media** panel is to use **List** view (click **More** and choose **View, List**) and sort the stills alphanumerically by clicking the word **Name** at the top of the media list. (Click **Name** a second time to reverse the sort order.)

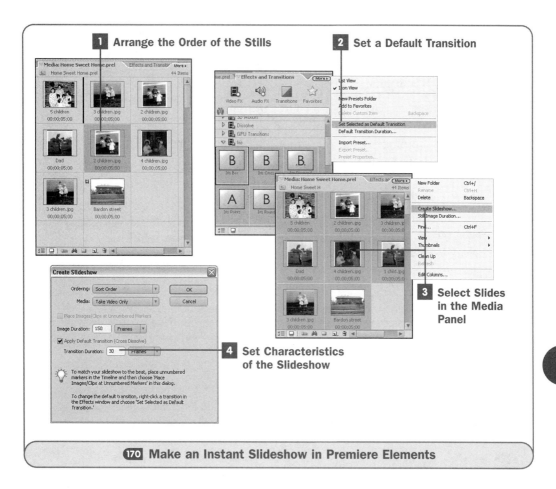

1 Arrange the Order of the Stills

2 Set a Default Transition

3 Select Slides in the Media Panel

4 Set Characteristics of the Slideshow

170 Make an Instant Slideshow in Premiere Elements

170

▶ **TIP**

You can easily change the names of your clips or stills so this sorting method puts them in the order you prefer. To do so, click the name of any clip, pause a moment, and then click again (or right-click and select **Rename**). The still or clip's name becomes an editable field. Type the new name and press **Enter**. Changing the name of a clip in the **Media** panel does not change the name of the file on your computer's hard drive. The only things that change are how the clip is displayed in Premiere Elements and, ultimately, how that clip is sorted by the **Media** panel.

2 Set a Default Transition

Your slideshow can be set to generate with a transition between each slide on the **Timeline**. If you choose this option, the default transition placed between each slide is initially a **Cross-Dissolve**.

To change the default transition, open the **Effects and Transitions** panel and browse to your preferred transition (see 🔲 **Add a Video Transition**). Note that clicking any transition starts a thumbnail preview of that transition. The current default transition will be outlined.

When you have selected your preferred transition, click the **More** button in the **Effects and Transitions** panel and select **Set Selected as Default Transition**. A blue box appears around the transition indicating that it is now your program default.

③ Select Slides in the Media Panel

Select the stills or clips you want to use in the slideshow either by holding down the **Shift** key and selecting the first and last of the series (all clips between are automatically selected) or by holding down the **Ctrl** key and clicking to select individual clips in the **Media** panel.

▶ TIP

As an alternative to ordering the clips in the **Media** panel as described in step 1, you can hold down the **Ctrl** key and click in the **Media** panel to select the clips or stills in the order you want them to appear.

170

▶ NOTE

The **Create Slideshow** feature loads your clips or stills to the **Timeline** in the order you have arranged them in the **Media** panel or by the order in which you select them.

④ Set Characteristics of the Slideshow

With all your stills or clips selected, click the **More** button in the **Media** panel and choose **Create Slideshow**. The **Create Slideshow** dialog box opens.

If the **Ordering** option is set to **Sort Order**, the slides appear on the **Timeline** in the order they are arranged in the **Media** panel. If, rather than ordering the clips in the **Media** panel, you selected them in the order you want them to appear in your slideshow, choose the **Selection** option to instruct the program to sort your clips in the order you selected them.

Disable the **Place Images/Clips at Unnumbered Markers** option and enable the **Apply Default Transition (Cross Dissolve)** option, which you specified in step 2, if you want to use a transition and set the duration of the transition in frames or seconds. You can also set the **Image Duration** in frames or seconds.

Click **OK**. A slideshow is automatically generated on your **Timeline**, beginning at the position of the current time indicator (CTI).

171 Change Slides to the Beat of Music

✔ BEFORE YOU BEGIN	→ SEE ALSO
84 Add Media with the Adobe Media Downloader	86 Trim Clips in the Media Panel
88 Prepare a Still for Video	119 Pan and Zoom Still Images a la Ken Burns
89 Scale and Position a Still	146 Set DVD Chapter Markers
170 Make an Instant Slideshow in Premiere Elements	

Video is a medium of motion ("movies move"). It is also a medium of both visuals and sound. Ideally, neither should happen independently of the other—rather, both should work together to tell the story you want to tell.

Just as there should be meaning to the motion added to your still images onscreen (see 119 **Pan and Zoom Still Images a la Ken Burns**), any marriage of your visuals to your sound makes the experience of watching your video much more interesting.

One simple way to marry sound and visuals is to synchronize the cuts in your video or your slideshow to the beat or rhythm of a music track. Although this can be, and often is, done manually on the **Timeline**, Premiere Elements contains tools in its **Create Slideshow** dialog box that enable you to sync the cuts in your slideshow to your music almost automatically.

1 Place a Music Clip on the Timeline

Drag your desired music clip from the **Media** panel to the **Timeline**. The audio track is displayed as a series of sound peaks and valleys. Occasionally, you can actually *see* the beat displayed in these peaks—most likely, though, you'll have to find the beat manually.

Click the **Play** button in the **Monitor** panel or press the **spacebar** on your keyboard to play the audio clip. As the music plays, watch the movement of the current time indicator. By listening for a drum beat, guitar riff, or other repeating element, you'll soon get a feel for the rhythm of the music. By watching the CTI, you can soon estimate the time interval between each beat.

In the example shown here—Blind Melon's "No Rain"—I noted that rhythmic slide changes should happen approximately every second.

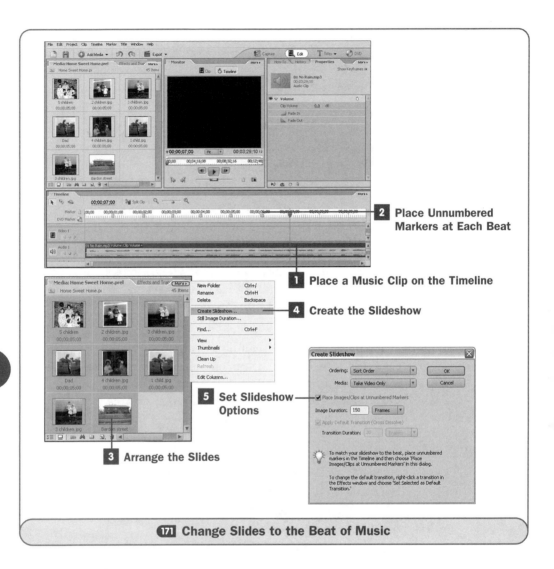

171 Change Slides to the Beat of Music

2 Place Unnumbered Markers at Each Beat

You should place an unnumbered marker at each beat in the audio file. The markers indicate where the slides will change. To place an unnumbered marker, click the **Marker** icon at the upper-left corner of the **Timeline**. (The **DVD Marker** is used in **146 Set DVD Chapter Markers**.)

Create a series of unnumbered markers by clicking the **Marker** icon and moving the CTI down the **Timeline**. The markers can be easily repositioned and don't have to be in their final positions when you create them. Create markers on the **Timeline** until you have one for every slide you plan to add to your slideshow.

Slide the markers into position on the **Timeline** at the approximate locations of the beats in your music. Reset your CTI and play the music clip again, watching the movement of the CTI over your markers and adjusting their positions as necessary.

You might find it more intuitive to play the music, clicking the **Marker** icon at each beat. The program drops an unnumbered marker at the CTI position each time you click the icon.

Spend some time getting these markers positioned as accurately as possible. Doing so will save you a lot of tweaking and trimming of your clips later.

3 Arrange the Slides

Ordering your slides in the **Media** panel ensures that they'll be in the correct order when you create your slideshow. You might want to create a new folder in this panel and move your still images into the folder so you can better manage the image files.

Rearrange the order of your slides by dragging and dropping them in the **Media** panel while in the **Icon** view. The order the slides are in the **Media** panel when you select them for your slideshow is the order they will appear on the **Timeline** when you create your instant slideshow.

▶ **NOTE**

Although we usually think of slides as still images, the **Create Slideshow** feature can also load video clips that play at the intervals and duration you designate. You can also set your video clips to change in time with the rhythm of a music clip, just as you can still images.

4 Create the Slideshow

Select the stills or clips you want to use in the slideshow by either holding down the **Shift** key and clicking the first and last clip (the first, last, and those clips in between are selected) or by holding down the **Ctrl** key and clicking to select one clip or image at a time.

When all the clips are selected, click the **Media** panel's **More** button and select **Create Slideshow**. The **Create Slideshow** dialog box opens.

5 Set Slideshow Options

Enable the **Place Images/Clips at Unnumbered Markers** option.

You can also place the default transitions between your clips, although doing so might minimize the effect of cutting the images in rhythm to your music clip.

171

Click **OK** to close the dialog box; your slideshow is created. Beginning at the first unnumbered marker, each slide changes in rhythm with the beat of the music.

Play your musical slideshow; if you're a little off the beat, you can lengthen or shorten the individual slides accordingly on the **Timeline** by dragging the edge of each slide to make it a bit longer or shorter as needed (see **95** **Trim a Clip on the Timeline**). You might find it helpful to use the slider at the top of the **Timeline** to zoom in so you can make precise adjustments.

If the whole slideshow is off the beat slightly, adjust its entire position by dragging to lasso the entire range of slides as a group and then dragging to move the group of slides up or down the **Timeline** a frame or two. You might find it helpful to use the + key to zoom into the **Timeline** as close as possible when making very fine adjustments.

171

29

Using DVD Menu Templates

IN THIS CHAPTER:

DVD menus provide a nice introduction to your DVD before your movie actually starts playing. Although you can have an auto-play DVD without a menu, most people like having a menu that lets them navigate through the DVD. A DVD menu provides options in the form of buttons that allow the person viewing the movie to make some choices. These buttons can include **Play, Scene Menu, Main Menu, Next**, and **Previous**. If you have played a commercial DVD, you have probably noticed all the options available from the DVD menu. Much of what you see in the menu system of a commercial DVD is available to you in the Photoshop Elements **DVD Template Editor**.

Premiere Elements has more than 70 DVD menu templates grouped in categories such as **Entertainment, General, Birthday, New Baby, Party Celebrations, Seasons, Sports, Travel**, and **Wedding**. The templates are not very customizable in Premiere Elements, but they can be completely customized in Photoshop Elements. If you have ever watched a commercial DVD movie, you have seen a DVD menu, which is used to navigate through the many DVD options. A DVD menu is usually divided into a main menu and a scene menu. The main menu contains buttons that take you to various options and might include Play, Next, Previous, Scenes, and Special Features, to name a few. The scene menu also contains buttons, but these buttons take you to a particular spot in the movie (the scene menu also typically includes navigation buttons such as Next, Previous, and a button to return to the main menu).

The DVD menu templates contain one main menu and a single scene menu that can be duplicated as many times as necessary to hold buttons for all your movie's *scene markers*. The scene menu templates vary, with some having room for more scene buttons than others. However, the maximum number of scene buttons a scene menu can include is six because of available space. If you use one of the DVD menu templates and have 12 scene markers in your movie, Premiere Elements creates one main menu and two scene menus. Each scene menu then has six scene buttons for a total of 12 scenes.

Premiere Elements allows you to make some changes to the menu; you can add a different background, specify menu audio, and decide whether the menu will have motion. That is about it. If all you want to do is change the background, you can do that in Premiere Elements without using the Photoshop Elements **DVD Template Editor**. The **DVD Template Editor** has nothing to do with the audio on your DVD menu, which is controlled by Premiere Elements. Changing menu text and buttons (not the text on the buttons but the style and position of the buttons), on the other hand, can be done only in the Photoshop Elements **DVD Template Editor**. What you want to do with your menu dictates which program you will use to do it. To get familiar with the DVD menus and what can be done to them, **172 About the DVD Template Editor** goes through the DVD menu options for both programs. When you have a good understanding of what can be changed and what program to use, you can move on to **173** **Modify an Existing DVD Menu Template** and learn to create new templates from scratch in **174** **Create a DVD Menu Template from Scratch**.

---

172 About DVD Menus and the DVD Template Editor

✔ BEFORE YOU BEGIN	→ SEE ALSO
1 Import Media from a Folder, CD-ROM, or DVD	**150** Customize a Menu with Any Background
149 Customize a DVD Menu Screen Template	**151** Create a Motion Menu
156 About Sharing Files	**175** Use Your DVD Menu Templates in Premiere Elements

---

First, we will take a look at the DVD workspace in Premiere Elements. Some elements of your DVD menus can be changed only in this workspace (the Photoshop Elements **DVD Template Editor** is of no use if that is the case). Audio and motion menus are handled only in the Premiere Elements DVD workspace. You can use either program to change a background. Depending on how much you want to change, the DVD workspace in Premiere Elements might be all you need.

- The **DVD menu preview window** shows an example of what your DVD menu will look like. There is only one thing you can do in the preview window: change the button text. Do this by double-clicking the button and typing into the text box that appears.

- The **Menu Background Properties** panel includes all the things you can change or add in regard to the DVD menu background. Here you can add a new menu background, such as a video clip or still image, by dragging clips from the **Media** panel to the small box labeled **Drag Media Here**. You can also drag clips to the media box from Windows Explorer or click the **Browse** button to search for a clip. You can set the in point (the place in the video clip where the clip starts playing) or use just one frame (a still image from the video). Click the **Play** arrow button to watch the selected clip, helping you locate the exact in point. You can also click and drag the **In Point** location numbers to the right or left, moving the clip forward and backward. If the video clip has to loop (that is, if the video clip ends before the viewer clicks a menu button, the clip replays until the viewer clicks a menu button), you can choose to add the default video transition to the loop. The **Reset** button reverts your menu to its default appearance.

172

DVD Menu Preview Window

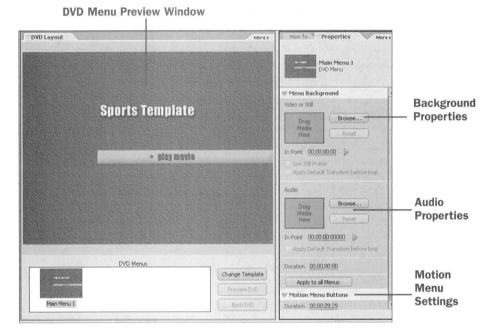

172

The DVD workspace in Premiere Elements.

▶ **NOTE**

The video transition with the blue border in the video transitions group, located in the **Effects and Transitions** panel, is the current default video transition. You can change the default video transition by right-clicking the transition you want to use as the default and selecting **Set Selected as Default Transition** from the context menu.

• The **Audio Properties** panel includes all the audio properties available to your DVD menu. Just like you did for the menu's background, you can drag audio clips into the small media box, set the audio clip's in point, play the audio file, and apply the default audio transition to the loop. The **Reset** button resets the menu audio to its default state. The **Duration** value, located below the **Audio Properties** panel, is the setting for the background video as well as for the audio; it is the length of time that the video and audio will play. The maximum duration is 29 seconds and 29 frames, at which point the audio and video loops back to the beginning. The **Apply to all Menus** button does just what it says: it applies the same background and audio to all your scene menus as well as the main DVD menu.

▶ **NOTE**

The audio transition with the blue border in the audio transitions group, located in the **Effects and Transitions** panel, is the current default audio transition. You can change the default audio transition by right-clicking the transition you want to use as the default and choosing **Set Selected as Default Transition** from the context menu.

- The **Motion Menu Buttons Properties** panel controls the scene menu buttons. The scene menu buttons can show a short clip, up to 29 seconds and 29 frames, of the video to which the scene marker points. You set the duration of the video clips used on the scene buttons here. A zero duration turns off the motion menu buttons; any value greater than that permits motion in the scene menu buttons.

▶ **TIP**

One added note about all this cool stuff you can add to your menus in Premiere Elements: the more background activity, audio, and motion menus you add, the more space it will all take up when you burn the project to a DVD. To get the most video as possible onto a DVD, at the highest possible quality, keep your extras to a minimum.

Eight steps are involved in modifying or creating a DVD menu template in the Photoshop Elements **DVD Template Editor**. The steps take you through selecting a template, choosing a main menu background, selecting main menu buttons, specifying main menu text, choosing the scene menu background, selecting scene menu buttons, specifying scene menu text, and saving your template. The following list details each of these steps.

172

1 On the first screen of the **DVD Template Editor**, choose the DVD format you prefer (**NTSC** or **PAL**). If you want to create your own menu template, choose the **Start from Scratch** option and refer to **174 Create a DVD Menu Template from Scratch**. If you want to use one of the many existing menu templates, choose the **Start from an Existing Template** option and refer to **173 Modify an Existing DVD Menu Template**. If you choose **Start from an Existing Template**, you can select from the list of templates you see on the screen or browse for more templates.

2 The second screen of the **DVD Template Editor** is where you start modifying the main menu. Here you see the DVD template preview and work area, where all the template details appear. Notice the navigation buttons in the lower-right corner of the screen: **Back** takes you to the previous step, **Next** takes you to the next step, **Finish** takes you to the last step, and **Cancel** takes you back to the Photoshop Elements **Editor**. Here in step 2, you choose the background for your menu; you can select from the list or browse for more backgrounds. Any image, even a photograph, can be a background as long as it is in a Photoshop-compatible format (see **156 About Sharing Files** for more information about file formats).

Start from
Scratch

Select NTSC or
PAL Format

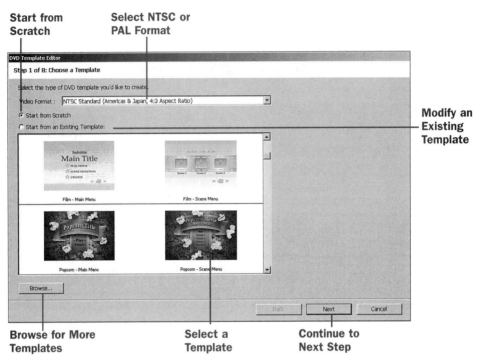

Modify an
Existing
Template

172

Browse for More
Templates

Select a
Template

Continue to
Next Step

*The first screen of the **DVD Template Editor**.*

Background
Selection List

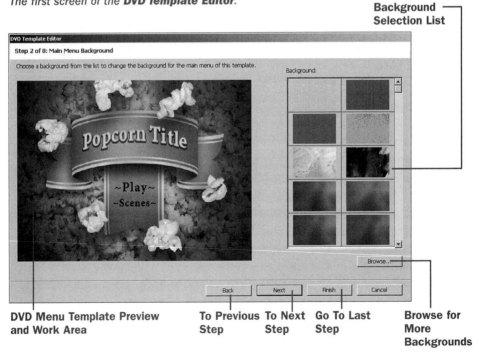

DVD Menu Template Preview
and Work Area

To Previous
Step

To Next
Step

Go To Last
Step

Browse for
More
Backgrounds

*The second screen of the **DVD Template Editor**.*

3 In the third screen of the **DVD Template Editor**, you add, modify, select, and delete the main menu buttons. Click the **Add** button to add a new button to the main menu, or click the **Delete Selections** button to delete the buttons from the main menu. The familiar **Back, Next, Finish,** and **Cancel** buttons appear as well. You can choose from six button types: **Home, Previous, Next, Play, Scene menu,** and **Main Menu Marker.** After you select the type of button, the button selection list is updated to show a wide range of button styles.

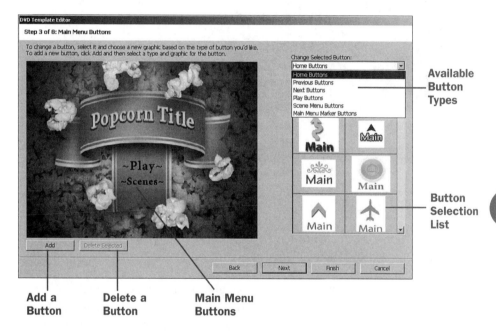

Add a Button   Delete a Button   Main Menu Buttons

*The third screen of the **DVD Template Editor**.*

4 In the fourth screen of the **DVD Template Editor**, you can add text to your menu and change the default button text. Click the **Add Text** button to add text; when you do so, a text box appears on the preview screen. Click the **Delete Selected** button to delete the selected text. The familiar **Back, Next, Finish,** and **Cancel** buttons appear in the lower-right corner of the screen. The **Text Properties** area gives you the ability to change the selected text characteristics. Change the actual menu text by typing in the **Change Selected Text** box. You can also change the text's font, change the **Font Characteristics** (**Bold, Italics,** and so on) by using the drop-down menu or by clicking the style buttons, change the text size, change the text's color, and choose a **Text Effect** from the drop-down list (which includes a variety of text effects such as **Drop Shadow, Outer Glow,** and **Gradient Overlay** to name a few).

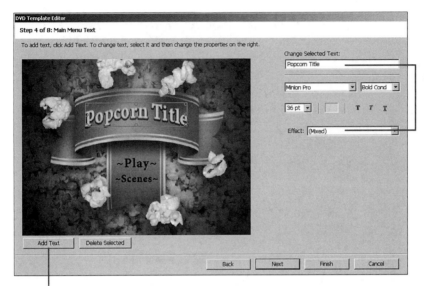

Add Text

The fourth screen of the ***DVD Template Editor.***

172

5 In steps 5–7 of the **DVD Template Editor**, you repeat steps 2–4, this time for a scene menu. The scene menu contains buttons for each scene marker in the movie; if your movie has more scene markers than will fit on a single scene menu, additional scene menus are created and the scene menus also have Next and Previous buttons; the scene menu always has a button to return to the main menu. Other than these details, the steps for creating scene menu buttons and main menu buttons are identical. After the menu template is created, you can add video and motion to your scene menu buttons when creating the DVD menu in Premiere Elements.

The scene menu can be repeated as many times as necessary to show all your movie's chapter/scene markers (refer to **146** **Set DVD Chapter Markers**).

8 The final screen of the **DVD Template Editor** is where you name and save your DVD menu template. The screen is very simple—it gives you a **Template Name** text box in which you type the name of the template, as well as **Back**, **Save**, and **Cancel** buttons.

When you save the template, it is automatically saved with the rest of the DVD menu templates and is available from the DVD menu template selection list in Premiere Elements.

Now that you have a good idea of what is involved in modifying DVD menu templates in both Premiere Elements and Photoshop Elements, you are ready to let your menu-creating adventure begin. In the tasks that follow, you learn how to modify an existing DVD menu, create a DVD menu from scratch, and finally use the menus you create in your Premiere Elements DVD project.

---

173 **Modify an Existing DVD Menu Template**

✔ BEFORE YOU BEGIN	→ SEE ALSO
172 About DVD Menus and the DVD Template Editor	**149** Customize a DVD Menu Screen Template
	151 Create a Motion Menu
	153 Add Audio to a Menu
	175 Use Your DVD Menu Templates in Premiere Elements

Now that you have learned about the DVD menu templates in **172** **About DVD Menus and the DVD Template Editor**, you are ready to take an existing template and make it your own. You can change as little or as much about the template as you like—whatever suits your taste.

173

▶ **NOTE**

In preparation for this task, you might want to take a quick look through the various templates available in Premiere Elements (see **149** **Customize a DVD Menu Screen Template**.) There you can get a larger view of the templates and choose the one you want to make changes to. Remember the name of the menu template so you can find the menu template again when you are on the **Step 1 of 8** screen of the **DVD Template Editor**.

In this example, I'll use the **Toy Train** template for modification. In this task, you will modify the existing background, buttons, and text for both the main menu and the scene menus. Open the Photoshop Elements **Editor** to get started.

1 **Open the DVD Template Editor**

From the main menu in the Photoshop Elements **Editor**, select **File**, **New**, **DVD Template**. The **DVD Template Editor** opens to Step 1 of 8: Choose a Template.

2 **Select Start from an Existing Template**

Because this task modifies an existing template, select the **Start from an Existing Template** radio button. If you want to create a template from scratch, see **174** **Create a DVD Menu Template from Scratch**.

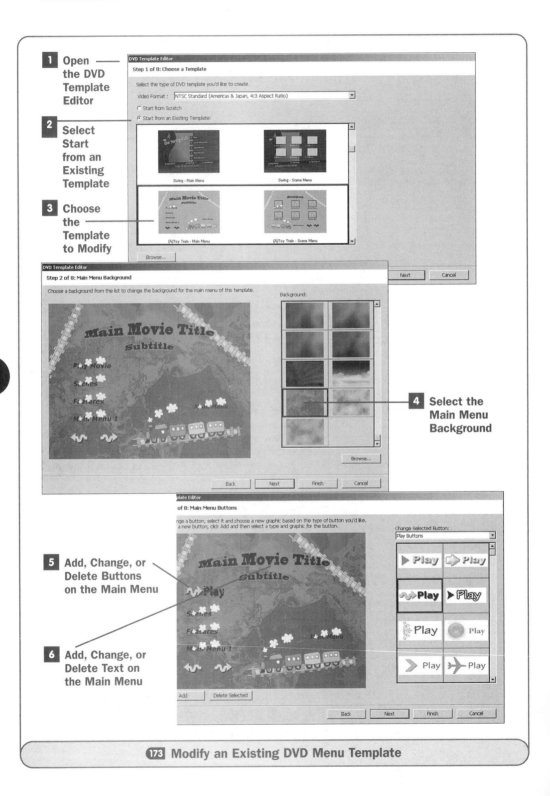

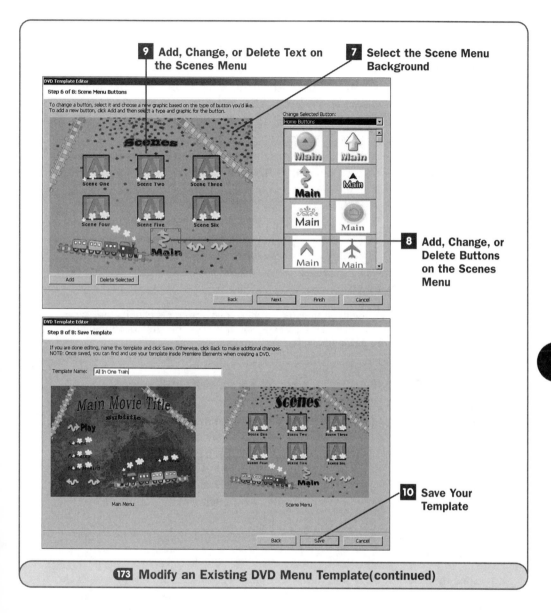

9 Add, Change, or Delete Text on the Scenes Menu

7 Select the Scene Menu Background

8 Add, Change, or Delete Buttons on the Scenes Menu

10 Save Your Template

173

173 Modify an Existing DVD Menu Template(continued)

3 Choose Template to Modify

Select the template you want to modify. If you had one in mind before starting the task, find it now using the scrollbar on the right side of the template selection area. If you don't have any particular template in mind, find and select the **Toy Train** template I used in the examples. When you have selected your template for editing, click the **Next** button to move to the **Step 2** screen.

4 ## Select the Main Menu Background

The **Step 2 of 8: Main Menu Background** screen appears. You have arrived at the place where the fun begins. To the right of the preview and work area are a number of backgrounds from which you can choose. Click one in the list to change the current background of the template in the preview window. Every time you click another background, the background in the preview window changes. If you want to use an image stored on your hard drive for the menu background, click **Browse** and browse to the file. You can use any Photoshop Elements-compatible file (photos or graphics) as a background for your DVD menu template. When you have found the right background, click the **Next** button to move to the **Step 3** screen.

▶ ## TIPS

You don't have to make changes to the template in a particular step. If you like the way that part of the template looks, just click the **Next** button without making any changes, and you move to the next step.

There is no reason to go through all the steps if all you want to do is change the background or some text. At any point in the process, you can click the **Finish** button and move to step 8, where you name and save your template.

173

5 ## Add, Change, or Delete Buttons on the Main Menu

The **Step 3 of 8: Main Menu Buttons** screen appears, where things get a bit trickier. Now it is time to add, change, or delete buttons.

To the right of the preview window is a list of button choices. Above that list is the **Change Selected Button** drop-down menu. Use the drop-down menu to select the type of button you want to add or change—for example, **Home** or **Main**, **Previous** or **Back**, **Next**, **Play**, **Scene**, and **Main Menu Marker**. Changing the type of button in this list changes the choices in the selection list below it. From the second list, you can choose from many styles of the selected button type.

Click the **Add** button to add a new button to your menu screen. (Before clicking **Add**, be sure you have selected the correct button type from the drop-down list and the desired button style from the selection list.)

To change a button you've already placed in the preview window, click the button in the work area and then click a new selection in the selection list. Click and drag any button you've placed on the menu screen to reposition it, or click a button and drag its sizing handles to make the button larger or smaller. When you have your buttons laid out the way you want them, click the **Next** button to move to the **Step 4** screen.

▶ **TIP**

At any time you need to, click the **Back** button to go back to the previous step.

6 Add, Change, or Delete Text on the Main Menu

The **Step 4 of 8: Main Menu Text** screen appears. In this step, you can add, change, or delete text from the menu template. There are basically two types of text on a menu template: button text and menu text. To add a text box for simple menu text, click the **Add Text** button; a text box appears on the work area. Type the desired text into the box, drag it into the proper position, and scale it to the proper size. If you want to change the text on an existing button, click the button and use the **Change the Selected Text** box in the **Text Properties** area to make your changes.

▶ **NOTE**

The button functionality cannot be changed. A **Play** button only plays the movie, and a **Scene** button only takes you to a scene. Changing the text on a button has no effect on the function the button performs.

The **Text Properties** area allows you to do many things with the text on the menu screen. For example, I changed the font of the *Main Movie Title* text to the **Bookman Old Style** font and added a **Stroke** effect. If you want to delete existing text, select the text and click the **Delete Selected** button. After making any text changes, additions, or deletions, click the **Next** button to move to the **Step 5** screen.

173

7 Select the Scene Menu Background

The **Step 5 of 8: Scene Menu Background** screen appears. Steps 5–7 are just like the last three steps, with the exception of the **Step 6 of 8** screen. In the **Step 5 of 8** screen, select the background for the scene menu just as you did for the background of the main menu in the **Step 2 of 8** screen. To keep the main menu and scene menu screens looking uniform, choose the same or a similar background for the scene menu as you choose for the main menu. After you have selected your scene menu background, click the **Next** button to move to the **Step 6 of 8** screen.

8 Add, Change, or Delete Buttons on the Scenes Menu

The **Step 6 of 8: Scene Menu Buttons** screen appears. The only differences between this step and the **Step 3 of 8** screen are the button types you can add. In the scene menu, you have fewer options for the types of buttons you can add, but you also have the scene marker buttons (the buttons that show a small thumbnail of each scene or chapter on your finished DVD, as explained in ⑭ **Auto Generat Scene Markers**, ⑭ **Set DVD Chapter Markers**, and ⑭ **Customize an Image As a Chapter Marker**. You can add, change, or delete these buttons in the same way you did the main menu buttons in the **Step 3 of 8** screen. When your buttons are just right, click the **Next** button to move to the **Step 7 of 8** screen.

⑨ Add, Change, or Delete Text on the Scenes Menu

The **Step 7 of 8: Scene Menu Text** screen appears. Here you have the opportunity to add, change, or delete text on the scene menu as well as the text characteristics. The process is identical to what you did in the **Step 4 of 8** screen: Click the text to select it; change the text in the **Change Selected Text** box in the upper-right corner of the screen; and make any desired changes to the text's font, size, and attributes. When your scene menu text is the way you like it, click the **Next** button to move to the final step.

⑩ Save Your Template

The **Step 8 of 8: Save Template** screen appears, showing both the main menu template and the scene menu template you just modified. Just above the view of the templates is a text box where you will enter a new name for your template.

After typing a name for your template, click the **Save** button. The template is saved along with all the other Premiere Elements templates. The next time you are in Premiere Elements, go to the **DVD Menu Template** selection list to see your new template listed along with all the other templates. If you would like to find the template you just created and use it for a DVD, see ⑰ **Use Your DVD Menu Template in Premiere Elements**.

▶ **NOTE**

To open the **DVD Menu Template** selection list from inside your Premiere Elements project, refer to ⑭ **Customize a DVD Menu Screen Template**.

---

174 Create a DVD Menu Template from Scratch

✔ BEFORE YOU BEGIN	→ SEE ALSO
⑫ About DVD Menus and the DVD Template Editor	⑭ Customize an Image as a Chapter Marker
	⑮ Create a Motion Menu
	⑮ Add Audio to a Menu

173

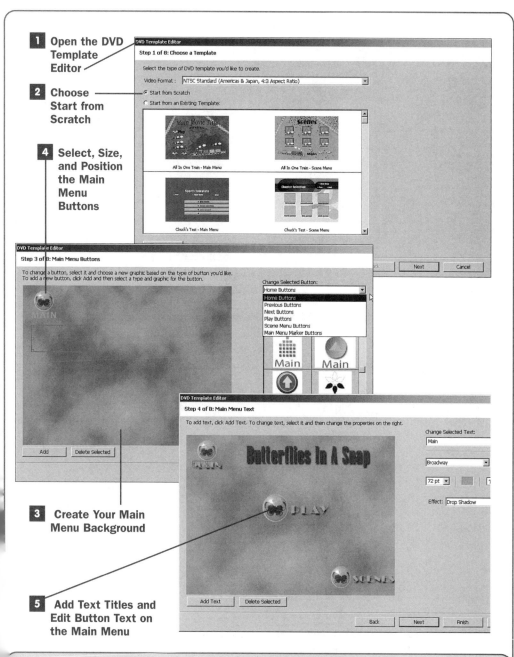

1 Open the DVD Template Editor

2 Choose Start from Scratch

4 Select, Size, and Position the Main Menu Buttons

3 Create Your Main Menu Background

5 Add Text Titles and Edit Button Text on the Main Menu

174

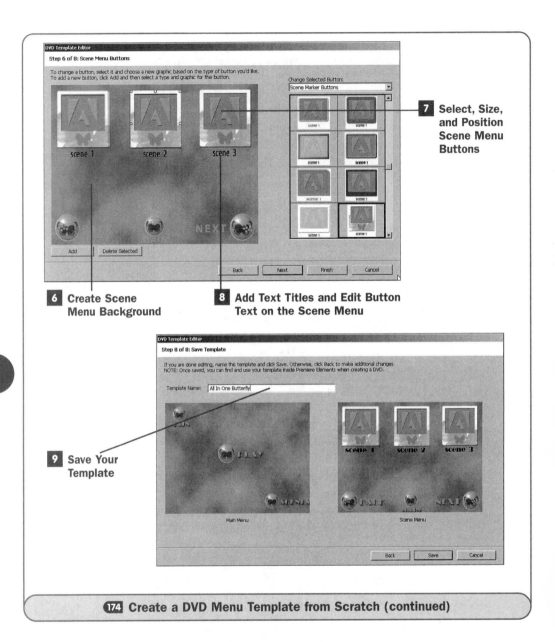

174

174 Create a DVD Menu Template from Scratch (continued)

If you have already read **173** Modify an Existing DVD Menu Template, this task will be easy for you. If you have not read the previous task, this current task will be something totally new. When you create a DVD menu from scratch, you start with a blank canvas instead of modifying an existing template. Creating your own DVD menu template takes a bit more creativity and design know-how. In the previous task, everything was laid out for you and all you had to do was change what was there. When you start from scratch, you have to build the whole thing.

In this example, I chose a butterfly theme and used existing items from the background selection list and button selection list. All the items I used in this example are available to you because they are part of what comes with the **DVD Template Editor.**

▶ **TIP**

You might want to jot down some notes or play around with some ideas on paper before you start creating your DVD menu in this task. Whenever you are ready, open the **Photoshop Elements Editor** to get started.

1 Open the DVD Template Editor

From the Photoshop Elements **Editor's** main menu choose **File, New, DVD Template.** The **DVD Template Editor** opens to the **Step 1** screen.

2 Choose Start from Scratch

Choose the file format in which you want to play the DVD you will ultimately create (**NTSC** or **PAL**), select the **Start from Scratch** radio button, and click the **Next** button. A blank template opens in the template work area.

3 Create Your Main Menu Background

The **Step 2 of 8: Main Menu Background** screen appears, where you can select the background for your main menu screen. (In the **Step 5 of 8** screen, you repeat what you do here when you add a background to your scene menu.) To the right of the work area is a list of available backgrounds. Click any of the background selections to apply that background to the blank template. Click another selection to replace the current background. If you want to use an image file stored on your hard disk as the background for this menu screen, click the **Browse** button and search for other files. You can use any Photoshop Elements-compatible file as a background for your template. After you have selected a background, click the **Next** button to move to the **Step 3** screen.

▶ **TIP**

At any time, you can click the **Back** button to go back to the previous step.

4 Select, Size, and Position the Main Menu Buttons

The **Step 3 of 8: Main Menu Buttons** screen appears. In this step, you add buttons to your main menu. Make sure you have at least a **Play** button and a **Scene Menu** button. First, select the **Home Buttons** option as the type of button you want to add from the **Change Selected Button** drop-down list.

174

Click the **Add** button located under the work area to put an empty box on your work area. Click any one of the buttons in the selection list to fill the empty box you added to the work area with the button you selected. Drag the button you just added to move it to the desired position on the screen.

▶ **NOTE**

If you are not going to set any scene markers for your movie, the scene menu is unnecessary. The scene menu exists solely for the purpose of taking the viewer to a particular scene(s) in the movie. However, if you think you will use this template again in another project, you should add the scene menu now, rather than going back to edit the template later.

From the **Change Selected Buttons** drop-down list, choose **Play Buttons** as the type of button you want to add and again click the **Add** button. Another blank box appears; when you click one of the buttons in the selection list, the box is filled in with the button you selected.

Repeat this process one more time to add a **Scene Menu Button**. If you make a mistake, click the erroneous button and click the **Deleted Selected** button. The selected button is deleted. When all the buttons for the main menu are in positions you like, click the **Next** button to move to the **Step 4** screen.

174

5 **Add Text Titles and Edit Button Text on the Main Menu**

The **Step 4 of 8: Main Menu Text** screen appears. In this step, you can add, change, or delete text from the template. There are basically two types of text on a menu template: button text and menu text. To add a text box for simple menu text, click the **Add Text** button; a text box appears on the work area. Drag the text box where you want it on the screen and use its sizing handles to scale it to the proper size. Change the text for a button by clicking the button in the work area and using the **Change Selected Text** box in the upper-right corner of the screen to make your changes. For both menu text and button text, you can make changes to the selected text only from the **Text Properties** area in the upper-right corner of the screen.

You can change many of the properties of your text. In this example, I changed the font of the three buttons to **Broadway** and added a **Drop Shadow** effect.

If you want to delete existing text (from the menu itself or from a button), select the text and then click the **Delete Selected** button. After making any desired text changes, additions, or deletions, click the **Next** button and move to the **Step 5** screen.

▶ **NOTE**

If you do not require a scene menu, you can skip the **Step 5–Step 7** screens by clicking the **Finish** button to move to the final step of saving the template. Not having a scene menu means that any chapter markers you created (refer to **146** Create DVD Chapter Markers) will not appear on the DVD when this template is used—that is, you will have only a main menu.

6 Create Scene Menu Background

Steps 6–8 (the **Step 5–Step 7** screens) are somewhat of a repeat of the previous three steps. In the previous steps, you were working with the main menu; now you are working with a blank scene menu. You must add a background, buttons, and text—just as you did for the main menu.

As you did for the main menu in the **Step 2** screen, select the background for your scene menu. When you are satisfied with your selection, click the **Next** button to move to the **Step 6** screen.

7 Select, Size, and Position Scene Menu Buttons

The **Step 6 of 8: Scene Menu Buttons** screen appears. As you did in the **Step 3** screen, choose the type of button you want to add to your scene menu screen from the **Change Selected Button** drop-down list and then choose the actual button from the selection list. The scene menu is repeated as many times as necessary to show all your movie's chapter/scene markers (refer to **146** Set DVD Chapter Markers).

174

▶ **NOTE**

If you have already set your scene/chapter markers and you know how many there are, you can make them fit evenly across the scene menus. Premiere Elements repeats the single scene menu until it can display all the scenes for which you have set markers. If you have 15 scenes, for example, you can spread those out over three or five scene menus. To spread them out over three scene menus, you need five scene buttons on the master scene menu; to spread the scene buttons out over five scene menus, you need only three scene buttons on the master scene menu.

You should ensure that the person viewing your movie can easily navigate through the scene menus. To make this possible, be sure to add a **Next** button, a **Back** button, all the scene buttons you will need, as well as a **Main Menu** button so the viewer can get back to where she started.

To insert scene marker buttons on the scene menu screen, first select **Scene Marker Buttons** from the **Change Selected Button** drop-down list. (You should create one scene marker button for each chapter marker you created in the DVD movie project.) Click the **Add** button to place a blank box in the work area. Click a button in the selection list to fill the box with that button. Notice that the scene marker buttons are a bit larger than the navigation buttons because each scene marker button holds a thumbnail image of the clip that will play when the person viewing the video clicks the button, see **148 Customize an Image as a Chapter Marker.**

If your video project has 12 chapter markers and your scene menu screen can hold 4 scene marker buttons, Premiere Elements automatically repeats the scene menu 3 times (3 screens × 4 button per screen = 12 scenes). You might not be able to display all 12 scene buttons on one scene menu screen because of the limited space available on each screen. Remember that, in addition to the scene buttons themselves, you must also include navigation buttons (such as **Next**, **Previous**, and **Main**). If you don't add the navigation buttons, the person viewing the DVD will get stuck in a scene menu with no way to get back to the main menu or to the next scene menu. When you have added all the buttons you want to this menu screen, click the **Next** button to move to **Step 7** screen.

▶ **NOTE**

174

After you set your scene markers for your movie in Premiere Elements, the scenes show up in chronological order from left to right on the scene menu, starting with your first scene marker. The first marker is the first scene button on the left, the second marker is the next button, and so on. If you have four scene markers and a scene menu with only three scene buttons, the first marker is the button farthest left on the first menu, the second marker is the middle button, and the third marker is the button on the left. Premiere Elements automatically duplicates the scene menu with only one scene button for the remaining marker. In the DVD workspace in Premiere Elements, you can easily see which button is attached to which scene marker by double-clicking the scene button. You can also choose the thumbnail image for the button and whether it is a motion menu button.

8 **Add Text Titles and Edit Button Text on the Scene Menu**

The **Step 7 of 8: Scene Menu Text** screen appears, where you have the opportunity to add, change, or delete text and the text characteristics for the menu items. The process is identical to what you did in the **Step 4 of 8** screen. When the scene menu text and scene menu button text are the way you want, click the **Next** button to move to the final step.

▶ **NOTE**

After you have created your template and added it to your Premiere Elements project, you can edit the button text. If you cannot remember the specific scene names while creating your template, you can use generic names such as **scene 1**, **scene 2**, and so on. When you get to the DVD workspace in Premiere Elements, you can add more meaningful names to your scene menu buttons.

9 Save Your Template

Congratulations, you have made it to the final step of creating your DVD menu template from scratch. On the **Step 8 of 8: Save Template** screen, give your template a name by typing the name in the **Template Name** box provided. The screen also shows what your finished DVD template looks like.

If you want to make changes to any part of the template, click the **Back** button in the lower-right corner of the screen as many times as necessary to return to the appropriate step in the **DVD Template Editor**. When you are satisfied with the way your template looks, click the **Save** button. Your custom-built template is saved with all the other templates in Premiere Elements. To learn how you can now use this template in a Premiere Elements project, see **175** Use Your DVD Menu Templates in Premiere Elements.

---

175 Use Your DVD Menu Templates in Premiere Elements

✔ BEFORE YOU BEGIN	→ SEE ALSO
149 Customize a DVD Menu Screen Template	**146** Set DVD Chapter Markers
156 About Sharing Files	**148** Customize an Image As a Chapter Marker
159 Move Images Between Premiere Elements and Photoshop Elements	**151** Create a Motion Menu
172 About DVD Menus and the DVD Template Editor	**153** Add Audio to a Menu
	154 Preview and Test Drive a DVD Movie

If you have not yet done so, modify or create a DVD menu template as explained in **173** Modify an Existing DVD Menu Template or **174** Create a DVD Menu Template from Scratch. If you have not yet created a custom menu, there will be nothing to select from later in this task.

After you have modified a DVD menu template or created one from scratch, I am sure you would like to start using it in your Premiere Elements DVD project. Maybe you have been busy and have a number of modified or created templates—the more, the better. Customizing your DVDs to show your design skills and personality is part of what Premiere Elements and Photoshop Elements are all about.

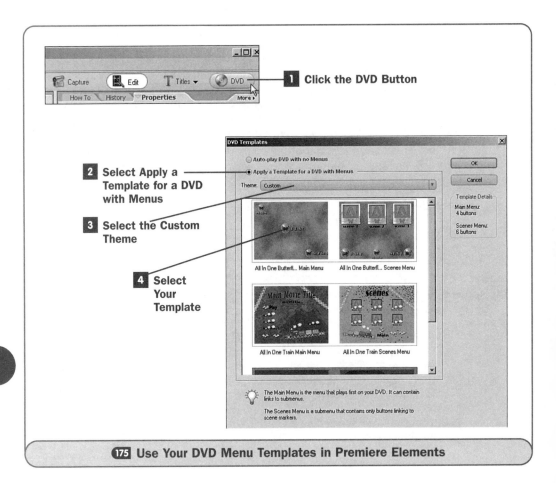

175 Use Your DVD Menu Templates in Premiere Elements

■ Click the DVD Button

In Premiere Elements, open a project to which you would like to add one of your custom DVD menu templates. From the **Edit** workspace, click the **DVD** button in the upper-right corner of the screen. The **DVD Templates** dialog box opens.

■ Select Apply a Template for a DVD with Menus

Click the **Apply a Template for a DVD with Menus** radio button.

■ Select the Custom Theme

From the **Theme** drop-down list, select the **Custom** option. The selection list is updated to display only those DVD menu templates you have modified or created yourself. None of the ready-made templates that come with Premiere Elements appear in the **Custom** list.

4 Select Your Template

From the list of custom templates, select the one you want to use with the current project by clicking the template's image. Then click the **OK** button. Your DVD menu template opens in the DVD workspace. To learn more about DVD menus and the DVD workspace, see **149** **Customize a DVD Menu Screen Template** and **172** **About DVD Menus and the DVD Template Editor**. Now go have fun with the menus you have created using the **DVD Template Editor!**

If you have not set your scene markers in your movie yet, the only menu that appears in the DVD workspace is the main menu. Premiere Elements asks whether you want to have the markers automatically placed for you (see **147** **Auto Generate Scene Markers**). You can manually set the scene markers on the timeline at any time. After the scene markers are set, the scene menu appears in the DVD workspace along with the main menu. If there are more scene markers than one scene menu can hold, the scene menu is automatically duplicated as many times as necessary to accommodate all the scene markers.

175

NUMBERS

A

C

D

E

F

H

J – K

L

M

Q – R

S

X – Y – Z

Key Terms

Don't let unfamiliar terms discourage you from learning all you can about Photoshop Elements and Premiere Elements. If you don't completely understand what one of these words means, flip to the indicated page, read the full definition there, and find techniques related to that term.